Maternal, Neonatal, and Women's Health Nursing

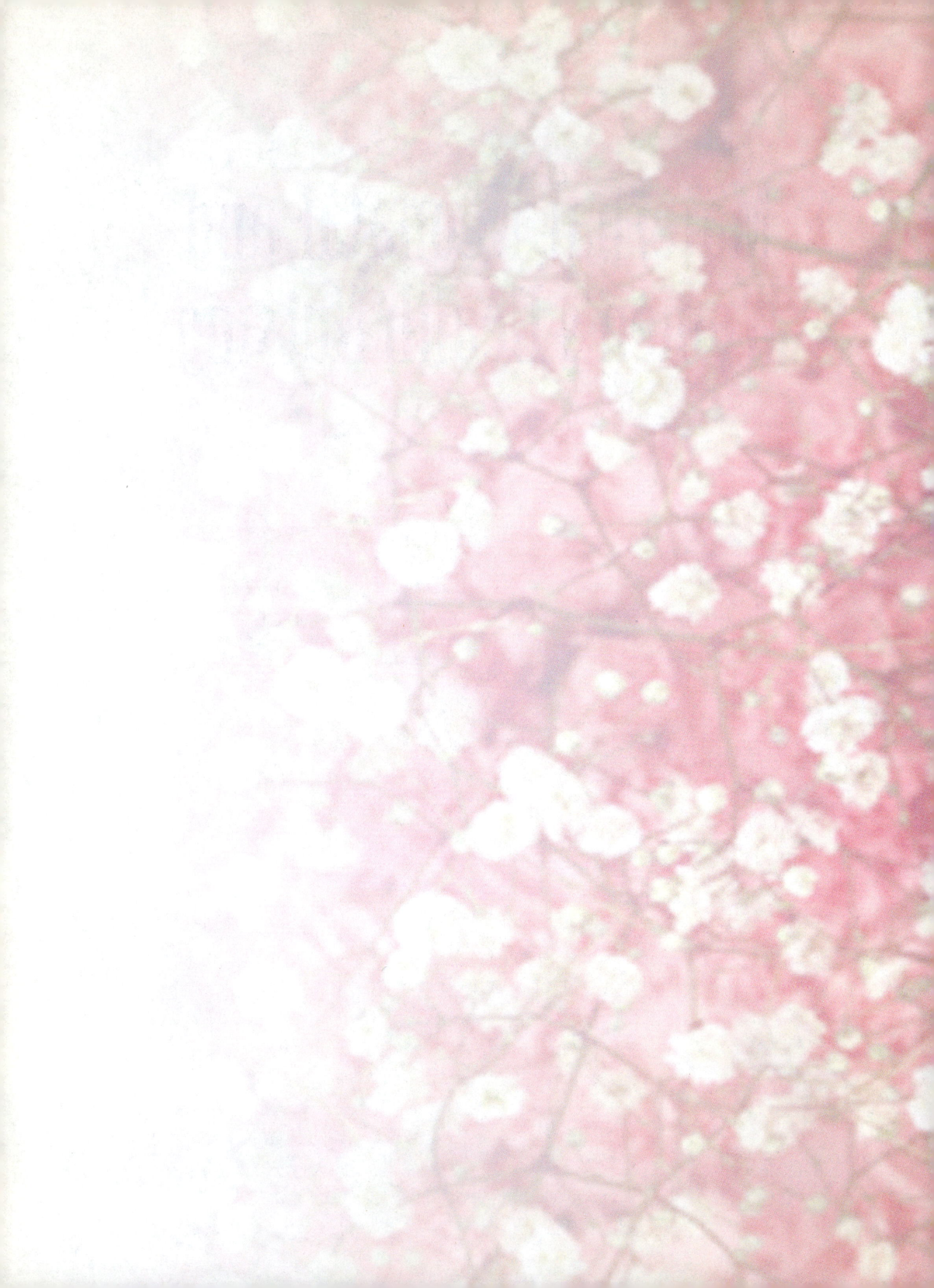

Maternal, Neonatal, and Women's Health Nursing

Lynna Y. Littleton, RNC, PhD

Director of the Women's Health Care Nurse Practitioner Program
Women's Health Nurse Practitioner
Associate Professor of Clinical Nursing
University of Texas Health Science Center at Houston
Houston, Texas

and

Joan C. Engebretson, RN, DrPH, HNC

Associate Professor
Nursing for Target Populations/Head of Division of Women and Childbearing Families
University of Texas Health Science Center at Houston
Houston, Texas

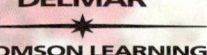

DELMAR

THOMSON LEARNING ™

Australia   Canada   Mexico   Singapore   Spain   United Kingdom   United States

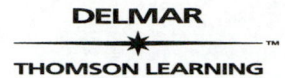

Maternal, Neonatal, and Women's Health Nursing

Lynna Y. Littleton, RNC, PhD
Joan C. Engebretson, RN, DrPH, HNC

Health Care Publishing Director:
William Brottmiller

Executive Editor:
Cathy L. Esperti

Acquisitions Editor:
Matthew Kane

Senior Developmental Editor:
Elisabeth F. Williams

Executive Marketing Manager:
Dawn F. Gerrain

Production Editor:
James Zayicek

Project Editor:
Maureen M. E. Grealish

Art/Design Coordinator:
Jay Purcell

Editorial Assistant:
Shelley Esposito

For permission to use material from this text or product, contact us by
Tel   (800) 730-2214
Fax (800) 730-2215
www.thomsonrights.com

Library of Congress Cataloging-in-Publication Data
Littleton, Lynna.
   Maternal, neonatal, and women's health nursing/Lynna Littleton and Joan Engebretson.
      p. cm.
Includes bibliographical references and index.
ISBN 0-7668-0121-7 (alk. paper)
   1. Maternity nursing. 2. Infants (Newborn)—Diseases—Nursing.
3. Infants (Newborn)—Care. 4. Gynecologic nursing. I. Engebretson, Joan. II. Title.
RG951.L563 2001
610.73′678–dc21   2001032460

NOTICE TO THE READER

CONTENTS

CONTRIBUTORS

Janet M. Banks, RN, PhD CPNP
Coordinator, Pediatric Nurse Practitioner Program
Assistant Professor, Department of Family Nursing Care
University of Texas Health Science Center at San Antonio
School of Nursing
San Antonio, Texas
Chapter 32: Assessment and Care of the Normal Newborn

M. Colleen Brand, RNC, MSN, NNP
Clinical Instructor
Neonatal Nurse Practitioner Program
University of Texas Health Science Center at Houston
School of Nursing
Houston, Texas
and
Neonatal Nurse Practitioner
Neonatal Nurse Practitioner Program
Texas Children's Hospital
Houston, Texas
Chapter 34: Newborns at Risk Related to Birth Weight and Premature Delivery

Nancy H. Busen, RN, PhD CFNP
Associate Professor
University of Texas Health Science Center at Houston
School of Nursing
Houston, Texas
Chapter 19: Pregnancy in Special Populations

Kathy Clarke, RNC, MS
Director, Women's Services
Memorial Hermann Hospital
Houston, Texas
Chapter 15: Normal Pregnancy

Miguel F. da Cunha, PhD
Professor
University of Texas Health Science Center at Houston
School of Nursing
Houston, Texas
Chapter 13: Genetics and Genetic Counseling

Diana Reyna Delgado, RN, MSN
Assistant Professor
Nursing Department
University of Texas Pan American
Edinburg, Texas
Chapter 35: Newborns at Risk Related to Congenital and Acquired Conditions

Judy Freidrichs, RN, MS
Death Educator and Grief Support Facilitator
Education and Quality Coordinator
Rush—Presbyterian—St. Luke's Medical Center
Chicago, Illinois
Chapter 37: Grief and the Family in the Perinatal Experience

Patricia G. Grantom, RNC, MS, CNS, NP
Perinatal Nurse Practitioner
Private Practice
Pasadena, Texas
Chapter 26: High-Risk Births and Obstetric Emergencies

Chris Hawkins, RN, PhD
Associate Professor and M.S. Program Coordinator
College of Nursing—Houston Center
Texas Woman's University
Houston, Texas
Chapter 16: Management and Nursing Care of the Pregnant Woman

Judith Headley, RN, PhD
Assistant Professor
University of Texas Health Science Center at Houston
School of Nursing
Houston, Texas
Chapter 4: Complementary and Alternative Therapies

Lori Hinton, RN, DrPH
Assistant Professor
University of Texas Health Science Center at Houston
Houston, Texas
and
President
American Case Management
Houston, Texas
Chapter 9: Health Care Issues for Women Across the Life Span

Nancy M. Hurst, RN, MSN, IBCLC
Director, Lactation Support Program and Milk Bank, Texas Children's Hospital
Instructor in Pediatrics
Baylor College of Medicine
Houston, Texas
Chapter 33: Newborn Nutrition

Margaret H. Kearney, RNC PhD
Women's Health Nurse Practitioner
and
Associate Professor
Boston College School of Nursing
Chestnut Hill, Massachusetts
Chapter 21: Environmental Risks Affecting Fetal Well-Being

Bonnie Kellogg, RN, DrPH
Professor
California State University—Long Beach
Long Beach, California
Chapter 20: Fetal Development

Elizabeth King, CNS, PhD
Assistant Professor of Clinical Nursing
University of Texas Health Science Center at Houston
School of Nursing
Houston, Texas
Chapter 25: Intrapartum Nursing Care

Karren Kowalski, RN, PhD, FAAN
President, Kowalski and Associates
Maternal Child and Women's Health Consultants
Castle Rock, Colorado
Chapter 37: Grief and the Family in the Perinatal Experience

Lynn L. LeBeck, CRNA, MS
DNSc student, Rush University
Chicago, Illinois
and
Assistant Director
Oakland University—Beaumont Hospital
Graduate Program of Nurse Anesthesia
Royal Oak, Michigan
Chapter 24: Analgesia and Anesthesia in Labor and Delivery

Terry Leicht, MSN, CNS, PNNP
Labor and Delivery
John Sealy Hospital
University of Texas Medical Branch at Galveston
Galveston, Texas
Chapter 18: Management and Nursing Care of the High-Risk Client

Dorothy Lemmey, RN, PhD
Associate Professor of Nursing
Lakeland Community College
Kirtland, Ohio
Chapter 11: Violence and Abuse

Harriet Linenberger, RNC, PhD
Vice President of Patient Care Sevices
Memorial Hermann Hospital—Southwest
Houston, Texas
Chapter 12: Sexual and Reproductive Function

Marilyn J. Lotas, RN, PhD
Associate Professor
Frances Payne Bolton School of Nursing
Case Western Reserve University
Cleveland, Ohio
Chapter 31: Physiologic and Behavioral Transition to Extrauterine Life
Chapter 36: Developmental Care of the Infant at Risk

Jeanne B. Martin, RD, PhD, FADA, LD
Associate Professor and Director, Dietetic Internship
University of Texas Health Science Center at Houston
School of Public Health
Houston, Texas
Chapter 8: Nutrition for Women Across the Life Span

Yondell Masten, RNC, PhD, WHNP, CNS
Professor
Texas Tech University Health Sciences Center
School of Nursing
Lubbock, Texas
Chapter 10: Common Conditions of the Reproductive System

Barbara McFadden, RNC, MSN, NNP
Clinical Instructor
Neonatal Nurse Practitioner Program
University of Texas Health Science Center at Houston
School of Nursing
Houston, Texas
and
Neonatal Nurse Practitioner
Neonatal Nurse Practitioner Program
Women's Hospital of Texas
Houston, Texas
Chapter 34: Newborns at Risk Related to Birth Weight and Premature Delivery

Cynthia L. Milan, RN, MSN, EdD
Assistant Professor
Nursing Department
University of Texas Pan American
Edinburg, Texas
Chapter 35: Newborns at Risk Related to Congenital and Acquired Conditions

Major Lourie R. Moore, RNC, MSN, CNS
Nurse Manager/Element Chief
Obstetrical Unit
56th Medical Group
Luke Air Force Base
Glendale, Arizona
Chapter 28: Normal Postpartum Nursing Care

Carol A. Norman, MEd, MSN
Instructor
University of Texas Health Science Center at Houston
School of Nursing
Houston, Texas
Chapter 29: Postpartum Family Adjustment

Jacquelyn Normand, RNC, MSN
Women's Health Care Nurse Practitioner
Southwest Clinic
Houston, Texas
Chapter 23: Processes of Labor and Delivery

Deborah A. Raines, RNC, PhD
Assistant Professor
College of Nursing
Florida Atlantic University
Boca Raton, Florida
Chapter 22: Evaluation of Fetal Well-Being

Faun G. Ryser, RN, PhD, CNS
Assistant Professor of Clinical Nursing
University of Texas Health Science Center at Houston
School of Nursing
Houston, Texas
Chapter 30: Lactation and Nursing Support

Janine Sherman, RNC, MSN
Instructor
University of Texas Health Science Center at Houston
School of Nursing
Houston, Texas
Chapter 23: Processes of Labor and Delivery

Maureen E. Sintich, RNC, MSN, CS, FNP
Administrator
Women's Health Service Line
North Carolina Baptist Hospitals, Inc.
Wake Forest University Baptist Medical Center
Winston-Salem, North Carolina
Chapter 7: Development of Women Across the Life Span

Jan Weingrad Smith, CNM, MS, MPH
Assistant Professor
Boston University School of Public Health
Department of Maternal and Child Health Program
Nurse Midwifery Education Program
Boston, Massachusetts
Chapter 27: Birth and the Family

Lene Symes, RN, PhD
Adjunct Faculty
Texas Woman's University
College of Nursing
Houston Center
Houston, Texas
Chapter 3: Theoretical Perspectives on the Family

Karen Trierweiler, MS, CNM
Nurse Consultant
Women's Health Section
Colorado Department of Public Health and Environment
Denver, Colorado
Chapter 6: Home Visiting Programs and Perinatal Nursing

Christine J. Valentine, RD, MD
Pediatric Resident, Neonatal Nutrition Consultant
Baylor College of Medicine
Houston, Texas
Chapter 33: Newborn Nutrition

Elias Vasquez, PhD, NP, FAANP
Associate Professor of Clinical Nursing
Director, Neonatal Nurse Practitioner Program
University of Texas Health Science Center at Houston
School of Nursing
Houston, Texas
*Chapter 38: Community and Home Health Care Nursing
for the High-Risk Infant*

Marlene Walden, RNC PhD NNP CCNS
Assistant Professor
School of Nursing
University of Texas Medical Branch at Galveston
Galveston, Texas
*Chapter 31: Physiologic and Behavioral Transition to
Extrauterine Life*
Chapter 36: Developmental Care of the Infant at Risk

Pam Willson, RN, PhD, FNP-C
Veterans Affairs Medical Center
Houston, Texas
Chapter 11: Violence and Abuse

Anne Young, RN, EdD
Associate Professor and Doctoral Program Coordinator
Texas Woman's University
College of Nursing
Houston, Texas
Chapter 5: Ethics, Laws, and Standards of Care

REVIEWERS

Maternal, Neonatal, and Women's Health Nursing was created from an understanding that effective nurse-client interaction is a foundation of proper care. Both nurse and client enter the relationship with knowledge bases of values and experiences, which inevitably shape the views and goals of each. While experience includes formal and theoretical knowledge for the nurse, each client brings a belief system that can vary by culture, religion, and education, which affects behavior and understanding about health. Acknowledging these differences and learning how to achieve a partnership of nurse and client is a goal of this text.

The framework of this book utilizes a holistic model of health care delivery that acknowledges traditional medical care, nursing roles at various levels of practice, and alternative health care modalities as complementary components of the individual's health care resources. Special attention is paid to changes in the health care system and the role of nursing as the site of delivery expands from the hospital into the community. Ultimately, the focus is on nursing care as it is delivered to women, neonates, and their families in the context of culture and the communities in which they live.

Maternal, Neonatal, and Women's Health Nursing will provide the instruction and application skills for the undergraduate nursing student to learn about maternity nursing in preparation for the NCLEX-RN™ exam. More importantly, the information and tools within will foster the development of a caring and professional nurse who is technically and ethically responsible. This text will also serve as an excellent reference for the practitioner, who can consult its pages as a clinical resource.

ORGANIZATION

The text consists of 38 chapters, organized into 9 units:

Unit I, Foundations of Nursing Care, analyzes the expectations, challenges, and rewards of contemporary practice in a number of ways. The unit begins with a discussion of modern issues pertinent to maternal, neonatal, and women's health nursing, including theoretical perspectives on the family. It then progresses to complementary and alternative therapies with regard to women's health, followed by a study in ethics, laws, and standards of care. Finally, home visiting programs and perinatal nursing are covered in a separate chapter.

Unit II, Health Care of Women, addresses the development of women and emphasizes wellness across the life span. Maintenance of health through proper nutrition and a balanced lifestyle are discussed, followed by specific factors that jeopardize women's health, such as chronic conditions and violence and abuse.

Unit III, Human Sexuality Across the Life Span, provides discussion on sexual and reproductive function with a focus on planning to affirm health. The role of genetics and genetic counseling and family planning is also explored in this context.

Unit IV, Pregnancy, describes how to manage care of the pregnant woman and her family in various settings, within special populations, and under normal and high-risk conditions. With close attention to the nurse-client relationship, education is stressed for both childbirth preparation and perinatal health.

Unit V, Assessment of Fetal Well-Being, presents normal fetal development and the environmental risks that can play a role in preventing normal growth. Tools are provided to monitor and evaluate fetal maturation.

Unit VI, Childbirth, focuses on the expected and unexpected aspects of labor and delivery. The unit moves from the process of normal childbirth to high-risk births and obstetric emergencies. Anesthesia, intrapartum nursing care, and the role of the family are discussed in-depth.

Unit VII, Postpartum Health and Nursing Care, explores the true spirit of nursing during this emotional period of adjustment for the woman and her family. Professional care is delivered within the framework of encouragement and assistance in addition to an entire chapter on lactation and nursing support.

Unit VIII, Newborn Development and Nursing Care, explains the physiologic and biological changes manifested in the transition to extrauterine life. Tools are offered to assess and care for the newborn, including the importance of good nutrition to maintain newborn health. In addition, nursing care of newborns at risk is explored in detail, with special attention to premature delivery, congenital and acquired conditions, and developmental care of the infant at risk.

Unit IX, **Special Considerations**, analyzes grief and the family as it relates to the perinatal experience and explores the unique challenges associated with caring for a high-risk infant in community and home care settings.

FEATURES

You will find a variety of special features in *Maternal, Neonatal, and Women's Health Nursing* designed to encourage self-reflection, caring, and application of knowledge. These complements to the text material support the developmental transition of student to practitioner:

- **Competencies** are included at the beginning of each chapter to present an outline of the material to follow. They call attention to the knowledge that will be expected upon reading of the content.

- **Key Terms** bolded in the chapters denote significant terminology in the subject matter. These terms are defined in the Glossary for easy reference.

- **Research Highlights** provide details of research findings in maternal, neonatal, and women's health nursing. These great resources also provide the necessary guidelines to formulate a research proposal.

- **Nursing Tips** are pearls of wisdom from experienced nurses that may prove useful for making decisions and taking action in a clinical setting.

- **Nursing Alerts** advise the reader to be aware of situations that may be dangerous to the client or nurse.

- **Client Education** boxes demonstrate how to equip clients with necessary health promotion information so they can take charge of their own well-being.

- **Reflections From Nurses And Families** are anecdotes from the experiences of nurses, clients, and their families. They are intended to stress the importance of caring at all times.

- **Critical Thinking** boxes challenge the reader to analyze the subject matter beyond rote memory and apply it to practice.

- **Case Study/Care Plans** present descriptions of potential clients and their conditions, reflecting a variety of cultural, religious, and sociological variables.

Care Plans demonstrate the appropriate nursing process approach for each case.

- **Photo Stories** furnish the reader with a full-color visual supplement to text material by demonstrating step-by-step techniques and events. These can be found in chapters 23, 24, 25, and 32.

- **Web Activities** direct the reader to additional sources of information that may prove useful in writing research papers or in clinical practice.

- **Key Concepts** direct attention toward information of considerable consequence in the text.

- **Review Questions and Activities** can be found in each chapter in intentionally varied formats that tap into different learning styles and strengths. Multiple choice, short answer, and critical thinking formats will be found.

STUDENT RESOURCES

Student Activity Software, a highly-interactive and enjoyable learning tool, is a free addition to *Maternal, Neonatal, and Women's Health Nursing*. Found on the inside back cover of the textbook, this exciting resource features 750 challenging questions delivered in a variety of formats and in a chapter-by-chapter outline. Games that test knowledge and comprehension of textbook material are included along with the capability of additional "players" for joint study.

Student Study Guide (order # 0-7668-0122-5), a print guide for self-directed learning, is available for purchase. Organized by chapter, it consists of Learning Objectives, Reading Assignments, Activities, Key Terms, and a Self-Assessment Quiz. All answers are in the back of the manual to encourage a programmed approach to learning.

INSTRUCTOR RESOURCES (ORDER # 0-7668-0123-3)

The Electronic Classroom Manager (ECM) was designed as a complete teaching tool for *Maternal, Neonatal, and Women's Health Nursing*. It assists instructors in the transition of class notes, preparing readings, creating lectures, constructing quizzes and tests, and developing presentations. This complementary item for adopters of the textbook is a two CD-ROM resource housed in a DVD package. The ECM consists of:

- **Instructor's Guide**, which provides suggestions for the direction of classroom lecture. Chapter Objectives, Student Learning Activities, Instructional Approaches, and Web Activities are presented in one format for viewing and another for personalized editing.

- **Computerized Testbank**, which consists of 1000 multiple choice and true-false questions relating to the content in the text to aid in the development of quizzes and tests.
- **PowerPoint** slides designed as a visually-appealing way to draw from key points of the textbook to en-

hance classroom lecture. This consists of approximately 450 slides developed for the Electronic Classroom Manager.

- **Image Library**, which is an extensive collection of over 600 pieces of art and photographs from the text; it is located on separate CD-ROM of the ECM. The electronic format allows the instructor to use these images to customize lectures.

ACKNOWLEDGMENTS

The following individuals should be acknowledged because without their support and skill this book would not have been possible. We are eternally grateful to these people and many more.

Earl Littleton, my husband of 35 years, who supported, encouraged, and provided unconditional love. My sisters, Carla Funderburg, Dorris Petrey, and Melva Fizeseri and my brother, John Petrey, who have been patient with my work and kind in my absence. Wentworth Eaton MD, longtime friend and mentor.

—L.L.

David Cohen, my husband, who has patiently dealt with very late dinners and frenzied weekends, and still provided support for this project. My three sons, Andrew, Adam, and Ethan, and daughter-in-law, Sarah, who being involved with their own higher education, appreciate the time and energy that has been diverted to this project. To my colleagues at UTHS School of Nursing who have heard the frustrations and elations, and steadily kept us afloat during the deadlines.

—J.E.

The many contributors to this text from all over the country. Harriett Linenberger for approving incredible photographic access. Carol Kanusky for making things happen at the hospital. Matt Kane for his organizational ability. Tom Stock for his photographic skill. Jay Purcell for his artistic design. Shelley Esposito for her attention to detail. Joe Chovan for his incredible artistic talent. Jim Zayicek for his production skill. Maureen Grealish for her editorial skill. Silvia Freeburg for her editorial skill and patience. The many students and faculty that provided input into the development of the book. And, finally, to Beth Williams, our developmental editor, who has nursed this project from beginning to end. She has demonstrated great patience and attentiveness to detail, and developed the vision of the completed product that was, at times, nebulous to us through the process.

—L.L. & J.E.

ABOUT THE AUTHORS

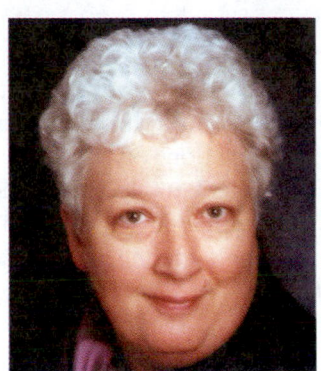

Lynna Y. Littleton

Lynna Y. Littleton has a diploma from City of Memphis Hospitals School of Nursing, with a BS, MS, and PhD in nursing from Texas Woman's University. She has worked in numerous women's health care settings, including labor and delivery, postpartum, and antepartum units in hospitals. She has also worked in ambulatory care settings. She is a women's health care nurse practitioner, an Associate Professor of Clinical Nursing, and Program Director of the Women's Healthcare Nurse Practitioner program at University of Texas Health Science Center at Houston. She has taught both undergraduate and graduate courses related to maternal and child health as well as women's health. She maintains a clinical practice as a nurse practitioner. She has won numerous teaching and clinical awards.

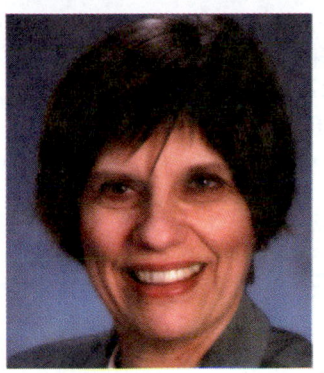

Joan C. Engebretson

Joan Engebretson received a BSN from St. Olaf College in Northfield, Minnesota, an MS from Texas Women's University, and a PhD at University of Texas Health Science Center at Houston School of Public Health. She is Associate Professor at University of Texas Health Science Center at Houston School of Nursing with an adjunct position at the School of Public Health. She has a clinical background in community health nursing, with a focus on maternal-child health. She has taught graduate and undergraduate courses in maternal-infant and women's health. She has conducted research on complementary therapies, touch therapies, and menopause. She also collaborated in the development of the Wee Thumbie, a pacifier for low-birth-weight infants. She is active in the Council of Nurse Anthropologists, the American Holistic Nurses Association, and The Holistic Nursing Credentialing board and other professional organizations.

HOW TO USE THIS TEXT

The presentation of the subject matter was designed to foster an understanding of maternal, neonatal, and women's health nursing from a variety of levels and perspectives. The following suggests how each engaging and confidence-building feature can be used to develop competency and professionalism.

CHAPTER OPENING BOX

Unique to other products within the discipline, each chapter of *Maternal, Neonatal, and Women's Health Nursing* begins on a personal note. In preparation of the content to come, the reader is challenged to examine his/her own thoughts, feelings, and experiences that might help him/her relate to the client before care is delivered. This feature serves as an introduction towards developing a solid nurse-client relationship.

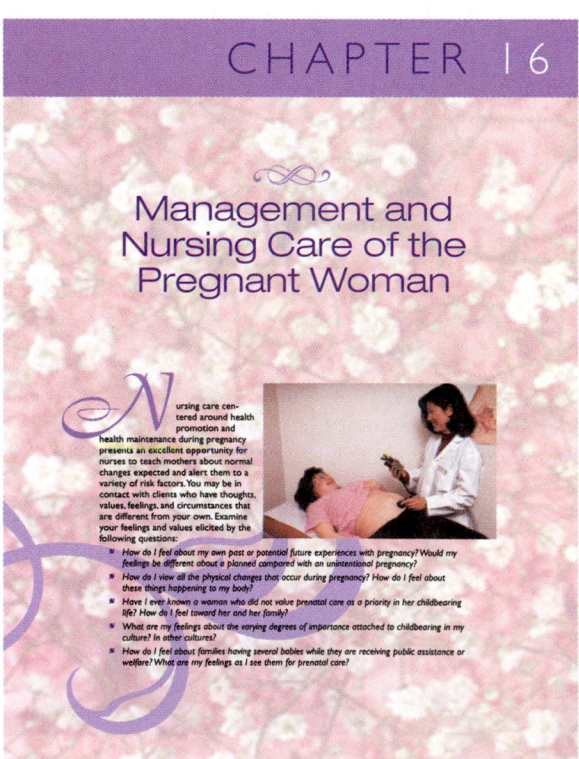

COMPETENCIES

Answering the question "What am I about to learn?" best describes the purpose behind the chapter-opening competencies. By the completion of the chapter, the reader should have a working knowledge of the material presented and be able to apply it to practice. These should be used as a structure for targeting and extracting the most significant points for study.

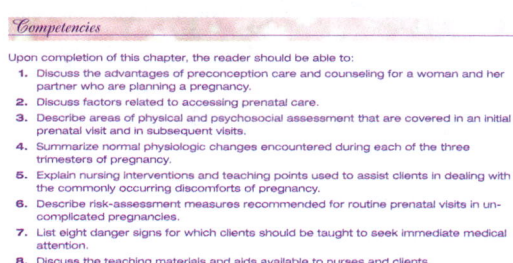

KEY TERMS

Calling attention to new terminology before first usage within the book, these chapter-opening elements are initially listed, then provided with a definition in context, and repeated with a definition in the glossary. Terms are bolded within the chapters at first usage for easy identification. Familiarize yourself with these words, as they must be understood to assimilate the chapter material.

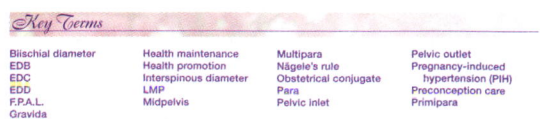

RESEARCH HIGHLIGHTS

These sections emphasize the importance of clinical research by linking theory to practice. Offering details of purpose, methods, findings, and nursing implications, the format also serves as a guide in constructing focused and accurate research proposal abstracts. Use the information

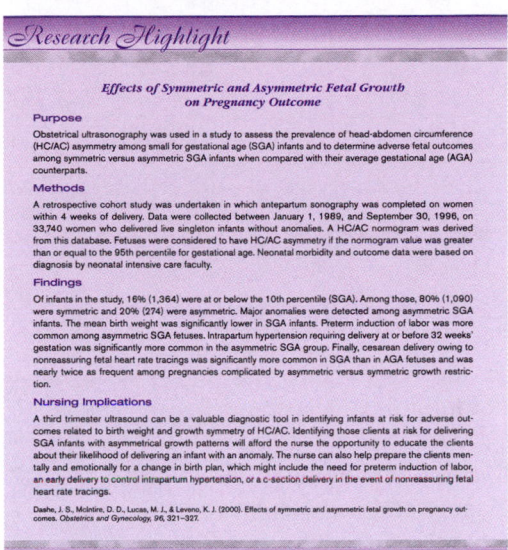

Research Highlight

Effects of Symmetric and Asymmetric Fetal Growth on Pregnancy Outcome

Purpose

Obstetrical ultrasonography was used in a study to assess the prevalence of head-abdomen circumference (HC/AC) asymmetry among small for gestational age (SGA) infants and to determine adverse fetal outcomes among symmetric versus asymmetric SGA infants when compared with their average gestational age (AGA) counterparts.

Methods

A retrospective cohort study was undertaken in which antepartum sonography was completed on women within 4 weeks of delivery. Data were collected between January 1, 1989, and September 30, 1996, on 33,740 women who delivered live singleton infants without anomalies. A HC/AC normogram was derived from this database. Fetuses were considered to have HC/AC asymmetry if the normogram value was greater than or equal to the 95th percentile for gestational age. Neonatal morbidity and outcome data were based on diagnosis by neonatal intensive care faculty.

Findings

Of infants in the study, 16% (1,364) were at or below the 10th percentile (SGA). Among those, 80% (1,090) were symmetric and 20% (274) were asymmetric. Major anomalies were detected among asymmetric SGA infants. The mean birth weight was significantly lower in SGA infants. Preterm induction of labor was more common among asymmetric SGA fetuses. Intrapartum hypertension requiring delivery at or before 32 weeks' gestation was significantly more common in the asymmetric SGA group. Finally, cesarean delivery owing to nonreassuring fetal heart rate tracings was significantly more common in SGA than in AGA fetuses and was nearly twice as frequent among pregnancies complicated by asymmetric versus symmetric growth restriction.

Nursing Implications

A third trimester ultrasound can be a valuable diagnostic tool in identifying infants at risk for adverse outcomes related to birth weight and growth symmetry of HC/AC. Identifying those clients at risk for delivering SGA infants with asymmetrical growth patterns will afford the nurse the opportunity to educate the clients about their likelihood of delivering an infant with an anomaly. The nurse can also help prepare the clients mentally and emotionally for a change in birth plan, which might include the need for preterm induction of labor, an early delivery to control intrapartum hypertension, or a c-section delivery in the event of nonreassuring fetal heart rate tracings.

Dashe, J. S., McIntire, D. D., Lucas, M. J., & Leveno, K. J. (2000). Effects of symmetric and asymmetric fetal growth on pregnancy outcomes. Obstetrics and Gynecology, 96, 321–327.

contained in these boxes to learn the systematic research process and apply it to the field of nursing.

NURSING TIPS

In any profession, there are benefits to learning from more experienced professionals. You can be better prepared and more efficient when receptive to the helpful tips, hints, and strategies presented here from skilled nurses. Study, share, and discuss them with your colleagues.

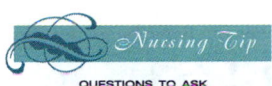

Nursing Tip

QUESTIONS TO ASK ABOUT STALKING

- Are you being followed or spied on by your intimate partner (or previous partner)?
- Does your intimate partner wait outside or show up unexpectedly at your home, school, or workplace?
- Do you receive unwanted phone calls from your intimate partner, or are you receiving many hang-up calls?
- Has your intimate partner sent or left you unwanted notes, letters, or other items of communication that frighten you?
- Has your intimate partner threatened to harm you, the children, or family members?
- Has your intimate partner caused damage to your personal property, for example, cut up your clothing, torn up photographs, slashed your car tires, tried to break down your door, or killed a pet?

NURSING ALERTS

As a nurse, it is important to react quickly in some cases to ensure the safety and health of your clients. This is a reminder that pitfalls exist and will train you to effectively identify and respond to critical situations on your own. Remember these important pieces of information so you can draw from them in practice.

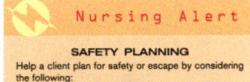

Nursing Alert

SAFETY PLANNING

Help a client plan for safety or escape by considering the following:

- Is it safe for the woman and her children to go home?
- Are there weapons in the home?
- Has there been an increase in the frequency or severity of the violence?
- Has the woman been hospitalized in the past as a result of the intimate partner violence?
- Has the abuser threatened to kill the woman or himself?
- Has the woman thought of committing or tried to commit suicide?
- Does the abuser hurt the children?
- Has the woman attempted or is she planning to leave the relationship?

CLIENT EDUCATION

Health promotion and prevention serve as a cornerstone to a healthy society. Clients will count on you to offer your

knowledge of self-care so they can maintain their own health. Client Education boxes demonstrate how to equip clients with the proper information to take charge of their own well-being or to prepare for certain procedures or outcomes. Use these boxes to think of additional ways clients can assume responsibility for their own health and self-care.

Client Education

Fatigue in Pregnancy

Find a comfortable and reasonably quiet place and try meditation. Close your mind to external sensation and outside stimulation. Pick one of the following five methods to achieve a single focus:

1. Meditative repetition: repeat a rhythmic chant, most commonly called a mantra, that is chanted over and over
2. Visual concentration: stare at an image, such as a candle, flower, or fruit
3. Repetitive sounds: listen to a sound, such as a drum, chimes, or a waterfall
4. Physical repetitive motion: perform motions such as rhythmic breathing or a rhythmic aerobic exercise
5. Repeated tactile motion: hold or manipulate a small object, such as a rosary or tumble stone

REFLECTIONS FROM NURSES AND FAMILIES

An historic strength of the nursing profession is the manner of compassion with which nurses have undertaken their responsibilities. Reflections boxes have been added as a forum for families and other nurses to share personal experiences, encouraging respect for individual uniqueness and promoting self-awareness and introspection. Try to identify with the thoughts and emotions expressed in these stories as they serve as positive reminders that nursing is not just about treating conditions, but rather caring for people.

REFLECTIONS FROM A LABORING MOTHER

"When I got to the hospital I was 4 cm dilated. Although I had managed pretty well so far, I knew what was coming. With my first baby, once I got to be 6 cm the contractions started to hurt a lot worse and that's when I got the epidural. Talk about the difference between day and night! I felt the contractions as pressure, but they were not as painful as they had been before the epidural. With my second baby, I asked for the epidural as soon as I just got into the labor-delivery room. I didn't want to miss getting one because my labor was moving too fast."

CRITICAL THINKING

Making sound clinical decisions is imperative as a nurse. These real-world scenarios with accompanying thought-provoking questions will encourage refined judgment and reinforce the elements that play a role in learning and sharpening this skill. They serve as a reminder that application of knowledge is more significant than its acquisition.

Critical Thinking

Successful Role Adaptation

Rosie is a teen who is pregnant with her first baby, and she is approaching her eighth month. She is in the office for her prenatal visit and has brought her girlfriend; they are going to a party at a friend's house later that night.

1. How can you determine if Rosie has accepted her pregnancy?
2. What behaviors would you expect Rosie to report to indicate that she is successfully adapting to her impending role as mother?
3. What questions will you ask to determine if Rosie understands the changes that she will have to make in her lifestyle to care for her infant?

CASE STUDY/CARE PLAN

To practically apply presented material into the nursing process framework, Case Studies have been included with appropriate Care Plans. The real-world scenarios exem-

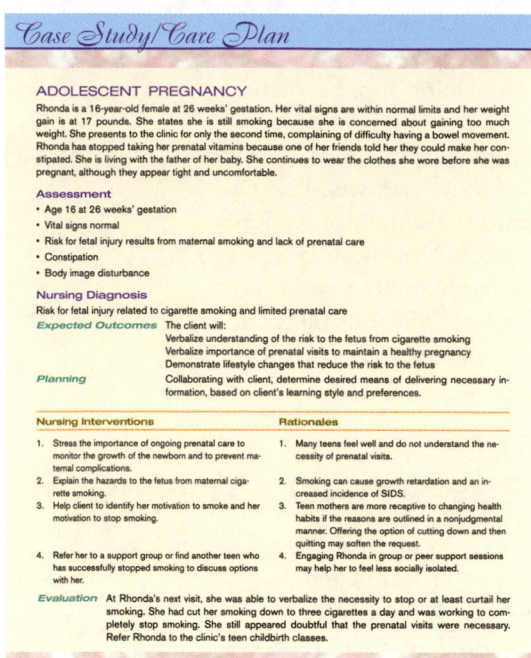

Case Study/Care Plan

ADOLESCENT PREGNANCY

Rhonda is a 16-year-old female at 26 weeks' gestation. Her vital signs are within normal limits and her weight gain is at 17 pounds. She states she is still smoking because she is concerned about gaining too much weight. She presents to the clinic for only the second time, complaining of difficulty having a bowel movement. Rhonda has stopped taking her prenatal vitamins because one of her friends told her they could make her constipated. She is living with the father of her baby. She continues to wear the clothes she wore before she was pregnant, although they appear tight and uncomfortable.

Assessment
- Age 16 at 26 weeks' gestation
- Vital signs normal
- Risk for fetal injury results from maternal smoking and lack of prenatal care
- Constipation
- Body image disturbance

Nursing Diagnosis
Risk for fetal injury related to cigarette smoking and limited prenatal care

Expected Outcomes The client will:
Verbalize understanding of the risk to the fetus from cigarette smoking
Verbalize importance of prenatal visits to maintain a healthy pregnancy
Demonstrate lifestyle changes that reduce the risk to the fetus

Planning Collaborating with client, determine desired means of delivering necessary information, based on client's learning style and preferences.

Nursing Interventions	Rationales
1. Stress the importance of ongoing prenatal care to monitor the growth of the newborn and to prevent maternal complications.	1. Many teens feel well and do not understand the necessity of prenatal visits.
2. Explain the hazards to the fetus from maternal cigarette smoking.	2. Smoking can cause growth retardation and an increased incidence of SIDS.
3. Help client to identify her motivation to smoke and her motivation to stop smoking.	3. Teen mothers are more receptive to changing health habits if the reasons are outlined in a nonjudgmental manner. Offering the option of cutting down and then quitting may soften the request.
4. Refer her to a support group or find another teen who has successfully stopped smoking to discuss options with her.	4. Engaging Rhonda in group or peer support sessions may help her to feel less socially isolated.

Evaluation At Rhonda's next visit, she was able to verbalize the necessity to stop or at least curtail her smoking. She had cut her smoking down to three cigarettes a day and was working to completely stop smoking. She still appeared doubtful that the prenatal visits were necessary. Refer Rhonda to the clinic's teen childbirth classes.

Review Questions and Activities

1. Why is it important for the home visitor to be culturally sensitive?
2. List two important principles of home visiting and give examples of how these might be put into operation by the nurse during the home visit.
3. List three tasks the nurse should perform before making a home visit.
4. Identify three strategies to promote communication during a home visit.
5. You are visiting a pregnant woman at home. Identify three nursing observations that might be made to assess the following: living necessities, coping and stress tolerance, and nutritional status.
6. List three strategies for ensuring personal safety during a home visit.
7. You have just completed a home visit where you provided extensive breast-feeding education and support to a new mother. How can the outcomes of this visit be evaluated?
8. Identify important areas for documentation after the home visit.
9. Discuss two limitations of home visits.
10. Discuss the challenges involved in terminating the home visiting relationship.

WEB ACTIVITIES

To offer additional helpful resources of information, Web Activities provide direction to sites that will aid in the writing of research papers and assignments. Related questions promote analysis of findings. Take advantage of the suggestions to continue your own education in maternal, neonatal, and women's health nursing.

Web Activities
- Locate your state's Visiting Nurse Association (VNA). Does it have a web site? What type of professional information is offered regarding regulations for home visits in your state? Compare these regulations with those listed for a neighboring state.
- Visit a local hospital's web site for information on its home visiting program.

plify the holistic approach of cultural, spiritual, and psychosocial aspects of nursing care and incorporate collaborative efforts in multiple settings. Take note of the care plan construction process for maternal, neonatal, and women's health and the number of variables that can play a role in its design.

PHOTO STORIES

In select chapters, step-by-step photo stories are included to advance your understanding of content and procedures. The full-color visual depictions are also intended to stress the caring involved in the nurse-client relationship.

KEY CONCEPTS

Key Concepts summarize the main points presented in each chapter and provide a framework to recall the material. Use these tools as a review guide or a checklist to structure your studying.

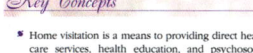

Key Concepts
- Home visitation is a means to providing direct health care services, health education, and psychosocial support to clients and families.
- The growth of social reforms and the expansion of the field of social work contributed to the rise of home care programs in the early 20th century.
- The home as the site of delivery provides the nurse with a unique opportunity to assess the client and family in their own environment.
- Home care can be provided by home health care agencies, hospitals, public health departments, schools, and other institutions.
- Cost savings in the form of reduced inpatient hospital stays is one of the many benefits of home care.
- The home visit consists of three phases: previsit preparation, the visit, and postvisit activities.

REVIEW QUESTIONS AND ACTIVITIES

At the end of each chapter, exercises encourage your application and synthesis of presented material to test your understanding and assimilation of the content. Answer the questions and follow the instructions to promote further discussion of key points from each chapter.

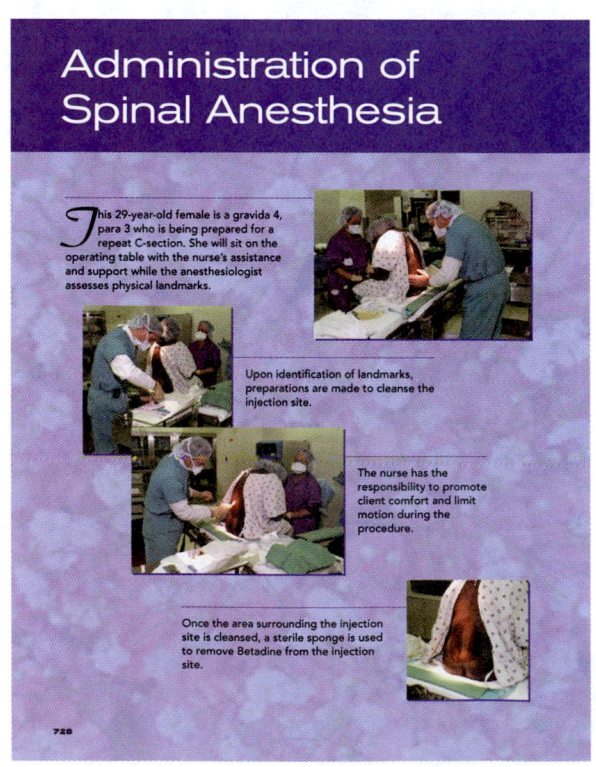

Administration of Spinal Anesthesia

This 29-year-old female is a gravida 4, para 3 who is being prepared for a repeat C-section. She will sit on the operating table with the nurse's assistance and support while the anesthesiologist assesses physical landmarks.

Upon identification of landmarks, preparations are made to cleanse the injection site.

The nurse has the responsibility to promote client comfort and limit motion during the procedure.

Once the area surrounding the injection site is cleansed, a sterile sponge is used to remove Betadine from the injection site.

728

HOW TO USE THE STUDENT ACTIVITY SOFTWARE

The Student Activity Software was designed as an exciting enhancement to *Maternal, Neonatal, and Women's Health Nursing* to help you learn difficult terms and concepts. As you study each chapter in the text, be sure to explore the corresponding unit on the CD-ROM.

Each chapter is divided into two major sections: exercises, and fun and games. Exercises can be used for additional practice, review, or self-testing. Fun and games provide an opportunity to play and practice through a variety of activities.

Getting started is easy. Follow the simple directions on the CD label to install the program on your computer. Then take advantage of the following features:

MAIN MENU

The main menu follows the chapter organization of the text exactly, which makes it easy for you to find your way around.

Just click on the button for the chapter you want, and you'll come to the chapter opening screen.

TOOLBAR

The Back button at the top left of every screen allows you to retrace your steps, while the Exit button gets you out of the program quickly and easily. As you navigate through the software, check the toolbar for other features that help you use individual exercises or games.

ONLINE HELP

If you get stuck, just press F1 to get help. The online help includes instructions for all parts of the Student Activity Software.

THE CHAPTER SCREEN

Here you have the opportunity to choose how you want to learn. Select one of the exercises for additional practice, review, or self-testing. Or click on a game to practice the concepts for that chapter in a fun format.

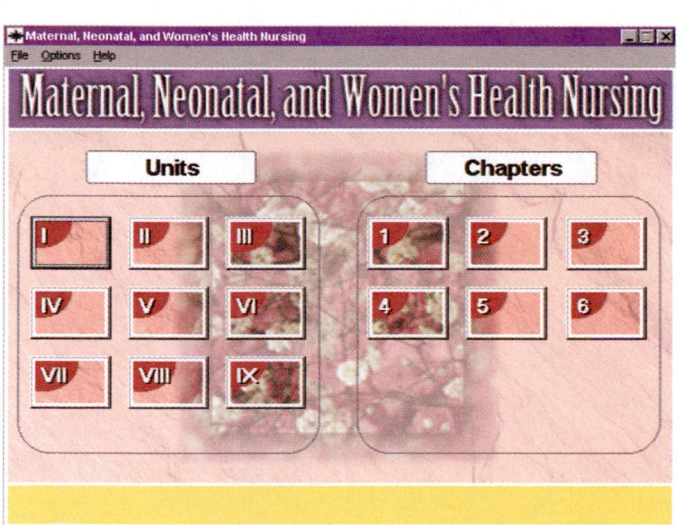

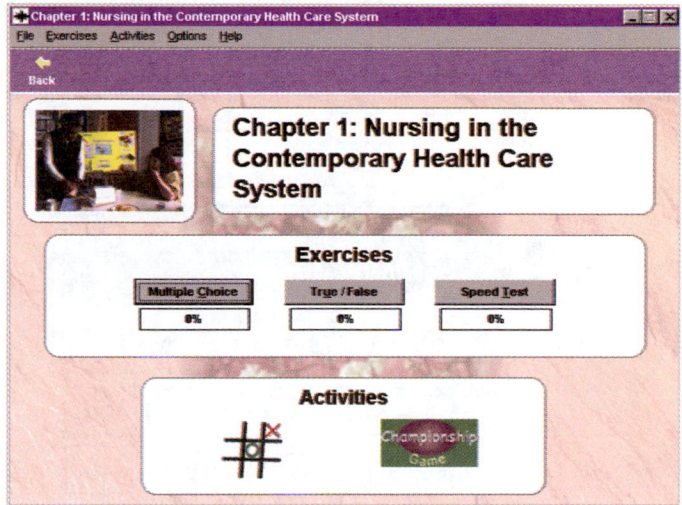

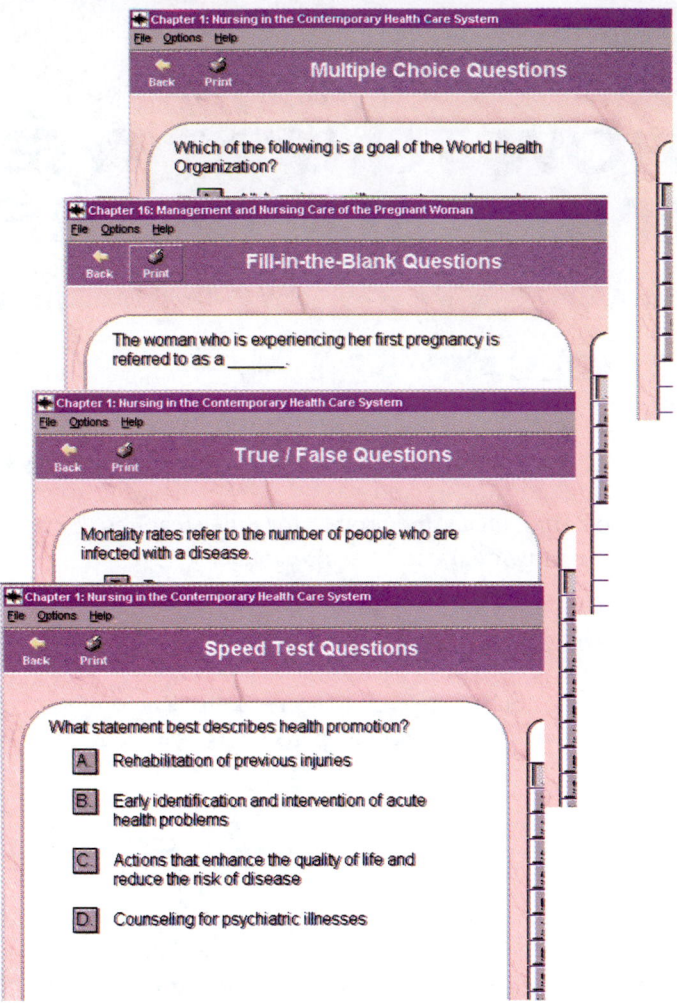

EXERCISES

The Student Activity Software acts as your own private tutor. For each exercise, it chooses from a bank of questions covering all 38 chapters. Putting these exercises to work for you is simple:

- Choose a true/false, multiple choice, or fill-in-the-blank exercise, whichever one appeals to you.
- You'll encounter a series of questions for each exercise format; each question gives you two chances to answer correctly.
- Instant feedback tells you whether you're right or wrong—and helps you learn more quickly by explaining why an answer was correct.
- The Student Activity Software displays the percentage of correct answers on the chapter screen. An on-screen score sheet (which you can print) lets you track correct and incorrect answers.
- Review your previous questions and answers in an exercise for more in-depth understanding. Or start an exercise over with a new, random set of questions that gives you a realistic study environment.
- When you're ready for an additional challenge, try the timed Speed Test. Once you've finished, it displays your score and the time you took to complete the test, so you can see how much you've learned.

FUN AND GAMES

To have fun while reinforcing your knowledge, enjoy the simple games on this disk. You can play alone, with a partner, or on teams.

- **Tic-Tac-Toe:** you or your team must correctly answer a question before placing an X or an O.
- **Championship Game:** challenge your classmates and increase your knowledge by playing this Jeopardy-style, question-and-answer game.

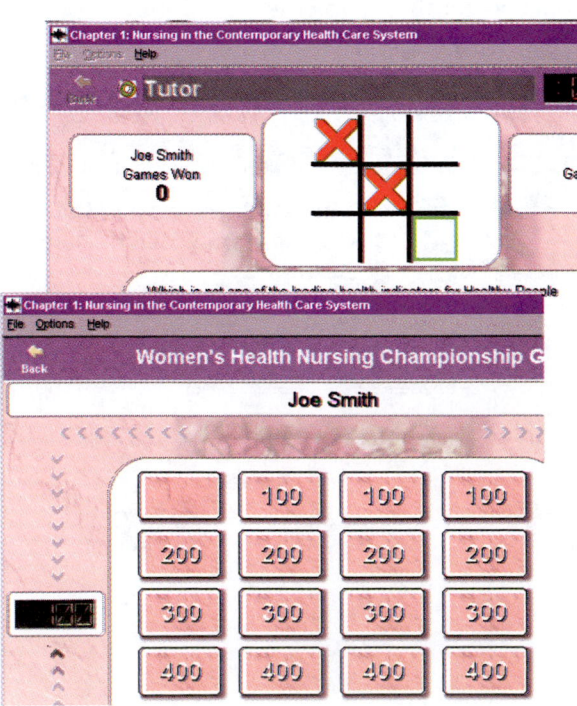

UNIT I

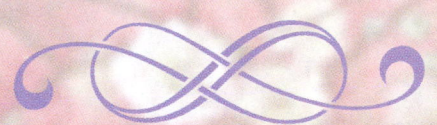

Foundations
of Nursing Care

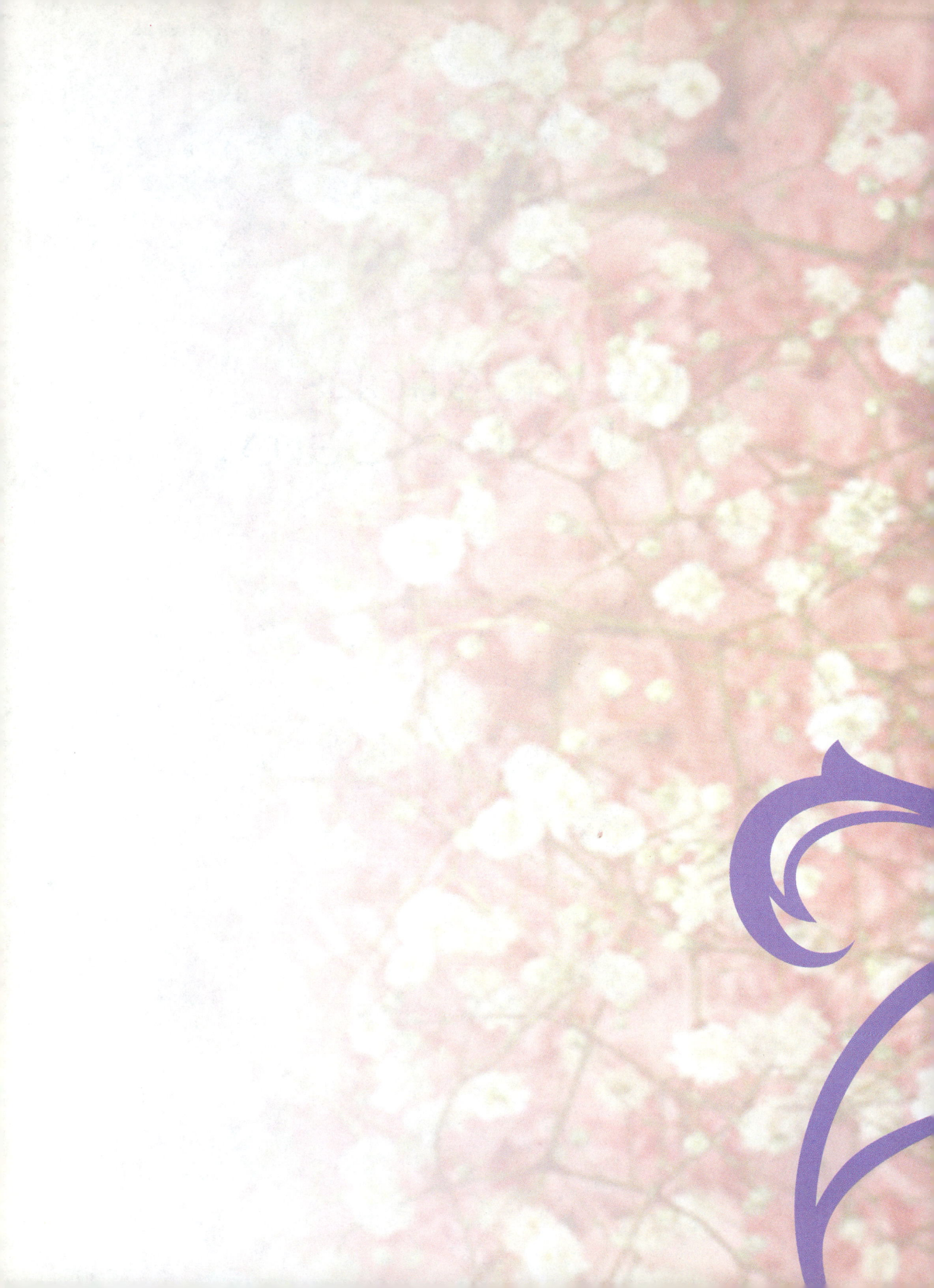

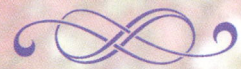

CHAPTER 1

Nursing in the Contemporary Health Care System

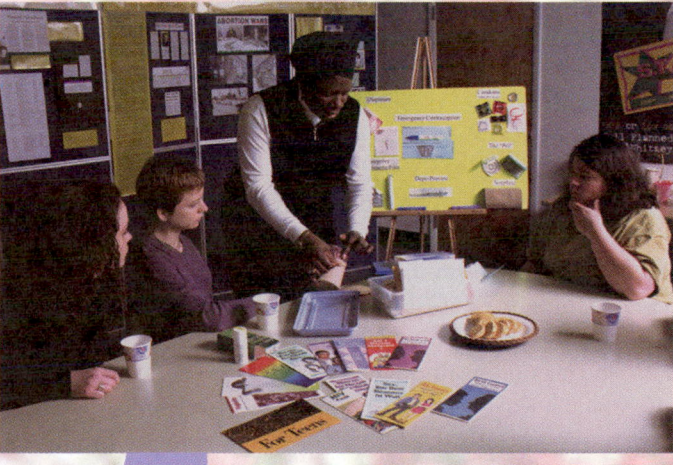

*U*nderstanding the contemporary health care system is vital to providing effective and appropriate nursing care. Understanding how your personal beliefs and values may influence your interpretation of the system is also important. Consider the following:

- *Have I ever wondered what health means?*
- *How does the health care system help keep clients healthy?*
- *If I am sick and see a clinician in Idaho, would I receive the same quality of care as I would in Connecticut?*
- *What are the things that affect my health?*
- *Who pays for expensive methods of diagnoses and treatments?*
- *How do people in other cultures think about health, illness, and disease?*

Key Terms

Behavioral medicine	Cultural competence	Health promotion	Objectives
Cost-benefit analysis	Disease prevention	Managed care	Risk assessment
Cost-effectiveness analysis	Evidence-based practice	Interdisciplinary teams	Social assets
Critical thinking	Goals	Morbidity rates	
	Health care informatics	Mortality rates	

Competencies

Upon completion of this chapter, the reader should be able to:

1. Describe the shift in health care delivery to encompass health outcomes.
2. Identify national goals and guidelines that direct the health care industry.
3. Discuss measures that have been undertaken to contain health care costs.
4. Apply evidence-based practice and best practice to clinical situations.
5. Discuss seven discoveries that are changing our understanding of health, illness, and disease.
6. Describe some contemporary challenges facing all health care providers.
7. Apply skills necessary for nurses to participate fully on health care teams.

Health care is affected by many factors both within the health care industry and external to it. Health care has expanded the focus beyond disease treatment to disease prevention and health promotion. A dual emphasis of cost containment and prevention has moved much of health care delivery into the community and even into client's homes. Nurses are now functioning on multidisciplinary teams.

In response to health care disparities, national objectives have been established and outcomes are being tracked. Guidelines are available to assist the clinician in providing the best care. A number of discoveries are changing our understanding of health, illness, disease, and treatment. These discoveries also have raised ethical issues and stirred controversy as they challenge some of the previous ideas about health. Nurses need specific skills to practice in the current health care system.

CURRENT STATE OF HEALTH CARE DELIVERY

Throughout history, most models of health care have been focused on diagnosis and treatment of diseases and disorders. In the late 20th century the delivery of health care, especially in the United States, underwent changes related to scientific and technologic advances. In addition to more sophisticated methods of diagnosing and treating disease,

these advances expanded the focus of health beyond disease and treatment of the person to the broader concepts of health maintenance and the health of populations. The delivery of health care also was becoming very expensive, and therefore, economics was a major factor in the changes made in health care.

Technologic Advancement for Diagnosis and Treatment

For most of the 20th century medical advances were related to the ability to diagnose and treat diseases. Biomedicine is strongly rooted in scientific discovery and therefore is profoundly influenced by the development of technology. Technologic development is constantly progressing and has transformed the way diseases are diagnosed and treated; however, medical advances often increase the costs of health care. Computerized technologies and microtechnology have allowed for more accurate monitoring and for management of intricate dynamic physiologic systems. For example, diagnostic tests and surgery can be performed on a fetus in utero to determine and limit future health problems. Complex physiologic systems can be managed and regulated by the use of pumps and other such means. As computers are developed further, more computerized technologies and microtechnology will be applied to health care.

The impact of technology on communications through the electronic means of the World Wide Web and Internet has allowed providers to access information and communicate with each other at great speeds. Clients can be diagnosed and treated over great distances through interactive television or other media. "Telehealth" has allowed clients and providers in rural areas to optimize expertise from large medical centers. The health-related information available to the public also has expanded.

Health Care Expansion

Since the late 1970s, advances in statistical analysis and epidemiology in public health have allowed for better analysis of the health of populations on international, national, and local levels. At the Alma Alta Conference (Russia) in 1978, the World Health Organization (WHO), put forth a **goal** (a broad statement of a desired outcome) that all the citizens of the world would attain a level of health that will permit them to lead a socially and economically productive life by the year 2000 (WHO, 1981). This emphasis broadened the focus of health care beyond specific diseases of individuals or public health concerns of containing or preventing epidemics. This broadened focus took three forms: early detection and treatment of disease, disease prevention, and health promotion.

Early Detection and Treatment

More sensitive and specific screening techniques became available to identify the early stages of a disease, when early treatment may reduce its development. Blood pressure and cholesterol screenings are good examples, in which disease can be detected in the early stages and thus lifestyle changes, medications, or a combination can be initiated to prevent or control development of the disease (Figure 1-1).

Disease Prevention

Disease prevention consists of measures taken to prevent the onset of a disease or disorder. Immunization is a good example of a successful effort in preventing disease. A number of public health measures have been enacted to protect public health by preventing epidemics and the spread of disease.

Health Promotion

Health promotion is a broad concept and includes actions that enhance the quality of life and reduce the risk of disease such as developing good stress management skills. Health promotion was defined by the WHO (WHO, 1986) to include not only individual well-being but also partnerships between lay and professional participants, professional and community groups, and other multilevel institutions and formal and informal groups.

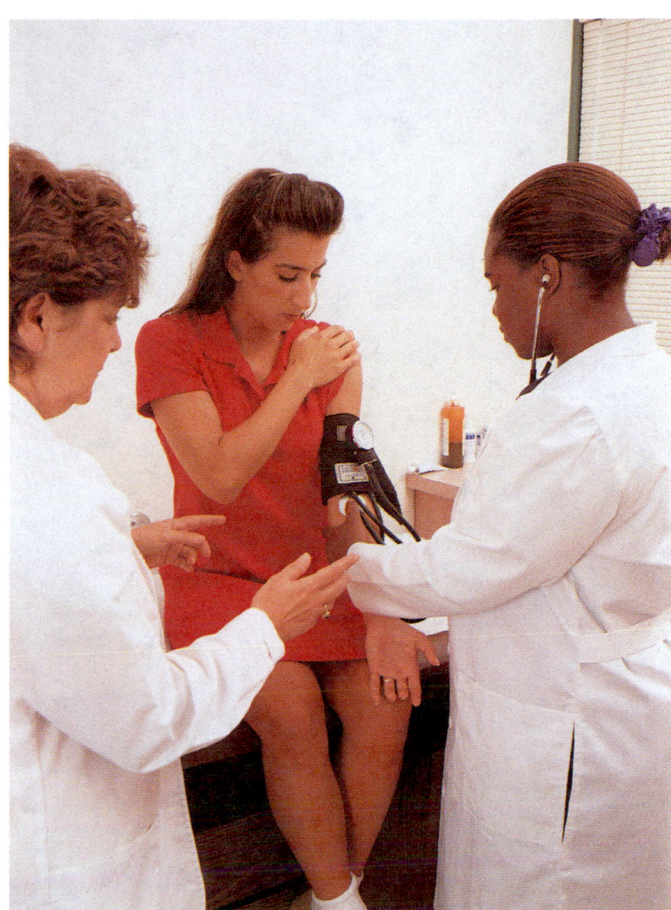

Figure 1-1 Routine blood pressure measurements are useful for early detection of some health problems.

The emphasis on disease prevention and health promotion has permeated most of health care. Government agencies and private foundations have been developing recommendations to move the health care system toward promoting better health for the entire population. Health indicators have been identified that allow more accurate evaluation of the health of the U.S. population and identify risk factors that may be targeted for better health outcomes. Awareness of disparities in the health of different groups of people has been the impetus for developing programs to improve the availability and quality of health care for all (Figure 1-2). With the emphasis on health, health care services and programs are increasingly being provided in community settings, with individuals and communities engaged as partners in the pursuit of health.

Risk Assessment and Management

Through epidemiologic studies, associations were made between diseases and certain conditions, exposures, or behaviors. Thus, factors were identified that could predict with some degree of probability that a person might

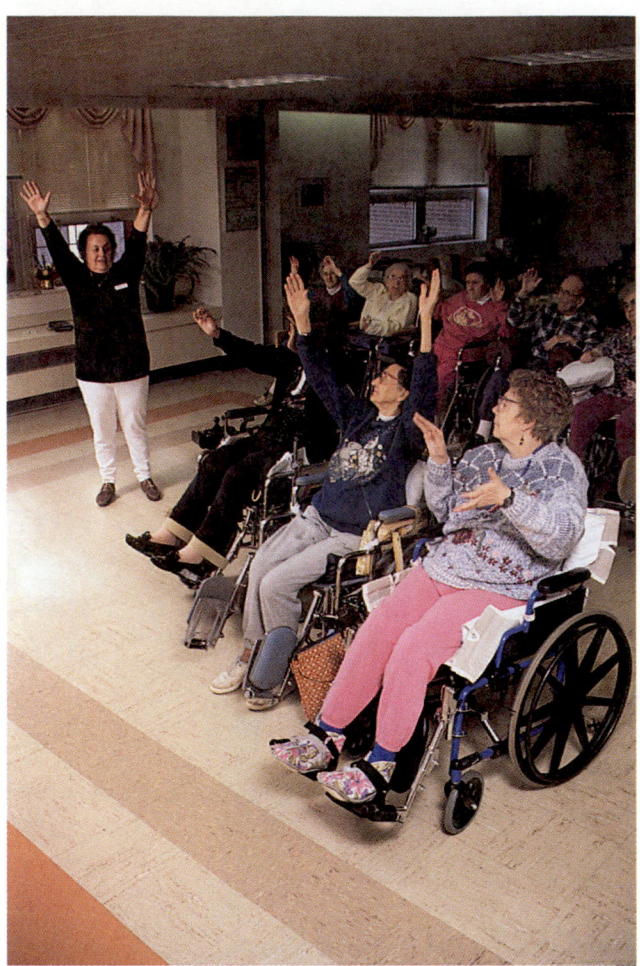

Figure 1-2 Health promotion activities may include exercises appropriate to the client's age and ability.

develop a disease in the future. **Risk assessment** is the process of examining the risk factors that place a person at risk for disease. For example, epidemiologic studies demonstrated an association between cigarette smoking

Nursing Tip

ANA POSITION STATEMENT
The American Nurses Association (ANA) issued a position statement supporting the promotion of health and prevention of disease and illness and disability. This position advocates comprehensive primary, secondary, and tertiary levels of prevention and engaging client participation. Prevention has long been within the scope of nursing as nurses work toward wellness with clients, families, and communities (ANA, 1995).

and a number of diseases. This association is for populations and cannot predict whether a certain person will develop a disease. These studies, however, do show that someone who smokes cigarettes is statistically more likely to develop a disease such as lung cancer compared with someone who does not smoke cigarettes. In many cases, biomedical research has strengthened the association by revealing physiologic links between risk factors and disease such as those between cigarette smoking and cardiovascular disease. Risk assessment and management are now part of basic clinical care.

Some of these risk factors can be altered, thereby decreasing the probability of acquiring a disease. Changing dietary and exercise behaviors are examples of initiating change to lower cholesterol levels, thereby reducing the risks of coronary artery disease. Other lifestyle changes, such as taking vitamins, avoiding smoking, and maintaining a healthy weight, may be undertaken to promote health rather than prevent a specific disease. With improved general health, the probability of getting a disease also may be reduced. Preventive and health-promoting efforts are relatively inexpensive. Health screenings, immunizations, and health education and counseling are low in cost when compared with the cost of complex acute care. Chronic debilitating diseases are costly, especially when the client needs long-term personal care. Many diseases, such as osteoporosis, can be very debilitating and require extensive nursing and medical care.

Movement of Health Care to the Community

Consistent with the shift in emphasis toward health, interventions have also shifted from large hospitals into the community in which the holistic approach has come to be recognized as increasingly important. New types of care delivery are emerging, such as day hospitals, day surgery, and transitional care, to move clients from the hospital to the home or other community setting. Nurses are finding positions in facilities for short-stay convalescence. Many centers that serve the chronically ill and geriatric populations are employing nurses for client education and other facets of nursing care. Home health care agencies employ nurses to provide care in the home to clients across the life span. Nurses are frequently providing both high-risk perinatal and neonatal care in the home as well as in hospitals and clinics. Nurses have had to incorporate interdisciplinary knowledge and cognitive skills to respond to this change in focus. As risk factors become better understood, psychologic, social, and environmental factors frequently are being implicated as contributors to health.

Primary care has been a growing area for health care and has expanded opportunities for nurses in all areas of practice. *Primary care* is the provision of integrated accessible health care by clinicians who address a large majority of personal health care needs, developing a sustained partnership with clients in the context of family and community (Institute of Medicine, 1996).

In addition to providing services to promote health and provide early detection and treatment of health problems, many nurses are beginning to work with local groups to promote the health of the community. Nurses often work with schools, churches, senior citizen centers, and other community organizations (such as the United Way and March of Dimes) to improve community health. Some of these collaborative efforts have resulted in building new clinics or health centers that may be run primarily by advanced practice nurses (APNs) and nurses at other levels. Other nurses may be involved in developing safe recreational areas for children and adults to exercise. Nurses' roles in the community have expanded and are predicted to expand even more as communities build their capacity for health environments.

Change in Philosophy

A substantially different relationship between client and clinician is required when dealing with health issues. In the traditional medical model, the clinician generally plays the active role and the client is the passive recipient of care. The need for a modification in that relationship has been addressed by two major advisory groups on health care change in the United States, the Robert Wood Johnson Foundation (1992) and the Pew Charitable Trust Commission on Health Professions (1995). In keeping with the goals for the nation, both groups have recommended restructuring of the relationship between the health care provider and client to one that emphasizes partnership rather than one of physician's orders and client compliance. These recommendations specify that the accomplishment of these goals requires a shared responsibility among individuals, families, communities, health professionals, media, and the government (Public Health Service, 1990). The Pew report also recommends that health care providers collaborate with clients and work together for health goals. These guidelines are based on the tenet that relationships among people constitute the foundation of all therapeutic activities (Pew, 1995).

An emphasis on health promotion and disease prevention relies on client participation and engagement in the therapeutic process, as does management of chronic illness. These modifications in the therapeutic relationship are congruent with nursing philosophy. Nursing interventions often have been health related such as instruction on a healthy diet, proper exercise, and other health-enhancing behaviors involving self-care. The current health care climate encourages the nurse-client relationship to be one of a partnership of mutual respect and setting of goals.

The American Holistic Nurses Association (AHNA) has described this relationship through the nursing process (Dossey, Keegan, & Guzzetta, 2000). In the Standards of Practice for Holistic Nurses, the nurse collaborates with the client and other health care team members. The nurse partners with the client in a mutual decision-making process to create a plan and engages the client in problem-solving. The nurse supports the client's participation in the plan, thus facilitating the client's efforts in health-seeking behaviors.

Cost Containment

As a social institution, the health care industry has a mission to develop the science and art of medicine and make health care services accessible to the public. The mission of healing has a long history and is the foundation for health care ethics. The mission of service recognizes the vulnerability of the client and thus is different from the motive of profit. The friction between these two coexisting missions is beneficial because they act as checks and balances within the system.

The costs of health care have continued to increase. Much of the increase is related to the high cost of technology and the expense of educating and training personnel to operate and interpret this technology. The health care sector constitutes more than 14% of the Gross National Product (GNP), and this percentage is projected to increase (Institute of Medicine, 2001). In 1970, the National Academies of Sciences (NAS) established the Institute of Medicine (IOM) to advance and disseminate scientific knowledge to improve human health. The IOM examines policy matters pertinent to the health of the public and acts as advisor to the federal government to identify issues of medical care, research, and education (IOM, 2001). The IOM issues reports to direct health policy and was asked by the U.S. Congress to address increasing health care costs.

Nurses must have some understanding of the economic forces that are now driving much of the organization of health care delivery such as managed care, cost containment, privatization, and the focus on prevention and efficiency. Emphasis now is on health care as a business and thus on the need to balance cost containment with competitive client satisfaction. The emphasis has increased the need to streamline health care delivery services to be more cost-effective and to compete for market shares, which has affected nursing roles. It was the streamlining of health care, for example, that led to the development of advanced practice roles. More often today, nurses are being asked to consider the cost-benefit ratio of their actions.

Cost-benefit analysis is the process of comparing the monetary cost (input) of doing something with the cost of the outcomes. The goal is to see if the benefits are greater than the costs. One of the most important concepts in the economics of health care is a cost-effectiveness analysis. **Cost-effectiveness analysis** compares the cost of doing something and measures the outcomes in non-monetary terms such as diseases or risks found, lives saved, or extra years lived (Gorin & Arnold, 1998). Effectiveness approaches allow the inclusion of issues such as quality of life, patient satisfaction, and comfort. This expanded definition allows for the inclusion of many nursing interventions. Nurses, however, must always be concerned about cost-benefit analyses because they often are used by administrators.

ACTIVITIES TO IMPROVE HEALTH

With the expanded focus and the shifts in emphasis discussed previously, the health care industry has established indicators to track the health of the U.S. population and has published goals and prevention guidelines for clinicians. Efforts are under way to address and better understand disparities in health. A number of adjustments in the organization of health care have addressed the economic issues of spiraling costs.

Identify Health Indicators

With the focus shifting to health, it has been necessary to identify determinants of health. Health indicators often have relied on **mortality rates**, the ratio of the number of deaths in various categories to a given population. These numbers often are written as rates; for example, the infant mortality rate (IMR) is the number of infants who die over the number of live births. The IMR often has been used to determine the quality of health in a country or population. For example, in the United States the IMR had decreased from 10/1,000 births to nearly 7/1,000 births in 1997, indicating that the target objective for the year 2000 would be met (National Center for Health Statistics, 1999). Specific signs and symptoms generally define disease. Thus, statistics can be collected on the number of people who have a disease, or the **morbidity rate**.

Whereas mortality and morbidity rates can be said to measure the absence of health, other indicators of health have been more difficult to measure. Health indicators have been established and evaluated by the U.S. Department of Health and Human Services (DHHS) in collaboration with the Centers for Disease Control and Prevention (CDC) and the National Center for Health Statistics (NCHS). These indicators are specifically stated in the published **objectives** (specific short-term achievements expected to result in the accomplishment of a goal) and are used to measure and evaluate progress toward the goals.

Establish Health Goals

The emphasis on health was reflected in the 1979 publication of "Healthy People: The Surgeon General's Report on Health Promotion and Disease Prevention" (DHHS, 1979). This document outlined goals and strategies to improve the health of the nation. These goals have been evaluated and new goals and specific objectives toward are established each decade. The first "Healthy People" document outlined three broad strategies: **disease prevention** (activities that prevent a disease or disorder), health promotion, and health protection (DHSS Department of Health & Human Services, 1979). These categories were subdivided into areas of concern with subsequent objectives.

"Healthy People 2000" established three main goals: Increase the span of healthy life, reduce health disparities, and achieve access to preventive services for everyone. Priority areas were established and over 300 measurable objectives identified (Public Health Service, 1990).

The U.S. Public Health Service (PHS) is responsible for coordinating activities directed toward attainment of the objectives. A midcourse review was put in place to provide an ongoing evaluation. These reviews generally are published shortly after the midpoint of the decade, for example, 1985, 1995, and so on, and these reports are available on the Internet at http://odphp.osophs.dhhs.gov/pubs/hp/2000/prog_htm. Currently, the progress toward meeting the goals is tracked and may be found through the NCHS (NCHS, 2001).

The current overall goals for "Healthy People 2010" are to increase quality and years of healthy life and to eliminate health disparities that are associated with race, ethnicity, and socioeconomic status. Community partnerships with persons, organizations, health care systems, and other partners are required to achieve these goals. The current objectives are listed under 28 focus areas (NCHS, 1999). Health indicators have been identified, objectives can be linked to these indicators, and data will be collected to determine the extent to which the objectives have been met. The leading health indicators for "Healthy People 2010" are given in Box 1-1. In addition to the goals for the nation described previously, state and local health departments have established goals, many of which are modeled after the "Healthy People" goals.

Address Health Disparities

Some U.S. populations had greater morbidity and mortality than did others. On multiple health indicators, ethnic, racial, and socioeconomic disparities exist (Moss, 2000; Lillie-Blanton et al., 2000). Research is being conducted to better understand issues related to the populations with poorer health such as access to care, social issues, and the

Box 1-1 Leading Indicators for "Healthy People 2010"
- Physical activity
- Overweight and obesity
- Tobacco use
- Substance abuse
- Sexual behavior
- Mental health
- Injury and violence
- Environmental quality
- Immunization
- Access to health care

effects of poverty. Currently, the large number of uninsured is an area of great concern. Disparities among population groups exist even when racial and ethnic disparities in income and health insurance coverage are eliminated (Weinick, Zuvekas, & Cohen, 2000).

A second aspect of disparities in health is the variation in practice patterns and the gap between what is known scientifically about medical treatment and what is practiced. The disparities in health led to an evaluation of access to health care services and redirecting resources to expand access. The Agency for Health Care Policy and Research (AHCPR) was created in 1989 to respond to concerns about the health care system (AHCPR, 1998). Its mission is to support, conduct, and disseminate research that improves access to care and the outcomes, quality, cost, and utilization of health care services (AHCPR, 1998). Decision makers at all levels are targeted by this agency: clinicians, clients, and policymakers. The agency has been renamed and is now the Agency for Healthcare Research and Quality (AHQR). The AHQR supports a rigorous research program that focuses on health care quality and the outcomes of health care services. The IOM also has issued a report that lays out a strategy to reduce medical errors that is directed toward government, industry, consumers, and health providers. The strategy was initiated because of reports of death and injury as a result of medical errors. The goal is to reduce medical errors by 50% in the next 5 years (Richardson, Kohn, Corrigan, Donaldson, 2000).

Institute Evidence-Based Practice or Best Practice

Evidence-based practice is a systematic approach that uses existing research for clinical decision processes (Westhoff, 2000). Reports are developed through epidemi-

ologic studies or rigorous syntheses and analyses of relevant scientific literature. Many of these reports use meta-analysis and cost analysis (AHQR, 2001). *Meta-analysis* is a process in which the published research studies on a particular topic are analyzed and results compiled when possible. Often, more than one research study or a very large study is required to warrant a recommendation for practice. This process allows for analyses of a group of small studies, and the findings can then represent a larger number of participants. Many times, however, published studies may not include all the necessary information for inclusion and therefore do not meet the criteria for inclusion in the meta-analysis. These reports are available to clinicians and are helpful in bringing the most well-informed up-to-date knowledge to clinical practice. With the use of the World Wide Web and Internet and connections to large information centers and databases, clinicians can access these reports and apply them to practice. Many of the guidelines now available have been generated from these systematic analyses. To initiate the process, a clinical question must be formulated and a search conducted. Two sources for published reviews are the Cochrane Database of Systematic Reviews and MEDLINE. Knowledge of research is necessary to critically appraise these studies. These reviews quickly give clinicians an idea about the current state of research so they can apply that knowledge to clinical practice. Good clinical practice in any discipline combines a knowledge of the latest clinical evidence to complement clinical assessment, clinical skills, and experience and clinical judgment (Westhoff, 2000). *Best practice* has been described in the nursing literature as a combination of evidence-based practice, clinician's judgment, and client preference (Hickey, Ouimette, & Venegoni, 2000).

Organizations are striving to provide cost-effective care based on the best evidence. Health care administrators are increasingly monitoring the outcomes of delivery of care in their organizations. This process involves gathering data on the status of client outcomes. For example, an organization may want to look at outcomes of deliveries and then compare them (e.g., the rate of cesarean sections or postpartum infections) with other institutions that are of similar size and have similar clientele. This process is called benchmarking. The organizations would evaluate their practice with guidelines, standards, and the literature on evidence-based practice. The organizations would then attempt to implement these guidelines, standards, and recommended practices and may alter the way care is delivered to meet those standards and improve outcomes. Many hospitals hire nurses for positions of outcomes managers. These nurses gather and analyze data from outcomes and may be involved in problem-solving techniques, such as continuous quality improvement, to achieve or improve on the benchmark standards.

Research Highlight

Caregiver Support for Women during Childbirth

Purpose

To systematically assess the effects of continuous support during labor on mothers and babies.

Method

Systematic search of the Cochrane Pregnancy and Childbirth Group Trials Register and the Cochrane Controlled Trials Register through April 2000. The review included 14 trials involving more than 5,000 women. Accompanied and unaccompanied women were compared. Persons accompanying the woman varied—nurses, midwives, family members, or lay persons. Varying designs of the included studies were discussed.

Findings

Continuous support reduced the likelihood of administration of pain medications (odds ratio, 0.59; 95% confidence interval; 0.52, 0.68), operative vaginal delivery (odds ratio, 0.77; 95% confidence interval, 0.65, 0.90), cesarean delivery (odds ratio 0.77, 95% confidence interval; 0.64, 0.91) and a 5-minute Apgar score less than 7 (odds ratio, 0.50; 95% confidence interval; 0.28, 0.87).

Nursing Implications

Intrapartum support has clear benefits and no known risks. Providers should encourage the provision of continuous presence, hands-on support, and encouragement to women in labor, which may come from a nurse, midwife, or lay person. Nurses could be involved in the education of labor support persons.

Hodnett, E. D. (2000). Caregiver support for women during childbirth. *The Cochrane Database of Systematic Reviews, 4,* (4). Available: http://gateway.ovid.com/server. Accessed February 7, 2001.

Develop and Publish Guidelines

The PHS convened the U.S. Preventive Services Task Force (PSTF) in 1984 to make recommendations over a range of clinical preventive services (Hickey, Ouimette & Venegoni, 2000). National guidelines to help health care providers implement preventive care were established and published in the *Guide to Clinical Preventive Services* (PSTF, 1996). These guidelines suggest age- and gender-specific screening tests, immunizations, and health advice. The second edition (PSTF, 1998) presents practical instructions for incorporating prevention into office and clinic routines. Guidelines are updated, and many are available on the AHQR website. Many of these updated topics relate to maternal, infant, and women's health.

Other guidelines have been established by consensus panels through the National Institutes of Health (NIH) to examine the research and current knowledge about a specific problem or treatment and make recommendations for practice. The National Guideline Clearinghouse is a publicly available database of evidence-based clinical practice guidelines, updated weekly, that is available over the Internet (www.guideline.gov). AHQR also publishes guidelines for practice.

Other guidelines are established for specific populations or specific medical conditions. These often are disseminated and published through professional organizations such as the American College of Obstetricians and Gynecologists (ACOG). This group has issued a number of guidelines in their technical bulletins and committee reports.

Nursing organizations also have published guidelines for practice. The Association of Women's Health, Obstetrics, and Neonatal Nurses (AWHONN) has guidelines for nurses on several issues related to maternity care, perinatal education, neonatal care, and women's health. Other professional groups, such as the National Association of Neonatal Nurses (NANN) and the AHNA, have standards of practice; the ANA has guidelines and position papers to guide practice. Other groups such as the March of Dimes and American Cancer Society publish guidelines for professionals and the public related to health promotion and disease prevention.

Work Toward Cost Containment

In an effort to provide the most cost-effective care, a number of changes in the organization of health care delivery and payment structures have been instituted. Best practice takes into account the most cost-effective way of delivering services and ways to make best care accessible to all persons.

Appropriate Technology

The most appropriate technology is often the most cost-effective kind. The most appropriate technology should be used to diagnose and treat illness. For example, critics have cited that using expensive technology, such as screening clients with magnetic resonance imaging for potential health problems, incurs excessive costs. Conversely, not using technology when it could prevent further health problems also is costly. For example, not monitoring fetal heart sounds during labor could result in prolonged hypoxia that, in turn, would result in chronic problems for that child (Figure 1-3). These illnesses often are very costly. Consensus reports and specialty guidelines have been developed to guide practice in the most cost-effective manner.

Another area of appropriate technology is using a variety of providers. In many cases a generalist is more appropriate and hence more cost-effective than is a specialist. Nurses prepared as APNs have been used in many cases to provide cost-effective management of patients.

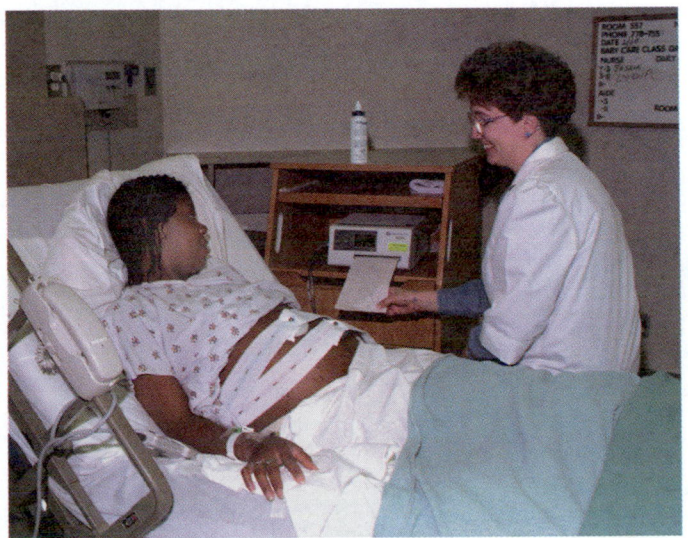

Figure 1-3 Fetal monitoring during labor is a good example of the appropriate use of technology.

Many of these APNs first provided primary care to low-risk clients. The role has expanded to providing specialized care in acute-care settings. Many managed care facilities have used APNs as the most effective technology, which has impacted the nursing profession by defining differentiated levels of practice to ensure that nurses are prepared to practice within the scope of their license. These certifications document the nurse's experience and mastery of a specialized body of knowledge. The effort to differentiate practice has impacted nurses at all levels. In many cases, roles between ADNs and nurses with a Bachelor of Science in Nursing (BSN) degree also are beginning to be differentiated. Baccalaureate-prepared nurses also are being certified to practice in specialties. One certification available to BSNs is Holistic Nurse Certification. This certification documents that the nurse has demonstrated mastery of a body of knowledge based on holistic autonomous care to clients which is based on research and nursing theory.

Managed Care

The advent of managed care has had a major impact on the U.S. health care delivery system in the last decade of the 20th century. **Managed care** refers to health care plans with a selective list of providers and institutions from which the recipient is entitled to receive health care that is reimbursed by the insurer (Committee on the Future of Primary Care, 1996). Typically, managed care plans also control the nature, amount, and site of services provided. Access to specialists may be restricted through the use of primary care providers as gatekeepers to the system (Mezey & McGivern, 1999).

Managed care in the United States has evolved over time and continues in its evolution. Growth of managed care plans varies according to region but predominates in large- to medium-sized markets (Committee on the Future of Primary Care, 1996). Evolution of managed care plans includes numbers of persons served, types of plans, and investment of providers.

In the 1960s and 1970s, health care costs became a major focus of attention in this country because they were becoming an ever-increasing portion of the national budget. There also were indicators suggesting that, without intervention, the escalation of health care costs would continue. Clearly, some measures needed to be implemented to control costs. By 1994, 180 million people were insured by private insurance plans and 115 million people were enrolled in some type of managed care plan (Bailit, 1995).

Three types of managed care plans currently exist: preferred provider organizations (PPOs), health maintenance organizations (HMOs), and point-of-service plans (POS). PPOs allow the consumer to see any provider or use any health care institution. The rate of reimbursement, however, is better when a provider or institution within the network is used.

Health maintenance organizations offer the consumer fewer options. Consumers must identify a primary care provider from a list of providers. When specialist care is sought, there must be a referral from the primary care provider or the expenses will not be reimbursed. The incentives for consumers to use this type of care usually are that the plan requires only a small copayment ($10 to $25) and all other expenses are covered by the plan. In HMO plans, hospitalization is usually covered by insurance, with a small copayment ($10 to $25).

Point-of-service plans are more flexible but more expensive for the consumer than are the other plans. PPOs allow the insured to be a member of an HMO but also seek health care outside the HMO at increased cost.

All three types of managed care plans offer advantages and disadvantages for the client, physician, and health care agency. The client is the primary concern for nurses. Managed care has changed the focus from institutional care to community care, with prevention and early detection as goals. Thus interest has moved toward primary care in the community. Many clients see this as an advantage; however, the result has been that when clients are admitted to the hospital they generally are sicker and have shorter stays.

Health maintenance organizations operate on the philosophy of providing preventive and early treatment. The care plans usually are set on capitated rates. The implications for physicians are that they must see more clients in a given period of time to break even. In general, this increase in flow rate has increased waiting time for appointments and time in the waiting room. The increased flow rate also has meant that physicians can no longer spend time with clients to answer questions or give explanations, which has led to disgruntled physicians and clients.

The major disadvantages clients see in managed care plans include relinquishment of choice of and limited access to health care providers. Many times it is the employer who initiates the managed care contract. Consumers provide little or no input. It may be necessary to relinquish excellent health care providers that have been clients' physicians or nurse practitioners for years because the managed care plan will not pay for their care. The private health care provider also seemingly had more time and was more available to the client.

Managed care has produced major effects on hospitals. Because the managed care plan makes contracts with hospitals and providers, these companies are very powerful. A managed care company contracting with a hospital for 500 deliveries per month results in a huge financial resource for the hospital. Losing the contract may be devastating to the economics of that hospital. It is especially stressful for the institution when the managed care company then awards the contract to the competition. The results on hospitals have been closings, mergers, and cost-containment measures.

Initially, cost-containment measures focused on early discharge. Later, care maps, critical pathways, guidelines, and protocols were developed to streamline patient care and make it cost-effective. Because nursing salaries are one of the major costs, many times hospital administrators have chosen to reduce staff or substitute licensed vocational nurses or technicians as a means of cost reduction. Later, administrators realized the lack of wisdom in this decision and are looking at the necessity of having more highly prepared nurses on staff.

Develop Collaboration with Multidisciplinary Teams

With the broader focus on health and the simultaneous concerns of improving effective care for all while containing costs, collaborative efforts from a variety of disciplines are necessary (Figure 1-4). *Multidisciplinary care* has been described as sequential provision of discipline-specific health care by various persons, whereas *interdisciplinary care* includes coordination, joint decision-making, communication, shared responsibility, and shared authority (Dossey, Keegan, & Guzzetta, 2000).

Three national foundations have addressed the health care system and made recommendations for health care delivery and provider education. The Pew Health Commission, Rockefeller Foundation, and Robert Wood Johnson Foundation have made recommendations and sponsored programs that foster interdisciplinary approaches to health (Hickey, Ouimette, & Venegoni, 2000). These organizations also have supported efforts in curricular reform to educate providers to an orientation to population health, primary care, and community health. Projects were spon-

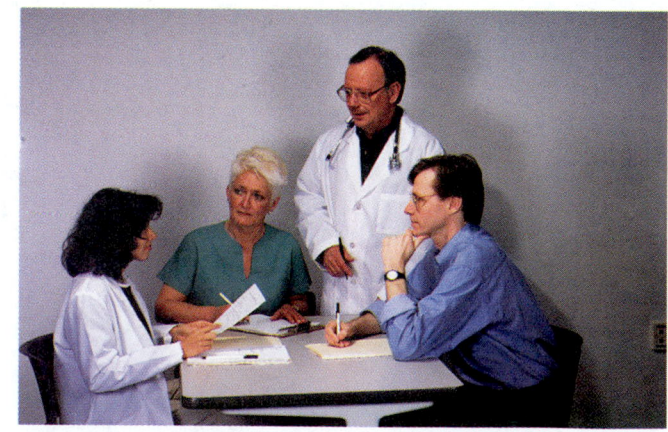

Figure 1-4 Multidisciplinary care involves coordination and joint decision-making with members of other health disciplines.

sored in which nurses, physicians, social workers, and nutritionists collaborated to provide comprehensive family-oriented care in a community setting. Before disbanding in 1999, the Pew Health Professions Commission proposed a

set of 21 competencies for all health professionals (Pew 1998); these are found in Box 1-2. These 21 competencies were further differentiated for various practice levels of nursing: Licensed Practical Nurse, AND, BSN, and those with a Master of Science in Nursing (MSN) degree (Brady et al., 1999).

Working closely on **interdisciplinary teams** (health care delivered by persons from various disciplines who share responsibility, authority, and decision-making) has allowed professionals from different disciplines to understand other disciplines and appreciate their contributions to client care as well as better understand different perspectives. Ideally, this approach offers the most comprehensive care to clients; however, it also requires good communication skills. Most disciplines have developed their own language, perspectives, and unique body of knowledge. It may not be easy to understand the perspective of persons in another discipline or their contribution to care. Conversely, nurses sometimes find it challenging to articulate the perspective and contribution of nursing.

The Pew Commission also made a number of recommendations on scope of practice and regulation of professions that would inform and protect the public against the actions of health care professionals outside of their scope of practice (Pew, 1995). Nurses often find that they are collaborating with other nurses and with nurses at other levels of practice. For example, a Baccalaureate-prepared nurse may be working with an APN. It is important to be clear on the unique professional perspective of nursing and the scope of practice at each level to effectively collaborate.

CHANGING VIEWS IN UNDERSTANDING HEALTH, ILLNESS, AND DISEASE

Recent discoveries and advances in knowledge from many disciplines have enhanced our understanding of health, illness, and disease. Some of the older approaches to health care are being challenged by advances in biologic research, behavioral medicine, and environmental medicine combined with advances in the social sciences related to the social and cultural aspects of health. Clients also have sought out complementary and alternative therapies to augment their health. Many of these therapies have been incorporated into health care delivery.

Biologic Science

Advances in the biologic sciences, such as breakthroughs in genetics and the mechanisms that connect the mind and body, are changing the understanding of many diseases and risk factors.

Box 1-2 Twenty-one Competencies for the 21st Century

1. Embrace a personal ethic of social responsibility and service.
2. Exhibit ethical behavior in all professional activities.
3. Provide evidence-based, clinically competent care.
4. Incorporate the multiple determinants of health in clinical care.
5. Apply knowledge of the new sciences.
6. Demonstrate critical thinking, reflection, and problem-solving skills.
7. Understand the role of primary care.
8. Rigorously practice preventive health care.
9. Integrate population-based care and services into practice.
10. Improve access to health care for those with unmet health needs.
11. Practice relationship-centered care with individuals and families.
12. Provide culturally sensitive care to a diverse society.
13. Partner with communities in health care decisions.
14. Use communication and information technology effectively and appropriately.
15. Work in interdisciplinary teams.
16. Ensure care that balances individual, professional, system, and societal needs.
17. Practice leadership.
18. Take responsibility for quality of care and health outcomes at all levels.
19. Contribute to continuous improvement of the health care system.
20. Advocate for public policy that promotes and protects the health of the public.
21. Continue to learn and help others learn.

Adapted from the Pew Health Professions Commission. (1998). *Recreating Health professional practice for a new century. The Fourth Report of the Pew Health Professions Commission.* San Francisco, CA: Pew Health Professions Commission.

Genetics

The Human Genome Project, a collaborative coordinated research effort through the NIH and Department of Energy, was funded by the U.S. Congress in 1988 (Jenkins, 2000). A second private organization, Celera Genomics, concurrently worked on decoding the human genome. This scientific breakthrough has made headlines and is predicted to radically change the diagnosis, risk assessment, and treatment of many diseases. These discoveries raise ethical, economic, and clinical issues at all levels of client care. Implications exist for medical management of predicted disease risks based on genetic profiles. Nurses will need to understand genetics to interpret information for and communicate it to clients. Professional nursing organizations (such as the International Society of Nurses in Genetics) exist that are dedicated to the scientific, professional, and personal development of nurses in the management of genetic information (Jenkins, 2000).

Ethical issues include protection of client confidentiality, which is among one of the foremost issues for providers and consumers (Jenkins, 2001). The impact that genetic screening may have on family relationships is another ethical impact. The potential uses of genetic information, fetal stem cells, and cloning are current topics of ethical discussion. Nurses in maternity and women's health need to be aware of the difficult ethical issues in making decisions related to fetal outcomes based on genetic knowledge available through prenatal screenings (Grant, 2000).

The National Coalition for Health Professional Education in Genetics (NCHPEG) has proposed a set of core competencies in genetics for all health care professionals (NCHPEG, 2001). Need exists for health professional curricula to incorporate genetic information so that professionals will be able to provide appropriate and accurate information for their clients.

Neuropsychology

Understanding of the physiologic mechanisms of thoughts and emotions has radically changed our understanding of many diseases. Selye's (1956) general adaptation syndrome described the systemic response of humans to stressors. Up until that time it was thought that specific diseases had specific causes. Selye's work generated a shift in thinking to the possibility of a person's resistance to disease being altered by the generalized effects produced by a variety of stressors. Continued research identified the neurologic and endocrine pathways by which humans respond to emotions such as fear, anger, and appreciation (Copstead, 1995). These pathways were further illuminated with the discovery of neuropeptides and neurotransmitters that connect a thought or emotion to physiologic changes (Pert, 1997). The pathways involved in anger and hostility and the way in which these emotions can result in

Critical Thinking

Competencies in Genetics

The National Coalition for Health Professional Education in Genetics (NCHPEG, 2001) has put forth a set of core competencies in genetics essential for all health care professionals. All health care professionals should, at minimum, be able to:

- Appreciate the limitations of their expertise in genetics.
- Understand the social and psychologic implications of genetic services.
- Know how and when to make a referral to a professional in genetics.

What do you think the role of a professional nurse is related to the criteria above?

How would you prepare yourself to function responsibly in the area of genetics?

How would you keep current in this area?

---

cardiovascular disease are fairly well understood (Rundell and Wise, 1996). This knowledge has been translated into stress management interventions in many areas of health care such as cardiac rehabilitation programs. Depression also has been associated with many diseases and has clear associations with heart disease (Rundell & Wise, 1996). Theoretical mechanisms related to emotions and the immune system are being developed as is a body of research on psychoneuroimmunology. This area has particular implications for nurses because they are in a position to facilitate coping and stress management in clients.

Environmental Medicine

With the excitement of the Human Genome Project, it is crucial to recognize that genes are only a part of complex disease processes. Very few diseases are the consequence of only genes or a single environmental event. Generally, diseases result from a combination of individual differences in susceptibility to diseases and dysfunctions that are linked to environmental exposure (Environmental Health Perspectives, 1997). Figure 1-5 illustrates the interaction of genetic predisposition, environment, and human behavior.

The DHHS, in collaboration with several private agencies including the Pew Charitable Trusts, has published guidelines to promote the development of a stronger public health system to protect citizens from environmental

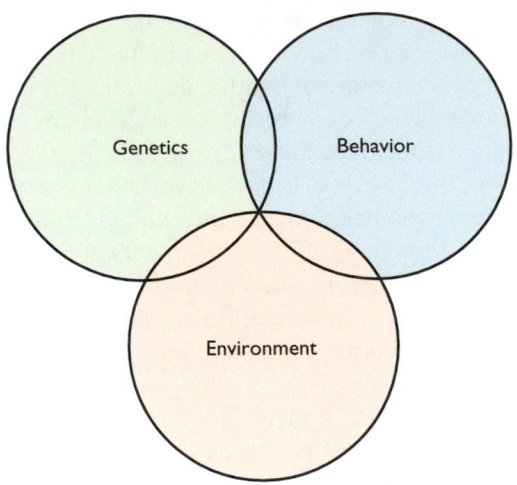

Figure 1-5 The interaction of genetics, behavior, and the environment.

threats to health (PEHC, 2000). The effects of environmental toxins are of particular interest in the area of maternity nursing because prenatal exposure to some toxins has been linked with birth defects.

Behavioral Medicine

Behavioral medicine is a branch of medicine that focuses on behavior and the cognitive, emotional, motivational, and biobehavioral interactions that result in behavior. A growing awareness exists regarding the behavioral underpinnings of disease. Many risk factors are involved in human behavior, and these behaviors interact with biologic factors to influence health outcomes. Human behavior is a critical avenue for prevention and treatment. The NIH has defined the term *behavioral* in various ways: overt actions; underlying psychologic processes such as cognition, emotion, temperament, and motivation; and biobehavioral interactions (Kirschstein, 2000). All these factors are part of our understanding of human behavior. Human behavior and its relationship to health outcomes have implications for nurses counseling clients about health promotion.

Research in the neurosciences has advanced the treatment of many brain and neurologic disorders from sleep disorders to dementia. Understanding of the connections between anger, hostility, and other emotions has been incorporated into cardiac rehabilitation programs. Progress in understanding the mind and immune system promise to have implications in many diseases.

A large area of research is ongoing in the area of better understanding of motivation and behavior change. This type of research is crucial if one is to modify behaviors to improve health. Some of the major areas of behavior with implications for health outcomes include nutrition, exercise, stress management, violence, smoking, the use of other harmful or addictive substances, and sexual behavior resulting in sexually transmitted diseases and unwanted pregnancies.

Social Aspects of Health

All societies have social structures, referring to the organized patterns of relationships between persons and groups in society. One social structure is the family. The roles that family members play and the effects of family dynamics on health are beginning to be addressed in health care (Figure 1-6). The effects of single-parent families on children, domestic violence, and isolation of older persons from family members are some of the social issues with medical consequences. Socioeconomic status and gender issues also are important social factors in health care, and their relationships to disparities in health outcomes are being examined.

Socioeconomic Status

Recent research is uncovering the impact that social inequities have on health. Risks of morbidity and mortality are increased with lower socioeconomic status (Wilkinson, 1996; Evans, Barer, & Marmor, 1994). This discovery has opened the frontier of medicine that examines health determinants embedded in the social structure of society. Social status generally is measured by income, education, employment, or housing. Research suggests that one's position in the social hierarchy affects one's health, with those at the lower end having poorer health. Although the mechanisms are unclear, much interest exists in the concept of social capital or one's **social assets** (benefits to health related to social position and socioeconomic status) and its relationship to health outcomes (Hawe & Shiell, 2000). Social networks and social relationships are increasingly

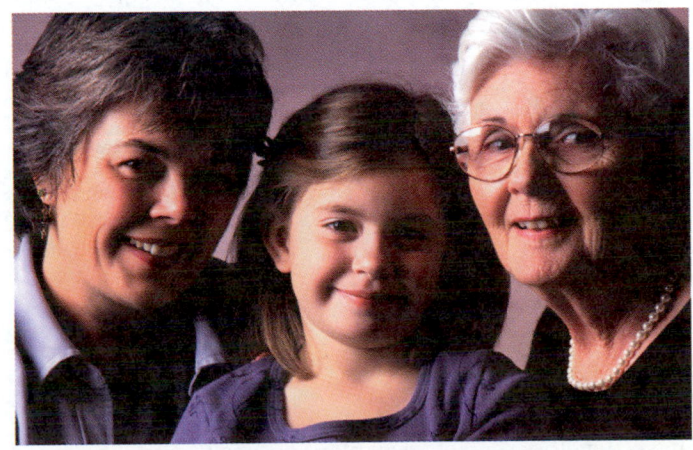

Figure 1-6 Family dynamics may have a significant impact on health.

being documented as being important in all aspects of health. Healthy egalitarian societies are more socially cohesive, have stronger community lives, and generally have better health indicators of lower mortality and morbidity than do societies with broad social disparity (Wilkinson, 1996).

Gender Issues

Women and men have gendered social roles and expected behavior in society. Gendered stereotypes also exist in the health care system. Most of medical research and approaches are based on knowledge about men. Women are biologically different from men and exist in a different social position in society. Women have higher incidences of certain diseases, such as depression, than do men. Women have different patterns of health care use than do men (Loustaunau & Sobo, 1997). A series of workshops known as the Hunt Valley workshops, in 1991, recommended an agenda to advance research in women's health (NIH, 1999). That same year, the NIH established the Office of Research on Women's Health (ORWH). Researchers and clinicians are now beginning to understand how differences in gender culture and socioeconomic backgrounds influence the causes, diagnosis, progression, and treatment of disease. The ORWH ensured that clinical trials addressed issues regarding women's health and that there was appropriate participation of women in clinical trials. An additional goal of ORWH was to increase opportunities for women in biomedical research careers. The research agenda has been evaluated and updated in 1996–1997. The new agenda targeted specific areas of medical research and addressed the following overarching issues (NIH, 1999):

1. Women are important sources of new information that will correct essentially male models of normal functions and pathophysiology.
2. Research into women's health must include physical, mental, and emotional changes that occur over the full biologic life cycle.
3. Multidisciplinary research is essential.
4. Social research and behavioral research are necessary and need to be integrated into mainstream medical disciplines.
5. Collection of research data on women to better understand female function and pathophysiology should continue.

Cultural Issues and Health

Systems of health care exist in all cultures. All cultures have developed ways of explaining health and illness and have given names to particular disorders called diseases. These schema are called explanatory models and contain a name for a condition or disorder, an understanding of what that disorder is, how one acquired it, what the course of the disorder would be, and suggestions for treatments (Kleinman, 1980). Biomedicine is one system of health care with a specific explanatory model and a scientific method of uncovering knowledge. Other systems may have different names and understandings of the disorder and may ascribe very different treatments. If the client and provider are based in discordant explanatory models, communication is impeded and the client is less likely to adhere to the recommendations given by the biomedical provider.

Kleinman (1980), a medical anthropologist, described three classic sectors of health care that are present in all cultures: professional, popular, and folk. Science-based biomedicine is the foundation of the professional sector that, in the United States and Canada, is synonymous with the health care system. This sector includes all the associated professions that work in collaboration with medicine such as nursing, physical therapy, occupational therapy, nutrition, psychology, and social work. These professions are greatly influenced by the biomedical approach to health and treatment of disease based on empirical science and sophisticated technology.

The second sector, the popular sector, is the largest. This sector incorporates the health care and health information provided by family, friends, and other social networks. Most health decisions are made and most health-related behaviors occur in this sector. That is, it is within the family and social networks that orientations toward health and lifestyle practices, such as eating, exercising, and simple remedies, take place. This sector also is the one in which the decision to seek help from other sectors occurs, as well as decisions regarding when, for which purposes, and from whom to seek additional care. This sector also determines if and how the person adheres to recommended treatments or advice.

The third sector, folk or traditional medicine, includes all the sacred and secular healers practicing outside the professional sector. This sector has recently gained great popularity in countries in which biomedicine has been well established. Sacred and secular healers have emerged in North America and Europe having a variety of complementary and alternative therapies. Many of these therapies have gained popularity outside of their original ethnic group, and many health care plans are moving to integrate some of these therapies into the mainstream health care system. For example, acupuncture is being researched and incorporated into some health care plans.

Recognition of these three sectors and the interaction among them is necessary for the nurse to facilitate clients from culturally diverse backgrounds to negotiate the health care system. **Cultural competency** describes a process of integrating cultural awareness in the delivery of culturally appropriate clinical care. Cultural competency is becoming a more recognized skill for all health care providers.

Complementary and Alternative Therapies

Increasingly, the public has been employing various strategies to enhance health and in some cases treat disease. Some of these strategies are massage and other forms of body work, use of food supplements and herbal remedies, and various forms of psychologic and spiritual techniques. Providers of these treatments comprise one of the more rapidly growing sectors of the work force. Many of these treatments are being researched, and the NIH has a center for studying them. Most of these treatments are used as adjuncts to biomedical health care, and many are being integrated into health care systems. The popularity of these treatments, and in some cases their proven effectiveness, has opened new approaches to promoting the health of clients. This popularity is of particular interest to those in the nursing profession because many of these strategies have been reported on in the nursing literature and have been practiced as autonomous nursing interventions. These strategies are facilitating health care providers to broaden their view of disease processes to the illness experience. In doing so, providers can begin to better understand and provide help and support to clients in their experience with illness or their attempts to stay healthy.

CONTEMPORARY CHALLENGES IN HEALTH CARE DELIVERY

A number of issues and challenges exist for clients and for anyone working in health care. Many of these concerns are associated with the recent trends and advancements in health care. Technologic advances bring not only increased ability to extend care and access information but raise new challenges. Changing U.S. demographics raise issues of meeting cultural competence and dealing with issues of age and gender. Cost containment remains an issue. One of the strategies in cost containment is differentiated practice on multidisciplinary teams, which is of particular interest to nurses because we have several levels of practice.

Rapidly Changing Technology

Technology is increasing in all areas. Technology in diagnosing, monitoring, and treating clients is changing almost daily. The most radical changes in our culture have been the technologic developments in how we attain, process,

and communicate information. The term for these developments is informatics and specifically **health care informatics** (integration of computer science, information science, and health care professionals involved in collecting, processing, and managing data). The ANA defined nursing informatics as a specialty that integrates nursing science, computer science, and information science in identifying, collecting, processing, and managing data and information to support nursing practice, administration, education, research, and the expansion of nursing knowledge (ANA, 1994).

Technology in Diagnosis and Treatment of Disease

Technologic breakthroughs in health care are coming from scientific research at many levels: the systems, molecular, and genetic levels. Technologic devices (such as miniaturized surgical instruments that allow intricate surgeries to be done with minimal trauma to clients) have reduced hospital stays. Understanding how to use and interpret these new technologies is a continuing challenge for nurses. Keeping abreast of new advances in areas of medicine such as genetics calls for continuing study on the part of every professional.

"Telemedicine" allows for assessment, monitoring, and treatment of clients at a distance. For example, while the mother is at home the heart rate of her fetus can be monitored and conveyed electronically to the hospital or clinic for interpretation. These technologic advances require that nurses be adept in using the latest technology.

Technology in Communication and Health Informatics

The nursing profession has been engaged in developing a common language for nursing practice and in defining a nursing minimum data set (NMDS) to reflect the common core of data that describes nursing practice. The four classification systems generally used for nursing and supported by the ANA are North American Nursing Diagnosis Association (NANDA) Nursing Diagnosis Taxonomy, the Omaha System, Home Health Care Classification (HHCC), and Nursing Intervention Classification (NIC) (Romano, 2000). The ANA has issued a position statement in support of the development of national nursing databases and establishment of a uniform language for nursing practice (ANA, 1994). The ANA has recognized NANDA as a body to be used for development, review, and approval of nursing diagnoses.

One of the major ethical issues concerning the use of computers in health care and electronic medical records is that of client privacy and confidentiality. Nurses are frequent processors of client information and must be accountable for the accuracy of data and maintenance of security to protect client confidentiality. The ANA position paper on privacy and confidentiality (ANA 1999) addresses these issues and states that nurses should contribute to the development of standards, policies, and laws that protect patient privacy and the confidentiality of health records and information. New legislation is slated to take effect in 2001 to protect the privacy of client's medical records. Many in the health care field are concerned that putting systems in place to comply with these regulations will be difficult and costly.

Client Access to Health-Related Information

Clients can now access much of the same health-related information as can health care providers. Many government websites with clinical guidelines and medical information are open to the public. Web browsers can access medical journals and scientific information. Nurses and other health care professionals are familiar with peer-reviewed journals and the research process to help evaluate health information. Clients may not have the appropriate background to interpret this information and may become needlessly worried or misinterpret appropriate actions.

Client Education

Using the Internet

The following are some questions that can guide clients in evaluating information on the Internet:

- Does the information seem logical?
- Is the information consistent with information from their health care provider?
- Is the website trying to sell a product or service?
- Are unrealistic or unsubstantiated claims being made?
- Is the information extremely biased against biomedicine or a different complementary therapy?
- Is the information documented and researched?
- Are there links to reputable sites?
- Do the creators of the site have credentials, institutional affiliations, or sponsorship?

Clients also are exposed to many helpful organizations that may have chat rooms that serve as self-help groups. Clients may find many valuable resources for health problems by searching the Internet. Much misinformation also is available on the Internet, and nurses may be in the position to help clients interpret the information they receive and sort out accurate information from useless or potentially harmful information. Without help, clients may be subject to fraudulent claims and inaccurate information.

Changing Demographics

The U.S. demographics are changing. Trends in ethnic distribution and the projected increases in the population of older persons have implications for health care provision.

Ethnic Pluralism

A dramatic increase has occurred in U.S. ethnic and minority populations. The U.S. census has classified people according to race as African American, Caucasian, other races, and people of Hispanic origin (Census gov, 2001). According to census projections, European Americans are the majority; however, African Americans, Hispanics, and other ethnic groups are increasing at a faster rate. Projections of the increase in population between 1995 and 2050 are as follows: Caucasians are expected to increase by 35.1%, African Americans by 82.8%, other races by 233.9%, and Hispanics by 258.3% (Administration on Aging, 2001). As a result, health care providers are providing care to clients who often do not speak the same language and have beliefs, values, and traditions that differ from their own. Cultural competence and linguistic competence are needed to respond effectively to health care encounters with these clients.

The Office of Minority Health (OMH) has published recommendations for national standards and an outcomes-focused research agenda regarding ensuring cultural competence in health (OMH, 2001). These recommendations are clustered into those pertaining to linguistic competence and the provision of appropriate interpreters and translation of written materials and those that relate to cultural competence. Several recommendations were made for organizations to promote competencies of the staff, engage the communities, and promote accountability. Formal certification for interpreters now exists in a few states (Cross Cultural Health Care Program, 2001).

It is important to recognize not only how to communicate with clients but how cultural differences may affect their health. Some biologic differences exist among cultures that affect certain diseases, such as Tay-Sachs disease in Ashkenazi Jews or the way some groups react to medications. Cultural beliefs, values, and traditions are the bases for most human behavior such as diet and exercise habits. *Culture* refers to integrated patterns of human behavior that include language, thought, communication, actions, customs, beliefs, values, and institutions of racial, ethnic, religious, or social groups.

Aging of the Population

In addition to changes in ethnic and racial makeup of the country, the population of older persons is projected to increase by 17% in 2010, 75% from 2010 to 2030, and 14% from 2030 to 2050 (AOA, 2001). This population will increase to about 79 million. From 2010 to 2030, the rate of growth will exceed that of the population under the age of 65 years; therefore, the proportion increases to 20%. This increase is related to low fertility rates, maturing of the baby boomers, and a decrease in mortality rates of adults in older age groups. Older women generally outnumber older men. The health concerns related to the aging population are the dependency burden of this large number of elderly if they are in poor health. Thus, it is an important public health concern and a humane objective to help the aging population maintain good health (Figure 1-7).

Balancing Cost with Best Practice

Contemporary health care continually balances the best practice and best use of technology with the attempt to keep costs from escalating. In addition to other technologic factors that increase costs, litigation adds to the costs of delivering health care. Differentiated practice has been discussed as a means to streamline care.

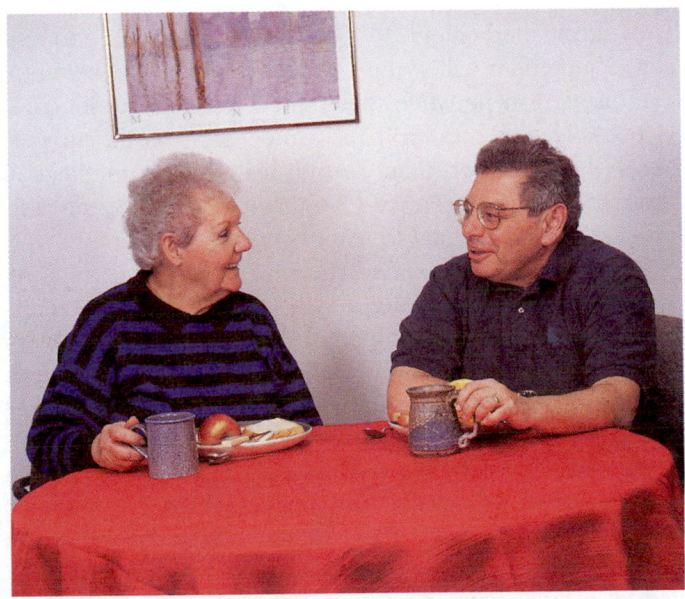

Figure 1-7 Good health, a positive attitude, and healthy behaviors are important at all ages.

Litigation

Litigation in health care has increased. With the increase in technology, providers often feel they need to use expensive tests, even if not medically necessary, to avoid being sued. As clients become more knowledgeable about health issues, they are demanding more tests and sometimes treatments. Providers feel they must practice defensively to avoid lawsuits, which often adds to the costs of health care.

Differentiated Practice and Regulatory Issues

Differentiated practice focuses on the structuring of roles and functions of nurses according to education, experience, and competence. Several models have been used to redesign nursing practice in institutions to use nurses most efficiently and effectively (Koerner et al., 1995). Many of these models also used clinical pathways. These pathways were designed as interdisciplinary plans of care to manage client populations by diagnosis or medical procedure. For example, a normal delivery with no complications might follow a clinical pathway. In one example (Koerner et al., 1995), a clinical specialist with an MSN would serve as case manager to coordinate the care based on holistic knowledge and familiarity with research and theory. The nurse, generally with an associate degree, would provide care for specified periods of time in structured settings with well-established policies and procedures and for clients who do not deviate from the clinical pathway. The primary nurse, generally with a BSN, would provide integrated health care from admission to discharge in both structured and unstructured settings. Many hospitals have instituted some form of differentiated practice and the use of clinical pathways.

NURSING IMPLICATIONS

Nurses must understand the environment of the health care system to function as a member of the health care team and adapt the environment to benefit the client. The holistic approach corresponds well with the changing orientation of health care delivery. Holistic nursing care is based on the view that an integrated whole has a reality independent of and greater than the sum of its parts (Dossey, Keegan, & Guzzetta, 2000). Holistic nursing involves understanding the interrelationships of the biologic, psychologic, sociocultural, and spiritual dimensions of the person who is interacting with the internal and external environments. This philosophic approach is consistent with most nursing theories (Stevens-Barnum, 1994; Mariner-Tomey, 1994) and has been used to differentiate autonomous nursing practice from that of other disciplines such as medicine, nutrition, and psychology. The holistic approach is the foundation of contemporary nursing practice and provides for delivery of the most comprehensive nursing care. This philosophy also enables nurses to assume a proactive role and become leaders in the new health care system.

NURSING SKILLS FOR PROFESSIONAL PRACTICE

In the current health care system, it is not sufficient for the practicing nurse to simply follow physician's orders. As an important member of the health care team, the contemporary nurse is required to participate in planning and implementing effective, cost-efficient health care. This role requires a nurse who has good cognitive abilities and who is able to reason and apply sound clinical judgment. As health care and information technology continue to advance, the nurse must have adept technical skills, which include the efficient use of technology. Nurses also need excellent communication skills for counseling and educating clients and communicating professionally with the interdisciplinary team. Self-reflection also is an important skill for the nurse to advance professional and personal development. These skills are learned throughout the nurse's career; however, the foundation must be laid during basic nursing education. Obtaining refined and sophisticated nursing skills requires practice; however, theoretical concepts must be socialized into the basic nursing curriculum.

Cognitive Skills

Cognitive skills, frequently referred to as critical thinking skills, include attainment of knowledge, ability to reason, analytic processing, clinical judgment, problem-solving, and critiquing. Attainment of knowledge is the focus of preparatory formal education and professional continuing education. The ability to reason is the foundation of any professional role. *Reasoning* is the act of discovering, formulating, or concluding by the use of reason or thought. Reasoning is an essential skill for practicing nurses and is the basis for proficiency in clinical judgment. Although reasoning is considered to be an ability all humans have to some degree (often called common sense), a more formal type of reasoning is required for the practice of nursing, which has been labeled critical thinking. Critical thinking skills can be very difficult to teach and more difficult to learn because they involve using abstract thought, judgment, and logic. **Critical thinking** is a formal and structured type of reasoning used in nursing as the foundation for sound clinical judgment. It involves reasoning, processing data, analyzing, and evaluating. The first step in the

learning process is to define and describe these concepts involved with reasoning.

All reasoning has a purpose, and usually it is to try to understand a phenomenon, settle a question, or solve a problem. The holistic nurse uses reasoning to understand the client, analyze and interpret information about the client, and engage in problem-solving.

Reasoning can be very complex because it is based on assumptions and reflects a certain point of view. Reasoning involves organization of data, information, and evidence shaped into concepts or ideas. Analytical processing must take place. Conclusions are drawn when the process is complete and some meaning is placed on the conclusions. All reasoning therefore leads to outcomes that have implications or consequences, which may be positive, negative, or unexpected. It is therefore important for the nurse to practice self-reflection and develop critiquing skills.

Critical thinking uses a structured type of reasoning. When used properly, critical thinking goes beyond stating personal preferences and opinions. This type of thinking allows the nurse to think independently of cultural and experiential knowledge and, at the same time, critique and integrate these sources of knowledge. Critical thinking involves more than simply restating facts; it involves an active use of formal knowledge.

Critical thinking allows one to distinguish among three different types of questions, that is, those with:

1. One right answer (factual questions)
2. Better or worse answers (well-reasoned or poorly reasoned answers)
3. As many answers as there are human preferences (opinion answers)

Only the second category of questions is amenable to reasoned judgment following critical thought. Unless nurses can distinguish between these three types of questions, it is possible that they will make decisions based on personal views rather than sound reason and intellectual thought (Elder & Paul, 1996). Successfully using this process is fundamental to sound clinical judgment.

Vickers (1997) clarified the need for critical thinking by asserting that there are a very large number of beliefs about health, some of which are contradictory. It is very unlikely that all commonly held health beliefs are both valid and useful. For example, when a woman becomes pregnant, it is a widely held belief that she needs to increase her dietary intake sufficiently to maintain the health of two entities, the mother and unborn child. The reality is that if a woman adopts this attitude and does not manage her diet conservatively, her risks for obesity, pregnancy-induced hypertension, and gestational diabetes are increased. It is through the process of logical reasoning and critical thinking that these conflicts are resolved.

Several components are necessary to begin to successfully use critical thinking. A specific formal knowledge base and experience are required to develop competencies in this area (Kataoka-Yahiro & Saylor, 1994). The knowledge base is begun during prenursing courses and is built on throughout the nursing career. Technical skills also are established during basic education but need to be refined with experience. As technology advances, the focus on clinical decision making, client-focused data, and client-appropriate solutions will radically alter the way concepts are defined and decisions in nursing are made (Turley, 1996). The ability to adapt to unforeseen elements of change requires flexibility.

Kataoka-Yahiro and Saylor (1994) described attitudes of nurses that are considered essential for the development of critical thinking skills: self-confidence, independence, fairness, responsibility, risk-taking ability, discipline, perseverance, creativity, curiosity, integrity, and humility. Critical thinking and intellectual thought are expressed through professional and personal communication. Certain standards are used to judge intellectual thought; these are clarity, precision, accuracy, relevance, depth, breadth, and logic (Paul & Elder, 1996). The degree to which these standards are met determines how logical the thought is and how valid the conclusions are that are based on that thought. These standards apply equally to critical thinking.

Clarity refers to having purpose of thought. Clarity involves differentiating the nurse's purpose from related purposes, and it requires periodic evaluation to ensure that thinking stays on target. To act on thought that lacks clarity exposes clients to unnecessary health risks and the clinician to unnecessary medical and legal risks.

Precision involves understanding the scope and meaning of the issue at hand. When issues are complex, they may need to be broken down into components to identify which type of question is to be resolved. To lack precision of thought increases the risk of unneeded therapy for the client.

Accuracy is ensured by identifying assumptions to determine if they are justifiable. Another factor involved in accuracy of reasoning is self-evaluation by the reasoner of personal beliefs and values that may influence reasoning outcome. Seeking the opinions of others is a method that promotes accuracy through an overt attempt to consider all points of view related to the issue before making decisions.

Many times problems are very complex, and whether all data surrounding the issue are relevant may be unclear. A determination must be made as to which data are sufficient and necessary to use in finding a solution. Analysis of the information until it is reduced to component parts may be useful. Sufficient depth and breadth must be considered to avoid missing important details or related issues. Caution must be advised to avoid reduction to oversimplification. When oversimplification occurs, important contextual factors may be eliminated from the decision-making formula, leading to unacceptable outcomes for the client or health care provider.

Cognitive skills necessary for critical thinking include interpretation, analysis, evaluation, inference, explanation, and self-regulation (Pless & Clayton, 1993). To interpret data necessitates the ability to categorize, recognize the significance of, and clarify the meaning of concepts. Through the process of analysis the reasoner is able to examine ideas, identify arguments, and determine the components of those arguments. Evaluation skills are required to assess claims and determine the validity of arguments. It is only through analysis, synthesis, and evaluation that inferences can be made to develop hypotheses and draw conclusions. The ability to articulate is required of the skilled reasoner to explain the findings, share the results, and justify the procedures, and then to present arguments that are reasonable. Self-awareness is required by the reasoner to evaluate the logical process.

Optimal nursing care depends on the nurse's ability to use logical reasoning and critical thinking skills throughout the nursing process. Reasoning is used to identify and conceptualize problems in terms of the nursing process through analysis of the problem, synthesis of this information into a plan of intervention, and identification of outcomes to facilitate modification of the plan of care to meet client needs (Table 1-1).

Technical Skills

As health care becomes more efficient and with continual technical changes in medical equipment, nurses must keep their technical skills current. Basic technical skills related to the operation of technology generally are part of the nurse's foundational education; however, these skills must be developed and expanded in practice. Nurses need to know how to operate, appropriately use, understand, and maintain technical equipment. Technologic proficiency

Table 1-1 Critical Thinking Skills Applied to the Nursing Process

Critical Thinking Skill	Nursing Process Element
Attainment of knowledge	Assessment
Integration of knowledge	Nursing diagnosis
Ability to reason through	Outcome identification
Analytic processing	Planning
Clinical judgment and	Nursing intervention
problem-solving	
Critiquing	Evaluation

goes beyond knowing how to operate a particular machine or execute a procedure. Nurses must be adept in interpretation of technology. It is not sufficient to record technologic data; nurses must understand and interpret that data and integrate that understanding into the nursing process. Nurses' participation in the health care arena and their close relationship with clients' experiences place nurses in a position to develop devices to facilitate their work and for client use.

Information technology is changing rapidly, and electronic communication is the technology of the future. Nurses must be adept at using this technology both to keep their own information up to date and to ensure that appropriate nursing data are part of clients' records. Opportunities also exist for nurses to use this media creatively to educate clients.

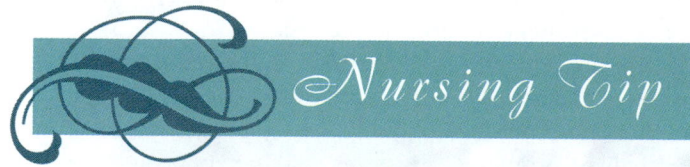

TECHNICAL SKILLS FOR THE CONTEMPORARY NURSE

1. Use of Technology
   - Operation of equipment and supplies
   - Maintenance of equipment and supplies
2. Interpretation of technology
3. Application of technologic expertise

Communication Skills

Communication skills are vital to the entire nursing process, and they are important to the nurse's ability to engage in interrelationships. All communication involves a sender and receiver. The nurse must be clear and accurate in both roles. Thus, nurses need to be astute in various types of communication: verbal, nonverbal, written, and virtual. Nurses also are senders of nonverbal communication; through self-awareness, nurses develop insight into subtle forms of communication.

A strategy of communication often used in client care includes client teaching and counseling. Client teaching follows the nursing process and must be anchored in a mutually derived diagnosis of lack of knowledge. Teaching is done with individual clients, families, and groups. Nurses are expected to develop client education programs and teach groups of clients (Figure 1-8). Skills in sequencing material and presentation of information appropriately to the selected audience are useful, and expert knowledge of the topic is essential.

COMMUNICATION SKILLS

1. Mastery of various types of communication
   - Verbal
   - Nonverbal
   - Written
   - Virtual
2. Application of specific methods of communication
   - Teaching
   - Counseling
   - Formal presentations
3. Domains for communication
   - Inter- and intraprofessional communication
   - Nurse-client communication

A nurse may conclude the problem or nursing diagnosis is lack of knowledge when, in fact, it may be that the recommended intervention is in conflict with the client's value system or the client does not have access to resources to adhere to the recommendations. In these cases, client counseling may be the more appropriate intervention. This skill includes working with the client in mutual problem-solving and developing creative solutions that are uniquely suited to the needs of the client and situation.

Nurses communicate in a number of domains that include different audiences and various media. In addition to communicating with clients, nurses must communicate effectively with professionals from multiple disciplines. To do so, nurses must be familiar with the scientific process and the perspectives of other members of the health care team.

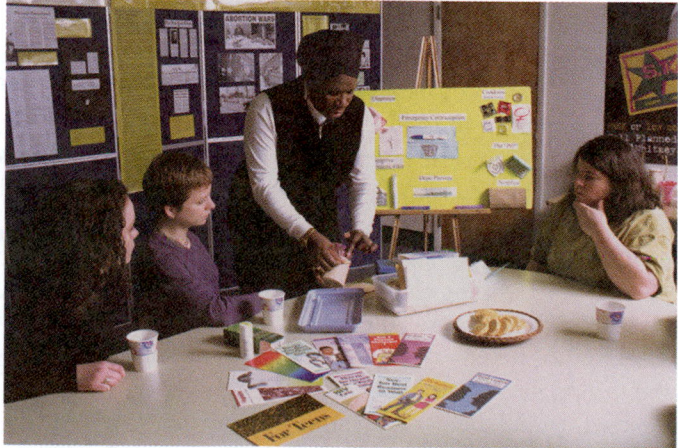

Figure 1-8 Client teaching often takes place in a group setting such as in this seminar on family planning.

Writing skills are the hallmark of intellectual and professional credibility. Nurses are increasingly writing in charts, correspondence, and client education. Many also are writing books and journal articles for professional and lay audiences. The written word allows for precision and inclusiveness that are not available through oral communication. Writing and formal speaking are venues by which nurses' intellectual and critical thinking skills are evaluated by others within and outside of the profession. The aforementioned criteria are the standards by which professional work often is judged.

Electronic or virtual types of communication are the media that nurses need to master in the future. It is vital for the viability of the profession that nurses develop the skills to communicate through this media. This media allows for avenues of expression that go beyond words and the two-dimensional printed page. This technology allows three-dimensional and animation effects that afford enormous potential for new types of communication. Nurses can communicate through mass media such as television, radio, local periodicals, and presentations using multimedia. Competence in the use of various media therefore is valuable.

Collaborative Skills

The nurse of the 21st century must develop collaborative skills. These skills are necessary to function as a member of the health care team required to meet the needs of the client, family, and community. It has been suggested that personal objectives are suppressed to meet the objectives of the team (Eddy, 1996). The need for collaborative skills is best illustrated through application of the concept of continuity of care for clients across settings. Although health care providers may be specialists, communication and evaluation must occur across disciplines. The nurse is in an excellent position to communicate client needs across disciplines (Hunt, 1998). The nurse must collaborate with physicians, families, third-party payers, attorneys, and members of other disciplines to meet the health care needs of the consumer (Carnevali & Thomas, 1993). As technology advances, collaboration among disciplines is likely to become increasingly important (Lasker et al., 1997). In fact, Roger J. Bulger, president of the Association of Academic Health Centers, suggested that no covenant among health care providers would be complete without acknowledgment of the need for collaboration among all the members of the team (Bulger, 1998).

Cultural Competency

Cultural competency is a skill that is developed through continual exposure, reflection, and awareness of cultural differences. This process begins with a recognition of the importance that cultural heritage plays in any human interaction. An understanding of one's personal heritage provides a platform from which to understand the culture of others. Cultural heritage refers to those beliefs and values that guide and orient our behavior, many of which are so integrated into daily life that one is generally unaware of one's own cultural perspective. Nurses may focus on the culture of the patient when it is different from their own but are unaware of the cultural heritage of their own beliefs. This lack of awareness then takes the form of prejudices, assumptions, and expectations. Decisions may be made from this cultural basis and may therefore create ethical conflicts. Thus, it is important for nurses to be aware of their own beliefs to avoid imposing them on others. Value clarification is a strategy to increase personal awareness and make some of the beliefs explicit.

Because cultural competency is a dynamic process, a defined level at which the nurse is competent does not exist. Rather, the competent nurse is one who continually engages in the process of increasing competency. Barry (1996) and Kavanaugh and Kennedy (1992) describe the following five steps in developing cultural competency:

1. Awareness and acceptance of cultural differences, which requires an open mind about other views of the world.

2. Awareness of one's own biases and attitudes, which can become barriers in interacting with others.

3. Recognition of dynamic differences among cultures without promoting the superiority of one culture over another.

4. Developing basic knowledge about other cultures through literature, observation, participation, interaction, and communication with people from diverse cultures.

5. Adaptation of clinical practice by being receptive to different cultures, actively seeking consultation from persons from that culture, and incorporating those ideas into one's practice. Skills also include articulating an issue from another's perspective, recognizing and reducing resistance to different ideas, and admitting mistakes and learning from them.

Economic Expertise

As the nursing profession advances and individual nurses work on interdisciplinary teams, nurses will need to understand the importance of economic issues in the delivery of health care. Nurses need to be able to justify their own participation in health care. They also are held accountable for keeping unnecessary costs under control. Nurses acting as case managers must understand the health care payment system to be able to direct client interventions

Critical Thinking

Values Clarification to Develop Cultural Awareness

Recognition of personal values includes assessing, exploring, and determining the ideals, principles, and behaviors that give meaning to our lives. Effective value clarification allows the nurse to be aware of personal values before being confronted with different values in the clinical setting. The purpose is not to change personal values but to become aware of personal beliefs and values. The following are three strategies for this exploration. Select a number of positional statements and identify if you strongly agree, agree, do not care, disagree, or strongly disagree. (There are no right or wrong answers.)

- Women should have the right to abortion on demand.

- Mentally retarded people should be sterilized.

- Women should not use anesthesia during labor.

- Teenagers should not be taught about birth control measures in public schools.

- Menopausal women should not take hormonal replacement therapy because it is against nature.

Complete the following sentences:

- If I were pregnant and unmarried, I would . . .

- Sexually active teenagers should . . .

- If I were a parent of a teenager, I would . . .

- If I were having a baby, I would want . . .

Rank these priorities. With limited resources, which clients should be given care?

- Preterm infants weighing less than 2 pounds at birth.

- Infants born with the human immunodeficiency virus.

- Antepartal clients with complications of pregnancy.

- Family planning agencies.

Web Activities

- Use a search engine to look up a particular health-related topic.

- Search a medical library site for evidence-based practice.

- Visit the website of the American Nurses Association, and examine some of the position statements.

- Visit the website of the Office of Women's Health at the National Institutes of Health, and explore the research agenda concerning women.

- Visit the websites of the Centers for Disease Control and the Agency for Healthcare Research and Quality, and search for guidelines for practice.

Self-Awareness and Reflective Practice

One of the most overlooked skills is that of self-awareness. This skill is important in the development of one's intuitive ability and the integration of personal knowledge. The skills used to develop this ability are self-reflection, value clarification, intuition, and cultural competency. Self-reflection is a practice that is useful in the nurse's ability to reflect on actions, thoughts, and beliefs and critique these for further development. This activity develops awareness and integration of personal and professional experience. Value clarification is important in understanding one's personal belief system as it pertains to professional ethics. Reflective practice is a deliberate process of discussing, reflecting, and even keeping a journal about one's practice. These activities are a systematic way to gain new insight, understanding, and compassion about one's clinical practice.

Development of Intuition

Historically, nurses have worked in a biomedical environment that has been greatly influenced by scientific reasoning. The traditional nursing process has focused on this type of analytic thinking. In practice, however, as the nurse moves from a beginner to an expert practitioner, other types of skills are integrated. In a study of the development of clinical excellence in nursing, Benner (1984) linked the expert's ability to move beyond simple application of rules and analytic processes to the development of an intuitive grasp of complex situations. Intuition, according to Rew (1996) has three attributes: the knowledge is

that are economically feasible. Many nurses have moved into administrative roles that rely on a good knowledge of business operations. Some advanced degree programs combine an MSN with a master's degree in business administration. Other programs have a strong economic component in the curriculum.

immediate, it is received as a whole and goes beyond the obvious, and it can occur in the absence of the conscious analytic process.

Beginners often choose to focus on technical skills and analytic reasoning until they develop proficiency. These skills often are emphasized in the beginning of formal education programs for nurses. In some cases, practicing nurses do not continue to develop the more holistic skills. The full range of these skills can be integrated into the nursing process so that the beginner may progress to expert through the integration of knowledge, experience, and intuition.

Rew (1996) discussed the need for the holistic nurse to develop not only the empirical or scientific skill, but also aesthetics, ethics, and a personal way of knowing that engages the development of intuitive thinking. A nurse with developed aesthetics skills attends to feelings and things that are pleasing to the senses (Rew, 1996). This nurse is very aware of sounds, sights, smells, taste, and touch and intervenes by creatively altering these elements in the environment. The professional expert nurse also is aware of values and employs this awareness in ethical practice.

Key Concepts

- An understanding of population health and the need to cut costs have shifted the emphasis of the health care delivery system from treatment of disease to prevention and health promotion. The concepts of risk assessment and management have pervaded all of health care.

- This shift has moved much of health care to the community setting and engaged multidisciplinary teams of providers, with both individuals and communities as active partners in the pursuit of health.

- Concerns for cost-effectiveness have affected the organization of health care delivery and required differentiated practice on the part of nurses.

- Health care providers are being more accountable for evidenced-based practice and for use of various guidelines to ensure the best quality health care practice.

- The ways of understanding health and illness are changing related to the following: advances in biologic science, environmental medicine, and behavioral medicine; the social aspects of health; cultural understanding; and complementary and alternative therapies.

- Contemporary issues include dealing with technology and informatics, changing demographics, and economic issues.

- The nursing profession historically has valued and described a holistic approach that is congruent with the changes in health care delivery.

- The nurse needs not only to develop content knowledge but also cognitive skills, technical skills, communication skills, cultural competence, collaborative skills, and a practice of self-reflection to fully enact the professional role.

Review Questions and Activities

1. One of the most fundamental shifts in health care delivery in the United States in the late 1900s has been:
   a. Lowering of costs of providing care
   b. Expansion to a focus on health
   c. Emergence of nurses to positions of power in health care delivery
   d. Advancement of isolated specialties

   The correct answer is b.

2. The United States has been tracking health goals since:
   a. 1949
   b. 1959
   c. 1970
   d. 1979

   The correct answer is d.

3. Which governmental agency was established to reduce disparities in the delivery of health care?
   a. National Institutes of Health
   b. Food and Drug Administration
   c. Health Care Financing Agency
   d. Agency for Healthcare Research and Quality

   The correct answer is d.

4. The Office of Research on Women's Health was established to:
   a. Reduce medical costs
   b. Standardize care to minorities
   c. Promote research on women's health
   d. Gain political equity for women

   The correct answer is c.

5. Which of the following is a true statement regarding cultural competency?
   a. One can be certified by taking a short course
   b. One must go to foreign countries to learn this
   c. One must understand one's own culture
   d. One must learn this from certified experts

   The correct answer is c.

6. Holistic theories in nursing are most congruent with which of the following issues in contemporary health care?
   a. Managed care
   b. A focus on health promotion
   c. Multidisciplinary teams
   d. Alternative systems of health care

   The correct answer is b.

References

Administration on Aging (AOA). (2001). *Demographic changes.* Available: www.aoa.dhhs.gov/aoa/aging21/demography. Accessed January 31, 2001.

Agency for Health Care Policy and Research (AHCPR). (1998). *AHCPR strategic plan,* Rockville, MD: Author. Available: www.ahrq.gov/about/stratpln.htm.

Agency for Health Care Policy and Research (AHCPR). (1998). *Background and purpose of the U.S. Preventive Services Task Force. Fact sheet.* Rockville, MD: Author. Available: www.ahrq.gov/clinicuspsfact.htm.

Agency for Healthcare Research and Quality (AHRQ). (2001). *Evidence-based Practice Centers.* Rockville, MD: Author. Available: www.ahrq.fov.clinic/epc. Accessed February 13, 2001.

American Nurses Association (ANA). (1994). *Position statement: A national nursing database to support clinical nursing practice.* Available: www.nursingworld.org/readroom/position/practice. Accessed February 13, 2001.

American Nurses Association (ANA). (1999). *Position statement: Privacy and confidentiality.* Available: www.nursingworld.org/readroom/position/ethics. Accessed February 13, 2001.

American Nurses Association (ANA). (1995). *Position statements: Promotion and disease prevention.* Available: www.nursingworld.org/readroom/position. Accessed February 13, 2001.

American Nurses Association (ANA). (1994). *Scope of practice for nuring informatics* (NP-90, 7.5M, 5/94) Washington, DC.

Bailit, H. L. (1995). Market strategies in managed care. In *Academic Health Centers in the Managed Care Environment.* D. Kour, C. J. McLaughlin & M. Oster Weis, Eds. Washington, DC: Association of Academic Health Centers.

Barry, P. D. (1996). *Psychosocial nursing: Care of physically ill patients and their families.* Philadelphia, PA: J. B. Lippincott.

Benner, P. (1984). *From novice to expert: Excellence and power in clinical nursing practice.* Menlo Park, CA: Addison-Wesley.

Brady, M., Leuner, J. D., Bellack, J. P., Loquist, R. S., Cipriano, P. F., & O'Neil, E. H. (1999). *A framework for differentiating the 21 Pew competencies by level of nursing education.* The Center for the Health Professions. Available: http://futurehealth.uscf.edu/pewcomm/competenciesRNs.htm. Accessed February 6, 2001.

Bulger, R. J. (1998). *The quest for mercy.* Charlottesville, VA: Carden Jennings.

Carnevali, E. L., & Thomas, M. D. (1993). *Diagnostic reasoning and treatment decision making in nursing.* Philadelphia, PA: J. B. Lippincott.

Committee on the Future of Primary Care (1996). *Primary Care: America's Health in a New Era.* Washington D.C.: National Academy Press.

Copstead, L.C. (1995). *Perspectives on pathophysiology.* Philadelphia, PA: W.B. Saunders.

Cross Cultural Health Care Program (CCHCP). (2001). *Recent news: Ask CCHCP: Question: What are the issues nationally in Certification of Medical Interpreters?* Accessed February 7, 2001. http://www.xculture.org.

Dossey B. M., Keegan, L., & Guzzetta, C. E. (2000). *Holistic nursing: A handbook for practice.* Gaithersburg, MD: Aspen.

Eddy, D. M. (1996). *Clinical decision making: From theory to practice.* Boston, MA: Jones & Bartlett.

Elder, L., & Paul, R. (1996). *The role of questioning.* Available: www.sonoma.edu/think. Accessed February 1, 1999.

Evans, R. G., Barer, M. L., & Marmor, T. R. (1994). *Why are some people healthy and others not?* New York: Aldine De Gruyther.

Grant, S. (2000). Prenatal genetic screening. *Online Journal of Issues in Nursing, 5,* (3). Available: www.nursingworld.org/ojin. Accessed February 13, 2001.

Gorin, S. S., & Arnold, J. (1998). *Health promotion handbook.* St. Louis, MO: Mosby.

Hawe, P., & Shiell, A. (2000). Social capital and health promotion: A review. *Social Science and Medicine, 51,* (6), 871–885.

Healthy people 2010. (2000). Available: www.health.gov/healthy-people. Accessed February 10, 2001.

Hickey, J., Ouimette, R.M., & Venegoni, S.L. (2000). *Advanced practice nursing: 2nd edition.* Philadelphia, PA: J. B. Lippincott.

Healthy People 2010: *Understanding and improving health 2nd ed.* (November 2000) Washington D.C.: US government printing office.

Hodnett, E. D. (2000). Caregiver support for women during childbirth: Review. *The Cochrane Database of Systematic Reviews, 4,* (4). Available: (Issue 4) http://gateway.ovid.com/ server. Accessed February 7, 2001.

Hunt, R. (1998). Community based nursing: Philosophy or setting? *American Journal of Nursing, 98,* (10), 44–48.

Institute of Medicine (IOM). (1996). *Primary care: America's health in a new era.* Washington, D.C.: National Academy Press.

Institute of Medicine (IOM). (2001). *Informing the future: Critical issues in health.* Washington, D.C.: National Academy of Sciences.

Jenkins, J. (2000). An historical perspective on genetic care. *Online Journal of Issues in Nursing,* Available: www.nursingworld.org/ojim. Accessed Feb. 7, 2001. September 30, 2000.

Jenkins, J. (2001). Ethical implications of genetic information. *Online Journal of Issues in Nursing,* Available: www.nursingworld.org/ojin. Accessed Feb 7, 2001. Feburary 9, 2001.

Kataoka-Yahiro, M., & Saylor, C. (1994). A critical thinking model for nursing judgment. *Journal of Nursing Education, 33,* (8), 351–356.

Kavanaugh, K. H., & Kennedy, P. H. (1992). *Promoting cultural diversity: Strategies for health care professionals.* Newbury Park, CA: Sage.

Kirschstein, R. L. (2000). *Description of Behavioral and Social Sciences* Washington, DC: Research Department of Health and Human Services: National Institutes of Health.

Kleinman, A. (1980). *Patients and healers in the context of culture.* Berkeley, CA: University of California Press.

Koerner, J., Bunkers, L., Gibson, S. J., Jones, R., Nelson, B., & Santema, K. (1995). Differentiated practice: The evolution of a professional practice model for integrated client care services. In D.L. Flarey (Ed.). *Redesigning nursing care delivery: Transforming our future.* Philadelphia, PA: J. B. Lippincott.

Lasker, R. D., & Committee on Medical and Public Health. (1997). *Medicine and public health: The power of collaboration.* Available: www.nyam.org./pubhlth.

Lillie-Blanton, M., Brodie, M., Rowland, D., Altman, D., & McIntosh, M. (2000). Race, ethnicity, and the health care system: Public perceptions and experiences. *Medical Care Research Review 57,* (Suppl. 1), 218–235.

Loustaunau, M. O., & Sobo, E. J. (1997). *The cultural context of health, illness and medicine.* Westport, CT: Bergin & Garvey.

Mariner-Tomey, A. (1994). *Nursing theorists and their work* (3rd ed.). St. Louis: Mosby.

Mezey, M. D. & McGivern, D. O. (1999). *Nurses. Nurse Practitioners: Evolution to Advanced Practice.* New York, NY: Springer.

Moss, N. (2000). Socioeconomic disparities in health in the US: An agenda for action. *Social Science and Medicine, 51,* (11), 1627–1638.

National Center for Health Statistics. (XXXX). Available: www.cdc.gov/nchs. Accessed February 13, 2001.

National Center for Health Statistics (NCHS). (1999). *Healthy people 2000 review, 1998–99.* Hyattsville, MD: Public Health Service.

National Coalition for Health Professional Education in Genetics (NCHPEG). (2001). *Core competencies in genetics essential for all health-care professionals.* Available: www.nchpeg.org/news-boxcorecompetencies000.html. Accessed February 7, 2001.

National Institute of Environmental Health Services (NIEHS). (1997). Understanding gene-environment interactions. *NIEHS News, 105,* (6). Available: http://ehpnet1.niehs.nih.gov. Accessed February 6, 2001.

National Institutes of Health. (1999). *Agenda for research on women's health for the 21st century, Vol. 1. Executive summary* (NIH Publication No, 99-4385) Bethesda, MD: Author.

Office of Minority Health (OMH). (2001). *Assuring cultural competence in health: Recommendations for national standards and an outcomes-focused research agenda.* Washington, DC: Public Health Service. Available: www.omhrc.gov/CLAS. Accessed January 16, 2001.

Paul, R., & Elder, L. (1996). *Fundamentals of critical thinking.* www.sonoma.edu/think accessed 2-1-99.

Pert, C. (1997). *Molecules of emotion.* New York: Scribner.

Pew Health Professions Commission. (1993). *Health professions education for the future: Schools in service to the nation.* San Francisco, CA: Pew Charitable Trust.

Pew Health Professions Commission. (1998). *Recreating health professional practice for a new century. The Fourth Report of the Pew Health Professions Commission.* San Francisco, CA: Pew Health Professions Commission.

Pew Environmental Health Commission at the Johns Hopkins School of Public Health. (Update Winter 1999–2000). *PEHC report exposes weaknesses in public health system.* Available: http://perwenvirohealth.jhsph.edu. Accessed January 31, 2001.

Pew Charitable Trust Commission on Health Professions. (1995). *Critical challenges in revitalizing the health care professions for the twenty-first century.* San Francisco, CA: UCSF Center for Health Professions.

Pless, G. S., & Clayton, G. M. (1993). Clarifying the concept of critical thinking in nursing. *Journal of Nursing Education, 32,* (9), 425–428.

Rew, L. (1996). *Awareness in healing.* Albany, NY: Delmar. Kohn, L., Corrigan Jr., Donaldson, M. (Eds.). (2000). *To err is human: Building a safer health system.* Washington D.C., The National Academies of Science Press.

Robert Wood Johnson Foundation. (1992). *Medical education transition. Commission on medical education: The sciences of medical practice.* Princeton, NJ: Robert Wood Johnson Foundation.

Romano, C. (2000). Nursing Informatics. In J. Hickey, R. Ouimette, & S. Venegoni (Eds.). *Advanced practice nursing* (2nd ed.). Philadelphia, PA: J. B. Lippincott.

Rundell, J. R. & Wise, M. G. (1996). *Textbook of Consultation-liasion psychiatry.* Wash D.C. America Psychiatric Press Inc.

Selye, H. (1956). *The stress of life.* New York: McGraw Hill.

Stevens-Barnum, B.J. (1994). *Nursing theory: Analysis, application, evaluation* (4th ed.). Philadelphia, PA: Lippincott.

Turley, J. (1996). Toward a model of nursing informatics. *Image: Journal of Nursing Scholarship, 28,* (4), 309–313.

U.S. Department of Health and Human Services (DHHS). (1979). *Healthy people: The Surgeon General's report on health promotion and disease.* Washington, D.C.: U.S. Government Publication.

U.S. Public Health Service (PHS). (1990). *Healthy people 2000* (DHHS Publication PH591-50213). Washington, DC: U.S. Government Printing Office.

U.S. Preventative Services Task Force (PSTF). (1996). *Guide to clinical preventive services,* (2nd ed.). Baltimore, MD: Williams & Wilkins.

U.S. Preventative Services Task Force (PSTF). (1998). *Guide to preventive services.* Available: www.ahcpr.gov/clinic/uspst. Accessed February 2, 2001.

Vickers, A. (1997). A proposal for teaching critical thinking to students and practitioners of complementary medicine. *Alternative Therapy in Health and Medicine, 3,* (3), 57–62.

Westhoff, C. L. (2000). Evidence-based medicine: An overview. *International Journal of Fertility, 45,* (Suppl 2), 105–112.

Weinick, R. M., Zuvekas, S. H., & Cohen, J. W. (2000). *Medical Care Research Review, 57* (Suppl. 1), 36–54. Racial and ethnic differences in access to and use of health care services, 1977–1996.

Wilkinson, R. G. (1996). *Unhealthy societies.* New York: Routledge.

World Health Organization (WHO). (1981). *Global strategies for health for all by the year 2000.* Geneva: Author.

World Health Organization (WHO). (1986). *Ottawa charter for health promotion.* Copenhagen: World Health Organization Regional Office for Europe.

U.S. Census (2001) http://www. census.gov. Accessed Feb. 2001.

Suggested Readings

Agency for Healthcare Research and Quality (AHRQ). (2000). *The National Guideline Clearinghouse. Fact sheet* (Publication No. 00-0047). Rockville, MD: Author. Available: www.ahrq.gov/clinic/ngcfact.htm.

American Nurses Association (ANA). (1980). *Nursing: A social policy statement*. St. Louis, MO: ANA.

Angier, N. (1999). *Woman: An intimate geography*. New York: Anchor Books.

The Center for the Health Professions.(2000). *Future health: Views from the Center*. San Francisco: Univeristy of California. Available: http://futurehealth.ucsf.edu. Accessed January 31, 2001.

Niessen, L., Grijseels, E. W. M., & Rutten, F. F. H. (2000). The evidence-based approach in health policy and health care delivery. *Social Science and Medicine, 51*, (6), 859–869.

Olshansky, E. (2000). *Integrated women's health: Holistic Approaches for comprehensive care*. Gaithersburg, MD: Aspen.

Resources

American College of Obstetricians and Gynecologists, 409 12th Street, SW, P.O. Box 96920, Washington, DC 20090-6920, www.acog.org

American Nurses Association, 600 Maryland Avenue, SW, Suite 100 West, Washington, DC 20024, 800-274-4262, www.nursingworld.org

Association for Women's Health, Obstetric, and Neonatal Nursing, 2000 L Street, NW, Suite 740, Washington, D.C., 20036, 800-673-8499, www.awhonn.org

The Center for the Health Professions, www.futurehealth.ucsf.edu

Centers for Disease Control and Prevention, www.cdc.gov

Medscape, www.medscape.com

National Association of Neonatal Nurses, 4700 W. Lake Avenue, Glenview, IL 60025-1485, 800-451-3795, www.nann.org

National Institutes of Health, www.nih.gov

Nursing index to journal articles, www.cinahl.com

Search medical and health related journals, www.pubmed.com

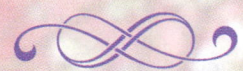

CHAPTER 2

Issues in Maternal, Neonatal, and Women's Health

*T*he practice of maternal, neonatal, and women's health care nursing is very complex. Many of the issues related to this nursing practice can be associated with strong emotional reactions.

- *As a nurse, which issues would I place as most important to be resolved related to women's health?*

- *Do I ascribe to the philosophy that a pregnant woman is one client or two clients?*

- *Do I think additional services are needed to meet the nation's needs and resolve issues related to maternal, neonatal, and women's health?*

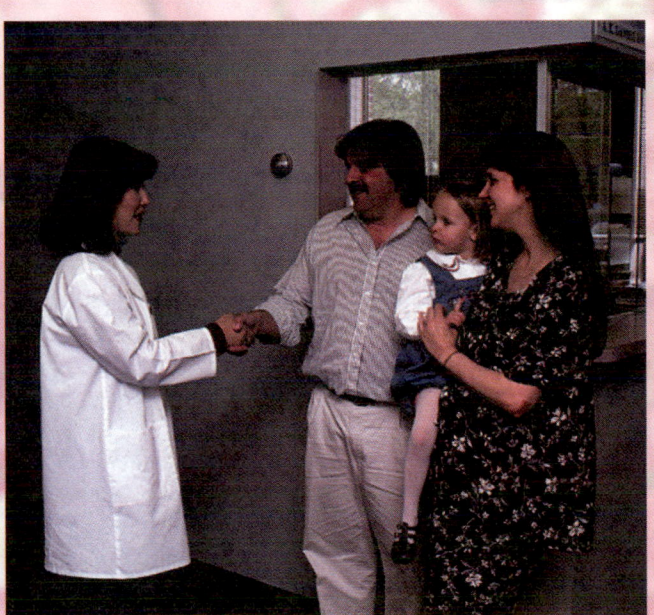

Key Terms

Cost containment   Evidence-based practice   Position statement   Risk-benefit analysis

Competencies

Upon completion of this chapter, the reader should be able to:

1. Discuss pertinent issues related to maternal, neonatal, and women's health.
2. Describe how these issues have developed in recent history.
3. Detail technologic advances in the field of maternal, neonatal, and women's health.
4. Analyze the importance of goals and guidelines for the practicing nurse.
5. Describe how health policy affects the practice of maternal, neonatal, and women's health.

Nursing in maternal, neonatal, and women's health care is very challenging and very rewarding. Some of the complexities of today's practice are discussed along with the social, economic, medical, and legal challenges facing nurses who practice in this field.

CHANGES IN MATERNAL, NEONATAL, AND WOMEN'S HEALTH CARE

Many factors have affected the course and practice of women's health care over the past few years and decades. Some of the most important influences are discussed.

Advances in Diagnosis and Treatment

Many advances in diagnosis and treatment have been made in the 20th century. These advances have included use of new technology, better methods of prenatal screening, better methods for management, and recognition of new entities affecting health. Examples of advances in women's health are the routine use of Pap tests, mammography, and the advent of laser technology for treatment of gynecologic conditions.

In the 1960s $Rh_0(D)$ immune globulin (RhoGAM) made an important contribution to maternal and newborn health by greatly reducing the number of cases of Rh isoimmunization. Before the introduction of RhoGAM, women who were Rh-negative and pregnant with an Rh-positive fetus were at risk for having an infant with hy-

drops, and that risk increased with each succeeding pregnancy. Since the routine administration of RhoGAM the incidence of this condition has decreased sharply, with the exception of women who have had an early spontaneous

REFLECTIONS FROM A NURSE

"I have been in nursing for almost 40 years and in maternal, neonatal, and women's health for most of that time. Expectations of nurses have changed radically during my career to the extent that the practice of nursing today requires much more responsibility and accountability for tasks that were not in the nursing domain when I went into practice. I wish I could predict how maternal, neonatal, and women's health nursing will change over the next 40 years. As I near retirement, if I were asked what advice I would give new graduates into the profession, I would say to never be afraid of taking risks or accepting change. In taking risks, however, be sure that you practice within your scope of practice, within the law, and within your personal ethics—and always consider the best interests of your clients."

abortion and are unaware of the need for antibody testing and immunization.

Fetal monitoring first became available in the 1970s for general use. When fetal monitoring was first developed, it promised to drastically reduce or eliminate the incidence of fetal intrauterine hypoxic ischemic events that occurred during labor. As a result, the number of children born with brain damage and the incidence of unnecessary cesarean sections would be decreased. Although the technology has flaws, it is still widely used. The American College of Obstetricians and Gynecologist (ACOG) and the American Academy of Pediatrics (1997) suggest that there is no difference between use of the electronic fetal monitoring and auscultation for assessment of fetal heart tones, if the equipment is used and documented properly. Much of the accuracy of fetal monitoring relates to the ability of the health care provider to interpret the monitor readings. In 1996, a consensus panel of experts met to begin to standardize the terminology related to fetal monitoring to clarify some of the ambiguity in interpretation (National Institute of Child Health and Human Development Research Planning Workshop, 1997). This panel of experts decided that the major weakness of the use of fetal monitoring was the lack of standardization of definitions and terminology among users. This panel made recommendations that should increase the reliability and validity of fetal monitoring results in practice and research.

In the 1970s, ultrasonography became an important tool in the diagnosis of maternal, neonatal, and women's health conditions (Callen, 1994). This technology has been important in identifying ectopic pregnancy before rupture. Ultrasonography has been instrumental in performing other tests such as amniocentesis and chorionic villus sampling. This technology has been widely accepted and performed in pregnancy to establish gestational age, fetal anomalies, and multiple gestation. In the neonatal arena, ultrasonography has become an important tool in assessing the infant for intraventricular hemorrhage. In the women's health arena, ultrasonography has been used to screen for ovarian cancer, uterine fibroids, and endometrial cancer. This technology has advanced to the degree that three-dimensional ultrasonography is now available. An expert nurse with special training may be the provider that conducts the ultrasound evaluation (Huffman & Sandelowski, 1997).

The biophysical profile (BPP) was developed to provide additional information about fetal well-being. The BPP uses ultrasonography in combination with fetal monitoring technology to increase the reliability of prediction of negative fetal outcome. The BPP has increased the likelihood that the health care provider will identify the fetus at risk. The incidence of negative fetal outcome, however, has still not been reduced to zero.

Endoscopy has been a major advance in the diagnosis and treatment of women's health problems and has elimi-

nated the need for major surgery in many cases. The laparoscope has been used for salpingectomy, myomectomy, and oophorectomy (Schenk & Coddington, 1999). The hysteroscope has been used for menstrual ablation to treat intractable uterine bleeding, with few risks and side effects. Most recently the endoscope has been used in a transcervical, transvaginal approach to visualize the fallopian tube from the uterotubal junction to the fimbria (Surrey, 1999).

Advancement in diagnosis and treatment has been made with the Human Genome Project. The advancement has significant implications for diagnosis and treatment. Two examples of application of knowledge obtained by the Human Genome Project follow. Research has been done on the Y chromosome. Until recently, scientists had great difficulty determining its role. It was thought that the Y chromosome played a limited role in fertility (Jegalian & Lahn, 2001). New findings demonstrate that the history of this sex chromosome has been strikingly dynamic. These findings have assisted in the explanation of some infertility problems in males. If deletions occur in any of three significant areas on the Y chromosome, infertility results. This type of azoospermia may be successfully treated with intracytoplasmic sperm injection.

Another example of application of knowledge discovered from the Human Genome Project is the technology in which gene and stem cell transplantations are used to treat disease. The earliest use of this technology was to treat genetic disorders such as cystic fibrosis and Duchenne muscular dystrophy (Kaji & Leiden, 2001). Geneticists have identified human genes involved in many disorders involving single genes and some cancers.

Health Indicators

In 2000, a national state-by-state survey was completed and a report card developed (National Women's Law Center, FOCUS/University of Pennsylvania & The Lewin Group [FOCUS/Lewin], 2000). The report card provides indicators that measure women's access to health care services; the degree to which women receive preventive health care and engage in health-promoting activities (Figure 2-1); the occurrences of key health conditions in women; and the extent to which the communities in which women live enhance their health and well-being. The indicators are displayed in Box 2-1.

This survey further identified 27 benchmarks related to the indicators that should be met. The results indicate that performance by the nation is unsatisfactory because some of the states or the District of Columbia have only met five of the benchmarks. The single benchmark met by all states and the District of Columbia is women aged 50 years and older receiving mammograms. The benchmarks missed are shown in Box 2-2.

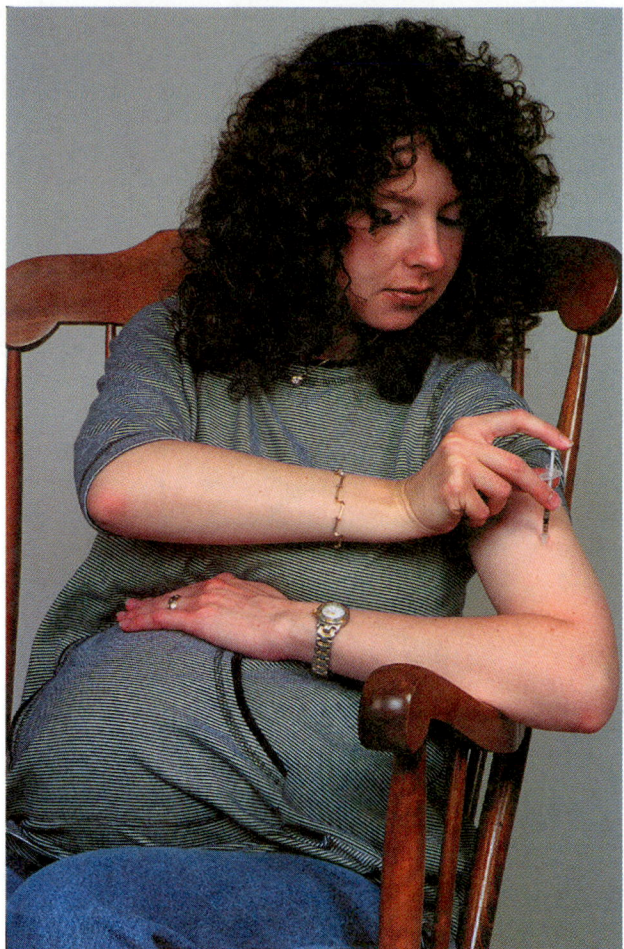

Figure 2-1 This woman is managing her diabetes successfully during pregnancy by following her insulin injection schedule and keeping all regular prenatal health appointments.

Box 2-1 National Indicators of Women's Health
- Women without health insurance
- First trimester prenatal care
- Women in a county without an abortion provider
- Pap smears
- Mammograms
- Colorectal screening
- Eating five fruits and vegetables per day
- No physical activity during leisure time
- Overweight
- Smoking
- Binge drinking
- Heart disease death rate
- Lung cancer death rate
- Breast cancer death rate
- High blood pressure
- Diabetes
- Rate of acquired immunodeficiency syndrome
- Rate of chlamydia
- Maternal mortality rate
- Poverty
- Wage gap
- High-school completion

Adapted from National Women's Law Center, FOCUS/University of Pennsylvania & The Lewin Group. (2000). *Making the grade on women's health: A national state-by-state report card.* Washington DC: National Women's Law Center.

Box 2-2 National Benchmarks Missed by All States and the District of Columbia
- Women without health insurance
- First trimester prenatal care
- No physical activity during leisure time
- Overweight
- Eating five fruits and vegetables per day
- High blood pressure
- Diabetes
- Life expectancy
- Poverty
- Wage gap

Adapted from National Women's Law Center, FOCUS/University of Pennsylvania & The Lewin Group. (2000). *Making the grade on women's health: A national state-by-state report card.* Washington DC: National Women's Law Center.

Findings of this study further indicate that women's access to health care is seriously compromised by inadequate health care coverage. Approximately 14% of women are uninsured. The percentage of uninsured women varies by state. Hawaii provides the best coverage, with 7.5% of women uninsured. Texas provides the worst, with 28% of women aged 18 to 24 years uninsured (FOCUS/Lewin, 2000).

Neither the nation nor the states have met the challenge of helping women secure better access to key health care services and increasing the availability of health care providers. No state met the national goal of 90% for women receiving first trimester prenatal care. The degree to which each state met the goal varied. Maine was closest with 89.9% of pregnant women receiving first trimester prenatal care, New Mexico had a 69.7% rate, and the rate in the District of Columbia was even lower at 64.6%.

The key indicators of health and causes of death vary by state. Thirty states met the national goal for reduction of the number of women who died from heart disease. Disparities exist among states. Minnesota has the best record, with 65.4 per 100,000 deaths from coronary heart disease; Mississippi has the worst record, with 141.2 per 100,000 deaths.

Infant mortality rates reflect the health of society. Eighteen states met the national goal for the infant mortality rate. Disparity exists between states. Massachusetts had the lowest rate, with 5.2 deaths per 1,000 live births. The District of Columbia had 15.9 deaths per 1,000 live births (FOCUS/Lewin, 2000).

This study further found that income levels and educational attainment are major factors associated with disparity in occurrences of illness and death. A wage gap still exists between men and women. On national average, women are paid 72.3% of what men are paid. This disparity also varies by state.

Risk Assessment and Management

Risk assessment, early identification, and prevention of complications apply to maternal, neonatal, and women's health. In the case of pregnant women, risk assessment is used to identify those women who have factors that contribute to having negative maternal or fetal outcomes. The risk can be biologic, behavioral, environmental, psychologic, or social. Assessments of maternal and fetal risks are completed and documented at the first visit and each additional client interaction with the health care system.

Providing neonatal care risk assessment is essential because the infant is unable to discuss signs and symptoms. Risk assessment may be the only tool available to the health care provider to predict adverse reactions and conditions. As we obtain more information about genetic makeup, risk assessment will become even more important as a tool.

Women's health care risk assessment is used to screen for cancer, domestic violence, eating disorders, and chronic diseases. Early identification and treatment can prevent illness, facilitate recovery, and prolong life.

Cost

Health care costs have excalated. New technology usually is very expensive, which adds to the costs of health care. In 1900, a woman's life expectancy was 48.3 years. In 1997, a woman's life expectancy had increased to 79.4 years (Office of Women's Health, 2000). The attempt to make this life extension of good quality has increased costs. Perinatal costs have escalated as a result of increasingly expensive intensive care as neonatal techniques have improved and resulted in fetal viability at decreasing gestational ages.

In women's health care, the number of women having hysterectomies has increased so much that hysterectomy is now the second most common major operative procedure performed in the United States. Of these procedures, 90% are performed for benign conditions (Summitt, 2000). Each year in the United States 590,000 hysterectomies are performed. The only operative procedure performed more commonly is cesarean section (Rosenfeld, 1997).

In the past decade much attention has been focused on the costs of health care. This focus has led to questions such as should a hysterectomy in the woman over 35 years of age include oophorectomy because of the risk for subsequent ovarian cancer? These kinds of questions increasingly are being asked, and the term risk-benefit analysis is being seen more frequently in the medical literature (Podszaski, Mortel, & Ory, 2001). **Risk-benefit analysis** is the determination of whether the risks of a certain procedure outweigh the benefits to the client of performing that procedure. One of the risk factors now being considered more commonly is cost.

Goals and Guidelines

Cost containment refers to the reduction of expenses by working more efficiently. Cost containment has come to the forefront as a factor in delivery of health care. Thus, it has become very apparent that it is no longer acceptable for individual health care providers to act without considering health care costs. Practice must become standardized, and a number of goals and guidelines have been established to guide health care providers.

The Agency for Healthcare Research and Quality (AHRQ), formerly known as the Agency for Health Care Policy and Research (AHCPR), is a federal agency that focuses on health care quality and outcomes of health care services. The AHRQ supports research on all aspects of health care provided to women, including quality, access, cost, and outcomes. The AHRQ has a number of ongoing studies investigating heart disease, stroke, breast cancer, and the health care practices of women. The findings of these studies will be used to determine and set federal policy. These studies also will assist in identifying strategies to improve health care provided to women.

The Centers for Disease Control and Prevention (CDC) set forth health goals in "Healthy People 2010" (CDC, 2000) that provide health care providers with benchmarks to attain in health promotion and disease prevention. These goals assist health care providers in conceptualizing health at a population rather than an individual level. Each individual outcome, however, contributes to the population statistics.

Each profession sets forth guidelines for members of that profession. The American Nurses Association (ANA) sets forth policies and position statements to help guide nurses. For example, the ANA has set forth a **position statement** (formalized statement by a professional organization to express the opinion of its membership) on home care for the mother, infant, and family following birth (ANA, 1995). This position statement strongly supports individualized postpartum care provided to the family in the home environment.

In a 1991 position statement, the ANA crafted a statement concerning physical violence against women (ANA, 1991). This statement formalized support for the education of nurses, health care providers, and women in the skills necessary to prevent violence against women.

Agencies have issued guidelines for care in maternal, neonatal, and women's health, including the American Academy of Pediatrics (AAP); American College of Obstetricians and Gynecologists (ACOG); Association of Women's Health, Obstetric, and Neonatal Nurses (AWHONN); and National Association of Neonatal Nurses (NANN). It is important that nurses gain familiarity with these guidelines because a national standard of care is being developed based on them. This means that the individual nurse is expected to provide the same services with the same degree of skill as is any other nurse. Standardization of care is a way of protecting against negative outcomes and reducing costs.

TRENDS IN MATERNAL, NEONATAL, AND WOMEN'S HEALTH CARE

The nurse in maternal, neonatal, and women's health nursing must be aware of trends that affect practice. Whereas many trends are affecting today's health care system, some of the major factors are described in this chapter.

Medicalization and Demedicalization

During the 19th century and early part of the 20th century, most persons received health care in their homes or community settings (Hawkins & Bellig, 2000). Public health nurses provided much of this community care. These nurses provided well-child care, prenatal care, and postpartum care in a number of settings, including schools and homes. It was not unusual at the turn of the 20th century for a pregnant woman to deliver her child at home under the care of a lay midwife or a nurse, especially in rural areas.

As medicine evolved as a profession in the 20th century, physicians decided it was more appropriate for their clients to deliver in hospitals (Rinker, 2000) (Figure 2-2). It was thought that advances in technology, equipment, anesthesia, and medication would reduce maternal and infant morbidity and mortality.

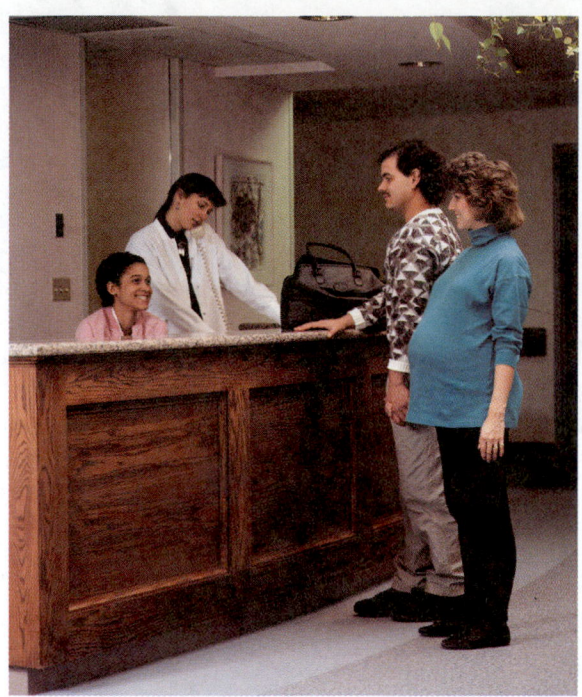

Figure 2-2 Most births in the United States today occur in a hospital setting.

The incubator was developed in the late 1800s, which provided warmth and protection for preterm infants. As this technology has advanced, it has enabled the survival of preterm infants at earlier gestational ages. This technology provided another argument that delivery in the hospital was safer than it was at home.

As medical specialties developed in the 19th and 20th centuries, specialty hospitals were built to provide the skilled care required for women to birth their children. Medication use became common in obstetric care delivery. Some women received so much sedation that they did not remember delivering their infants. Visitors were not allowed in the labor or delivery rooms because it was thought they posed the threat of infection for the mother and infant. Fathers were considered visitors.

Other practices related to childbirth were equally as rigid. When delivery was imminent, women were moved from their labor bed to a stretcher and transferred to the delivery room. Once there, they were moved again to the delivery table. Here, women's hands were often restrained with leather straps so they would not put their hands in the sterile field during delivery.

Anesthesia is another area in which advances were made. Home delivery usually was without anesthesia. In the hospital, however, women were given general or spinal anesthesia. When general anesthesia was given, women had no memory of the birth. Particular care had to be taken in administering anesthesia to avoid sedation of the neonate. If the neonate was sedated, resuscitation was required. Ether as an anesthetic agent posed additional dangers of explosion; inhalation of fumes by health care providers; and maternal hemorrhage, which frequently occurred because of uterine atony. The dangers of general anesthesia led to the popularity of spinal anesthesia.

The saddle block was the most frequently used type of spinal anesthesia. It was administered when delivery was imminent, as determined by the crowning of the baby's head. After the woman was transferred to the delivery room, she was required to sit up for administration of the saddle block. She also was required to be very still so the anesthesiologist would have a stable and sterile field for insertion of the needle. This process sometimes required 15 to 20 minutes, and the client continued to have contractions throughout the procedure as well as feeling the urge to push. Because saddle block anesthesia did not impair the woman's memory or produce uterine atony, it was preferred over general anesthesia. Still, no visitors were allowed in the delivery room, including the husband (Zwelling, 2000).

In the 1960s women became more empowered and began to insist that childbirth was a natural process and many of the medical interventions that had become customary were not necessary. Women began taking childbirth education classes in an effort to understand the processes of labor and strategies for pain relief that did not involve anesthesia or sedation. Childbirth education classes flourished, and many of these classes were taught by nurses (Figure 2-3). It was because of childbirth classes that women began to ask their physicians why husbands and other family members could not be present for labor and delivery. As client requests mounted, physicians became advocates for loosening hospital policies.

Nurses continue to support, teach, and value childbirth education classes even when clients plan to receive an epidural. Epidural anesthesia became very popular in the 1970s and 1980s. It offered the advantage of pain relief that could be administered early in the labor process. It allowed the woman to be awake and participate in her delivery and did not have some of the adverse effects of general and spinal anesthesia. Continuous epidurals became popular because the tube could be inserted and anesthetic agent injected when the client was approximately 4 to 5 cm dilated. Thus, when the pain returned, the agent could be injected again through the tubing that remained in place.

In summary, the past century of maternity care has been one of medicalization as physicians increasingly made decisions for women, and demedicalization as women decided they wanted control of this natural process. Today, more births outside of hospitals are occurring, and more women are choosing midwifery care as opposed to physician care for their childbirth experience.

Decreased Hospital Stay

Decreased hospital stays have been a major source of cost reduction in the past 10 years. In the 1980s, a 3-day hospital stay was standard for a normal delivery and a 5-day hospital stay was standard for major operative procedures such as a hysterectomy or cesarean section. In the 1990s, however, the 24-hour discharge of mother and newborn became common. After many complaints from health care professionals and clients and some tragic outcomes, Congress stepped in and federally mandated that insurance companies must cover a 48-hour hospitalization after delivery. Women may return home sooner if they request. If complications occur, the hospital stay may be extended past 48 hours. Clients having hysterectomy or cesarean section typically return home 3 to 4 days after surgery.

Reduction in Intervention

In the practice of maternal and child health care, reduction in intervention has been a major issue in the past decades. Many women consider birth a natural process. Yet when they were admitted to the hospital, they had to experience childbirth under the control of physicians. Induction of labor was widespread, use of Lamaze was discouraged in many facilities, and forceps deliveries and cesarean sections were commonplace. Some of these interventions were undertaken as first choices under the advice of physicians. As women have become more verbal and cost-containment more of an issue, some interventions have been reduced.

Family-Centered Care

In 1994, Celeste Phillips, a maternity nurse, and Dr. Loel Fenwick worked together to develop the concept of family-centered maternity care. Family-centered maternity care is

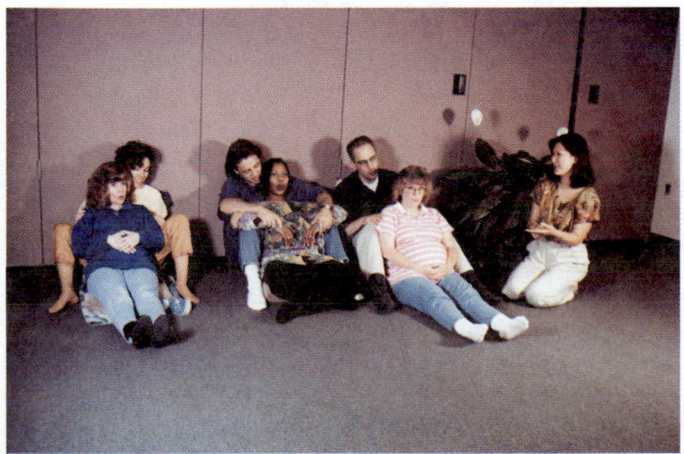

Figure 2-3 Childbirth education classes are a means for women and their partners to learn about pain management and the birth process.

Research Highlight

Evidence-based Protocol

Purpose

To develop an evidence-based protocol for initial evaluation and treatment of urinary incontinence and to design procedures to facilitate implementation of the protocol in clinical practice.

Method

A review of the literature was conducted, including a descriptive report from the Association of Women's Health, Obstetric, and Neonatal Nurses (AWHONN) Continence for Women Project. Twenty-one public, private, and other women's health sites were identified to collect data from 1,474 women. A protocol was developed, sites were selected, site co-coordinators were trained to collect the data, and the process was evaluated. The participation of a representative sample was the first outcome measure. Feedback from the site coordinators was the second outcome criterion. Feedback from the site coordinators was in the form of feedback about the orientation session and on the experience of implementing the protocol.

Findings

Of the original 36 sites, 15 participated in the study. The settings met criteria for diversity of patient population. The site coordinators provided positive feedback.

Nursing Implications

The Continence for Women Project demonstrated potential for development and testing of an evidence-based protocol for clinical practice. Nurses are in an ideal position to perform utilization research and develop protocols that can standardize treatment of many issues related to the health care of women. The nurse of the 21st century will have to develop the skills of evidence-based practice analysis and decision-making.

Sampselle, C.M., Wyman, J.F., Thomas, K.K., Newman, D.K., Gray, M., Dougherty, M., & Burns, P.A. (2000). Continence for women: Evaluation of AWHONN's third research utilization project. *Journal of Obstetric, Gynecologic, and Neonatal Nursing, 29,* (1), 9–17.

---

based on 10 principles that reverse many of the restrictive policies and practices and return choices about the childbirth process to families (Figure 2-4). This philosophy has been adopted across the country as women decide they want to be in control of their bodies and reproductive processes (Zwelling, 2000).

Community-Centered Care

There has been a trend to move maternity care away from major medical centers and to community-based facilities. The effect of this change has been twofold. Being in the community enables better family interaction in the birth process because of convenience. This practice also has caused the maternity facilities in major cities to gain a higher percentage of high-risk maternity clients, changing the client demographics of and increasing the costs to these facilities.

Evidence-Based Practice

Evidence-based practice is a systematic approach to finding, appraising, and judiciously using research results as a basis for clinical decision-making (Westhoff, 2000). This type of systematic approach to decision-making is becoming more popular in health care in general but specifically in maternal, neonatal, and women's health. Westhoff (2000) provides a detailed description of the processes of appraising evidence found through meta-analysis of studies based on the development of research questions related to this topic. Evidence is appraised and categorized based on the level of research available. The approach has proven so useful that in 1997 the AHRQ established 12 5-year contracts to institutions across the United States to serve as evidence-based practice centers. Several of these topics are related to women's health. Duke University, Durham, North Carolina, is studying cervical cytology and treatment of uterine fibroids. MetaWorks, Inc., Boston, Massachusetts, is studying management of breast disease. Oregon Health Science Center is studying diagnosis and treatment of osteoporosis. The University of Texas Health Science Center at San Antonio, Texas, is studying management of chronic hypertension in pregnancy and management of chronic fatigue syndrome, a condition seen more commonly in women (AHCPR 2000).

UNDERSTANDING WOMEN'S HEALTH

The many elements that overall comprise women's health are discussed.

Biologic Health

Until the 1990s it was assumed that the biology of men and that of women were identical and therefore what worked in the treatment of men should work for women. In the 1990s, the public began to question the validity of this assumption. As a result of this questioning, the Women's Health Initiative was begun to study parameters of women's health. It became apparent that women metabolize alcohol, experience heart disease, and metabolize medications differently than do men. The Women's Health Initiative currently is studying other biologic differences between men and women. One area of investigation is the interrelationship of hormones and mental health.

Behavioral Health

Behavior is a very important component of health. It is becoming increasingly apparent that obesity is a particular problem in our society. Being overweight contributes to the development of chronic diseases such as diabetes, hypertension, and cardiovascular disease. The negative health effects of being overweight can be prevented by early identification and treatment. Overeating in pregnancy contributes to the development of gestational diabetes, increases the risks for negative fetal outcomes because of macrosomia and hypoglycemia, and increases the woman's risk of developing adult onset diabetes later in life. Because gestational diabetes is a major health problem in the United States the Centers for Disease Control and Prevention, or CDC (1986), issued guidelines for enhancing diabetes control through maternal and child health programs. Despite these guidelines the incidence of gestational diabetes has not decreased.

Environmental Health

Rural women face unique and specific health challenges regarding health care access as a result of geographic and occupational circumstances. Many women in the United States are farmworkers. An estimated 313,000 farmworkers may suffer from pesticide-related illnesses each year and from 800 to 1,000 farmworkers die each year as a direct result of pesticide exposure (Gaston, 2001).

Women are exposed regularly to teratogens in the workplace, as are men. Manicurists are exposed to inhalants that may be toxic. Nurse anesthetists have a higher rate of spontaneous miscarriage that does the normal population. There may be numerous other examples of workplace exposure to teratogens. A detailed discussion can be found in Chapter 21.

Social Health

In the exploration of the differences between women's and men's health, a leading question is that of biology compared with sociocultural determinants to explain these patterns. An attempt to differentiate between these factors was discussed in the Agenda for Research on Women's Health for the 21st Century (U.S. Department of Health and Human Services, 1999). One suggestion was to use the terms *sex* and *gender,* respectively, to refer to biologic and sociocultural differences. This differentiation is similar to the one between race and ethnicity, which refer to biologic and sociocultural factors, respectively. These definitions are controversial and the overlap between these factors is very complex.

Two classic studies described women's thought processes as different from but not inferior to those of men. Gilligan (1982) described women's complex process of moral reasoning as being rooted in relationships rather than purely rational principles. Men generally are more concerned with individual rights, justice, autonomy, and independence; women generally are more concerned with relationships and principles of caring for and connection with others. Belenkey et al. (1986) described women's different ways of knowing, opening up a number of avenues of women's thinking and behavior that contrasted with some of the male models of knowing.

As we come to understand more about the effects of socioeconomic status on health, we find that many of the issues disproportionately affect women. Greater numbers of women live at low income or poverty levels, both in single-parent families and among older persons (Administration on Aging, 2001). Poverty affects not only access to health but also many of the resources needed to promote health such as a healthy diet and places to exercise. Lack of power and social status creates additional stressors that can be damaging to one's health over time. Women have different patterns of health care use than do men; women use health care services more than do men and, on average, live longer than men.

Women's social roles and expectations also impact their health. Women's roles as mothers may make them more aware of health and more receptive to health education because they are eager to promote the health of their families (Loustaunau & Sobo, 1997). In many families, however, women may play a subservient role to their male partners. If the family is prone to domestic violence, women are more likely to be the victims. Women may be reluctant to leave an abusive relationship because of the role expectations of wife and mother. Women also may relate to their doctor or nurse practitioner in a different manner than do men relevant to their social roles.

In industrialized countries as women joined the labor force, generally their fertility rates declined. In developing countries, this relationship is much more complex (Sargent & Brettell, 1995). In many cases women see clear, concrete advantages to reducing their own fertility; however, social pressures may make it impossible for them to do so. This contradiction between beliefs and reality may lead to physical and emotional overburdening of women, posing health threats to these women and their children.

Cultural Health

Women's roles are determined by culture. In many cultures, women make decisions about their health and that of their family. Culture also determines many activities of women that have health implications. Cultural beliefs and values underlie the basic assumptions about biomedicine and the delivery of health care.

Cultural Influences in Women's Health

Women often are the decision-makers regarding nutrition, daily health practices, and treatment of minor illnesses. These decisions arise from cultural heritages and the attendant beliefs, values, and practices related to health and health-seeking behaviors. For example, dietary habits, food choices, and food preparation are based on cultural practices. Pregnancy and birth are special transition times, with particular customs and beliefs that direct activities and behaviors. These beliefs direct behavior throughout a woman's life span. For example, cultural beliefs and traditions influence who gives information about menses and reproduction to a pubescent girl. These factors also influence the type of information given to the young woman and the circumstances under which this information is shared. Feminine hygiene practices, such as douching, bathing, and acceptable activities during menses, are culturally related.

Cultural beliefs also will influence a woman's social roles and her relationship with her husband and other family members. Those things that constitute appropriate activities and decision-making roles within and outside of the family generally are determined by culture.

In many cultures, women do not have social authority to access health care outside of the family (Sargent & Brettell,

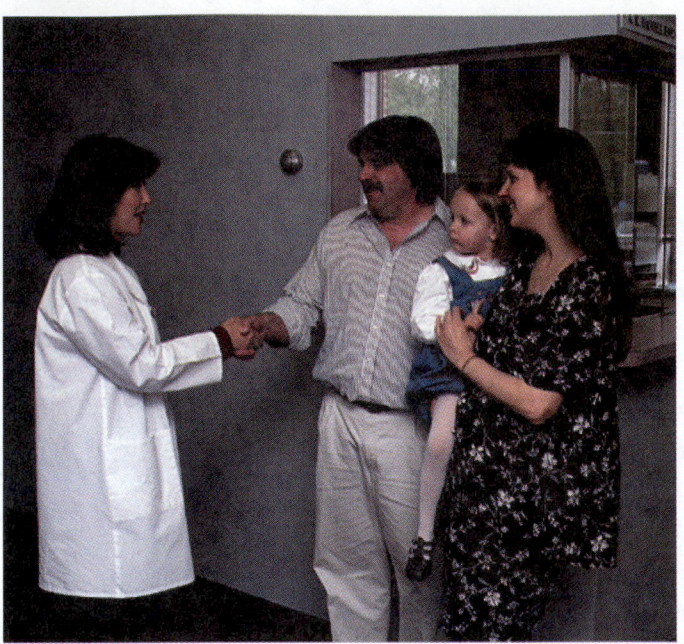

Figure 2-4 Family-centered care involves family members, in addition to the pregnant woman, in decision-making processes.

1995). Other family members, generally the woman's husband, must make the decision to go to a health care provider and whether to adhere to the provider's recommendations. These cultural practices may be minor and involve the woman's husband coming with her to the clinic; in contrast, they may be extreme, and may involve a husband refusing to bring the woman or children to receive health care or not permitting the woman to use contraception.

Mattson (1993) discussed the impact of culture on childbearing women. She describes the cultural nature of beliefs regarding the antepartum period such as preparation for birth, taboos, practices to ensure a safe delivery, and who transmits knowledge about birth. During the intrapartum period cultural beliefs influence who controls the labor and delivery process, who attends the birth, the location of the birth, positions for laboring and delivery, and degree and type of interventions at birth. Cultural beliefs during the postpartum period have an impact on birth rituals, allowable maternal activities, dietary patterns, norms for maternal and child contact after birth, and who controls postnatal care.

Menopause is another example of a biologic transition, the management of which is significantly affected by cultural beliefs. Use or nonuse of hormone replacement therapy during perimenopause, for instance, is highly influenced by cultural beliefs and values.

Culturally Influenced Behaviors with Health Implications

American cultural values of what a woman should be also reflect predominantly male values. Despite women's acceptance of these values, they can lead to poor health for women. Images of beauty and acceptable appearance often lead to poor dietary habits as increasingly younger women are attempting to lose weight in the pursuit of a cultural ideal. Many women seek out cosmetic treatments and even surgery to attain cultural standards of beauty. Breast augmentation, liposuction, and other cosmetic surgeries may carry considerable health risks. Naomi Wolf (1992) provided an in-depth description of these behaviors, noting that the images of beauty are political and cultural ideas that perpetuate the position of women as ornamental, whose value and self-worth is dependent on their physical beauty and sexual allure.

Cultural Influences on Biomedical Care

Another cultural aspect of health care of women is the cultural perspective of biomedicine. Before the emerging awareness with the establishment of the Office for Research on Women's Health (ORWH), most biomedical knowledge was based on studies and understanding of men. Women's health consisted of gynecologic and obstetric issues. Research generally was not conducted on women because the hormonal changes during the menstrual cycle were considered variables that would be difficult to control. (It has since been discovered that men also experience hormonal fluctuations.) As we begin to learn more about the biologic differences between men and women, we are discovering that all systems may be different and treatments resulting from studies in men may not always be generalized to women.

The use of language influences the way we react to the world and behave in it. Anthropologists have studied biomedical metaphors and found them to be predominantly military, economic, or other masculine models (Martin, 1987). In examination of biomedical and scientific texts, females are depicted as body and emotion, equated with nature, and considered inferior to males. Males are depicted as having culture, mind, and reason. These metaphors reflect a cultural approach to health in which women's bodies, associated with nature, are to be controlled. Another anthropologist, Davis-Floyd (1992), studied biomedical birth practices as a ritual response to contemporary society's extreme fear of natural processes and the use of technology as an expression of American cultural beliefs of the superiority of technology over nature.

Complementary and Alternative Therapies

Women often use complementary and alternative therapies. Because of their focus on health promotion, these therapies may be particularly appealing to women. Women may be more inclined to use these therapies because women traditionally are in positions to nurture the health of their family members. More women also are taking control of their own health needs and those of their families (Olshansky, 2000). Many of these therapies are gentle and nourishing and therefore more in keeping with women's social roles. Several herbs have shown some efficacy in relieving menstrual and menopausal discomforts. Many of these therapies also facilitate relaxation and reduce stress, and they may be appealing because women and others with limited social power frequently have additional stress.

ISSUES RELATED TO MATERNAL, NEONATAL, AND WOMEN'S HEALTH CARE

As trends in maternal, neonatal, and women's health have developed, issues have evolved that have affected practice in the field. Among those issues are cost containment, access to care, medical errors, reproductive ethical issues, medical-legal issues, and issues related to the philosophy of care provision.

Cost Containment

Cost containment involves reduction of cost through efficiency. One of the common procedures in discussing cost is cost-effectiveness. In fact, there are individuals whose sole purpose in employment is determining the cost-effectiveness of certain procedures. This process is a very sophisticated one by which models are developed to determine whether outcomes for two procedures are equivalent and whether the cost is more or less, depending on the procedure chosen. The cost-effectiveness model looks at many factors related to choosing the procedure that has the best outcome at the lowest price. Nurses have taken the lead in conducting some of these cost-effectiveness studies.

For example, Heaman et al. (2001) studied preterm birth. Five categories of health determinants were identified related to preterm birth: social and economic factors, physical environment, personal health practices, individual capacity and coping skills, and health services. These categories were used in design of a program to provide health strategies for women to help prevent preterm labor.

Fleschler et al. (2001) studied severity and risk adjustment related to obstetric outcomes, diagnosis-related group (DRG) assignments, and reimbursement. The impetus for this study was that risk and variation in condition were not adequately considered when determining reimbursement. These nurses assisted in determining correct benchmarks for high-risk obstetric clients, especially those experiencing preterm labor. The results were that cost-appropriate, quality care was being provided.

Roberts and Sward (2001) studied birth outcomes reported through automated technology. This study examined whether birth center clinical outcomes could be efficiently reported using an automated birth log. It was determined that the automated birth log was a good communication tool that provided an excellent means of data storage.

As long as costs remain an issue in health care, there will be a need for nurses to perform studies such as those mentioned. Numerous benchmarks exist in this field that have yet to be established and measured.

Access to Care

Access to care remains a very important issue related to maternal, neonatal, and women's health. An estimated 48 million Americans lack access to health care, and 44 million have no health care insurance (Gaston, 2001). Many of the uninsured are women. When a person does not have insurance, access to health care may be delayed and treatment may be less effective or ineffective. In addition, access to care involves the availability of appropriate health care services in the community, transportation, and childcare—and many other factors. Ensuring affordability of health care continues to be a major issue in the United States as is evidenced by public attention, congressional rhetoric, and the impairment present when some women finally do receive the needed care.

Reduction of Medical Errors

Increasingly, medical errors have gained attention as being major causes of morbidity and mortality. The Institute of Medicine, or IOM (2000), indicates that errors usually represent plans in which the system failed and the breakdown resulted in harm. Further, the IOM suggests that errors depend on two kinds of failure: actions do not go as intended, or the intended action is not the correct one. These two types of errors are commonly referred to as error of execution or error of planning, respectively. Contrary to popular belief, errors usually are not caused by incompetence (Dickenson-Hazard, 2001). In many instances, downsizing and re-engineering, which are facts of life in contemporary health care organizations, are found to be at the root of the problem (Knox et al., 1999). In some instances, organizational changes undertaken to increase productivity or cut operational costs result in systems that break down, and often, client safety is not a primary consideration.

Nurses have been an easy target on which to place blame for medical errors. In reality, nurses are doing their jobs in a health care system that is in turmoil. Individual nurses and nursing organizations across the country are committed to improving health care by developing practice standards, developing system improvements, and recruiting additional workers to the profession (Dickenson-Hazard, 2001).

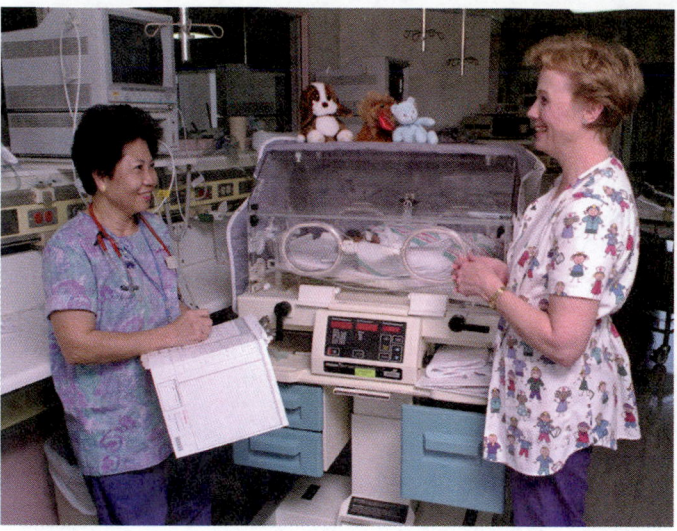

Figure 2-5 Charting is a responsibility of the entire interdisciplinary care team.

Reducing the occurrences of medical errors must be a collaborative effort on the part of doctors, nurses, administrators, and all other health care workers (Underwood, 2001). Nurses are an important part of the solution (Figure 2-5). Client outcomes are better in hospitals with higher staffing levels and higher ratios of registered nurses in the staffing mix than in hospitals with lower levels and ratios. Nurses are fiercely committed to quality client care (Kincaide, 2001).

The AHRQ recommends that clients become involved in their health care as a means to reduce medical errors. The AHRQ provides 20 tips in a client education fact sheet, an adaptation of which is included in the Client Education box.

Ethical Issues

Many potential ethical issues are related to maternal, neonatal, and women's health. Chapter 5 discusses these issues in some detail. Gene and stem cell therapies are just two areas representative of these concerns. Several ethical concerns have been raised about gene and stem cell therapies. Many members of the public are troubled by perceived and actual problems associated with altering the genetic composition of humans. Specific concerns have been raised about the appropriate traits to be selected for genetic modification. Concern also exists about the potential for inadvertently altering the genetic composition of germ cells. Finally, there has been concern about the use of fetal tissue in the treatment of disease (Kaji & Leiden, 2001).

Medical-Legal Issues

The major medical-legal issue in nursing today is malpractice. *Malpractice* is a specific kind of negligence that

Client Education

Preventing Medical Errors

The AHRQ (2000b) recommends these 20 tips for clients to help prevent medical errors:

1. The single most important way you can prevent errors is to be an active member of the health care team.

2. Make sure all doctors know about everything you are taking, including prescription medications, over-the-counter medications, vitamins, and herbs.

3. Make sure your doctor knows about allergies and adverse reactions you may have had to medications.

4. When your doctor writes a prescription, make sure you can read it.

5. Ask about your medications in terms you can understand at the time of prescription and the time of administration.

6. When you pick up your medications from the pharmacy, ask: Is this the medicine that my doctor prescribed?

7. If you have any questions about the directions on your medication label, be sure to ask them.

8. Ask your pharmacist for the best device to measure your liquid medicine.

9. Ask for written information about the side effects your medicine could cause.

10. If you have a choice, choose a hospital at which many patients have the procedure or surgery you need.

11. If you are in a hospital, consider asking all health care workers who have direct contact with you whether they have washed their hands.

12. When you are being discharged from the hospital, ask the doctor to explain the treatment plan you will use at home.

13. If you have surgery, make sure you, you doctor, and the surgeon agree and are clear on exactly what will be done.

14. Speak up when you have questions or concerns.

15. Make sure that someone, such as your personal doctor, is in charge of your care.

16. Make sure that all health professionals involved in your care have important health information about you.

17. Ask a family member or friend to be there with you and to be your advocate.

18. Know that "more" is not always better.

19. If you have had a test, do not assume that no news is good news.

20. Learn about your conditions and treatments by asking your doctor and nurse and by using other reliable resources.

Following these AHRQ recommendations does not guarantee clients will avoid experiencing medical errors. By participating in their own care, however, clients can reduce this possibility.

---

occurs when the standard of care that reasonably can be expected is not performed (Aiken & Catalano, 1994). Four elements are required to prove liability for malpractice:

1. Duty
2. Breach of the standard of care
3. Proximate cause
4. Harm to the client

Further discussion of the concepts involved with proving malpractice will help clarify the meaning of these elements and make them more easily understood. All four components must be present for malpractice to occur.

The concept of duty is a legal term that means that the nurse has or should have undertaken the care of the client in the capacity of a nurse. Duty may be independent of payment for services (Hall, 1996). For example, a nurse comes to the labor and delivery unit to deliver a message to another nurse. As she enters the unit, it is very apparent there is a crisis situation because the nurses are engaged in preparing for an emergency cesarean section. As the nurse passes a client's room, the client calls out: "Nurse. Can you help me?" The nurse is from the neonatal unit and has no experience in dealing with laboring women. She has no duty to assist this client. If the nurse enters the room, the care provided must meet the same standard of what a reasonable prudent nurse would do under the same or similar circumstances. If this standard is not met and harm to the client results as a result of the nurse's action or inaction, then malpractice can be proven.

If the nursery nurse, rather than entering the room, explained to the client that she was not a labor and delivery nurse and therefore was not qualified to deliver nursing care to the laboring client, she has not taken on the duty to provide such care. The ethical nurse, however, should find the appropriate nurse to assist the client.

Many of the malpractice cases in maternal, neonatal, and women's health nursing involve poor pregnancy outcomes. Some examples of negative outcomes are infants born with low Apgar scores in the face of nonreassuring fetal heart monitoring patterns and shoulder dystocia. Shoulder dystocia is an emergency condition in which the fetal shoulders become entrapped in the maternal bony pelvis after the head has been delivered. Immediate action is required to prevent permanent damage to the infant or death. Many times these infants experience nerve damage if there is too much traction placed on the neck in an attempt at vaginal delivery. The nerve damage can cause a paralysis of the affected upper extremity.

In the past, physicians were primarily the target of malpractice suits. As the status of nursing has involved, however, professional responsibility has increased and so has legal accountability (Aiken & Catalano, 1994). Currently, when a malpractice action is taken, the nurse is usually involved as an employee of the hospital. The involvement may be as simple as not maintaining adequate documentation or as complex as failing to intervene on the client's behalf when the physician does not perform a timely cesarean section.

Hagedorn & Gardner (1997) suggest there are several ways nurses can reduce their risks of being a defendant in a lawsuit. Nurses must develop caring relationships with clients, because a failed relationship between a health care provider and the client and family is a major source of malpractice claims. The key to good relationships is good communication.

Nurses must maintain clinical competence (Hagedorn & Gardner, 1997). It is not acceptable to practice based on yesterday's knowledge. In this age of change, nursing is not the same profession it was 10 or even 5 years ago. The only way to remain clinically competent is to continue to practice and continue to learn.

Nurses must know their legal responsibility (Hagedorn & Gardner, 1997). It is no longer safe to assume the nurse will not be sued because the physician and hospital have more financial resources. Knowing responsibility also refers to being familiar with standards, guidelines, and institutional policies and procedures.

The nurse must define appropriate assignments (Hagedorn & Gardner, 1997). As costs are being reduced, nurses are being asked to take on more responsibility with the aid of assistive personnel. The nurse is accountable for assignments given to assistive personnel and the outcome of that care. The nurse also should be cognizant of the fact that unsafe assignments can be declined.

Nurses must take action when the client's condition deteriorates (Hagedorn & Gardner, 1997). In the physician's absence, the nurse is responsible and accountable for attempting to provide the health care the client requires. If the client decompensates, it is the nurse's responsibility to call another physician if the client's physician is not available to provide the needed intervention or is unable to provide the needed intervention because of policy or condition. For example, if the hospital has a policy that a family physician may perform a delivery in a low-risk pregnancy, when the client's condition changes the nurse has a duty to discuss making a referral with the family physician. If the physician refuses to make the referral, the nurse has a duty to advocate for the client and institute action by what is called the chain of command. The chain of command is a method of providing care when the physician is not following policy or is placing the client in danger. The staff nurse usually notifies her immediate supervisor, who notifies the chief of obstetrics. The chief of obstetrics ordinarily will resolve the issue. In case of nonresolution, however, the chain of command further involves hospital administration and the chief of the medical staff. Any such intervention should be documented.

Nurses should defensively document client care, treatment, and intervention (Hagedorn & Gardner, 1997). Accuracy is of paramount importance. Additionally, all legally relevant material should be documented (Figure 2-6). In nursing documentation, several important considerations should be made (Box 2-3).

Moores (1997) indicates that proactive risk management begins with the nurse at the bedside. The nurse should feel empowered to be proactive. Organizations that want to reduce their risks of being sued will empower nurses to work in a proactive manner to advocate for the client and prevent client dissatisfaction and harm.

Philosophy of Care

Philosophy of care refers to the values the nurse places on certain interventions regarding client care. For example, much discussion is occurring about whether it is more important for the nurse to ensure the technology is working correctly and the documentation is flawless or whether it is more important for the nurse to concentrate on those aspects of practice that are related to touch. Touch in this context means communicating with the client, ensuring comfort, and ensuring the client's individual needs are met. Traditionally, nursing has been a high-touch disci-

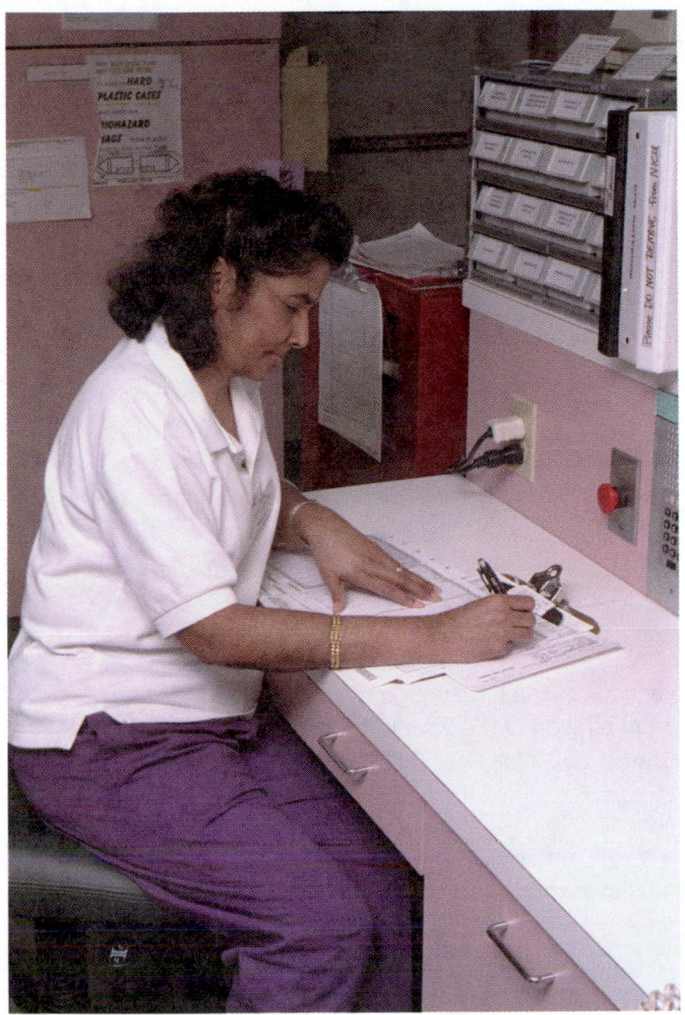

Figure 2-6 Accurate and timely documentation is a strong defense against legal action.

pline. There are those who insist that the concept of caring is what makes nursing different from other professions and why nurses are held in high esteem by the public. In maternal, neonatal, and women's health, the high touch philosophy is very much required to meet the client's needs. The nurse in this specialty must be very skilled to manage the high-tech versus high-touch dilemma.

Box 2-3 Considerations in Nursing Documentation

- Accuracy
- Thoroughness
- Compliance with standards
- Individualized nursing care based on client need
- Appropriate goals and interventions that are timely in completion
- Discharge planning

NURSING IMPLICATIONS

Changing trends in maternal, neonatal, and women's health nursing have implications for nursing practice, education, and research. These implications will be discussed in some detail.

Nursing Practice

Nursing practice is affected by trends in the health care industry. These trends help determine which skills will be required of practicing professional nurses. The acquisition of these skills will determine successful licensure and credentialing.

Skills Required for Practice

As the profession continues to develop, the skills required to practice maternal, neonatal, and women's health care nursing will change. Nurses must know the parameters within which they can practice so as not to exceed that which is legal. To practice beyond one's scope of practice is illegal. Currently, the skills required are those discussed in Chapter 1 and some competencies specific to the specialty. The nurse in maternal, neonatal, and women's health nursing is required to have strong assessment skills. In this field, in particular, nurses are asked to care for the fetus in utero and the newborn in the nursery. Neither of these clients can communicate verbally to let their needs be known. Technologic skills are required to use fetal monitoring equipment, ultrasonography, and fetal pulse oximetry. Other technologic advances also are certain to occur.

Credentialing and Licensure

Licensure is a requirement of state law to perform the services of a registered nurse and to call oneself a registered nurse. To become licensed, the person must graduate from a school that is approved by the Board of Nursing in the state in which the school is located. Licensure has been classified as defining the minimal acceptable standard for the practice of professional nursing.

Credentialing is a process that the individual nurse undertakes beyond basic education and licensure. Credentialing is sought to illustrate expertise in an area of practice. At this time in the United States, credentialing is required for advanced practice in nursing. There has been overture, however, to make certification more broadly applicable to the general practice of nursing. Certification is the process by which a nurse becomes credentialed as an expert. In maternal, neonatal, and women's health nursing there are a number of advanced practice specialties that require certification, including nurse midwife, women's health care nurse practitioner, and neonatal nurse practitioner. Each of these specialties requires a certification

Research Highlight

Improving Outcomes for Newborn Twins

Purpose

To compare newborn outcomes and costs of hospital stays for twins.

Methods

A prenatal clinic in central Texas. A retrospective historical cohort study was completed of women pregnant with twins—one group of 30 women received care in a specialized twin clinic with a research-based care protocol and one consistent caregiver; the other group of 41 women received standard prenatal care.

An advanced practice nurse provided prenatal care, including weekly clinic visits, home visits, and 24-hour availability for telephone support.

Data on gestational age at birth, birth weight, length of stay in the neonatal intensive care unit (NICU), and hospital charges for newborn care were obtained.

Findings

No newborns of less than 30 weeks' gestation were born and the mean birth weight was 249 g higher in the specialized care group. Days in the NICU were reduced from a mean of 17 days in the standard group to 7 days in the group receiving specialized care. Charges were $30,000 less per infant in the specialized care group.

Nursing Implications

Neonatal outcomes were improved, and costs and hospital stays were reduced significantly in the group receiving specialized care.

Ruiz, R.J., Brown, C.E.L., Peters, M.T., & Johnson, A.B. (2001). Specialized care for twin gestations: Improving newborn outcomes and reducing cost. *Journal of Obstetric, Gynecologic, and Neonatal Nursing, 30,* (1), 52–60.

examination and specific criteria, which are designed to provide information about continued competency.

Nursing Education

Nursing education must continually change and develop as does the practice of nursing. There has been a push from licensure agencies to include jurisprudence in the undergraduate nursing curriculum. Core competencies have been developed to integrate the study of genetics into the curriculum of nursing schools. Technologic advances, such as fetal monitoring and ultrasonography, have mandated that nurses develop skills in maternal, neonatal, and women's health nursing that were beyond the scope of nursing practice a decade ago.

Nurse educators must remain competent practitioners, which may mean that the faculty member must find opportunities to practice in addition to teaching responsibilities. Competency also requires that faculty update their

knowledge through continuous learning, reading, and formal and informal educational programs.

Nursing Research

Nursing research related to maternal and child health has developed over the last decade. Research utilization projects sponsored by AWHONN have studied the use of upright versus recumbent position for the second stage of labor to reduce fetal compromise and maternal pain; and the use of exhalatory versus sustained bearing down during the second stage of labor to reduce abnormal fetal heart rate patterns and low Apgar scores. Other research utilization projects have included "Transition of the Preterm Infant to the Open Crib" (Medoff-Cooper, 1994) and "Second Stage Labor Management" (Niesen & Quirk, 1997). The scope and diversity of research related to mothers, fathers, infants, and families over the past 25 years is vast (Moore, 2000). Much more research is still to be done.

Collaboration within the Profession

Collaboration within nursing will become a necessity for nursing research. Many research questions require large samples to provide meaningful results. This type of research requires multiple investigators and multiple sites. Evidence exists that some of this type of research is ongoing. An example of this type of research is Lund et al. (2001) who undertook a study to develop and evaluate an evidence-based protocol for assessment and routine neonatal skin care to educate nurses about the protocol and design procedures for implementation of the project in 51 hospitals across the United States.

Interdisciplinary Collaboration

Collaboration with other professions for research is equally important for nursing. This type of collaboration opens up possibilities for answering research questions in settings and in populations that otherwise would be unavailable. The nurse brings very important skills to the research team as a team member and as a principal investigator.

Web Activities

- Using the Internet, which sites can you find that are related to maternal, neonatal, and women's health?
- Determine what the agenda is for the Women's Health Initiative.
- What is the average cost per day in a neonatal intensive care unit?
- Which resources are available to the pregnant woman who is homeless?
- Which resources are available to the woman who cannot afford the expense of milk and dairy products during her pregnancy?

Key Concepts

- Maternal, neonatal, and women's health care nursing is very complex and poses unique challenges to nurses who practice in this field.
- Nursing in maternal, neonatal, and women's health care is influenced by societal trends.
- Cultural and societal trends must be acknowledged and understood by nurses who practice in the field.
- A number of professional organizations guide nurses in determining the most cost-effective and beneficial interventions for the best practices in a given situation.

- Evidence-based practice results in less liability for malpractice.
- Many ethical considerations arise when trends in practice change. As members of a collaborative interdisciplinary team, nurses are in a unique situation to have input into practice changes.
- Nurses must develop an open attitude toward politics because politics are involved in all institutions and practices.

Review Questions and Activities

1. Name 5 factors that are instrumental in determining whether a woman has access to health care.
2. What is the origin of practice standards and guidelines? What is the purpose of standards and guidelines?
3. Why has great emphasis been placed on prenatal care for women?
4. Why is neonatal ICU care so expensive?
5. What are the risks and benefits of managed care?

References

Administration on Aging. (2001). *Demographic changes.* Available: www.aoa.dhhs.gov/aoa/aging/21 demography. Accessed January 31, 2001.

Aiken, T. D., & Catalano, J. T. (1994). *Legal, ethical, and political issues in nursing.* Philadelphia, PA: F.A. Davis

Agency for Healthcare Research and Quality (AHRQ). (2000a). *Evidence-based practice centers.* Available: www.ahcpr.gov/clinic/epc. Accessed February 15, 2001.

Agency for Healthcare Research and Quality (AHRQ). (200b). Available: www.ahcpr.gov/consumer/20tips.htm.

American College of Obstetricians and Gynecologists (ACOG) and the American Academy of Pediatrics (1997). *Guidelines for perinatal care* (4th ed.). Washington DC: American Academy of Pediatrics and American College of Obstetricians and Gynecologists.

American Nurses Association (ANA). (1995). *Position statement: Home care of the mother, infant, and family following birth.* Available: www.nursingworld.org. Accessed February 15, 2001.

American Nurses Association (ANA). (1991). *Position statement: Physical violence against women.* Available: www.nursingworld.org. Accessed February 15, 2001.

Callen, P. W. (1994). *Ultrasonography in obstetrics and gynecology* (3rd ed.). Philadelphia, PA: W. B. Saunders.

Belenky, M., Clinichy, B., Goldberger, N., & Tarule, J. (1986). *Women's ways of knowing.* New York: Basic Books.

Centers for Disease Control and Prevention (CDC). (2000). *Healthy people 2010.* Washington DC: U.S. Government Printing Office.

Centers for Disease Control and Prevention (CDC). (1986). Perspectives in disease prevention and health promotion public health guidelines for enhancing diabetes control through maternal- and child-health programs. *Morbidity and Mortality Weekly, 35,* (13), 201–208, 213.

Davis-Floyd, R. B. (1992). *Birth as an American rite of passage.* Berkeley, CA: University of California Press.

Dickenson-Hazard. (2001). Wrongly blaming nurses: A response from Sigma Theta Tau. *Lifelines, 4,* (6), 11.

Fleschler, R. G., Knight, S. A., & Ray, G. (2001). Severity and risk adjusting relating to obstetrical outcomes, DRG assignment, and reimbursement. *Journal of Obstetric, Gynecologic, and Neonatal Nursing, 30,* (1), 98–109.

Gaston, M. H. (2001). 100% access and 0 health disparities: Changing the health paradigm for rural women in the 21st century. *Women's Health Issues, 11,* (1), 7–16.

Gilligan, C. (1982). *In a different voice.* Cambridge, MA: Harvard University Press.

Hagedorn, M. I., & Gardner, S. L. (1997). Accountability for professional practice. In *Legal aspects of maternal-child nursing.* Menlo Park, CA: Addison-Wesley.

Hall, J. K. (1996). *Nursing ethics and law.* Philadelphia, PA: S. L. Gardner & M. I. Hasedoneds W. B. Saunders.

Hawkins, J. W., & Bellig, L. L. (2000). The evolution of advanced practice nursing in the United States: Caring for women and neonates. *Journal of Obstetric, Gynecologic, and Neonatal Nursing, 29,* (1), 83–89.

Heaman, M. I., Sprague, A. E., & Stewart, P. J. (2001). Reducing the preterm birth rate: A population health strategy. *Journal of Obstetric, Gynecologic, and Neonatal Nursing, 30,* (1), 20–29.

Huffman, C., & Sandelowski, M. (1997). The nurse-technology relationship: The case for ultrasonography. *Journal of Obstetric, Gynecologic, and Neonatal Nursing, 26,* (6), 673–682.

Institute of Medicine (IOM). (2000). *To err is human: Building a safer health system.* Washington DC: National Academy Press.

Jegalian, K., & Lahn, B. T. (2001). Why the Y is so weird. *Scientific American, 284,* (2), 56–61.

Kaji, E. H., & Leiden, J. M. (2001). Gene and stem cell therapies. *Journal of the American Medical Association, 285,* (5), 545–550.

Kincaide, G. G. (2001). Create a responsible discussion: A response from AWHONN. *Lifelines, 4,* (6), 11–12.

Knox G. E., Kelley M., Hodgson S., Simpson K. R., Carrier L. & Berry D. (1999). Downsizing, reengineering and patient safety: numbers, newness, and resultant risk. *Journal of Healthcare Risk Management, 19,* (4), 18–25.

Loustaunau, M. O., & Sobo, E. J. (1997). *The cultural context of health, illness and medicine.* Westport, CT: Bergin & Garvey.

Lund, C. H., Osborne, J. W., Kuller, J., Lane, A. T. Lott, J. W., & Raines, D. A. (2001). Neonatal skin care: Clinical outcomes of the AWHONN/NANN evidence-based clinical practice guideline. *Journal of Obstetric, Gynecologic, and Neonatal Nursing, 30,* (1), 41–51.

Mattson, S. (1993). Ethnocultural considerations in the childbearing period. In S. Mattson & J. Smith (Eds.). *Core curriculum for maternal-newborn nursing.* Nurses Association of the American College of Obstetricians and Gynecologists Philadelphia, PA: W. B. Saunders.

Medoff-Cooper, B. (1994). Transition of the preterm infant to the open crib. *Journal of Obstetric, Gynecologic, and Neonatal Nursing, 23,* 329–335.

Moore, M. L. (2000). Perinatal nursing research: A 25 year review 1976–2000. *The American Journal of Maternal-Child Nursing, 25,* (6), 305–310.

Moores, P. (1997). Empowering women in the practice setting. In M. I. Hagedorn & S. L. Gardner (Eds.). *Legal aspects of maternal-child nursing practice.* Menlo Park, CA: Addison-Wesley.

National Women's Law Center, FOCUS/University of Pennsylvania & The Lewin Group. (2000). *Making the grade on women's health: A national state-by-state report card.* Washington DC: National Women's Law Center.

National Institute of Child Health and Human Development Research Planning Workshop. (1997). *Journal of Obstetric, Gynecologic, and Neonatal Nursing, 26,* (6), 635–640.

Office of Women's Health. (2000). *Women's health issues overview.* Available: www.4woman.gov/owh.

Olshansky, E. (2000). *Integrated women's health.* Gaithersburg, MD: Aspen.

Podszaski, E., Mortel, R., & Oty, S. J. (2001). Should hysterectomy in the woman over 45 include oophorectomy? *Contemporary Obstetrics/Gynecology 46,* (1), 15–19.

Rinker, S. D. (2000). The real challenge of obstetric nursing history. *Journal of Obstetric, Gynecologic, and Neonatal Nursing, 29,* 100–105.

Roberts, L., & Sward, K. (2001). Birth center outcomes reported through automated technology. *Journal of Obstetric, Gynecologic, and Neonatal Nursing, 30,* (1), 110–119.

Rosenfeld, J. A. (1997). *Women's health in primary care.* Baltimore, MD: William and Wilkins.

Ruiz, R. J., Brown, C. E. L., Peters, M. T., & Johnston, A. B. (2001). Specialized care for twin gestations: Improving newborn outcomes and reducing cost. *Journal of Obstetric, Gynecologic, and Neonatal Nursing, 30,* (1), 52–60.

Sampselle, C. M., Wyman, J. F., Thomas, K. K., Newman, D. K., Gray, M., Dougherty, M., & Burns, P.A. (2000). Continence for women: Evaluation of AWHONN's third research utilization project. *Journal of Obstetric, Gynecologic, and Neonatal Nursing, 29,* (1), 9–17.

Schenk, L. M., & Coddington, C. C. (1999). Laparoscopy and hysteroscopy. *Obstetric and Gynecology Clinics of North America, 26,* (1), 1–22.

Sargent, C. & Brettell, C (1995) Gender and Health: An international perspective. New York: Prentice Hall.

Summitt, R. L. (2000). Laparoscopic assisted vaginal hysterectomy: A review of usefulness and outcomes. *Clinical Obstetrics and Gynecology, 43,* (3), 584–593.

Surrey, E. S. (1999). Falloscopy. *Obstetric and Gynecology Clinics of North America, 26,* (1), 53–62.

Underwood, P. (2001). Flawed care delivery system: A response from ANA. *Lifelines, 4,* (6), 12–13.

U.S. Department of Health and Human Services (DHHS). (1999) *Agenda for research on women's health for the 21st century.* Executive summary (NIH Publication No. 99-4385). Bethesda, MD.

Westoff, C. L. (2000). Evidence-based medicine: An overview. *International Journal of Fertility, 45,* (Suppl. 2), 105–112.

Zwelling, E. (2000). Trendsetter: Celeste Phillips, the mother of family-centered maternity care. *Journal of Obstetric, Gynecologic, and Neonatal Nursing, 29,* (1), 90–94.

Wolf, N. (1992). *The beauty myth: How images of beauty are used against women.* New York: Anchor Press.

Suggested Readings

Martin, E. (1987). *The woman in the body: A cultural analysis of reproduction.* Boston, MA: Beacon Press.

Niesen, K. M., & Quirk, A. G. (1997). The process for initiating nursing practice change in the intrapartum: Findings from a multisite research utilization project. *Journal of Obstetric, Gynecologic, and Neonatal Nursing, 26,* (6), 709–719.

Resources

American College of Obstetricians and Gynecologists, 409 12th Street, SW, P.O. Box 96920, Washington, DC 20090-6920, www.acog.org

American Nurses Association, 600 Maryland Avenue, SW, Suite 100 West, Washington, DC 20024, 800-274-4262, www.nursingworld.org

Association for Women's Health, Obstetric, and Neonatal Nursing, 2000 L Street, NW, Suite 740, Washington, DC 20036, 800-673-8499, www.awhonn.org

National Association of Neonatal Nurses, 4700 W. Lake Avenue, Glenview, IL 60025-1485, 800-451-3795, www.nann.org

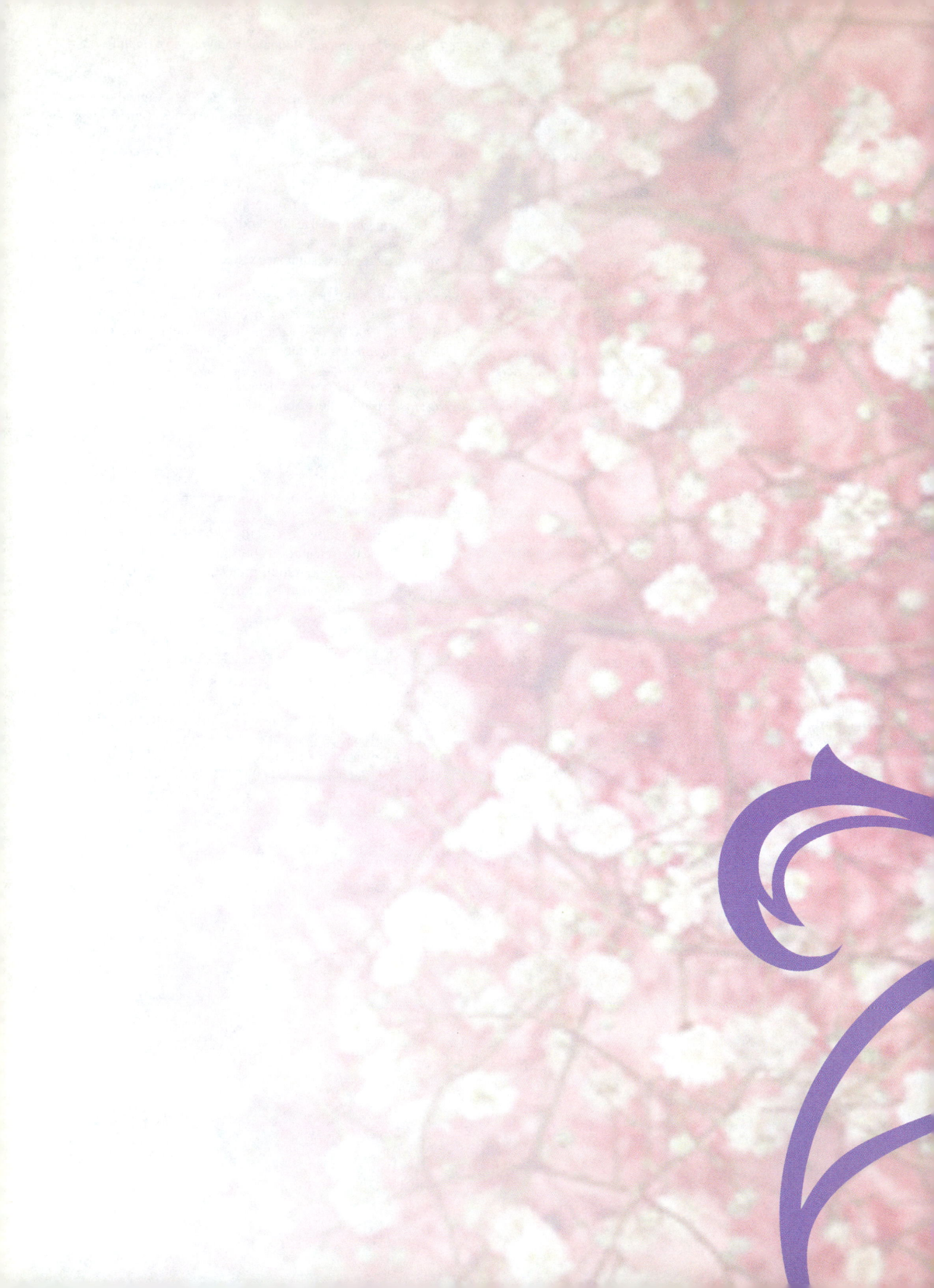

CHAPTER 3

Theoretical Perspectives on the Family

Nurses who work with families or clients who have families often respond as if these families were similar to or should be like their own. These responses make it difficult to understand and respect the diverse cultural and personal values and needs of clients' family units or family members. Use the following questions to examine your personal feelings:

- *How do families change over time? For example, how is a family with an adolescent different from that same family when the child was a newborn?*

- *How do you feel about families that are structurally different from your own?*

- *Have you spent time with a communal family or a couple who is homosexual who have children?*

- *How do you think nurses can incorporate families into their care of clients?*

- *Which strengths do you appreciate about your family?*

- *Which concerns do you have about your family?*

Key Terms

Blended family
Cohabitation
Communal family
Culture

Dyad
Empowering
Enabling
Extended family

Family
Family boundaries
Family dynamics
Family structure

Medical model
Nuclear family
Proactive

Competencies

Upon completion of this chapter, the reader should be able to:

1. Identify various family structures.
2. Discuss some of the common issues related to specific family structures.
3. Discuss theoretical frameworks of families that are relevant to the nursing profession.
4. Discuss the developmental theories of family as they pertain to the childbearing family.
5. Discuss how systems theories apply to family dynamics.
6. Identify contemporary social and cultural issues that impact families.
7. Apply the Resiliency Model of Family Stress, Adjustment and Adaptation to the childbearing family.
8. Describe how a nurse might incorporate the Proactive Model for Enabling and Empowering Families into professional care.

Nurses provide care to clients who are members of families, to aggregates of clients who form families, or to families as units. A common definition in nursing identifies the **family** unit as a group consisting of an adult or adults, and living and unborn children linked by kinship or social bonds whose function is to provide for the physical, psychological, and cultural needs of its members. Family units are estimated to provide 75% of all the health care received by family members, including health promotion, disease prevention, early intervention, and rehabilitation (Duffy, 1988). In cross-cultural studies of health care, Kleimann (1980), an anthropologist, found that the family was consistently the key in determining health-related behaviors. Nurses provide care to the family unit to maintain or enhance the family's ability to provide for the needs of its members.

Nurses, beginning with Florence Nightingale, have explicitly or implicitly accepted responsibility for caring for the family unit. Nightingale (1858, 1863) called for improved living conditions and health care for soldiers' children and wives. In 1904, Wald established general principles for home nursing. These included assessing the family's ability to care for an ill member, evaluating the family support system, including neighbors and community agencies, and making referrals to community agen-

cies. These principles are in the American Nursing Association standards of community health practice (Whall, 1993).

The family, as a unit, has been the domain of community health. Community or public health nurses have considered the family—not the individual—the unit of service in the context of their larger goal, facilitating the health of the community. Maternal-child nursing has focused on family-oriented care beginning with the need to care for mother and infant together. Maternal-child nurses later expanded their sphere to care for the entire family unit as it prepared for and then incorporated a new member. Throughout nursing, nurses now include in their sphere of responsibility the care of the family.

Nurses' understanding of family as a concept varies with the patient care situation and also over time. At one time, nurses viewed the family as an aggregate of persons of different ages. Using that frame of reference, nurses assessed the family because it was the context for providing care to the client. Nurses now understand the concept of family to mean a unit, which may be their client. To care for the family unit the nurse is concerned with family development, dynamics, interaction, and the health of the family as a whole. An understanding of family development, dynamics, and interaction enables the nurse to work effectively with the family in crisis and to facilitate the

Critical Thinking

Definition of Family

Think of the families you know. Describe them to yourself.

- What do you think a typical family is?
- Do you know any typical families?

health of the family in various health situations. A developmental approach and an understanding of parental role attainment also allow the nurse to provide anticipatory guidance to the childbearing family.

This chapter includes descriptions of the structure and function of the family system, treatment frameworks for caring for the family unit, current issues affecting families, provider models, nursing implications, and a care plan.

FAMILY SYSTEM OF STRUCTURE AND FUNCTION

For the purposes of this section **family structure** refers to family form (e.g., single- or two-parent) and marital patterns (e.g., communal or homosexual). In North America in the 1950s and 1960s, a family generally consisted of heterosexual parents in a long-term marriage raising their biologic offspring. In the intervening years, divorce, remarriage, same-sex relationships, and different kinds of adoption have become more common. Our ideas of what makes a family unit encompass much more than the traditional family with the homemaker mother, working father, and their biologic children (Okun, 1996).

Traditional or Nuclear Family

The traditional family is a **nuclear family** composed of two generations, parents and their children. Their **extended family** includes members of other generations, such as grandparents, great grandparents, aunts, uncles, nieces, and nephews, or perhaps even a second nuclear family. In the classic family, the father provided for the economic needs of the family and the mother was a homemaker. In 1998, in the United States, only 25% of all households were composed of married couples with their children under 18. This is compared to 27% of families that are maintained by one parent (U.S. Census, 1998).

Myths of Idealization, Harmony, and Effortlessness

Family members may experience unnecessary anxiety if they hold idealized expectations of so-called normal family life or family traditions that are in conflict with their actual experience (Walsh, 1993). Families are in a continual state of change. The members are aging, and experiencing the need to accomplish different developmental tasks and move on to new stages. Emotional, physical, and economic resources of a family are limited to a greater or lesser extent, and always to some extent. At times, family members have competing not complementary needs. For example, a husband may desire to spend time alone reading after a busy day at work. However, his wife, excited by changes at her workplace, wants to tell him about her day. At the same time, the two toddlers demand attention because one is tired and the other is hungry. Each family member may feel some anger and resentment toward the others. Some angry words may be exchanged: "You never listen to me anymore." "You don't show any consideration for me." Do you think this family is in trouble? The answer probably is no, that is, if the family members know that families are not perfect and that it is almost impossible to get through daily life without some stress. If all goes well the toddlers will be asleep in a couple of hours, the wife will have told her news, and the husband will have some time to read.

If the couple has unrealistic expectations of what marriage and family should be like, the family may be in trouble. Does the wife still have expectations about romantic love that are not always met in the context of a busy family life? Does the husband resent the interest his wife takes in her work? Perhaps the wife believes that a good mother is never angry, tired, or crabby and becomes overwhelmed

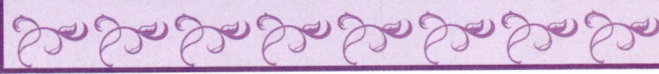

Critical Thinking

Nostalgia for Family Traditions that Never Existed

"Nostalgia for a lost family tradition that never existed has distorted our perceptions and fueled the myth that any deviation from the idealized normal family is inherently pathological" (Walsh, 1993).

- What do you think of the preceding statement?
- What do you think Walsh meant by the words "idealized normal family"?
- Why are families important?

by the demands this idealized notion of motherhood places on her.

Myths of Egalitarianism and Fairness

Perhaps in an ideal world men and women (parents, marital partners) would receive equal pay for equal work and would contribute time, energy, and ability equally in caring for the family. The world is changing but is not ideal. Many persons still view the family as the woman's domain, and often, the woman has primary responsibility for children and the elderly. The roles of men and women in the family often lag behind the roles they have in the work world. For example, although women participate in the work force they continue to do most of the housework (Walsh, 1993).

Myths of Rigid Gender Roles

In the narrow definition of the classic family, the father worked outside the home to provide economically for the family and the mother was responsible for home making, including childcare. The classic family was the norm for only a few unusually prosperous years in the 1950s, when three fifths of families conformed to the classic model. In pre-industrial times "families functioned as a workshop, school, church, and asylum. Most work took place in the household, with children considered economic assets and members of the work force" (Walsh, 1993). Women had limited time for child rearing because of the work they did to meet their obligations to the family economy. Fathers, older siblings, and extended family participated in child rearing (Walsh, 1993).

Myth of Treating All Children Equally

Imagine a family in which one child has congenital heart problems, another lacks coordination but loves music, and another has natural athletic abilities. What would you think of parents who did not differentiate among these three children? You would probably think that they were bad parents. This is an extreme example of treating all children equally because one of the children has heart problems. What would your reaction be if only the second and third children were in the family? Should not their individual interests and abilities be honored and supported? Parents who ignore their children's individual differences decrease opportunities to highlight the unique qualities each child brings to the family. Nevertheless, parents often say, "I treat all my children equally," the implication being that doing so is a good thing. Children are not the same, however, and each child has individual needs. Responding to each child as an individual may make the already com-

Critical Thinking

Each Child is Unique

"Each child, then, presents an opportunity to his parents for a unique adventure as he unfolds and develops" (Satir, 1972, psychologist).

Think of children you know.

- How are they alike?
- How are they different?
- In what ways should they be treated the same?
- In what ways should they be treated differently?

plicated job of parenting even more complicated but certainly more rewarding.

Childless Dyads

Couples, also called **dyads**, may be childless by choice, because of infertility, or because of spontaneous abortions. Nurses should not assume they know why a couple is childless or what being childless means to a couple. Childless couples are sensitive to the intrusion by others into their personal lives and possibly painful issues. Bradt (1989) states that a couple's decision not to have children is influenced by many cultural changes. A woman may choose not to become a mother for many reasons. Women today have greater educational and professional opportunities. A woman may need to work for financial reasons or may not want to bear the responsibilities of parenthood. A woman may take into account the high divorce rate when deciding whether to have a child. Moreover, women today have access to birth control and abortion. About 5% of women who have been married are childless by choice (Friedman, 1992).

Nurses who successfully counsel childless couples are aware of the many avenues that couples may take in resolving issues related to being childless. Couples who are not childless by choice may be struggling with whether to accept being childless, pursue fertility treatments, or adopt.

Extended Family

Extended families are of two main types. Three, four, or even five generations may live in one household or two or more nuclear families may live in households located near each other (Figure 3-1). Even when members of the extended family do not live together, they may give and

REFLECTIONS FROM CLIENTS

Tom and Jill pursued fertility treatments. When the treatments were unsuccessful, they decided to remain childless and now say, "We like having time for each other and feel very close. We also enjoy relationships with our nieces and nephews."

Philip and Sue pursued fertility treatments unsuccessfully and now are the proud parents of two adopted children. They say, "We wish we had decided to adopt right away because we love being parents."

Steve and Mary thought about having children but have successful careers that bring them into daily contact with young adults whom they mentor. They say, "We are happy with our lives the way they are. We don't want to change a thing."

receive social support and exchange goods and services. Even in families separated by great distances the availability of transportation and communication permit extended kinship ties (mainly to parents and siblings) that provide support to nuclear families (Friedman, 1992). Families may have an extensive support network or extended family that includes kin and nonkin, for example, godparents, neighbors, and fellow church members.

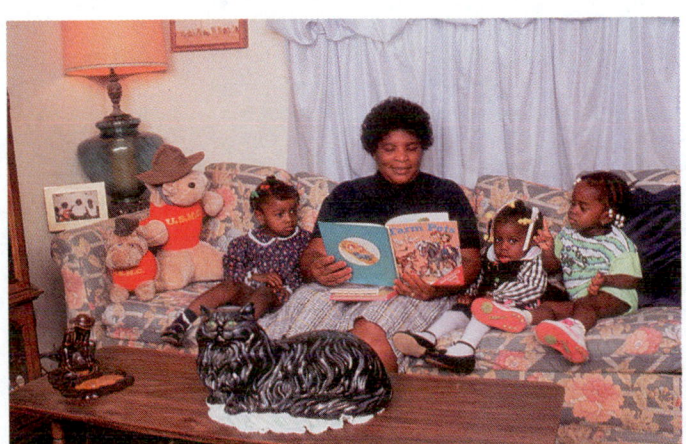

Figure 3-1 Grandparents often assume some childcare responsibilities in extended families.

Relationships Within the Extended Family and Parenting

Various dyads form within all families. These dyads may lead to weakening of the bonds of the extended family. For example, the couple may focus on each other to the exclusion of children and parents, leading to neglect of their children and elderly parents. Parents may focus on their relationships with their children or with their own parents, leading to a decline in the marital bonds. Ideally, extended family members will provide additional resources of time, energy, and psychosocial connections to all the members. Grandparents, aunts, and uncles may be involved in nurturing children and supporting their parents (Bradt, 1989).

Communal Family

A **communal family** forms when individuals, couples, or families live together and jointly carry out family functions. Couples may or may not be monogamous. Child rearing responsibilities may be shared or parents, perhaps particularly mothers, may retain responsibility for rearing their biologic children. Polygamous families, in which one husband has several wives, are a variant of communal families.

Unmarried Heterosexual (Cohabitation) Family

Increasingly, couples are living together without entering into marriage. They may have children that they bring to the relationship or they may have children together. Recently, there has been an increase in older couples choosing to cohabitate. Couples may enter into these relationships to meet needs for love and belonging. They may view **cohabitation** as a temporary stage, a trial period before entering a legal marriage. Older couples may choose cohabitation to avoid disturbing existing inheritance plans for children from other relationships or to avoid reduction in social security or pension benefits.

Homosexual Family

Homosexual families are diverse, as are all families. The household may be headed by a single parent or a couple. In either case the parent or parents may be gay or lesbian. The children may be adopted, biologic, foster, or some combination.

Persons who are gay or lesbian and know they want to become parents may select mates partly on that basis. They may achieve parenthood by adoption, artificial insemination, or heterosexual activity. Gay persons may use a surrogate mother. Adoption remains difficult for homosexual couples, although it does occur. These families face

Critical Thinking

Couples who are Homosexual Becoming Parents

Describe the financial, societal, and cultural hurdles faced by same-sex parents. Ask yourself how you feel about couples who are gay or lesbian becoming parents. Will your personal feelings influence the care you provide?

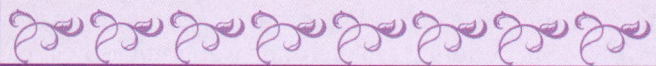

some challenges. For example, how will they ensure that the nonlegal or nonbiologic parent has an ongoing parenting role if the couple separates, or if the legal or biologic parent dies? Parents who are gay may experience the bias against men being the primary caregivers. Parents who are gay or lesbian who have children from heterosexual marriages may remain single to avoid custody disputes with their former spouses (Okum, 1996).

Single-Parent Family

The single-parent family has only one parent, mother or father. Single-parent families are formed in numerous ways: when adults without marital partners choose to have a child, when teenagers become pregnant, when parents in traditional families divorce or separate, and when a spouse dies. Single-parent families are most likely to be headed by mothers. In the United States, only 3% of children live in father-only families, whereas 22% of children live in mother-only families (Levy, 1995). In the early 1990s, almost 3 of every 10 births were to single mothers, many of them teenagers (Farley, 1995; Friedman, 1992). Poverty and teenage motherhood increase the potential for problems in single-parent families; however, when these factors are not present, single-parent families are as successful as are two-parent families (Seibt, 1996).

Single-Parent Families and Poverty

Single-parent families are more likely to be financially disadvantaged than are two-parent families. A higher incidence of poverty exists in families headed by women. The gap between the earnings of men and women has narrowed in recent decades; nevertheless, in 1990, for those working full-time, the average woman earned only 16 cents for every dollar earned by the average man (Levy, 1995). Children in single-parent families are at higher risk

for dropping out of school, premarital teen birth, and being out of school and unemployed than are children in two-parent families (Levy, 1995). There is some indication that these risks are related to poverty rather than to having a single parent. Children of mothers who have high-school diplomas are more than twice as likely to complete requirements for high-school diplomas compared with children of mothers who do not have high-school diplomas (Mare, 1995).

REFLECTIONS FROM A CLIENT

"As a single mother, I often felt ambivalent about leaving household chores undone to spend time with my children or to take time for myself. As a solution, I decided to ask myself if the chore would matter in 50 years. When the answer was no, the chore could wait—and almost always did."

Role Overload: Flexibility and Social Support

Single parents are responsible for the economic, physical, spiritual, and emotional care of the family. Single parents may be overwhelmed if they try to perform all family functions well. They may find it particularly difficult to neglect household chores to provide physical and emotional care for their children. Single parents may benefit from help in setting priorities. Single parents also may worry about having enough time to spend with their children and may need help balancing work and family responsibilities (Seibt, 1996).

Single parents may feel cut off from social activities that meet their needs for affection and companionship.

Nursing Tip

SINGLE PARENT SUPPORT

Nurses may refer single parents to support groups, such as Parents Without Partners, that provide help with parenting and also act as a source of social support for single parents.

Research Highlight

Maternal Employment and Parent-Child Relationships in Single-Parent Families of Low-Birth-Weight Preschoolers

Purpose

This study explores the differences in parent-child and family relationships of single mothers of low-birth-weight and full-term preschool children. Family environmental factors, such as employment of the mother, employment history, and employment attitude-behavior consistency were studied in relation to family relationships.

Methods

Data regarding employment, the Parenting Stress Index, Feetham Family Functioning Survey, and Home Observation for Measurement of the Environment were gathered on single mothers with low-birth-weight and full-term preschool children, 60 and 61 mothers, respectively.

Findings

Employed mothers provided more stimulating home environments and had more positive perceptions of their children. These results could be related to other related effects such as education, income, and number of children. Mother-child relationships and family functioning were similar for families of preterm and full-term children.

Nursing Implications

Employment and gestational status had little effect on mother-child relationships. It is unclear whether the early intervention often provided by nurses and other health care professionals to families having preterm infants may have prevented family dysfunction.

Youngblut, J. M., Singer, L. T., Madigan, E. A., Swegart, L. A., & Rodgers, W. L. (1998). Maternal employment and parent-child relationships in single-parent families of low-birth-weight preschoolers. *Nursing Research*, 47, (2), 114–121.

Parents with well-established sources of support outside the family will be less likely to deprive their children of parenting by turning to their children for emotional support (Seibt, 1996). Social support provides family members with emotional support, a communication network, feedback, and good will from others; social support also enhances self-esteem (Danielson, Hamel-Bissell, & Winstead-Fry, 1993).

Emotional Climate for Resolution of Losses

Members of single-parent families are likely to experience a sense of loss, even in families in which a single person chose to be a parent. Children will fantasize about how their lives would be different if they had a second parent. Parents will find themselves wishing for help or support from a partner. In families in which children express these feelings and are listened to, the children are likely to realize that some of these fantasies are unrealistic. They will also, with the help of the parent and the social support system, be able to identify solutions to meet their needs. If there is no father to coach the little league team, perhaps a grandfather, uncle, or family friend will step in. Single parents who have open communication with other adults similarly will be able to voice and resolve their sense of loss.

In single-parent families formed after divorce, the feelings of loss may be more intense. The family will experience a period of destabilization. Divorce is a crisis for the nuclear family and also for the extended family. The effect of divorce on the family varies with the ages of the children and length of the marriage. Families at greatest risk for divorce are those with preschool and school-aged children. Children in these groups may respond to divorce by regressing developmentally, adding to their parents' stress. When divorce occurs while the children are adolescents

Critical Thinking

Children in Single-Parent Families

"The children raised by single parents can be just as healthy and normal as those raised in the traditional two-parent family. In fact, despite the obstacles, children in most single-parent families are provided with the love and nurturing that all children need and deserve" (Seibt, 1996).

- What do you think Seibt means by the term normal?
- Which needs are met when a child is loved and nurtured?
- Can you think of ways to evaluate whether a child's needs for love and nurturing are being met?

the problems of completing the developmental tasks of adolescence are compounded and frequently the process is prolonged. After divorce the family may take from 1 to 3 years to stabilize (Friedman, 1992). The process of family stabilization is aided when the parents meet their financial responsibilities, continue to talk with each other about parenting issues, and support the other parent's relationship with the children. Parents also need to find ways to rebuild or maintain their separate financial resources and social networks (Carter & McGoldrick, 1989).

In all families, good communication helps the members resolve their sense of loss. Good communication is characterized by the ability of the family members to listen attentively, share feelings about themselves and their relationships, state clearly what they think and feel, stay on topic, speak for themselves and not for others, and have respect and regard for the feelings of others (Olson, 1993).

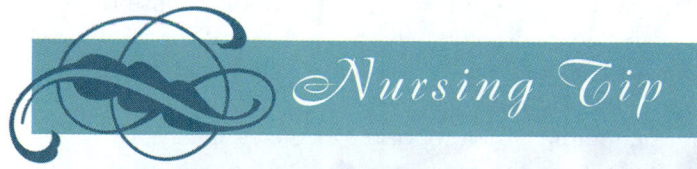

SINGLE-PARENT FAMILY

"After a death or divorce, the reorganized, single-parent family often bonds itself into a very close unit emotionally." (Seibt, 1996).

Reconstituted Family

A **reconstituted family** differs from a traditional family. These differences are described subsequently. Authors use various terms to label the reconstituted family, including remarriage family, stepfamily, and **blended** family. These terms are used interchangeably herein.

Born of Losses

The reconstituted family forms because the earlier marriage or partnership of one or both of the parents ended. Usually the marriage ended in divorce or, less frequently, a spouse died. When members of the reconstituted family have recovered emotionally from the loss of the earlier marriage and have accepted their own and the other's fears about forming a new family, they can begin imagining and planning for the new family. Ideally, they will accept that it will take time and patience for all the family members to take on new roles in the reconstituted family. There will be a period of confusion as they decide where to spend holidays and what their relation is to people to whom other members of the reconstituted are biologically related (e.g., their stepfather's sister). They will have to work through the issues of who belongs where, who has authority for what, and how space and time will be apportioned to various members. They will need to deal with emotional issues, including guilt, loyalty conflicts, a desire

RECONSTITUTED FAMILIES: THE MOST TYPICAL

"Following divorce about 75% of men and 65% of women go on to remarry. By the year 2000, remarried families were predicted to become the predominant family form—the most normal, in the sense of typical" (Walsh, 1993).

- One out of every 3 Americans is a member of a stepfamily.
- 52%–62% of all first marriages end in divorce and 75% of all divorced persons remarry.
- 43% of all marriages are remarriages for one of the adults.
- 60% of all remarriages eventually end in divorce. This makes stepfamilies one of the more typical family structures. (Stepfamily Association of America, 2001) http://www.stepfam.org

for mutuality, and the fact that some past hurts may never be resolved. The family that successfully negotiates these tasks will develop a family that permits children to move from the household of one biologic parent to another and engages in the ongoing work to keep lines of communication open between the parents, grandparents, and children (Carter & McGoldrick, 1989). The family members also will have twice as many sources of support, four sets of aunts and uncles and grandparents.

Family Members' Histories

Members of the remarried family join the family at different points of their individual, marital, and family life cycles. Adults and children may have experienced differing parenting and housekeeping styles and differing traditions in previous families. As a result they may vary in their developmental stages, values, and convictions. For example, a man who has never been married or has never been a parent may marry a woman who has two children, an adolescent daughter and a preschool-aged son, from an earlier marriage. The teenager is developmentally at the stage of moving away from close family ties to peer relationships. Her mother may be dealing with issues related to letting her begin to separate from the family while her stepfather is trying to establish a relationship with her (Visher & Visher, 1993).

Parent-Child Relationship

The reconstituted family may have a very different meaning for children and adults. Adults may view the new family as an opportunity for happiness. In contrast, the children are likely to experience the new family as a threat to their relationship with their biologic parent. In the reconstituted family, children are likely to act out because their sense of security is threatened. When biologic parents and stepparents understand that their relationship threatens the child's feeling of security, the stepparent can avoid taking on a parental role until the child shows readiness. The stepparent can act as a caring adult friend to the child and as a support person to the biologic parent (Seibt, 1996).

The bond between the couple and the bond between the stepchild and stepparent to a large extent are formed independently of each other. The couple's bond, however, usually precedes and provides a foundation for satisfying the child-stepparent bond. Both are needed to establish a successful family (Papernow, 1993).

Influential Biologic Parents

Noncustodial parents, that is, biologic parents who do not live with the children, may have a great impact on the reconstituted family. Children may continue to fantasize about their biologic parents getting back together long after the marriage has ended. The children may see their parent's marriage to a new partner as a betrayal of the former spouse, especially if the former spouse died. Children struggle with divided loyalties when choosing who to invite to important events and with whom to spend time. When parents are hostile and living in separate houses, children are more likely to be successful at causing rifts. They gain power from threats, such as "I'll go live with my dad if you don't let me go out," or from comparing their mother and stepmother, "My real mother lets me go out." These problems are minimized when the adults are able to maintain cordial relationships and open communication around parenting issues (Visher & Visher, 1993).

Members of Two Households

Although the marriage ends when parents with children divorce, the family does not end. Parents continue to have a parenting relationship with each other and with their children. The family takes on new forms, often with children moving back and forth between two homes, with different customs, foods, and ways of doing things. Family members are likely to experience tension when the children prepare to leave one home and when they arrive at the other home. At each transition the children may struggle with feeling left out of one home and needing to become an insider in the other home. Children may not have an identifiable space or may find their space intruded on by stepsiblings. Finding ways to deal with the ongoing transitions is difficult but important. When families do not find ways to manage the transitions, children who experience repeated feelings of being excluded, intruded on, or rejected may develop strong feelings of anger and depression (Visher & Visher, 1993).

Legal and Social Relationships

Stepparents may have an ongoing parenting role that is not recognized legally or socially in their community. Stepparents may not be able to sign for medical care, may not receive invitations to graduation ceremonies, and may be forgotten when biologic parents are asked to join the parent-teacher association at school or other child-centered volunteer activities.

Financial Issues

Finances are likely to take on meanings beyond the intrinsic value of money. To a child, knowing that child-support payments are arriving intermittently or late may add to feelings of vulnerability ("Will I lose my home and end up homeless?"), abandonment ("If she cared, she would send the money on time"), and guilt ("Having to send money to support me is hurting her"). The anger and resentment of former spouses toward each other also are likely to influence their financial dealings. The spouse paying child support may wonder if the money is being spent to meet the needs of the child. The custodial parent may feel anger that the noncustodial parent's living standard has not been affected by the divorce, whereas the custodial parent and the children have a lower standard of living. Stepsiblings may receive differing levels of support from the non-custodial parent, which adds more tension to their relationship. In contrast, having child-support payments arrive routinely may enhance the child's sense of security and decrease tension between the former spouses. The noncustodial parent who routinely pays child support may feel satisfaction and be more likely to remain involved with the children in other ways, maintaining the parenting role.

Additional Relatives

If each of the marital partners has been married before and brings children to the family, they will each have experienced at least three previous family systems: the family of origin, the first marital family, and the single-parent family. The children will have experienced at least two previous family systems (Visher & Visher, 1993). The reconstituted family may have a total of four sets of grandparents and step-grandparents. There will likely be aunts, uncles, and cousins from all the previous families. All these persons may add to the support system available to the family.

Myth of the Wicked Stepmother

Stepmothers and families in which the woman is the stepparent (stepmother families) are likely to experience more stress than are stepfathers or families in which the father is the stepparent. This extra stress on these families may be partly related to the fact that women are still expected to set the emotional tone for the family. More probably, the additional stress in stepmother families is related to the father having custody of the children. Mothers generally are expected to retain custody of their children. These social expectations may add to the mother's and the children's stress. Tension between the mother and stepmother also may add to the stress (Visher & Visher, 1993). Children may wonder what is wrong with them, thinking that their own mother does not want them, no matter what the circumstances of the custody agreement. The mother also may experience anger, frustration, and guilt. Her feelings may exacerbate the children's difficulties dealing with a sense of divided loyalties between mother and stepmother (Engebretson, 1982). A number of children's stories describe stepmothers as evil and wicked. These stereotypes may create additional tension for the stepmother.

Myth of Instant Love

In stepfamilies there are many relationships and not all persons entering the family do so by choice. Remarried parents and stepparents, however, may cling to the myth of "instant love" in the hope that the new family will end the pain that they and their children feel as a result of past losses. The implicit demands that everyone be friendly and feel good can lead to anger, guilt, and tension. Not all stepfamilies are the same; families with a stepfather and a mother and her children tend to experience less stress than do other stepfamilies. Families with a stepmother and father with his children experience more stress, as described previously. Families with the greatest likelihood of divorce are families to which both parents bring children. The larger the family the more difficult the task of forming emotional bonds between all members. Families in which the members can give up the myth of instant love and let relationships develop slowly and naturally will be the most successful (Visher & Visher, 1993).

Papernow (1993) has described emotional and developmental stages that families go through in the process of developing an integrated stepfamily household. Members fantasize about what the family will be like, immerse themselves in the family, become aware of differences, and ally along biologic lines during times of tension. Adults become aware that changes need to be made, lead-

Critical Thinking

Establishing a Family Unit

"Slowly, former alliances and ways of doing things become transformed, as stepfamily members move from having little or no emotional connections between them to the establishment of bonds that give them a sense of belonging together as a family unit" (Visher & Visher, 1993).

As a nurse you understand that it may take time for members in a stepfamily to establish a strong sense of bonds. How would you respond to a mother who is holding a newborn and looking somewhat sad when she says, "I've never had these feelings for my stepdaughter. I love this baby so much"? Would the following statements support the mother's bonds with both children? "This baby is so precious. Having a new baby can be an exciting time in a family. What is your stepdaughter's name? Will she see her baby sister soon?" What else could you say?

ing to mobilization and then action. During these stages the family may find the tension intolerable and may divorce because they cannot work as a team. It may take the adults 5 or 6 years to bond as a team to meet family stressors. In successful families, contact and resolution are the stages of deepening stepparent-stepchild relationships and recognition that the family has achieved stability as a unit.

Myth of the Re-Creation of Another Nuclear Family

Although the family members may fantasize that they are creating a nuclear family with two parents and their children, the stepfamily or remarried family is a more complicated unit. To function successfully, family members must negotiate the complicated issues related to helping children move between two households. When successful the family will have semipermeable boundaries, allowing the adults to communicate about parenting issues and the children to establish a sense of belonging in both households while, at the same time, maintaining a sense of separateness, cohesion, and unity within the household (Engebretson, 1982; Visher & Visher, 1993).

Conflicts

Conflicts may occur between the stepparent and parent of same sex, the spouse and former spouse, biologic groups, stepparents and stepchildren, and parents and biologic children. Of course, conflict may occur between any and all members of the extended family. Sources of conflict include discipline, finances, and sexuality.

Discipline

Discipline issues can be a source of much conflict in all families, but stepfamilies have some unique concerns. It is unlikely that any two people agree completely on discipline. In a family where both parents care for the child from birth, they have an opportunity to develop their discipline styles from infancy. While this does not mean that both parents will agree on discipline styles, they do have an opportunity to work out some of the conflicts while the child is very young. In stepfamilies, one of the parents has an established discipline style and relationship with the child. The new partner must establish a relationship as well as a discipline style with that child. Often the child will resent and challenge the discipline from the stepparent. In some cases, the custodial parent also resents the stepparent's discipline and emerging relationship with the child. This can be a source of much distress in the family. The best advice is for the parents to agree on some disciplinary rules and then present a united front to the child. This avoids overt conflict between the parents and provides more security for the child.

REFLECTIONS FROM A STEPMOTHER

Seth was 6 years old and had lived with his stepmother since he was 4 years old, when his biologic mother had died. He had known his stepmother since he was a toddler. He saw little of his biologic mother's mother. He called his stepmother's parents grandma and grandpa. His grandpa thought he was wonderful, and he and Seth loved being together. However, when his grandpa learned that his daughter, Seth's stepmother, was pregnant, he said, "Finally a real grandchild." His wife quickly turned to him and said, "Don't ever say that again." Fortunately, Seth was not present, and his bond with his grandpa was not harmed. Years later, when Seth and his younger half-brothers were adults, his stepmother recounted that scene, saying, "There were so many feelings of guilt and anger, but we were enriched. It didn't just happen. Our lives have been so much richer than if we were just a nuclear family."

How could you respond if your client spoke of having "real" grandchildren? What makes a family relationship real?

Finances

Parents who are providing financial support to both their stepfamily and their biologic children may feel like "walking wallets," who have had their personal control and power taken from them. Women who have learned to survive as the head of a single family may resent losing their sense of control or power in a new relationship. Both adults are likely to equate money with power and may keep financial matters secret from each other. Finances may serve as the focus for both parents when the family is dealing with power issues and may exacerbate other power issues in the relationship (Visher & Visher, 1993).

60 UNIT I **Foundations of Nursing Care**

Sexuality

Sexuality is likely to be a source of tension in a stepfamily. The newly married couple may exhibit overt sexual behavior that is stimulating to their children. The new family may include teenagers who find themselves attracted and stimulated by their proximity to each other more overtly than siblings who have grown up together and who repressed similar feelings at a young age. Stepfathers and stepdaughters may be attracted to each other. Incest taboos that apply to biologic relatives may be weakened. Daughters generally compete with the mother for the attention of the father. Sons generally resent the father who they view as competing for attention from the mother. These issues are heightened in stepfamilies (Visher & Visher, 1993).

Nursing Implications

The goals of counseling are based in the numerous issues that stepfamilies are likely to be coping with, discussed previously. Helping the couple establish a strong primary bond, which will determine the stability of the family, is the primary task of counseling. The couple will need to establish and support their individual roles in issues related to discipline. Family members will need to establish new alliances that go beyond biologic ties. They will need to resolve issues of loss, anger, grief, and guilt so that they can be assertive in meeting their own needs and defining limits within the new family. Children will need to have a sense of personal space as they come and go between two households. Communications about parenting relationships need to be established and maintained between ex-spouses and stepparents. All members need to be flexible in adapting and readapting to the multiple and complex relationships within the family (Visher & Visher, 1993).

Visher and Visher (1993) give specific guidelines for working with stepfamilies or members of stepfamilies.

🌱 Avoid holding to an ideal family model. The stepfamily does not and will not fit the nuclear family model.

🌱 Stepfamilies may experience extreme stress related to culture and to their structural complexities. They therefore may exhibit more emotional distress than do members of traditional families. This may not indicate a need for in-depth therapy but rather a need for support and validation of their experiences. As they gain in confidence and experience a sense of

---

Critical Thinking

How Family Members Are Connected

When Seth was 8 years old and his brothers were 2 and 3 years old, his aunt (his biologic mother's sister), came to stay with the family for a week. His stepmother recalled her thoughts and feelings as she anticipated the visit. "This person is only related to one of my children. How will she treat the younger children who don't have biologic aunts?" She wondered: "What is my relation to her? I don't have a name for how we are connected. She is family but she is an alien element." The visit started with the two women treating each other politely but formally. Their relation began to change when the aunt bought presents for each of the boys. The visitor was becoming an aunt to all of the boys. Then the women could talk about their anxiety and find common ground.

How can a nurse support the transformation of awkward relationships into supportive relationships?

Client Education

Working with Reconstituted Families

The following tips might be useful in working with a reconstituted family:

- All members of the family need to realize that establishing family rituals, traditions, and relationships will take time.

- Parents must take the time and energy to nurture their own relationship because it is pivotal for the health and stability of the family.

- All members of the family need to establish dyadic relationships and learn to function as a family unit.

- Parents need to work together to establish mutual rules related to discipline.

- Parents should help make noncustodial children feel they are a permanent part of the family. When they visit, make sure they have their own space to keep personal items.

- Parents should take extra time for holiday planning because there are additional relatives to consider.

- All members of the family must be flexible.

mastering the tasks of their unique family, the chaos will probably decrease.

🐚 The most beneficial interventions for counseling stepfamilies include validating experiences, educating family members about the issues related to integrating the stepfamily, reducing family members' sense of helplessness, and strengthening the couple's bond.

🐚 There may be times when family counseling meetings should include other significant adults, for example, adult friends, grandparents, or ex-spouses. The purpose of such meetings should be clearly defined before they occur and limited to issues involving the children to avoid undermining the couple's bond.

🐚 Nurses who counsel the family may have strong feelings (countertransference) both positive and negative, about stepfamily situations. It is therefore important to consult with others while counseling families.

THEORETICAL FRAMEWORKS

Several theories related to family are found in the disciplines of psychology and sociology. Four theoretical frameworks applicable to the nursing professions, particularly nursing with childbearing and child rearing families, are the developmental, interaction (or structural-functional), role, and systems frameworks. The first three allow the nurse to assess the family as a unit; an understanding of role theory is necessary to evaluate individual roles within the family.

Developmental Theories

Developmental theories look at families as they develop over time. Common to developmental theories, each stage has specific tasks. The tasks are represented by the development of the family. For example, the birth of a child presents the tasks of caring for an infant. Successful mastery of the tasks at each stage prepares the family to master the tasks of subsequent stages and maximize the health of the family. Many developmental frameworks exist with various numbers of stages. One of the classic developmental frameworks describes eight stages through which a family progresses from marriage of the couple to death of both (Duvall & Miller, 1985). Duvall orients the stages around the development of the traditional family structure. It is important to note that each stage has tasks for the couple-family unit and for the development of the children. Often, families in traditional structures fail to acknowledge the need to nourish the spousal relationship. Other family

development theorists, such as Carter & McGoldrick (1989), have identified stages that are not limited to traditional family structure. The family progresses through these stages led by the oldest child. Duvall identifies the source of developmental tasks as biologic and physical maturation, cultural and social expectation, and individual aspirations and values.

Family Tasks

The tasks that society expects of the family at different stages and the focus on childbearing-rearing families is most relevant to nurses who care for women and families perinatally. According to Duvall (1977), certain tasks are incumbent on all families:

🐚 Providing physical maintenance: food, shelter, and health care.

🐚 Allocating resources: physical, time, and space.

🐚 Dividing labor to support the home and family.

🐚 Socializing family members.

🐚 Communicating and appropriately expressing feelings.

🐚 Bearing and rearing children.

🐚 Relating to the community.

🐚 Maintaining morals, values, and cultural beliefs.

Eight Stages of Family Development with Tasks

1. *Beginning Family:* This stage spans the start of the marriage to the birth of the first child, including establishment of a new household and the beginning of the nuclear family. The following tasks are important for the new couple to perform:
   🐚 Establishing a mutually satisfying marriage.
   🐚 Planning for the possibility of having children.
   🐚 Relating harmoniously to kin.

2. *Childbearing Family:* This stage begins with the birth of the first child and lasts until the child is 30 months of age. The tasks are the following:
   🐚 Having, adjusting to, and encouraging development of the infant.
   🐚 Establishing a satisfying home for parents and infant.
   🐚 Expanding kinship roles to include the grandparents of the child.

3. *Family with Preschool Children:* This period covers the years from the time the oldest child is 2.5 years old until the youngest child is 5 years old (Figure 3-2). The tasks are the following:
   🐚 Adapting to critical needs and interests of preschool children.

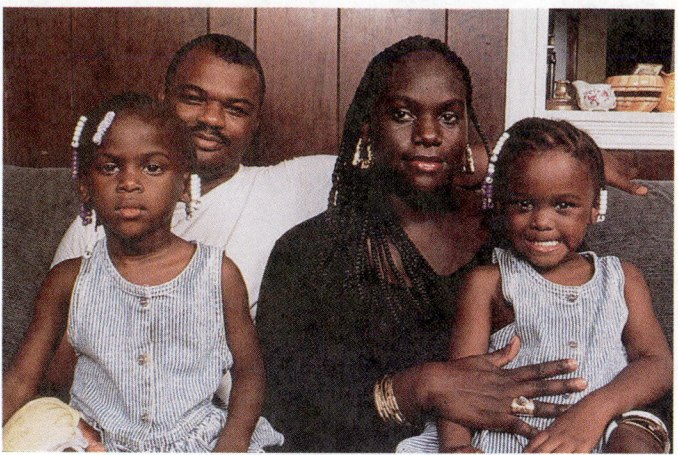

Figure 3-2 Families go through predictable growth stages as members are challenged to adapt to developmental transitions of the family unit combined with changing needs of individual members.

- Meeting the needs of additional children while continuing to meet those of the firstborn.
- Coping with energy depletion and lack of privacy.

4. *Family with School-Aged Children:* The time from when the oldest child is 6 years of age until the child turns 13 years of age is considered the school-aged stage. The tasks are the following:
  - Constructively fitting into the community of families with school-aged children.
  - Encouraging the child's educational achievement.
  - Meeting the physical health needs of all family members.
  - Maintaining a satisfying marital relationship.

5. *Family with Teenagers:* This time period begins when the oldest child is 13 years of age and ends when the youngest child is 20 years of age or leaves home. The tasks are the following:
  - Balancing teenagers' freedom with responsibility as they mature and emancipate from the family.
  - Establishing postparenting interests and careers.

6. *Launching Center Family:* This period covers the years between the time the first child leaves home and the last child leaves home. The tasks are the following:
  - Releasing young adults into lives of their own with appropriate rituals and assistance.
  - Maintaining a supportive home base.
  - Building a new life together as a couple.
  - Assisting with aging or ill parents.

7. *Middle-Aged Family:* This phase refers to the years from the time the last child leaves home to the retirement or death of one of the spouses. The tasks are the following:

FAMILY DEVELOPMENTAL TASKS
Family members engage in individual developmental tasks simultaneously with family developmental tasks. Sometimes these tasks may create conflict. For example, meeting the family task of adapting to needs and interests of a preschool child may create tension with the needs of the young adults to establish intimacy.

- Rebuilding the marriage relationship.
- Maintaining ties with older and younger generations.

8. *Aging Family:* This period lasts from the retirement of one or both members of the couple through the death of one of the spouses, ending with the death of the remaining spouse. The tasks are the following:
  - Adjusting to retirement.
  - Closing the family home, or adapting it for the physical limitations associated with aging.
  - Coping with bereavement and living alone.

Interactional or Structural-Functional Theory

The structural-functional approach to family theory generally understands the family as a subsystem of society. This approach is important to nursing because it allows the nurse to evaluate the family system as a whole, the parts of the family system, and the family system as it interacts with other systems. Friedman (1992) uses the structural-functional theory along with the general systems and developmental theories to provide a "comprehensive and holistic perspective" for assessing family dynamics and the internal and external forces that influence families. When assessing the family using the structural-functional approach the nurse considers the family's structure or organization and how it allows the family to carry out its goals or functions.

Structure

The structure of the family is the way the family is organized. Is the family traditional, a single-parent family, a family resulting from remarriage, and so on? Where is the power in the family? What are the subsystems of the family group? What is the family lifestyle (values, communication, roles, and power)? (Friedman, 1992). If the family structure or organization is functioning well, then the family will carry out its functions.

Function

Functions are those things the family does to meet the needs of its members and of society. Friedman (1992) lists five family functions that are important in assessing and intervening with families:

1. Affective Function: Promotes the stability of family members by meeting their psychologic needs.

2. Socialization and Social Placement Function: Socializes children to become contributing members of society and gives social status to family members.

3. Reproductive Function: Allows the family to acquire and allocate adequate financial resources to meet their needs.

4. Economic Function: Allows the family to acquire and allocate adequate financial resources to meet their needs.

5. Health Care Function: Allows the family's physical needs to be met.

Role Theory

Role theory is based on the understanding that certain behaviors and responsibilities are identified with certain positions. Every person has numerous positions. For example, a man may be a father, husband, son, bricklayer, gardener, neighbor, and so on. Each of these positions has related roles or behaviors associated with it. One of the man's roles as father is to provide childcare. He is likely to share this role with the child's mother and, perhaps, with extended family members and childcare workers. Friedman (1992) stresses that understanding role theory is essential for all nurses who care for families to allow nurses to support healthy role behaviors and determine role problems. This is particularly relevant for childbearing families as they learn parenting roles. Some of the issues surrounding role theory are discussed next.

Conflicting, difficult, or impossible demands may place strain on family members. Examples include a single mother who is expected to provide childcare, work full-time, cook three meals a day, and keep a clean, tidy home. The successful single parent will modify these expectations to manage her role. A mother whose job is vital to her family's economic well-being may find herself having to choose between the needs of a sick child and the requirements of work. Having the support of others may be vital to her in meeting the conflicting demands on her time. Some mothers will have others who can take over her role when needed. For example, the mother and father in a family are likely to share in nurturing children. Extended family members, teachers, members of the religious congregation, and others also may participate in caring for the children.

Individuals never have roles in isolation. Roles are reciprocal, and the role partners influence and adapt to each other constantly. For example, the parent and child roles are continually being modified as the child makes developmental gains and the parent responds. In families, roles are allocated by someone in a leadership role. That person is assigned the role by culture and social class. Roles may be assigned by what the family needs done, by individuals and may also seek satisfactory roles within the family. Families use regulatory mechanisms to maintain equilibrium. The regulatory mechanisms are adaptations of roles to meet the family's needs for outside resources and internal cohesiveness. When family members do not meet their expected roles, both formal and informal, the family may experience difficulty or loss of homeostasis. For example, if the mother's formal role is to provide income the family may experience stress if she becomes ill and unable to work until or unless another family member, perhaps a grandparent, comes to their aid. If the mother's informal role was as peacekeeper between her husband and son and her illness prevents her from carrying out this role, the father and son may have difficulty resolving disputes.

In families in which roles are complementary, compatible with family and social norms, meeting the psychologic needs of family members, flexible in responding to change, and not overloading one or more members, then all family functions probably are being carried out. The family is said to be coping adequately to meet its needs (Friedman, 1992).

Systems Theory

Systems theory has its roots in the physical sciences. Sociologists adapted the understanding that systems can be explained in terms of how they interact with their environment and with their subsystems to evaluate social systems. Friedman (1992) described systems theory as inclusive and powerful. Understanding the family as a system allows the nurse to view the family as a client to be assessed and treated as a whole rather than as an aggregation of individual clients.

Family as a System

A nurse who takes the family systems approach to evaluating a family thinks of the family as a goal-directed unit made up of interdependent and interacting parts that endure over a period of time (Figure 3-3). The family is a relatively open or closed system; that is, the family interacts, to a greater or lesser extent, with other systems. **Family boundaries** establish the family's separateness from the environment and regulate input and output. Families with rigid boundaries are relatively closed and limit family members' interaction with others, who may be potential

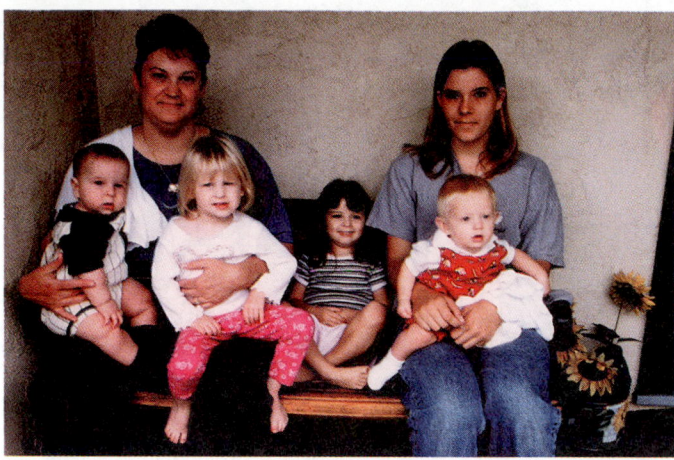

Figure 3-3 The nurse must understand a family's system and structure to provide appropriate care and guidance.

sources of support. Families with few boundaries may have members who are so focused outside the family that they neglect the needs of other family members. An overly closed family system (self-contained) gives little output (energy, material, and information) to the environment and receives little input (energy, material, and information) from the environment. An overly open family system gives so much output and receives so much input from the environment that it is in danger of losing its sense of being a unique, intact entity.

Family subsystems include individuals, such as the husband, who interacts with another individual subsystem, the wife. Subsystems may include more than one individual. One subsystem, the marital couple, may interact with another subsystem, the children in the family. The focal system is the system or subsystem that is of particular interest. For example, the mother-infant pair is the focal system when the nurse is teaching the mother to bathe her newborn child. The nurse also may be interested in the family suprasystem, that is, the extended family or the community to which the family belongs. The nurse may be evaluating the relationship of the mother to others in her extended family or to the community to determine the level of support available to the new mother.

Family systems experience adaptation when they adjust to changing demands and resources from the environment or to internal needs and changes. Self-regulation is the process of adaptation that occurs when the system adjusts internally by modifying subsystems, or externally by controlling its boundaries. It can accept or reject input, and it can modify its structure to accommodate changes.

Family Systems Concepts that Guide Nursing Interventions

Nurses who assess and intervene in family systems are guided by understanding the following:

- The members of a family system are interdependent. The interrelationships are so intrinsically bound that if one member changes, changes will occur in the entire system.
- The family system is greater than and different from the sum of its parts. This is called nonsummativity. One aspect of the family cannot be understood apart from the rest of the family system, and the family as a whole cannot be understood from one of the members.
- The assessment of a family's interactional patterns may be approached from various vantage points. The process is more relevant than is the content. This is known as equifinality.
- Understanding family structure, organization, and transactional patterns aids in understanding the behavior of family members. A major strength of family systems theory is that it naturally allows for incorporation of developmental, interaction, and role theories.

CULTURAL ISSUES THAT INFLUENCE FAMILIES

Many forces affect families. These forces include better health care and public health systems that lead to longer life spans and lower infant mortality rates. The economy of the community in which the family lives influences the family's economic status. Families in the United States and Canada belong to diverse cultures. The role of women in the workplace has changed a great deal since the 1950s and 1960s. These issues are discussed in the subsequent sections.

Lower Birth Rate and Longer Life Span

Fewer children are being born into most American families, and older family members are living longer. The U.S. Census Bureau (2000) estimates that the birth rate per 1,000 persons decreased from 16.7 in 1990 to 14.6 in 1998 (NCHS, 2001). By 2030, 21% of Americans will be 65 years of age or older. Middle-aged adults may find themselves responsible for aging parents, with few siblings to share the caregiving responsibilities. In contrast, the family generations may offer mutual support. The older generation may provide financial support and other services to the younger generations, and the older generation may receive support during times of illness.

Economics

Financial status influences the type of housing, food, health care, and education families can provide for their members. In late adolescence and early adulthood, decisions are made about education, career, marriage, and childbearing that may determine long-term economic well-being. Individuals make these decisions in the context of family expectations, family economic status, as job availability, and social norms (Farley, 1995).

Numerous factors influence the financial status of families. Elderly families (with members over 65 years of age) were half as likely to have income levels below the poverty rate in 1989 (12%) as they were in 1969 (25%) because Social Security benefits were indexed to the rate of inflation in 1971, ensuring that Social Security income kept pace with inflation. The increase in home prices and the expansion of the system of private pension funds also contributed to the decrease in impoverished elderly families. Older persons could sell their increasingly valuable homes and purchase smaller homes or rent and have a substantial amount of money left over to augment their income. Older persons also were more likely to have contributed to pension plans and thus were more likely to have income available in the form of a pension.

In contrast with older persons, children are more likely to live in families with incomes below the poverty level. In 1997, 19% of children lived in families with incomes below the poverty level compared with 17% in 1975. During those years the poverty level increased from 12% to 15% for Caucasian children and decreased from 41% to 37% for African American children. Hispanic children also experienced an increase in the likelihood that they would live in families with incomes below the poverty level. In 1990, 14% lived in poverty compared with 16% in 1997. From 1985 to 1993, the percentage of children living in poverty increased. In 1994, as the economic conditions in the country improved and more jobs became available, paying higher wages, the percentage of children living in poverty decreased.

The growing numbers of families that are headed by women are likely to be among the 20% of American families with the lowest income, because women often have low incomes. Families with dual incomes are more likely to be among the 20% of Americans with the highest income (Levy, 1995). From 1975 through 1997, the median income of mother-only families was never more than 35% of the median income of two-parent families (U.S. Department of Health and Human Services, 1999). In 1997, 32.4% of all births in the United States were to unmarried women, up from 5.3% in 1960 and 28% in 1990 (U.S. Department of Health and Human Services, 2000).

Although an increasing percentage of children are born into single-parent families with low incomes many families with children benefited from social changes, including generally better-educated parents and smaller family size. In 1970, 70% of all children lived with two or more siblings (at least three children). In 1990, more than 50% of children lived with one or no siblings (no more than two children). Parents were more likely to have a higher education and therefore a higher income. From 1969 to 1989,

the proportion of children living in families with incomes above $50,000 (in 1989 dollars) increased (Levy, 1995). On average, family incomes increased from 1979 to 1996, primarily because women were in the work force.

Most families, however, are not average. (Remember when you add 10 + 3 + 2 and divide by 3 the average is 5 but none of the numbers you started with is 5.) The economic status of families often is discussed using income distribution. To determine income distribution all families are ranked by income, then divided into five groups, with 20% of all the families in each group. Economists can then determine how much of the total annual income of a country each group receives. The groups are called quintiles, or simply fifths, for example, the top or bottom fifth. In the United States, the distribution of income has changed over the past twenty years. The lowest quintile accounted for less of the aggregate income: 5.3% in 1980 down to 4.3% in 1999 (U.S. Census, 2001). The top quintile

Critical Thinking

Cultural Practices

At a recent social gathering a group composed of two Muslim couples from Egypt, a Coptic Christian from Africa, a nonreligious couple from China, a nonreligious couple from South America, and two nonreligious North American couples discussed how their mates were chosen. The parents of the couples from Egypt, Africa, and China had arranged marriages. All the couples whose parents had arranged marriages expressed satisfaction with this process of finding a mate. The North and South American couples expressed opposition to arranged marriages and emphasized the importance of finding their own mate. All the couples expressed satisfaction with their mate and the process they had experienced.

- What do you think about how a marital partner is chosen?
- Can you imagine getting to know and love someone before you marry?
- Can you imagine getting to know and love someone only after you marry?
- Which values do you have that make it easier to imagine one situation over the other?
- Do you value individual autonomy more than family, or do you value family more than individual autonomy?
- How might your values get in the way of working with people who have different values?

accounted for 41.1% of the income in 1980 and up to 47.2% in 1999. As a matter of fact, the top 5% of the population accounts for more than two times the income of the bottom two quintiles. Thus, only 20% of the population account for nearly ½ of the total income. The rest is distributed over 80% of the population.

Cultural Diversity

Culture is used here to mean the customs, ideas, beliefs, values, social structure, and language that a family transmits to successive generations. A given family's cultural behaviors and beliefs are based on membership in larger groups, often ethnic or national. Shared language, nationality, or ethnic group, however, does not necessarily indicate shared culture. Cultures often include subcultures. For instance, the European-American cultural group includes German, Italian, Scandinavian, and many other subgroups. Subculture membership may be based on religious practices, educational level, and socioeconomic status. Different cultural groups continually interact, resulting in changes when members of the interacting cultural groups respond to different ideas or behavior patterns. Therefore cultures are dynamic, changing constantly (Cuellar & Glazer, 1996).

In most cultures the family has three social functions. Society expects the family to provide food, shelter, clothing, and medical care to meet the physical needs of its members. The family also is the primary source of communication and emotional support, providing the individual with both preparation for and respite from the demands of society. Finally, the family transmits its cultural values, beliefs, and traditions from the older to the younger generations, thereby providing for continuity of the society.

Immigration increases the diversity of cultures in the United States. Before the mid-1920s there was little restriction on immigration to the United States. From that time until 1965, however, immigration was greatly limited from all regions except Northwestern Europe. This restriction was removed beginning in 1965. From 1965 to 1999, an estimated 27 million persons immigrated to the United States. In the 1950s, immigrants were primarily from

CULTURAL SENSITIVITY
Many sources are available regarding cultural diversity. Nurses must remember not to stereotype clients. Great diversity exists within a culture as well as between cultures.

ACCULTURATION
When families immigrate to a new culture, a process of acculturation occurs. This process may progress faster with younger generation than older generations. For example, a Chinese family immigrating to the United States may have some internal conflict because adolescents begin to acculturate to popular American youth-oriented culture and fail to offer respect to their aging relatives, which is a traditional Chinese value.

Europe. Late in the 20th century, immigrants were primarily from Asia and Latin America (Doyle, 1999).

Cultural variations can be seen in families. Organizational structure and role flexibility within families varies from culture to culture. In some cultures, the males make all instrumental decisions. For example, in Hispanic families, often the male must be included in any decision regarding birth control. In other cultures, women make that decision independently.

Cultures modulate the nuclear (parents and children only) family's relationships with extended (nuclear family and grandparents, aunts, uncles, and cousins) family and the family's relationships to society. For example, a Mexican family may expect unmarried adult children to live in the family home until marriage. In contrast, a middle-class family in the United States likely expects adult children to move out on their own after their formal education is completed. It is not a universal family norm for young adults to live apart from their nuclear family for long periods.

Choice of Marriage Partner

People choose marital partners to meet their needs for love and belonging, companionship, emotional and economic stability, and procreation, among other reasons. Mate selection is greatly influenced by place of birth, current residence, and the social control exerted in one's culture (Okum, 1996). In the dominant North American culture, persons are expected to choose their own mates. In other cultures, parents or matchmakers may select mates.

Generally, first-generation immigrants (those born elsewhere who immigrate) retain the patterns of mate selection dominant in their original culture. The second generation (children born to first-generation immigrants), however, often takes on the values of the dominant culture. When the second generation reaches dating and marital age, conflicts between the two generations may arise.

People may choose mates of differing races, cultures, and religions. These differences sometimes increase difficulties within the marriage. Their difficulties may include knowing less about each other's cultures than people who are in same race, culture, and religion marriages do. These persons also may have to deal with racism and prejudice within their families and communities. There may be a disparity in their level of knowledge about the other's culture. For example, because the dominant culture is more likely to be depicted in popular media, a partner who is African American will probably know more about the culture of a partner who is Caucasian than the other way around (Okum, 1996). When these difficulties can be resolved, the couple may have a satisfying and emotionally rich marriage.

Same-Sex Partners

With a few exceptions, marriages of same-sex couples are not culturally or legally established. Thus, long-term same-sex couples face unique challenges. In many places throughout the world, same-sex couples and their supporters have been working to change existing laws to ensure that their relationships are afforded the same rights and obligations available to married couples under the law. Economic benefits that generally have not been available to same-sex couples include health care insurance for dependents and rights of inheritance. The dependent partner in a same-sex relationship does not have the right to alimony, an obligation on the part of the supporting partner in a heterosexual common-law or married relationship. In a heterosexual marriage if one of the marriage partners becomes extremely ill and is unable to make health care decisions, the other partner is able to do so legally. This has not been true for same-sex couples and is one of the rights they desire.

At present only one country, Cambodia, extends equal marriage rights to homosexuals. The Netherlands passed a bill authorizing same-sex marriage in 2000 that is expected to take effect in 2001. Once the bill is in effect, same-sex partners who marry will have all the same rights as do heterosexual married couples except for the right to adopt. In Brazil, a bill passed in 1996 gives same-sex partners rights, including inheritance, joint-income declaration, and joint income consideration in purchasing a house. In Canada, the Human Rights Act was changed in 1996 to eliminate discrimination based on sexual orientation. In the Canadian province of British Columbia, in 1997, legislators passed laws giving same-sex couples the same rights as common-law heterosexual couples. In Denmark, since 1984, same-sex couples have had equality with heterosexual couples under laws governing inheritance and taxation. Beginning in 1999, Danish same-sex couples could adopt their partner's children but could not adopt outside

the partnership. Norway, Sweden, and Spain have laws similar to those of Denmark. In France, in 1998, unmarried same-sex and heterosexual couples were given many of the tax breaks and legal benefits married couples have. Although adoption became easier for unmarried heterosexual couples, this option was not extended to same-sex couples. In Hungary, in 1996, registered same-sex couples gained the same rights as common-law couples, except the right to adopt. In Iceland, same-sex couples have had the same rights and responsibilities as other couples since 1996, except that they cannot adopt, practice artificial insemination, or have church weddings. However, doing so has little, if any, legal impact. In Hawaii, same-sex marriages were permitted for a few hours in early 1996. A stay of the court ruling was granted to the state; subsequently, voters in Hawaii passed a constitutional amendment prohibiting same-sex marriages. However, same-sex couples can register in Hawaii as reciprocal beneficiaries. Recently, in Vermont, the house has passed a bill that will create a system that gives same-sex couples the same rights, obligations, and benefits as heterosexual couples. A similar bill is currently in the U.S. Senate (Robinson, 2000).

Changing Role of Women

In 1970, 42% of women marrying for the first time were teenagers. By 1990, that figure was 17%. In 1970, 46% of women marrying for the first time were 20 to 24 years of age. By 1990, that number was 41%. In 1970, 8% of women marrying for the first time were 25 to 29 years of age. By 1990, that number was 27%. A similar shift was seen in the age of first-time marriage for men (Clark, 1995). Several social changes are related to the delay in marrying. Young adults spend more years in school, women participate in the labor force, and sexual experiences outside of marriage are more likely to be considered permissible.

Women Working Outside the Home

Men and women work to meet economic needs and goals. They may also work to meet needs for belonging, interesting activities, and a sense of purpose. Although significant differences remain between gender experiences regarding participation in the work force, educational level, and occupation, these differences have been lessening since the beginning of the industrial economy early in the 19th Century. In recent decades, delays in marrying and childbearing and laws making discrimination on the basis of gender and marital status illegal have contributed to increased participation in the work force by women. Because many women can meet their financial needs adequately, women are now more likely never to marry, or if they marry, to divorce and never remarry. A woman who marries and remains married is likely to outlive her spouse and, therefore is likely to depend greatly on her earnings and pension entitlements during widowhood. The real wages of semi-skilled men in the work force have decreased. Therefore, to have adequate income to support a family, the spouses of semi-skilled men need to be employed (Wetzel, 1995).

Any participation in the work force by married mothers with children under 18 years of age increased from 51% in 1970 to 73% in 1990, and full-time participation increased from 16% to 34%. For the same years, any participation in the work force by married mothers with children aged 6 to 17 years increased from 58% to 78%, and full-time participation increased from 23% to 40%. For married mothers with children under 6 years of age any participation increased from 44% to 68%, and full-time participation increased from 10% to 28% (Wetzel, 1995).

Divorce

From 40% to 50% of first marriages by women (the woman's first marriage may be the man's second or third marriage) are likely to end in divorce. Women of African American descent are more likely to divorce than are Caucasian women. Women of Hispanic descent are less likely to divorce than are women in the other two groups. Several additional factors are associated with divorce. Women who marry before 20 years of age, persons who have begun but not completed an educational degree or diploma, and women whose firstborn child was conceived before her first marriage are more likely to divorce (U.S. Bureau of the Census, 1992).

Children and Childcare

The increase in mothers working outside the home has led to a need for accessible, affordable, and high-quality childcare. Parents desire childcare that protects their children's health and safety and provides developmental stimulation. Finding childcare may be difficult, time-consuming, and frustrating for all families. Poor families have a particularly hard time finding high-quality childcare because of the expense involved. Some parents work opposite shifts to care for their children. Grandparents, siblings, and other relatives may care for children. Children are cared for by unrelated adults in the child's or the adult's home, in schools, and in organized childcare facilities. Families may combine various sources of care to meet their childcare needs (Hayes, Palmer, & Zaslow, 1990).

PROVIDER MODELS

Family-focused nurses may focus on an individual within the context of the family or on the family system. When the nurse provides care to an individual client in the context of the family, the individual is understood to be a sub-system of the complete family system. The complete family system is the individual's environment, shared with the other individual family members. Others in the family system support the identified client. The nurse teaches subsets of the family to care for the family member if indicated or to provide support to the client (Friedemann, 1993).

Nurses who care for the family as a unit (the master system) promote changes in the family system. To accomplish for change goals, nursing interventions may extend to the community or environment of the family. Nurses use provider models based in psychoanalytic, general systems, and stress and family coping theories. Nurses also incorporate their understanding of family development, family function, education, learning, and social support to formulate and carry out family-system nursing interventions (Friedemann, 1993).

To carry out interventions in the family system, nurses first assess the system to determine which if any changes are needed. The assessment includes evaluation of family-system processes, individual factors, interaction between family members, and interaction of family and interpersonal systems with the environment. Goals for changes in the family system are established based on analysis and synthesis of the assessment data. Nurses are more likely to be effective when they set goals that are congruent with family needs and values. After goals are established, interventions are planned and implemented to meet the goals. Throughout the entire process the nurse evaluates the family changes and modifies goals and interventions as indicated by the family response (Friedemann, 1993).

In this section concepts or models for caring for families are introduced. These include the concept of family dynamics based in psychoanalytic therapeutic models, the biopsychosocial model based in general systems theory, and the resiliency model based in earlier models of stress and coping. The proactive model for enabling and empowering families is described. A case study that uses the nursing process in accordance with the proactive model follows.

Family Dynamics

The concept of family dynamics is rooted in psychoanalytic therapeutic models. Psychoanalysts originally focused on the impact a mother's role during early childhood has on determining an individual's future development. **Family dynamics** means the ongoing emotional processes within the family (a social unit) over time, as the individuals and the family unit develop (Walsh, 1993). Friedman (1992) emphasizes the importance of evaluating family power to understand the relationships between family members and between the family and its environment. Answers to questions such as those that follow give the nurse information about family dynamics:

Critical Thinking

Care of Families as Individuals or as a Unit

In *First, Do No Harm,* Lisa Belkin (1993) described 15-year-old Patrick, his family, and the hospital community where he had spent much of his life. Patrick was born with Hirschsprung disease. The severity of the disease and the more than 20 surgeries that gradually removed his intestine had left Patrick dependent on intravenous (IV) nutrients dripped directly into his heart. His veins were too damaged by numerous previous IV lines to be useful for the IV feedings. Patrick had survived longer than most children with this disease but was entirely dependent on this type of feeding. Patrick was on a ventilator and had a feeding tube. The feeding tube was intermittently clogged as a result of chronic infections.

Patrick's biologic family consisted of his mother, Oria, and his grandmother. His father had left his mother before he was born. When not at the hospital, Patrick slept at his grandmother's home, which was next door to his mother's home. His mother often worked three poorly paying jobs. To encourage her to spend more time with her son, social workers found her a job in the hospital cafeteria. They included her in meetings about his care, although often she was late or simply did not come. The nurses were angry with her because she often slept or sat silently during her short and infrequent visits to her son. The grandmother who provided most of Patrick's care at home did not visit the hospital.

In the hospital the play therapist, a primary nurse, and many others constituted Patrick's surrogate family. When the primary nurse who cared for him for the first 10 years of his life left the hospital to take another job, she "gave" Patrick to the primary nurse, Kay. Kay remained involved in Patrick's care until his death. Both Kay and the play therapist, Richard, took Patrick on outings. Patrick called Kay at home in the middle of the night when he was scared, anticipating surgical procedures. Celebrities visited Patrick, and he participated in hospital celebrations of major holidays.

Patrick was re-admitted to the hospital with another serious infection of his feeding tube. It was later discovered that Patrick had contaminated his line with feces and dirt to ensure that he would be admitted to the hospital. He had done this previously. Patrick admitted that he did not want to die but was fearful of being outside the hospital. After Patrick's death, his mother stated that she was "bone tired" and that she was not a bad mother, although she felt that the staff did not understand that Patrick had been seriously ill for 15 years and the whole family was tired.

Throughout Patrick's life the professionals who cared for him viewed him, not his family, as the focus of care. They did not ignore his mother but limited their assessments and interventions to attempts to change the ways she mothered. Patrick's mother had long ago decided that the doctors and nurses were better parents to Patrick than she could ever be. They were better educated, more sophisticated, wealthier, and could ease his pain better than she could.

- Did the nurse's role harm or help Patrick?
- Was it helpful for the staff to take Patrick on outings and allow him to call them at home?
- Do you think Patrick's family was addressed?
- Would viewing the family unit rather than Patrick as the focus of care have improved Patrick's life?
- How do you think the nurses viewed the mother's lack of response?
- How did it happen that the nurses gave good care to the child and wonderful attention to the mother but missed the family?

- Who made the decision?
- What was the effect of the decision on individual family members and on the family as a whole?
- Is the power to make decisions shared or does it reside with one family member?
- What does the decision-making say about the family's values?

Understanding a family's dynamics may help the nurse predict areas in which the family may experience difficulty (Figure 3-4). For instance, in families in which decision-making rests with the father and mother, and the children do not participate in decision-making, the children may experience difficulties as adolescents and young adults. Perhaps they will rebel, acting out their need for power and autonomy. Conversely, they may

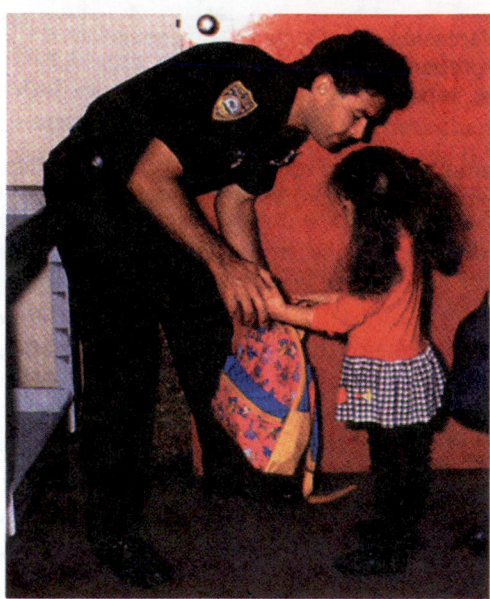

Figure 3-4 Family dynamics and role responsibilities will vary from family to family.

have difficulty carrying out adult roles, demonstrating a sense of incompetency and powerlessness.

Biopsychosocial Model

The biopsychosocial model is based on general systems theory. It illustrates the interaction and boundaries between the systems in which a person exists, for example, those between a person and family subsystems and those between a person and his or her nervous system. The person is part of, yet separate from, the family. The family is part of, yet separate from, the community. The biopsychosocial model strengthens the case for evaluating and treating the family as part of providing health care (McCubbin & McCubbin, 1993).

The **medical model** or **traditional model** of health care is based on the assumption that illness can be understood in terms of the person who is ill and biologic processes. The biomedical model has been very successful at treating persons with specific diagnoses. The emphasis is on the cause and effect of the illness, as explained using medical science, and on concrete signs and symptoms. Generally, the psychological, social, and behavioral aspects of an illness have been ignored or considered beyond the professional's responsibilities in caring for a person. The health care provider whose understanding of illness is limited to the biomedical model is unlikely to perceive a need to evaluate a family as a whole or to explore emotional and psychological stressors in a person's life. The profession of nursing, however, maintains a holistic perspective compatible with the biopsychosocial model.

Resiliency Model of Family Stress, Adjustment, and Adaptation

The Resiliency model of family stress, adjustment, and adaptation was developed from earlier models of stress and family coping by McCubbin and McCubbin (1993). The resiliency model focuses on family adaptation to acute or cumulative stress. Interventions follow evaluation of family functioning and diagnosis of a problem. The goal of nursing intervention is to support the family to enhance their coping skills to facilitate family adjustment and family adaptation. The nursing interventions are most likely to be effective when nurses recognize family strengths and resiliency (McCubbin & McCubbin, 1993).

A family's response to stress is partly determined by the number and severity of the stressors. If the illness stressors are few and relatively minor the family will probably experience a process of adjustment, which is described in the model as the adjustment phase. If the illness stressors are more severe the family is likely to undergo more extensive changes, which is the adaptation phase of the model.

Adjustment Phase

McCubbin and McCubbin (1993) define a **stressor** as a demand placed on the family that produces, or has the potential of producing, changes in the family system. The more threatening the stressor is to the family as a unit, to the family resources, or to the family's coping abilities, the greater the severity of the stress. Families are more or less vulnerable to stress. The degree of vulnerability is related to the number of stressors and to the difficulties family members may be experiencing in the current life cycle stage.

Family types also influence family response to stressors. Families that are of the resilient type have bonds within the family that follow established patterns and allow for flexibility. Resilient families generally are better able to deal with adversity and to maintain or enhance family functioning than are other family types.

Family resistance resources refer to the resources that affect the family's ability to respond to a stressor, without having to make major changes to established family functioning patterns. Families with more resources are more likely to be able to avoid a major crisis when a stressor occurs. Resources may be spiritual, psychological, economic, or material.

Family appraisal of the stressor is the family's understanding of the illness. The culture and community of the family members influence their understanding of a given stressor. Family appraisal of the stressor refers to the family's expectations about the stressor. For example, a family whose child is diagnosed with a severe visual impairment may view this as an overwhelming hardship that will lead to family breakdown or as an opportunity to develop new skills to support the child to develop fully.

Family problem-solving and coping refer to the family's ability to identify and respond effectively to manageable problems related to the stressor and to the multitude of coping behaviors that the family uses as it responds to stress. Coping behaviors have as their goal maintaining or enhancing family equilibrium.

Family response to stress and distress refers to the family's tension in response to the stressor. Reducing or managing the tension avoids stress. Family stress is experienced when the demands placed on the family exceed the family resistance resources and coping abilities.

Family bonadjustment, maladjustment, and crises refer to the extent of the hardship a family experiences in response to the stressor. Bonadjustment is responding to a stressor by making only minor changes that have a positive outcome. Maladjustment may occur in response to severe stressors and results in a state of crisis. Families in crisis are disorganized and, despite repeated attempts to adjust, are unable to restore stability to the family. A family crisis may be necessary to identify and make the major adaptive changes needed to restore stability. Therefore a family crisis may indicate a functional and not dysfunctional family system.

Adaptation Phase

The family adaptation phase occurs when adjustment has not been successful and the family is in crisis. Illnesses in family members often require changes in the family system. The family adaptation phase includes adaptation within the family and between the family and its community. The process of adaptation occurs in response to an accumulation of stressors. The more severe the stressor accumulation and the greater the family's vulnerability, the more difficult will be the task of adapting.

Family types and newly instituted patterns of functioning refer to the categorization of families based on processes they use to maintain a bonded and ongoing family unit. In the family adaptation phase, the family has realized that existing processes are not adequate for the demands placed on the family system and that new patterns of functioning are required to maintain a bonded and ongoing family unit. Families with an ill member may need to change the way they use their time, share work at home and in the work force, and develop closer relationships with health care professionals and, perhaps, with extended family.

Family resources, strengths, and capabilities refer to the family's capabilities or potential to meet the demands with which it is faced. Two important capabilities are the

family's strengths and resources. These may be personal, social, and familial. For example, family members may consistently communicate clearly with each other, a source of family strength.

Family appraisal includes the family's understanding of the stressor and assessment of the family's ability to cope with the stressor. This appraisal allows the family to determine which changes in family functioning are necessary to meet the demands imposed by the stressor. Appraisal also includes schema and meaning. Families assign meaning to an illness based on an evaluation of the family's past and future. A family's schema includes shared values, beliefs, expectations, goals, and so on.

Problem-solving and coping refer to actions taken by the family to manage the demands of a stressor. Actions may be taken to reduce the demands placed on the family by the illness, obtain needed resources, manage tension, and appraise the situation with the goal of understanding it in such a way that it is more positive and therefore more manageable.

Bonadaptation, maladaptation, and crises refer to the outcome of the adaptation process. When family stability and satisfaction are restored, bonadaptation is achieved. When stability and satisfaction do not occur, the family experiences maladaptation. A crisis situation then occurs, forcing the family to attempt to find a new way to adapt.

Proactive Model for Enabling and Empowering Families

The proactive model for enabling and empowering families is based on the assumption that a given family is competent or able to become competent (Dunst, Trivette, & Deal, 1994). If the social system had not failed to provide opportunities for the person to develop or display competencies, the person would be acting competently (Figure 3-5). Effective intervention results in family members developing and displaying competent behaviors and being empowered to acknowledge their own roles in making changes in behavior.

Those using the proactive model hold that the family is a social unit within other formal and informal social support systems and networks. Those who provide care based on the proactive model act from a proactive stance with the goal of enabling or empowering their clients. The three terms are defined below.

1. **Proactive stance:** Belief that people are, or have the capacity to become, competent.
2. **Enabling:** The creation of opportunities for competencies to be displayed or developed.
3. **Empowering:** The help seeker or client acknowledges that the behavior changes he or she has made were due, at least in part, to his or her own actions.

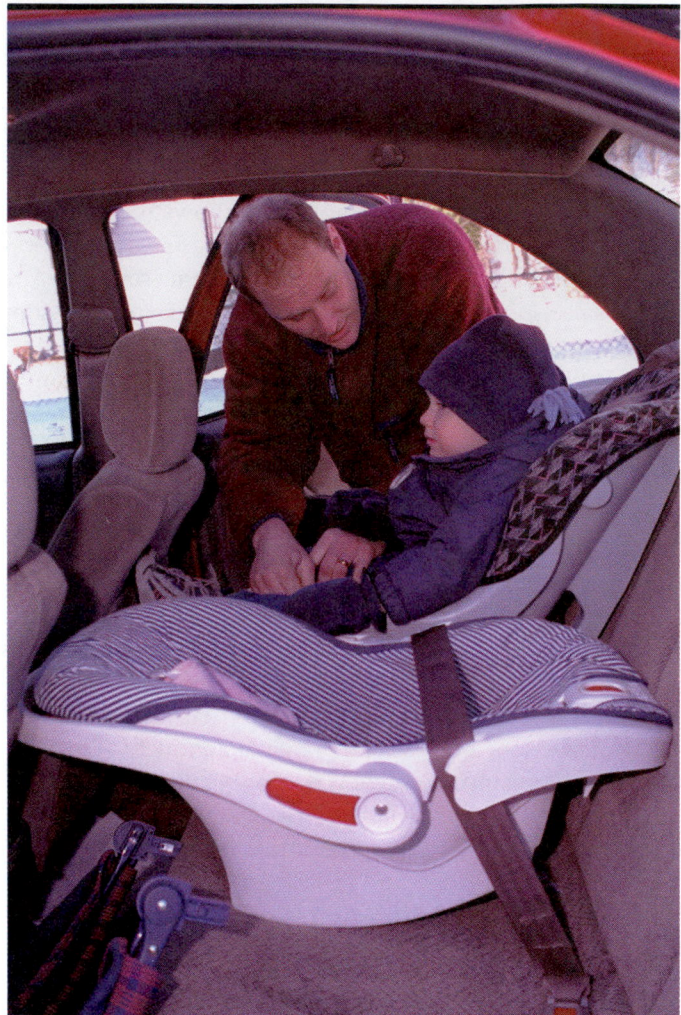

Figure 3-5 Each family member brings a unique set of competencies to the family system.

There are four major components of the model.

1. Family Needs and Aspirations: Nurses who use the proactive model want to help the family members identify their own needs and aspirations, not to superimpose the nurses needs and aspirations onto the family. To meet this goal the nurse will act as a partner, not a parental figure, to the family members. The nurse will learn about the family's strengths, including sources of social support and other resources available to them.

2. Family Functioning Style: This includes the family's beliefs and values, interactional behaviors, and competencies. These are the characteristics that indicate the family's strengths. The family uses these to respond to crisis situations, cope with normative life events, and promote growth and development in all family members. It is most important to acknowledge family strengths and resources that can be mobilized to meet needs. Building on existing strengths facilitates family functioning.

3. Support and Resources: These are sources of support and resources that are outside the family but that may be called on in times of need. Support refers to emotional, physical, informational, and instrumental resources and includes the immediate family, relatives, professionals and agencies, and the larger society.

4. Help-Giving Behaviors: The behaviors of professionals are most effective when they are positive, non-threatening, and support and enhance the autonomy and self-esteem of the help-seeker. The relationship between the nurse and the help-seeker is a partnership.

Case Study/Care Plan

IMPLEMENTING THE NURSING PROCESS USING THE PROACTIVE MODEL

The nurse who works in labor and delivery sees Joel nervously pacing in the waiting room. Earlier, during his wife's labor with their second child, he had left the room quickly if she seemed distressed or if a procedure was being carried out. He had chosen not to be present during the delivery of the couple's first child. Now, when his child is about to be born, he says, "I don't know anything about babies. I've never even held one." The nurse says, "Lots of men have been in your shoes, and they did fine. Fathers are important people. I will help you the first time." The father quietly says, "Thank you." Later, the nurse from the newborn nursery wheels out the baby in the isolette. When the father reaches out to the baby, the nurse says, "You aren't allowed to walk with the baby. You might drop him." She then wheels the baby into the mother's room, with the father following some distance behind.

The labor and delivery nurse is in the room with the mother. As the father enters the room the mother turns to her and says, "What does he know about it? He didn't go through it." The nurse says, "No, he doesn't get to be a mother but I bet he'll be a great father. He is so concerned and anxious about the two of you." The father is standing awkwardly near the door. Turning to him the nurse says, "Sit down in that chair. Arrange your arm to make a cradle to hold your baby." She then places the baby in the father's arms, making sure the baby is well supported. Then, after making sure the baby is awake and alert, she says, "Look at him. He wants to see your face. Good. Now talk to him. Keep watching. Did you see him respond? Your baby knows you. He likes to hear your voice. He knows it." The baby had turned to the sound of his father's voice. The father then settled back more comfortably in the chair and smiled. He kept looking at the baby and started touching his face. The nurse turned to the mother and said, "You have a great family." The mother smiled.

Assessment

During her assessment of the family, the labor and delivery nurse noted the father's pacing, his comment about never having held a baby, and the mother's comment that suggested she did not think he knew much about parenting. The nurse's informal assessment was that the father was not sure how to father and the mother also was insecure and doubtful about his abilities.

Nursing Diagnosis

If she had formalized her diagnosis it might be the following: potential for family maladaptation to the baby owing to lack of experience caring for infants.

Expected Outcomes

Family members will begin to understand and accept the differing roles they play and the unique attributes each brings to the family unit.

Planning

Throughout the process, the labor and delivery nurse collaborates with the family as she plans her intervention.

Interventions

The father shares his lack of experience with a newborn, and the nurse suggests a plan. She offers to help him; he accepts. All her actions are geared to helping this family function as a unit. She acknowledges the mother's role in giving birth and her roles as wife and mother in this family. The nurse stresses the positive aspects of the father's behavior and, through teaching and encouragement, empowers him to become an active parent and partner with his wife. The family unit is strengthened. The nurse does not side with either parent at the expense of the other.

(continued)

Evaluation

The nurse needs to observe the interaction of the family unit. The manner in which the father interacts with the infant reveals a lot about his relationship with the infant, his wife, and their adaptations to the new infant. The way the couple interact with each other also is important. For example, when the father brings flowers to the wife and tells her how proud he is of her, this would be one indicator of a positive adjustment to the birth of a child.

NURSING IMPLICATIONS

When applying the nursing process to a family, the nurse follows the usual steps of the process but for the family as a whole and not for an individual client. During the assessment, information is gathered about the structure, interrelationships, and dynamics of the family. The strengths, resources, and concerns of the family also are assessed. A diagnosis is then made based on the assessments. A plan is developed through a mutual process. For the plan to be successful, the family members must act as collaborators. Nursing interventions should follow the proactive-empowering model. The outcomes are on the level of the family and not on the level of the individual client.

Key Concepts

- Many types of family structures exist: traditional, extended, single-parent, reconstituted, unmarried heterosexual, homosexual, and communal structures. These need to be understood to adapt nursing care to an individual family.

- Many families hold family myths that often direct their relationships. These myths often are not based on facts.

- Family functions of providing for its members, child rearing, and transmitting cultural values are found across cultures. The beliefs, values, and manner in which the functions are carried out, however, are highly dependent on culture.

- Several theoretic models related to function are used in nursing. Some of the most common are developmental, interactive structural-functional, systems, and role theory models.

- Health care providers approach the family based on provider models or orientations. Nursing uses holistic and empowerment models.

Review Questions and Activities

1. In general, health care providers tend to have expectations regarding families that are predicted on which family structure?
   a. Traditional
   b. Single-parent family
   c. Reconstituted family
   d. Communal

   The correct answer is a.

2. Traditional families who believe the mother is responsible for the happiness and well-being of all family members are ascribing to which family myth?
   a. The myth of instant love
   b. The myth of treating all children equally
   c. The myth of rigid gender roles
   d. The myth of egalitarianism

   The correct answer is c.

3. Which task do single-parent families and reconstituted families have in common?
   a. They have significant losses to resolve
   b. They have additional family members to incorporate into the family
   c. They need to combine divergent family histories into a harmonious unit
   d. Legal relationships are ambiguous

   The correct answer is a.

4. Which is an example of an approach to families that uses the empowerment model?
   a. The nurse discerns the diagnosis after a brief assessment of the problem
   b. The nurse conducts her intervention in collaboration with other health care professionals
   c. The nurse begins the process by having the family identify their own strengths, needs, and aspirations
   d. The family is expected to solve their own problems independently

   The correct answer is c.

5. In the resiliency model, which of the following describes the adaptation phase?
   a. A period of rapid decline related to the inability to deal with the accumulation of stressors

   b. A response to an accumulation of or prolonged stressors
   c. Family maladjustment is an inevitable outcome
   d. Problem-solving is left to health care providers

   The correct answer is b.

6. Who are the most likely to live in poverty?
   a. Homosexual families
   b. Communal families
   c. Families with children
   d. Reconstituted families

   The correct answer is c.

References

Belkin, L. (1993). *First, do no harm*. New York: Fawcett.

Bradt, J. O. 1989. Becoming parents: Families with young children. In B. Carter & M. McGoldrick (Eds.) *The changing family life cycle,* 2nd ed. (pp. 235–254). Boston, MA: Allyn and Bacon.

Carter, B., & McGoldrick, M. (Eds.). (1989). *The changing family life cycle* (2nd ed.). Boston, MA: Allyn and Bacon.

Clark, S. C. (1995). Advance report of final marriage statistics, 1989 and 1990. Monthly Vital Statistics Report. National Center for Health Statistics.

Cuellar, I., & Glazer, M. (1996). The impact of culture on family. In M. Harway (Ed.). *Treating the changing family.* (pp. 17–38). New York: John Wiley.

Danielson, C. B., Hamel-Bissell, B., & Winstead-Fry, P. (1993). Families, health, and illness. Boston, MA: Mosby.

Doyle, R. (1999). U.S. immigration. *Scientific American.* www.sciam.com/1999.

Duffy, M. E. (1988). Health promotion in the family: Current findings and directives for nursing research. *Journal of Advanced Nursing, 13,* 109–117.

Dunst, C. J., Trivette, C. M., & Deal, A. G. (Eds.). (1994). *Strengthening and supporting families. Volume 1: Methods, strategies, and practices.* Cambridge, MA: Brookline.

Duvall, E. M., & Miller, B. C. (1985). Marriage and family development (6th ed.). New York: Harper and Row.

Engebretson, J. C. (1982). Stepmothers as first-time parents: Their needs and problems. *Pediatric Nursing, 8,* (6), 387–390.

Farley, R. (1995). *State of the Union: America in the 1990s. Volume one.* New York: Russell Sage Foundation.

Friedman, M. M. (1992). *Family nursing theory and practice.* (3rd ed.). Norwalk, CT: Appleton and Lange.

Friedemann, M. L. (1993). The concept of family nursing. In G. D. Wegner & R. J. Alexander (Eds.). *Readings in family nursing.* Philadelphia, PA: J. B. Lippincott.

Harway, M. (Ed.). (1996). *Treating the changing family.* New York: John Wiley.

Hayes, C. D., Palmer, J. L., & Zaslow, M. J. (Eds.). (1990). *Who cares for America's children? Child care policy for the 1990s.* Washington, DC: National Academy Press.

Kleimann, (1980). *Patients and healers in the context of culture.* Berkeley, CA: University of California Press.

Levy, F. (1995). Incomes and income inequality. In R. Farley (Ed.). *State of the Union: America in the 1990s Volume one.* (pp. 1–58). New York: Russell Sage Foundation.

Mare, R. D. (1995). Changes in educational attainment and school enrollment. In R. Farley (Ed.). *State of the Union: American in the 1990s. Volume one.* (pp. 155–214). New York: Russell Sage Foundation.

McCubbin, M. A., & McCubbin, H. I. (1993). Families coping with illness: The resiliency model of family stress, adjustment, and adaptation. In C. B. Danielson, B. Hamel-Bissell, & P. Winstead-Fry, (Eds.). *Families, health, and illness.* (pp. 21–64). Boston, MA: Mosby.

National Center for health statistics NShs, http:www.cac.gov. nchs, accessed March 2001.

Nightingale, F. (1858). *Notes on matters affecting the health, efficiency, and hospital administration of the British Army.* London: Harrison and Sons.

Nightingale, F. (1863). *Notes on hospital.* London: Longman, Green.

Okum, B.F. (1996). *Understanding diverse families.* New York: The Guilford Press.

Olson, D. H. (1993). Circumplex model of marital and family systems: Assessing family functioning. In F. Walsh, (Ed.). *Normal family processes.* (2nd ed.). (pp. 185–207). New York: The Guildford Press.

Papernow, P. (1993). *Becoming a stepfamily: Patterns of development in remarried families.* San Francisco, CA: Jossey-Bass.

Robinson, B. A. (2000). Countries and companies which have taken action on same sex relations. Ontario Consultants on Religious Tolerance. www.religioustolerance.org

Seibt, T. H. (1996). Nontraditional families. In M. Harway, (Ed.). *Treating the changing family.* (pp. 39–61). New York: John Wiley.

Stepfamily, Association of American (2001) http://www.stepfam.org, accessed March 2001.

U.S. Bureau of the Census, Current Population Reports. (1992). *Marriage, divorce, and remarriage in the 1990's.* (pp. 23–180). Washington, DC: U.S. Government Printing Office.

U.S. Department of Health and Human Services. (1999). Economic security. Trends in the Well-Being of America's Children and Youth.

U.S. Department of Health & Human Services. (2000). Family structure. In E. B. Visher, & J. S. Visher (Eds.). 1979 *Stepfamilies: A guide to working with stepparents and stepchildren.* Secaucus, NJ: The Citadel Press.

Visher, E. B., & Visher, J. S. (1993). Remarriage families and stepparenting. In F. Walsh (Ed.). *Normal family processes.* (2nd ed.). (pp. 235–253). New York: The Guildford Press.

Walsh, F. (Ed.). (1993). *Normal family processes* (2nd ed.). New York: The Guildford Press.

Wetzel, J. R. (1995). Labor force, unemployment, and earnings. In R. Farley, (Ed.). *State of the Union: America in the 1990s Volume one.* (pp. 59–106). New York: Russell Sage Foundation.

Whall, A. L. (1993). The family as the unit of care in nursing: A historical review. In G. D. Wegner & R. J. Alexander (Eds.). *Readings in family nursing.* (pp. 3–12). Philadelphia, PA: J. B. Lippincott.

Youngblut, J. M., Singer, L.T., Madigan, E. A., Swegart, L. A., & Rodgers, W. L. (1998). Maternal employment and parent-child relationships in single-parent families of low-birth-weight preschoolers. *Nursing Research, 47,* (2) 114–121.

U.S. Census (1998) Current Populations Survey http://www.cache.census.gov, accessed March 2001.

U.S. Census (2001) http://www.census.gov, accessed March 2001.

Suggested Readings

Feethan, S. L., Meister, S. B., Bell, J. M., & Gilliss, C. L. (1993). *The nursing of families.* Newbury Park, CA: Sage.

Wilson, N. L., & Trost, R. (1993). A family perspective on aging and health. In G. D. Wegner & R. J. Alexander (Eds.). *Readings in family nursing.* (pp. 141–150). Philadelphia, PA: J. B. Lippincott.

Wright, L. M., & Leahey, M. (2000). *Nurses and families.* Philadelphia, PA: F. A. Davis.

Zeller, J. M., McCain, N.L., & Swanson, B. (1996). Psychoneuroimmunology: An emerging framework for nursing research. *Journal of Advanced Nursing, 23,* (4), 657–664.

Resources

American Association for Marriage and Family Therapy, www.aamft.org

Parents Without Partners, www.parentswithoutpartners.org

Stepfamily Association of America, www.stepfam.org

CHAPTER 4

Complementary and Alternative Therapies

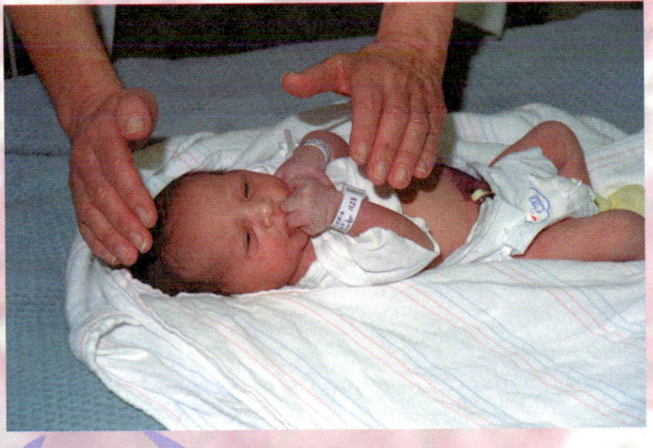

K im is a 52-year-old nurse who was diagnosed with breast cancer. She was treated surgically with a modified radical mastectomy, followed by chemotherapy for 6 months and radiation therapy for 6 weeks. Having grown up on a farm, Kim felt that proper nutrition might reduce the side effects of chemotherapy and radiation and decrease the chance of a recurrence. She consulted a nutritionist who put her on a diet of all organic foods, including a juice consisting of celery, carrots, parsley, lettuce, and beets. After her treatments, she continued to restrict her diet and incorporated yoga, exercise, writing in a journal, and meditation into her daily routine. Kim feels that the most difficult part of her experience was dealing with the fear of cancer recurrence.

Have you ever wondered how you would react to a life-threatening diagnosis? Engaging in complementary therapies (CTs) may improve one's sense of well-being and control throughout such an experience. Some CTs have been reported to decrease the side effects of standard treatments. However, CTs may be expensive in terms of time, energy, and money, and the degree to which they may interfere with standard biomedical therapy or yield toxicities of their own often is not known. Nurses can influence the decisions clients make regarding the use of CTs, which often are widely advertised and easily available.

Key Terms

Acupressure	Biomedicine	Culture	Meridian
Acupuncture	Chi	Dosha	Moxibustion
Allopathy	Chi gong	Healing	Phytotherapy
Alternative therapies	Complementary	Holism	Prana
Ayurvedic medicine	therapies	Integrated medicine	Vitalism

Competencies

Upon completion of this chapter, the reader should be able to:

1. Differentiate between complementary and alternative therapies.

2. Discuss the evolution of traditional healing systems and their influence on healing approaches in the 19th century.

3. Identify the influencing factors for the contemporary use of complementary therapies by clients and their families.

4. Describe a classification of complementary modalities of healing.

5. Evaluate research related to complementary therapies.

6. Discuss legal, regulatory, and ethical issues encountered by nurses with regard to complementary therapies.

7. Discuss the use of complementary therapies for health promotion.

8. Identify indications and contraindications for complementary therapies in women with health deviations.

9. Recognize resources for further education or certification to incorporate complementary therapies into the client's plan of care.

The popularity of complementary and alternative medicine (CAM) increased in the 1990s. The terms alternative, complementary, and unconventional medicines have been used interchangeably in the literature and in health care practice. Because the range of modalities and the purposes for using them are complex, clarification of the terms is warranted. The term **alternative therapy** implies outside of or apart from **biomedicine** (the scientific-based professional medicine taught in medical schools and generally practiced in the United States and Canada) and is best reserved for the therapies used instead of biomedical treatment. In the literature, the term alternative therapy has been used to describe many of the popular activities to enhance health, including nutrition, exercise, massage, and use of vitamin supplements. Because many of these therapies are used as a complement to biomedical treatment or for health promotion, **complementary therapy (CT)** is a more appropriate term. These modalities are used along with biomed-

ical treatment for comfort, pain reduction, and symptom relief. Many CTs also facilitate coping and promote or maintain general health.

Many health care providers, health maintenance organizations, and third-party payers are advocating **integrated medicine**, which combines biomedicine with CTs to provide holistic care. This change in health care delivery has come about largely because of consumer demand for holistic health care services. Consumers want emphasis on health promotion, self-care, and attention to the human experience of health and illness.

This consumer movement has large implications for the nursing profession, which has a conceptual basis oriented toward holism, with a focus on health. Biomedicine has had a historic focus on the diagnosis and treatment of disease, whereas nurses have focused on the experience of the person along the health-illness continuum. Many modalities currently identified as popular CTs have previously been described as independent nursing interven-

REFLECTIONS FROM A NURSE

"As an oncology nurse caring for women with breast cancer, I became interested in complementary and alternative therapies (CAMS) as I noted that more and more clients were seeking these therapies. Many of these women had metastatic disease and were coming to the major comprehensive cancer center where I worked as a clinical nurse specialist with the hope of a cure, only to be disappointed that they had exhausted all treatment options. Other women who were without evidence of active disease wanted to do all that they could to prevent cancer from recurring. Women were consuming large doses of vitamins and herbs, sometimes with evidence of toxicity. One client was admitted for severe electrolyte imbalances resulting from coffee enemas, and another with thrombocytopenia and bleeding related to the combination of chemotherapy and ginseng. Young women receiving adjuvant chemotherapy were experiencing disabling hot flashes from the toxic effect of the drugs on the ovaries. This was particularly distressing because hormone replacement therapy is contraindicated in women with breast cancer, and there were no known effective alternatives. Little was known about CAM use and its effects in clients with cancer prior to the 1970s and 1980s. It was apparent, however, that women with breast cancer were desperate for anything that might offer some degree of hope and control over this ravaging disease."

tions (Snyder & Lindquist, 1998). Nurses are in a position to provide or help the client access many of these services. Nurses also should assess client interest in and use of such services to help clients safely integrate complementary modalities into their health care.

CONTEMPORARY USE OF COMPLEMENTARY THERAPIES

As health care providers it is important to understand consumer changes in health care use. The surfacing of public interest and demand for complementary therapies is a change in the consumer culture for health care. This interest has stimulated much research on the efficacy of these treatments in the United States, Canada, Europe, and worldwide. Research also has focused on better understanding of who uses CTs, why and how they are used, and satisfaction with their use.

Surveys have indicated that CT use increased in the 1990s. Many surveys indicate that about half the U.S. population uses some form of CT. Some well-known surveys have found that the rate of use of CT increased from 33% in 1992 to 42% in 1997 (Eisenberg et al., 1993, 1998). Other surveys have found similar or higher rates of use (Landmark Report, 1998; Villaire, 1998). The rate increases in clients with chronic diseases; for example, one survey in clients with cancer found the use rate was 83% (Richardson et al., 2000). Women account for two thirds of the use of CTs, which is consistent with their more frequent use of conventional health care services (Beal, 1998). These surveys may underestimate use because they generally ask respondents to identify from checklists modalities they have used in the past year. Therefore, if the respondent has used a modality not listed on the form or not within the past year, the response does not get tabulated. Other surveys have described CT users as highly educated, relatively affluent, and often having a holistic orientation toward health (Astin, 1998; Eisenberg et al., 1998; McGuire, 1988). Most respondents paid for these services themselves, spending collectively more than $27 billion annually in the United States. The amount spent was comparable to all U.S. physician services. In one survey of consumers, 44% used CTs in the past year, 60% of these perceived the treatments to be as effective as traditional ones, and 89% would recommend CT to others (Oldendick et al., 2000). In many cases, consumers do not tell their physicians nor are physicians aware of the use of CTs. Problems can result from treatment contraindications, interactions, and poor communication patterns between client and provider.

Because little was known regarding the efficacy of CAM, Congress mandated the National Institutes of Health (NIH) to set up an Office of Alternative Medicine (OAM), which was started in 1992. This office was later upgraded to the National Center for Complementary and Alternative Medicine (NCCAM), which was established to study nonconventional therapies for potential efficacy and to disseminate information to providers and the public. Centers have been established around the United States to study

Research Highlight

Alternative Medicine Use in Older Adults

Purpose

To determine the use of complementary and alternative medicines in Americans aged 65 years and older.

Method

Secondary analysis of data collected in a nationally representative, randomized telephone survey of adults regarding alternative medicine use in the past 12 months. The sample comprised 311 adults over the age of 65 years.

Findings

Of those surveyed, 30% reported they had used at least one alternative medicine, most commonly herbal preparations. Nearly 20% had visited an alternative medicine provider in the past year, most often a chiropractor. The older persons who had a primary care provider were more likely to use alternative therapies than were those with no such provider. Over half of all seniors who used such therapies, however, did not tell their physicians.

Nursing Implications

1. Use of alternative therapies in older adults is of particular concern because many have multiple medical problems and are likely to be taking prescription medicines as well, thus increasing the risk of adverse interactions.

2. Nurses should ask clients which medications they are taking, including all over-the-counter preparations, vitamins, minerals, and herbs.

3. Nurses should encourage clients to discuss alternative medicine use with their physicians.

Foster, D. F., Phillips, R. S., Hamel, M. B., & Eisenberg D. (2000). Alternative medicine use in older Americans. *Journal of the American Geriatrics Society, 48,* 1560–1565.

various aspects of alternative and complementary healing. CAM practices have been cataloged into seven broad categories: mind-body interventions, bioelectromagnetic applications, alternative systems of medical practice, manual healing methods, pharmacologic and biologic treatments, herbal medicine, and diet and nutrition in the prevention and treatment of chronic disease (National Institutes of Health, 1994) (Box 4-1). Some modalities have been recommended for incorporation into general health care. For example, integration of behavioral and relaxation therapies such as meditation, hypnosis, and biofeedback into medical management of chronic pain and insomnia was recommend by a NIH consensus panel of experts (Chilton, 1996).

Several peer-reviewed journals have been established to focus exclusively on CAM therapies. A number of research studies and articles related to CAM also have been published in most medical and specialty journals across

Box 4-1 Classification of Complementary and Alternative Practices

- Alternative systems of medical care: acupuncture and homeopathic medicine
- Bioelectromagnetic applications: electromagnetic fields and electrostimulation
- Diet, nutrition, and lifestyle changes: macrobiotics and nutritional supplements
- Herbal medicine: echinacea and ginseng root
- Manual healing: chiropractic and therapeutic touch
- Mind-body control: art therapy, meditation, and music therapy
- Pharmacologic and biologic treatments: antioxidizing agents and chelation therapy

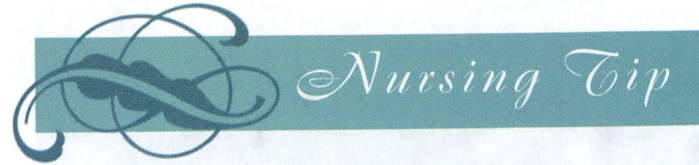

Nursing Alert

CANCER RECURRENCE

For women with a personal history of breast cancer, all exogenous hormonal preparations, including hormone replacement therapy (all oral, patch, vaginal, and injectable forms) and oral contraceptive agents, are contraindicated owing to the potential for such agents to stimulate recurrence of breast cancer. Some biologics are sold that contain ground animal ovaries and other hormonal agents. Phytoestrogens also should be avoided because their influence on cancer recurrence has not been validated scientifically.

Nursing Tip

DISADVANTAGES OF COMPLEMENTARY AND ALTERNATIVE MEDICINE THERAPY

Some disadvantages associated with some complementary and alternative therapies are the following:

- May be based on anecdotal evidence and testimonials
- Lack scientific data
- Lack standardization
- May be costly
- May interfere with the effectiveness of standard therapies

health care disciplines. According to one survey, 64% of medical schools have added courses covering CAM (Wetzel, Eisenberg, & Kaptchuk 1998).

The American Holistic Nurses Association, which focuses on incorporating select complementary modalities into nursing care, is one of the fastest growing nursing organizations. The American Holistic Medical Association is a comparable organization of physicians who advocate incorporating select CAM into holistic health care.

National commissions related to health care delivery have made recommendations related to CAM. Both the Robert Wood Johnson Foundation and the PEW Charitable Trust called for the following recommendations: cost containment, focus on health, use of innovative and diverse provisions for health care, and engaging the client as an active agent in health care (Marston & Jones, 1992; PEW, 1995). The Hastings Center for Bioethics established goals for medicine in 1996, calling for more research on alternative therapies (Callahan, 1996). The Institute for Alternative Futures (1998 http://www.altfutures.com) anticipates that two thirds of the population will use some form of CAM by 2010. Many of these complementary modalities are well-matched with the changing health care focus on health promotion and healthy lifestyles.

DIFFERENTIATING ALTERNATIVE FROM COMPLEMENTARY THERAPIES

It is important for nurses to distinguish between treatments used in place of biomedical care and those therapies used to complement biomedical treatment or to promote health and well-being. Cassileth (1998) differentiates between alternative treatments, which are used in place of biomedical treatments and lack scientific proof of efficacy, and

CTs, which are helpful and applicable during illness and in health. These CTs are noninvasive, gentle, pleasant, often natural, and have stress-reducing effects. A number of biologic treatments for serious diseases such as cancer, acquired immunodeficiency syndrome, and heart disease would best fall into the alternative category. These therapies are primarily ones that have not undergone rigorous clinical trials for safety and efficacy; however, in many cases, research is currently under way. These alternative therapies often are invasive and may contain active biologic or chemical agents; thus, while having potential benefits, they may have inherent toxic or harmful effects. In other instances, the treatment itself may not be toxic but can be dangerous if used in place of or if its use delays effective medical treatment. Sometimes these treatments may be effective in certain circumstances, and anecdotal accounts may add to their appeal to potential users. Professional nurses should be aware of the potential dangers of unconventional therapies and follow the code of practice of their state and professional ethical codes in using or endorsing these treatments. This information generally can be found through the Board of Nurse Examiners of each state.

This chapter focuses on CTs. These generally gentle, natural, noninvasive, holistic treatments are used as supplements to biomedical treatments or to enhance health and well-being. Many CTs are used to reduce stress, enhance coping, and engage the natural healing of the body. Their use parallels the public interest in self-help, human potential movements, and consumer interest in enhancing health and wellness. Although some clients may abandon biomedical treatment to pursue these treatments, most use these therapies in conjunction with

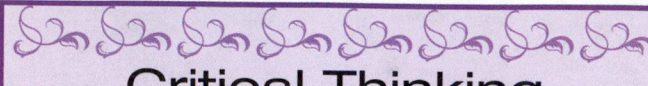

Critical Thinking

Complementary and Alternative Medicine Literature

As a responsible health care provider, you search the literature related to alternative and complementary therapies. You find a variety of reports about a particular modality. Being a critical consumer of the literature, you ask yourself the following questions:

- Are the authors uncritically enthusiastic?
- Do they make unsubstantiated claims?
- Do they have a vested interest in promoting a service or product?
- Do they make general comments against biomedicine?
- Are the authors uncritically dismissive of the modality?
- Do they make unsubstantiated claims disapproving of the modality?
- Do they make general comments against complementary therapies?
- Do they have any knowledge about the modality?

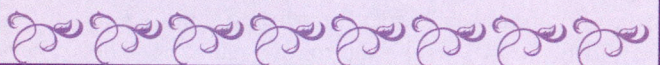

biomedicine or to enhance their health and sense of well-being.

BACKGROUND AND CLASSIFICATION OF MODALITIES

Many of these modalities have their origins in ethnic traditional healing or the historical healing practices of Europe and America. Because many of these modalities are used to improve or maintain health and to cope with illness, they can be viewed as part of the client's or family's actions toward health and reflect cultural orientations and understandings about health. Therefore, when caring for clients from diverse cultures, it is important to understand some of their traditional health beliefs and practices. Practices of traditional cultural systems of healing, such as acupuncture, traditional Chinese medicine (TCM), yoga, or traditional Indian Ayurvedic medicine are becoming popular with clients of diverse backgrounds. As clients are exposed to health care modalities from other cultures, many are incorporating those practices into their own use. In Europe and America, before the use of anesthesia and antibiotics, a number of healing practices were used that were

intended to bolster the body's natural healing. Many of these are resurfacing now as clients search for natural means of promoting health and healing, incorporating physical, psychological, social, spiritual, and environmental health.

Systems of Healing

Systems of healing generally employ several modalities under an organizing unified framework. For example, biomedicine is the system of scientifically based professional medicine taught in medical schools. It is the system of healing with which most persons are familiar. Biomedicine uses many modalities of physical manipulation, such as surgery, ingested and applied medications, therapeutic diets, and other therapies (such as psychotherapy) within one system. **Healing** systems reflect a way to classify disease, determine causes, and provide treatment based on an understanding of health and illness. Healing systems also provide for the education and preparation of practitioners and the delivery of the practice to the public. Differing systems have existed across cultures and over time. Some of the currently popular healing modalities, such as acupuncture and yoga, are derived from healing systems that have evolved over thousands of years.

Healing systems are dynamic and culturally embedded. Many of these systems have developed over time and have incorporated techniques adapted from the environment and interaction with other cultures. (**Culture** is the knowledge, beliefs, art, morals, customs, laws, and other characteristics of persons and members of society [Andrews & Boyle, 1995]). All these systems have components of treatment, prevention, and wellness. Cultural beliefs, values, and worldviews are reflected in the way in which persons understand illness. Five traditional healing systems are discussed briefly: TCM, Ayurvedic, yoga, shamanic, and ritual healing systems.

Traditional Chinese Medicine

Traditional Chinese medicine is a complete health system that is thousands of years old. It encompasses exercise, herbal medicine, massage, nutrition, and a holistic approach to healthy living. (**Holism** is the philosophy of integration of body, mind, and spirit within a dynamic environment.) TCM also includes treatments using herbs, acupressure, and acupuncture. The TCM system is based on the interrelatedness between the whole person and nature. The philosophy of health is based on a balance of opposites. The popular symbol for the union of yin and yang in a circle reflects one aspect of this complex philosophy. The philosophies of Taoism, Confucianism, and Buddhism underlie these ancient healing arts (NIH, 1994; Kaptchuk, 1983; Micozzi, 1996). Assessment of the client includes examination of the characteristics of the radial pulse, skin, and mucous membranes; a thorough health history also is obtained.

The concept of energy is described in Oriental healing systems as chi, ki, or qi. **Chi** is best translated as the point at which matter converts to energy or energy to matter (Kaptchuk, 1983). Chi is understood to flow through various energy channels of the body called **meridians** that have been mapped out over centuries of Oriental medical practice. Illness is a disturbance of chi within the body that may be caused by external factors (environmental influences), internal factors (mental states), and factors other than these (Ergil, 1996). Treatment modalities aim to restore balance and the unimpeded flow of chi through the meridians. Specific points along the meridians correspond with various organs or aspects of the body. **Acupuncture** and **acupressure** are applied at the meridians to facilitate the smooth flow and balance of chi. In acupuncture, fine needles are inserted into the skin and rotated; in acupressure, physical pressure is applied to specific points along the meridians. **Moxibustion** is the application of heat, herbs, or both to the energy points. Various forms of massage and touch, both contact and noncontact, also are used to manipulate and balance energy. **Chi gong** ("working the chi"), tai chi, and other Oriental movement techniques use breathing, movement, and meditation to cleanse, strengthen, and circulate the vital life energy and blood. Chinese medicine has developed a text describing the complex practices of preparing and administering herbs. The most common Oriental practices currently used in the West are acupuncture, acupressure, and forms of chi gong, including tai chi.

The efficacy of these treatments currently is being studied. A NIH consensus panel of experts (co-sponsored by the OAM and the Office of Medical Applications of Research [OMAR]) evaluated scientific and medical data on the uses, risks, and benefits of acupuncture procedures for a variety of conditions. Acupuncture was recommended as an effective treatment for nausea caused by chemotherapy drugs, surgical anesthesia, and pregnancy; for pain resulting from surgery and dental procedures; and for a variety of musculoskeletal conditions (CAM Newsletter, 1998). Most Chinese herbal preparations are individually mixed and specific for each client. The efficacy of Chinese herbal therapies has not been researched in Western scientific trials and may defy the type of clinical trial research used in biomedicine that standardizes dosages and measures disease and treatment-specific outcomes.

Many practitioners of TCM have a lengthy period of schooling and apprenticed practice and many can legally practice in the United States under a state waiver that allows ethnic groups to obtain medical services from a traditional healer. More recently, several states have enacted legislation regulating and licensing acupuncturists, ensur-

ing sterile needles are used and practitioners have met certain standards. Use of Oriental herbal medicine is not regulated, however, and caution should be used because many of the herbs are imported directly from the Orient and may contain contaminants. Because these herbs are not mass-produced, they do not need to pass U.S. standards of clean preparation for consumers. Various combinations of herbs often are used, increasing the likelihood of drug interactions.

Ayurvedic Medicine

Ayurvedic medicine originated in India and means knowledge of life or science of longevity. These ancient teachings have been passed on through the Vedas, a body of ancient Sanskrit literature. Modern Ayurvedic medicine has been revived by Maharishi Mahesh Yogi and is known as Maharishi Ayurveda (Micozzi, 1996). It is holistic and based on the concepts of balance and a vital life force. Ayurvedic medicine in India is centered on the concept of **prana**, a type of vital energy. Health is based on well-being, prevention of disease, and aligning lifestyles with one's individual constitution and personal medical history. Harmony with the environment is sought through understanding and balancing circadian rhythms, seasons, behavior, emotions, and other sensory experiences. Diet, herbs, yoga, meditation, and internal cleansing preparations are addressed in the concept of health. Three **doshas** or metabolic types of people exist: kapha, pitta, and vata, with one being dominant. For optimal health, all doshas need to be in balance; however, the dominant dosha determines the types of foods and other lifestyle practices one should incorporate. This ancient and complex system, with its focus on prevention and holistic integration, is of interest as Western biomedicine focuses more on prevention and holistic health. Transcendental meditation, often practiced in Ayurvedic medicine, has been used by many Westerners.

Yoga

Yoga is a classic Indian practice dating back 5,000 years. It is a philosophy of ethics and personal discipline. Although Yoga is an entire system of life practice with a spiritual philosophy, many Westerners use the techniques without ascribing to the entire practice that includes a philosophy of living. Aspects of the practice of hatha yoga, which focuses on fitness, have become the most popular. Various stretches and postures are used to relieve mild aches and pains, increase flexibility and coordination, and reduce stress while promoting deep relaxation. Breathing, stretching, taking various body postures, and meditating are incorporated in yoga. The purpose of these exercises is to improve circulation, stimulate the internal organs, stretch the body and restore normal alignment, and facilitate proper

REFLECTIONS FROM A CLIENT

"When I developed a nagging pain in my left thigh and hip in 1988, I went to many physicians in search of a cause and treatment. Finally, 17 doctors and 1 year later, a neurosurgeon, who insisted on a myelogram (despite the multiple MRI films I carried with me to the consultation with him), diagnosed a meningioma impinging on my thoracic spine. After a laminectomy to resect the benign tumor, my pain was partially relieved enough so that I was able to discard my cane and gradually wean myself off opioid analgesics. The pain did not go away entirely, however, despite extensive physical therapy, rehabilitation, and nerve blocks.

My long-established faith in the medical model as a health care practitioner was seriously challenged as I slowly realized that there was no cure for the pain. Once I accepted that fact, however, I was able to mobilize other resources for dealing with the pain. Over the past decade, I have engaged in a number of complementary therapies, including acupuncture, neuromuscular massage, yoga, biofeedback, and healing touch. I find that I am best able to manage the pain with regular massage, meditation, and yoga, and with healing touch sessions as needed. Having this experience with pain has enabled me to look beyond the biomedical community for self-care and holistic approaches to enhance my sense of health and well-being, even though the pain is still present."

breathing. Yoga has been shown to reduce blood pressure, reduce heart rate, improve circulation, enhance memory, and release endorphins, the body's natural opiates.

Shamanic Healing

Shamanic healing systems refer to many traditional cultural healing systems. Many of these systems have multi-

ple components and providers such as midwives, bone-setters, herbalists, seers, massagers, and spiritual healers. Medicine and religion are fused in these systems; the medicine person also may be the religious and, in some cases, the political leader. Often, the healer is called a shaman. The shaman's healing powers are related to the ability to communicate with the spiritual world for direction in healing. The shaman enters a controlled trance or altered state of consciousness by drumming, making repetitive sounds, meditating, or using plant extracts. This state of ecstasy, in which the shaman is able to transcend the physical body and sojourn into the spirit world, is one of the most characteristic elements of shamanic systems (Kinsley, 1996). The healing practices may involve physical manipulation, ingestion or application of natural substances, and supranormal actions. A shaman learns these skills through an apprenticeship with an elder shaman. A special marking at birth, exhibition of special healing skills as a child, or overcoming a personal illness or hardship identifies future shamans. The calling is a life-long commitment to healing the members of the community (National Institutes of Health, 1994; Micozzi, 1996). Shamanic systems most familiar to American nurses are Native American healing systems, Curanderisimo, Espiritisimo, Santeria, and African folk healing systems such as hoodoo, voodoo, and rootwork (Gordon, Nienstedt, & Gesler, 1998). Many popular healers incorporate shamanic practices.

Ritual Healing

Spiritual or religious healing has been part of most cultures. Laying on of hands, prayer, and other religious rituals are fairly universal parts of healing practice. These types of healing practices need to be approached in the context of the religious belief and practice. Healing has been a strong emphasis in Judeo-Christian practice and beliefs. Numerous accounts of ritual or spiritual healing are recorded in the Bible and the literature about the saints (Kinsley, 1996). In some Christian denominations, such as Pentecostalism, healing is a central practice. A charismatic healing revival has been evident in the Catholic Church over the past 25 years (Csordas, 1994). One of the Sacraments of the Catholic Church has been changed from being called Last Rites to Anointing of the Sick. Healing rituals also have become more evident in Protestant and Jewish religious practices. Recently, medical and scientific investigators have begun to look at the healing power of faith and religious ritual practices (Dossey, 1993; Koenig, 1999). Levin (1994) found positive health benefits associated with participation in church activities. Some religious ritual practices include penance, forgiveness, meditation, and prayer. Some religious ritual practices also include primal religious experience, which is a physical, psychological, and spiritual experience of ecstasy.

Nursing Implications

The traditional healing practices mentioned previously reflect cultural heritages and beliefs about health, illness, and life in general. These systems also reflect the fundamental cosmologies or philosophic beliefs about the structure of the universe that are intertwined with religious heritage. Nurses should approach the use of these practices as part of culturally competent care. When the practices are not harmful and do not interfere with medical treatments, nurses should support and facilitate clients in their use and practice. Clients determine which practices are congruent with their belief system; nurses should never impose a ritual or symbolic healing system on clients.

Recently, many people in Western cultures have become very interested in varying systems of health and healing. Often the yoga teacher or the shamanic healer is a person of European-American descent who has developed an interest in this system without being from the traditional culture. Many times these healers or teachers have studied extensively with a healer or expert and have adapted the practice or part of the practice for contemporary Western use. Nurses should be cautious about making referrals because a certification process rarely exists in these healing systems and one does not usually know much about the individual practitioner. Word of mouth or other referral sources often are helpful in locating good resources. Some organizations, such as the American Holistic Nurses Association, may be useful in providing information and resources.

Healing Approaches Congruent with Self-Healing

In the 19th century, several approaches to healing were developed. While having some efficacy and continuous practice, many of these approaches were eclipsed by the technologic advances of the 20th century. Modern biomedicine changed dramatically in the 20th century with the discovery of anesthesia that made surgery possible, development of antibiotics and, most recently, understanding the human genome. Some of the 19th-century approaches have experienced a resurgence in popularity. Some of these popular approaches are discussed. The commonality is the underlying purpose of facilitating the body in healing itself or maximizing health.

Vitalism has been an underlying belief in many cultural healing practices and in many of the following self-healing approaches popular in the 19th century. Vitalism refers to a "vital energy" or spiritual force. This force or energy is necessary to explain life and health, which cannot be reduced to physical and mechanical function. This philosophy describes the ways in which many therapeutic techniques were thought to aid in healing, such as those used in Christian Science, chiropractic medicine, osteopathy, naturopathy, homeopathy, hydrotherapy, acupuncture, and in hypnosis, crystals, and other types of psychic healing. The philosophy of vitalism has been integrated into health care in many approaches that use a holistic approach to healing. Some of the more popular approaches are discussed: osteopathy, chiropractic medicine, homeopathy, and naturopathy.

Osteopathic Medicine

Osteopathy, founded in America by Andrew Taylor Still in 1892, is a healing art that places emphasis on the structural integrity of the body. A comprehensive system of diagnosis and therapeutics was based on this interrelationship between anatomy and physiology. The principles are holistic and include the unity and self-regulation of the body. When it is in normal structural relationship and has favorable environmental conditions and adequate nutrition, the body is capable of making its own remedies against disease and other toxic conditions (Wagner, 1996). Currently, there are 15 schools of osteopathy in the United States. Graduates earn a doctor of osteopathy degree, or DO. Doctors of osteopathy are licensed to practice all recognized branches of clinical medicine, having much the same education as do medical doctors. Doctors of osteopathy have additional training and emphasis in diagnosis and treatment of the musculoskeletal system and osteopathic manipulative therapy. Somatic dysfunction is based on local asymmetry, restriction of motion, or fixed postural tension. Treatments include medication, surgery, physical therapy, osteopathic manipulative therapy, and education about nutrition and lifestyle. The American Osteopathic Association has a research institute that has focused on the techniques and principles behind osteopathic manipulative therapy. With the convergence of osteopathic medicine and biomedicine, today many of these techniques are used in standard medical practice (www.am-osteo-assn.org).

Chiropractic Medicine

Chiropractic medicine is a manual healing art that originated in the American Midwest in late 1895, founded by Daniel Palmer, a self-educated healer. He based the profession on two premises: vertebral subluxation (a spinal misalignment causing abnormal nerve transmission) is the cause of virtually all disease; and chiropractic adjustment or manual manipulation of the subluxated vertebra is the cure. Chiropractors treat primarily musculoskeletal conditions, principally back and neck pain and headaches. Although criticized for their one cause–one cure approach and marginalized by biomedicine, the American Medical Association (AMA) was recently found guilty of antitrust violations in banning interprofessional cooperation between medical doctors and chiropractors. The Agency for Health Care Policy and Research (AHCPR) endorsed spinal manipulations for back pain in the 1994 Guidelines for Acute Lower Back Pain. Chiropractors are licensed throughout the English-speaking world and educated in accredited schools. They have a professional code of ethics and standards of practice. Four years of course work builds on science prerequisites in college. Several research studies have shown chiropractic treatments to be effective in low back pain and headaches. Additional trials have begun to demonstrate efficacy in a number of organ disorders, and in hypertension and infant colic (Redwood, 1996).

Homeopathy

Samuel Hahnemann, a German physician and chemist, developed homeopathy in the early 1800s (Jacobs & Moskowitz, 1996). He adhered to a belief in holism in which the totality of symptoms is interrelated, and remedies need to be individualized to the unique experience of the client. All healing was essentially self-healing. He felt that symptoms were the body's attempt to self-heal. Based on these observations, he developed a process of provings in which a substance that produced the same symptoms in a well person could be used to augment the body's efforts in combating disease. This practice of using medications producing symptoms similar to those of the disease contrasts with the standard practice of **allopathy** (traditional or established medical or surgical procedures, both invasive and noninvasive, used in the diagnosis and treatment of mental or physical illnesses), or using medicines to counteract the symptoms. Hahnemann believed that spirit was more powerful than matter; therefore, the essence (spirit) of the medicine was more important than the substance. He innovated a rigorous system of experimentation and established a *Materia Medica,* which now has over 2,000 remedies. Medications are prepared by a series of dilutions and agitations, and the end result is more essence and less matter. These preparations, some diluted beyond Avogadro's number, are so dilute that not even a molecule of the substance can be found in the solution (Jacobs & Moskowitz, 1996). This fact has been puzzling to many biomedical scientists who have difficulty accepting the possible efficacy of a medication without substance.

Homeopathy is practiced widely in Europe, India, Mexico, and other parts of the world; it flourished in the United States until the early 20th century. In 1914, the Flexner Report standardized medical education in the United States and led to a ban on homeopathic medicine by the AMA (Starr, 1984). Practitioners of homeopathic medicine currently are adding homeopathic practice to an existing legal practice license. Many medical doctors and chiropractors also practice homeopathy. Hahnemann's original research in the provings was conducted with rigor that set the stage for much medical research, including in-

oculations. Current research has demonstrated efficacy in a number of chronic conditions, such as asthma, allergies, and other conditions not involving advanced tissue damage.

Naturopathy

Naturopathy is concerned with a philosophy of life rather than a particular type of disease treatment. Naturopathy is holistic and focuses on health. It was founded in the late 1800s from the European nature cures, with roots back to the time of Hippocrates. Benedict Lust brought the concept to the United States in the late 1800s (Pizzorno, 1996). Lust integrated osteopathic medicine, chiropractic, hydrotherapy, and homeopathy as an alternative to the biomedical system. Naturopaths believe that most disease is the result of ignoring or violating the laws of nature. Naturopaths espouse natural treatment, healthy nutrition (primarily vegetarian), fresh air, and natural light as natural healing. This philosophy of healing has become popular because it combines a critique of the established pharmaceutical emphasis with a focus on nutrition, exercise, and the environment. The principles of naturopathy are holistic; the whole person is treated, with a focus on preserving health, preventing disease, avoiding harm, and using the inherent natural healing systems of harmony to correct the underlying cause of disease (Pizzorno, 1996). The practitioner is a teacher whose major focus is to educate the client toward natural health.

The establishment of three colleges of naturopathy in the United States and related research in nutrition, environmental medicine, and clinical ecology have contributed to the rise of naturopathy in contemporary health care. Naturopathic physicians are licensed in some states and practice as primary care providers. They use a variety of natural therapies and diagnostic methods. Required education is a bachelor's degree in biologic science that is similar to a premedicine program and a 4-year accredited graduate program.

COMPLEMENTARY MODALITIES

A host of complementary therapies and therapists currently is available. These are discussed in the following general categories: physical movement and manipulation, ingested and applied substances, energy-based therapies, psychologic or mind-body therapies, and spiritual healing.

Physical Manipulation

Manipulation of the physical body is a common type of modality and includes those body movements a person performs and therapeutic manipulations performed by a therapist on the client. Physical manipulations in biomedicine include surgery, physical therapy, and other physical treatments. Complementary modalities include exercise and physical movements, and various types of body work.

Exercise and Physical Movements

Exercise and physical movements have a well-established link to health and well-being. A number of specific techniques and approaches currently is available. Exercise programs are designed to do one or a combination of the following. Flexibility exercises are planned and deliberate actions taken to enhance range of motion using a combination of stretching and relaxation techniques, such as yoga and calisthenics. Endurance exercises are used to build stamina and general conditioning. They often are aerobic and are helpful in maintaining cardiovascular health and losing weight. Aerobic exercises aim to increase cardiac endurance and include fast walking, jogging, cycling, and swimming. Strengthening exercises often use weights or machines, with repetitions to build muscle. Sports and athletics often are good methods to achieve a variety of exercise benefits.

Exercise is important for women of all ages. The type of exercise, however, may need to be modified for age and physical condition (Figure 4-1). Exercise should continue during pregnancy to maintain strength and stamina. Stretching also is a good preparation for labor. Pregnant women should avoid leg lifts that may put strain on abdominal muscles after the 4th month. Women should engage in weight-bearing exercise throughout life to maintain bone calcium to help prevent osteoporosis. Swimming and cycling are good aerobic and strengthening exercises but do not strengthen bone. In choosing an exercise program, women need to follow the type of activities they enjoy and to which they are able to adhere. For example, some women are motivated by the social aspects of sports and group exercises, whereas others find a solitary jog is a welcome time alone each day. Many sports and fitness clubs have trainers, kinesologists, or exercise physiologists available for individualized exercise programs.

Specific Exercise or Movement Techniques

A number of specific body techniques is available from teachers who have special training or certification in a particular technique. Some examples are found in Table 4-1.

Body Work

Body work techniques are types of physical manipulation that require a trained therapist. Some of the more popular techniques, such as craniosacral manipulations, massage

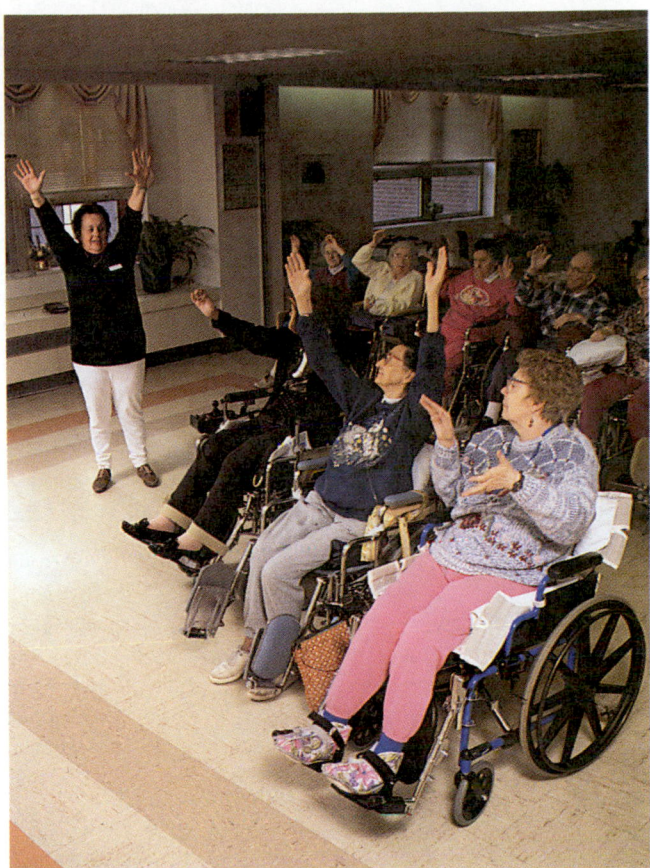

Figure 4-1 All exercise should be tailored to the individual's lifestyle and physical abilities.

therapy, Rolfing, and Trager, are described in Table 4-2. Some nurses have acquired additional training and can offer these types of body work to clients.

Nursing Implications

Body work and exercise are very popular and generally have few risks. Most body-work therapists are certified in their training and have been educated to avoid medical risks. It is generally a good practice to ask about certification or preparation of the provider. For women with chronic illnesses and the frail elderly, it is a good idea to consult the physician or nurse practitioner before having body work performed.

Ingested and Applied Substances

Pharmaceuticals are the most commonly applied and ingested substances and are the major focus of biomedical treatment. Many medical pharmaceuticals are derived from plants, and plant-derived products are found in all healing systems. Foods and dietary supplements along with *phytomedicines* (plant-based medicines) are among the most

Table 4-1 Select Exercise and Movement Techniques

Technique	Description	Uses and History	Providers and Availability	Information
Alexander technique	Form of body technique or postural therapy that works on proper alignment of head, neck, and spine. This alignment is thought to improve physical and psychologic well-being. Relearning better alignment and posture has been associated with reduction in chronic pain from previous injuries or poor posture.	Developed by Frederick Alexander, an actor, to help him project his voice. Became popular with dancers, singers, and other performers.	Classes are available in many cities taught by certified instructors who have completed a 3-year training program.	www.alexandertechnique.com
Feldenkrais	Awareness through movement, this method focuses on various parts of the body while sequencing simple movements. It has been helpful in clients with neuromuscular disorders, such as multiple sclerosis, musculoskeletal pain, cerebral palsy, and stroke, and in older persons and those with spinal injuries (Rosenfeld, 1996).	Developed by Moshe Feldenkrais who investigated various sciences to treat his knee injuries.	Certified Feldenkrais instructors have training throughout the country.	www.feldenkrais.com
Pilates	Method that aims to create balance, flexibility, and coordination by focusing on specific muscles. Very individualized technique. Also is useful for rehabilitation from injury.	Developed by Joseph Pilates in the early 1900s to assist dancers' performance and help recovery from injuries.	Local trainers and classes.	www.pilates.net

popular forms of CTs. An estimated 60 million Americans used herbal therapies. In 1996, Americans spent approximately $3.24 billion on these products.

Numerous dietary plans to lose weight, improve health, and cure diseases are available by way of the popular media. A number of proposed curative diets are popular with the public. Many have not been researched, and nurses should exercise caution in providing dietary advice that may interfere with a therapeutic diet or guidelines for healthy nutrition. (See Chapter 8 for basic nutritional guidelines and information about vitamins, minerals, and micronutrients.) Another popular health practice is fasting, which is relatively safe for healthy people for a short duration (less than 3 days). Frequent or long-term fasting may deprive the client of adequate nutrients.

Dietary Supplements

Other ingested or applied substances include various enzymes, hormones, and other biologic products. These generally are not recommended unless under a physician's di-

Table 4-2　Select Body Work Techniques

Technique	Description	Uses and History	Providers and Availability	Information
Craniosacral manipulations	Based on theory that unimpeded flow of cerebrospinal fluid (CSF) is key to good health. Gentle pressure applied on the client's head to lengthen spine and facilitate flow of CSF. Reported to help with cognition, concentration, and learning disabilities.	Originally described by William Sutherland, OD, in the early 1900s; further developed over the past 30 years by John Upledger, OD.	May be practiced by osteopaths, chiropractors, physical therapists, body workers, and some massage therapists.	www.upledger.com
Massage: may employ a variety of techniques. It is generally safe, except in cases of specific physical conditions, such as bleeding disorders, phlebitis, and some skin conditions.	Massage therapy has long been popular with athletes and recently has gained more general popularity. The American Massage Therapy Association (AMTA) endorses various techniques. • Deep tissue and friction massages release chronic patterns of tension using slow strokes and deep finger pressure on contracted areas. • *Effleurage*, a smooth gliding stroke used to relax soft tissues, is taught in childbirth classes as a relaxation technique for labor. • Sports massage focuses on muscle groups related to particular sports. • Swedish massage uses long strokes, kneading, and friction on superficial muscle layers. • *Tapotement* incorporates percussion-type movements. • Trigger-point massage applies pressure to active and latent trigger points in muscles; then muscles are stretched to help relaxation.	Various techniques of massage are used for health maintenance and relief of pain from muscle strain and stiffness. Massage is widely used to treat minor sports injuries because it reduces muscle spasms, increases circulation, and allows for elimination of lactic acid after physical activity. Massage also is useful in hospitalized or immobilized clients because it relieves pain and discomfort, increases circulation, and enhances relaxation. Infant massage has been introduced in many hospitals and often is taught to parents to soothe infants.	Massage therapists are registered and licensed as Registered Massage Therapists (RMT) by state or local boards or Nationally Certified in Therapeutic Massage and Bodywork (NCTMB). Some nurses also are RMTs and certified to provide massage therapies.	www.amtamassage.org
Myofascial release	Form of body work that seeks to rebalance the body and facilitate inherent ability to correct soft tissue dysfunction. This interactive stretching technique uses feedback from client's body to determine force, duration, and direction of therapist's strokes. It releases tension in *fascia*, (weblike connective tissue within the body), allowing the body to realign to reduce future injury. It helps restore musculoskeletal function, relax contracted muscles, increase circulation, and increase venous and lymphatic drainage.	Originated in the osteopathic literature of the 1950s and is founded on neurophysiologic function.	Many physical therapists are trained in this technique.	www.myofascialrelease.com

(continued)

Table 4-2 Continued

Technique	Description	Uses and History	Providers and Availability	Information
Rolfing	Rolfing, or structural integration, uses various body manipulations to work on fascia. Chronic stress and inactivity cause the normally loose, mobile fascia to become thick and fused. Muscles react by painful spasms. Rolfing stretches the fascia to re-establish proper alignment and thus improve function. Treatment usually involves a series of 10 2-h sessions 1–2 wk apart.	Developed by Ida Rolf. Some studies have demonstrated efficacy in range of motion, general body movement, posture, and pain.	Certified Rolfers who have completed a course of classroom and practicums can be found through the institute. They are licensed in some states but requirements vary.	www.rolf.org
Trager	Approach that uses simple self-induced movements and passive movement, guided by a practitioner, to assist clients in recognizing and unlearning physical and mental habits that limit movement, cause pain, and prevent optimum function. It consists of gentle rhythmic body work to loosen stiff joints and muscles, and dancelike exercises to increase awareness of body movement.	Developed by Milton Trager, MD, an American physician, in the 1940s. It was used to release deep-seated physical and mental patterns to facilitate deep relaxation and improve function.	Certified by the Trager Institute.	www.trager.com

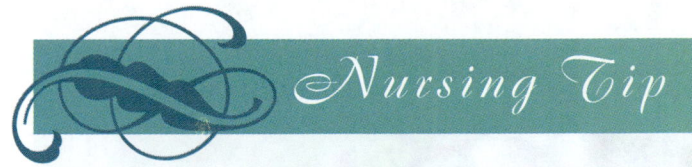

Nursing Alert

HERBAL THERAPY PRECAUTIONS

There are many species for one genus, which may have various therapeutic or side effects. Keep in mind the following:

1. Not all parts of the plant are active.
2. The levels of active ingredients vary with growing conditions (e.g., soil and climate).
3. The amounts of active ingredients vary among and within brands.
4. A lack of standardized manufacturing exists.
5. Some plant ingredients are toxic.

Nursing Tip

HEALTH HISTORY AND HERBAL SUBSTANCES

You should always assess clients for use of other ingested and applied substances because clients often will not relate this information when asked about medications. Many of these herbs have biologic effects that may interfere with or add to the effect of medications and produce complications to medical treatment. Always ask clients directly about herbs, vitamins, or other dietary supplements they are taking. Neglecting to ask this question may subject clients to harmful drug interactions and side effects.

rection. A number of products are sold for weight loss. The active ingredient in many of these products is *ephedera* (as in Ma Huang), a pharmaceutical drug that acts as a stimulant. Some persons have suffered elevated blood pressure and strokes while using products that contain ephedera without medical supervision. Other effects that have been reported are seizures, kidney stones, myocarditis, vasculitis, and cardiovascular events. Deaths have been associated with the use of these products. Currently, these products are marketed as nutritional supplements and thus do not come under the regulatory arm of the FDA.

Herbal Medicine or Phytotherapies

The World Health Organization estimates that over 80% of the world's population uses herbal medicine for some aspect of primary care (National Institutes of Health, 1994). **Phytotherapy** refers to the therapeutic use of plants, often meaning herbal remedies. A number of herbal medicines currently are available and can be ingested or applied in a variety of preparations. Fresh plant parts, including roots, leaves, seeds, and flowers, may be used in cooking or the preparation of foods. Plant parts, often the

dried leaves or flowers, may be crushed and placed in gelatin capsules. Dried leaves, flowers, or roots may be loose or finely ground and used in infusions or teas. The plant parts may be prepared in tablets or liquids for ingestion or in poultices, lotions, salves, or oils for topical application. There are few risks with the culinary use of herbs, other than individual sensitivities or allergic reactions; however, potentially harmful amounts may be ingested when herbs are concentrated in pill or capsule form. Many consumers, thinking that these are natural products, do not feel there are risks. Many consumers also feel that because a product is natural, it cannot be harmful. Thus, they will take exceptionally large amounts. Herbal products may have therapeutic effects but also can have toxic effects if taken at the wrong time, in the wrong amount, in the wrong combination, or by the wrong person.

An overview of the more popular herbs, their known actions, and uses are given in Tables 4-3 and 4-4. Although nurses generally should not recommend herbs, it is important for nurses to be knowledgeable about them to advise

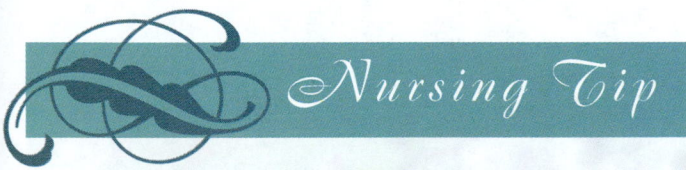

Nursing Tip

INFORMED CONSUMERS

Nurses can help clients be prudent consumers by teaching them to read labels carefully and avoid taking excessive doses of potentially dangerous products.

Nursing Alert

RESTRICTION OF HERBAL PREPARATIONS

Clients taking anticoagulants or antiplatelet agents should be cautioned against using certain herbal preparations. Bioflavonoids found in feverfew, ginkgo biloba, grape seed extract, and bilberry possess antiplatelet activity. These clients also should avoid herbal preparations of ginger, garlic, and ginseng (Glisson, Crawford, & Street, 1999).

Table 4-3 Herbs of General Use for Women

Name	Actions and Uses	Side Effects	Contraindications	Classification	Research
Bilberry (*Vaccinium*)	Vasoprotective, antidiarrheal, and astringent actions. Used for circulatory and eye disorders and healthy eye function. Used for dyspepsia and diarrhea.	None known		Commission E–approved AHPA Class 1	
Capsicum (cayenne pepper, chili pepper)	**External:** acts as counter-irritant, increasing blood flow; used for peripheral neuropathies and herpes zoster. **Internal:** acts as an antispasmodic and antiflatulent; used for GI disorders and hyperlipidemia.	Irritant and hypersensitivity	Do not use on injured skin.	Commission E–approved FDS-GRAS Approved as over-the-counter drug (capsaicin, Zostrix) AHPA Class 1 (Internal) AHPA Class 2d (External)	
Chamomile	**Internal:** digestive aid sometimes used for inflammatory bowel disease. **Oral:** used as mouthwash for mouth irritations. **Topical:** used for inflammatory eczema, insect bites, and poison ivy.	None known	Avoid if allergic to ragweed, asters, and chrysanthemums.	Commission E–approved	
Cranberry (*Vaccinium macrocarpon*)	Antibacterial and acidifier. Used for prophylaxis and treatment of UTIs.	Diarrhea (with large doses)		Not evaluated by Commission E Not rated by AHPA	Reduces bacteriuria and pyuria and lowers pH of urine.
Echinacea (*Echinacea angustifolia* and *E. purpurea*)	Immune stimulant, antibacterial, antiviral, and anti-inflammatory. **Internal:** used for colds, respiratory infections, and arthritis. **External:** used for eczema, herpes, and burns. **Oral:** used for vaginal yeast infections.	Tongue numbness Allergic reactions	Autoimmune diseases and some systemic disease, such as MS and TB. Avoid if allergic to daisies.	Commission E–approved FDA-GRAS	Equivocal; some studies show efficacy and decreased incidence and severity of colds and flu, whereas others show little difference.

Herb	Actions/Uses	Adverse Effects	Cautions	Regulatory Status	Research
Evening Primrose (fever plant)	Essential fatty acid (omega-6) and prostaglandin precursor. Decreases inflammation and dilates coronary arteries. Used for eczema, PMS, menopausal symptoms, psoriasis, MS, asthma, diabetic neuropathy, and cancer.	GI disturbances Headaches		Not evaluated by Commission E FDA dietary supplement AHPA Class 1	Promising use of essential fatty acids in decreasing PMS symptoms, pain in mastalgia, symptoms of psoriasis, and cholesterol in hyperlipidemia.
Feverfew (*Tanacetum parthenium*)	Migraine prophylactic, anti-inflammatory, antipyretic, and antispasmodic. Used for prevention and treatment of migraine, fever, arthritis, and menstrual cramps. Long-term treatment required: 4–6 wk.	Rebound migraine Mouth ulcers GI irritation	Avoid if allergic to daisies. Avoid in pregnancy.	Not evaluated by Commission E FDA-GRAS AHPA Class 2b	Some studies indicate reduction in number of migraines.
Garlic (Kwai)	Allicin is the active ingredient. Used for hyperlipidemia, prophylaxis of atherosclerosis, hypertension, and respiratory infection. Lowers cholesterol, triglycerides, and BP; decreases intermittent claudication; and increases resistance to infection and possibly stomach and colorectal cancers. Similar to dicyclomine (Benocol) and some of the new butter substitutes. Enteric coating enhances allicin availability.	Nausea and vomiting Flatulence GI burning	Use caution because of possible interaction with anticoagulants. Avoid in lactation. Avoid in pregnancy.	Commission E–approved FDA-GRAS AHPA Class 2c	Several studies found mild effectiveness in lowering low-density lipoprotein cholesterol; long-term protection against cardiovascular disease is inconclusive.

(continued)

Table 4-3 Continued

Name	Actions and Uses	Side Effects	Contraindications	Classification	Research
Ginger	Volatile oil promotes secretion of saliva and gastric juices. Used as antiemetic, especially for morning and motion sickness. Used in India for years as antiemetic and digestive aid.	In large doses, may cause heartburn	May interact with warfarin (antiplatelet). May interfere with antidiabetic agents. Avoid with gallstones. Avoid prolonged and excessive use in pregnancy.	Commission E–approved FDA-GRAS AHPA Class 1	Inconsistent. results.
Chinese ginseng (*Panax schinseng*)	Expensive. Has long history as general tonic, stimulant, and antioxidant. Used for stress, fatigue, debility, diabetes, depression, hyperlipidemia, and to improve physical performance and enhance immunity. **Note:** Be sure to distinguish from American ginseng (*P. quinquefolius*)	Hypertension Irritability Hypoglycemia Diarrhea Rash	May interact with antipsychotics, monoamine oxidase inhibitors, stimulants, and anticoagulants. Avoid with hypertension.	Commission E–approved FDA-GRAS AHPA Class 2d	Not effective as an exercise enhancer; in reviewing the literature be sure to clarify which type of ginseng was used.
Ginkgo biloba	Active ingredients 6% lactones and 24% glycosides. Improves circulation and acts as antioxidant. Used for dementia, memory enhancement, cardiovascular insufficiency, intermittent claudication, peripheral neuropathy, depression, tinnitus, retinopathy, and in early Alzheimer's disease. Need to build up dosage over time for effects.	Nausea and vomiting Headache	May interact with anticoagulants.	Commission E–approved FDA-GRAS	Some efficacy in controlled trials for treatment of dementia and memory deficit.
Goldenseal (*Hydrastis canadensis*)	Used for upper respiratory conditions, flu, and menorrhagia.	GI effects Uterine contraction Blood vessel contraction Hypoglycemia	Avoid with diabetes. Avoid with hypertension. Avoid in pregnancy.	Not evaluated by Commission E FDA-GRAS AHPA Class 2b	None for URIs.

	Uses/Action	Side effects	Regulatory status	Comments
Grape seed extract	Antioxidant and anti-inflammatory. Used for inflammatory conditions and circulatory disorders. Used as antioxidant for disease prevention.	None known	Not evaluated by Commission E FDA dietary supplement Not rated by AHPA	No human studies.
Kava kava (*Piper methysticum*)	Similar to valerian. Active ingredient is kava lactones (70% kava lactones in standard preparation). Used as antianxiety and tension-reducing agent. Currently very popular with teenagers.	Yellowing of skin Allergic reactions	Commission E–approved	Acts as sedative and may interfere with driving and other types of performance. May interact with antidepressants and barbiturates. Avoid with depression. Avoid in pregnancy.
Milk thistle (*Silybum marianum*)	Used as liver tonic since the days of Pliny. Used to treat viral hepatitis, hepatitis C, and other liver diseases, and for exposure to environmental toxins.	Transient laxative	Commission E–approved	
St. John's wort (*Hypericum perforatum*)	Increases neurotransmitter levels of serotonin and norepinephrine. **Internal:** used for depression, anxiety, and dyspepsia. **External:** used for wounds and burns. May have mild antiviral activity.	GI disturbances Photosensitivity	Commission E–approved FDA-GRAS AHPA Class 1	Interacts with antidepressant drugs, and when used together could alter dosage. May require dietary restriction of tyramine. May interfere with AIDS medications. May increase size of cataracts. Avoid in pregnancy. In a meta-analysis found to be effective in treating mild to moderate depression.
Valerian root (*Valeriana officinalis*)	Action of binding benzodiazepine receptors Used for insomnia, nervous excitability, hysteria, rheumatic pain, and dysmenorrhea.	Sedation and paradoxical reactions	Commission E–approved FDA-GRAS AHPA Class 1	Should not be paired with other drugs or herbal preparations with the same effects. Some efficacy in clinical trials.

The authors thank the following persons for their advice and help with the preparation of this table: Sherri Konzem, PharmD, University of Houston, College of Pharmacy and Memorial-Hermann SW Family Practice Residency Program, Houston, Texas; and Roberta Anding, MS, RD/LD, CDE, Instructor, Section of Adolescent Medicine, Baylor College of Medicine and Texas Children's Hospital, Houston, Texas.
GI–gastrointestinal; UTIs–urinary tract infections; MS–multiple sclerosis; TB–tuberculosis; PMS–premenstrual syndrome; BP–blood pressure.
American Herbal Products Association (AHPA) Botanical Safety Rating: Class 1, internal use. Class 2nd, avoid in pregnancy. Class 2c, avoid in lactation. Class 2d, external use. Commission E–approved, FDA-GRAS, Food and Drug Administration

Table 4-4 Herb Use in Perimenopause

Name	Actions and Uses	Side Effects	Contraindications	Classification	Research
Black cohosh (*Cimicifuga racemosa*), also called snakeroot and squawroot	Action appears to reduce luteinizing hormone and may potentiate hormonal production with a mild estrogenic action and uterine tonic. Used for reduction in menopausal symptoms, such as hot flashes, sleep disturbances, and irritability. Was one of the primary ingredients in Lydia Pinkham's woman's tonic, popular remedy in the early 20th century.	Headaches Increased menstrual bleeding Central nervous system depressant	Avoid in pregnancy because may cause uterine contractions.	Commission E–approved	Some studies show effectiveness in reducing perimenopausal symptoms.
Chaste berry (*Vitex agnus-castus*) also called chaste tree	Assumed to increase progesterone if insufficient. Thought to act as hormonal balancing agent during hormonal fluctuations. May affect anterior pituitary and increase progesterone production in luteal phase. Used for premenstrual syndrome (PMS), menopausal problems, especially for heavy menstrual flow and to reduce hot flashes caused by high levels of follicle-stimulating hormone.	None known	Concomitant use with oral contraceptives may result in diminished effect. Avoid in pregnancy.	Commission E–approved	
Dong Quai (*Angelica sinensis* or *A. phymorpha maxim*)	Contains phytoestrogens (plant estrogens). Acts as coumarin and affects blood clotting and hematopoiesis. Is a uterine relaxant. Used for menopausal symptoms.	Photosensitivity May cause heavy menstrual bleeding May cause heart palpitations	Avoid in women with heavy menstrual periods, spotting, or uterine fibroids. Avoid taking blood-thinners. Avoid during menstruation. Avoid in pregnancy.	Not evaluated by Commission E AHPA Class 2b	No more effective than placebo in some studies; more research needed.
Motherwort	Mild cardiotonic and aid to female reproductive system. Used for menopausal symptoms, PMS, menstrual cramps, and sleep disturbances.	May cause heavy menstrual bleeding	Avoid in pregnancy.	Commission E–approved	
Sage (*Salvia officinalis*)	Contains bioflavonoids and phytoesterols for weak estrogenic and progesteronic effects. Mild antibacterial and antifungal properties. Used for excessive perspiration and relief of hot flashes, night sweats, and mood swings.	May dry mucous membranes in mouth and vagina	Excessive use may cause kidney or liver problems. Avoid in pregnancy.	Commission E–approved	

Learn, C. D., & Higgins, P. G. (1999). Harmonizing herbs: Managing menopause with help from Mother Earth. *AWHONN Lifelines*, Oct–Nov, 39–43, and Hardy, M. L. (2000). Herbs of special interest to women. *Journal of American Pharmaceutical Association*, 40, 2, 234–242.
American Herbal Products Association (AHPA) Botanical Safety Rating: Class 2b, avoid in pregnancy.
Commission E–approved.

clients of risks or alert other members of the medical team about potential problems. Because research information is being published rapidly, the nurse should look for updates on descriptions of herbs, official classifications, labeling statements, possible uses, dosages, preparation, research, and risks. Additional information may be found in *The Commission E Monographs* and *The Physicians Desk Reference (PDR) for Herbal Medicine*.

Regulatory Issues and Herbal Remedies

Recognizing a need to standardize approval of herbal medicines, the European Economic Community developed guidelines for quality, quantity, production, and labeling of herbal preparations. In Germany, over 70% of physicians use phytomedicines as supportive medicines for chronic diseases and minor illnesses. Herbal production is more regulated in Germany than in the United States. The *Commission E Monographs* (Commission E was appointed by the German Federal Health Office to investigate the scientific literature regarding herbal products and identify herbal products approved for use) recently have been translated into English and are available in the United States (Blumenthal et al., 1998). *The Commission E Monographs* are one of the best resources on safety and efficacy of herbal products. *The Physicians Desk Reference (PDR) for Herbal Medicine* also is a good resource for clinicians. Medical journals also are publishing more reports of research on herbs.

Biomedical pharmaceuticals often are derived from plants used in folk medicine. Isolating active ingredients and chemically synthesizing them in a laboratory ensures purity and dose standardization. Some herbal preparations involve complex mixtures of several plants or several parts of a plant. One of the beliefs of herbalists is that the whole plant, rather than extracted or synthesized ingredients, includes substances that modify side effects and may potentiate therapeutic action. This controversy remains unresolved for both researchers and practitioners. These additional ingredients, however, pose problems for researchers and for standardization of products on the market.

Currently, the FDA regulates most herbal products in the United States under the classification of food supple-

ments. The 1994 Dietary Supplement Health and Education Act (DSHEA) allows manufacturers to advertise benefits of the products as long as they do not claim the products cure or prevent specific illnesses. The products are regulated by safe handling and labeling; however, because they often are natural products, considerable dosage variation may occur. Currently in the United States, the Food and Drug Administration (FDA) classification for use generally is recognized as safe and effective (FDA-GRAS). The current DSHEA regulation allows for labeling that includes structure and function claims without going through full FDA review. Labels can claim that the product affects the structure or function of the body but cannot make disease claims that involve treatment, cure, mitigation, or diagnosis of a medical condition without FDA evaluation. The manufacturer needs to be able to substantiate all claims it makes, and the label needs to state that the product is a supplement and has not been evaluated by the FDA. The FDA has proposed a limit on the amount of ephedra that can be present in supplements or purchased at one time and has issued warnings on potentially dangerous herbs, including chaparral, comfrey, yohimbe, lobelia, germander, willow bark, Jin Bu Huan, and magnolia (Harvard Health Letter, 1997). The herbal industry has attempted to regulate itself. A classification system has been proposed by the American Herbal Products Association (AHPA) Botanical Safety Rating to address safety issues in the use of herbal products, ranging from Class I (no restrictions) to Class I–V (insufficient data on safety), that can be accessed on the AHPA website. During pregnancy, a conservative approach is best, as many of the effects of herbal ingestion are unknown; some herbs that should not be used in pregnancy and lactation are found in Box 4-2. They are classified as follows:

Class 1 considered safe—no restrictions

Class 2 safe but with restrictions
    2a external use only
    2b avoid use in pregnancy
    2c avoid use in lactation
    2d miscellaneous restrictions

Class 3 recommend to be used only under guidance of an expert

Class 4 Insufficient data available

(McGuffin, M, Hobbs, C, Upton, E, Goldberg A [Eds] [1997] *American Herbal Products Association's Botanical Safety Handbook,* Boca Raton, FL CRC Press.)

The Food and Drug Administration has a classification: Generally Regarded as Safe (GRAS). Commision E—approved means that they were reasonably safe when used according to the dosage, contraindications, and other warnings specified in the monographs. Efficacy was based on reasonable verification of historical use.

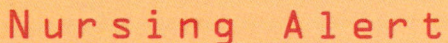

Nursing Alert

DRUG REACTIONS

If a client has an adverse effect or drug interaction to an herbal product, you should report it to the Food and Drug Administration's MEDWATCH (1-800-FDA-1088).

Box 4-2 Herbal Use in Pregnancy and Lactation

Pregnancy

The most conservative approach is to avoid all but ginger because the purity and dosages of products cannot be ensured.

The following *should not* be used in pregnancy:

- Pennyroyal*
- Tansy*
- Rue*
- Black cohosh* and any of the herbs that cause uterine contractions
- Ma Huang
- Cascara sagrada and other harsh laxatives

Lactation

A number of herbs have been used in folk culture to enhance or reduce milk flow. The following *should not* be used during lactation:

- Aloe
- Black cohosh
- Buckthorn
- Cascara sagrada
- Cocoa[†]
- Coffee[†]
- Kava kava
- Ma Huang
- Sage
- Senna
- Tea[†]
- Wintergreen

---

*Abortifacients and should be avoided by childbearing women.
[†]Avoid excessive consumption.
Hardy, M. L. (2000). Herbs of special interest to women. *Journal of the American Pharmaceutical Association*, 40, (2), 234–242.

Nursing Alert

MEDICAL SUPERVISION REQUIRED

The following herbs are considered dangerous and should not be used without medical supervision:

- Borage
- Coltsfoot
- Life root
- Germander
- Ma Huang
- Calamus
- Comfrey
- Chaparral
- Licorice (herbal, not the candy form)

---

haled by placement in a diffuser where they are heated by a light bulb. Many are placed in carrier oils of high-quality vegetable oil, such as almond, grape seed, or sesame oil. Essential oils are very concentrated and should not be used without dilution in a carrier oil. Once diluted, the oil may then be used directly on the skin, in bath water, or in a diffuser. Flower essences, such as Bach Flower Remedies often are diluted with brandy or an alcoholic base and taken by dropper sublingually. These oils should be stored away from extreme heat and often are kept in colored glass containers to maintain freshness. Essential oils are highly concentrated and therefore one can get a very high dose. In certain oils, a high dose can be very toxic. Aromatherapists advise not using undiluted oils on the skin. Lavender or tea tree oil, however, can be used on burns and skin eruptions as long as one does not have extremely sensitive skin. Testing for sensitivities, with a patch test of a 2% dilution and observing for 12 hours, is recommended. Citrus oils can cause uneven pigmentation with sun exposure. Contact with the eyes and sensitive mucous membranes should be avoided when using certain oils, and most should not be ingested. Caution should be exercised when used in preg-

Negative results were given where there was no plausible evidence of efficacy or safety and weighed potential benefits (Blumenthal, 1998).

Applied Substances

Essential oils have been used for centuries and are used in perfumes and in body and bath products. Essential oils can be applied to the skin through lotions, salves, oils, poultices, plasters, or taken sublingually; these oils also are in-

Nursing Alert

DRUG ABSORPTION

Another risk of using essential oils is an allergic reaction that can be very severe because many oils are very concentrated. In addition, substances taken sublingually are absorbed into the bloodstream very quickly.

nancy because some oils may contribute to miscarriage. Oils that are considered safe in pregnancy are rose, neorli, lavender, ylang-ylang, chamomile, citruses, geranium, sandalwood, spearmint, and frankincense (Kevile & Geeen, 2000). The American Holistic Nurses Association, (AHNA) has endorsed educational programs in aromatherapy such as the Pacific Institute of Aromatherapy and the National Association for Holistic Aromatherapy.

Energy-Based Therapies

Energy is a concept that is used to explain forms of healing touch, therapeutic touch, Reiki, and laying on of hands. These treatments may involve actual touching or noncontact touch, such as placing the hands several inches from the body. The focus is the "energy field" rather than the physical body. The proposed theoretic basis for this modality is electromagnetic fields or quantum physics.

Magnetic Healing

Magnetic healing includes use of magnets for pain relief and the use of transcutaneous electrical nerve stimulation (TENS), which involves passing low-voltage current through pads applied to the skin. Some research has demonstrated efficacy in pain reduction. A number of magnetic products is available on the market, and many pain clinics use magnets therapeutically. TENS has been used to aid in the start of healing of fractured bones, promote healing and tissue regeneration, and reduce pain. TENS has been used with some effectiveness in reducing labor pain (Kemp, 1996). Magnetic and electromagnetic therapies have been used in a number of treatments and are sometimes used to provide electrical stimulation of acupuncture points to reduce pain.

One theoretic framework on which magnetic therapies are based is that they stimulate the body's production of endorphins and close the pain gate, as proposed by Melzack and Wall (1965). Reversal of effects from the use of naloxone, which is an opiate antagonist, has supported this theory. Another theoretic framework is the principle that magnets alter the orientation of the chromosomes within cells, which has been observed under electron microscopes (Rosenfeld, 1996). This shift is thought to relieve acute and chronic pain.

Touch Therapies

Touch therapies have been used historically and across cultures. The use of human touch for healing has been recorded in early records and archeological data across cultures. Healing by laying on of hands is a key element in many spiritual traditions, including Judeo-Christian scriptures. Touch has been shown to be vital to human devel-

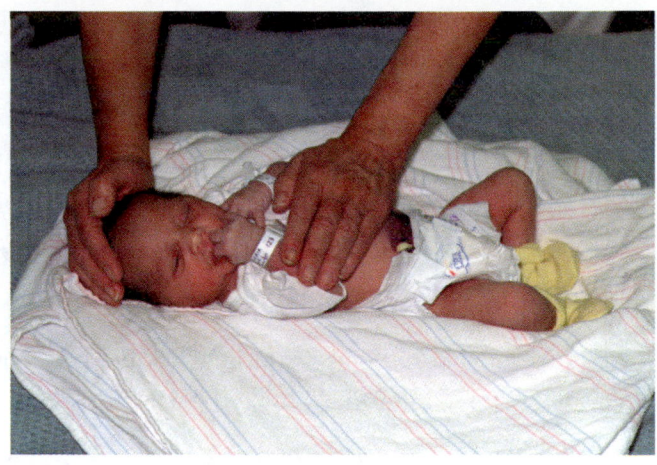

Figure 4-2 Laying on of hands is one means of touch therapy.

opment (Figure 4-2). Infants and young children may develop pathologies and may even stop eating and die if they do not receive caring touch. Nurses have embraced touch as integral to caring for clients.

The therapeutic use of touch has been understood as operating through universal healing, life energy, or by means of spiritual intervention. Slater (1996) has linked these earlier descriptions of prana, chi, and vital energy with physicists' descriptions of quantum and electromagnetic fields. A number of physicists (Bohm, 1980; Capra, 1984; and Zukav, 1979) have written about quantum physics, compared it with Eastern mysticism, and challenged the existence of matter as being distinct from energy. As touch therapies began to be taught within nursing, these theories and the vocabulary of frequencies, waves, energy, vibration, and balanced or congested fields were commonly used.

Two groups have promoted touch therapies within the nursing profession: Therapeutic Touch (TT), founded by Dolores Krieger; and Healing Touch International (HTI), founded by Janet Mentgen. Both these groups provide education and training for nurses interested in practicing this modality. Reiki is another form of touch therapy that is practiced by both nurses and laypersons.

Therapeutic Touch

Therapeutic touch was brought into nursing by Dolores Krieger, PhD, RN. She had worked with healers Oskar Estebany and Dora Kunz. Kreiger's research on the increase of hemoglobin after therapeutic touch was one of the first studies conducted on this modality. In learning this technique, the practitioner is taught to enter a calm state through a process of "centering" and to hold an "intention" of desiring to help the client. The practitioner is taught to assess the client's energy field and then modulate or correct the deficient, congested, or unbalanced areas. The practitioner's hands are placed a few inches above the

Research Highlight

Electroacupuncture for Control of Myeloablative Chemotherapy-Induced Emesis: A Randomized Controlled Trial

Purpose

To determine the efficacy of acupuncture plus antiemetic drugs in controlling nausea and vomiting from chemotherapy in women with breast cancer compared with antiemetic drugs alone.

Method

Randomized controlled trial.

Findings

Among the 104 women undergoing high-dose chemotherapy for breast cancer, those randomized to the acupuncture plus antiemetic drugs group experienced less than half the number of nausea and vomiting episodes over the 5 days of treatment compared with women receiving antiemetic drugs alone.

Nursing Implications

1. The complex and multifactorial nature of chemotherapy-induced nausea and vomiting suggests that no single treatment will completely control these side effects.

2. Acupuncture may provide a degree of control of nausea and vomiting by affecting chemicals of the central nervous system. This may be particularly helpful in women who experience significant toxicity from antiemetic agents or in whom such agents render ineffective control of nausea and vomiting.

Shen, J., Wenger, N., Glaspy, J., Harys, R. D., Albert, P. S., Choi, C., & Shekelle, P. G. (2000). Electroacupuncture for control of myeloablative chemotherapy-induced emesis. *JAMA, 284,* 2755–2761.

physical body, which is felt to be the optimal area to work with the energy (Figure 4-3).

Healing Touch

Healing touch also uses touch to influence energy. Along with touch, it employs a number of additional techniques the practitioner can use in working with clients. These techniques are used to align and balance the energy field, thus facilitating the client's self-healing. Proponents claim that these techniques are healing in a holistic manner because they act on physical, emotional, and spiritual domains. This program is taught in a series of classes as the practitioner advances to different levels. The program is available to nurses as well as laypersons. HTI is one of the most rapidly growing healing organizations in this country.

Reiki

Reiki is based on the Tibetan Sutras (ancient sacred texts) and was reintroduced into Japan by Usui in the 1800s (Stewart, 1995). Takawa, a Japanese woman who moved

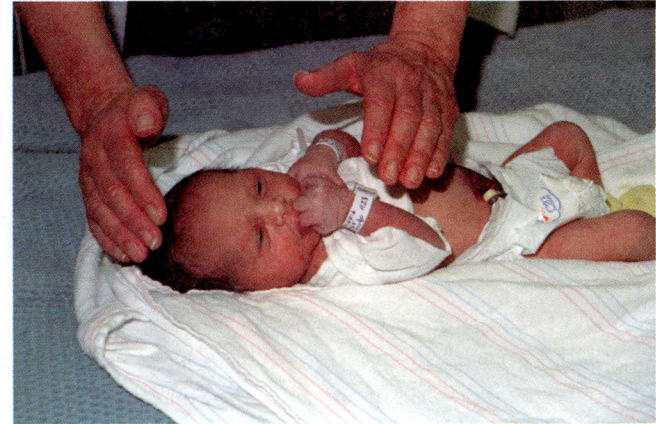

Figure 4-3 Therapeutic touch involves centering and assessing the client's energy by placing the hands a few inches above the client's body.

to Hawaii, trained several healers who then brought the technique to the United States. Novice practitioners are initiated through a ritual involving ancient symbols. The healer channels universal healing energy through the hands, which can be placed directly on or held at a distance from the client. The healer does not direct the energy, but holds the intent to heal. The energy then goes to where it is needed. This modality also uses a technique for distance healing. Preparation is through weekend seminars and work with a Reiki Master. The Master level involves a lifelong commitment to healing and to Reiki. Many nurses and laypersons are Reiki healers.

Nursing Implications

Nurses and clients often cite anecdotal reports of the benefits of touch therapies; however, relatively few research studies have established their efficacy. Most nursing research into touch therapies has been conducted in therapeutic touch. Research supports decreased anxiety and increased relaxation; results on wound healing are equivocal. Some recent studies demonstrate that exposure to touch therapies may increase humoral immunity; however, results are preliminary (Wardell & Engebretson, 2001; Olsen et al., 1997). The lack of a testable theory and the references to energy alien to biomedical thinking may explain the difficulty in understanding this modality and identifying appropriate research designs to capture effectiveness. Touch modalities are of particular interest to the profession of nursing and warrant further study and theoretic development. They remain low-cost and low-risk strategies that many clients claim have benefit. Many hospitals have integrated these modalities into their care delivery and have sponsored nurses' preparation in them.

Although little research has been done on the use of touch therapies in pregnancy and labor, many nurses have used these techniques to aid in comfort and relaxation. Touch therapies also have been used in infants. Noncontact or light touch may be particularly useful in infants in the neonatal intensive care unit for whom rigorous physical contact, such as massage, may lead to overstimulation (Figure 4-4). These areas currently are under research.

Psychologic or Mind-Body Therapies

Psychologic therapies are related to cognitive thought or the function of the brain. Mind-body medicine recently has become established in health care with the understanding of the effect of thoughts and emotions on the body and the effect that the physical body has on emotions. The recent understanding of psychophysiologic mechanisms has provided a firm base for many of these strategies to be well researched. Much of the research has been based on

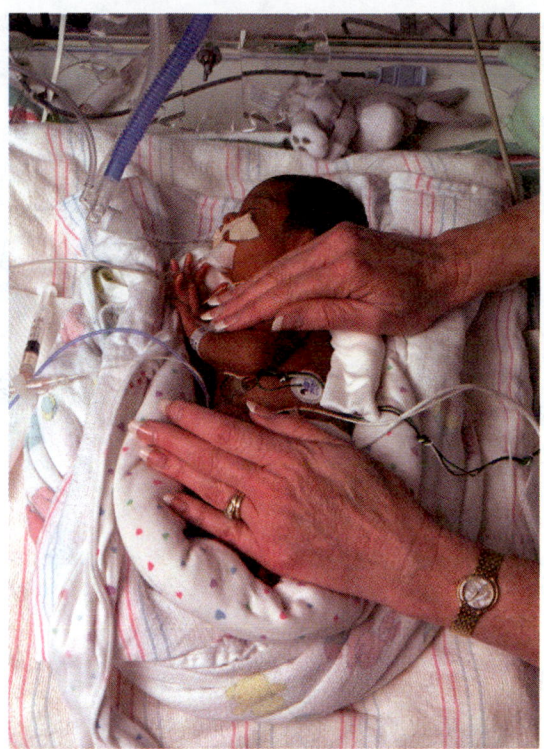

Figure 4-4 Infants in the NICU can benefit from calm, warm, nondisruptive touch therapy.

stress reduction and relaxation. Other strategies include cognitive repatterning, behavioral modification, psychotherapy, group therapy, and coping strategies. Many of these techniques are incorporated into the therapeutic relationship that nurses establish with clients and use in wellness counseling.

Additional clinical interventions of stress reduction are being tested. Relaxation strategies, such as autogenic training, progressive muscle relaxation, distraction techniques, and paced breathing, have been used in the care of women during pregnancy and in preparation for labor over the past 40 years (Figure 4-5). Many of these techniques may be used to promote general relaxation other than in labor.

In addition to the relaxation strategies taught in childbirth preparation, some additional techniques that nurses can use to promote relaxation are biofeedback, mindfulness, self-reflection, mental imagery, affirmations, and music therapy. Research has demonstrated such techniques to be effective adjuncts in reducing pain and anxiety related to surgery or invasive procedures, and with symptom control related to specific treatment side effects. The AHNA has described several practices that are part of holistic nursing care, many of which are felt to facilitate stress reduction and relaxation. *Holistic Nursing: A Handbook for Practice* (Dossey, Keegan, & Guzzetta, 2000) is a good reference for additional guidance on how to develop and use these skills in clinical practice.

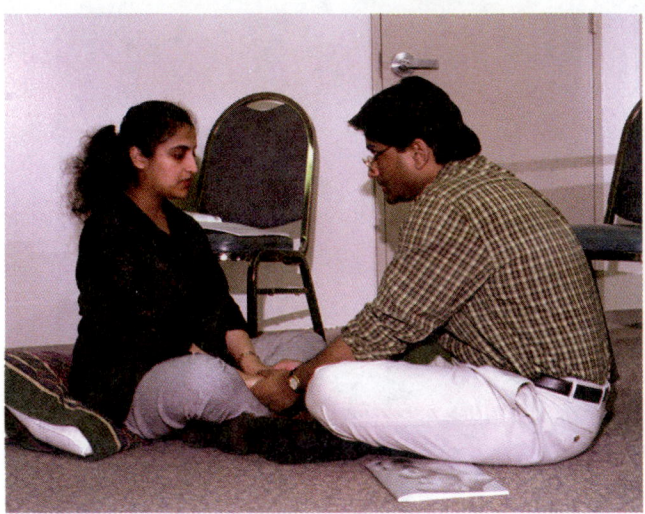

Figure 4-5 Childbirth preparation classes often include techniques wherein the partner helps the woman to relax, focus, and breathe deeply.

Mental imagery, a therapeutic process in which imagination and memory are used to mentally taste, smell, see, and hear images that suggest a state of health are used for promoting both health and healing. AHNA endorses a program for learning the techniques of visual imagery, which is directed by nurses and offers certification.

Spiritual Healing

The literature is clear that spirituality and religion are not synonymous, although spirituality often is described in terms of religious belief or practice. *Spirituality* is the essence of who we are as human beings and includes but is not limited to the process of discovering purpose, meaning, and inner strength throughout life's journey. Spirituality is experienced and expressed in many ways outside the context of *religion,* which can be identified as an organized system of beliefs and practices shared by a group of people. According to Burkhardt and Jacobsen (2000), elements of spirituality can include connectedness to an Absolute or Higher Power, to nature, to others, and to self.

Both illness and wellness activities have been derived from spiritual practices. Spiritual issues often concern suffering, redemption, forgiveness, faith, hope, grace, and love. Within the context of spirituality, healing is much more than the recovery from illness and absence of disease. Healing can imply a restoration of wholeness, establishment of internal and external resources, a sense of transcendence, or a feeling of interconnectedness (Burkhardt & Jacobsen, 2000). Many rituals and health practices have been described that focus on the attainment or restoration of balance between mind, body, and spirit. Some of these may seem quite appropriate within Judeo-Christian traditions, such as worship and prayer; whereas others from

Native American or Southwestern cultures, such as chanting or use of a medicine wheel, may be unfamiliar.

Religious practices, such as participating in church activities, have demonstrated positive health benefits (Levin, 1994). Other religious practices, such as forgiveness, have historically been used as a means of spiritual purification. Meditation has been used in many spiritual traditions as a way of attaining balance both internally and with the environment. Meditation also has been researched for its efficacy in relaxation and stress reduction. Prayer and primal religious experiences are spiritual actions found in many cultures and are associated with healing. Many CAMs have their roots in spiritual traditions and practices (Kinsley, 1996).

Because no consensus exists on the definition, scope, and measurement of spirituality, it is vital that nurses recognize all forms of spiritual expression to provide professional and holistic care. The connectedness inherent in the therapeutic nurse-client relationship is an avenue of nurturing spiritual awareness for both the nurse and client. Spiritual elements of health and illness can be expressed through story (Cohen, Headley, & Sherwood, 2000), presence, touch, listening, creative expression, ritual, and use of sacred space. Instruments and guides are available to aid the nurse in spiritual assessment, although story sharing often provides a vehicle through which clients gain insight and meaning for emotions, issues, and conflicts (Burkhardt & Jacobsen, 2000; Liehr & Smith, 2000).

Client Education

Questions for Consideration for Clients Interested in Taking or Engaging in Complementary Therapies

- Do they make claims to cure cancer, enhance treatment, or relieve symptoms or side effects?
- What are credentials of those supporting the therapy?
- Have they published or referenced trustworthy journals?
- What are the costs of the treatment?
- Is it widely used in the health care community, or is access limited?
- Is it used in place of standard therapies and if so will the delay affect a chance for effective treatment?

Adapted from the American Cancer Society.

NURSING IMPLICATIONS

Nurses must be aware of the types of health-related activities in which their clients may be engaged. This awareness is important for safety and to assess the interaction of these activities with biomedical care. Nurses can conduct their assessment in a manner that engages clients in the most appropriate planning and incorporation of complementary strategies. If the nurse is knowledgeable about complementary therapies, appropriate referrals may be made that can help clients augment their treatments, cope with symptoms and unpleasant side effects from treatments, and maintain and promote their health. A number of strategies that currently are labeled as CTs have been part of nursing care and are well documented in the nursing literature. Table 4-5 lists some of these interventions described by Snyder and Lindquist (1998) and listed in the *Nursing Interventions Classification* (McCloskey & Bulechek, 1996).

Implications for Women's Health

Women seek care more frequently than do men from both CTs and traditional medicine. In many cultures, women are central to the physical and emotional health of the family. Women prepare most of the food, purchase dietary supplements, and provide the majority of childcare. Women generally are the caregivers and tend to the sick of the family, both old and young. Many CTs are likely to be well received by women and meet many of their needs and those of their families. Promoting the health of women over the life span improves not only the client's health but also that of the entire family.

Implications for Research

Because many of these modalities mirror autonomous nursing actions, nurses should welcome interdisciplinary interest in researching these modalities. It is important for nurses to keep abreast of the research not only published in nursing journals but in medical, psychological, public health, and specialty journals for alternative and complementary medicine. Because many of the modalities present challenges to biomedical research methods, nurses must read the research critically.

Implications for Practice

As they incorporate these complementary therapies into practice, nurses must ensure they have adequate education, training, and experience. Nurses attempting to engage in these interventions may need additional training or certification for some techniques. Nurses not educated in the

Client Education

Complementary Approaches for Women

Nausea in Pregnancy

- Acupuncture
- Sea bands
- Ginger
- Vitamin B_6
- Visualization
- Relaxation techniques

Premenstrual Syndrome

- Good nutrition: reduce intake of sugar, caffeine, dairy products, and animal fats
- Exercise
- Body work
- Herbal: chaste berry, black cohosh, wild yam, ginkgo biloba, and progesterone creme
- Supplements: vitamin B_6, vitamin E, magnesium
- Acupuncture

Menopause

- Good nutrition
- Exercise: strengthening, flexibility, weight-bearing, and mild aerobic
- Movement therapies: Pilates, Feldenkrais, Alexander technique, and yoga
- Body work: massage and various therapeutic techniques
- Mind-body: Stress reduction, relaxation, and biofeedback
- Spiritual: prayer, meditation, and religious rituals
- Social: connections with family, friends, and other groups
- Herbal: black cohosh, vitex, and other herbs, depending on symptoms
- Acupuncture and acupressure

technique have the professional responsibility to obtain the proper preparation, either from the literature or from continuing education. The AHNA website provides a current listing of endorsed educational and certificate programs. All clients should be assessed regarding supplements or substances they may be taking. Nurses must be very

Table 4-5 Complementary Modalities in the Nursing Literature

Relaxation	Relationships	Therapeutic Use of Self	Exercise	Energy-Based Technique	Cognitive Therapies	Spiritual	Other
Anxiety reduction	Advocacy	Active listening	Body work techniques	Biomagnetic healing*	Decision-making support	Meditation	Aromatherapy*
Autogenic relaxation training*	Assertiveness training	Caring or healing presence*	Exercise promotion	Healing touch*	Guided imagery (simple)	Prayer*	Art therapy
Biofeedback training	Family support	Humor	Tai chi*	Therapeutic touch	Hypnosis	Spiritual counseling	Environmental management
Breathing techniques*	Group support	Presence	Yoga*	Touch	Self-awareness	Spiritual support	Herbal remedies*
Progressive muscle relaxation	Pet or animal therapy				Self-esteem enhancement		Music therapy
					Self-reflection*		Nutritional counseling
					Storytelling*		Pain management
					Values clarification Writing in journal*		

*Interventions discussed in the literature but not officially recognized by the Nursing Interventions Classification Code. Compiled with information from Snyder M., & Lindquist R. (Eds.). (1998). *Complementary/alternative therapies in nursing* (3rd ed.). New York: Springer, and Dossey B., Keegan, L., & Guzzetta, C. E. (Eds.). (2000). *Holistic nursing: A handbook for practice* (3rd ed.). Gaithersburg, MD: Aspen Publishers.

HOLISTIC NURSE-CERTIFIED

Registered nurses with a baccalaureate degree (BSN) or higher can become certified as holistic nurses (HNC). This certification acknowledges nurses' knowledge of holistic practices and complementary therapies. This certification *does not* certify the nurse to practice specific modalities, which generally require separate certificates. More information may be obtained by calling American Holistic Nurses Certification Corporation headquarters at 1-877-284-0998.

cautious in recommending herbal remedies. It is imperative that nurses be in compliance with the Board of Nurse Examiners scope of practice regulations of their state.

NURSING PROCESS

The nursing process can be applied to clients seeking or engaging in alternative and complementary therapies.

Assessment

In assessing clients, it is important to ask specifically what they are taking in the way of vitamins, minerals, herbs, and over-the-counter medications in addition to prescribed medications. Clients also should be asked about therapies that they are considering taking, their financial resources for such therapies, and modalities that they would consider acceptable or unacceptable.

Nursing Diagnoses

North American Nursing Diagnosis Association (NANDA) –approved nursing diagnoses for clients seeking or engaging in CTs might include the following (NANDA, 2001):

- Deficient knowledge regarding the potential benefits and applicability of CTs.
- Deficient knowledge regarding the types and availability of CTs.
- Deficient knowledge regarding the potential risks associated with CTs.
- Decisional conflict related to the accessibility and efficacy of standard therapies and CTs.
- Chronic pain.
- Ineffective coping.
- Hopelessness.
- Powerlessness.

- Anxiety.
- Fear.
- Spiritual distress.
- Fatigue.
- Ineffective health maintenance.
- Interrupted family processes.

Specific nursing diagnoses in women may include the following:

- Stress urinary incontinence.
- Imbalanced nutrition.
- Sexual dysfunction.
- Disturbed sleep pattern.
- Caregiver role strain.
- Impaired parent-infant attachment.
- Risk for constipation.
- Rape-trauma syndrome.
- Ineffective breastfeeding.
- Ineffective thermoregulation.

Outcome Identification

In partnership with the client, the nurse should outline the desired results of care and therapy. Targeted goals should be prioritized according to the client's physical and emotional state and needs and to the client's wishes. Family members and significant others can be included in the goal-setting as requested by the client.

Planning

In planning interventions, it is important to engage the client in mutual planning of appropriate use of CTs and discuss expected outcomes. Referral sources for certified practitioners of specific modalities with regard to the client's financial resources are crucial. Integration of selected CTs into the medical plan of care also is advised.

Nursing Intervention

Appropriately prepared nurses may provide the intervention, particularly for CTs that may relate to client education for self-care. Many nurses are able to guide clients in relaxation techniques or provide touch therapies. Nurses need to be knowledgeable about the risks, benefits, and indications of specific CTs. Clients should be informed that behavioral interventions take practice and lifestyle changes are most effective when accomplished gradually. Efficacy of such therapies, as well as those of ingested and applied substances, may not be apparent for several weeks.

Case Study/Care Plan

USE OF COMPLEMENTARY THERAPY

Mary is a 55-year-old married woman who is having mood swings, fatigue, insomnia, vaginal dryness, hot flashes, and muscular stiffness related to perimenopause. After discussing the issue with her health care provider, she has decided not to take hormone replacement therapy. Mary approaches you for advice regarding nondrug therapies for her symptoms, which are interfering with her daily living and ability to perform her work as a professional seamstress.

Assessment

- Mary has no difficulty in falling asleep but wakes up several times at night perspiring and tossing off her bed covers. She is often too tired to complete her usual workload or engage in social activities.
- Mary is taking no medications other than a daily multivitamin and occasionally an over-the-counter laxative. Her medical history is unremarkable, and she denies having allergies.
- Mary has numerous hot flashes daily, which interrupt her work and ability to concentrate.
- Mary states that she often is irritable about situations that previously would not have bothered her and has also had regular episodes of feeling "down."
- Mary is increasingly reluctant to engage in sexual intercourse owing to dyspareunia.
- Mary has noted increasing muscular stiffness, especially when the weather is cold; she denies joint pain.
- Mary is interested in therapies other than prescribed estrogens or progesterones and a regular exercise routine.

Nursing Diagnosis

Disturbed sleep pattern related to night sweats, hot flashes, and muscular stiffness.

Expected Outcomes   In 3 weeks, Mary will report decreased frequency and severity of hot flashes, decreased muscular stiffness, and decreased awakening during sleep.

Planning   Work with Mary to plan sleep and exercise activities that will fit into her routines and lifestyle.

Nursing Interventions	Rationales
1. Inform Mary of herbal preparations such as black cohosh, Evening Primrose oil, and vitamin E supplements, and to use soy-based dairy products.	1. Use of these preparations may relieve her hot flashes.
2. Instruct Mary in forms of exercises such as yoga, tai chi, or Pilates along with resources for certified instruction in such methods.	2. These exercises will reduce muscle tension and diminish muscle stiffness.
3. Assist Mary in planning daily activities to allow for intermittent rest periods.	3. Rest periods during the day will help diminish fatigue; they also can help make up for lost sleep at night, until Mary's nighttime sleep routine is re-established.

Evaluation   Goal will be evidenced by client self-report on a list of menopausal symptoms, including symptoms for insomnia, and hot flashes.

(continued)

Nursing Diagnosis

Ineffective role performance related to fatigue, irritability, decreased mental concentration, and diminished sexual activity.

Expected Outcomes   In 2 months, Mary will report decreased irritability, re-establishment of usual work routine, and overall improved quality of life.

Planning   Help Mary identify those areas in which she has positive role involvement and those areas (such as work and spousal relationship) where she feels there is a need to improve.

Nursing Interventions	Rationales
1. Instruct Mary in deep breathing exercises to use regularly and when feeling irritable.	1. Controlled breathing releases tension and has a calming effect.
2. Advise Mary of the need to continue social and other activities that are enjoyable for her.	2. Maintaining social contacts will reinforce a sense of normalcy and help Mary keep a balanced perspective on her life.
3. Advise Mary to use a water-based lubricant for sexual intercourse and as needed in between, and to engage in regular intercourse as desired.	3. Lubricant will reduce feeling of vaginal dryness.

Evaluation   Progress will be evidenced by a self report of fewer menopausal symptoms including irritability and fatigue, and by work productivity and client report of quality of life rating of 8 or more on a 1 to 10 scale.

Evaluation

Evaluation of the effectiveness of the intervention depends on the therapeutic indications and goals. Evaluation can be obtained by client follow-up reporting, although many self-reporting instruments are available for clients to document changes in symptoms in the interim and over time. Nurses should keep in mind that many behavioral interventions have therapeutic effects beyond symptom relief in that effectiveness of biologic response to medical treatments sometimes improved.

Web Activities

- Search the Internet for alternative therapies for the discomforts of pregnancy. Critically analyze the source, information, and potential effect the information might have on clients.

- Go to the AHNA website. Explore the endorsed programs and other information.

- Pick a modality that interests you, and search the Internet.

- Go to the National Institutes of Health Center for Complementary and Alternative Therapies website and read about current research.

Key Concepts

- Complementary therapies are those used in conjunction with biomedical therapy, whereas alternative therapies are those used in place of standard biomedical therapy.

- Traditional healing systems are closely tied to cultural and religious influences and are generally thousands of years old.

- Biomedicine is an example of a healing system.

- Many complementary therapies are congruent with autonomous nursing interventions in that they support self-care and self-healing of the client.

- The complexity and technology of modern medicine, lack of effective standard therapies for chronic illnesses, the crisis in health care delivery in Western society, and increasing availability and advertising are factors contributing to the use of complementary therapies by clients and their families.

- The lack of an established theoretic basis for many modalities, such as energy-based modalities, or the limitations of quantitative methodology may account for the difficulty in applying standard biomedical research to document the effectiveness of complementary therapies. Outcome-based research is needed for such therapies to become reimbursable, affordable, and accepted by the medical community.

- Some complementary therapies have been accepted as nursing interventions, such as relaxation, therapeutic use of self, range-of-motion exercise, spiritual support, touch therapies, cognitive therapies, and nutritional counseling. Other techniques may require additional training and certification. It is vital that nurses are in compliance with the Board of Nurse Examiners scope of practice regulations of their state.

- Complementary therapies can be helpful and should be permitted if they are not harmful in general or do not interfere with standard biomedical treatment. It is important that nurses familiarize themselves with indications and contraindications before encouraging or recommending these therapies to clients.

- Resources for further information include the American Holistic Nurses Association, National Institutes of Health, Center for Complementary and Alternative Therapy, and American Botanical Council.

Review Questions and Activities

1. Which one of the following reasons might *best* explain the appeal of alternative therapy to women with chronic illnesses?
   a. Alternative therapies are generally health-oriented
   b. Alternative therapies are relatively inexpensive
   c. Alternative therapies usually are efficacious and nontoxic
   d. Alternative therapies generally involve self-care

   The correct answer is d.

2. Many clients use alternative and complementary therapies in addition to standard treatments. Which of the following clients who are using such therapies might you be most concerned about?
   a. A healthy perimenopausal woman who is taking black cohosh for relief of hot flashes.
   b. A woman using acupuncture for control of nausea related to morning sickness.
   c. A woman receiving standard chemotherapy for ovarian cancer who is taking weekly colonic irrigations.

   d. A woman who has had an uncomplicated pregnancy continuing her yoga classes into her third trimester.

   The correct answer is c.

3. Which is the nursing diagnosis *most* applicable to an adolescent girl who is concerned about her weight, although she is within normal range for her height, and is considering taking an ephedra-based herbal product to lose weight?
   a. Deficient knowledge related to risks and benefits of complementary therapies
   b. Imbalanced nutrition, more than body requirements
   c. Ineffective health maintenance related to adequate nutrition
   d. Deficient knowledge related to availability of complementary therapies

   The correct answer is a.

4. Which of the following statements is true regarding the role of the nurse in recommending or administering complementary therapies?
    a. Nurses should recommend only herbs and vitamin or dietary supplements that have been approved by the Food and Drug Administration
    b. Nurses should recommend or practice only those complementary therapies whose efficacy has been scientifically documented
    c. Nurses should encourage the use of alternative therapies that do not interfere with biomedical treatment
    d. Nurses should seek additional education or certification before recommending or practicing complementary therapies that are unfamiliar

    The correct answer is d.

5. How can the efficacy of mind-body therapies best be measured?
    a. By measurement of biochemical markers of immune function
    b. By self-reporting of symptom relief
    c. By the absence of disease states
    d. By measurement of clients' performance accuracy for such therapies

    The correct answer is b.

6. Body work is most likely to be contraindicated in which women?
    a. Those with a history of degenerative joint disease
    b. Those with the human immunodeficiency virus
    c. Those with bleeding disorders
    d. Those with osteopenia

    The correct answer is c.

7. Which persons are most likely to use complementary and alternative therapies?
    a. Those with limited education
    b. Those with an acute life-threatening illness
    c. Those with access to practitioners of such therapies
    d. Those with higher income

    The correct answer is d.

8. Visit a local holistic health center, natural food store, or book store and explore the offerings for complementary or alternative health.

References

Andrews, M. M., & Boyle, J. S. (Eds.). (1995). *Transcultural concepts in nursing care*. Philadelphia, PA: J.B. Lippincott.

Astin, J. A. (1998). Why patients use alternative medicine. *JAMA, 279,* 1548–1553.

Beal, M. (1998). Women's use of complementary and alternative therapies in reproductive health care. *Journal of Nurse Midwifery, 43,* 224–234.

Blumenthal, M., Busse, W. R., Goldberg, A., Gruenwald, J., Hall, T., Riggins, C. W., & Rister, R. S. (Eds.). (1998). *The complete German commission E monographs: Therapeutic guide to herbal medicines*. Austin, TX: American Botanical Council.

Bohm, D. (1980). *Wholeness and the implicate order*. London: ARK.

Burkhardt, M. A., & Jacobsen, M. G. N. (2000). Spirituality and health. In B. M. Dossey, L. Keegan, & C. E. Guzzetta (Eds.). *Holistic nursing: A handbook for practice (3rd ed.)*. Gaithersburg, MD: Aspen Publishers.

Callahan, D. (1996). The goals of medicine. *Hastings Center Report: Special supplement. Nov–Dec,* S1–26.

CAM Newsletter. (1998). http://odp.od.nih.gov/consensus/statements/edc. (Website accessed August 5, 1998.)

Capra, F. (1984). The Tao of physics: An exploration of the parallels between modern physics and Eastern mysticism (2nd ed.) Toronto: Bantam.

Cassileth, B. R. (1998). *The alternative medicine handbook: The complete guide to alternative and complementary therapies*. New York: W.W. Norton.

Chilton, M. (1996). Panel recommends integrating behavioral and relaxation approaches into medical treatment of chronic pain, insomnia. *Alternative Therapies in Health and Medicine, 2,* 18–28.

Cohen, M. Z., Headley, J., & Sherwood, G. (2000). Spirituality and bone marrow transplant: When faith is stronger than fear. *International Journal for Human Caring, 4, (2),* 40–46.

Csordas, T. (1994). *The sacred self: A cultural phenomenology of charismatic healing*. Berkeley, CA: University of California Press.

Dossey, L. (1993). *Healing words: The power of prayer and the practice of medicine*. San Francisco, CA: Harper.

Dossey, B., Keegan, L., & Guzzetta, C. E. (Eds.). (2000). *Holistic nursing: A handbook for practice (3rd ed.)*. Gaithersburg, MD: Aspen Publishers.

Eisenberg, D. M., Kessler, R. C., Foster, C., Norlock, F. E., Calkins, D. R., & Delbanco, T. L. (1993). Unconventional medicine in the United States: Prevalence, costs and patterns of use. *The New England Journal of Medicine, 328,* 252–256.

Eisenberg, D. M., Davis, R. B., Ettner S. L., Appel, S., Wilkey, S., Van Rompag, M., & Kessler, R. C. (1998). Trends in alternative medicine use in the United States, 1990–1997. *JAMA, 280,* 1569–1575.

Ergil, K. V. (1996). Chinese Medicine/China's Traditional Medicine. In M. S. Micozzi (Ed.). *Fundamentals of complementary and alternative medicine*. New York: Churchill Livingstone.

Foster, D. F., Phillips, R. S., Hamel, M. B., & Eisenberg, D. (2000). Alternative medicine use in older Americans. *Journal of the American Geriatrics Society, 48,* 1560–1565.

Glisson, J., Crawford, R., & Street, S. (1999). Review, critique and guidelines for the use of herbs and homeopathy. *The Nurse Practitioner, 24,* (4) 44–67.

Gordon, R. J., Nienstedt, B. C., & Gesler, W. M. (1998). *Alternative therapies: Expanding options in health care*. New York: Springer.

Hardy, M. L. (2000). Herbs of special interest to women. *Journal of the American Pharmaceutical Association,* 40, (2), 234–242.

Harvard Health Letter. (1997). *Alternative medicine: Time for a second opinion, 23,* (1), 1–3.

Jacobs J., & Moskowitz, R. (1996). Homeopathy. In M. S. Micozzi (Ed.). *Fundamentals of complementary and alternative medicine.* New York: Churchill Livingstone.

Kaptchuk, T. J. (1983). *The web that has no weaver: Understanding Chinese medicine.* New York: Congdon and Weed.

Kemp, T. (1996). The use of transcutaneous electrical nerve stimulation on acupuncture points in labour. *Midwives, 109,* (1307) 318–320.

Keville, K., & Green, M. (2000). Aromatherapy: Guidelines for using essential oils and herbs. Health World Online. www.healthy.net. (Website accessed July 2, 2000).

Kinsley, D. (1996). *Health, healing, and religion: A cross-cultural perspective.* Upper Saddle River, NJ: Prentice-Hall.

Koenig, H. G. (1999). *The healing power of faith.* New York: Simon & Schuster.

Landmark Report on Public Perceptions of Alternative Care. (1998). Landmark Healthcare. Http://landmarkhealthcare.com. (Website accessed August 5, 1998.)

Levin, J. S. (1994). Religion and health: Is there an association, is it valid and is it causal? *Social Science and Medicine, 29,* 589–600.

Liehr, P., & Smith, M. J. (2000). Using story theory to guide nursing practice. *International Journal for Human Caring, 4,* (2), 13–18.

Marston, R. Q., & Jones, R. M. (Eds.). (1992). *Medical education in transition.* Princeton, NJ: The Robert Wood Johnson Foundation.

McCloskey, J. C., & Bulechek, G. M. (1996). *Nursing interventions classification (NIC).* St. Louis, MO: Mosby.

McGuire, M. B. (1998). *Ritual healing in suburban America.* New Brunswick, NJ: Rutgers University Press.

Melzak, R. and Wall, P. (1965) Pain mechanism: A new theory. *Science, 150* (3699), 971–979.

Micozzi, M. S. (Ed.). (1996). *Fundamentals of complementary and alternative medicine.* New York: Churchill Livingstone.

North American Nursing Diagnosis Association (NANDA). (2001). www.nanda.org. (Website accessed December 12, 2000.)

National Institutes of Health. (1994). *Alternative medicine: Expanding medical horizons.* A Report to the National Institutes of Health on Alternative Medical Systems and Practices in the United States (Publication No. 017-040-00537-7). Washington, DC: U.S. Government Printing Office.

Nurse's handbook of alternative and complementary therapies. (1999). Springhouse, PA: Springhouse.

Oldendick, R., Coker, A. L., Wieland, D., Raymond, J. I., Probst, J. C., Schell, B. J., & Stoskoph, C. H. (2000). Population-based survey of complementary and alternative medicine usage, patient satisfaction and physician involvement. *Southern Medical Journal, 93,* (4) 375–381.

Olsen, M., Sneed, N., LaVia, M., Virella, G., Bonadonna, R., & Michel, Y. (1997). Stress-induced immunosuppression and therapeutic touch. *Alternative Therapies in Health and Medicine, 3,* 68–74.

PEW Health Professions Commission. (1995). *Critical challenges: Revitalizing the health profession for the twenty-first century.* San Francisco, CA: PEW Health Professions Commission.

Pizzorno, J. E. (1996). Naturopathic medicine. In M. S. Micozzi (Ed.). *Fundamentals of complementary and alternative medicine.* New York: Churchill Livingston.

Redwood, D. (1996). Chiropractic. In M. S. Micozzi (Ed.). *Fundamentals of complementary and alternative medicine.* New York: Churchill Livingston.

Richardson, M. A., Sanders, T., Palmer, J. L., Greisinger, A., & Singletary, S. E. (2000). Complementary/alternative medicine use in a comprehensive cancer center and their implications for oncology. *Journal of Clinical Oncology, 18,* 2505–2514.

Rosenfeld, I. (1996). *Guide to alternative medicine.* New York: Random House.

Shen, J., Wenger, N., Glaspy, J., Harys, R. D., Albert, P. S., Choi, C., & Shekelle, P. G. (2000). Electroacupuncture for control of myeloablative chemotherapy-induced emesis. *JAMA, 284,* 2755–2761.

Slater, V. (1996). Healing touch. In M. S. Micozzi (Ed.). *Fundamentals of complementary and alternative medicine.* New York: Churchill Livingston.

Snyder, M., & Lindquist, R. (Eds.). (1998). *Complementary/alternative therapies in nursing (3rd ed.).* New York: Springer.

Starr, D. (1984). *The Social Transformation of American Medicine.* New York: Basic Books.

Stewart, J. C. (1995). *Reiki touch.* Atlanta, GA: The Reiki Touch.

Villaire, M. (1998). Popularity of alternative medicine still growing in US, Canada, polls find. *Alternative therapies in health and medicine, 4,* 29.

Wagner, G. N. (1996). Osteopathy. In M. S. Micozzi (Ed.). *Fundamentals of complementary and alternative medicine.* New York: Churchill Livingston.

Wardell, D. & Engebretson, J. (2001). Biological correlates of Reiki touch healing. *Journal of Advanced Nursing, 33* (4), 439–445.

Wetzel, M. S., Eisenberg, D. M., & Kaptchuk, T. D. (1998). Courses involving complementary and alternative medicine at US medical schools. *JAMA, 280,* 784–787.

Zukav, G. (1979). The Dancing Wu Li Masters: An overview of the new physics. New York: Quill.

Suggested Readings

National Institute of Health. *Alternative Medicine: Expanding Medical Horizons.* (1994). Chantilly Report. Washington DC, US Government Printing Pub #017-040-00537-7

Cassidy, C. M. (1996). Cultural context of complementary and alternative medicine systems. In M. S. Micozzi (Ed.). *Fundamentals of complementary and alternative medicine* (pp. 9–34). New York: Churchill Livingstone.

Collinge, W., Duhl, L., (1996). *The American Holistic Health Association complete guide to alternative therapies.* NY: Warner Books.

Cox, H. (1995). *Fire from heaven.* Boston, MA: Addison-Wesley.

Dossey, B. (Ed.). (1997). *Core curriculum for Holistic Nursing.* Gaithersburg, MD: Aspen Pub.

Engebretson, J. (1996). Comparison of nurses and alternative healers. *Image: Journal of Nursing Scholarship, 28,* 95–99.

Engebretson, J. (1997). A multiparadigm approach to nursing. *Advances in Nursing Science 20,* 22–34.

The Burton Goldberg Group. (1994). *Alternative medicine: The definitive guide.* CA. Future Medicine Publishing.

Goodwin, M. (1997). A health insurance revolution. *New Age Journal 1997–1998 Special edition,* 66–69.

Kaptchuk, T. J. (1996). Historical context of the concept of vitalism in complementary and alternative medicine. In M. S. Micozzi (Ed.). *Fundamentals of complementary and alternative medicine.* New York: Churchill Livingstone.

Learn, C. D., & Higgins, P. G. (1999). Harmonizing herbs: Managing menopause with help from mother earth. *AWHONN Lifelines, Oct-Nov,* 39–43.

Lovallo, W. R. (1997). *Stress and health: Biological and psychological interactions.* Thousand Oaks, CA: Sage.

Machover, L., Drake, A., & Drake, J. (1993). *The Alexander technique birth book.* New York: Sterling.

Moore, N. G. (1997). The Columbia-Presbyterian complementary care center: Comprehensive care of the mind, body and spirit. *Alternative Therapies in Health and Medicine, 3,* 30–32.

Ray, P. H. (1997). The emerging culture. American demographics. www.demographics.com.

Resources

Advances: The Journal of Mind-Body Health
Alternative Therapies in Health and Medicine
Herbalgram
Holistic Nursing Practice
Journal of Alternative and Complementary Medicine
Journal of Holistic Nursing
Acupuncture www.acupuncture.com
Alternative Health News Online www.altmedicine.com
American Botanical Council www.herbalgram.org

American Holistic Health Association www.healthy.net/ahha
American Holistic Nurses Association www.ahna.org
Healing Touch International www.healingtouch.net
National Center for Homeopathy www.homeopathic.org
National Institutes of Health Consensus Reports www.nih.gov.consensus
Office of Complementary and Alternative Medicine at the National Institutes of Health http://www.altmed.od.nih.gov/oam

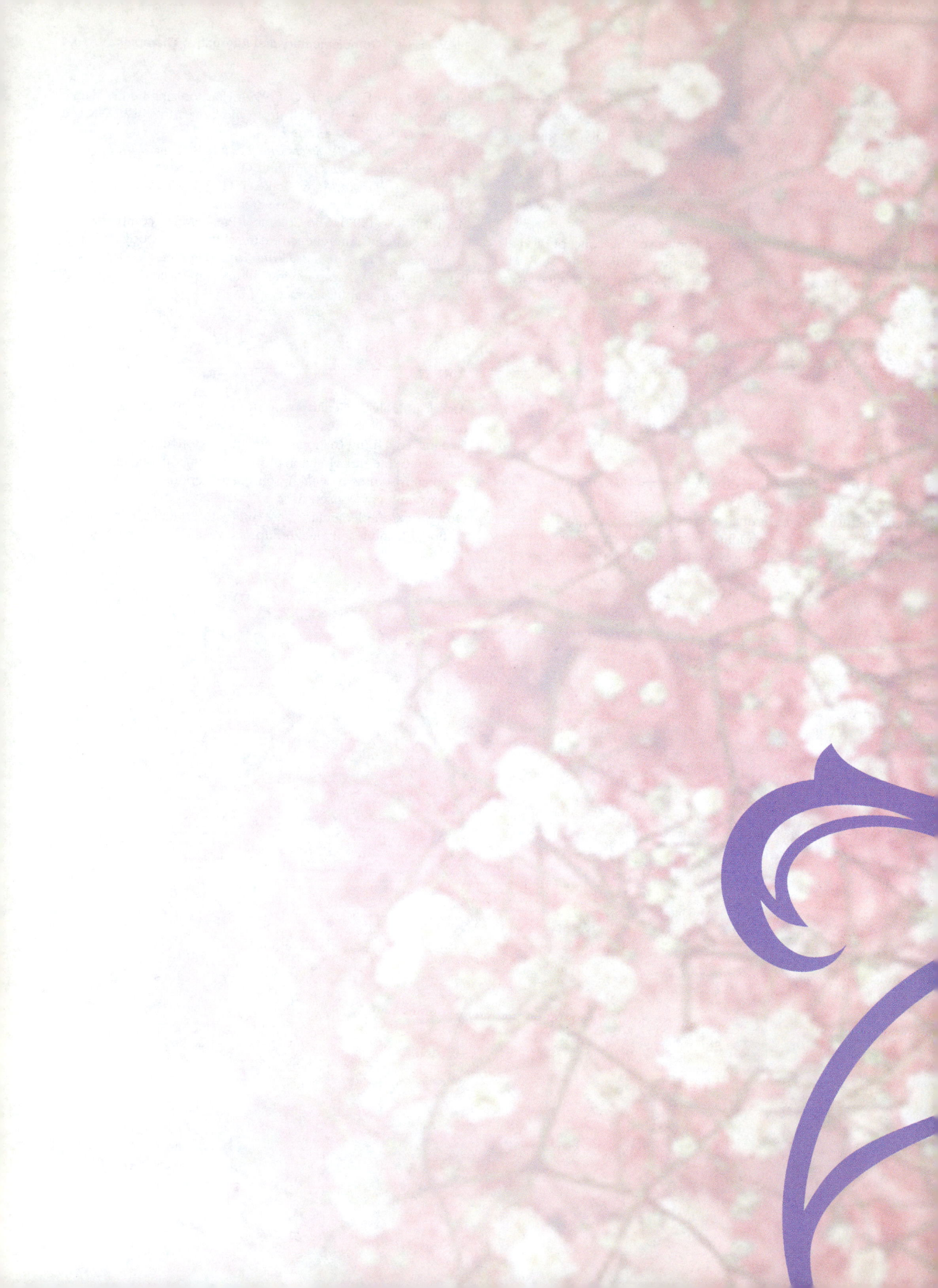

Ethics, Laws, and Standards of Care

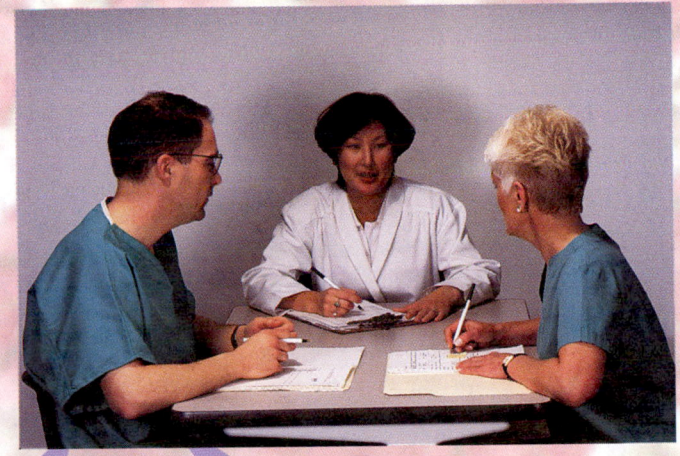

hile ethical and legal issues are present in many aspects of nursing practice, special issues exist when working with childbearing clients. An awareness of personal and professional values facilitates discussion of issues related to caring for perinatal clients. Ask yourself how you would respond to the following questions:

- *What values do I hold to be important in my life?*
- *What beliefs about professional nursing serve as a basis for my practice?*
- *How do I respond when a client's value system is different from mine?*
- *What happens when I find I have conflicting ethical responsibilities?*

As you read this chapter, continue to think about how your values influence practice decisions. Special boxes raise specific questions about your values and experiences when caring for perinatal clients.

Key Terms

Autonomy
Beneficence
Categorical imperative
Civil law
Criminal law
Code
Deontology
Dilemma
Doctrine of the golden
  mean

Due care
Ethics
Ethic of care
Fidelity
Harm
Informed consent
Justice
Law

Liability
Malpractice
Material principles of
  justice
Negligence
Nonmaleficence
Paternalism
Prima facie

Standards of care
Tort
Universalizability
Utilitarianism
Veracity
Virtue
Virtue ethics

Competencies

Upon completion of this chapter, the reader should be able to:

1. Describe common ethical and legal issues in maternal-child nursing.
2. Discuss basic ethical theories that potentially guide decision making, including utilitarianism, deontology, virtue ethics, and nursing ethics.
3. Identify four ethical principles that can be applied in ethical thinking.
4. Use the basic steps that lead to dilemma resolution.
5. Describe documentation safeguards that should be used to adequately document care for childbearing clients.
6. Discuss standards of care commonly used in maternal-child nursing.

Who has more rights during a pregnancy—the mother or the fetus? Can anything be legally done to make pregnant women stop using illicit drugs during their pregnancies? Do all women have a right to prenatal care? What measures should be taken so that care given to clients during the perinatal period is safe and appropriately documented? What care standards should guide care given during the perinatal period?

While ethical and legal considerations are a component of all aspects of nursing care, some unique issues exist in maternal-child nursing. Many of these issues occur because two parties, inextricably linked, are involved—the mother and the developing fetus. This chapter focuses on basic concepts related to ethical and legal considerations, including relevant ethical theories and principles; a method for dilemma resolution and specific dilemmas that nurses may encounter; legal concepts, standards of care for maternal-child nursing, and guidelines for practicing within legal boundaries. Readers will find guidance for practice issues that nurses face in maternity nursing.

What is meant when the term "ethics" or "laws" is used? **Ethics** refers to the branch of philosophy that pro-

vides rules and principles that can be used for resolving ethical dilemmas. **Laws** are rules that govern the behavior of individuals and represent the minimum standard of morality (Hall, 1996).

Since this chapter concerns both ethical and legal issues, a good beginning would be to examine the similarities and differences between law and ethics. The relationship between ethics and laws includes similarities and differences. First, both laws and ethics identify social sanctions and provide guidance for actions. In fact, many laws are derived from ethical considerations. Laws generally define the minimum ethical principles that must be followed (Hall, 1996). Both laws and ethics provide mechanisms through which disputes can be settled. However, laws and ethics can differ in important ways. Laws are rules that are external to an individual and that members of society must obey. On the other hand, ethics tend to be personal and involve values, beliefs, and interpretations to guide behavior. Laws are written with the interests of society as the major consideration, whereas ethics focus on the interests of an individual within the society. Laws are enforced through law enforcement agencies and the judicial system. Ethical decisions are more reflective, and ethics commit-

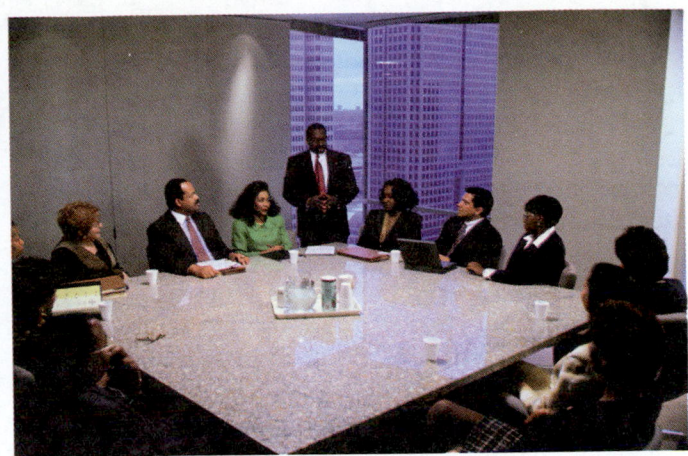

Figure 5-1 Many institutions have ethics committees designed to provide guidance and support in the critical issue of client care. (Photo courtesy of Photodisc.)

tees often serve as a forum for discussion, persuasion, and recommendations for action (Figure 5-1).

Some actions are both ethical and legal. For example, informed consent of clients is an ethical obligation for health care providers as well as a legal one. Some actions are legal, but may not be considered ethical. One possible example of an ethical and legal conflict, depending on the individual's point of view, would be abortion; an individual who feels abortion is unethical may have difficulty with its legality. Finally, some actions that are illegal might be considered ethical. An example of this situation would be assisted suicide. Although some care providers consider assisted suicide to be within the realm of ethical behavior, such assistance is currently illegal.

ETHICAL ISSUES

Nurses frequently encounter ethical dilemmas. In a survey by the American Nurses Association Center for Ethics and Human Rights, 79% of nurses reported encountering ethical issues in practice on either a daily or weekly basis (Scanlon, 1994). Many of these issues were related to cost containment that jeopardized client welfare, end-of-life issues, breaches in confidentiality, and incompetent or unethical practices of colleagues. Unfortunately, 59% of the nurses surveyed indicated that their educational programs had not sufficiently prepared them for managing ethical issues found in practice. This section focuses on some basic ethical theories and principles and suggests a method that nurses can use for resolving ethical dilemmas in practice.

Bandman and Bandman (1995) suggest that ethics are concerned with doing good and avoiding harm. Certainly, nurses have opportunities to promote client welfare and prevent harm. However, just what constitutes good and what can be defined as harmful is open to interpretation.

For example, is it better to promote fetal health at the expense of overriding the expectant mother's right to make decisions about her care?

Why are some dilemmas considered to be ethical dilemmas? Ethical dilemmas can arise out of a conflict in duties. For example, nurses have obligations to many parties—their clients, their employing institution, physicians, and most importantly, themselves. Unfortunately, these obligations sometimes conflict. Clients may demand one thing, a hospital or clinic another, and the profession of nursing another. It can be difficult to identify the obligation that is the most important and act on it. Ethical dilemmas deal with human concerns. Making an ethical decision is different from determining what kind of car you might like to buy or which color is your favorite. A dilemma sometimes encountered in practice is how to protect the health and safety of a fetus while promoting a mother's right to make choices about her pregnancy. Perhaps the most apt description of a **dilemma** is that it is making a choice between two unsatisfactory alternatives (Davis, Aroskar, Liaschenko, & Drought, 1997). Regardless of the choice, the desired happy ending cannot occur. Nonetheless, ethical dilemmas are resolvable situations that demand attention and thoughtful reasoning. Understanding ethical theories and principles can be useful in helping to resolve dilemmas and in discussing the rationale for our actions with others. Each of the ethical theories presented below offers different perspectives about how a dilemma may be viewed and how right actions can be selected.

Basic Ethical Perspectives

The concept of bioethics, or the application of ethics to health care, was popularized in the late 1960s and early 1970s because care providers felt a need to have better methods to resolve dilemmas. Ethical conflicts have always existed, but increased use of technology in health care has increased the number and visibility of dilemmas. Initially, two major classes of theories, derived from existing studies of ethics, were used: utilitarianism and deontology. As the field of bioethics began to grow, providers were concerned that while these perspectives provided guidance for ethical decision making, they did not reflect the characteristics of care providers. Another class of ethics was revived: virtue ethics, an ancient theoretical perspective. Nursing theorists also began to explore the unique relationships that nurses have with clients and to examine the basis for their care. Out of this tradition, an ethic of care, linked to nursing ethics, was proposed to encompass some of the unique perspectives that nurses bring to the health care arena. Because nurses work collaboratively in health care, they must understand the perspectives that each of these theories brings to ethical decision making, because these perspectives can guide thinking and provide a mechanism for explaining and justifying actions. Although these theoretical perspectives can serve as a guide for action, each has some shortcomings.

Utilitarianism

Utilitarianism is a type of ethical theory focusing on the consequences of actions. Individuals who were prominent in the development of utilitarian theory during the 19th century included Jeremy Bentham, a social reformer, and John Stuart Mill. Although the theories they produced were not exactly identical, the overarching themes are similar. In utilitarianism, acts are right if they produce the greatest possible balance of good when everyone is considered (Mappes & DeGrazia, 1996). No action in itself is considered to be right or wrong. Rather, right actions are those that produce the best possible outcomes.

Utilitarian thinking involves a certain amount of calculation. Whenever a decision is being considered, an individual tries to predict all of the possible good and bad consequences arising from each action that could potentially be taken. Once those are identified, the decision-maker would weigh the outcomes and select the action that would produce the best results and the least number of bad results for everyone involved. Utilitarian theory requires that the decision-maker be impartial and the decision not be based on personal interests. Utilitarian theory is sometimes classified as "act utilitarian," in which the principle of utility is applied to each specific act considered, or as "rule utilitarian," in which rules are developed that, if followed consistently, usually provide the greatest good. Act utilitarianism is sensitive to individual cases, but rule utilitarianism holds that following the rules produces the greatest degree of social utility, but not necessarily individual good (Beauchamp & Childress, 1994). One difficulty with utilitarian theory is that it might permit the interests of the majority group to override the interests of a minority group (Beauchamp & Childress, 1994). A positive aspect of utilitarianism is that it works to promote good.

For example, it is good for women to receive prenatal care during pregnancy because it helps both mothers and their babies to be healthier. We also have technology available to provide care for low-birth-weight babies. However, resources are limited and there is not enough funding to pay for both prenatal care for all pregnant women and high-technology care for all low-birth-weight infants. From a utilitarian perspective, this problem would be weighed to find a solution that would promote the best outcomes for the greatest number of individuals. In this situation, would better outcomes for more people be produced by provision of early prenatal care to all expectant mothers or by provision of "high-tech" care to a smaller number of low-birth-weight infants? Based on the benefits to the greatest number of individuals, a utilitarian solution would be to provide prenatal care to all expectant mothers.

Deontology

Deontology is another type of ethical theory that is concerned with people doing the right thing. The word "deontology" is derived from *deon,* which means duty. Rather than focusing on whether or not actions bring about the best outcome, deontology strives to identify the best possible action directed by one's duty or obligations, without considering rather than based on the consequences of actions.

The utilitarian theory previously discussed had many critics. Immanuel Kant considered utilitarianism as providing a "wavering and uncertain standard" for action (Mappes & DeGrazia, 1996; p. 16). To remedy this situation, Kant proposed what is known as the **categorical imperative**, or supreme rule, that should govern actions. Simply expressed, the categorical imperative is to act only on that maxim (or rule) that can be willed to become universal law (Kant, 1981). In other words, the rule used to guide actions should be one that could be followed in all other similar situations. This concept is called **universalizability** because it refers to the concept that the rule should be generalizable to other situations. For example: Is telling a lie to a client ever acceptable? To answer this question, an individual would have to decide if telling lies to clients was acceptable in other situations. Since telling the truth is better in most situations, lying would not be acceptable in any specific instance.

Kant identified several formulations of the categorical imperative. Another formulation that is of interest to health care providers is to always act to treat humanity, either yourself or others, as an end rather than as a means (Kant, 1981). This formulation recognizes that because of their rationality, human beings have inherent worth and dignity. Therefore, we should have respect for all persons, including ourselves. Also, we should never use others simply as a means to an end. For example, clients are a means to our livelihood as nurses. If we care for clients simply as a means to earn a paycheck, we are treating them as only a means. However, if we treat clients with the respect they deserve because they are human beings with inherent worth, then even though clients help us earn a living (means), we are also treating them as an end as well. While Kant's theory provides clear guidelines for action in many situations, it is sometimes criticized for offering such a rigid system of choice that it is difficult to follow.

Other deontologists feel that a supreme rule, such as the categorical imperative, is insufficient to guide decision making in all ethical situations, particularly when a conflict of duties exists. W. D. Ross (1994) proposed the concept of conditional duties, or *prima facie* duties, as a guide for correct action. Rather than asserting that there is a supreme duty, a ***prima facie*** duty is a conditional duty that can be overridden by a more stringent duty. Ross suggests that some duties are derived from previous acts, such as a promise; acts done by others for which we may owe an obligation; special relationships to families or employers; or acts that serve as a mechanism for personal growth or for benefit to others. From the perspective of Ross, the moral decision-maker would decide which obligation or duty was the most important and then act accordingly. For example, as nurses, we have an obligation to follow hospital policies. However, we also have a professional obligation to render safe care for clients. When working in an understaffed environment, a nurse may feel that safe care cannot be given, potentially putting clients at risk for harm. The nurse would then have to choose which obligation was the most stringent, either following the institutional policy of accepting assignments given or rendering safe care to clients. The nurse would act on the basis of which obligation was perceived to be the most important.

Virtue Ethics

A **virtue** is a character trait that is valued; a moral virtue is a trait that is morally valued. **Virtue ethics** focus on the personal characteristics of the moral agent or person and the way in which these virtues guide moral action. Virtue ethics are attributed to Aristotle (Singer, 1994), the ancient Greek philosopher who believed that a virtuous life would be a happy one. According to Aristotle, all living things are endowed with certain capacities or potentialities. For human beings to live a happy life, they must live a life that is distinctive from other creatures through the development of intellectual and moral virtues. Intellectual virtues enable humans to discover and recognize rules of life that should be followed. Moral virtues deal with feelings, emotions, and impulses that make the effective use of intellect possible.

Virtues are not attributes that humans are born with, but characteristics that are perfected. Aristotle proposed the **doctrine of the golden mean** as a guide for virtue development. This doctrine suggests that many virtues develop at the midpoint between extremes of less desirable characteristics. For example, one is not born brave, but becomes brave by conquering fear. However, if fear is diminished too much, then dangerous risks may be taken. The virtue of courage demonstrates the doctrine of the golden mean: too little courage would make us excessively fearful, but too much would place us in extreme danger. The virtue of courage would be the midpoint between those two extremes. Virtues that may be useful for health care providers to embrace include compassion, benevolence, respectful, honesty, and kindness. Beauchamp and Chil-

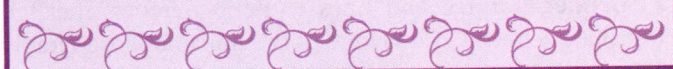

Critical Thinking

Virtue Ethics and Respect for Clients

Virtue ethics suggests that respectfulness is a worthwhile virtue to be embraced by nurses. How would acting on the virtue of respectfulness make a difference in the way you treat clients and their partners during the perinatal period? Would you listen to client concerns or suggestions differently? What special considerations might be needed for clients with different cultural backgrounds?

dress (1994) suggest that virtue ethics can serve as a useful adjunct to other theories and principles of ethics that enable individual perspectives on both the right action and the right motive.

Nursing Ethics

As bioethics has developed, nursing has begun to question whether there is a unique set of ethics for nursing and how those ethics might be embodied. Based on the work of Noddings (1984), who helped to link caring to ethics; Benner and Wrubel (1989), who linked caring and nursing in a very practical sense; and others, an ethics of caring that is applicable to nursing practice has emerged. The **ethic of care** is a perspective that recognizes the personal concerns and vulnerabilities of clients in health and illness. Nurses, operating under the tenets of an ethic of care, would be willing to provide care to achieve therapeutic goals without expectation of reciprocity, because of a desire to be a caring individual.

Gadow (1988) suggests that nurses have a covenant to care by alleviating another's vulnerability. Wicker (1988) indicates caring may help bring clients lives into balance, even if curing cannot occur. Benner and Wrubel (1989) propose that caring creates possibility because it focuses on others and identifies personal concerns. To be considered moral, caring must be an overriding value to guide action and apply to all persons in similar circumstances. Additionally, caring considers the welfare of others and incorporates empathy, support, and compassion (Fry, 1988). An ethic of care enables nurses to respond to others as worthy, with no expectation of reciprocity (Benner, Tanner, & Chesla, 1996). Bishop and Scudder (1996) propose that rather than merely applying principles, the moral sense of nursing is articulated through the "caring presence of nurses that achieves the therapeutic intent of nursing practice" (p. xi).

According to Noddings (1984), the ethical self exists in relationship with others. Caring relationships are grounded in an ideal vision, in which we hold our best selves. Caring involves reciprocity; our desire to care is rooted in previous relationships, where others have cared for us and we have cared for others. Moral behavior arises from a natural impulse to care, preserving the fundamental goodness of these experiences. Ethical caring occurs because of the desire to be a caring person. Caring relationships permit the caregiver to view the world from the perspective of the recipient of care. From that perspective, the one caring is able to set aside personal agendas and place herself or himself at the disposal of the recipient.

Benner, Tanner, and Chesla (1996) perceive that the ethical and clinical knowledge of the nurse are inseparable and are learned experientially. Through experience, nurses develop an ethical comportment that encompasses a practical "know-how" of relating to clients in a respectful and supportive way. The ethical comportment aids in protecting those who are vulnerable, promoting growth and health, or fostering a peaceful death. These skills can be developed within a socially based practice, through the stories of others, and through other experiences, permitting nurses to move from the status of a novice to that of a skilled practitioner (Figure 5-2).

Nursing ethics are therapeutic in the sense that they promote the well-being of clients "Nursing ethics should evoke thinking about concrete practice in ways that help nurses individually and collectively to fulfill the moral sense of nursing" (Bishop & Scudder, 1996; p. 135). Nurses, working from a framework of caring, should consider the individual needs of clients and attempt to respond in a caring, personalized manner. Advocacy on behalf of clients should be an example of engaging in a therapeutic ethic of nursing. Treating clients holistically—

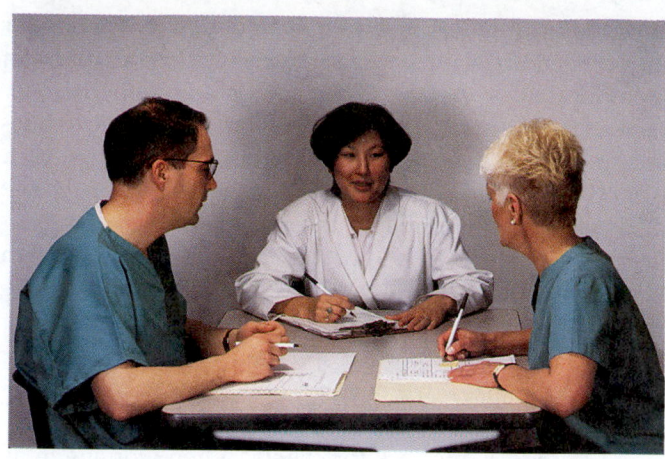

Figure 5-2 Consultation with health care team members is an important part of maintaining an autonomous practice. Good communication promotes safe care and facilitates discussion of ethical issues.

not simply as a body in need of repair—is another way of engaging in ethical nursing practice. Recognizing that nursing is practiced in a context with many players, including administrators, physicians, and other care providers, nurses should feel a particular sense of commitment to clients and their families and be an advocate on their behalf.

Ethics and Holism

Holistic ethics is a philosophical perspective that merges the concept of unity and wholeness of all people and nature (Keegan, 1995). Acts are performed by people who have a desire to do good and to contribute to the unity of the self and the universe. Correct acts are ones that reflect the enlightened consciousness of the individual and are judged by the effects that the act has on the nature of the individual and the larger self. From this perspective, holistic ethics encompasses elements of both utilitarian and deontological thinking. Outcomes are important, but there is also a concern for the intrinsic nature of the act.

The *Code of Ethics for Holistic Nurses* provides guidance for action and identifies responsibilities for self and others (American Holistic Nurses Association, 1995). The code expresses that nurses have fundamental responsibilities for health promotion, facilitation of healing, and alleviation of suffering. It suggests that nurses have an obligation to self, demonstrated by modeling health behaviors and achieving harmony in life. Nurses have a primary responsibility to clients that reflects an awareness of the holistic nature of human beings. Nurses are responsible for cooperating with co-workers and maintaining competence. Nurses practicing within a holistic framework should work to meet the health-related and social needs of

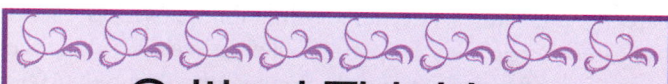

Critical Thinking

Caring and Personal Agendas

According to the tenets of an ethic of care, nurses should be able to set aside their personal agendas when caring for clients. This may be difficult to achieve. Is it possible to put aside personal agendas and focus on the needs of the client? How might you go about leaving your personal agenda behind when giving care? What are the risks of setting aside a personal agenda? What are the potential rewards?

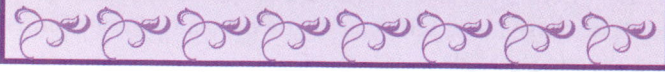

the public and facilitate healing by manipulating the environment to promote peace, harmony, and nurturance.

Ethical Principles

Four major principles guide ethical thinking in nursing practice. These include respect for autonomy, nonmaleficence, beneficence, and justice. These principles may be used in conjunction with the theoretical perspectives discussed as guidelines to help resolve ethical dilemmas. Each of these ethical principles is equally important in the consideration of ethical dilemmas, although some dilemmas may cause us to focus more emphasis on one principle than another.

Respect for Autonomy

Autonomy refers to individual independence in holding a particular view, making choices, and taking action based on values and beliefs (Beauchamp & Childress, 1994). Respect for autonomy requires that others be treated in a way, such as noninterference in decision making or actions, that enables autonomous action. The concept of respect for autonomy recognizes the inherent worth of the individual and that a competent human being is qualified to make decisions in his or her own best interests. Autonomy should encompass aspects of free action, which are voluntary and intentional, and authenticity, in which choices are congruent with the person's attitudes, values, and life plans (Miller, 1981). For autonomous choice to occur, individuals must be aware of the alternatives and consequences. The concept of informed consent is firmly rooted in the principle of respect for autonomy and is discussed later.

Although respect for autonomy implies that individuals have the right to make choices, it also focuses on the relationship of individuals to the communities in which they live (Figure 5-3). For example, while individuals can

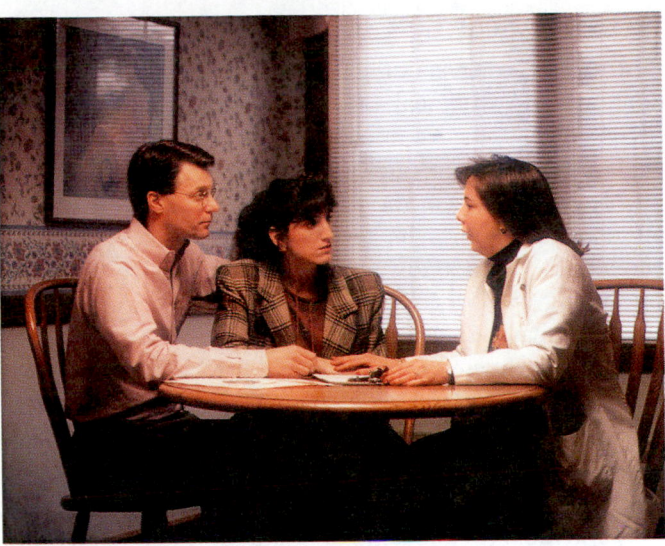

Figure 5-3 Providing information plays a significant role in promoting the autonomy of pregnant women and their families. (Photo courtesy of Bellevue, The Women's Hospital, Niskayuna, NY.)

anticipate that community members will respect their autonomy, they also must respect the autonomy of others. We are not given license to perform any act simply because we have autonomous choice. In fact, there are some specific instances where autonomy may be limited. Autonomy of children is routinely restricted because parents believe a child's welfare is promoted by making decisions on behalf of the child. An individual may not be competent to make decisions. For example, clients who are confused or lack the mental capacity to make decisions may have limited autonomy. Another reason for limiting autonomy is when an action could generate harm or when benefit would be derived from restricting autonomy (Mappes & DeGrazia, 1996).

Nonmaleficence

Nonmaleficence refers to the concept of preventing harm to others and is an important principle for nurses. **Harm** is the interference with the mental or physical well-being of others (Beauchamp & Childress, 1994). Many basic rules are nonmaleficent, including not killing, not causing pain, not disabling, and not depriving of freedom. Nonmaleficence encompasses both harm and the risk of harm. The harm may be either intentional or unintentional. As nurses, we have the obligation to exercise due care in professional practice so that unintentional harms do not occur. **Due care** is a legal and ethical standard of performance by which professionals abide. As professionals, nurses must possess sufficient knowledge and skills and render care that is cautious, diligent, and thoughtful.

Critical Thinking

Autonomy

Sometimes competent clients make decisions that may be potentially harmful. When this situation occurs:

- Can health providers ever overrule the client's decision? If so, under what circumstances?
- How would you work to promote this client's autonomy?

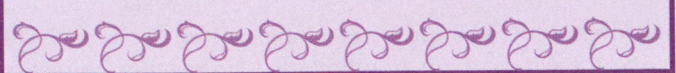

Beneficence

Beneficence means doing good and may include: prevention of harm, removal of evil, and promotion of good (Frankena, 1973). As nurses our goal is to promote the welfare of clients in our care, so beneficence is a key to our actions. Because the goods and services we have to offer are sometimes limited by our resources, unlimited beneficence is not always possible. In these instances, combining the principle of beneficence and the principle of justice may be helpful.

An issue related to beneficence is what happens when the health care provider's desire to promote client welfare clashes with the client's autonomous decisions. **Paternalism** is the interference with the liberty of another in which the interference is justified by promoting the well-being of that individual (Beauchamp & Childress, 1994). One example of paternalism would be a situation in which a person coerces another to do something that is perceived to be beneficial. This situation frequently causes conflict in health care. For example, maternal-child nurses possess knowledge and expertise about care during and after pregnancy. Education and experience allow these nurses to make suggestions to clients about behavioral modification that should be made to promote a healthy pregnancy. These might include recommendations regarding diet, exercise, smoking, and alcohol intake. How should nurses respond when clients fail to make the changes suggested, even when clients know the potential consequences of failing to modify behavior? The principle of autonomy would suggest that nurses support the client's choices, whereas the principle of beneficence would suggest that nurses override the mother's autonomy to ensure that sug-

gested changes are made. The second choice could be considered paternalistic in nature.

Justice

Justice refers to how we divide benefits and burdens in our society (Beauchamp & Childress, 1994). For example, health care is a benefit that promotes the health and well-being of individuals in our society. However, paying for health care is a burden. Because our health care resources are not unlimited, we must decide on the fairest system for allocation of both the benefit and resources of health care and the burden of paying for care. A basic principle of justice is that, in distribution of resources, equals should be treated equally and nonequals treated unequally. In health care, pregnant women need access to prenatal care. So all pregnant women should be treated equally in terms of access to care. However, some pregnant women experience greater complications during their pregnancy, causing them to need more sophisticated care. According to this rule, these women would receive additional care not given to women who do not need them (i.e., nonequals are treated unequally).

Depending on the benefit or burden to be divided, the material principles of justice may be invoked to decide how to distribute society's goods. The **material principles of justice** provide a set of guidelines that can be used to justify the distribution of benefits. They offer the following concepts to defend distribution decisions:

- Equality, in which everyone receives an equal share
- Need, for which those who need more receive more
- Contribution, in which goods are received in proportion to productive labor
- Effort, in which the amount of work is rewarded
- Merit, for which rewards are given according to achievement
- Free market exchange, in which wealth and income would be derived from a natural distribution of talent and abilities (Beauchamp & Childress, 1994)

Veracity and Fidelity

Other principles or rules that affect ethical decision making and conflict resolution include veracity and fidelity, both important concepts for nurses. **Veracity** is truthfulness: nurses are truthful with clients in their care. **Fidelity** is keeping promises: if nurses make promises to clients, they keep them. Both these rules reflect respect for others and are essential for establishing trust in relationships.

Code for Nurses

Another guide for nurses in making ethical decisions is the *Code for Nurses with Interpretative Statements* published

Critical Thinking

Client Request for Information about Treatment Options

A client who is in her second pregnancy has been told by her physician that she must have a second cesarean section with this pregnancy because she had one for her first birth. She asks you if repeated cesarean sections are always done for subsequent births. You know that her physician always does this without giving clients an option. Other physicians you know do not do this. What would you tell her? How would the principle of respect for autonomy influence your thinking?

Research Highlight

The "Real World" of Hospital Nursing Practice as Perceived by Nursing Undergraduates

Purpose

This study investigated expectations of senior nursing students regarding the ethical dimensions of their nursing role. Nurses who are able to maintain their personal and professional integrity are less likely to burn out. However, new graduates are vulnerable to role compromise.

Methods

Twenty-three senior baccalaureate students completing their program were interviewed and asked to complete written clinical logs regarding professional values, guidelines for conduct, application of a professional code, and thoughts about the nature of future nursing practice. Data collected were subjected to the grounded theory methodology of constant comparison and refinement of interview questions based on prior data analysis.

Findings

Most students were realistic about their future practice but felt relatively powerless as they entered practice. Students indicated a commitment to the principle of respect for clients, which they would promote through listening, accepting clients, providing information, and providing a climate for self-determination. Students felt guilty if they did not advocate for clients and also expressed disappointment when other nurses failed to do so.

Nursing Implications

New graduates lack confidence in their role as ethically competent nurses who can advocate for clients. To reduce the frustration that might result from compromise of integrity, a supportive environment that permits students to build their skills and confidence in their capabilities would be beneficial. Constructive feedback and a transition to greater self-reliance on self-evaluations would assist new nurses in accepting professional responsibility and accountability.

Kelly, B. (1993). The "real world" of hospital nursing practice as perceived by nursing undergraduates. *Journal of Professional Nursing, 9*(1), 27–33.

by the American Nurses Association (1985). **Codes** represent people's acceptance of the obligations and responsibilities entrusted to them by society. The purpose of codes is to provide guidance for action, although codes are not necessarily binding. The *Code for Nurses* has evolved over the past 40 years and currently includes 11 principles for nursing practice: The American Nurses Association Code (Box 5-1) clearly identifies that the fundamental principle of respect for persons is central to nursing practice. According to the code, nurses are to support human dignity and to safeguard the client's welfare.

Ethical Decision-Making Model

Many ethics texts or articles suggest a series of steps that can be used to resolve an ethical dilemma (Davis et al., 1997; Thompson & Thompson, 1990; Silva, 1990; Waithe, et al., 1989). These steps encourage individuals to focus on the situation, gather information, apply ethical theories and principles to guide reasoning, and propose actions for dilemma resolution. By engaging in critical thinking, guided by the model, dilemma resolution can occur.

Box 5-1 American Nurses Association Code for Nurses

1. The nurse provides services with respect for human dignity and the uniqueness of the client, unrestricted by considerations of social or economic status, personal attributes, or the nature of health problems.

2. The nurse safeguards the client's right to privacy by judiciously protecting information of a confidential nature.

3. The nurse acts to safeguard the client and the public when health care and safety are affected by the incompetent, unethical, or illegal practice of any person.

4. The nurse assumes responsibility and accountability for individual nursing judgments and actions.

5. The nurse maintains competence in nursing.

6. The nurse exercises informed judgment and uses individual competence and qualifications as criteria in seeking consultation, accepting responsibilities, and delegating nursing activities to others.

7. The nurse participates in activities that contribute to the ongoing development of the profession's body of knowledge.

8. The nurse participates in the profession's efforts to implement and improve standards of nursing.

9. The nurse participates in the profession's efforts to establish and maintain conditions of employment conducive to high-quality nursing care.

10. The nurse participates in the profession's effort to protect the public from misinformation and misrepresentation and to maintain the integrity of nursing.

11. The nurse collaborates with members of the health professions and other citizens in promoting community and national efforts to meet the health care needs of the public.

Reprinted with permission from *Code for Nurses with Interpretive Statements,* © 1985. American Nurses Publishing, American Nurses Foundation/American Nurses Association, 600 Maryland Avenue, SW, Suite 100W, Washington, DC 20024-2571, p. 1.

Although the number and sequence of steps may vary, similarities exist among models. A composite framework incorporating common aspects of decision-making models can be found in Box 5-2. One of the things that the framework requires is ascertaining which ethical theories and principles are to be applied for dilemma resolution. Additionally, the decision-maker must determine how to weight the theories and principles, i.e., which theory or principle should be the most influential in deciding the correct action? This process is necessary because theoretical perspectives or ethical principles may be in conflict with one another.

To apply the model to a dilemma, nurses should review the case with which they are dealing by responding to the suggested questions. Sometimes nurses feel impatient with having to stop and answer questions, particularly when they are in a situation that may be emotional or frustrating. However, efforts will be rewarded because issues will be clarified, and reasoning based on ethical principles and theories offers perspectives to approach the problem and helps provide a rationale for action. Unfortunately, nurses sometimes find themselves engaged in dilemmas that require resolution over short periods—from seconds to minutes. For this reason, it is helpful to discuss case scenarios with others and practice using the ethical decision-making framework, to increase awareness of is-

Nursing Tip

GETTING SUPPORT WHEN AN ETHICAL DILEMMA OCCURS

Sometimes you may find yourself dealing with an ethical dilemma. In addition to using the dilemma resolution format suggested in this chapter, you may feel that you need some additional support. Support may come from several places.

- There may be administrative support on your nursing unit or clinic.

- Some institutions have a nursing ethics committee for the purpose of providing a forum for nurses to discuss ethical dilemmas they encounter.

- Many institutions have more generalized ethics committees, which are multidisciplinary bodies that discuss and make recommendations about actions that would be appropriate to resolve a dilemma.

Find out what resources your institution has and how nurses can use them.

Client Education

Advance Directives

Ordinarily, nurses specializing in women's health care do not think about teaching clients about advance directives. However, completion of these documents helps clients ensure that their wishes are carried out in circumstances in which they are no longer considered competent. Knowledge of advance directives helps both providers and clients to consider the encompassing totality of the life cycle from birth to death. Consider the following teaching points:

- A Living Will, or a Directive to Physicians and Family or Surrogates—as it is known in some states, permits individuals to indicate their wishes about the medical care that they want to receive in the event of a terminal illness or irreversible condition.

- A medical power of attorney (sometimes known as a durable power of attorney for health care) permits individuals to appoint someone to make decisions regarding medical care when he or she is no longer able to do so.

- Each state has specific laws regarding completion of advance directives. Information regarding specific regulations regarding advance directives can be obtained from health care institutions or from organizations, such as Choice in Dying.

- Copies of a living will or medical power of attorney should be given by the client to the person designated as the decision-maker and to health care providers.

- Having these documents in place helps to ensure that wishes are followed, even if client is no longer competent.

Box 5-2 Ethical Decision-Making Framework

Context

- Who is involved and how are they involved?
- What is the setting of the situation?
- What other information is needed for dilemma resolution?
- What personal beliefs of the nurse may have an impact on this situation?

Clarification of Issues

- What are the ethical issues involved?
- Who should decide the issue?

Identification of Alternatives and Potential Outcomes

- What are the possible alternatives and the potential outcomes of each?

Ethical Reasoning

- What ethical theories and principles have bearing on this situation? How?
- Should some principles or theories be given greater weight in the decision-making process? Why?
- What legal or social constraints are factors in this decision?
- What special obligations might be present in my role as a nurse?

Resolution

- Based on the reasoning above, what is the best action in this situation?
- What would be the best strategy for carrying out this action?

Evaluation

- What were the outcomes of the action?
- Should the same action be chosen when a similar dilemma arises in the future? Why or why not?

sues and potential resolutions. A case study applying the decision-making framework is provided later in this chapter.

Selected Dilemmas in Maternal-Child Practice

Several dilemmas and controversial issues relating to maternal-child practice are now discussed.

Abortion

Abortion, the willful or purposeful termination of a pregnancy, usually within the first trimester, is a controversial issue. The ethics of abortion have been debated, especially considering the question: "up to what point of fetal development and under what circumstances is abortion morally acceptable, if ever?" Individuals with a conservative view toward abortion would propose that abortion is always wrong. A more liberal perspective suggests that abortion should be available to those who desire to terminate their pregnancies, while a moderate view would advocate abortion in selected instances.

Consider some of the following situations: Mary G., an unmarried 16-year-old, discovers she is pregnant; after amniocentesis disclosed the presence of Down syndrome, Shirley B., a 38-year-old woman, is considering terminating her pregnancy; although she did not report it, Fay C. was raped 3 months ago and is now pregnant. Each of these is a scenario in which a woman might want to consider an abortion. However, decision making in this process can be complex and lonely to navigate. Maternal-child nurses often find themselves in a position of providing support for women who are making decisions about whether to terminate a pregnancy. The client education box suggests interventions for nurses working with clients who are considering abortion.

Since the 1973 U.S. Supreme Court decision in the case of *Roe v. Wade,* the right of women to choose abortion has been available in the United States and the debate over the ethical implications has continued. The *Roe v. Wade* decision permitted women to choose abortion within the first trimester, but permitted states the option to regulate abortion to protect the life of the mother during the second trimester. States were also permitted to regulate or prohibit abortion after 28 weeks of pregnancy—the age of fetal viability. Subsequent Supreme Court decisions (*Beal v. Doe* and *Maher v. Roe)* suggested that states were not required to spend federal funds to pay for elective abortions, thereby restricting access to abortion for women who do not have money.

Despite persistent efforts to limit abortion through denial of Medicaid funding for abortions, gag rules prohibiting care providers who are working in clinics that receive federal funding from offering abortion as an option to pregnant women and (unsuccessfully) proposed legislation to limit late-term abortions, abortion remains a legal option for women in this country. Although the U.S. Supreme Court recognized personal privacy derived from constitutional amendments as a legal basis for permitting women and physicians to elect pregnancy termination, ethical debate continues to be divisive. Some opponents of abortion feel that life begins at conception, and therefore, it deserves protection similar to that extended to other humans. Opponents feel abortion is killing and deprives the victim (fetus) of the basic right to life, including the experiences, activities, and enjoyment constituting an individual's future (Marquis, 1996). Those who support the right to choose abortion argue that the fetus does not necessarily have the right to use a woman's body during pregnancy (Thompson, 1996). Another argument supporting the right to choose abortion suggests that there are two senses of being human—a biologic one derived from genetics and a moral one that is contingent on being a full-fledged member of the moral community. If one uses the moral sense of being human, a fetus would never qualify for equal protection of life (Warren, 1996).

Maternal-Fetal Conflict

The following situations are examples of maternal-fetal conflict:

- Annie Z., a pregnant client in your care, continues to use cocaine in spite of education about the harmful effects on the fetus and referrals to a drug abuse program.

- Bess Y. is still smoking during her pregnancy even though she is aware the habit can adversely affect her pregnancy.

- As a result of extended labor, Betty O. has been scheduled for a cesarean section; however, Betty wishes to continue with the labor process and have a vaginal delivery.

- During her second trimester, Nancy D. has been told that she needs to have intrauterine fetal surgery. She considers the procedure risky and wants to refuse.

In each of these instances, pregnant women are being asked to modify behavior or to submit to treatment to benefit their developing fetus. Although most pregnant

Client Education

Working with Clients Considering An Abortion

- Provide relevant information about the pregnancy when it becomes available.

- Remember that religious beliefs and effects on other family members may influence abortion decisions.

- Allow clients time to make the decision. A clinic or office visit is usually not sufficient time for most clients.

- Identify potential sources of client support and assess the adequacy of these sources.

- If clients choose to have an abortion, help them recognize that it is normal to feel a sense of loss after the procedure.

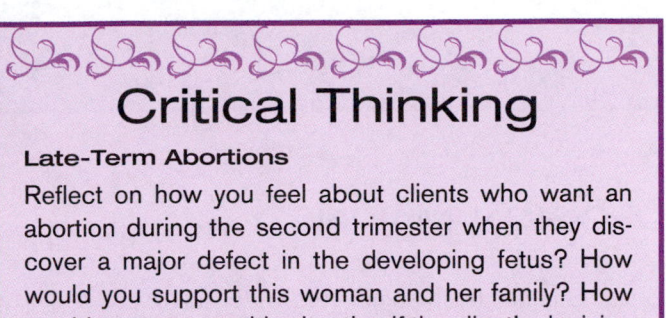

Critical Thinking

Late-Term Abortions

Reflect on how you feel about clients who want an abortion during the second trimester when they discover a major defect in the developing fetus? How would you support this woman and her family? How would you manage this situation if the client's decision was different than the decision you would make?

women would say they want a healthy baby, modifying behaviors or submitting to unwanted intervention during pregnancy is not easy. Maternal-fetal conflict occurs when the interests of a pregnant woman are divergent from the interests of the fetus. For example, a client who smokes may have difficulty stopping a habit that she knows is unhealthy for her fetus. One role of health care providers is to make recommendations that in their opinion are beneficial to the pregnancy. When the pregnant woman disagrees, conflict is inevitable. One way of describing this situation is that there is a conflict between the ethical principles of respect for autonomy (the pregnant mother's decision) and beneficence (what health care providers perceive as beneficial to the fetus). Maternal-fetal conflict has become a more prominent problem with the advent of technology that enables fetal diagnosis and management. The ethical question becomes whether a pregnant woman and her fetus represent one client, and the pregnant woman serves as the decision-maker, or the mother and fetus are really two clients, each with rights and privileges that may compete with one another. In a two-client model, decision-making control could be removed from a pregnant woman and given to another individual who would be responsible for making decisions on behalf of the fetus.

Consider the situation in which a physician has told a woman that she must have a cesarean section and she refuses the intervention. In such a time-limited and potentially risky situation, attempts to use the legal system for problem resolution have ensued. In fact, court-ordered cesarean sections have occurred (Lindgren, 1996). Unfortunately, such court-ordered treatments are coercive and create a conflict between the perceived interests of the woman and the fetus (Lindgren, 1996).

Three competing values may be present in maternal-fetal conflicts: autonomy of the pregnant woman, protection of the fetus, and protection of the common good (Andrews & Patterson, 1995). Ordinarily the right of the person to make autonomous decisions is the most highly

valued. The principles of nonmaleficence and beneficence are used to justify mandating intervention for protection of the fetus. Another argument supporting fetal intervention is that if a woman has chosen to continue a pregnancy, then she has a responsibility to make her pregnancy and therefore her fetus as healthy as possible. A woman's failure to do so may leave her open to more coercive tactics. An argument to support the mother's autonomy is that the fetus maintains its life though the woman's body and as such is inseparable from it. Therefore, a pregnant woman should have sufficient autonomy to make decisions on her own behalf and on behalf of the fetus. Pregnant women do have a responsibility to protect their fetuses, but it does not follow that coercive public policies should force them to do so. Chervenak and McCullough (1992) suggest that a combined approach, based on the viability of the fetus, be a guide in consideration of maternal-fetal conflict. Viable fetuses that could survive outside the uterus should be treated under a beneficence-based obligation to promote fetal welfare. However, if the fetus was pre-viable because of gestational age or not viable because of the severity of a defect, then the mother's autonomy should prevail in decision making.

Whether nurses support the one-client or two-client model of the pregnant woman and fetus, they should work to maximize the client's understanding of behaviors that support good fetal outcomes. They should continue to work to get substance abusers into treatment programs. If a woman is refusing a cesarean section, care providers should seek to find out why. A better understanding may facilitate a resolution that is agreeable to both mother and care provider. Mishkin and Povar (1993) suggest that health care decision making is a joint enterprise between

REFLECTIONS FROM FAMILIES

"It was like a nightmare. I found out that my pregnancy might not be normal and then had to have an ultrasound. Waiting to find out the results was really hard . . . I couldn't sleep. Once I knew for sure there was a problem, I had to decide what to do—whether to keep the pregnancy—and that was even harder than waiting. I wanted to do the right thing, but making the decision to terminate the pregnancy was hard, even though I always have thought of myself as pro-choice."

Case Study/Care Plan

APPLICATION OF AN ETHICAL DECISION-MAKING FRAMEWORK

Marcella G. is a 26-year-old woman who is 5 months pregnant. She has been coming to your clinic for prenatal care since her third month of pregnancy. On her initial visit, another nurse identified that Marcella has a history of active cocaine use. At that time, counseling was given regarding the destructive effects that cocaine could have on the fetus and mother, and a referral to a drug treatment program was made. Now, 2 months later, you discover that the referral appointment has not been kept and that Marcella continues to use cocaine.

Context

Marcella, the client, and the nurse are the primary players. The fetus may be considered a player, if the two-client model, consisting of the fetus and the mother, is used, rather than the one-client model, in which the mother is responsible for decisions on behalf of both herself and the fetus. There may be other health care providers, such as a nurse practitioner, physician, or social worker, who would also be concerned about the continued drug use. The setting is a prenatal clinic. Your personal beliefs are also important: you may feel that maintaining the autonomy of pregnant clients is important or that protection of the fetus has priority.

Clarification of Issues

You must decide your action based on the information that drug use continues. You feel that expectant mothers should make autonomous decisions, but you also recognize that the fetus is at physiologic risk if drug use continues. While the client is a participant in the dilemma, the nurse should decide what her (own) next actions should be.

Identification of Alternatives and Potential Outcomes

1. The nurse could do nothing and let the clinic visits continue, with Marcella using drugs throughout her pregnancy. The potential outcome is that Marcella would continue her prenatal care but the fetus would suffer harm because of the drug use. Also, Marcella would not receive help for her addiction.

2. The nurse can try to persuade Marcella to enter a drug treatment program for the remainder of her pregnancy. This action would support Marcella's autonomy and promote a better pregnancy outcome. Trust for the nurse-client relationship would be maintained.

3. The nurse could report Marcella's continued drug use and see if she could force Marcella to enroll in a treatment program. Coercive behaviors would negate Marcella's right to privacy and autonomy. Trust in the nurse-client relationship would be eroded. However, the fetus would benefit from a drug-free environment.

(continued)

Critical Thinking

Maternal-Fetal Rights: One-Client Or Two-Client Model

Do you perceive pregnant women to fit the one-client or the two-client model? Why?

caregivers and their clients, in which client autonomy and professional standards of care are complementary. In the instance of refusal of fetal surgery, procedures are not routine and involve risk thus the maternal considerations should be thoroughly addressed. Care providers should seek to provide accurate information and support the mother's autonomous decision.

Genetic Mapping

As mapping of the human genome continues, rapid advances are being made in the nature and amount of information that is available to health care consumers. Genetic

Ethical Reasoning

If a two-client model—where the mother and fetus have an equivalent moral status—is assumed, arguments would center around the obligation the mother has to the fetus. If you approached this problem from a utilitarian perspective, you would try to examine the action that would produce the best possible outcome for all concerned, but with a real concern that the mother meet her fetal obligations. Using a one-client model, the autonomy of Marcella in promoting the welfare of the fetus would be important. The nurse favoring a fetal-rights stance would believe that if Marcella wanted to procreate, then she has a special obligation to the fetus. Reporting Marcella and forcing drug program enrollment would probably improve fetal outcome. However, the outcome would be better for all three parties—mother, fetus, and nurse—if the nurse could convince Marcella to enroll in the program on her own volition. The principle of respect for autonomy would help to focus on the unity of the mother and fetus and their mutual welfare. The body of the mother is integral to maintaining fetal safety. Doing nothing to intervene in the process would be the worst option because both the welfare of the mother and the fetus are negated. From a deontologic perspective, the nurse would have to decide the correct action that promotes the autonomy and welfare of pregnant women who use drugs. If the virtue of integrity is considered paramount for practice, the nurse must intervene. The second option of voluntary entry into a drug program would preserve professional integrity of the nurse as well as support maternal autonomy and promote maternal and fetal welfare. Using an ethic of care, the nurse would feel an obligation to promote client well-being and advocate on behalf of the client. This action would be further supported by the *Code for Nurses,* because the nurse would act on behalf of the client to promote the welfare of mother and fetus in the context of respecting client choices. Coercion would be difficult under these circumstances. One legal consideration would be Marcella's parental status if she has positive results on a drug screen at the time of delivery. Potentially, the child could be placed in custody until drug rehabilitation is successfully completed. In this circumstance, if Marcella does not remain drug-free, she could permanently lose custody of her baby.

Resolution

The second option of voluntary entry into the drug program is the best option of the three. To try and coercively modify behavior would be counterproductive. Efforts to maintain the nurse-client relationship should continue. Blaming and hostility on the part of the nurse discourages further efforts to seek help.

Evaluation

Ideally, the outcome would be that Marcella entered the treatment program. Even if Marcella did not initially agree to enroll, the nurse should continue to monitor her pregnancy and continue to encourage help-seeking behaviors. Care should include education, treatment referral, complication prevention, and promotion of optimal parenting.

---

mapping identifies individual genes, their function, and DNA sequences. It is estimated that mapping of the human genome will be completed by the year 2005, with a complete identification of 70,000 to 100,000 genes (Jones, 1996). Many benefits can potentially be derived from this newfound knowledge. Preventive treatments may be available in more instances, and cures for lethal diseases may be found. For example, parents at risk for Huntington's disease—a progressive neurologic disorder—could elect to have preimplantation genetic testing. In this testing, an embryo developed through *in vitro* fertilization would have a genetic analysis completed on one or two cells before cell differentiation. Only embryos without the gene for Huntington's disease would be implanted.

However, genetic information could also be used to great detriment. Insurance agencies or employers may discriminate against individuals or groups who carry particular genes. A central ethical issue in genetics is how to balance the need for genetic information with an individual's right to privacy, particularly when the health care system is moving toward a client-based longitudinal electronic health record (Gostin, 1995). A longitudinal health record would be an electronic database containing all data

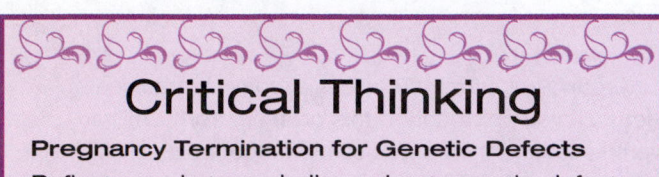

Critical Thinking

Pregnancy Termination for Genetic Defects
Reflect on what you believe about genetic defects. Are there defects that should always be terminated? Are there other genetic defects that never should be terminated?

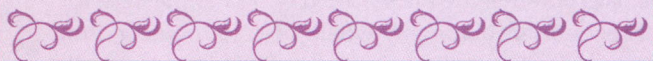

relevant to an individual's health status over a lifetime. Such a database would be available to a wide variety of individuals or institutions, permitting a loss of confidentiality regarding personal health information. Potentially, an individual could lose health benefits or employment or face stigmatization if sensitive genetic information were disclosed.

In addition to privacy, there are other issues related to genetic testing. If testing resources are inadequate—which is often the case with a new technology—it may be difficult to determine who should have priority for testing. Should testing be done for genetic disorders that are currently untreatable? Or should testing be done for parents who wish to choose the gender of their child? Prenatal testing can also create agonizing choices, such as when parents face the choice of whether to terminate a pregnancy because genetic screening indicates the presence of a defect (Penticuff, 1996).

Although many of these questions are difficult to answer, some suggestions about how to approach genetic screening are offered (Penticuff, 1996). Before screening, consideration should be given to the benefits that will be derived and the therapeutic capabilities of treating identified disorders. Laboratory facilities must be adequate and tests should be reliable. Counseling should be available before and after testing so that the need and appropriateness for testing can be explained and the explanation of the findings and their implications can be given. Genetic screening should be voluntary, done with the informed consent of the individual. Findings should remain confidential, disclosed only with the consent of the person tested. However, to ensure confidentiality of information, rigorous safeguards must be legislated; otherwise, insurance providers could secure information and deny coverage (Penticuff, 1996; Gostin, 1995).

Reproductive Technology

The availability of reproductive technologies has produced a new set of ethical dilemmas. These technologies encompass a broad range of techniques, including *in vitro* fertil-

ization, gamete intrafallopian transfer, zygote intrafallopian transfer, ovum transfer, embryo adoption, embryo hosting, and surrogate parenting (see Chapter 14 for a discussion of these techniques). Questions about the use of reproductive technologies have produced a number of court cases because ethical resolution of issues is lacking. The Roman Catholic Church has rejected many of these techniques because of the belief that procreation is the function of marriage and because multiple zygotes must be developed to secure a viable one (Hall, 1996). An alternate perspective supporting the use of technology in insemination is that sexual intimacy and procreation are separate activities (Bandman & Bandman, 1995).

Surrogate motherhood, in which one woman contracts to carry a pregnancy to term for another woman, also poses many problems. Cases have ended in court proceedings, with the surrogate mother not wanting to give up the newborn to the biologic father and his wife. In another instance, none of the contracting parties wanted to keep a newborn with multiple disabilities. Who should be responsible for the emotional welfare and cost of care for this child? At issue is the surrogate mother's right to make an agreement to bear a child and whether that agreement can be broken. Beneficence is a useful ethical principle when considering the welfare of the child born into a surrogate situation.

Unanswered questions surrounding reproductive technologies include:

- To whom should reproductive technologies be available—all who request them or only to married individuals or to those with adequate financial resources?

- Who has ownership of the remaining frozen embryos—the father, the mother, or the potential infant who would be represented through state protection? Lawsuits have occurred during divorces to prevent one spouse from obtaining ownership of frozen embryos.

- Should donors remain anonymous and can they be compensated?

HIV Status Determination

During pregnancy, women infected with untreated human immunodeficiency virus (HIV) have a 25% to 35% chance of transmitting the infection to their unborn child. Transmission can potentially occur via the placenta, during delivery, or through breastfeeding. While many states have instituted anonymous testing of all newborns to establish the prevalence of HIV infection, prenatal testing is not mandated. Prenatal testing has become a more urgent issue since treatment with the antiviral drug zidovudine (AZT or ZDV) has decreased perinatal transmission of HIV (Downes, 1995).

Critical Thinking

HIV Testing for Pregnant Clients
The issue of HIV testing for all pregnant women is controversial. One issue surrounding mandatory testing is what would be done for women who are found to be HIV-infected. Treatment with AZT has been found to reduce the incidence of perinatal transmission. Should pregnant women who are infected be required to submit to treatment to reduce the possibility of HIV transmission to the fetus? What consideration should be given to the wishes of the pregnant woman regarding treatment preferences?

The ethical conflict of HIV screening is related to the client's right to privacy and autonomy to make decisions regarding care versus the benefit that might potentially be derived from accurate knowledge regarding HIV status of the population. Advantages to knowing HIV status include knowing that infected mothers could be at greater personal risk because the pregnancy may alter cell-mediated immunity. Knowledge of HIV status during pregnancy could promote correct diagnosis and treatment, which would decrease complications and the risk of perinatal transmission. However, diagnosis of HIV infection has special social and financial considerations. In addition to the emotional impact of such a diagnosis, employment and insurance may be lost once the diagnosis is disclosed. Also, fear of being tested may prevent some women from seeking prenatal care. Although it may be medically beneficial to establish the diagnosis, policies mandating HIV testing may deter women from receiving care. Insisting that testing be done would undermine the client's autonomy, her right to privacy, and restrict her liberty to control her body.

Nurses need to maintain an open mind when counseling HIV-infected pregnant women. The risk of HIV transmission must be considered in light of the significance of the pregnancy to this woman and the availability of treatment. Women should be informed about the risks of HIV and counseled accordingly. Nurses must be careful to listen to client concerns about testing and treatment options. Treating clients with respect and developing trusting relationships may facilitate testing and treatment (Downes, 1995; Schmeltzer & Whipple, 1991).

Female Circumcision

As more women from other countries immigrate to North America, nurses are seeing a greater incidence of female circumcision, which is also sometimes termed "female genital mutilation" (Gibeau, 1998). Female circumcision is a cultural practice that can involve removal of the prepuce and clitoris or may extend to excision of the labia minora, excision of the labia majora, and closure of the vagina, leaving a small opening (infibulation). Sometimes considered a rite of passage or a mechanism for socialization into the role of a woman, the practice has persisted, particularly in Northern Africa. Female circumcision is considered by some to be a sign of purity and is essential to maintain family honor and to be a desirable mate for marriage (Lane & Rubinstein, 1996; Lightfoot-Klein & Shaw, 1991). Opposition to female circumcision has occurred because it is perceived as subjugation of women.

Female circumcision has also come under criticism because of significant short- and long-term health implications. Short-term complications include hemorrhage, shock, infection, and damage to urethra, vagina, and anus. Long-term complications include recurrent vaginitis and urinary tract infections, keloid scar formation, persistent infection, cysts, vulvar abscesses, dysmenorrhea, painful intercourse, and increased morbidity and mortality related to childbirth (Gibeau, 1998; Lightfoot-Klein & Shaw, 1991). During childbirth, the infibulation must be cut and then resutured following delivery.

National and international groups (including the World Health Organization and UNICEF) have opposed female genital circumcision on the basis of it being a health risk and a human rights violation (Gibeau, 1998). In 1997, federal laws became effective that prohibit female genital surgeries from being performed in the United States on girls under age 18. Yet, the dilemma remains: how can nurses be sensitive to cultural beliefs and also promote practices that enhance the well-being of clients? Nurses may encounter clients who request to be reinfibulated following delivery or may have clients who request female circumcision for their daughters.

The cultural significance of practices must be recognized, even when they differ from the nurse's cultural norms. Women who practice female circumcision come from cultures in which the practice is considered to be normal. While Western concerns make ending female genital surgeries a priority, in the context of other cultures, other priorities, such as ending physical abuse, education, or economics, may prevail (Lane & Rubinstein, 1996). Nurses should recognize that practices exist in Western culture that could be considered equally destructive. For example, breast augmentation to meet a Western cultural standard that large breasts are desirable may be considered abnormal. Often, the principle of autonomy guides the care that nurses provide. However, when cultural practices are physically harmful, such practices are difficult to support. One strategy to resolve the ethical dilemmas of this issue is to express respect for cultural practices but also work to shed new light on the negative health outcomes of female genital surgeries (Lane & Rubinstein, 1996).

Alternative or Complementary Therapies

Alternative or complementary therapies are health-related techniques and practices that are meant to promote healing and, in some instances, complement mainstream medical practices. The focus of these therapies is to treat the person holistically, recognizing that the mind, body, and spirit interact with the environment as a whole. Examples of complementary therapies can include, but are not limited to, healing touch, acupuncture, massage therapy, use of guided imagery, nutrition, yoga, dance, aromatherapy, and folk remedies. The use of complementary and alternative therapies is increasing in health care, and some nurses now incorporate these care modalities into their practices (Simon, 1999). Although client use of alternative therapies is increasing, clients do not necessarily inform their care providers that they are undergoing these therapies, because these practices have been devalued in the past (Nash, 1999). Nurses must be sensitive to client needs with respect to alternative therapies. The principle of respect for autonomy indicates that clients have a need to be informed about potentially useful therapies and make decisions regarding their use. The principle of beneficence indicates that positive acts to improve the welfare of clients should be supported; the principle of nonmaleficence indicates that care should be taken so that harm is not done to patients through either the provision of or withholding of potentially therapeutic opportunities (Nash, 1999). Nurses need to investigate client use of alternative therapies and explore how these practices may be beneficial.

LEGAL ISSUES

As professionals, nurses are both ethically and legally accountable for their practices. Care of pregnant women and newborns requires specialized knowledge, communication, and teamwork among health care providers. Accurate assessment, reporting, and documentation are essential to safe and effective nursing care. When pregnancy and childbirth are involved, most people anticipate normal deliveries and healthy babies. However, adverse events resulting from poor nursing care in the labor room accounted for 128 (17.4%) of a total of 747 malpractice cases in a study conducted by Beckmann (1996). In these cases, poor nursing assessment and medication errors contributed to maternal injuries and death. The purpose of this section is to examine basic aspects of the laws and standards that govern nursing practice, including suggestions for promoting quality care throughout pregnancy.

Basic Legal Concepts

We live according to laws that set minimum standards for behavior. Laws are derived from federal, state, or local sources and provide a necessary order for individuals living within a society. Laws also extend to professional nursing practice that have developed along with laws governing medical practice.

There are two major divisions of law: criminal and civil. **Criminal law** addresses public concerns and punishes the wrongs that threaten a group or society; **civil law** is concerned with and punishes wrongs against the individual (Hall, 1996). Laws are derived from three major sources: statutory law, or those laws passed through legislative process; regulations, which are established by the executive branch (such as President or Governor); and case law, sometimes referred to as common law, which is derived from judicial decisions on specific cases. Some laws from each of these sources concern nurses. Statutory laws, through nurse practice acts, define what constitutes the scope and practice of nursing and determine educational qualifications and titling for registered nurses. The Board of Nurse Examiners for each state helps to establish regulations governing nursing practice and can make decisions regarding issuing or suspending licenses for practice (Figure 5-4). Case law may identify a minimum standard to which a health care provider is expected to adhere. For example, the need for institutions to identify an effective chain of command for dealing with emergencies has been set through case law (Mahlmeister, 1996).

A **tort** is a civil wrong that may be caused either intentionally or unintentionally. **Negligence** occurs when there is an unintentional wrong caused by the failure to act as a reasonable person would under similar circumstances (Mahlmeister, 1996). **Malpractice** is a type of negligence

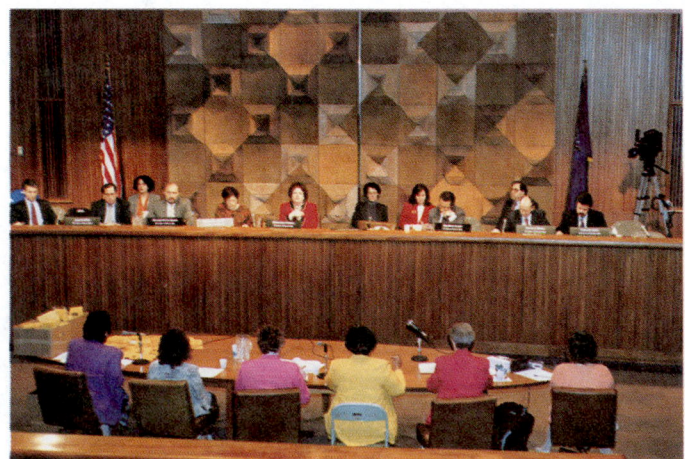

Figure 5-4 Nurses must be involved in legislative activities that are a means of regulating nursing practice. (Photo courtesy of the New York State Nurses Association)

involving the actions of professionals who failed to perform as other competent professionals would in the same set of circumstances. Four components must be present to demonstrate malpractice, including duty, breach of duty, client injury, and proximate cause (Hall, 1996; Mahlmeister, 1996). In a case of malpractice, the defendant must have a duty toward the injured person. For example, a nurse has a duty to provide safe care for a client. That duty must have been breached. In other words, the professional must have failed to act in such a way that the standards of practice were upheld. A common question asked in cases of a breach of duty is: Did the nurse act in a way that a reasonable, prudent nurse would act in a similar situation? Next, an injury must have occurred. The potential for injury is not adequate for establishing malpractice, there must have been an actual injury. Last, the resulting injury must be directly caused by the negligence that occurred. Consider the example of a postpartum client, who had an epidural block, and, while under the influence of the drug, fell and sustained a head injury, because the nurse left the bed rails down and had not instructed the client to seek assistance in walking. The nurse would be considered negligent for not providing safeguards that a reasonable and prudent nurse would have provided under similar circumstances.

Another way of looking at causation is through proving the injury would not have occurred except that the nurse failed to act in a reasonable and prudent manner. As professionals, nurses are expected to possess specialized knowledge and are liable for their actions. The concept of **liability** means that each person is accountable for his or her acts that fail to meet the standards of the profession (Mahlmeister, 1996).

Standards of Care

In addition to laws, standards of care also guide nursing practice. **Standards of care** are documents developed by professional groups to establish a level of practice agreed upon by members of the profession. In many instances, these standards reflect the minimum expectations required of professionals for a safe practice. Because standards are based on current knowledge, they are dynamic and may be subject to change as new information becomes available. Standards of care are sometimes used in legal situations as a yardstick for determining if negligence occurred. Nurses should be knowledgeable about professional standards of practice in their specialty and practice within those guidelines. This professional accountability serves nurses well when issues of liability arise (Mahlmeister, 1996).

A standard used in women's health is published by the Association of Women's Health, Obstetric, and Neonatal Nurses (AWHONN, 1998). These standards are divided into standards for care and professional performance; guidelines for women's, perinatal, and newborn health; acute care; community and home care; and administration. The standards of care section uses the nursing process format and addresses assessment, diagnosis, outcome identification, planning, implementation, and evaluation. The section on professional performance addresses quality of care, performance appraisal, education, collegiality, ethics, collaboration, research, resource utilization, practice environment, and accountability (AWHONN, 1998). The guidelines suggest actions appropriate to nursing practice in specific areas of maternal-child nursing.

Additional sources of standards are the scope and standards for nursing practice developed by each state's Board of Nurse Examiners, and standards developed by individual institutions and found in policy and procedure manuals. Sometimes it is difficult for nurses to assess whether they are practicing within the scope and standards of nursing. Suggested questions that nurses may ask to determine the acceptability of their practices or any given activity include (Flores, 1997, pp. 6–7):

- Is the activity consistent with the state's Nurse Practice Act and rules and regulations of the Board of Nurse Examiners?
- Is the activity in accordance with established policies and procedures of the institution?
- Is the act supported by research or in the scope and standards of practice statements?
- Does the nurse possess the required knowledge and demonstrated competency in performing the activity?
- Would a reasonable and prudent nurse perform the activity in this setting?
- Is the nurse prepared to assume accountability for the provision of safe care and the outcomes rendered?

If nurses are knowledgeable and able to respond affirmatively to each of these questions, then the activity in question should be within the scope and standards of practice. Flores suggests that referring to a decision-making model such as this one becomes more automatic with routine use, ensuring more critical thinking about practice issues and empowering nurses to be proactive.

Practicing Safely in Perinatal Settings

A holistic, interpersonal approach to care and adequate documentation are essential components of safe nursing practice and serve to reduce the risks of liability. Competent care requires a team approach, with nurses playing a key role in assessment and communication (Fiesta, 1995).

McMullen and Philipsen (1995) offer suggestions to decrease litigation and to improve care throughout a client's pregnancy (Philipsen & McMullen, 1994a; 1994b). Believing that interpersonal care and communication are important factors in reducing liability, McMullen and Philipsen (1995) suggest that nurses must establish good rapport with clients and their families. Nurses should encourage input from clients and families, allowing sufficient time for questions and dialogue. These measures enhance communication, health teaching, and interpersonal relationships. Good rapport with clients helps them to feel respected and well cared for during pregnancy (Philipsen & McMullen, 1994b). These measures also improve continuity of client care and reduce potential liability.

Policies and procedures are also an important factor in safe nursing practice. Policies and procedures should be updated regularly and should be realistic within the framework of practice (McMullen & Philipsen, 1995). When new practices become accepted, institutions should revise existing policies to reflect correct practice guidelines so that nurses are not left in the position of trying to implement updated practices that are not in the hospital procedure manual. Nurses also should be able to perform the outlined procedures within the context of the work setting. Otherwise, the policy should be examined and a safe, but more feasible, policy substituted. Nurses should be aware of what constitutes safe practice and know how policies are changed in their institution.

As institutions cut costs, the skill mix of the nursing staff may change, leading to greater use of unlicensed assistive personnel (UAPs) for providing client care. To efficiently practice, registered nurses are responsible for delegating selected care tasks to UAPs. The function of UAPs is to complement performance of nursing functions rather than to substitute for the registered nurse. To promote safe

practice, nurses should be familiar with state regulations governing delegation, so that appropriate tasks are delegated for UAPs to carry out. The *Standards and Guidelines for Professional Nursing Practice in the Care of Women and Newborns* (AWHONN, 1998) suggest that task delegation should be based on client needs and the knowledge and skill of the provider designated to perform the task.

During pregnancy, the prenatal care offered should meet nationally established standards and be documented accordingly. An area of particular concern during the first trimester of pregnancy is giving adequate information to the client regarding the availability of prenatal tests, such as chorionic villus sampling, amniocentesis, triple screen of alpha-fetoproteins, and screens for some teratogenic communicable diseases (Philipsen & McMullen, 1994a). Not only should this information be given to clients, but their response should also be documented in the medical record. If testing is done, findings should be communicated to the client and, if necessary, options explored. Once again, this information, including options and the client's response, should be documented. Another area of concern during the first trimester is that pregnancy and possible risks be correctly diagnosed so that early intervention can begin. Remember when working with all women of childbearing age to consider the possibility of pregnancy, especially women presenting with abdominal pain and a potential ectopic pregnancy.

Later in pregnancy, testing remains a significant issue. Once again, nurses should be careful to inform clients about the availability of specific testing, including the potential risks and benefits, and record the expectant mother's response (Philipsen & McMullen, 1994b). Even routine test results, such as those from urinalysis, blood cell counts, and blood pressure measurement, should be documented. Other common tests include nonstress, contraction stress, oxytocin challenge, and biophysical profiles. Communication of results, assessment of client understanding, provision of health education, and documentation of client response remain important. When there is a lack of documentation and an adverse outcome, it is difficult to demonstrate that standards of care have been met, creating an opportunity for liability to be assessed.

Another legal issue centers around antepartum clients being discharged from labor and delivery because they are not yet ready to deliver. Before discharge, there should be documentation of at least two assessments, noting any change in client condition and a baseline fetal monitor strip from 20 to 30 minutes of observation. Assessment should include vital signs and examination of the cervix. The physician or nurse-midwife must be notified of the client's presenting condition and reassessment before discharge (Rommal, 1996). If clients are discharged before delivery, written discharge instructions should be re-

Critical Thinking

Unrealistic Hospital Policy

You are a nurse working in labor and delivery. One of the policies of your institution is that all women in the first stage of labor be monitored every 15 minutes and a charted entry regarding their status be made. Checks may include vital signs, assessment of fetal heart rate, and vaginal examination. While you feel that frequent checks are important, the staffing of your unit does not allow nurses sufficient time to meet this policy. Consequently, nurses do not follow this policy. How would you respond to this situation?

viewed, signed by the mother, and a copy given to the mother (McMullen & Philipsen, 1995). This opportunity presents an excellent chance to answer any questions a mother may have.

Nurses must be knowledgeable about the expected practices of physicians and question the appropriateness of physician orders when deviations from standards occur. These activities can be called affirmative duty actions, in which nurses are expected to protect clients from harm (Mahlmeister, 1996). In the process of reporting emergencies, nurses must be familiar with the established chain of command in the institution. For example, the chain of command for a staff nurse may begin with the nurse manager and then the nurse supervisor. If the complaint concerns an obstetrician and cannot be resolved at that level, then the Chief of Obstetrics may be called. The hospital administrator may be a part of the chain of command. Nurses should know when to activate the chain of command and when it is appropriate to move up the chain of command (Mahlmeister, 1996). When seeking help, nurses should remember that prompt reporting facilitates problem resolution and that persistence can help ensure that clients

Research Highlight

Informed Consent for Maternal Serum Alpha-Fetoprotein Screening

Purpose

To determine if pregnant women who received information regarding measurement of maternal serum alpha-fetoprotein (MSAFP) levels understood information sufficiently to sign an informed consent.

Methods

Fifty-three inner-city pregnant women were given an explanation of screening for MSAF by a care provider and viewed an explanatory videotape. An interview using open-ended questions to assess understanding of the screening process followed the information-giving process.

Findings

Although most women were able to correctly identify that MSAFP required a blood sample and had no risks, only 74% were able to correctly identify that it tested for "birth defects" and 62% could identify what MSAFP was and what the tests are used for. Only 45% recognized that a positive test result required follow-up, and only 22% respectively could identify what a high-positive and low-positive MSAFP test result meant.

Nursing Implications

These findings revealed that women in this study met only part of the criteria for informed consent. While the consent may have been voluntarily given by a competent woman who had been given information regarding the test, a substantial portion of the women did not understand the meaning and implications of the test. Nurses should request information from clients to ensure their understanding. Suggested questions might include:

What do you call your condition?

Which treatment is being recommended?

What is the treatment supposed to do for you?

Are there risks associated with the treatment?

What alternatives are there to the treatment?

Freda, M., DeVore, N., Valentine-Adams, N., Bombard, A., & Merkatz, I. (1998). Informed consent for maternal serum alpha-fetoprotein screening in an inner city population: How informed is it? *JOGNN, 27*(1), 99–106.

receive appropriate care. Following these guidelines should promote safe client care and reduce opportunities for negligence to occur.

Legal Issues in Maternal-Child Practice

Two issues that nurses often encounter in maternal-child practice are informed consent and the right to privacy.

Informed Consent

Informed consent is an issue that has well-defined legal and ethical foundations. Based on a client's right to self-determination, **informed consent** demands that information regarding treatment procedures be given to clients and their consent secured. To obtain a valid consent, clients must be presented with information regarding the course of treatment; methods by which the treatment is carried out; any alternative forms of treatment available, including the inherent risks and benefits of each option; and risks of nontreatment. If any of these areas is not included, then the consent process is incomplete.

The amount of information clients must be given to consider the consent to be informed varies according to the standard used. The most commonly used standard is the community standard in which the amount of information given would be similar to what other health care professionals would give in similar circumstances. Another option, the reasonable client standard, requires the amount of information given be sufficient for a hypothetical reasonable client to make a decision. The reasonable client standard is becoming more commonly accepted. A third standard, the individual client standard, asks what information this individual client needs to make a decision (Bernzweig, 1996); this subjective standard tends to be the least used.

Physicians are responsible for determining the competency of clients and providing information to clients for consent. If permissible by hospital policy, nurses can witness consent documents, but should witness the physician obtaining the signature on the form (Figure 5-5). If nurses feel that a valid consent is lacking, then the nursing supervisor or physician should be notified (Fiesta, 1994). For example, clients facing a cesarean section should be informed of the nature of the procedure, the risks involved, and options before signing a consent. Nurses should work to ensure that clients are well-informed.

Closely related to informed consent is the right of competent individuals to refuse treatment. In maternal-child nursing, treatment refusal carries particular significance because the well-being of the fetus may be affected by maternal decisions. The issue of viewing pregnant women by a one-client or two-client model affects the

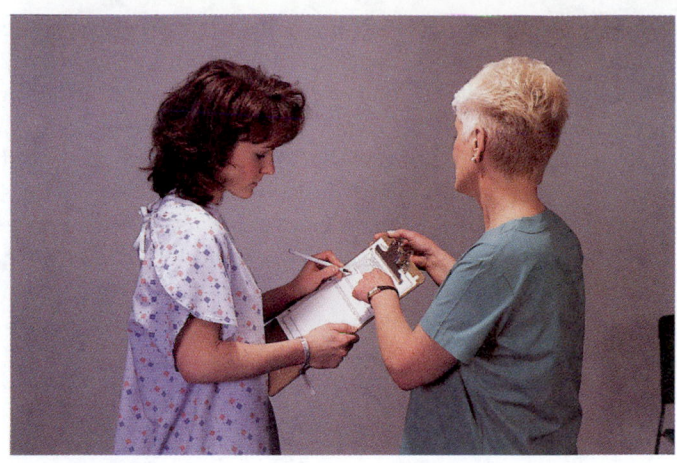

Figure 5-5 Nurses can play an important role in a client's informed consent.

right of refusal. Every effort should be made to ensure that pregnant women are well-informed of their options and that treatment decisions are not coercive.

Right to Privacy

In recognition of care providers having access to sensitive information about clients, certain legal, professional, and ethical standards have been developed to help ensure a client's right to privacy. A client's right to privacy means that nurses should not unnecessarily expose a client's body or disclose information to unauthorized parties. During labor and delivery, many personnel may be in and out of the client's room. To protect privacy, only those responsible for care should have room access. Measures, such as drawing a

REFLECTIONS FROM NURSES

"In the United States, fathers are encouraged to play an active role during pregnancy and the birth process. However, in other cultures men do not participate in the event of birthing. As a nurse, I find it challenging to manage family dynamics when caring for a family whose values differ from mine. To provide sensitive care, I make an effort to ask the pregnant woman if she will have a partner or coach during the labor and delivery process. Her answer helps me better understand her expectations of support during the childbirth experience."

curtain or closing doors during examinations, should be taken to afford privacy. Casual conversation in the hall or elevators about clients under care should be avoided. Health care providers should access information only for clients in their care. It is often tempting to review a chart of a friend or colleague receiving care. However, a client's right to privacy would prohibit securing this information.

PRACTICE IMPLICATIONS FOR MATERNAL-CHILD NURSING

Maternal-child nurses face a complex array of ethical and legal issues in practice. With some reflection and planning, nurses can prepare themselves to manage difficult clinical situations proactively. First, nurses need to identify their practice values and identify the ethical stances that are the most compatible with practice and think about how these can be incorporated into daily practice. Would a utilitarian perspective focusing on outcomes be the best decision guide? Or is a primary goal of practice to deliver care that maintains a sense of personal and professional integrity? Consider the implications of being a caring advocate for clients. Remember that even though nurses are charged with promoting the client's best interest, not all clients share the same value system.

Nursing Tip

BUILDING KNOWLEDGE AND EXPERIENCE

Knowledge and experience are powerful tools in practice. Be knowledgeable about maternal-child nursing and about the standards of care and policies that govern practice. Make critical analysis of client care part of a daily routine. Find expert practitioners who integrate ethical practice and promote high standards of care. These tasks strengthen the quality of your practice and provide a mechanism for you to become an experienced nurse.

Nurses also need to function within the context of a legal framework. Nurses should be familiar with regulations governing their practice and should incorporate an understanding of the regulations of the Board of Nurse Examiners, have a thorough grounding in delegation, and be familiar with the Standards of Practice for Maternal-Child nurses.

Web Activities

- Explore the Internet Encyclopedia of Philosophy: http://www.utm.edu/research/iep/. Many of the selections here reflect a more theoretical aspect of ethics. Review the portion of this chapter that discusses ethical theories and principles. What more can you discover about these areas on this website?

- Visit and explore the website for advanced directives: http://www.choices.org. How might this information be useful to you personally as well as to you in your role as a nurse working in women's health?

- Visit the American Nurses Association website: http://www.nursingworld.org. Click on the ethics site. What kind of position statements do you find there that are related to the topic of ethics and women's health? Think about women's health from a broad perspective and remember to include issues such as childbearing, violence against women, genetics, HIV, and eldercare.

- Explore the health law resource: http://www.netreach.net/%7Ewmanning/. Click onto the bioethics section. What topics here might provide useful knowledge regarding women's health nursing practice?

Key Concepts

- Ethics provides rules and principles that can be used for resolving ethical dilemmas. Ethical decisions tend to be reflective and may be influenced by values, beliefs, and personal interpretations.

- Laws are rules that represent the minimum standard of morality and govern the behavior of individuals. Laws are written to promote the welfare of society.

(continued)

- Standards of care are developed by professional groups to establish a level of practice agreed upon by members of the profession.

- Utilitarianism is an ethical theory that focuses on the consequences of action. Actions bringing about good consequences are considered the best.

- Deontology is an ethical theory that is concerned with doing the right action rather than with the consequences of the action. Actions selected should be ones that could be followed in other similar situations.

- Virtue ethics focus on developing desirable personal attributes and acting in a manner that is congruent with those attributes.

- An ethic of care is a nursing perspective that recognizes the personal concerns and vulnerabilities of clients in health and illness. Nurses, operating under the tenets of an ethic of care, would be willing to provide care to achieve therapeutic goals without expectation of reciprocity.

- In holistic ethics there is a concern both for the outcome of a decision and the intrinsic nature of the act itself. Acts are selected based on a desire to do good and to contribute to the unity of the self and universe.

- Respect for autonomy recognizes the right of competent individuals to make informed choices on their own behalf.

- Nonmaleficence suggests that health care providers must exercise due care to prevent client harm.

- Beneficence is an ethical principle focusing on promoting the welfare of others.

- Justice provides a mechanism for making decisions about dividing benefits and burdens within society.

- The American Nurses Association *Code for Nurses* supports the concept of respect for persons and safeguarding a client's welfare. The code offers guidance for nursing actions.

- Ethical decision making is best when conducted in a systematic manner that carefully examines characteristics of the situation and uses ethical theories and principles as tools.

- Malpractice occurs when professionals are negligent and fail to perform as other professionals would in a similar set of circumstances. Malpractice consists of a breach of duty, resulting in client injury that is directly related to the negligence.

- Interpersonal care and good communication are key factors in reducing the risks of liability.

- Nurses should be proactive in their care approach, i.e., be knowledgeable about perinatal nursing practice, legal issues, and standards of care. Adequate patient assessment, communication with other care providers, and documentation are essential to safe practice.

Review Questions and Activities

1. Discuss informed consent with your classmates. Have one group describe the kinds of information that might be disclosed about a cesarean section when using the reasonable person standard. Another group can describe the information that might be given when using the community standard. The third group should describe information to be given when using the individual client standard. Share your information with the other groups and compare the nature of the information divulged. What ethical principles support the concept of informed consent?

2. Review the case study. What other arguments or viewpoints might be considered for trying to persuade Marcella to enter the drug rehabilitation program or for coercing her into the program? In this situation, what type of actions would the one-client model support? What actions would a two-client model permit? Which would the best model to use in your ethical thinking? Why?

3. The ethical perspective focusing on a sense of commitment to clients and advocacy on their behalf is:
   a. Virtue ethics
   b. Deontology
   c. Ethic of caring
   d. Utilitarianism
   The correct answer is c.

4. The ethical principle concerned with distributing benefits and burdens is:
   a. Respect for autonomy
   b. Justice
   c. Nonmaleficence
   d. Beneficence
   The correct answer is b.

5. Due care is both an ethical and legal concept that indicates that care providers should:
   a. Encourage client decision making
   b. Promote client autonomy
   c. Divide benefits carefully

d. Exercise caution to prevent unintentional harms
The correct answer is d.

6. A health care provider interferes with the decisions of a competent person for the purpose of promoting the competent person's welfare. This statement is an example of:
a. Paternalism
b. Beneficence
c. Autonomy
d. Due care
The correct answer is a.

7. While a client was in labor, health care providers failed to note early signs of fetal distress, although a later review of fetal-monitor readouts clearly indicated that distress occurred. Following delivery, the baby appears to be healthy and has Apgar scores that are within normal limits. As a nurse, you are being pressured to omit those sample monitor strips from the labor and delivery record. What legal and ethical obligations should you consider as you respond to this situation? How will these obligations influence your response? Are there ever circumstances where modifying the medical record would be appropriate? Why or why not?

References

American Holistic Nurses' Association. (1995). *Code of ethics for holistic nurses*. Raleigh, NC: Author.

American Nurses' Association. (1985). *Code for nurses with interpretative statements*. Washington, DC: Author.

Andrews, A., & Patterson, E. (1995). Searching for solutions to alcohol and other drug abuse during pregnancy: Ethics, values, and constitutional principles. *Social Work, 40,*(1), 55–64.

AWHONN. (1998). *Standards and guidelines for professional nursing practice in the care of women and newborns* (5th ed.). Washington, DC: Author.

Bandman, E., & Bandman, B. (1995). *Nursing ethics throughout the lifespan* (3rd ed.). Norwalk, CT: Appleton & Lange.

Beauchamp, T., & Childress, J. (1994). *Principles of biomedical ethics,* (4th ed.). New York: Oxford University Press.

Beckmann, J. (1996). *Nursing negligence: Analyzing malpractice in the hospital setting*. Thousand Oaks, CA: Sage.

Benner, P, & Wrubel, J. (1989). *The primacy of caring: Stress and coping in health and illness*. Menlo Park, CA: Addison.

Benner, P., Tanner, C., & Chesla, C. (1996). *Expertise in nursing practice: Caring, clinical judgment and ethics*. New York: Springer.

Bernzweig, E. (1996). *The nurse's liability for malpractice,* (6th ed.). New York: Mosby.

Bishop, A., & Scudder, J. (1996). *Nursing ethics: Therapeutic caring presence*. Boston: Jones & Bartlett.

Chervenak F., & McCullough, L. (1992). Fetus as patient: An ethical concept. *Contemporary OB/GYN, 37,*(10), 11–16, 22.

Davis, A., Aroskar, M., Liaschenko, J., & Drought, T. (1997). *Ethical dilemmas in nursing practice* (4th ed.). Stamford, CT: Appleton & Lange.

Downes, J. (1995). The ethical dilemmas of mandatory prenatal and newborn HIV testing. *Nursing Connections, 8*(4), 43–50.

Fiesta, J. (1995). Assessment and communication. *Nursing Management, 26*(6), 22, 24.

Fiesta, J. (1994). *Twenty legal pitfalls for nurses to avoid*. Albany, NY: Delmar.

Flores, K. (1997). Scope of practice, Part III: The decision-making model. *RN Update, 28*(4), 6–7.

Frankena, W. (1973). *Ethics* (2nd ed.). Englewood Cliffs, NJ: Prentice Hall.

Freda, M., DeVore, N., Valentine-Adams, N., Bombard, A., & Merkatz, I. (1998). Informed consent for maternal serum alpha-fetoprotein screening in an inner city population: How informed is it? *JOGNN, 27*(1), 99–106.

Fry, S. (1988). The ethic of caring: Can it survive in nursing? *Nursing Outlook, 36*(1), 48.

Gadow, S. (1988). Covenant without cure: Letting go and holding on in chronic illness. In J. Watson & M. Ray, (Eds.) *The Ethics of Care and the Ethics of Cure: Synthesis in Chronicity*. New York: National League for Nursing.

Gibeau, A. (1998). Female genital mutilation: When a cultural practice generates clinical and ethical dilemmas. *JOGNN, 27*(1), 85–91.

Gostin, L. (1995). Genetic privacy. *Journal of Law, Medicine, & Ethics, 23,* 320–330.

Hall, J.K. (1996). *Nursing ethics and law*. Philadelphia: W.B. Saunders.

Jones, S. (1996). Genetics: Changing health care in the 21st century. *JOGNN, 25*(9), 777–783.

Kant, I. (1981). *Grounding for the metaphysics of morals* (J. Ellington, trans.). Indianapolis, IN: Hackett Publishing. (Original work published 1785).

Keegan, L. (1995). Holistic ethics. In B. Dossey, L. Keegan, C. Guzzeta, & L. Krolkmeier, (Eds.) *Holistic nursing: A handbook for practice*. (pp. 137–151). Gaithersberg, MD: Aspen.

Kelly, B. (1993). The "real world" of hospital nursing practice as perceived by nursing undergraduates. *Journal of Professional Nursing, 9*(1), 27–33.

Lane, S., & Rubinstein, R. (1996). Judging the other: Responding to traditional female genital surgeries. *Hastings Center Report, 26*(3), 31–40.

Lightfoot-Klein, H., & Shaw, E. (1991). Special needs of ritually circumcised women patients. *JOGNN, 20*(2), 102–107.

Lindgren, K. (1996). Maternal-fetal conflict: Court-ordered cesarean section. *JOGNN, 25*(8), 653–656.

Mahlmeister, L. (1996). The perinatal nurse's role in obstetric emergencies: Legal issues and practice issues in the era of health care redesign. *Journal of Perinatal and Neonatal Nursing, 10*(3), 32–46.

Mappes, T., & DeGrazia, D. (1996). *Biomedical ethics* (4th ed.). New York: McGraw-Hill.

Marquis, D. (1996). Why abortion is immoral. In T. Mappes & D. DeGrazia (Eds.). *Biomedical ethics* (4th ed.) (pp. 441–444). New York: McGraw-Hill.

McMullen, P., & Philipsen, N. (1995). Fetal well being III: Strategies to diminish liability and improve client care in all trimesters. *Nursing Connections, 8*(1), 50–53.

Miller, B. (1981). Autonomy and the refusal of lifesaving treatment. *Hastings Center Report, 11*(4), 22–28.

Mishkin, D., & Povar, G. (1993). Decision making with pregnant patients: A policy born of experience. *Journal on Quality Improvement, 19*(8), 291–302.

Nash, R. (1999). The biomedical ethics of alternative, complementary, and integrative medicine. *Alternative Therapies, 5*(5), 92–95.

Noddings, N. (1984). *Caring: A feminine approach to ethics and moral education.* Los Angeles, CA: University of California Press.

Penticuff, J. (1996). Ethical dimensions of genetic screening: A look into the future. *JOGNN, 25*(9), 785–789.

Philipsen, N., & McMullen, P. (1994a). Fetal well being I: The health care provider's responsibility in the first trimester. *Nursing Connections, 7*(2), 32–33.

Philipsen, N. & McMullen, P. (1994b). Fetal well being II: Health care providers' responsibility in late pregnancy. *Nursing Connections, 7*(3), 52–54.

Rommal, C. (1996). Risk management issues in the perinatal setting. *Journal of Perinatal and Neonatal Nursing, 10*(3), 1–31.

Ross, W. D. (1994). The personal character of duty. In P. Singer (Ed.). *Ethics.* (pp. 332–337). New York: Oxford University Press.

Scanlon, C. (1994). Ethics survey looks at nurses' experiences. *The American Nurse. 26,* 1, 22.

Schmeltzer, S., & Whipple, B. (1991). Women and HIV infection. *Image, 23*(4), 249–255.

Silva, M. (1990). *Ethical decision making in nursing administration.* Norwalk, CT: Appleton & Lange.

Singer, P. ed. *Ethics.* (pp. 185–188). New York: Oxford University Press.

Simon, J. (1999). The explosion of complementary and alternative therapies. *Nursing Diagnosis, 10*(3), 91.

Thompson, J. (1996). A defense of abortion. In T. Mappes & D. DeGrazia (Eds.). *Biomedical ethics* (4th ed.) (pp. 445–452). New York: McGraw-Hill.

Thompson, J., & Thompson, H. (1990). Ethical decision making: Process and models. *Neonatal Network, 9*(1), 69–70.

Waithe, M., Duckett, L., Schmitz, K., Crisham, P., & Ryden, M. (1989). Developing case situations for ethics education in nursing. *Journal of Nursing Education, 28*(4), 175–180.

Warren, M.A. (1996). On the moral and legal status of abortion. In T. Mappes & D. DeGrazia (Eds.). *Biomedical ethics* (4th ed.) (pp. 434–440). New York: McGraw-Hill.

Wicker, P. (1988). Discussion group summary: When caring doesn't mean curing. In J. Watson & M. Ray, Eds. *The Ethics of Care of the Ethics of Cure: Synthesis in Chronicity.* New York: National League for Nursing.

Suggested Readings

Dossey, B., Keegan, L., Guzzeta, C. & L. Krolkmeier, C. (1995). *Holistic nursing: A handbook for practice.* Gaithersberg, MD: Aspen.

Resources

Advanced directives: Choice in Dying, 1035 30th Street, NW, Washington, DC 20007, 1-800-989-9455, http://www.choices.org

American Nurses Association: 600 Maryland Avenue, SW, Suite 100 West, Washington, DC 20024, 1-800-274-4ANA, http://www.nursingworld.org/

The Association of Women's Health, Obstetric, and Neonatal Nurses (AWHONN): 700 14th Street, NW, Suite 600, Washington, DC 20005-2019, (202)662-1600

Health law resource: http://www.netreach.net%7Ewmanning/

Internet Encyclopedia of Philosophy, http://www.utm.edu/research/iep/

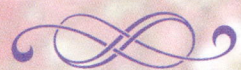

CHAPTER 6

Home Visiting Programs and Perinatal Nursing

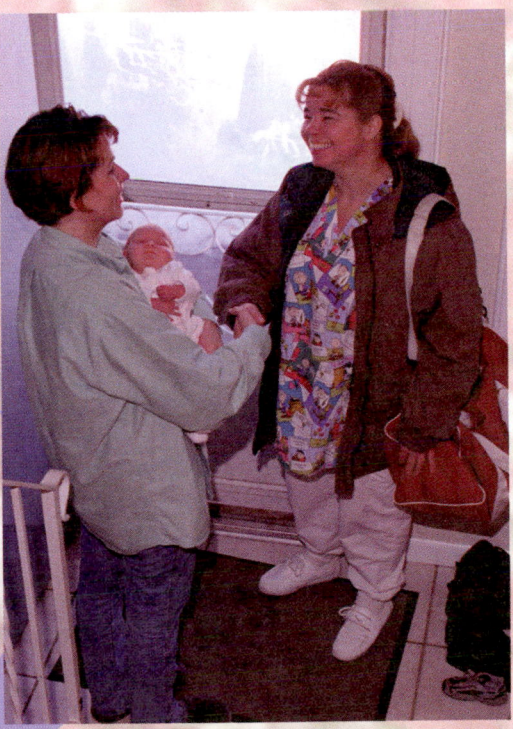

*N*urses working in home care develop a unique and special relationship with the clients and families they serve. For many nurses, this helping relationship is particularly memorable.

- *How do I feel about entering a stranger's home to provide care?*

- *How do I provide nursing care in the home compared with the hospital or clinic setting?*

- *What are my feelings about cultural and spiritual differences in family life?*

- *What can I do if I cannot address the client's needs in the home?*

- *What can I do if my clients become too attached to me?*

- *How do I terminate a long-term home visiting relationship?*

Key Terms

Case management, care coordination	Empowerment Enablement	Enhancement Home visit

Competencies

Upon completion of this chapter, the reader should be able to:

1. Discuss the history of home visitation, and describe how current trends in home visitation parallel or differ from the historical effort.
2. Define home visiting.
3. List at least three principles of home visiting, and discuss how they might be incorporated into home visiting practice.
4. List three advantages and disadvantages of home visiting.
5. Discuss the process of providing a home visit in terms of assessment, nursing diagnosis, outcome identification, planning, intervention, and evaluation.
6. List three essential skills for home visitation, and discuss how these skills might be integrated into each phase of the home visiting process.
7. Describe at least two proven outcomes from home visitation, and apply this research to the development of an evaluation plan for a home visiting program.
8. Discuss termination of the home visiting relationship, and describe how the nurse can set the stage for termination throughout each phase of the home visiting process.

Home visitation has long been used as a strategy to provide direct health care services, health education, and psychosocial support to clients and families. Recent changes in the health care environment, emphasizing cost containment and shifting of care to nonhospital settings, have resulted in an even larger number of clients receiving services in their homes for a variety of reasons. Home visiting interventions frequently are employed to care for women and newborns during the postpartum period and to provide education and support to new families. Proponents believe that this service delivery strategy offers unique benefits to clients and their families.

Owing to the increase in home-based services, nurses must be familiar with home care concepts. This chapter focuses on the *process* of serving clients and families in their homes, emphasizing the nursing process in terms of assessment, nursing diagnosis, expected outcomes, planning, intervention, and evaluation.

HISTORICAL BACKGROUND

Informal home visiting efforts have been ongoing throughout time as family members, friends, and significant others have helped care for sick and less fortunate persons. In the late 1800s, home visiting efforts became more organized in response to the increase in immigration and industrialization in the United States. Lay women, known as "friendly visitors," visited immigrants and the poor to provide friendship and "moral and behavioral guidance" (Hoover et al., 1996). These charitable efforts, aimed at what was perceived as the need to improve the character of poor people, were seen as a way of resolving the pervasive societal problems caused by urban poverty, personal irresponsibility, and classism (Boyer, cited in Weiss, 1993). The need for a more organized approach to these issues led to the development of settlement houses designed to provide more formal assistance to new immigrants in acculturating to American life. Indeed, these settlement programs can be viewed as a precursor to current nationwide home visitation efforts to promote family support (Klass, 1996).

The 20th century brought a firm commitment to social reform and the field of social work. In 1909, Theodore Roosevelt convened the first White House Conference on Children, which focused on the necessity of maintaining a good home environment for children (Bremner, 1971). This conference led to the development of the Child Welfare League of America. The League sanctioned the use of public funds for home visiting for the purpose of fostering

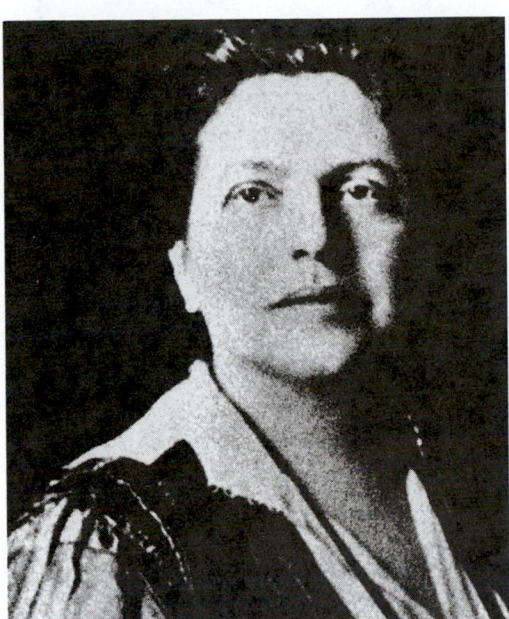

Figure 6-1 Lillian Wald. (Photo courtesy of the American Nurses Association.)

family life. This era of social reform lasted well into the 1920s, when a focus on efficiency led to a shift from home to office-based services (Wasik, Bryant, and Lyons, 1990). The War on Poverty in the 1960s again saw home visiting being promoted as a means of assisting low-income families to overcome the multigenerational problems associated with poverty (Klass, 1996). In the child welfare arena today, home visitation often is the cornerstone of efforts to promote family preservation and support.

The nursing profession has a long history of involvement in home care. Florence Nightingale, as well as others, argued that nurses should be trained to provide care to the sick in their homes (Wasik, 1993). Lillian Wald (Figure 6-1) established the Henry Street Settlement House in the 1890s where nurses provided both preventive and acute health care to the needy. By 1910, visiting nurse associations (VNAs) had developed in urban areas focusing primarily on maternal-child health. VNAs continued to thrive, in many cases functioning as a cornerstone for community health efforts in large cities and towns. Today, home health care is emerging as one of the fastest-growing specialties in nursing. Nurses continue to provide an increasing array of acute care services in the home for adult and pediatric clients and to use the home as a base for delivering preventive health services and health education to pregnant and parenting families.

COMMUNITY HEALTH CONCEPTS

For the most part, traditional nursing practice focuses on health maintenance and disease prevention for an individual client. Community health practice moves beyond this focus on the individual to encompass the health of the entire community. Health is defined quite broadly to include not only the absence of disease but the promotion and maintenance of wellness in the physical, emotional, social, cultural, and spiritual domains. Community or public health practice ensures a high-level of wellness and quality of life for all members of a given population. A report by the Institute of Medicine entitled "The future of public health" (1988) describes this function as "assuring conditions in which people can be healthy."

Given this focus, it is not surprising that most efforts in community or public health are preventive in nature, because the best way to *be* healthy is to *stay* healthy. The three levels of community health prevention can be defined as primary, secondary, and tertiary. Preventive efforts can target the individual or the community as a whole. *Primary prevention* describes interventions that promote general health or well-being or those that prevent the development of health problems (Woods & Mitchell, 1997). Primary prevention related to maternity care can include education about folic acid use preconceptually and during early pregnancy to decrease the incidence of neural tube defects in the fetus and promotion of early access to and use of prenatal care. These interventions can be initiated at both the individual and community level. For example, every woman of childbearing age should be counseled by her health care provider about the benefits of folic acid. At the community level, a local or state health entity may initiate a campaign to inform the community at large about the benefits of folate. Secondary prevention focuses on early diagnosis and treatment of existing health problems with the goal of preventing serious sequelae (Woods & Mitchell, 1997). Efforts relative to secondary prevention include screening a prenatal client for signs and symptoms of preeclampsia at every home visit (individual level) or initiating a series of smoking cessation classes for pregnant women in the community (community level). *Tertiary prevention* consists of efforts to reestablish a high level of wellness after amelioration of a health problem or to prevent recurrence of a previous health problem (Woods & Mitchell, 1997). Recommending prenatal diagnosis and genetic counseling to a family with a previous history of Down syndrome illustrates tertiary prevention at the client level. At the community level, an example of this third level of presentation would be the development of a public information campaign about the importance of genetic counseling that targets women who have delivered babies with congenital anomalies.

Home visitors intervene at both the individual and community level. At the client level, the visitor usually has a specific purpose or indication for the visit, whether it is to examine the new mother and infant during the early postpartum period or to provide ongoing support and anticipatory guidance to new families during the first 2 years of the child's life. Home visiting programs, as a whole, may be part of a community-implemented intervention to decrease low-birth-weight infants or child abuse and neglect within a given region or health district. The home visitor provides services and education to clients to impact individual health outcomes but also intervenes as a member of the community in an attempt to maintain, and hopefully improve, health status indicators for the community as a whole.

DEFINING HOME VISITATION

Any discussion of home visitation must focus on the unique aspects of providing care in the home for pregnant and parenting women and families. The nature of home visiting can be further explored by focusing on the home as a site of service delivery and by examining the development of a special helping relationship between the client and visitor.

Site of Service Delivery

A **home visit** occurs in the family's place of residence or in any such facility at which a family may be housed, such as a homeless shelter, group home, church, or halfway house (Gomby, Larson, Lewit, and Behrman, 1993). Having services provided in the home is convenient for clients. Lack of transportation and childcare along with language barriers can make accessing care difficult, especially for low-income populations. In addition, some clients are physically or emotionally incapable of leaving home, making them unlikely to receive care in other settings. Ambulatory care settings typically feature an appointment-only structure, with moderate to lengthy waiting times, that many times is designed to meet the needs of providers and not clients. Home visiting also brings nurses in contact with client groups who, for whatever reason, might not have accessed health care in more traditional settings. This case finding aspect, then, is a particularly important function of home visitation; nurses have contact not only with the client or family initially referred for service but also with neighbors, extended family, and friends.

The home as a site of service delivery also provides a unique opportunity to assess the client and family in their own environment. The nurse can observe how physical, psychosocial, and spiritual factors (such as housing, interpersonal relationships, and religious beliefs), resources (such as finances and support systems), and potential environmental hazards (such as improper food storage and faulty electrical wiring) relate to and impact health status. Health-related issues can be evaluated within the context of daily life. Given this opportunity to fully assess the environment and the way in which the client interacts within

it, the nurse can more readily understand the needs, strengths, motivations, and desires of the client and family. This knowledge allows the nurse and client, in partnership, to formulate an appropriate nursing diagnosis and develop a more effective plan for intervention. Services also can be personalized and individualized more than is possible in the clinic or hospital setting, using the family, significant others, and the surrounding community as sources of assistance or referral. Finally, the nurse can subsequently evaluate the success of the intervention strategy within the same setting. For example, a pregnant client with an inadequate weight gain may relate a diet history in the clinic that is consistent with standard prenatal recommendations. When the nurse visits the home and finds no food in the refrigerator, the problem of inadequate weight gain becomes attributable to an issue much different from simple knowledge deficit. The nurse can then mobilize the client and community resources (food banks, food stamps, and community food share programs) to address the real problem. In like manner, the client may report in clinic that she is taking supplemental iron tablets regularly. When questioned about the unopened bottle of tablets during a home visit, however, she admits being unable to swallow large pills.

Relationship Building

At the core of home visiting is the relationship between the client and family and the home visitor (Klass, 1996). In the home visiting situation, control is in the hands of the client. At all times, the nurse is a guest in the client's home (Hoover et al., 1996). This concept can be a difficult one for health care providers who often perceive themselves as experts, confident in their ability to solve other people's problems. Mutuality is key. The client and nurse must work together as a team to develop the care plan (Figure 6-2).

One of the primary purposes of any home visiting program is to foster the client's and family's ability to eventually provide self-care and make decisions independently. The nurse, recognizing that the client is in control, **empowers** the client and family. **Empowerment** is the process of assisting the client and family to care for themselves. Through the use of **enhancement**, the nurse identifies and builds on the client's and family's existing strengths to increase their ability to solve problems and provide self-care. Finally, the nurse functions as an enabler. **Enablement** is the process of assisting the client and family in locating and accessing the services and resources necessary for success, in short, helping clients help themselves. The nurse and the client-family unit function as a team, within a relationship that is collaborative, not authoritative, resulting in a plan for intervention that is developed jointly. This team approach is more likely to be successful.

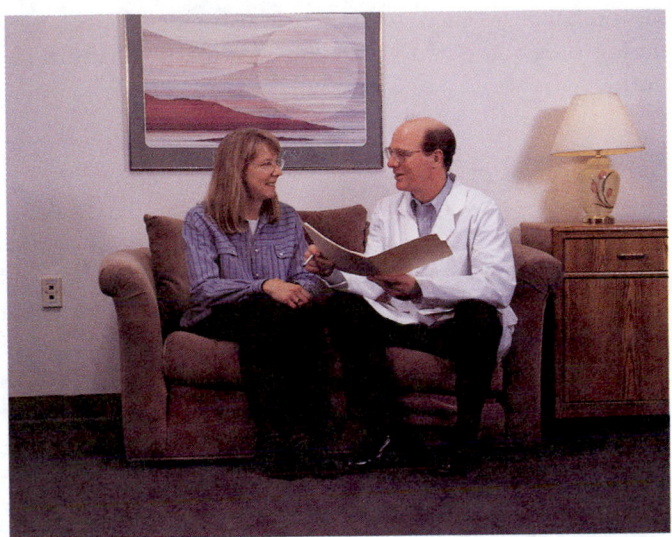

Figure 6-2 The client and home care nurse will work collaboratively to develop a plan of care.

Owing to the nature of their work, home visitors form a special helping relationship with their clients that is based on trust, especially when home visiting intervention is ongoing. Because clients feel at ease in their own environment, communication flows more easily and often is more truthful. Many times, nurses learn more about a client and family in a 2-hour home visit than a provider might learn during 7 months of prenatal care. Given the potential richness of this service setting, good assessment and communication skills are paramount.

INDICATIONS FOR HOME VISITATION

Home visitation is undertaken for a variety of purposes to meet a variety of goals. Home care is provided by independent home health care agencies, hospitals, public health departments, schools, and other institutions as a single intervention or as an adjunct to other types of care. For the purposes of this discussion, indications for home visiting will be classified as acute care focused or health promotion/disease prevention focused. The acute focus is one in which the provision of medical and nursing care is paramount. Health education, family preservation and support, and case management fall under the broader rubric of health promotion. In many cases, however, these indications overlap. It is difficult to administer any type of nursing care without providing health education. Conversely, the need for acute care might arise during a home visit initially indicated for health promotion. While accepting that this is true, home visitation still will be characterized according to these broader indications for purposes of discussion.

Provision of Acute Care

Regardless of the indication, home health nursing practice requires a broad base of skills. Knowledge of assessment (physical, psychosocial, and spiritual), communication, case management, health education, teaching and learning principles, and community resources are paramount. For women of childbearing age, provision of direct health care services during the prenatal or postpartum period often is the primary indication for a home-based nursing encounter. In response to increasing health care costs and third-party payment for home health care, the field of perinatal home care has developed over the past few years (Association of Women's Health, Obstetric, and Neonatal Nurses [AWHONN], 1994). Perinatal home care focuses most commonly on the provision of acute care services to women before conception, during pregnancy, and after delivery, along with care for their neonates (AWHONN, 1994). Fiscal considerations usually dictate that services be restricted to high-risk populations, although perinatal home care nurses can potentially serve all childbearing women. Encounters may be single or multiple, and the number of visits is dictated by client need and the insurer. For example, women who are at risk for preterm labor can access perinatal nurse specialists to assess contractions, evaluate the condition of the cervix, monitor fetal well-being, and manage medications that cause tocolysis, such as terbutaline delivered by pump. In response to early hospital discharge after delivery, a perinatal home care nurse may visit in the first 24 to 48 hours postpartum to assess maternal-newborn physical status and adjustment. AWHONN has developed a set of suggested clinical skills for professional nurse providers of perinatal home care; activities should be "philosophically directed" toward the following (AWHONN, 1994):

- Assisting women in optimizing their state of health before conception.

- Assessing and managing actual or potential problems of pregnancy that can be managed safely on an outpatient basis.

- Facilitating postpartum physical restoration and adaptation to parenthood.

- Promoting the achievement of maximal health for the neonate and family.

Interventions usually involve single or multiple encounters on a short-term basis. Whereas the visit care is focused on acute care, the nurse still focuses on issues germane to health promotion and disease prevention, such as environmental assessment, health education, and anticipatory guidance.

HEALTH PROMOTION

In the public health arena, home visitation has been used as a strategy for delivering both preventive and interventive services. Visitation programs with a focus on health promotion and disease prevention may use home contacts as a means of identifying clients and families in need of medical care or services (case finding). Referrals to existing resources usually follow. In the childbearing age population, visitors can provide social support and health education to promote optimal pregnancy outcomes and healthy parent-child relationships, and to prevent future child abuse. Home visitation also is employed as an intervention strategy once risks have been identified, such as substance abuse during pregnancy or child abuse and neglect. Health promotion or public health home visitation programs rarely focus on the provision of acute health care. Interventions usually involve multiple encounters on a long-term basis. For instance, a community-based program may provide nurse home visits to families identified at risk for child abuse and neglect on a regular basis for the first 2 years postpartum to teach and model appropriate parenting skills. Similar programs have been initiated for pregnant women who abuse substances, beginning during pregnancy and extending into the postpartum period.

PRINCIPLES OF HOME VISITATION

In order to be effective, home visiting programs should conform to existing standards. The Colorado Department of Public Health and Environment has proposed a set of Home Visiting Program Standards (1994) for programs providing these services:

1. Home visiting services are community-based and designed with the demographic and cultural characteristics of the community in mind.

2. Home visiting services are purposeful and goal-oriented. These services relate directly to the defined mission of the home visitation program.

3. Home visiting programs have a focus that recognizes the strength of families and promotes self-sufficiency of clients.

4. Home visiting programs utilize appropriate community services and resources to promote coordination and avoid duplication of services.

5. Home visiting programs ensure that the discipline and background of the home visitor is identified and that adequate training and oversight are provided.

In designing programs, consideration should be given to the language and cultural characteristics of the community being served. For example, programs serving a primarily non–English-speaking Latino community should employ nurses who are bilingual in English and Spanish and, ideally, bicultural. Similarly, services should target identified needs within a community. For example, developing services for childbearing women is probably not a priority in a small retirement community. Knowledge of the needs and cultural characteristics of the community is important in determining whether health needs can be adequately addressed by home visiting.

Home visiting programs should have a sense of purpose and be goal-oriented. Clear, written guidelines are key. Such guidelines should articulate the goals and purposes of the program, the population targeted, eligibility criteria (if applicable), content of services, and frequency and intensity of the home visiting intervention. Expected outcomes and criteria for evaluating outcomes also should be stated.

Skilled home visiting program staff should be able to promote self-sufficiency for the clients served, helping clients learn to help themselves. In order to meet this goal, the client must be involved and invested in the process.

REFLECTIONS FROM FAMILIES

"I didn't pay much attention to this program at first. My nurse came over to my home just to talk, to see how I was doing, to see what was up and how I felt. I thought, 'Okay, well I get it now, they are actually here to help me.' I never encountered anything like that—ever! People don't just come to your home and say, 'How are you? How do you feel? Are you living in a safe environment? Is your home stable? Do you have something to cook on? If you don't, we need to help. We need to make this pregnancy as stress-free as possible so if we can be a support system and be there for and with you, it will make this pregnancy easier for you.' I was blown away to see someone care like that."

Trierweiler, K., Ricketts, S., Kent, H., & Albert, S. (1994). *The helping moms program: A case management approach to delivering enhanced prenatal services.* Denver, CO: Colorado Department of Public Health and Environment.

The visitor and client-family unit work jointly as a team to develop a set of goals and a plan for intervention. Given this blueprint, it is best if client participation is voluntary, not mandatory. Plans tend to be one-sided when the client is compelled to participate as in cases of court-ordered visitation for child abuse and neglect. In order to ensure a successful intervention, every effort should be made to address goals that the client and family may have for themselves along with goals that the home visitor has for the client. For instance, a pregnant client may agree that smoking cessation is desirable during pregnancy; however, this goal may not be realistic for the client who, at the same time, is struggling to pay her rent. In this case, a program that is narrowly focused on prenatal smoking cessation may not be able to address the client's more urgent needs for housing. Smoking cessation during pregnancy along with adequate housing are short-term goals that impact the long-term goal of a healthy pregnancy outcome. Programs offering a broad range of services that encompass the client's needs as well as the nurse's objectives enhance the chance for mutual success. As illustrated in the previous example, once the client has adequate housing, energies may be better focused on behavior change, thus satisfying the goals of both the client and the home visitor. However, the nurse must always recognize that the client and family are the ultimate decision-makers regarding care. Doing so is relatively easy when the client makes decisions that seem rational. In contrast, it may be difficult for the nurse to support a decision she thinks may be "wrong." A client may simply decide that she cannot or will not stop smoking during pregnancy. In this case, efforts may be better focused on helping the client decrease the number of cigarettes smoked each day.

A client's value system forms the basis for decision-making. When the client's values differ from those of the mainstream or the providers, difficulties can arise. For example, a 36-year-old pregnant woman may decide against having an amniocentesis during pregnancy because she says she would not terminate her pregnancy no matter what the test results show. This viewpoint is not in line with current medical recommendations regarding amniocentesis during pregnancy and may clash with the provider's own personal values. Clients have every right to refuse testing and treatment. The nurse must first determine that the client fully understands the recommendations. If so, the client's decision should be documented and respected. Nurses also should reflect on their own feelings and prejudices relative to the issue. Any legal (e.g., violation of the nurse practice act) or ethical implications (e.g., violation of client confidentiality) to the client's decision also should be considered.

Along these lines, home visiting programs should focus on the strengths of clients and families, not their weaknesses. Doing so can be challenging given that risk status usually is based on a deficits model. For example, the nurse may determine that a pregnant woman is at psychosocial risk because she is an unmarried high-school dropout with two children and three jobs changes in the past year. Her lack of education and work inconsistency might initially be viewed as weaknesses. However, further assessment may reveal mitigating factors. The client may have changed jobs frequently to finish her high-school education and enroll in junior college. Working at a place located closer to her childcare provider may have necessitated a job change. When deficits are evaluated in this fashion, strengths may emerge. In this example, the client is completing her education, from which new job opportunities can arise. She also has supportive family available to ease the stresses of single parenthood and to assist with a new baby. Identifying her motivation to finish school and her solid support network serves as a cornerstone in developing a plan of intervention for self-sufficiency during pregnancy and the postpartum period.

Identification of client strengths is helpful in determining the need for community resources and referrals. In the example above, based on deficits only, the client appears to be in need of a variety of resources, such as job training, subsidized childcare, and possibly parenting classes. In actuality, given the client's motivation and support system, few resources are needed. Referrals and resources also may have been provided by another provider. The popularity of home visiting as an intervention strategy gives rise to the possibility that a client or family may be working with multiple home visitors. In these cases, collaboration is key. All who provide care and services to the client and family should communicate regularly, including the medical care provider. In order to facilitate this process, one home visitor should be designated as the case manager, who coordinates the activities of all caregivers. Case

Critical Thinking

Immunizations

A pregnant client tells you at a home visit that she is planning on refusing all newborn and pediatric immunizations for her infant.

- How would you respond?
- What additional information do you need, if any?
- How does this make you feel?
- What are your feelings toward this client?
- What are your responsibilities as a care provider in this situation?

management will be discussed in more detail subsequently.

The staff of the home visiting program must have access to adequate training, consultation, and supervision. Supervision should be available in accordance with the discipline and experience level of the visitor and the complexity of the client's case. New staff should receive an ex-

tensive orientation on the goals, objectives, and purposes of the home visiting program as well as on the program's guidelines and expectations for providing care and services to clients and families. New staff should make several home visits under the watchful eye of a mentor or supervisor until the desired skill level is achieved and documented. All home visitors should be aware of the re-

Research Highlight

Long-term Effects of Home Visitation on Maternal Life Course and Child Abuse and Neglect

Purpose

To determine the long-term effects (15 years) of nurse home visitation during pregnancy and postpartally for the first 2 years relative to maternal life course and child abuse and neglect.

Methods

A randomized controlled trial was conducted in a semirural town in upstate New York in which women received an average of 9 home visits during pregnancy and approximately 23 home visits postpartally for the first 2 years. Of 400 women originally enrolled in this study, 324 participated in a follow-up investigation when their children were 15 years old.

Findings

Compared with a control group, women with low incomes who received home visitation during pregnancy and postpartally

- Were less likely to be reported for child abuse and neglect during the 15-year period after delivery: 0.29 reports compared with 0.54 reports in the control group ($P = 0.001$).

- Who also were single had fewer additional children, with longer periods between having children: 1.3 children compared with 1.6 children in the control group ($P = 0.02$), and 65 months compared with 37 months in the control group ($P = 0.001$).

- Received public assistance for a shorter amount of time: 60 months compared with 90 months for the control group ($P = 0.005$).

- Had less substance-related misbehavior: 0.41 reports compared with 0.73 reports in the control group ($P = 0.03$).

- Had fewer arrests as verified by state records: 0.16 arrests compared with 0.90 arrests in the control group ($P = 0.001$).

Nursing Implications

Prenatal and postpartum home visitation by nurses to women who are single with low incomes can lead to a decrease in the incidence of child abuse and neglect, a longer interconceptional period, fewer months on welfare, a decrease in behavior problems related to substance use, and less frequent criminal behavior for up to 15 years after the birth of the index child. Consideration should be given to wider implementation of long-term nurse home visitation.

Olds, D., Eckenrode, J., Henderson, C., Kitzman, H., Powers, J., Cole, R., Sidora, K., Morris, P., Pettitt, L., Luckey, D. (1997). Long-term effects of home visitation on maternal life course and child abuse and neglect. *Journal of the American Medical Association, 278,* 637–643.

sources available for consultation in the event high-risk medical or psychosocial conditions develop. Agency-specific systems for continuing education and quality assurance are paramount. Peer review and chart review should be ongoing quality assurance measures taken by the home visiting program. Opportunities for continuing education must be made available to all staff on a regular basis.

EFFICACY OF HOME VISITATION

The effectiveness and cost benefits of providing acute medical and nursing care services in the home for perinatal clients are subjects of ongoing investigation. Cost savings as measured by a reduction in inpatient hospital days

has been postulated. Findings from several recent studies support this notion. Cooper et al. (1996) noted that newborns in the inner city whose mothers received at least one postpartum home visit from a nurse had fewer emergency room visits during the first 3 months after delivery. A universal postpartum nurse home visiting program resulted in a twofold reduction in acute care visits during the first 2 weeks of the postpartum period (Braveman et al., 1996). The effectiveness of perinatal in-home interventions in terms of health outcomes, however, has not been proven.

Research supporting the benefit of public-health–related home visitation also is limited. Until recently, the results have been somewhat mixed. When looking at home-based health promotion activities, researchers have noted differences in pregnancy outcomes, parenting and

Research Highlight

Effects of Prenatal Home Visitation by Nurses

Purpose

To determine the effect of home visits made by nurses during pregnancy and postpartally for 2 years on the incidence of pregnancy-induced hypertension (PIH), preterm birth, maternal life, childhood behavior and development, immunizations, and injuries.

Methods

A randomized controlled trial was conducted in 1,139 women receiving care within the public health system in Memphis, Tennessee, the majority of whom were African American, at less than 29 weeks' gestation, without a previous live birth, who exhibited at least two of the following risk factors: unemployment, unmarried, and less than 12 years of education. Each participant received an average of 7 home visits during pregnancy (total number of visits ranging from 0 to 18) and 26 visits from birth and postpartally for 2 years (total number of visits ranging from 0 to 71).

Findings

Compared with a control group, women and their infants were visited by nurses during pregnancy and postpartally for 2 years. It was found that

- The women were less likely to have PIH: 13% compared with 20% in the control group ($P = 0.009$).
- The women were less likely to become pregnant again during that time: 36% compared with 47% in the control group ($P = 0.006$).
- The women had fewer medical visits during that time: 0.43 visits compared with 0.55 visits in the control group ($P = 0.05$).
- The infants had fewer hospital days for childhood injuries: 0.03 days compared with 0.16 days in the control group ($P < 0.001$).

There were no effects on preterm delivery, maternal life course, child cognitive development or behavior problems, or maternal education and employment.

(continued)

Research Highlight continued

Nursing Implications

This study replicates an earlier randomized controlled trial of home visiting conducted in a rural, Caucasian population in Elmira, New York. While prenatal effects were noted only for PIH, the postpartum results for this minority urban population found a decrease in children's medical visits and hospitalizations for injuries as well as fewer subsequent pregnancies among the study participants. These results were not as dramatic as were those in the Elmira study; however, long-term nurse home visitation programs can result in measurable differences in selected postnatal outcomes in different populations. Wider dissemination of public-health–related home visiting efforts deserves consideration.

In addition, a review of the literature has shown that successful public-health–related home visiting programs do have several characteristics. Successful programs address a broad range of client and family needs as opposed to having a single narrow focus (Gomby, Larson, Lewit, and Behrman, 1993). Using home visitation as an adjunct to other intervention strategies, such as medical care, peer counseling, and drug and alcohol treatment, also appears to enhance outcomes. Broad-based programs usually offer services that are ongoing and intense. Olds and Kitzman (1993) feel that at least four home visits must be made before any gains can occur; and more if a major change in health or behavioral status is desired. These authors also believe that using nurses instead of lay or paraprofessional home visitors leads to more efficacious outcomes. This assumption has been supported in Olds' most recent research (see Research Highlights: Long-Term Effects of Home Visitation). Currently, a randomized clinical trial in Colorado is investigating the effectiveness of professional compared with lay or paraprofessional home visitors in serving women during pregnancy and early postpartum. Finally, high-risk populations appear to benefit more from home interventions than do low-risk groups. In other words, women at high risk for delivering low-birth-weight infants should benefit more from programs designed to decrease or ameliorate this risk than would the general population (Olds & Kitzman, 1993).

Kitzman, H., Olds, D., Henderson, C., Hanks, C., Cole, C., Tatelbaum, R., McConnochie, K., Sidora, K., Luckey, D., Shaver, D., Engelhardt, K., James, D., & Barnard, K. (1997). Effect of prenatal and infancy home visitation by nurses on pregnancy outcomes, childhood injuries, and repeated childbearing. *Journal of the American Medical Association, 278,* 644–652.

caregiving, child development, prevention of child abuse, and enhancement of maternal personal development (Graham, as cited in Hoover et al., 1996). An additional study suggests a relationship between nurse-community worker team home visiting during the first year postpartum and decreased postneonatal mortality (Barnes-Boyd et al., 1996). Two recent randomized, controlled trials have demonstrated benefits in reducing pregnancy-induced hypertension (PIH) along with a long-term reduction of child medical and hospital visits related to injuries.

ESSENTIAL SKILLS FOR HOME VISITING

The home visitor uses a variety of skills in providing home care. Good communication is key along with proficiency in the nursing process: assessment, nursing diagnosis, outcome identification, planning, intervention, and evaluation. The home visitor also often functions as a case manager, or care coordinator, and therefore familiarity with community resources is imperative.

Nurses must be good communicators. Speaking clearly, directly, honestly, and nonjudgmentally should be second nature. Communication skills are particularly important in home visiting because the nurse must fully engage the client to set the stage for the development of trust and mutuality throughout the course of the home visiting relationship. Each nurse develops a particular personal style of communication; however, certain principles are universal (Figure 6-3).

Listening provides the means for good communication. Novices often are so concerned with their response that they fail to hear what the client is saying and fail to

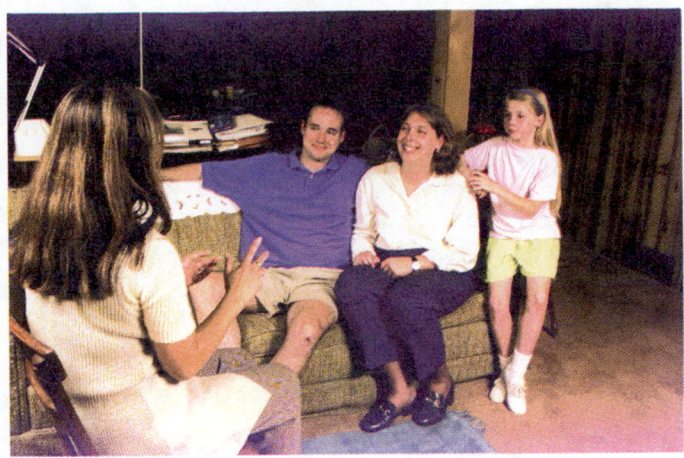

Figure 6-3 The seeds of trust and a good working relationship are planted during the first encounter between the client and visiting nurse.

observe nonverbal cues. True listening is difficult, requiring utmost attention to what is being said verbally and nonverbally. The nurse must attempt first to understand, then to respond. Listening can be put into operation by maintaining good eye contact and facing the client with an open and accepting posture with arms uncrossed and the body leaning slightly forward. Attention is centered on the client, not the chart. Focused, caring attention, especially in the home environment, can enhance the client's self-concept and put a client at ease so that a richness of information results. Listening is a learned skill that often is underemphasized; however, listening is vital in establishing rapport and creating a climate of caring concern.

Listening often is impaired by the fear of silence, especially when the nurse is practicing in an environment that may not be completely comfortable, such as the home. The power that silence can bring to the communication process should not be underestimated. Frequently, the client's words are only half acknowledged as the nurse uses this time instead to plan a response. Employing silence after the client stops speaking allows an opportunity for the client to clarify without any further prompting from the nurse. Often, more will be expressed if another question is not asked immediately. Silence also can be affirming, especially when accompanied by gestures on the part of the nurse, such as head shaking or touching. These techniques reflect empathy or an understanding of the client's viewpoint. Silence also gives the nurse an opportunity to process the information and briefly plan a response.

When more information is needed, the nurse may elect to paraphrase what the client has said to validate understanding and encourage additional dialog. Using open-ended questions or statements also is effective. For example, the nurse might respond, "I heard you express your concerns that this pregnancy will be normal. Tell me about your last pregnancy." Acknowledging the client's feelings is helpful. "You seem scared about being pregnant."

Body language and nonverbal cues speak loudly. Experienced home visitors attend to what is not verbalized by observing the client's expression, posture, and gestures. The client may state that her partner would never strike her, while nervously looking over her shoulder to see if he can hear her response. A question or comment here may elicit the truth.

The development of rapport and trust occurs over time. Good communication fosters the development of a long-term therapeutic relationship (Figure 6-4). Employing these techniques consistently while working with a client

Critical Thinking

Personal Opinion

A client who is in her first trimester of pregnancy confides to you during a home visit that she has decided to have an abortion. You feel that abortion is morally wrong.

- How would you respond?
- What additional information do you need, if any?
- How does this make you feel?
- What are your feelings toward this client?
- What are your responsibilities as a care provider in this situation?
- How is this situation similar or different from the one in Critical Thinking: Immunizations?

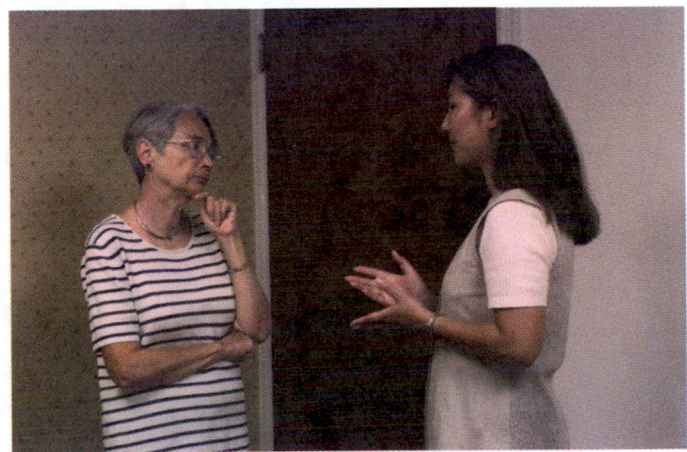

Figure 6-4 Active listening, concentrating on the needs of the client, will enhance communication.

or family can lead to the development of the rapport and eventually the trust necessary for the successful completion of goals. Rapport, however, is difficult to establish in a single home visit. Good communication will result in the efficient use of the time available for home assessment.

Many barriers exist to good communication. In the interest of time, some providers may anticipate what the client will say and thus may finish the client's sentences. The client may interpret this action as an attempt to wade through what the nurse sees as extraneous information to get to "the point." A respectful approach dictates that the client be allowed to speak without interruption. Similarly, the nurse may interject advice and counseling after each client comment. It is important to note that assessments, including data gathering, must be completed before a plan can be developed and initiated. Giving information this readily does not allow for client-generated or mutually derived solutions.

Nurses may also attempt to validate a client's experience by relating a similar personal experience of their own. This technique can be helpful when used in brief (e.g., the nurse can say, "I had that same problem with my baby."); however, it is important to remember that the focus is on the client, not the provider.

Being judgmental is a powerful deterrent to communication and future interaction. Further data gathering is useless because the nurse has already made a determination about the client. Judging influences the nurse's ability to arrive at an appropriate nursing diagnosis and thus influences the subsequent plan for intervention. For example, a pregnant woman may refuse to have blood drawn for testing during pregnancy and this action may result in the nurse initially labeling her as a "bad mother." Further probing may reveal that the client is actually afraid of needles. Being judgmental is damaging. Nurses in their roles as client advocates must guard against being judgmental by making objectively based client assessments.

NURSING PROCESS

Nurse home visitors must be skilled in using the nursing process; each of the steps is discussed as they relate to the process of home visitation.

Assessment

Home-based activities should be individualized based on an assessment of the physical, psychosocial, spiritual, and cultural attributes of the client or family (Hoover et al., 1996). These detailed assessments form a database from which a nursing diagnosis and ultimately a plan for intervention can be developed. Assessment information is derived from subjective sources (e.g., the client's medical history, chief complaint, feelings, and perceptions) and objective sources (e.g., the client's physical examination and laboratory data and the nurse's observations).

Nursing Diagnoses

For a client receiving home visits as a result of being on complete bedrest for placenta previa, relevant nursing diagnoses might include impaired physical mobility, ineffective role performance, and deficient diversional activity. These diagnoses will be reevaluated at each encounter and most likely will continue to be applicable until the client delivers the infant. The diagnosis in this case also indicates a need for health teaching and counseling. The client may exhibit deficient knowledge relative to labor and delivery information because her imposed bedrest precludes attendance at childbirth education classes.

Outcome Identification

Once a diagnosis is made, both short- and long-term outcomes should be identified. In preceding examples, the short-term outcome is avoidance of preterm labor and birth and the long-term outcome is a healthy, full-term infant.

Planning

Based on the diagnosis, the plan is developed in collaboration with the client and family (Figure 6-5). Their needs and desires must be prioritized. Issues identified by the client should take precedence unless clear threats to safety are present. For instance, a pregnant client may be concerned

---

Critical Thinking

Making Judgments

Some people feel that women with low incomes should not become pregnant and access federal entitlement programs such as Medicaid to finance their health care.

- How does this situation make you feel?
- What is your responsibility as a nurse caring for this population?

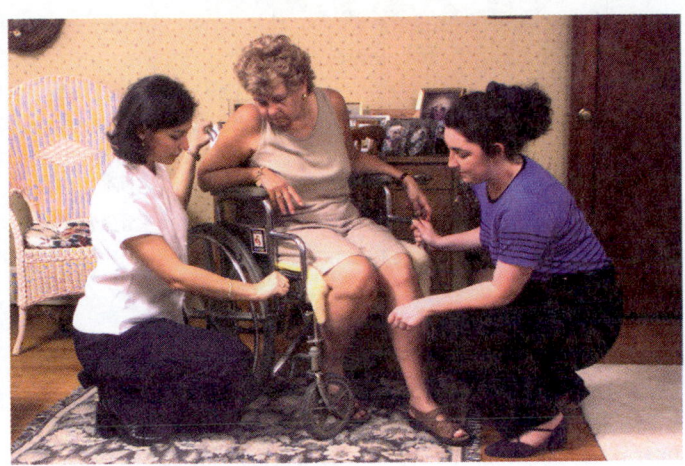

Figure 6-5 The plan of care for a client often includes instructions to family members.

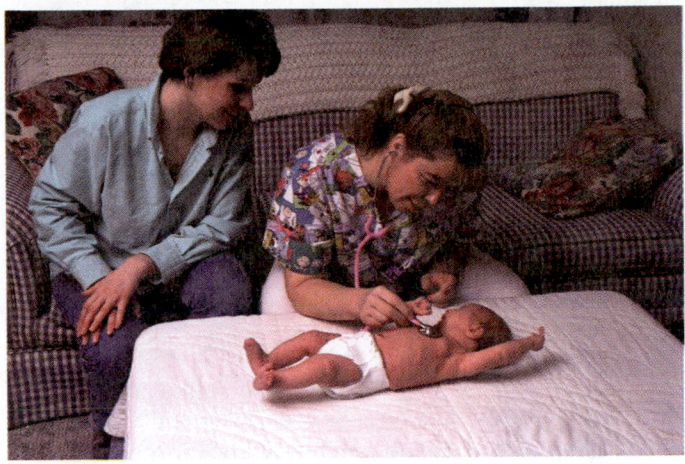

Figure 6-6 Postpartum home visits will include physical assessment of the mother and newborn.

about job training but may first need a restraining order against her abusive ex-husband. The client will be more receptive to addressing other concerns if her priority needs are met first. Other issues can then be ranked in order of importance according to mutual agreement. Prioritizing will result in interventions being developed for the most important issues first, leaving others for later follow-up.

Once priority needs have been agreed on, the nurse must ascertain that the plan reflects both short- and long-term expected outcomes. In the preceding example, the long-term outcome is for the client to live without fear of abuse and the short-term outcome might be achieving success in obtaining a restraining order.

Nursing Interventions

Nursing interventions may be preventive, such as providing anticipatory guidance or health education. Interventions may address specific health concerns, such as performing nursing procedures in response to a specific physician order. Interventions also may take the form of referrals, especially in the home visiting program. Home visiting done during the early postpartum period includes activities pertinent to all three types of interventions. For example, the new mother receives information from the nurse about normal newborn care, behavior, feeding, and parenting. The nurse also performs a physical assessment of both the mother and baby to rule out abnormalities (Figure 6-6). When a problem is discovered, such as noting that the newborn has significant jaundice, an appropriate intervention would be a referral to the pediatrician for bilirubin screening. Similarly, the mother may be referred to a new mothers' group to increase her social support systems.

Evaluation

Evaluation is probably the most underused step of the nursing process in home-based care. Criteria established before initiating the intervention must be analyzed to evaluate the effectiveness of the intervention employed relative to the nursing diagnoses identified. For example, in the example cited previously, the woman on bedrest needed childbirth education owing to a knowledge deficit regarding labor and delivery information. If the nurse provides this teaching and notes that the client is subsequently more knowledgeable, the intervention can be deemed successful. On a larger level, nurses should be involved in setting overall home visiting program evaluation criteria. For example, an agency providing home-based services to pregnant and postpartum women might attempt to increase breast-feeding initiation and continuation rates or attempt to reduce the incidence of unintended pregnancy within their population.

When reviewing the efficacy of the plan and activities initiated, the nurse must assess progress in meeting both the short- and long-term outcomes identified earlier. For example, the pregnant client with an abusive ex-husband decided, in consultation with the home visitor, to obtain a restraining order. The nurse may phone the client several days later to verify that she has contacted legal aid. At the next encounter, the nurse will again ask if the client has spoken to the lawyer and filed the paperwork. Follow-up is ongoing until the restraining order is filed and the short-term outcome achieved. Further analysis will determine whether or not the existence of the restraining order enables the client to function without fear of abuse, which is the long-term outcome.

The efficacy of home visitation as a service delivery strategy for use with a particular client also should be evaluated. Was home visiting the best strategy for addressing the issues? Was the nurse prepared with the appropriate information to assist the client? Would referral to a social worker have been more effective? In some cases, client needs may be better served in the ambulatory or inpatient setting. The nurse is responsible for determining which site of service would be most effective.

CASE MANAGEMENT

The nursing process shares many similarities with the process of case management. Nurse home visitors may find themselves functioning as case managers, or care coordinators, for clients and families. **Case management**, or **care coordination**, refers to the process of coordinating care and services to ensure that clients receive appropriate care and services in a timely manner. The case manager performs a comprehensive assessment, develops a plan of care, assists the client to access needed care and services, and follows up to evaluate the success of these strategies in meeting client needs (Trierweiler, Ricketts, Kent, & Albert, 1994). Underlying the process is a commitment to an active partnership between the client and case manager, with the ultimate goal of self-sufficiency.

Over 40 states have approved funding through Medicaid for prenatal case management programs for high-risk pregnant women. Case managers assist pregnant women in addressing all aspects of their life that may affect pregnancy outcome and maternal and child health in general (Trierweiler, Ricketts, Kent, & Albert, 1994). These care coordinators ensure that clients attend prenatal medical visits; assist clients in accessing nutrition and social work counseling as needed; and ensure client access to transportation, childcare, and health education.

The home is an ideal site for case management. Because the steps of the case management process are similar to the nursing process, nurses can use their full professional role to ensure that client needs and desires are identified and met.

MAKING THE HOME VISIT

The home visit consists of three phases: previsit preparation, visiting the home, and postvisit activities. The previsit and postvisit phases are as important as the visit itself. Without adequate planning and follow-up, the nurse may miss the opportunity for successful interaction and intervention. Careful preparation is paramount.

Previsit Preparation

The nurse must be familiar with the population served by the home visiting program in terms of demographics, culture, language, and religion. Agency orientation should include these vital issues; however, the nurse should review these issues again before entering the home. Further planning includes reviewing the chart and the indication for referral, assembling necessary equipment and supplies, and contacting the client or family to schedule an appointment. Familiarity with community resources is required. The issues of dress and personal safety also require careful consideration before visiting the home.

Chart Review

First, the nurse must be familiar with the indication for the home visit. Careful review of all available client information is recommended, with attention to basic client demographics, such as age, gravity, parity, number and age of children in the home, and presence of the partner and significant others. When provision of acute care is the purpose of the visit, review of the hospital discharge summary will highlight the client's physical status. When the client will be receiving a postpartum home visit, labor and delivery data (date, time and type of delivery, complications, postpartum course, and date and time of discharge) as well as newborn status (date and time of birth, birth weight, weight at hospital discharge, type of feeding, circumcision status, and problems or complications during hospitalization) are crucial. Frequently, the nurse will receive paperwork from the referring agency that addresses most of this information. Access to this data enables the nurse to begin assessing the potential needs of the client and family based on the information assembled to date.

When the client has been receiving home care services, the current home health chart should be reviewed before the visit. In this way, the new home visitor is aware of previously initiated goals, objectives, plans, and interventions and can continue following the current plan of care. The client will not be required to repeat information to a new practitioner.

Chart review is especially important in scheduling the amount of time needed for the visit, in planning potential activities or interventions, and in assembling the equipment that may be needed. For example, the assessment and plan will likely be different when a home visit is to be made to a 14-year-old primipara with premature twins compared with a 34-year-old multipara with a term newborn and supportive partner. Given this information, the nurse may anticipate spending more time visiting the teen mother than the multipara mother. The potential activities and interventions also will differ. The adolescent may be in need of extensive teaching about newborn care and a discussion of available resources, whereas the older mother may need only reassurance about infant health and reinforcement of parenting information. Flexibility is key because this situation may not play out as expected. It could be that the older mother is experiencing a problem with postpartum depression while the adolescent is receiving the help and support of her extended family.

Assembling Equipment and Supplies

Necessary equipment and supplies must be assembled before the home visit. Knowing something about the family demographics (e.g., if any children will be present), the physical environment (e.g., if there are running water and a private space for talking or performing an examination) along with the indications for the home visit will allow the nurse to gather adequate supplies. The nurse should always carry rudimentary medical and nursing supplies, even if the purpose of the home visit is primarily oriented toward education. A stethoscope, blood pressure cuff, thermometer, small light source, sterile and unsterile examining gloves, paper towels, Handiwipes, and alcohol swabs are supplies that should be routinely carried. Other medical supplies may be needed, depending on the indication for the visit (e.g., a baby scale or medications). A supply of commonly used teaching materials and brochures also should be assembled. Veteran home visitors often carry a resource or referral directory containing the names, addresses and phone numbers of neighborhood health care providers, health and human services agencies, and support groups. The ability to supply the family with the appropriate contact information at the time of the visit enhances follow-through.

When children will be present in the home, the nurse may bring a small assortment of age-appropriate toys. These should be easy to clean and should be disinfected after each home visit. Toys distract children, allow evaluation of growth and development, and provide opportunities for assessment of parent-child interaction and teaching regarding age-appropriate play and stimulation.

Scheduling the Visit

Once the referral has been received and the preparatory data collected, the nurse contacts the client and family to establish a mutually acceptable time for the home visit. Timing of the visit is important. In cases in which acute care will be provided, the timing must be such that critical medical needs are addressed and the scheduled regimen of care initiated. For example, in the case of a postpartum family experiencing a hospital stay of 18 to 24 hours, it is crucial to visit during the first 24 to 48 hours after discharge because newborn jaundice or feeding problems may be evident at this time. This fact should be emphasized when phoning the family to set an appointment time. Similarly, the nurse may need to visit a pregnant woman on bedrest for PIH daily or every other day to closely monitor her condition and response to bedrest. When the home visit has a preventive health or psychoso-

SCHEDULING THE HOME VISIT

1. When calling to schedule an appointment, give your name and title and identify the agency you represent.

2. Discuss how and when the client was referred and the purpose of the home visit.

3. Briefly outline what will be done during the visit and estimate the amount of time required.

4. Write down detailed directions to the client's house. Consult a map before leaving the office if you are uncertain about the location.

5. End the phone call by verifying the date and time of the visit. Confirming the visit the day before will help avoid missed appointments.

6. Plan to keep your scheduled appointments and arrive on time. Notify the client as soon as possible if you will be late or if you need to reschedule the home visit.

cial focus, it is best to visit when the client and family are responsive and ready to accept the home visitor. In this situation, the nurse may call and discuss the home visiting program with the client and family and then allow them to suggest appropriate times and schedules. It is best to give a deadline for a response, such as a week or 10 days. An example of such a program might be one in which a pregnant woman at psychosocial risk agrees to receive home visits during pregnancy and postpartally to promote optimal pregnancy outcome and increase parenting skills.

Dress

The home visitor should dress professionally and appropriately. Although a uniform or laboratory coat is not necessary (but often is supplied by the employer), it is important to avoid being underdressed or overdressed for the occasion. Jeans, shorts, and revealing clothing are as inappropriate as are dressy, designer ensembles. In general, casual slacks or skirts with low-heeled shoes should be worn. Jewelry should be kept to a minimum. Expensive personal items should not be taken into the client's home. An identification badge with a photograph should always be worn, listing the visitor's name, title, and agency affiliation. The nurse should also attend to the client's own standard of dress, which may vary according to culture. The nurse may decide to dress more formally or casually based on her observations during the initial visit.

Safety

Being knowledgeable about maintaining personal safety is paramount. Safety issues should be taken into consideration when planning for the home visit. The agency and supervisor should be aware of the visitor's schedule for the day. A copy of the appointment schedule can be posted centrally within the agency, including clients' names, addresses, telephone numbers, visit times, and estimated times of completion. Cellular phones should be available for staff use. Gather information about the neighborhood to be visited. If the area is potentially unsafe, working in pairs may be an option. In addition, a call to the police or sheriff's department might result in an escort. While driving to the client's home, the nurse should look for public places where aid could be requested if necessary, such as gas stations, grocery stores, and police or fire stations. Some agencies supply an identification card that can be mounted on the dashboard when the car is parked outside the client's home, alerting others to the car's official status. Activity near the home, such as groups gathering, shouting, and fighting, or a complete absence of activity should be observed while approaching. When leaving, the visitor should pay attention to how these activities might have changed. Client input also can be helpful when assessing threats to personal safety. Clients may advise visits at certain times to avoid potential confrontations. If the visit is to take place in a high-rise building, the nurse should try to ride the elevator either alone or with a group of peo-

Nursing Tip

PERSONAL SAFETY ON A HOME VISIT

1. Keep your car in good working order and the gas tank filled. A flashlight, first aid kit, emergency flares, and items appropriate for a weather emergency should be kept in the trunk. If car trouble develops, raise the hood and stay inside the car with the doors locked. Use a cellular phone if available to call a local gas station or towing service. If someone stops to help, ask the person to call the closest gas station.

2. Park as close to the client's home as possible, ideally in a space that is visible from the home. Avoid dark streets, concealed driveways, and alleys. Keep the car doors locked at all times. Remember where your car is parked.

3. Make certain that all supplies and client records are stored in the trunk or out of view.

4. Carry as little money as possible but keep change for a pay phone handy or carry a cellular phone. Carry your purse close to your body, or conceal it in a briefcase or file. If possible, avoid carrying a purse at all; carry your wallet in a coat pocket.

5. Request that pets be restrained before you arrive at the home. Be cautious about entering the yard, even if an animal is restrained.

6. Avoid walking close to buildings, doorways, dumpsters, or any place that could conceal a person. Walk confidently, with your head up, scanning the area for possible threats. If you are being followed, cross the street or zig-zag back and forth. Walk toward people or lighted areas.

7. When returning to the car after the visit, have car keys ready to quickly unlock the doors and start the engine. Look in the back seat and on the floor to ensure no one has broken into and is hiding in your car.

8. Watch for any cars that might be following you as you leave the home. If you are being followed, proceed to a well-lit public area or a police station. Never stop, even if someone indicates they are having a medical problem.

9. If you are accosted, use any means possible to get away including biting; scratching; kicking the shins, groin, or instep; screaming; yelling "Fire"; or blowing a rape whistle attached to a key ring. Carrying concealed weapons is not recommended.

10. If a situation feels unsafe, it probably is unsafe. Promptly leave any situation that may pose a threat to personal safety.

Sometimes, a threat to safety develops after the nurse has entered the home. Potentially dangerous situations might involve an abusive spouse or family member or the presence of weapons or illicit substances. Again, the nurse should quickly assess the situation and leave as circumstances dictate. The nurse may need to report these instances to the proper authorities, depending on the dictates of agency policy and state or federal laws.

ple. Stairwells often are safer than elevators. The home or apartment should not be entered if there are safety concerns. Most agencies have policies addressing safety issues.

Visiting the Home

The initial visit to the home sets the stage for future interactions between the client, family, and nurse. The home visitor confronts the unknown at this first encounter, entering into an environment controlled by others. The client also may be apprehensive about inviting a "stranger" inside, concerned about what the nurse may say and do while in the home. Thus, it is vital that the visit be conducted in a professional fashion to set the client and fam-

ily at ease and to allow the nurse to meet both agency and client objectives for the visit.

Initiating the Encounter

On arrival, the nurse should always knock before entering, even if the door is open. The visit begins with introductions (Figure 6-7). The nurse should identify herself by title and the agency represented, state the purpose of the visit, and estimate the amount of time required for the encounter. Giving the client a business card also is a good practice, reinforcing the nurse's position as a professional as well as providing a means for future contact. The client usually will introduce children and any other family members or friends who may be present. If not offered, these additional introductions should be requested.

Consent for services must be obtained before any services are performed. Most agencies require that the client sign a release of medical information request, allowing home visit data to be shared with other agency

BLOODBORNE PATHOGENS AND HOME VISITING

The nurse home visitor must use precautions in providing nursing care in the home to protect against exposure to bloodborne pathogens. Precautions (Occupational Health and Safety Administration, 1991) for home visiting include the following:

1. Wearing gloves when exposure to blood or body fluids is possible.

2. Washing hands immediately after any contact with potentially infectious materials.

3. Using eye or mouth protection when splashes, splatters, or droplets of potentially infectious materials may pose a hazard to the eyes, nose, or mouth.

4. Using the proper procedures with needles. Used needles should not be recapped, bent, or otherwise manipulated after injection. Used needles must be placed in a puncture-resistant container that has been brought into the home for this purpose. This container should be removed from the home for disposal at the agency.

5. Discarding items contaminated with blood or bodily fluids appropriately. Dressings, bandages, gloves, eyewear, and so on, that have been contaminated with blood or bodily fluids during the home visit should be discarded in appropriately marked biohazard bags and removed from the home by the nurse.

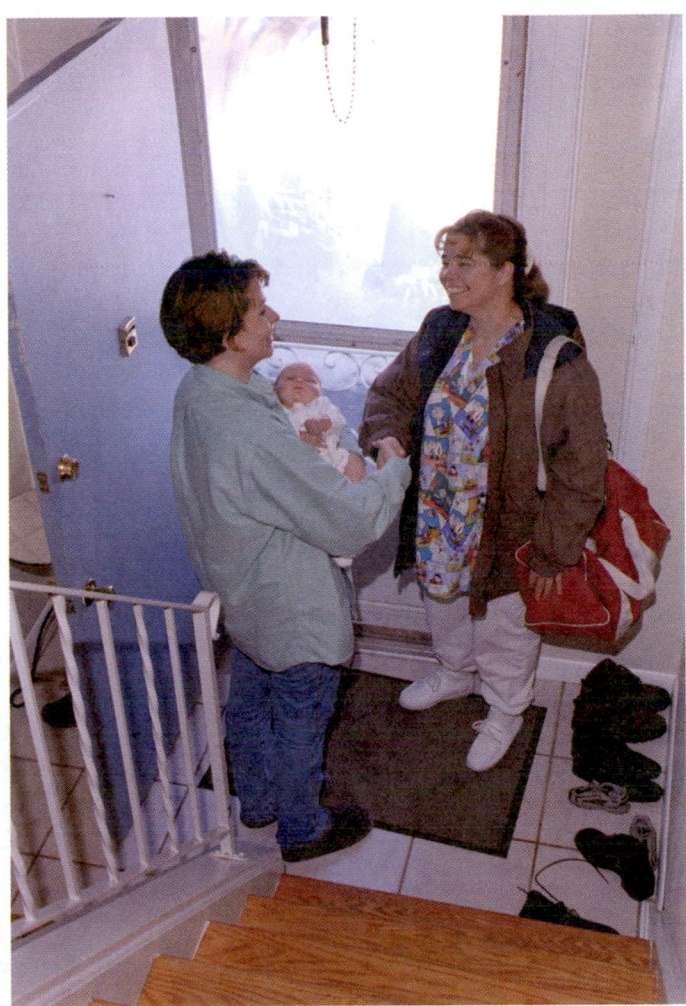

Figure 6-7 A warm greeting sets the tone for a positive house visit.

Critical Thinking

Performing Physical Assessments in the Home

Some nurses feel uncomfortable examining a client in a nonmedical setting. Ask yourself how you could best facilitate an examination in the client's home.

- Should you use the client's bed or would the couch suffice?
- How will you deal with children if they need to be present while the examination is being done?
- Could any supplies, such as pillows, screens, or drapes, be brought into the home to facilitate this process?
- Should you practice examining clients in the clinic to feel more confident of your skills before attempting a home visit?
- Would observing another nurse's technique be helpful?

providers, referral sources, and third-party payers. The client and family should be assured that all information, except as indicated, will remain confidential. Families must be informed of the nurse's responsibility as a health care provider, under most state laws, to report any cases of suspected child abuse or neglect. Any other discussions about the client or family with program staff, health care providers, or referral sources should occur solely for the purpose of client or family assistance.

A discussion of the purpose and goals of the visit, the role and responsibilities of the home visitor, and the rights and responsibilities of the client should occur early on. Client and family expectations should be elicited and clarified. The nurse then will attend to the business at hand by employing the nursing process, as discussed previously, in collaboration with the client's input to develop a mutually derived plan.

Distractions

The efficiency and effectiveness of home visiting can be compromised by distractions. The television or radio may need to be turned off to enhance attentiveness. If other family members are present, the visit may need to be moved to another room to allow for more privacy. The needs of small children cannot be ignored. Having toys available can facilitate uninterrupted conversation. It may be more efficient to schedule the visit at a specific time, for

example, when the baby usually is napping or the 3-year-old is at preschool.

The client may respond to distractions to avoid talking with the nurse, especially if she is apprehensive about the reason for the visit. This behavior often can be prevented by a careful explanation of the intent and purpose of the visit at the beginning of the encounter. As rapport and trust develop over time, this behavior should be less of an issue. However, the nurse should explore these feelings with the client and family when they surface.

The nurse may be distracted during the encounter for other reasons. There may be a perceived threat to personal safety, which inhibits or halts the interaction. The nurse also may be overwhelmed by the volume of work to be accomplished at the visit and may not be attending to client input regarding needs, wants, and desires. For example, the visitor may only be able to provide one visit to a new postpartum mother. In this time, complete maternal-newborn physical assessments and maternal-newborn teaching must be accomplished; the client, however, may be focused solely on breast-feeding and sore nipples.

The client's lifestyle, culture, and value system may be in such contrast to those of the nurse that meaningful interaction is difficult. These situations usually are rare if the nurse has taken time to inventory her own values, beliefs, and biases. Once these issues can be put aside and rational assessments made, the nurse should be able to distinguish a situation that is potentially hazardous from one that is simply different. Developing a familiarity with the culture and values of the population that is being served can foster a nonjudgmental approach.

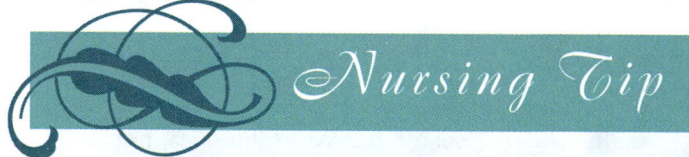

Nursing Tip

WHEN A NURSE'S VALUES AND BELIEFS ARE IN CONFLICT WITH THOSE OF A CLIENT

1. Clarify your feelings. Why are you reacting to the client's decision and lifestyle? Is the decision or behavior dangerous or different from that of your own belief system?

2. Identify your legal, moral, and ethical responsibilities to the client.

3. Recall your role as client advocate.

4. Consult with other professionals about your feelings and responsibilities.

5. Maintain a nonjudgmental attitude.

Ending the Visit

At the end of the visit, the nurse should reiterate the specific plans for follow-up, highlighting the responsibilities of the nurse and the client and family. For example, if the mutually derived plan includes the client deciding to cut down on her smoking during the next week, the nurse should remind the client that she agreed to smoke one fewer cigarette each day for the next week. The nurse should mention that the client will receive a phone call in a few days to support her efforts. Ascertaining that the client knows how to contact the agency if necessary also is recommended. If additional home visits are planned, another appointment should be scheduled at this time and plans for the next encounter reviewed. If only one home visit is planned, the nurse should make certain that the client is aware of other resources for medical care, support, and education as needed.

Postvisit Activities

Postvisit activities include evaluation and documentation. Evaluation is important for measuring whether goals have been met or need revision. Documentation is essential for providing seamless provision of care by the health care team.

Evaluation and Follow-up

Some time usually is spent reflecting on the success of the visit in terms of progress in meeting short- and long-term goals. As discussed previously, progress may be slow, especially early in the home visiting process. In cases in which single encounters are the rule there is no opportunity to see progress. Nonetheless, it is still important to review the success of any interventions implemented. In like manner, the nurse also may examine the effectiveness of home visitation as an intervention strategy given the indications for client service. For example, the nurse may have visited the home to provide instruction in childbirth education to a pregnant woman on bedrest for preterm labor. The client may have been better served by watching a video series on childbirth education, with subsequent telephone follow-up to answer any questions. The most effective method may need to be determined by a research project studying the results of both methods. Evaluation often points to a need for follow-up. To use an earlier example, the pregnant woman who agrees to stop smoking during pregnancy needs close follow-up in addition to her scheduled home visits to be successful. The nurse may need to phone the client three to four times each week to check on progress or provide encouragement. Similarly, a client who is trying to parent preterm twins may need a great deal of assistance in accessing medical care and re-

sources. Frequent phone contact and coordination with other service providers may result in the client keeping her appointments and accessing additional resources.

Follow-up often is neglected or lacking in intensity because nurses may feel that the client should take responsibility for her part of the care plan. Unless the client has the skills to act independently, however, her situation will remain unchanged. Follow-up helps address a client's dependency needs. In order to be successful, the client must have experienced success in the past and thus feel confident of her ability to succeed again. This sense of confidence and competence allows the client to act independently. Follow-up provides the ongoing encouragement and advice that is needed to nudge the client along the continuum of self-sufficiency. Once the client realizes that resources for assistance are available and success is possible, progress toward independence will result.

Documentation

Documentation provides a clinical and legal record of the home visit and serves as a means of communicating with other service providers. Reimbursement is tied to appropriate recording. Payers often designate which services need to be documented for maximum reimbursement to be approved. Most agencies designate specific forms and formats for documentation. All aspects of the nursing process should be recorded.

Organizing information according to a SOAP format (subjective, objective, assessment, and plan) leads to a coherent entry. Each note should begin with the date of the encounter along with the reason for the referral. The goals and objectives for this particular visit are recorded. Subjective data consists of the client's historical information, data collected from other sources (e.g., other health care providers and extended family), and statements made by the client. Objective data consists of data directly observed by the nurse on the date of the encounter. Physical examination data and laboratory results fall into this category. Under assessment, the nurse records the nursing diagnosis or impression based on the subjective and objective data relative to the client's condition. Evaluation data may be included here initially. Subsequently, evaluation data are relegated to the subjective or objective domains, depending on whether the evaluation criteria are reported on by the client or directly observed by the nurse. The plan category details interventions performed during the visit as well as those planned or recommended for the future. Any referrals made or consultations initiated would be documented here along with plans for follow-up. In addition, mutually agreed on goals may be recorded in this section to allow for follow-up at the next encounter. The note concludes with the date of the next encounter. If only one visit will occur, the plan should note that the client received information about other resources. Each entry must be signed with the complete name and title of the home visitor.

Documentation can be accomplished during or after the visit. Nurses may record assessment information as they interview the client and family. The entire entry is completed once the visit is concluded. Making some rudimentary notes during the visit ensures that all pertinent information is included in the final entry. Keep in mind that the client may review the chart at any time. All entries should be professional in nature, using objective information to arrive at a logical and nonjudgmental assessment.

The chart also is a legal record. Complete documentation protects the nurse and the agency in the event of litigation. The health care provider may have provided the standard of care but may have failed to comprehensively record the information. For legal purposes, an intervention that is not recorded did not occur. Thus, careful attention to charting is crucial.

CHALLENGES OF HOME VISITATION

Despite the benefits of home-based care and services, challenges also exist. Clients and families often present with multiple needs and issues. In addition, home visitors struggle with the issues of dependency versus self-sufficiency in working with clients and families. Home visitors primarily work alone, having fewer on-site resources available than might be accessible in the ambulatory or inpatient setting. The emotional investment required to build a relationship between the client and nurse may make it more difficult to maintain a healthy distance. Home-based interventions, in particular, must be highly individualized to address the cultural, social, and economic diversity among clients within their own environment. Finally, in some cases, the length and intensity of home-based services are dictated by cost and reimbursement issues and not necessarily by client needs or outcomes.

Meeting Multiple Needs

Home visitors providing acute home care services or interventions focused on health promotion often are confronted with a group of clients that are at high risk. Currently, clients are being released from the inpatient setting earlier than ever before in the course of recovery. Consequently, they have more health care needs that require home-based convalescence. As a result, nursing care and procedures in the home are more complex, often requiring longer and more frequent visits. In the face of an overwhelming number of medical and physical care needs, the client's psychosocial issues often are not being addressed. Nurses visiting the home to provide public-health–oriented interventions face similar challenges, as discussed in Chapter 38. In certain situations, clients and families may face multiple economic and psychosocial hardships so that the predominant mode of care becomes ongoing crisis intervention. Proactive planning and the setting of mutual goals rarely occur because the pressing needs of the moment always take precedence.

Fostering Self-sufficiency

In both acute care and public health settings, overall goals consistently emphasize recovery and self-sufficiency. Most interventions attempt to move the client along the continuum of care to meet these goals. Dependence is viewed as undesirable; however, dependency needs must be met before the client can assume responsibility for self-care. The initial assessment takes these issues into consideration. By mutually deriving a plan of care, the nurse and client can identify overall goals for recovery or self-sufficiency, highlighting specific areas in which assistance is needed to meet those goals. Initially, more assistance is given by the nurse, who provides a role model for the skills and behaviors necessary for independence. Frequently, however, these steps are skipped because the pressures of time and reimbursement limitations push providers toward an end to the intervention. The client outcome or the home visiting strategy as a whole may be viewed as being unmet or unsuccessful when, in fact, the process was simply too short to result in significant behavioral change.

Physical and Emotional Overload

The home care nurse faces more isolation than do other health care providers. In the hospital or ambulatory area, other staff is available for assistance, support, and consultation. In the home, the nurse works alone. The nurse experiences physical and psychological stressors. Clients receiving acute home care often require much from the nurse in terms of physical assessment and monitoring. Their emotional needs are such that social support also is a necessity. Similarly, with health promotion activities, ongoing psycho-emotional issues can be time-consuming for the nurse and difficult to resolve. This isolation coupled with the volume of work and the emotional investment required to establish trust and mutuality can lead to frustration, depression, and feelings of guilt or low self-esteem on the part of the nurse. Home visitors need an opportunity to discuss their case load with peers, supervisors, and other providers. Regularly scheduled case conferences and staff meetings provide an outlet to express feelings and a chance to obtain peer support. Peer support also decreases staff burnout and turnover. However, administrators sometimes view these non–revenue-producing activities as superfluous. Time allotted for consultation and oversight is critical to the provision of quality care.

Responding to Client Diversity

Home visitors interact with populations of great cultural, social, and economic diversity. The nurse must be familiar with the cultural practices of a variety of groups and respond sensitively and appropriately (Wasik, 1993). Home visitors must be aware of the characteristics of the communities that they serve and demonstrate an understanding and appreciation for cultural differences. For example, assigning a male nurse home visitor to provide care for a Muslim woman would be culturally inappropriate because religious tenets forbid Muslim women to receive care from male providers. In some cases, administrators have been slow to authorize recruitment and hiring of bilingual or bicultural personnel. An interpreter should always accompany the nurse on a home visit if bilingual professional staff is not available.

Cost and Reimbursement

Appropriately, with the advent of managed care, the health care arena has been called on to demonstrate a cost-effective approach to client care and service. A balance must be achieved between management of costs and provision of quality service. Third-party reimbursement is tied primarily to the provision of technical and procedural nursing care rather than health promotion, health education, and support. Nurses find themselves providing preventive health services while attending to the acute health care needs of the client, the so-called billable service. Many agencies use reimbursement from acute home health care to fund health promotion and education in the home. Additional outcomes-based research is necessary to establish the cost benefits of preventive home care to ensure reimbursement solely for these valuable activities. Given the recent research of Olds et al. (1997) supporting the long-term cost-effectiveness of these types of home visit interventions, however, focused on prevention reimbursement.

TERMINATING THE HOME VISITING RELATIONSHIP

Home visiting services are terminated when the service plan has been accomplished, the strategy is not resulting in problem resolution and alternatives are available, reimbursement is exhausted, or the client no longer desires or needs care. The process of termination often is difficult for both the client and the nurse, especially if the relationship has been a long one. Because the nurse-client relationship has involved a great degree of trust and mutuality, a sense of loss may ensue for both the nurse and the client-family. Preparation for termination best begins at the initial encounter. The client must be made aware of the expected length of service, which may vary according to agency or reimbursement policies; the amount of special funding or grant funds available; and the amount of time estimated to accomplish the stated goals and objectives. The termination date should be reiterated at regular intervals throughout the home visiting relationship. The last few encounters should focus on identifying other resources for care and services and planning for follow-up once visitation ends. This information also should be completely documented.

It is helpful to discuss the affective aspect of the home visiting process with the client to facilitate a successful termination. The client should be encouraged to voice her feelings and reflect on the process and the home visiting relationship. The nurse should verbalize the positive aspects of the relationship.

Termination issues are virtually nonexistent with single encounters or when clients refuse services. The nurse may feel a sense of responsibility if the home visiting intervention is terminated for ineffectiveness. When a case is not progressing smoothly, it is helpful to review the plan of care with a peer or supervisor to confirm that the plan is a valid one. A therapeutic relationship usually is not terminated without consultation and discussion by the staff involved.

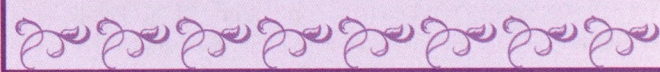

Critical Thinking

Terminating the Home Visiting Relationship
A client for whom you provided ongoing home visitation services continues to call you several times a week approximately 2 months after the relationship was terminated owing to reimbursement limitations.

- How would you respond to this client on the phone?
- Which problems might arise if this relationship were to continue?
- What is your professional responsibility in this case?

When the relationship is terminated as a result of reimbursement limitations, the client may feel abandoned, especially if care ends before goals and objectives have been accomplished. In this situation, the nurse must ensure that the client is well acquainted with existing resources and service alternatives. Termination, if planned and executed proactively, can provide a fitting end to a satisfying and hopefully successful helping relationship.

Web Activities

- Locate your state's Visiting Nurse Association (VNA). Does it have a web site? What type of professional information is offered regarding regulations for home visits in your state? Compare these regulations with those listed for a neighboring state.

- Visit a local hospital's web site for information on its home visiting program.

Key Concepts

- Home visitation is a means to providing direct health care services, health education, and psychosocial support to clients and families.

- The growth of social reforms and the expansion of the field of social work contributed to the rise of home care programs in the early 20th century.

- The home as the site of delivery provides the nurse with a unique opportunity to assess the client and family in their own environment.

- Home care can be provided by home health care agencies, hospitals, public health departments, schools, and other institutions.

- Cost savings in the form of reduced inpatient hospital stays is one of the many benefits of home care.

- The home visit consists of three phases: previsit preparation, the visit, and postvisit activities.

Review Questions and Activities

1. Why is it important for the home visitor to be culturally sensitive?

2. List two important principles of home visiting and give examples of how these might be put into operation by the nurse during the home visit.

3. List three tasks the nurse should perform before making a home visit.

4. Identify three strategies to promote communication during a home visit.

5. You are visiting a pregnant woman at home. Identify three nursing observations that might be made to assess the following: living necessities, coping and stress tolerance, and nutritional status.

6. List three strategies for ensuring personal safety during a home visit.

7. You have just completed a home visit where you provided extensive breast-feeding education and support to a new mother. How can the outcomes of this visit be evaluated?

8. Identify important areas for documentation after the home visit.

9. Discuss two limitations of home visits.

10. Discuss the challenges involved in terminating the home visiting relationship.

References

Association of Women's Health, Obstetric, and Neonatal Nurses (AWHONN). (1994). Didactic content and clinical skills verification for professional nurse providers of perinatal home care. Washington, D.C.: AWHONN.

Barnes-Boyd, C., Norr, K. F., Kayon, K. W. (1996). Evaluation of an interagency home visiting program to reduce postneonatal mortality in disadvantaged communities. *Public Health Nursing, 13,* (3), 201–208.

Braveman, P., Miller, C., Egerter, S., Bennett, T., English, P., Katz, P., Showstack, J. (1996). Health service use among low-risk newborns after early discharge with and without nurse home visiting. *Journal of the American Board of Family Practice, 9,* (4), 254–260.

Bremner, R. H. (1971). *Children and youth in America: A documentary history.* Cambridge, MA: Harvard University Press.

Cooper, W. O., Kotagel, U. R., Atherton, H. D., Lippert, C. A., Bragg, E., Donovan, E. F., Perlstein, P. H. (1996). Use of health care services by inner-city infants in an early discharge program. *Pediatrics, 98,* (4), 686–691.

Gomby, D., Larson, C., Lewit, E., & Behrman, R. (1993). Home visiting: Analysis and recommendations. In *The future of children: Home visiting,* (pp. 6–19). Los Altos, CA: The David and Lucille Packard Foundation.

Hoover, T., Johnson, F., Wells, C., Graham, C., & Biddleman, M. (1996). *A guest in my home: A guide to home visiting that strengthens families and communities.* Tallahassee, FL: Florida Department of Health and Rehabilitative Services.

Institute of Medicine. (1988). *The future of public health.* Washington, DC: National Academy Press.

Kitzman, H., Olds, D., Henderson, C., Hanks, C., Cole, R., Tatelbaum, R., McConnochie, K., Sidora, K., Luckey, D., Shaver, D., Engelhardt, K., James, D., & Barnard, K. (1997). Effect of prenatal and infancy home visitation by nurses on pregnancy outcomes, childhood injuries, and repeated childbearing. *Journal of the American Medical Association, 278,* 644–652.

Klass, C. (1996). *Home visiting: Promoting healthy parent and child development.* Baltimore, MD: Paul H. Brookes Publishing.

Occupational Health and Safety Administration (OSHA). (1991). *Occupational exposure to bloodborne pathogens.* (vol. 56, no. 235). Federal Register.

Olds, D., Eckenrode, J., Henderson, C., Kitzman, H., Powers, J., Cole, R., Sidora, K., Morris, P., Pettit, L., & Luckey, D. (1997). Long-term effects of home visitation on maternal life course and child abuse and neglect. *Journal of the American Medical Association, 278,* 637–643.

Olds, D., & Kitzman, H. (1993). Review of research on home visiting for pregnant women and parents of young children. In *The Future of Children: Home Visiting* (pp. 6–19). Los Altos, CA: The David and Lucille Packard Foundation.

Trierweiler, K., Ricketts, S., Kent, H., Albert, S. (1994). *The helping moms program: A case management approach to delivering enhanced prenatal services.* Denver, CO: Colorado Department of Public Health and Environment.

Wasik, B., Bryant, D., & Lyons, C. (1990). *Home visiting: Procedures for helping families.* Newbury Park, CA: Sage Publishing.

Wasik, B. (1993). Staffing issues for home visiting programs. *The future of children: Home visiting* (pp. 140–157). Los Altos, CA: The David and Lucille Packard Foundation.

Weiss, H. (1993). Home visits: Necessary but not sufficient. *The future of children: Home visiting* (pp. 113–127). Los Altos, CA: The David and Lucille Packard Foundation.

Woods, N. F., & Mitchell, E. S. (1997). Preventive health issues: The perimenopausal to mature years (45–64). In K. Allen & J. Phillips, J. (Eds.). *Women's health across the lifespan* (pp. 39–54). Philadelphia, PA: Lippincott-Raven Publishers.

Suggested Readings

Byrd, M. E. (1995). A concept analysis of home visiting. *Public Health Nursing, 12,* (2), 83–89.

Byrd, M. E. (1997). A typology of the potential outcomes of maternal-child home visits: A literature analysis. *Public Health Nursing, 14,* (5), 3–11.

Ciliska, D., Hayward, S., Thomas, H., Mitchell, A., Dobbins, M., Underwood, J., Rafael, A., Martin, E. (1996). A systematic overview of the effectiveness of home visiting as a delivery strategy for public health nursing interventions. *Canadian Journal of Public Health, 87,* (3), 193–198.

Doherty, M. (1994). Suburban home care: Cost, financing and delivery. *Nursing Clinics of North America, 29,* (3), 483–493.

Narayan, M. C., Tennant, J., Larose, P., Grumble, J., Marchessault, L. (1996). Achieving success in home care through the self-directed work group approach. *Home Healthcare Nurse, 14,* (11), 865–872.

Struk, C. M. (1994). Women and children: Infant mortality, urban programs and home care. *Nursing Clinics of North America, 29,* (3), 395–408.

Zink, M. R. (1994). Nursing diagnosis in home care: Audit tool development. *Journal of Community Health Nursing, 11,* (1), 51–58.

Zotti, M. E., & Zahner, S. J. (1995). Evaluation of public health nursing home visits to pregnant women on WIC. *Public Health Nursing, 12,* (5), 294–304.

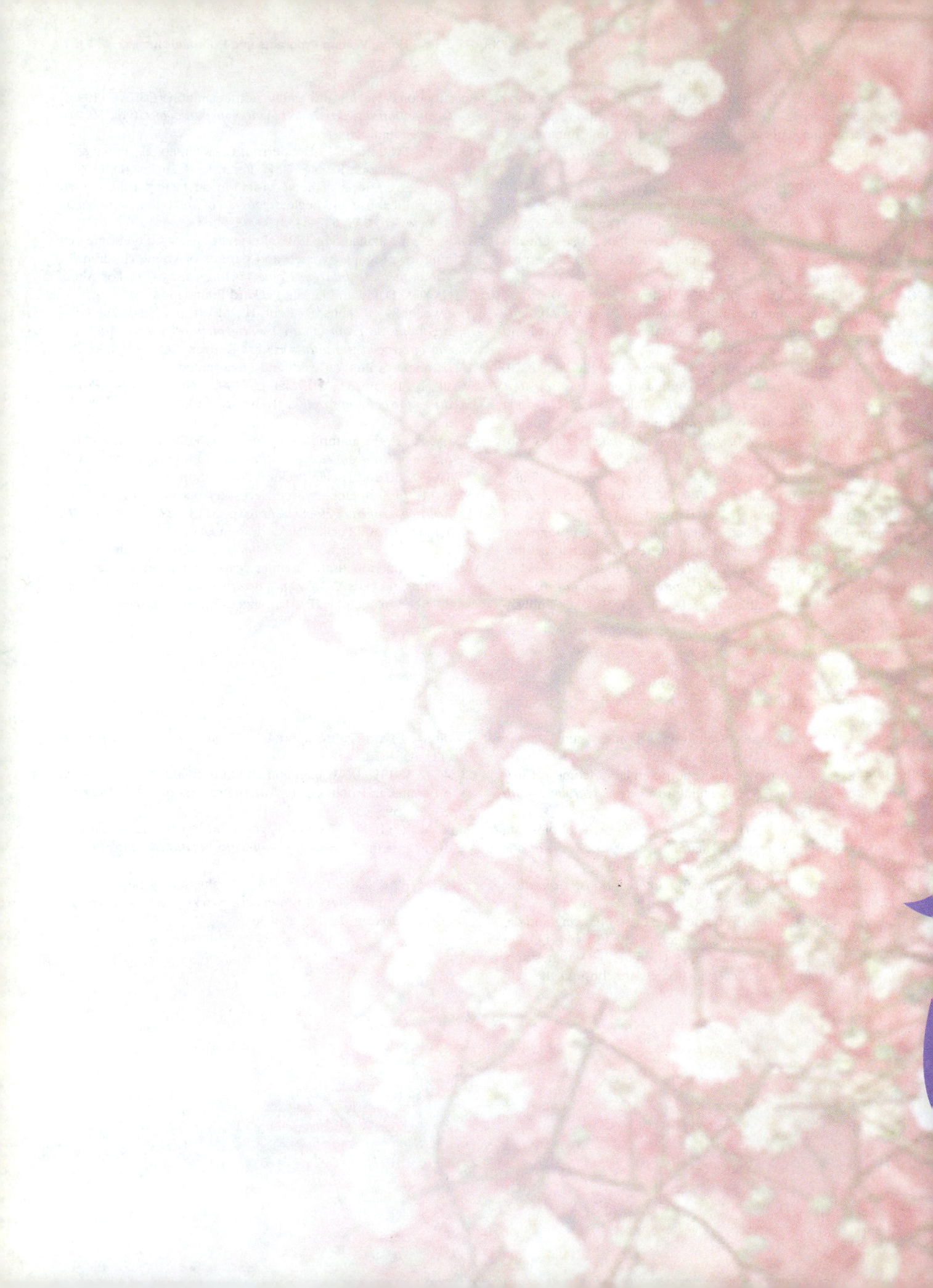

UNIT II

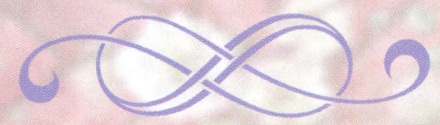

Health Care of Women

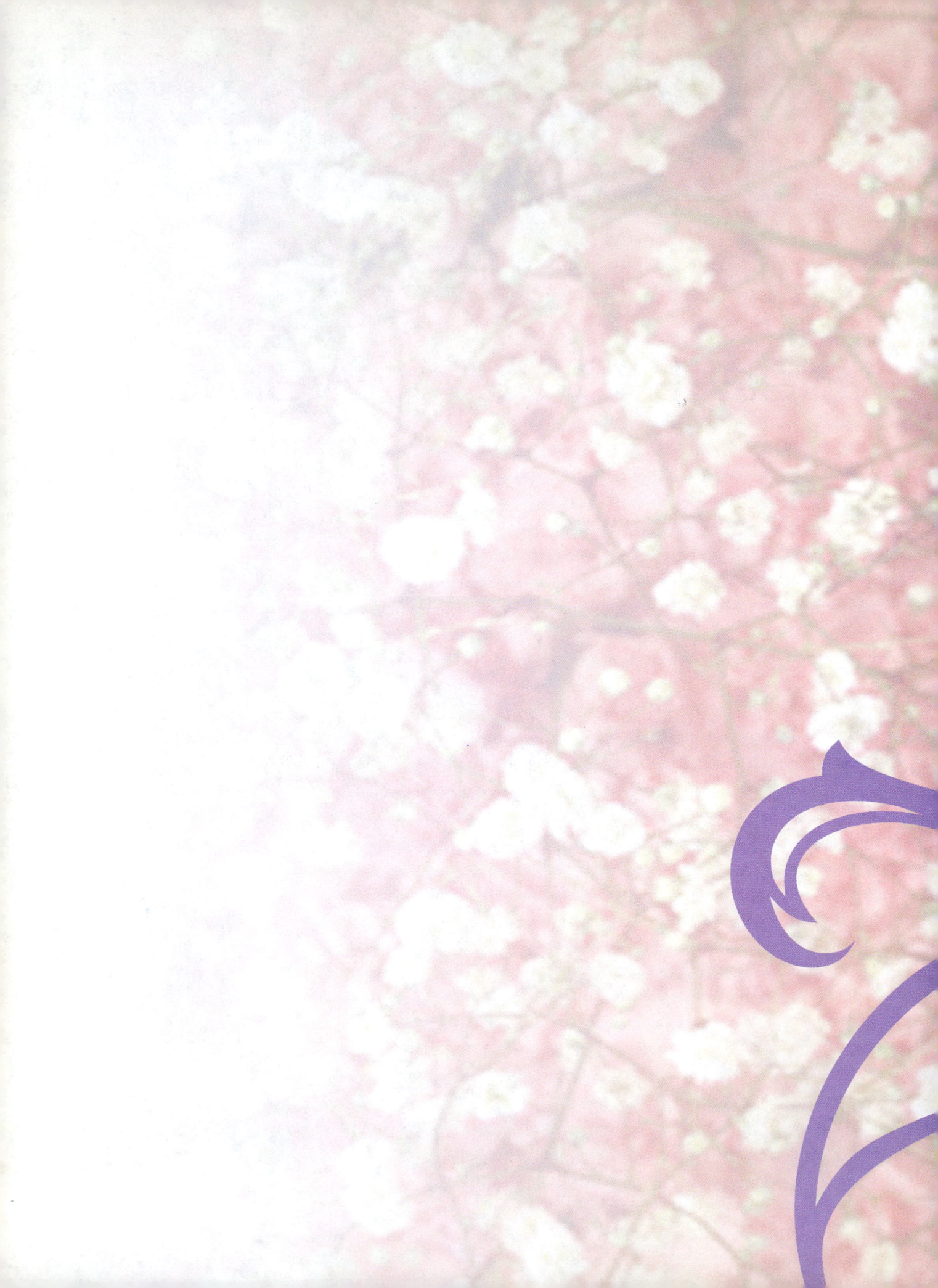

CHAPTER 7

Development of Women Across the Life Span

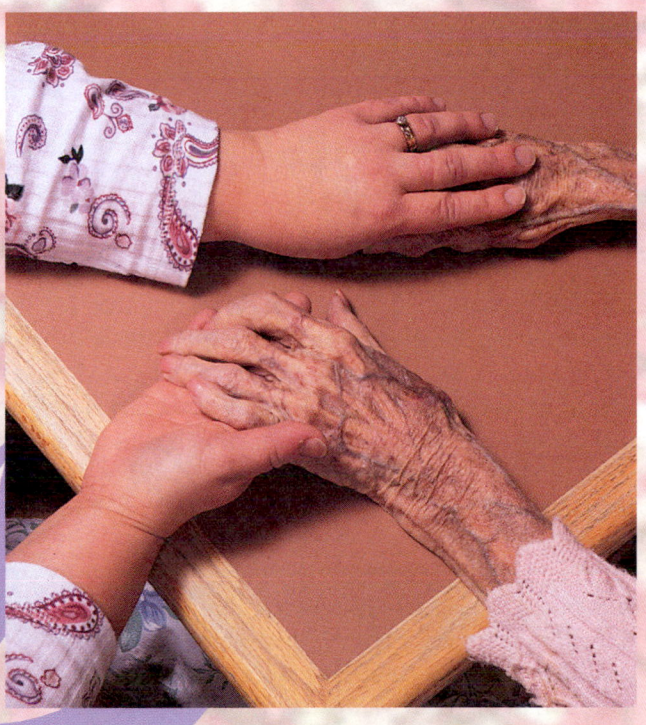

"So much has happened during the past 40 years. I feel as though I've been through so many changes; something was always happening. When I was in my teens, I had a hard enough time dealing with my changing body, let alone the relationships that were constantly changing with friends, boyfriends, parents, and grandparents. Now that I'm a parent, I understand why my parents acted as they did. They were looking out for my interests. I think that the best years are yet to come. I'm finally comfortable with myself, and my body. I feel good. I love my job, and I am very happy with my relationships. I know that I have to manage my stress, exercise, and eat right to take proper care of myself, but overall, I'm very pleased with my development as a woman."

Key Terms

Adolescence
Anovulatory cycle
Corpus luteum
Hypothalamic-pituitary-
  ovarian axis

Menarche
Menopause
Osteoporosis
Ovulation

Perimenopause
Pseudomenstruation
Puberty
Stress incontinence

Tanner Stages
Thelarche
Urge incontinence

Competencies

Upon completion of this chapter, the reader should be able to:

1. Describe the hypothalamic-pituitary-ovarian axis.
2. Determine physiologic development using the Tanner Stages.
3. Understand the three phases of the menstrual cycle.
4. Discuss the rationale behind adolescent risk-taking behavior.
5. Discuss adolescent emotional development.
6. Describe the hormonal and physiologic changes during pregnancy.
7. Understand the psychosocial changes that occur during pregnancy.
8. Name three cultural differences in women across the lifespan.
9. Discuss the physiologic changes of the peri- and postmenopausal periods.
10. Name five psychosocial issues of the aging woman.
11. Describe self-care methods across the lifespan.

Women experience many changes throughout their lives. Women learn behaviors in the context of their experiences in their cultural environments that affect socialization of the roles they participate in and their choices with respect to their lives, including choices relating to health care. Their environment and responsibilities may affect their ability to access the health care system for preventive care, health education, and prenatal care compared with their ability to access emergent care for acute onset and late-stage illnesses.

As women age, their health care choices may be abundant or dependent on lifestyles and careers. Resources may be limited by fixed incomes, chronic illness, and loss of family and life partners. There are more women in the U.S. population than there are men, and a woman's life expectancy is 79 years compared with 72 years for men (Commonwealth Fund, 1997). As a result, additional health resources are used by women. By understanding the physiologic and psychosocial needs of women who are aging, nurses can better direct clients to the most appropriate resources available.

This chapter focuses on female development in utero through senescence. The discussion begins with the cellu-

lar changes that differentiate the female from the male reproductive system and continues to the hormonal effects at birth. Next, the female adolescent's physical, emotional, and cultural development are examined. The discussion proceeds to the young adult, the woman during midlife, and the mature woman. Included are specific self-care and cultural cues to assist the nurse in providing culturally appropriate health care to women throughout their lives.

PRENATAL THROUGH EARLY ADOLESCENT YEARS

Initial differentiation between genders begins at fertilization at the time in which the genetic sex is determined by chromosomes XX (female) or XY (male). After the female genetic sex is determined, development of the reproductive system occurs in three phases: ovarian development, duct development, and the development of the external genitalia. By 10 weeks' gestation, the ovaries can be identified. By approximately 16 weeks' gestation, the cells that will later make up the ovarian follicles can be identified (Blackburn & Loper, 1992).

Genital duct development leads to the development of the uterus, fallopian tubes, and vagina. The embryo has two pairs of ducts, the mesonephric duct (wolffian) and the paramesonephric (müllerian) duct. The ducts develop side by side. The paramesonephric ducts are dominant in the female embryo and continue to develop, while the mesonephric ducts degenerate. The opposite occurs in the male embryo. The paramesonephric ducts develop into the fallopian tubes, uterus, and vagina by 16 weeks' gestation (Blackburn & Loper, 1992).

The development of the external genitalia is complete before that of the internal reproductive organs. Differentiation of male from female external genitalia occurs in the absence of androgens. The clitoris develops. The urethra and vaginal orifice open into the vestibule. The labia majora and labia minora develop from the surrounding connective tissue. The development of the external genitalia is complete at approximately 12 weeks' gestation (Blackburn & Loper, 1992).

During the newborn assessment shortly after birth, both female and male infants may exhibit signs of circulating maternal estrogens. The newborn's breasts may seem slightly swollen and enlarged, with nipple size ranging from 1.0 to 1.5 cm. The swelling will resolve in time and rarely lasts beyond the first month of life.

Not only is the breast tissue affected by maternal hormones, the female genitalia also are affected by maternal estrogens. The labia minora and labia majora appear engorged, and the labia minora may be more prominent than is the labia majora. A pinkish-white mucoid vaginal discharge also may be noted in the diaper. This is termed **pseudomenstruation** and is a sign of maternal transfer of estrogen. On resolution of the maternal hormonal effects, the childhood hormonal values are maintained at a static level until the nighttime changes that occur just before the onset of puberty.

ADOLESCENCE

Adolescence can be defined as the passage from childhood to maturity. Adolescence begins with the appearance of secondary sex characteristics and ends with cessation of growth and lasts from approximately ages 11 to 18 years. **Puberty** is the onset of the process of physical maturity. At puberty the secondary sex characteristics begin to develop and the capability of sexual reproduction is attained. The events leading to puberty occur in a timed sequence that is initiated with the secretion of the gonadal hormones and the development of the secondary sexual characteristics (Stedman, 1995). As girls move through adolescence, they become concerned with appearance, beauty, and their changing bodies. As adolescent females begin to mature physically, they look to their peers for recognition and val-

idation. They begin to make choices based on the interaction of the social group and peer relationships rather than on family recommendations. Emotional maturity is related to life experiences and the ability to make appropriate life choices and therefore often occurs many years after physical maturity. The cultural influences of the family and peer group in turn influence the life choices of the adolescent.

The age of pubertal growth ranges from 8 to 14 years. Any visible sign of pubertal development before age 8 years in girls is considered precocious and needs further medical investigation (Rosenfeld, 1997). The age of puberty may be determined by health status, genetics, and nutrition. Theories suggest that a minimum body weight of 48 kg and a minimum percent of body fat, 17%, are necessary for **menarche**, the onset of menstruation, to occur (Speroff, Glass, & Kase, 1999).

Physiologic Changes

The onset of puberty and menarche occur as a physiologic response to hormonal pulses associated during the sleep cycle. The pulses are cues of the **hypothalamic-pituitary-ovarian axis**, which is the transport mechanism of a hormone from the hypothalamus that stimulates the release of gonadotropins that, in turn, stimulates the ovaries to release estrogen and progesterone. The pulses begin between the ages of 6 and 8 years with the nighttime release of **gonadotropin releasing hormone (Gn-RH)** from the hypothalamus. Gn-RH flows to the anterior pituitary gland by way of the portal circulation, causing the release of the gonadotropins, or luteinizing hormone (LH) and follicle stimulating hormone (FSH). Gonadotropins such as LH and FSH are released from the anterior pituitary gland. LH and FSH stimulate the ovary to release estrogens, progestins, and androgens. Early hormonal stimulation precipitates the developing changes in the female reproductive organs: the breasts, labia, vagina, and uterus. Changes in the reproductive organs typically occur 2 years before the onset of menstruation (Blackburn & Loper, 1992). Hormonal stimulation also leads to rapid growth of the axial skeleton, resulting in the so-called growth spurt frequently experienced before the onset of menses.

External Development

The **Tanner Stages** are the five stages of female and male development developed by Tanner (1981) and recognized today as the standard in adolescent physical development (Tables 7-1 and 7-2). Stage one is the state of preadolescence, in which there are no signs of physical maturity. Stage five represents full maturity of the breast and pubic hair development. The initial visible sign of puberty is **thelarche**, or the prominence of glandular tissue in the breast behind the nipple, also called the breast bud.

Table 7-1 Sexual Maturity Rating for Female Breast Development

Developmental Stage	Description
	1. Preadolescent stage (before age 10) Nipple is small, slightly raised.
	2. Breast bud stage (after age 10) Nipple and breast form a small mound. Areola enlarges. Height spurt begins.
	3. Adolescent stage (10–14 years) Nipple is flush with breast shape. Breast and areola enlarge. Menses begins. Height spurt peaks.
	4. Late adolescent stage (14–17 years) Nipple and areola form a secondary mound over the breast. Height spurt ends.
	5. Adult stage. Nipple protrudes; areola is flush with the breast shape.

Table 7-2 Sexual Maturity Rating for Female Genitalia

Developmental Stage	Description
Stage 1	No pubic hair, only body hair (vellus hair)
Stage 2	Sparse growth of long, slightly dark, fine pubic hair, slightly curly and located along the labia (ages 11 to 12)
Stage 3	Pubic hair becomes darker, curlier, and spreads over the symphysis (ages 12 to 13)
Stage 4	Texture and curl of pubic hair is similar to that of an adult but not spread to thighs (ages 13 to 15)
Stage 5	Adult appearance in quality and quantity of pubic hair; growth is spread to inner aspect of thighs and abdomen

Simultaneously, or shortly thereafter, the first sign of pubic hair development is noted sparsely on the labia majora and mons pubis. This is indicative of Tanner Stage two. Stage three reveals further enlargement of the breast mound (the areola and breast as one unit). A slight darkening of the areola pigment may be noted. Sparse, dark, curly hair is noted over the mons pubis. In Stage four, separation of the areola-nipple unit above the breast occurs. The pubic hair appears adultlike but is limited to the mons pubis and labia. The final stage, Stage five, reveals further nipple-areola development, with increased pigmentation and the enhancement of Montgomery's tubercles and

ducts on the areola. The pubic hair is adultlike, with extension to the inner thighs. By Tanner Stage 5, the labia majora increases to twice the size of the labia minora. The vaginal orifice becomes more prominent, and the urethral

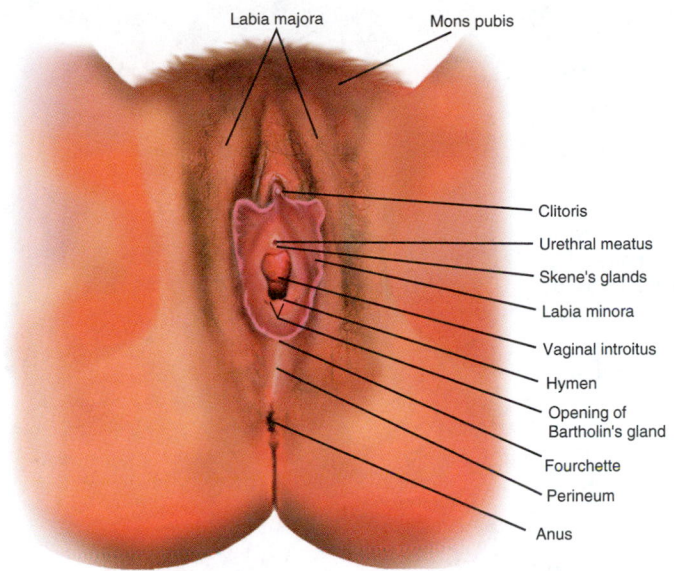

Figure 7-1 External structures of the female genitalia

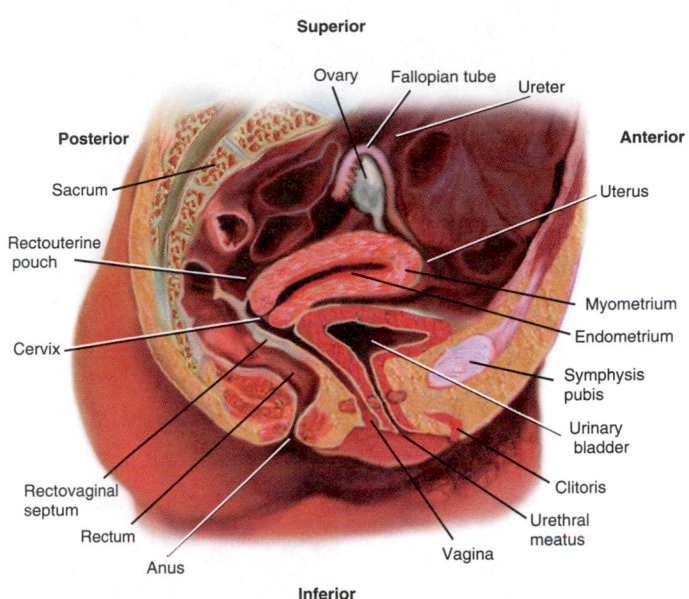

Figure 7-2 Female internal pelvic organs

orifice becomes less prominent (Blackburn & Loper, 1992). The external structures of the female genitalia are shown in Figure 7-1. The Tanner Stages are of great assistance in educating adolescents about the chronologic stages of their physical development.

Internal Development

As the external physiologic characteristics change, the internal structures of the female organs also develop. The vagina lengthens and increases in size. The pH of the vaginal secretions decreases to an acidic pH (pH of 5), and the amount of the vaginal secretions increases. The acidic pH and increase in secretions support conception. The uterus also increases in size and length to prepare for fertility. The ovary increases in size but at a slower rate than does the uterus. The internal structures of the female pelvis are illustrated in Figure 7-2.

As estrogen is released, the ovary develops a complex vasculature network in preparation for ovulation. Once the vasular compartments are fully developed, and a sufficient amount of estrogen is released, the estrogen stimulates the anterior pituitary to release LH that, in turn, causes ovulation to occur.

Breast Development

Breast development is the first visible sign of puberty. The breast is made up of 15 to 20 lobes of glandular tissue supported by fibrous connective and adipose tissues. Within each lobe of glandular tissue there are 20 to 40 lobules lined with epithelial cells called acini cells, which produce milk in lactating women. The lobules are connected by lactiferous ducts that empty into a lactiferous sinus near the nipple. Montgomery's tubercles are located on the lat-

eral edges of the areola and provide natural secretions for the lactating breast. The fibrous tissue provides support to the glandular tissue of the breasts, as do the suspensory ligaments know as Cooper's suspensory ligaments. Figure 7-3 depicts the internal anatomic structures of the breast. It is not unusual for breasts to develop simultaneously. However, the breasts may develop in an asynchronous manner, with one breast developing faster than the other. As the breasts develop to Tanner Stage 5, it is not unusual for a woman to have one breast that is slightly larger in caliber than the ipsilateral breast.

Menarche

Menarche is the beginning of the menstrual function, or the onset of the first menstrual period as a result of the hypothalamic-pituitary-ovarian axis. The mean age of menarche is approximately 12 years. The age range varies from 9 to 17 years (Speroff, Glass, & Case, 1999). Menarche may be delayed in adolescents who have a very lean habitus owing to physical exertion. Conversely, girls who are obese, that is, whose body weight is 20% to 30% more than their ideal weight, may begin menses early (Wilson, 1998). Initially, menstruation is irregular and sporadic. The duration of the menstrual cycle ranges from 21 to 45 days, with an average of 28 days. The bleeding may vary from very light to very heavy and last from 2 to 7 days. Menstrual bleeding that lasts longer that 10 days is considered abnormal or dysfunctional. Anovulatory cycles account for 90% to 95% of all dysfunctional bleeding that occurs. An **anovulatory cycle** is a menstrual cycle that occurs in the absence of ovulation. An adolescent may have anovulatory cycles for the first several years of menstruation. The cause of anovulatory cycles in the adolescent usually is an

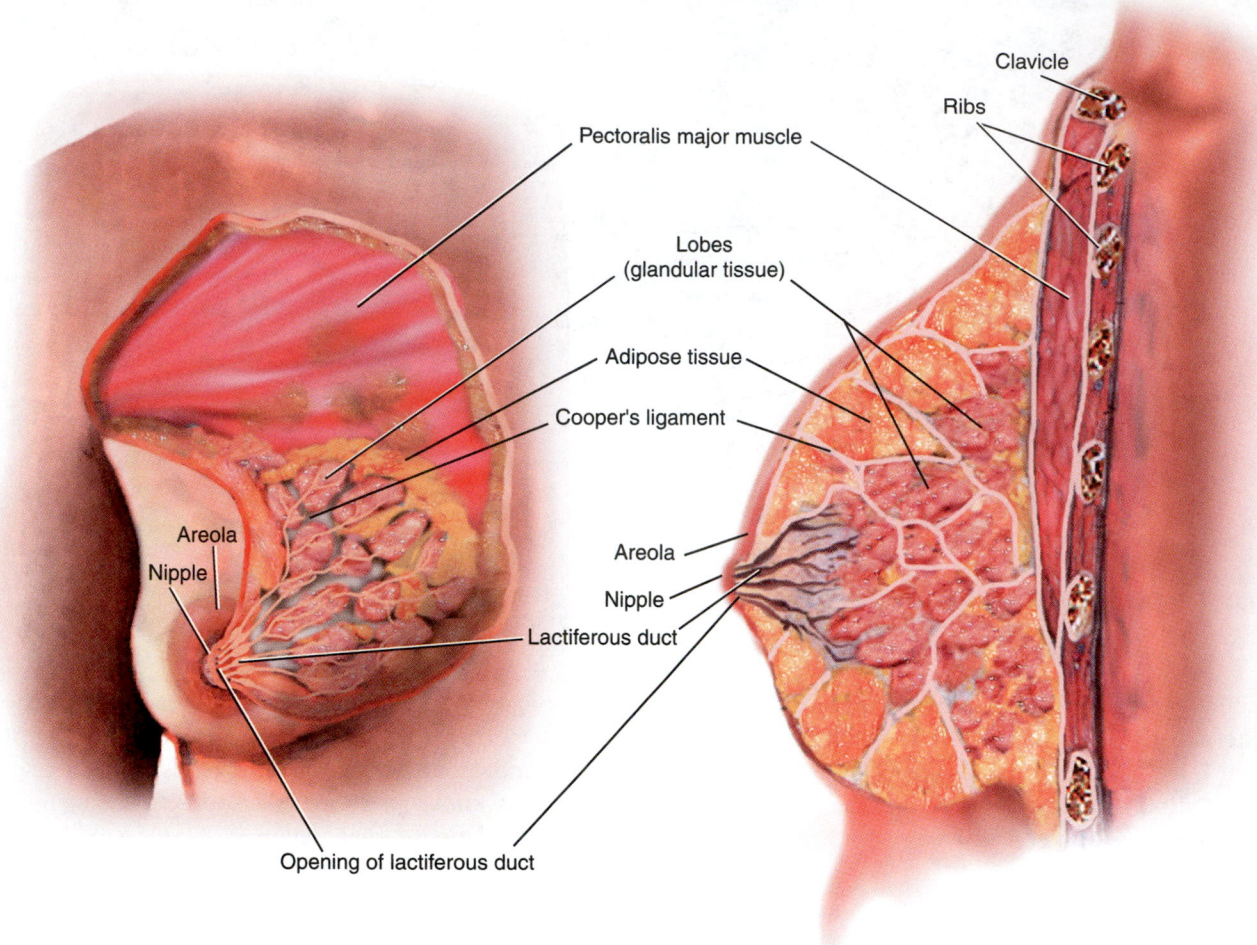

Figure 7-3 Anatomical structures of the female breast

immature hypothalamic-pituitary-ovarian axis; however, in some cases, a pathological cause may be established (Dealy, 1998).

The Menstrual Cycle

There are three phases of the menstrual cycle. The phases occur as a result of the effects of hormonal influence on the ovaries and uterus (Figure 7-4). As menarche approaches, the Gn-RH pulses increase in frequency and intensity. The pulses occur throughout the day rather than solely at nighttime. The first day of the menstrual bleeding is considered day 1 of the cycle and is considered the menstrual phase, or phase one. At this time, levels of estrogen, progestin, LH, and FSH are relatively low. Gn-RH continues to stimulate the anterior pituitary to release FSH, which acts as a stimulus on the ovary to release estrogen in preparation for the developing follicles and provides thickening of the uterine lining.

By day 5 to 7, a single follicle has assumed dominance (Hatcher et al., 1998). This is phase two, also termed the proliferative-follicular phase. Estrogen levels in the blood begin to increase, sending a message to the anterior pituitary gland to decrease the circulating levels of FSH. As the woman approaches day 14, or midcycle, the continued increase in estrogen stimulates the release of LH from the anterior pituitary. The LH surge is responsible for **ovulation**, or the release of the dominant follicle in preparation for conception, which occurs within the next 10 to 12 hours after the levels of LH have peaked.

Phase three, or the secretory-luteal phase, begins after ovulation. Once the dominant follicle is released the remnant cyst of the follicle releases estrogens, progesterone, and androgens. The remnant cyst of the dominant follicle left behind in the ovary is termed the **corpus luteum**. The corpus luteum is a yellow mass in the ovary formed by an ovarian follicle that has matured and discharged its ovum. The estrogen levels begin to decrease after the surge in LH, and progesterone levels begin to increase. There is a second increase in estrogen levels that coincides with the release of progesterone from the corpus luteum. The endometrial lining changes in substance to provide a glycogen-

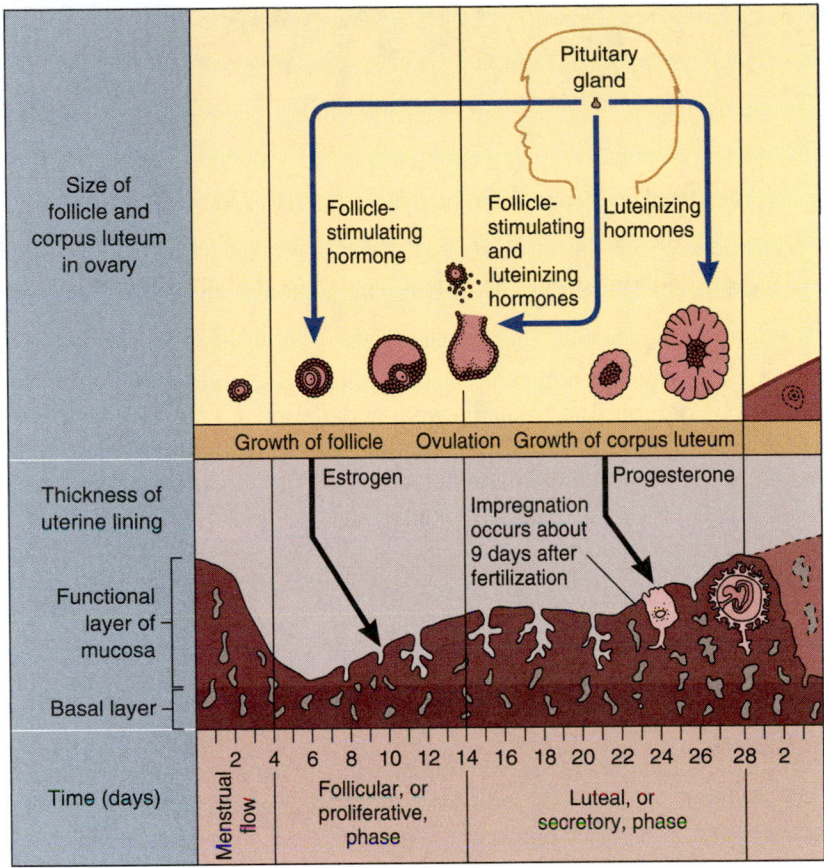

Figure 7-4 Events of the menstrual cycle

rich environment to foster implantation. FSH and LH levels decrease as a result of the increasing estrogen and progesterone levels. If implantation, fertilization, or pregnancy do not occur, the corpus luteum regresses and the estrogen and progesterone levels decrease, which results in menstruation returning to day 1 of the cycle (Hatcher et al., 1998). If pregnancy (implantation) occurs, the corpus luteum continues to produce estrogen and progesterone, thus prohibiting menstruation.

Psychosocial Changes

A young woman approaches normal physical development over a span of years. Her emotional development also occurs as a lengthy process. Changes in body image, function, the onset of menses, and relationships play a role in the perception of what is normal in her eyes. Girls are socialized in the context of their environment and relationships. Erikson (1950) identified the adolescent developmental task as "identity versus role confusion" in his developmental theory. This developmental phase supports the premise that emotional maturity is based on separation and independence, meaning that the adolescent must detach herself from current relationships to be able to grow and develop a new, productive adult identity. Erikson's theory has been challenged by feminist theorists, such as Belenkey et al. (1986) and Gilligan (1993), for the lack of inclusion of girls in his research, yet the research continues to be legitimized to both genders. According to Gilligan's (1993) psychological theory of women's development, girls are socialized and develop through relationships and the maintenance of those attachments rather than through separation. A young woman who develops without the benefit of relationship-building may feel isolated and would therefore not achieve emotional maturity.

Critical Thinking

Teenage Sexual Behavior

Nearly half of all teenaged girls admit to being sexually active. How accurate do you think these figures are? Given this high percentage, should adolescents have access to contraception without parental consent?

Research Highlight

Teen Mothers' Perceptions of Parenting

Purpose

To describe the parenting perceptions of African American teen mothers based on their own experiences.

Methods

Descriptive, qualitative design was used in data collection. Using a moderator, 17 African American teens were interviewed in 10 focus groups. The sessions were audiotaped. Of the 17 teens, 8 were pregnant and 9 were parenting. The topics discussed came from a school-based teen parenting program and were infant feeding; comforting a crying infant; bathing, diapering, and dressing the infant; infant and child safety; childhood illnesses; an infant's need for play and stimulation; an infant's need for holding and cuddling; childhood discipline; and identification of the teen mothers' needs.

Findings

Seven themes emerged from the data:

1. Artifacts. Items considered necessary to parenting, for example, disposable diapers and the television remote control.

2. Sources of information. The teens received traditional health care information from nurses and doctors; however, the teens depended on family members to validate the instructions. If there was no validation, the teens took the advice of family members.

3. Problems. Special events of concern. The mothers of the teens were very involved in the infant's lives and the teens did not like it if the child referred to the grandmother as mother and the mother as sister. They also voiced concerns of the grandmothers spoiling the child by "picking the child up too much."

4. Strategies or remedies. How the teens solved a specific problem, specifically how they stop the baby from crying. Examples included giving a bottle, picking up the child, sleeping with the child, and playing music. The teens also discussed home remedies such as olive oil for skin care and flour browned in a pan on top of the stove for diaper rash.

5. Unique language. Terms the teens used consistently that had no meaning to the researchers. Additional dialogue was pursued to gain an understanding of the teens' perceptions.

6. Lack of information. Information seeking from the teens regarding infant feeding; breast-feeding; and baby care, such as use of the emergency department for care.

7. Misinformation. The teens believed that their babies were already spoiled. The teens did not participate in safe behaviors with their infants, such as using car seats.

Nursing Implications

Teen mothers need appropriate information as to the expectations of parenting after delivery. Involvement of family members would enhance educational processes and provide a sense of support to the teens.

Wayland, J., & Rawlins, R. (1997). African-American teen mothers' perceptions of parenting. *Journal of Pediatric Nursing, 12,* (1), 13–20.

Peer acceptance is extremely important. Behaviors related to dress, activities, and habits follow individual peer norms. Weight is also a factor in development of self-concept. An average weight is valued most by teens. Second is thinness, and least valued is being overweight (Fogel & Woods, 1995). As the peer group becomes more powerful, girls emphasize their own self-worth in the context of their relationships, further enhancing self-esteem. They see problems differently from being either right or wrong, and will work together to resolve conflicts. Girls are socialized to establish relationships through creative mechanisms. Even in play, girls will adapt change into games to make them more appropriate for the play group whereas boys play strictly by the rules (Gilligan, 1993).

Adolescent girls often define themselves in response to the reactions of their peers. Feelings of connectedness and intimacy support self-esteem throughout a woman's life (Belenky, Clinchy, Goldberger, & Tarule, 1986). Belenky's research also has revealed that as women learn, they do not segregate their feelings. Women tend to "think what they feel." Nurses providing care for female adolescent clients must gain understanding of the uniqueness of female psychological development as well as physiologic development.

Cultural Influences

The adolescent's sense of self also is dependent on the cultural context in which she lives. Based on data from the Centers for Disease Control and Prevention (as cited in Rosenfield, 1997), adolescent girls' self-esteem varied based on ethnicity. African American girls cited higher levels of self-esteem than did Hispanic or Caucasion girls. Hispanic girls had the greatest decrease in self-esteem and were most likely to report emotional distress. The decrease in self-esteem may be due to discrimination; inadequacy of the education received; and the influence of additional factors, such as poverty and gang involvement.

Self-Care Considerations

The opportunity to provide self-care knowledge to adolescents is tremendous. Through anticipatory guidance and trusting relationships, health information and education can be provided to the adolescent. Because adolescents generally are healthy, the focus should be on primary and secondary preventive practices. Primary preventive practices target those diseases and maladies that can be prevented. Primary prevention consists of practices such as wearing seat belts, receiving immunizations, and following instructions for safe sex. Secondary prevention includes screening for diseases. Secondary prevention practices include breast self-examination and Pap smear screening.

As the adolescent matures psychologically, she will begin making independent choices and pursue a degree of autonomy establishing her identity. Risk-taking behavior is most prevalent during adolescence. Some degree of risk taking during adolescence signifies autonomy and independence. Serious forms of risk taking, however, can lead to disaster. Accidental and unintentional injury is the leading cause of death in adolescents. The second and third causes are homicide and suicide, respectively (Commonwealth Fund, 1997). Risk-taking behavior may occur with or without knowledge of the potential aftermath. The

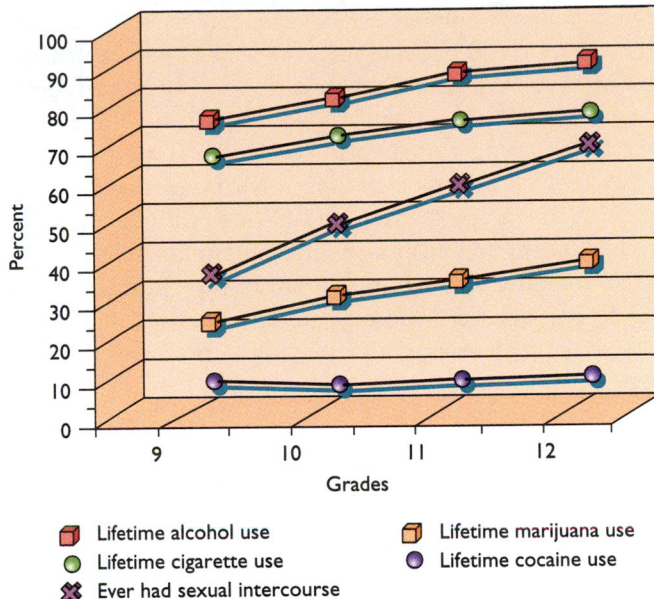

Figure 7-5 Female Adolescent Risk Behaviors. (J. Rosenfeld, Women's Health in Primary Care, Lippincott Williams & Wilkins, 1996.)

most serious forms of risk-taking behavior in adolescents are substance abuse and sexual activity. Figure 7-5 depicts female adolescent risk behaviors from grades 9 through 12.

Adolescents report binge drinking as early as the eighth grade (14%), with 23% of high-school seniors admitting to binge drinking. Binge drinking is defined as four to five or more drinks once in a 2-week period of time (Commonwealth Fund, 1997). Alcohol use in adolescents also is related to poor academic performance, early sexual activity, and troubled social environments (Rosenfield, 1997). Cigarette smoking is on the rise in young women compared with young men. One in four women admit to smoking. This year, more women will be smoking than men (Centers for Disease Control and Prevention [CDC], 1995). Teens underestimate the power of nicotine addiction and find quitting difficult. In providing anticipatory guidance to adolescents, nurses should focus on the benefits of abstaining from tobacco products such as fresh breath, whiter teeth, and increased exercise and performance ability (Wallis, Kasper, Reader, & Brown 1998).

Engaging in early sexual activity is another form of risk-taking behavior in adolescents. In young women, early sexual activity can lead to pregnancy, sexually transmitted diseases, and pelvic inflammatory disease. Nearly 50% of all high-school students report engaging in sexual activity, which is a decrease from 70% in 1995 (CDC, 1999). On average, 48% of high-school girls admit to "ever having" sexual intercourse and 52% of high-school boys admit to "ever having" sexual intercourse (CDC, 1999). Although the rate at which U.S. teenagers engage in sexual intercourse is on the decline, as is teen pregnancy, the

United States continues to have the highest teen pregnancy rates of the developed nations. Teen pregnancy continues to be a major health care issue for adolescents.

Adolescence is a time of discovery. In finding a sense of self, the young woman also will find a sense of responsibility. With the support of their environment, adolescents prepare for a productive adulthood through positive choices, accepting responsibility, and ultimately psychological maturity through their relationships. If they are unable to achieve their identity, adolescents will have difficulty making decisions and playing a productive role in society.

YOUNG ADULTHOOD TO PERIMENOPAUSAL YEARS

This period spans roughly the years between 15 and 44, although the childbearing years are typically considered to be from ages 18 to 39 years. Pregnancy outside of this age window historically has been considered high risk. During this time period, a woman often makes major life decisions and seeks independence. She may go to college and leave the nuclear family for the first time. Choices regarding career and potential life partners also are made. Extensive psychosocial development occurs during the childbearing years as women take on new roles and leave former roles behind.

Physiologic Changes

The young adulthood years are typically characterized by good health and further maturity of the body. Nursing care and interventions are geared toward promoting optional health through healthy diet, exercise, and good habits. The specific physiologic changes of pregnancy are outlined in detail in Chapter 15.

Psychosocial Changes

Further social and moral development occurs during the young adult years. Again, there are differences in the theoretic explanations of social and moral development between men and women. Lawrence Kohlberg (1969) developed the theory of moral development. Kohlberg's theory was based on the premise that individuals progressed through three levels in their moral development: preconventional (selfish and egocentric), conventional (based on shared and societal norms), and postconventional (forward thinking and individualistic). The developmental tasks of each stage must be achieved before moving on to the next stage. According to Kohlberg, most individuals do not aspire to the postconventional status. In contrast, Gilli-

gan (1993) questions Kohlberg's theory of moral development that is law- or principle-based, with a theory that is care- or relationship-based. Gilligan's research has revealed that women's moral development is based on the care and acknowledgement of responsibilities in addition to the further development of relationships and that the self and others are interconnected (Gilligan, 1993). Gilligan's theory explains the ease in which women make transitions between roles of wife, mother, daughter, and career person.

The psychosocial changes that occur during pregnancy should be considered from the point of view that pregnancy is a cycle of change in women's lives. Even as partners plan for their pregnancies, ambivalence is present as the woman imagines the new challenges as a mother. As women anticipate their labor and delivery, they ask themselves questions. "Will I be a good parent?" "Will I be able to provide an adequate home?" During the first trimester, a woman must adjust to being pregnant. Some of the physiologic effects of early pregnancy, such as nausea and vomiting, provide a negative experience that may be difficult to understand when the pregnancy is not yet visible. Multiple emotions prevail as a woman discovers she is pregnant and throughout gestation. Women who are not typically prone to mood swings and crying find their moods extremely labile.

Pregnancy has been described as a developmental crisis and a situational crisis, especially if it is high-risk pregnancy or coincides with other family issues such as moving to a new home or changing jobs. Regardless of how strongly the pregnancy is desired, the woman may experience ambivalence when she discovers she is pregnant. Nichols and Humenick (2000) have summarized the work of Rubin and others in discussing the changes during the pregnancy experience. The woman experiences dreams and fantasies throughout the pregnancy that help her prepare for the maternal role and assist her in accepting the pregnancy. Emotional liability is increased throughout pregnancy.

In the second trimester of pregnancy, emotional issues focus on fetal embodiment and altered body image. The mother's mental image of the baby often starts as an older child and regresses through the pregnancy to an infant. The woman becomes more introverted as she accomplishes the maternal tasks of pregnancy and adapts to meet the requirements of motherhood. Her becoming introverted may create confusion among her family and friends. It is important that family and friends accept the pregnancy so the baby will come into a safe and loving environment. If the mother perceives disapproval, she will become even more introverted.

In the third trimester, the pregnant woman often focuses on preparation for the delivery. She may begin to prepare space in the home for the infant. She may also

REFLECTIONS FROM FAMILIES

"I knew that I wanted to be pregnant, but at times I had overwhelming anxiety and fear of the unknown. It was the right time in our lives to have a baby. I thought we were prepared, but I wasn't sure. Initially, I was nauseated and felt bad all of the time. I thought it was some kind of sign that the pregnancy was in trouble. My health care provider explained to me that what I was going through both physically and emotionally was normal. I never realized that pregnancy could be such a time of great joy and anxiety at the same time."

begin to focus on the event of labor and delivery. When her due date approaches, she becomes eager for birth to occur and may become frustrated if she does not deliver by her due date.

Throughout the pregnancy, during the birth process, and immediately postpartum, the mother will further develop the capacity to give and care for her infant. Being cared for by others—family, friends, and health care providers—assists her in making this transition.

The pregnant woman may feel more comfortable asking questions of the nurse rather than other health care providers. It is important to assess for any emotional discomfort or anxiety that the woman or her partner may be feeling. Development of a birth plan may provide a feeling of control and decision-making for the client. Cases of extreme anxiety should be referred to social services (Davis, 1996).

Cultural Influences

The cultural patterns and behaviors the woman had assimilated during earlier years will continue in this period. She may prefer to spend time with friends who share her cultural practices or may seek out those with different ideas as a means of expanding her own viewpoint.

As to pregnancy, it usually is considered a time of expectancy, joy, and hope. Childbearing is a similar process in all parts of the world; however, beliefs, customs, and practices differ.

Jordan's (1982) research on birth practices in different cultures led her to write the following: "Childbirth is an intimate and complex transaction whose topic is physiologi-

cal and whose language is cultural." In providing care for clients in the childbearing years, nurses have the opportunity to gain the wisdom to better provide support when they understand clients in the context their own cultures. Additional insights are offered in Chapters 15 and 17.

Self-Care Considerations

Self-care considerations for women in young adulthood center on achieving and maintaining health. Good health is promoted through practices such as a healthy diet, stress management, exercise, reduced caffeine and alcohol intake, monthly breast self-examination, and yearly Pap tests.

The birth plan is an appropriate form of self-care during pregnancy. A birth plan usually is a written document that outlines the desires of the client and partner or family as she progresses through the trimesters of pregnancy. The plan details the client's desires for antenatal testing, medication use, anesthesia choices, and postpartum care. A broad plan with alternate options has the best opportunity for success. A rigid plan does not allow the opportunity for change. The plan offers the care provider a concise view of the concerns of the client to better tailor the care.

PERIMENOPAUSAL TO MATURE YEARS

The middle years, generally considered to be from 45 to 64 years, may be the most challenging and productive years of a woman's life. She may have completed her childbearing and is now focusing on a career, or she may have initially focused on her career and is now considering childbearing. If her children are young, their demands on her time may need to be balanced with the demands of her career. Her parents may be aging and may require more care and assistance. The woman's physiologic and hormonal changes demand attention; however, many women no longer feel the need to regularly see a care provider. Women may struggle with self-image and physical appearance of staying young, although trends are changing in that there is a resurgence of focus on the woman in midlife. Health education programs are focusing on health risks during this developmental phase to better provide women with the tools to care for themselves and their families. This time also is one in which women are accessing health care for physical changes and perimenopausal symptoms. Women may feel excited or confused by the extensive health care options available with respect to stress management, hormone replacement therapy, and complementary and alternative medicine. There is an abundance of health information available to women on the Internet and in other media sources. The nurse should assist and support women in their quest for valid knowledge. An example would include the ability to provide assistance in the interpretation of the most recent research findings, because frequently the media will provide a sensational interpretation.

Physiologic Changes

The physiologic and hormonal changes that occur during midlife have also been called perimenopause. **Perimenopause** is the time before cessation of menses or menopause. A woman may be considered to be in perimenopause for 5 to 10 years, or until cessation of menses for 1 year. During this time period, the woman may have normal menses, spotting, or absence of a monthly menstrual cycle. A woman who has not had a menstrual period for 1 year is considered to be in **menopause**. As a woman approaches her 40s, she begins to have fewer ovulatory cycles. The ovary may only have several thousand follicles remaining at this time and may be less sensitive to go-

nadotropin stimulation (Speroff, Glass, and Kase, 1999). In turn, the follicles, by way of the feedback system, produce less estrogen. The decrease in estrogen does not provide for maturation of the endometrial lining, and therefore, menses may not occur. Eventually, estrogen production decreases sufficiently to affect estrogen-dependent tissues, such as the breasts, bone, mucous membranes, heart, neuroendocrine system, and reproductive organs.

The glandular tissue of the breasts atrophies with the loss of circulating estrogen. The glands and lobules are replaced with fat. The skin becomes less elastic, and the breasts become soft and pendulous. The best demonstration of the difference is in the mammographic interpretation of the breast of a premenopausal woman and that of a postmenopausal woman. Figure 7-6 distinguishes the differences between dense breast tissue and breast tissue replaced by fat. The glandular tissue is very dense and appears white on the mammogram. Breast lesions are difficult to visualize in the white glandular tissue. The fatty

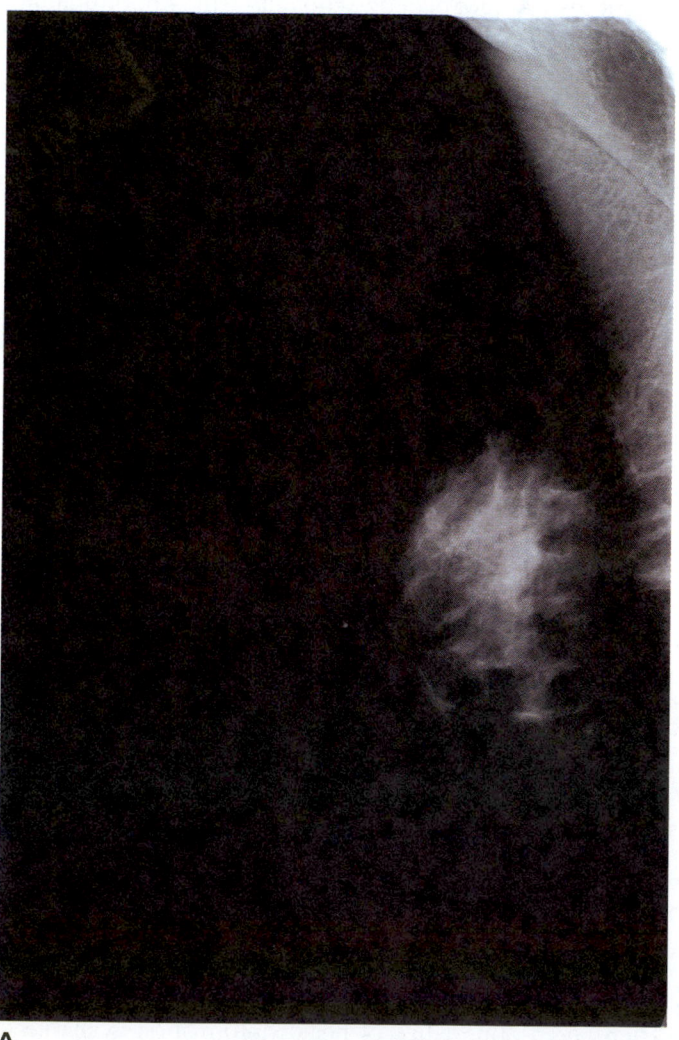
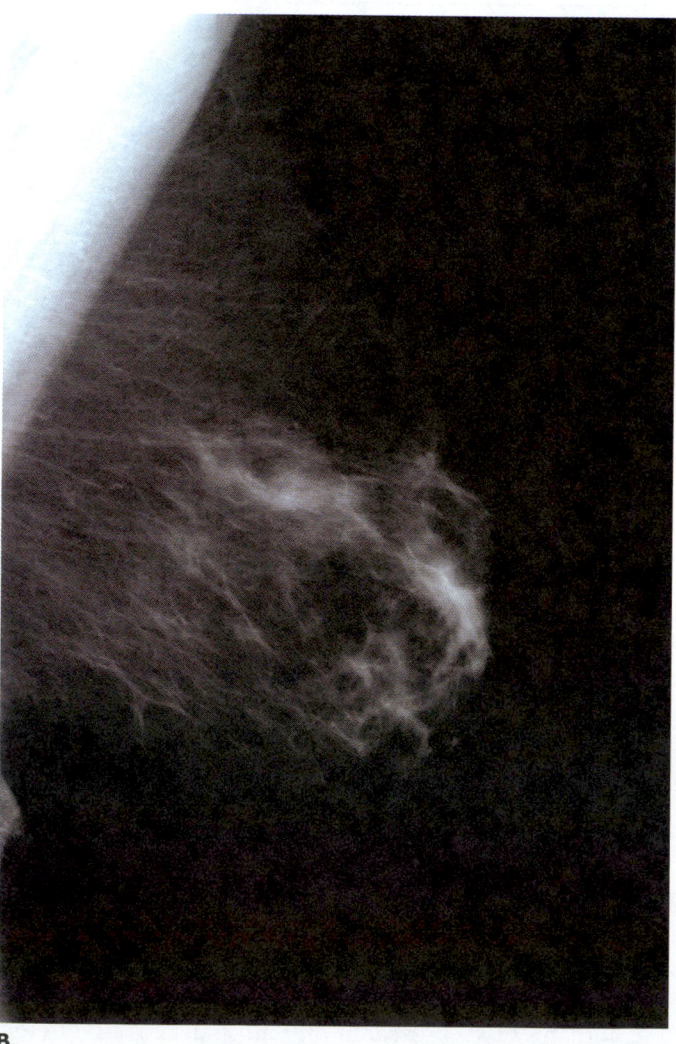

A.

B.

Figure 7-6 Mammogram of breast tissue A. Premenopausal B. Postmenopausal

tissue is darker and much less dense, making it easier to see abnormalities.

Women lose calcium from the bone as a normal process of aging. With the loss of estrogen during the peri- and postmenopause periods, the bone loss is dramatic. Decreased levels of calcium intake and high levels of physical activity that results in less than 10% body fat also contribute to bone loss before the midlife years. A woman may lose 1% of her bone density per year for 5 to 10 years after menopause (Cook, 1993). The bone loss may result in back pain and compression. Fractures also may occur with bone stress. When women lose bone either naturally or pathologically, they are diagnosed with **osteoporosis**. **Osteoporosis** is bone loss owing to a decrease in calcium absorption or the loss of estrogen. Osteoporosis can be a devastating disease, leading to fractures, loss of independence, and potentially death (Society for Women's Health Research, 1999). Although education about prevention of osteoporosis should begin in childhood or adolescence, during the time of bone formation, it is important to continue to provide education to women about their risk for osteoporosis and to develop a plan for prevention (Figure 7-7). An osteoporosis prevention plan would include a diet high in calcium (approximately 1,000 mg for pre-menopausal women and 1,500 mg for postmenopausal women) and weight-bearing exercise 3 to 4 times a week. Hormone replacement therapy also may be an option for women experiencing menopause.

Heart disease is the leading cause of death in women and is responsible for more deaths than breast, ovarian, and uterine cancers combined (Society for Women's Health Research, 1999). As a woman approaches menopause, her risk for heart disease becomes equal to that of a man's risk. The current thinking is that estrogen provides protection against heart disease because of its

Nursing Alert

RISK FACTORS FOR HEART DISEASE

- Age over 60 years
- Obesity
- Cigarette smoking
- Hypertension
- Diabetes mellitus
- Sedentary lifestyle
- Family history

American Heart Association. (1999). *2000 Heart and stroke statistical update.* Dallas, TX: American Heart Association.

positive effects on serum lipids in reducing cholesterol. Because a decrease in estrogen occurs at menopause, there is an increased risk for heart disease. Additional risk factors for heart disease also must be considered when providing nursing care to the woman in midlife.

Diminished estrogen levels are responsible for atrophy of the skin and mucous membranes of the mouth, urethra, vagina, and bladder. The skin becomes less elastic and taut. It may appear dry and loose, which may lead to increased wrinkling. There is also drying and thinning of the mucous membranes around the mouth and within the urogenital system. Women may notice a change in the appearance of their lips and mouths in that the tissue supporting the lips becomes less taught.

The effects of estrogen loss on the urinary system can be quite disturbing for women. Decreasing circulating levels of estrogen cause a loss of elasticity of the urethra, resulting in frequency and urgency of urination. An overall loss of muscular support within the pelvis may add to the woman's urinary tract symptoms. Complaints of stress incontinence and urge incontinence may occur in this phase of life. Stress incontinence is the most common type of incontinence in women under 60 years of age. **Stress incontinence** is an involuntary discharge of urine with a cough, sneeze, or laughter owing to the loss of muscular support at the neck of the urethra. Urge incontinence is less common than is stress incontinence. **Urge incontinence** occurs when the urge to void is present but the bladder is unable to empty normally. As a result, the bladder can become distended, which results in an uncontrolled loss of urine (Johnson, Johnson, Murray, & Apgar, 1996). Women with urge incontinence cannot postpone urination for more than a few minutes once the need to urinate is sensed. Although nonsurgical and surgical interventions are available, many

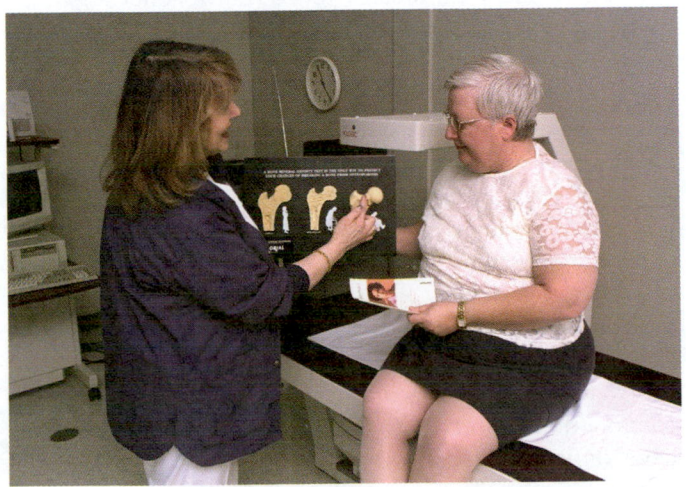

Figure 7-7 As women approach menopause, osteoporosis prevention education is critical in promoting optimal health.

women may be uncomfortable initiating a discussion about incontinence. The nurse-client relationship provides a non-threatening mechanism to bring that information forward through the educational process.

The reproductive organs also are affected by the loss of circulating estrogen. The vagina decreases in depth and the uterus decreases in size. The ovaries shrink. The vaginal skin thins, and the rugae diminish. There is an increase in vaginal pH from an acidic state to a neutral or alkaline state, which increases the risk of infection in the perimenopausal woman (Cook, 1993). Sexual intercourse frequently is uncomfortable, and trauma may occur as a result of thinning vaginal epithelium. Water-soluble lubricants may provide comfort during sexual intercourse.

Changing estrogen levels also result in vasomotor instability, causing hot flashes or flushing. The instability occurs as a result of the altered balance of norepinephrine and dopamine. Sympathetic activity increases, resulting in a rapid heart rate. Skin temperature also increases, resulting in a flash or sensation of warmth. When the flash progresses to vasodilation of the skin, it is termed a flush (Cook, 1993). Night sweats may occur as a result of the flushing. Nighttime wakening as a result of night sweats may cause sleep deprivation. Hot flashes or flushes are the most common symptoms of menopause.

Psychosocial Changes

Women's perceptions of the midlife period have changed over the past 20 years. Past studies focused on women's

---

Critical Thinking

Menopause

A 45-year-old woman is beginning to notice changes in her menstrual cycle. Her cycles are increasingly longer (approximately 45 days), with a shortening duration. She is concerned about how these changes may affect her lifestyle and her health. Some of her friends at work have told her that they felt their health was negatively impacted when they went through menopause. As the nurse involved with this client's primary care:

- How would you initiate anticipatory guidance?
- In what key areas would you provide health education?
- How would you address the "concerns of friends"?

---

roles in terms of their launching their children into independence or on the time left in their lives. In the past, many women identified their sense of self with the child rearing or spousal role. More recent studies have revealed an understanding of stressful life events, such as physical changes, physical limitations, empty nest concerns, and changes in interpersonal relationships; however, the women are positive in their overall outlook (Woods & Mitchell, 1997). The traditional emotional effects of perimenopause are rooted in physiologic processes. Symptomatology related to sleep disturbances, decreased libido, and mood swings can be associated with decreased estrogen levels. Currently, women's psychosocial issues related to midlife are attributed to managing the busy demands of daily life (Woods & Mitchell, 1997).

Cultural Influences

Cultural perceptions of midlife are not clearly understood. Women's lifestyles and social interactions influence health. Based on culture, as a woman ages her social status may increase and she may be valued as a life expert. In contrast, her social status may decrease and she may be devalued because of her culture. Obermeyer (2000) questioned the symptomatology associated with and leading up to menopause as having cultural differences. The author's findings revealed that there are cultural differences in self-reported descriptions of the menopause process. The difficulty is in the interpretation because there are not validated descriptions of menopause symptoms across cultures. Further cross-cultural research is clearly needed in comparing women's experiences in menopause (Woods, 1994).

Self-Care Considerations

Nurses are ideal candidates to educate clients regarding the self-care measures that can be taken during midlife. As physiologic symptoms begin to occur, the nurse may have the first contact with the client. Clients experiencing nighttime flushing should be advised to wear light-weight cotton clothing to bed to decrease diaphoresis.

In an effort to maintain bone density, all clients should be advised to perform weight-bearing exercises and maintain a minimum calcium intake of 1,000 mg/d of elemental calcium. Bone density testing may be advised to determine a baseline bone density, as well as to determine the client's risk for fracture (Figure 7-8).

Water-soluble lubricants can be used to reduce discomfort during intercourse. Be advised that woman may have difficulty in expressing sexual difficulties. Because nurses are excellent counselors and educators and because communication is a core component of nursing curriculum, nurses should have less difficulty eliciting a sexual history than would most physicians. Nurses also may have a greater comfort level with this discussion.

Women should also be reminded to perform monthly breast self-examinations and have annual mammograms after the age of 50. As a woman ages, her risk for breast cancer increases, with the majority of breast cancers being diagnosed after age 50 (American Cancer Society, 1999). Educational information regarding hormone replacement therapy or alternatives should be provided at this time. Women should feel comfortable and confident in performing their own self-examinations. Questions about or clarification of their examination should be referred to the health care provider.

MATURE YEARS

The perceptions of mature women (aged 65 and older) regarding health are not determined by the number of chronic illnesses they might have but by how the women feel. Perry and Woods (1995) asked a group of women ranging in age from 70 to 91 years, "What does being healthy mean to you?" The research of these authors led them to write the following quote about health and women of advanced age (Perry and Woods, 1995, p. 55): "Health involves the appreciation of life, experiencing joy and happiness. To be free from sickness does not guarantee health. Likewise, health can be experienced despite chronic illness and disability, because being healthy is a philosophy or way of living."

Physiologic Changes

Physiologic concerns of the aging woman are multifocal and affect all body systems (Figure 7-9). Some changes in the integumentary system, for example such as wrinkles, spots on the skin and graying hair may have a different social and psychological effect on women than on men related to the expectations and values that our culture has placed on youth and beauty in women. A brief review of systemic of physiologic changes follows.

- Pulmonary System: The rib cage and its accessory muscles become less flexible making older women more susceptible to respiratory disorders:

- Cardiovascular System: Heart rate slows, cardiac output and recovery time decline. Blood flow to organs decreases, veins dilate and arterial elasticity decreases, which may result in a rise in blood pressure and peripheral vascular disease. The effect of the use of estrogen supplementation for cardiovascular health is under debate and is currently is being researched.

- Gastrointestinal System: Dental problems related to thinning of tooth enamel and periodontal disease

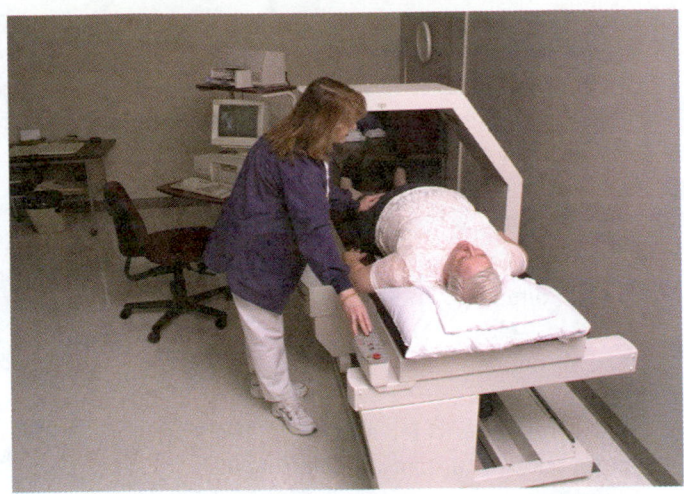

A.

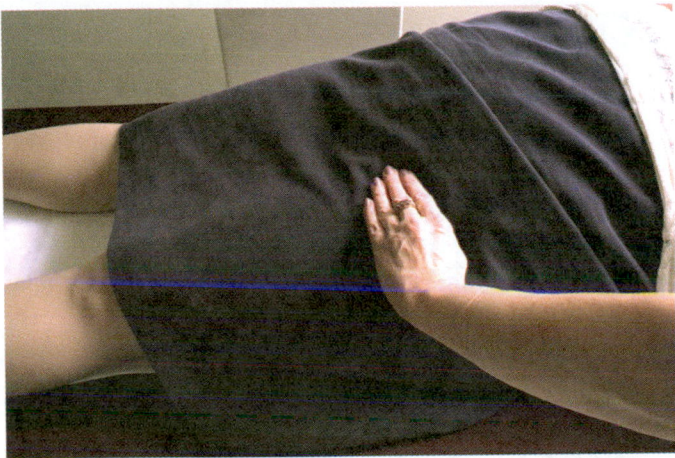

B.

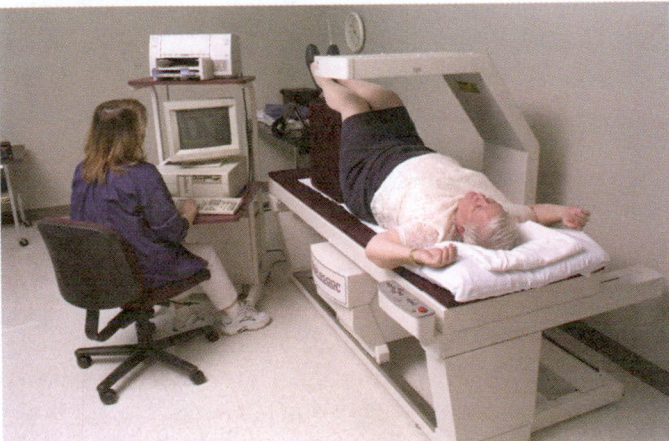

C.

Figure 7-8 A bone density scan should be done to determine a baseline as well as to determine a client's fracture risk. A. Positioning the client B. Aligning the scanner C. Reading the results.

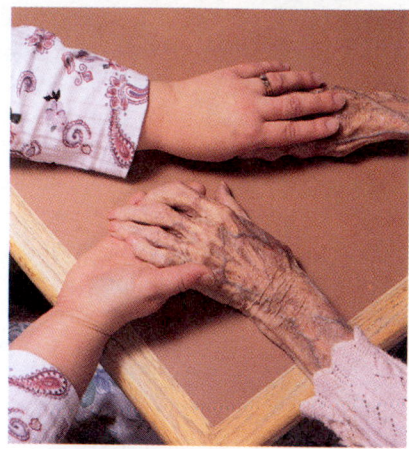

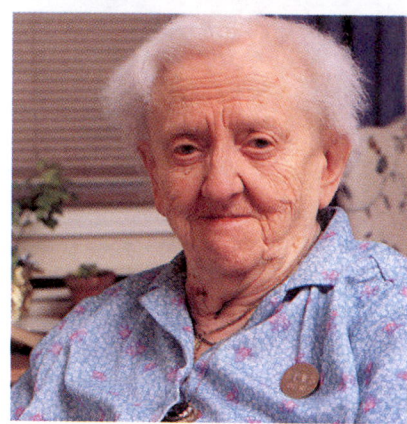

Figure 7-9 Changes in the skin and hair are some of the more visible effects of aging.

increases. Risks of choking increase related to decreased effectiveness of the gag reflex. Gastric emptying time and peristalsis slows, resulting in constipation. Gallbladder lessens in efficiency, resulting in greater incidence of gallstones. Liver enzymes decrease, slowing drug metabolism and detoxification.

🌀 Reproductive System: Estrogen decreases and ovaries, uterus decrease in size. The vagina shortens and secretions decrease and become more alkaline, which can increase the risk of atrophic vaginitis. The supportive musculature of the reproductive organs weakens, increasing risk of uterine prolapse. Breast tissue diminishes and breast cancer risk increases with age. Libido and need for intimacy remains unchanged.

🌀 Endocrine System: Changes occur in both the production of hormones and reception of hormones. Thyroid changes may lower basal metabolism. Release of insulin slows, causing an increase in blood sugar. The most common endocrine disorder related to aging is Type II Diabetes.

🌀 Musculoskeletal System: Muscle mass and elasticity diminish. Reduced strength, endurance, coordination

are decreased with aging. Bone demineralization occurs leading to osteoporosis. This is a particularly significant problem for post-menopausal women. Exogenous estrogen and avoidance of smoking can reduce the risk or extent of osteoporosis. Joints often degenerate causing pain, stiffness, and loss of range of motion.

🌀 Integumentary System: Subcutaneous tissue and elasticity diminish, therefore the skin becomes thinner and less elastic. Melanocytes are less able to produce even pigmentation resulting in hyperpigmentation on hands and wrists, commonly called liver spots. Skin becomes drier and nails become more brittle. Cutaneous sensitivity decreases. Risks of skin cancer, herpes zoster (shingles), and pressure ulcers increase with age.

🌀 Nervous System: Cerebral blood flow decreases, the time to carry out motor and sensory tasks increases, short-term memory diminishes more than long-term memory. Night sleep disturbances are more likely with aging.

🌀 Urinary System: Kidneys decrease in their ability to filter, excrete, and reabsorb. The reduction in filtration rate decreases in the renal clearance of drugs. Bladder capacity decreases and bladder and perennial muscles weaken. These may contribute to stress incontinence and cystitis.

🌀 Sensory System: Presbyopia (trouble seeing object up close) is a common vision problem with aging. Incidence of cataracts and glaucoma increases. Pupil size accommodation decreases, decreasing the adjustment to variations in lighting. Lacrimal secretions decrease, causing dryness itching and increasing risks for infection. Cochlea degenerates and impairment of hearing is often accompanied by a loss of tone discrimination, with loss of high frequency tones first.

Psychosocial Changes

The physiologic processes that occur as a result of aging directly affect the psychological health and social interactions of women who are aging. The woman must make adjustments in her own life owing to changes in functional status; in many cases, the woman also must provide care for an aging partner. Considerations are made for retirement that may cause lifestyle changes for the woman living on a fixed income. The aging woman may choose to either identify with a social group or isolate herself. Independent living may not be an option for some women, yet alternatives may be unsatisfactory. Responsibilities for grandchildren may lie with the aging woman, causing increased stress that may result in added health risks (Rosenfeld, 1997).

Depression is more common in women than in men. The lifetime risk for major depression in women is 20% to 25%; at any point in time, 5% to 10% of women are suffering from a depressive disorder (Byyny & Speroff, 1996). Depression is not related only to physiology but to the social and economic factors unique to women. Because of decreased physical abilities related to aging, social isolation, and economic problems, older women should be screened for depression.

Rosenfeld (1997) outlined some of the sociologic tasks of older women, including the following:

- Adjusting to declining physical strength and health.
- Adjusting to retirement and its reduced income.
- Adjusting to changes in the health of one's spouse.
- Establishing an explicit affiliation with one's age group.
- Adopting and adapting social roles in a flexible way.
- Establishing satisfactory physical living arrangements.

Cultural Influences

Although aging in American society often has been devalued, in some cultures women gain social status after childbearing and as they age. This may be a source of conflict. For instance, researchers have suggested a sense of fatalism within the aging African American and Hispanic populations (Haynes, 1996). Some may say, "Why seek health care? You're going to die from something." Unfortunately, women in the United States who are aging and belong to a minority group have had little choice in their health care decisions in the past. Negative experiences have led them to a lack of understanding and fear of health care and the provider (Haynes, 1996). The negative experiences may contribute to inadequate or inappropriate use of health care. Hispanic women are more likely to value the care provided when the family is involved. In the case of women who are aging, instructions and health education must be delivered in a trusting personal manner. When provided respectfully, the information is more likely to be valued and the advice followed (Caudle, 1993). Health information and education relayed in a kind, caring, and respectful way can be successful in breaking down cultural barriers.

Self-Care Considerations

Safety is a major self-care focus for mature women. Nurses providing care for the aging population must become proficient in assessing functional and cognitive status. Clients with osteoporosis are at risk for fractures. Initial assessments of the aging woman can be done from the waiting room as she walks to the exam room.

HEALTH CARE VERSUS FAMILY CARE

It is important to consider culture and familial influence when carrying out nursing interventions. Individuals are more likely to adhere to nursing care instructions and health education when their family members also are instructed and believe in the process.

During the interview/health history for an office visit or admission to the hospital, a medication history should be taken. Because of the nature of many chronic illnesses, multiple medications may be prescribed. Self care education should be provided in an easy to understand format using printed materials with a large font. The instructions must extend beyond prescription medication to include over the counter medications as well. The client can be encouraged to use a single pharmacy with computerized records to reduce the risk of adverse drug interactions.

NURSING IMPLICATIONS

There are many gender-related issues in the development of women. These are physiologic, psychological, and social in nature. A number of health-related issues surround reproduction and nurses should be sensitive to the multifaceted processes by which women become mothers. The hormonal changes in women from menarche through

Web Activities

- Where would you find information specific to nursing care of women with incontinence? Which nursing resources are available for practice as well as client education?

- Which resources can you locate on the Internet for families of women who have breast cancer? Is there a listing of support groups in your local area?

- Where would you find information specific to the risk for osteoporosis on the Internet in an effort to better educate your midlife clients on their risks?

menopause have manifestation beyond the reproductive organs. Nurses are in a position to educate women about these developmental changes and to provide counseling and support. Many times women may be more comfortable discussing these issues with a nurse than other health care providers. Nurses can apply their understanding about women's developmental issues to female clients in whatever arena they encounter clients. It does not need to be restricted to maternity care. Nurses can provide information and support about these issues for individual clients or to groups of clients. Many times nurses are asked to speak to community groups about woman's issues. This is an excellent opportunity to give sound health information about women's development.

Key Concepts

- Physiologic gender differentiation occurs at fertilization at the time in which the genetic sex is determined by chromosomes XX or XY.

- The maternal transfer of estrogen causes changes in the newborn's breast tissue and genitalia that resolve shortly after birth.

- Physical maturity and emotional maturity do not occur simultaneously, which frequently leads to adolescent conflicts.

- Female adolescent emotional and moral growth differs from that of males because females mature through their relationships rather than their separations.

- The early trimester physiologic effects of pregnancy are sometimes difficult for the expectant mother to understand when the pregnancy is not yet visible.

- Individual cultural beliefs may impact the care of the woman throughout pregnancy.

- Hormonal changes during the midlife years bring on additional physiologic changes to most organ systems.

- The physiologic changes that occur during midlife also may have a negative psychological impact.

- Health education and self-care measures are key in providing positive support to women during the midlife years.

- Physiologic and psychosocial issues continue to affect women as they age. Functional assessment is key in providing self-care and maintaining a safe environment for the client.

Review Questions and Activities

1. What causes dysfunctional uterine bleeding during adolescence?
   a. abnormal periods
   b. anovulatory cycles
   c. poor diet
   d. poor grades

   The correct answer is b.

2. What is the most visible sign of puberty?
   a. social withdrawal
   b. weight gain
   c. enlargement of the breast bud
   d. anger

   The correct answer is c.

3. How can the Tanner Stages be defined?
   a. emotional changes of the aging woman
   b. thelarche
   c. stages of adolescent physical development
   d. menarche

   The correct answer is c.

4. What is the second phase of the normal menstrual cycle?
   a. ovulation
   b. secretory-luteal phase
   c. menstruation
   d. proliferative-follicular phase

   The correct answer is d.

5. The corpus luteum regresses with decreases in estrogen and progestin, resulting in menstruation, when what does not occur?
   a. ovulation
   b. cysts
   c. menarche
   d. implantation

   The correct answer is d.

6. Which type of theory of development in women was identified by Gilligan?
   a. psychological
   b. physiologic

c. questionable

d. activity

The correct answer is a.

7. In what context are women socialized?

a. families

b. colleagues

c. friends

d. all of the above

The correct answer is d.

8. What is the Birth Plan?

a. list of birthing centers

b. a document that outlines the desires of the client and partner during pregnancy

c. postpartum contraceptive choices

d. a list of anesthesia choices in the delivery room

The correct answer is b.

9. On what does a reduction in circulating estrogen have an effect?

a. heart

b. breast

c. bones

d. all of the above

The correct answer is d.

10. Which is not a major focus for the aging woman?

a. safety

b. retirement

c. social interaction

d. Internet access

The correct answer is d.

References

American Cancer Society. (1999). *Breast cancer facts and figures 1999/2000.* Atlanta, GA: American Cancer Society.

American Heart Association. (1999). *2000 Heart and stroke statistical update.* Dallas, TX: American Heart Association.

Belenky, M., Clinchy, B., Goldberger, N., & Tarule, J., (1986). *Women's ways of knowing: The development of self, voice and mind.* New York: Harper Collins.

Blackburn, S., & Loper, D. (1992). *Maternal, fetal, and neonatal physiology: A clinical perspective.* Philadelphia, PA: W.B. Saunders.

Byyny, R., & Speroff, L. (1996). *A clinical guide for the care of older women* (2nd ed.). Baltimore, MD: Williams & Wilkins.

Caudle, P. (1993). Providing culturally sensitive health care to Hispanic clients. *The Nurse Practitioner: The American Journal of Primary Care, 18,* (12), 40–51.

Centers for Disease Control and Prevention (CDC). (1995). Tobacco use and usual source of cigarettes among high school students. United States. *MMWR, 45,* 413–418.

Centers for Disease Control and Prevention. (1999). Youth behavioral risk surveillance. *MMWR,* 1999: *49,* (SS05), 1–96.

Commonwealth Fund. (1997). *Selected facts on U.S. women's health.* New York: Columbia University.

Cook, M. (1993). Perimenopause: An opportunity for health promotion. *JOGGN, 22,* (3), 223–228.

Davis, D. (1996). The discomforts of pregnancy. *JOGNN, 25,* (1), 73–81.

Dealy, M. (1998). Dysfunctional uterine bleeding in adolescents. *Nurse Practitioner: The American Journal of Primary Health Care, 23,* (5), 12–23.

Erikson, E. (1950). *Childhood and society.* New York: W. W. Norton.

Fogel, C., & Woods, N. (1995). *Women's health care: A comprehensive handbook.* London: Sage Publications.

Gilligan, C. (1993). *In a different voice: Psychological theory and women's development.* Cambridge, MA: Harvard University Press.

Hatcher, R., Trussel, J., Stewart, F., Cates, W., Stewart, G., Guest, F., Kowal, D. (1998). *Contraceptive technology.* New York: Ardent Media.

Haynes, M. (1996). Geriatric gynecologic care of minorities. *Clinical Obstetrics and Gynecology, 39,* (4), 946–958.

Johnson, C., Johnson, B., Murray, J., & Apgar, B. (1996). *Women's healthcare handbook.* Philadelphia, PA: Hanley & Belfus.

Jordan, B. (1982). Studying childbirth: The experience and methods of a woman anthropologist. In S. Romalis (Ed.) (pp. 181–215).*Childbirth alternatives to medical control.* Austin, TX: University Press.

Kohlberg, L. (1969). Stage and sequence: The cognitive-developmental approach to socialization. In D. Goslin,(Ed.). *Handbook of socialization theory and research.* Chicago, IL: Rand McNally.

Nichols, F. & Humenick, S. (2000). Childbirth Education: Practice, Research and Theory. 2nd Edition. Philadelphia: W.B. Saunders Co.

Obermeyer, C. (2000). Menopause across cultures: A review of the evidence. *Menopause: Journal of the North American Menopause Society, 7,* (3), 184–192.

Perry, J., & Woods, N. (1995). Older women and their images of health: A replication study. *Advanced Nursing Science, 18,* (1), 51–61.

Rosenfeld, J. (1997). *Women's health in primary care.* Baltimore, MD: Williams & Wilkins.

Society for Women's Health Research. (1999). *What do women suffer from?* Washington, DC: Society for Women's Health Research.

Speroff, L., Glass, R., & Kase, N. (1999). *Clinical gynecologic endocrinology and infertility* (6th ed.). New York: Lippincott Williams & Wilkins.

Stedman, T. (1995). *Stedman's medical dictionary.* New York: Lippincott Williams & Wilkins.

Wallis, L., Kasper, A., Reader, G., & Brown, W. (1998). *Textbook of women's health.* New York: Lippincott Williams & Wilkins.

Wayland, J., & Rawlins, R. (1997). African-American teen mothers' perceptions of parenting. *Journal of Pediatric Nursing, 12,* (1), 13–20.

Woods, N., & Mitchell, E. (1997). Women's images of midlife: Observations from the Seattle midlife women's health study. *Health Care for Women International, 18,* 439–453.

Woods, N., & Perry, J. (1995). Older women and their images of health: A replication study. *Advances in Nursing Science, 18,* (1), 51–61.

Woods, N. (1994). Menopause: Challenges for future research. *Experimental Gerontology, 29,* (3/4), 237–243.

Suggested Readings

Callister, L. (1995). Cultural meanings of childbirth. *JOGGN, 24,* (4), 327–331.

De Sevo, M. (1997). Keeping the faith: Jewish traditions in pregnancy and childbirth. *Lifelines, 1,* (4), 46–49.

Hill Collins, P. (1991). *African American feminist thought: Knowledge, consciousness, and the politics of empowerment.* London: Routledge, Chapman and Hall.

Romeo, K. (1995). The female heart: Physiological aspects of cardiovascular disease in women. *Dimensions of Critical Care Nursing, 14,* (4), 170–177.

Siedel, H., Ball, J., Dains, J., & Benedict, G. (1999). *Mosby's guide to physical examination.* 4th ed. St. Louis, MO: Mosby Year Book.

Tanner, J. (1981). Growth and maturation during adolescence. *Nutrition Reviews, 39,* (2), 43–55.

Wilson, J. (1998). *Williams textbook of endocrinology* (9th ed.). Philadelphia, PA: W.B. Saunders.

Resources

Association of Women's Health Obstetric and Neonatal Nurses (AWHONN), 2000 L Street, NW, Suite 740, Washington, DC 20036, 800-673-8499, www.awhonn.org

American Cancer Society, 1599 Clifton Road, Atlanta, GA 30329, 800-ACS-2345, www.cancer.org

American Heart Association, 7272 Greenville Avenue, Dallas, TX 75231. For Women's Health information call 1-888-MY-HEART, www.americanheart.org

National Coalition for Women with Heart Disease, 1718 M Street, NW, Washington, DC 20036, 202-736-1770, www.womenheart.org

National Osteoporosis Foundation, 1232 22nd Street, NW Washington, DC 20037-1292, 202-223-2226, www.nof.org

YIN, "A Women's Guide to the Best Web Sites", www.yin.org. Based in Seattle, this website includes health links as well as career, nature, and political information.

CHAPTER 8

Nutrition for Women Across the Life Span

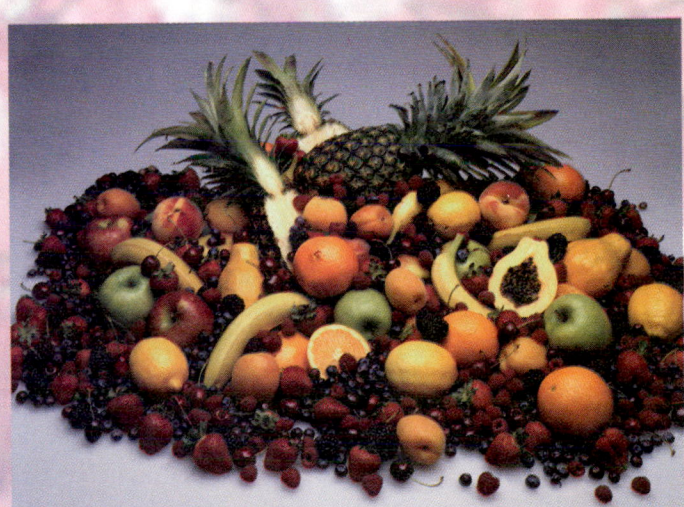

The Malone family consists of Sam and Julie and two children, ages 5 and 9. Julie is pregnant with her third child. Sam is a truck driver and Julie is active in the children's school and other activities. Their eating patterns are typical of their community. A meal commonly consists of meat, potatoes, canned vegetables, and dessert. Many of their meals contain fast foods, which are convenient when they are busy with other activities. Julie was 25 pounds overweight before this pregnancy. She is in her second trimester and has gained an additional 20 pounds.

- *What nutritional concerns do you think this family has?*
- *What implications does this nutritional pattern have for Julie's pregnancy?*
- *How does this family's diet differ from your diet?*
- *How do you think a family can change its eating patterns?*
- *What do you think a nurse can do to facilitate a change in nutritional patterns?*

Key Terms

Amylophagia
Anencephaly
Anorexia nervosa
Basal metabolism
Binge eating
Body mass index (BMI)
Botanicals
Bulimia nervosa
Calorie
Carotenoids
Daily Reference Values (DRVs)

Dietary Guidelines for Americans
Encephalocele
Food Guide Pyramid
Geophagia
Heme iron
Hemochromatosis
Hemosiderosis
Herbs
Hypochromic anemia

Isoflavones
Insoluble fiber
Microcytic anemia
Nonheme iron
Nutrition Facts Food Label
Obesity
Pagophagia
Phytochemicals
Pica

Plubism
Recommended Dietary Allowances (RDA)
Reference Daily Intakes (RDIs)
Soluble fiber
Spina bifida
Upper intake level (UL)
Vegan

Competencies

Upon completion of this chapter, the reader should be able to:

1. Describe the common nutritional guidelines used to advise normal, healthy women on recommended eating practices to provide optimum nutrition.
2. Use the Food Guide Pyramid to plan a healthy, culturally appropriate meal for a Hispanic woman, an African American woman, an Asian American woman, a woman of Mediterranean descent, and a vegetarian.
3. State the three most important factors to consider when evaluating a woman's dietary pattern.
4. Identify key nutrients of importance in a woman's dietary intake pattern.
5. Calculate the average ideal body weight and body mass index (BMI) for a woman.
6. Classify a woman's body size based on her BMI.
7. Calculate the average caloric needs for a woman, based on her ideal body weight.
8. Calculate a woman's prepregnancy BMI and set optimum weight gain goals for the pregnancy.
9. State the additional caloric requirements for pregnancy and describe food selections to meet those needs.
10. State the additional caloric requirements for lactation and describe food selections to meet those needs.
11. Give four of the dietary guidelines for cancer prevention.

Nutrition is a vital aspect of the health of women at all ages and is particularly important during the childbearing years because it affects the health and development of the child. Nutrition has also been identified as an area of lifestyle that can be modified to reduce risks for chronic diseases. Nurses have long been engaged in nutritional counseling interventions, and a good nutritional assessment and appropriate interventions should be a part of every nursing plan. Nurses who are providing care to women should be especially concerned with this area, because women generally procure and prepare the food for the entire family. Nutrition during pregnancy has implications for both the mother and the fetus. The mother's nutrition before pregnancy is also important for the health of the fetus.

Healthy People 2010 is the disease prevention agenda for the United States. This document has set the overall health goals for the nation. The two all-encompassing goals are:

- Goal 1: Increase quality and years of healthy life
- Goal 2: Eliminate health disparities

One of the sections relevant to all Americans and of particular significance to women across the life span is related to nutrition. The nutrition and overweight section has as its goal to promote health and reduce chronic disease associated with diet and body weight. There are 18 key objectives in this section dealing with healthy weight, optimum food and nutrient intakes, locations where food is most commonly consumed, and safety in food preparation. Six of the top 10 leading causes of death in the United States in 1997 had a direct link to nutritional practices. These causes included heart disease, cancer, stroke, diabetes mellitus, kidney disease, chronic liver disease, and cirrhosis. Osteoporosis, another disability affecting millions of Americans, is influenced by dietary and lifestyle choices. Truly optimal nutrition is a positive factor for our health status and fights disease.

This chapter focuses on the nutritional concerns of women throughout their life cycle, with a major focus on needs during pregnancy. Emphasis is placed on the factors contributing to healthy lifestyles during the stages of a woman's life. Nutrients of special concern to women and nutritional needs during select times of a woman's life are highlighted. Prevention of major illnesses is the focus. Finally, there is a brief discussion of the major nutritional concerns related to the primary causes of morbidity and mortality in women.

NUTRITIONAL GUIDELINES

Nutritional guidelines can come in different forms. The Dietary Guidelines for Americans, the Food Guide Pyramid, culturally adapted food guides, and Nutrition Facts food labeling are discussed here.

Dietary Guidelines

Dietary Guidelines for Americans was the first joint publication effort of the Department of Health and Human Services and the Department of Agriculture. They are mandated by public law to be revised every 5 years (USDA, 2000). *Dietary Guidelines for Americans* provides guidance on diet and health to the general population with practical recommendations that meet nutritional requirements, promote health, support an active lifestyle, and reduce the risk of chronic disease.

Dietary Guidelines for 2000 includes the following 10 recommendations:

- Aim for a healthy weight.
- Let the food pyramid guide your food choices.
- Eat a variety of grains daily, especially whole grains.

- Eat a variety of fruits and vegetables daily.
- Keep food safe to eat.
- Choose a diet low in saturated fat that is also low in cholesterol and moderately low in total fat.
- Choose beverages and foods that limit intake of sugar.
- Choose and prepare foods with less salt.
- Drink alcoholic beverages in moderation.
- Be physically active each day.

Food Guide Pyramid

The **Food Guide Pyramid** was first introduced in 1992, published by the Department of Agriculture and Department of Health and Human Services (USDA/HS, 1992). This guide is an easy way to recommend adequate servings from the various food groups every day for the entire population. The Food Guide Pyramid translates the dietary guidelines for Americans into practical eating portions that meet the dietary guidelines and, if foods are chosen carefully, they also meet the recommended daily allowances (RDA) and Dietary Reference Intakes (DRI). The National Academy of Sciences Food & Nutrition Information Center is in the process of replacing RDA with DRIs (Nutrient Data Laboratory, 2001).

The Food Guide Pyramid was designed to graphically illustrate the dietary guidelines for Americans, emphasizing balance, moderation, and variety. The Food Guide Pyramid can be modified to fit the cultural preferences of clients by using foods customary to their culture and to fit differing age groups by modifying the types of foods, and the serving sizes. Depending on cultural food preferences, food groupings may be modified to adequately adjust for a client's nutrient requirements. Figure 8-1 presents the traditional Food Guide Pyramid.

Culturally Adapted Food Guides

While the basic nutritional requirements and guidelines generally apply to all people, nutritionists and nurses have long been aware of cultural differences in eating patterns and food preferences. Translating nutritional requirements into cultural food practices has sometimes been challenging. The Oldways Preservation and Exchange Trust, (1994, 1995, 1996) the World Health Organization (WHO) European regional office, and Food and Agricultural Organization (FAO) Collaboration Center in Nutritional Epidemiology at Harvard University's School of Public Health have adapted the food pyramids to be used with clients from various cultures or with specific dietary practices, such as those common to Asian, Mediterranean, and Latin American diets (Townsend & Roth, 2000).

**The Food Guide
Pyramid
A guide to daily food choices**

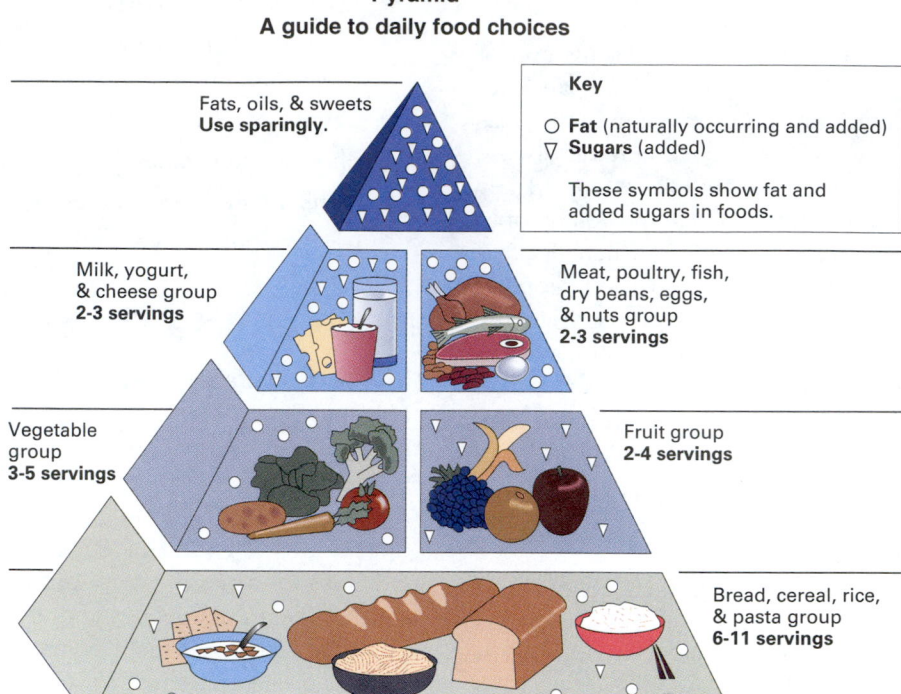

Fats, oils, & sweets
Use sparingly.

Key
○ **Fat** (naturally occurring and added)
▽ **Sugars** (added)

These symbols show fat and
added sugars in foods.

Milk, yogurt,
& cheese group
2-3 servings

Meat, poultry, fish,
dry beans, eggs,
& nuts group
2-3 servings

Vegetable
group
3-5 servings

Fruit group
2-4 servings

Bread, cereal, rice,
& pasta group
6-11 servings

Figure 8-1 Food Guide Pyramid. *(Courtesy of United States Departments of Agriculture and Health and Human Services (1992). The food guide pyramid: A guide to daily food choices. Washington, DC, (leaflet no. 572).*

All of the pyramids limit saturated fats to protect against heart disease. The Asian, Mediterranean, and Latin American plans give greater daily predominance to heart-healthy monounsaturated fats. As *Dietary Guidelines for Americans* (USDA, 2000) suggests, the fat content of the diet should be kept low: total fat, saturated fat, and cholesterol. The total daily fat intake should be no more than 30% of the total calories, and saturated fats should comprise no more than 10% of total calories.

The following section briefly discusses some food patterns typical of various cultures and regions. While enormous variations exist within any classification, some culturally influenced patterns are recognizable.

Native American

Approximately half of the edible plants commonly eaten in the United States today may have origins in the Native American diet. Examples are corn, potatoes, squash, cranberries, pumpkins, peppers, beans, wild rice, and cocoa beans (Figure 8-2). In addition, Native Americans used wild fruits, game, and fish. Foods were commonly prepared as soups and stews or were dried. The original Native American diets were probably more nutritionally adequate than are current diets, which frequently consist of a high proportion of sweet and salty, snack-type foods that are low in nutrient density. Native American diets today

may be deficient in calcium, vitamins A and C, and riboflavin.

Southern United States

Hot breads, such as corn bread and baking powder biscuits, are common in the South because the wheat grown in the area does not make good-quality yeast breads. Grits and rice are also popular carbohydrate foods. Favorite vegetables include sweet potatoes, squash, green beans,

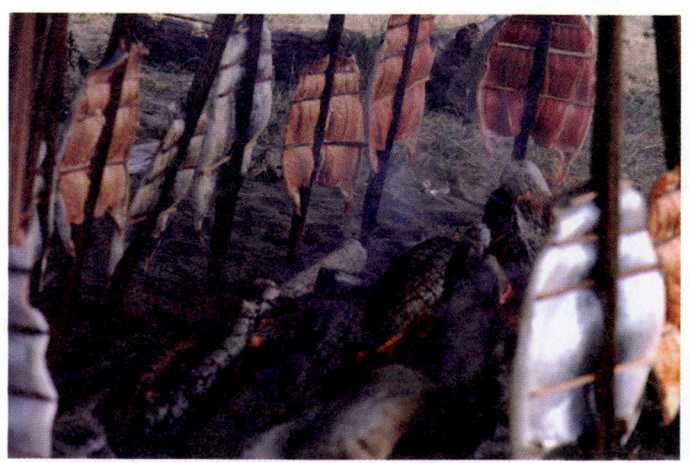

Figure 8-2 Traditional Native American food

and lima beans. Green beans cooked with pork are commonly served. Watermelon, oranges, and peaches are popular fruits. Fried fish is served often, as are barbecued and stewed meats and poultry. These diets have a great deal of carbohydrate and fat and limited amounts of protein, in some cases. The diet may be deficient in iron, calcium, and vitamins A and C.

Mexican

Mexican food is a combination of Spanish and Native American foods. Beans, rice, chili peppers, tomatoes, and corn meal are favorites. Meat is often cooked with vegetables, as in chili con carne. Cornmeal or corn flour is used to make tortillas, which serve as bread. The combination of beans and corn makes complete protein. Corn tortillas filled with cheese (called enchiladas) provide some calcium, but the consumption of milk should be encouraged. Additional green and yellow vegetables and vitamin C–rich foods would also improve these diets.

Puerto Rican

Rice is the basic carbohydrate food in Puerto Rican diets. Vegetables include beans, plantains, tomatoes, and peppers. Bananas, pineapple, mangoes, and papayas are popular fruits (Figure 8-3). Favorite meats are chicken, beef, and pork. Milk is not used as much as would be desirable from the nutritional point of view.

Italian

Pastas with various tomato and cheese or fish sauces are popular Italian foods. Fish and highly seasoned foods are common to southern Italian cuisine; meat and root vegetables are common to northern Italy. The eggs, cheese,

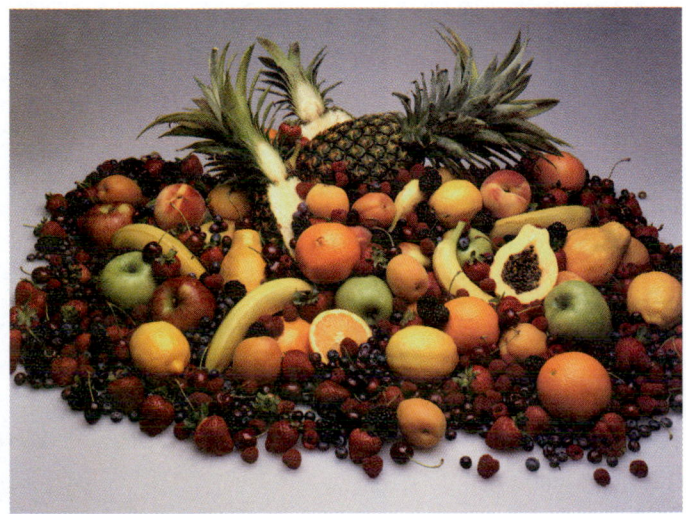

Figure 8-3 Traditional Puerto Rican food

tomatoes, green vegetables, and fruits common to Italian diets provide excellent sources of many nutrients, but additional fat-free milk and low-fat meat would improve the diet.

Northern and Western European

Northern and Western European diets are similar to those of the U.S. Midwest, but with greater use of dark breads, potatoes, and fish, and fewer green vegetable salads. Beef and pork are popular, as are various cooked vegetables, breads, cakes, and dairy products. The addition of fresh vegetables and fruits would add vitamins, minerals, and fiber to these diets.

Central European

Citizens of Central Europe obtain the greatest portion of their calories from potatoes and grain, especially rye and buckwheat. Pork is a popular meat. Cabbage cooked in many ways is a popular vegetable, as are carrots, onions, and turnips. Eggs and dairy products are used abundantly. Limiting the number of eggs consumed and using fat-free or low-fat dairy products would reduce the fat content in this diet. Adding fresh vegetables and fruits would increase vitamins, minerals, and fiber.

Middle Eastern

Grains, wheat, and rice provide carbohydrates in Middle Eastern diets. Chickpeas, in the form of hummus, are popular. Lamb and yogurt are commonly used, as are cabbage, grape leaves, eggplant, tomatoes, dates, olives, and figs. Black, very sweet coffee is a popular beverage (Figure 8-4). There may be insufficient protein and calcium in this diet, depending on the amounts of meat and calcium-rich foods eaten. Fresh fruits and vegetables should be added to the diet to increase vitamins, minerals, and fiber.

Chinese

The Chinese diet is varied (Figure 8-5). Rice is the primary energy food and is used in place of bread. Foods are generally cut into small pieces. Vegetables are lightly cooked, and the cooking water is saved for future use. Soybeans are used in many ways, and eggs and pork are commonly served. Soy sauce is extensively used, but it is very salty and could present a problem for clients on low-salt diets. Tea is a common beverage, but milk is not. This diet may be low in fat.

Japanese

Japanese diets include rice, soybean paste and curd, vegetables, fruits, and fish. Food is frequently served fried. Soy sauce (shoyu) and tea are commonly used. Current

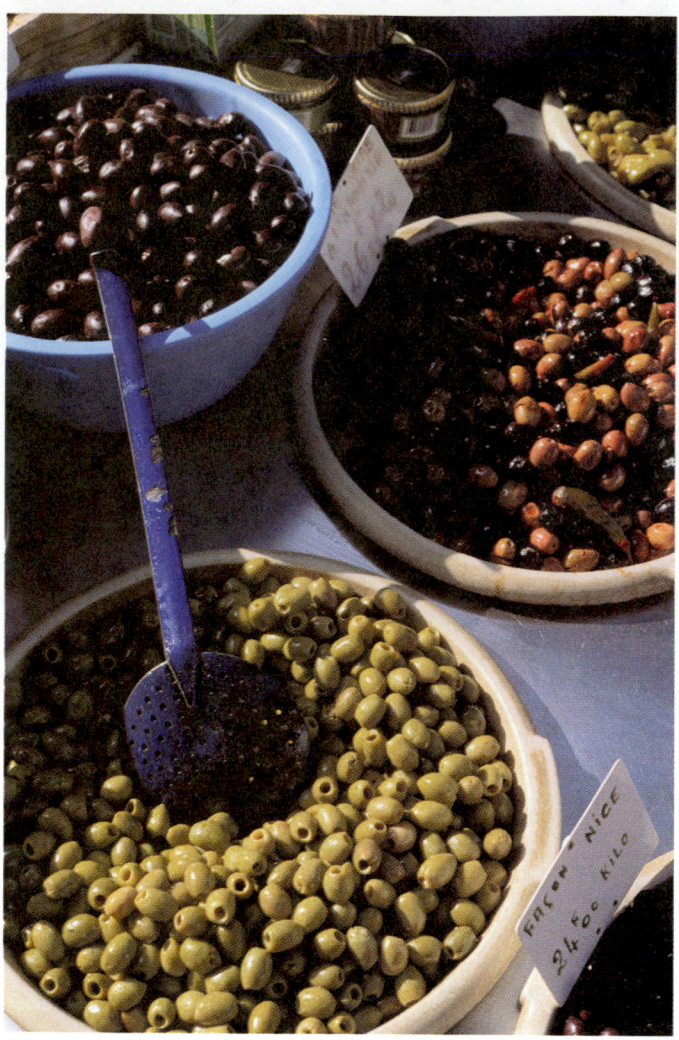

Figure 8-4 Traditional Middle Eastern food

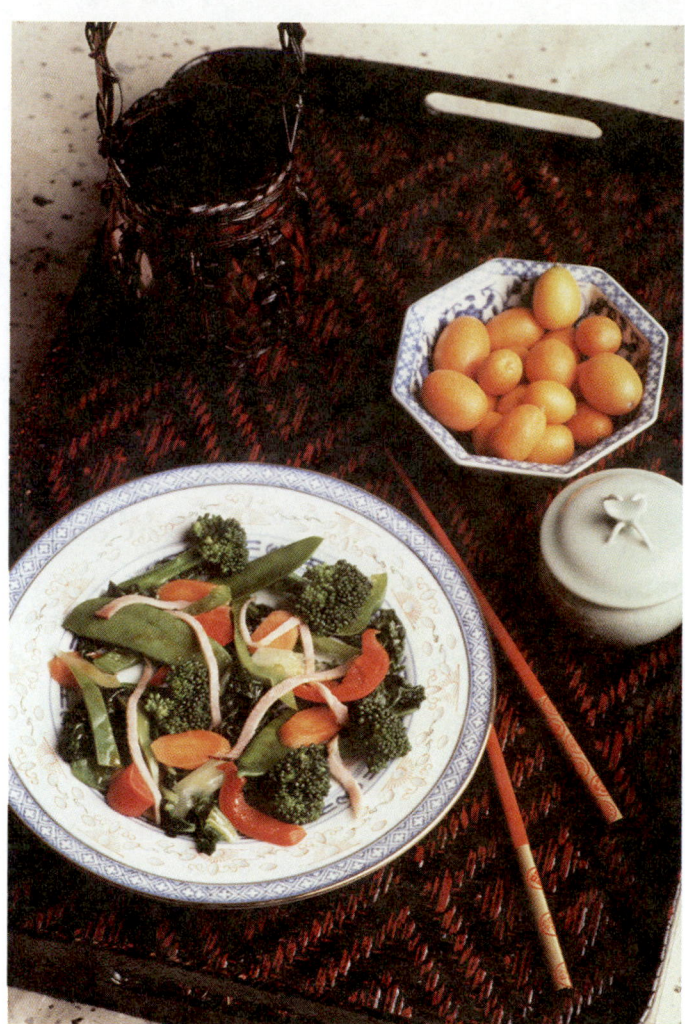

Figure 8-5 Traditional Chinese food

Japanese diets have been greatly influenced by Western culture. Japanese diets may be deficient in calcium, given the near total lack of milk in the diet. Although fish is eaten with bones, it may not supply sufficient calcium to meet needs. Japanese diets may contain excessive amounts of salt.

Indian

Many Indians are vegetarians who use eggs and dairy products. Rice, peas, and beans are frequently served. Spices, especially curry, are popular. Indian meals are not typically served in courses, as Western meals are. The meals generally consist of one course with many dishes.

Thai, Vietnamese, Laotian, and Cambodian

Rice, curries, vegetables, and fruit are popular in Thailand, Vietnam, Laos, and Cambodia (Figure 8-6). Meats and fish are used in small amounts. The wok (a deep, round pan)

is used for sautéing many foods. A salty sauce made from fermented fish is commonly used. These diets may contain inadequate amounts of protein and calcium.

Nutrition Facts Food Label

Another tool designed to aid people in selecting a healthy diet is the **Nutritional Facts food label**, which was introduced in 1993 (FDA, 1993). Nutrition labeling on processed packaged foods includes credible health and nutrient content claims and standardized serving sizes (FDA, 1999).

The items, with amounts per serving, that must be included on the food label are:

- Total calories
- Calories from fat
- Total fat
- Saturated fat
- Cholesterol
- Sodium

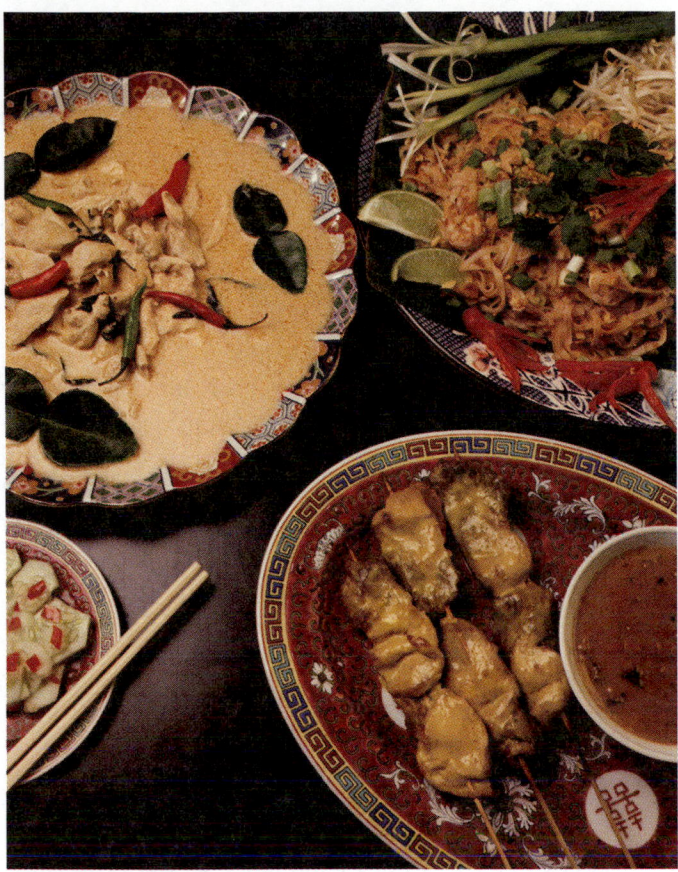

Figure 8-6 Traditional Thai food

* Total carbohydrates
* Dietary fiber
* Sugars
* Protein
* Vitamin A
* Vitamin C
* Calcium
* Iron

The food manufacturer can voluntarily include additional information on food products. Figure 8-7 shows a sample food label. The percent daily values (DV) are based on a 2000-calorie diet. Clients must adjust their intake of nutrients based on their estimated caloric consumption each day and on the serving size they consume. The DVs are based on two sets of standards. One is based on the **Daily Reference Values (DRVs)**, which are the standards for daily intake of total fat, saturated fat, cholesterol, total carbohydrate, dietary fiber, and protein. The total fat DRV is based on diets that provide 30% of total calories as fat; saturated fat is set at 10% of total calories. The DRV for total carbohydrates is based on 60% of the total calories, and for protein, on 10%.

Nutrition Facts

Serving Size 1/2 cup (114g)
Servings Per Container 4

Amount Per Serving

Calories 90	Calories from Fat 30

	% Daily Value
Total Fat 3g	**5%**
Saturated Fat 0g	**0%**
Cholesterol 0mg	**0%**
Sodium 300mg	**13%**
Total Carbohydrate 13g	**4%**
Dietary Fiber 3g	**12%**
Sugars 3g	
Protein 3g	

Vitamin A	80%	•	Vitamin C	60%
Calcium	4%	•	Iron	4%

• Percent Daily Values are based on a 2,000 calorie diet. Your daily values may be higher or lower depending on your calorie needs:

	Calories	2,000	2,500
Total Fat	Less than	65g	80g
Sat Fat	Less than	20g	25g
Cholesterol	Less than	300mg	300mg
Sodium	Less than	2,400mg	2,400mg
Total Carbohydrate		300g	375g
Fiber		25g	30g

Calories per gram:
Fat 9   •   Carbohydrate 4   •   Protein 4

Figure 8-7 Sample nutrition facts food label

The other standard used to calculate percent daily values on nutrition labels is the **Reference Daily Intakes (RDIs)** Nutrient Data (2001). This standard addresses the vitamin and mineral content of foods. It provides legal standards set by the U.S. Food and Drug Administration (FDA) for labeling foods and supplements uniformly. The RDIs generally represent the highest values of vitamins and minerals in the 1968 **Recommended Dietary Allowances (RDA)** (Food & Nutrition Board, 1989) tables for nutrients in any age group over age 4, excluding pregnant and breast-feeding women. The RDA lists the average daily nutrient intake levels recommend for healthy Americans. The Nutrition Facts labels make it possible for consumers to compare products easily, based on the product's contribution of fat, cholesterol, sodium, and other major nutrients.

NUTRITIONAL NEEDS ACROSS THE LIFE SPAN

Nutritional needs vary with age, gender, and reproductive status. These nutritional variations generally reflect additional needs, such as the need for additional Kcal and nutrients during pregnancy and lactation and concerns for eating patterns that may be prevalent at certain stages, such as adolescence. Nutritional needs for newborns and infants are discussed in detail in Chapter 33. The nutritional needs for girls during childhood do not differ from those for boys.

Adolescence

For women, adolescence is a special time of growth and development. In this discussion, adolescence covers ages 11 to 18.

Nutritional Needs

Nutrient requirements increase greatly during this time as a result of rapid growth, the onset of puberty, and an increase in body mass. Sufficient dietary calories must be provided so that protein is available for growth. Adequate calcium intake is another main concern for the adolescent because 45% of the skeletal mass is formed during this period; calcium is also important in the prevention of future osteoporosis. The new Daily Reference Intake (DRI) Adequate Intake (AI) for calcium is 1300 mg/day for girls aged 9 to 18 (Food & Nutrition Board, 1997). This is equal to at least four and one-half servings of calcium-rich foods each day.

The typical food habits of adolescents are characterized by an increased tendency toward skipping meals, snacking, inappropriate consumption of fast foods, dieting, and fad diets (Table 8-1). Adolescence is a time when peer influence is often greater than parental influence. The teen's search for independence, challenge of existing values, concern about body image, search for self-identity, and coping with the pressures of a quickly changing world enter in to the milieu of factors influencing dietary behavior.

Nutritional Concerns

Eating disorders frequently begin during adolescence in girls. When dealing with the rapid physiologic and psychologic changes experienced in this stage of life, adolescent females tend to alter their eating behavior to gain control over this aspect of their life (Giannini, Newman, & Gold, 1990). The medical community's attention to eating disorders increased in the mid-1970s. The groups affected by eating disorders have expanded from the traditional young, Caucasian, affluent girl or woman, whose illness is a reflection of disturbed family relationships, to include women and men of all ethnic backgrounds. The national chapters of Anorexia Nervosa and Related Eating Disorders, Inc. (ANRED) and Anorexia Nervosa and Associated Disorders (ANAD) estimate that 20% of the population between ages 12 and 30 is experiencing a major eating disorder. Today's society promotes the ideal physique for males and females as being thin with a high lean body mass ratio. Western society's media images and high fashion industry perpetuate and reinforce these often unattainable body images, which stereotype slim and obese people. The incidence of anorexia nervosa and bulimia in a society is proportional to the value placed on thinness by that society. The disparity between what is seen as ideal and what is normal for the individual leads to great emotional discontent. Many normal-weight teens and women are not satisfied with their weight.

Anorexia Nervosa

Anorexia nervosa is self-starvation motivated by excessive concern with weight and an irrational fear of becoming fat; it was first reported as early as 1868 (Frisch & Frisch, 1998). People with anorexia excessively control and restrict their caloric intake and have an unrealistic view of their body fat stores and body shape. They are often perfectionists in their daily lives. The medical complications of anorexia nervosa are similar to those seen in starvation: slow resting heart rate, low blood pressure, amenorrhea (disruption of the menstrual cycle), and hypothermia (complaints of being cold). The skin is often cool and there may be a loss of scalp hair. Soft lanugo (fine, soft, blonde) hair may appear on the face and trunk area. The normal amount of body fat for females (20% to 25%) decreases to an extremely low level (7% to 13%).

The most serious medical complications of anorexia nervosa are damage to the cardiovascular system and sudden death (Kaplan and Sadock, 1998). Irregular heart rhythms may occur, especially with deficiencies in potassium, magnesium, or phosphorus. Treatment for anorexia nervosa is successful in about 50% of cases. The focus of treatment is on gradually restoring body weight, improving self-esteem and attitudes about weight and body shape, and normalizing eating and exercise patterns and behavior. Antidepressant medications and family therapy are often used.

Bulimia Nervosa

Bulimia nervosa is characterized by behaviors that are the opposite of those seen in anorexic clients. Binge eating, which is excessive consumption of calories over a short period of time; purging by self-induced vomiting; use of laxatives or diuretics, or both; excessive exercise; and periods of severe caloric restriction are the typical patterns

Table 8-1 Nutrient and Calorie Content of Some Fast Foods Compared with Recommended Daily Allowances (RDA) for 16-Year-Old Girl

	Weight (oz)	Calories	Protein (g)	Fat (g)	Calcium (mg)	Iron (mg)	Sodium (mg)	Vitamin A (RE)	Thiamin (mg)	Riboflavin (mg)	Niacin (mg)	Vitamin C (mg)
Hamburger	3½	250	12	11	56	2.2	463	14	0.23	0.24	3.8	1
French fries	2	160	2	8	10	0.4	108	0	0.09	0.01	1.6	5
Chocolate milk shake	10	335	9	8	374	0.9	314	59	0.13	0.63	0.4	0
Pizza	4	300	15	9	220	1.6	700	106	0.34	0.29	4.2	2
Soda	12	160	0	0	11	0.2	18	0	0	0	0	0
Doughnut	2	210	3	12	22	1.0	192	5	0.12	0.12	1.1	0
Potato chips	2	315	3	21	15	0.6	300	0	0.09	0	2.4	24
Chocolate bar with peanuts	1½	225	6	16	75	0.6	30	12	1.0	1.0	2.1	0
RDAs for 16-year-old girl		2,200	44	73	1,200	15	500	800	1.1	1.3	15	60

of the bulimic client. The client with bulimia often eats in secret, is depressed, and is a substance abuser. In contrast to the close-knit, orderly, often rigid family of clients with anorexia, instability and conflict characterize the families of clients with bulimia. Clients with bulimia appear impulsive and out of control and usually have a normal body weight or are slightly overweight. Bulimia is more common in athletes and ballet dancers than in other groups. The medical complications related to the anatomic and physiologic changes characteristic of bulimia are often severe. The body is constantly adjusting to the feast or famine cycle. As a consequence of self-induced vomiting, severe erosion of the dental enamel, loss of teeth, esophagitis, hiatal hernia, esophageal tear or rupture, hypochloremic alkalosis, hypokalemia, shock, and other symptoms may occur. If ipecac is used to induce vomiting, myocardial ipecac toxicity may develop, causing fatal dysrhythmias and potentially fatal myocarditis. Laxative abuse may result in chronic hypokalemia, along with renal tubular damage. Binge eating may also create marked gastric dilation, gastric rupture, or post-binge pancreatitis. Enlargement of the parotid glands may occur and can become disfiguring. Treatment for bulimia consists of nutritional counseling to replace the disordered eating patterns with regular meals and snacks and psychologic counseling to improve self-image and attitudes toward body weight. Antidepressants are often useful in the treatment plan.

Binge Eating

Binge eating is a disorder of periodic binge eating that is not normally followed by vomiting, the use of laxatives, or excessive exercise. Several thousand calories are consumed within a short period of time. Binge eating twice a week for 6 months is usually required for diagnosis. Stress, depression, anger, anxiety, and other negative emotions usually prompt the binge eating episodes. Nutrition and psychologic counseling help focus on the disordered eating pattern and the underlying feeling or circumstances surrounding the event. Antidepressants may again be part of the treatment plan.

Eating disorders are often seen in fashion models, wrestlers, figure skaters, gymnasts, dancers, drill teams, competitive athletes, flight attendants, actors, and persons training to be dietitians, all of whose careers may depend on their ability to maintain a particular body weight. Close attention should be given to the degree of body-size conformity placed on adolescents by their coaches, agents, peers, or parents. The evaluation and treatment of clients with eating disorders often requires an interdisciplinary team approach that includes professionals in psychiatry, psychology, general medicine, nutrition, nursing, and social work. The family must be involved in the treatment and care of the patient over an extended period.

Adulthood and Childbearing Years

The nutritional needs of women in the reproductive phase of their life are set forth in the Recommended Dietary Allowances and the Dietary Reference Intakes (Food & Nutrition Board, 1997, 1998, 2000). Updates to the nutrient needs of all individuals are continually being reviewed and periodically published. The key nutrients of concern to women are addressed in the following section, with specific nutritional concerns for pregnancy, lactation, and old age. Therefore, periodic review of the nutritional literature is essential to keep practice and guidance current.

The body weight of a client reflects her past history of nutritional habits. The current recommendations are to determine a client's ideal body weight based on the **body mass index (BMI)**. The BMI represents a ratio of the relationship between height and weight. BMI is calculated by the formula:

$$BMI = \frac{\textbf{weight (kg)}}{\textbf{height (m}^2)}$$

$$\textbf{or weight (lb)} \times \frac{700}{\textbf{height (in}^2)}$$

Conversions: 2.2 pounds = 1 kg; 1 inch = 2.53 cm

Example: For a 125 lb (56.8 kg), = 5'6" (66 inches, or 167 cm) woman:

$$\frac{56 \text{ kg}}{(1.67 \text{ m}^2)} = \frac{56}{2.7889} = 20.007 \text{ BMI}$$

or

$$\frac{125 \text{ lb} \times 700}{(66 \text{ in}^2)} = \frac{875000}{4356} = 20.087 \text{ BMI}$$

The interpretation of the BMI calculation is as follows: less than 18, severe underweight; 18 to 20, low body weight; 20 to 25, normal body weight; 30 to 40, overweight; and more than 40, gross obesity. Tables are available for a quick calculation.

Nutritional Needs

The Food and Nutrition Board, National Academy of Sciences Institute of Medicine, and National Research Council, published the Recommended Dietary Allowances (RDA), revised in 1989, and the Dietary Reference Intakes, in 1997, 1998, and 2000. These values reflect the new Dietary Reference Intakes (DRIs) published by the National Academy of Sciences in 1997, 1998 and 2000. The DRIs include two sets of values from the Recommended Dietary Allowances (RDA) and Adequate Intakes (AI). The tolerable **upper intake level** (UL) for selected daily nutrients is also provided. Table 8-2 presents these recommendations for women in the childbearing years and for pregnancy, lactation, and postmenopausal women. Overall, a pregnant woman's nutritional needs increase by 15% during the second and third trimesters of pregnancy.

Calories or Energy Needs

A kilocalorie is unit of measure for energy; it is the amount of energy needed to raise the temperature of 1 kilogram of water from 1° C. The amount of energy provided to the body by food is measured in calories. Kilocalorie is the proper term, but calorie is commonly used. The body uses the energy from foods for growth, tissue repair, maintenance; to fuel muscular activity; to process nutrients; and to maintain body temperature. **Basal metabolism** is the energy used to support the body functions while the body is at rest. To calculate the basal metabolic rate (BMR) for females, multiply body weight by 10. Physical activity also requires calories. The activity level can be multiplied by a factor to determine the calories usually expended in activity.

The final category of energy needs of the body is dietary thermogenesis, also called specific dynamic action (SDA) of foods, diet-induced thermogenesis, and thermic effect of foods, which is the heat or energy expended during digestion of food and the absorption and use of nutrients. Dietary thermogenesis requires approximately 10% of the body's total energy needs. By adding these three categories of energy needs by the body, a good estimate of caloric needs can be determined.

The composition of energy nutrients found in foods determines their caloric content. Each gram of carbohydrate or protein contains four calories. Each gram of fat contains nine calories. Alcohol contains seven calories per gram. The information in Nutrition Facts food labels assists consumers in determining the number of calories per serving of food.

The average caloric requirement of a full-term pregnancy is 55,000 calories, which is consumed throughout the course of the pregnancy. There is no increased requirement during the first trimester, unless there was severe starvation before conception or the woman has severe hyperemesis gravidarum, which would deplete the bodily nutrient reserves. A 200- to 300-calorie per day increase over prepregnancy caloric needs is recommended during the second and third trimesters of pregnancy for women entering pregnancy at a normal BMI. The calculation is 200 calories/day × 7 days/week × 40 weeks' gestation = 56,000 calories.

The increased nutritional needs of pregnancy can be met by consuming one additional serving of a skim milk product, one additional serving from the bread and cereal group, one additional serving of fruit or vegetable, or one additional ounce of meat or meat substitute beyond the basic food guide plan for adult women. Pregnant adolescents should add one additional serving of dairy foods for increased calcium requirements, because their own skeleton is still forming.

Protein

The protein requirement for adult women is 0.8 kg body weight. The need for increased protein for the pregnant woman is 30% greater than when nonpregnant. This translates into an increase of 10 to 14 additional grams of protein per day during the last half of pregnancy. The increased need should be expected as a result of the increase in both maternal and fetal tissue formation. Adequate calories must be consumed so that protein can be used for the body's building and synthetic processes (Table 8-2). If calories are not consumed in adequate amounts, the protein in the diet is used to meet the energy needs of the body, rather than the building and synthesizing needs. Additional calories provide protein-sparing effects that are greater than in the nonpregnant woman.

Calcium

Calcium is a mineral needed for strong bones and teeth, neural transmission, and muscle contractions; it also plays

---

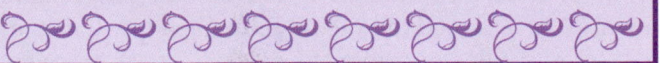

Critical Thinking

Determining Caloric Needs

The following formula may be used to determine caloric needs:

130 lb woman × 10   = 1300 calories for BMR

+ 1300 calories × 30% (average activity level)
                            = 390 calories for activity

+ 1690 calories × 10% (SDA)
                            = 169 calories

Total caloric needs/day   = 1859 calories

Therefore, approximately 1859 calories per day would be necessary for this woman to maintain her body weight. Since each pound of body weight equals 3500 calories, to lose 1 pound a week, this woman would need to consume 500 fewer calories per day or to consume 250 fewer calories per day and increase her activity expenditure by 250 calories per day. If this woman desired to gain 1 pound of weight per week, she would need to increase her caloric intake by 500 calories per day. What are the caloric needs for a woman weighing 145 lb?

Table 8-2 Recommended Dietary Allowances During Pregnancy and Lactation

Age	Weight (kg)	Weight (lb)	Height (cm)	Height (in)	Protein (g)	FAT-SOLUBLE VITAMINS Vitamin A (µg RE)	Vitamin D (µg)	Vitamin E (µg α-TE)	Vitamin K (µg)	WATER-SOLUBLE VI Vitamin C (mg)	Thiamin (mg)
11–14 years											
Not pregnant	46	101	157	62	46	800	5	8	45	50	1.1
Pregnant					60	800	5	10	65	70	1.5
Lactating											
1st 6 months					65	1,300	5	12	65	95	1.6
2nd 6 months					62	1,200	5	11	65	90	1.6
15–18 years											
Not pregnant	55	120	163	64	44	800	5	8	55	60	1.1
Pregnant					60	800	5	10	65	70	1.5
Lactating											
1st 6 months					65	1,300	5	12	65	95	1.6
2nd 6 months					62	1,200	5	11	65	90	1.6
19–24 years											
Not pregnant	58	128	164	65	46	800	5	8	60	60	1.1
Pregnant					60	800	5	10	65	70	1.5
Lactating											
1st 6 months					65	1,300	5	12	65	95	1.6
2nd 6 months					62	1,200	5	11	65	90	1.6
25 years +											
Not pregnant	63	138	163	64	50	800	5	8	60	60	1.1
Pregnant					60	800	5	10	65	70	1.5
Lactating											
1st 6 months					65	1,300	5	12	65	95	1.6
2nd 6 months					62	1,200	5	11	65	90	1.6

Source: Institute of Medicine. *Nutrition During Pregnancy*. Washington, D.C.: National Academy Press, 1989.

a role in cells and cell membranes, blood clotting, and other functions. Nearly 99% of the body's calcium is in the bones and teeth. Calcium is in a dynamic state in the body, always being moved from the bloodstream to the bones, according to the body's needs. The remaining 1% of calcium is found in body fluids. Calcium is required to maintain normal blood pressure and for the absorption of vitamin B_{12}. In 1997, the Food and Nutrition Board recommended that the adequate intake level for females ages 19 to 50 remain the same at 1000 mg/day of calcium, even during pregnancy and lactation. This may seem strange, but this represents an increase of 400 mg/day over the 1989 RDA. The calcium recommendations were increased primarily because of the increase in recognition of osteoporosis in women. The Food and Nutrition Board, in 1997, increased the calcium recommendations for adequate intake to 1300 mg/day for ages 9 through 18 and 1000 mg/day for ages 19 to 50, for both males and females. The benefit of increased calcium intake on weight-bearing

sites, such as the hip, is enhanced in women with high levels of physical activity. Urinary calcium loss is increased by excessive intake of sodium or protein. This is especially true of animal proteins, which are high in the sulfur amino acids, methionine and cysteine. Epidemiologic studies demonstrate that countries with the highest consumption of animal protein have the highest rate of hip fractures.

It is recommended that pregnant and lactating girls less than age 18 consume 1300 mg of calcium per day. Women should be encouraged to consume three to four servings from the dairy group daily. If women are lactose-intolerant, they should be advised to use lactase tablets or drops with dairy products; drink lactose-digested milk; use fermented milk products, such as buttermilk or yogurt; or take calcium supplements. Table 8-3 offers an overview of calcium needs.

If a woman does not regularly consume dairy products or other foods high in calcium each day, a calcium supplement of at least 600 mg/day is recommended. Calcium in the form of calcium carbonate, calcium citrate, or calcium

WATER-SOLUBLE VITAMINS			MINERALS							
Vitamin B$_6$	Folate (µg)	Vitamin B$_{12}$ (µg)	Calcium (mg)	Phosphorus (mg)	Magnesium (mg)	Fluoride (mg)	Iron (mg)	Zinc (mg)	Iodine (µg)	Selenium (µg)
1.4	150	2.0	1,300	1,055	200	2.0	15	12	150	45
2.2	400	2.2	1,300	1,055	200	2.0	30	15	175	65
2.1	280	2.6	1,300	1,055	200	2.0	15	19	200	75
2.1	260	2.6	1,300	1,055	200	2.0	15	16	200	75
1.5	180	2.0	1,300	1,055	300	2.9	15	12	150	50
2.2	400	2.2	1,300	1,055	335	2.9	30	15	175	65
2.1	280	2.6	1,300	1,055	300	2.9	15	19	200	75
2.1	260	2.6	1,300	1,055	300	2.9	15	16	200	75
1.6	180	2.0	1,000	580	255	3.1	15	12	150	55
2.2	400	2.2	1,000	580	290	3.1	30	15	175	65
2.1	280	2.6	1,000	580	255	3.1	15	19	200	75
2.1	260	2.6	1,000	580	255	3.1	15	16	200	75
1.6	180	2.0	1,000	580	265	3.1	15	12	150	55
2.2	400	2.2	1,000	580	300	3.1	30	15	175	65
2.1	280	2.6	1,000	580	265	3.1	15	19	200	75
2.1	260	2.6	1,000	580	265	3.1	15	16	200	75

phosphate, in supplements that carry the United States Pharmacopoeia (USP) symbol, have been shown to be highly absorbable. Each client should discuss possible interactions among calcium supplements and prescription or over-the-counter medications with their doctor or pharmacist.

Vitamin D

Vitamin D plays an important role in calcium absorption and bone mineralization. Vitamin D allows calcium to leave the intestines and enter the bloodstream to be absorbed and allows the bones to release more calcium and the kidneys to retain more calcium in the body. It is essential to have sufficient quantities of this vitamin on a regular basis. Because it is a fat-soluble vitamin, it is stored in the liver. Vitamin D intake is recommended at 5 µg (200 IU) per day for adults over age 19, even during pregnancy and lactation. For adults between ages 51 and 70, the (Daily Recommended Intake) is 10 µg (400 IU) per day, increas-

ing to 15 µg (600 IU) per day for individuals over age 70. The tolerable upper intake level for vitamin D is 50 µg/day (Table 8-2).

Sources of vitamin D include vitamin D–fortified cow's milk or margarine, eggs, and butter. Most commercial yogurts are not fortified with vitamin D. Complete vegetarians who consume no animal products at all should consider supplementation if their exposure to sunlight is limited. Not all soy-containing products are fortified with vitamin D. Reading labels is important. Adequate exposure of the skin to sunshine, i.e., about 30 minutes of direct sunlight on the hands and face without sunscreen two to three times weekly, may be enough for the body to produce an adequate amount of vitamin D. Synthesis of vitamin D may be reduced in winter months, in darker-pigmented individuals, and in those living with high concentrations of atmospheric ozone. For women in northern climates or those with little exposure to sunlight, such as office workers, nursing home residents, and house-

Research Highlight

Food Consumption by Americans

Purpose

To examine the contribution of energy-dense, nutrient-poor (EDNP) foods to the diet of Americans and to examine the relationship between EDNP food intake and the availability of macronutrients and micronutrients.

Method

Twenty-four-hour recall data from the National Health and Nutrition Examination Survey (NHANES) were analyzed (n = 1561, ages $\geq$ 20). Linear logistical regressions were used to examine relationships with serum profiles of vitamins, lipids, and carotenoids.

Findings

EDNP foods accounted for 27% of the total energy intake; alcohol accounted for another 4%. One third of the population consumed an average of 45% of energy from EDNP foods. The relative odds of consuming foods from all five food groups and meeting the RDA for protein and micronutrients decreased with increased EDNP intake. Serum concentrations of vitamins A, E, C, and B_{12}; folate; several carotenoids; and HDL cholesterol were inversely related ($P \leq 0.0005$). Serum homocysteine was positively related to EDNP food intake ($p = 0.002$).

Nursing Implications

This study indicates that assessing for EDNP foods, such as visible fats, nutritive sweeteners and sweetened beverages, desserts, and snacks may be a good indicator of more general nutritional problems. As these foods tend to substitute for, rather than supplement, more nutrient-dense foods, clients who consume them in large amounts are at risk not only for obesity and problems of fat and caloric excess, but for nutrient deficiencies as well.

Source: Kant, A. K. (2000). Consumption of energy-dense, nutrient-poor foods by adult Americans: Nutritional and health implications. The 3rd National Health and Nutrition Examination Survey, 1988–1994. *American Journal of Clinical Nutrition*, 72(4), 929–936.

---

bound persons, supplementation should be considered if the diet is inadequate. In addition, women with closely spaced, multiple pregnancies; people with fat malabsorption syndromes; or individuals who regularly use topical sunscreens are in a group with higher needs. Vitamin D_3, synthesized in the skin from 7-dehydroxycholesterol with ultraviolet radiation, is the naturally occurring form and is needed by the body to absorb calcium and phosphorus and deposit these minerals in the teeth and bones to maintain skeletal integrity. The recommended intake of vitamin D for individuals with osteoporosis may be increased by the physician to 10 µg (400 IU) per day. Rich sources of vitamin D include fortified milk (400 IU per quart), high-fat fish (250 to 800 IU per serving), canned fish (200 to 500 IU per serving), and cod liver oil (400 IU per teaspoon). Table 8-3 provides an overview of vitamin D.

Folate

Folate, sometimes referred to as folacin or folic acid, is a B vitamin found in many vegetables, beans, fruits, whole grains, and fortified breads and cereal products. Routine supplementation with folate should occur at least 1 month before conception through the first trimester of pregnancy. All women in the reproductive years should consume at least 400 µg of folic acid per day from fortified foods, vitamin supplements, or a combination of the two, in addition to a varied, healthful diet. Since January 1, 1998, the FDA and the Department of Health and Human Services (DHHS) have required the enrichment of all cereal and grain products to provide 10% of the RDA per serving, or 1.4 mg folate per kilogram of flour or cereal or grain product (1.4 µg folate per gram of cereal or grain product), and not to exceed the recommended maximum of 1 mg/day

Table 8-3 Overview of Selected Vitamins and Minerals

Nutrient	Function	Sources	Deficiency	Toxic Effects
Calcium (Ca)	• Aids in bone and teeth formation • Promotes muscle contraction and relaxation • Aids blood clotting • Aids in nerve transmission • Promotes normal heart rhythm • Needs vitamin D for absorption	• Milk • Cheese • Sardines • Salmon • Green leafy vegetables • Whole grains	• Rickets • Osteoporosis • Tetany • Poor tooth formation	• Kidney stones • Deposits in joints and soft tissue • May inhibit iron and zinc absorption
Vitamin D	• Stimulates absorption of calcium and phosphorus for good bone mineralization	• Yeast • Fish liver oils • Fortified milk and cereals	• Rickets • Malformed teeth • Bone deformities	• Hypercalcemia • Kidney stones • Cardiovascular damage
Folate (folic acid)	• Is necessary for synthesis of RNA and DNA • Promotes amino acid metabolism, red and white blood cell formation	• Green leafy vegetables • Meat • Eggs • Yeast	• Glossitis • Diarrhea • Macrocytic anemia	• None known
Vitamin B_{12} (cobalamin)	• Promotes normal function of all cells, especially of the nervous system • Promotes blood formation • Promotes carbohydrate protein, and fat metabolism • Aids in synthesis of RNA and DNA • Is necessary for folate metabolism	• Fresh shrimp, oysters, meats, milk, eggs, and cheese	• Pernicious anemia • Anorexia • Indigestion • Paresthesia of hands and feet • Poor coordination • Depression	• None known
Iron	• Aids in formation of hemoglobin • Aids in antibody formation	• Meat • Whole grains • Egg yolk • Legumes • Prunes • Raisins • Apricots	• Iron deficiency anemia	• Hemochromatosis • GI cramping • Vomiting • Nausea • Shock • Convulsions • Coma

intake of folic acid. Synthetic folic acid has been shown to be twice as absorbable as dietary folate. The folic acid fortification of widely consumed cereal and grain products should have a remarkable effect in reducing the number of pregnancies affected by neural tube defects (NTD), when these products are consumed with synthetic supplements of folic acid (Lewis, Crane, Wilson, & Yetley, 1999). The incidence of occlusive vascular diseases may also be decreased by higher intakes of folic acid lowering plasma or serum homocysteine concentrations. Clients should be evaluated for pernicious anemia and vitamin B_{12} deficiency before being given large doses of folate.

Dietary sources of folate include meat, fish, poultry, eggs, fortified whole-grain breads, fortified cereals, peanuts, leafy green vegetables, and yeast extract. Liver is an excellent source, with 3.5 ounces of chicken livers containing 770 µg of folic acid and 3.5 ounces of beef liver containing 217 µg of folic acid.

Sufficient body supplies of folic acid before and during conception and for up to 13 weeks after conception help guard against birth defects of the brain and spine (NTDs) that occur when the neural tube does not close completely, as in spina bifida (in which the spinal canal does not close and protrudes out of the back), **encephalocele**

REFLECTIONS FROM A YOUNG ADULT

"My grandmother recently fell and broke her hip for the second time. All her life she's been a heavy smoker and coffee drinker and not very big on dairy products, especially milk. I guess I never really appreciated the link among good dietary habits, a healthy lifestyle, and overall physical health and well-being. Most of my life I've done what I've wanted and been very healthy, but seeing my grandmother's troubles really motivates me to watch my habits and consider their impact on my long-term health."

(in which the brain protrudes through a defect in the skull), and **anencephaly** (a fatal condition in which a baby is born with a severely underdeveloped brain and skull and dies shortly after birth). In the United States, more than 3000 infants per year are born with NTDs, about 4 of every 1000 births. Babies with the other NTDs live longer, with paralysis, neurologic damage, and possibly bowel and bladder incontinence. Women who have had one infant with an NTD are considered to be at high risk for having another infant with an NTD. Four mg of folate per day is recommended for these women, beginning at least 1 month before pregnancy and throughout the first trimester of pregnancy. This treatment has been shown to reduce the risk of the mother having another NTD-affected child by about 70%.

As a coenzyme, folate serves a role in the synthesis of ribonucleic acid (RNA) and deoxyribonucleic acid (DNA) and, therefore, is necessary for the proliferation of cells and the transmission of inherited characteristics. Folic acid also functions in the formation and maturation of red and white blood cells and the synthesis of enzymes. Folate deficiency results in macrocytic or megaloblastic anemia, which is characterized by immature, large red blood cells. Glossitis, gastrointestinal irritation, depression, and other neuropsychiatric disturbances are also found in children of women with folic acid deficiency. Alcohol also interferes with folate use by the body and thus increases folate requirements even more. Anticonvulsants, some antacids, antihypertensive agents, and aspirin also interact with folic acid. Adequate body stores of folic acid and vitamins B_6

and B_{12} may protect against high blood levels of homocysteine, a chemical that, at an elevated level, has been linked to damaging arteries and setting the stage for atherosclerosis and stroke (Mills, McPartlin, Kirke, Lee, Conley, Weir, & Seoth, 1995).

Without an adequate amount of folic acid, women, especially those who are poorly nourished and from low-income groups, have a higher proportion of premature, low birth weight babies. Currently, researchers are studying the role of genetics in how women metabolize food folates and how folic acid is transferred from the placenta to the fetus (Locksmith & Duff, 1998). Identifying women who are at risk for having babies with NTDs before conception and improving ways to treat them are long-term goals.

The (Bailey, 1998) DRI expresses the new recommended intakes for individuals for folate in dietary folate equivalents (DFEs). The DFEs account for the difference in the absorption of naturally occurring food folate and synthetic folic acid, which is more bioavailable. The following formula was used to calculate DFEs of sources of folate.

Folic acid content = total folate content of fortified food − food folate content.

Dietary folate equivalents = μg of food folate + (1.7 + μg folic acid)

The Nutrition Facts label is based on a recommended daily 400 μg of folic acid. To find out the number of micrograms of folic acid per serving size, multiply the percentage of the daily value times 400 μg (the daily value for folic acid). Then, multiply the result by 1.7 to obtain dietary folate equivalents.

As stated in Table 8-2, women aged 19 and older need 400 μg of DFE per day. One DFE = 1 μg food folate = 0.6 μg folic acid (from fortified food or supplement) consumed with food = 0.5 μg of synthetic (supplemental) folic acid taken on an empty stomach. During pregnancy, the recommendations increase by 200 μg per day to equal 600 μg DFE per day. During lactation, the recommendations increase by 100 μg over the basic recommendations per day to equal 500 μg DFE per day. Table 8-3 gives an overview of folate needs.

Vitamin B_{12}

Vitamin B_{12} is needed to build red blood cells and to keep the nervous system healthy. It is also essential for the normal use of folate and helps protect against the risk factors characteristic of heart disease and atherosclerosis. This vitamin is only found in animal food sources. The best sources of this vitamin are meats, fish, poultry, shellfish, eggs, milk, and milk products. Some brands of soymilk products are fortified with vitamin B_{12}. Vegetarians consuming no animal products (vegans) need 2.4 μg per day of vitamin B_{12}. Care should be taken to get adequate amounts of this vitamin, either through the diet or a multivitamin and mineral supplement. Vitamin B_{12} is absorbed in the ileum and requires intrinsic factor (IF), produced and secreted in the parietal cells of the stomach mucosa, for absorption. IF is a glycoprotein that protects vitamin B_{12} from degradation as it moves through the intestinal tract to the ileum, the site of absorption. Impaired absorption of this vitamin accounts for more than 95% of the cases of vitamin B_{12} deficiency in the United States. With adequate intake, the liver can store vitamin B_{12}, which is somewhat unique for the B vitamins.

Deficiency of vitamin B_{12} in the diet or in individuals lacking the intrinsic factor can mean the development of pernicious anemia. The name was given to this deficiency disease in 1822 when pernicious meant "to lead to death." This deficiency causes macrocytic, megaloblastic anemia, in which red blood cells have delayed and abnormal nuclear maturation.

Vitamin B_{12}, known as cyanocobalamin, was the last water-soluble vitamin to be isolated and have its structure identified. It is required in very small amounts in comparison to other water-soluble vitamins. The RDA is 2.4 μg per day for this vitamin, for both adolescents and adults. In pregnancy, the recommendation increases to 2.6 μg/day, and in lactation to 2.8 μg/day. The next lowest recommended intake for a B vitamin is for folate, for which the requirement is 167 times greater than that of vitamin B_{12} for women. Strict vegetarians (vegans), breastfed infants of vegans, vegan children, elderly persons, and individuals with past gastrointestinal surgeries are at high risk for vitamin B_{12} deficiency.

Vitamin B_{12} is involved in the conversion of homocysteine to methionine (Gerhard, Malinow, DeLoughery, Evans, Sexton, Connor, Wander, & Connor, 1999). If there is inadequate vitamin B_{12}, of methylenetetrahydrofolate (THF), or lowering level reduced folate, which is needed for nucleic acid metabolism than this causes a combination of events that is responsible for the megaloblastic anemia, characteristic of both vitamin B_{12} and folate deficiency. The red blood cells look identical in both types of deficiency. Symptoms accompanying pernicious anemia include weakness, indigestion, abdominal pain, constipation alternating with diarrhea, sore and glossy tongue, and damaged nerve fibers. Treating individuals with folate supplementation may reverse the megaloblastic anemia, although the B_{12} deficiency may worsen. Prolonged deficiency can result in irreversible nervous system damage. The determination of folate and vitamin B_{12} deficiency is therefore necessary before initiating treatment. Deoxyuridine suppression tests differentiate between folate and vitamin B_{12} deficiency. Serum levels reflect early reduction in tissue stores. Macrocytic anemia appears months or years after depletion. Doses of up to 1000 μg/day are used to treat deficiency. Doses greater than this can mask more

obvious signs of vitamin B_{12} deficiency. If the deficiency is caused by inadequate absorption, such as a client with gastrectomy, monthly injections of 100 μg are appropriate. Such clients should have their serum vitamin B_{12} levels monitored every 6 to 12 months. Table 8-3 provides an overview of vitamin B_{12} needs.

Iron

Iron is a trace mineral that functions to transport oxygen to the cells as a component of hemoglobin and myoglobin. Iron is also a required by several enzyme systems and helps convert energy for normal cell activities. Iron is stored intracellularly as ferritin and hemosiderin, primarily in the liver, spleen, bone marrow, and other organs. Table 8-2 lists the recommended intake of iron for each age group. In general, for menstruating females, the iron recommendation is 15 mg/day. The recommendation decreases past the age of 51 to 10 mg/day. For pregnancy, the recommended level doubles to 30 mg/day, and during lactation, the recommended level returns to the menstruating female level of 15 mg/day.

If dietary intake is inadequate, the stored iron is used to meet the body's need for iron. Only after depletion of iron stores do hematocrit levels begin to fall. Signs of iron deficiency are the depletion of the iron stores, microcytic (small cell size) anemia, **hypochromic** (lacking in color) anemia. Iron deficiency anemia is the most common nutritional deficiency in the United States. The incidence in high-risk populations ranges from 10% to 50%: in menstruating women, 5% to 14%; in males in early adolescence, 4% to 12%; in children, ages 1 to 2, 9%. There is currently an interagency group, consisting of the Micronutrient Initiative and the University of Toronto, presenting the technology to fortify salt with iron, in addition to iodine, to address the severe levels of iron deficiency anemia existing worldwide.

Because women are consuming fewer calories and losing iron during menstruation, they often enter pregnancy with depleted iron stores. During pregnancy, the increased blood volume and fetal requirements reduce the iron stores even further. The fetal tissues take predominance over the mother's tissues with respect to use of the iron stores. During the last trimester of pregnancy, when the iron stores are being laid down in the fetus, 3 to 4 mg of iron is transferred to the fetus from the mother daily.

Ferrous iron supplements of 30 to 60 mg/day are recommended for the general population of pregnant women beginning the 12th week of pregnancy and continuing throughout the pregnancy, assuming an omnivorous diet with adequate intake of vitamin C. The proper dose of iron may be provided by 150 mg of ferrous sulfate, 300 mg of ferrous gluconate, or 100 mg of ferrous fumarate. Iron supplements should be continued for 2 to 3 months postpartum. Full-term neonates do not require

ORAL CONTRACEPTIVE AGENTS

Millions of women use oral contraceptive agents (OCAs), commonly known as "the pill," to prevent unplanned pregnancy. The effect of OCA use on nutritional status is that OCAs reduce menstrual flow by approximately half, therefore conserving nutrients normally lost during menstruation, especially iron. The different OCAs affect the absorption or excretion rate of nutrients according to the hormone types and concentrations of the pill. For some OCAs, the rate of metabolic conversion changes the nutrient status in the body. Most women can correct these changes by paying close attention and eating a well-balanced and varied diet. Supplements are indicated only if a deficiency exists and symptoms are apparent.

Women are advised to stop taking oral contraceptive agents 6 or more months before planning to become pregnant, because oral contraceptives can alter nutritional status. Table 8-4 presents the effect of these agents on the nutritional status of women. When women stop taking OCAs before trying to conceive, alternate methods of birth control are recommended while the woman's body is rebuilding and readying for conception. Some other forms of birth control methods commonly used are the condom, rhythm method, diaphragm, intrauterine device, and morning-after pill. Intrauterine devices double the menstrual loss, and consequently, also affect nutrient stores in the body.

Table 8-4 Effects of Oral Contraceptive Agents on Nutritional Status

Nutrient	Effect of Agent	
Vitamin B_6	↑ requirement	↓ blood levels
Riboflavin	↑ requirement	↓ blood levels
Folic acid	↓ absorption	↓ blood levels
Vitamin B_{12}	↑ requirement	↓ blood levels
Vitamin C		↓ blood levels
Vitamin A	↓ carotene	↑ blood levels
Calcium	↑ absorption	
Iron	↑ serum levels	
Copper	↑ serum levels	
Magnesium	↓ blood levels	
Zinc	↑ erythrocyte levels	

Compiled and copyrighted by Jeanne B. Martin, PhD, RD, FADA, LD.

iron supplementation until 4 months of age, but should have iron supplements as long as they are fed from the breast or with formula without iron supplements in it. Premature infants should begin iron supplementation earlier.

Iron in the diet consists of two forms. **Heme iron** (iron from animal sources) constitutes about half of the iron in the diet animal sources. **Nonheme iron** (dietary iron sources other than from meats, in which the iron is not bound to hemoglobin). comprises the remaining half of the iron found in animal sources and all of the iron found in plant sources, including grains and cereals. There is greater absorption of nonheme iron when it is taken with a good dietary source of ascorbic acid, like orange juice or oranges. Nonheme iron is less absorbable when taken with tea (tannic acid), dairy products (calcium phosphate), many cereals (phytates), bran, oxalates, and antacids. Heme iron is absorbed four to five times better than nonheme iron. Nonheme iron accounts for a larger percentage of total human iron intake. On the average,

about 10% of iron consumed is absorbed. The rate of absorption varies with need and the form of the iron consumed.

Administration of the iron supplement between meals or at bedtime increases absorption rates. If a client has iron-deficiency anemia and therapeutic levels of iron (more than 30 mg/day) are given to treat the anemia, the client should also be given 15 mg of zinc and 2 mg of copper because of the interference of iron with the absorption and use of these trace minerals.

Hemochromatosis (a rare genetic defect in iron metabolism, in which excess iron is deposited in the tissues, causing skin pigmentation, hepatic cirrhosis, and decreased carbohydrate tolerance, which eventually ends in multiple-system organ failure) and **hemosiderosis** (increase in iron stores without associated tissue damage) are iron-storage diseases that result from iron toxicity. Alcohol consumption enhances iron absorption, sometimes by as much as 50%, which may also result in a toxic overload of iron. Signs and symptoms of acute iron poisoning include gastrointestinal cramping and pain, vomiting and nausea, convulsions, and coma (Table 8-3).

Fiber

Dietary fiber is a complex carbohydrate, mainly composed of the indigestible parts of plant cell walls. Dietary fiber is connected to better colon health, a reduced incidence of type 2 diabetes mellitus, lower blood pressure and cholesterol levels, and less risk of cardiovascular disease. Individuals who eat a lot of whole grain cereals and bread products and fruits and vegetables with the skins seem to have less constipation and diverticulitis. Although no dietary recommendations exist for fiber for pregnant women, they should consume the same amount as recommended for the general population. This is 20 to 35 g/day of dietary fiber from a wide variety of food sources, such as fruits, vegetables, legumes, and whole grains. When fiber intake is increased, it should be done gradually. In addition, 1 to 2 quarts of additional fluid should be consumed with the additional fiber. This helps with possible constipation problems characteristic of supplemental iron intake and normal pregnancy. Participating in regular physical exercise is recommended to manage constipation.

There are two types of fiber: insoluble and soluble. **Insoluble fiber** resists absorption into the body. It moves quickly through the digestive tract, absorbing water and making the stools softer and bulkier. The rapid passage of food through the intestines is believed to reduce the potential for carcinogens to interact with the intestinal surface. However, this hypothesis is under study. Insoluble fiber is found primarily in whole grains, nuts, seeds, vegetables, cooked dried beans, and dried peas or legumes.

Soluble fiber reduces blood cholesterol levels. It can bind bile acids or coat the intestines, thus inhibiting the absorption of cholesterol. Soluble fiber includes pectins, gums, and mucilages that dissolve in water. Some key sources of soluble fiber are oat bran, barley, apples, fruits, seaweed, and cooked dried beans and peas (legumes).

Water

Water is an essential, vital nutrient, often overlooked in recommendations. It is an essential nutrient because it is required in amounts that exceed the body's ability to produce it. It is necessary for the transport of nutrients in the body and for body temperature maintenance and serves as a solvent for minerals, vitamins, amino acids, and glucose. Water provides a means for the elimination of waste materials and toxins from the body in urine. Approximately 60% of the adult's body is composed of water with two-thirds of this water distributed intracellularly and one-third extracellularly. Water accounts for 50% to 80% of body weight, depending on the level of lean body mass. Usual recommendations for adults are to drink 8 to 10 cups (1 cup = 8 oz = 237 mL) of water per day, or 30 mL/kg of body weight, with a minimum of 6 cups (1500 mL) for small individuals. Another way to calculate water needs is based on 1 mL/kcal of energy consumption per day (2200 kcal diet = 2200 mL/day of water = approximately 9.28 cups/day of water). More daily fluid is required: (1) in hot, dry climates or high altitudes; (2) with a high-fiber diet; (3) with a diet high in alcohol or caffeine; and (4) with increased activity. Early symptoms of dehydration include headache, fatigue, loss of appetite, flushed skin, heat intolerance, lightheadedness, dry mouth and eyes, a burning sensation in the stomach, and dark urine with a strong odor.

Because the pregnant woman's blood volume is expanding, water and other fluids should be increased. The pregnant woman needs an additional daily 30 mL of water per kilogram of body weight gained. Alternate sources of water should be obtained if there is concern about the lead content of the water pipes. Lead intake has been linked to decreased stature and deficient neurocognitive development of the fetus. The local or state public water department can direct clients to facilities for testing the lead content in their household water supply.

Vegan Diets

Vegans are "pure" vegetarians who do not consume any animal-containing product, including eggs, milk, or milk products in addition to meats, poultry, or fish. Vegans can get enough calcium from plant sources alone, with careful diet planning, by including sufficient quantities of calcium-rich foods, such as tofu processed with calcium, calcium-fortified soy beverages, broccoli, seeds, nuts, legumes, some dark greens (kale, collards, mustard greens), okra, rutabagas, bok choy, dried figs, tortillas made from lime-processed corn, and calcium-fortified orange juice and breakfast cereals. Some plant foods (e.g., beet greens, rhubarb, spinach, Swiss chard, and amaranth) contain oxalates and some grain products contain phytates, which bind to calcium and block its absorption. Therefore, these foods should not be relied on as the sole source of absorbable calcium in the diet.

Pregnancy and Lactation

The nutritional status of women entering the reproductive phase of life may be one of the most important nutritional stages of life. The mother's nutritional history plays a direct role in the development of the fetus. Women must plan nutritionally for their pregnancy to help achieve healthy full-term newborns. There are many events outside a woman's control during the conception and development of the fetus, but the woman's capacity to conceive should motivate her to follow sound nutritional advice from health professionals to ensure a successful outcome of pregnancy. This is critical to the mother's health, her baby's prenatal development, and the development of the child long after its birth. All women in their teens and throughout their 40s should be cognizant of their potential to conceive, and therefore, optimize their nutritional status prior to conception. Health professionals in any setting should try to help women in all age groups form sound, lifetime nutritional practices.

Prepregnancy nutritional status is most easily evaluated in the clinical setting using the prepregnancy weight-for-height index. The measurement is easy to make and provides systematic methods for evaluating women's weight. The health care professional can use a chart for estimating BMI or can use the formula: weight (kg)/height (m^2) to determine BMI. This can help the woman and health care professional set realistic, appropriate weight-gain goals. Table 8-5 provides the recommended ranges

Table 8-5 Recommended Total Weight Gain Ranges for Pregnant Women in Second and Third Trimesters According to Prepregnancy BMI

Prepregnant BMI	Total Weight Gain (kg)	Gain in 4 Weeks (kg)	Total Weight Gain (lbs)	Gain in 4 Weeks (lbs)
Underweight (BMI < 19.8)	12.7–18.2	2.3	28–40	5.0
Normal (BMI = 19.8–26.0)	11.4–15.9	1.8	25–35	4.0
Overweight (BMI = 26.1–29.0)	6.8–11.4	1.2	15–25	2.6
Obese (BMI > 29.0)	6.8	0.9	<15	2.0
Twin gestation	15.9–20.4	2.7	35–45	6.0

BMI, body mass index = weight (kg)/height (m^2)
Source: Institute of Medicine. *Nutrition During Pregnancy*. Washington, D.C.: National Academy Press, 1990.

for total weight gain for pregnant women, based on their prepregnancy BMI.

The first 6 weeks after conception are extremely important for optimum fetal development. Therefore, the woman must be aware of and avoid as many as possible of the nutritional risk factors that are related to poor pregnancy outcome. These include consumption of alcohol, tobacco, and prescription, over-the-counter, and illegal drugs. Currently the recommendation is for supplementation of folic acid prior to conception to lower the risk of neural tube defects (Cuskelly, McNulty, & Scott, 1999). A well-planned pregnancy should ideally include an initial health examination 8 to 12 weeks before conception. This period is critical for establishing a prepregnancy baseline weight.

Weight Gain in Pregnancy

At the first prenatal visit, the health professional should measure height and weight, determine the prepregnancy BMI, and explain the importance of adequate weight gain during pregnancy. The weight gain of the pregnant woman should be recorded, plotted, and monitored at

Box 8-1 Weight Gain Distribution During Pregnancy

5.0 kg (11 lbs)	Fetus, placenta, and amniotic fluid
0.9 kg (2 lbs)	Uterus
1.8 kg (4 lbs)	Increase in blood volume
1.4 kg (3 lbs)	Breast tissue
2.3 to 4.5 kg (5 to 10 lbs)	Maternal stores

Total = 11 to 13 kg (25 to 30 lbs) gained
For women at their ideal BMI at conception

Adapted from Cunningham. et. al., 1997

each prenatal visit. Weight gain during the first half of the pregnancy is reflective of increasing maternal stores. In the second half of gestation, the weight gain is primarily attributable to fetal growth (Box 8-1).

Under no circumstances should a woman lose weight during her pregnancy. If this happens, or if an excess rate of weight gain occurs, the cause should be assessed and referral made to a registered dietitian. During the second and third trimesters of pregnancy, underweight women (prepregnancy BMI of less than 19.8) should gain slightly more than one pound per week. Women with normal or moderate prepregnancy BMI of 19.8 to 26.0 should gain about 1 lb/wk. Women with a high prepregnancy BMI of 26.1 to 29.0 are encouraged to gain two-thirds of a pound per week. Very obese women (prepregnancy BMI of more than 29.0) should have their total weight gain determined on an individual basis. The date of the office visit, the weeks of gestation, the mother's weight, and any significant findings should be recorded at each visit. Weight should be plotted at each visit to assure no weight loss is occurring and, if it does, an explanation for the loss can be found. A copy of this information should also be given to the mother, if she also wants to keep track of this.

Weight gain for pregnant women under the height of 62 inches (less than 157 cm) should be toward the lower end of the recommended range for BMI. Adolescents should try to achieve the upper recommended range of weight gain for their BMI because their bodies are still growing and need additional nutrients for this as well as for their pregnancy. The recommended range for a twin pregnancy is 35 to 45 pounds (16 to 20 kg). In a 1997 (Suitor, 1997) review of the Institute of Medicine's (IOM) report, *Nutrition During Pregnancy,* an expert group recommended that, contrary to the 1990 report (Institute of Medicine, 1990), which suggested that African-American women should strive for the upper end of the recommended range of weight gain because of their higher likelihood of delivering low-birth-weight babies, African American women should be advised to stay within the IOM-recommended BMI-specific weight-gain range for optimum pregnancy outcome. This was recommended because African American women had an increased likelihood of low prenatal weight gain in each BMI category and a decreased likelihood of gaining more weight than recommended overall (Suitor, 1997).

In 1992 the Committee on Nutritional Status During Pregnancy and Lactation proposed eight recommendations in their book, *Nutrition Services in Perinatal Care,* 2nd edition (Institute of Medicine, 1992). These key recommendations are relevant today and are listed below.

1. Basic, client-centered, individualized nutritional care should be integrated into the primary care of every woman and infant—beginning prior to conception and extending throughout the period of breast-feeding.

2. All primary care providers should have the knowledge and skills necessary to screen for nutritional problems, assess nutritional status, provide basic nutritional guidance, and implement basic nutritional care.

3. Nutritional care should be documented in the permanent medical record.

4. When health problems that benefit from special nutritional care are identified, there should be consultation with and often referral to an experienced registered dietitian or other appropriate specialists.

5. Attention should be directed toward aspects of nutritional care that have been seriously neglected in the past: providing care prior to conception and in support of breast-feeding and ensuring the continuity of nutritional care despite changes in providers.

6. Action should be taken to make appropriate policy and structural changes for the promotion and support of breast-feeding.

7. Where not already in place, mechanisms should be established to pay for basic and special nutrition services in both the public and the private sectors.

8. Cost-effective strategies for implementing the nutritional care recommended in the report should be developed and tested.

Dietary Supplements in Pregnancy

For pregnant women who are unable to consume an adequate daily diet and for those in high-risk categories, the Subcommittee on Nutritional Status and Weight Gain During Pregnancy and on Dietary Intake and Nutrient Supple-

Table 8-6 Recommended Daily Prenatal Multivitamin and Mineral Supplement for Pregnant Women at Increased Nutrient Risk

Iron	30–60 mg	Vitamin B_{12}	2 µg
Zinc	15 mg	Folate	400 µg
Copper	2 mg	Vitamin C	50 mg
Calcium	250 mg	Vitamin D	10 µg (400 IU)
Vitamin B_6	2 mg		

Source: Morgan, S.& Weinsier, R. L. (1998). *Fundamentals of Clinical Nutrition.* 2nd Ed. St. Louis: Mosby.

ments During Pregnancy recommends a daily multivitamin and mineral preparation containing the nutrients listed in Table 8-6, beginning in the second trimester. Pregnant women who are considered to be at high risk for vitamin and mineral deficiency would include the following: those who smoke or are alcohol or drug abusers; those who have frequent, closely spaced, or multiparous births; those who are carrying more than one fetus; those who experience hyperemesis gravidarum; those who have an eating disorder or are obese or underweight; and those who are adolescents or strict vegetarians.

Over-the-counter prenatal vitamn and mineral supplements are readily available. Generic brands should be compared with name brands for price and nutrients.

Nutritional Needs during Lactation

Breast-feeding should be strongly encouraged. Breastfeeding only is adequate for the first 4 to 6 months in almost all healthy infants. Lactation is the physiologic completion of the reproductive cycle. An adequate volume of breast milk with optimal nutrient composition can be produced, even with suboptimal dietary intake, by drawing on the maternal nutrient stores and tissue reserves. Nutrient needs of the client are increased during lactation, according to the volume of breast milk produced and the duration of breast-feeding.

For the vegan breast-feeding mother, vitamin B_6 and vitamin B_{12} supplements are needed because meat, eggs, and dairy products are the primary source for these B vitamins. The lactating woman needs to replace the fluid lost in breast milk. The increased fluid need of the lactating woman is 750 to 1000 mL/day above the basic requirement.

Well-nourished breast-feeding women need an additional 200 calories per day over pregnancy energy requirements to adequately initiate and maintain lactation. Therefore, 500 calories more than the nonpregnant calorie intake must be consumed. Young adolescents, underweight women, and women who gained an inadequate amount of weight during their pregnancy or who are highly active physically will require greater energy intakes while lactating; an additional 650 calories per day are needed.

At least 1800 calories are needed per day from the major food groups for a well-balanced diet that provides the increased protein and nutrients needed (Table 8-2). The increase can be met by consuming one additional serving each from a skim milk product, from the bread and cereal group, and from the fruit or vegetable group. Some dietary guidelines for lactating women include the following:

- Consume enough fluids (especially milk, juice, water, and soup) to keep from getting thirsty.
- Try to keep intake of coffee, tea, cola drinks, or other sources of caffeine to two servings or less per day.
- Avoid alcohol consumption, and be aware that beer drinking does not aid lactation.
- If you use beverages containing sugar substitutes, use moderation and do not use them to substitute for more nutritious foods, such as milk or fruit juices.
- Continue the multivitamin and mineral supplement prescribed during pregnancy.

Breast-feeding has many positive benefits for the mother and the infant besides offering the infant ideal nutrition. Besides the beneficial nutritional aspects of breast milk (e.g., increased antibodies, ideal protein content, ideal profile of amino acids for the neonate's developing brain, and appropriate lipids and cholesterol levels), breast-feeding an infant offers increased maternal-infant bonding, immunologic protection, allergy prophylaxis, more rapid maternal postpregnancy weight reduction, and suppression of ovulation.

Nutritional Concerns in Pregnancy

Many substances pose a risk to the mother or fetus during pregnancy and should therefore be avoided. Nutritional disturbances of pregnancy and suggested remedies are discussed in this section.

Mercury. Contaminated grains and fish may contribute to mercury toxicity, which has been associated with cerebral palsy, mental retardation, and multiple organ failure in newborns. If mercury contamination is suspected, the pregnant woman should wash all vegetables and fruits (if the skin is eaten) with a weak soap solution and scrub the skin with a brush and rinse well. Otherwise, the skin should be peeled and disposed of before consumption. Likewise, raw fish (e.g., sushi) or fish caught in contaminated waters should be avoided during pregnancy.

Toxic Doses of Vitamin A. A pregnant or lactating woman should not take high doses of retinol (preformed vitamin A) or a potentially teratogenic medication, such as isotretinoin (Accutane) (a vitamin A analog used to treat severe acne). Large doses of vitamin A can cause sponta-

neous abortion or fetal anomalies. Excessive intake (over 10,000 IU per day of vitamin A) from food and supplements should be avoided. No apparent toxicity or teratogenicity exists for beta carotene: harmless yellow skin pigmentation occurs with higher doses. One retinol equivalent (RE) = 1 μg retinol = 6 μg beta carotene.

Alcohol. Women and elderly persons have lower levels of total body water and, therefore, intake of smaller amounts of alcohol achieve higher blood alcohol concentrations than in men. Moderate drinking is defined as 1 or 2 drinks per day for men and 1 drink a day for women and persons over age 65. One alcoholic drink is defined as a 12-ounce bottle of beer or wine cooler, a 5-ounce glass of wine, or 1.5 ounces of 80-proof distilled spirits. These quantities of alcoholic beverages contain approximately 17 grams of alcohol, equal to 119 calories.

Women should avoid alcohol consumption during pregnancy. All alcoholic beverages display the Surgeon General's warning regarding the possible ill effects on the fetus. An absolutely safe minimum limit has not been established. Alcohol increases the urinary excretion of zinc.

Consumption of even small amounts of alcohol during pregnancy may cause fetal alcohol syndrome (FAS) in the newborn. Babies with FAS are abnormally small at birth and have less brain tissue (smaller head circumference) than normal infants. Babies with FAS may have severe mental retardation, may have heart defects, and other alcohol-related birth defects. Therefore, clients should be advised to avoid alcohol consumption beginning at least 1 month before attempting to conceive and throughout pregnancy to protect their unborn child. The severity of FAS depends on how much alcohol was consumed during pregnancy and whether excessive intake occurred early or late in pregnancy. The incidence of FAS in the U.S. varies between 0.4 and 2.6 births per 1000 live births (Mattson, Riley, Gramling, Delis, & Jones, 1997). FAS is characterized by the following:

1. Prenatal or postnatal growth retardation and weight, length, or head circumference below the tenth percentile on growth charts. Unlike other small-for-gestational age infants, infants with FAS do not experience normal "catch-up" growth.

2. CNS involvement, with neurologic abnormality, developmental delay, or intellectual impairment, including:
   Delayed gross motor development
   Low IQ   Hyperactivity
   Poor coordination   Fine motor problems
   Irritability   Extreme nervousness

3. Characteristic facial disfigurations, including:
   Underdeveloped groove in center of upper lip below nose

Low nasal bridge	Short eyelid opening
Small midface	Thin, reddish upper lip
Short nose	Small head circumference

Fetal alcohol effects (FAE) are detectable effects of maternal alcohol consumption but to a more limited extent than seen in FAS.

Caffeine.
Again, there is no definite recommendation about caffeine consumption levels for pregnant women. The research is ambiguous regarding the relationship of caffeine intake to pregnancy outcome. Caffeine acts as a CNS stimulant but does not appear to affect a woman's fertility or her ability to conceive. The fetus does not metabolize caffeine. Recent studies show that caffeine does not increase the risk of spontaneous abortions, fetal growth retardation, or birth defects. The infants of breast-feeding mothers do not metabolize the caffeine either.

The FDA recommends that pregnant women reduce their caffeine intake from coffee, tea, colas, and cocoa to not more that two to three servings per day, for a total of 300 mg of caffeine per day. More than 1000 over-the-counter drugs have caffeine as an ingredient, in addition to prescription drugs that contain caffeine. Caffeine can have a diuretic effect, increasing water loss. Therefore, caffeine-containing beverages should not be counted in tallying the daily fluid recommendations for the pregnant or lactating woman. One tablespoon of milk in coffee offsets the interference of caffeine with calcium absorption. Latte or cappuccinos are better choices than expresso brews for the pregnant woman because of the diluting effect of the milk (Table 8-7).

Artificial Sweeteners.
Moderation in the consumption of artificial sweeteners is recommended for pregnant and lactating women. Women who do not have phenylketonuria (PKU) generally have sufficient phenylalanine hydroxylase activity in their livers to keep phenylalanine levels in the blood at reasonable levels. Women with elevated serum phenylalanine levels or with PKU should avoid aspartame during pregnancy. The use of saccharine is not recommended because studies have been inconclusive about its safety.

Herbal Supplements
Herbal medicines are often referred to as herbs or botanicals. **Herbs** refer to leafy plants that do not have woody stems; **botanicals** are all parts of the plant that have medicinal value: roots, rhizomes, leaves, stems and flowers. The key concern with herbal medicine is the lack of consistent potency in the active material in any given batch of product. The reputable manufacturers try to ensure quality, purity, safety, and reliability. "Natural" does not always mean "safe."

Worldwide, more than 80% of people use botanicals as medicine. More than $3.87 billion is spent per year in

Table 8-7 Caffeine Content of Beverages and Chocolate

Food	Quantity	Caffeine (mg)
Brewed coffee	6 fl. oz.	103
Ground coffee, Folgers	1 Tbsp.	59
Instant coffee powder		
Decaffeinated	1 rd. tsp.	2
Freeze-dried	1 rd. tsp.	57
With chicory	–	37
Tea, brewed 3 min	6 fl. oz.	36
Instant	1 tsp.	30
Chocolate chips, semi-sweet	6 oz.	105
Milk chocolate, Cadbury	1 oz.	15
Cocoa mix, Carnation	1 oz.	3
Coca Cola	12 fl. oz.	46
Dr. Pepper	12 fl. oz.	41
Kick	12 fl. oz.	58
Mello Yello	12 fl. oz.	52
Mountain Dew	12 fl. oz.	55
RC Cola	12 fl. oz.	18
7-Up Gold	12 fl. oz.	46

Compiled and copyrighted by Jeanne B. Martin, PhD, RD, FADA, LD.

the United States on the herbal therapy industry, with 25% to 50% rate of growth per year. At least 73 out of 440 herbs in the *Physicians' Desk Reference (PDR) for Herbal Medicine* (Gruenwald, Brendler, and Jaenicke, 1998) are common foods or culinary herbs, such as soy, tomatoes, basil, or mint. Since the Dietary Supplement Health Education Act (DSHEA) of 1994 was passed, there has been an explosion in the number and variety of herbal medicines available. Health care practitioners should inquire which, if any, herbal supplements are consumed by their clients on a regular basis and which ones are used on an as-needed basis. Interactions among nutrients, drugs, and herbal supplements must be evaluated by the health care practitioner.

Herbal supplementation should be avoided during pregnancy and lactation because scientific studies that have been conducted have had inadequate results regarding the consequences of use during this time. Class 2 is the safety classification given to herbs that are not to be used during pregnancy and lactation, unless otherwise directed by an expert qualified in the use of the described substance, according to the American Herbal Products Association's (AHPA, 2000) Herbal Safety Rating. The *Botanical Safety Handbook* (BSH), published by AHPA, lists nearly 600 herbs and botanical products sold in the U.S. market with a relative safety rating for each herb formulation. The

BSH's rating classes for the standardization of the safety of herbal products are:

- Class 1: Herbs which, when used appropriately, can be consumed safely without specific use restrictions.
- Class 2: Herbs for which the following use restrictions apply:
  - 2a. For external use only, except under the supervision of an expert qualified in the appropriate use of this substance.
  - 2b. Not to be used during pregnancy, except under the supervision of an expert qualified in the appropriate use of this substance. No other restrictions apply, unless noted.
  - 2c. Not to be used while nursing, except under the supervision of an expert qualified in the appropriate use of this substance. No other restrictions apply, unless noted.
  - 2d. Other specific use restrictions as noted.
- Class 3: Herbs for which enough significant data exist to recommend the following labeling: "To be used only under the supervision of an expert qualified in the appropriate use of this substance." Labeling must include proper use information: dosage, contraindications, potential adverse effects, drug interactions, and any other relevant information related to the safe use of this substance.
- Class 4: Herbs for which insufficient data is available for classification.

The usual recommendation for pregnant and lactating women is not to ingest medicinal amounts of any herb because of possible harm to the fetus. Most herbal digestive aids are antispasmodic, relaxing the smooth muscle lining of the intestinal tract. If medicinal amounts are taken, uterine stimulation occurs, which may lead to contractions.

HERBAL MEDICINES

The German Federal Health Agency established scientific commissions to review various categories of drugs in 1974. Commission E was charged with reviewing herbal medicines to determine the safety and effectiveness of each (Blumenthal et al., 1998). Their monographs have recently been translated into English. These can serve as a useful tool for the health care professional to use in evaluating herbal supplements taken by clients.

MORNING SICKNESS

For treatment of motion sickness or morning sickness, if there is no history of miscarriage, the following may be tried, with the approval of the obstetrician:

A 12-ounce glass of ginger ale, provided it contains ginger and not artificial flavor, or a prescribed preparation of 500 to 2000 mg ginger, taken 30 minutes before travel. Ginger may be used in the form of capsules, ginger tea infusions, or ginger ale. For ginger tea, add 2 teaspoons of powdered or grated ginger root to one cup of boiling water. Steep 10 minutes.

Ginger has been shown to be safe in the treatment of morning sickness, at a dose of less than 1 g, but causes uterine contractions and triggers menstruation when given at a dose that is 20 times the stomach-settling dose. Women who are attempting to conceive and pregnant women may use culinary amounts of digestion-enhancing herbs, but must have the approval and supervision of their obstetrician or health care provider for any herb used medicinally.

Over-the-Counter Drugs. Drugs taken during pregnancy can cause serious congenital malformations. Potentially more than 500,000 over-the-counter drugs are on the market. Health care providers should be made aware of all such drugs taken intermittently or on a regular basis by women desiring to conceive and after conception.

The effects of these substances on the fetus include low birth weight, CNS disturbances, pulmonary hypertension, neonatal bleeding, renal failure, growth and mental retardation, inhibition of bone growth, discoloration of teeth, drug addiction, FAS, congenital malformations, spontaneous abortions, and fetal death.

Nursing Alert

MEDICATION AND PREGNANCY

Pregnant women must use extreme caution in taking or using any herb, over-the-counter or prescription drug; illicit drug; excessive amounts of caffeine; or alcohol or nicotine immediately before conception and throughout the pregnancy.

Pica. **Pica**, a psychobehavioral disorder, is the persistent ingestion of substances having little or no nutritional value or the craving for nonfood articles as food (Rainville, 1998). There are several hypotheses regarding the causes of pica. One is that a deficiency of an essential nutrient, such as calcium or iron, results in ingestion of nonfood substances that contain these nutrients. Another theory is that the behavior is based on superstitions, customs, traditions, or practices passed down through generations. Pica may indicate anemia, for which the client should be evaluated if the behavior is known to the practitioner, but it is more likely to be a consequence of family traditions.

Commonly ingested nonfood substances include dirt or clay (**geophagia**); laundry starch or cornstarch (**amylophagia**); lead paint flakes (**plumbism**); ice or ice frost (**pagophagia**); and chalk, mothballs, baking soda, coffee grounds, or cigarette ashes. Some of these items contain toxic compounds or untolerated substances. Eating these items usually displaces the intake of nutritious foods or interferes with nutrient absorption. Other potential complications vary with the items ingested and include lead poisoning, fecal impaction, parasitic infections, prematurity of the infant, and toxemia. Laundry starch and cornstarch consumption can lead to excessive intake of calories and contribute to excessive weight gain. These substances have 4 calories per gram, just as other forms of carbohydrates do. There may be contaminants in laundry starch, since it is not intended for human consumption.

When evaluating a pregnant client's dietary intake, inquiring about pica behavior is essential. The health care practitioner should always inquire about unusual nonfood cravings, even if there is no suspicion of pica. Being culturally sensitive and nonjudgmental when discussing this topic is key to obtaining information about the practices of clients. It is important to know if a woman is consuming these substances, for the safety of herself and her unborn child.

Nausea and Vomiting. Nausea is a common phenomenon during pregnancy; 60% of women experience it during the first trimester of gestation (Lenders & Henderson, 1996). The increased levels of human chorionic gonadotropin (hCG) hormone, which double every 48 hours in early pregnancy, are thought to contribute to nausea. Nausea and vomiting may also be related to hypoglycemia, decreased gastric motility, relaxation of the cardiac sphincter, or anxiety.

Heartburn. Heartburn or indigestion is caused primarily by the reflux of gastric contents up the esophagus after a large meal or upon reclining. Several physiologic changes may contribute to heartburn in pregnant women. A decrease in gastric motility, relaxation of the cardiac sphinc-

Client Education
Relieving Nausea and Vomiting

Women experiencing nausea and vomiting in early pregnancy could try a few of the following ideas:

- Eat small, low-fat meals and snacks, every 2 to 3 hours.
- Eat slowly.
- Drink soups and liquids between meals, rather than with meals, to avoid dehydration.
- Slowly sip a carbonated beverage when nauseated.
- Avoid citrus and tomato products, spearmint, peppermint, and caffeine. For some, peppermint is not nauseating and helps to alleviate nausea.
- Avoid or limit intake of spicy and high-fat foods; avoid greasy or fried foods.
- Avoid eating or drinking for 1 to 2 hours before lying down.
- Avoid aromatic foods and cooking odors that may trigger nausea.
- Avoid drinking coffee or tea.
- Inhale the scent of fresh-cut lemon to refresh the senses.
- Get plenty of fresh air and rest.
- When rising from bed or couch, get up slowly.
- Eat more pasta, bread, and potatoes.
- Eat a few bites of a soda cracker before getting out of bed in the morning.
- Take a walk after meals to help with digestion of food.
- Wear loose-fitting clothing.
- Sleep or rest with head elevated.
- Never take medicines for nausea without first consulting with a health care professional.
- Ginger capsules or herbal tea infusions help some clients with nausea. Consult a health care professional on type, quantity, and safety. Do not exceed 1 g/day.

ter, and pressure of the uterus on the stomach may contribute. The guidelines for dealing with nausea and vomiting also apply here. In addition, avoiding bending over immediately after eating may help.

Constipation and Hemorrhoids. Constipation has been associated with the smooth-muscle relaxation of the gastrointestinal tract, increased progesterone levels, and pressure of the fetus on the intestines. Other causes may include inadequate fluid and fiber intake or a decrease in physical activity. Iron supplements may also contribute to constipation. Constipation often causes gastrointestinal discomfort, a bloated feeling, exacerbated hemorrhoids, and, sometimes, decreased appetite. Strategies to combat constipation and hemorrhoids include increasing fluid intake to 2 to 3 quarts per day; eating high-fiber cereals, whole grains, legumes, fruits, and vegetables daily; and engaging in physical activity. Laxatives and herbal products with laxative effects should be used only with a physician's approval.

Mature Years

The age group that is most rapidly gaining members in the United States is elderly persons (over 65); those over age 85 are in the fastest-growing subgroup. In 1995, there were 3.6 million persons over age 85. By 2040, over 12 million people may be over age 85; and by 2050, two thirds of all Americans over age 85 may be women (Administration on Aging, 2000).

As aging occurs, the nutrients needed to maintain optimal nutritional status stay relatively high, but the caloric needs decrease because of lower levels of activity and decreased rates of metabolism. The diet of aging individuals should be nutrient-dense to obtain essential nutrients in a limited number of calories. Emphasis should be placed on consuming a diet high in fruit and vegetables, low-fat meats, fortified dairy products, and enriched and fortified high-fiber breads and cereals. Limited consumption of fats, sweets, and alcohol is advised, because these foods are high in calories but low in other essential nutrients. The older adult usually needs about 1600 calories daily. The daily calcium intake should increase to 1200 mg/day and vitamin D, to 10 µg/day for women age 50 and older.

The proportion of lean body mass decreases and relative total body fat increases during aging. Usually between ages 25 and 75, the amount of total body fat doubles. Exercise programs assist in slowing the decrease in lean body mass. If muscle decreases, a decrease in the energy requirements also occurs. The elderly client needs to keep well-hydrated by consuming at least 8 cups of water or other fluids a day, with a minimum intake of 25 mL/kg daily. As people age, there is a greater risk for dehydration. Physiologically, there is a decreased thirst perception and a decrease in the kidney's ability to concentrate water, and antidiuretic hormone (ADH) may be less effective. The elderly may decrease their fluid intake because of incontinence and may take drugs that increase their fluid loss (e.g., diuretics or laxatives). The physical symptoms of dehydration should be especially carefully monitored in the elderly.

Women should determine their nutritional health by watching for signs of poor nutrition. Anyone with three or more risk factors should consult a doctor, registered dietitian, or other health care professional. The risk factors can be remembered by the following mnemonic:

- **D**isease
- **E**ats poorly
- **T**ooth loss or mouth pain
- **E**conomic hardship
- **R**educed social contact
- **M**any medicines
- **I**nvoluntary weight loss or gain
- **N**eeds assistance in self-care
- **E**lderly, over age 80

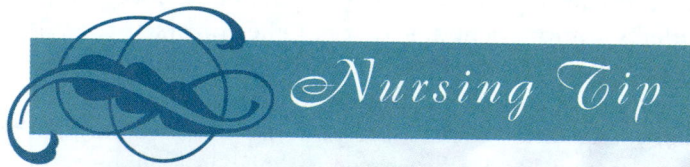

SOY FOODS AND MENOPAUSE

Soy products contain phytoestrogens, in the form of isoflavones, genistein, and daidzein. Much research has been conducted on the beneficial effects of including soy in the diet. Soy foods are commonly consumed in Asian countries. Asian women typically consume 10–100 times more isoflavones per day than Western women (Somekawa, Chiguchi, Ishibaski, & Aso, 2001) Japanese women rarely report symptoms of perimenopause, such as hot flashes, night sweats, insomnia, vaginal dryness, or headache, which are commonly reported in women from Western countries. These symptoms are believed to result from fluctuating levels of estrogen.

In menopause, the decline in estrogen production increases a woman's risk for cardiovascular disease and osteoporosis. It has been suggested that soy foods may be able to replace or enhance hormone replacement therapy (HRT), which is commonly prescribed to prevent negative health effects of menopause (Ramsey, Ross, & Fischer, 1999). Although epidemiologic studies do indicate an association between phytoestrogen intake and a decreased incidence of osteoporosis, cardiovascular disease, breast, ovarian, and endometrial cancer, and perimenopausal symptoms, research on the effect of the soy isoflavone is equivocal (Lissin & Cook, 2000; Somekawa, Chiguchi, Ishibashi, & Aso 2001; Wangen, Duncan, Merz-Demlaw, & Marcus, 2001).

NUTRITION-RELATED HEALTH CONCERNS

Nutritional status affects a woman's overall health and quality of life. Many health alterations are directly or indirectly tied to dietary practices.

Physical Activity

Physical inactivity characterizes most Americans—be they children, adolescents, adults, or elderly persons. Physical activity is defined as any bodily movement produced by skeletal muscles that requires energy expenditure and produces overall health benefits. Physical activity protects against many morbidities and possibly against mortality, especially from cardiovascular disease, high blood pressure, elevated blood lipid levels, insulin resistance, and obesity. Many factors affect an individual's ability to exercise, among them are socioeconomic status, cultural influences, age, and health status. Environments should support exercise activity—schools, work sites, health care settings, and homes.

National surveillance programs have documented that one of every four adults (more women than men) currently have sedentary lifestyles, with no leisure-time physical activity. Girls become less active than boys do as they grow older. Children become less active as they progress through adolescence. Obesity and type 2 diabetes mellitus are increasing in children. These health problems are related to the energy imbalance of overconsumption of food with inadequate amounts physical activity. A pound of body adipose tissue is equal to 3500 kilocalories. The recommended rate of weight loss is 1 to 2 pounds per week. If a 1-pound weight loss is desired over 1 week, then it would require reducing the daily caloric intake by 500 kcal/day, increasing the amount of energy spent in physical activity by 500 kcal/day or reducing the daily caloric intake by 250 kcal/day and increasing the amount of energy expended in physical activity by 250 kcal/day. If 2 pounds of weight loss per week is desired, then doubling the amount of this would be required.

Most individuals who are successful at long-term weight maintenance combine food intake monitoring with engagement in a physical activity program. Dieting alone does not have lasting positive results in weight maintenance after weight loss. With at least 12 weeks of exercise training, a beneficial rise in high-density lipoprotein (HDL) cholesterol levels has been detected. Likewise, decreases in systolic and diastolic blood pressure, improved insulin sensitivity, and a decreased incidence of osteoporosis and some cancers have been noted with increases in endurance exercise. Reduction in the symptoms of anxiety and depression and improvement in mood and feelings of well-being are seen with regular physical exercise.

The frequency, intensity, and duration of the physical activity are interrelated. The individual's preferences and what is sustainable with their unique lifestyle and circumstances best determine the appropriate type of activity. The National Institutes of Health (NIH, 1995) Consensus Statement on Physical Activity and Cardiovascular Health proposed the following guidelines for adopting and maintaining a physically active lifestyle. The client must:

- Perceive a net benefit.
- Choose an enjoyable activity.
- Feel competent doing the activity.
- Easily access the activity on a regular basis.
- Feel that the activity does not generate financial or social costs that he or she is unwilling to bear.
- Experience a minimum of negative consequences, such as injury, loss of time, negative peer pressure, and problems with self-identity.
- Be able to successfully address issues of competing time demands.

Recognizing the need to balance the use of labor-saving devices (e.g., power lawn mowers, golf carts, automobiles) and sedentary activities (e.g., watching television, use of computers) with activities that involve greater physical exertion is important to maintain good activity levels. Support for behavior change from family and friends is very helpful. Policy change and education are critical in increasing physical activity at schools and at the work place.

Obesity

Obesity is defined as a body weight that is 20% over the ideal. Obesity is increasing in the United States at an alarming rate. Many common health conditions are increasing along with overweight and obesity. Recent studies show that 50% of adults in the United States are overweight or obese: this reflects a 25% increase over the past 30 years (Mokdad, Serdula, Dietz, Bowman, Marks & Kaplan, 1999).

Excess weight has been seen in conjunction with increased rates of cardiovascular disease, type 2 diabetes mellitus, hypertension, stroke, hyperlipidemia, osteoarthritis, and some cancers. Concerted initiatives need to be undertaken to prevent and treat overweight in children and in adults, or the health care system will be more and more overwhelmed with individuals seeking treatment for obesity-related health conditions. The physical, social, environmental, and psychologic factors contributing to this malady must be assessed and addressed by a multidisciplinary health care team of doctor, nurse, psychologist, dietitian, social worker, and others.

Heart Disease

One in every ten women aged 45 to 64 has some form of cardiovascular disease. Heart disease is the number 1 cause of death in women and accounts for one-third of all

Client Education

Controlling Food Intake

Controlling food intake can be enhanced by using the following tips:

- Eat slowly; chew your food.
- Put your fork down between bites.
- Keep food intake records as food is consumed. Reflect on the amount of food consumed daily.
- Eat only in one location in your home or office, preferably at a table with no distractions.
- When it is time to eat, do only that.
- Don't overfill your plate.
- Eat off smaller plates than you usually do.
- Try doing something else if you have a food craving. Cravings usually fade after 30 minutes.

deaths. The five major risk factors for heart disease can be changed by changing diet and exercise habits. These factors are high blood cholesterol levels (over 200 mg/dL) especially high LDL cholesterol (over 160 mg/dL); high blood pressure (over 140/90 mm Hg); smoking; inactive lifestyle; and overweight or obesity. Other changeable risk factors are: low blood levels of high-density lipoprotein (HDL) cholesterol (less than 35 mg/dL), high blood level of triglycerides (over 250 mg/dL). Unchangeable risk factors for heart disease include age, sex, race, and family history. Those individuals at greater risk are:

- Elderly persons
- Women after menopause
- African American women
- Persons with close relatives who developed heart disease at an early age

Coronary heart disease (CHD) is responsible for more than 65% of cardiovascular disease (CVD). Environmental determinants, cigarette smoking, diet, and activity levels play a prominent role in CHD morbidity and mortality. General recommendations for a heart-healthy nonmedical therapeutic lifestyle, which is a combination of dietary and other lifestyle habits that reduce CHD, are as follows:

- Eat a diet with not more that 30% of calories from fat and less than 10% of calories from saturated fat.

- Limit average intake of dietary cholesterol to less than 300 mg/day.
- Reduce dietary salt intake.
- Increase intake of fruits and colored vegetables.
- Take antioxidant vitamins if recommended by your health care professional.
- Stop smoking.
- Increase physical activity; take part in regular, moderate exercise.

In addition to the above, water-soluble fiber, a component of many fruits, vegetables and grains, is more effective in lowering serum cholesterol than insoluble fibers. The soluble fibers increase fecal elimination of bile acids and cholesterol. These actions stimulate hepatic uptake of low-density lipoproteins (LDLs), thus lowering serum cholesterol. High-fiber diets also displace higher fat foods in the diet, indirectly affecting the total cholesterol intake.

Soy protein tends to lower total serum cholesterol by 12 mg/dL when 20 to 30 g/day are consumed. The phytoestrogen of importance in soy products is isoflavone. Genistein from soy inhibits smooth-muscle cell proliferation, and soy protein inhibits oxidation of LDL cholesterol. Both of these effects help reduce the risk of atherosclerosis. Genistein also inhibits platelet aggregation, interfering with clot formation, and thus, may reduce the risk for stroke and heart attack.

The FDA authorized the use of a health claim connecting the consumption of soy protein to a reduced risk of coronary heart disease on October 20, 1999. This health claim can appear on product packages of foods that contain at least 6.25 g of soy protein per serving. Soy products include soy milk, tofu, soy flour, textured vegetable protein, tempeh, soybeans, and others.

Folic acid's role in lowering homocysteine levels has already been discussed. There is a high association of high serum levels of homocysteine with CHD, because of its adverse effects on endothelial cells, abnormal clotting, and platelet adhesiveness and aggregation. Increasing intake of vegetables, legumes, and fortified grains and cereals is recommended.

There is a growing number of studies that suggest phytochemical antioxidants (e.g., vitamins C and E, carotenoids, selenium) may inhibit LDL oxidation, which decreases atherosclerosis and its clinical sequelae. Prospective studies have revealed a 77% decrease in the risk of nonfatal heart attacks with consumption of 400 to 800 IU of vitamin E in supplements over 18 months. Women have a reduction in risk with as little as 10 IU of vitamin E per day. Studies also show that people eating more fruits and vegetables containing these antioxidants have a lower rate of cancer.

Finally, garlic supplements may have significant effects on reducing total cholesterol without affecting HDL cholesterol levels. The benefits of the allium compounds contained in garlic and vegetables in the onion family are being studied extensively.

Osteoporosis

Osteoporosis is a systemic skeletal disease, characterized by decreased bone mass that results in a markedly increased risk for traumatic fractures. The consequences can include fractures, pain, and disability, which may result in loss of independence. In most cases, osteoporosis can be prevented and treated. It occurs when too much old bone is removed and not enough new bone is formed to replace it. Even as we age, bone tissue continues to renew itself: bone is a dynamic tissue undergoing constant remodeling throughout life. Some bone loss is normal during aging, but osteoporosis and the fractures it causes are not a normal part of aging. Loss of bone and the changing geometric pattern of bone contributes to a loss of bone strength. Osteoporosis is often called the "silent thief," because there are no symptoms and women often do not know they have osteoporosis until a fracture occurs.

Osteoporosis affects approximately 28 million Americans, 80% of whom are women. The loss of ovarian estrogens at menopause is accompanied by an accelerated rate of bone loss, so the incidence of osteoporosis greatly increases after menopause. Twenty percent of American women have, by the age of 65, experienced a bone fracture resulting from osteoporosis. The health care costs of fractures caused by the disease are in excess of $10 billion annually. Women are protected from rapid bone loss before menopause by estrogen, which keeps the bones strong. Postmenopausal osteoporosis begins without notice. Over time, symptoms, such as a curved spine, rounded shoulders, or loss of height as the spine compresses, may occur. Broken hips and wrists are the most common fractures.

Risk factors for osteoporosis include prolonged amenorrhea before menopause, early menopause (before age 45), excessive alcohol consumption, extremely short or tall stature, small body size (less than 127 pounds), a small body frame, and Caucasian race (Wangen, Duncan, Merz-Darlow, Xu, Marcus, Phipps, & Kurzer, 2000). Other risk factors include lack of regular weightbearing exercise or resistance; cigarette smoking; poor nutritional intake, especially minimal intake of calcium-rich foods; and high protein consumption levels. Medically, women who have had a history of fractures as an adult, use glucocorticoid medicines, and are in poor health are more likely to have osteoporosis than others. Glucocorticoid medications often are used to treat rheumatoid arthritis, lupus, and other inflammatory diseases. They decrease the bone mass with prolonged use. Women needing glucocorticoids should talk with their physician about the safest dosage. Five mg/day has a minimal effect on bone structure.

If a client develops osteoporosis, taking 1200 mg of calcium per day with 400 μg of vitamin D is the current recommended treatment. The health care provider should also assess calcium absorption (Prince, Devine, Dick, Criddle, Kern, Kent, Price, & Randall, 1995). Calcitonin, a hormone produced by the parathyroid gland, is believed to reduce the activity of the osteoclasts, the cells that remove old bone. This allows the osteoblasts to continue to create new bone tissue, and thus, an increase in bone mass is seen. Calcitonin from salmon, now available in nose sprays, has been shown to slow the rate of bone loss and increase the density or thickness of bone in women with postmenopausal osteoporosis. This treatment works best with adequate amounts of calcium and vitamin D in the diet (Table 8-2).

There have been preliminary studies showing that dietary soy protein containing isoflavones prevents bone loss when ingested in sufficient quantity (Somekawa, Chiguchi, Ishibashi, & Aso, 2001). Bone estrogen receptors are largely of the beta type, which has an affinity for genistein. This might explain why diets high in soy protein offer a protective effect against osteoporosis, as seen in Asian women. The phytoestrogens, such as isoflavone, in soy foods mimic the protective effect of circulating estrogen in premenopausal women. The bioavailability of calcium from soybeans is equal to that of milk (Table 8-6).

The following four diagnostic categories have been established for describing bone mineral density (BMD) in women (WHO, 1994):

- Normal: BMD or bone mineral content (BMC) within 1 standard deviation (SD) of the young adult mean.
- Low bone mass (osteopenia): BMD or BMC more than 1 but less than 2.5 SD below the young adult mean.
- Osteoporosis: BMD or BMC 2.5 SD or more below the young adult mean.
- Severe osteoporosis: BMD or BMC more than 2.5 SD below the young adult mean along with one or more fragility fractures.

Cancer

The World Cancer Research Fund and the American Institute for Cancer Research (AICR) published *Food, Nutrition, and the Prevention of Cancer: A Global Perspective* in 1997. The report reviewed over 4500 research studies. Their recommendations to individuals on the best ways to prevent cancer through diet and lifestyle are summarized in the following list. Sixty to 70% of all cancers can be prevented through lifestyle choices that are made every day. The AICR diet and health guidelines for cancer prevention are:

- Choose a diet rich in a variety of plant-based foods.

- Eat plenty of vegetables and fruits (at least 5 servings a day).

- Maintain a healthy weight and be physically active (BMI should be between 18.5 and 25).

- If occupational activity is low, take an hour for brisk walking or similar exercise daily and also exercise vigorously for a total of at least 1 hour per week.

- Drink alcohol in moderation, if at all. (Men, two or fewer drinks per day; women, one or less. A drink is defined as 12 oz. of regular beer, 5 oz. of wine, or 1.5 oz. of 80-proof distilled spirits.)

- Select foods low in fat and salt. (Fat consumption should be equal to 15% to 30% of total calories; salt consumption should be less than 6 g/day.)

- Prepare and store food safely. Wash, refrigerate, and freeze by food safety guidelines. Do not char food.

- Do not use tobacco in any form, i.e., smoke or chew.

There is an especially strong scientific basis for using plant-based foods, especially fruits and vegetables, to reduce the risk of developing cancers of the gastrointestinal and respiratory tracts, particularly colon and lung cancer. Fruits and vegetables are complex foods, and scientists do not know which of the nutrients or other constituents in these foods are offering the protective effect. The specific vitamins and minerals, fiber, and **phytochemicals** (plant-based chemicals), which include **carotenoids** (a group of pigments in fruits and vegetables, including alpha carotene, beta carotene, lycopene, lutein, and many other compounds), flavonoids, terpenes, sterols, indoles, and phenols, offer possibilities for investigation of their protective effects (Ames, 1999). Until more is known, the recommendation to eat five or more servings of fruit and vegetables each day should be heeded. Do not substitute vitamin pills or supplements for the real food, because it is not known which substance in the food offers the protective effect.

The role of soy foods in cancer prevention is still being elucidated. Epidemiologic studies show that populations that consume a traditional Asian diet have lower incidences of breast, prostate, and colon cancers than those consuming a traditional Western diet. The Asian diet is low in fat and animal foods and high in legumes, fruits, vegetables, and rice. Japan has a 75% lower mortality rate for breast and prostate cancers than the United States.

The compounds in soybeans, which have been identified as anticarcinogenic, include isoflavones, saponins, phytates, protease inhibitors, and phytosterols. Soy is the only significant source of isoflavone, a weak phytoestro-

gen. Isoflavones function as antiestrogens by binding the estrogen receptor (ER) in place of estrogens. Thus, cancers stimulated by estrogen are reduced. Geistein, an isoflavone in soy foods, has been found to inhibit the growth of human prostate and breast cancer cells and tyrosine kinases and, thus, block the growth and proliferation of cancer cells. It also inhibits angiogenesis, the growth of new blood vessels, and is a strong antioxidant, blocking the formation of oxygen free radicals, which are involved in cancer promotion (Ames, 1999). Soy added to the diets of premenopausal women in a recent study decreased serum levels of hormones that might regulate breast cell proliferation, but it also increased the level of prolactin, which increases breast cell proliferation. Thus, it is premature to prescribe moderate consumption of soy to prevent breast cancer. A balanced, varied diet, with soy foods as a component, is still the recommendation for the general public.

NURSING IMPLICATIONS

Women entering the childbearing years enter a phase of life in which their body undergoes many changes. The miracle of birth is unfolded with the delivery of the newborn, but forethought about good nutrition practices before conception and during the pregnancy leads to healthier newborns. The role of nutrition in the mother and infant's lives remains of utmost importance after the birth: the nurse should encourage breast-feeding for up to 6 months. Sound dietary practices learned during pregnancy and lactation can serve as guides for the rest of the mother's and the child's lives.

Women who are past the years of fertility have similar recommended nutrient allowances. Because of a slightly decreased level of recommended calories, the B vitamins also decrease proportionately in relation to calorie intake. Because of the cessation of menses, iron losses are minimized; therefore, the recommendations for iron intake also decrease. The older woman should select nutrient-dense foods to maximize intake of essential nutrients, while slightly reducing caloric consumption. The Food Guide Pyramid is a useful tool to nutritionally guide the aging woman. By adhering to sound nutritional intakes in adolescence, young adulthood, pregnancy, lactation, and adulthood, the woman of today can enter her golden years with an adequate store of nutrients to avoid debilitating disorders.

Many times the nurse has the best opportunity to discuss nutritional issues with clients. To effectively counsel clients about nutritional changes, the nurse must be aware of nutritional needs and be able to assess for nutritional risks of deficiency or excess. In nutritional counseling, the entire family must be considered, as most meals are prepared for the entire family rather than for individual members. Women are crucial in nutritional counseling because they generally make all the food choices as they shop, plan menus, cook, and serve the family's food. Eating patterns are infused with cultural beliefs and practices, and these practices are passed on from generation to generation. Eating patterns are also heavily influenced by social networks and activities. For example, teenagers are likely to adopt eating patterns of their peers rather than their family. However, as adults they will revert back to family eating patterns. The availability of food and economic resources are also important in a family's dietary decision making. All of these factors illustrate the complexity of nutritional patterns and the consequent difficulty of instigating dietary changes.

Nurses can follow the nursing process, beginning with an assessment that includes a 24-hour recall of dietary intake, validation of whether this is a typical eating pattern, and assessment of resources for getting and preparing foods. Cultural beliefs and eating patterns should also be assessed. These data should be analyzed for nutritional adequacy. Interventions may consist of connecting the family with available resources for acquisition of food or nutritional services. Providing the family with information about healthier eating behaviors is an important intervention. However, interventions to alter a family's dietary choices

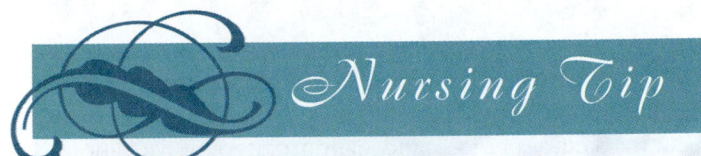

MODEL FOR READINESS FOR CHANGE

Health professionals should keep in mind the stage of readiness for changes their client is in before overwhelming her with dietary recommendations. Prochaska, Norcross, and DiClemente in *Changing for Good* (1994), identifie five stages that individuals must go through before making behavior changes. Dietary change is definitely a behavioral change. Consider each step outlined below in assessing what stage your client is in before asking her to change too many behaviors at once. Success will be slower, perhaps, but more enduring, if change is addressed when the client is ready to make the behavioral modification required to adhere to new dietary plans. Remember to encourage a few small, slow changes at a time and give a lot of reinforcement and positive support (Prochaska, Norcross, & DiClemente, 1994).

The stages of change are as follows:

1. Precontemplation: Before the client has thought about the behavior change. There is no intention to change behavior in the next 6 months. (Example: The client does not consider consuming dairy foods.)

2. Contemplation: The client is "thinking" about making a behavior change, or intending to change, but not too soon. (Example: The client is thinking about purchasing low-fat milk and yogurt to consume daily and is discussing this with her family.)

3. Preparation: The client is preparing to implement the behavior change within the next month. (Example: Foods are being bought, recipes modified, and plans made to adjust to the new recommendations.)

4. Action: The client begins implementing the behavior change. (Example: The client purchases low-fat milk and vanilla yogurt regularly, for at least the past 6 months. The client includes three servings each day from the dairy group in her meal plan. She consumes the servings in their entirety.)

5. Maintenance: The client maintains the new behavioral change for at least 6 months and, hopefully, indefinitely. (Example: The client consumes at least three servings from the milk group daily or eats other foods containing a high level of calcium.)

Client Education

Resources for Food Programs

If clients have difficulty managing their food budget to meet food costs, refer them to a registered dietitian or social worker who can assist them. There are several federal nutrition programs designed to improve the nutritional status of pregnant and lactating women, their infants, and children up to age 5. The Special Supplemental Food Program for Women, Infants, and Children (WIC) certifies individuals meeting the current federal guidelines to be at nutritional risk and living on a household income of 185% or less of the federal poverty level income. Other supplemental nutrition programs may also be available for the client, such as food stamps and the Cooperative Extension—Expanded Food and Nutrition Education Program (EFNEP). These are for lower-income individuals who need to enhance their access to adequate nutrition and receive sound nutrition education.

and methods of food preparation involve more than providing information. The Readiness for Change Model is helpful in working with families over time to promote healthy dietary choices and eating patterns. Evaluation of interventions is necessary and should be undertaken for referrals to community agencies and educational interventions and should be incorporated into an ongoing engagement with the family.

Web Activities

- Visit the U.S. Department of Agriculture website. Use it to plan a daily menu for a: (a) 15-year-old girl; (b) pregnant 31-year-old woman; (c) 65-year-old woman.

- Visit the National Dairy Council home page. Do they outline calcium needs for pregnancy and lactation? What foods do they recommend as the best sources for calcium?

Key Concepts

- A woman's overall health throughout the life span is greatly affected by her nutrition and lifestyle choices.

- Adolescents need to strive for a balanced diet while keeping consumption of junk foods to a minimum.

- Eating disorders are most prevalent in the adolescent years and stem from an unhealthy, distorted body image.

- Women of all ages should work toward a target weight for their height and body type.

- Balancing intake of necessary nutrients and taking a vitamin supplement as prescribed by a health care provider are important steps in maintaining a healthy pregnancy.

- As a woman ages, the nutrient needs to maintain optimal nutritional status stay relatively high but the caloric needs decrease as a result of lower activity level and decreased metabolic rates.

- Many diseases, such as heart disease, osteoporosis, and cancer, are linked to suboptimal nutrition.

Review Questions and Activities

1. Record all the food that you eat for 24 hours.
   a. Analyze it and compare it to the recommended daily intakes for your age group.
   b. Calculate your body mass index (BMI).
   c. Make nutritional recommendations for yourself based on the above data.

2. Design a healthy diet for an Asian woman who is pregnant.

3. On your next trip to the grocery store, check labels and identify 15 popular foods that have over 10 grams of fat per serving. Note the serving size on the label.

References

Blumenthal, M., Busse, W. R. Goldberg, A., Gruenwald, J., Hall, T., Riggins, C. W., & Rister, R. S. (Klein, S., & Rister, R. S., trans.). (1998). *The complete commission E monographs: Therapeutic guide to herbal medicines. (English Translation)*. Austin, TX: American Botanical Council; Boston: Integrative Medicine Communications.

Cunningham, F. G., MacDonald, P. C. Gant, N. F., Leveno, K. J., Gilsap, L. C., Hankins, G. DV., and Clark, S. L. (1997) *Williams Obstetrics* 20 ed. Stanford, CT: Appleton & Lange.

Dietary Supplement Health and Education Act of 1994. (Public Law 103-417), October 25, 1994.

Food and Nutrition Board, National Academy of Sciences, Institute of Medicine. (1997). *Dietary reference intakes, 1997*. Washington, DC: National Academy Press.

Food and Nutrition Board, National Academy of Sciences, Institute of Medicine. (1997). *Dietary reference intake for calcium, phosphorous, magnesium, vitamin D, and fluoride*. The Standing Committee on the Scientific Evaluation of Dietary Reference Intakes. Washington, DC: National Academy Press.

Food and Nutrition Board, National Academy of Sciences, Institute of Medicine. (1998). *Dietary reference intakes; thiamin, riboflavin, niacin, vitamin B6, folate, vitamin B12, pan-*

tothenic acid, biotin, and choline. Washington, DC: National Academy Press.

Food and Nutrition Board, National Academy of Sciences, Institute of Medicine. (2000). *Dietary reference intakes for vitamin C, vitamin E, selenium, and carotenoids.* Washington, DC: National Academy Press.

Food and Nutrition Board, National Academy of Sciences, National Research Council. (1989). *Recommended dietary allowances, revised 1989,* 10th Ed. Washington, DC: National Academy Press.

Frisch N. C. & Frisch L. E. (1998). *Psychiatric mental health nursing.* Albany: NY Delmar.

Gerhard, G. T., Malinow, M. R., DeLoughery, T. G., Evans, A. J., Sexton, G., Connor, S. L., Wander, R. C., & Connor, W. E. (1999) Higher total homocysteine concentrations and lower folate concentrations in premenopausal Black women than in premenopausal white women. *Am J Clin Nutr,* 70, 252–260.

Giannini, J. A., Newman, J., & Gold, M. (1990). Anorexia and bulimia. *American Family Physician,* 41, 169–176.

Gruenwald, J., Brendler, T. & Jaenicke, C. (1998). *The physicians's desk reference for herbal medicines.* Montvale: Medical Economics Company.

Institute of Medicine. (1992). *Nutrition during pregnancy and lactation: An implementation guide.* Washington, DC: National Academy Press.

Kaplan H. I., & Sadock B. J. (1998). *Synopsis of psychiatry Baltimore:* Williams & Wilkins.

Lewis, C. J., Crane, N. T., Wilson, D. B., & Yetley, E. A. (1999). Estimated folate intakes: Data updated to reflect food fortification, increased bioavailability, and dietary supplement use. *Am J Clin Nutr,* 70, 198–207.

Lission L. W., & Cook, J. B. (2000). Phytoestrogens and cardiovascular health. *Journal by the American College of Cardiology* 35, (6), 1403–1410.

Locksmith, G. J., & Duff, P. (1998). Preventing neural tube defects: the importance of periconceptional folic acid supplements. *Obstetrics & Gynecology,* 91, 1027–1034.

McGriffin, M., Hobbs, C., Upton, R., & Goldberg, A. (Eds.) (1997). *American Herbal Product Association's botanical safety handbook: Guidelines for the safe use and labeling for herbs of commerce.* Baco Raton, FL: CRC Press.

Mattson, S. N., Riley, E. P., Gramling, L., Delis, D. C., & Jones, K. L. (1997). Heavy prenatal alcohol exposure with or without physical features of fetal alcohol syndrome leads to IQ deficts. *J Pediatrics,* 131,718–721.

Mills, J. L., McPartlin, J. M., Kirke, P. N., Lee, Y. J., Conley, M. R., Weir, D. G., & Scott, J. M. (1995). Homocysteine metabolism in pregnancies complicated by neural-tube defects. *Lancet* 345, 149–151.

Mokdad, A. H., Serdula, M. K., Dietz, W. H., Bowman, B. A., Marks, J. S., & Koplan, J. P. (1999). The spread of the obesity epidemic in the U.S., 1991–1998. *JAMA* 282, 1519–1522.

Morrison, G., Hark, L. (1996). *Medical nutrition and disease.* Cambridge, MA: Blackwell Science.

National Institutes of Health, Office of the Director (1995). *NIH consensus statement: Physical activity and cardiovascular health,* Vol. 13, No. 3. December 18–20.

Prince, R., Devine, A., Dick, I., Criddle, A., Kerr, D., Kent, N., Price, R., & Randell, A. (1995). The effects of calcium supplementation (milk powder or tablets) and exercise on bone density in postmenopausal women. *J Bone Miner Res,* 10, 1068–1075.

Prochaska, J. O., Norcross, J. C., & DiClemente, C. C. (1994). *Changing for good.* New York: Avon.

Rainville, A. J. (1998). Pica practices of pregnant women are associated with lower maternal hemoglobin level at delivery. *J Am Diet Assoc,* 98, 293–296.

Townsend, C. E. and Roth, R. A. (1999) Nutrition and Diet Therapy. Albany, NY: Delmar Pub.

U.S. Departments of Agriculture & Department of Health and Human Services. (1992). *The food guide pyramid.* Home and Garden Bulletin No. 252.

United States Department of Agriculture (2000). 2000 Guidelines for Americans. (5th ed.) Washington DC: U.S. Government.

Wangen, K. E., Duncan, A. M., Merz-Demlow, B. E., Xu, X., Marcus, R., Phipps, W. R., & Kurzer, M. S. (2000). Effects of soy isoflavones on markers of bone turnover in premenopausal and postmenopausal women. *Journal of Clinical Endocrinology & Metabolism* 85, (9), 3043–3048.

World Cancer Research Fund and American Institute for Cancer Research. (1997). *Food, nutrition, and the prevention of cancer: A global perspective.* Washington, DC: American Institute for Cancer Research.

World Health Organization. (1994). *Assessment of fracture risk and its application to screening for postmenopausal osteoporsis. WHO technical report series 843.* Geneva Switzerland: World Health Organization.

Suggested Readings

Administration on Aging. (2001). *Aging into the 21st Century.* Washington, D.C.: U.S. Bureau of Census.

Allen, K. M., & Phillips, J. M. (1997). *Women's health across the life span: A comprehensive perspective.* Philadelphia: Lippincott-Raven.

American Cancer Society. (1996). *Cancer facts and figures.* New York: NY ACS.

American Dietetic Association & American Diabetes Association. (1989). *Ethical and regional food practices: A series. Mexican American food practices, customs, and holidays.* Chicago: American Dietetic Association.

American Dietetic Association & American Diabetes Association. (1995). *Ethical and regional food practices: A series. Soul and traditional Southern food practices, customs, and holidays.* Chicago: American Dietetic Association.

Ames, B. N. (1999). Micronutrient deficiencies: A major cause of DNA damage in cancer prevention. Novel nutrient and pharmaceutical developments. (Bradlow, H. L., Fishman, J., and Osborn, M. P., Eds.). *Annals of the New York Academy of Sciences,* 899, 87–107.

Anliker, J., Damron, D., Ballesteros, M., Langenberg, P., Havas, S., Mettger, W., & Feldman, R. (1999). Using the stages of change model in a 5-a-day guidebook for WIC. *J Nutr Educ,* 31, 175A–176A.

Bailey, L. B. (1998). Dietary reference intakes for folate: The debut of dietary folate equivalents. *Nutr Reviews,* 56, 294–299.

Blumenthal, M., & Riggins, C. W. (1997). *Popular herbs in the U.S. market. Therapeutic monographs.* Austin, TX: American Botanical Council.

Brown, J. E. (1999). *Nutrition now. 2nd Ed.* Belmont: West/ Wadsworth.

Castleman, M. (1995). *The healing herbs: The ultimate guide to the curative power of nature's medicines.* New York: Bantam.

Chernoff, R. (1991). *Geriatric nutrition: The health professional's handbook.* Gaithersburg: Aspen.

Chitwood, M. Botanical therapies for diabetes: On the cutting edge. *Diabetes Care and Education,* Winter, 1–20.

Cuskelly, G. J., McNulty, H., & Scott J. M. (1999). Fortification with low amounts of folic acid makes a significant difference in folate status in young women: Implications for the prevention of neural tube defects. *Am J Clin Nutr,* 70, 234–239.

Davidow, J. (1999). *Infusions of healing: A treasury of Mexican-American herbal remedies.* New York: Fireside.

Dudek, S. G., (1997). *Nutrition handbook for nursing practice.* Philadelphia PA: Lippincott-Raven.

Duyff, R. L. (1996). *The American Dietetic Association's complete food & nutrition guide.* Minneapolis: Chronimed.

Finn, S. C. (1997). *The American Dietetic Association guide to women's nutrition for healthy living.* New York: Berkley.

Farnsworth, N. R. Akerele, Bengel A., Asaurta, D. P., Eno, Z. (1985). *Medical plants in therapy.* Bull World Health Organization 63, (6), 965–981.

Food and Drug Administration. (1993). *FDA Consumer* Special Issue. FDA (1999). The Food Label FDA Background, May 1999.

Foster, S., & Tyler, V. E. (1999). *Tyler's bones herbal: A sensible guide to the use of herbal and related remedies,* 4th Ed. New York: Haworth Press.

Gerber, J. M. (1993). *Handbook of preventive and therapeutic nutrition.* Gaithersburg: Aspen.

Greene, G. W., Rossi, S. R., Rossi, J. S., Velicer, W. F., Fava, I. L., & Prochaska, J. O. (1999). Dietary applications of the stages of change model. *J Am Diet Assoc,* 99: 673–678.

Hagen, P. T. (1997). *Mayo health quest: Guide to self-care.* Rochester, MN: Mayo Clinic.

Jacobson, M. S., Rees, J. M., Golden, N. H., & Irwin, E. (Eds.) (1997). *Adolescent nutritional disorders: Prevention and treatment. Annals of the New York Academy of Sciences,* 817.

(AMA, 1999). Patient page: Benefits and dangers of alcohol. *JAMA,* 281, (1) 104.

Kleiner, S. M. (1999). Water: An essential but overlooked nutrient. *J Am Diet Assoc,* 99, 200–206.

Kristal, A. R., Glanz, K., Curry, S. J., & Patterson, R. E. (1999). How can stages of change be best used in dietary interventions? *J Am Diet Assoc,* 99, 679–684.

Krummel, D. A., & Kris-Etherton, P. M. (1996). *Nutrition in women's health.* Gaithersburg: Aspen.

Landis, R. (1997). *Herbal defense: Positioning yourself to triumph over illness and aging.* New York, NY: Warner.

Lenders, C. M., & Henderson, S. A. (1996) Nutrition in pregnancy and Lactation. In G. Morrison & L. Hark (Eds.). *Medical Nutrition and disease.* Cambridge MA: Blackwell Science.

McMann, M. C. (1999). *Taking control: Women and health. A primer on women's health.* Houston: Women's Fund for Health Education and Research.

Morgan, S. L., & Weinsier, R. L. (1998). *Fundamentals of clinical nutrition,* 2nd Ed. St. Louis, Missouri: Mosby.

Must, A., Spadano, J., Coakley, E. H., Field, A., Colditz, G., & Dietz, W. H. (1999). The disease burden associated with overweight and obesity. *JAMA,* 282, 1523–1529.

Nagell, K., & Jones, K. (1993). Eating disorders: Prevention through education. *J of Home Econ,* 85, 55–56.

Nutrient Data Laboratory. (2001). Recommended dietary intakes. http://www.nal.usda.gov/fnig. Accessed 3-16-01.

Ody, P. (1993). *The complete medicinal herbal.* New York, NY: DK.

Oldways Preservation & Exchange Trust. (1996). *Healthy traditional Latin American diet pyramid.* Cambridge, MA: Oldways Preservation & Exchange Trust.

Oldways Preservation & Exchange Trust. (1995). *The traditional healthy Asian diet pyramid.* Cambridge, MA: Oldways Preservation & Exchange Trust.

Oldways Preservation & Exchange Trust. (1994). *The traditional healthy Mediterranean diet pyramid.* Cambridge, MA: Oldways Preservation & Exchange Trust.

Pennington, J. A. T. (1998). *Bowes and Church's food values of portions commonly used,* 17th Ed. Philadelphia, PA: Lippincott.

Pfeiffer, C. M., Rogers, L. M., Bailey, L. B., Gregory, III, J. F. (1997). Absorption of folate from fortified cereal-grain products and supplemental folate consumed with or without food determined by using a dual-label stable-isotope protocol. *Am J Clin Nutr,* 66, 1388–1397.

Poppy, J. (Ed.) (1999). *The essential woman's health guide 2000.* San Francisco, CA: Time.

(1999). Position of the American Dietetic Association and Dieticians of Canada: Woman's health and nutrition. *J Am Diet Assoc,* 99, 738–751.

Ramsey, L. A., Ross, B. S., & Fischer, K. G. (1999). Phytoestrogens and management of menopause. *Advanced Nurse Practitioner,* 7, (5), 26–30.

Pronsky, Z. M. *Food medication interactions,* 11th ed. (2000). Birchrunville: Food-Medication Interactions.

Rakowski, W. (1996). The transtheoretical model of behavior change: Applications to clinical practice. *Mind/Body Medicine,* 1, 207–220.

Rossi, S. R., Rossi, J. S., Rossi-DelPrete, L. M., Prochaska, J. O., Banspach, S. W., & Carleton, R. A. (1994). A process of change model for weight control for participants in community-based weight loss programs. *Int J Addict,* 29, 161–177.

Sandmaier, M. (Revised, July 1997). *Healthy heart handbook for women.* U.S. Department of Health and Human Services, Public Health Service, National Institutes of Health, National Heart, Lung and Blood Institute, Office of Prevention, Education and Control. NIH Publication No. 97-2720.

Sarubin, A. (2000). *The health professional's guide to popular dietary supplements.* American Dietetic Association.

Scholl, T. O., Hediger, M. L., Schall, J. I., Khoo, C. S., & Fischer, R. L. (1996a). Dietary and serum folate: Their influence on the outcome of pregnancy. *Am J Clin Nutr,* 63, 520–525.

Shils, M. E., Olson, J. A., Shike, M., & Ross, A. C. (Eds.) (1999). *Modern nutrition in health and disease,* 9th Ed. Baltimore, MD: Lippincott/Williams & Wilkins.

Sigman-Grant, M. (1996). Stages of change: A framework for nutrition interventions. *Nutr Today,* 31, 162–170.

Somekawa, Y., Chiguchi, M., Ishibashi, T., & Aso, T. (2001). Soy intake related to menopause symptoms, serum lipids, and bone mineral density post menopausal Japanese women. *Obstetrics & Gynecology,* 97, (1), 109–115.

Suitor, C. W. (1997). *Maternal weight gain: A report of an expert work group.* Arlington, VA: National Center for Education in Maternal and Child Health.

Suitor, C. W., & Bailey, L. B. (2000). Dietary folate equivalents: Interpretation and application. *J Am Diet Assoc, 100,* 88–94.

Tamura, T. (1997). Bioavailability of folic acid in fortified food. *Am J Clin Nutr, 66,* 1299–1300.

Tyler, V. E. (1993). *The honest herbal: A sensible guide to the use of herbs and related remedies.* New York, NY: Haworth Press.

United States releases health goals for 2010. (2000). *Epimonitor, 21,* 1, 3.

Van Way, III, C. W. (1999). *Nutrition secrets.* Philadelphia: Hanley and Belfus.

Wiederman, M. W., & Pryor, T. (1996). Substance use and impulsive behaviors among adolescents with eating disorders. *Behaviors, 21,* 269–272.

Wildman, R. E. C., & Medeiros, D. M. (2000). *Advanced human nutrition.* Boca Raton, FL: CRC Press.

Wilkening, V. L. (1993). FDA's regulations to implement the NLEA. *Nutrition Today,* September/October, 13–20.

Wolinsky, I., & Klimis-Tavantzis, D. (Eds.) (1996). *Nutritional concerns of women.* Boca Raton, FL: CRC Press.

Yanovski, J. A., & Yanovski, S. Z. (1999). Recent advances in basic obesity research. *JAMA, 282,* 1504–1506.

Resources

www.cfsan.fda.gov/~dms/supplmnt.html
U.S. Food & Drug Administration Center for Food Safety & Applied Nutrition provides voluntary dietary supplement adverse event reporting, and product information, such as labeling, claims, package inserts, and accompanying literature, www.nnfa.org/quality/(July, 1999).

National Nutritional Foods Association's (NNFA) principal voice on issues of, research, technology and quality in the health foods industry, the Science and Quality Assurance Department also serves as an information resource on scientific issues, www.health.gov/dietsupp

The Commission on Dietary Supplement Labels—established by Congress in the Dietary Supplement Health and Education Act of 1994 and appointed by President Clinton, www.ificinfo.health.org

The International Food Information Council Foundation (IFIC). IFIC's purpose is to bridge the gap between science and communications by collecting and disseminating scientific information on food safety, nutrition and health, www.nal.usda.gov/fnic/etext/fnic.html

Food and Nutrition Information Center. Food and nutrition topics listed alphabetically. Great web site for clients, www.healthfinder.gov

Healthfinder. Useful website for clients to conduct searches for specific health conditions, health news, and useful health resources. Also available in Spanish, www.hedc.org

The world-renowned Harvard Eating Disorders Center conducts research, mentors developing scientists, and expands knowledge about eating disorders, their detection, treatment, and prevention, www.anad.org

National Association of Anorexia Nervosa and Associated Disorders (ANAD) is the oldest national non-profit organization helping eating disorder victims and their families. In addition to its free hotline counseling, ANAD operates an international network of support groups for sufferers and families, and offers referrals to health care professionals who treat eating disorders, across the U.S. and in fifteen other countries, www.health.org

SAMHSA's National Clearinghouse for Alcohol and Drug Information. SAMHSA is the Federal agency charged with improving the quality and availability of prevention, treatment, and rehabilitative services in order to reduce illness, death, disability, and cost to society resulting from substance abuse and mental illnesses, www.alcoholics-anonymous.org

Alcoholics Anonymous is a fellowship of men and women who share their experience, strength, and hope with each other that they may solve their common problem and help others to recover from alcoholism. Resource for practitioners and clients, www.americanheart.org

The official website for the American Heart Association. Useful to practitioners and clients, www.nhlbi.nih.gov

Division of the Department of Health and Human Services: The National Heart, Blood, and Lung Institute. Offers basic health information as well as clinical guidelines, www.eatright.org

American Dietetic Association—Your Link to Nutrition and Health! Offers food tips and dietitian services, www.usda.gov/fcs/cnpp.htm

Food, Nutrition, and Consumer Services FNCS) ensures access to nutritious, healthful diets for all Americans. Through food assistance and nutrition education for consumers, FNCS encourages consumers to make healthful food choices, www.medscape.com/

Medscape offers daily news and updates concerning health and medicine. Easy search option beneficial to clients, www.merck.com

Home medical reference book online, www.cancer.org

Cancer Resource Center provided by the American Cancer Society. Answers to questions about the nature of cancer, its causes, and risk factors, www.diabetes.org

Everything you need to know, from nutrition to exercise to who's at risk for diabetes presented by the American Diabetes Association, www.cdc.gov

Official site for the Centers for Disease Control and Prevention (CDC). CDC serves as the national focus for developing and applying disease prevention and control, environmental health, and health promotion and education activities designed to improve the health of the people of the United States, www.fda.gov

U.S. Department of Health and Human Services, Food and Drug Administration (FDA). News, drug updates, and search options.

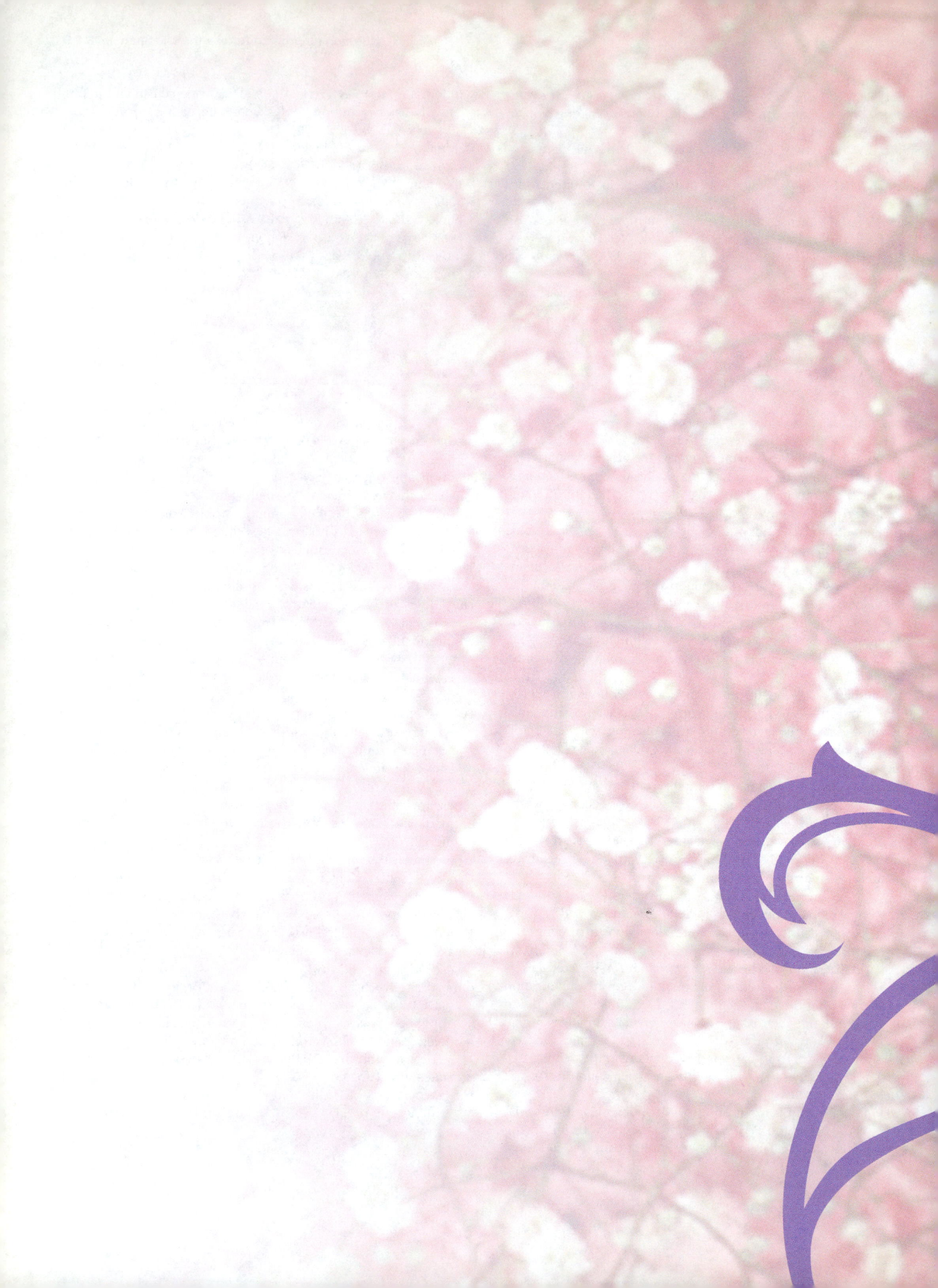

CHAPTER 9

Health Care Issues for Women Across the Life Span

A more comprehensive view of women's health has recently emerged, which includes not only reproductive health conditions but also other health conditions that affect women over the life span. These health conditions include those that affect both men and women, such as cardiovascular disease, although these diseases may affect women differently than men. Use the following questions to examine your personal feelings.

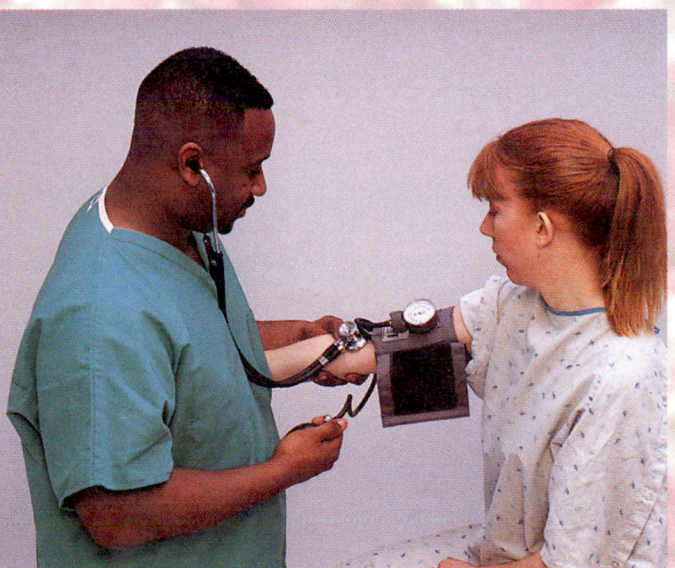

- *Are women my age likely to live longer than men?*

- *Are women likely to be healthier in later years than men?*

- *Is there anything wrong with women taking drugs for which efficacy was based on research that included only male subjects?*

- *Are more women apt to die from breast cancer or heart disease?*

- *Am I doing all I can to help women reduce their risk of breast cancer, lung cancer, heart disease, and HIV infection?*

Key Terms

Birth rate	Fertility rate	Life expectancy	Osteoporosis
Carcinoma in situ	Health promotion	Morbidity	Race
Culture	Invasive cancer	Mortality	Screening
Ethnic group			

Competencies

Upon completion of this chapter, the reader should be able to:

1. Discuss the historical perspective of women's health in the U.S.
2. Describe demographic data for American women.
3. Describe the leading causes of death (mortality) and disease (morbidity) in women from childhood to old age.
4. Discuss the factors that put women at an increased risk of death and disease over the life span and describe methods of health promotion, disease prevention, and screening.

omen's health care has become a priority in the United States in the last two decades. This is evidenced by consumer activism and major commitment by governmental agencies, research institutions, and service delivery systems to redefine women's health care, expand the research focus on women's health issues, and implement expanded prevention and intervention programs. Historically, women's health care involved reproductive conditions and diseases of the reproductive system only. Now, women's health involves not only reproductive conditions and issues but also diseases or conditions unique to, more prevalent in, or more serious among women or some subgroups of women as well as diseases or conditions for which the factors or interventions are different for women than for men. Women with different ethnic, cultural, and religious backgrounds have different health beliefs and behaviors that affect their overall health status. Health-seeking behaviors, compliance, prevention and health promotion behaviors, risk factors, and the incidence and prevalence of both gynecologic and nongynecologic diseases also differ among the various groups.

HISTORICAL PERSPECTIVE OF WOMEN'S HEALTH

Until recently, there was no such entity as women's health care. Women received care as adults who happened to have additional health conditions relating to childbearing

and diseases of the reproductive system. This care relied primarily on a disease model in which diagnosis and treatment of reproductive health problems were the focus. Little attention was given to prevention, health promotion, risk factors, and nonreproductive health conditions of women across the life span, including the years before or after the reproductive years. For nongynecologic issues, females received care according to the male disease model. The male disease model used information obtained from teaching, research, and clinical trials that were based on diagnosis, treatment, and outcomes reported from studies on males.

History of Reproductive Health Care in the U.S.

Historically, women's health care revolved around reproduction. Women's gynecologic health care was focused on women of reproductive age and postmenopausal age, involving primarily birth control, pregnancy, delivery, infertility, and diseases of the reproductive system.

Over the centuries, midwives provided most reproductive care. This represented the model of care in most civilizations, in which women, who through experience and handed-down knowledge, cared for the women in their community during pregnancy and childbirth. In the United States, midwifery was a respected profession until the mid-1800s. At about that time, the profession of medicine became better organized, and care of pregnant women became the province of physicians, most of whom were men. Physicians considered midwives ignorant and unskilled because they received no formal education. In the late 1800s and early 1900s, the medical community, in many states, convinced public health authorities that midwifery should be abandoned. The medical profession blamed immigrant midwives for the high maternal and infant mortality rate of the immigrant population. This was not justifiable, because new immigrants had no or limited access to medical care and were living in extremely unhealthy environments. In reality, the high maternal and infant mortality rate was the result of unsanitary housing, water, food, and living conditions, not inadequate care by midwives (Wertz & Wertz, 1977).

The medical profession's rejection of midwifery denied poor women access to reproductive health care. Women had little political influence on health policy and legislation. The decrease in the influence of midwifery occurred at approximately the same time that the movement towards women's suffrage began. Unfortunately, the suffrage movement did not address the health needs of the poor or immigrant women. One outcome of the suffrage movement was that women began to move into the occupations of social work, nursing, and education but not medicine. Midwifery did not become an academic discipline. The study of medicine incorporated the role of reproductive health care. As a result, reproductive health care became the domain of the male-dominated medical profession, with little input from women in society, women as patients, or female physicians.

In the early 20th century, medical schools began to emphasize the basic sciences as prerequisites for admission, making it difficult for women to enter the medical profession. Women were not encouraged to take science prerequisites in high school or college and were discouraged from entering medical school. As a result, women did not enter the profession of medicine in any great numbers until the late 1970s. It was not until the 1990s that women entered medical school in about the same proportion as men. Concurrent with the increase in enrollment of women in medical schools was the demand for an expanded concept of women's health, a resurgence of the profession of midwifery, expansion of the role of nursing, and support for advanced practice nurses to provide primary health care. In addition, many individuals, groups, and organizations were effective in increasing the focus of the scientific community on women's health. Some of these included the National Women's Health Network, the Society for the Advancement of Women's Health Research, and the Boston Women's Health Book Collective. All these factors helped fuel the demand to address women's health care separately from men's.

Today, women's health care is provided by a broad array of health disciplines, including nursing, medicine, public health, social work, and midwifery. While preventive health care has been viewed as important to the overall health and welfare of society for the past 30 years, little focus has been on women's preventive health care issues. Health care providers have intuitively understood the value of prevention and health promotion but implementation of effective services for women has lagged. It is known that many health problems can be prevented or postponed by immunizations, accident prevention, healthier lifestyles, or detected earlier through screening leading to early treatment. Women's health problems are different than men's and must be addressed appropriately in prevention, early detection, and treatment.

Some reasons for inadequate preventive health care include lack of health care provider time, inadequate reimbursement, lack of provider interest and knowledge, lack of client involvement and knowledge, and lack of delivery systems to promote preventive care (U.S. Department of Health and Human Services [DHHS], 1994).

Current View of Women's Health Care

A newer view of women's health includes not only the reproductive years, but also the years before and after, including the nonreproductive health conditions that occur over the life span. The foundation for the physical and emotional health of adult women occurs in childhood, during which gender differences in diet, exercise, values, and roles have an impact on the biologic and psychological development of women. Diet and exercise affect bone density, growth, and body image in later life. Values and roles affect health-seeking behaviors, economic status, prevention behaviors, nutrition and exercise habits, fertility rates, and potential for domestic abuse. **Fertility rate** is defined as the number of births per 1,000 women, ages 15 to 44. Educational experience affects socioeconomic status, self-esteem, and access to care. Given a normal life expectancy, one-third of a woman's life is lived after menopause. **Life expectancy** is defined as the average number of years for which a group of individuals of the same age are expected to live. Health status after menopause is affected not only by the previous biologic factors but also by psychological development, sociocultural environment, and economic status. Many reproductive and gynecologic issues are intrinsically related to biologic factors. Social Roles, economic level, race, culture, psychological development, and religious beliefs also affect biologic factors. **Race** is a system of classifying people into groups according to physical features, such as skin color, facial features, and texture of body hair. **Culture** is defined as an individual's way of looking at life, encompassing their feelings, beliefs, attitudes, and practices, which in turn affect how the individual views such things as health, nutrition, and health policies.

Women's health encompasses conditions that are not specific to the reproduction system, including those found in both men and women, but which may be expressed differently in women. Some diseases, such as osteoporosis, occur more frequently in women than in men. Some diseases, such as HIV infection, historically occurred more frequently in men, but manifest differently in women; some diseases, such as heart disease, occur commonly in both genders but manifest differently in women (Cohen, 1997).

Generally, women's health care providers have been physicians with training in internal medicine, cardiology, obstetrics and gynecology, family practice or another specialty, who used the male disease model. More recently, a recognition of the effects of biology, genetics, culture, economic level, gender roles, education, and psychological development on women's health status has caused a major shift in the scope of women's health, including research methods, health care delivery systems, prevention, early identification of disease and training of nurses, physicians, and other health care workers (Magrane & McIntyre-Seltman, 1996). The Office on Women's Health, a part of the U.S. Public Health Service, has outlined a strategic plan to develop educational programs to expand the education and training of health care workers to incorporate this new approach to women's health (Blumenthal, 1994).

Sensitivity to gender issues, racial and cultural backgrounds, sexual orientations, personality types, marital status, economic status, patterns of risk-taking behaviors, genetic and environmental risk factors, and age are now considered essential to providing comprehensive health care to women. A newer approach to women's health includes health promotion and health protection throughout the life span (Foster, 1994). Health promotion includes consideration of adequate nutrition intake, development and maintenance of physical fitness, development and use of stress management skills, attainment and maintenance of optimal bone density, and avoidance of hazardous substances, including tobacco, alcohol, and drugs (Figure 9-1). Health protection includes provision of safe childbearing through adequate prenatal and postnatal care, safe delivery, and effective family planning for child spacing and desired family size; it also includes prevention, early diagnosis, and appropriate treatment for infections, cancer, cardiovascular and respiratory disease, diabetes, and other chronic illnesses (Foster).

Sociocultural Influences

Women's health concerns reflect the diversity of women's cultural, economic, and physical environments, which affect the duration and quality of life. Unfortunately, women continue to experience serious threats to their physical and mental well-being. Despite living an average of 6 years longer than men, women have poorer health and

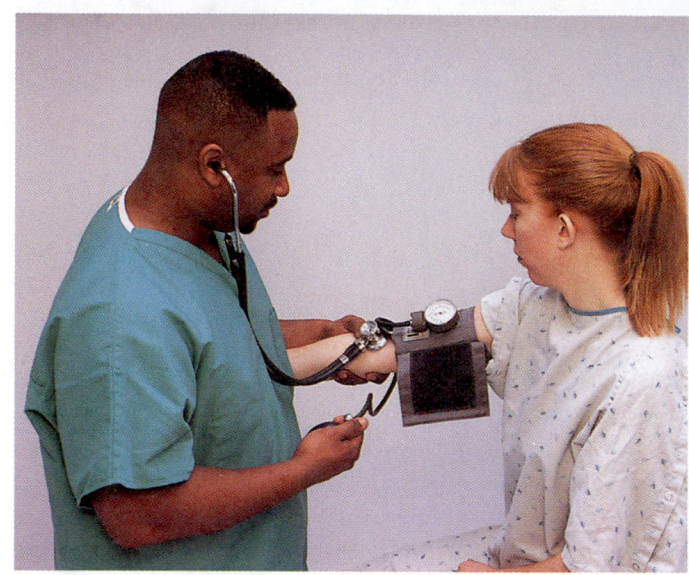

Figure 9-1 Health promotion for women of all ages includes regular physical exams.

greater disability from disease than men (U.S. Bureau of the Census, 1998). Some factors that may account for women's poorer health relate to the fact that women are frequently victims of poverty, experience unequal access to care, and receive less income for similar work than men. Women who live in poverty and are poorly educated have shorter life spans, higher rates of illness and death, and more limited access to health care services. The majority of single heads of households in the U.S. are women, putting them at a greater risk for poverty. Also, more women live in poverty than men. Women participate in the work force in greater numbers than ever before. Women have less ability to pay for health care, even though they use health care services more frequently than men. Women, in general, have greater problems obtaining access to primary health care. Overall, women have a poorer quality of life and have more acute symptoms, chronic conditions, and disabilities from health problems than do men (Wentz, 1994).

A positive factor influencing women's health care is the growing number of women who are developing political power and consumer interest in changing national policy regarding women's health. Women have become more involved in promoting reproductive choices, which give them control over their bodies and life choices. The availability of the birth control pill in the 1960s gave women the power to make their own choices about when to have children, spacing children, number of children, and combining a career with motherhood. Today, more women are demanding participation in health care decisions on an individual level and in health care policy at local, state, and national levels.

Women's Health as a National Priority

There has been considerable interest in reproductive women's health issues as a result of recent public awareness of advances in scientific knowledge and technology. A number of factors in the last two to three decades have caused major changes in the scope of women's health care. Political, social, and cultural influences have contributed to the emergence of a new perspective toward the study of women's needs. In the 70s and 80s, women entered the work force in record numbers and became more active in politics and policy making. Women became more visible in the public and economic life of the nation. Employers began to pay more attention to the economic and social consequences of women's health care. Women in medicine and other health care professions became more vocal and influential in health care policy development and implementation. As a result, women demanded a change in their medical care.

National Response to Women's Health Issues

In the last 20 years, a variety of federal agencies responded to the national concern that women's health issues were not being adequately addressed. The first major effort was the establishment of the Public Health Service Task Force in 1983 to study women's health issues. In 1985, this task force recommended that biomedical and behavioral research should be expanded to focus on conditions and diseases unique to or more prevalent in women in all age groups (Women's Health Report of the Public Health Task Force on Women's Health Issues, 1985). In 1986, the National Institute of Health (NIH) established a policy to encourage inclusion of women in clinical trials. The major reason women were previously excluded was the potential risk to the fetus if the woman became pregnant while participating in a study or unknown risks for subsequent pregnancies. In 1989, members of the U.S. Congress requested the General Accounting Office (GAO) to investigate NIH to determine whether women were being included in clinical trials as dictated by policy. The GAO found that women continued to be excluded from large scale studies. Examples included the U.S. Physicians Health Study, the Health Professionals Follow-Up Study (Hennekens, 1989), and the Multiple Risk Factor Intervention Trials (MRFIT, 1990). In 1990, the GAO reported to Congress that NIH had made little progress in implementing its policy to encourage the inclusion of women in research. Even when women were included in research, gender analysis was not completed (Wentz, 1994). The publication of the GAO report caused considerable reaction in the popular media, women's groups, and Congress.

In 1990, NIH created the Office of Research on Women's Health (ORWH) in reaction to the public reaction to the GAO findings. The ORWH was established to strengthen and enhance the prevention, diagnosis, and treatment of illness in women and to enhance research related to diseases and conditions that affect women. The mission of ORWH was to:

- Ensure that women's health issues were addressed
- Ensure appropriate participation of women in clinical research
- Increase the number of women scientists in biomedical research and their decision-making authority
- Oversee and coordinate all activities related to women's health including delivery of services, education, and public policy in national and regional offices of the U.S. Public Health Service

Agencies affected by this policy included NIH Centers for Disease Control and Prevention CDC, Food and Drug Administration (FDA), Health Resources and Service Administration, Indian Health Service, Substance Abuse and Mental Health Services Administration (SAMHSA), and Agency for Health Care Policy and Research (ACPR).

The year 1991 was pivotal in the scientific, political, and public arenas for women's health. In 1991, Dr. Bernadine Healy became the first woman director of NIH. Under her leadership, a research agenda was established to include women and minorities in adequate numbers in research and to address the diseases and disorders that affect women. A new policy was issued requiring inclusion of women and minorities in research unless there were scientifically sound reasons for exclusion. To encourage the inclusion of women and minorities in research, factors such as child care and transportation for women subjects were to be addressed in all research.

In 1992, at the request of Congress, the GAO issued a report regarding the FDA's policy of excluding and restricting women of childbearing age from participating in drug studies. The GAO report concluded that gender-related differences in response do exist for some drugs and that drug trials must include sufficient members of women to permit analysis of these gender-related differences (U.S. General Accounting Office [GAO], 1992). In 1993, Congress passed the NIH Revitalization Act, which mandated the inclusion of women in NIH-funded clinical trials. It did not require studies of enormous populations, but rather that analysis by gender occur or sample sizes of statistical significance be chosen when the existence of gender differences is unknown. In 1993, the FDA lifted its ban on the inclusion of women in clinical trials (FDA, 1993).

In 1992, the NIH undertook the Women's Health Initiative, which is a 15-year study of major diseases and conditions, including heart disease, stroke, breast cancer, colon and rectal cancer, depression, and osteoporosis, in a sample of 160,000 postmenopausal women at 45 centers across the country. This is the largest clinical study ever undertaken in the U.S., with $625 million appropriated for the initiative. The Women's Health Initiative includes three major types of study:

- Surveillance study to identify specific risk factors for disease

- Clinical trial, involving 45,000 individuals, to study the role of diet modification and hormone replacement therapy in the prevention of cardiovascular diseases, cancer, and osteoporosis

- Prevention study, carried out in 60 communities, to determine effective methods for incorporation of health-promoting behaviors

The Women's Health Initiative provided recognition that women have many nonreproductive years of life, during which they are at great risk for cardiovascular disease, cancer, osteoporosis, and depression. This is the first major study that recognized that heart disease is the leading cause of death for women and that heart disease develops later in life in women than men. The study's premise is that understanding the role of risk factors for cancer, osteoporosis, and cardiovascular disease will provide future treatment recommendations for the care of women who are postmenopausal (National Institutes of Health [NIH], 1994).

In 1993, ORWH was given an expanded mission and mandate. Their mission included the following:

- Coordinating and implementing of the National Breast Cancer Action Plan

- Establishing links between research institutions and service organizations in communities throughout the nation

- Promoting healthy behavior in young women

- Improving the health of minority women

- Preventing domestic violence

- Providing greater access to health services

- Fostering research and education by innovative methods

- Instituting strategies to recruit and promote women in science and health care careers

In 1996, ORWH convened a series of meetings to address women's health for the 21st century. This resulted in the recommendations of the 1997–1998 Task Force for Beyond Hunt Valley, Research on Women's Health for the 21st Century, to determine the most fruitful and useful directions for medical research conducted by NIH. Current research of importance for women includes the following:

Neuroscience and Brain Biology

- Development and degeneration of neurons

- Therapeutic effects of St. John's wort

- Nature of pain

- Behavioral research on obesity, substance abuse, and nicotine addiction

- Development of new drugs for treatment of alcoholism and drug addiction

- Project on molecular anatomy of the brain

Cardiovascular Disease

- Role of hypertension in accelerating vascular disease

- Role of plaque in atherosclerosis and mechanism of formation

- Role of genes in progression and experience of disease of the heart and blood vessels

Asthma

- Prevalence of asthma in women, particularly Hispanic women

- Prevention of environmentally induced asthma in children

Infectious Diseases

- Search for novel approaches to treatment of infectious disease

- Work on genome of the HIV virus

Diabetes

- Role of nutrition and obesity in development diabetes

- Efforts to regenerate insulin-producing cells

- Enhanced methods of drug delivery

- Cause of various types of diabetes

Outreach to Special Populations

- Health promotion for cardiovascular health among Hispanics

- Treatment of hypertension and dyslipidemia for African Americans

- Inducements to increase participation of women and underrepresented minorities in research

Themes revealed in the task force findings and scientific reports include the following:

- Women's health is expanding into the larger concept of gender-specific medicine; it is no longer considered a feminist issue or isolated phenomenon. Studies of women are important sources of new information, which will help to convert male models of normal function and pathophysiology of disease to accommodate women's needs.

- Women have changing needs over the course of the life span. Research must take into consideration the biologic life cycles and the physical, mental, and emotional changes that occur over the life cycle.

- Multidisciplinary research is essential.

- Social and behavioral science is essential in research on women's health.

- Collection of first-hand information on women is essential to correct male models of normal function and the pathology of disease.

One outcome of the increased interest in and emphasis on women's health was the emergence of a broader concept of women's health. It incorporates cellular, systemic, individual, and societal prospectives. Rather than perceiving women's health narrowly as reproductive health, the current model integrates basic and social sciences that describes the health of women across the life span from birth to old age and considers other factors, such as ethnicity, race, culture, and religion. This integrated approach use the biochemical, physiologic, social, behavioral, and environmental sciences to develop and integrate an effective approach to women's health.

DEMOGRAPHIC DATA FOR AMERICAN WOMEN

The overall health of both men and women has improved in the 20th century. Life expectancy has increased for both genders, with life expectancy of women exceeding that of men. A century ago, many women died during their reproductive years from complications of childbearing and infections. Early deaths in men also resulted from infections, but fewer men died of infection than women because of infections from complications of childbirth. Advancements in maternity care, antibiotic therapy, public sanitation, and biomedicine have been major factors in increasing the life expectancy of women. It is estimated that, in the next century, the life expectancy for both genders will continue to increase (Table 9-1). Longevity will result from technological advances and more effective prevention and treatment of acute and chronic disease. In addition, the intensity of research on the biology of aging, including the study of the cellular aging process, may increase life expectancy in the future. As women live longer, chronic conditions that affect older women will be more prevalent. Health care providers and delivery systems must be prepared for the increased numbers of women needing preventive and restorative care in the future.

Life Expectancy

Life expectancy has increased for both males and females. Life expectancy is defined as the average number of years for which a group of individuals of the same age are expected to live. It is derived from summary measures of mortality and is calculated from age-specific death rates for a population at a particular time (Harper & Lambert, 1994). Even though men and women have different causes of death overall, women outlive men by an average of 5.7 years, based on 1998 mortality data (Table 9-2). Women born in 1900 had a life expectancy of 48 years, approximately 2 years longer than men. In 1998, women had a life expectancy of 79.5 years, whereas all men had a life expectancy of 73.8 years (U.S. Bureau of the Census [USBC], 1998).

African Americans had a lower life expectancy than Caucasians, with African American women having a life expectancy of 74.8 years and African American men 67.6 years in 1998. Caucasian women continue to have the highest life expectancy (79.5 years), followed by African American women (74.8 years), Caucasian men (74.5 years), and African American men (67.6 years). In general, the Caucasian population is expected to outlive the African American population born in the same year by an average of 6.0 years (USBC, 1998). Currently, women make up 51% of the total U.S. population. More than 60% of the population over age 65 are women, and more than 70% of the population over age 85 are women. (USBC, 1996).

Table 9-1 Projections of Life Expectancy, for People Born 2000–2010

Year	Caucasian (yrs) Female	Male	African American (yrs) Female	Male	All Other Races (yrs) Female	Male
2000	80.5	74.2	74.7	64.6	77.5	68.3
2005	81.0	74.7	75.0	64.5	78.1	69.1
2010	81.6	75.5	75.5	65.1	78.7	69.9

Adapted from Table No. 118, Statistical Abstract of the United States, 1996.

Table 9-2 Life Expectancy: in Years, by Race, Sex, and Age, 1998

Age	All Races Female	All Races Male	Caucasian Female	Caucasian Male	African American Female	African American Male
At Birth	79.5	73.8	80.0	74.5	74.8	67.6
10	70.2	64.6	70.6	65.2	66.6	59.0
20	60.3	55.0	60.8	55.5	56.2	49.5
30	50.6	45.7	51.0	46.1	46.7	40.6
40	41.1	36.4	41.4	36.8	37.5	31.9
50	31.8	27.6	32.0	27.9	28.8	23.9
60	23.2	19.6	23.3	19.7	21.0	17.1
70	15.5	12.8	15.6	12.8	14.1	11.5
80	9.2	7.5	9.1	7.5	8.7	7.1
85 & over	6.7	5.5	6.6	5.4	6.6	5.5

Adapted from Table No. 5, National Vital Statistics Report, Vol 48, No 11, July 24, 2000.

Race and Ethnicity

Ethnic and racial diversity has varied over time in the United States. In the early 1990s, approximately 84% of the women living in the United States were Caucasian, 13% were African American, 8% were Hispanic, and 3% were of other races. Projections indicate a continuing change in racial diversity over time, with increases in African American and Hispanic populations. The National Center for Health Statistics (NCHS, 1992) reported that the number of babies born to Hispanic women reached record highs; births to Hispanic women comprised 18% of the total births across the nation in 1995. This increase in births is the result of high fertility rates among Hispanics, particularly recent immigrants. The increased Hispanic birth rate contrasts with birth rates of other groups that have been stable or have declined (NCHS, 1998). **Birth rate** is defined as the number of births per 1,000 population.

Also, there were sharp increases in births among Hispanic teenage girls from 1989 to 1995. There were 106.7 births per 1,000 Hispanic teenage girls in 1995, compared to 100.8 in 1989. In the same period, the birth rate among African American teenage girls dropped from 84.8 births per 1,000 to 74.5. However, Hispanic teenage girls who give birth are more likely to be married than African American teenage girls are (NCHS, 1998).

Population Shift

As the baby boom generation (persons born between 1946 and 1964) reaches age 65, there will be major economic and sociologic changes, resulting in increased demands for health care, fewer workers to support the Medicare program, a large aging population, and an increased interest in healthy living. A major proportion of this generation will be made up of women, who will live longer than men but not necessarily healthier. Women significantly outnumber men in the over-age-65 group because premature deaths are almost twice as high for men in earlier decades than for women. Men die in earlier years as a result of motor vehicle accidents, homicides, suicides, heart attacks, and AIDS (CDC, 2000). This results in a higher age-adjusted mortality rate for males than females. This trend has been observed throughout the 20th century and results in approximately 70% of persons over age 85 being women. (USBC, 1999). The major shift in the population is the increasing number of elderly women.

Employment

Historically, there have always been more men than women in the labor force. This trend continued throughout the 1990s. However, in the last several decades, more women are participating in the labor force than ever before in the history of the United States. In 1962, 43% of women, aged 25 to 54, were in the labor force and 55% were keeping house full-time. In 1990, 75% of women, aged 25 to 54, were in the labor force; 20% were keeping house full-time (DiMona & Herndon, 1994). This represents an increase of 32% of working women.

Men earn more than women, even when men and women work in the same occupations. Women earn between 60% and 80% of what men in comparable positions earn, regardless of race and ethnicity, although this gap appears to be closing in some areas. On average, men who have completed high school earned $28,742 compared with $17,898 for women who have completed high school. The same disparity exists at all levels of education for women. African American and Hispanic women earn less than Caucasian, African American, and Hispanic men.

A portion of that improvement in women's income is the result of the downward trend in men's income (Tauber, 1992). Even when women have a higher level of education, the earning gap is not overcome. However, both men and women are less likely to experience poverty if they are educated. Level of employment and earning power are closely correlated with level of education. Poverty is strongly correlated with a low level of education.

Education

The more education, the better the health status, for both men and women. Educational attainment is defined as the highest grade or degree completed. Education has an important influence on socioeconomic status. The overall trend in the U.S. reflects a more educated population, with the younger population being more educated than the older population (USCB, 1999). In 1999, 83% of all adults, aged 25 or older, had completed at least high school and 25% had at least a bachelor's degree (USBC, 1999). Men and women had the same rate of high school completion (83%). Men had a slightly higher rate of completion of a bachelor's or higher degree, with 27.5% of men and 23.1% of women earning these degrees (USBC, 1999). The percentages of high school completion vary by race. Among Caucasians, 87.7% had earned high school degrees or higher; among African Americans, 77.4%; among non–Hispanic Asian and Pacific Islanders, 84.7%, and among Hispanics, 56.1% (USBC, 1999). At high school, some college, and college graduate levels, the Hispanic population had the lowest proportion of completed education in comparison to all other races. The Hispanic population increased the proportion of the population aged 25 and over with a high school diploma or higher degree by about 5% from 1989 to 1999, and the proportion who had some college increased about 6% during that time. However, the proportion with a bachelor's degree or higher did not change significantly (USBC, 1999). There were fewer foreign born persons with a high school diploma than U.S. citizens, but interestingly, the percentage of these with a bachelor's degree was approximately the same. Of particular importance, the incidence of foreign-born Hispanics with less than a high school education was almost twice that of Hispanics born in the U.S. (56% of foreign-born Hispanics versus 30% U.S. born Hispanic). (USBC, 1999)

Since 1970, there has been a steady increase in the number of women who have completed college. In 1970, 8.1% of women completed college compared to 19.3% in 1993. However there is great variation among racial groups. In 1993, Asian women were most likely to be college-educated, with 27% had college educations in comparison to 12.4% African American women and 8.5% Hispanic women. In 1995, 18.3% of the population did *not* have a high-school degree, 33.9% had graduated from high school,

17.6% had some college but no degree, 7.1% had an associate degree, 15.2% had a bachelor's degree, and 7.8% had a graduate degree. Slightly more females than males are high-school graduates (35.7% females versus 31.9% males). However, there is great disparity on the basis of race for those not completing high school, with 46.6% of Hispanic persons, 26.2% of African Americans, and 24.6% of other races who have not completed high school compared with 17% of Caucasians (USBC, 1996). Educational attainment is higher for employed persons then unemployed persons. Ninety percent of employed persons have completed high school or a higher level (USBC, 1999).

Since education is positively associated with health status, persons who have not completed at least high school are at higher risk for poor health. Lower levels of education are seen in conjunction with poorer nutrition, decreased access to health care, and increased likelihood of risk behaviors, such as smoking.

Marital Status

Both men and women are marrying later in life. They are delaying marriage from the early 20s to late 20s or 30s. In 1993, 30% of women ages 25–29 had never married, compared with only 11% in 1990 (Tauber, 1992). In conjunction with the trend of later marriages, both married and unmarried women are having children later. In 1950, the marriage rate was 11.1 per 1,000 population as compared to 9.9 in 1999 (USDHHS, 2000). As the marriage rate has decreased, the divorce rate has increased from 2.6 per 1,000 in 1950 to 4.1 in 1999 (USDHHS, 2000).

Fertility and Birth Rates

The fertility rates of women in the U.S. have declined from 87.9 per 1,000 women in 1970 to 65.9 per 1,000 in 1999 (National Vital Statistics Reports, 2000). The overall birth rate has decreased from 24.1 in 1950 to 14.5 in 1999 (USDHHS, 2000).

Trends in childbearing differ among women of various ages and are reflected in age-specific birth rates. Women are having children later in life than before. There has been an increase in the birth rate for women aged 30 to 34, from 61.9 per 1,000 in 1980 to 85.4 per 1,000 in 1997, and in women aged 35 to 39 years, from 19.8 per 1,000 in 1980 to 31.7 per 1,000 in 1990 (USBC, 1999). Clearly there has been a trend toward more women giving birth later, when they are in their thirties and forties. Some reasons for this are:

- Ability to control the timing of childbearing through the use of contraception
- Starting careers before having children
- Later marriages
- Development of technology to enhance fertility

The Fertility, Family Planning and Women's Health: New Data From the 1995 National Survey of Family Growth (Abma, Chandra, Mosher, Peterson, 1997) reported that 89.3% of all women aged 15 to 44 had been sexually active. Older women were more likely to be sexually active than younger women. Of the women interviewed, 22.1% were sexually active at age 15, 38% at age 15, 51.1% at age 17, 65.4% at age 18, and 75.5% at age 19. Of women aged 20 to 24, 88.6% were sexually active; of those aged 25 to 29, 95.9%; of those aged 30 to 44, 98.2% (Abma et al, 1997). In the ages 15 to 19 range, African American women were most sexually active (59.5%), followed by Hispanic women (55%), then Caucasian women (49.5%). Mean age at first intercourse for women who were ages 20 to 24 years at the time of the survey was 17.5; for women ages 30 to 34, 17.8; for women ages 35 to 39, 18; and for women ages 40 to 44, 18.6 (USHHSS, 2000). This demonstrates that women are having first intercourse at a younger age and that availability of education about sex, family planning, and prevention of sexually transmitted diseases (STD) is essential for teenagers before their first sexual experience to prevent unplanned pregnancy and STDs.

Birth Rates for Adolescent Mothers

Birth rates for adolescent mothers rose from 1980 to a high in 1992 and dropped from 1992 to 1997. The birth rate for adolescents ages 15 to 17 in 1980 was 32.5 per 1,000; in 1992 was 37.8; and in 1997 was 32.6 (USBC, 1999). The birth rate for adolescents ages 18 to 19 was 82.1 per 1,000 in 1980, 94.5 in 1992, and 84.4 in 1999 (USBC, 1999).

The Centers for Disease Control and Prevention (CDC) reported in 1997 that there had been a decrease in sexual intercourse by teenagers from 1990 to 1995. About 50% of teenagers ages 15 to 19 reported that they had ever had sexual intercourse in 1995 compared with 55% in 1990. This is consistent with the downward trend in the birth rate for teen mothers between 1990 and 1999.

The 1995 National Survey of Family Growth found that 55% of Hispanic, 49.5% of Caucasian, and 59.5% of African American women aged 15 to 19 years had had sexual intercourse. As women age from 15 to 24, sexual intercourse increases (Abma, Chandra, Mosher, Peterson, & Piccinino, 1997):

The percentage of women reporting sexual intercourse for each age are as follows:

- 22.1% at age 15
- 38.0% at age 16
- 51.1% at age 17
- 65.4% at age 18
- 75.5% at age 19
- 88.6% at ages 20 to 24

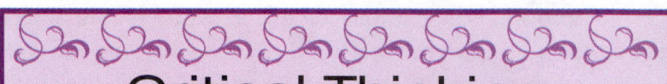

Critical Thinking

Sexually Active Adolescents

You may feel anxious about asking adolescents if they are sexually active. Before you can help an adolescent make good decisions about prevention of STDs or pregnancy, you need to know what your beliefs and feelings are about sex. What are your beliefs about sex before marriage, sexual activity by adolescents, abstinence from sex, and the role of family, spirituality, and religion in dealing with sexuality? Working through your feelings will reduce your reluctance to discuss sexual experiences with adolescents. Some activities you can do to reduce your reservation or anxiety include:

- Learn current teen slang and lay terms
- Practice asking questions with a friend or family member
- Do some extra readings on the topic, attend a seminar on sexuality
- Talk to an experienced nurse practitioner or other nurse
- Learn how other professionals ask questions and how they approach their clients

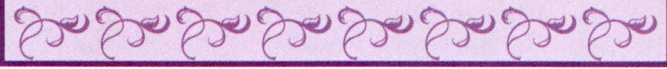

Birth Rates for Unmarried Women

Births to unmarried women in the U.S. have dramatically increased, from a total of 399,000 in 1970 to 1,260,000 in 1996 (USCB, 1999). Births to unmarried adolescents under age 15 increased from approximately 10,000 in 1970 to 12,000 in 1994, then decreased to 10,000 in 1996. Births to unmarried adolescents ages 15 to 19 increased from 190,000 in 1970 to a high of 381,000 in 1994, and then decreased to 373,000 in 1996. There has been a dramatic increase in the number of births to women age 20 and older. This is because of the increase in the proportion of women in the population over age 20. In 1970, women over age 20 accounted for 199,000 births, while in 1993, they accounted for 872,000 births. In 1970, 50.2% of all births were to women age 19 or under, in 1993 only 29.7% of all births were to women age 19 or under. The birth rate for Caucasian unmarried women has increased from 43.9% of women in 1970 to 59.8% in 1993. In contrast, the birth rate for African American unmarried women has decreased from 54% in 1970 to 36.5% in 1993 (USBC, 1996).

Unmarried mothers and their children are of concern. Statistically, they are at greater risk for poverty, limited education, poor health, and social problems, such as dropping out of school, behavior problems, and delinquency. Unmarried women under age 25 are at greater risk than their married counterparts as a result of living below the poverty line, not completing high school, having poorer health, and less access to care.

MORTALITY AND MORBIDITY

One way to measure the health of the nation or subgroups within the population is to examine mortality and morbidity data. **Mortality rate** refers to the total number of deaths in a population over a specific period of time. **Morbidity rate** refers to the total number of persons in a population who currently have a specific disease or condition.

Leading Causes of Death

The leading causes of death for both men and women in the U.S. according to the U.S. Bureau of the Census (1999) are:

- Heart disease
- Malignant neoplasms (cancer)
- Cerebrovascular diseases (stroke)
- Chronic obstructive pulmonary disease (COPD)
- Accidents
- Pneumonia and influenza
- Diabetes mellitus
- Suicide
- Nephritis, nephrotic syndrome, and nephrosis
- Chronic liver disease and cirrhosis

The two leading causes of death in women, cardiovascular disease and cancer, occur in women at different ages and in different ways than in men. Women tend to be protected from cardiovascular disease until menopause. Cancer mortality incidence and prevalence for women differ from men and varies over the lifespan.

Of these diseases, more men than women die from heart disease, cancer, COPD, accidents, suicide, and chronic liver disease. More women die from cerebrovascular disease, pneumonia, diabetes, and nephritis (USBC, 1999). For both men and women, with all ages combined, heart disease is the leading cause of death, regardless of race. Cancer is the second leading cause of death for men and women, and stroke is the third. Together, heart disease, cancer, and stroke account for two-thirds of all deaths for both sexes (Table 9-3)

Table 9-3 Leading Causes of Deaths for Females and Males, 1998

Cause of Death	Deaths Per 100,000 Population		
	Both Sexes	Female	Male
All causes	864.7	853.5	876.4
Heart disease	268.2	268.3	268.0
Cancer	200.3	189.7	213.6
Stroke	58.6	70.4	46.3
COPD	41.7	40.2	43.2
Accidents	36.2	25.2	47.7
Pneumonia	34.0	36.8	31.0
Diabetes	24.0	25.4	22.4
Suicide	11.3	(NA)	18.6
Nephritis	9.7	9.9	(NA)
Chronic liver disease	9.3	(NA)	12.4

Adapted from Table No. 8, National Vital Statistics Report, Vol. No. 11, July 24, 2000.

Cardiovascular Disease

Cardiovascular disease is the leading cause of death for both men and women in the United States. Approximately one of every two female deaths in the U.S. results from cardiovascular diseases. Forty-nine percent of women die within 1 year of a heart attack compared with 31% of men. This may be because cardiovascular disease presents differently in women than in men and is not recognized by health care providers when an emergency situation occurs. Even though there has been a major reduction in the number of deaths from heart disease in the United States, heart disease remains the major overall health problem facing women today.

Even though cardiovascular disease is the leading cause of death for both sexes, there has been a decrease in deaths from cardiovascular disease in the past three decades. Deaths caused by cardiovascular disease have dropped dramatically since 1970, from 496.4 deaths per 100,000 population to 268.2 in 1998 for both sexes (USDHHS, 2000). In 1998, 370,962 women died of heart disease compared with 353,897 men (DHHSKDCP, 2000). There are more than three times more deaths from heart disease than from breast and lung cancer combined.

The prevalence of heart disease increases as women age. The increased risk for cardiovascular disease in women may be the result of the decrease in estrogen at menopause. The prevalence increases to one in three at age 65 and older. Cardiovascular disease typically develops in women 10 to 15 years later than in men. The risk of coronary artery disease for younger women is less than for men the same age, but as women age, mortality from heart disease increases. By age 75, the incidence of heart disease is essentially the same in both sexes. The prevalence of heart disease varies by race and ethnicity. For both men and women, African Americans have a higher death rate (317/100,000) from cardiovascular disease than Caucasians (285/100,000). Caucasian women have a higher death rate (286.8/100,000) than African American women (224.6/100,000) (DHHSCDCP, 2000).

Most treatment of cardiovascular disease in women is based on the male disease model, since the majority of cardiovascular studies have been conducted predominantly or exclusively on middle-aged men. In the past, women have not been included in studies for several reasons, including potential risks to a developing fetus and the potential for other medical conditions and diseases that would confound study design. As a result, information regarding prevention, screening, diagnosis, treatment, and prognosis for cardiovascular disease in women have been based on the male disease model, even though there are major differences in disease expression and mortality between the sexes.

There has been pervasive inattention by both health care providers and women themselves to the importance of cardiovascular disease in women. Women tend to fear having a heart attack less than having breast cancer. Women who have heart attacks are twice as likely as men to die because they lack access to appropriate medical care, are less aware of symptoms that could be related to cardiovascular disease, and are not provided with appropriate medical interventions. A recent study showed that women, minorities, and elderly clients experiencing a heart attack are less likely than middle-aged Caucasian men to receive potent clot-busting drugs and other advanced procedures to restore blood flow during a heart at-

tack. Women also were found to be less likely than men to undergo bypass surgery and angioplasty (Wong, Froelicher, Bacchetti, Burron, Gee, Selly, Lundstrom, Swain, and Truman, 1997).

Stroke is the third leading cause of death for women. It kills more than twice as many women annually as breast cancer. Three percent of strokes occur in women, and 61% of stroke deaths are women. Stroke and heart disease cause almost twice as many deaths in women than all types of cancer combined (DHHS, 2000).

Cancer

Cancer is uncontrolled growth or spread of abnormal cells, resulting from malfunction of genes that control cell growth and cell division (American Cancer Society [ACS], 2000). The majority of cancerous diseases result from gene mutation; heredity accounts for only for 5% to 10% of cancers (ACS, 2000). Cancer is the second leading cause of death for both men and women living in the United States (ACS, 2000). One of every four deaths results from cancer, with more than 1,500 cancer deaths occurring each day (ACS, 2000). However, when specific age groups are considered, cancer is the leading cause of death in women ages 25 to 64 but not in men. For all types of cancer combined, cancer incidence rates decreased an average of 0.7% per year from 1990 to 1995 in contrast to an increasing trend in earlier years (Wingo, 1998). From 1990 to 1996, cancer incidence decreased for Caucasians by 1.2% per year, Hispanics by 1.7% per year, Native American by 0.7% per year, and remained stable for Asian or Pacific Islanders and African Americans (ACS, 2000).

Mortality and morbidity rates vary according to gender (Figure 9-2).

Among the ten leading cancers, a similar reversal in trends was apparent for lung, prostate, colorectal, bladder, and blood cells cancers. Breast cancer rates increased significantly from 1973 to 1990 but were level from 1990 to 1995. Death rates for the four major cancers (lung, breast, prostate, and colorectal) decreased significantly from 1990 to 1995 (Wingo, Ries, Rosenberg, Miller, & Edwards, 1998). The decline in mortality rates was greater in men than women, largely because of the decrease in male lung cancer rates. There were greater decreases in rates in young males than in older males and greater decreases in African Americans than in Caucasians, although mortality rates remain higher in African Americans (ACS, 1998). As people get older, their cancer risk increases. Americans aged 55 and older receive nearly 80% of all cancer diagnoses (ACS, 2000) (Figure 9-3). Some inroads in prevention and health promotion have been made, which reduces mortality rates. Some of these include reduction in tobacco use, diet modification, cancer screening procedures, and progress in treatment based on research (Wingo, 1998).

Nursing Tip

PREVENTING CARDIOVASCULAR DISEASE

- Quit smoking
- Follow a low-fat, low-cholesterol diet
- Exercise at least three times per week
- Maintain a normal body weight
- Have periodic blood pressure checks
- Consider hormone replacement therapy at menopause

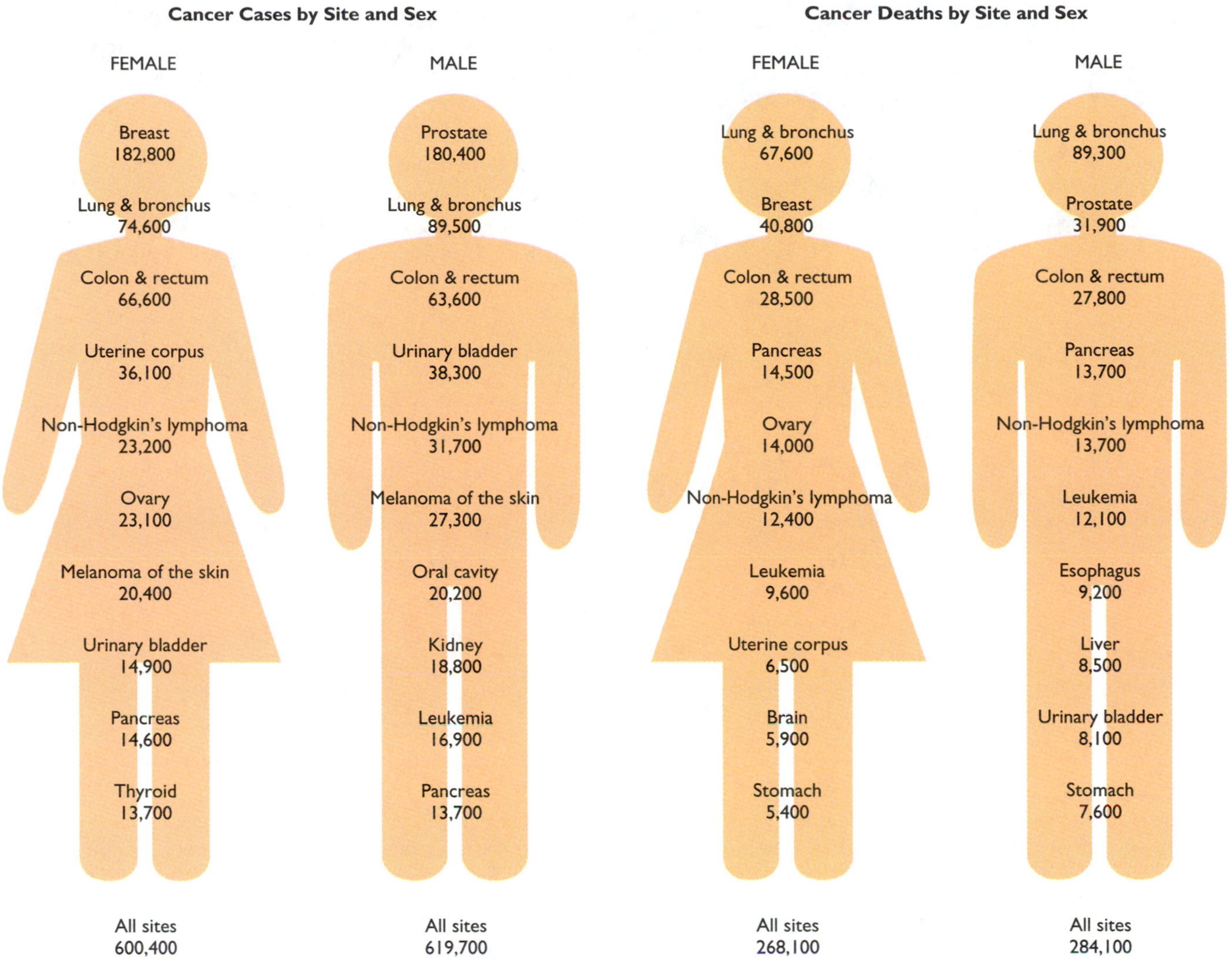

Cancer Cases by Site and Sex

FEMALE

Breast
182,800

Lung & bronchus
74,600

Colon & rectum
66,600

Uterine corpus
36,100

Non-Hodgkin's lymphoma
23,200

Ovary
23,100

Melanoma of the skin
20,400

Urinary bladder
14,900

Pancreas
14,600

Thyroid
13,700

All sites
600,400

MALE

Prostate
180,400

Lung & bronchus
89,500

Colon & rectum
63,600

Urinary bladder
38,300

Non-Hodgkin's lymphoma
31,700

Melanoma of the skin
27,300

Oral cavity
20,200

Kidney
18,800

Leukemia
16,900

Pancreas
13,700

All sites
619,700

Cancer Deaths by Site and Sex

FEMALE

Lung & bronchus
67,600

Breast
40,800

Colon & rectum
28,500

Pancreas
14,500

Ovary
14,000

Non-Hodgkin's lymphoma
12,400

Leukemia
9,600

Uterine corpus
6,500

Brain
5,900

Stomach
5,400

All sites
268,100

MALE

Lung & bronchus
89,300

Prostate
31,900

Colon & rectum
27,800

Pancreas
13,700

Non-Hodgkin's lymphoma
13,700

Leukemia
12,100

Esophagus
9,200

Liver
8,500

Urinary bladder
8,100

Stomach
7,600

All sites
284,100

*Excluding basal and squamous cell skin cancer and in situ carcinomas except urinary bladder.

Figure 9-2 Leading sites of new cancer cases and deaths—2000 estimates *(Reprinted from American Cancer Society Cancer Facts and Figures, 1999)*

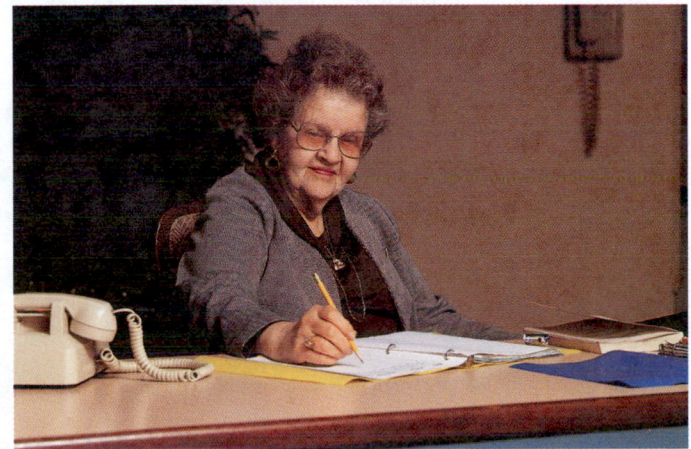

Figure 9-3 Nearly 4/5 of all cancer cases occur in adults over the age of 55.

More men than women die of cancer annually. The cancer death rate for men was 222.1 per 100,000 in 1993 compared with 189.8 for women. In 1993, out of 2,268,553 total deaths in the United States, 250,529 women and 279,375 men died of cancer (USBC, 1996). African Americans are more likely to develop cancer than any other ethnic or racial group (ACS, 2000). Overall cancer rates per 100,000 from 1990 to 1996 were 442.9/100,000 for African Americans, 402.9 for Caucasians, 275.4 for Hispanics, 279.1 for Asian and Pacific Islanders, and 153.4 for Native Americans (ACS, 2000). Most types of cancer can be treated and cured if detected early. Yet the death rates from cancer have been increasing for both men and women. In 1970, there were 69,500 deaths from lung cancer. In 2000, the American Cancer Society estimated that there were 156,900 lung cancer deaths, which is 28% of all cancer deaths.

Client Education

Recommendations for Early Cancer Detection

- Tell clients that persons ages 20 to 40 should have a cancer-related checkup every 3 years, and clients over age 40 should be seen yearly. Examination should include counseling as well as examinations of the thyroid, lymph nodes, and skin.

- Encourage women age 40 and older to have a mammogram and a clinical breast examination each year. Women ages 20 to 39 should have a clinical breast examination every 3 years.

- Teach clients how to perform a breast self-examination.

- Provide breast self-examination information (appropriate for age, language, and culture of client).

- Teach your client the appropriate time of month for breast self-examination.

- Explain to the client that people age 50 older should be screened for colorectal cancer every 5 to 10 years (depending on the recommendation of their physician).

- Inform all sexually active women and women age 18 and older of the importance of having an annual pelvic examination and Pap Smear.

- Explain to your client what to expect during a pelvic examination, particularly before your client's first pelvic examination.

- Encourage your client to schedule routine office visits for screening.

- Schedule an appointment with your client to reinforce the discussion of the importance of follow-up for early cancer detection and breast self-examination (ACS, 2000).

For women, the increased cancer mortality has occurred primarily in women over age 55. Mortality rates for 1990 to 1996 show that more African American men and women die annually from cancer (223,400) than Caucasian men and women (167,500). Annual Hispanic deaths from cancer were 104,900; American Indian deaths, 104,000; and Asian and Pacific Islander deaths, 103,400 per year. The incidence of most types of cancer in women is also higher for Caucasian women than for African American women. Caucasian women have a higher incidence of

breast, uterine, and ovarian cancer; African American women have a slightly higher incidence of lung and cervical cancer. While there is a higher incidence among Caucasian women, African American women have poorer survival rates (ACS, 2000). Reasons for poorer survival rates of African American women are unclear. One long-held hypothesis has been that poorer survival rates for African American women are caused by lack of access to care, which delays early detection and successful treatment. A recent study conducted at military hospitals, where supposedly everyone has the same access to care, found a gap between the breast cancer death rate of Caucasian and African American women that persisted even when they had equal access to care (Wojeik, 1998). Other factors that may contribute to differing survival rates, include genetic factors, diet, culture, and lifestyle, such as use of alcohol and tobacco (Wojicik, 1998).

Lung Cancer

Since 1985, lung cancer has been the leading cause of cancer death among women in the United States. Over the past 30 years, the lung cancer death rate among American women has increased nearly 400%, almost exclusively from cigarette smoking. From 1992 to 1996, mortality rates from lung cancer decreased significantly in men (down 1.7% per year), but rates for women increased (up 0.9% per year) (ACS, 2000). The dramatic increase in smoking among women has caused lung cancer to surpass breast

Client Education

Promoting a Healthy Lifestyle

- Obtain family history, nutrition history, and exercise or activity history
- Encourage a healthy diet
- Limit intake of high-fat foods
- Promote intake of high-fiber foods
- Limit consumption of alcoholic beverages
- Instruct client to keep a nutrition or diet record
- Encourage physical activity
- Encourage establishing or maintaining a healthy weight
- Discuss stress reduction activities
- Provide access to healthy lifestyle information (appropriate to age, language and culture)
- Schedule a follow-up visit

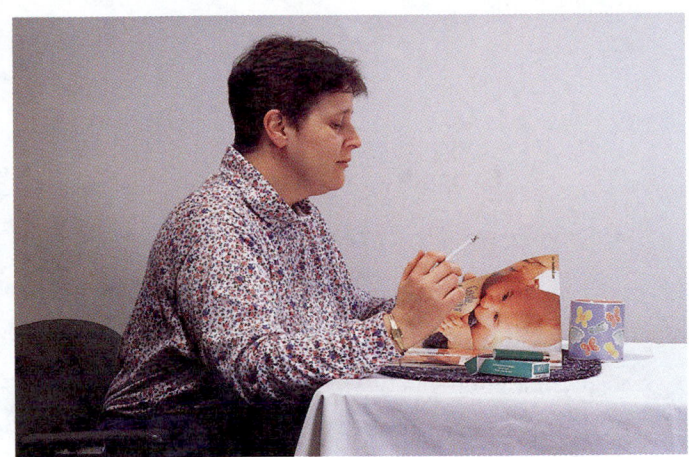

Figure 9-4 Lung cancer is the leading cause of cancer death in women.

cancer as a cause of death in women. Since 1987, more women have died from lung cancer than breast cancer, which was the major cancer killer of women for more than 40 years (ACS, 2000).

The death rate for lung cancer has risen despite medical advances and early diagnosis, which may be related to women lagging behind men in quitting smoking. Lung cancer symptoms of persistent cough, chest pain, bronchitis, sputum with bloody streaks, and recurring pneumonia usually do not appear until the advanced stages of the disease (Figure 9-4). An additional concern is the increasing use of tobacco among youth. Lung cancer from smoking is the most preventable cause of death today (ACS, 2000). Tobacco use in the United States causes the death of nearly one in every five Americans.

Society is beginning to mount an all-out effort at a major reduction in smoking habits, including legislation and policy regarding elimination of environments where smoking is permitted, public education regarding risks to health, and cigarette advertising targeted to minors. Litigation against tobacco companies and the surrounding publicity has increased the public's awareness of the addictive properties of nicotine and the risks of continued use. The litigation activity has spurred increased efforts at development of a national policy to discourage cigarette smoking. From 1978 to 1995, the prevalence of smoking among Caucasian, African American, Hispanic, and Asian or Pacific Islander men and women decreased, while the prevalence among Native Americans and Native Alaskan men and women did not change (ACS, 2000). The prevalence of cigarette smoking from 1991 to 1997 among high school students increased by 32%, which included an 80% increase among African American students, an increase of 39% among Hispanic students, and 28% among Caucasian students (ACS, 2000). Targeting of specific populations by the tobacco industry has led to an increase in teenage

smoking, with adolescent females for the first time surpassing adolescent males in the rates of starting smoking. Teenage girls' smoking rates have increased from 27% to 37% between 1991 and 1997 (USDHHS, 2000b).

Damaged lung tissue often returns to normal in persons who stop smoking when precancerous changes are found. After 10 years of abstinence, the risk of lung cancer is 30% to 50% lower than that of continuing smokers (ACS, 2000). In 1990, The U.S. Department of Health and Human Services published *The Health Benefits of Smoking Cessation,* in which the Surgeon General of the United States outlined the benefits of smoking cessation:

- People who cease to smoke, regardless of age, live longer than people who continue to smoke.
- Smokers who cease to smoke before age 50 have half the risk of dying within the next 15 years compared with those who continue to smoke.
- Smoking cessation substantially decreases the risk of lung, laryngeal, esophageal, oral, pancreatic, bladder, and cervical cancers.
- Smoking cessation lowers the risk for other major diseases, such as coronary heart disease and cardiovascular disease.

Nurses and other health care providers have both the opportunity and the means to help clients modify smoking behavior. About 70% of the 45 million adult smokers in the United States could be counseled by a health care worker during their ongoing care but often are not (CDC, 1994). The U.S. Preventative Services Task Force (1996) identified, in order of effectiveness, the key elements of effective counseling as follows:

- Providing reinforcement through consistent and repeated advice to stop smoking
- Setting of a specific "quit date"
- Scheduling follow-up contact or visits
- Providing self-help materials
- Making referral to group counseling
- Arranging for advice from more than one health care provider
- Including chart reminders to identify clients who smoke
- Prescribing nicotine-containing products to aid cessation

Historically, smoking prevention efforts have not focused on women, and women tend to be less successful in smoking cessation than men. Women are beginning to smoke in adolescence in greater numbers than ever. Antitobacco messages should be included in health promotion counseling of children, adolescents, and young adults (U.S. Preventive Services Task Force, 1996).

Critical Thinking

Lung Cancer in Women

More women die of lung cancer than breast cancer in the United States. Yet most women are far more frightened of breast cancer than they are of lung cancer. Cigarette smoking is the No. 1 risk factor in the development of lung cancer. Other risk factors include exposure to industrial substances, radiation, air pollution, tuberculosis, and second-hand smoke (ACS, 2000).

With lung cancer, early detection is difficult because symptoms often do not appear until the disease is advanced. Diagnosis of cancer is done primarily through chest x-ray films, analysis of sputum cells, and bronchoscopy, which a fiberoptic examination of the bronchial tubes. Treatment for lung cancer is determined by the specific type and stage of the disease. Treatment options include surgery, chemotherapy, or radiotherapy, or a combination of these. Often by the time lung cancer is diagnosed, it has metastasized.

We know that approximately 75% of lung cancer is caused by smoking. Yet most of the attention in the media and by health professionals is given to breast cancer. All health care providers who care for women must be far more diligent in assessment of smoking status. Women who smoke require counseling, support, and information regarding smoking cessation programs and smoking risks. Far more attention should be given to the dangers of smoking in the public media and from health professionals. Increased public attention is needed for programs to decrease the number of adolescents who are beginning to smoke and the availability of smoking cessation programs that work. Assessment of each client's smoking status is important and counseling regarding cessation is part of nursing practice.

Survival rates for lung cancer have increased. The American Cancer Society (2000) note that 1-year relative survival rates have increased (between 1975 to 1995) from 34% to 41%, but the 5-year relative survival rate for all stages of lung cancer is 14%.

Client Education

Smoking Cessation

- Obtain smoking history from every client regardless of the reason for health care
- Encourage every client who smokes to stop smoking
- Identify benefits of smoking cessation
- Identify risks of smoking
- Help client to set a specific date to stop smoking
- Schedule follow-up visits with client to reinforce cessation
- Provide smoking cessation literature that is appropriate for age, language, and culture
- Develop appropriate collection of literature for client population served and knowledge of community smoking cessation programs
- Reinforce advice to client by arranging for other health care providers to also counsel client
- Chart smoking history and counseling given at each client visit
- Provide access to nicotine patch or other products to reduce nicotine addiction

of computing risk assumes that every woman has an equal chance for breast cancer and that every woman will live to be 110 years old; therefore, the risk cited can be misleading. The chance of developing breast cancer for an average 40-year-old woman is 1 in 1,000. The risk increases as women get older. In 1998 it was projected there would be 178,700 new cases of invasive breast cancer and 43,500 deaths from breast cancer (ACS, 1998). Incidence of new cases of breast cancer increased by about 4% per year during the 1980s, but has leveled off in recent years. The increase in new cases was attributed in part to the earlier detection of breast cancer through increased use of breast self-examination, clinical breast examination, and diagnostic screenings, including mammography (NCHS, 1992).

In the year 2000, approximately 182,800 new cases of invasive breast cancer will affect women in the U.S. and 1,400 men will be diagnosed with breast cancer (ACS, 2000). Early detection and advances in medical treatment of breast cancer have helped to decrease mortality rates in African American women. The incidence of breast cancer is highest in Caucasian woman (113.2 per 100,000) and lowest among Native American women (11.6 per 100,000).

Breast Cancer

Breast cancer is the second most prevalent cancer in women. The American Cancer Society estimates that one of every eight women in the United States will develop breast cancer during her lifetime (ACS, 1998). This method

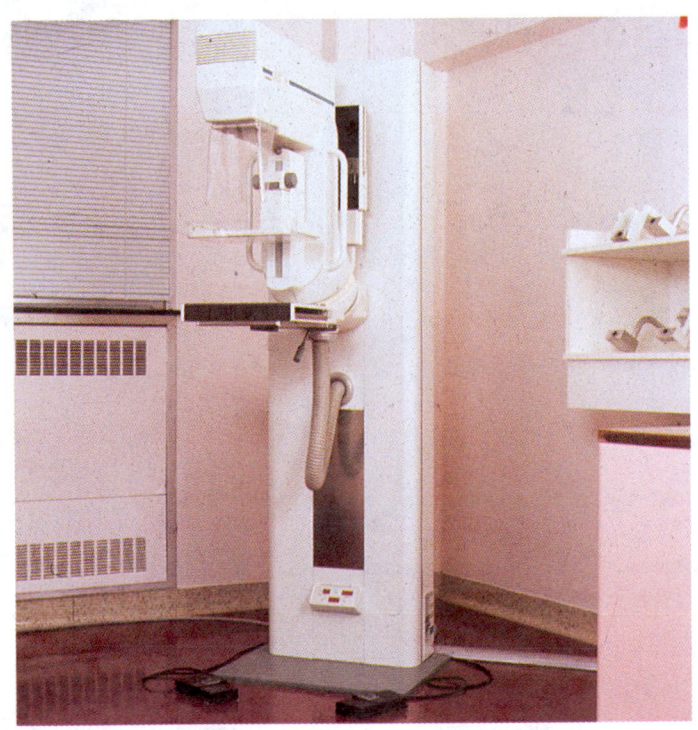

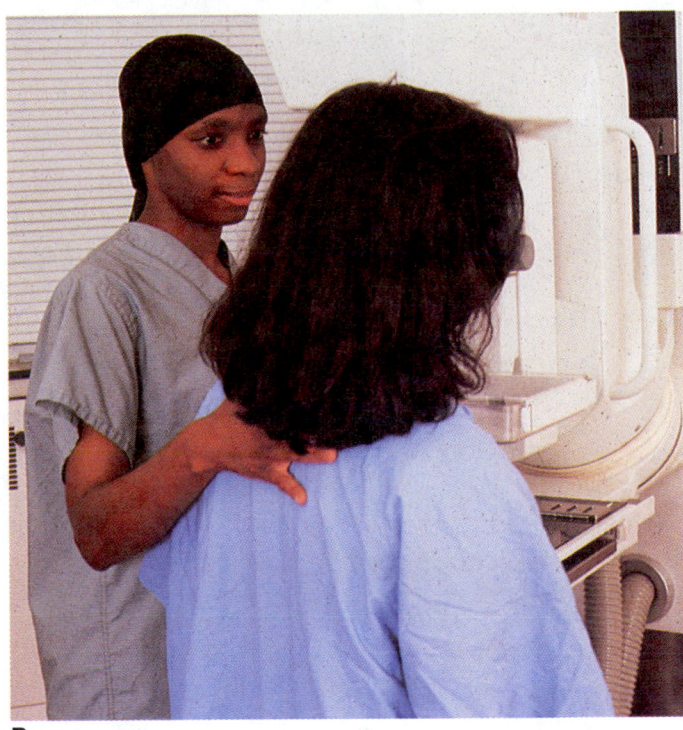

A.   B.

Figure 9-5 A. Mammographic x-ray unit. B. Client positioning for mammography.

Mortality rates continue to decline with the largest decrease occurring in younger women. These decreases have occurred in both Caucasian and African American women. These decreases are likely due to earlier detection and improved treatment (ACS, 2000). Mammography is the best method for early detection of breast cancer and has attributed to the decrease in breast cancer deaths due to early detection (Figure 9-5).

Breast self-examination is important for detecting physical signs and symptoms of breast cancer. Women can examine their own breasts to detect a breast lump, swelling, distortion, dimpling, nipple pain, scaliness, or retraction (ACS, 2000). Many women experience breast pain or tenderness, which is often seen in conjunction with benign conditions of the breast. Breast pain is not normally the first symptom of breast cancer. The American Cancer Society recommends that women ages 20 to 39 have a clinical breast examination every 3 years and a monthly self-examination.

The risk of breast cancer rises as women age, most notably after age 40. Breast cancer occurs more frequently in Caucasian women over age 35 than in African American women of comparable age. Risk factors for breast cancer include personal or family history of breast cancer, biopsy-confirmed atypical hyperplasia, early menarche, late menopause, recent use of oral contraceptives or post-menopausal estrogens, never having children or having the first live birth at a late age, and a higher level of education and socioeconomic status (ACS, 1998). Alcohol consumption of as many as two to five drinks per day has been associated with an increased risk of breast cancer that is comparable to that associated with having a family history of breast cancer or starting to menstruate before age 12 (ACS, 2000). Alcohol use and poor diet are risk factors that can be modified with lifestyle change, including smoking cessation, regular exercise before menopause, and a low-fat diet. International variability in breast cancer rates sug-

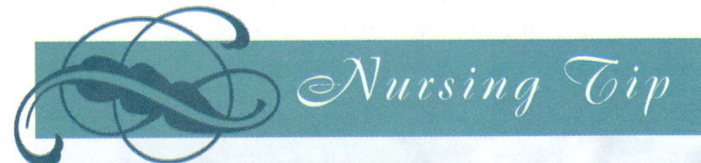

BREAST SELF-EXAMINATION (BSE)

First assess if your client performs monthly BSE. If your client reports to you that she is doing monthly BSE, have her demonstrate to you how she does it. This will tell you whether she is doing it correctly. If she is not doing it correctly, view this as an opportunity to help her learn it correctly. Also, when asking her to show you how she does BSE, she might be more willing to tell you if she is not doing it on a regular basis. You also have an opportunity to explore her reasons for not doing monthly BSE. You may find that she has negative feelings about touching her body, or incorrect information.

Research Highlight

Risk of Breast Cancer with Oral Contraceptive Use in Women with a Family History of Breast Cancer

Purpose

To determine whether the association with oral contraceptive use and the risk of breast cancer are influenced by a family history of breast cancer.

Methods

Historical cohort study of 426 families of women with breast cancer that was diagnosed between 1944 and 1952. Follow-up data on family members were collected by telephone interviews between 1991 and 1996. Follow-up family members included 394 sisters and daughters of the women in the initial study, 3002 granddaughters and nieces, and 2754 women who married into the families.

Findings

There was a significantly increased risk of breast cancer for sisters and daughters of the original group of women with breast cancer if they had ever used oral contraceptives; however, there was no significant increase for granddaughters, nieces, and marry-ins. The elevated risk among women with a first-degree family history of breast cancer was most evident for oral contraceptive use before 1975, when formulations were likely to contain larger amounts of estrogens and progestins.

Nursing Implications

Findings indicate that women who have used earlier formulations of oral contraceptives (before 1975) and who have a first-degree relative with breast cancer may be at a significant risk for breast cancer.

Grebick, D.M., et al. (2000). Risk of breast cancer with oral contraceptive use in women with family history of breast cancer. *JAMA*, 248 (14), 1791–1798.

gests that high-fat diets may correlate with an increased risk of breast cancer. Other factors that may be associated with increased risk include pesticide and other chemical exposures, weight gain, induced abortion, and physical inactivity. Some of the possible risk factors are amenable to lifestyle changes, such as poor diet, lack of exercise, and alcohol use. Because most of the established risk factors are not amenable to change through lifestyle or prevention strategies, the major focus has been on early detection and early treatment. A small percentage of breast cancers (1% to 5%) are associated with a genetic predisposition (genes BRCA-1, BRCA-2 and possibly other as yet unidentified genes).

Genetic screening and gene therapy may be beneficial interventions in the future for women at risk for breast cancer. Genetic screening for the general population is not currently recommended (ACS, 2000).

The American Cancer Society's recommendations for early breast cancer detection include (ACS, 2000):

- Women aged 40 and older should have a screening mammogram every year.

- Between ages 20 and 39, women should have a clinical breast examination by a health professional every 3 years and after age 40, every year.

- Women age 20 or older should perform BSE every month (Figure 9-6). By doing BSE regularly, one learns how one's breasts normally feel and can more readily detect signs or symptoms.

- If a change occurs, such as development of a lump or swelling, skin irritation or dimpling, nipple pain or retraction (turning inward), redness or scaliness of the nipple or breast skin, or a discharge other than breast milk, the health care provider should be seen as soon as possible. However, most of the time, these breast changes are not cancer.

- Although there are some features of a mass that suggest whether it is likely to be benign or cancerous, women examining their own breasts should discuss any new lump with their health care professionals.

Experienced health care professionals can examine the breast and determine whether the changes are benign or a breast cancer. They can determine when additional tests are appropriate to rule out cancer and when follow-up examinations are the best strategy. If there is any suspicion of cancer, a biopsy should be done.

The American Cancer Society believes the use of mammography, clinical breast examination, and BSE, according to the recommendations outlined above, offers women the best opportunity for reducing the breast cancer death rate through early detection. This combined approach is clearly better than any single examination. Without question, physical breast examination without mammography would miss many breast cancers that are too small for a woman or her doctor to feel. Although mammography is the most sensitive screening method, a small percentage of breast cancers do not show up on mammograms but can be felt by a woman or her doctor.

Colorectal Cancer

Colorectal cancer ranks third as a cause of cancer deaths in women and is three times more prevalent than uterine or ovarian cancer. In 2000, there were an estimated 130,200 new cases, including 93,800 cases of colon cancer and 36,400 of rectal cancer. Invasive colorectal cancer is the most preventable visceral cancer. Most cases arise from adenomatous polyps that take approximately 10 years to progress to an invasive stage.

The incidence of colon cancer declined from 1992 to 1996 by 2.1% per year (ACS, 2000). This decline in colon cancer has been suggested by research to be related to the increases in screening and the removal of polyps. Rectal bleeding, changes in bowel habits, and blood in the stool are symptoms of colon cancer.

Colon cancer was estimated to be responsible for 11% of all cancer deaths in the year 2000. Risk factors include family history, ulcerative colitis, first-degree family history of adenomas or colorectal cancer, and a personal history of adenomas or of ovarian, endometrial, or breast cancer.

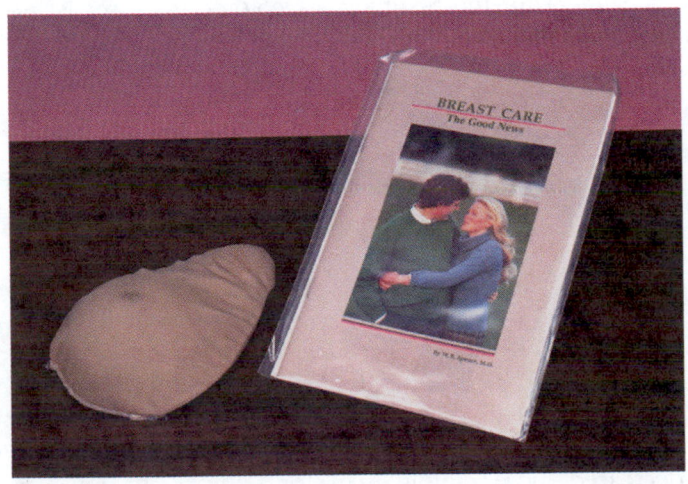

A.

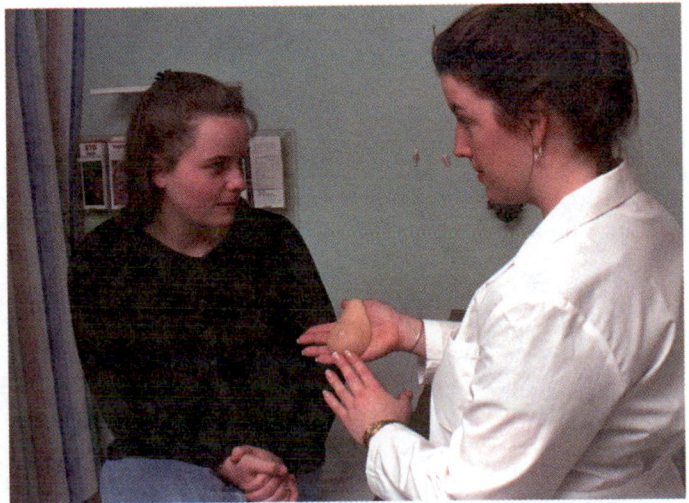

B.

Figure 9-6 A. Breast exam materials. B. Nurse teaching client breast exam techniques on a model.

Client Education

Breast Self-Examination (Recommendations of the American Cancer Society)

By regularly examining her own breasts, a woman is likely to notice any changes that occur. The best time for BSE is about a week after your period ends, when your breasts are not tender or swollen. Of you are not having regular periods, do BSE on the same day every month. Women who are pregnant, breast-feeding, or have breast implants also need to do regular breast self-examinations (BSE).

Lying Down

- Lie down with a pillow under your right shoulder and place your right arm behind your head (Figure 9-7A).
- Use the finger pads of the three middle fingers on your left hand to feel for lumps in the right breast.
- Press firmly enough to know how your breast feels. A firm ridge in the lower curve of each breast is normal. If you're not sure how hard to press, talk with your doctor or nurse.
- Move around the breast in a circular, up-and-down line or wedge pattern (Figure 9-7B). Be sure to do it the same way every time, check the entire breast area, and remember how your breast feels from month to month.

- Repeat the examination on your left breast, using the finger pads of the right hand. (Move the pillow to under your left shoulder.)

Standing Before a Mirror

- Repeat the examination of both breasts while standing, with your one arm behind your head (Figure 9-7C). The upright position makes it easier to check the upper and outer part of the breasts (toward your armpit). This is where about half of breast cancers are found. You may want to do the standing part of the BSE while you are in the shower. Some breast changes can be felt more easily when your skin is wet and soapy.
- Gently squeeze the nipple to check for discharge (Figure 9-7D)
- For added safety, you can check your breasts for any dimpling of the skin, changes in the nipple, redness, or swelling while standing in front of a mirror right after your BSE each month (Figure 9-7E).
- Raise your arms over your head to visualize the breast contour and the lower quadrants (Figure 9-7F).
- Place your hands on your hips and press inward to flex the pectoral muscles, which may enhance skin dimpling or puckering (Figure 9-7G).
- Repeat the examination on the alternate side.
- If you find any changes, see your doctor right away.

Possible additional risk factors include inactivity, high-fat diets, low-fiber diets, and inadequate intake of fruit and vegetables (ACS, 2000).

If detected at an early stage, colorectal cancer can be successfully treated with surgery (US Preventive Services Task Force, 1996). Recommendations for early detection for both men and women, beginning at age 50, include:

- Performing a fecal occult blood test (FOBT) and flexible sigmoidoscopy; if normal, repeat the FOBT annually and the sigmoidoscopy every 5 years, or
- Performing a colonoscopy; if normal, repeat every 10 years, or
- Performing a double-contrast barium enema; if normal, repeat every 5 to 10 years, and
- Performing a digital rectal examination in addition to the above diagnostic tests

Surgery for the treatment of colorectal cancer is frequently curative for cancers that have not spread. Treatment for clients whose cancer has deeply perforated the bowel wall or spread to the lymph nodes includes chemotherapy or chemotherapy plus radiation in addition to surgery. Treatment can be performed before or after surgery.

Cervical Cancer

Rates of cervical cancer have decreased steadily over the past several decades. The rate dropped from 14.2 per 100,000 in 1973 to 7.8 per 100,000 in 1994. The American Cancer Society notes that in the year 2000, there were an estimated 12,800 new cases. Rates for African Americans decreased more rapidly than for Caucasians; however, from 1992 to 1996, the mortality rate for African American continued to be more than twice that for Caucasian

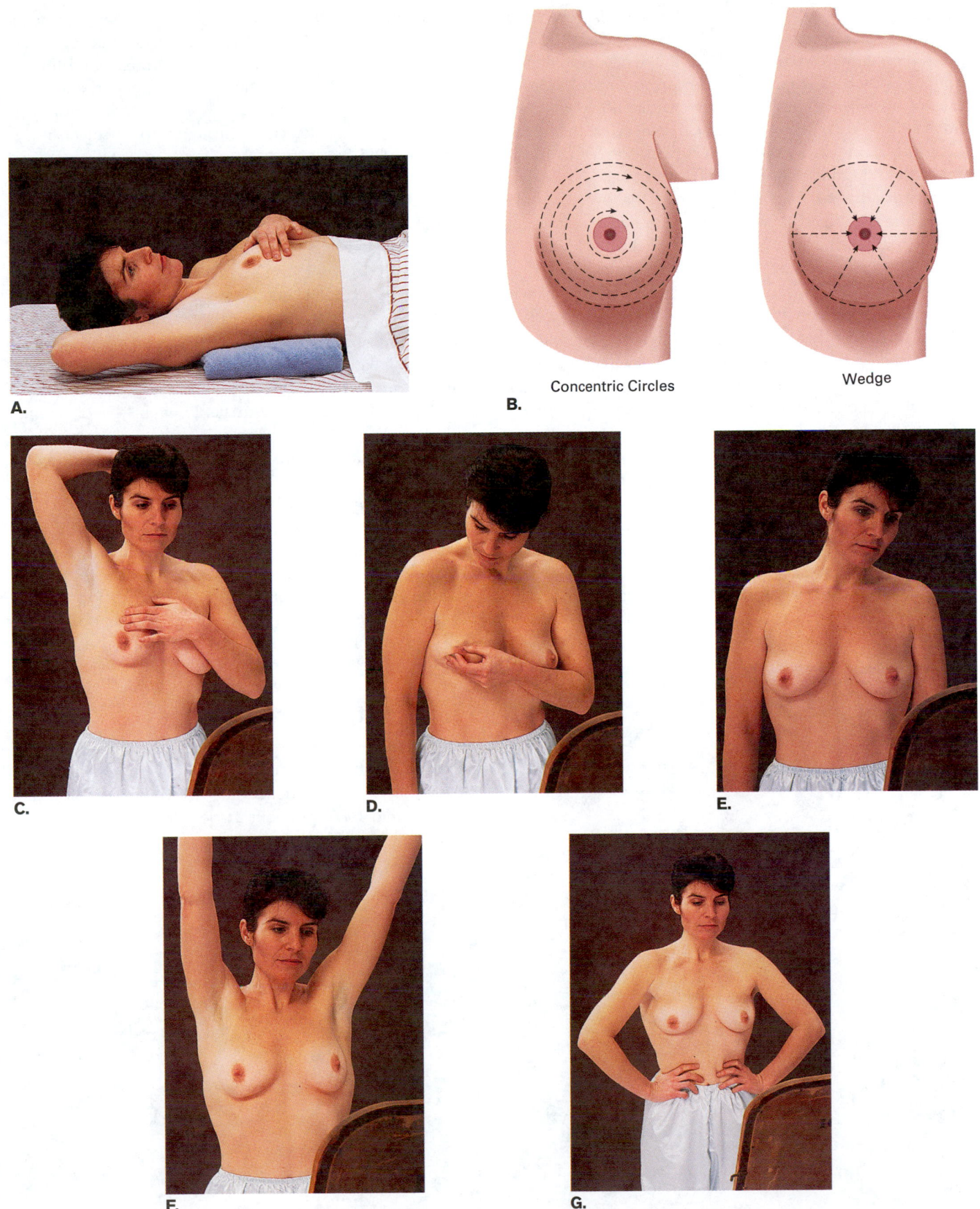

A.

B.

Concentric Circles   Wedge

C.

D.

E.

F.

G.

Figure 9-7 Breast Self-Examination.

women (ACS, 2000). This decrease results largely from early detection through the use of the Pap smear. Hispanic and Native American have higher incidence and higher death rates than Caucasian women. Approximately 15,000 cases of invasive cervical cancer were diagnosed in 1994, and 4,600 women died of cervical cancer in that year. Rates for carcinoma in situ reach a peak for both African American and Caucasian women between ages 20 and 30. **Carcinoma in situ** is defined as cancer that involves only the cells in the organ in which it began and that has not spread to any other tissue. After age 25, the incidence of invasive cancer in African American women increases dramatically with age, while in Caucasian women, the incidence rises more slowly (ACS, 1998). **Invasive cancer** is defined as cancer that has spread or infiltrated beyond the original site or organ. Over 25% of invasive cervical cancers occur in women older than age 65, and 40% to 50% of all women who die from cervical cancer are over age 65 (ACS, 1998). Invasive cervical cancer is defined as cancer that has spread from the surface of the cervix to the deeper tissues of the cervix.

Signs and symptoms for cervical cancer include abnormal vaginal bleeding or spotting and abnormal vaginal discharge. Pain is known as a late symptom for cervical cancer.

Risk factors for cervical cancer include early age at first intercourse, multiple sexual partners or partners who have had multiple sexual partners, smoking, and low socioeconomic status (ACS, 2000). Cervical cancer risk is closely linked to sexual behavior and sexually transmitted human papillomavirus (HPV) infection. Early detection and treatment has caused a marked decrease in mortality from cervical cancer. Early detection through Pap smear testing is recommended because 8 to 9 years is generally required for development of precancerous changes to progress to invasive carcinoma, also known as infiltrating cancer. Almost all early-stage cancers can be effectively treated. Pap smears can detect precancerous changes years before invasive cancer sets in.

Most cervical cancers are treated with surgery, radiation therapy, or both. In situ cancers may be treated with cryotherapy, which destroys cells with extreme cold, or electrocoagulation, which destroys cells with intense heat that is generated by an electric current (ACS, 2000).

Cervical cancer is very treatable, with 91% of women with localized cervical cancer surviving 5 years (ACS, 2000). Caucasian women are more likely to have cervical cancer detected at an early stage.

It is recommended that all women who are or have been sexually active or have reached age 18 should have annual Pap smears (Figure 9-8). This recommendation has been adopted by the major organizations (U.S. Preventive Services Task Force, 1996). The recommendation permits Pap testing less frequently after three or more normal annual test results, at the discretion of the health care provider and client.

Endometrial Cancer

An estimated 36,100 cases of cancer of the body of the uterus, usually of the endometrium, were diagnosed in 2000 (ACS, 2000). Incidence has been relatively constant since the mid-1980s at about 21 per 100,000 women (ACS,

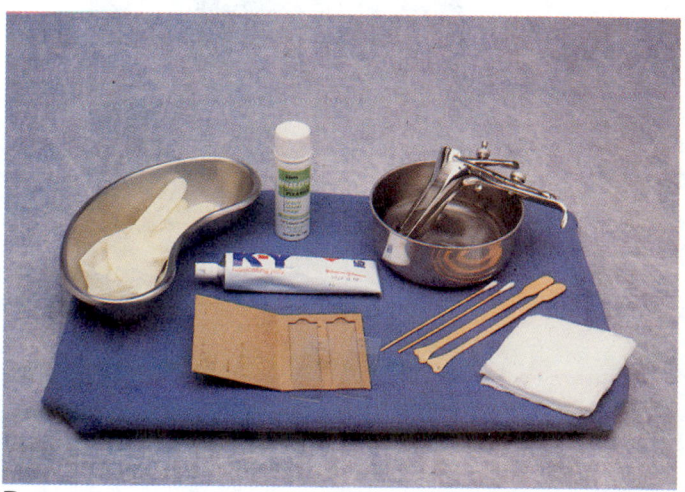

A.   **B.**

Figure 9-8 A. The nurse and client prepare for a pelvic exam. B. Materials needed for a gynecologic exam.

Nursing Alert

RISK FACTORS FOR CERVICAL CANCER

- Early age at first intercourse
- Multiple sex partners
- Sex with partners who have had multiple sexual partners
- Smoking
- History of HPV infection
- Low socioeconomic status

1998). Incidence is higher among Caucasian woman than African American women. Mortality rates were also relatively constant in the mid-1990s at about 3 per 100,000 women and about 6,300 deaths in 1998 (ACS, 1998). Although incidence of endometrial cancer is higher for Caucasian women than African American women, African American women have mortality rates that are nearly two times higher (ACS, 2000).

Endometrial cancer is rarely seen in women under age 50, but the risk rises sharply in women in their late 40s to mid-60s. The incidence of endometrial cancer increased rapidly during the years when unopposed estrogen was commonly used to treat postmenopausal women for symptomatic relief. Estrogen replacement therapy (ERT) was more common among Caucasian women, resulting in higher rates of endometrial cancer for Caucasian women than African American women. Unopposed estrogen therapy for menopause is no longer recommended because of the increased risk of endometrial cancer.

Signs and symptoms for endometrial cancer are similar to that of cervical cancer: abnormal uterine bleeding or spotting. Late manifestations of the disease include pain and systemic symptoms (ACS, 2000).

Risk factors for uterine cancer include those factors that expose the endometrium to estrogen, including (ACS, 1998):

- Unopposed estrogen therapy
- Therapy with tamoxifen
- Early menarche (before age 12)
- Never having children
- Late menopause (after age 55)
- History of failure to ovulate
- Infertility
- Diabetes

- Gallbladder disease
- Hypertension
- Obesity

There is preliminary evidence suggesting that a high-fat diet increases the risk of developing uterine cancer. Factors associated with a lower risk of endometrial cancer are having multiple children, use of oral contraceptives that combine both estrogen and progestin, and use during menopause of ERT combined with progesterone therapy. A genetic syndrome known as heredity non–polyposis colon cancer has been associated with endometrial and ovarian cancer (ACS, 2000). Endometrial cancer is treated by surgery, radiation therapy, hormonal therapy, chemotherapy, or a combination of these treatments, depending on the stage of the cancer (ACS, 2000).

Survival rates women with for uterine cancer are good when the disease is treated early. The 5-year survival rate for early-stage endometrial cancer is 95%; for regional (later-stage) cancer, it is 64% (ACS, 2000). The survival rates for Caucasian women are at least 18% better at every stage than for African American women (ACS, 2000).

Ovarian Cancer

One in seventy women develop ovarian cancer. Approximately 23,100 new cases of ovarian cancer occurred in 2000, with an estimated 14,500 deaths (ACS, 2000). The average age at diagnosis is 63. Approximately 90% of cases occur in Caucasian women. Risk factors for ovarian cancer include a family history of ovarian cancer (in first-degree relatives, such as mother, sister, daughter), nulliparity, older age at the time of first pregnancy or live birth, fewer pregnancies, use of fertility drugs, high-fat diet, and a personal history of breast, endometrial, or colorectal cancer. Women who have had breast cancer or have a family history of breast or ovarian cancer are at increased risk. Alteration in BRCA-1 or BRCA-2 genes has been noted in women with ovarian cancer, and the use of oral contraceptives and pregnancy appear to reduce the risk of ovarian cancer (ACS, 2000). The American Cancer Society (2000) notes that industrialized countries, except for Japan, have the highest incidence of ovarian cancer.

Ovarian cancer usually shows no signs or symptoms until late in development. Enlargement of the abdomen from accumulation of fluid is the most common sign (ACS, 2000). Usually ovarian tumors are of considerable size by the time they are detectable by pelvic examination. Women over age 40 who present with persistent symptoms of vague digestive disturbances (stomach discomfort, gas, distention) that cannot be explained by any other cause may need an ovarian cancer evaluation, including a thorough pelvic examination (ACS, 2000).

As of 2000, the only screening test available for ovarian cancer is an annual pelvic examination, which includes bimanual palpation of the ovaries. Even this method may not detect ovarian cancer early enough for adequate treatment. The Pap test rarely detects ovarian cancer, since it samples only cervical cells. Improvements in diagnostic methods continue, including identification of the breast and ovarian cancer gene on chromosome 17.

Only 25% of ovarian cancers are diagnosed early in the localized stage, with the survival rate at this stage being 95% for 5 years (ACS, 2000). For women with regional ovarian cancer, the survival rate is 79%; the survival rate for progressive disease is 28% (ACS, 2000).

Malignant Melanoma

Malignant melanoma is increasing faster than any other cancer. It is now more common than ovarian or cervical cancer. The incidence and mortality rates for women are rising and are greater than for men. Between ages 20 and 25, melanoma is the most common cancer in women and exceeds breast cancer and lung cancer. Between ages 30 and 39, melanoma is second to breast cancer in incidence.

Incidence is 10 times greater in Caucasians than African Americans, with an estimated 7,000 deaths in the year 2000 (ACS, 2000). Signs and symptoms include changes in the color or size of a mole or darkly pigmented spot on the skin, scaliness, oozing, bleeding, or a change in the appearance of a bump or nodule (ACS, 2000). Risks include fair skin, exposure to ultraviolet radiation, occupational exposures to chemical compounds, and family history (ACS, 2000).

The use of sunscreen and limiting exposure to the midday sun are important steps for prevention. The most common treatment is excision of the growth. The 5-year survival rate for malignant melanoma in the early stage is 95%; for regional disease, it is 58%; and for distant metastates, it is 13% (ACS, 2000).

Cancer Prevention

Cancer prevention in women has focused on smoking cessation, reduction of unprotected sex with multiple sex partners, low-fat diets, moderation in alcohol consumption, exercise, and elimination of unopposed estrogen use for menopause. Early detection and treatment has focused on periodic screening, including Pap smears, mammograms, gynecologic examinations, fecal occult blood tests, and sigmoidoscopy.

Chronic Conditions

Women live longer than men, but they are not necessarily living better. This is particularly true during later life, when they are more likely to have chronic disease (Rodin & Ick-ovics, 1990). Chronic diseases that women are more likely to be effected by include arthritis, osteoporosis, os-

teoarthritis, diabetes mellitus, obesity, urinary incontinence, Alzheimer's disease, fibromyalgia, chronic fatigue syndrome, orthopedic impairments, and vision and hearing problems (DHHS, 2000). In every age group, more women than men experience and seek care for illness and disability. During the reproductive years (ages 15 to 45), women seek care for acute conditions and short-term disabilities more frequently than men. Women in this age group may experience acute illness more frequently than men because women are exposed to school children with childhood infections to a greater degree than men (ORWH, 1992). Also, women are more likely than men to seek care for chronic conditions in middle and late life.

Osteoporosis

Osteoporosis is a disorder characterized by excessive loss of bone density. Osteoporosis affects over 25 million Americans; more than 80% of them are women. This disease affects one-third to one-half of postmenopausal women. The rates for osteoporosis increase dramatically for women as they age (ORWH, 1992). Hip fractures are the most serious consequence of osteoporosis, with more than 250,000 people hospitalized with hip fractures annually. About one-third of these become totally dependent, and one-half never walk again. Risk factors include (Bonnick, 1994):

- Caucasian woman
- Premature menopause
- Lack of exercise
- Excessive caffeine intake
- Regular alcohol use
- Excess dietary phosphate and sodium
- Post-menopause
- Insufficient dietary calcium
- Smoking
- Family history of osteoporosis

Prevention of osteoporosis should span the entire lifetime. Approximately 60% of a woman's bone mass develops by age 18, and peak bone density is achieved by age 35. To build and maintain bone density, women should eat calcium-rich foods, get regular exercise, and avoid tobacco and excessive consumption of alcohol or caffeine. Treatment includes calcium and vitamin D supplementation, estrogen replacement at menopause, and medications to strengthen bone structure.

Alzheimer's Disease

Alzheimer's disease occurs more frequently in women than in men and increases with age—dramatically so after age 85. In 1998, there were 22,725 deaths from Alzheimer's disease, with most deaths occurring after age 75 (DHHS, 2000). The disease usually begins after age 65, and the risk goes up with age. Younger people may have Alzheimer's disease, but it is less common. About 3% of the population aged 65 to 74 have Alzheimer's disease. Alzheimer's disease is not a normal function of aging, although about 50% of the population over age 85 years may have the disease.

Immune Disorders

Immunologic diseases occur more frequently in females than males. Autoimmune thyroid disease occurs fifteen times more frequently in women than men. Rheumatoid arthritis occurs three times more frequently in women than men, and leads to disability and decreased life expectancy. Systemic lupus erythemathosus (SLE) occurs nine times more frequently in women than men and is three times more prevalent in African American women than in Caucasian women. Systemic sclerosis affects women four times as frequently as men. Diabetes mellitus and multiple sclerosis occur more frequently in women (DHHS, 2000b).

Urinary Incontinence

Eleven million older women in the United States have urinary incontinence. Women are more frequently affected than men; approximately 2 million men experience the condition. Approximately 50% of persons residing in nursing homes are incontinent. Urinary incontinence is the tenth leading cause of hospitalization. More diapers are sold in the United States to women over age 65 than are used for babies. Although half of all elderly people experience episodes of incontinence, it is a problem of younger women also. 10–30% of women in 15–65 age group develop incontinent as a result of weakened pelvic muscles or pelvic trauma (Shint & Peggs, 2000). Table 9-4 outlines five types of urinary incontinence.

Urinary Tract Infections

Urinary tract infections are common in women of all ages and account for an estimated 8 million physician visits annually, costing over $4 billion. Urologic disorders in women have not been studied well. Research in women's urologic disorders lags far behind research in bladder and prostate cancer and urologic disorders of men.

HIV Infection

The risk of becoming infected with HIV has increased in certain populations of women. The number of women who progress from undetected HIV infection to AIDS may be a major contributor to death among young women in certain risk groups. Before 1992, the majority of HIV-infected women were drug users or sex partners of drug

Table 9-4 Types of Urinary Incontinence

Type	Characteristics
Functional	Bladder emptying is unpredictable but complete. Incontinence is related to impairment of cognitive, physical, or psychological functioning or to environmental barriers.
Urge	Incontinence occurs immediately after the sensation to void is perceived.
Reflex	Incontinence is related to neurogenic bladder and central nervous system or spinal cord injury. Bladder fille, and uninhibited bladder contractions cause loss of urine.
Stress	Increased abdominal pressure is higher than urethral resistance. Stress associated with coughing or laughing causes incontinence.
Total	Unpredictable, involuntary, continuous loss of urine.

users. However, because of the dramatic increase in the number of women infected through heterosexual transmission, the number of women with HIV infection is rapidly increasing. Women infected with HIV are predominantly from minority groups (75%) and are likely to have dependent children, be on welfare, and have inadequate access to health care. HIV infection and AIDS present a different clinical course in women than men. Because women have not been included in AIDS clinical trials, understanding of HIV infection in women is inadequate. This results in less effective early identification and treatment of women with HIV infection and AIDS. To prevent HIV infection, the CDC promotes safer-sex behaviors that include postponing sexual activity among youth, restricting sexual contact to a mutually monogamous relationship with an uninfected partner, and consistently and cautiously using latex condoms during intercourse. For drug users who inject, the CDC encourages participation in a drug treatment program and avoiding use of needles used by another person.

Mental Illness

Mental health is crucial to a woman's well-being. Some of the most common mental disorders, including depression and anxiety, occur in approximately twice as many women as men. It is estimated that there are currently 7 million women in the United States with clinical depression. An estimated 12% of women experience a major form of depression at some time in their lives, compared with 7% of men. Women are twice as likely as men to suffer from clinical depression. Suicide was the fourth leading cause of death among women aged 25 to 44 in 1998 (DHHSa, 2000). Women are more likely than men to attempt suicide but are far less likely to die as a result, primarily because men are more likely to use a firearm. Of women who have depression, about 75% are untreated. Most drugs to treat depression have been studied in clinical trials on men. The effects of hormones on depression and their interaction with psychotropic drugs have not been well-studied and are therefore largely unknown. At least 90% of the eating disorders anorexia nervosa and bulimia nervosa occur in women. Anorexia nervosa causes death in approximately 5% of those affected. It is believed that a combination of biologic, genetic, psychological, social, and environmental factors contribute to the reason women experience these illnesses at a higher rate than men. Women who have had a history of substance abuse or physical or sexual abuse are particularly at risk for depression, eating disorders, and anxiety orders.

Substance Abuse

The abuse of alcohol and other legal and illicit drugs is a serious and growing problem among U.S. women. There are approximately 10 million alcoholics in the United States, of which 30% to 50% are women. Women are less likely to use or abuse alcohol than men but have a 50% to 100% higher death rate from alcoholism than men. Alcohol use during pregnancy poses a serious threat to the developing fetus. Heavy drinking during pregnancy has clearly been implicated in severe birth defects, including mental retardation, abnormal face and neck features, nervous system disorders, and delayed growth. Use of alcohol during pregnancy occurs more frequently in single women, smokers, teenagers, and those with little education. In 1998, approximately 4.5 million women aged 15 to 44 were currently illicit drug users, of which one-third were raising children. Women tend to be more easily addicted to tranquilizers than men.

Smoking in women has increased as a result of the tobacco industry's aggressive marketing to women, particularly to teenage girls. Smoking contributes substantially to deaths and disability from cancer, lung disease, heart disease, and stroke. Smoking rates have decreased 35% from their peak in 1965. However, over 22 million (22%) of women were smoking in 1997. The number of female teenagers who smoke has increased 10%, from 27% in 1991 to 37% in 1997, which is more than the percentage of male teenagers who smoke. Smoking is the leading cause of premature births and increases the risk of miscarriage, mental retardation, and low birth weight. Exposing children to secondhand smoke increases the risk of sudden infant death syndrome (SIDS), recurrent otitis media, and severe respiratory illness. Smoking cessation programs have been more successful in males than in females. By age 25, one in three women is a smoker. The number of women who are heavy smokers has also increased in the last two decades.

AGE-SPECIFIC ISSUES

Certain health alterations are more prevalent in certain age groups, and are grouped accordingly in the following discussion.

Infancy to Young Adulthood

Less than 1% of all deaths of females occurs in girls aged 1 to 4. Accidents are the leading cause of death in this age group, followed by congenital anomalies, cancer, homicide, heart disease, pneumonia, septicemia, perinatal disease, stroke, and benign neoplasms (DHHS, 2000a) (Table 9-5).

Between ages 5 and 14, the death rate for female children drops by 50%. Accidents continue to be the leading cause of death, followed by cancer, homicide, congenital anomalies, heart disease, suicides, chronic obstructive pulmonary disease (COPD), pneumonia, benign neoplasms, and stroke (Table 9-6). In this age group, boys have almost twice the death rate from accidents that girls do (National Vital Statistics Report, 2000).

The major cause of death and illness among all children is injury, both intentional and unintentional. Injury accounts for over half of all deaths in this age group (Figure 9-9). Chronic illness is rare and is usually related to the increase in sex hormones during puberty. Women are also

Table 9-5 Leading Causes of Death by Age and Sex for Ages 1–4: 1998

Cause of Death	Deaths Per 100,000 Population		
	Both Sexes	Female	Male
All causes	34.6	31.4	37.6
Accidents	12.7	10.5	14.9
Congenital anomalies	3.7	3.7	3.7
Cancer	2.4	2.4	2.4
Homicide	2.6	2.4	2.9
Heart disease	1.4	1.3	1.5
Pneumonia and influenza	1.0	1.0	0.9
Septicemia	0.6	0.5	0.7
Perinatal-related	0.5	0.5	0.5
Stroke	0.4	0.4	(NA)
Benign neoplasms	0.3	0.3	(NA)

Adapted from Table No. 8, National Vital Statistics Report, Vol. No. 11, July 24, 2000.

Table 9-6 Leading Causes of Death by Age and Sex for Ages 5–14: 1998

Cause of Death	Deaths Per 100,000 Population		
	Both Sexes	Female	Male
All causes	19.9	16.2	23.4
Accidents	8.3	6.1	10.4
Cancer	2.6	2.3	2.9
Homicide	1.2	1.1	1.3
Congenital anomalies	0.9	0.9	1.0
Heart disease	0.8	0.7	1.0
Suicide	0.8	0.4	1.2
COPD	0.4	0.4	0.4
Pneumonia and influenza	0.3	0.3	0.3
Benign neoplasms	0.2	0.2	0.2
Stroke	0.2	0.2	0.2

Adapted from Table No. 8, National Vital Statistics Report, Vol. No. 11, July 24, 2000.

prone to autoimmune diseases, including systemic lupus erythematosus (SLE), juvenile rheumatoid arthritis, and thyroid disease.

Areas for research that have been recommended by NIH in the infancy and childhood years include calcium intake; diet and physical activity; tobacco, alcohol, and other drug abuse; child mistreatment; growth and development; interaction between girls and their parents; hormonal influences; environment; asthma; mental health and depression; and oral health (NIH, 1999).

Young Adulthood to Perimenopausal Years

As girls, ages 15 to 24, become adolescents and young adults, the leading cause of death continues to be accidents. The leading causes of death for this age range are listed in Table 9-7. During this period, males have almost three times the risk of dying of females, with most deaths attributable to accidents, homicide, and suicide (USBC, 1999).

For adult women between ages 25 and 44, the risk of dying is more than double that of the previous age range. For the first time in their lives, cancer is the leading cause of death. The remaining causes of death in this age group are accidents, heart disease, suicide, AIDS, homicide, stroke, chronic liver disease, diabetes, pneumonia, summarized in Table 9-8. In contrast, the leading cause of death for men in this age group is accidents. AIDS and accidents are

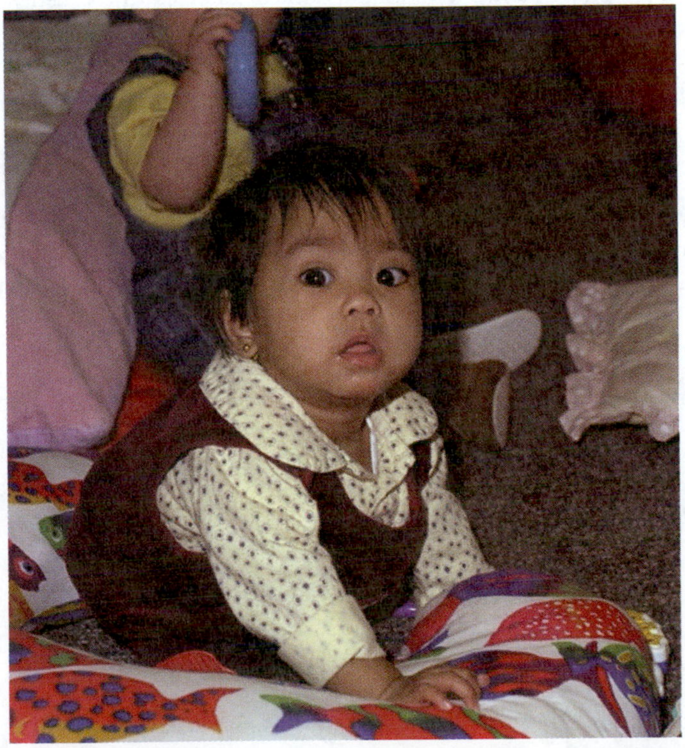

Figure 9-9 Injury is the major cause of morbidity and mortality in young children.

Table 9-7 Leading Causes of Death by Age and Sex for Ages 15–24: 1998

Cause of Death	Deaths Per 100,000 Population		
	Both Sexes	Female	Male
All causes	82.3	43.5	119.3
Accidents	35.9	19.1	51.9
Homicide	14.8	3.0	24.8
Suicide	11.1	3.3	18.5
Cancer	4.6	3.7	5.4
Heart disease	2.8	2.1	3.5
Congenital anomalies	2.8	1.1	1.3
COPD	0.6	0.5	0.8
Pneumonia and influenza	0.6	0.6	0.6
AIDS	0.5	0.6	0.6
Stroke	0.5	(N/A)	0.6

Adapted from Table No. 8, National Vital Statistics Report, Vol. No. 11, July 24, 2000.

Table 9-8 Leading Causes of Death by Age and Sex for Ages 25–44: 1998

Cause of Death	Deaths Per 100,000 Population		
	Both Sexes	Female	Male
All causes	157.7	107.4	208.8
Accidents	32.6	16.5	48.9
Cancer	25.7	28.0	23.4
Heart disease	20.2	11.9	29.0
Suicide	14.6	6.0	23.5
AIDS	10.4	5.1	15.7
Homicide	9.8	4.6	15.0
Chronic liver disease	4.7	2.9	6.5
Stroke	4.0	3.9	4.1
Diabetes	3.0	2.4	3.6
Pneumonia and influenza	2.3	1.9	2.7

Adapted from Table No. 8, National Vital Statistics Report, Vol. No. 11, July 24, 2000.

more than three times more frequently causes of death in men than women. Homicide and suicide are more than four times more common causes of death in men than women during this period of life (USBC, 1999).

From ages 15 to 44, accidents, cancer, heart disease, suicide, and AIDS are the most frequent causes of death in both genders (Figure 9-10). The most frequent causes of ill health among women are eating disorders, autoimmune diseases, depression, alcohol and tobacco use, STDs, reproductive problems, homicide, and sexual abuse. Intervention strategies that can reduce or prevent serious illness or death in this age group address women at risk and risky

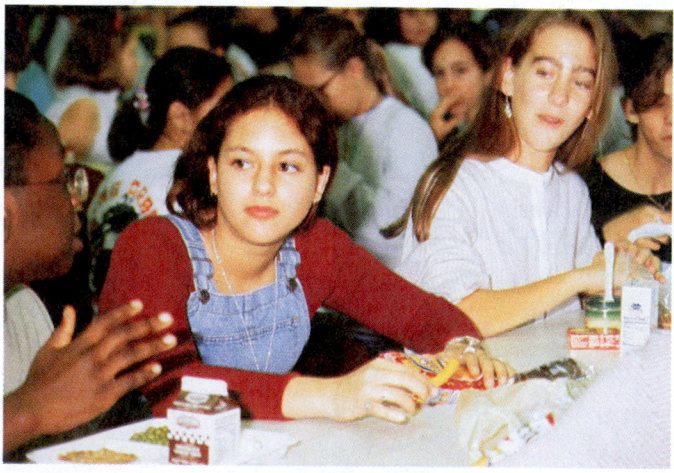

Figure 9-10 Adolescents are most at risk for mortality from accidents, cancer, heart disease, suicide, and AIDS.

behaviors associated with the diseases and illnesses. Alcohol is often a causative factor in motor vehicle accidents and violence that ends in homicide and suicide. Risky sexual behavior puts women at risk for STDs, HIV infection, cervical cancer, unwanted or unplanned pregnancies, pelvic inflammatory disease (PID), atopic pregnancy, and infertility. Smoking puts women at risk for lung and other cancer, heart disease, and COPD.

Perimenopausal to Mature Years

For mature women, ages 45 to 64, the risk of dying is more than five times that of women aged 25 to 44. Approximately 14% of all female deaths occur in this age range. The leading causes of death for men and women are summarized in Table 9-9.

Women in the menopausal to mature years are a fast-growing segment of the population because of the aging of the baby boom generation. These years are important because of menopause and the fact that many chronic conditions first appear. More than 10% of women in this age group have chronic conditions, including arthritis, hypertension, chronic sinusitis, skeletal deformity, and heart disease. Approximately 5% of these women have hearing impairments, chronic bronchitis, hemorrhoids, asthma, and diabetes. Another 1% to 3% of these women have visual impairments, cataracts, ulcers, abdominal hernias, and emphysema (National Center of Health Statistics, 1992). The rates of some of these chronic conditions in-

Table 9-9 Leading Causes of Death by Age and Sex for Ages 45–64: 1998

Cause of Death	Deaths Per 100,000 Population		
	Both Sexes	Female	Male
All causes	664.0	501.9	836.9
Cancer	231.9	209.9	255.3
Heart disease	174.9	101.5	253.2
Accidents	31.9	18.0	46.8
Stroke	26.8	23.3	30.6
Diabetes	22.9	21.1	25.8
COPD	22.7	21.2	24.3
Chronic liver disease	19.3	10.1	29.0
Suicide	14.1	6.4	22.4
Pneumonia and influenza	10.5	8.2	13.0
AIDS	7.2	(NA)	12.1

Adapted from Table No. 8, National Vital Statistics Report, Vol. No. 11, July 24, 2000.

crease markedly in the population between the ages of 45 to 64. During these years, one out of seven women has heart disease. Lung cancer is the leading cause of cancer deaths; breast cancer is the second most common cause. By age 54, one-third of women have had a hysterectomy (National Center for Health Statistics, 1992). Approximately 3% of women in this age group have a major depressive episode. Major reasons for hospitalization of women in this age range include heart disease, cancer, gall bladder disease, benign tumors, psychosis, and diabetes. The most common surgical procedures are hysterectomy, oophorectomy and salpingo-oophorectomy, cholecystectomy, cardiac catheterization, spinal fusion, dilatation and curettage, and biopsies (National Center for Health Statistics, 1992).

The three major risk factors for the diseases that relate to morbidity and mortality during this period are smoking, obesity, and a sedentary lifestyle. The drop in estrogen levels at menopause is a factor in the increased incidence of heart disease and osteoporosis. The Women's Health Initiative is conducting the largest and most expensive clinical trial ever conducted to determine whether women should begin hormone replacement therapy at menopause, how long it should be continued, and whether it will reduce the incidence of heart disease and osteoporosis.

Prevention strategies are aimed at identification of risk factors and avoiding or stopping risky behaviors that can be changed. Avoiding or stopping risky behavior, such as smoking, drinking, overeating, and a sedentary lifestyle, can reduce the risk of chronic disease and mortality in this age range. Smoking has been linked with lung cancer, coronary artery disease, cerebrovascular disease, peripheral vascular disease, cervical cancer, hypertension, osteoporosis, and respiratory diseases. High-fat diets may contribute to colon cancer, obesity, coronary artery disease, and possibly breast cancer. Excessive alcohol use may cause cirrhosis of the liver, alcoholism, accidents and injuries, suicides, homicides, hypertension, obesity, anemia, malnutrition, and gastrointestinal hemorrhage. The moderate intake of alcohol and its possible protective effects against cardiovascular disease remain controversial.

Research topics recommended by NIH regarding women of childbearing and middle age include contraception, infertility, osteoporosis, chronic pain, and cancer as well as the effects of ethnicity, culture, sexual orientation, socioeconomic status, and disability. Research in the effects of access to screening, fitness and health education, contraception, infertility, low birth weight babies, infant mortality rates, premature labor, infectious diseases and STDs, premenstrual syndrome, substance abuse, mental health, pharmacodynamics of drugs in women, postpartum depression, violence, endometriosis, in different racial and ethnic groups is recommended. In addition, research

on poverty, health of urban women, and women with disabilities are priorities (NIH, 1999).

Mature Years

While many women aged 65 and over lead full and productive lives, statistics show that women in this age group die at a rate that is almost seven times higher than women 45 to 64 years of age. Death of women aged 65 and over accounts for 8 of 10 female deaths annually. Heart disease is the major killer of both men and women, followed by cancer, stroke, COPD, pneumonia, diabetes, accidents, nephritis, Alzheimer's disease, and septicemia (Table 9-10).

Older women experience a significant number of chronic illnesses, including hypertension, diabetes, arthritis, digestive disorders, thyroid diseases, neurologic degenerative diseases, dementia, osteoporosis, and incontinence. Frequently, older women have multiple health problems that can be compounded by social and psychological problems including loneliness, isolation, and loss of independence (Figure 9-11). Research topics recommended by NIH regarding women in the postmenopausal years are summarized in the accompanying nursing tip. NIH research recommendations concerning the older woman include the effects of chronic diseases and disability on quality of life; longitudinal multigenerational effects of diethylstilbestrol; action and side effects of drug in relation to age, race, and ethnic group, and gender of client; the interactions of food, alcohol, tobacco, and other substances with drugs; impact of estrogen on immune, endocrine, and cardiovascular systems and on cognitive and affective

Table 9-10 Leading Causes of Death by Age and Sex for Ages 64 and Over: 1998			
Cause of Death	Deaths Per 100,000 Population		
	Both Sexes	Female	Male
All causes	5096.4	4754.9	5582.4
Heart disease	1760.6	1658.4	1906.1
Cancer	1116.8	912.7	1407.2
Stroke	404.5	438.2	356.5
COPD	284.6	240.2	347.8
Pneumonia and influenza	241.2	233.6	252.1
Diabetes	142.4	139.1	146.9
Accidents	95.9	83.2	113.9
Nephritis	65.8	59.9	74.2
Alzheimer's disease	65.2	76.7	48.7
Septicemia	55.3	56.1	54.1

Adapted from Table No. 8, National Vital Statistics Report, Vol. No. 11, July 24, 2000.

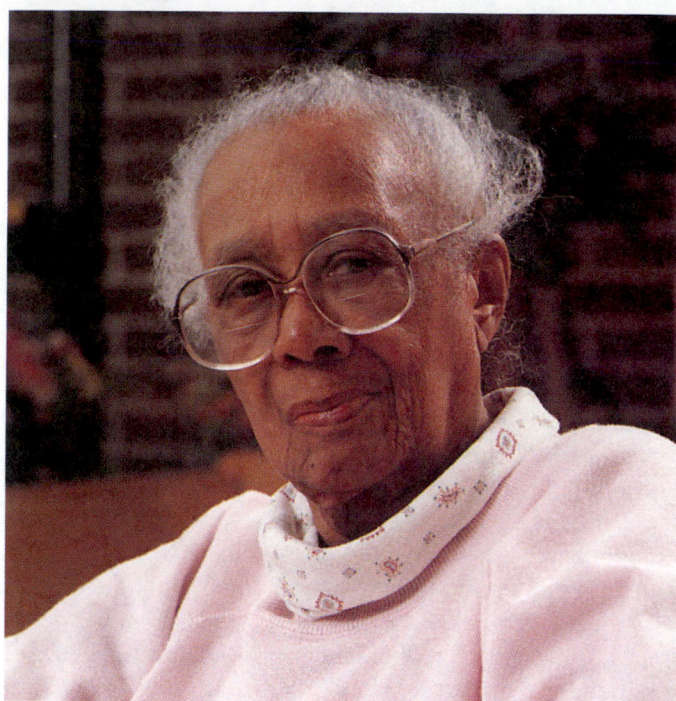

Figure 9-11 Despite health alterations, older adults often embody grace and dignity.

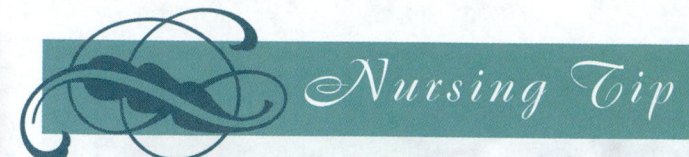

NIH RECOMMENDATIONS FOR RESEARCH CONCERNING WOMEN IN THE POSTMENOPAUSAL YEARS

- Health status of special populations
- Environmental exposures
- Epidemiology on risk factors & diseases
- Characteristics influencing health status & behaviors
- Health outcome differences in racial subgroups
- Quality of life with chronic disease
- Factors effecting breast cancer risk
- Role of menopause in aging
- Gender differences in surgical & pharmacologic treatments
- Risk factors for stroke
- Differences in prevalence of diabetes subgroups of women
- Screening tests & follow up in minority & underserved women
- Action of natural hormones in post menopausal women
- Drug use and misuse
- Gender differences in pain threshold tolerance and sensitive
- Gender & age differences in mental health effects of racism on health

processes; impact of oral health on quality of life; evaluation of effectiveness, benefits, risks and costs of alternative and complementary medicine; multisensory impairment; relationship between self-efficacy and positive self-image; functional independence and self-care; influences of spirituality on health outcomes in diverse groups; causes, consequences, and interventions related to physical and emotional violence, abuse, and traumatic stress; influence of age, culture, and socioeconomic status on health practices and receptivity to lifestyle interventions; effectiveness of health behavior interventions in different population groups; impact of living arrangements (independent, group, familial, or institutional) and health care decisions; effectiveness of interventions for incontinence, falls, depression, anxiety, cognitive impairment, insomnia, and violence; medication use and polypharmacy; patterns of alcohol and drug abuse of subpopulations across the sociocultural spectrum; models of providing care and caregivers; interactions among women and caregivers of different culture, age, socioeconomic status, and racial and ethnic group; barriers to care of the homebound and disabled; inclusion of the oldest old and institutionalized clients in studies; attitudes toward death as a function of ethnicity, culture, and age; end-of-life decisions, including end-of-life care; cultural and ethnic backgrounds and their influences on end-of-life decisions; managing death and ethnic and cultural differences regarding pain management, family support, place of death, dignity, and assisted dying; and quality of dying and ways to improve the end of life for women and caregivers (NIH, 1999).

HEALTH PROMOTION AND DISEASE PREVENTION

In recent years, health promotion has become a major goal for the U.S. and many other countries of the world. The World Health Organization defines **health promotion** as a process, action, program, or endeavor to obtain the goal of complete physical, mental, and social well-being. Other definitions have included concepts of self-care, health-promoting behaviors, empowerment, development of healthy lifestyles, maintenance or enhancement of well-being, and healthy environments.

Not only are there many definitions of health promotion and disease prevention, there are differing sets of preventive services recommended by government agencies, professional organizations, voluntary associations, and academic experts. However, in spite of this, there seems to be basic agreement among authorities on recommendations for the major types of preventive care. The U.S. Preventive Services Task Force (1996) published its report in the *Guide to Clinical Services,* which is widely regarded as the premiere reference source on the effectiveness of clinical preventive services, including screening tests for early detection of disease, immunizations to prevent infections, and counseling for risk reduction (U.S. Preventive Services Task Force, 1996). Recommendations of the major U.S. authorities are also summarized (USPHS, 1994). The following is a summary of the major findings and recommendations contained within the report.

Delivery of Preventive Services

Even for those services in which there is agreement that the services are necessary among all major U.S. authorities, the delivery of preventive services is less than satisfactory. In some cases, the rate of delivery of services is less than 20%. Some of the reasons for these poor rates include lack of clinician time, inadequate reimbursement, lack of clinician interest and knowledge, lack of client involvement and knowledge, and lack of office or clinic systems to promote preventive care. Effective delivery of clinical preventive services includes establishment of a preventive care protocol and implementation plan.

Types of Preventive Services

The three major types of preventive services include screening, immunization, and counseling.

Screening

Screening is the process of completing a test or examination to detect the most characteristic sign or signs of a disorder or disease that may require further investigation. Screening sensitivity and specificity and positive predictive value must be considered when evaluating and selecting screening tests. There is little value in performing screening tests without close tracking of results and the necessary follow-up testing. Analysis of screening tests must adhere to national standards for accuracy in testing and reporting of results. Clients should be clearly informed of the potential cost and side effects of necessary follow-up testing and treatment as appropriate.

Immunizations

Immunizations can prevent or postpone serious disorders. The National Vaccine Advisory Committee has set standards for childhood immunization practices, and the National Coalition for Adult Immunization has developed standards for adult immunization practices.

Counseling

The third method to implement preventive care is counseling. The U.S. Preventive Services Task Force described 10 principles for client education and counseling with which all health care professionals should be familiar. These principles include:

1. Develop a therapeutic alliance
2. Counsel all clients
3. Insure that clients understand the relationship between behavior and health
4. Work with clients to assess barriers to behavioral change
5. Gain commitment from clients to change
6. Involve clients in selecting risk factors to change
7. Use a combination of strategies
8. Design a behavior modification plan
9. Monitor progress through follow-up contact
10. Involve office staff

In addition, the counseling should be culturally appropriate. Information and services should be presented in a style and format that is sensitive to the culture, values, and traditions of the client. The services should be provided at a level of comprehension consistent with the age and learning skills of the client.

The following are recommendations for development of preventive services.

- Preventive services must become an integral part of all health services, including nursing
- Protocols for prevention must continue to be developed

Web Activities

- Visit some of the websites listed in the Resources section, such as the American Cancer Society and the American Heart Association. Using the health promotion guidelines that they post, develop a teaching plan for a woman at risk for cervical cancer and cardiovascular disease.

- Search the CDC's website for statistics on various conditions discussed in this chapter. Is geographic information also included?

- Screening must be useful, i.e. have the ability to detect conditions that are treatable, and be completed at the right time
- Screening must be acceptable to the client
- Prevalence of a condition must be sufficient to justify the cost of the screening
- Immunizations can prevent or postpone serious disorders

- Counseling is an integral component of prevention
- Nurses must continue to strive for excellence and sensitivity in providing prevention education, counseling, and screening
- Counseling must be culturally appropriate

Key Concepts

- Historically, health care research has used male subjects with little attention to health issues or conditions that affect postmenopausal women.
- Because of technologic advances and more effective prophylactic treatment for acute and chronic diseases, both women and men will live longer in the next century.

- The leading cause for mortality in women is heart disease, followed by cancer and stroke, which account for two-thirds of all deaths among women.
- Factors that put women at increased risk of mortality and morbidity are smoking, obesity, and sedentary lifestyle. Prevention strategies to minimize these factors are essential.

Review Questions and Activities

1. Women's health relates to all of the following except:
   a. Reproductive conditions of women
   b. Diseases and conditions unique to women or more prevalent, more serious, or differently expressed in women than in men
   c. Prevention, risk assessment, health promotion, early diagnosis, treatment based on genetics, culture, biology, economics, and psychological development of women
   d. Socioeconomic status of men

   The correct answer is d.

2. The Office of Research and Women's Health has as its mission all of the following except:
   a. Promotion of healthy behavior in women
   b. Improvement of health of minority women
   c. Recruitment of women for legislative positions
   d. Provision of greater access to health services for women

   The correct answer is c.

3. The Women's Health Initiative is a:
   a. 10-year study of breast cancer
   b. Clinical trial to study cardiovascular drugs in women
   c. Longitudinal study of nurses
   d. 15-year study of major diseases and conditions of postmenopausal women

   The correct answer is d.

4. Life expectancy in the U.S. is:
   a. Decreasing faster in the last 10 years than ever before
   b. Longer for men than women
   c. Longer for women than men
   d. Higher for African American women than Caucasian women

   The correct answer is c.

5. Birth rates in the United States are:
   a. Increasing in married adolescents
   b. Increasing since 1950
   c. Increasing in women over 30 years of age
   d. Similar for African American and Caucasian women

   The correct answer is c.

6. The highest birth rates are occurring in:
   a. African Americans
   b. Caucasians
   c. Hispanics
   d. Asians

   The correct answer is c.

7. The two leading causes of death for both sexes are:
   a. Heart disease and stroke
   b. Cancer and stroke
   c. Heart disease and cancer
   d. Heart disease and accidents

   The correct answer is c.

8. Heart disease in women:
   a. Occurs more frequently than in men at all ages
   b. Decreases slightly after age 65
   c. Increases after menopause, with an incidence similar to that in men by age 75
   d. Occurs more frequently in Caucasian women than African American women

   The correct answer is c.

9. Knowledge about cardiovascular disease in women is deficient because:
   a. Most studies on heart disease were completed in the 1960s and 1970s
   b. Lipid levels in women have never been standardized
   c. Women refused to participate in drug studies
   d. Most studies have been conducted on middle-aged men

   The correct answer is d.

10. Accidents are the leading cause of death in women in all of these age groups except:
    a. 5 to 14 years
    b. 15 to 24 years
    c. 25 to 44 years
    d. 45 to 64 years

    The correct answer is d.

11. Cancer deaths in the United States are:
    a. Increasing in men and decreasing in women
    b. Decreasing in men and increasing in women
    c. Increasing in both men and women
    d. Decreasing in both men and women

    The correct answer is d.

12. The leading cause of cancer deaths in women is:
    a. Lung
    b. Cervical
    c. Ovarian
    d. Breast

    The correct answer is a.

13. Lung cancer in women is:
    a. Decreasing because of a decrease in smoking habits of women
    b. Increasing because of an increase in smoking habits of women
    c. Difficult to treat, but easy to detect
    d. Less important as a cause of death in women than breast cancer

    The correct answer is b.

14. Risk factors for breast cancer include:
    a. Family history
    b. History of HPV infection
    c. Early menopause

    d. Low-fat diet

    The correct answer is a.

15. Most women with breast cancer are all of the following except:
    a. Over the age of 50
    b. Likely to have no known risk factors
    c. Likely to have a good prognosis if the cancer is detected early
    d. Likely to have another type of cancer before the diagnosis of breast cancer

    The correct answer is d.

16. Ovarian cancer is:
    a. Common among young African American women
    b. Easy to detect with the pap smear
    c. Likely to carry a good prognosis once it is detected
    d. Frequently detected late in its course

    The correct answer is d.

17. Cancer prevention programs for women include all of the following except:
    a. Smoking cessation
    b. Periodic screening
    c. Bone density index measurement
    d. Elimination of unopposed estrogen use for menopause

    The correct answer is c.

18. Chronic diseases that women experience more frequently than men are:
    a. Diabetes, osteoporosis, arthritis
    b. HIV infection, homicide, pneumonia
    c. Alcoholism, cirrhosis, COPD
    d. Asthma, ulcers, bronchitis

    The correct answer is a.

19. The following statements are true regarding osteoporosis *except:*
    a. It effects one-third to one-half of postmenopausal women
    b. It increases as women age
    c. It puts women at high risk for hip fractures
    d. It occurs as a result of arthritis

    The correct answer is d.

20. Depression in women:
    a. Occurs less frequently than in men
    b. Tends to be treated in only about 75% of women with the condition
    c. Is twice as likely to occur in women than men
    d. Is easy to treat with psychotropic drugs developed in research on women

    The correct answer is c.

References

Abma, J. C., Chandra, A., Mosher, W. D., Peterson, L., & Piccinino, L. (1997). Fertility, family planning, and women's health: New data from the 1995 National Survey of Family Growth. National Center for Health Statistics, Vital Health Statistics, 23(19).

American Cancer Society. (1998). *Cancer facts and figures—1998*. Atlanta, GA: Author.

American Cancer Society. (2000). *Cancer facts and figures—2000*. Atlanta, GA: Author.

Blumenthal, S. J. (1994). Advancing women's health. Washington, DC: Public Health Service.

Bonnick, S. L. (1994). *Every women's guide to prevention and treatment: The osteoporosis handbook.* Dallas, TX: Taylor Publishing Co.

Center for Disease Control and Prevention. (2000) National Vital Statistics. Vol 48, 11 July 2.

Centers for Disease Control and Prevention. (1994). Mortality patterns: U.S., 1992. *Morbidity and Mortality Weekly Report, 43,* (40), 916–920.

Cohen, M. (1997). Natural history of HIV infection in women. *Obstetrics and Gynecology Clinics of North America, 24,* (8), 743–758.

DiMona, L., & Herndon, C. (1994). Work. In L. DiMona & C. Herndon (Eds.), *Women's Source Book,* (p. 47–131). Boston: Houghton Mifflin.

Food and Drug Administration. (1993, July 22). Guidelines for the study and evaluation of gender differences in clinical evaluation of drugs. *Federal Register, 58* (139), 39406–39414.

Foster, J. C. (1994). A woman's health agenda. *Holistic Nurse Practice, 8,* 74–88.

Grabrick, D. M., Hartmann, L. C. Cerhan, J. R., Vierkant, R. A., Therneau, T. M., Vachon, C. N., Olsen, J. E. Couch, F. J., Anderson, K. C., Pankratz, V. S. & Sellers, T. A. (2000). Risk of breast cancer with oral contraceptive use in women with family history of breast cancer. *The Journal of the American Medical Association, 284,* (14), 1791–1798.

Harper, A. C., & Lambert, L. J. (1994). *The health of population: an introduction.* (2nd ed.) New York: Springer.

Hennekens, C. H. (1989). Steering Committee of the Physicians' Health Study Research Group: Final report on the aspirin component of the ongoing physicians' health study. *New England Journal of Medicine, 321,* 129–135.

Magrane, D. M., & McIntyre-Seltman, K. (1996). Women's health care issues for medical students: An education proposal. *Women's Health Issues, 6,* 4, 184–191.

National Center for Health Statistics. (1992). *Health, United States, 1990* (DHHS Pub No. (PHS) 91-1232) Hyattsville, MD: Public Health Service.

National Centers for Health Statistics. (1998). *Births of Hispanic origin, 1989–1995.* Washington, DC: Author.

National Institutes of Health. (1994). *Women's health initiative.* Bethesda, MD: Author.

National Institutes of Health. (1999). *Agenda for research on women's health for the 21st century.* Bethesda, MD: Author.

Office of Research on Women's Health. (1992). *Report of the National Institutes of Health: Opportunities for research on women's health.* (NIH Publication No. 92-3457). Washington, DC: Author.

Rodin, J., & Ickovics, J. R. (1990). Women's health: Review and research agenda as we approach the 21st century. *American Psychologist, 45,* 1018–1034.

Tauber, C. (1992). *Statistical handbook on women in America.* Phoenix, AZ: Oryx Press.

Shimp, L. A., & Peggs, J. F. (2000). Urinary incontinence. In *Women's Health Care* M. A. Smith & L. A. Shimp Eds. New York: McGraw-Hill.

The Multiple Risk Factor Intervention Trial. (1990). Mortality rates after 10.5 years for participants in the Multiple Risk Factor Intervention Trial: Findings related to a prior hypotheses of the trial. *Journal of the American Medical Association, 2* (63), 1795–1801.

U.S. Bureau of the Census. (1996). *Statistical abstract of the United States: 1996* (116th ed.), Washington, DC: Author.

U.S. Bureau of the Census. (1999). *Statistical abstract of the United States: 1999* (119th ed.), Washington, DC: Author.

U.S. Department of Health and Human Services. Public Health Services. (1994). *Women's health:* report of the Public Health Service Task Force on women's health issues. Vol. II. Washington, DC: Author.

U.S. Department of Health and Human Services, Center for Disease Control and Prevention, National Center for Health Statistics. (2000). *Deaths: Final data for 1998.* Vol. 48, Number 11. Washington, DC: Author.

U.S. Department of Health and Human Services. Office on Women's Health. (2000). *Women's health issues: An overview.* Washington, DC: Author.

U.S. Preventive Services Task Force. (1996). *Guide to clinical preventive services.* 2nd ed. Baltimore: Williams & Wilkins.

U.S. General Accounting Office. (1992). Report to Congressional requesters. *Women's health: FDA needs to ensure more study of gender differences in prescription drug testing.* Washington, DC: Author.

Wentz, A. C. (1994). Women's health issues. In *Advances in internal medicine.* Vol. 40. (pp. 1–28). St Louis: Mosby Year Book, Inc.

Wingo, P. A., Ries, L. A., Rosenberg, H. M., Miller, D. S., & Edwards, B. K. (1998). Cancer incidence and mortality, 1973–1995. *Cancer, 82:*1197–1207.

Wojcik, B. E. (1998). Breast cancer survival varies by race. *Cancer, 82:*1310–1318.

Women's Health Report of the Public Health Task Force on Women's Health Issues. (1985). *Public Health Report, 1:*74–106.

Wertz, R. W. & Wertz, D. C. (1977). *Lyinginia is a history of childbirth in America.* New York: Schoken Books.

Suggested Readings

Mosca, L., Manson, J. E., Southerland, S. E., Lange, R., Manolio, T., & Barret-Conner, E. (1997). American Heart Association Medical/Scientific Statement. *Cardiovascular disease in women: A statement for healthcare professionals from the American Heart Association. Circulation, 96:*(7), 2468–2482.

Wong, C., Froelicher, E., Bacchetti, F., Barron, H., Gee, L., Selby, J., Lundstrom, R., Swain, B., & Truman, A. (1997). Influence of Gender on Cardiovascular Mortality in Acute Myocardial Infarction Patients with high indications for Coronary Angiopathy. *Circulation, 96,* (9 Supplement) 51II–57II.

Resources

Agency for Health Care Research and Quality, 2101 E. Jefferson St., Suite 501, Rockville, MD 20852, Ph: 301-594-1364, Address: http://www.ahcpr.gov

American Cancer Society (ACS), 1599 Clifton Road, NE., Atlanta, GA 30329-4251, Ph: 404-320-333, 1-800-227-2345, Address: http://www.cancer.org

American Heart Association, 7272 Greenville Ave., Dallas, TX 75231-4596, Ph: 214-373-6300, 1-800-242-1793, Address: http://www.amhrt.org

Cansearch: A Guide to Cancer Resources, Address: http://www.cansearch.org/canserch/canserch.htm

Centers for Disease Control and Prevention, 1600 Clifton Rd., Atlanta, GA 30333, Ph: 404-639-3311, 1-800-311-3435, Address: http://www.cdc.gov

Food and Drug Administration, FDA, HFI-40, Rockville, MD 20857, Ph: 1-888-463-6332, Address: http://www.fda.gov

Health and Human Services, 200 Independence Avenue, S.W., Washington, DC 20201, Ph: 202-619-0257, 1-877-696-6775, Address: http://www.os.dhhs.gov

HealthSeek, Address: http://www.healthseek.com

Journal of the National Cancer Institute, Oxford University Press, Journals Subscription Department, Great Clarendon Street, Oxford OX2 6DP, U.K., Address: http://jnci.oupjournals.org

Medical/Health Sciences Libraries, Hardin Library for the Health Sciences, 600 Newton Rd., University of Iowa, Iowa City, IA 52242-1098, Ph: 319-335-9871, Address: http://www.arcade.uiowa.edu/hardin-www/hslibs.html

MEDLINE Search Tools, Address: http://www.medsitenavigator.com/medicine/medline.html

Morbidity and Mortality Weekly Report, John W. Ward, M.D., Editor Epidemiology Program Office MS C-08, Centers for Disease Control and Prevention, 1600 Clifton Rd., Atlanta, GA 30333, Fax: 404-639-4198, Address: http://www.cdc.gov/mmwr/

National Cancer Institute (NCI) CancerNet, Public Inquiries Office, Building, 31, Room 10A03, 31 Center Drive, MSC 2580, Bethesda, MD 20892-2580, Ph: 301-435-3848, 1-800-4-Cancer, Address: http://www.icic.nci.nih.gov/patient.html

National Center for Health Statistics, National Center for Health Statistics, Division of Data Services, 6525 Belcrest Road, Hyattsville, MD 20782-2003, Ph: 301-458-4636, Address: http://www.cdc.gov/nchs

National Institutes of Health, 9000 Rockville Pike, Bethesda, MD 20814, Ph: 301-496-4000, Address: http://www.nih.gov

National Library of Medicine, 8600 Rockville Pike, Bethesda, MD 20894, Ph: 888-346-3556, Address: http://www.nlm.nih.gov

NursingNet, Address: http://www.nursingnet.org

Occupational Safety and Health Administration, Office of Public and Consumer Affairs, US Department of Labor, Room N3637, 200 Constitution Ave NW, Washington, DC 20210, Ph: 202-523-8148, Address: http://www.osha.gov

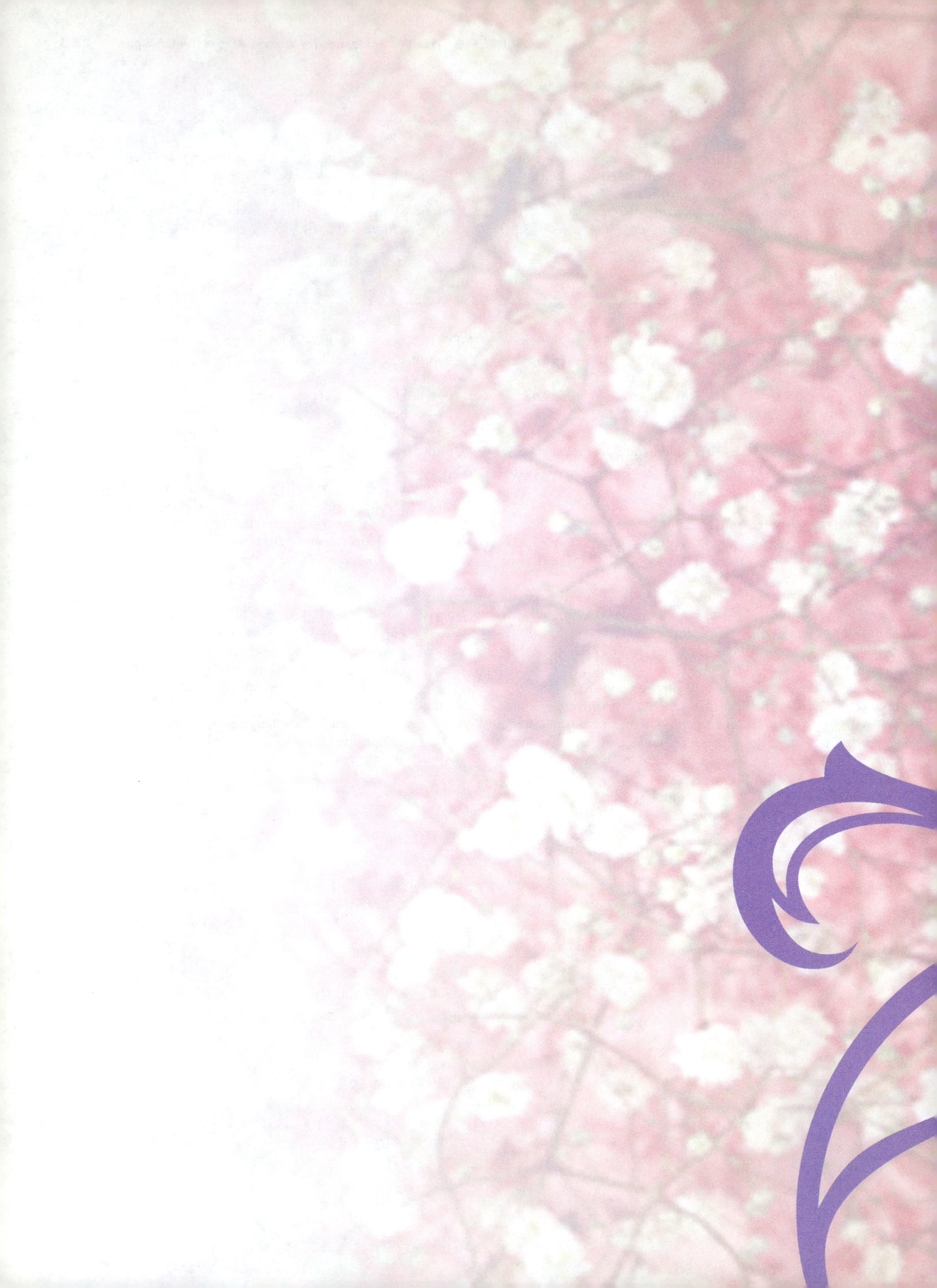

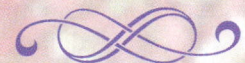

CHAPTER 10

Common Conditions of the Reproductive System

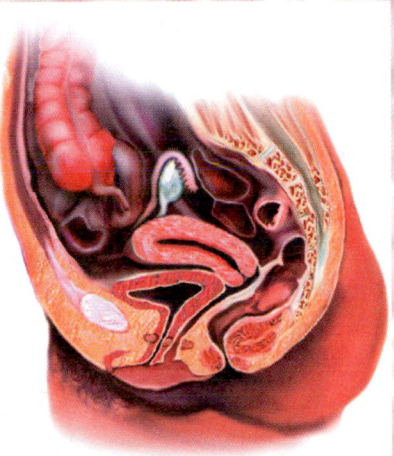

Working with women who have conditions affecting the reproductive system is both challenging and rewarding. The process is challenging because creative solutions to daily health care concerns are required, and rewarding because helping women focus on individual health promotion activities enables families to focus on health promotion. To get the most out of each encounter with a woman in your care, you should gauge the awareness of her home environment, gauge your comfort level with her decision making regarding her health care, and be content to work on one condition or concern at a time. You may find the following questions helpful in determining your feelings and values regarding these conditions:

- *How do you feel toward a woman who repeatedly has sexually transmitted infections?*

- *What is your reaction toward a woman who chooses to purchase cigarettes instead of an annual "Pap" smear or healthy food?*

- *How will you provide high-quality care to a woman who is a single mother with several children, all of whom have a different father?*

- *Are you willing to facilitate health promotion for a woman who does not make the same choices for her health as you would?*

- *How would you react toward a woman who says she must ask her husband or partner if she can undertake a prescribed therapy?*

- *What is your reaction toward a woman who repeatedly comes into the health care facility with the same modifiable health problem, such as a vaginal infection, because of poor hygiene habits?*

Key Terms

Amenorrhea	False discharge	Nipple discharge	Premature ovarian failure
Cervical cancer	Fibroadenoma	Osteoporosis	Premenstrual syndrome
Cervical infection	Fibrocystic changes	Ovarian cancer	(PMS)
Dysfunctional uterine	Fibroid tumor	Pathologic discharge	Primary amenorrhea
bleeding (DUB)	Invasive breast cancer	Pelvic inflammatory	Primary dysmenorrhea
Dysmenorrhea	Lactational discharge	disease (PID)	Secondary amenorrhea
Endometrial cancer	Localized breast cancer	Pelvic relaxation	Secondary
Endometriosis	Mastectomy	Physiologic discharge	dysmenorrhea
Estrogen deficiency	Menopause	Polycystic ovarian	Vaginal infection
vulvovaginitis	Metastatic breast cancer	syndrome	

Competencies

Upon completion of this chapter, the reader should be able to:

1. Define each woman's reproductive health issue as addressed in the chapter.
2. Describe subjective and objective data, laboratory test results, and procedure result data for women's reproductive health conditions.
3. Discuss usual therapeutic interventions for women's reproductive health conditions.
4. Identify risk factors for women's reproductive health conditions.
5. Discuss the nursing process steps appropriate for each women's reproductive health condition.

omen are living longer now than ever before. Thus, a woman can expect to experience a variety of health conditions resulting from the aging process, as well as the normal physiologic "wear and tear" that occurs on a daily basis. Women can realistically expect to live into their 80's, and they want to have a high quality of life throughout their life span. Women traditionally have been the "keepers" of health for themselves and family members. Although women may have tended to ignore personal health conditions in the past, more women are now recognizing the need to attend to personal health, especially if conditions prevent them from maintaining their quality of life or from being able to meet the responsibilities of caring for loved ones. Nurses can facilitate the achievement of women's goals for quality of life by assessing their clients' health conditions and developing an individualized plan to reduce the adverse effects of disease. Conditions of the female reproductive system can be classified as common deviations from the usual pattern and occur from puberty to beyond menopause. Conditions addressed in this chapter include menstrual, mammary, pelvic, and menopausal conditions.

MENSTRUAL CYCLE ABNORMALITIES

In general, abnormal conditions of the menstrual cycle are deviations from what is normal for an individual woman. The condition may occur in the frequency or length of the cycle, volume or length of menstrual flow, or the total number of years of menstruation.

Menstrual cycle conditions are a readily noticeable concern. Common conditions may be classified as amenorrhea, dysfunctional or abnormal uterine bleeding, dysmenorrhea, endometriosis, or premenstrual syndrome. Refer to Table 10-1 for a list of menstrual cycle conditions and to Table 10-2 for therapeutic interventions for menstrual cycle conditions. Box 10-1 lists additional alterations in menstrual cycle function.

Amenorrhea

Amenorrhea is the absence or lack of menses during the reproductive years. Normal causes of amenorrhea include pregnancy, lactation, and menopause. Other causes can be pathologic and may include stress, excessive exercise, eating disorders, weight loss, a low body mass index (BMI),

Table 10-1 Menstrual Cycle Conditions

Condition	Data		
	Subjective	Objective	Laboratory or Procedure
Amenorrhea			
Primary amenorrhea	No menarche	Secondary sex characteristics	Thyroid function tests
			Blood glucose level
		Reproductive tract anomalies	Karyotype (Turner syndrome)
			Laparoscopy (ovarian pathology)
Secondary amenorrhea	3 or more missed menstrual periods	Previous gynecologic procedures or problems	Decreased thyroid function tests
	Menstrual pattern	Weight gain or loss	Increased Blood glucose level
		Major life events	Increased Serum prolactin level
		Exercise level	Laporoscopy to detect polycystic ovary syndrome
		Thyroid size	Ultrasound to detect ovarian cysts
		Exophthalmia	
		Moon facies	
		Hirsutism	
		Delayed deep tendon reflexs	
		Breast atrophy	
		Thinning hair	
		Temporal baldness	
Abnormal or Dysfunctional Uterine Bleeding			
Bleeding between menstrual periods	Possible uterine abnormality	Anemia	Low thyroid function, pituitary function (FSH or LH)
	Irregular bleeding	Pregnancy test	hCG studies (for anovulation)
	Heavy bleeding	CBC, Complete Blood Count for anemia or infection	Increased prolactin level
	Prolonged bleeding	Ultrasound	
	Light bleeding	Endometrial biopsy to rule out endometrial cancer	
	Short or long cycles		
Dysmenorrhea			
Primary dysmenorrhea	Mild to severe cramping, lasting from 2–4 days before menses to third day of menses	Nulliparity	Ultrasound
	GI symptoms: bloating, nausea, vomiting	Age (adolescence to early 20s)	
	Back, thigh, and headache pain	Normal results on physical examination	
	Family history		
Secondary dysmenorrhea	Increasingly painful menses	Third or fourth decade of life	Elevated WBC count if STD or PID is present
	Dyspareunia	Endometriosis	Cultures for Gonorrhea and Chlamydia
	Painful defecation	PID, STD	Ultrasound
	Rectal pressure	Increased uterine size	Laparoscopy (endometriosis)
	Heavy or irregular bleeding	Endometritis	
		Salpingitis	
		Leiomyomata	

(continued)

Table 10-1 Menstrual Cycle Conditions (*continued*)

Condition	Data Subjective	Objective	Laboratory or Procedure
Endometriosis			
Dysmenorrhea	Infertility Cyclic dyspareunia Dyschezia GI symptoms Pelvic heaviness Chronic pelvic pain (may radiate to thighs) Abnormal bleeding	Uterus may be fixed Possible adenexal mass(es) Pelvic tenderness	Ultrasound monitoring of implants Laparoscopy
Premenstrual syndrome			

Cluster of symptoms
  at luteal phase
	Depressed mood
	Mood swings
	Irritability
	Difficulty in concentration
	  or coping
	Fatigue
	Edema
	Breast tenderness
	Headache (premenstrual)
	Sleep disturbances
	Abdominal bloating
	Increased appetite
	Weight gain
	Food cravings
	Acne
	Heart palpitations
	Anxiety
	Hostility
		Signs of stress
		Emotional lability
			None

or other potentially life-threatening disorders. Amenorrhea can be classified as primary or secondary.

Primary Amenorrhea

Primary amenorrhea is the absence of menarche until age 16 or the absence of the development of secondary sex characteristics and menarche until age 14 (Keene, 1999). Causes of primary amenorrhea may involve hypothalamic, pituitary, enzymatic, or chromosomal abnormalities; genitourinary tract abnormalities; or drug therapy. The primary symptom is failure to experience menarche when there has been development of secondary sex characteristics or without such development as in Turner syndrome. Therapeutic intervention depends on the cause of primary amenorrhea and usually includes estrogen replacement therapy (ERT) to prevent osteoporosis or to stimulate development of secondary sexual characteristics.

Secondary Amenorrhea

Secondary amenorrhea is the absence of menses for at least 6 months or for three cycles after menarche (Keene, 1999; McGee, 1997). Secondary amenorrhea is more common than primary amenorrhea and is often caused by physiologic responses to pregnancy, lactation, or anovulation. (Keene, 1999). In addition to absence of menses, the woman may have diseases related to endocrine dysfunction that are causing the secondary amenorrhea, such as hypothyroidism, hyperthyroidism, adrenal disease, chronic hepatic disease, chronic renal disease, or polycystic ovary syndrome. Women athletes who train vigorously or women with anorexia often experience secondary amenorrhea because of the affects of the relationship of height and weight, percentage of body fat, and malnutrition on the hypothalamic-pituitary-ovarian axis. Therapeutic intervention for secondary amenorrhea includes cyclic proges-

Table 10-2 Management of Menstrual Conditions

Condition	Usual Therapeutic Interventions
Amenorrhea	
Primary amenorrhea	Hymenectomy for imperforate hymen
	Nutritional correction of low BMI
	Hormone replacement for endocrine dysfunctions
Secondary amenorrhea	Nutritional correction for high or low BMI
	Estrogen and/or progesterone replacement therapy
	Thyroid hormone replacement therapy
Dysfunctional or abnormal uterine bleeding	
	Hormone replacement therapy (OCPs, combined estrogen and progestin therapy, progestin therapy alone)
	Iron supplements for anemia
	Possible laser ablation of endometrium
Dysmenorrhea	
Primary dysmenorrhea	NSAIDs or prostaglandin synthetase inhibitors
	OCPs
Secondary dysmenorrhea	Antibiotics for infection
	Treatment specific to underlying cause
Endometriosis	
	NSAIDs
	Surgical removal or ablation of endometrial implants
	GnRH agonists
	Medroxyprogesterone (Provera)
	Continuous OCP therapy
Premenstrual syndrome	
	Education regarding syndrome
	Stress reduction techniques
	Regular exercise
	Smoking cessation
	Regular sleep habits
	Support groups
	Regular, balanced meals with low intake of sodium and caffeine
	Diuretic agent at time of symptoms
	NSAIDs
	Prostaglandin synthetase inhibitors
	Selective serotonin reuptake inhibitors (SSRIs)
	OCPs
	GnRH agonist (extremely severe symptoms)

terone, when the cause is anovulation; oral contraceptives, for the woman who desires contraception; bromocriptine, when the woman is experiencing hyperprolactinemia; gonadotropin-releasing hormone (GnRH), when the cause is hypothalamic failure; and thyroid hormone replacement therapy, when the cause is hypothyroidism. In addition, the woman who is hypoestrogenic is given calcium and ERT to prevent development of osteoporosis.

Dysfunctional Uterine Bleeding

Dysfunctional uterine bleeding (DUB) is "any significant deviation from the usual menstrual pattern" (Keene, 1999, p. 75). DUB occurs more often in adolescents and perimenopausal women. An estimated 20% of women seek therapeutic intervention at some point in their lives for

Box 10-1 Menstrual Cycle Alterations

- Hypermenorrhea or menorrhagia: Excessive menstrual bleeding, either in duration or amount, during regularly occurring menstrual cycles
- Hypomenorrhea: Decreased menstrual bleeding, either in duration or amount, occurring at regular intervals
- Intermenstrual bleeding: Irregular vaginal bleeding, usually not caused by menses and not excessive in amounts, occurring between regular menstrual cycles
- Menometrorrhagia: A combination of menorrhagia and metrorrhagia. Irregular, frequent, possibly excessive, or prolonged vaginal bleeding, which may or may not be menstrual.
- Oligomenorrhea: Light menstrual bleeding or infrequent menses, which occur in cycles at least 35 days apart
- Polymenorrhea: Frequent menses that occur in cycles no more than 21 days apart

DUB (Smith, 1998). The differences from the usual bleeding pattern may include hypermenorrhea and menorrhagia, intermenstrual bleeding and metrorrhagia, menometrorrhagia, oligomenorrhea, polymenorrhea, or hypomenorrhea.

Causes of DUB include hormonal abnormalities, such as anovulation; pregnancy-associated events; pelvic inflammatory disease (PID); trauma; neoplasm; endometriosis; and anatomic or systemic disease.

A woman may report characteristics of oligomenorrhea when she experiences a scant amount of menstrual bleeding or cycles more than 35 days apart. Therapeutic interventions include:

- Oral contraceptives for menstrual cycle control
- Administration of high doses of estrogen and progesterone to produce therapy withdrawal bleeding (pharmaceutical dilation and curettage)
- Cyclic progesterone therapy for chronic anovulatory bleeding
- Nonsteroidal anti-inflamatory drugs (NSAIDS) to reduce the amount of menstrual bleeding
- Endometrial ablation to decrease or eliminate menstrual bleeding by eliminating the tissue sloughing
- Hysterectomy, when abnormal uterine bleeding cannot be corrected by more conservative methods

Dysmenorrhea

Dysmenorrhea is painful menses or cramping during menstruation. Typically dysmenorrhea begins up to 48 hours before onset of menses and resolves within 2 to 4 days of onset or by the end of the menstrual period (Ugarriza, Klinger, & O'Brien, 1998). Dysmenorrhea can be classified as primary or secondary.

Primary Dysmenorrhea

Primary dysmenorrhea is painful menses with a uterine cause, but without pelvic pathology, and usually occurs within 1 to 3 years of menarche (Ugarriza et al., 1998). Painful uterine contractions stimulated by prostaglandin produced by the endometrium during menses are most often identified as the cause for primary dysmenorrhea. Symptoms of primary dysmenorrhea may include sharp, intermittent suprapubic pain radiating to the back or thighs; headache; fatigue; backache; flushing; dizziness; and syncope. Typically, adolescents do not experience dysmenorrhea until menstrual cycles become ovulatory. Women often experience reduction in dysmenorrhea after pregnancy. Therapeutic intervention for primary dysmenorrhea are directed toward reduction of symptoms and include NSAIDs started 1 to 3 days before the onset of menstrual flow (to decrease prostaglandin production) and oral contraceptives, to decrease endometrial proliferation and, therefore, the amount of prostaglandin produced by the endometrium.

Secondary Dysmenorrhea

Secondary dysmenorrhea is painful menses resulting from a pathologic process, such as pressure from outside the uterus, tissue ischemia, cervical stenosis, congenital abnormality (imperforate hymen), endometriosis, ovarian cysts, PID, or uterine fibroid tumors (Ugarriza et al., 1998). Symptoms may begin earlier in the cycle and last longer than the symptoms of primary dysmenorrhea, with specific symptoms other than pain. These symptoms can include breast tenderness and a change in bowel habits. Therapeutic intervention usually involves correction of the cause.

Endometriosis

Endometriosis is a chronic disorder resulting from the implantation of endometrial tissue outside the uterus. Pelvic sites of endometrial tissue implantation include the cervix, cul-de-sac, ovaries, fallopian tubes, pelvic peritoneum, uterine broad ligaments, and bowel (Figure 10-1) (Corwin, 1997). Distant sites of endometrial tissue implantation occur less commonly and can include the abdominal wall, kidneys, spleen, gallbladder, diaphragm, lung, stomach, or breasts. Each of these sites will bleed during the menstrual cycle. The disorder affects nearly one in seven women of childbearing age. Endometrial tissue, regardless of location, responds to cyclic ovarian hormone fluctuations. However, there is no place for the endometrial tissue to be sloughed off; blood shed from the endometrial tissue implants accu-

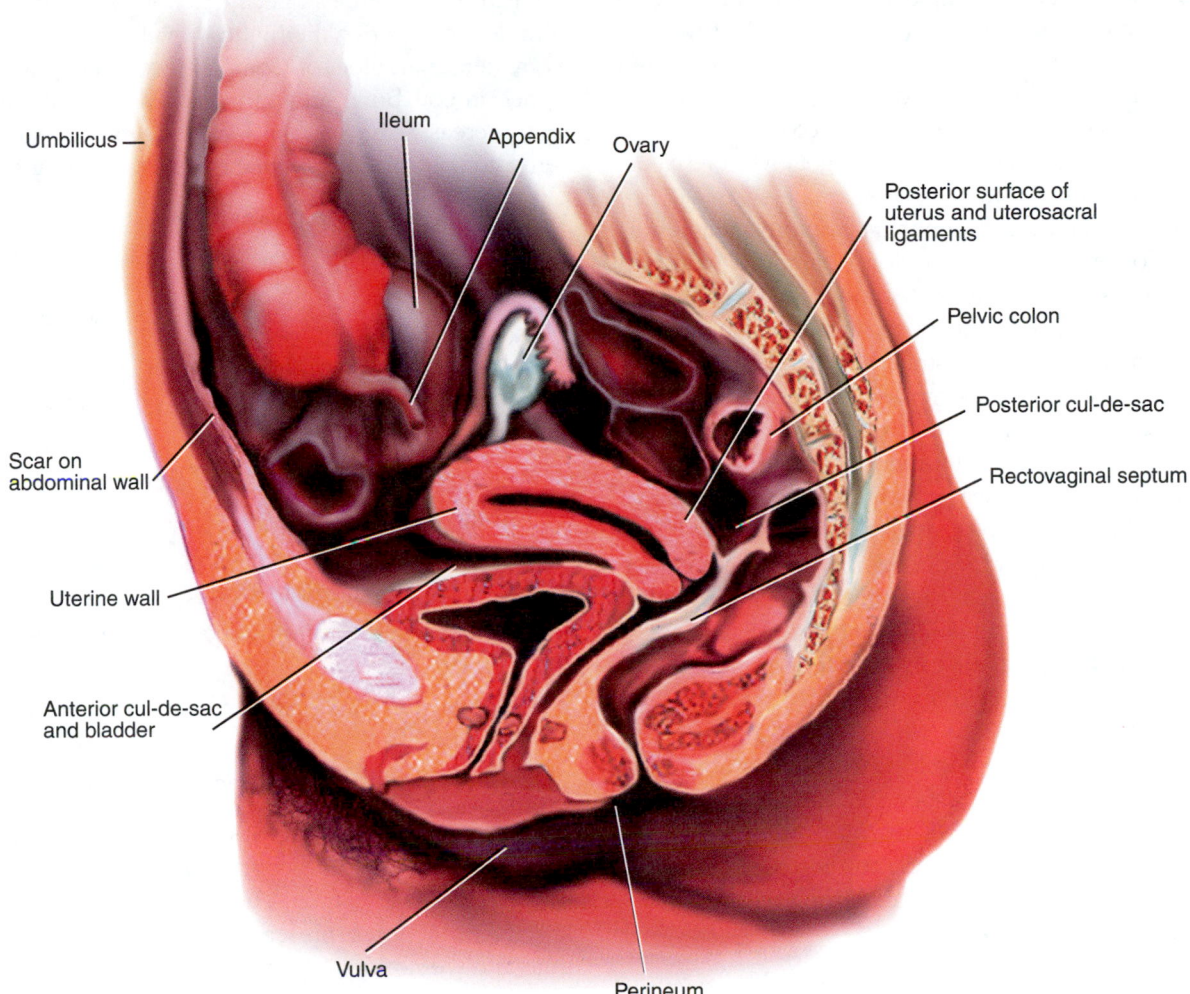

Figure 10-1 Common sites of endometriosis.

mulate locally during menses. Often, women experience short menstrual cycles (less than 28 days), increased duration of bleeding (7 days or more), excessive bleeding (for at least 5 days), and significant cramping (Corwin, 1997). The woman experiences symptoms of pain, inflammation, or pelvic heaviness, depending on the duration of the disorder, location of endometrial tissue implants, and the phases of the menstrual cycle. The intensity and duration of symptoms seem to be greater in women with more advanced disease. Such women may experience chronic pelvic pain, frequent low back pain and heaviness, dyspareunia, cyclic painful defecation or rectal bleeding, cyclic diarrhea, cyclic flank pain, or cyclic hematuria or dysuria.

Therapeutic intervention is focused on stopping the progressive destruction of pelvic organs caused by the progression of endometrial implants and preserving fertility options for the woman. Endometrial implants are removed surgically or ablated with laser or electrocautery to preserve childbearing capability. NSAIDs aid in pain control by reducing prostaglandin production by the endometrial implants during menses. In addition, temporary relief can be

achieved by continuous administration of gonadotropin-releasing hormone (GnRH) to prevent release of luteinizing hormone (LH) and thus cause temporary cessation of menstruation. If suppression of menstrual cycles lasts longer than 6 months, low-dose ERT or estrogen and progesterone replacement therapy is usually begun to prevent bone loss and alleviate symptoms of menopause.

Premenstrual Syndrome

Premenstrual syndrome (PMS) is a cyclic cluster of behavioral, emotional, and physical symptoms that occur during the luteal phase of the menstrual cycle. The symptoms must be sufficiently severe to interrupt normal activity before the diagnosis can be made (Ugarriza et al., 1998). The cause is unknown but is thought to be related to hormonal changes. Since 1987, PMS has been recognized as a mental disorder (Ugarriza et al., 1998). For most women with PMS, symptoms are noticed from 2 to 12 days before the onset of menses and resolve within 24 hours of the onset of menses and vary in severity. An estimated

30% to 40% of women of childbearing age are believed to experience PMS to some degree (Ugarriza et al., 1998).

Women may experience one or more of the recognized symptoms, which can be classified as affective, autonomic, behavioral, neurologic, cognitive, dermatologic, a result of fluid or electrolyte imbalances, neurovegetative, or algetic. Affective symptoms include sadness, anxiety, anger, irritability, and mood swings. Cognitive symptoms manifest as decreased concentration, indecision, paranoia, rejection sensitivity, and suicidal ideation. Autonomic symptoms include nausea, diarrhea, palpitations, and perspiration. Behavioral symptoms are demonstrated by decreased motivation, poor impulse control, decreased efficiency, and social isolation. Clumsiness, seizures, dizziness, paresthesias (numbness or tingling), and tremors are the neurologic symptoms. Dermatologic symptoms are acne or greasy or dry hair. Fluid or electrolyte imbalances may cause bloating, weight gain, oliguria, or edema. Neurovegetative symptoms include insomnia, hypersomnia, anorexia, fatigue, lethargy, agitation, and libido change. Pain experienced by women with PMS can manifest as headaches, breast tenderness, and joint and muscle pain.

Therapeutic interventions for PMS are designed to achieve alleviation of symptoms, since PMS is not a disease. No single treatment has been effective. Women are taught to modify diet, increase exercise, alleviate stress, and change activities of daily living to reduce the intensity of symptoms, reduce fatigue, enhance the ability to sleep, and reduce stress.

Nursing Implications

Nursing assessment for menstrual conditions involves careful medical and gynecologic history taking, assessment of symptoms, and assessment for specific suspected conditions. The interview should begin with a discussion of medical and gynecologic history and lifestyle behaviors, which permit establishment of rapport before asking more personal questions specific to characteristics of the menstrual cycle. The physical assessment focuses on collection of data regarding the suspected menstrual cycle abnormality, including collection of laboratory test samples and specimens.

The nursing diagnosis can be formulated once the condition is identified. Nursing diagnoses are individualized for the client and her condition. Applicable nursing diagnoses may include:

- Pain related to a specific menstrual condition
- Fear related to the medical diagnosis
- Anxiety related to unknown outcomes
- Deficient knowledge related to limited experience (or information) regarding (specific menstrual cycle condition)

Planning includes specific actions the woman should complete to achieve the highest level of wellness. There is a greater guarantee of compliance when plans are designed in collaboration with the client. Collaborative planning increases the woman's self-esteem and supports her sense of control. Sample planning goals may include:

- Consume correct proportions of foods recommended in the food pyramid, as evidenced by a 24-hour diet recall.
- Exercise by walking 30 minutes each day.
- Take any prescriptive medications as written.
- Understand instructions regarding prescriptive medications.
- Return to the health care facility as scheduled for follow-up visits.
- Call the health care provider if adverse effects of prescriptive medications occur.
- Call the health care provider if symptoms do not improve.
- Have questions answered to satisfy need for information.
- Understand health promotion counseling.

Nursing interventions involve educating the woman regarding the specific condition and its consequences, therapeutic intervention choices and recommendations, specific procedures, prescription medications ordered, and outcomes; emotional support; reduction of fear, anxiety, stresses, and concerns; and relief of pain, if it accompanies the condition. Nursing actions are based on knowledge of the usual symptoms, consequences, outcomes, therapeutic interventions, counseling needs, and responses of women diagnosed with the condition.

Women diagnosed with endometriosis may experience loss of self-esteem because of being unable to fulfill various role expectations (e.g., work, family, social) during cyclical periods of intense pain. In addition, such women may be concerned about retaining childbearing capabilities. Educating women with endometriosis about coping strategies, such as guided imagery, relaxation and breathing exercises, massage therapy, and exercise can improve their sense of control and self-esteem (Corwin, 1997) and reduce intensity of symptoms.

Women with PMS can be counseled to keep a calendar to identify the timing of symptoms, so that they can plan to reduce other stresses during PMS, implement strategies to reduce severity of symptoms, and develop positive coping mechanisms. Some strategies that are beneficial can include dietary changes, such as reducing intake of salt, refined sugar, chocolate, and red meat; increasing intake of complex carbohydrates (fruit and vegetables); increasing aerobic exercise (walking, aero-

Case Study/Care Plan

CLIENT WITH ENDOMETRIOSIS

A 21-year-old undergraduate student comes to the health service with the chief complaint of painful menstrual periods that require bed rest at least 1 to 2 days each cycle. The client states, "When I have my period, it hurts so bad I have to go to bed for 1 or 2 days. I can't think straight or move. I have to finish school before I can have a baby, but I don't want to wait too late to have one." Following a physical examination, she is referred for laparoscopy. The diagnosis of endometriosis is established by the laparoscopic results. The client indicates the desire for childbearing in the future.

Assessment

Nulliparity, dyspareunia, dyschezia (painful or difficult bowel movements), and irregular bleeding; laparoscopy findings show extrauterine endometrial implants.

Nursing Diagnosis

Chronic pain, related to physiologic response, secondary to endometriosis.

Expected Outcomes Client will describe the physiologic source of pain.
Client will identify days of cycle when pain begins and ends or is most intense.
Client will discuss the impact of the disease process on her life.
Client will discuss therapeutic options.

Planning Assist client in outlining care measures that will be accommodated by her lifestyle.

Nursing Interventions	Rationales
1. Explain endometriosis in simple terms.	1. Simple terms are less likely to confuse the client. More complex terms can be added later based on her knowledge.
2. Assist client in recording the intensity and timing of pain (e.g., continuous, cyclical, dull, sharp, mild, moderate, exruciating).	2. Planning must be individualized to the client to be useful and must include the client in the process.
3. Encourage discussion of the effects of the disease process on her life (class attendance, full time employment, daily activities).	3. Determining the severity of the pain facilitates useful planning and improves compliance.
4. Explain effects, side effects, indications, and outcomes of usual medications (NSAIDS, GnRH agonists, progestin, OCPs), and surgical interventions (surgical removal of implants, laser ablation of implants).	4. The nurse is responsible for providing information for the client's decision making process.

Evaluation

• Client understands that endometrial implants respond to ovarian hormones like uterine endometrium.

• Client knows to expect continuous heaviness and most intense pain during menses and for 2 days following menses.

• Client expresses frustration, nonacceptability of pain as excuse for class absence, timing of most intense pain on inconvenient days (e.g., on examination day), desire to delay childbearing until career established.

• Client states that her first treatment choice is continuous oral contraceptives and second choice is surgical removal of implants.

Client Education

Women's Health Problems

For the client to successfully achieve her outcome goals, she must know the following:

1. Expected, unexpected, and adverse effects of her medication.
2. Correct scheduling of medication according to her daily schedule.
3. Convenient reminders for taking medication (i.e., when she brushes her teeth or some other routine activity).
4. Rationale for change in lifestyle behaviors as they affect her treatment regimen.
5. Effects, outcomes, and physical sensations for all assessment procedures and treatment procedures.
6. Rationale for and recommended schedule for followup assessments.
7. Reinforcement that all medication must be taken, leftover medication must be discarded, primary provider must be informed when medication is discontinued before scheduled end of therapy, and medication must not be shared among family members or friends.

---

bics, jogging, bicycling, or swimming for 45 to 60 minutes three or four times per week); and restricting tobacco, caffeine, and alcohol intake (Ugarriza et al., 1998).

Women experiencing primary or secondary amenorrhea are at risk for premature development of osteoporosis at a time when they should be enhancing bone development for protection against postmenopausal osteoporosis. Thus, assessment of the lifestyle choices contributing to amenorrhea and subsequent counseling regarding calcium intake are essential nursing actions. Women can be taught creative ways of adding calcium to their diet while avoiding increased intake of fats. For example, skim milk, tofu, and reduced-fat or fat-free cheeses can be added to a variety of dishes, and nonfat powdered milk can be added to food (even to skim milk). Fat-free yogurt is an excellent source of calcium as well as a healthy snack.

All women can benefit from counseling regarding:

- Nutritional intake based on the food pyramid
- Exercise for cardiovascular health
- Osteoporosis prevention and maintenance of normal BMI

- Positive coping strategies for stressful situations
- Lifestyle choices to prevent disease and promote health
- Enhancement of knowledge regarding choices for therapeutic interventions

Nurses are in the ideal position to provide counseling each time a client seeks care.

Women may feel that the interventions and counseling are more personalized when the nurse takes the time to write a brief note that gives instructions specific to that woman's needs. She is more likely to read and follow those instructions.

BREAST CONDITIONS

Women's breast conditions are intimately connected with personal and social images of women. Thus, breast conditions have the potential to generate significant emotional and physiologic effects. Breast conditions tend to cause intense fear and anxiety. Some women even refuse to practice monthly breast self-examination (BSE) because of the fear of "finding something." Breast conditions can be categorized as benign or malignant. Table 10-3 lists data related to breast conditions and Table 10-4 lists therapeutic interventions.

Benign Breast Conditions

Benign breast conditions are noncancerous changes in the breast and account for the majority of breast conditions.

Client Education

Women's Health Promotion

For the client to achieve an optimal health outcome, she must be instructed regarding the following:

1. Breast self-examination (BSE), vulvar self-examination (VSE) and skin examination monthly.
2. The best time for her to perform BSE, based on her menstrual cycle status.
3. Rationale for performing BSE, VSE, and skin examinations (for skin cancer).
4. Convenient reminders to perform these examinations.
5. Strategies to protect skin from sun damage.
6. Rationale for avoiding tanning beds.

Table 10-3 Common Conditions of the Breast

Condition	Data — Subjective	Data — Objective	Data — Laboratory or Procedure
Benign Conditions			
Fibrocystic changes	Lump(s) Pain Tenderness Bilateral	Palpable, movable, rubbery, firm, smooth, distinct mass(es) Bilateral	Mammogram Ultrasound examination Fine-needle aspiration for biopsy Possibly excisional biopsy
Fibroadenoma	Lump(s) Nontender	Firm, smooth, discrete mass(es) Often bilateral	Mammogram Ultrasound examination Possibly excisional biopsy
Nipple discharge	Unilateral or bilateral discharge Pain (duct ectasia)	Multicolored or gray, thin-to-thick discharge (must be expressed) Nipple fixation Discharge from multiple ducts	Cytologic examination of discharge Hemostix (blood detection strip)
	Spontaneous discharge most often from one nipple only (intraductal) Papilloma (if multiple papillomas, discharge can be bilateral)	Serosanguinous discharge Usually one duct (unless multiple papillomas)	Cytologic examination of discharge Hemostix Surgical biopsy
	Bilateral milky discharge (galactorrhea)	Milky color From multiple ducts Possibly signs of hypothyroidism or pituitary enlargement	Visual field testing Pituitary MRI Hemostix
Malignant Conditions			
Localized cancer	Lump(s) Possibly unilateral nipple discharge	Palpable, nondiscrete, movable or fixed mass(es) Abnormal results on mammogram Nipple discharge that is bloody, serous, serosanguinous, or watery	Mammogram Ultrasound examination Biopsy Hemostix Cytologic examination of discharge
Invasive cancer	Lump(s) Possible nipple discharge	Hard, nondiscrete, fixed mass(es) Dimpling Nipple flattening or deviation (unilateral)	Mammogram Ultrasound examination Biopsy with cytologic examination Hemostix and cytology (for any discharge)
	May also incude: nipple skin change, such as itching, burning, "weeping," bleeding ulceration (Paget's disease)	Nipple discharge Peau d'orange (Figure 10–2) appearance Nipple skin changes Venous prominence (unilateral) Swelling (unilateral)	
Metastatic cancer	Lump(s) Skin changes Arthralgia Bone pain Shortness of breath Possible spontaneous nipple discharge	Masses of varying size Hard, fixed lymph nodes Dimpling the skin Skin erythema Bloody, serous, serosangiunous, or watery discharge from single duct	Biopsy Bone scan Chest x-ray film Hemostix Cytologic studies

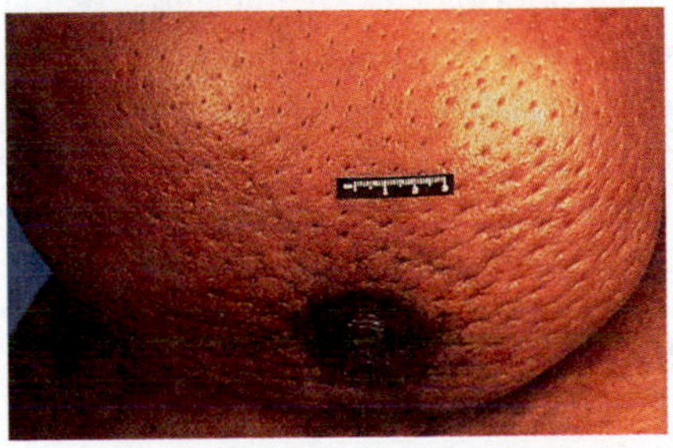

Figure 10-2 Peau d'orange

Table 10-4 Management of Conditions of the Breast

Condition	Usual Therapeutic Interventions
Benign Conditions	
Fibrocystic changes	Consider avoiding methylxanthine (caffeine) Avoid tobacco Wear well-fitting bra Diuretic agent for premenstrual symptoms Clinical breast examination annually (every 6 months if there is a familial risk for breast cancer) Baseline mammogram at age 35, every 1 to 2 years from age 40 to age 50, annually after age 50
Fibroadenoma	Excisional biopsy for solid lumps not clearly identified as benign by other methods Follow-up clinical breast examinations and mammograms (see fibrocystic changes)
Nipple discharge	Evaluation for possible malignancy Follow-up clinical breast examinations and mammograms (see fibrocystic changes) Bromocriptine (Parlodel) for galactorrhea Surgery (depending on cause)
Malignant Conditions	
Localized cancer	Radiation Lumpectomy (breast-conserving surgery)
Invasive cancer	Surgery Combination therapy: chemotherapy, hormone therapy, radiotherapy
Metastatic cancer	Combination therapy: chemotherapy, hormone therapy, radiotherapy Possibly autologous marrow transplant Consider thoracentesis and paracentesis, if shortness of breath is a symptom

For the most part, benign breast conditions are related to physiologic changes and include fibrocystic changes, fibroadenoma, and nipple discharge. Evaluation and characteristics of breast masses are outlined in Tables 10-5 and 10-6.

Fibrocystic Changes

Fibrocystic changes are age-related changes most commonly involving cyst formation and thickening of breast tissue: the result is "lumpy" breasts. The "lumps" may be tender or painful. The tenderness may be present throughout the cycle or episodic. Women who report fibrocystic changes often experience cyclic, bilateral nodularity, usually in the upper outer quadrant of the breast or in the axillia, and increased tenderness or pain before the onset of menses (Baron & Walsh, 1995). The nodularity feels like fibrous thickening or lumpiness without a clear outline and may disappear after the menstrual period. The changes are thought to be caused by estrogen and progestin changes, imbalances, or fluctuations and occur in premenopausal women or chronically in women aged 35 to 50. When the changes result from atypical hyperplasia, the woman's risk for development of breast cancer increases (White, Griffith, Nenstiel, & Dyess, 1996). There does not seem to be an association between fibrocystic nodularity and increased risk of breast cancer. Therapeutic interventions are limited to differentiating between fibrocystic changes and breast cancer. Screening interventions include clinical breast examination, mammography, and ultrasonography. Contents of fluid-filled cysts are aspirated and evaluated to determine if neoplastic cells are present. Aspiration of the cyst often eliminates the cyst, but the cyst may reform.

Fibroadenoma

Fibroadenoma is a painless solid breast mass or tumor, which has well-defined borders, is mobile, often feels oval-shaped, frequently feels "rubbery," tends to reach a size of 1 of 3 centimeters, and does not change in response to cycling hormone levels (Brucker & Scharbo-DeHaan, 1991). The woman may report a discrete, mobile, seed-sized, or marble-sized "lump" (with no nipple discharge) in one or both breasts. The cause of fibroadenoma is an overgrowth of breast tissue, which occurs most often between the ages of 20 and 40; however, it may not be discovered until the perimenopausal or postmenopausal period (Brucker & Scharbo-DeHaan, 1991). Therapeutic interventions are focused on establishing the benign diagnosis. Screening techniques include mammogram and ultrasound. The mass may be evaluated using fine-needle aspiration biopsy or excision biopsy.

Table 10-5 Evaluation of Breast Mass Characteristics

If a breast mass is noted during palpation, the following information should be obtained regarding the mass. Always note if one or both breasts are involved.

LOCATION

Identify the quadrant involved or visualize the breast with the face of a clock superimposed on it. The nipple represents the center of the clock. Note where the mass lies in relation to the nipple, e.g., 3 cm from the nipple in the 3 o'clock position.

SIZE

Determine size in centimeters in all three planes (height, width, and depth).

SHAPE

Qualify the mass as round, ovoid, matted, or irregular.

NUMBER

Note if lesions are singular or multiple. Note if one or both breasts are involved.

CONSISTENCY

Qualify the mass as firm, hard, soft, fluid, or cystic.

DEFINITION

Note if the mass borders are discrete or irregular.

MOBILITY

Determine if the mass is fixed or freely mobile in relation to the chest wall.

TENDERNESS

Note if palpation elicits pain.

ERYTHEMA

Note any redness over involved area (Figure 10-3).

DIMPLING OR RETRACTION

Observe for dimpling (Figure 10-4) or retraction (Figure 10-5) as the client raises arms overhead and presses her hands into her hips.

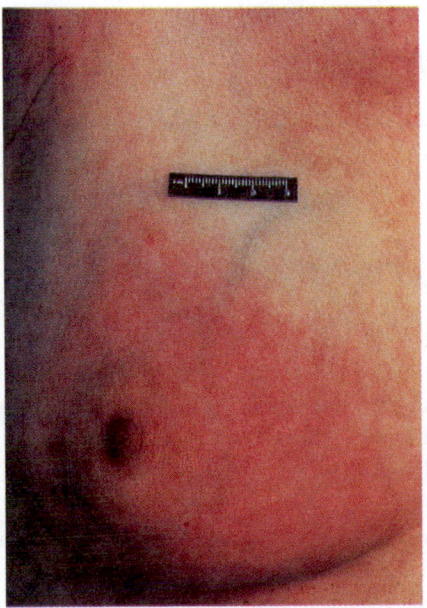

Figure 10-3 Erythema with Abnormal Vascular Pattern Secondary to Inflammatory Breast Cancer (Courtesy of Dr. S. Eva Singletary, University of Texas, M.D. Anderson Cancer Center)

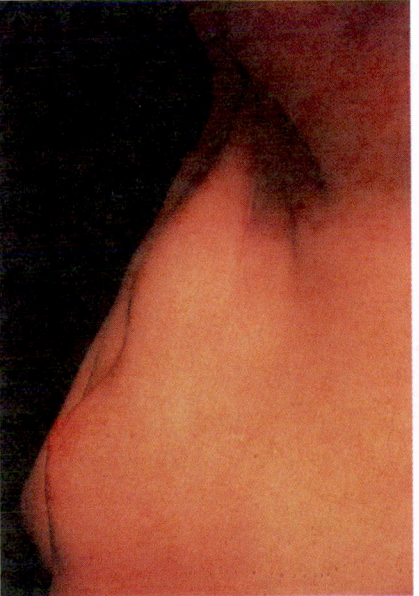

Figure 10-4 Dimpling of Left Breast Tissue (Courtesy of Dr. S. Eva Singletary, University of Texas, M.D. Anderson Cancer Center)

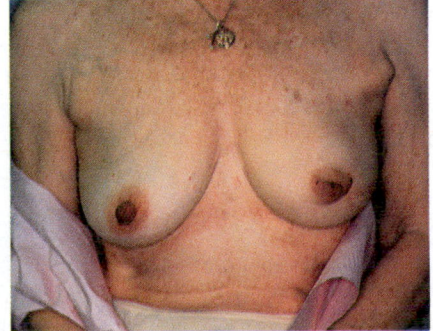

Figure 10-5 Nipple Retraction on Left Breast (Courtesy of Steven M. Lynch, M.D.)

Table 10-6 Characteristics of Common Breast Masses

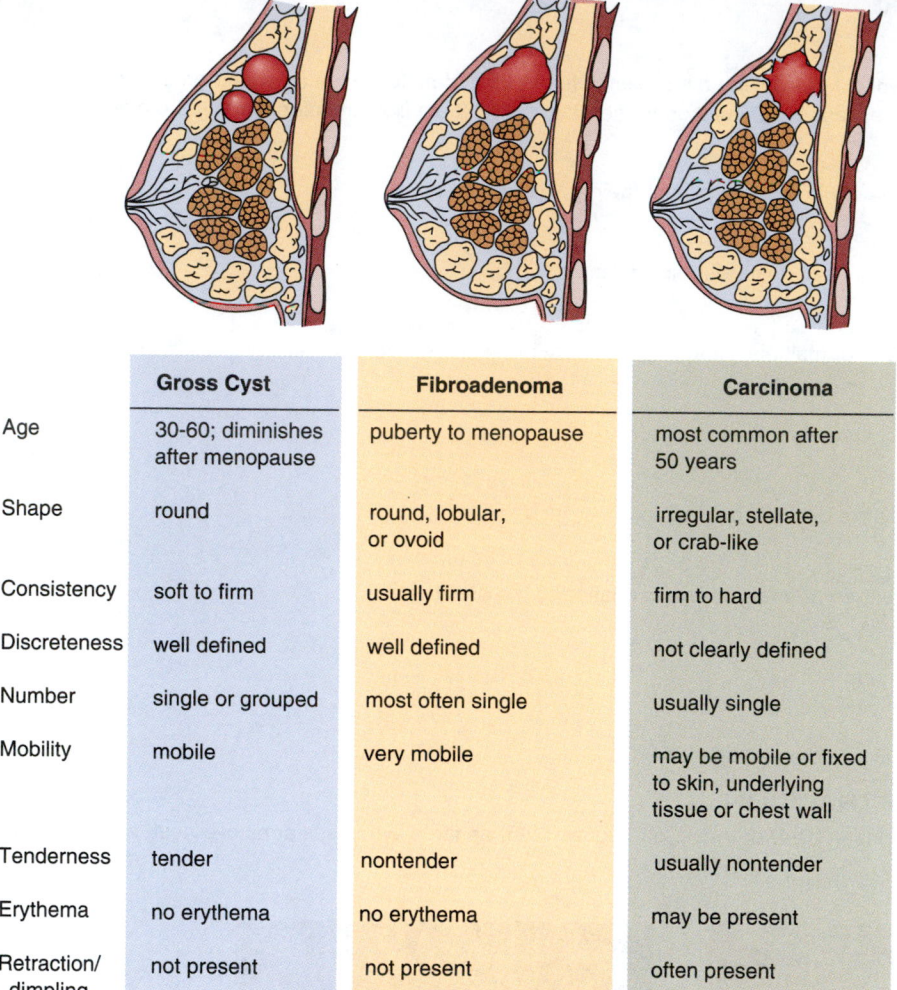

	Gross Cyst	Fibroadenoma	Carcinoma
Age	30-60; diminishes after menopause	puberty to menopause	most common after 50 years
Shape	round	round, lobular, or ovoid	irregular, stellate, or crab-like
Consistency	soft to firm	usually firm	firm to hard
Discreteness	well defined	well defined	not clearly defined
Number	single or grouped	most often single	usually single
Mobility	mobile	very mobile	may be mobile or fixed to skin, underlying tissue or chest wall
Tenderness	tender	nontender	usually nontender
Erythema	no erythema	no erythema	may be present
Retraction/ dimpling	not present	not present	often present

Nipple Discharge

Nipple discharge is fluid produced by and accumulating within a secretory unit of the breast and exiting through the nipple (Arnold & Neiheisel, 1997). The woman may notice nipple discharge on her bra or night clothing. Nipple discharge can be categorized as lactation, physiologic, pathologic, or false discharge.

Lactation Discharge

Lactation discharge is any secretory discharge occurring as a physiologic response to the normal hormonal stimulation of pregnancy, postpartum, or the period following weaning of the infant (Arnold & Neiheisel, 1997). The discharge is usually thin and white and discharged from both breasts. With continued stimulation, the woman may continue to experience lactation discharge for several weeks to years after weaning the infant. The lactation discharge is

not harmful. Therapeutic interventions involve education regarding the cause of the discharge and the recommendation to limit or avoid stimulation of the breasts.

Physiologic Discharge

Physiologic discharge is the result of physiologic conditions affecting all breast tissue equally (i.e., bilaterally), involving secretory tissue in each breast, and resulting in milky-white or multicolored (yellow, green, or gray) fluid. Usually milky, nonlactation nipple discharge is referred to as galactorrhea. Occurrences or practices that are characteristic of galactorrhea include hyperprolactinemia (an elevated serum prolactin level); menarche or menopause; intake of exogenous estrogens or progestins, dopamine antagonist medications, or opiates; sexual or mechanical nipple stimulation; and traumatic anterior thoracic nerve stimulation. Thus, the discharge is not part of a disease process. Therapeutic interventions include reassurance and counseling.

Research Highlight

The Breast Cancer Prevention Trial: Evaluating Tamoxifen's Efficacy in Preventing Breast Cancer

Purpose

To review literature regarding tamoxifen and breast cancer with a focus on the Breast Cancer Prevention Trial (BCPT).

Methods

A sample of 16,000 women who were at least 35 years of age and were considered to be at risk for breast cancer were recruited to participate in a randomized, prospective, double-blind, placebo-controlled clinical investigation. Women who were pregnant, who had a history of breast cancer or a history of clinical depression, were taking oral contraceptives, ERT, HRT, or Warfarin (Coumadin) were excluded from the investigation. Women in the experimental group took 20 mg of tamoxifen once a day, and women in the control group took a placebo once a day. Each woman is seen for follow-up visits, initially at 3 months and then every 6 months for at least 7 years. The treatment continues for at least 5 years.

Findings

Preliminary findings after 4 years of study were reported McKeon (1998) showing 45% fewer diagnoses of invasive breast cancer in subjects who were randomly assigned to the experimental group (daily intake of 20 mg of tamoxifen) than in the subjects randomly assigned to the control (placebo) group. There were 85 women diagnosed with invasive cancer in the experimental group versus 154 in the control group. In addition, only 31 women in the experimental group were diagnosed with noninvasive cancer, while 59 were diagnosed with noninvasive cancer in the control group. Only 47 bone fractures occurred in women in the experimental group compared with 71 in the control group.

Nursing Implications

The findings can be used to gain knowledge regarding the effectiveness of tamoxifen in preventing breast cancer in women at risk. Additional studies should be conducted to provide information regarding prevention for women who are not at risk for breast cancer.

Note: McKeon, V.A. (1997). The Breast Cancer Prevention Trial: Evaluating tamoxifen's efficacy in preventing breast cancer, *Journal of Obstetric, Gynecologic, and Neonatal Nursing*, 26(1), 79–90.

Pathologic Discharge

Pathologic discharge is the result of pathologic conditions affecting the hypothalamic-pituitary axis, prolactin levels, or breast diseases, and, thus, may affect both breasts (Arnold & Neiheisel, 1997). Pathologic conditions that cause hyperprolactinemia include tumor of the pituitary gland, Addison's disease, and hypothyroidism. The nipple discharge associated with such conditions is thin and milky (Arnold & Neiheisel). Most of the causes of pathologic galactorrhea are benign and include intraductal papilloma (benign epithelial neoplasm), duct ectasia (inflammatory response to stagnation of breast duct secre-

tions), and breast infections. Nipple discharge caused by intraductal papillomas tends to be serous or bloody and may be secreted from only one breast, unless one or more intraductal papillomas are present in each breast. The color of the nipple discharge caused by ductal ectasia can be bloody, brown, cream-colored, gray, green, purulent, or white and can vary from thin to extremely thick. Breast infections usually result in purulent nipple discharge. Therapeutic interventions involve individualization of treatment to the cause of the discharge. Lactogenic medications can be eliminated or the dose reduced, antibiotics are administered for infectious processes, exercise habits causing the discharge can be altered, and referral for biopsy for suspected malignant discharge establishes the cause of the discharge (Arnold & Neiheisel, 1997).

Of greatest concern is diagnosis of the pathologic discharge accompanying breast cancer. Fortunately, the majority of pathologic nipple discharges are caused by benign pathologic processes, but occasionally, pathologic nipple discharge is caused by breast cancer (Arnold & Neiheisel, 1997). In such cases, the discharge is most often spontaneous, associated with a breast mass, and a "classically unilateral, single-duct discharge" (Arnold & Neiheisel, 1997, p. 109). Usually, the discharge associated with breast cancer is bloody, serous, and watery: the bloody discharge ranges from bright red to black and the serous discharge is thin, sticky, and yellow to light orange (Arnold & Neiheisel, 1997).

False Discharge

False discharge refers to fluid appearing on the nipple or areolar surface that is not secreted by breast tissue (Arnold & Neiheisel, 1997). Conditions associated with false nipple discharge include any dermatologic disease (eczema, bacterial or viral dermatitis), nipple trauma, or Paget's disease (inflammatory, malignant neoplasm). The fluid appearing on the nipple or areola may be bloody, clear, colored, purulent, serous, or viscous. Management includes treatment of the disease causing the discharge (e.g., antibiotics, topical dermatologic medication).

Malignant Breast Conditions

Malignant breast conditions are life-threatening and life-altering, both emotionally and physically. The cancer most

frightening to many women is breast cancer. In 2000, Johnson predicted, "An estimated 175,000 new cases of breast cancer among women will be diagnosed (in 2000), and 43,000 women will die of this disease". The primary risks for development of breast cancer are female gender and increasing age (Thomas & Greirzu, 2000). Risk factors have been categorized as major (age and genetic factors), minor (reproductive status and lifestyle), and suspected, based on research studies (White, Griffith, Nenstiel, Dyess, 1996).

Hereditary breast cancer tends to occur before age 45, accounts for only 5% to 10% of all breast cancer development, and is thought to be related to a variety of lifestyle, environmental, and genetic factors (McCance & Jorde, 1998). Thus, most women who have breast cancer do not have familial risk factors. All people (male and female) the breast cancer genes, *BRCA*-1 and *BRCA*-2. Familial premenopausal breast cancer risk is increased when a woman inherits mutations of the genes. Inheritance of "normal" *BRCA*-1 and *BRCA*-2 genes means the woman has a reduced risk for familial breast cancer and the same risk for breast cancer caused by other factors as other women. Some mutations of the *BRCA*-1 and *BRCA*-2 genes result in an increased risk for breast cancer, and other mutations increase the risk for ovarian cancer (McCance & Jorde). Women can inherit mutations of *BRCA*-1 and *BRCA*-2 genes from either parent. A man who inherits a mutation of the *BRCA*-2 gene has a higher risk for development of breast cancer than other men in the general population, and a man who inherits mutations in the *BRCA*-1 gene has an increased risk for prostate cancer (McCance & Jorde, 1998).

Malignant breast conditions arise from genetic (*BRCA*-1 and *BRCA*-2) mutations or spontaneous abnormal epithelial cell growth and most often occur in ductal or lobular epithelial cells. In the presence of abnormal epithelial cell growth (atypical hyperplasia), the woman is at risk for development of ductal or lobar carcinoma. Malignant breast

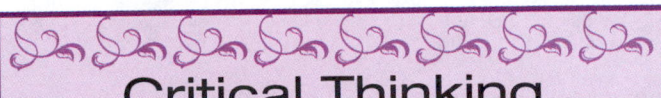

Critical Thinking

Oral Contraceptives and Cancer Risk

There have been recent studies indicating a correlation between estrogen-based oral contraceptive use and breast cancer, with a two- to fourfold increased risk noted for some populations. During the breast assessment, the client asks you about the association between oral contraceptives and increased breast cancer risk because she is considering switching from oral contraceptives to another method of birth control. How would you respond?

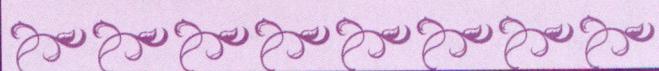

Nursing Alert

RISK FACTORS FOR BREAST CANCER

Age and Genetic Risk Factors

Over age (50)

Female

Personal history of breast cancer

Personal history of ovarian or endometrial cancer

Personal history of breast hyperplasia

History of two or more first-degree relatives (mother, sister, daughter) with breast cancer

History of a first-degree relative with bilateral cancer before age 50

Reproductive Status and Lifestyle Behavior Risk Factors

Delayed childbirth (age 30 or older first completed pregnancy)

Early menarche (age 11 or younger) and late natural menopause (age 55 or older)

Nulliparity

Exposure to ionizing radiation (before age 40)

Factors Needing More Research to Establish Risk

Obesity (postmenopausal)

Magnetic field exposure

Environmental exposure to pesticides

Excessive alcohol intake (nine or more drinks per week)

Smoking

High-fat diet

---

conditions can be categorized as localized (ductal or lobar), invasive (ductal or lobar), or metastatic.

Localized Breast Cancer

Localized breast cancer has not metastasized, is usually less than 2 centimeters in size, is considered noninvasive beyond the breast, and has potential for the best client outcome. The lower the stage of breast cancer at diagnosis, the better the outcome. According to the tumor, nodal involvement, and metastasis (TNM) method of staging cancer, localized ductal or lobar breast cancer meets the criteria for TNM stage 0 or stage 1. Stage 0 criteria include cancer *in situ*, confined to the milk duct or the lobe, and with no occurrence of metastases and stage 1 criteria include size less than 2 centimeters, infiltration to surrounding breast tissue, and no lymph node involvement (Thomas & Greizu, 2000).

Management of localized breast cancer, where the cancer is confined to one area, can include lumpectomy (to remove the tumor and a small amount of surrounding tissue) and adjunctive radiation therapy. Adjacent lymph nodes may be removed. The woman is not a candidate for lumpectomy if she has more than one tumor, tumors in more than one quadrant of the breast, or diffuse calcifications; has had previous radiation therapy to the area; has large breasts; has a tumor located under the nipple; or has small breasts with a large tumor mass–to–breast mass ratio (Thomas & Greifzu, 2000).

Invasive Breast Cancer

Invasive breast cancer has extended beyond the local epithelium and has the potential to spread (metastasize) from the breast to other parts of the body. Invasive breast cancer meets TNM criteria for stages II and III. TNM stage II criteria are size between 2 and 5 centimeters and tumor cells that have spread to adjacent axillary lymph nodes; stage 3A criteria include size less than 5 centimeters and fixed (attached to each other or to surrounding tissue) adjacent axillary lymph nodes; and stage 3B criteria include tumor of any size; spread to the skin, chest wall, or mammary lymph nodes; and no metastases to distant organs (Thomas & Greizu, 2000).

Management depends on the size of the tumor, involvement of lymph nodes, and type of tumor cells (positive or negative estrogen receptors). The usual treatment includes mastectomy, radiation, chemotherapy, or a combination of these (Thomas & Greizu, 2000). Adjuvant hormone therapy may be added to the treatment plan.

Case Study/Care Plan

CLIENT WITH BREAST CANCER

A 51-year-old, single, mildly retarded woman visits a community women's health clinic with a chief complaint of a lump in her left breast. Client states, "I am afraid of cancer. I am afraid I will die." The woman wrings her hands, eyes dart back and forth and she looks toward her sister as if for help.

Physical examination reveals a 3-cm solid mass with an irregular, dimpled surface in the inner quadrant of the left breast in the 10 o'clock position. Mammography indicates a potentially malignant mass, and she is referred for biopsy. Biopsy reveals the mass is malignant, and a mastectomy is scheduled.

Assessment

Nulliparity, sporadic practice of BSE, and sporadic use of the health care system.
Mammography results indicate malignant breast cancer.
Biopsy results document diagnosis of malignant breast neoplasm.

Nursing Diagnosis

Fear related to breast cancer diagnosis.

Expected Outcomes

Client will:

1. Identify emotional feelings related to diagnosis of breast cancer.
2. Relate understanding of usual medical and surgical treatments for breast cancer.
3. Discuss perception of effect of mastectomy, radiotherapy, and chemotherapy on her life.
4. List coping strategies for incisional pain, radiation discomfort, and chemotherapy side effects.

Planning

The nurse must ensure that all information is presented at the client's level of understanding, with involvement of family and support persons as needed or appropriate.

(continued)

Metastatic Breast Cancer

Metastatic breast cancer is breast cancer that has spread to other parts of the body. It meets the criterion for TNM stage 4, which is metastasized tumors of any size (Thomas & Greizu, 2000). Once metastases occur, there is no cure and life expectancy is short. Thus, therapeutic intervention is primarily futile.

Nursing Implications

Nursing assessment for breast conditions involves careful medical and gynecologic history taking, with special emphasis on breast history, including results of and frequency of BSE (e.g., several times per day versus once per month), breast trauma, breast stimulation, and assessment for symptoms of specifically suspected breast conditions. Physical assessment focuses on the collection of data regarding the suspected breast condition, including necessary laboratory test and collection of biopsy specimens.

Nursing diagnoses may include the following:

- Pain related to screening, diagnostic procedures, surgical procedures
- Fear related to medical condition and selected therapeutic intervention
- Grief, related to body image change or prognosis
- Deficient knowledge related to specific breast condition, screening, diagnosis, or intervention procedures

Nursing plans include specific actions that the client completes to achieve the highest level of wellness possible or to achieve peace regarding prognosis. Sample goals include the following:

- Consume food portions according to the daily recommendations in the food pyramid or as required on the basis of medical diagnosis from 24-hour diet recall; intention to consume suggested foods and intention to modify detrimental food intake.

Nursing Interventions	Rationales
1. Discuss client's emotional feelings regarding breast cancer diagnosis. Facilitate client's use of support system. Refer client to local breast cancer support group.	1. Acknowledging client's feelings is supportive of her emotional response and demonstrates caring and a concerned attitude. Diagnosis of breast cancer is a shock, and she will need a support system to help her cope. The local breast cancer support group has volunteers who have experienced breast cancer and support clients through all stages of the grieving, treatment, and recovery phases.
2. Explain the anticipated level of discomfort, physical sensations, anticipatory grieving, procedures, and outcome for mastectomy (loss of breast, removal of lymph nodes), radiotherapy (fatigue, itching or peeling skin).	2. Information facilitates understanding and acceptance of condition; anticipatory guidance reduces fear.
3. Discuss client's perception of the effect of mastectomy, radiotherapy, and chemotherapy on her life (e.g., job, family, friends).	3. Women's perception affects planning and compliance.
4. Describe potential coping strategies for incisional pain (pain medication, relaxation techniques), radiation effects (sunscreen, protective cotton clothing to decrease additional skin irritation), and chemotherapy effects (antiemetic medication, cap to decrease hair loss, balanced nutrition to decrease fatigue). Provide client with choices for coping strategies.	4. Anticipatory guidance decreases fear and increases compliance. Providing woman with choices increases sense of control and enhances self-esteem.

Evaluation

- Client states that she can expect to have her breast and lymph nodes under her arm removed.
- Client states that she will need to come for radiation treatments after surgery each day for 5 to 6 weeks.
- Client states that she may have skin irritation and will have chemotherapy, possibly for 3 to 8 months, depending on the schedule chosen by her oncologist.
- Client states that she may have some nausea, vomiting, fatigue, and hair loss, and she will be given medication to control her nausea.
- Client states that she will not be able to work as a dishwasher at the café while she is recovering and undergoing radiation and chemotherapy.
- Client states that she will move in with her sister while she is recovering and taking radiation and chemotherapy treatments.
- Client states that she can take medication for pain and nausea.

- Complete daily exercise (walking 30 minutes per day, any prescribed exercise required for restoration of function after surgery).
- Understand instructions regarding prescriptive medications.
- Return to the health care facility for scheduled follow-up visits.
- Call the health care provider regarding adverse effects of prescriptive medications as instructed.
- Call health care provider regarding any adverse symptoms of breast condition as instructed.
- Have all questions answered to her satisfaction.
- Understand health promotion counseling.

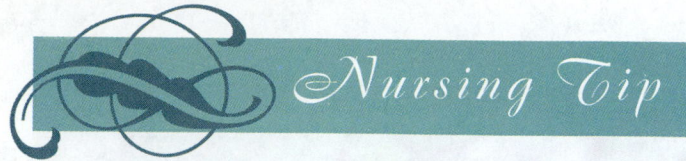

Nursing Tip

THE CLIENT AFTER MASTECTOMY

There are four types of **mastectomy** (excision of the breast). In a simple mastectomy, only the breast is removed. In a modified radical procedure, the breast and lymph nodes from the axilla are removed (Figure 10-6). In a radical mastectomy, the breast, lymph nodes from the axilla, and pectoral muscles are removed (Figure 10-7). This procedure is rarely performed. In a subcutaneous mastectomy, the skin and nipple are left intact, but the underlying breast tissue and lymph nodes are removed. The client who has undergone a simple, modified radical, or radical mastectomy has had the breast amputated from the chest wall.

Reconstruction techniques include synthetic implants, tissue expansion techniques (in which a temporary device is placed in a subpectoralis-subserratus position between the anterior chest wall and skin and is then inflated with saline over a period of weeks), and latissimus dorsi myocutaneous flap breast reconstruction. A myocutaneous flap reconstruction involves transferring skin from the back or the abdomen to the anterior chest wall.

Assessment of the client who has had a mastectomy is guided by the type of mastectomy and the presence or absence of reconstructive surgery. Follow the standard assessment procedures and modify your technique to suit the amount of breast tissue and the presence, if any, of a nipple. Always begin the assessment on the unaffected breast. Mastectomy clients should continue to perform monthly breast self-examinations to determine if masses have returned to the excised area. Annual clinical evaluations and mammograms are also recommended.

Nursing interventions involve educating the woman regarding the diagnosis, consequences, interventions, specific procedures; her choices; counseling regarding expected outcomes; emotional support; reduction of fears, anxiety, stresses, and concerns; advocacy; and relief of current or future pain.

Women who seek care for breast conditions are demonstrating concern and are usually ready to learn about protecting the health of their breasts. Breast and general health promotion and disease prevention strategies include recommendations for regular exercise and for diet from the food pyramid to maintain normal BMI; avoiding or stopping smoking; performing self-assessments; and scheduling provider assessments and screenings as necessary. The nurse can use such interventional moments to assess the woman's practice of BSE, including the frequency, technique, and related concerns. Most women are concerned about being able to "tell the difference" between cancer and "normal" changes. Thus, the nurse needs to assure the woman that the purpose of the monthly BSE is not to determine whether or not she has breast cancer but to determine whether or not she feels anything different in her breast than she felt in the previous monthly BSE. The key is for her to identify anything she has not felt before and make an appointment with her provider for a clinical breast examination and screening. Caution her that most of the "differences" noted on BSE and clinical breast examinations are normal physiologic changes, and the reason for practicing BSE is to notice any problematic changes early. Diagnosis of breast cancer is facilitated best by the combination of attention to changes during the BSE, annual clinical breast examinations, followup screening (i.e., mammogram, ultrasound), and diagnostic procedures.

To ensure the woman can differentiate normal changes related to hormonal fluctuations, she should perform her BSE on the same day of her menstrual cycle each month, about a week after her menses. To help her remember, she can perform BSE on the day after her last day of menstrual flow.

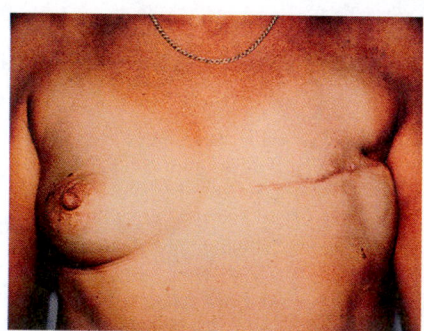

Figure 10-6 *Modified Radical Mastectomy.*

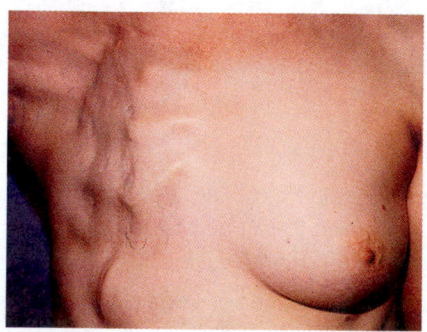

Figure 10-7 *Radical Mastectomy.*

Women who seek care for breast conditions tend to be frightened and anxious. They are fearful of both the diagnosis and treatment. Thus, initial nursing actions are focused on reducing fear and anxiety. Acknowledgement of concerns and a careful history can begin to reduce the fear and anxiety.

Once the medical diagnosis is made, the nurse assesses the woman's understanding and the affect of the diagnosis on her life and support system. Nursing actions must include clarification, explanation, and education.

If the woman requires surgery, she needs to be educated regarding pain reduction interventions, anticipated appearance of the surgical wound, wound care, nutrition, postoperative exercises, recovery, and health promotion. She may need to be taught when to take medication, expected side effects of the medication, and adverse effects. If therapy involves radiation, she needs instruction on skin appearance and sensation after radiation therapy, how to reduce trauma to the site (i.e., wearing loose-fitting cotton clothing, avoiding additional trauma to the area, such as shaving, sun exposure), use of mild soap with lukewarm water, and avoidance of creams or lotions containing alcohol or oil (Thomas & Greizu, 2000).

PELVIC CONDITIONS

Pelvic conditions can be categorized as infectious, benign, or malignant conditions. Infectious conditions include vaginal, cervical, and pelvic inflammatory infections. Benign conditions may affect the cervix, uterus, and ovaries. Malignant conditions can be cervical, uterine, or ovarian. Table 10-7 lists criteria for pelvic conditions, and Table 10-8 lists usual therapeutic interventions for pelvic conditions.

Infectious Conditions

Infectious conditions of the pelvis include vaginal infections, cervical infections, and PID. Infections may be caused by bacterial, viral, fungal, or protozoal organisms.

Vaginal and Cervical Infection

A **vaginal infection** is inflammation of the vagina, and a **cervical infection** is inflammation of the cervix. Many of the infectious organisms are sexually transmitted (chlamydia, gonorrhea, trichomoniasis, herpes simplex infection, human papilloma virus infection), while others are overgrowth of organisms normally or frequently found in the vagina (yeast, Döderlein's bacillus, beta-hemolytic streptococci). Postmenopausal women who are not receiving ERT or hormonal replacement therapy may experience atrophic vaginitis caused by the response of the vaginal environment to decreased estrogen levels. Bacterial vaginosis (inflammation caused by an overgrowth of anaerobic bacteria) accounts for 40% to 50% of vaginitis, vulvovaginal candidiasis (yeast infection) accounts for 20% to 25%, and vaginal trichomoniasis (a sexually transmitted protozoal infection) accounts for 15% to 20% (Cullins, Dominguez, Guberski, Secor, & Wysocki, 1999).

Women who come for treatment of vaginal infection typically relate symptoms of vaginal discharge (amount, odor, and color); pruritus; local irritation; dysuria; and dyspareunia. If the woman has bacterial vaginosis, she often complains of a "fishy" odor of the vaginal discharge, especially after sexual intercourse. If the vaginitis is caused by *Candida* species, pruritus, dysuria, and vulvovaginal irritation tend to be the primary complaints. The woman who has trichomoniasis usually complains of copious yellowish or greenish discharge with a foul odor, pruritus, vulvovaginal irritation, and dysuria. Table 10-9 contains a description of vaginal discharges. Women should be taught how to perform a self-inspection of the external genitalia (Figure 10-8).

Based on the Centers for Disease Control and Prevention (CDC) recommendations, therapeutic intervention for bacterial vaginosis is intravaginal metronidazole or clindamycin cream (Cullins, et al., 1999). CDC recommendations for vulvovaginal candidiasis are intravaginal terconazole cream or suppositories. Oral metronidazole is the CDC recommendation for treatment of trichomoniasis (Cullins et al., 1999) Since trichomoniasis is considered a sexually transmitted disease (STD), the woman's partner must be treated simultaneously and she must avoid sexual intercourse until the disease is cured.

Pelvic Inflammatory Disease

PID is inflammation of the uterus, fallopian tubes, or ovaries, or a combination, caused by ascent of vaginal flora or bacteria. At least 1 million women, 70% of whom are younger than age 25, are estimated to have PID annually (Mott, 1998). The majority of PID infections are caused by STD organisms, especially chlamydia and gonorrhea, ascending from the vagina. High-risk women are age 25 or younger, single or divorced, have multiple sex partners without barrier protection, who douche, and use intrauterine devices. PID is often undiagnosed and the treatment is delayed, which increases the risk for infertility, ectopic pregnancy, and chronic pelvic pain. The CDC criteria for diagnosis of PID are at least three symptoms of lower abdominal tenderness, adnexal tenderness, cervical motion tenderness, an oral body temperature of 38.3°C (101°F), abnormal vaginal or cervical discharge, elevated erythrocyte sedimentation rate, elevated C-reative protein levels, and laboratory evidence of chlamydial or gonorrheal infection (Mott, 1998). Therapeutic intervention includes cefoxitin and doxycycline or clindamycin and gentamycin, if the woman is hospitalized, and cefoxitin or ceftriaxone and doxycycline or ofloxacin and metronidazole, for outpatient treatment.

Table 10-7 Pelvic Conditions

Condition	Data		
	Subjective	**Objective**	**Laboratory or Procedure**
Infections			
Cervicitis	Spotting (especially after sexual intercourse) Increase in vaginal discharge May be asymptomatic	Yellowish-white discharge Red, edematous, friable cervix Cervical motion Tenderness Grayish-green discharge, with cervix having strawberry-like appearance (trichomoniasis)	Wet mount for WBCs count, trichomonads Cultures for *C. trachomatis, N. gonorrhoeae* HSV Numerous white blood cells
Bacterial vulvovaginosis	Increased vaginal discharge Odor after sexual intercourse	Homogenous gray-white discharge Musty or fishy odor	pH of discharge using pH sensitive strips Wet mount (clue cells) Positive amine test
Monilial vulvovaginitis	Itching, burning Discharge Dyspareunia	Thick, curd-like vaginal discharge Vulvar or vaginal erythema Edematous cervix Possibly friable cervix	Wet mount (budding hyphae, leukocytes)
Atrophic vulvovaginitis	Vaginal dryness Vaginal irritation and burning Itching Postcoital spotting	Vulvar and vaginal atrophy Pale, thin, friable vaginal mucosa Sparse pubic hair	No lab test is reliable. A maturation index can be done with the pap smear to provide some data
Pelvic inflammatory disease	Lower abdominal pain or tenderness Chills and fever Nausea and vomiting Increased vaginal discharge Irregular bleeding Malaise Dysmenorrhea Dyspareunia Postcoital spotting Dysuria	Lower abdominal rebound tenderness Cervical motion tenderness Hypoactive bowel sounds Adenexal fullness, tenderness Mucoprurulent cervical discharge Cervical friability Body temperature of over 100.4°F	C-reactive protein Erythrocyte sedimentation rate Positive Gonorrhea and chlamydia cultures Ultrasound for fluid in cul-de-sac or pelvic mass or abscess Wet mount
Benign Conditions			
Pelvic relaxation			
Uterine prolapse	Backache Pelvic pressure or heaviness	Cervix descended into vagina or through introitus	Bimanual pelvic exam
Cystocele	Urinary frequency, urgency, incontinence Dyspareunia Vaginal pressure Urinary tract infections Incomplete bladder emptying	Bulging of anterior vaginal wall	Postvoid urinary retention Postvoid analysis of urinary retention determines the severity of the condition
Rectocele	Difficult defecation Vaginal pressure Rectal fullness	Bulging of posterior vaginal wall	Rectal exam reveals the severity of rectocele
Enterocele	Vaginal pressure Abdominal pain Loose stools	Bulging of cul-de-sac or posterior vaginal wall	

(continued)

Table 10-7 Pelvic Conditions (*continued*)

Condition	Subjective	Objective	Laboratory or Procedure
Functional Conditions			
Polycystic ovary syndrome	Often asymptomatic Amenorrhea or oligomenorrhea Dysfunctional uterine bleeding Infertility Irregular menstrual cycles	Obesity Hirsuitism Acne Enlarged ovaries Enlarged clitoris Voice changes Alopecia	Elevated LH Level Ultrasound examination of ovarian size and follicles Endometrial biopsy for hyperplasia Hyperinsulinemia Serum gluclose Serum Prolactin level Testosterone level
Premature ovarian failure	Amenorrhea Hot flashes Night sweats Vaginal dryness Dyspareunia	Vaginal atrophy Vulvar atrophy Uterine atrophy	↑FSH and LH levels ↓Thyroid function tests ↑Prolactin level
Structural Conditions			
Fibroid Tumors	Most are asymptomatic Possible pressure discomfort Possible hypermenorrhea Pain if tumor is twisted Pelvic pressure Deep pelvic pain Dyspareunia	Abnormal results on pelvic examination Anemia from hypermenorrhea Palpation of painless, mobile, smooth uterine mass or nodule	Ultrasound examination Pelvic magnetic resonance imaging (MRI) These tests identify the location and size of fibroids
Malignant Conditions			
Cervical cancer	Blood-tinged, watery vaginal discharge Abnormal vaginal bleeding Postcoital spotting or bleeding Dyspareunia Abdominal, back, or flank pain	Enlarged cervix Foul smelling discharge Anemia Leg edema	Pap smear Colposcopy, cervical, and endocervical sampling for cytology
Endometrial cancer	Metrorrhagia (premenopausal) Pelvic pain or bloating (advanced disease) Postmenopausal bleeding	Uterus may be an abnormal palpation	Endometrial biopsy for cytology
Ovarian cancer	Changes in bowel or bladder function Abdominal fullness, discomfort Dyspareunia Irregular bleeding Fatigue Back pain Shortness of breath Pelvic pressure	Ascites Possible pelvic mass Weight loss	Blood level of CA-125 Vaginal ultrasound Ba Enema MRI or CT scan with contrast Laparotomy

Nursing Implications

Nursing assessment for infections includes assessment for risk, symptoms, medical history, gynecologic history, and lifestyle behaviors. Physical assessment focuses on data and specimen collection to aid diagnosis of the specific infection (Table 10-7).

Nursing diagnoses are formulated after diagnosis of infection. Applicable nursing diagnosis may include the following:

- Pain related to infection.
- Fear related to the diagnosis.

Table 10-8 Management of Pelvic Conditions

Condition	Usual Therapeutic Interventions
Structural Conditions	
Fibroid Tumors	Iron and progestins (small tumors and minimal symptoms)
	Surgery (myomectomy, hysterectomy)
	GnRH agonists (short-term therapy only)
	Annual pelvic ultrasound to monitor size of tumors
Pelvic Relaxation	
Uterine prolapse	Kegel exercises, ERT, vaginal pessaries (mild prolapse)
	Hysterectomy
Cystocele	Kegel exercises, vaginal pessaries for uterine prolapse, ERT
	Surgical repair
Enterocele	Weight reduction
	Vaginal pessary
	Surgical repair
Rectocele	High-fiber diet
	Regular bowel habits
	Increased fluid intake
	Stool softeners
	Vaginal pessary
	Surgical repair
Functional Conditions	
Polycystic ovary syndrome	Diet modification (obesity)
	Weight reduction
	Stress management (decrease excess androgen)
	Hair removal (hirsutism)
	Medroxyprogesterone for cyclic withdrawal bleeding
	Clomiphene for ovulation induction
	ERT or oral contraceptives (for hyperandrogenism)
	Possible ovarian wedge resection
Premature ovarian failure	Hormone replacement therapy

(continued)

❧ Deficient knowledge related to limited experience regarding the disorder.

Nursing plans include specific actions the client completes to achieve the highest level of wellness possible. Sample goals may include the following:

❧ Take prescriptive medication as written.

❧ Understand instructions regarding prescriptive medication(s).

❧ Return to health care provider as scheduled for follow-up assessment of infection status.

❧ Notify health care provider of adverse effects of prescribed medication(s).

❧ Notify health care provider of failure of symptoms to improve as expected.

❧ Adopt recommended change in lifestyle behavior to prevent recurrence of infection.

❧ Have questions answered to her satisfaction.

❧ Understand health promotion counseling.

Nursing interventions involve teaching, counseling for prevention, and explaining prescribed medications. Women with multiple sexual partners should be counseled about:

❧ The risks for infection

❧ Recommendations for annual screening for chlamydial and gonorrheal infections

❧ Testing for chlamydial and gonorrheal infections 3 to 6 months after starting a relationship with a new sexual partner

Table 10-8 Management of Pelvic Conditions (*continued*)

Condition	Usual Therapeutic Intervention

Infection

Cervicitis	Medication specific to the causative organism (metronidazole for trichomoniasis, acyclorir for herpes simplex virus, ceftriaxone for gonorrhea, doxycycline for chlamydia)
Vaginitis	
Bacterial vulvovaginosis	Metronidazole, clindamycin
Monilial vulvovaginitis	Terconazole
Trichomoniasis	Metronidazole
Pelvic inflammatory disease	Cefoxitin or cefotetan and doxycycline; or clindamycin and ofloxin; or clindamycin and gentamicin
	ERT or hormone replacement therapy
	Vaginal lubricant (K-Y Jelly, Replens)
	Atrophic Vaginitis

Malignant Conditions

Endometrial cancer	Surgery: total abdominal hysterectomy and bilateral salpingo-oophorectomy (TAH-BSO) or TAH-BSO followed by radiotherapy or intrauterine radiation followed by TAH-BSO (depends on stage of cancer)
	Chemotherapy and/or progestin therapy for distant metastases
Cervical cancer	Cryosurgery, loop electrosurgical excision procedure (LEEP), cone biopsy, laser surgery, or hysterectomy for pre-invasive dysplasia
	Total vaginal hysterectomy
	TAH, radical hysterectomy with lymph node dissection (depending on size of lesion)
	Radiation (advanced disease)
Ovarian cancer	Surgery (from unilateral oopherectomy to TAH-BSO) and/or node excision (depends on stage of cancer)
	Radiotherapy
	Chemotherapy

Table 10-9 Description of Vaginal Discharges

Characteristic	Normal	Nonspecific Vaginitis	Trichomonal	Candidal	Gonococcal
Color	White	Gray	Grayish yellow	White	Greenish yellow
Odor	Absent	Fishy	Fishy	Absent	Absent
Consistency	Nonhomogenous	Homogenous	Purulent, often with bubbles	Cottage cheese–like	Mucopurulent
Location	Dependent	Adherent to walls	Often pooled in fornix	Adherent to walls	Adherent to walls
Anatomic Appearance					
Vulva	Normal	Normal	Edematous	Erythematous	Erythematous
Vaginal mucosa	Normal	Normal	Usually normal	Erythematous	Normal
Cervix	Normal	Normal	May show red spots	Patches of discharge	Put in os

Reproduced with permission, from Estes, M.E.Z. (2002). *Health Assessment & Physical Examination,* 2nd ed. Albany, N.Y.: Delmar.

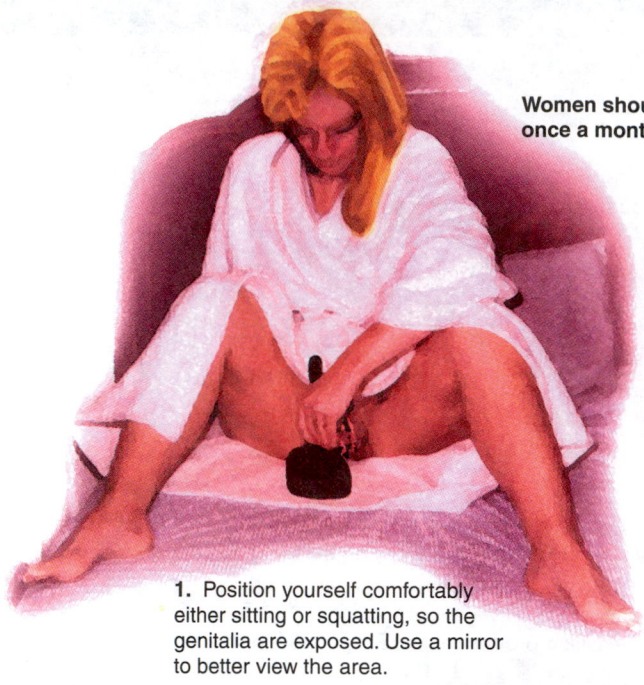

Women should be encouraged to examine their external genitalia once a month, following these steps:

1. Position yourself comfortably either sitting or squatting, so the genitalia are exposed. Use a mirror to better view the area.

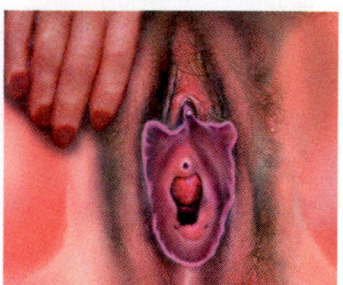

2. Inspect for symmetry, moles, growth, changes in skin color, inflammation, irritated areas, and infestations.

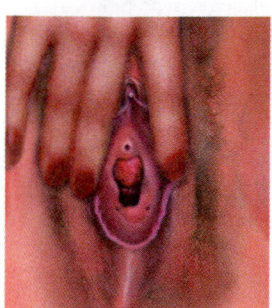

3. Using the index and middle fingers, gently spread the labia to inspect the clitoris and inner sides of the labia.

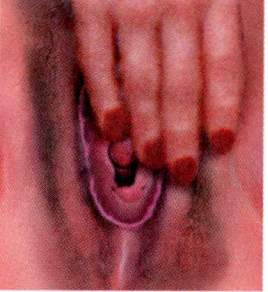

4. Using the finger pads, gently palpate the vulvar region, noting any lumps, nodules, irregularities, or tenderness.

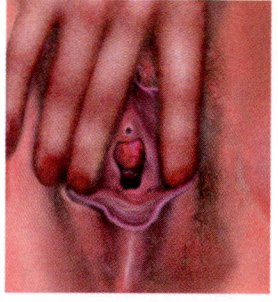

5. Using the index and middle fingers, spread the vaginal opening slightly and palpate the tissue for moistness, elasticity, lumps, nodules, irregularities, or tenderness.

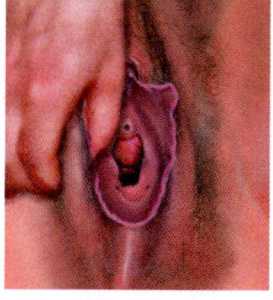

6. Insert the thumb inside the labia and gently compress the tissue between the thumb and index finger, noting any lumps, lesions, or tenderness.

Figure 10-8 Steps to follow to perform vulvar self-examination.

- The need for sexual partners to be treated each time chlamydial and gonorrheal infections occur
- Eliminating douching, because such practices destroy the lactobacilli residing in the vagina and may force bacteria from the vagina into the uterus
- Distinguishing between normal vaginal discharge and discharge characteristic of vaginal infection

Educational nursing intervention includes explaining the dangers of self-diagnosis of vaginal infection and use of over-the-counter or herbal therapies instead of seeking early diagnosis and therapeutic intervention at the first sign of a vaginal infection. Nurses should provide emotional support and therapeutic communication to over-

come a client's embarrassment regarding vaginal infections and to help clients understand that the delicate balance of the vaginal ecosystem can be disturbed by a variety of factors (Cullins, 1999).

When a woman presents with a pelvic infection, the nurse can use such a moment to explain the vulvar self-examination to her. The woman can be encouraged to perform the vulvar examination at the same time of the month as she performs BSE. To perform the vulvar examination, she lies down, spreads and flexes her knees, and prepares to palpate the inguinal area and vulva with the flat surface of her hand to detect enlarged lymph nodes. Then, using a mirror, she inspects the entire vulvar surface (the area between her legs from the top of her pubic hair to the rectum), looking for any growths or discolorations. She inspects surfaces of both the labia majora and labia minora. Then she spreads the labia with her index and middle fingers, looking for growths or discolorations. Lastly, she looks for discharge and, if present, evaluates for odor, amount, and color.

Benign Pelvic Conditions

Benign pelvic conditions can be categorized as structural or functional. Common structural conditions include pelvic relaxation and uterine fibroid tumors. Common functional conditions include polycystic ovary syndrome and premature ovarian failure.

Structural Conditions

Structural conditions are changes in the size or position of the pelvic organs, including the bladder, uterus, ovaries, and rectum. Common structural changes involving the pelvic organs are known collectively as pelvic relaxation.

Pelvic Relaxation

Pelvic relaxation is the loss of pelvic muscle support of the pelvic organs, which may result in development of a cystocele (bulging of the posterior wall of the bladder into the anterior vaginal wall), enterocele (bulging of the bowel into the posterior cul-de-sac and vaginal wall), rectocele (bulging of the anterior wall of the rectum into the posterior vaginal wall), or uterine prolapse (protrusion of the uterus into the vaginal canal). The causes of pelvic relaxation include permanent damage to connective tissue or muscular structure during the stretching and trauma of vaginal birth, chronically increased intraabdominal pressure (from heavy lifting, obesity, straining with constipation, ascites, coughing with obstructive respiratory disease), aging-related muscle atrophy (estrogen deficiency), and congenitally weak connective-tissue strength (elasticity). The woman may experience urinary incontinence, urgency, or frequency; constipation or difficult defecation; pelvic pressure; dyspareunia; walking or sitting discomfort; or protrusion of an organ through the introitus (Lucas, 1999).

Therapeutic interventions for pelvic relaxation depend on the stage of relaxation. First-degree prolapse consists of descent of the cervix into the lower third of the vagina; second-degree is descent of the cervix to the introitus or less than 1 centimeter through the introitus; third-degree is descent of the cervix 1 centimeter beyond the introitus; and fourth-degree is descent or prolapse of the uterus and cervix through the introitus (Lucas, 1999). Women with first- or second-degree stages may increase muscle support for the pelvic organs by performing Kegel exercises several times per day or using a vaginal pessary to provide support for the pelvic organs. For the woman with a third-

or fourth-degree prolapse, weakness of the pelvic musculature is irreversible and hysterectomy is usually the treatment of choice (Lucas, 1999).

Fibroid Tumors

Fibroid tumors (leiomyomas) are benign tumors arising in the myometrium, which can protrude into the uterine cavity (submucous leiomyomas), bulge through the outer uterine layer (subserous leiomyomas), or grow within the myometrium (intramural leiomyomas). The cause is proliferation of smooth-muscle cells. The tumors usually do not grow more than 1 to 2 centimeters per year; thus, the tumor growth can be watched until the uterus reaches a 4- to 5-month gestation size as a result of tumor growth (Lucas, 1999). By the time the uterus reaches this size, the woman may be experiencing excessive urination, backache, pelvic pressure, abdominal discomfort, hypermenorrhea, anemia, or pressure on the ureters (Lucas, 1999). The tumors are dependent on estrogen for growth and, thus, grow more rapidly during pregnancy. The tumors are found more often during the fourth or fifth decades of life, affect 1 out of 5 Caucasian women, affect 1 of 3 African American women, and occur more often in nulliparous, nonsmoking women who take oral contraceptive pills (Grabo, Fahs, Nataupsky, & Reich, 1999). Anovulatory menstrual cycles (unopposed estrogen) are thought to be the cause of fibroid tumor growth during the perimenopausal period (Grabo et al., 1999). The resulting distortion of uterine shape and size contributes to interference with conception, pregnancy maintenance, and fetal growth and development (Grabo et al., 1999).

Therapeutic intervention depends on the woman's desire for future childbearing. If she does not desire future pregnancies and the tumors are large (at least 4-months' gestation size), she may choose to have a hysterectomy (Lucas, 1999). If she desires future childbearing, she may have a myomectomy to remove submucosal tumors before conception. GnRH agonists may be used for short-term intervention to decrease the size of the fibroid tumors (Lucas). However, the woman will experience menopausal symptoms and is at risk for osteoporosis if the intervention is continued for more than 6 months (Lucas, 1999).

Functional Conditions

Functional conditions include changes in function of the pelvic organs, such as polycystic ovary syndrome and premature ovarian failure.

Polycystic Ovary Syndrome

Polycystic ovary syndrome (PCOS) is "a complex endocrine disorder associated with long-term anovulation and an excess of androgens circulating in the blood . . . [and] characterized by formation of cysts in the ovaries, a

REFLECTIONS FROM A NEWLEYWED

"I was vacationing at the beach with my new husband. The first day, we went for a long walk on the beach and I developed a little pain and stiffness in my lower back, which I attributed to the car ride, sleeping on a thin mattress, and walking in soft sand. About 3 AM the next morning, I was awakened by cramping and nonspecific pain in my lower pelvis. Thinking it was gas, I got up to go to the bathroom and could barely stand upright. After another half hour, the pain was no better—even a little worse. I was sweating and then was chilled and had a loose bowel movement. We called the ambulance, having no idea where the nearest hospital was. On the way, I vomited, my pulse was erratic, and I was generally miserable. When we arrived at the hospital, they drew blood, took a urine sample, and gave me a Cat scan. After considering everything from gas to kidney stones to appendicitis, they discovered through ultrasound that I had an ovarian cyst that had swollen and caused the ovary to twist around. Laparoscopic surgery proved that ovarian torsion was present, causing the cessation of blood flow that basically killed the ovary. I also had a cyst on the other ovary, but the doctor was pretty sure that was a "functional" cyst, which is pretty normal. During the surgery they removed the cyst, the ovary, and the fallopian tube.

I was 33, newly married, and had just stopped taking oral contraceptives and was looking forward to starting a family. I had always had an annual pelvic examination and Pap smear and had never before experienced any irregularity or cysts. We were very concerned about how having only one ovary would affect our ability to conceive, but we've been reassured it should be no problem."

process related to the failure of the ovary to release an ovum" (Marantides, 1997). PCOS is the leading cause of amenorrhea in premenopausal women. It is the cause for amenorrhea in 30% of all women, oligomenorrhea in 75% of women, and hirsutism in 87% of women. Causes of PCOS are the results of anovulation, such as ovarian failure, hypothalamic or pituitary suppression, and adrenal enzyme dysfunction. The syndrome begins with an imbalance of LH and follicle-stimulating hormone (FSH), with LH levels elevated and FSH levels low-to-normal. The result of the imbalance of LH and FSH is continued follicular development, elevated estrogen levels, anovulation, and formation of multiple ovarian cysts. Endocrine involvement results in hyperestrogenemia, adrenal androgen excess, ovarian abnormalities, hyperprolactinemia, and hyperinsulinemia. Women typically seek health care for amenorrhea or irregular menstrual cycles, infertility, hirsutism (excessive hair growth), acne, or obesity.

Medical management for PCOS is targeted to the woman's primary concern (e.g., amenorrhea, hirsutism, infertility, obesity) (Marantides, 1997). Combination oral contraceptives or GnRH agonists can be used for hyperandrogenic effects (e.g., male-pattern hair growth and acne). A weight-loss program must be established, or symptoms will return when medication is discontinued. Amenorrhea and anovulation associated with PCOS place the woman at increased risk for endometrial cancer at a young age and for postmenopausal breast cancer. Medroxyprogesterone (Provera) can be used for treatment of the PCOS amenorrhea.

Premature Ovarian Failure

Premature ovarian failure is failure of ovarian estrogen production and ovulation after the menarche and before age 40, in which the woman experiences the symptoms of menopause. The cause can be an endocrine imbalance (gonadal failure, hypothalamic-pituitary-ovarian disorder, Cushing's syndrome, Addison's disease, rigorous physical stress or training). Common causes of secondary amenorrhea are investigated. Medical management includes treatment for any causes of secondary amenorrhea identified or hormone replacement therapy.

Malignant Pelvic Conditions

Malignant pelvic conditions are considered collectively as gynecologic cancers. The most common gynecologic cancers are cervical, endometrial, and ovarian. In this group, only cervical cancer can be screened for early detection.

Cervical Cancer

Cervical cancer is a neoplasm of the uterine cervix. Because of the introduction of the Papanicolaou (Pap) smear in 1942 by Dr. George Nicholas Papanicolaou and Herbert Traut, the annual number of deaths of women resulting

Nursing Alert

RISK FACTORS FOR CANCER OF THE FEMALE GENITALIA

Evaluate each client for risk factors, and counsel the client regarding diminishing risk factors that are behavior dependent. Suspected carcinoma of the female genitalia requires an immediate referral.

Cervical Cancer

- Early age at first intercourse
- Multiple sex partners
- Prior history of human papillomavirus
- Tobacco use
- Family history

Endometrial Cancer

- Early or late menarche (before age 11 or after age 16)
- History of infertility
- Failure to ovulate
- Unopposed estrogen therapy
- Use of tamoxifen
- Obesity
- Family history

Ovarian Cancer

- Advancing age
- Nulliparity
- History of breast cancer
- Family history of ovarian cancer

Vaginal Cancer

- Daughters of women who ingested diethylstilbestrol during pregnancy

Source: Reproduced, with permission, from Estes, M.E.Z. (2002). *Health Assessment & Physical Examination*, 2nd ed. Albany: Delmar.

from cervical cancer have dropped significantly. However, invasive cervical cancer affects 16,000 women per year, and 5,000 women die of this cancer annually (Klingman, 1999). Cervical cancer is most prevalent in women aged 40 to 55 (Bristow and Montz, 2000). If detected early, cervical cancer is curable. Thus, screening by Pap smear is an essential health care assessment for every woman who is sexually active or age 18 or older.

The Pap smear is a screening device for cervical cancer; the results identify women at risk. Cervical cancer is detected by evaluating a biopsy specimen of abnormal cervical epithelium. Risk factors for cervical cancer include initiation of sexual activity before age 18 years; multiple sexual partners; sexual partners who have had multiple sexual partners; history of STDs, including human papilloma virus (HPV); smoking; failure to use a barrier method of contraception; and exposure to diethylstilbesterol in utero (Foulks, 1998).

The cause of abnormal Pap smear results in approximately 25% of women is HPV infection; 80% of cervical cancers occur in the presence of HPV infection; and 50% of women are thought to be infected with HPV by age 30 (Klingman, 1999; Higgins, 1997). There are more than 100 HPV types. However, not all types of HPV have been seen in conjunction with development of cervical cancer. HPV types 6 and 11 cause genital warts, and types 16, 18, 31, and 33 are seen in conjunction with cancerous cervical lesions (Carson, 1999).

Medical management for abnormal cervical cell development or cervical cancer includes local excision, cryotherapy, electrocoagulation, or carbon dioxide laser therapy to destroy the abnormal cells (Bristow & Montz, 2000). Surgery, radiotherapy, or radiotherapy and chemotherapy combined are the usual therapeutic interventions when cervical conditions have progressed to invasive cervical cancer (Carson, 1999).

Endometrial Cancer

Endometrial cancer is a malignant neoplasm of the uterine lining. Endometrial cancer occurs most often in women aged 60 to 74; comprises 13% of all cancers in women in the United States, with 35,000 new cases found annually; and 25% of these cases have progressed to invasive cancer at the time of diagnosis (Carson, 1999). There is no screening method to identify women with atypical cellular changes before development of endometrial cancer. The Pap smear does not screen for this type of cancer. Risk factors for endometrial cancer include age over 50, postmenopausal status, irregular menses (because of potential anovulation caused by unopposed estrogen stimulation of the endometrium), polycystic ovary disease, diabetes mellitus, hypertension, and unopposed ERT with an intact uterus (Bristow & Montz, 2000). Endometrial cancer occurs most often in the perimenopausal or postmenopausal woman and tends to grow slowly.

Medical management for endometrial cancer includes endocervical curettage in a postmenopausal women with vaginal bleeding or in a perimenopausal woman with heavy menses. The type of intervention depends on the stage of the cancer development and may include surgery, radiotherapy, chemotherapy, or hormone therapy.

Ovarian Cancer

Ovarian cancer is a malignant neoplasm of the ovary. Over 30 types of ovarian neoplasms have been identified, involving the epithelium, germ cells, or stromal cells, with epithelial ovarian tumors accounting for 80% of ovarian cancers (Shurpin, 1997). Because there is no screening method for identification of early cellular changes, the cancer has usually spread beyond the ovary to the peritoneum by the time of diagnosis in 75% of cases. Only 20% to 25% of affected women survive longer than 5 years. Ovarian cancer is considered to be the "silent killer". In addition, the first symptoms the woman may notice are vague (abdominal discomfort or fullness, pelvic pressure, urinary frequency, constipation, and dyspepsia as the tumor grows). Many women associate these symptoms with midlife changes or responses to stress rather than a "serious" disease process. Ovarian cancer occurs most often in women aged 40 to 70, is diagnosed in 24,000 women in the United States each year, and 13,600 women die of the disease each year (Averette & Nguglen, 1995).

Risk factors for ovarian cancer include family history (especially a first-degree relative); personal history of breast, colon, or endometrial cancer; ovulation for more than 40 years; and presence of an abnormal *BRCA*-1 gene, which is considered responsible for 80% of inherited ovarian cancers. In high-risk women, transvaginal ultrasonography can detect ovarian enlargement and color Doppler ultrasonography can differentiate malignant and benign growths.

Medical management includes surgery, followed by radiotherapy or chemotherapy, or a combination of the two (Carson, 1999). Continued monitoring of blood levels of the tumor marker CA 125 and regular follow-up pelvic examinations are required after therapeutic interventions.

If woman is undergoing chemotherapy, recommend eating small, frequent, low-fiber, high-calorie, high-protein meals to reduce nausea, vomiting, anorexia, and diarrhea and to prevent malnutrition. In addition, taking an antiemetic before meals may enhance the ability to keep food down. Skin exposed to radiotherapy can be protected by avoiding the use of cosmetics, powder, soap, and sun (or infrared lamps) on the affected areas; wearing loose cotton clothing next to the skin of the affected area; avoiding shaving the affected area; carefully patting affected skin dry after bathing; and avoiding exposure of affected skin to extremes of heat and cold (Campbell & Pruitt, 1996).

Nursing Implications

Nursing assessment for pelvic conditions involve assessing risk factors for benign and malignant pelvic conditions, current symptoms, and medical and gynecologic history. Physical assessment focuses on the collection of data to rule out or confirm a benign pelvic condition and identification of the need to collect specimens for laboratory tests and for additional diagnostic procedures (Table 10-7).

Nursing diagnoses are formulated after the pelvic condition is identified. The diagnoses are individualized for the client and based on the identified pelvic condition. Applicable nursing diagnoses may include the following:

- Pain related to pelvic conditions
- Fear related to procedures and treatment
- Anxiety related to effects of condition or treatment on future childbearing
- Deficient knowledge regarding (specific pelvic condition)

Nursing plans include specific actions that the client will complete to achieve the highest level of wellness possible. Sample goals may include the following:

- Develop strategies for coping with pain.
- Consume recommended foods, based on the food pyramid, daily.
- Reduce stress and promote wellness by exercising at least 30 minutes daily (e.g., walking, swimming, biking).
- Take prescriptive medication as written.
- Understand instructions regarding prescriptive medication(s).
- Return to health care provider for follow-up visits as scheduled.
- Notify health care provider of adverse effects of medications.
- Notify health care provider of failure of symptoms to improve.
- Answer questions to her satisfaction.
- Become informed about choices for medical management.
- Understand expected outcomes of therapy.
- Understand health promotion activities.

Nursing intervention involves education, consequences and prevention of the condition (if possible), specific procedures in and the outcomes of the therapeutic intervention plan, prescription medications, and consequences of "doing nothing," assisting the woman with informed decision making and serving as client advocate. Nurses must provide emotional support for each woman, especially the woman who is embarrassed.

Pain assessment includes rating the severity of pain (such as on a scale of 1 to 10, with 1 being no pain and 10 being the most excruciating pain possible), factors that relieve or reduce the pain, and factors that intensify the pain. The pain must be treated before it becomes severe. The nurse should avoid negating the woman's perception of pain and help the woman select pain control options appropriate for her, her family, and her environment. The

Case Study/Care Plan

CLIENT WITH BACTERIAL VULVOVAGINOSIS

A 19-year-old with a complaint of "another vaginal infection" is being examined in the nurse practitioner clinic at the city health department. Client states, "I've got another infection. There's lots of discharge on my pants and it smells bad when I have sex." Her latest Pap smear (after a period of 2 years of failure to keep her scheduled appointments) reveals an abnormal result, suggestive of HPV infection. Her history indicates that she is single, never married; gravida 4, para 4 (each child has a different father); has had multiple sex partners; delivered her first baby at age 14; has been treated numerous times in the STD clinic; and has smoked 1 to 2 packs of cigarettes daily since age 10. On examination, copious, homogenous, gray, malodorous discharge is observed. A wet-mount examination of the discharge shows clue cells and the "whiff" test is positive for amine odor. The diagnosis is bacterial vulvovaginosis.

Assessment

- Positive results on "whiff" test.
- Wet-mount examination reveals copious clue cells (epithelial cells covered with bacteria), no lactobacilli present, and WBCs too numerous to count.

Nursing Diagnosis

Ineffective health maintenance related to risk-taking behaviors, as evidenced by chief complaint and subjective, objective, and laboratory data.

Expected Outcomes   Client will:

1. Describe risk factors for cervical cancer.
2. Identify cervical cancer risk factors specific to herself.
3. Relate strategies she is willing to use to reduce her personal cervical cancer risk.

Planning   The nurse should take into account the client's developmental maturity and target education and materials to a level the client understands.

Nursing Interventions	Rationales
1. Discuss cervical cancer risk factors (cigarette smoking, early age at first sexual intercourse, first childbirth before age 20, history of STDs (especially HPV infection), multiple sexual partners.	1. Teaching is more effective when it builds on a woman's existing knowledge base. Official list of risk factors may help late adolescent accept reality of vulnerability to cancer.
2. Assist client in relating risk factors to herself.	2. Awareness of the reality of risk increases the likelihood that the woman will change lifestyle behaviors.
3. Discuss potential strategies to decrease risk for cervical cancer (i.e., stop smoking, "safe sex"). Fascilitate implementation of cervical cancer reduction strategies.	3. Information permits informed decision making. Verification of woman's understanding permits correction of misinformation. Her involvement in planning increases compliance.

Evaluation

- Client is able to state cervical cancer risk factors in her own words.
- Client identifies cigarette smoking, young age at first sexual intercourse and first childbirth, multiple sexual partners, frequent STDs and HPV infection, abnormal Pap smear results.

Client Education

Kegal Exercises

Every woman should be taught to use Kegel exercises every day to prevent or improve urinary incontinence. Kegel exercises contract the pubococcygeus muscle (the muscle supporting the pelvic organs) by alternately contracting and relaxing the muscle controlling the rectum. The client is instructed to first relax the muscle as she would for defecation. She may visualize the process better if she conceptualizes her pelvic floor muscle as an elevator. When the elevator is in the basement, the muscle is relaxed. She contracts (or squeezes) the muscle enough to raise the elevator to the first floor, then contracts the muscle a little more to raise the elevator to the second floor, and contracts the muscle a little more to raise the elevator to the third floor, where she holds it for 3 seconds at first and gradually increases the time each week by 2 to 3 seconds, until she sustains the contraction for 10 seconds. She then relaxes the muscle by descending the elevator to the second, then first, and finally the basement floor. She maintains relaxation for 3 seconds (increasing the relaxation time as she increases the contraction time) and repeats the process 10 times. She is instructed to complete 6 to 8 sets of 10 repetitions per day. She can use a variety of triggers to remind her to complete a set of Kegel exercises. Some events used as triggers include a stop at a red light or stop sign while driving, the ringing of the telephone, or a commercial while watching television.

nurse should teach nonpharmacologic methods of coping, such as guided imagery, breathing and relaxation techniques, massage, cold or hot baths, and diversional activities. Assist the client in controlling as many factors regarding her care and pain control as possible by providing support and advocacy for the client's choices. Reduce the woman's fears by providing sufficient information in a form that she can understand to make informed choices.

MENOPAUSE

Menopause is the result of the decline in ovarian function (estrogen production). **Menopause** refers to the end of mensus, just as menarche refers to the beginning of men-

sus. Menopause is determined when the woman experiences no menstrual periods for 12 months. At the beginning of the 1990s, there were approximately 1.3 million women who had reached the age of 50, making about one-third of the United States' female population menopausal (Moore & Noonan, 1996). Because many women today live well into their 80's, and if they experience natural menopause in their early 50's, they can expect to live a large portion of their lives after menopause.

If she lives long enough, every woman will experience menopause at some point in her life, most often at about ages 49 to 51, and thus, experience the physiologic effects of estrogen deficiency in tissues containing estrogen receptors. Even though the severity of symptoms varies from woman to woman, most women experience menopausal symptoms, with some of these symptoms persisting for decades. Typical menopausal symptoms are related to vasomotor instability, urogenital atrophy, psychological discomforts, and long-term effects, such as development of cardiovascular disease and osteoporosis (DeMasters, 2000).

Vasomotor Instability

Vasomotor instability is commonly known as "hot flashes" or "hot flushes." The hot flash is uncontrollable, unpredictable, uncomfortable, and embarrassing and prompts many women to seek relief. Women experience the hot flash as an intense heat sensation, beginning in the upper chest or neck, progressing to the head, and demonstrated by a reddening of the skin. It occurs either occasionally (one or two a day) or frequently (several in an hour) (LeBoeuf & Carter, 1996). For many women, hot flashes are more severe at night, resulting in night sweats and contributing to insomnia. In addition, women report the increased occurrence of hot flashes during periods of stress.

The cause of hot flashes is unknown and the response of the brain to surges of LH levels is not well understood. A hot flash is known to coincide with an LH level surge, including a measurable increase in body surface temperature with a measurable drop in core body temperature. There is speculation that the fluctuating estrogen levels may alter the balance between norepinephrine and dopamine; thus creating the hot flash. Other professionals speculate that the low estrogen levels result in a malfunction of the temperature control system in the brain and cause an overproduction of heat in general or that a drop in body temperature may stimulate the body to readjust its temperature (Crandall, 1997).

Intervention for vasomotor instability responses most often includes ERT. An additional nonprescription intervention may include vitamin E therapy (DeMasters, 2000). Nursing interventions frequently include recommendations to wear nonsynthetic fabrics (cotton or silk) and loose clothing, dress in layers for easy removal of clothing during a hot flash, place two sets of cotton sheets on the bed for easy removal of damp sheets during the night, maintain normal blood glucose levels (small, frequent, nutritious meals), drink at least 6 to 8 glasses of water per day to maintain fluid balance, and avoid intake of substances associated with hot flashes (such as spicy foods, alcohol, and caffeine) (Crandall, 1997).

Urogenital Atrophy

Urogenital atrophy is the response of the estrogen receptor tissues to loss of estrogen. Such responses typically include a thinning and decreased elasticity of the vaginal epithelium and walls; change in color of vaginal epithelium to pale, almost whitish-pink; vaginal narrowing and shortening; progressive decrease in vaginal rugae and vaginal secretions; increased vaginal pH; vaginal dryness and itching; dyspareunia; and lower urinary tract symptoms (LeBoeuf & Cartz, 1996). With loss of estrogen, the genitourinary tract epithelium loses peripheral blood flow, resulting in loss of tone and development of urinary incontinence and a shortened urethra. This loss of tone may result in development of cystocele and rectocele (Crandall, 1997). In addition, cystocele increases urinary incontinence and rectocele increases constipation. Vaginal dryness results in dyspareunia, a risk for tearing the vagina during sexual intercourse, and development of atrophic vulvovaginitis (inflammation of the vulva or vaginal epithelium).

ERT as a therapeutic intervention successfully reverses the physiologic responses of the urogenital tissues to loss of estrogen (DeMasters, 2000). Since oral or transdermal ERT can take several weeks to reverse urogenital atrophy, some providers prescribe topical estrogen for the woman to apply for a short time, along with oral or transdermal ERT.

Nonprescriptive nursing interventions often include recommendations to increase vaginal moisture by using a lubricant (K-Y Jelly, Replens), continue sexual activity to increase blood flow to the genitourinary tissues, spend more time in foreplay to increase vaginal lubrication, and try to find a position during sexual intercourse that decreases the discomfort of dyspareunia (Crandall, 1997). Performing six to eight sets of 10 repetitions of Kegel exercises daily can reduce episodes of urinary incontinence and increase structural support to pelvic organs. In addition, eliminating substances known to cause frequent urination and bladder irritation, such as caffeine, artificial sweeteners, and even some fruit juices, may decrease episodes of urinary incontinence. Increasing water and fresh vegetable intake and walking for exercise can decrease constipation.

Psychological Conditions

Psychological disturbances of menopause include the mood swings, irritability and changes in short-term memory thought to be related to declining estrogen levels. Decreases in circulating estrogen directly affects neurotransmitters responsible for regulating mood, appetite, sleep, and pain perception (Washa, & Angelopoulos, 1996; Crandall, 1997). The changes in mood are responses similar to the psychological and emotional responses of premenstrual syndrome and postpartum blues, conditions related to the decrease in hormone levels. In addition, the menopausal woman is usually experiencing the role and lifestyle changes (retirement, widowhood, caring for sick parents, caring for grandchildren, beginning a career or second career) characteristic of the aging process, along with the accompanying insomnia. Thus, the combination of such changes and the decline in circulating estrogen can intensify psychological and emotional responses to both processes.

Alzheimer's disease is a chronic, progressive disease of mental deterioration and disability, the incidence of which increases from 5% of women over age 65 to 25% to 50% of women over age 85 (Cotter, 1997). ERT has demonstrated an effect of delaying the onset of Alzheimer's disease (Cotter, 1997).

Long-Term Considerations

Long-term effects of menopause are linked to estrogen loss and, if progression is undetected, may cause irreparable damage (Crandall, 1997). These effects include cardiovascular disease and osteoporosis. Estrogen fosters new bone growth and helps prevent cardiovascular disease.

Cardiovascular Disease

Cardiovascular diseases are collectively known as heart disease. Cardiovascular disease is the leading cause of death in the United States. Men have three times more risk for death than women at age 50 or younger, but women have an equal risk for death by age 65 (LeBoeuf, 1996). The increased cardiovascular disease risk for women is related to pathologic increases in cholesterol and triglyceride levels because of estrogen loss after menopause. Thus, after menopause, cardiovascular disease becomes the leading cause of disability and death in postmenopausal women (Crandall, 1997). More than 500,000 women die annually of cardiovascular disease (DeMasters, 2000). Although women are more frightened of dying of breast cancer, only 1 postmenopausal women in 28 dies of breast cancer annually, while 1 in 2 dies of cardiovascular disease. Other factors related to cardiovascular disease development include smoking, diabetes mellitus, excess weight, and genetic factors.

Therapeutic interventions for postmenopausal cardiovascular disease include medication, lifestyle changes, and ERT. The Postmenopausal Estrogen/Progestin Interventions (PEPI) trial has demonstrated the cardioprotectiveness of ERT and hormone replacement therapy (HRT) for women with and without existing cardiovascular disease. The PEPI findings reveal an *increased* number of cardiac events in women *with* existing cardiovascular disease (Byyny and Speroff, 1996) when they begin ERT or HRT in comparison to women without existing cardiovascular disease; these women require closer evaluation by their clinicians.

Osteoporosis

Osteoporosis includes the progressive bone loss, increased bone fragility, and increased risk for bone fractures that occur in postmenopausal women. Symptoms (atraumatic skeletal fractures, height loss, spinal deformity) do not occur until significant bone loss has occurred. One in 10 Caucasian women will experience an osteoporostic fracture; 400,000 people are admitted to hospitals and 44 million to nursing homes as a result of osteoporosis at an annual cost of approximately $14 billion; 20% of hip fractures and hip fracture–related complications result in death, killing more women than breast cancer (DeMasters, 2000). Osteoporosis has been diagnosed in approximately 28 million people in the United States, and the number is expected to continue to increase (Kessenich, 2000).

Risk factors for osteoporosis include the following (Licata, 1999; McClung, 1999):

- Caucasian ancestry (Northern European)
- Family history of osteoporosis (especially maternal family)
- Sedentary lifestyle
- Low intake of dietary calcium
- Small-boned frame
- Low body weight
- Excessive alcohol intake
- Smoking
- Late menarche and early menopause
- History of amenorrhea
- Excessive intake of certain medications (glucocorticoids, thyroid hormone, tetracyclines)
- Chronic illness (kidney, bowel, or liver disease; Cushing's syndrome; hyperthyroidism, hyperparathyroidism; hyperprolactinemia; hypogonadism)

Women achieve peak bone mass in the third decade of life and then begin losing 1% to 1.5% of bone mass per year until menopause, when the loss is accelerated up to 5% during the first 5 menopausal years as a result of estrogen loss (Crandall, 1997). Thus, women can lose approximately 40% to 50% of their bone mass after the third decade of life. Throughout life, bone tissue is remodeled on a cyclic basis by osteoblasts (bone cells that cause bone growth) and osteoclasts (bone cells that cause bone breakdown and resorption) (Kessenich, 2000). After menopause, the remodeling process is altered: osteoclast activity (bone breakdown) exceeds osteoblast activity (bone growth).

Therapeutic interventions for osteoporosis prevention and treatment include adequate calcium and vitamin D intake, weightbearing exercise, and consideration of ERT or HRT (DeMasters, 2000). In addition, bisphosphonates— etidronate (Didronel), alendronate (Fosamax), risedronate (Actonel) act to inhibit osteoclast activity. Studies document the benefit of bisphosphonates in the treatment and prevention of osteoporosis.

Nursing interventions include emphasizing the need for girls and women to consume at least 1000 mg of dietary calcium daily until age 50 and to increase the consumption after age 50 to 1500 mg daily (Crandall, 1997). Calcium-rich foods include dairy products, green leafy vegetables, and calcium-fortified foods such as cereal and orange juice). If the woman is unable to consume sufficient calcium from food, she can take calcium supplements in divided doses (1250 mg of calcium carbonate provides 500 mg of absorbable calcium; 1500 mg of calcium citrate provides 315 mg of absorbable calcium) (Crandall, 1997). Calcium is absorbed more readily when stomach acidity is increased and adequate vitamin D (400 IU daily) is available. Nurses need to remind women that smoking and caffeine and alcohol intake interfere with osteoblast cell activity and that weightbearing exercise (such as walking, cycling, tennis, dancing, weightlifting, or low-impact aerobics) increases osteoblast cell activity.

Nursing Implications

Nursing assessment for menopausal conditions involves careful personal and family history taking, and assessment for personal and familial risk factors, symptoms, and how the client has been coping with the symptoms. Physical assessment is focused on data collection for a diagnosis of the menopausal condition. Identification of necessary laboratory tests and diagnostic procedures also must be done.

Nursing diagnoses are individualized to each woman and her specific menopausal condition. Applicable diagnoses may include the following:

- Pain (mild or moderate) related to (specific menopausal condition)
- Grief related to mid to late life losses

- Deficient knowledge related to limited experience (or information) regarding (specific menopausal condition)
- Ineffective coping related to lack of acceptance of prognosis for (specific menopausal condition)

Nursing plans include specific actions the woman and her family will complete to achieve the highest possible level of wellness. Sample goals may include the following:

- Consume recommended foods based on the food pyramid in serving sizes to meet body requirements, including intake of calcium from foods or supplements.
- Exercise 30 minutes per day at least 3 to 4 times per week.
- Take prescriptive medication(s) as written.
- Understand instructions regarding prescriptive medication(s).
- Understand therapeutic intervention plan.
- Notify health care provider of adverse effects of medication(s).
- Notify health care provider of failure of symptoms to improve.
- Return to health care provider for scheduled follow-up visits.
- Have questions answered to her satisfaction.
- Understand health promotion counseling.

Nursing interventions for menopausal conditions include education regarding reduction of risk factors for

Critical Thinking

ERT and Cancer Risk

Research has been completed that focuses on the relationship of ERT and the risk for breast cancer. Some of the research identifies a slightly increased risk for clients on long-term ERT. Others do not support this finding.

Your client is an 84-year-old woman with severe osteoporosis (bilateral hip fractures, vertebral fractures, microfractures of the bones in the feet). After her second hip replacement, she began taking estradiol. She now has a suspicious result on her mammogram and is scheduled for a biopsy. She asks you if she should continue to take her estradiol. How would you respond?

Client Education

Hormone Replacement Therapy

The client who is at risk for osteoporosis should be taught the following:

1. Perform weight bearing exercise at least 5 days per week.
2. Consume 1200 mg of calcium with 400 IU of vitamin D per day if premenopausal.
3. Consume 1500 mg of calcium with 400 to 800 IU of vitamin D per day if postmenopausal and not on hormone replacement therapy.
4. Consume 1200 mg of calcium with 400 to 800 IU of vitamin D per day if postmenopausal and on hormone replacement therapy.
5. Consider hormone replacement therapy if she is postmenopausal. (Note: The client who has not had a hysterectomy must take both estrogen and progesterone to prevent an increased risk for endometrial cancer caused by unapposed estrogen therapy.)
6. Avoid smoking.

each woman, emphasizing prevention strategies, and explaining therapeutic interventions to ensure successful compliance. Nursing interventions for each menopausal condition described must be explained, encouraged, and evaluated. In addition, education should focus on health-promoting nutrition, maintenance of appropriate weight for height (BMI), and exercise: these can prevent many osteoporotic conditions.

Many women are frightened to take ERT or HRT because of conflicting news reports of research findings. Nurses can help women evaluate the research studies and recommend the benefits of ERT or HRT in comparison to the adverse potential of each woman's risk for each menopausal condition. For example, is a particular woman's risk of death from cardiovascular disease greater than her risk for death from breast cancer? In addition, the woman can be reminded that the increased risk of developing breast cancer from taking HRT must be weighed against post menopause breast cancer that occurs postmenopausally, which is less aggressive, typically takes longer to develop than aggressive cancer, responds to early diagnosis and treatment, and carries a better survival rate among HRT users than those not taking HRT (DeMasters, 2000). Women without a uterus who use ERT seem to have a lower risk of developing postmenopausal breast cancer than women who use estrogen plus progestin (HRT) (DeMasters, 2000).

Research has shown the risk for endometrial cancer is almost eliminated by adding progestin to estrogen (DeMasters, 2000). Some research findings indicate women who use HRT may have a lower endometrial cancer risk than women who do not. Other research findings seem to indicate that ERT and HRT are protective against colorectal cancer, delay Alzheimer's disease, and may help prevent osteoporosis and cardiovascular disease. Several long-term research studies in the woman's health initiative, will be completed in the next few years that may provide answers to many of the questions and concerns of women and, most likely, create new questions.

Web Activities

- Visit the American Cancer Society's website. What are the 5-, 10-, and 20-year survival rates for the cancers discussed in this chapter?

- Search for information on some of the disorders in this chapter, such as endometriosis. Are there websites available? Do they offer "healthy-living" guidelines? Can you volunteer to be part of a clinical trial if you have some of these conditions?

Key Concepts

- Menstrual cycle alterations relate to frequency and length of cycle, amount of flow, and number of years cycles are experienced.

- Endometriosis is a chronic disorder caused by implantation of endometrial tissue outside the uterus; it affects 1 in 7 women of childbearing age.

- Premenstrual syndrome affects 30% to 40% of women of childbearing age and is characterized by behavioral, emotional, and physical symptoms.

- Common benign breast conditions include fibrocystic changes, fibroadenoma, and nipple discharge.

- Risk factors for breast cancer include age over 50, female gender, history of ovarian or endometrial cancer, and history of first-degree relatives with breast cancer.

- Infections in the pelvic area include vaginal, cervical, and pelvic inflammatory diseases, which may be caused by bacteria, viruses, fungi, or protozoa.

- Benign pelvic conditions affect the vagina, cervix, uterus, and ovaries.

- Cancers of the pelvic region include cervical, endometrial, and ovarian.

- Menopause may be accompanied by hot flashes, urogenital atrophy, mood swings, irritability, and estrogen loss, which may increase the risk of cardiovascular disease and osteoporosis.

Review Questions and Activities

1. You are counseling a perimenopausal client regarding prevention of osteoporosis. You recommend that she increase her dietary intake of which of the following?
   a. Milk and iron
   b. Calcium and vitamin D
   c. Magnesium and vitamin C
   d. Magnesium and phosphorus

   The correct answer is b.

2. You are explaining the intervention strategies for PMS to a 28-year-old client. You recommend that during the latter part of her cycle she limit which of the following:
   a. Exercise
   b. Fluid intake
   c. Fruits and vegetables
   d. Salt and caffeine intake

   The correct answer is d.

3. You are completing the chief complaint interview for a 17-year-old with dysmenorrhea. You will assess for which of the following symptoms:

a. Food cravings

b. Heart palpitations

c. Abnormal bleeding

d. Duration of her pain

The correct answer is d.

4. You are counseling a 40-year-old who has come to the clinic because she found a "lump" in her breast last night. She is frantic because she believes she has cancer. The clinical breast examination reveals firm, smooth, discrete masses in both breasts. You reinforce the physician's impression that what she is feeling is most likely a noncancerous "lump" and that she should have which of the following evaluation procedures first:

a. Lumpectomy

b. Mammogram

c. Excisional biosy

d. Stereotactic biopsy

The correct answer is b.

5. You are collecting data from a 37-year-old client who you suspect may have fibroid tumors. You expect her subjective data to include which of the following symptoms:

a. Urinary urgency

b. Difficult defecation

c. Cyclic migraine headaches

d. Deep pelvic pain dyspareunia

The correct answer is d.

6. You are completing the chief complaint interview with a client who states that she has a continuous blood-tinged, watery discharge; postcoital bleeding; and dyspareunia. Based on her subjective data, you suspect which of the following medical diagnoses:

a. Cervical cancer

b. Hypermenorrhea

c. Pelvic relaxation

d. Polycystic ovary disease

The correct answer is a.

7. The chief complaint interview on a client reveals vaginal discharge with itching and burning. The client also reveals she experiences dyspareunia. If her diagnosis is monilial vulvovaginitis, you would expect the wet mount slide to contain which of the following:

a. Bacteria

b. Clue cells

c. Trichomonads

d. Budding hyphae

The correct answer is d.

8. You are conducting the discharge teaching session for a client with bacterial vulvovaginosis. You instruct her regarding which of the following medications:

a. Cefoxitin

b. Gentamicin

c. Doxycycline

d. Metronidazole

The correct answer is d.

References

Arnold, G. C., & Neiheisel, M. B. (1997). A comprehensive approach to evaluating nipple discharge. *Nurse Practitioner, 22,* (7), 96, 98–102, 105–111.

Averette, H. E., & Muyen, H. (1995) Gynecologic Cancer In G. Murphy, W. Lawrence, & R. Lonhard Eds. Clincial Oncology. Atlanta Ga. American Cancer Society.

Baron, R. H., & Walsh, A. (1995). Nine facts everyone should know about breast cancer. *American Journal of Nursing, 95,* (7), 29–33.

Bristow, R. & Montz, F. (2000). Cervical Cancer in S.B. Ranson Ed. Practical Strategies in Obstetrics & Gynecology, Philadelphia, PA. WB Saunders.

Brucker, M. C., & Scharbo-DeHaan, M. (1991). Breast disease: The role of the nurse midwife. *Journal of Nurse-Midwifery, 36,* (1), 63–73.

Byyny, R. and Speroff, L. (1996). A clinical guide for care of older women. (2 ed) William and Wilkins, Baltimore, M.D.

Campbell, M. K., & Pruitt, J. T. (1996). Radiation's Therapy: Protecting your patient's skin: *RN, 59,* (1) 46–47.

Corwin, E. J. (1997). Endometriosis: Pathophysiology, diagnosis, and treatment. *American Journal of Primary Health Care, 22,* (10), 35–36, 38–42, 45–46, 48–51, 55.

Cotter, V. T. (1997). Hormonic convergence: Finding balance through hormone replacement therapy. *AWHONN Lifelines, 1,* (1), 37–42.

Crandall, S. G. (1997). Menopause made easier. *RN, 60,* (7), 46–50.

Cullins, V. E., Dominguez, L., Guberski,Dominguez, L., Guberski, T., Secor, R. M., & Wysocki, S. J. (1999). Treating vaginitis. *Nurse Practitioner, 24,* (10), 46–63.

DeMasters, J. (2000). A clinician's guide to understanding the dilemma. *AWHONN Lifelines, 4,* (2), 26–35.

Foulks, M. J. (1998). The Papanicolaou smear: Its impact on the promotion of women's health. *Journal of Obstetric, Gynecologic, and Neonatal Nursing, 27,* (4), 367–373.

Grabo, T. N., Fahs, P. S., Nataupsky, L. G., & Reich, H. (1999). Uterine myomas: Treatment options. *Journal of Obstetric, Gynecologic, and Neonatal Nurses, 28,* (1), 23–31.

Higgins, P. G. (1997). Assessing cervical cancer risk. *Lifelines, 1,*

(6), 43–47; Carson, S. (1997). Human papillomatous virus infection update: Impact on women's health, *The Nurse Practitioner, 22,* (4), 24–37.

Johnson, C. L. (2000). Update on breast and cervical cancers, *AWHONN Lifelines, 4,* (1), 20–21.

Keene, G. F. (1999). Office gynecology: Common reproductive tract disorders. *Clinician Reviews, 9,* (1), 58–80.

Kessenich, C. R. (2000). Risedronate: A new bisophosphonate for the treatment of osteoporosis. *Nurse Practitioner, 25,* (3), 106–108.

Klingman, L. (1999). Assessing the female reproductive system. *American Journal of Nursing, 99,* (8), 37–43.

LeBoeuf, F. J., & Carter, S. G. (1996). Discomforts of perimenopause. *Journal of Obstetric, Gynecologic, and Neonatal Nursing, 25,* (2), 173–180.

Licata, A. A. (1999). Update on osteoporosis: Strategies for prevention and treatment. *Women's Health in Primary Care, 2,* (3), 229–244.

Lucas, B. D. (1999). Five reasons to consider a hysterectomy. *Patient Care for the Nurse Practitioner, 2,* (9), 28–50.

Marantides, D. (1997). Management of polycystic ovary syndrome. *Nurse Practitioner, 22,* (12), 34–41.

McCance, K. L., & Jorde, L. B. (1998). Evaluating the genetic risk of breast cancer. *Nurse Practitioner, 23,* (8), 14–27.

McClung, B. L. (1999). Using osteoporosis management to reduce fractures in elderly women. *Nurse Practitioner,* 26–47.

McGee, C. (1997). Secondary amenorrhea leading to osteoporosis. *Nurse Practitioner, 22,* (5), 38–64.

Moore, A. A., & Noonan, M. D. (1996). A nurse's guide to hormone replacement therapy. *Journal of Obstetric, Gynecologic, and Neonatal Nurses, 25,* (1), 24–31.

Mott, A. M. (1998). Prevention and management of pelvic inflammatory disease by primary care providers. *American Journal for Nurse Practitioners, 2,* (6), 7–15.

Shurpin, K. M. (1997). Clinical snapshot: Ovarian cancer. *American Journal of Nursing, 97,* (4), 34–35.

Smith, C. B. (1998). Pinpointing the cause of abnormal uterine bleeding. *Women's Health Primary Care,. 1,* (10), 835–844.

Thomas, S., & Greirzu, S. P. (2000). Oncology today: Breast cancer, *RN, 63,* (4), 41–45.

Ugarriza, D. N., Klinger, S., & O'Brien, S. (1998). Premenstrual syndrome: Diagnosis and prevention. *Nurse Practitioner, 23,* (9), 40–58.

Wasaha, S., & Angelopoulos, F. M. (1996). What every woman should know about menopause. *American Journal of Nursing, 96,* (1), 24–33.

White, G. L., Griffith, C. J., Nenstiel, R. O., & Dyess, D. L. (1996). Breast cancer: Reducing mortality through early detection. *Clinician Reviews, 6,* (9), 77–102.

Suggested Readings

Baker, S. (1998). Menstruation and related problems and concerns. In Youngkin, E. Q., & Davis, M. S. (Eds.) *Women's health: A primary care clinical guide.* Stamford: Appleton & Lange, 139–160.

Bosarge, P. M. (1995). Hormone therapy: The woman's decision. *Supplement: Contemporary Nurse Practitioner, 11,* (4), 3–10.

Bristow, R. & Montz F. (2000) Cervical Cancer in S. B. Ransom and Practical Strategies in Obstetrics & Gynecology Philadelphia PA. W. B. Saunders.

Burke, T. W., Tortolero-Luna, G., Malpica, A., Baker, V. V., Whittaker, L., Johnson, E., & Mitchell, M. F. (1996). Endometrial hyperplasia and endometrial cancer. *Obstetrics & Gynecology Clinics of North America, 23,* (2), 411–456.

Clark-Coller, T. (1991). Dysfunctional uterine bleeding and amenorrhea: Differential diagnosis and management. *Journal of Nurse Midwifery, 36,* (1), 49–62.

Davis, K. M., & Schlaff, W. D. (1995). Medical management of uterine fibromyomata. *Obstetrics & Gynecology Clinics of North America, 22,* (4), 727–738.

Dest, V., & Fisher, S. (1994). Breast cancer: dreaded diagnosis, complicated care. *RN, 57,* (6), 49–54.

Edwards, C. L., Tortolero-Luna, G., Linares, A. C., Malpica, A., Baker, V. V., Cook, E., Johnson, E., & Mitchell, M. F. (1996). Vulvar intraepithelial neoplasia and vulvar cancer. *Obstetrics & Gynecology Clinics of North America, 23,* (2), 295–324.

Fiorica, J. V. (1994). Nipple discharge. *Obstetrics & Gynecology Clinics of North America, 21,* (3), 453–460.

Galsworthy, T. D., & Wilson, P. L. (1996). Osteoporosis: it steals more than bone. *American Journal of Nursing, 96,* (6), 27–33.

Garner, C. (1997). Endometriosis: What You Need to Know. *RN, 60,* (1), 27–31.

Hutchins, F. L., Jr. (1995). Uterine fibroids: Diagnosis and indications for treatment. *Obstetrics & Gynecology Clinics of North America, 22,* (4), 659–665.

Igoe, B. A. (1997). Symptoms attributed to ovarian cancer by women with the disease. *Nurse Practitioner, 22,* (7), 122–143.

Isaacs, J. H. (1994). Benign tumors of the breast. *Obstetrics & Gynecology Clinics of North America, 21,* (3), 487–497.

Kelsey, B., & Freeman, S. (1997). Identifying and treating pelvic inflammatory disease. *American Journal of Nursing, 97,* (11), 17–22.

Klemm, P. R., & Guarnieri, C. (1996). Cervical cancer: A developmental perspective. *Journal of Obstetric, Gynecologic, and Neonatal Nursing, 25,* (7), 629–634.

McMullin, M. (1992). Holistic care of the patient with cervical cancer. *Nursing Clinics of North America, 27,* (4), 847–858.

Mogus, M. (1997). Pelvic floor surgery. *RN, 60,* (4), 36–41.

Poma, P. A. (1997). A simple strategy for managing perimenopausal bleeding. *Contemporary Nurse Practitioner, 2,* (3), 21–26.

Rush, C. B., & Entman, S. S. (1995). Pelvic organ prolapse and stress urinary incontinence. *Medical Clinics of North America, 79,* (6), 1473–1479.

Shapiro, T. J., & Clark, P. M. (1995). Breast cancer: What the primary care provider needs to know. *Nurse Practitioner, 20,* (3), 36–53.

Sharts-Hopko, N. C. (1997). STDs in women: What you need to know. *American Journal of Nursing, 97,* (4), 46–54.

Siris, E. S., & Schussheim, D. H. (1998). Osteoporosis: Assessing your patient's risk. *Women's Health in Primary Care, 1,* (1), 99–106.

Spiegel, K. K. (1997). On your markers: Research advances in breast cancer in women. *AWHONN Lifelines, 1,* (5), 33–38.

Resources

American Cancer Society, 1599 Clifton Road, NE Atlanta, GA 30329, (800) ACS-2345, www.cancer. org

Breast Cancer Information, www.breastcancernews.com

Centers for Disease Control and Prevention, 1600 Clifton Road, NE, Atlanta, GA 30333, (404) 329-1819, (404) 329-3286, www.cdc.org

National Alliance of Breast Cancer Organizations, 9 East 37th Street, 10th Floor, New York, NY 10016, (800) 719-0145, www.nabco.org

National Breast Cancer Coalition, P.O. Box 66373, Washington, DC 20035, (800) 935-0434, (202) 296-7477, www.natbcc.org

National Cancer Institute, (800) 4-CANCER, www.nci.nih.gov

Susan G. Komen Breast Cancer Foundation, (800) I'M AWARE or (462-9273)

Y-ME National Breast Cancer Organization, (800) 221-2141 (9 AM to 5 PM CST), (312) 986-8228 (24 hours), www.y-me.org

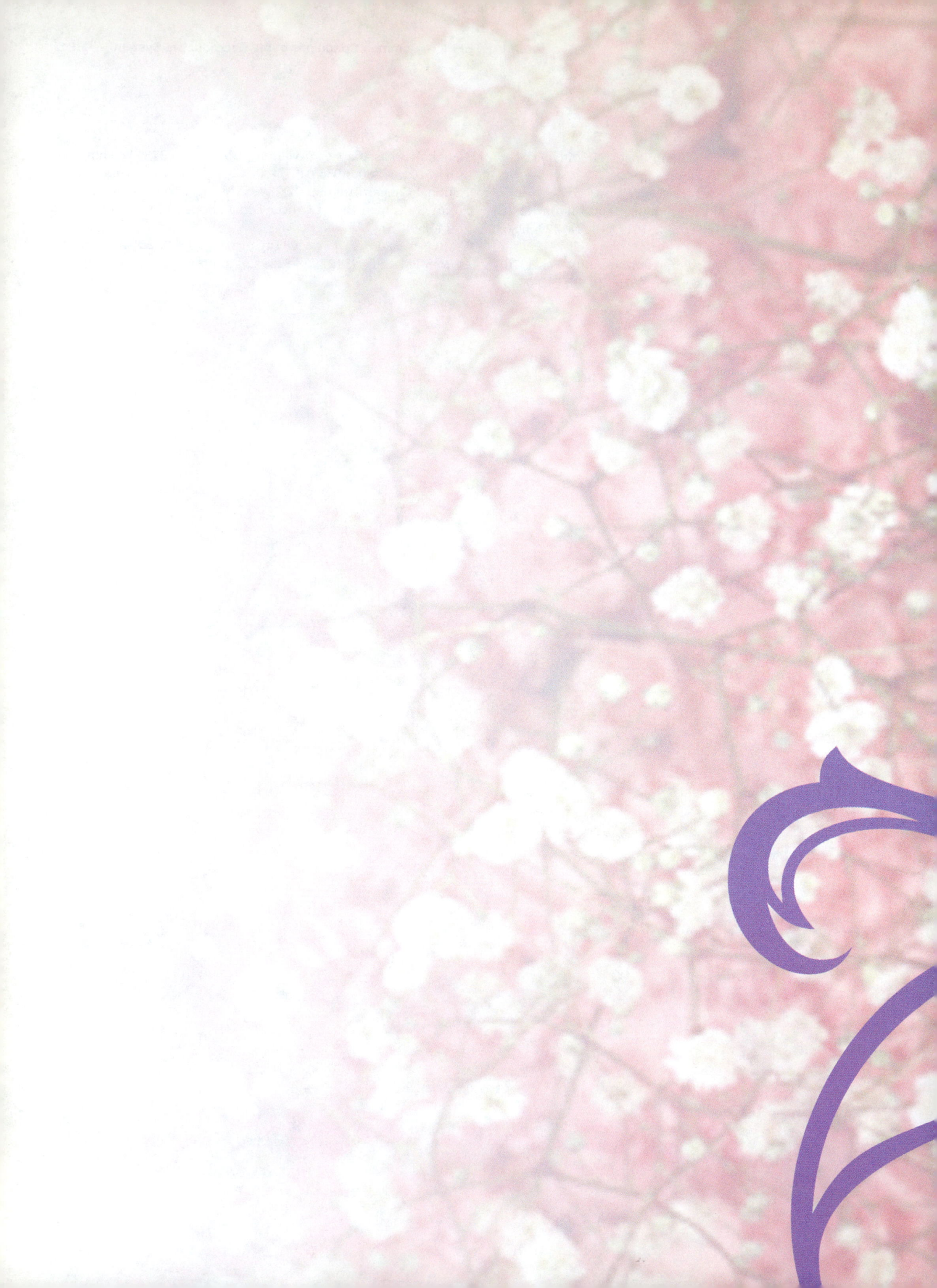

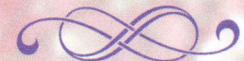

CHAPTER 11

Violence and Abuse

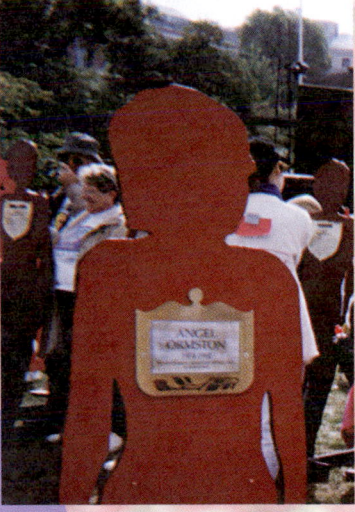

*N*urses who work with clients who are abused may experience strong personal emotions because providing supportive counseling to these clients is often difficult. The following questions are designed to help caregivers of these women and children clarify their personal feelings and increase their awareness of the far-reaching consequences of physical and emotional abuse.

- *How do I feel when I see a woman in the emergency department or office with injuries such as bruises or broken bones sustained from a beating by her husband?*

- *Have I personally experienced emotional, physical, or sexual abuse?*

- *Am I emotionally distressed when I interview and care for children or older persons who are abused?*

- *What are my feelings about women who return to their abusers after a severe beating?*

- *What do I believe about sexual harassment, date rape, and forced sex? Do I believe that women are responsible for bringing these acts on themselves, or do I think they are victims of a crime?*

- *Have I ever seen a woman with a gunshot or knife wound? How did I feel when caring for her? How did I react when she was discharged from the hospital? How did I react when one of these women died?*

Key Terms

Acquaintance rape
Adult maltreatment
   syndrome
Assault

Child abuse
Date rape
Femicide
Incest

Neglect
Perpetrator
Rape
Stalking

Stranger rape
Supine hypotension
   syndrome
Wife rape

Competencies

Upon completion of this chapter, the reader should be able to:

1. Identify factors that may support a system in which abuse of adults, children, or older persons occurs.
2. Define categories of violence: physical and psychological violence, sexual abuse, and neglect.
3. Identify risk factors for abuse or neglect of adults, children, and older persons.
4. Describe the legal responsibilities of the nurse involved with mandatory reporting and documentation of abuse.
5. Describe the cycle of abuse of an intimate partner.
6. Utilize community resources to aid in the prevention and treatment of persons in abusive relationships.

iolence against women in the United States is a serious threat to their health and welfare (Paluzzi & Houde-Quimby, 1996). This chapter focuses on interpersonal violence and abuse against women of all ages and their children.

INTIMATE PARTNER VIOLENCE

Intimate partner violence is sometimes referred to as *intimate partner abuse, domestic violence, domestic abuse, spouse abuse,* or *wife battering,* all of which describe intentional violent or controlling behavior by a current or former intimate partner. In 1996, some 840,000 women experienced aggravated **assault** (the intentional act of inflicting physical injury on another person), rape, and assaultative victimization by their current or former spouses, boyfriends, or girlfriends (Greenfield et al., 1998). On average, each year from 1992 to 1996, 8 of every 1,000 women received nonfatal injuries from willful or intentional abusive acts by their intimate partners. In addition, women are eight times more likely than are men to be assaulted by intimate partners (Greenfield et al., 1998). Each abusive interaction has the potential to be deadly. From 1976 through 1996, 29.7% of women victims of murder were killed by husbands, ex-husbands, and nonmarital partners compared with 5.9% of male victims (Greenfield

et al., 1998). Among murder victims for every age group, females are much more likely than are males to have been murdered by intimate partners (Cooper & Eaves, 1996). Thousands of deaths occur as a result of repeated assaults over many years (Hodges, 1993). Coercive behaviors of the **perpetrator** (the person accused of a criminal offense), such as belittlement, physical assaults, and stalking, can escalate to **femicide** (murder of a female). Of murders attributed to intimate partners, 75% were female victims. Femicide is the major cause of death for African American women aged 15 to 34 years and the seventh leading cause of premature death for all women in the United States (Hambleton, Clark, Symaya, Weissman, & Horner, 1997). According to the Federal Bureau of Investigation, in 1996, 30% of all women victims of murder were slain by husbands or boyfriends (Uniform Crime Reports for the United States, 1996).

Sexual Assault

Rape is defined as sexual penetration of another by force or threat of force, without consent. Abuse by an intimate partner accounts for half of all rapes of women over 30 years old (Jones, 1994). In one study, Murdoch and Nicholand (1993) found that one in four women in the military under the age of 50 had been physically abused within the past year. Of enlisted women, 31% had been forced to have nonconsensual sex.

REFLECTIONS FROM NURSES

In 1990, the first silent witnesses were produced (see Resources for information on the Silent Witness National Initiative). The silent witnesses are free-standing life-size wooden figures painted red (Figure 11-1). They bear the name and story of a woman murdered in domestic violence, honoring her life and memory. Each figure is carried by two persons in a demonstration march, or the figure is placed on a stand for display. In 1997, Washington, DC, was the site of the Silent Witness National Initiative, where representatives from all 50 states and several countries brought their witnesses for a silent march to Capitol Hill.

During this rally one of the speakers, Laura Katzif, shared her story. Her husband attacked her and cut her face, requiring 17 stitches. As she lay on the gurney in the emergency room thinking to herself, "What did I do to deserve this?," an attending nurse came up to her, leaned toward her head, and whispered in her ear, "You don't deserve this. No one does." Hearing the nurse's poignant words of validation helped her to make changes to leave this dangerous situation.

Critical Thinking

Risks of Being Raped

- What would you say to a woman who asks if it is possible to contract AIDS or gonorrhea as an outcome of being raped?
- What are her options for sexually transmitted disease testing?
- What are her options for preventing conception?

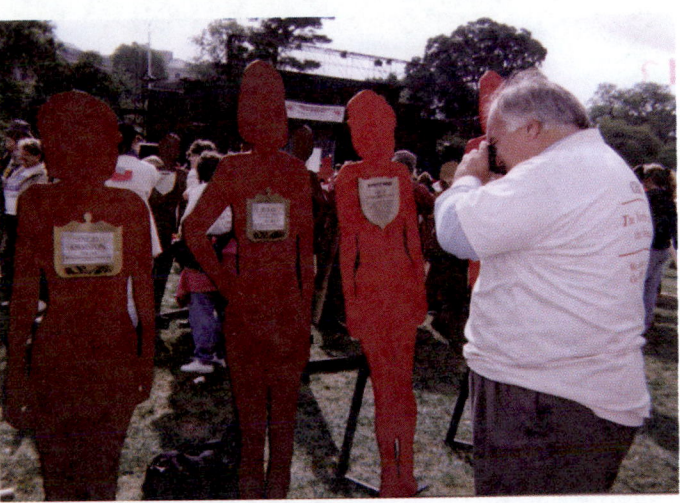

Figure 11-1 The Silent Witness National Initiative demonstration in Washington, DC, in 1997 has focused national attention on the many women who have lost their lives as a result of abuse.

Two major categories of rape exist: acquaintance rape and stranger rape. **Acquaintance rape** occurs when a perpetrator with whom the victim has had a previous nonviolent relationship uses deceit and coercion to obtain sex. Two types of acquaintance rape are wife rape and date rape. **Wife rape** is a forced sexual experience with a common-law or legally married spouse; **date rape** is rape that occurs between a dating couple without consent of one of the participants. **Stranger rape** is a nonconsensual sexual experience between a victim and an assailant who are strangers. Stranger rape is sudden and often involves weapons (Marx, Wie & Gross, 1996). By 1993, all 50 states had passed laws making marital rape a crime. Studies have estimated that 14% to 25% of wives are forced by their spouses to have sexual intercourse against their will at some time during the course of their marital relationship (Resnick, Kilpatrick, Walsh, & Vernonen, 1991; Russell, 1990).

To assess and provide care to a person who experiences rape, nurses must first understand the psychological effect of rape trauma syndrome. This syndrome is characterized as a response to the extreme stress and profound fear of death, which most survivors experience (Figure 11-2). Rape trauma syndrome begins with an acute or immediate phase of disorganization followed by a long-term process of reorganization that occurs as a result of attempted or forcible sexual assault. The majority of women report symptoms of avoidance and denial, which may prevent them from seeking help and participating in legal prosecution (Kramer & Green, 1991). Nurses may use information on the prevalence of symptoms of post-traumatic stress disorder (PTSD) to help in identification and provision of anticipatory guidance to survivors of sexual assault. PTSD is discussed later in this chapter.

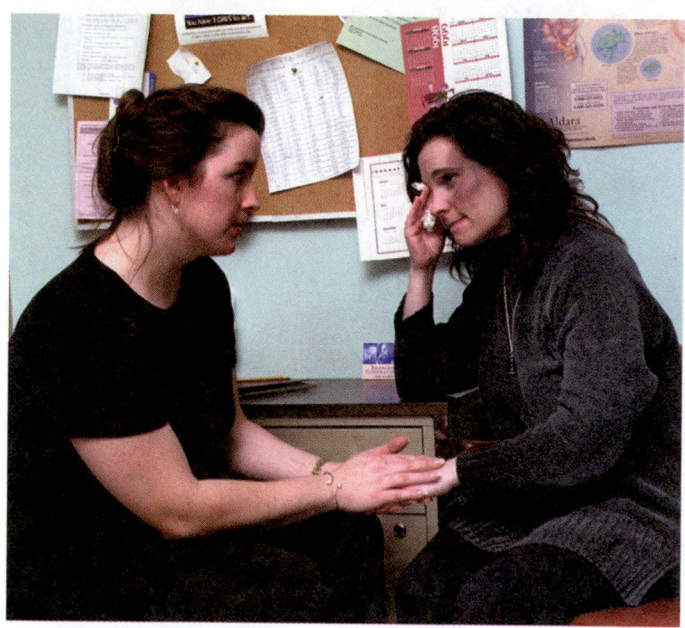
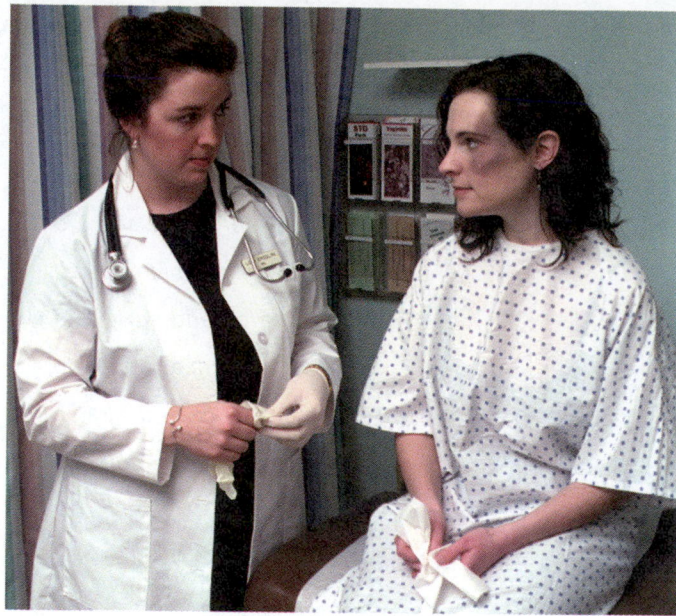

Figure 11-2 Caring for a woman who has survived an assault requires compassion and sensitivity during both the interview and physical examination.

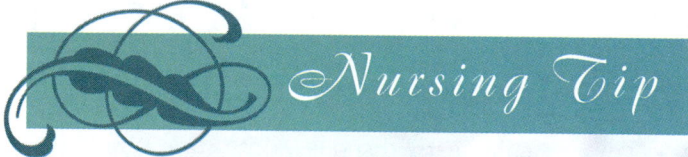

HELPING SURVIVORS OF RAPE

What you can say to a survivor of intimate partner violence or rape:

- I am afraid for the safety of you and your children.
- Violence only gets worse over time.
- You know when it would be safest to leave, and we are here for you when you are ready.
- You do not deserve to be hit.
- It is not your fault.
- Let me help you figure out a safety plan for you and your children.

Violence During Pregnancy

Abuse during pregnancy occurs at rates of 9% to 20% (Paluzzi & HoudeQuimby, 1996; Rodriguez, Quiroga, & Bauer, 1996). McFarlane, Parker, Soeken, and Bullock (1992) reported a 60% recurrence rate of abuse among pregnant women who are battered. Abuse is associated with the following complications of pregnancy: low weight gain, anemia, infections, increased incidence of first and second trimester bleeding, and increased rates of maternal depression and attempted suicide. Abuse also is associated with increased use of tobacco, alcohol, and illicit drugs during pregnancy.

The normal physiologic changes of pregnancy can mask the severity of battering and thus the extent of injury to the mother and fetus. Therefore, the nursing assessment for the traumatized client who is pregnant must include an understanding of a woman's altered body systems (i.e., cardiovascular, respiratory, and gastrointestinal systems) during pregnancy. As cardiac output increases, the hormone progesterone lowers systemic vascular resistance. This lowered resistance can cause a hypervolemic state that could mask hypovolemic shock until nearly a 30% blood loss has occurred. At that point the uterus would not have adequate uteroplacental perfusion, and decreased fetal oxygenation would result. The enlarging uterus may further compromise perfusion by compressing the vena cava, decreasing venous blood return to the heart. This phenomenon is referred to as **supine hypotension syndrome**. Severe shock can occur when blood loss is coupled with supine hypotension syndrome.

During pregnancy, respiratory function creates a state of chronic respiratory alkalosis to provide adequate fetal oxygenation. Lower levels of arterial carbon dioxide pressure and serum bicarbonate decrease the buffering capacity of the woman's body and allow for hypoxic tissue damage to occur more rapidly in the traumatized client. Gastric motility is encumbered by the size of the uterus, and the hormones of pregnancy relax the gastroesophageal sphincter. These normal changes make the woman more likely to aspirate food and liquids, and bowel sounds are less audible. Because it is displaced anteriorly by the developing fetus, the urinary bladder is at greater risk for injury.

The abdomen and trunk areas are frequent targets of assaultive blows. A leading cause of fetal death from blunt abdominal trauma is placenta abruption, which is most likely to occur within 48 hours of an assault. Separation of the placenta can be complete (total dislodgment) or incomplete (partial separation). Hemorrhage caused by the abruption will be either concealed (confined within the uterine cavity) or, more frequently, external. If external, blood will drain through the cervix. Women experiencing placental abruption will have unremitting uterine or back pain, a tender and irritable uterus, and visible or concealed hemorrhage. Signs of fetal distress, disseminated intravascular coagulation, and hypovolemic shock may or may not occur. Placental separation may be detected early by fetal monitoring. Monitoring will show increased uterine tonus, contractions, and a rapid fetal heart rate. The fetus has a better prognosis if the abdominal trauma occurs late in the third trimester and results in only a small, partial separation of the placenta.

Maternal and fetal morbidity risks increase with each additional episode of battering. Campbell (1995b) has found that as the severity of battering increases, so does the woman's risk of death.

Research Highlight

Nurses Assessing for Domestic Violence at Prenatal Visits

Purpose

To determine the extent of violence during pregnancy experienced by Hispanic women receiving prenatal care at an urban public health department.

Methods

During the routine prenatal intake interview the clinic nurse screened all prenatal clients for abuse at the first visit to the maternity clinic. Abuse screening procedures were based on the March of Dimes protocol and included administration of the Abuse Screen questionnaire, developed by Judith McFarland, PhD. If the women had been abused in the year before or during the current pregnancy by their current or former male partners, the women were referred to the on-site abuse counselor. The counselor obtained consent and administered the Severity of Violence Against Women Scale (SVAWS) (Marshall, 1992).

Findings

During a 12-month period, 329 Hispanic women were identified as having been abused. SVAWS scores were high: 30% of women had been threatened with death, 18% had been threatened with a knife or gun, 40% had been punched, 33% had been kicked, and over 20% had been coerced or forced into having sexual relations. Of these women, 80% had been shaken or roughly handled, 71% had been pushed or shoved, and 64% had been slapped on the face and head. Hispanic women who were abused during pregnancy experienced violence of sufficient severity to pose a risk to maternal and fetal health.

Nursing Implications

This study demonstrates the importance of screening healthy women regularly for abuse and if abuse is present, for injury to the unborn child. Nurses should always ask these four prenatal abuse screening questions:

1. During any pregnancy were you ever pushed, shoved, slapped, hit, kicked, or otherwise physically hurt by anyone?
2. During this pregnancy have you been pushed, shoved, slapped, hit, kicked, or otherwise physically hurt by anyone?
3. Before you were pregnant had anyone ever forced you to engage in sexual activity?
4. Since this pregnancy began has anyone forced you to engage in sexual activity?

Wiist, W. H., & McFarlane, J. (1998). Severity of spousal and intimate partner abuse to pregnant Hispanic women. *Journal of Health Care for the Poor and Underserved, 9,* 248–261.

Emergency Department Visits

Bureau of Justice Statistics (1997) show that of 243,000 American women who were abused, 199,260 (82%) were treated in hospital emergency departments for injuries sustained as a result of intimate partner violence and 32% of the women who went to the police did not seek medical treatment. Between 22% and 35% of women seeking medical treatment at an emergency department received their injuries from partners in an ongoing abusive relationship (Anderson & Taliaferro, 1997). These data show that the injuries caused by intimate partner violence are not merely minor bruises, contusions, or excoriations. Of all women needing emergency surgery, research shows that 20% were battered (Jones, 1994).

The self-report study by Straus and Gelles (1986) has estimated that about 16% of women experienced violence at the hands of intimate partners, which included punching, kicking, and attacks with an object or weapon. Another national survey by Greenfield and co-workers (1998) has shown that 51% of abused women reported their injuries to the police. One in five of these women sought professional medical treatment, with 7% going to an emergency department, and 32% were not treated (Greenfield et al., 1998). Serious injuries (4%) included broken bones,

Research Highlight

Physical Abuse During Pregnancy

Purpose

To determine the prevalence of physical abuse among an ethnically stratified group of pregnant women experiencing vaginal bleeding and reporting to an emergency department.

Methods

This study was a cross-sectional survey using two screening tools: the Abuse Assessment Screen (Stark et al., 1981) and the Danger Assessment (Campbell, 1986). The study sample consisted of 261 African American, Hispanic, and Caucasian pregnant women seen for vaginal bleeding in private and public emergency departments in a large metropolitan area. The women were interviewed in private rooms and were informed about community resources regarding domestic violence. Pregnancy status was determined by urine or serum beta human chorionic gonadotropin tests. A discharge diagnosis was obtained from emergency department records.

Findings

Of the 261 pregnant women interviewed, 33% reported abuse: of these, 27% were African American women; 25% were Hispanic; and 58% were Caucasian. Overall, Caucasian women reported significantly more abuse than did non-Caucasian women. No differences were found among diagnostic groups, and no significant differences among ethnicities were seen.

Nursing Implications

Pregnant women who are abused commonly report to an emergency department and can be readily identified using the following two-question 5-minute screening process:

1. Have you ever been hit, slapped, kicked, or otherwise physically hurt by your partner?
2. Have you ever been forced to engage in sexual activity by your partner?

A "yes" response to either question identifies the need for further abuse assessment. The Danger Assessment (Campbell, 1986, 1995b) is one such tool that can be used to identify whether the woman is at high risk for escalating violence that might be life-threatening.

Greenberg, E. M., McFarlane, J., & Watson, M. G. (1997). Vaginal bleeding and abuse: Assessing pregnant women in the emergency department. *Maternal Child Nursing, 22,* 182–186.

internal injuries, loss of consciousness, and any other injury requiring 2 or more days' hospitalization; other injuries (41%) consisted of bruises, black eyes, lacerations, chipped teeth, and injuries requiring less than 2 days' hospitalization. Of injuries reported to the police, 6% resulted from rape or sexual assault, whereas 0.05% resulted from gunshot or knife wounds (Greenfield et al., 1998).

Recognizing the importance of health care providers in the care of persons experiencing domestic violence, the Joint Commission for the Accreditation of Healthcare Organizations (JCAHO, 1997) requires accredited emergency departments to have policies, procedures, and staff education on the treatment of adults who are battered. Utilization of the ICD-9 diagnostic code of **adult maltreatment syndrome** (995.81) for all clients who have a current history of abuse greatly aids in the monitoring for both JCAHO site review and the prevalence and recidivism of violence by clients using the facility. Some states require nurses to have received continuing education on the topic of domestic violence to renew their nursing license. Use of nationally prepared training materials and programs are helpful in meeting these requirements. Much progress has been made in identifying abuse and implementing interventions to ensure the safety of the client and her family.

Primary Care of Abused Women

Neufeld (1996) reported that 23% of women seen in a family practice setting had experienced domestic violence within the past 12 months. Other researchers showed abuse rates from 14% to 32% in ambulatory care practices (Cohen, DeVos, & Newberger, 1997; Rodriguez, Quiroga, & Bauer, 1996). All this violence by intimate partners adds up to 100,000 days in the hospital, 30,000 emergency department visits, and 40,000 health care visits each year (Felder, 1996).

Forensic nursing is a specialty area of practice that advocates for abused clients by providing clear, precise, detailed descriptions of the abuse. This documentation can be used legally to help obtain a protective or restraining order or assist in the prosecution for assault or murder. Included in the forensic nursing process is an assessment of the client's immediate danger and the creation of a safety plan. These steps are the responsibility of every nurse. Sexual assault examinations involve collecting oral, vaginal, and anal swabs; performing external and internal genital examinations (speculum and colposcopic or endoscopic procedures); combing pubic hairs; and inspecting the skin surfaces of the body for sperm using Wood's light (ultraviolet light) (Figure 11-3). The clinician collects and preserves the integrity of the evidence. While providing examinations to obtain legal evidence, the trained clinician

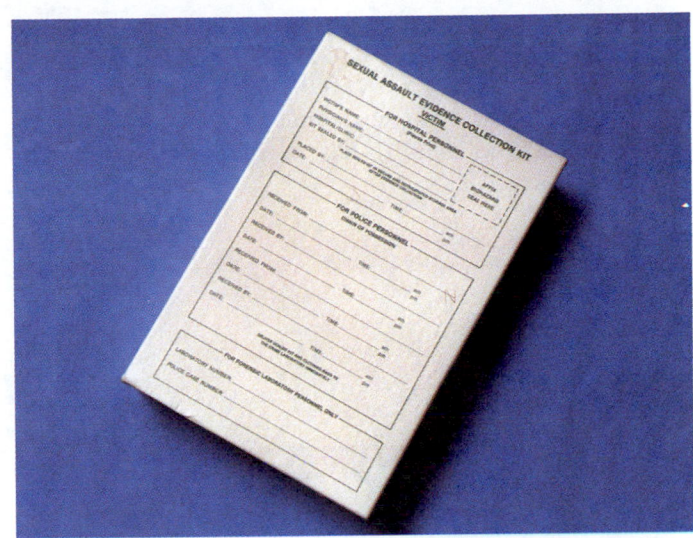

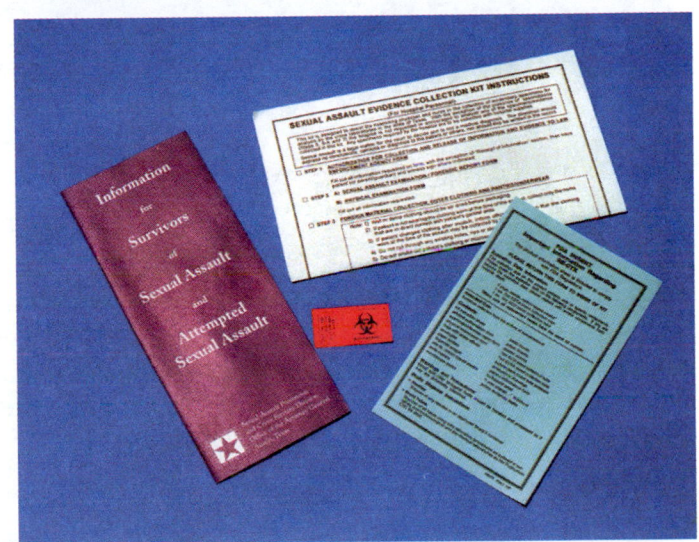

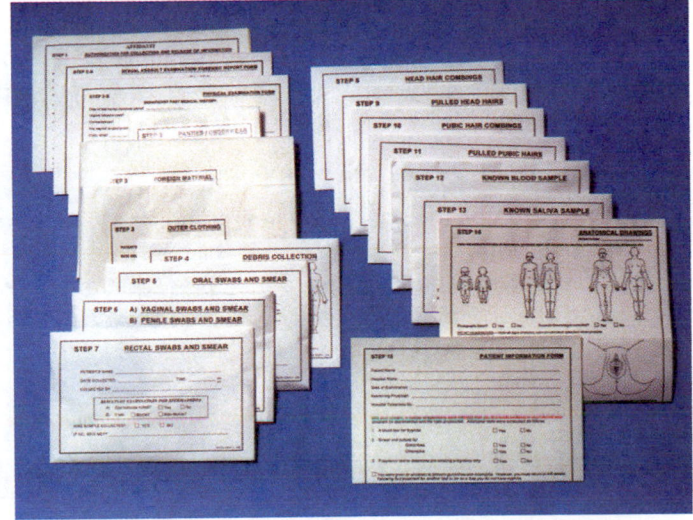

Figure 11-3 A sexual assault evidence collection kit contains detailed instructions on paper evidence collection and labeling.

always must be aware that these invasive procedures are highly traumatic to the survivor. Some survivors have even referred to the process as a "second rape." Nonjudgmental support, therapeutic listening, and an individualized safety plan can help the client to take steps toward ending the cycle of abuse.

Safety Planning

Minimum components of a safety plan include preparatory steps for ensuring safety during violent episodes, or details about how the woman who is being abused will leave the relationship. Community resources (e.g., women's shelters, the police, the district attorney's office, women's centers, and hotline phone numbers) are reviewed, and referrals are offered or made at the time of the visit. The nurse should assess the client's risk of danger privately, maintaining confidentiality, and must maintain a nonjudgmental demeanor. Each encounter with a client can foster disclosure of the extent of intimate partner violence and empower the client to develop strategies that increase her safety. The nurse should discuss methods of limiting the

Research Highlight

Retaliation after Reporting Abuse

Purpose

To describe the amount of violence experienced by women after they have sought help from the police for violence committed by intimate partners.

Methods

Nurse researchers interviewed 90 consecutive women at a family violence unit of an urban police department after the women sought to file assault charges. Threats of violence, physical assault, stalking, and danger for homicide were measured by interview questionnaires on the day charges were filed and again 3 and 6 months after filing. The women were assigned a counselor and then a police officer who counseled them on the legal process, the cycle of violence, safety planning, and community resources.

Findings

Of these women, 33% had enough evidence to file assault charges, 15% did not, and 11% dropped charges previously accepted by criminal justice officials. Of the perpetrators, 37% were arrested, and 4% were fugitives. Mean violence scores for each outcome were calculated for each time frame using one-way analysis of variance. Only one group was statistically different. The danger of homicide at 3 months was higher in women who had insufficient evidence to file assault charges. The act of attempting to file assault charges by the women, whether or not the charges were accepted or the abusers were arrested, resulted in equally lower levels of future violence.

Nursing Implications

During safety planning, two fears commonly arise: retaliation by the perpetrator because the woman has sought police assistance and inability of the police to provide safety for the woman being abused. In this study, some women reported that the perpetrator knew she had gone to the police. This action demonstrated that she intended to put a stop to the violence and that she had legal support to make it happen. The perpetrators were deterred by the criminal justice system and the prospects of "going to jail" for their crimes. In addition to experiencing less violence after partnering with the criminal justice system, women being abused gained knowledge of their legal rights and how to use the legal system for their protection.

McFarlane, J., Willson, P., Lemmey, D., & Malecha, A. (2000). Women filing assault charges on an intimate partner: Criminal justice outcome and future violence experienced. *Violence Against Women, 6* (4), 396–408.

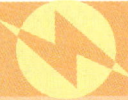

Nursing Alert

SAFETY PLANNING

Help a client plan for safety or escape by considering the following:

- Is it safe for the woman and her children to go home?
- Are there weapons in the home?
- Has there been an increase in the frequency or severity of the violence?
- Has the woman been hospitalized in the past as a result of the intimate partner violence?
- Has the abuser threatened to kill the woman or himself?
- Has the woman thought of committing or tried to commit suicide?
- Does the abuser hurt the children?
- Has the woman attempted or is she planning to leave the relationship?

danger, such as removing guns from the house and attempting to avoid arguments in high-risk rooms, such as the kitchen, garage, or any room with objects that are potential weapons. The nurse should help the client prepare a decisive escape plan. First, the client should consider how she will exit the house, for example, by which door or window. Second, the client needs to plan what to take with her when leaving: purse, car keys, cash, and important papers. The client should know to keep these items nearby. She should gather together important documents and be sure they are secure and easy to access. Personal

SEQUELAE OF ABUSE

Abuse of women is likely to be the precursor of chronic disease, substance abuse, and mental health problems, which affect women of all ethnic backgrounds and socioeconomic classes (Grisso & Ness, 1996). All those who experience or witness abuse suffer psychological consequences; some are so traumatized they develop PTSD (Bohn & Holz, 1996).

documents she will need include birth certificates, social security cards, and her driver's license; medical documents include health insurance identification cards and policies; and financial information includes bank account numbers.

A safety plan includes seeking out supportive family members or friends who will assist the woman in leaving the relationship, provide shelter, and call the police when violence is suspected. Integral to all safety planning is referral to community agencies that assist women who are abused. It is important to discuss the woman's concerns about using community agency resources. Fear of physical retaliation after reporting the abuse to the police is a common concern. Does filing assault charges against one's partner stop the abusive behaviors or just make them worse? Some research findings indicate that police intervention is associated with decreased levels of abuse. Research-based clinical practice can assist the nurse in helping the abused woman overcome her fears by building on knowledge and dispelling myths.

Threats of abuse, physical assaults, and the increased risk of homicide experienced by women who are abused affect their health and carry a tremendous amount of morbidity. Campbell and Lewandowski (1997) identified multiple violence-associated illnesses that ranged from minor difficulty with mental concentration and headaches to irritable bowel syndrome and PTSD.

Post-Traumatic Stress Disorder

Post-traumatic stress disorder may develop when an event outside the range of normal human experience occurs that produces marked distress in the person. Violence-related events that may result in PTSD in women include rape, sexual molestation, attempted sexual assault, and witnessing such events. Most typically the triggering event is either aggravated assault with or without a weapon (physical attacks or threats made with the intent to injure) or simple assault, such as pushing, shoving, hitting, kicking, or punching. This traumatic event (or events) coupled with characteristic symptoms that may include intrusive thoughts, nightmares, and flashbacks are frequently and persistently relived by survivors. They experience intense psychological or physiologic distress, or both, when they are re-exposed to environmental stimuli that resemble aspects of their traumatic event. Hence, clients with PTSD try to avoid stimuli that are painful or that cause anxiety by avoiding thoughts or conversations associated with the trauma; avoiding persons, places, or activities that remind them of the trauma; or blocking out memories of the trauma. Women experiencing PTSD from abuse may have a combination of panic disorder and major depression.

Cultural Influences

No ethnic or socioeconomic group of women is immune to domestic violence. The National Victims Survey found no significant difference in the rates of severe abuse among Caucasian, African American, or Hispanic American women (Campbell, Masaki, & Torres, 1997). Unfortunately, women belonging to minority groups often face racism and anti-immigrant sentiment that create additional barriers to ending the abuse. Male batterers may use culture and immigration status to control their partners (e.g., claiming that battering is an acceptable cultural practice or threatening to report the woman for deportation if she does not do as told). Fewer services and less information are available to battered women of color, primarily because of economic restraints. Awareness of cultural influences on the abusive ex-

OVERCOMING CULTURAL BIASES

Culturally astute nurses are aware of their own biases and how they may affect their perceptions and relationships with clients from other cultures. You should seek information about other cultures through interactions with clients and community experts, and through reading.

perience can assist nurses in approaching and individualizing services for the client in a more caring manner.

Research studies suggest that African American women are more likely than are Caucasian women to report abuse and other violent crimes to the police (Bachman & Coker, 1995; Hutchison, Hirschel, & Pesackis, 1994).

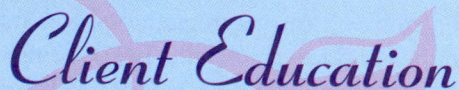

Culturally Appropriate Solutions

For clients experiencing violence, refer to the following:

- Bilingual and bicultural programs within the community.
- Support groups that meet in predominantly local areas (e.g., shelters and churches), which provide shared experiences for persons of the same race.
- National African American Women's Health Project, which uses model community-based self-help programs, community-based health centers, films, and publications.
- Immigrant and Refugee Women, Immigrant Assistance Line: English and Spanish, 415-554-2444; Cantonese, Mandarin, and Vietnamese, 415-554-2454.
- Native Americans, Women of Nations: 612-222-5830.
- Additional sources, which can be found by looking in the blue or white pages of your local telephone directory under Domestic Abuse Information and Treatment Centers, Social Service Organizations, Human Service Organizations, Shelters, Women's Organizations, or Family Services.

Stalking

Stalking is repeated harassing or threatening behavior, such as following a person, appearing at a person's home or workplace, making harassing phone calls, leaving written messages or objects, or vandalizing personal property. Stalking includes behavior that would cause fear in a reasonable person: repeated occasions of visual or physical proximity; nonconsensual communication; or verbal, written, or implied threats (Tjaden & Thoennes, 1998). Like sexual assault, stalking is almost exclusively a crime against women and often is perpetrated by ex-husbands or ex-boyfriends (DeBecker, 1997; Jordan, 1995; Patton, 1994; Tjaden & Thoennes, 1998). The National Violence Against Women Survey (Tjaden & Thoennes, 1998) collected information from 8,000 men and women on violence and found that 8% of women and 2% of men had been stalked at some time in their lives. Tjaden and Thoennes found that 1.4 million Americans are stalked yearly and that women are four times more likely to be victims of stalking and twice as likely to be stalked by intimate partners. Stalking affects the health of victims by causing fear and anxiety, which stimulates 30% of women to seek help through counseling and 55% to seek police protection (Tjaden & Thoennes, 1998).

The Bureau of Justice (National Criminal Justice Association, 1996; Greenfield et al., 1998) proposed the following three broad classifications for stalkers based on their relationship to victims: (1) intimate or former intimate persons, (2) acquaintances, or (3) strangers (frequently involving celebrities). By far the most common category of stalking is by intimate partners, and it is the most likely to

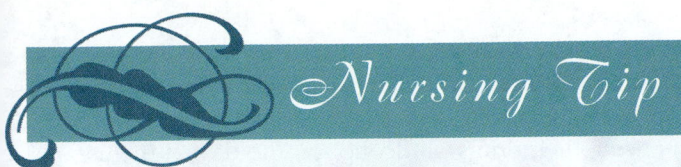

QUESTIONS TO ASK ABOUT STALKING

- Are you being followed or spied on by your intimate partner (or previous partner)?

- Does your intimate partner wait outside or show up unexpectedly at your home, school, or workplace?

- Do you receive unwanted phone calls from your intimate partner, or are you receiving many hang-up calls?

- Has your intimate partner sent or left you unwanted notes, letters, or other items of communication that frighten you?

- Has your intimate partner threatened to harm you, the children, or family members?

- Has your intimate partner caused damage to your personal property, for example, cut up your clothing, torn up photographs, slashed your car tires, tried to break down your door, or killed a pet?

have a serious or fatal outcome (DeBecker, 1997; Lingg; 1993; Meloy, 1997).

Interpersonal violence and stalking often are interrelated and may indicate an increased risk of severe violence or fatal outcome (Lingg, 1993; Perez, 1993; Sanford, 1993). A national survey found that 81% of stalked women also were assaulted physically by the same partner (Tjaden & Thoennes, 1998). This finding confirms results of other studies that report a stalker is more likely to be violent if there has been an intimate relationship with the victim (Coleman, 1997; Meloy, 1998). When stalking occurs in conjunction with intimate partner violence, it is likely to end in severe violence and possibly murder (DeBecker, 1997; Perez, 1993). Experts believe that most (70%) women murdered by intimate partners had been stalked by the murderers (DeBecker, 1997; Lingg, 1993; Meloy, 1997; Perez, 1993).

California enacted the first anti-stalking law in 1990, and today comprehensive stalking laws modeled after the Model Stalking Code (National Institute of Justice, (1993) have been adopted by other states (Wallace, 1999; Westrup, 1998). The effect that anti-stalking laws have had and will have on the health and safety of women and children will remain unknown until evaluative studies have been conducted. Most states stipulate that to be classified as an offense the following must have occurred:

- *Course of Conduct.* The person must commit an act on more than one occasion (the acts included vary from state to state).

- *Threat Requirement.* The person must commit actions that would cause a reasonable person to be fearful (the threat need not be written or verbal to instill fear).

- *Intent of the Stalker.* Most states require that the perpetrator know the conduct will cause the other person to perceive said behavior to be threatening (National Criminal Justice Association, 1996). Many states do not require proof of intent to cause fear, rather, merely the intent to commit the act is sufficient.

Impact in the Workplace

Workplace violence is a growing concern in the United States. The employment setting is often the site of an attack by an intimate partner. Several surveys of women who are abused report that high percentages of women experienced harassment or stalking while at work (Riger, et al., 1998; Shepard & Pence, 1988). The workplace is the leading site for homicide of employed women. Most working women are killed in the course of a robbery or other crime. However, Department of Labor statistics show that from 1992 to 1994, 17% of alleged murderers of women in the workplace were current or former husbands or boyfriends. For African American women, the figure was 28%; for Hispanic women, it was 20% (U.S. Department of Labor, 1996).

The effects of domestic violence impact employment productivity. Working women who are being abused at home reported being harassed by their abusive partners in person or by telephone while at work. These women reported being late for work, having to leave work early, and missing work because of the abuse. Some women reported having their cars vandalized by their abuser so that they would have no way of getting to work. In addition, women reported being reprimanded by their employers for problems associated with the behavior of the abusers (Shepard & Pence, 1988). These women also reported losing at least one job because of the violence in their lives. In an attempt to escape or cover up the abuse, women may be compelled to frequently change jobs or accept low-salary positions.

In a study conducted by EDK Associates (1997), 37% of women who had experienced domestic violence reported that the abuse had an impact on their work performance. One in four (24%) victims of domestic violence said the abuse caused them to arrive late for work or to miss days of work. Of these women, 15% had a difficult time keeping a job, 20% said the abuse affected their

Nursing Alert

WARNING SIGNS FOR POSSIBLE WORKPLACE VIOLENCE

The following are indicators of possible violent behavior in a co-worker:

- Keeping away from others.
- Failing to take responsibility for personal actions.
- Behaving in a rigid and controlling manner.
- Acting out anger, or seeing only one point of view.
- Talking one way and acting another.
- Engaging in addictive behavior, which is used to escape reality.
- Acting out of character, which is done to shock others.

ability to advance their careers, and 12% reported that a current or former intimate partner harassed them at work.

Employers have begun to recognize that domestic violence is a threat to employee safety and productivity. Companies now are actively implementing policies and procedures that support a "no tolerance" attitude toward domestic violence.

Domestic Violence in the Workplace

The cost of domestic violence to businesses is enormous. Statistics show that the yearly medical costs of domestic violence total $3 to $5 billion (Bureau of National Affairs, 1990). Businesses forfeit another $100 million owing to lost wages from sick leave and absenteeism and to the costs of nonproductivity, turnover, and retraining (Colorado Domestic Violence Coalition, 1991). Domestic violence has negatively impacted many aspects of employee performance, most notably psychological well-being (56%), productivity (49%), and attendance (47%) (Roper Starch Worldwide, 1994). It is clear that physical abuse, harassment, and stalking by intimate partners affect quality of work and even the ability to be employed.

Portrait of an Abuser

Chronic alcohol use and illicit drug use are among the most prevalent risk factors for being an abuser (Fagan, Barnett, & Patton, 1988; Greenfield et al., 1998; Hotaling & Sugarman, 1986: Kantor & Straus, 1989; Ptacek, 1998). Roberts (1988) found that at the time of the assault, 70% of perpetrators were under the influence of drugs, alcohol, or

both; 32% used only drugs, 17% used only alcohol, and 22% used both. Even higher rates of drug and alcohol use were seen in a study by Brookoff (1997): 92% of perpetrators used illicit drugs or alcohol on the day of the assault, and 45% had been intoxicated daily for the past month. Coleman and Strauss (1983) reported rates of violence almost 15 times higher for husbands who were "often" versus "never" drunk in the past year. Men's drinking patterns, especially binge drinking, are associated with marital violence across all ethnic groups and social classes (Kantor, 1993).

Battering is more than an isolated case of the person "blowing up." It is a process of deliberate intimidation intended to coerce the person being abused (i.e., girlfriend or boyfriend, spouse, significant other, child, or older person) into doing the will of the abuser. It is enacting behavior that shows an established set of control skills. In reality the man who abuses his wife and children is not "out of control," rather, he is very much "in control." The perpetrator enforces control in a way that compares to brainwashing. Coercive techniques are used to set up a regulating situation for domestic violence. These techniques include isolation, monopolization of perception, induced debility and exhaustion, threats, occasional indulgences, demonstration of the abuser's omnipotence, degradation,

Client Education

Business Interventions Against Intimate Partner Violence

- Provide safety training sessions on the telltale signs of domestic abuse to aid in recognizing abuse and providing help for employees who are being abused.
- Post hotline numbers for violence prevention information in rest rooms where they can be written down discreetly.
- Provide cellular phones to employees who are being abused for rapid access to emergency police intervention.
- Assign parking spaces close to front doors to employees who are being abused to allow them to avoid isolated parking areas.
- Alter the workplace or work pattern of employees who are being abused by temporarily reassigning them to a different branch of the company or by initiating a flexible time schedule.

Research Highlight

Indicators of Intimate Partner Domestic Violence in Women's Employment

Purpose

To better understand the effects of violence committed by an intimate partner on employee productivity.

Methods

Nurse researchers surveyed 90 consecutive women applying for protection orders against intimate partners (current or former) at the district attorney's office of a large county.

Findings

The researchers found that 87% of women interviewed had been employed at one time and 89% had experienced harassment by intimate partners related to their work. The most common outcome (65%) of work-related harassment was being late for work or leaving work early as a result of abuse. Lost productivity and reduced performance also were indicated by findings that these women missed work (58%), lost a job (21%), or were prevented from working (47%) because of intimate partner violence. When these women were asked how the abusers prevented them from working, almost half (44%) stated the abusers left them without transportation to work by disabling the car or hiding the car keys.

Nursing Implications

This study shows the need for nursing intervention in intimate partner violence in the workplace. Nurses should help women who are abused to develop personal safety plans, which include safety issues at the workplace. Nurses should also develop community interventions through corporate and business public education projects by working collaboratively with occupational health nurses, company safety committees, and concerned employees.

McFarlane, J., Malecha, A., Gist, J., Schultz, P., Willson, P., & Fredland, N. (2000). Indicators of intimate partner violence in women's employment: Implications for workplace action. *Journal of Occupational Health Nursing*.

and enforcement of trivial demands (Jones, 1994; Willson, 1998). Perpetrators of abuse use these same techniques over a broad spectrum of victims (i.e., intimate partners; older persons; special populations, such as persons who are disabled or homeless and immigrant persons; and children).

- Isolation of the person being abused from support systems makes that person solely dependent on the person committing the abuse. For example, women frequently say, "He moved me away from my friends, he didn't want me to go anywhere unless he was with me, or he would eavesdrop on my telephone conversations."

- Monopolization of perception is the total perceptual concentration of the person being abused on not upsetting the person committing the abuse. For exam-

ple, this technique is expressed by the comment, "I was always scared the abuser would blow up." This technique causes the victim to concentrate on the immediate situation, be introspective, and decrease competing input that frustrates (or eliminates) all actions that are not in compliance with the wishes of the controller (Jones, 1994; Willson, 1998).

- Induced debility and exhaustion occurs when the person committing the abuse physically or emotionally debilitates the victim and acts to create a state of exhaustion in that person. Examples of this technique are keeping the victim awake at night by starting a fight and not allowing access to a health care provider for injuries the victim receives from battering or other types of abuse. The exhaustion or debilitated physical condition weakens the victim's ability to resist the will of the controller.

- Threats also are used to induce anxiety and despair. For example, the person committing the abuse may threaten to take away something of great value to the victim (e.g., children from a mother; a car or home from an older person; an ambulatory aid, such as a wheelchair, from a person with a disability; or a special pet, toy, or person from a child). Perpetrators also exact their control by making threats such as "I'll find you wherever you go."

- Occasional indulgences (e.g., flowers; a vacation; special gifts; or treats, such as dining out, going to a movie, or visiting a friend) are positive motivators for compliance with the controller's wishes. Because the victim is very isolated, these occasional indulgences may be the only signs of kindness or love she receives (Jones, 1994; Willson, 1998).

- Demonstration of omnipotence often is manifested in physical signs of abuse and seems to prove to the victim the total futility of resistance (Jones, 1994; Willson, 1998). For example, the abuser often beats the victim or withholds food, assistance with personal care regimens, or mobility (e.g., transportation; or if the victim is a person with a disability, a wheelchair, braces, or ambulatory assistance).

- Degradation is another tactic used by the controller (Jones, 1994; Willson, 1998). Degrading words and actions beat down the victim's spirit and self-confidence. Victims are left with an eroded sense of self-worth and no belief in their own capabilities.

- Enforcement of trivial demands (e.g., "You'll wear your hair long or else!") by the controller is used to develop the habit of compliance in the victim. A behavioral pattern of obedience occurs because every victim knows what "or else" means in their relationship with an abuser.

By using the behavior clues listed previously, abusers succeed in turning victims into obedient isolated persons with low self-esteem. Victim are restricted emotionally and often socially and financially. Victims are fearful of leaving because the threats made by the person committing the abuse may be carried against them and possibly their loved ones. Victims fear for their lives!

Nursing Implications

Women who are abused seek health care interventions at emergency departments; prenatal clinics; general medicine practices; and social support agencies, such as women's shelters (Klein, Campbell, Soler, & Ghez, 1997). When the abusive relationship becomes eminently violent, women most often seek help and protection from legal enforcement agencies (McFarlane, Soeken, Reel, Parker, & Silva,

Nursing Alert

ABUSE ASSESSMENT SCREENING

Questions that help you screen for abuse:

- Has anyone ever hit, slapped, restrained, or hurt you physically or emotionally?
- Are you afraid of your partner at times? Of your previous partner?**
- Have you ever felt unsafe in your home situation?**
- Does your partner* like to boss you around?
- If your partner does not get his own way, how does he act?
- Have you been forced to have sexual relations or engage in sexual activities that you are uncomfortable doing?
- When arguing with your partner, does he threaten to hurt you or the children?
- Has your partner ever stopped you from leaving home, visiting family or friends, or going to work or school?
- Do you have a say in how to spend money?
- Are any of these things occurring now?

*Partner, spouse, boyfriend, ex-husband, or ex-boyfriend.
**Quick screening questions.

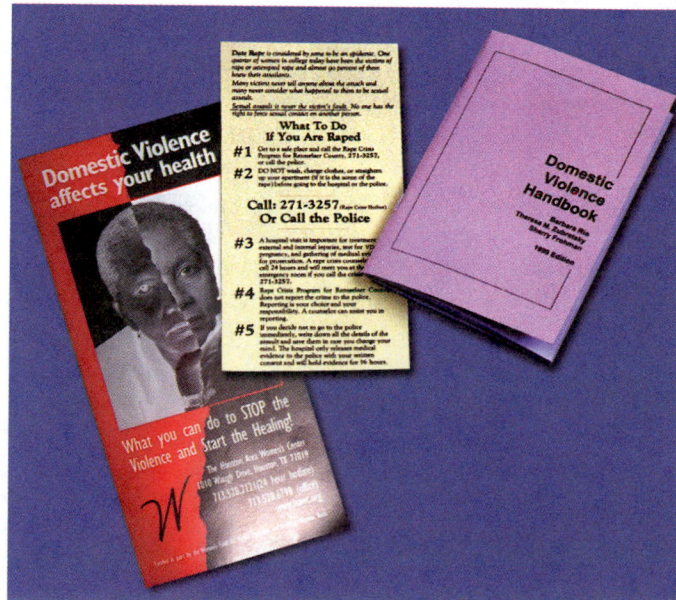

Figure 11-4 In addition to physical and emotional support, nurses can share literature and make referrals for clients who have experienced violence.

1997). In large urban police departments, specialty units have been established to facilitate services for domestic violence victims (Berry, 1998).

Violence against women creates a public health dilemma that mandates nurses to implement preventive strategies. Nurse clinicians are called on to assess the dangerousness of abusive relationships for their clients in a variety of settings and to offer care, resources, and referrals as appropriate (Figure 11-4). These assessments frequently are based on a history of abuse, the nurse clinician's intuition, and the clinician's knowledge of risk factors for homicide (Campbell, 1995b; Gondolf, 1998). Nurse clinicians refer or are mandated to report women who are abused to the criminal justice system, that is, the police or the district attorney's office.

THE CYCLE OF VIOLENCE

The cycle of violence was first described by Walker in 1962 (Paluzzi & Houde-Quimby, 1996). Walker (1984) identified family violence patterns as consisting of three phases: the tension-building phase, the acute battering phase, and the honeymoon phase. The cyclic behavior begins with a time of tension-building arguments, progresses to violence, and settles into a making-up or calm period. The time between the acute battering and honeymoon phases was identified by Curnow (1997) as the open-window phase, when the battered victim is most receptive to receiving help. With time, this cycle of violence increases in frequency and severity as it is repeated over and over again.

The traditional view of a woman who is battered is that of a dependent victim, one psychologically unable to take steps to stop the abuse (Campbell & Fishwick, 1993; Gondolf, 1998; Gondolf & Fisher, 1988). This traditional perspective fails to see the potential present in these women that enables them to survive. These women will seek help; and it behooves nurses to understand when that will occur, learn effective interventions, and provide empirical information as to the impact of those interventions.

Understanding Walker's cycle of violence can assist nurses in identifying the process and timing of interventions for women who are stalked and abused. In phase one, the tension-building phase, the perpetrator becomes irritated easily and increases demands and efforts to control the woman. She, in turn, increases her attempts to placate the abuser and denies awareness of impending danger. This phase may last for hours, day, weeks, or even years.

In phase two, the acute battering phase, perpetrators hit, slap, kick, or perform other acts of violence against the intimate partners. This phase also may last for hours or

days, and women are powerless to affect the outcome. Women who are battered initially may not perceive the reality of their situations and therefore ignore their intuition, cognitively minimize the danger and severity of the violence, or blame themselves (DeBecker, 1997; Graham et al., 1995). These women believe no alternatives to the violence exist and thus focus their attention on survival (Curnow, 1997; Landenburger, 1989; Walker, 1984). Women who are severely abused experience a loss of self and often become zombielike or numb (Graham et al., 1995; Vitanza, Vogel, & Marshall, 1995).

In phase three, the honeymoon phase (calm period), the perpetrator expresses sorrow and promises the abuse will never happen again. Denial permeates the cycle; the woman denies her partner is a batterer, denies being injured, and denies there are alternatives. She also defends herself by appealing to high loyalties, such as religion, marriage, and family values (Curnow, 1997). The denial of reality prevents her from seeking help during this phase.

A phenomenon observed in women who are severely abused is that they appear to lose their "observing self" and question their own perceptions (Gondolf & Fisher, 1988). It is the loss of self or an awareness of the reality of her situation that prevents a woman who is abused from seeking help. However, during the open-window phase the woman is most likely to see the reality of her situation, that is, she is a victim and is not able to stop the violence (Curnow, 1997). That is not to deny the fact that persons who are abused have innate strength, will work to change or improve their situation, and will seek help as the violence escalates (Gondolf & Fisher, 1988). Another perspective is that once the costs of living in a violent relationship (e.g., injuries) outweigh the benefits (e.g., loving contriteness), the woman will seek help if she perceives effective help is available (Walker, 1984).

Helpseeking in women who are abused may offer a narrow window of opportunity for nursing interventions to occur. Various actions indicate helpseeking: calling police; going to the emergency department or a clinic; contacting a lawyer; seeing her clergy; confiding in someone; talking about suicide, retaliation against the violence, and leaving the abuser (Curnow, 1997; Gondolf & Fisher, 1988; Greenfield et al., 1998). According to Curnow the open-window phase is the opportune time for nurses to intervene and educate these women as to the reality of their situation (Figure 11-5). Curnow (1997, p. 132) states that during this phase women make reality statements such as "I realized I couldn't take it anymore" or "I just woke up." When the woman seeks help, she is in less denial and open to validation of her current perceptions (Curnow, 1997). Nursing knowledge concerning abusive behaviors at the time of helpseeking and abusiveness after helpseeking can provide empirical knowledge to facilitate interventions at the most opportune time and may save the woman's life. It is

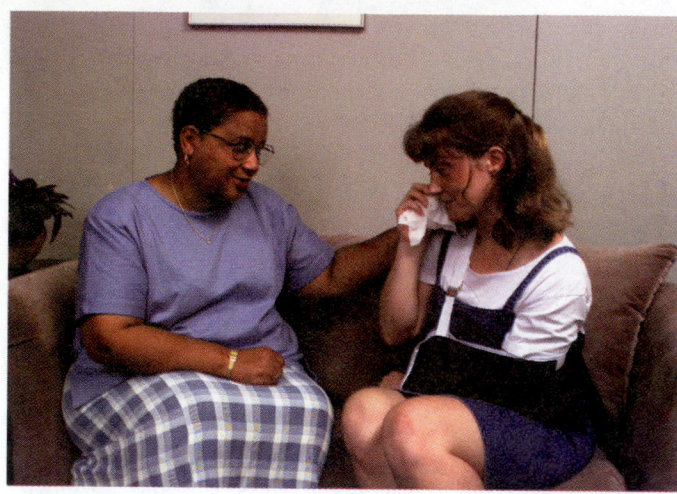

Figure 11-5 Nurses need to be skilled in recognizing when a client who is battered is most receptive to help and most likely to accept the reality of the abusive situation.

essential that nurses attain information to identify and strengthen protective mechanisms used by women who are abused (Woods & Campbell, 1993). This information is vital because researchers have indicated that the abused woman's continued helpseeking depends on the response she receives and the impact that response has on the violence (Dobash, Dobash, & Cavanagh, 1985).

VIOLENCE AGAINST CHILDREN

Children who are in an environment in which violence is occurring among adults are far more likely to be abused than are other children. Even if they are not abused, young children may receive serious injuries such as broken bones or loss of consciousness when objects are thrown, slammed, or overturned. Older children may sustain injuries while trying to intervene to end the assault. The witnessing of their mothers being assaulted by their partners—emotionally, physically, or sexually—causes children to live in fear and a state of instability. Children who witness battering often suffer from guilt, anger, depression, anxiety, and shyness; they have nightmares, are irritable, and have problems getting along with others. Frequently they "act-out," that is, they mimic aggressive and violent behaviors they have seen (e.g., slapping a younger sister, like Dad does Mom; or telling their mother to "shut up or I'll kill you").

A major modifier of human behavior is experience—not genetics—and it results in the critical neurobiologic factors associated with violence (Perry, 1997, p. 125). Family relationships during infancy and childhood determine how the neurologic pathways of the person are organized. In a study by Perry, Pollard, Blakley, and Baker (1995),

175 young children who were severely traumatized demonstrated both mental and physical adaptive responses that included hyperarousal and dissociation. These researchers theorized that the trauma of violence on the developing child disrupts the normal sequential order of brain development, leading to major abnormalities in neurodevelopment (Perry et al., 1995). For example, the child experiencing severe abuse may develop atypical or abnormal patterns of neuronal activity, such as an overactive "fight and flight" response that can be expressed as hypervigilance, difficulty sitting still or concentrating, and learning problems. Preschoolers from violent homes may develop aggressive behavior or PTSD.

Children who witness violence may internalize their stress. They frequently blame themselves for the violence. Considerable amounts of their energy are spent trying to figure out how to prevent their parents from fighting. Both physical and intellectual growth can be affected. These children routinely have been found to have higher blood pressure readings and higher pulse rates than children who do not witness violence. Children from violent homes experience more colds, sore throats, sleepless nights, and bed-wetting than do other children. In psychological development the child must first obtain a sense of safety before progressing to the higher developmental stages of self-esteem or self-actualization. Children reared in violent homes have difficulty expressing empathy. Typically the child's method of conflict resolution is learned from parental modeling; in a violent home this modeling consists of either passive (submissive) or aggressive (abusive) methods to resolve problems.

It can be difficult for health care workers to distinguish the normal injuries of childhood from those resulting from abuse. Children routinely sustain scratches, scrapes, cuts, bumps, and broken bones. Some of these injuries are serious enough for medical attention in a physician's office, a clinic, or hospital. However, some of these children with

Critical Thinking

Evaluating the Risks and Benefits of Leaving an Abusive Spouse because of the Children

- Is it better for a woman to leave an abusive spouse and rear the children in a single-parent home?
- What if the single parent has financial difficulties?
- What are the benefits and risks of keeping the family together "for the children's sake"?

injuries are victims of abuse. As a nurse, you will be on the front line in caring for these injured children. You must sort through the historical and physical data to implement a nursing care plan that ensures optimal health and safety for the young patient.

Child Abuse

Child abuse is any physical or mental injury, sexual abuse, exploitation, negligent treatment, or maltreatment of a child who is of the age designated by the particular state as being a child (usually 18 years old or younger). Mental abuse can damage a child's psychological, social, and intellectual well-being. Behavioral signs and symptoms include anxiety, depression, aggression, and withdrawal. Often, one or more behaviors are exhibited by a change in the child's behavior (e.g., the child drops out of extramural school activities), emotional response (e.g., the child behaves aggressively, or cognition (e.g., a sudden drop in the child's grades is seen). **Neglect** of a child occurs when the parent or guardian fails to provide adequate food, clothing, shelter or medical care expected within the family's financial means. The negligent acts endanger

REFLECTIONS FROM A NURSE

"The year was 1975. A neighbor boy's very tired stepfather came home from his auto repair shop one hot summer afternoon. He drank several beers as he rested while mom left to mind the shop. The 9-year-old boy did not jump to do something the stepfather instructed, so he took off his 2-inch leather belt and lashed the boy's back and even left a buckle mark by his ear. Some of the welts were bloody when the boy appeared on my doorstep for first aid, and I called the chief of police. The stepfather was arrested, went to trial, paid a fine, and was released. As a neighbor, nurse, and parent myself, I was shocked and angry that a 9-year-old child would be subjugated to such violence."

Nursing Alert

WARNING SIGNS OF CHILD ABUSE

- Bruises and welts that resemble the shape of the object that inflicted the injury, such as a belt buckle
- Cigarette burns on the soles of the feet, palms of the hands, back, or buttocks
- Immersion burns, that is, doughnut-shaped burns on the buttocks, or stocking or glovelike patterns without splash burns on the extremities
- Rope burns
- Lacerations or abrasions of the mouth, gums, lips, eyes, ears, or external genitalia
- Broken bones
- Abdominal injuries, that is, bruises, intestinal perforation, ruptured liver or spleen, renal or urinary bladder injury, pancreatic injury, or intramural hematoma of the bowel
- Subdural hematoma, subarachnoid hemorrhage, or cerebral infarction
- Retinal hemorrhage and other symptoms of suffocation
- Chemical abuse

the child's health. Physical abuse can be recognized by the nurse's assessment of subtle or obvious signs and symptoms.

The long-term physical and mental consequences of *corporal punishment* (use of physical force to discipline) are well documented in the literature and support the position of the scientific community on nonviolent discipline (Hemenway, Solnick, & Carter, 1994). These authors indicate that verbal abuse may have even more severe outcomes than does physical abuse. Verbal intimidation is the root of low self-esteem, poor conflict resolution skills, and lower intelligence.

Physical assaults, such as hitting the back of the hands with a ruler or strap, can cause permanent orthopedic deformities of the hands and subsequent loss of function (Chicarilli et al., 1997). Children can suffer PTSD from their abusive experiences. Spanking to the buttock invokes sexual physiologic responses. Johnson (1996) has indicated that the sexual nature of the buttocks is understandable by the close proximity to the genitals as well as the high concentration of nerve endings. When the buttock is spanked, blood flow to the genitals increases. This physiologic change coupled with the desire for intimacy with the parent can link an association of fulfillment of longing with the pain of spanking.

A common sense rule of moral code is "Do not injure." This rule would support preventing physical, sexual, and psychological injury to a child. Another, common sense rule is "Prevent an innocent person from being harmed." Class disruption and a poor learning environment may result in greater harm to more students than would a spanking to one child, especially if the corporal punishment was given in a timely manner, consistently, and without emotion. Societal rules for corporal punishment are in a state of flux and are weighted on the side of nonuse of corporal punishment. Nurses should offer other choices to parents to achieve nonviolent outcomes, such as a system that reinforces positive behavior (e.g., the parent gives the child praise for favorable behavior). Discipline need not be punitive to be effective. One common type of noncorporal punishment is "time-out" whereby the child's behavior causes the consequence of being made to "sit in a chair" or "go to bed" for a few minutes instead of receiving a "spanking." Nurses should discuss with parents different forms of discipline and help parents form clear discipline guidelines that aid in reinforcing their child's positive behavior. Parents must be comfortable with the guidelines they set forth for their children or the guidelines will be difficult to reinforce consistently.

Child Sexual Abuse

For decades child sexual abuse had been thought to be rare; however, growing research indicates the contrary. Salter (1992) reviewed child abuse studies from the 1920s through the 1980s and found that child sexual abuse was a substantial social problem. All the studies she analyzed reported sexual abuse prevalence rates of at least 20%. Child abuse often occurs in the form of *incest,* or sexual relations between blood relatives or surrogate family members.

The number of substantiated child sexual abuse cases in the United States was 126,095 per year (U.S. Bureau of Census, 1997). One national telephone survey of 1,042 boys and 958 girls aged 10 to 16 years revealed that 15.3% of girls and 5.9% of boys interviewed had experienced some form of sexual abuse (Finkelhor & Dziuba-Leatherman, 1994). These reports demonstrate the need for vigorous investigation of child sexual abuse as a public health problem. Sexual abuse occurred more frequently than did acquired immunodeficiency syndrome (71,547 cases), hepatitis A (31,582 cases), hepatitis B (10,805 cases), Lyme disease (11,700 cases), salmonellosis (45,970 cases), shigellosis (32,080 cases), primary and secondary syphilis (16,500 cases), and tuberculosis (22,860 cases) (Centers for Disease Control and Prevention, 1998).

When a sexually transmitted disease (e.g., gonorrhea, syphilis, or chlamydia) is diagnosed in a child after the neonatal period, sexual abuse must be considered in de-

termining the cause. Nurses are ethically and legally obligated to report suspected child abuse, including sexual abuse.

Some indicators of child sexual abuse are:

- Sexually transmitted diseases (STDs). STDs among children presenting for care after the neonatal period almost always indicate sexual abuse (Eng & Butler, 1997, p. 80).
- Anogenital injuries. Anogenital injuries often are absent in children who are sexually abused because these elastic tissues can return to their normal appearance after injury, bruises may take more than 24 hours to appear, and lubricants may have been used to prevent injury. It also is possible that penetration may not have occurred. Gross injury is seen in 25% to 40% of children who are sexually abused (De Jong, 1992). Colposcopy, tissue stains, and photographic evidence may aid in detection of anogenital injuries. Some of the injuries reported are labial agglutination, external injuries to the labia minora, posterior fourchette (indicative of penile penetration), irregular hymenal scarring, and swelling or bruising of the perineum (Bachman, Moeller, & Benett, 1988; De Jong, 1992). Indicators of anal trauma are anal sphincter relaxation, swelling, and bruising; anal fissures; loss of perianal fat; and venous engorgement after 2 minutes in a knee-chest position (De Jong, 1992; McCann, Voris, Simon, & Wells, 1990). The increased vascularity in the anal region may last from weeks to years.
- Other physical injuries. Other physical indicators of sexual abuse in children are enuresis, encopresis, sleep disturbances, eating disorders, and increased oral behavior, such as nail biting and thumb sucking (De Jong, 1992).

Children Witnessing Violence

Children witness violence on television, in sports, on the playground, in the classroom, on the streets, and in the home. Every year 3 to 10 million children observe their mothers being physically assaulted (e.g., punched, slapped, stabbed, shot, or burned) by their intimate partners (Humphreys, 1997; Jaffe, Wolfe, & Wilson, 1990). Children are more traumatized by witnessing such violence in their own homes than by witnessing violence that occurs outside the home, such as street fighting or gang violence (Groves, 1995; Groves, Zuckerman, Marans, & Cohen, 1993). Kalmuss (1984) has studied children who experienced physical violence and compared them with those who only witnessed violence within their family. Children who witnessed violence in their home were more likely to commit spousal abuse as adults than were those who did not. Intergenerational learned abuse is supported by an almost societal tolerance of violence—outbursts of fighting by sports celebrities, songs about abuse and killing of abusers, computer games emphasizing violence.

Children who exhibit violent behavior during their preschool years or who have learning disabilities, language delays, or attention deficit–hyperactivity disorder are at increased risk for conduct disorders when they are older. Youngsters who are physically aggressive before the age of 15 years have the strongest propensity for being perpetrators of violence.

Unfortunately, spousal and child abuse often occur together. Stark and Flitcraft (1988) reviewed the charts of children suspected of being abused or neglected and found that 45% of the mothers of these children were abused. A somewhat higher estimate was obtained in Straus and Gelles' 1985 national survey of over 8,000 American families (Straus & Smith, 1995). In a home in which the husband hit his wife, child abuse was 150% more likely to occur than in a home in which the husband did not do so (Straus & Getter, 1996). Not only are children at risk for injury, they also are at risk for death. Felix and McCarthy (1994) examined 67 child fatalities in families identified by the Massachusetts Department of Social Services and found that 29 (43%) of these deaths occurred in families in which the mother of the child also was beaten.

Child abuse sequelae are most often exhibited by the child's physical behavior (aggression and conduct problems) and the child's emotional behavior (withdrawal, anxiety, or fearfulness) (Kolbo, Blakely, & Engleman,

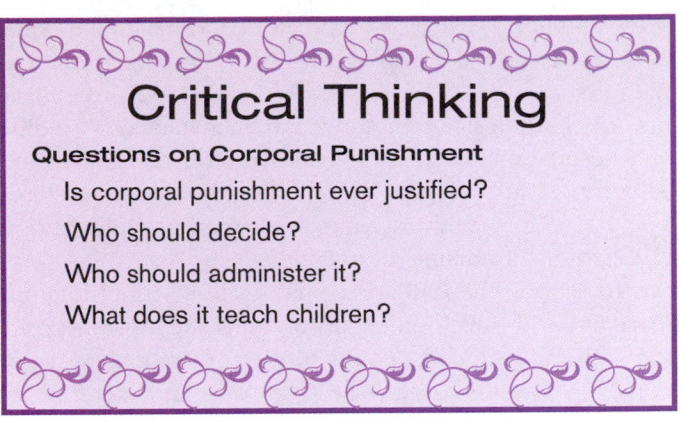

Critical Thinking

Questions on Corporal Punishment

Is corporal punishment ever justified?

Who should decide?

Who should administer it?

What does it teach children?

1996). Aggression has a common pattern of problematic behaviors (aggressive, antisocial, and oppositional actions), particularly among boys. Holden and Ritchie (1995) have found that children of women who are battered showed significantly more physical aggression toward their mothers than did children of women who were not battered. Role modeling may account for the high aggression rates among boys who observe their fathers hitting their mothers. Straus, Gelles, and Seinmetz (1980) found that boys who observed their fathers hitting their mothers were 1000% more likely to abuse their wives than were sons who did not witness this type of abuse.

Holden, Geffner, and Jouriles (1998) found that many children of women who are abused experience learning difficulties, PTSD, and social behavior problems. Exposure to domestic violence has negative mental health effects on children, with higher levels of conflict resulting in more severe dysfunction (Campbell & Lewandowski, 1997). Whereas even young children are sensitive to parental verbal aggression, it is the actual acts of abuse that have the most harmful effects (Kilpatrick & Williams, 1997; Laumakis, Margolin, & John, 1998).

Jaffe, Wolfe, and Wilson (1990) have suggested that the school problems of children who witness abuse may be due to anxiety surrounding imminent violence. These researchers noted that these children spend much of the school hours distracted and inattentive to classroom activity.

Nursing Responsibilities

Children living in abusive homes are at developmental risks as well as being at risk for physical abuse and ultimately death. Yet these children are difficult to identify because their symptoms can mirror behavioral problems unless viewed in the context of the conflict at home. For example, it may be abnormal for children to be concerned about the safety of their parents unless it is viewed in the context of the violence that the parent is experiencing in the home. Another reason it may be difficult to identify

Client Education

Recommendations of the American Academy of Pediatrics

The American Academy of Pediatrics (AAP) recommends that parents be taught:

- That homes without handguns reduce accidental and intentional injury or suicide.
- That they should monitor television content to avoid violence and limit viewing time to 2 hours daily (no TV before 2 years of age).
- That they should set limits for children, without spanking or hitting them.

Conference News Update: American Academy of Pediatrics 1999 Annual Meeting. Washington, DC. (2000). *Clinician Reviews*, *10*(1), 154–156.

these children by their symptomatology is that the aberrant behaviors, such as sleeping disorders, may be labeled as pathological conduct (Hughes & Barad, 1982). Identification of children living in abusive homes may also be difficult because these children are asymptomatic at the time. Therefore, nurses must remain cognizant that children being seen for health care may be living in a violent home and may need nursing intervention.

In school, these children may exhibit vision, hearing, learning, and developmental problems. Regression symptomatology in a child could trigger the school nurse to consider psychological testing or psychiatric referral for stress, trauma, alcohol or drug dependency, or depressed mood states. Indeed, these are important differential diagnoses; however, for the child witnessing violence in the home, health interventions may not ameliorate the problem. The child's situation can only be resolved by resolving the violence in the home.

Child health visits are perfect opportunities for nurses to detect and intervene for the entire family (Barkan & Gary, 1996). A woman who is battered may not seek health care for herself but will take her young children for routine preventive health care and for identified childhood issues such as encopresis, enuresis, or night terrors. Therefore, many professionals have encouraged routine screening of women who are battered within the pediatric setting

NURSING CARE OF THE CHILDREN OF WOMEN WHO ARE BATTERED

Indicators of Abuse in Children

- Difficulty sleeping, night terrors
- *Enuresis* (involuntary release of urine after the age of bladder control)
- *Encopresis* (watery colonic contents that bypass a hard stool)
- School problems: drop in grades, truancy, or dropping out of school
- Aggressiveness: hitting a parent or fighting with siblings or peers
- Unexplained weight loss or gain
- Loss of appetite lasting more than a month

Indicators of Abuse in Mothers

- Lack of eye contact
- Low tone of voice
- Inappropriate affect for the situation
- Visible injuries
- Expression of feelings of hopelessness or of being trapped
- Few support systems

Questions to Ask the Mother

- We all have conflict in our homes. How is conflict handled in your home?
- Are you being slapped, hit, punched, kicked, or beaten by your partner?
- Has your child witnessed this violence?

Plan of Action

- Develop a protocol for a plan of action before assessment.
- Advise the mother that no one deserves to be abused.
- Discuss the cycle of violence to diminish the mother's minimization of the problem.
- Encourage the mother to develop a safety plan: Have her find family and friends who will help her get out of the dangerous situation. She should

  Hide a suitcase packed with clothes, any insurance policies, her marriage license, her driver's license, and any bank account numbers.

  Hide money.

  Hide an extra set of house keys and car keys.

  Establish a secret code with her family and friends.

  Initiate role-playing about the secret code with her children.

- Offer to keep a photocopy of the children's social security cards, birth certificates, and immunization records in the chart for the mother.
- Address the presence of guns in the home; if present, encourage the mother to try to ensure the guns are not loaded.
- Refer the mother to the appropriate community services.
- Refer the mother to the social services department.

(American Academy of Pediatrics' Committee on Child Abuse and Neglect, 1998; Barkan & Gary, 1996; Wright, Wright, & Isaac, 1998).

Routine screening of battered women at all well-child visits allows mothers the opportunity to talk about this problem and gives advanced practice nurses the opportunity to educate families. Health care workers should interview women alone; ask questions such as "We all have disagreements at home—what happens when you and your partner disagree?"; provide information on community resources; and educate women about the dangerousness of domestic violence (American Academy of Pediatrics' Committee on Child Abuse and Neglect, 1998). Tested clinical nursing protocols exist for assessment and intervention (McFarlane & Gondolf, 1998; McFarlane & Parker, 1998) (Table 11-1). A unique form of child abuse called Munchausen Syndrome by Proxy is discussed in Box 11–1.

Current interventions are focused primarily on safety. Another concern is prevention of intergenerational transmission of aggressive behaviors, which can be accomplished by focusing on the safety of the victim and children.

Table 11-1 Tested Clinical Protocols for Abuse Assessment and Intervention

American College of Nurse-Midwives	www.midwife.org
Family Violence Prevention Fund	www.fvpf.org
National Coalition Against Domestic Violence	www.ncadv.org

VIOLENCE AGAINST OLDER PERSONS

Older persons usually are defined as those over 65 years of age; however, this definition may include persons aged 60 and older. This population often is further classified into two groups: the young-old, 65 to 75 years of age, and the old-old, over 75 years of age. The percentage of older persons in the population is increasing rapidly because of declining birth rates and increased life expectancy. Unfortunately, an alarming number of older persons are being abused or neglected. Domestic abuse of older persons remains a hidden and underreported crime. The National Center for Elder Abuse (NCEA, 1997) estimates that only 1 of 14 abuse incidents in this population is reported to adult protective agencies or the police. The U.S. national incidence and prevalence of abuse in older persons is unknown; estimated figures range from 820,000 to 2.5 million persons.

Characteristics

Most (67%) older persons who are abused and neglected are women, with a median age of 77.9 years for both men and women (NCEA, 1997). Of abused older persons, 66% are Caucasian, 19% are African American, and 10% are Hispanic. Ethnic groups with the lowest rate of abuse are Asian– Pacific Islanders and Native Americans. In addition, older persons who are abused often come from families with a pattern of violence for several generations or in which stress levels are high for a caregiver ill-prepared to fulfill the complex needs of an older person. No stereotypical set of characteristics exists for those who commit abuse against older persons: The perpetrators may be spouses, adult children, close friends, family members, guardians, or neighbors.

Signs

Abuse of older persons falls into five categories: neglect, physical abuse, psychological (emotional) abuse, financial abuse, and sexual abuse. Neglect is the most common form of abuse in older persons and results when the caregiver fails to provide adequate care. Neglect may be a

Box 11-1 Munchausen Syndrome By Proxy

Munchausen syndrome by proxy is a form of child abuse that can cause illness, disease, or even the death of a child. This syndrome is defined as the deliberate induction of symptoms of illness or reporting of physical symptoms in a child by the caregiver (often the mother) to solve some personal conflict. For these caregivers, their personal history of illness or family members' illness has taught them that sickness brings attention and love. This syndrome has four components:

- The caregiver first simulates the symptoms of illness in the child (e.g., bleeding, seizures, central nervous system dysfunction, apnea, diarrhea, vomiting, fever, or rashes) (Rosenberg & Fenley, 1991).

- The caregiver may stimulate symptoms by suffocating or poisoning the child or by contaminating laboratory specimens. Children are repeatedly brought for medical care, whereby the child is subjected to multiple diagnostic procedures in search of the cause of the illness.

- The caregiver appears as caring and overprotective; however, when the child and caregiver are separated, the child's symptomatology ends.

- The caregiver denies causing the symptoms that have stopped. In light of the caregiver's protective behavior, it is often a difficult diagnosis for the health care team to make.

willful act or the result of inadequate knowledge on the part of the caregiver; the latter is known as nonwillful failure to provide adequate care of the older person. Self-neglect is failure of older persons to care for themselves. Some indicators of neglect are poor personal hygiene, soiled clothing, misuse of medications, malnutrition, and isolation (being left alone).

Physical and psychological (emotional) abuse are the next most frequent types of abuse in this population. Physical abuse of older persons is like that in any age group: hitting, slapping, tripping, beating with an object (e.g., a belt or paddle), pushing or shoving, deliberate food or medicine deprivation (or overmedicating, overfeeding), or deliberate withdrawal of providing adequate personal hygiene. Psychological (emotional) abuse is withholding attention, inducing sensory deprivation, deliberately frightening the person by action or words, annoying the person by action or words (e.g., playing music known to irritate the person or making hateful remarks and threats), or abandoning the person for long periods of time without adequate provision of care.

Financial abuse or financial exploitation consists of misuse or misappropriation of assets. The crime may include theft or conversion of money or property by using force, misrepresentation, or other illegal acts that take advantage of the older person's partial or total lack of legal competency. Because many older persons have a fixed income, even minimal monetary loss could leave the person unable to afford the essentials of daily living, that is, adequate food, medications, or rent.

Sexual abuse of older persons is the least frequent category of reported abuse. Sexually transmitted diseases or any pain, itching, bleeding, or bruising in the genital area should raise the suspicion of sexual abuse.

Nursing Responsibilities

State laws mandate that doctors, nurses, social workers, police officers, fire fighters, and home care agency personnel report suspected abuse of older persons. State laws also designate which agency is to receive and investigate reports of abuse, neglect, and exploitation of older persons. The most frequently designated reporting agencies are state Adult Protective Service agencies, (APS) human service agencies, and law enforcement agencies. If an incident is witnessed the police or a law enforcement agency would be the most appropriate choice for a referral. A 24-hour hotline has been established through the Department of Elder Affairs, Department on Aging, or Commission on Aging for each state and depending on which state you are in, and this department receives reports from health professionals and citizens alike. In 1996, 64% of all suspected abuse reports were substantiated. In the 10 years from 1986 to 1996, a steady increase in abuse of older persons occurred, accounting for a 150% increase in abusive incidences reported (NCEA, 1997).

Protective service agencies initiate the following process once a report is received:

- Investigate allegations of abuse.
- Determine the severity and cause of the abuse.
- Initiate steps to alleviate the abuse.
- Arrange home care to relieve some of the burden on the caregiver(s).
- Assist the older person to obtain a restraining or protective order.
- Refer the case to the district attorney's office.

SPECIAL CASE: FEMALE CIRCUMCISION

Female circumcision is a practice steeped in cultural traditions but that often is viewed as a form of abuse by those of different cultural backgrounds. The statement of the Director-General to the World Health Organization's (WHO) Global Commission on Women's Health (1994) points out the lack of knowledge between the cultural norm in societies practicing female circumcision, sometimes referred to as female genital mutilation, and future outcomes for the young women subjected to this practice (WHO, 1996):

Experience shows for example that many people in the societies concerned do not naturally see the link between genital mutilation suffered by a woman in her childhood and the pain, infections

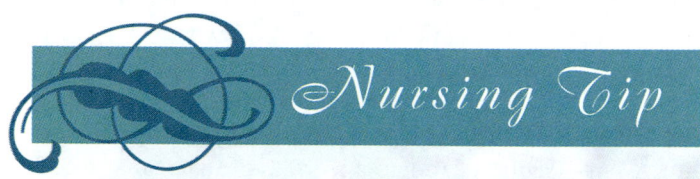

ASSESSING FOR ABUSE AND NEGLECT AMONG OLDER PERSONS

Some examples of questions you should ask to assess for abuse or neglect of the older person are

1. Does anyone hit you?
2. Are you afraid of anyone at home?
3. Does anyone take things that belong to you without asking?
4. Has anyone ever touched you without your consent?
5. Are you alone a lot?
6. Does anyone yell at you or threaten you?

and health problems she may suffer in her later years. Our first task must be to document this link, and then to inform people very simply and clearly about it.

The Council on Scientific Affairs of the American Medical Association (1995, p. 1714) defined **female genital mutilation** as "the medically unnecessary modification of female genitals." This procedure falls into four types of mutilation (Barstow, 1999):

1. Sunna, which is removal of the prepuce of the clitoris.
2. Clitoridectomy, which is removal of the prepuce and the clitoris.
3. Excision, which is removal of the prepuce, clitoris, upper labia minora, and some of labia majora.
4. Infibulation, which is removal of the prepuce, clitoris, labia minora, and labia majora.

Female circumcision is an ancient custom that has been practiced worldwide for 2,500 years (Barstow, 1999; Dire & Lindmark, 1991). Today, 100 to 130 million women in 40 countries have undergone female circumcision (Burstyn, 1995). Central Africa is the main area where different forms of female circumcision are performed, with the most severe forms in Sudan and Ethiopia (Kun, 1997). Various rationale are given for performing this surgery, from religious practice claimed to be endorsed in the Koran and the Bible, assurance of marriageability, cleanliness, enhanced sexual faithfulness, to protection from temptations by the devil, and protection from forcible rape and abortion (Barstow, 1999).

The surgery usually is carried out by a lay midwife, who uses a razor blade or broken glass and no anesthesia; the conditions often are unsanitary (Barstow, 1999; Odoi, Body, & Elkins, 1997). Infibulation involves the complete removal of the clitoris, labia minora, and inner surface of the labia majora. The two sides of the vulva are stitched together with either thorns or sutures made of silk or catgut. When the remaining skin of the labia majora heals, it forms a bridge of scar tissue over the vagina (WHO, 1996). A small opening is maintained by the insertion of a foreign body until the site heals to permit the passage of urine and menstrual blood. The girl's legs usually are bound closely together for several weeks until scar tissue forms over the wound (WHO, 1996).

Research Highlight

Prevalence of Female Circumcision

Purpose

To examine the prevalence of and motivation for female circumcision among an Egyptian village population.

Methods

A survey was conducted of all 819 households in a village in Upper Egypt near Assiut. The mothers of 1,732 girls under 20 years of age were interviewed to obtain information about their daughters' genital procedures.

Findings

Sixty-two percent of mothers said that their daughters had undergone female circumcision, most often at 5 to 9 years of age; 36.6% of mothers were planning for their daughter to undergo this procedure; and 1.1% of mothers had no plans for their daughters to have this procedure. The most prevalent (77%) reason given for female circumcision was that it followed customs and traditions.

Nursing Implications

The study raises a number of questions about the motivation for maintaining the practice of female circumcision and the kinds of interventions needed. Community health education and individualized counseling about the risks and complications may help change the prevalence of this practice.

Sayed, G. H., El-Aty, M. A. A., & Fadel, K. A. (1996). The practice of female genital mutilation in Upper Egypt. *International Journal of Gynecology & Obstetrics, 55,* 207–335.

The procedure of female circumcision became restricted in the United States on March 30, 1997, with enactment of the U.S. Federal Prohibition of Female Genital Mutilation Act of 1995. This practice is punishable by law, with prison sentences of up to 5 years for a person who "circumcises, excises, or infibulates the whole or any part of the labia majora or labia minora or clitoris of another person who has not attained the age of 18" (Robinson, 1998, p. 1).

Thousands of women who have had various forms of circumcision immigrate to the United States each year from countries in which this surgery is routinely performed (Feminist Majority Foundations, 1998). In order to acknowledge the cultural and religious diversity of these women and to meet their special health care needs, it is important that nurses know how to provide sensitive nonjudgmental care both for the woman and her spouse (Barstow, 1999). Culturally sensitive nursing care may include having the spouse be present at all his wife's procedures and having only female nurses participate in her care.

Circumcision can impact young girls both physically and psychologically. Immediate physical complications seen after this procedure include shock, hemorrhage, urinary retention, infection, tetanus, and death (Odoi, Body, and Elkins, 1997). Delayed complications may include chronic urinary tract infections, vulvar dermal cysts, vaginal stenosis, dysmenorrhea, and chronic pelvic inflammatory disease (Odoi, Body, and Elkins, 1997).

During labor and delivery the vaginal closure needs to be deinfibulated, or opened (Barstow, 1999). In the women's native country the closure would be reinfibulated after delivery, and this process would be repeated with each subsequent delivery. Multiparous women may have thick scarring and little redundant skin. Multiple complications of labor and delivery are seen in women with female circumcision: higher than normal incidences of maternal and neonatal mortality and morbidity, prolonged second stage of labor, more frequent postpartum hemorrhage, and a higher rate of episiotomies in primiparas (De Silva, 1989).

Web Activities

- Search the web for sites addressing abuse, violence, and rape. Do these sites offer information on the different types of assault (e.g., acquaintance rape versus date rape)? Are there resources for families as well as health care providers?

- Check the sites of some of the major nursing and health care organizations, such as NANDA, the National League for Nursing (NLN), and DSM (APA). Do these sites include information on abuse, violence, and rape?

- Search government web sites for support groups for survivors of violence and self-help programs for abusers. Are research studies available on-line?

Key Concepts

- Domestic violence is a public health problem with great consequences, including the physical, mental, and emotional pain of the victim.
- The economic cost of violence and abuse is felt by the health care industry, the legal system, and business communities.
- Health economists calculate that violent crime costs the United States $192 billion per year (Gladwell, 1997).
- The nurse is an essential provider of domestic violence prevention, screening, and referral to community resources.
- Children who witness violence are more likely to become abusers themselves.
- The implementation of an interdisciplinary community plan for prevention of domestic violence needs nursing leaders, educators, researchers, and practitioners to help design, develop, and implement it.
- Minimum components of a safety plan include a private interview, preparatory steps for ensuring safety or for leaving the relationship, and a listing of community resources.
- Subsequent client encounters are opportunities for nurses to re-question the client about abuse and her safety.

Review Questions and Activities

1. Outline appropriate nursing care for a rape survivor.
2. Which physical signs would you expect to find in a pregnant woman who is abused?
3. Suggest approaches to ensure that the physical examination of a woman who has experienced rape does not feel to her like a "second rape."
4. Develop an escape plan for a wife who is battered and has two school-age children.
5. Outline the different types of abuse experienced by older persons.

References

American Academy of Pediatrics' Committee on Child Abuse and Neglect. (1998). The role of the pediatrician in recognizing and intervening on behalf of abused women. *Pediatrics, 101,* 1091–1092.

Anderson, R. J., & Taliaferro, E. (1997). *Violence as preventable in the practice of medicine: Social and economic impact.* Proceedings of the Family Violence and Health Care Systems, Feb. 6-7, Houston, TX.

Bachman, G. A., Moeller, T. P., & Benett, J. (1988). Childhood sexual abuse and the consequences in adult women. *Obstetrics & Gynecology, 71,* 631–641.

Bachman, R., & Coker, A. L. (1995). Police involvement in domestic violence: The interactive effects of victim injury, offender's history of violence, and race. *Violence and Victims, 10,* 91–106.

Barkan, S. E., & Gary, L. T. (1996). Woman abuse and pediatrics: Expanding the web of detection. *Journal of the American Medical Women's Association, 51*(3), 96–100.

Barstow, D. G. (1999). Female genital mutilation: The penultimate gender abuse—female genital mutilation and the sexual blinding of women. *Child Abuse & Neglect, 23,* 405–522, 501–510.

Berry, D. B. (1998). *The domestic violence sourcebook: Everything you need to know.* Los Angeles, CA: Lowell House.

Bohn, D. K., & Holz, K. A. (1996). Sequelae of abuse: Health effects of childhood sexual abuse, domestic battering, and rape. *Journal of Nurse-Midwifery, 41,* 442–456.

Brookoff, D. (1997). *Drugs, alcohol, and domestic violence in Memphis.* NIJ Research Preview. Washington, DC: National Institute of Justice.

Bureau of Justice Statistics. (1997). *Violence-related injuries treated in hospital emergency departments* [On-line]. Available from www.ojp.usdoj.gov/bjs

Bureau of National Affairs. (1990). *Domestic violence in the workplace.* Washington, DC: Bureau of National Affairs.

Burstyn, L. (1995). Female circumcision comes to America. *The Atlantic Monthly, 10,* 28–35.

Campbell, J. C. (1986). Assessment of risk of homicide for battered women. *Advances in Nursing Science, 8*(4), 36–51.

Campbell, J. C. (1995b). Prediction of homicide of and by battered women. In J. Campbell (Ed.), *Assessing dangerousness: Violence by sexual offenders, batterers, and child abusers* (pp. 96–113). Thousand Oaks, CA: Sage.

Campbell, J. C., & Fishwick, N. (1993). Abuse of female partners. In J. C. Campbell & J. Humphreys (Eds.), *Nursing care of survivors of family violence* (pp. 68–104). St. Louis: Mosby.

Campbell, J. C., & Lewandowski, L. A. (1997). Mental and physical health effects of intimate partner violence on women and children. *Psychiatric Clinics of North America, 20,* 353–374.

Campbell, D. W., Masaki, B., & Torres, S. (1997). In E. Klein, J. Campbell, E. Soler, & M. Ghez (Eds.), *Ending domestic violence: Changing public perceptions/halting the epidemic* (pp. 64–87). Thousand Oaks, CA: Sage.

Centers for Disease Control and Prevention (1998). Summary of notifiable diseases, United States, 1997. *MMWR, 46,* 1–87.

Chicarilli, Z., Cullen, B. J., Harris, N. M., Kalenak, A., Lewis, J. R., McCarthy, R. E., McKinley, B., Oates, R. K., Poss, R., Schwentker, E. P., Shaw, A., & Taylor, L. A. (1997). *Corporal punishment to children's hands: A statement by medical authorities as to the risks* [On-line]. Available from http://silcon.com/~ptave/hands.htm

Cohen, S., DeVos, E., & Newberger, E. (1997). Barriers to physician identification and treatment of family violence: Lessons from five communities. *Academic Medicine, 72*(1), S19–S24.

Coleman, D. H., & Straus, M. (1983). Alcohol abuse and family violence. In E. Gottheil, K. A. Druley, T. E. Skoloda, & H. S. Waxman (Eds.), *Alcohol, drug abuse, and aggression* (pp. 104–124). Springfield, IL: Charles Thomas.

Coleman, F. L. (1997). Stalking behaviors and the cycle of domestic violence. *Journal of Interpersonal Violence, 12,* 420–432.

Colorado Domestic Violence Coalition. (1991). *Domestic violence for health care providers* (3rd ed.). Colorado Domestic Violence Coalition.

Conference News Update: American Academy of Pediatrics 1999 Annual Meeting, Washington, DC: (2000). *Clinician Reviews, 10*(1), 154–156.

Cooper, M., & Eaves, D. (1996). Suicide following homicide in the family. *Violence and Victims, 11*(2), 99–112.

Council on Scientific Affairs of the American Medical Association. (1995). Council report: Female genital mutilation. *Journal of the American Medical Association, 274,* 1714–1716.

Curnow, S. A. M. (1997). The open window phase: Helpseeking and reality behaviors by battered women. *Applied Nursing Research, 10*(3), 130.

DeBecker, G. (1997). *The gift of fear: Survival signals that protect us from violence.* Boston: Little Brown.

De Jong, A., (1992). Medical detection and effects of the sexual abuse of children. In W. O'Donohue & J. H. Greer (Eds.), *The sexual abuse of children: Clinical issues* (Vol. 2; pp. 71–99). Hillsdale, NJ: Lawrence Erlbaum.

De Silva, S. (1989). Obstetric sequelae of female circumcision. *European Journal of Obstetric Gynecological Reproductive Biology, 32,* 233–240.

Dobash, R., Dobash, R., & Cavanagh, K. (1985). The contact between battered women and social and medical agencies. In J. Pahl (Ed.), *Private violence and public policy: The needs of battered women and the responses of the public services* (pp. 142–165). London: Routledge & Kegan Paul.

EDK Associates for the Body Shop. (1997). *The many faces of domestic violence and its impact on the workplace.* New York: EDK Associates.

Eng, T., & Butler, W. (Eds.). (1997). *The hidden epidemic: Confronting sexually transmitted disease.* Washington, DC: National Academy Press.

Fagan, R. W., Barnett, O. W., & Patton, J. B. (1988). Reasons for alcohol use in maritally violent men. *American Journal of Drug and Alcohol Abuse, 14,* 371–392.

Felder, R. (1996). Domestic violence—should victims be forced to testify against their will? *American Business Association Journal, 5*(82), 213.

Felix, A. C., & McCarthy, K. F. (1994). *An analysis of child fatalities 1992.* Boston: Massachusetts Department of Social Services.

Feminist Majority Foundation's (1998). Associated Press article, 1998-FEB-16 [On-Line]. Available from www.feminist.org/news/newsbyte/february98/0218.html

Finkelhor, D., & Dziuba-Leatherman, J. (1994). Children as victims of violence: A national survey. *Pediatrics, 94,* 413–420.

Gladwell, M. (1997). *Violence* [On-line]. Available from www.iuma.com/RTV/violence.html.

Gondolf, E. W. (1998). *Assessing woman battering in mental health services.* Thousand Oaks, CA: Sage.

Gondolf, E. W., & Fisher, E. R. (1988). *Battered women as survivors: An alternative to treating learned helplessness.* Lexington, MA: Lexington.

Graham, D., Rawlings, K., Laltimer, D., Foliano, J., Thompson, A., Suttman, K., Farrington, M., & Hacker, R. (1995). A scale for identifying "Stockholm Syndrome" reactions in young dating women: Factor structure, reliability and validity. *Violence and Victims, 10,* 3–22.

Greenberg, E. M., McFarlane, J., & Watson, M. G. (1997). Vaginal bleeding and abuse: Assessing pregnant women in the emergency department. *Maternal Child Nursing, 22,* 182–186.

Greenfield, L. A., Rand, M. R., Craven, D., Klaus, P. A., Perkins, C. A., Ringel, C., Warchol, G., Maston, C., & Fox, J. A. (1998). *Violence by intimates: Analysis of data on crimes by current or former spouses, boyfriends, and girlfriends* (NCJ-167237). Washington, DC: U.S. Department of Justice, Bureau of Justice Statistics.

Grisso, J. A., & Ness, R. B. (1996). Update in women's health. *Annals of Internal Medicine, 125,* 213–214.

Groves, B. (1995). How does exposure to violence affect very young children? *Harvard Mental Health Letter, 11,* 8–13.

Groves, B., Zuckerman, B., Marans, S., & Cohen, D. J. (1993). Silent victims: Children who witness violence. *Journal of American Medical Association, 269,* 262–264.

Hambleton, B. B., Clark, G., Symaya, D. V., Weissman, G., & Horner, J. (1997). HRSA's strategies to combat family violence. *Academic Medicine, 72*(1), S19–S24.

Hemenway, D., Solnick, S., & Carter, J. (1994). Child-rearing violence. *Child Abuse & Neglect, 18,* 1011–1020.

Hodges, K. (1993). Domestic violence: A health crisis. *North Carolina Medical Journal, 54,* 213–216.

Holden, G. W., Geffner, R., & Jouriles, E. N. (1998). *Children exposed to marital violence.* Washington, DC: American Psychological Association.

Holden, G., & Ritchie, K. L. (1995). Linking extreme marital discord, child rearing, and child behavior problems: Evidence from battered women. *Child Development, 62,* 311–327.

Hotaling, G. T., & Sugarman, D. B. (1986). An analysis of risk markers in husband to wife violence: The current state of knowledge. *Violence & Victims, 1,* 101–124.

Hughes, H. M., & Barad, S. (1982). Changes in the psychological functioning of children in a battered women's shelter: A pilot study. *Victimology: An International Journal, 7,* 60–68.

Humphreys, J. (1997). Nursing care of children of battered women. *Pediatric Nursing, 23*(2), 122–128.

Hutchinson, I. W., Hirschel, J. D., & Pesackis, C. E. (1994). Family violence and police utilization. *Violence and Victims, 9,* 299–313.

Jaffe, P. G., Wolfe, D. A., & Wilson, S. K. (1990). *Children of battered women.* Newbury Park, NJ: Sage.

Johnson, T. (1996). *The sexual dangers of spanking children.* [On-line]. Available. http://silcon.com/~ptave/sexdngr.htm

Joint Commission on Accreditation of Hospitals and Healthcare Organizations. (1997). *Hospital standards—possible victims of domestic abuse and neglect.* Chicago: JCAHO.

Jones, A. (1994). *Next time she'll be dead: Battering and how to stop it.* Boston: Beacon.

Jordan, T. (1995). The efficacy of the California stalking law: Surveying its evolution, extracting insights from domestic violence cases. *Hastings Women's Law Journal, 6,* 363–383.

Kalmuss, D. (1984). The intergenerational transmission of marital aggression. *Journal of Marriage and the Family, 46,* 11–19.

Kantor, G. K. (1993). Refining the brushstrokes in portraits of alcohol and wife assaults. In S. E. Martin (Ed.), *Alcohol and interpersonal violence: Fostering multidisciplinary perspectives* (NIH Publication #93-3496, NIH Monograph 24; pp. 281–290). Washington, DC: National Institutes of Health.

Kantor, G. K., & Straus, M. A. (1989). Substance abuse as a precipitant of wife abuse victimizations. *American Journal of Drug and Alcohol Abuse, 15,* 173–189.

Kilpatrick, K. L., & Williams, L. M. (1997). Post-traumatic stress disorder in child witnesses to domestic violence. *American Journal of Orthopsychiatry, 67,* 639–644.

Klein, E., Campbell, J., Soler, E., & Ghez, M. (1997). *Ending domestic violence: Changing public perceptions/halting the epidemic.* Thousand Oaks, CA: Sage.

Kolbo, J. R., Blakely, E. H., & Engleman, D. (1996). Children who witness domestic violence: A review of empirical literature. *Journal of Interpersonal Violence, 11*(2), 281–293.

Kramer, T., & Green, B. (1991). Posttraumatic stress disorder as an early response to sexual assault. *Journal of Interpersonal Violence, 6*(2), 160–173.

Landenburger, K. (1989). A process of entrapment in and recovery from an abusive relationship. *Issues in Mental Health Nursing, 10,* 209–227.

Laumakis, M. A., Margolin, G., & John, R. S. (1998) The emotional, cognitive, and coping responses of preadolescent children to different dimensions of marital conflict. In G. W. Holden, R. Geffner, & E. N. Jouriles (Eds.), *Children exposed to marital violence* (pp. 257–288). Washington, DC: American Psychological Association.

Lingg, R. A. (1993). Stopping stalkers: A critical examination of antistalking statutes. *St. John's Law Review, 67,* 347–381.

Marshall, L. L. (1992). Development of the severity of violence against women scales. *Journal of Family Violence, 7,* 103–121.

Marx, B. P., Wie, V. V., & Gross, A. M. (1996). Date rape risk factors: A review and methodological critique of the literature. *Aggression and Violent Behavior, A Review Journal, 1*(1), 27–45.

McCann, J., Voris, J., Simon, M., & Wells, R. (1990). Perianal findings in prepubertal children selected for nonabuse: A descriptive study. *Child Abuse & Neglect, 13,* 179–193.

McFarlane, J., & Gondolf, E. (1998). Preventing abuse during pregnancy: A clinical protocol. *MCN. The American Journal of Maternal Child Nursing, 23,* 22–27.

McFarlane, J., Malecha, A., Gist, J., Schultz, P., Willson, P., & Fredland, N. (2000). Indicators of intimate partner violence in women's employment: Implications for workplace action. *Journal of Occupational Health Nursing.* 48(5), 215–220.

McFarlane, J., & Parker, B. (1998). *Abuse during pregnancy: A protocol for March of Dimes Nursing Monograph* (2nd ed.). White Plains, NY: March of Dimes.

McFarlane, J., Parker, B., & Soeken, K. (1996). Physical abuse, smoking and substance abuse during pregnancy: prevalence, interrelationships and effects on birthweight. *Journal of Obstetrical and Gynecological and Neonatal Nursing, 25,* 313–320.

McFarlane, J., Parker, B., Soeken, K., & Bullock, L. (1992). Assessing for abuse during pregnancy: Severity and frequency of injuries and associated entry into prenatal care. *Journal of the American Medical Association, 267,* 3176–3178.

McFarlane, J., Soeken, K., Reel, S., Parker, B., & Silva, C. (1997). Resource use by abused women following an intervention program: Associated severity of abuse and reports of abuse and reports of abuse ending. *Public Health Nursing, 14,* 244–250.

McFarlane, J., Willson, P., Lemmey, D., & Malecha, A. (2000). Women filing assault charges on an intimate partner: Criminal justice outcome and future violence experienced. *Violence Against Women, 6* (4), 396–408.

Meloy, J. R. (1997). The clinical risk management of stalking: "Someone is watching over me." *American Journal of Psychotherapy, 51,* 176–185.

Meloy, R. (1998). *The psychology of stalking. Clinical and forensic perspectives.* Boston: Academic Press.

Murdoch, M., & Nicholand, K. L. (1993). *Women veterans' experiences with domestic violence and with sexual harassment while in the military* [On-line]. Available from www.fvpf.org/fund/the facts/veteran.html

National Center for Elder Abuse (NCEA). (1997). [On-line information]. Available: www.gwjapan.com/NCEA/basic/p.3html

National Criminal Justice Association. (1996). *Domestic violence, stalking and antistalking legislation* (NCJ 160943). Washington, DC: U.S. Department of Justice, National Institute of Justice.

National Institute of Justice. (1993). *Project to develop a model antistalking code for states.* Washington, DC: National Institute of Justice.

Neufeld, B. (1996). SAFE questions: Overcoming barriers to the detection of domestic violence. *American Family Physician, 53,* 348–354.

Odoi, A., Body, S. P., & Elkins, T. E. (1997). Female genital mutilation in rural Ghana, West Africa. *International Journal of Gynecology & Obstetrics, 56,* 179–180.

Paluzzi, P. A., & Houde-Quimby, C. (1996). Domestic violence: Implications for the American college of nurse-midwives and its members. *Journal of Nurse Midwifery, 41,* 430–435.

Patton, E. (1994). Stalking laws: In pursuit of a remedy. *Rutgers Law Journal, 25,* 465–515.

Perez, C. (1993). When does obsession become a crime. *American Journal of Criminal Law, 20,* 263–280.

Perry, B. (1997). Incubated in terror: Neurodevelopmental factors in the "Cycle of Violence". In J. D. Osofsky (Ed.), *Children in a violent society* (pp. 124–149). New York: Guilford.

Perry, B. D., Pollard, R. A., Blakley, T. L., & Baker, W. L. (1995). Childhood trauma, the neurobiology of adaptation, and "use-dependent" development of the brain: How "states" become "traits." *Infant Mental Health Journal, 16,* 271–291.

Ptacek, J. (1998). Why do men batter their wives? In R. K. Bergen (Ed.), *Issues in intimate violence* (pp. 181–195). Thousand Oaks, CA: Sage.

Resnick, H., Kilpatrick, D., Walsh, C., & Vernonen, L. (1991). Marital rape. In R. Ammerman & M. Herson (Eds.). *Case studies in family violence.* New York: Plenum.

Riger, Stephanie, Ahrens, Courtney & Blickenstaff, Amy. (2000). Measuring interference with employment and education reported by women with abusive partners: Preliminary data. *Violence and Victims, 15,* (2), 161–172.

Roberts, A. (1988). Substance abuse among men who batter their mates: The dangerous mix. *Substance Abuse Treatment, 5,* 83–87.

Robinson, B. A (1998). Female & intersexual genital mutilation: In North America & Europe. [On-line]. Available from www.religioustolerance.org/fem cira.htm

Rodriguez, M. A., Quiroga, S. S., & Bauer, H. M. (1996). Breaking the silence—battered women's perspectives on medical care. *Archives of Family Medicine, 5,* 153–158.

Roper Starch Worldwide for Liz Claiborne. (1994). *Addressing domestic violence—A corporate response.* New York: Roper Starch Worldwide.

Rosenberg, M., & Fenley, M. A. (1991). *Violence in America. A public health approach.* New York: Oxford.

Russell, D. E. H. (1990). *Rape in marriage.* New York: MacMillan.

Salter, A. C. (1992). Epidemiology of child sexual abuse. In W. O'Donahue & J. H. Greer (Eds.), *The sexual abuse of children: Therapy and research, Vol. 1* (pp. 108–137). Hillsdale, NJ: Lawrence Erlbaum.

Sanford, B. S. (1993). Stalking is now illegal: Will a paper law make a difference? *Thomas M. Cooley Law Review, 10,* 409–442.

Sayed, G. H., El-Aty, M. A. A., & Fadel, K. A. (1996). The practice of female genital mutilation in Upper Egypt. *International Journal of Gynecology & Obstetrics, 55,* 207–335.

Shepard, M., & Pence, E. (1988). The effects of battering on employment status of women. *Affilia, 3*(2), 55–61.

Stark, E., & Flitcraft, A. H. (1988). Women and children at risk: A feminist perspective on child abuse. *International Journal of Health Services, 18,* 97–119.

Stark, E., Flitcraft, A., Zuckerman, D., Grey, A., Robison, J., & Frazier, W. (1981). *Wife abuse in the medical setting: An introduction for health personnel* (Monograph No. 7). Washington, DC: U.S. Department of Health and Human Services.

Straus, M. A., & Gelles, R. J. (1986). Societal change in family violence from 1975 to 1985 as revealed by two national surveys. *Journal of Marriage and the Family, 48,* 465–479.

Straus, M. A., Gelles, R. J., & Steinmetz, S. K. (1980). *Behind closed doors: Violence in the American family.* New York: Anchor Press/Doubleday.

Straus, M. A., & Smith, C. (1995). Family patterns and child abuse. In M. A. Straus & R. J. Gelles (Eds.), *Physical violence in American families: Risk factors and adaptation in 8,145 families.* New Brunswick, NJ: Transaction.

Tjaden, P. & Thoennes, N. (1998). *Stalking in America: Findings from the National Violence Against Women Survey* (Grant No. 93-IJ-CX-0012). Washington, DC: U.S. Department of Justice, National Institute of Justice and Centers for Disease Control and Prevention.

Uniform Crime Reports for the United States. (1996). *Who are the victims* [On-line]. Available from www.ojp.usdoj.gov/vawo/manual/who.htm

U.S. Bureau of Census. (1997). *Poverty 1997* [On-line]. Available from www.census.gov/hhes/www/povty97.html

U.S. Department of Labor, Women's Bureau. (1996). *Facts on working women* (No. 96-3). Washington, DC: U.S. Department of Labor.

Vitanza, S., Vogel, L., & Marshall, L. (1995). Distress and symptoms of post-traumatic stress disorder in abused women. *Violence and Victims, 10,* 23–34.

Walker, L. E. (1984). *The battered woman syndrome.* New York: Springer.

Wallace, H. (1999). *Family violence: Legal, medical, and social perspectives* (2nd ed.). Boston, MA: Allyn & Bacon.

Westrup, D. (1998). Applying functional analysis to stalking behavior. In J. R. Meloy (Ed.), *The psychology of stalking: Clinical and forensic perspectives* (pp. 275–294). San Diego: Academic Press.

Wiist, W. H., & McFarlane, J. (1998). Severity of spousal and intimate partner abuse to pregnant Hispanic women. *Journal of Health Care for the Poor and Underserved, 9(3),* 248–261.

Willson, P. (1998). Domestic violence: Are nurses hiding the facts? *The Internet Journal of Advanced Nursing Practice.* Vol. 2 (3): April [On-line]. Available from www.ispub.com/journals/ijanp.htm

Woods, S. J., & Campbell, J. C. (1993). Post-traumatic stress in battered women: Does the diagnosis fit? *Issues in Mental Health Nursing, 14,* 173–186.

World Health Organization. (1994, April 12). *Statement of the Director-General to the World Health Organization's Global Commission on Women's Health.* Geneva: World Health Organization.

World Health Organization. (1996). *Female genital mutilation: Information pack* [On-line]. Available from www.who.int/frh whd/FGM/infopack/English/fgm infopack.htm

Wright, R., Wright, R., & Isaac, N. (1998). Response to battered mothers in the pediatric emergency department: Call for an interdisciplinary approach to family violence. *Pediatrics, 99,* 186–192.

Suggested Readings

Campbell, J. C. (1995a). Making the health care system an empowerment zone for battered women: Health consequences, policy recommendations, introduction, and overview. In J. C. Campbell (Ed.), *Assessing dangerousness: Violence by sexual offenders, batterers, and child abusers* (pp. 3–22). Thousand Oaks, CA: Sage.

Campbell, J. C., & Campbell, D. W. (1996). Cultural competence in the care of abused women. *Journal of Nurse Midwifery, 41,* 457–462.

Carlson, B. E. (1984). Children's observations of interparental violence. In A. R. Roberts (Ed.), *Battered women and their families: Intervention strategies and treatment programs* (pp. 147–167). New York: Springer.

Dire, M. A., & Lindmark, G. (1991). A hospital study of the complications of female circumcision. *Tropical Doctor, 21,* 146–148.

Kun, K. E. (1997). Female genital mutilation: The potential for increased risk of HIV infection. *International Journal of Gynecology & Obstetrics, 56,* 153–155.

Parker, B., & McFarlane, J. (1991). Feminist theory and nursing: An empowerment model for research. *Advanced Nursing Science, 13(3),* 59–67.

Rorie, J-A. L., & Barger, M. K. (1996). Primary care for women: Cultural competence in primary care services. *Journal of Nurse Midwifery, 41(2),* 92–100.

Sheridan, D. (1998). *Measuring harassment of battered women: A nursing concern.* Unpublished doctoral dissertation. Oregon Health Sciences University.

Walker, L. E. (1979). *The battered woman.* New York: Harper & Row.

Resources

Abuse During Pregnancy: A Protocol for Prevention and Intervention Continuing Education Credits Available from the March of Dimes, 800-367-6630, www.modimes.org

Family Violence: A Self-Study Guide for Health Care Professionals in Primary Care, The Family Peace Project, Medical College of Wisconsin, 414-548-6903

Family Violence Prevention Fund, 383 Rhode Island Street, Suite 304, San Francisco, CA 94103-5133, www.fvpf.org

How to Identify and Document Genital and Non-Genital Injuries, Health Education Alliance, Monterey, CA 800-404-3258

Improving the Health Care Response to Domestic Violence: A Resource Manual for Health Care Provider, Family Violence Prevention Fund, San Francisco, CA 415-252-8900

National Coalition Against Domestic Violence (NCADV), P. O. Box 18749, Denver, CO 80218-0749, 303-839-1852, Fax: 303-831-9251, www.ncadv.org

Silent Witness National Initiative, 7 Sheridan Avenue South, Minneapolis, MN 55405, 612-377-6629, Fax: 612/374-3956, E-mail: info@silentwitness.net, www.silentwitness.net/html/talkous.html

U.S. Department of Labor, Women's Bureau, www.dol.gov/dol/wb

Violence Against Women Office, U.S. Department of Justice, 10th & Constitution Avenue, NW, Room 5302, Washington, DC 20530, 202-616-8894, www.raw.umn.edu

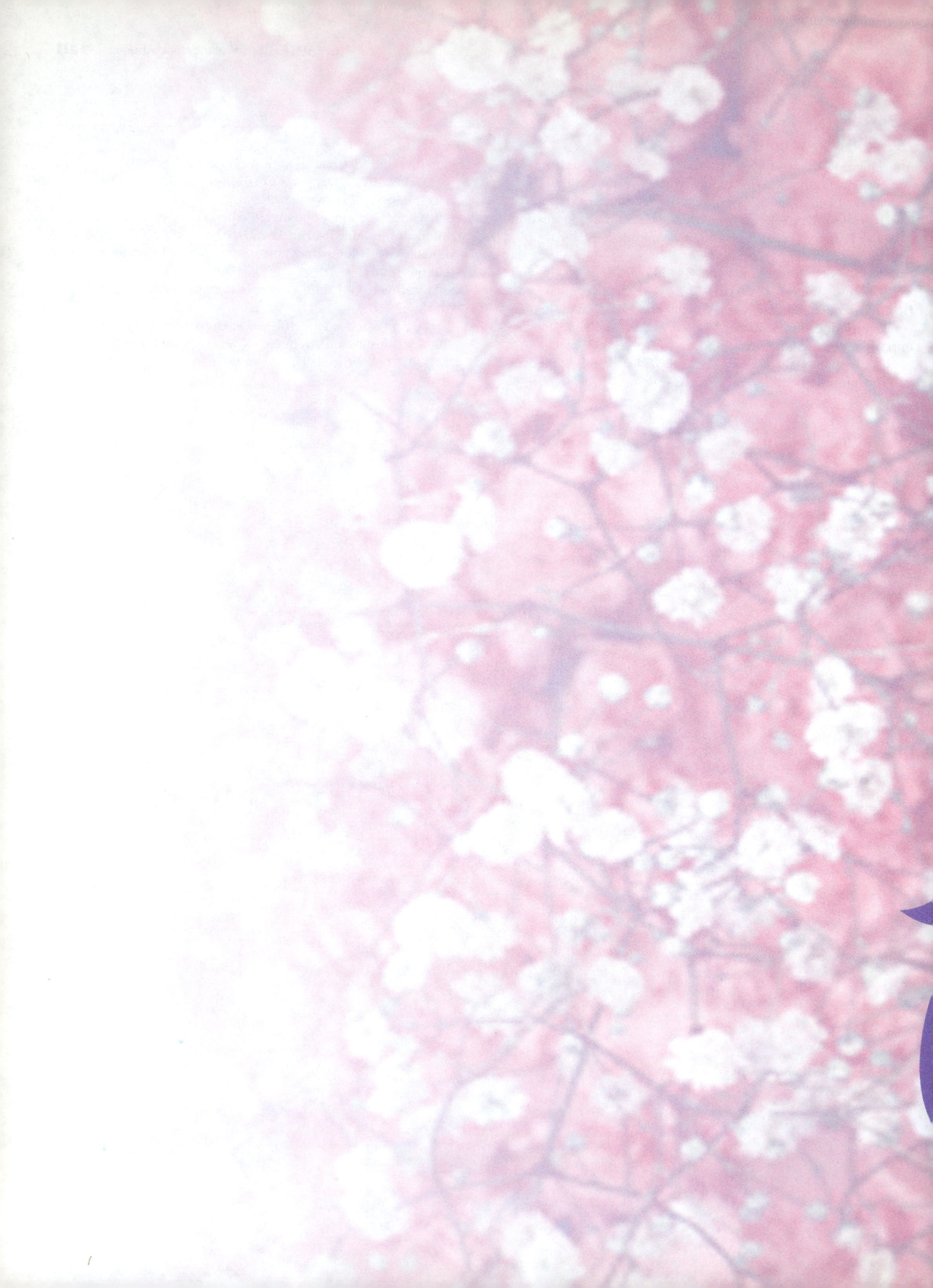

UNIT III

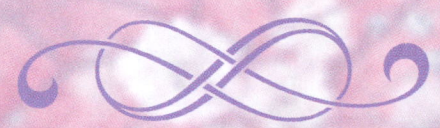

Human Sexuality Across the Life Span

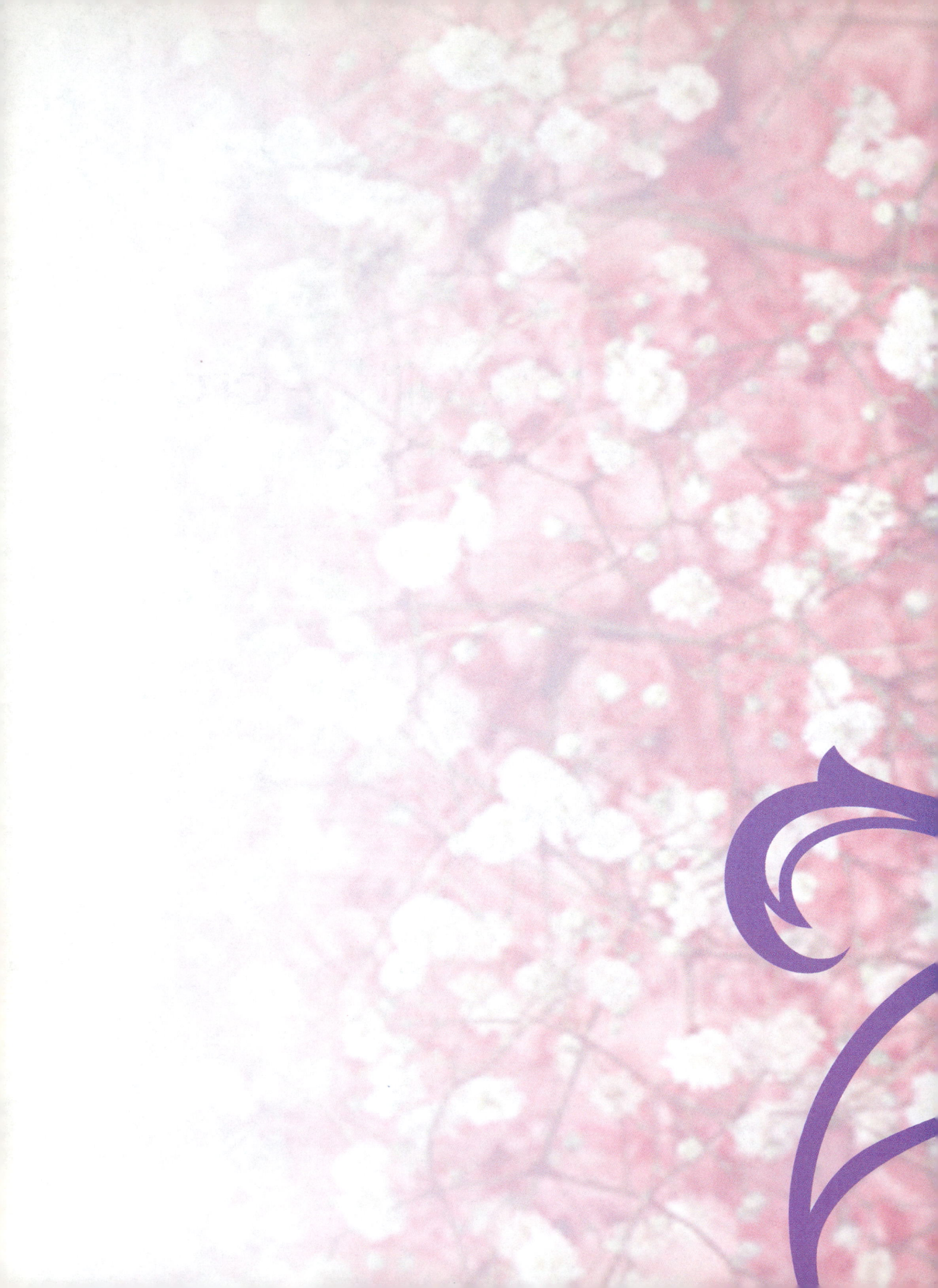

CHAPTER 12

Sexual and Reproductive Function

opics dealing with bodily functions and sexuality continue to be shrouded in secrecy and embarrassment. Often, health care providers and those seeking assistance find they are uncomfortable exploring issues that may affect reproductive functioning. Terms as diverse as the "monthlies" or the "curse" are used to refer to the menstrual cycle. These terms may indicate being uncomfortable with more specific technical terms or a negative attitude toward menses. Alternatively, these terms may merely have been acquired from the cultural milieu and are not indicative of a person's attitude toward menses. Terms dealing with menstruation and sexuality often are value-laden. The following questions can be used to explore personal knowledge, values, and beliefs that may affect your ability to care for women and their partners:

- Do I understand the interrelationship of menstruation and ovarian function? Can I explain the relationship clearly to clients of various ages and educational levels?

- How do I feel about men or women whose choices, such as drug use or sexual activity, may have affected their fertility?

- How do I feel about pregnancy, the decision to have children, and the decision not to have children?

- Which terms do I use to describe menses, sexuality, and body parts? Are these terms value-laden? Are they appropriate to the client's level of education and understanding? Which issues affect the use of certain terms?

- Do my attitudes toward sexuality influence my delivery of health care?

Key Terms

Androgen
Anovulatory
Corpus luteum
Desire phase
Dyspareunia
Endometriosis
Endometrium
Estrogen
Excitement phase
Follicular phase
Follicle-stimulating
hormone (FSH)
Galactorrhea
Germ cells

Gonadal
Gonadotropin-releasing
hormone (Gn-RH)
Graafian follicle
Hypothalamic-pituitary-
gonadal axis
Human chorionic
gonadotropin
Hydrocele
Impotence
Infertility
Leydig cells
Libido
Luteal phase

Luteinizing hormone
Menarche
Menopause
Menses
Menstrual phase
Mittelschmerz
Neurohormonal
Orgasmic phase
Ovulation
Perimenopause
Plateau phase
Precocious
Progesterone
Proliferative phase

Prostaglandins
Puberty
Refractory period
Resolution phase
Secretory phase
Seminiferous tubules
Serial monogamy
Sexual dysfunction
Spermatogenesis
Spermatozoa
Spinnbarkeit
Testosterone
Vaginismus
Varicocele

Competencies

Upon completion of this chapter, the reader should be able to:

1. Explain the menstrual cycle in terms of the ovarian, endometrial, and neurohormonal components.

2. Identify the normal ages of onset and cessation of menses and factors related to normal variations.

3. Describe normal menstruation in terms of length of cycle, flow, and quantity.

4. Describe spermatogenesis.

5. Discuss factors related to male and female infertility.

6. List key components of an infertility examination and a rationale for their inclusion.

7. Discuss the emotional impact of infertility.

8. Describe regimens to treat infertility, including assisted reproductive technology.

Considering the coordination of the complex body systems required for reproductive functioning, it is amazing that conception and birth occur. Yet within that complexity, finely ordered events produce cyclic changes that can be predicted. In women the most evident result of this neurohormonal interplay, the menstrual cycle, provides a basis for understanding the physiology of reproduction. (The term **neurohormonal** pertains to hormones formed by secretory cells and liberated by nerve impulses.) To grasp the usually predictable events, which are driven by the functioning of the ovary, it is helpful to start at the beginning of human sexual development. In men the physiology is not quite as complex; however, a number of organs and systems are involved with reproduction.

This chapter describes the physiology of the female and male reproductive systems. Normal parameters for

functioning are provided as guidelines for assessment. Sexuality and sexual dysfunction are discussed. Finally, infertility is discussed. Its emotional impact and clinical guidelines for assessment and treatment are presented.

NORMAL SEXUAL DIFFERENTIATION

In human embryos, sexual development is a product of genetic and hormonal influences, which determine the differentiation of the internal systems and formation of external genitalia. **Gonadal** (referring to the ovaries in the female and the testes in the male) development begins at 5 to 6 weeks' gestation, with testicular differentiation at 7 weeks' gestation. At this time the production of **testosterone**, a potent, naturally occurring androgen (male) hormone, begins. Testosterone regulates the development of the penis, testes, scrotum, seminal vesicles, prostate gland, and genital duct system.

Without the activity of the Y chromosome, ovarian development occurs 2 weeks later. In the female ovary, 5 to 7 million **germ cells**, the precursors of ova, are evident by 20 weeks' gestation. By birth, this number has already decreased to 1 to 2 million cells. By puberty, the number of germ cells is approximately 300,000. This decrease continues until menopause when only thousands are left. The ovaries provide varying amounts of **estrogen** (female sex hormone) and **progesterone** (antiestrogenic hormone) needed for the production of eggs (**oocytes**) from these germ cells. The ovaries coordinate the development and sloughing of the **endometrium** (lining of the uterus), resulting in the menstrual cycle. Thus, these two events, the ovarian and the endometrial cycles, occur at the same time and produce **ovulation** (release of a mature ovum) and **menses** (monthly bleeding from the lining of the uterus).

Female Reproductive Function

The onset of menstrual bleeding, or **menarche**, usually occurs between 9 and 16 years of age (Speroff, Glass, & Kase, 1999). The average age of menarche in the United States is 12.8 years. Several factors may affect the age of onset of menses including family history, geographic location, general health, and nutrition. Current information supports the importance of body weight in determining the time of menarche (Speroff, Glass, & Kase, 1999). Moderately overweight girls begin menstruation earlier than do those of normal weight. Girls with very low body fat, such as those having anorexia and girls who participate in strenuous athletics, may have delayed menarche.

For 12 to 18 months after menarche, menses may be irregular, often do not produce ovulation (**anovulatory**), and may be very heavy or very light. It is important to be aware that pregnancy can result during this time, and appropriate education should be provided. Parents may seek evaluation with concerns that their daughter may be experiencing early (**precocious**) puberty (Smith & Hornberger, 1997), irregular or heavy menses, or delayed menses. Often, explaining the wide range of what is considered to be normal is all that is required. Conversely, the child under 8 years of age who has pubertal changes, such as menarche, requires further evaluation because there may exist important growth implications or another underlying disease. Likewise, with delayed menses, a girl over the age of 17 years could have a genetic, hormonal, or hypothalamic-pituitary disorder. Anatomic defects of the uterus and vagina also must be ruled out.

A menstrual cycle refers to the time that passes from the first day of one menstrual period to the first day of the next menstrual period. The normal cycle length can range from 21 to 36 days, although 95% of women have cycles between 25 to 32 days. A working number used to describe a so-called normal cycle is 28 days. Timing the cycle

Client Education

Adolescence and Puberty

Puberty, the development of secondary sex characteristics and the ability to reproduce, can be a tumultuous time for parents and teens. It is quite common for the mother of an adolescent girl to have questions about when certain developmental events can be expected in her daughter's life. The nurse may be the person who is first approached to provide this information. The following is a synopsis of the range of normal events:

- The average age of menarche in the United States is 12.8 years.
- Menarche usually is a mid to late event in puberty and usually occurs after the development of pubic and axillary hair, breast buds, and genital changes.
- A young girl who has not developed secondary sex characteristics by the age of 14 years should be evaluated by a physician.
- A young girl who develops secondary sex characteristics but does not begin menses also should be evaluated by a physician.

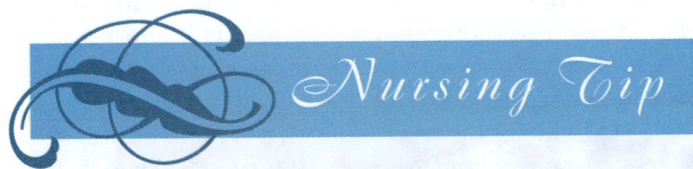

IRON AND MENSTRUATION

Blood loss from menstruation results in approximately 0.5 mg of iron being lost with each milliliter of blood, explaining why women tend to have lower hemoglobin levels than do men, especially women with heavy menses. These iron deficits can be overcome through dietary means by eating liver and other foods rich in iron or by taking a multivitamin with iron.

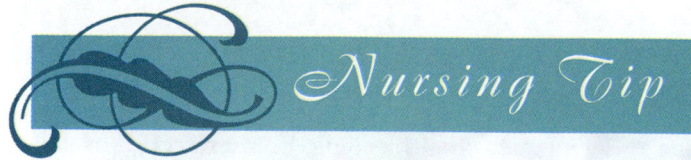

MENOPAUSE

It is important to realize that the diagnosis of menopause, and the end of reproductive functioning, is not made until 1 year after the last menses (Speroff, Glass, & Kase, 1999). Thus, it is wise to counsel women to continue contraception throughout the perimenopausal years.

begins on the first day of bleeding, day 1 of the cycle. Bleeding usually continues for 3 to 5 days, with 1 to 8 days considered to be within normal limits. The amount of blood lost averages 30 mL (1 oz) per cycle but ranges from 20 to 80 mL (0.67 to 2.67 oz). Blood loss usually is greater during the first 3 days of the cycle because the precise hormonal events leading to menses affect the entire **endometrium** (cellular lining of the uterus that is shed monthly at the time of menses) at the same time, resulting in generalized sloughing of the endometrial tissue.

Normally, menstruation continues until **menopause** (cessation of menses), which occurs between the ages of 35 and 60 years (Byyny & Speroff, 1996). Menopause is determined to be present when a woman has completed 1 year without menses. For as many as 15 years before the cessation of menses, women may experience changes in their cycle, such as heavier or lighter bleeding and changes in the length or duration of menses. This time is described as the **perimenopause** and is a result of changes in ovarian function. In the United States, 51 years of age is the average time of menopause (Speroff, Glass, & Kase, 1999).

Endometrial Activity

The activity of the endometrium during the menstrual cycle can be described as the menstrual, proliferative, and secretory phases. The endometrium is prepared for implantation of a fertilized ovum by the ovarian hormones. When implantation does not occur the tissue sloughs and new tissue begins to build for the next cycle. This cycle of growth and regression occurs approximately 300 to 400 times in the human adult. Specific changes in the endometrium occur in the various phases of the menstrual cycle.

The **menstrual phase** is the time during which the woman experiences vaginal bleeding. It begins with day 1 of the menses and continues for about 5 days, during which time almost two thirds of the endometrial tissue is lost. The lost tissue has been described as having evidence of necrosis and white cell infiltration as well as fragmentation of vessels and glands.

The **proliferative phase** describes the endometrium from the end of menses through ovulation, which occurs on or about day 14 of the normal 28-day cycle. The growth of the glands of the endometrium is associated with increased estrogen levels produced by the ovary. The tissue of the endometrium has changed and grown from being dense and approximately 0.5 mm thick to being spongy and 3.5 to 5.0 mm thick, an increase of 7 to 10 times in size.

The **secretory phase** continues from the time of ovulation (days 14 to 28) under the combined effects of estrogen and progesterone. The endometrium stops growing but increases in vascularity and the glycogen-producing glands occur. With the increased blood and glycogen, the tissue is ready for implantation. Without fertilization and implantation, estrogen and progesterone levels decrease, leading to decreased blood supply to the tissue. As blood vessels constrict and relax, leading to separation of the prepared endometrial layer, necrosis of the tissue results in menstruation. Even during menses, increasing estrogen levels produced by the ovary begin the healing process, and the endometrium begins to regenerate and prepare for the next cycle.

Ovarian Regulation

In the reproductive aspect of a woman's life there are baselines of all sex hormones. Fluctuations also occur that establish the menstrual cycle. The main organs of regulation are the hypothalamus and pituitary in the brain and the ovaries in the pelvis (Speroff, Glass, & Kase, 1999). These structures are termed the hypothalamic-pituitary-gonadal axis and form a feedback loop that controls hormone production. Although a delicate interplay and regulation between the brain and ovaries exist, the ovaries actually drive the process of ovulation. Two phases can be used to describe the functioning of the ovary as it regulates the menstrual cycle and the development of an egg, the follicular and the luteal phases.

The **follicular phase** refers to maturation of the follicle leading to the production of an egg and ovulation. The **luteal phase** refers to the secretion of hormones from the corpus luteum, which is formed from the follicle that produced the egg. The corpus luteum continues to secrete estrogen and progesterone. These hormones prepare and maintain the endometrium for implantation of the fertilized ovum. Again, it is important to remember that the menstrual cycle is driven or regulated by these ovarian hormones. Thus, the visible evidence of the hormone fluctuations and ovarian functioning is menses. When a woman's cycle is regular and predictable, without the aid of hormone therapy, she probably is ovulating.

As well as producing the steroid hormones estradiol and progesterone and small amounts of testosterone, the ovaries produce oocytes or eggs. At 4 to 6 days before menses, ovarian follicles begin to grow independent of hormonal stimulation. For most follicles, growth is limited, and they never reach maturity. Under the influence of hormones, a single follicle is chosen to reach maturity by day 5 to 7 in the cycle. Termed the *preantral* or *primary follicle,* the selected follicle continues to enlarge. It is surrounded by a membrane, the zona pellucida. The size and number of layers of the cells increase under the influence of estrogen, and follicular fluid begins to increase. The maturing follicle or **graafian follicle** continues growing until ovulation occurs. Typically, in a 28-day cycle, ovulation would be on day 14; however, the day of ovulation varies according to the number of days needed for maturation of the follicle. The follicular phase may vary in length from 7 to 22 days and determines the length of the cycle. That is, the follicular phase may vary in length but the luteal phase is consistently 14 days. Thus, menses will begin 14 days after ovulation.

Ovulation

Although not always considered a phase of the ovarian cycle, multiple important events occur at the time of ovulation that warrant special note. Physical and hormonal events take place to enhance the possibility of fertilization (Speroff, Glass, & Kase, 1999). The increased estrogen levels at this time have prepared the endometrium for implantation but also change the characteristics of the cervi-

cal mucus. The role of cervical mucus is to facilitate sperm transport into the uterus. Before ovulation, cervical mucus threads are 1 to 2 cm long, increasing to 12 to 24 cm and becoming thin, clear, and copious when ovulation occurs. The increased elasticity is called **spinnbarkheit** and facilitates sperm transport into the uterus (Figure 12-1). The cervix becomes softer and the os opens. Some women can determine the time of ovulation because they experience pain in the lower abdomen called **mittelschmerz.**

Hormonal events include an increase in androgen levels. Androgens are hormones derived from testosterone that increase libido and prepare the follicle for ovulation. **Prostaglandins** are chemicals produced by many bodily systems, including those of the female reproductive system. Prostaglandins increase and, although the exact action is not known, may act to thin the follicle wall and contract smooth muscle in the cell wall to facilitate release of the oocyte.

The luteal phase begins with ovulation as the cells of the ovary that produced the egg increase in size and accumulate lutein. Lutein is a yellow pigment that gives the name to the **corpus luteum** or *yellow body.* The corpus luteum continues to produce estrogen and progesterone. Progesterone levels increase rapidly for nearly 8 days as this hormone suppresses the growth of new follicles. The corpus luteum begins to degenerate on days 9 to 11 when not sustained by the hormone of early pregnancy, **human chorionic gonadotropin (hCG).** When pregnancy occurs, hCG prevents regression of the corpus luteum, which

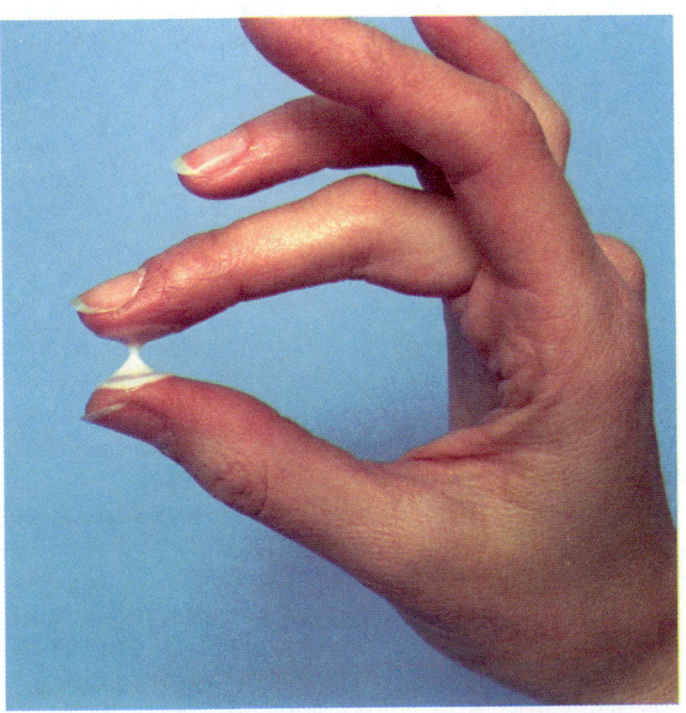
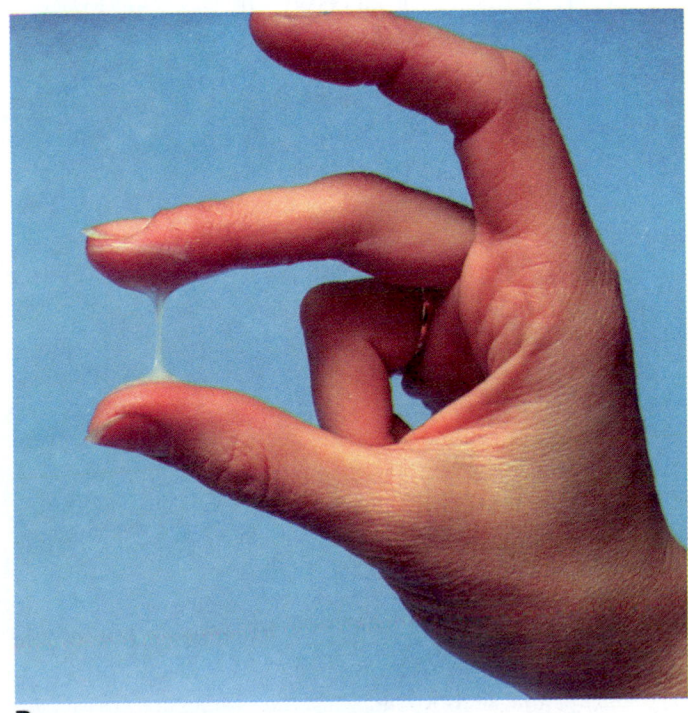

A.   B.

Figure 12-1 Spinnbarkheit test. A. Before ovulation, cervical mucus is thick, preventing transport of sperm. B. At ovulation, secretions become thinner and elastic, facilitating sperm transport.

continues to produce hormones until 9 or 10 weeks gestation. By this time the placenta has assumed production of the needed steroidal hormones estrogen and progesterone.

When pregnancy does not occur the corpus luteum begins to degenerate and the levels of estrogen and progesterone decrease, stimulating the start of a new cycle. This continuing cycle of events, although controlled by the follicle, which will ovulate, are under the direction of the anterior pituitary and hypothalamus. The **hypothalamic-pituitary-gonadal axis** is a triad of the hypothalamus, pituitary, and ovaries that regulates the hormones of reproduction and that must function in synchrony for conception to occur.

Hormonal Regulation

The hypothalamus functions similarly to a thermostat, sensing hormone levels in the blood (Speroff, Glass, & Kase, 1999). Depending on the set levels, the hypothalamus sends a message to the anterior pituitary to either increase or decrease the amounts of the specific hormone needed. As well as regulating the ovaries, the hypothalamus also plays a regulatory function in growth hormone, thyroid-stimulating hormone (TSH), and the adrenal hormones.

The hypothalamic hormone that controls the gonadotropins is called **gonadotropin-releasing hormone (Gn-RH)**. When the hypothalamus senses a decrease in the level of hormones produced by the ovary Gn-RH is released into the blood. The hypophyseal portal system provides a mechanism by which the hypothalamus and anterior pituitary communicate. The anterior pituitary receives the message that more or fewer hormones are needed and either stimulates or suppresses the release of hormones.

The hormones produced by the pituitary are **follicle-stimulating hormone (FSH)**, which stimulates the ovary to prepare a mature ovum for release, and **luteinizing hormone (LH)**, which is responsible for the release of the ovum. The anterior pituitary also produces the hormone prolactin, which regulates milk production. With the release of FSH and LH, events in the ovary are regulated to produce the hormones needed to support the development of the oocyte and for ovulation. As the ovary is preparing an egg for ovulation, the endometrium is being prepared to support the implantation and growth of the fertilized egg. Preparation of the endometrium is primarily under the influence of estrogen. Estrogen is the hormone responsible for the secondary sex characteristics of the female.

During the second phase of the cycle the corpus luteum produces progesterone, which stimulates the secretory phase and supports the continued growth of the endometrium. When fertilization does not occur 8 to 10 days after ovulation, the corpus luteum degenerates and progesterone levels rapidly decrease. This rapid decrease results in progesterone levels below those needed to sustain the endometrium, and menstruation begins. With the decrease in progesterone levels the hypothalamus is stimulated to increase secretion of Gn-RH, and the cycle begins again (Speroff, Glass, & Kase, 1999).

An understanding of the complexity and interrelatedness of the hypothalamic-pituitary-gonadal axis provides a basis for understanding and treating many of the problems related to the reproductive system. The diagnosis of problems such as dysfunctional uterine bleeding, amenorrhea, and infertility and the appropriate treatment can be determined based on this knowledge.

Male Reproductive Function

The genetic sex of the fetus is determined at conception. The male and female reproductive systems, however, are similar until differentiation begins at 5 to 6 weeks' gestation and testicular development occurs by 7 weeks' gestation. In utero, the fetal gonads are active and secrete either estrogen or testosterone. As noted previously, in the male the hormone testosterone regulates development of the penis, testes, scrotum, seminal vesicles, prostate gland, and genital duct system. During childhood, hormones are inhibited. During puberty, however, the hypothalamus begins to produce increased levels of Gn-RH, which stimulate the anterior pituitary to produce FSH and LH. Hormones produced in the hypothalamus, pituitary, and testes are responsible for **spermatogenesis**, or development of sperm cells. This system is analogous to the hypothalamic-pituitary-ovarian axis in the female, which produces an ovum.

Follicle-stimulating hormone stimulates the production of primary spermatocytes in the **seminiferous tubules**, which are the tubes that carry semen from the testes. Concurrently, LH stimulates the **Leydig cells** in the testes to produce testosterone. Testosterone encourages maturation of the **spermatozoa**, or sperm.

Testosterone is essential for spermatogenesis and also stimulates the production of seminal fluid. Testosterone is responsible for secondary sexual characteristics such as the distribution of body hair, increased muscle mass, and enlargement of the vocal cords. The sexual drive is thought to be controlled by testosterone. The action of testosterone continues throughout life, including the development of sperm. Levels of this hormone decrease as men age, however, resulting in decreased hair distribution, reduced body mass, and decreased sexual activity. This decrease in testosterone has led to the suggestion that men have a series of physical and emotional changes comparable with those that occur during menopause in women.

Development of sperm in the testes takes approximately 70 days. After leaving the testes the sperm remains in the epididymis for 12 to 26 days, during which time they mature. The semen, which forms the ejaculate, contains sperm and secretions from the prostate, vas deferens, and seminal vesicles. Being a complex system, it is apparent that many factors can affect male fertility, even events that occurred days to months before the sperm is developed. Some of the factors that affect male fertility can be as simple as wearing tight-fitting underwear, excessive use of hot tubs, or use of marijuana. A combination of events also may affect male fertility, including infection, a varicocele, and injury.

Once ejaculated, sperm can live from 2 to 3 days in the female genital tract but with decreasing activity after 24 hours, whereas an ovum is fertile only for 24 hours. The relative long life of sperm enhances the capacity for fertilization of an ovum.

In addition to the purely physiologic processes in men and women that regulate fertility, there are behaviors involved in procreation that society has termed *sexuality*.

SEXUALITY

Sex, sexual behavior, and sexuality are terms that often are used synonymously. In reality, they are different but related concepts. Sex is one of four primary drives, including thirst, hunger, and avoidance of pain. Sexual behavior refers to those practices involving sexual intercourse and other behaviors involving stimulation of the genitalia and other erogenous zones for the purpose of procreation or gratification. Sexuality is a complex concept that deals with the quality of being sexual, sexual activity, and sexual receptivity or interest. Sexuality encompasses issues related to human sexual response; sexual orientation; and beliefs, attitudes, and social and cultural patterns related to sexual matters. The expression of sexuality is influenced by ethical, spiritual, cultural, and moral factors.

Sexuality and sexual function are important to a woman's health and well-being. The nurse plays a significant role in assisting women to understand their sexual health, sexual development, and sexuality (Figure 12-2). In fact, the holistic framework requires that the nurse be able to assist clients with concerns related to sexuality. Nurses, like other health care providers, can be uncomfortable discussing such personal topics with their clients. This unease may stem from vulnerability related to inadequate experience in dealing with clients with sexual difficulty, lack of information, or misinformation on the part of the nurse. Sexual awareness is required on the part of the client; however, cultural influences may inhibit conversation about such matters.

Many women have questions about their sexuality or sexual function. In fact, it has been estimated that as many as 60% of women have questions related to their sexuality (Baram, 1996). Many times women are hesitant to discuss these personal problems with anyone. Women may be

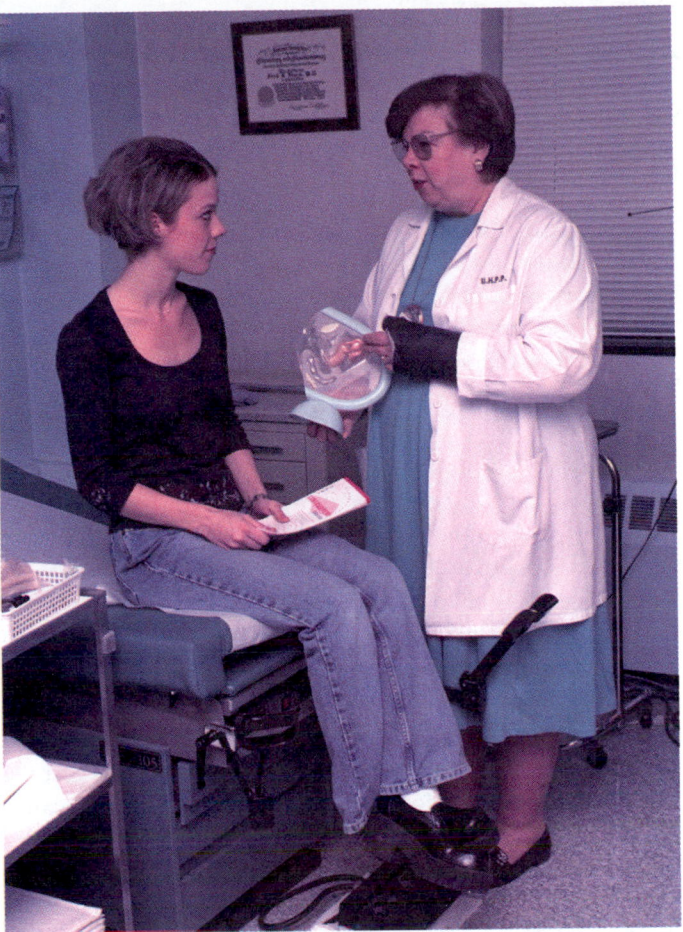

Figure 12-2 Nurses play an important role in helping clients understand their sexual health and development.

most uncomfortable asking questions related to sexuality when cared for by someone of the opposite sex. Because of the awkwardness of discussing personal issues with providers, there is a tendency to seek information from other women or from the lay press. Occasionally, this practice leads to myth and misinformation. The tendency to obtain partial information and misinformation makes it very important for the nurse to assess the client's perception of her situation before institution of a plan of care.

Sexual dysfunction can produce multifaceted and severe alterations in a woman's physical and mental health. Even if the question is one of health promotion, the nurse is in an excellent position to help women voice their questions and to dispel myths. Before these things can happen, the nurse must have an adequate understanding of the complexity of sexuality and the interaction of its components. Typically, this information is not high priority in educational programs and may not be discussed. In fact, it has been the practice at some institutions to relegate the study of sexuality to prenursing courses. The resulting general lack of information decreases the likelihood that the nurse will feel comfortable with this subject matter. Providing information about sexuality requires that the

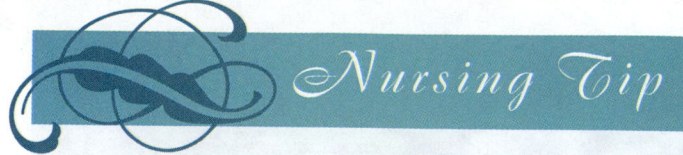

BEING NONJUDGMENTAL

In the United States, body piercing and tattooing currently are trends. It is common to see piercing of navels, nipples, tongues, and the clitoris. These practices have roots in sexuality and sexual mores. You have the duty to accept the client's practices even when they differ from your own values.

nurses have a nonjudgmental accepting attitude to allow women who have been enculturated never to discuss sex to do so in a public setting. Some women may not even have the vocabulary to voice their questions and concerns. The nurse may have to teach some women the names of body parts and their functions before being able to assist in answering questions or solving problems. Assistance may take many forms. A woman who has been sexually abused, for example, may have great difficulty tolerating a simple vaginal examination. A woman who is a lesbian may not participate in routine gynecologic care because she does not want her health care providers to know about her lifestyle. The young adolescent may not understand how to insert a tampon and may be very uncomfortable about seeking such information.

The nurse may be required to closely examine personal values through self-reflection and rely on cultural competence to assist women with their sexual concerns (Figure 12-3). It is important that the nurse does not inject personal biases and other factors into the nurse-client interaction that will produce negative outcomes.

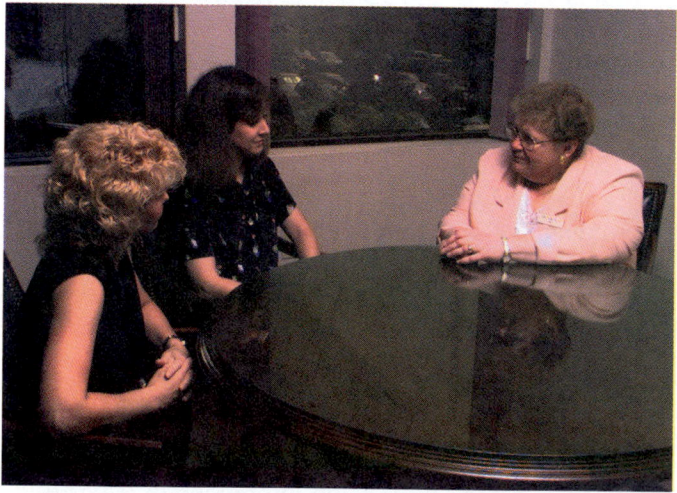

Figure 12-3 During the health history and interview, the nurse must remain nonjudgmental when discussing clients' practices and lifestyle choices.

Human Sexual Response

Masters & Johnson (1966) are renowned for their study of human sexual response. They conceptualized the human sexual response consisting of four phases: excitement, plateau, orgasmic, and resolution. These phases occur in men and women and are associated with a number of physiologic changes. Contemporary sources include a fifth phase, which has been identified as the desire phase. The **desire phase** is conceptualized as being present before the other four phases. The desire phase has been described as the motivation or inclination to be sexual. Baram (1996) indicates that internal cues, such as fantasies, or external cues, such as an interested partner, may trigger sexual desire. Baram further states that desire also depends on proper neuroendocrine function. Other influences include sexual orientation, sexual preferences, mind set, and the environment. All of these factors affect an individual's libido.

The **excitement phase** occurs as a result of internal or external cues. During this phase the woman experiences increased vaginal lubrication, engorgement of the blood vessels of the breast and pelvis, and a sense of muscular tension. She also experiences increased heart rate, respiratory rate, and blood pressure. Besides the increase in muscular tension, many women experience flushing of the skin over the chest, neck, and face known as *sexual flushing*. These skin changes are the result of surface vasodilation, which produces congestion of the vessels with blood. The woman's nipples also become erect. Because of pelvic vasocongestion, the clitoris and labia become swollen. The vagina becomes distended and elongated, and the vaginal opening constricts forming what is called an orgasmic platform (Kohn & Kaplan, 2000).

The man's response during the excitement phase includes changes in the scrotum, penis, and breasts. The scrotal sac becomes thickened and is elevated against the body owing to shortening of the spermatic cord. The penis becomes engorged with blood, which increases its circumference and length. This penile state is called an erection. As in the woman, the man's nipples become erect and he may experience the same sexual flushing of the chest, neck, and face.

The **plateau phase** of sexual response follows the excitement phase. During the plateau phase, women experience the most heightened sense of sexual tension. The labia become congested with blood to the extent that they may have a bluish hue. The change in color may be more difficult to recognize in dark skin types. There is full vaginal expansion as well as elevation of the uterus out of the pelvis in preparation for entry of the penis. By this phase, 75% of women experience sexual flushing. Tachycardia and hyperventilation occur as does a modest increase in blood pressure of 20 to 60 mm Hg (Cohen, Kenner, & Hollingsworth, 1991).

The man's response during the plateau phase includes an increase in coronal circumference of the penis with continued erection. The testicles increase in size and are elevated against the body. As in the woman, there is generalized muscular tension that increases in intensity as orgasm approaches. The man also experiences tachycardia, hyperventilation, and increased blood pressure. The systolic pressure increases by 20 to 80 mm Hg, and the diastolic pressure increases by 20 to 40 mm Hg (Cohen, Kenner, & Hollingsworth, 1991).

In the **orgasmic phase** the woman experiences elongation of the vaginal canal. There is an intense desire for sexual release as a result of blood vessel congestion. This sensation builds until the woman reaches orgasm. During this time the woman experiences an increase in blood pressure, tachycardia, and hyperventilation.

As the man enters the orgasmic phase, he experiences muscular contractions of the accessory reproductive organs, including the vas deferens, seminal vesicles, and ejaculatory duct. The sphincters of the bladder relax, and contractions of the urethra and perirectal muscles occur. Ejaculation occurs as the man achieves orgasm. As in the woman, the man experiences further tachycardia, hyperventilation, and blood pressure elevation.

During the **resolution phase** release of muscular tension occurs. The woman experiences a feeling of warmth and relaxation. Physiologic changes that took place in the previous phases of the response are reversed within 5 to 10 minutes (Baram, 1996). Resolution is slower when orgasm has not been achieved. Findings by Masters and Johnson suggest that women actually may experience a very short **refractory period**, that is, time before they are interested in experiencing intercourse again. Women are capable of multiple orgasms.

The man experiences a longer resolution phase. Immediate decrease in penile erection occurs after ejaculation, with partial decrease in vasocongestion. Over a few minutes after ejaculation, complete remission of erection occurs. There is a refractory period in which the man cannot achieve another erection. The time of the refractory period is somewhat variable; however, it is unusual for men to achieve multiple orgasms as do women.

Saks (1999) indicated there is a physiologic difference in the brains of men and women after orgasm. There is a hippocampal neurologic discharge in the brain that makes men sleepy. In women, there is no such discharge. Women may experience a spurt of energy after orgasm.

American Sexual Practices

The public image of sex in America bears very little resemblance to what occurs in reality. Television portrays men and women as sexual beings who must be thin, beautiful, and young. The results of these myths are false expectations, deficits in self-esteem, broken relationships, and perhaps even a decline in physical health. When one tries to untangle the reality of sexuality, however, it becomes apparent that a realistic picture is almost impossible to ascertain. Masters and Johnson spent their entire careers scientifically analyzing the human sexual response, and many questions still remain unanswered.

In the late 1960s and 1970s, federal agencies studied sexuality, sexual practices, and homosexuality in an attempt to uncover the truth about sexuality in America (Michael, Gagnon, Laumann, & Kolata, 1994). Many of these studies were flawed and biased, and therefore, myths sometimes were perpetuated.

In 1994, Michael, Gagnon, Laumann, & Kolata undertook a survey to study sexuality that was designed to eliminate some of the flaws in previous research. The survey consisted of a sample of 3432 Americans. Responses of the participants were compared with U.S. census data on the variables of gender, age, education, marital status, and race and ethnicity. The study group was found to represent 97.1% of American adults from 18 to 49 years of age. The following is a description of findings from the survey and may assist the nurse in making decisions about so-called normal sexuality.

When asked how many sexual partners they had had in the past 12 months, participants responded as follows: 11.1% of men and 13.7% of women denied having sexual partners, 67.6% and 75.5% had one partner, 9.6% and 6.3% had two partners, and 11% and 4.5% had three or more partners, respectively. These data support the notion that most American men and women participate in monogamous relationships. These data, however, do not address the concept of serial monogamy as a sexual practice.

Serial monogamy is a term used to describe the practice of having one sexual partner at a time but several partners during a lifetime. There has been speculation that a factor in the exceedingly high divorce rate in the United States is the great value Americans have placed on monogamy (Michael, Gagnon, Laumann, & Kolata, 1995). It is speculated that when a person become sexually dissatisfied with a relationship with a spouse, divorce enables that person to leave the relationship and still maintain the value of monogamy. This is a characteristic of serial monogamy. In reality, divorce is a much more complex phenomenon.

Sexual Preferences

The next question addressed by the survey (Michael, Gagnon, Laumann, & Kolata, 1994) related to gender preference. The question was "Have your sex partners in the past 12 months been exclusively male, male and female, or exclusively female?" In answer to this question, 98.3% of women and 96.3% of men reported heterosexual relationships; 1.0% of men and 0.5% of women reported bisexual relationships; and 2.6% of men and 1.2% of women reported homosexual relationships.

Frequency of intercourse is a factor that is commonly discussed among couples concerning what is normal and was addressed in the survey. Frequency of intercourse was analyzed based on gender, age, marital status, education, religion, and race and ethnicity. The norm for frequency of intercourse was several times monthly: 37% of men and 36% of women reported having intercourse several times monthly; 26% of men and 30% of women reported having intercourse 2 to 3 times weekly; and only 8% of men and 7% of women reported engaging in intercourse four or more times weekly. These findings suggest there is a wide range of what is considered normal behavior concerning frequency of intercourse. Frequency of intercourse becomes a problem for couples when expectations are different between the two members of the sexual dyad.

Age is a factor in frequency of participation in intercourse. Men under the age of 30 years reported engaging in intercourse more frequently (2 to 3 times per week). Men over 40 years of age more commonly (43%) reported engaging in intercourse several times per month. Women in all age categories most commonly reported intercourse several times per month. Similar findings were obtained concerning marital status, education, religion, and race and ethnicity. This group of variables can have immeasurable influence on one's sexuality and sexual behavior.

This study also examined sexual practices and preferences. Vaginal intercourse had the widest appeal for men and women. The least preferred sexual practice was forcing a partner to have sex or being forced to have sex of any type.

Masturbation was another sexual practice studied. Findings suggested that masturbation is not rare. It is a practice preferred by men more than women but common in both genders. In this study, fewer than 6 out of 10 (60%) of men in the 18- to 24-year-old age group and 7 out of 10 (70%) of all men reported masturbating in the past year. Fewer than 4 out of 10 (40%) of women in the 18- to 24-year-old age group and 3 out of 10 (30%) of women over 54 years of age masturbated. Nearly half of women in their 30s reported masturbating. It has been speculated that masturbation is not as common as once thought among young men because it is perceived by them to be an activity indicating immaturity. It also has been suggested that masturbation is controlled by social factors and cultural influences (Michael, Gagnon, Laumann, & Kolata, 1995).

Among the group of most sexually active persons, approximately 85% of men and 45% of women living with a sexual partner reported masturbating in the past year. Married persons were more likely to masturbate than were

those living alone. These findings led the researchers to conclude that masturbation is not a substitute for other sexual practices but is an activity that stimulates and is stimulated by other sexual activity.

A change has occurred in American culture involving the meaning and place of sexuality (D'Emilio & Freedman, 1997). The view that sex is a family-centered process with the aim of reproduction, as was conceptualized in the colonial era, has changed to the view that sex is for personal pleasure. In the 19th century, sexuality was focused more on intimacy and romance. In contemporary times the attitude exists that sexuality is linked to personal identity, individual desire, and personal fulfillment. The focus is away from procreation and continually is being reshaped by the nature of the economy, the family, and politics. For example, the availability of abortion for the woman with limited means may change depending on politics because funding for abortion may be decreased by the federal government in an administration having antiabortion sentiment.

One of the factors that has contributed greatly to the contemporary view of sexuality is contraception (Figure 12-4). In the 1920s and 1930s there was much resistance to the idea of contraception. When oral contraceptives became available in the 1960s, the social and sexual cultures had changed to the extent that contraceptive practices became acceptable. Sexual abstinence was less likely as marriage and childbearing were more likely to occur later in life after completion of education. It was considered more socially acceptable for couples to live together; however, childbearing was more likely to be delayed until marriage. Unintended pregnancy is sometimes the precipitating event that leads to marriage in cohabiting couples. In sex-

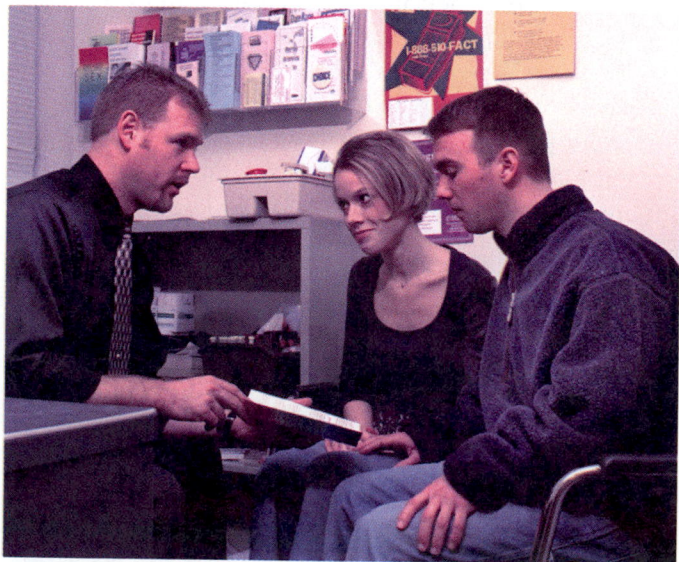

Figure 12-4 An important element in sex education and counseling is sharing information on contraceptive options.

ual relationships, contraception and conception may be the key to the relationship, especially when partners do not agree about sexual matters. In fact, some believe that women do not control their destiny until they control their fertility (D'Emilio & Freedman, 1997).

Media and advertising have contributed greatly to how women view their sexuality. For example, advertisements offer suggestions about clothing and a vast array of personal grooming products to make women feel more attractive sexually. The media has greatly influenced our sexuality, and increasingly so in the past few decades.

As sexuality has changed, so have attitudes about sexual preference. During the era of World War II, homosexuality was considered a psychiatric problem. In the decades since then, homosexuality has been viewed as sexual deviance and most recently as an alternative lifestyle. Even though homosexuality is not the predominant sexual preference in the United States, evidence exists that it is becoming more widely accepted culturally. Evidence of this acceptance can be seen in the laws that have changed to enable marriage and adoption of children by couples of the same gender. Even the rigid structure of the military is exhibiting some flexibility by no longer questioning service people about their sexual preference.

Pregnancy and Sexuality

Pregnancy is a time when sexual issues may come to the forefront. Couples may express concerns about maintaining a sexual relationship throughout their pregnancy. Certain changes may take place in normal sexual response that are related to the physiologic changes of pregnancy (Alteneder & Hartzell, 1997). In fact, there may be changes in each trimester. In the first trimester, the woman may be less interested in sex because of fatigue, nausea, or adaptation to pregnancy. In the second trimester, her interest may increase. As she nears term however, she may experience some discomfort unless there are position changes to allow for the increase in her abdominal size. Education and support may assist the couple in maintaining a positive sexual relationship.

Women who are sexually abused in childhood may develop gender and sexual identities that emphasize self-worth based on sexuality (American College of Obstetricians and Gynecologists, 2000). These women are likely to have particular problems with sexual issues during pregnancy.

Sexuality and Aging

There is not an abundance of evidence related to sexuality and aging. There are physiologic changes that occur with aging, as well as attitudinal factors, physical illnesses, and social factors that can affect sexuality as a woman ages. Two physiologic changes in women are likely to affect a

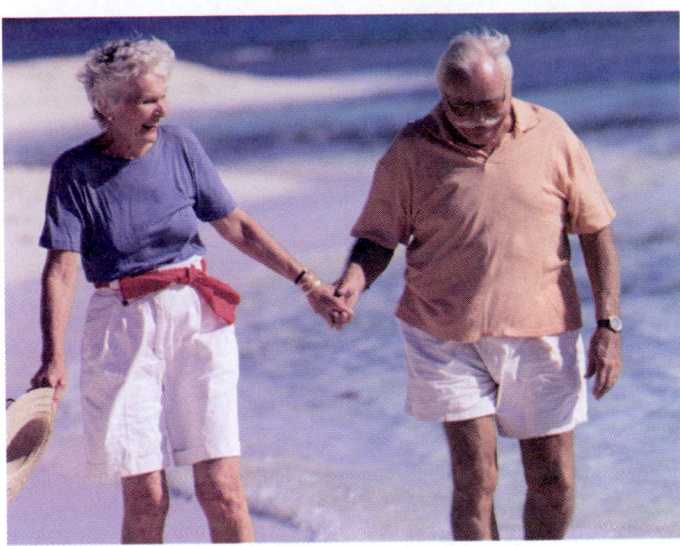

Figure 12-5 Sexual expression and intimacy are elements of partnerships throughout the life cycle.

woman's sexuality as she grows older. Decreases in the rate of production and volume of vaginal lubrication can lead to vaginal dryness and a sense of tightness, irritation, or burning after intercourse (Byyny & Speroff, 1996). Some loss of elasticity of the vaginal muscles also occurs that limits the woman's ability to tolerate deep or prolonged thrusting. These changes can result in postcoital spotting and soreness. These atropic symptoms can be relieved or eliminated by the use of lubricants, a change in coital position, or hormone replacement therapy.

Even after menopause women have sexual desire. Women in their 60s and 70s may continue to be sexually active depending on their health and social circumstances (Figure 12-5). Many times older women have outlived their husbands and thus their opportunity for sexual expression is limited.

Byyny & Speroff (1996) suggest that younger people and health care providers underrate the interest older people have in sex. These authors submit that the two most important factors influencing interest in sex are strength of the relationship and health of both partners. They further suggest that sexual activity among the aging is more influenced by culture and attitude than by nature and physiology.

SEXUAL DYSFUNCTION

Sexual dysfunction is the disturbance of one or more of the phases of human sexual response. The diagnosis is based on clinical judgment and must be evaluated in the biopsychosocial context in which it occurs (Vermillion & Holmes, 1997). In other words, sexual dysfunction may be biologic, psychologic, or social in nature or the result of a combination of any of these variables. Because the disturbance is so complex, a thorough assessment must be undertaken to determine the cause.

Epidemiologic data concerning sexual dysfunction are sparse and reflect the hesitancy to discuss such matters by clients and some health care providers. Sexual dysfunction can affect males and females; however, it is unclear statistically which gender is more greatly affected.

Female Sexual Dysfunction

Problems with female sexual dysfunction are not rare; however, precise data are not available concerning the incidence of specific disorders. Sarwer and Durlak (1996) suggest there is a lifetime prevalence of adult female sexual dysfunction that may be as high as 35%. Berman, Berman, & Goldstein (1998) submit the incidence may be as high as 76%. Hypoactive (significantly diminished) desire is considered the most prevalent sexual dysfunction and may affect as many as one in five women. It has been estimated that 5% to 10% of women experience inhibited orgasm (O'Donahue, Dopke, & Swingen, 1997). It also has been reported that 10% to 15% of women identify painful intercourse as a presenting complaint when seeking medical treatment (Meana, Binik, Khalife, & Cohen, 1997). An interaction of physical, psychologic, and relationship factors determine sexual responsiveness (Heiman & Meston, 1997).

Four types of female sexual disorders have been identified, including desire disorders, pain disorders, orgasmic disorders, and disorders related to other conditions. These disorders are described and discussed.

Desire Disorders

Desire disorders may be of two types. If the woman has a persistent deficiency or absence of sexual feelings and desire for sexual activity that is not accounted for by a psychiatric problem, it is classified as an hypoactive disorder. Hypoactive desire may be further classified as primary or secondary based on whether the disinterest has always existed or whether it is a new phenomenon. This disorder may result from physical or psychologic causes. Common organic causes of the disorder include decreased testosterone levels, use of medications, substance abuse, chronic disease, pregnancy, and malnutrition (Vermillion & Holmes, 1997). Psychogenic factors include relationship problems, loss of personal attractiveness, and situational disturbances such as personal tragedy, illness, and stress.

Sexual aversion disorder is the second type of sexual desire disorder. It is characterized by persistent or recurrent aversion to or avoidance of contact with a partner, not accounted for by other major psychiatric disorder (Vermillion & Holmes, 1997). This disorder is much rarer than are hypoactive sexual desire disorders. It is characterized by low sexual desire and occasionally vaginismus or dyspareunia. Women with this disorder exhibit inadequate lubrication and vasocongestion during the excitement phase. Sexual aversion disorder is common among women with a history of physical or sexual abuse. Extensive relationship problems may exist. Physical factors rarely are involved; however, significant related anxiety occurs.

Pain Disorders

Sexual pain disorders include vaginismus and dyspareunia. **Vaginismus** is painful spasm of the muscles of the introitus that can prevent penetration. When a woman experiences **dyspareunia**, that is, painful sexual intercourse, she has genital or pelvic pain before, during, or after intercourse. Its cause may be physical, psychologic, or a result of a combination of factors. Some physical factors that have been associated with dyspareunia are vaginitis, cystitis, hormone deficiency, endometriosis, uterine prolapse, cystocele, rectocele, pelvic cancer, pelvic inflammatory disease, gastrointestinal disease, and renal disease (Vermillion & Holmes, 1997). The most commonly cited characteristic in women with chronic pelvic pain is a history of sexual trauma (Holland & Finger, 1999).

Certain psychologic factors also have been associated with dyspareunia (Meana, Binik, Khalife, & Cohen, 1998). Predominant factors identified are phobic anxiety, negative attitudes toward sexuality, relationship conflicts, and childhood sexual abuse (Sarwer & Durlak, 1996).

Whatever the cause of dyspareunia, women with this problem tend to require a great deal of support when undergoing the childbirth experience or even when attaining routine gynecologic health care. These women may experience avoidance behavior or an anxiety attack linked to simple procedures such as obtaining a Pap smear and having a bimanual pelvic examination. Postmenopausal women may experience dyspareunia secondary to decreased lubrication.

Vaginismus is a pain disorder in which the woman experiences discomfort related to involuntary spasms of the muscles of the outer third of the vagina. These muscle spasms either interfere with or prevent penetration. Vaginismus is classified as primary or secondary dependent on timing of onset. Primary vaginismus usually manifests itself by an unconsummated marriage (Renshaw, 1994). Secondary or acquired vaginismus may arise from sources such as a conditioned response to vaginitis, a healing episiotomy, problems with the sexual experience, or adverse past sexual experiences.

Orgasmic Disorders

Women with orgasmic disorders experience delayed orgasm, or cannot experience orgasm. The woman may be unable to achieve orgasm with intercourse but may be able to achieve orgasm with a partner using noncoital methods. This disorder is found most commonly among young, less sexually experienced women and is often situational. The cause usually is psychological and may be related to discomfort or use of medications, especially selective serotonin reuptake inhibitors or other antidepressants.

Disorders Related to Other Conditions

Chronic medical conditions can affect sexual function. Many times this effect is associated with medications that are taken to treat the chronic condition. For example, antihypertensives, antiseizure medications, digoxin, diuretics, methyldopa, psychoactive drugs, sleeping pills, and tranquilizers can affect sexual response (Ringel, 1999). In fact, it has been suggested that many times noncompliance with medication regimens is related to the sexual side effects of drugs.

Substance abuse has been associated with sexual dysfunction. Alcohol can affect sexual desire. Cocaine has been associated with sexual promiscuity and sexually transmitted diseases. Other drugs have been linked to diminished sexual response, including antidepressants, antihypertensives, anti-inflammatory drugs, antiparkinsonian drugs, antiseizure medications, beta-blockers, cimetidine, digoxin, diuretics, methyldopa, psychoactive drugs, sleeping pills, and tranquilizers (Ringel, 1999).

Another factor associated with sexual dysfunction among women is sexual abuse in childhood. Sarwer & Durlak (1996) reported studying 359 married women who sought sex therapy with their spouses. In this study, 75% to 94% of women could be identified as having been victims of previous sexual abuse.

Male Sexual Dysfunction

The most common sexual dysfunction in men is erectile dysfunction, also called **impotence**. Until recently, this condition was not discussed publicly because there was no effective treatment (Bachman, Coleman, Driscoll, & Renshaw, 1999). It is estimated that 30 million men in the United States are affected by erectile dysfunction. The condition increases in incidence with aging, even in the absence of illness. Use of medications, chronic illnesses, and use of alcohol also have been implicated as causative agents. It has been estimated that half of cases of erectile dysfunction are related to atherosclerotic changes in men over the age of 50 years (Bachman et. al., 1999).

With the release of the drug Viagra (sildenafil) in 1998, it became apparent how pervasive the problem of erectile dysfunction is in the United States. The drug was adver-

tised as a cure for impotence. In the first 8 months on the market, 50 million prescriptions were written for sildenafil. It proved so popular and effective in men that women began taking it to see if it would improve their sexual function. There is no known benefit to women, and the Food and Drug Administration had not approved the drug for use in women. The popularity of sildenafil has stimulated discussion about how sexual response differs between men and women (Leiblum, 2000). Several deaths reportedly have been linked to the use of sildenafil.

Premature ejaculation is another form of sexual dysfunction in men. Commonly, this disorder is seen in very young men and men who have abstained from sex for long periods of time. It also is seen in men with chronic illnesses and multiple sclerosis (Bachman, Coleman, Driscoll, & Renshaw, 1999). If it persists, premature ejaculation can lead to other sexual problems, such as erectile dysfunction.

Priapism is a condition in which erection is sustained for several hours. This disorder may be associated with certain chronic diseases and with abuse of substances, such as cocaine. This situation is dangerous because persistent engorgement of the penile vessels causes cell death and fibrosis. Treatment of priapism usually consists of removal of blood from or injection of phenylephrine into the corpora cavernosa (Bachman, Coleman, Driscoll, & Renshaw, 1999).

Evaluation of Sexual Dysfunction

The nurse can make a major contribution to the care of couples with sexual dysfunction by providing an atmosphere that allows discussion of personal, highly emotional topics. The nurse often is the person with whom individuals share their feelings. Evaluation of sexual problems begins with taking a sexual history from both parties in the relationship (Van Sickle & Rosenstrock, 1999). Although it is not the nurse's role to treat sexual dysfunction, the practitioner should have enough knowledge to discuss normal compared with dysfunctional behavior and make appropriate referrals.

The PLISSIT model has been identified as a useful one in general care settings for discussing sexual concerns (Katz, 2000). PLISSIT is an acronym for permission, limited information, specific suggestions, and intensive therapy. The PLISSIT model also has been used successfully to address sexual concerns during pregnancy (Alteneder & Hartzell, 1997).

Permission

When taking a sexual history, the nurse should ask open-ended, nonjudgmental questions that identify what the woman considers to be her normal sexual activity. This ap-

Research Highlight

Impact of Hysterectomy on Sexual Functioning

Purpose

To examine changes in sexual functioning after hysterectomy.

Method

Of 1,299 women interviewed before hysterectomy, 1,101 (84.8%) completed the study with follow-up at 6, 12, 18, and 24 months postoperatively. The main outcome measures were frequency of sexual activity, dyspareunia, orgasm, vaginal dryness, and sexual desire.

Findings

Finding	Preoperatively (%)	12 mo Postoperatively (%)	24 mo Postoperatively (%)
Engaging in sexual activity	70.5	77.6	76.7
Decreased dyspareunia	18.6	4.5	3.6
Anorgasmia	7.6	5.2	4.9
Decreased libido	10.4	6.3	6.2
Vaginal dryness	37.3	46.8	46.7

Each of the outcome measures improved after surgery.

Nursing Implications

Many times nurses are asked questions about how hysterectomy will affect sexual function. This study lends support to teaching clients that many sexual factors may actually improve after surgery.

Rhodes, J.C., Kjerulff, K.H., Lagenberg, P.W., & Guzinski, G.M. (1999). Hysterectomy and sexual functioning. *Journal of the American Medical Association 282*, (20), 1934–1941.

proach gives the woman permission to express concerns and ask questions.

Limited Information

The nurse should be familiar with sexual terms and sexual norms and should be able to determine which limited information is needed to assist the woman with her problem. Many times information is all that is necessary to resolve the problem.

Specific Suggestions

The nurse should have enough knowledge to make suggestions for alleviation of client concerns. In pregnancy, for

example, women may have dreams that they find unacceptable. It may be sufficient to let them know that many pregnant women experience emotionally charged dreams. If this information is not sufficient, however, the nurse can make a suggestion for referral to another health care provider who has expertise in dealing with such problems.

Intensive Therapy

The nurse should know her limitations concerning time and expertise and should make referrals for complex or time-consuming cases. In making the referral, it is wise for the nurse to suggest that the client needs someone with more skill rather than insinuate there is something abnormal about the client's problem.

INFERTILITY

As noted previously, when one considers the complex physical and hormonal sequence of events required for conception and pregnancy, it is amazing that normal births ever occur. For pregnancy to occur the female ovary must produce a mature egg, capable of being fertilized, which must be transported through the fallopian tube into the uterus where the hormonally prepared endometrium supports implantation. The male testes must produce an adequate quantity of mature, motile sperm, capable of surviving the arduous trip through his reproductive system, into the vagina, through the cervical mucus, uterus, and fallopian tube to join with the ovum. With each normal ovulatory cycle, there is about a 25% chance of pregnancy resulting. For normal couples, pregnancy may not occur for 6 months to 1 year with unprotected intercourse.

Clearly, many factors affect fertility. The ability to have children, however, is considered a normal expectation of adult life. **Infertility** is defined as the inability to conceive after 1 year with appropriately timed coitus without the use of contraception. Infertility affects almost 15% of couples (Silverberg, 2000), with the risk increasing for women after 35 years of age. After this age, nearly one third of women desiring a child are unable to conceive (Wallach, Garcia, Rosenwaks, & Seifer, 1998). For those who have difficulty or are unable to conceive, infertility can be devastating.

It is estimated that there were 4.5 million women who reported infertility in 1982 (Stephen & Chandra, 1998) as compared with 4.8 million in 1988 and 6.2 million in 1995. This increase is thought to be multifactorial. Proposed factors include delayed childbearing by a number of baby-boomers in society, the decreased popularity of permanent sterilization as a means of contraception, and an advance in age limits beyond 35 years as a criterion to qualify for infertility treatment. The result has been that many couples wait until later in life to attempt a first pregnancy.

The financial and psychological costs of infertility can be immense (Jerka, Schuett, & Foxhall, 1996). Estimates of the financial costs of infertility treatment vary according to the technology used. However, Van Voorhis (1998) noted that "In 1992, the overall cost per delivery was $30,252." Psychologic sequelae described include depression, guilt, stress, loss, grief, disturbances of self-esteem, relationship problems, and even divorce. Estimates of financial costs often are inexact but include direct medical costs, such as drugs, ovulation prediction kits, physician fees, laboratory tests, hospitalizations, and radiologic examinations. Indirect costs may include expenses related to food and transportation when seeking care, lost wages, and extended care of children while the parents are undergoing testing. Other elusive costs may be incurred related to pain and grief or psychologic counseling.

Factors Affecting Fertility

Because of the complexity of determining the cause of infertility and its expense, it is important that both partners be involved in the process from the beginning. A thorough assessment, which can be time-consuming, expensive and emotionally burdensome, may be required to produce a live birth. For the infertile couple the evaluation and treatment may be positive experiences because they offer hope.

Female Factors

Approximately 40% of the time female factors are the cause of infertility. Within this group of women, for 40% the major reason is failure to ovulate (Rosenthal, 1997). Another 40% have either tubal or pelvic problems. The remaining 20% have unusual problems or unexplained infertility.

Perhaps the single most important factor in female infertility is aging (Sauer, 1998). Although the causes of infertility are many, the decision to delay childbearing may result in difficulty in achieving a pregnancy. The decline in fertility with age has several components. With increasing age, there is higher risk of spontaneous abortion. The incidence of pelvic or tubal problems increases. Finally, the endocrine changes that begin 10 to 15 years before menopause lead to decreased fertility. Factors related to infertility are presented subsequently and then a systematic method for evaluation is presented.

Problems of Ovulation

For most women (95% to 98%) the presence of monthly menstrual cycles with premenstrual symptoms indicates an ovulatory cycle. Although its value has become more controversial with more sophisticated test measures (Illions & Thompson, 1997), taking the basal body temperature (BBT) can be a helpful and inexpensive indicator of ovulation for the woman experiencing monthly menses. The BBT should be evaluated after two menstrual cycles. A biphasic temperature pattern suggests ovulation.

The woman who is having irregular or infrequent menses or who is not having menses should be evaluated for ovulatory dysfunction (Kaplan, 1996). Common signs of problems of ovulation other than alterations in menses are **galactorrhea** (nipple discharge); signs of androgen excess, such as facial hair or male pattern hair growth; alterations in thyroid or adrenal functioning; and weight changes.

Ovarian Abnormalities. Anovulation may be a result of ovarian abnormalities such as hypogonadism (Turner's syndrome), a genetic disorder, or external causes such as radiation or chemotherapy (Seaman, Telich-Vidal, & Sable, 1997). A cause that occasionally is overlooked is the use of oral contraceptives, which were initially prescribed to regulate menses or for the treatment of acne. Ovarian tumors or polycystic ovaries may prevent ovulation owing to changes in the feedback mechanism regulating ovarian function.

Hormonal Abnormalities. Abnormalities of hormonal functioning or ovarian failure may result in anovulation (Prior, 1997; Anasti, 1998). Irregularities in any of the sectors of the hypothalamus-pituitary-ovarian axis may alter the hormonal balance needed for ovulation. Appropriate levels of the adrenal, thyroid, and pituitary hormones also are needed. General poor health, inadequate nutrition, stress, and excessive exercise affect ovarian function.

Tubal Structural Problems

Fertilization usually occurs in the outer portion of the fallopian tube, which also provides transport for the embryo into the uterus for implantation. Obstruction or narrowing of the tube can lead to the inability to conceive or tubal pregnancies. Blockages may be a result of congenital defects or endometriosis (Spielvogel, Shwayden, & Coddington, 2000). Infection is the most common cause of scarring, however, and can result from organisms such as *Neisseria gonorrhoeae, Chlamydia trachomatis, Mycoplasma,* and *Mycobacterium tuberculosis.* Seemingly minor surgery such as appendectomy or laparoscopy also may cause infection or adhesions, with resultant infertility.

Structural Problems of the Uterus

Infertility related to uterine problems also usually of structural origin. Although fibroid tumors (leiomyomata) themselves usually are not a cause of infertility, they may obstruct the fallopian tubes or interfere with implantation. Although somewhat rare, congenital malformations may interfere with implantation or the ability to carry a fetus to term. An inadequate endometrium also may impede fertility because implantation may not be successful. An inadequate endometrium can result from Asherman's syndrome, a thinning of the uterine lining after surgical procedures, or inadequate hormonal preparation.

Endometriosis has gained the reputation for being the cause of many cases of infertility (Berube, Marcoux, Langenum, & Maheux, 1998). **Endometriosis** is the implantation of uterine endometrium outside the uterus. The exact mechanism is not known but a reflux through the tubes at the time of menses is thought to explain the unusual implantation sites. Although the most common sites for endometriosis are in the lower pelvis and bowel, it has been

seen on the diaphragm, lungs, and brain. Again, it is difficult to correlate the severity of the endometriosis with infertility because a woman with very few visible implants may be unable to conceive, whereas a woman with a severe case may have no problem conceiving. The exact reason for the resultant infertility also is not known. The infertility may be merely from obstructing implantation or adhesions, or it may be a result of a much more complex problem involving the body's response to foreign tissue (Seltzer & Pearse, 1995).

Structural Problems of the Vagina and Cervix

As the vagina and cervix are developing, a variety of congenital structural abnormalities may occur that could interfere with the transport, implantation, or growth of the embryo. There may be two vaginal vaults, two cervixes, imperforate hymen, irregularly shaped uterus or tubes, or the cavities within either may be misshapen. Although these structural problems may be determined by physical examination, other diagnostic tests such as ultrasonography may be needed.

In addition, infections may change the cervical mucus and vaginal secretions that aid sperm motility and viability. Historically, cervical mucus and vaginal secretions were of greater concern. The use of intrauterine insemination, however, has lowered the incidence of these problems.

Male Factors

Male factors account for 35% to 40% of infertility. The incidence of male reasons for infertility is summarized in Box 12-1.

A semen analysis, a simple noninvasive screening test, should be an early if not first step in assessing a couple experiencing infertility. It is important that the specimen be collected and analyzed properly. After at least 48 hours of abstinence, a specimen obtained by masturbation should be collected in a clean container. The specimen should remain at body temperature and be delivered to the laboratory in 30 to 45 minutes. Because of the variability between specimens, it is suggested that the test be repeated

Box 12-1 MALE FACTORS ASSOCIATED WITH INFERTILITY
- Idiopathic, 70%–75%
- Testicular disorders (surgery, trauma), 10%–13%
- Genital tract obstructions, 8%–10%
- Sperm autoimmunity, 4%–6%
- Hormonal disorders, 1%
- Ejaculation, sexual dysfunction, 1%

Table 12-1 Normal Semen Analysis	
Element	**Quantity or Quality**
Volume	2.0 mL or more
Sperm concentration	20 million/mL or more
Motility	50% or more with forward progression, or 25% or more with rapid progression within 60 min of ejaculation
Morphology	30% or more normal forms
Leukocytes	Fewer than 1 million/mL
Immunobead test	Fewer than 20% with adherent particles
SpermMar test	Fewer than 10% with adherent particles

in 2 to 4 weeks. Findings in a normal semen analysis are provided in Table 12-1.

Even the parameters in Table 12-1 are not necessarily predictive of fertility because there are many possibilities for error, including laboratory error, error in the way in which the specimen was collected, or events that occurred 3 months before the test that may have affected spermatogenesis, such as an illness or injury.

Many factors should be considered when the cause of a low sperm count seems to be idiopathic (Bigelow, et al., 1998). Increased scrotal heat owing to activities, such as frequent hot tub or sauna use, chronic infections causing increased body temperature, and sitting at a desk or in a car or bike riding for long periods, can cause a decreased sperm count. Sons of mothers who took diethylstilbestrol (DES) while pregnant have been shown to have reduced sperm counts. Trauma to the testes and surgery also can affect sperm production or cause adhesions resulting in obstructions (Silber, 2000). The use of drugs or alcohol is a factor that may cause low sperm count. Environmental factors such as exposure to toxic drugs, chemicals, and anesthetic gases also have been implicated in low sperm counts.

Testicular disorders account for approximately 10% to 13% of male infertility (Illions & Thompson, 1997). These disorders include cryptorchidism (undescended testes) and other congenital abnormalities. Obstructions of the genital tract (8% to 10%) can result from congenital abnormalities, trauma or surgery, and genital infections. Abnormalities in hormonal functioning, including the thyroid, pancreas, and pituitary, can impair fertility. Ejaculation or sexual dysfunction, which may be physical or psychologic, also may result in an inability to reproduce. Even when sperm count and mobility seem adequate, an immune response to the sperm in the male or female may decrease fertility.

Unexplained Infertility

For approximately 10% of infertile couples no specific causative problem can be identified. Possibly, each partner has minor problems that alone cannot explain the infertility but in combination prevent fertility (Guzick, 2000). For couples such as these, assisted reproductive technology may be of benefit. Often, however, these couples will require support and encouragement to seek other alternatives, such as adoption.

Assessment of the Infertile Couple

When a couple presents with concerns about infertility, it is important to understand that men and women possibly are very concerned and emotionally fragile. Many couples have read and tried many of the common folklore remedies to achieve pregnancy. Depending on their own values, or those of their culture, the ability to bear children can be very important. Entering a medical setting for evaluation is in itself, for some, an admission of failure. In addition, much concern can center on which partner is at fault. Before even beginning the medical aspects of care, it is important to understand and assist the couple to understand their motivation for pregnancy and be prepared to offer support. The couple should understand that the evaluation and treatment for infertility will be stressful and will involve both partners throughout the process. It is important to meet with the couple together. Some time also should be spent alone with each individual because there may be issues the person would prefer not to discuss in the presence of his or her partner.

The first and perhaps most valuable step in the evaluation for infertility is taking a detailed medical history from each partner. An outline for this history is shown in Box 12-2.

Client Education

Sperm Count

Several habits can reduce sperm count:

- Frequency of ejaculation
- Wearing tight-fitting clothing
- Overuse of saunas and hot tubs
- Marijuana use

Box 12-2 EVALUATION OF INFERTILITY

Female History

1. Age
2. Fertility history
   How long the pregnancy has been sought
   Prior pregnancies: age at conception, outcome of
      each pregnancy
   Prior contraception: method, complications, length of
      time without contraception
   Use of an intrauterine device
   Abortions: number, type
3. Menstrual history
   Date of last menstrual cycle
   Age of menarche
   Characteristics of menses: interval, duration,
      regularity, predictability (breast tenderness,
      bloating), dysmenorrhea
   Awareness of ovulation, change in cervical mucus,
      mittelschmerz (midcycle pelvic pain), midcycle
      spotting
   Polycystic ovaries, ovarian cysts
4. Medical history
   Major diseases: diabetes, tuberculosis, tumors
   Treatments for disease, including medications and
      chemotherapy
   Sexually transmitted infections: gonorrhea, syphilis,
      chlamydia, herpes
   Hormonal irregularities: adrenal, thyroid, pituitary
      (hyperprolactinemia)
5. Surgical history
   Laparoscopy or other reproductive surgery
   Appendectomy
   Endometriosis
   Any abdominal surgery
   Dilation and curettage
6. Medications
   In utero exposure to DES
   Hormones, including oral contraceptives
   Antibiotics
   Tretinoin (Retin-A)
7. Occupation
   Exposure to radiation, toxic drugs, chemicals,
      anesthetic gases
8. Personal and sexual habits
   Alcohol or drug use (cocaine, marijuana, inhalants,
      and so on)

Smoking
Extremes of weight gain or loss
Douching
Frequency of intercourse; use of lubricants
Timing of intercourse for optimum conception
Pregnancy with other partners
Number of other partners (risk of sexually transmitted
   infections and antibody reaction to sperm)

Male History

1. Fertility history
   Age
   Previous children
   Frequency of intercourse; difficulties associated with
      function, including erection and ejaculation
2. Medical history
   Major diseases: diabetes; tuberculosis; renal, thyroid,
      or adrenal diseases; other hormonal imbalances
   Mumps after childhood
   Abnormality or disease of the genital tract, tumors,
      epididymitis, prostatitis
   Acute illness in past 3 months
   Sexually transmitted infections and treatment
3. Surgical history
   Genital surgery, including hernia repair,
      retroperitoneal surgery, and prostate surgery
4. Medications
   List all drugs being taken, both prescription and over
      the counter (some may affect spermatogenesis,
      others function)
5. Occupation (sitting for long periods affects
      spermatogenesis)
   Exposure to radiation, toxic drugs, chemicals,
      anesthetic gases
6. Personal and sexual habits
   Alcohol or street drug use (cocaine, marijuana,
      inhalants, and so on)
   Smoking
   Wearing of tight underwear or biking shorts (elevates
      temperature)
   Use of hot tubs (temperature)
   Use of personal lubricants; condom use
   Frequency of intercourse (very frequent ejaculation
      can reduce sperm count)

Physical Assessment and Diagnostic Tools

In many infertility practices the medical history is completed by the nurse. Often the physician or nurse practitioner will complete the physical examination, with the nurse providing assistance and much of the education. An overview of tools commonly used in infertility assessment is given in Table 12-2. Typically, the woman's examination is done in the office of the infertility practice; however, the man may be referred to a urologist for evaluation. In the man's examination, the presence of secondary sexual characteristics and genital abnormalities should be noted. Key evaluations include undescended testes and absence of the vas deferens. Attention should be paid to the presence of a **varicocele**, or abnormal blood vessels in the scrotum. A varicocele and the presence of a **hydrocele**, fluid in the scrotum, may be related to infertility.

In the woman, attention is paid to secondary sexual characteristics, such as breast development, pattern of facial and genital hair distribution, and the presence of acne. These characteristics are indicators of sexual maturity and therefore the ability to conceive. The thyroid should be palpated carefully for enlargement or nodules. The breasts should be evaluated for normal development and the presence of discharge. Surgical scars may indicate abdominal surgery, with resultant adhesions affecting reproductive function. A complete pelvic examination, including inspection of the external genitalia, should be performed to rule out anatomic abnormalities and infection. With the pelvic examination, cultures should be taken and a Pap smear performed. The first visit is an ideal time to offer preconceptual counseling, including testing for blood type, Rh antibodies, and immunity to measles. Vaccines should be given as needed for measles, hepatitis B, and

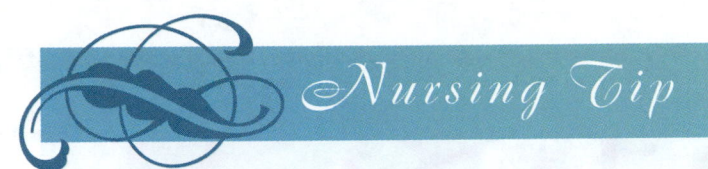

BASAL BODY TEMPERATURE

The basal body temperature (BBT) test has become less popular since the advent of the ovulation prediction kits because the BBT is less accurate.

REFLECTIONS FROM AN INFERTILE COUPLE

"We wanted to have a child very badly, but after 3 years of marriage and unprotected regular intercourse we had no pregnancy. After a long discussion with my husband, we decided to seek medical advice. We decided the best way to proceed was for me to visit my gynecologist.

We had no idea how impersonal and cold the whole process would be. You are asked to distance yourself from the emotional aspects of sexuality and focus on the mechanics of conception. My husband remembers the semen analysis as being the most challenging. He was given a sterile container, shown to a room, and told to produce a semen specimen. No further instructions were given. My most embarrassing time was when we had a postcoital test scheduled. The physician wanted me to be seen in his office within 2 hours after intercourse to examine my vaginal secretions under the microscope. On a bad traffic day, it can take 2 hours to travel from our home to his office. We had to rent a motel room near my husband's workplace and have intercourse during his lunch hour because we both had missed so much work. I'm not sure health care providers understand how stressful some of these tests can be."

UNDERSTANDING THE MENSTRUAL CYCLE

Many couples do not understand when the fertile time of the menstrual cycle occurs. Before considering an infertility workup, it is important to explore basic knowledge about sexuality and timing of intercourse. Helping the woman to be more aware of how her body functions, when ovulation occurs, and midcycle changes in the cervical mucus can assist couples in achieving conception.

Table 12-2 Tools Used to Assess Infertility

Test	Instructions	Findings
Semen analysis	Semen should be collected by masturbation after 2–3 days' abstinence. Collect in a clean, dry container. Be sure to collect entire ejaculate; do not use withdrawal or condoms for collection. Special sheaths can be used, if required. Specimen should be kept warm and delivered to the laboratory in 30–60 min. Two or three specimens may be collected over several months because spermatogenesis takes 2.5 months.	Normal values: Volume, 2–6 mL Viscosity, liquid within 30 min pH, 7–8 Count, more than 20 million/mL Motility, more than 40% moving Morphology, more than 50% mature and normal
Basal body temperature (BBT)	Used to confirm ovulation and time intercourse. Temperature can be taken orally or rectally with a regular thermometer, but special BBT thermometers or newer digital ones may be easier to read. Temperature must be taken on awakening, before any activity. The chart should be started on day 1 of the cycle. All events, such as intercourse, variations in normal activity, and illness, should be recorded.	Typically, the temperature decreases slightly (0.2 F) 24–36 h before ovulation and increases (0.4–0.8°F) 24–72 h after. Temperature stays elevated for 11–16 d. This biphasic pattern indicates ovulation. The most most fertile time is 3–4 d before ovulation and 1–2 d after. Coitus every other day during this time is suggested.
Postcoital test	Evaluates cervical mucus to determine adequacy of mucus and the ability of sperm to transverse it. Intercourse should occur after 48 hours of abstinence within 24–48 h of ovulation. Cervical mucus is examined by obtaining a sample during pelvic examination 2–8 h. after coitus.	The mucus should be described in terms of quantity, clarity, viscosity, pH, spinnbarkeit, and sperm characteristics of number, motility, and forms. Normal findings are described as 5–10 morphologically normal sperm with linear motility in thin, clear, copious, acellular mucus with spinnbarkeit >8 cm.
Ovulation predictor kit	A urine test used to predict ovulation based on luteinizing hormone (LH) be measured in the urine. Available over the counter, the kits cost $30–$40/mo and include 5–10 tests. LH triggers ovulation, which occurs 20–48 h after the LH surge. LH can be detected in the urine 8–12 h after its peak levels. Urine should be tested at the same time each day. Some tests require first morning voiding. Be sure to read instructions in the kit.	False-positive results can be obtained owing to menopause, pregnancy, and polycystic ovaries. Instructions in the kit will describe the findings.
Hysterosalpingogram	An X-ray study to determine if the uterine cavity and fallopian tubes are open and healthy. Performed 2–5 d after the end of menses. Special evaluation and possible alternative treatment should be considered if a history of pelvic inflammatory disease, pelvic mass, or sensitivity to iodine exists.	Abnormalities of the structure of the uterus or tubes may be identified. Narrowing or occlusion of the tubes can be seen.
Endometrial biopsy	A sample of the endometrial tissue lining the uterus to determine the uterine response to hormonal stimulation. Performed 2–3 d before an expected menstrual period. Danger of pregnancy loss exists, and a pregnancy test should be performed before this biopsy. Usually done in the physician's office with the use of a pipelle, a thin catheter inserted into the uterine cavity. Taking ibuprofen decreases possible cramping and discomfort. Helpful in diagnosing a luteal phase defect.	The pathology report will describe the influence of hormones on the uterus.

(continued)

Table 12-2 Continued

Test	Instructions	Findings
Ultrasonography	Sound waves used to evaluate the structure of the pelvic organs and monitor ovulation by identification of follicles and release of the ova. Used to evaluate the fetus during pregnancy. Identifies ectopic pregnancies, endometriosis, and submucosal fibroids. May be abdominal or vaginal.	Structural abnormalities can be identified. Size, development, and maturation of ovarian follicles can be monitored, and status for egg retrieval provided.
Laparoscopy	Surgical procedure using an endoscope to view the pelvic organs. Treatments may be performed as problems are identified. Uterine abnormalities such as fibroids, adhesions, and endometriosis may be identified and removed. Used to retrieve eggs for reproductive technology. May be abdominal or vaginal. Usually suggested when no other cause of infertility is found.	Depending on the findings, treatment usually is performed at the same time to correct abnormalities. Findings might include fibroids, endometriosis, adhesions, ovarian cysts, and tubal blockages.
Laboratory evaluations	Based on medical history and physical examination, additional blood or urine tests may be ordered to evaluate the function of ovaries, pituitary, adrenal, hypothalamus, thyroid, and other glands to determine the cause of infertility.	Test parameters vary and are determined by the laboratory. Abnormalities may require further testing or treatment.

other immunizations as recommended. Teaching should include the need to use contraception until the immunizations have been completed. This recommendation is not likely to be received positively by the couple who so desperately want to conceive a pregnancy.

Before any further evaluation is done, a semen analysis should be obtained. This is the easiest and least invasive test that can be performed and often is overlooked. The ordering of further diagnostic tests will depend on the findings of the medical history and physical examination.

After the first examination, couples who have not previously kept a BBT chart may be asked to keep this record for 1 or 2 months. With newer technology such as the ovulation predictor kit and hormonal assays, however, the BBT may not be required.

Management of Infertility

After the findings of the history, physical examinations, laboratory tests, and other diagnostic tests are reviewed, a therapeutic regimen to treat the underlying cause of the infertility is decided on with the couple. It is very important that the couple understand each treatment considered for their situation. In planning their care the health care provider also must take into consideration influences such as the ages of the partners, how long they have been trying to conceive, health care insurance coverage or financial resources, and any cultural or religious concerns. Generally, less invasive and less complex treatments are tried first, moving progressively to more involved procedures or combinations of therapies (Angard, 1999). Treatment decisions will depend on the couple's desires. Because of the expense of infertility treatment, both financial and emotional, communication about the proposed treatments, possible side effects, and potential effectiveness is very important.

Laparoscopy

Laparoscopy is one of the most important diagnostic and therapeutic tools used in infertility. It allows direct visualization of peritoneal structures and definitive diagnosis of endometriosis, adhesions, and abnormalities in structure or function of the pelvic organs. During the procedure, treatment of adhesions, ablation of endometriosis, and restoration of patency of the fallopian tubes may be accomplished. Occasionally, a myoma or fibroid may interfere with fertility and may be removed during laparoscopy. A general anesthetic typically is used and carbon dioxide gas is used to distend the abdomen for better visualization. It is important to inform the woman that there may be some discomfort, such as cramping from manipulation of the pelvic organs and shoulder pain as a result of the gas used.

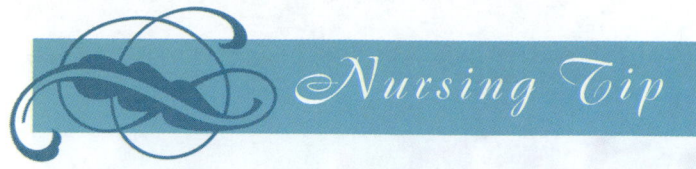

CANCER AND FERTILITY

As cure rates for cancer have improved, both men and women who have or have had cancer are considering the effects of the cancer and cancer treatments on their fertility. Although the cancer itself may affect the ability to conceive, treatment with surgery, chemotherapy, or radiation may damage reproductive capability. With increased awareness, more emphasis is being put on preserving reproductive function. Cryopreservation (freezing) of sperm, decreased toxicity of chemotherapy, and the use of shielding during radiation have been used. Hormonal suppression of gonadal activity has been suggested as a means of preserving gonadal function.

It is important to be aware of the implications of cancer on fertility and that couples may desire pregnancy after cancer therapy. Education, information, and emotional support can assist these clients in making treatment decisions.

Artificial Insemination

Artificial insemination, with either the partner's or donor's sperm, allows for semen to be placed in the vagina near the cervical os. This is most appropriate when infertility is a result of problems with sperm production or ejaculation. Intrauterine insemination provides a means to bypass cervical mucus problems when the tubes appear to be open, allowing for fertilization in the tubes. For this procedure, a washed sperm specimen is prepared and inserted high into the uterus at the appropriate time in the cycle.

The use of donor sperm presents health and ethical issues that should be discussed clearly with the person seeking insemination. Standards for testing, preparation, and storage of sperm have been established and reduce the possibility of infection with the human immunodeficiency and hepatitis viruses. The couple also has the option to describe criteria used for donor matching, such as ethnic and physical characteristics.

Hormonal Therapy

A disturbance in ovulation usually is treated with one or more hormones, depending on the cause of the problem. Many times medications are available to assist in the management of infertility (Table 12-3). Bromocriptine, clomi-

Table 12-3 Medications for Treatment of Ovarian Disorders

Drug	Purpose	Administration
Bromocriptine (Parlodel)	Inhibits prolactin secretion by the pituitary, which interferes with the secretion of gonadotropin-releasing hormone (Gn-RH). Used in the presence of galactorrhea or elevated prolactin levels.	2.5 mg, orally, twice daily (because of side effects, may start with 2.5 mg at bedtime increasing to twice daily).
Clomiphene (Clomid, Serophene, Milophene)	Induce ovulation. May produce multiple gestation. Incidence of twins may be slightly higher (Wolf, 2000).	50 mg, orally, starting day 5 of the cycle for 5 days. If no ovulation, increase dosage by 50 mg/mo to 200–250 mg. If no pregnancy by 3–4 mos, reevaluate.
Human menopausal gonadotropin or menotropins (Pergonal, Humegon, Repronex)	Stimulate follicle growth in the ovaries, often with multiple eggs. For women who fail to respond to clomiphene. Watch for hyperstimulation syndrome.	Made from equal amounts of follicle-stimulating hormone (FSH) and luteinizing hormone (LH). 75 or 150 IU injected intramuscularly daily starting day 3–5 for 7–14 d based on estrogen blood levels and ultrasound monitoring of follicles.
Gn-RH (Leuprolide, Lupron)	Reduces endometriosis of fibroids and suppresses LH surge.	May be given intravenously, intranasally, or subcutaneously; dose will vary according to method.
Purified FSH (Metrodin)	Induces ovulation in clomiphene-resistant women with higher levels of LH than FSH.	Daily intramuscular (IM) injections starting early in the cycle.
LGC (APL, Pregnyl, Profasi, Novarel)	Stimulates LH surge, and triggers ovulation. Used in conjunction with clomiphene, hMG, and FSH.	10,000 IU given IM.
Progesterone	For luteal phase defects.	Given as vaginal or rectal suppository.

Research Highlight

Efficacy of Intrauterine Insemination

Purpose

To examine the efficacy of intrauterine insemination and the baby take home rate in cases of infertility attributable to male factors with and without a woman's hormone factor.

Methods

A retrospective analysis was done of 78 long-standing involuntarily childless couples in Austria.

After the follicular phase, a Gn-RH analogue protocol with a menotropin (Pergonal) was undertaken to stimulate ovulation and a silica preparation (Percoll) and capacitation of the man's semen were completed. Intrauterine insemination was completed. Percoll is an isotonic fluid used to replace semen for intrauterine insemination.

Findings

Of 109 inseminations there were 53 pregnancies and 38 deliveries. Of these, 49 infants were live born and 47 remain alive.

When combined with ovarian stimulation, semen preparation, and sperm capacitation, intrauterine insemination is a feasible solution to male factor infertility.

Nursing Implications

Because of new technologic advances, such as those described in this study, more couples are able to conceive a pregnancy than would have been possible in the past.

Rammer, E., & Friedrich, F. (1998). The effectiveness of intrauterine insemination in couples with sterility due to male infertility with and without a woman's hormone factor. *Fertility and Sterility, 69*, (1), 31–36.

---

phene, human menopausal gonadotropins, Gn-RH, and purified FSH are used to induce ovulation. HCG stimulates ovulation. Progestins may be used to support the luteal phase of the cycle. Before these drugs are used, thyroid, pituitary, and adrenal disorder must be diagnosed and treated.

Assisted Reproductive Technology

Although many advances in the diagnosis and treatment of infertility have improved the chances of pregnancy, for some couples pregnancy would be impossible without the use of advanced technology. Assisted reproductive technology (ART) involves the use of in vitro fertilization (IVF), gamete intrafallopian transfer (GIFT), and embryo transfer (ET). Typically, ovulation is induced with the use of fertility drugs to produce several mature follicles from which eggs can be retrieved. In IVF and ET, the eggs are aspirated from the ovarian follicles and fertilized outside the woman's body. IVF is most appropriate when the tubes are absent or blocked. In this process the eggs are fertil-

ized, and after 48 hours the embryo is inserted into the uterus for implantation. In GIFT and ET, at least one tube must be open. In ET, the eggs are fertilized outside the body but placed in the tube and enter the uterus for implantation. In GIFT, the retrieved egg and prepared sperm are drawn into a catheter separately and injected into the tube so that fertilization can take place in the tube. These methods have been in use for almost 20 years and have been successful in many cases.

New technology has provided the means for retrieving sperm from the testes when ejaculation is not possible, injecting sperm into the ova (intracytoplasmic sperm injection, or ICSI), cryopreservation of embryos for future pregnancies, and surrogate pregnancies. Future advances may include cloning, chromosome manipulation, the transfer of cell components from one cell to another, and biochemically assisted hatching of the egg to improve the chances of fertilization (American Society for Reproductive Medicine, 1998). As technology has expanded, ethical and legal issues have emerged. The ethical issues that have arisen include the use of technology for sex selection, pregnancies in much older women, and the use of donor eggs and embryos. Legal issues defining parenthood, the use of embryos and sperm after death or divorce of the spouse, and the disposal of embryos cause concern. Nurses need to be aware of these issues and help clients address them as possible outcomes.

The use of technology is not without cost. ART can be very expensive, and pregnancy is not guaranteed (Angard, 1999). Many couples have undergone numerous cycles without success. Insurance companies have varying policies as to what will be covered, and often very little is included in the policy. Clearly, the financial and emotional impact can be immense, and nurses may be in the position to help couples deal with giving up the hope of having a biologic child.

NURSING IMPLICATIONS

All nurses should be familiar with the terminology and substance of information concerning sexuality, sexual dysfunction, fertility, and infertility. This information is essential in dealing with clients in any clinical setting. The nurse is viewed by the public as someone who has this knowledge and is very capable of taking very technical material and relaying it in terms that almost anyone can understand. Every nurse should be equipped with information to take an accurate and adequate sexual medical history. Every nurse should be aware of the PLISSIT model and be familiar with its use in screening for sexual dysfunction.

Every nurse should be able to identify resources that couples could refer to if they are having problems with sexuality or fertility.

Some nurses choose to work in the field of sexual counseling or infertility. These nurses need more extensive education and training to develop expertise. Sometimes these nurses actually participate in teams who undertake the infertility workup or in surgery where the ART is undertaken.

Web Activities

- What support groups, chat rooms, or resources can you locate for infertile couples?

- Search the Internet under the key words "fertility," "infertility," and "artificial insemination." What links can you find?

- Visit the website of a pharmaceutical company such as Glaxo or Mead Johnson. Do they offer information on their infertility drugs?

- Go to www.aasect.org. What three major sexual concerns can you identify using their on-line journal that are of importance to women?

Key Concepts

- Couples experiencing infertility or sexual dysfunction undergo a highly emotionally charged situation that also may be technically difficult.

- Many times a couple's problems with infertility or sexuality are multifactorial and may require prolonged interaction with the health care system for diagnosis and treatment.

- To some couples, conception is more important than most other things in their lives.

- With new advances in technology, conception is occurring in couples in whom it would not have been possible in the recent past.

- The new assisted reproductive technologies carry ethical considerations with which society must deal.

Review Questions and Activities

1. What is the most common male factor in infertility?
2. What is the most common female factor in infertility?
3. When fertility is in question, which factors must be evaluated and why?
4. Why is infertility sometimes difficult to diagnose and treat?

5. Which cultural practices do humans have related to fertility and sexuality?
6. Which components relate to the experience of sexual dysfunction?
7. What is serial monogamy, and how is it an important concept in American culture?

8. What are your ethical beliefs about freezing and storing fertilized ova?

9. How do you see the Human Genome Project relating to infertility?

10. With new information forthcoming, what reproductive technologies may be available in the coming century?

References

American College of Obstetricians and Gynecologists (ACOG). (2000). Adult manifestations of childhood sexual abuse. *ACOG educational bulletin.* Washington, D.C.: American College of Obstetricians and Gynecologists.

American Society for Reproductive Medicine. (1998). Induction of ovarian follicle development and ovulation with exogenous gonadotropins. Washington, D.C.: American Society for Reproductive Medicine.

Alteneder, R., & Hartzell, D. (1997). Addressing couples' sexual concerns during the childbearing period: Use of the PLISSIT model. *Journal of Obstetric, Gynecologic, and Neonatal Nursing, 26,* (6), 651–658.

Angard, N.T. (1999). Diagnosis infertility: These treatments can help couples achieve pregnancy. *AWHONN Lifelines, 3,* (3), 22–29.

Anasti, J.N. (1998). Premature ovarian failure: An update. *Fertility & Sterility, 70,* (1), 1–14.

Bachman, G. A., Coleman, E., Driscoll, C. E., & Renshaw, D. (1999). Patients with sexual dysfunction: Your guidance makes a difference. *Patient Care for the Nurse Practitioner, 2,* (4), 14–25.

Baram, D. A. (1996). Sexuality and sexual function. In *Novak's gynecology* (12th ed.). Baltimore, MD: William & Wilkins.

Berman, J.R., Berman, L.A., & Goldstein, I. (1998). Sexual dysfunction: Past, present, and future. *The Female Patient 23,* (12), 45–51.

Berube, S., Marcoux, S., Langenum, M., & Maheux, R. (1998). Fecundity of infertile women with minimal or mild endometriosis and women with unexplained infertility. *Fertility & Sterility, 69,* (6), 1034–1049.

Bigelow, P.L., Jarrell, J., Young, M.R., Keefe, T.J., & Love, E.J. (1998). Association of semen quality and occupational factors: Comparison of case control analysis and analysis of continuous variables. *Fertility & Sterility, 69,* (1), 11–18.

Byyny, R.L., & Speroff, L. (1996). *A clinical guide for the care of older women: Primary and preventive care* (2nd ed.). Baltimore, MD: William and Wilkins.

Cohen, S., Kenner, C., & Hollingsworth, A. (1991). *Maternal, neonatal, and women's health nursing.* Springhouse, PA: Springhouse.

D'Emilio, J., & Freedman, E.B. (1997). *Intimate matters: A history of sexuality in America* (2nd ed.). Chicago, IL: University of Chicago Press.

Guzick, D.S. (2000). When infertility can't be explained. *Contemporary Ob/Gyn, 45,* (9), 102–111.

Heiman, J.R., & Meston, C.M. (1997). Evaluating sexual dysfunction in women. *Clinical Obstetrics and Gynecology, 40,* (3), 616–629.

Holland, K.L., & Finger, W.W. (1999). Chronic pelvic pain and sexual trauma in women. *The Female Patient, 24,* (1), 13–18.

Illions, E.H., & Thompson, R.J. (1997). Office evaluation of the infertile couple. In *Women's Primary Health Care* (V.L. Seltzer & W.H. Pearse Eds.). New York, New York: McGraw-Hill.

Jerka, J., Schuett, S., & Foxhall, M.J. (1996). Loneliness and social support in infertile couples. *Journal of Obstetric, Gynecologic, and Neonatal Nursing, 25,* (1), 55–60.

Katz, A. (2000). Birds do it, bees do it, let's talk about it: The nurse's role in sexual counseling. *AWHONN Lifelines, 4,* (5), 40–41.

Kohn, I.I., & Kaplan, S.A. (2000). Female sexual dysfunction: What is known and what can be done. *Contemporary Ob/Gyn, 45,* (2), 25–46.

Leiblum, S.R. (2000). Redefining female sexual response. *Contemporary Ob/Gyn 45* (11), 120–126.

Masters, W.H., & Johnson, V.E. (1996). *Human sexual response.* Boston, MA: Little Brown.

Meana, M., Binik, Y.M., Khalife, S., & Cohen, D.R. (1998). Biopsychosocial profile of women with dyspareunia. *Obstetrics and Gynecology, 90,* (4) Part 1, 583–589.

Michael, R.T., Gagnon, J.H., Laumann, E.O.., & Jolata, G. (1994). *Sex in America: A definitive survey.* Boston, MA: Little Brown.

O'Donahue, W., Dopke, C.A., & Swingen, D.N. (1997). Psychotherapy for female sexual dysfunction: A review. *Clinical Psychology Review, 17,* (5), 537–566.

Prior, J. (1997). Ovulatory disturbances and amenorrhea: A physiologic approach to diagnosis and therapy. In J.A. Rosenfeld (Ed.). *Women's health in primary care.* Philadelphia, PA: William & Wilkins.

Rammer, E., & Friedrich, F. (1998). The effectiveness of intrauterine insemination in couples with sterility due to male infertility with and without a woman's hormone factor. *Fertility and Sterility, 69,* (1), 31–36.

Renshaw, D. (1994). Unconsummated marriage: A neglected aspect of sexual dysfunction. *The Female Patient, 19,* (5), 55–60.

Rhodes, J.C., Kjerulff, K.H., Lagenberg, P.W., & Guzinski, G.M. (1999). Hysterectomy and sexual functioning. *Journal of the American Medical Association 282,* (20), 1934–1941.

Ringel, M. (1999). Patients with sexual dysfunction: Your guidance makes a difference. *Patient Care for the Nurse Practitioner, 2,* (4), 14–24.

Rosenthal, M.R. (1997). Ovulatory disturbances and amenorrhea: A physiologic approach to diagnosis and therapy. In J.A. Rosenfeld (Ed.). *Women's primary health care.* Baltimore; MD: William & Wilkins.

Saks, B. (1999). Sexual dysfunction: Sex, drugs, and women's issues. *Primary Care Update for Ob Gyns, 6,* (2), 61–65.

Sauer, M.V. (1998). Motherhood at any age? Egg donation not intended for everyone. *Fertility & Sterility, 69,* (3), 187–188.

Sarwer, D.B., & Durlak, J.A. (1996). Childhood sexual abuse as a predictor of adult female sexual dysfunction: A study of couples seeking sex therapy. *Child Abuse and Neglect, 20,* (10), 963–972.

Seaman, E.K., Telich-Vidal, M., & Sable, D. (1997). Effects of cancer treatment on fertility. *Contemporary Ob/Gyn, 42,* (5), 31–52.

Seltzer, V.L., & Pearse, W.H. (1995). *Women in primary health care: Office practice and procedures.* New York, NY: McGraw-Hill.

Silber, S.J. (2000). Evaluation and treatment of male infertility. *Clinical Obstetrics and Gynecology, 43,* (4), 854–888.

Silverberg, K.M. (2000). Evaluation of the couple with infertility in a managed care environment. *Clinical Obstetrics & Gynecology, 43,* (4), 844–853.

Smith, K., & Hornberger, L. (1997). Rewards of caring for and the health promotion of women adolescents. In J.A. Rosenfeld (Ed.). *Women's health in primary care.* Baltimore, MD: William & Wilkins.

Spielvogel, K., Shwayden, J., & Coddington, C.C. (2000). Surgical management of adhesions, endometriosis, and tubal pathology n women with infertility. *Clinical Obstetrics and Gynecology, 43,* (4), 916–928.

Speroff, L., Glass, R.H., & Kase, N.G. (1999). *Clinical gynecological endocrinology and infertility.* Baltimore, MD: William & Wilkins.

Stephen, E.H., & Chandra, A. (1998). Updated projections of infertility. *Fertility and Sterility, 70,* (1), 30–34.

Van Sickle, M., & Rosenstrock, H. (1999). Taking a sexual history: Which questions to ask. *The Female Patient, 24,* (3), 33–40.

Van Voorhis, B.J. (1998). Infertility treatment: What is a cost-effective approach? *Drug Benefits Trends, 10,* (2), 22–29.

Vermillion, S.T., & Holmes, M.M. (1997). Sexual dysfunction in women. *Primary Care Update for Ob-Gyns, 4,* (6), 234–240.

Wolf, L.J. (2000). Ovulation induction. *Clinical Obstetrics and Gynecology, 43,* (4), 902–915.

Suggested Readings

Kaplan, C. R. (1996). Work-up of infertility: Diagnosis and treatment of anovulation. *The Female Patient, 21,* (3), 35–42.

Reichart, G.A. (1998). Female circumcision: What you need to know about genital mutilation. *AWHONN Lifelines, 2,* (3), 31–34.

Ullman, S.R. (1997). *Sex seen: The emergence of modern sexuality in America.* Berkley, CA: University of California Press.

Wallach, E.E., Garacia, J., Rosenwak, Z., & Seifer, D.K. (1998). Fertility over 35: Improving the odds. *Contemporary Ob/Gyn, 43,* (5), 106–118.

Resources

Infertility

American Society for Reproductive Medicine, 1209 Montgomery Highway, Birmingham, AL 35216, Office: 205-978-5000, http://asrm.com

Hannah's Prayer, a Christian network, P.O. Box 5016, Auburn, CA 95604-5016

International Council on Infertility Information Dissemination (INCIID), P.O. Box 6836, Arlington, VA 22206, Voice: 520-544-9548, Fax: 703-379-1593, INCIIDinfo@inciid.org, www.inciid.org

RESOLVE, 1310 Broadway, Somerville, MA 02144, Business office: 617-623-1156, Helpline: 617-623-0744, www.resolve.org

Sexual Dysfunction

American Association of Sex Educators, Counselors and Therapists (AASECT), P.O. Box 238, Mt. Vernon, IA 52314, www.aasect.org

American Psychological Association, 750 First Street, N.E., Washington, D.C. 20002, www.apa.org

American Psychiatric Association, 1400 K Street, N.W., Washington, D.C. 20005, www.psych.org, Society of Human Sexuality, University of Washington, www.sexuality.org/index.html

CHAPTER 13

Genetics and Genetic Counseling

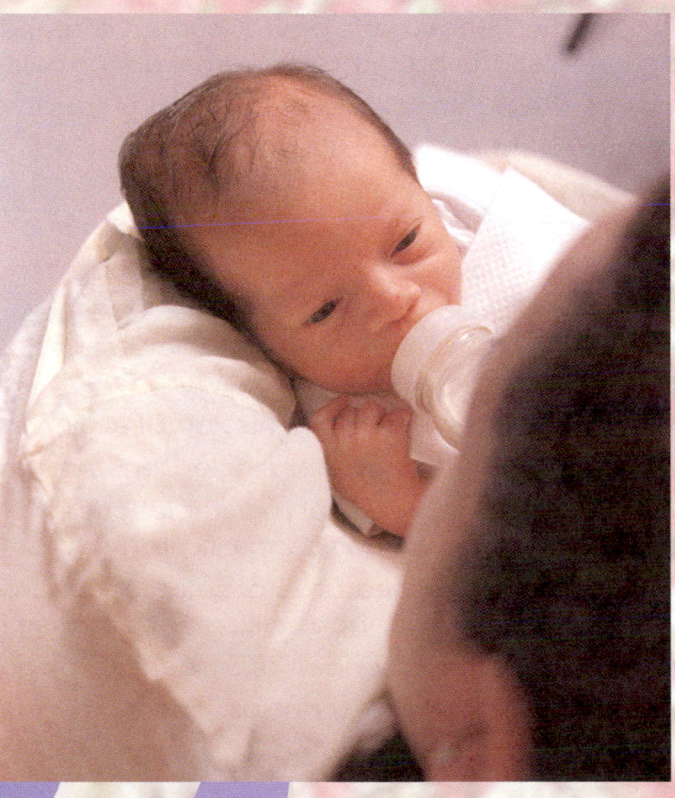

enetic counseling has been defined as a specialized type of family counseling. A great portion of nursing education is dedicated to the teaching and application of mental health methodology. Even if you are not a practicing psychiatric-mental health nurse, you have been exposed to these techniques and approaches during your education. They are extremely helpful in a genetic counseling situation and, as a member of a genetic counseling team, you are contributing invaluable expertise and experience to this process. However, the nurse in a genetic counseling team is often confronted with ethical issues that may evoke past personal and professional experiences. They require some preparation on the part of the practitioner, and you may want to review, before the occasion, some of your personal and ethical value systems. For example:

* How would you respond to the often-heard question: "Tell me what you would do in my place. Help me make this decision"?
* Could you maintain a strictly nondirective approach to counseling? Is it even desirable to be nondirective?
* Are you able to support the decision of a client (for example, not to have amniocentesis in a high-risk genetic situation) that goes against your moral values?
* How do you feel about giving a client referral information that may lead him or her to an outcome contrary to your beliefs?

Key Terms

Allele	Dominant	Heterozygote	Mutation
Alpha-fetoprotein (AFP)	Euploid	Homologous	Nondisjunction
Amniocentesis	Gamete	Homozygote	Pedigree (Genogram)
Aneuploidy	Gametogenesis	Karyotype	Phenotype
Autosome	Gene	Meiosis	Polygenic
Chromosome	Genetic counseling	Mitosis	Proband
Clastogen	Genotype	Monosomy	Recessive
Cytogenetics	Haploid	Mosaicism	Translocation
Deletion	Hemizygous	Multifactorial	Trisomy
Diploid			

Competencies

Upon completion of this chapter, the reader should be able to:

1. Discuss the genetic etiology of human disease, emphasizing the difference between gene alterations and chromosomal abnormalities.

2. Discuss the numerical and structural features of chromosomes.

3. Compare and contrast the stages of gamete formation in oogenesis and spermatogenesis.

4. Define and characterize meiotic and mitotic chromosome nondisjunction.

5. Differentiate between euploidy and aneuploidy, and discuss mechanisms that lead to aneuploidies.

6. Discuss the normal function of structural genes and analyze their derangements in Tay-Sachs disease, phenylketonuria, and Lesch-Nyhan syndrome.

7. Differentiate between transmission of alleles in dominant and recessive patterns.

8. Compare characteristics of single-gene and multifactorial inheritance.

9. Describe the major clinical manifestations of selected autosomal and X-linked disorders. Analyze their significance in prenatal testing.

10. Describe the major features of selected disorders that result from numerical and structural chromosomal abnormalities and discuss their effects on women's health care.

11. Analyze the consequences of screening for genetic diseases.

12. Discuss the various elements of genetic counseling and their effect on the family.

13. Compare and contrast various procedures and methods used in prenatal diagnosis.

edical genetics is a relatively new branch of an old science. Familial occurrences of specific traits have been cited in the literature for centuries. An early example of accurate genetic observation that illustrates the X-linked inheritance of hemophilia is provided in the Jewish Talmud. According to Jewish law, any newborn boy whose male maternal cousin had a bleeding disorder is exempted from circumcision.

However, it has been only since the turn of the 20th century, and especially after 1950, that formal knowledge about medical aspects of genetics has begun to flourish. The landmark work by Archibald Garrod (1902) on alkaptonuria introduced the concept of "inborn errors of metabolism" and established the grounds for the emerging science of biochemical genetics. Despite his limited knowledge of genetic mechanisms—the work of Gregor

Mendel was not yet widely disseminated—Garrod concluded that the existence of blood relatives among affected individuals in his study represented inherited human biochemical variations, a concept currently termed "polymorphism." He accurately predicted that the lack or dysfunction of some mediators of metabolic pathways was responsible for the disorders studied.

In the early 40s, research by Beadle and Tatum (1941) established the relationship between genotype and phenotype (a concept initially known as "one gene-one enzyme") and defined genes as the primary determinant in the control of protein synthesis. Their studies gave Garrod's work immediate validation by identifying enzymes as Garrod's missing mediators. The era of molecular genetics was marked by the discovery of a molecular defect in sickle cell disease, initially postulated by Linus Pauling in 1949 (Pauling, Itano, Singer, & Wells, 1949), and confirmed by Ingram in 1956. With these discoveries, the focus of genetic research was turned to identifying the protein (enzyme) products of specific genes and to relating them to disease process (Cox & Sinclair, 1997).

The field of **cytogenetics**, or the study of chromosomes with a special focus on chromosome abnormalities, was launched by the discovery of the first human chromosomal abnormality by Jerome Lejeune and coworkers in 1952, who identified trisomy 21 as the causative event in Down syndrome. Many other chromosomal disorders were subsequently defined, and cytogenetics was the standard working tool of geneticists for many years.

In the early 1960s, the technique of prenatal diagnosis was to be totally revolutionized by the development of genetic **amniocentesis**. In this technique, a sample of amniotic fluid is removed, and cells that were sloughed off by a developing fetus are studied, allowing geneticists to identify both biochemical defects and chromosome anomalies. The process of genetic counseling, which up to this point was based, at best, on statistical predictions and fixed-risk figures, now could be done on a personal level, as geneticists began to provide genetic information about a specific pregnancy. In the early 1970s, Sarah Lawrence University in New York began to offer the first master's degree program in genetic counseling, with a curriculum based on a strong foundation of genetics and psychology. The modern approach to genetics is based on the concept of reverse genetics, whereby genes are mapped and cloned before the identification of their (protein) products. The addition of gene cloning to the armamentarium of medical genetics set the pace for genetic engineering and potential gene correction of hereditary diseases.

The purpose of this chapter is to provide the reader with baseline essentials of genetics and to awaken an interest in further reading. A thorough glossary of genetic terms can be found on the Internet (see Resources).

CHROMOSOMAL BASIS OF INHERITANCE

A **gene** is a segment of nucleic acid that contains genetic information necessary to control a certain function, such as the synthesis of a polypeptide. A **chromosome** is a filament-like nuclear structure consisting of chromatin that stores genetic information as base sequences in DNA, and whose number is constant in each species. When attempting to generate a list of human genetic disorders, one soon discovers that some are classified under gene alterations (e.g., sickle cell disease, galactosemia, cystic fibrosis), while others represent chromosomal abnormalities (e.g., Turner syndrome; Down syndrome; cri du chat, or cat's cry syndrome). Although such numerical or structural chromosomal aberrations automatically affect large groups of genes, a small gene alteration does not alter chromosome structure and number. Alterations in single genes (single-gene disorders) or even in large groups of genes (polygenic disorders) may be a lesion too small to cause an alteration in chromosomal structure and cannot be identified by karyotype analysis. A **karyotype** is the chromosomal constitution of an individual, which is represented by a laboratory-made display, in which chromosomes are arranged by size and centromere position. This concept is easily understood when one considers that human somatic cells (nucleated cells, with the exception of ova and spermatozoa) contain approximately 100,000 genes, distributed in the form of tightly coiled DNA molecules along 46 **chromosomes**. If all chromosomes were the same size, each would carry approximately 2,300 genes. However, since human chromosomes vary in size, the larger the chromosome, the greater the number of genes carried. Therefore, the clinical manifestations of numerical chromosome alterations increase in severity in proportion to the increasing size of the involved chromosome. For example, a **trisomy** (a condition caused by the presence of an extra chromosome that is added to a given chromosome pair and results in a total number of 47 chromosomes per cell) in which the extra chromosome is one of the smallest size, group G (Down syndrome, or trisomy 21), produces malformations that are much more compatible with life than a trisomy involving a larger chromosome, group D (Patau syndrome, or trisomy 13).

Chromosome Number and Structure

When grouped in a karyotype (Figure 13-1) for cytogenetic analysis, somatic cell chromosomes, usually derived from small lymphocytes collected from circulating blood, are arranged according to size (groups A through G, in decreasing size) and position of the centromere (metacentric, submetacentric, and acrocentric chromosomes). Group A

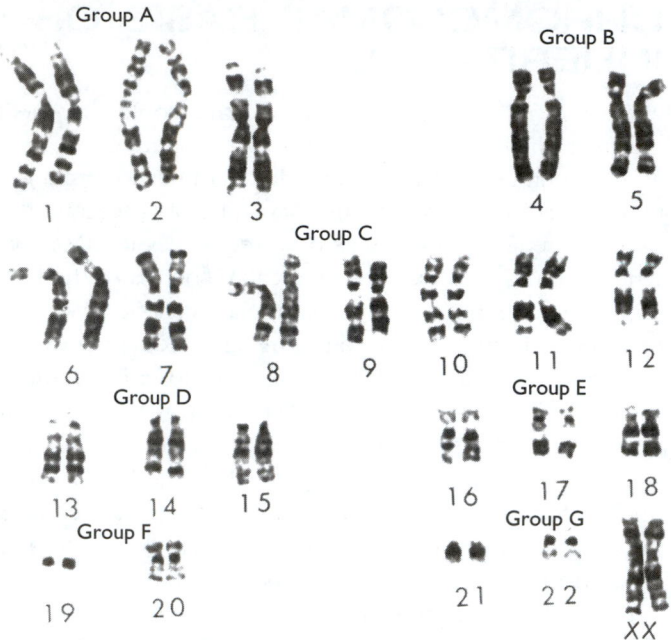

Figure 13-1 Karyotype of a human female cell. Chromosomes obtained from a peripheral blood lymphocyte culture. (Courtesy of Dr. David Ledbetter, Department of Human Genetics, University of Chicago)

chromosomes consist of pairs 1 through 3, group B include pairs 4 and 5, and group C encompass pairs 6 through 12; groups D (pairs 13 to 15) and G (pairs 21 and 22) are the large and small acrocentric chromosomes, respectively; group E contain pairs 16 to 18; and group F include pairs 19 and 20. The X chromosome approximates the size and shape of a group C pair, and the Y chromosome is similar to a group G chromosome. Short chromosome arms are designated as *p* (for *petit,* or small in French), long arms as *q*. This nomenclature allows for quick recognition of chromosomal structural features or abnormalities. For example, the designation 46, XX, B(5)p⁻ indicates a deletion (⁻) of a portion of the small arm (p) of chromosome pair number 5 of the B group, occurring in a female (XX) with a normal chromosome number (46). This is the typical chromosome pattern found in the cri du chat (cat's cry) syndrome. When stained with special techniques, each homologous chromosome pair displays a different, constant pattern of banding (e.g., Giemsa stain banding as depicted in Figure 13-1). Banding techniques, developed in the early 1970s, allow the exact classification of chromosomes in groups and the identification of alterations in chromosome structure, such as deletions and translocations. The term **deletion** refers to the loss of chromosomal material, and **translocation** is the misplacement of genetic material from one chromosome to another.

Patterns of Chromosome Anomalies

The normal structure of chromosomes is subject to alterations that result from breakage and rearrangement. Chromosome breakage has long been recognized as a significant source of genetic abnormalities. The term **clastogen** (i.e., chromosome-breaking agent, from *clastos,* to break, and the suffix, *gen,* an agent) was coined in the early 1970s to designate agents that could cause chromosome breakage. Many clastogens have been identified since then, including physical agents (e.g., ionizing radiation), chemical agents (e.g., chlorpromazine), and biologic agents (e.g., viral infections). However, the significance of clastogens as disease-causing agents has been questioned in many instances. For example, an infection with the influenza virus usually results in chromosome breakage in somatic cells (circulating small lymphocytes), but the chromosome structures return to normal in a few days. Chromosome breakage, therefore, becomes significant when: 1) it is permanent, or at best, long-lasting; and 2) these permanent changes, in addition to appearing in somatic cells, are also present in germ cells and thus have the potential of being transmitted to the offspring. Figure 13-2 depicts some of the possible consequences of chromosome breakage.

Chromosome breakage resulting in loss of the broken fragment is termed "chromosome deletion," which may have significant clinical consequences, such as cri du chat syndrome. In addition, chromosome breakage may also result in unstable end points ("sticky ends"), which predisposes chromosomes to a variety of rearrangements of the resulting fragments. One such rearrangement is a translocation, by which a chromosomal fragment reunites with another nonhomologous chromosome. Two types of translocations have clinical significance: reciprocal and robertsonian. In a reciprocal translocation, breaks occur in two different chromosomes and the fragments are mutually exchanged, resulting in derivative chromosomes. Robertsonian translocations occur when the short arms of two acrocentric chromosomes (pairs 13 to 15 of group D, and pairs 21 and 22 of group G) are lost, and the remaining long arms fuse at the centromere, forming a "single chromosome." Both types result in individuals who have the same amount of genetic information, although "rearranged," and therefore no clinical manifestations are expected. These persons are termed "balanced translocation carriers." However, if this person reproduces, there is a chance that the translocated chromosome will be present in the gamete that undergoes fertilization by a normal gamete. The resulting zygote will have a gene imbalance caused by the extra chromosomal (genetic) material, and the child will be at risk for physical and mental abnormalities.

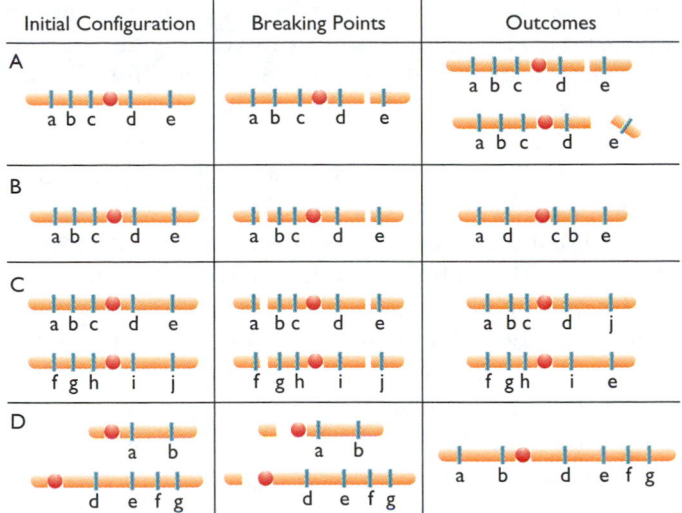

Initial Configuration	Breaking Points	Outcomes

Figure 13-2 Examples of structural rearrangements after chromosomal breakage. Initial chromosome constitution, breaking points, and consequences of the breaks and rearrangements are shown. In panel A, a break occurs between markers *d* and *e*. Three consequences are: the resulting chromosomes, bearing markers *a* through *d* have undergone a deletion. The severed fragment may stay aligned with the rest (top example), the space being narrower than the length of the fragment: chromosome gap. Or it may be lost (bottom example): chromosome break. In panel B, the initial chromosome suffers two breaks (between markers *a* and *b* and between *d* and *e*). The center portion undergoes a pericentric inversion, resulting in a newly arranged chromosome, in which the markers are sequenced *a, d, c, b,* and *e*. Panel C depicts an exchange of genetic material between chromosomes bearing markers *a* through *e* and *f* through *j*. Since no genetic material was lost, only rearranged, this is termed a balanced translocation. Panel D represents a robertsonian translocation between two acrocentric chromosomes (one from group G, the small chromosome, the other from group D, the large chromosome). Loss of the short arms and fusion at the centromere results in a translocated chromosome. If no significant genetic material is lost, this is also a balanced translocation, causing no clinical manifestations.

Distribution of Chromosomes During Cell Division

Human somatic cells are **diploid** (a cell which contains two copies of each chromosome). Such a diploid chromosome number is represented by the notation 2n=46. A **haploid** chromosome constitution (n=23) is found in germ cells, the male and female **gametes** (spermatozoa and ova). Somatic cell chromosomes are represented by 44 **autosomes** (the 22 pairs of chromosomes, which do not greatly influence sex determination at conception) and two sex chromosomes, XX in females and XY in males. As somatic cells multiply by **mitosis**, each daughter cell receives the same chromosome number as the initial cell. This equitable chromosome sharing results from a phenomenon termed "disjunction." During anaphase, chro-

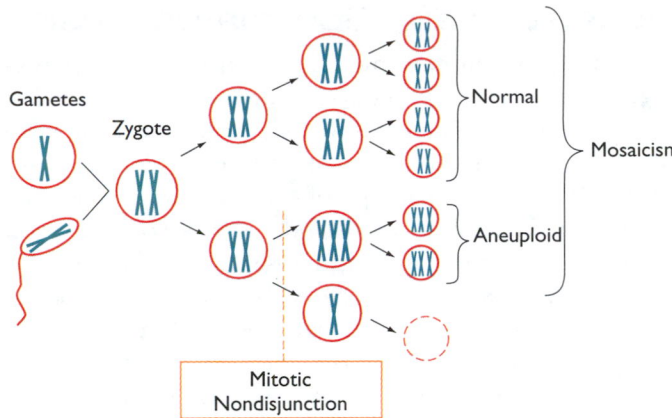

Figure 13-3 Consequences of chromosome nondisjunction occurring during mitosis, after a normal zygote was formed by fertilization of two normal gametes. (Only one chromosome pair is represented). Following the first mitosis, the upper cell originates a normal line of cells with the correct chromosome number. The bottom cell undergoes nondisjunction, resulting in a line of cells with one extra chromosome. (The monosomic cell is not viable and there are no further divisions.) The outcome is a mosaic individual with two cell lines, one containing the normal chromosome number, the other aneuploid.

matids of each chromosome separate and migrate to opposite poles of the cell, guided by microtubules of the mitotic spindle (Figure 13-3). Disruption of this orderly chromosome distribution occurs in **nondisjunction**. Through failure of homologous chromosomes or chromatids to separate properly during meiotic (meiosis I or II) or mitotic anaphase, daughter cells will have different chromosome numbers (e.g., 45 and 47, instead of 46 and 46). Cells that are **monosomic** (the aneuploid condition of having a chromosome represented by a single copy in a somatic cell) tend to degenerate and die, but those with the extra chromosome (trisomic) continue to divide and generate a complete line of trisomic cells.

Mitotic Nondisjunction and Mosaicism

When mitotic nondisjunction occurs during embryonic development, the trisomic cell line proliferates concomitantly with the normal cell line, and an individual with **mosaicism** for that particular chromosome results. Mosaicism, therefore, results in an individual (mosaic) with two or more genetically different cell populations. The chromosomal notation for a male with a mosaic type of Down syndrome, for example, is: 46, XY/47, XY, G(21)$^+$. The slash (/) indicates a dual cell population, in which one has the normal chromosomal constitution (46, XY), while the other carries the extra G(21) chromosome ($^+$) and has a total number of 47 chromosomes.

Oogenesis and Spermatogenesis

The halving of chromosome number that occurs in **gametogenesis** (a series of mitotic and meiotic divisions occurring in the gonads that leads to the production of gametes) takes place during the first division (meiosis I) of meiosis. **Meiosis** is a reductional type of cell division, in which the chromosome number is halved. The second division (meiosis II) is an equational, mitosis-like cell division. As somatic chromosomes are shared by the products of the first meiotic division, each daughter cell receives one member of each autosomal pair and one of the sex chromosomes (either the X or the Y). As a result, women can form only X-bearing ova, but men can produce X-bearing and Y-bearing spermatozoa.

Oogenesis

The process of oogenesis (Figure 13-4) begins during prenatal development and comprises three main phases: cell proliferation by mitosis, reduction of chromosome number and genetic recombination through meiosis, and maturation of oocytes. During fetal development, early germ cells divide by mitosis until the stages of oogonia and primary oocytes are reached. These cells still have a diploid chromosome number (2n=46). Primary oocytes then enter meiosis I and, at birth, they are found at an arrested stage, termed "dictyotene," which persists until puberty. Starting at menarche, shortly before each ovulation, the primary oocyte resumes cell division and completes meiosis I, now with the number of chromosomes reduced to the haploid number (n=23). The outcome of meiosis I is one secondary oocyte and one first polar body. At ovulation, the nucleus of the secondary oocyte initiates meiosis II (the first polar body degenerates). At this point, if fertilization does

not occur, the secondary oocyte degenerates and dies without completing meiosis II. However, if fertilization occurs, the nucleus of the secondary oocyte resumes and completes meiosis II as the male pronucleus approaches it. The product of meiosis II is one ovum and one secondary polar body (which later degenerates). The female pronucleus contained in the ovum now fuses with the (haploid) male pronucleus and forms a diploid zygote, which evolves into the embryo, fetus, and newborn infant.

Of the approximately 2 million oocytes present at birth, only about 300,000 are present at puberty, and of these, only approximately 400 reach full maturity, which culminates in monthly ovulation during reproductive years. The remaining follicular units undergo progressive atresia, by apoptosis, a physiologic phenomenon that persists throughout those years. From a genetic perspective, the long duration of the first meiotic division, while the oocyte continues its metabolic functions, may be responsible, at least in part, for the occurrence of meiotic errors, such as nondisjunction. From a teratogenic viewpoint, an ovum fertilized at an advanced age has remained in the ovaries since birth and therefore has been exposed to a variety of environmental (internal and external) influences. This long-term exposure may account for the linear relationship between maternal age and birth defects discussed later.

Spermatogenesis

Unlike oogenesis, in which oocytes are produced prenatally, the process of sperm production only begins at puberty (Figure 13-5). As in oogenesis, three sequential steps can be identified in spermatogenesis: intense cell prolifer-

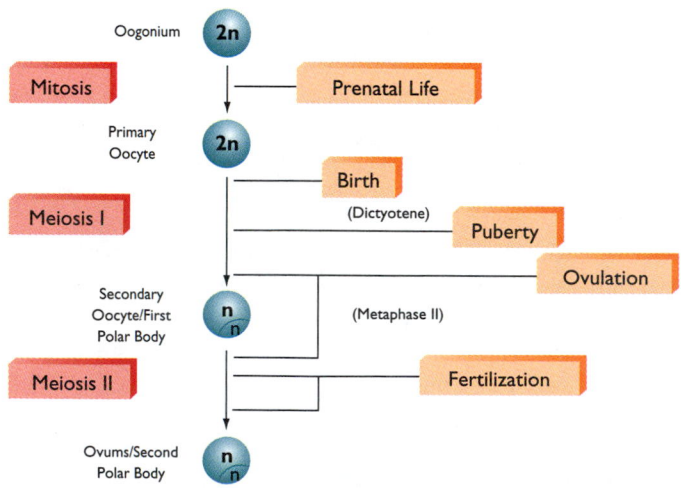

Figure 13-4 Oogenesis. Depicted here are the various types of cell division, the resulting cell types, and the time elapsed from primordial oogonium to mature ovum. First ovum is released at menarche, the last one immediately before menopause. Permanence of the latter in the ovary, approximately 52 years.

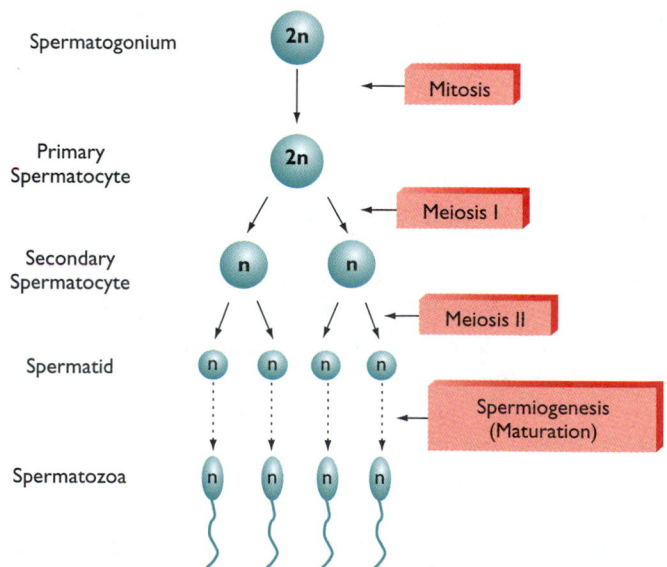

Figure 13-5 Spermatogenesis. Different cell divisions and resulting cells. Approximate time elapsed from spermatogonia to mature spermatozoa is 75 days, followed by a further 10 to 12 days of maturation in the epididymis.

ation by mitosis, the recombination and reduction events of meiosis, and spermiogenesis (maturation of spermatozoa). At puberty, testicular endocrine cells, called Leydig cells or interstitial cells, increase in number and begin to produce testosterone, which initiates spermatogenesis. The process of spermatogenesis is characterized by a series of mitotic divisions, followed by meiosis I and II. Reduction in the number of chromosomes occurs in meiosis I, between the stages of primary and secondary spermatocytes. Meiosis II converts secondary spermatocytes into spermatids. After this step, no further divisions occur, only a process of maturation (spermiogenesis), which results in mature spermatozoa. Unlike oogenesis, which produces only one viable gamete, each spermatogonium (early male germ cell) entering spermatogenesis produces four mature gametes. Spermatogenesis continues throughout a lifetime.

Meiotic Nondisjunction and Aneuploidy

Meiotic nondisjunction is a major cause of **aneuploidy**, an abnormal chromosome pattern in which the total number of chromosomes is not a multiple of the haploid number, n=23. Nondisjunction can occur during meiosis I and II, during both oogenesis and spermatogenesis, resulting in gametes with an aneuploid chromosome number (for example, 22 and 24, instead of 23 and 23) (Figure 13-6). As in the case of somatic cells, gametes lacking a chromosome are not likely to survive. The gametes with an extra chromosome are more viable, and on fertilization, a normal gamete will produce an aneuploid zygote. The most common aneuploidies in humans are trisomies. For example, as a result of meiotic nondisjunction, a spermatozoon carrying an extra G(21) chromosome, i.e., 24, X or Y, G(21)$^+$ may fertilize an ovum with a normal chromosomal constitution, 23, X. The result will be a zygote with 47 chromosomes, including the extra G(21), which will develop into an infant with Down syndrome, or G(21) trisomy. The chromosome notation for a female with free trisomy-type Down syndrome, for example, is 47, XX, G(21)$^+$. Unlike the mosaic case described, all somatic cells in this person contain the extra G(21) chromosome. The addition of one chromosome to one of the pairs (trisomy) creates a relatively small aneuploid alteration in the total chromosome number (46 to 47), which is usually quite compatible with life. However, the addition of one or more chromosomes to each pair (increments of the haploid number, 23) results in triploid cells with 69 chromosomes (46+23) or tetraploid cells with 92 chromosomes (46+23+23). The product of this uniform addition of chromosomes to all of the original pairs is termed euploidy, a **euploid** cell being one whose chromosome number is a multiple of 23. But even in the case of triploid individuals (3n=69) the genetic imbalance is of such magnitude that the few infants who are carried to term have severe multiple abnormalities that limit their life span to a few hours or days.

GENE STRUCTURE AND FUNCTION

Genes are sequences of DNA that determine a certain biologic function. Many are structural genes and carry the necessary information to promote the synthesis of proteins (polypeptides), others are regulatory and control the function of other genes or groups of genes. A **mutation** (alteration) of a structural gene may result in the synthesis of an abnormal protein (e.g., enzyme) with potential clinical consequences. The following four figures illustrate some mechanisms of gene-protein interaction. Figure 13-7 represents the normal metabolic conversion of a substance

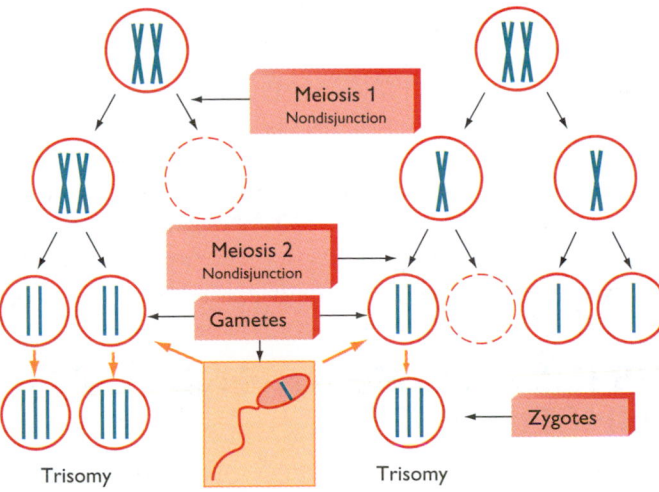

Figure 13-6 Outcomes of meiotic chromosome nondisjunction occurring during meiosis 1 (left) and meiosis 2 (right). (Only one chromosome pair is represented). Nondisjunction at meiosis 1 results in one aneuploid and one monosomic cell (which does not survive). Meiosis 2 produces two aneuploid gametes, which, on fertilization by normal, euploid gametes, will produce trisomic zygotes. Likewise, nondisjunction at meiosis 2 also results in aneuploid gametes, and subsequently in trisomic zygotes.

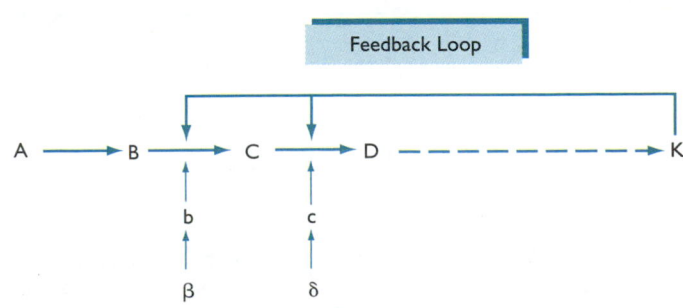

Figure 13-7 Normal sequence of events in the metabolic conversion of product *A* into end product *K*, mediated by enzymes *b* and *c*, which are encoded by genes β and δ respectively.

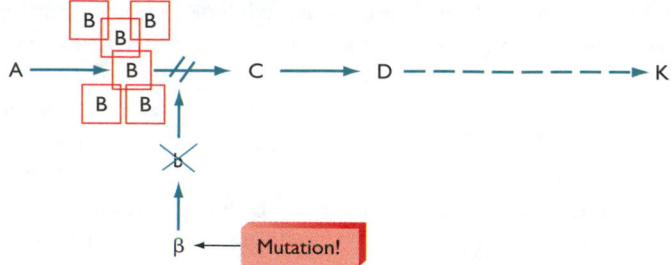

Figure 13-8 Consequences of a mutation in gene β, resulting in lack of enzyme b, interruption of the metabolic pathway, and accumulation of byproduct B. Prototype gene dysfunction in Tay-Sachs disease.

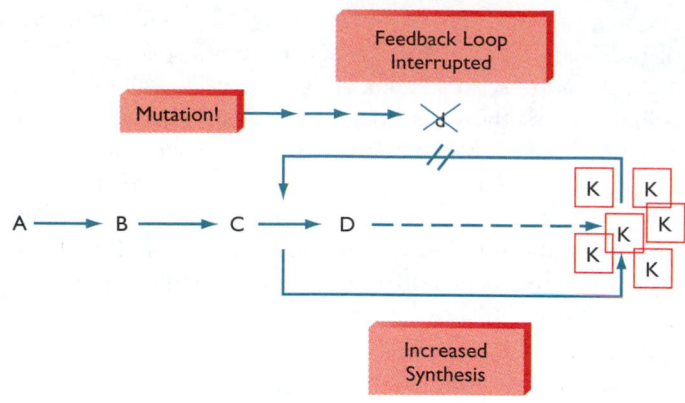

Figure 13-10 Consequences of a mutation in the gene encoding for enzyme d, which is involved in the feedback control loop for end-product K. As a result, increased synthesis of K is observed, eventually reaching toxic levels. Prototype gene dysfunction in Lesch-Nyhan syndrome.

A into an end-product K, via byproducts B, C, D, and so on. Enzymes b and c, whose synthesis is controlled by genes β and δ, catalyze steps B ⇒ C, and C ⇒ D, respectively. A feedback loop ensures physiologic levels of K.

In Figure 13-8, a mutation has occurred in gene β, preventing normal (quantitative or qualitative) synthesis of enzyme b, and the consequent interruption of the pathway between B and C. Continuous uptake of A will produce two results: accumulation of B, and depletion of all products beyond the block. An example of this situation is Tay-Sachs disease (a GM₂ gangliosidosis): mutation of the Tay-Sachs gene (β) causes the lack of the enzyme hexosaminidase A (HexA), represented by (b), and whose absence results in accumulation of ganglioside GM₂ (B) in nerve cells, producing all the clinical manifestations of this progressive neurologic disorder.

Figure 13-9 depicts a mutation in gene δ, blocking the synthesis of enzyme c, and interrupting the metabolic conversion of C into D. In this instance, an alternative pathway C ⇒ E ⇒ F is opened. This event may have two out-

comes: product F may eventually be converted into K, with no significant clinical consequences, or F may represent the end point to the alternative pathway and begin to accumulate until it reaches toxic levels. The example here is phenylketonuria (PKU), an inborn error of metabolism that creates an intolerance to the amino acid phenylalanine. The missing enzyme here (c), which results from mutation in the PKU gene (δ), is phenylalanine hydroxylase. The alternative pathway leads to the formation and accumulation of phenylketones (F), which, in combination with phenylalanine deficiency, prevents the postnatal completion of myelination of nerves and results in profound mental retardation.

Figure 13-10 represents a genetic alteration of the enzyme d, which mediates the feedback loop controlling ideal concentrations of K. As a result, K may accumulate to toxic levels. The prototype genetic disease here is Lesch-Nyhan syndrome, in which d is the enzyme hypoxanthine-guanine phosphoribosyl transferase (HGPRT) and K is uric acid. Accumulation of uric acid to extremely high levels, plus HGPRT deficiency, results in mental retardation and a tendency for self-mutilation in affected persons.

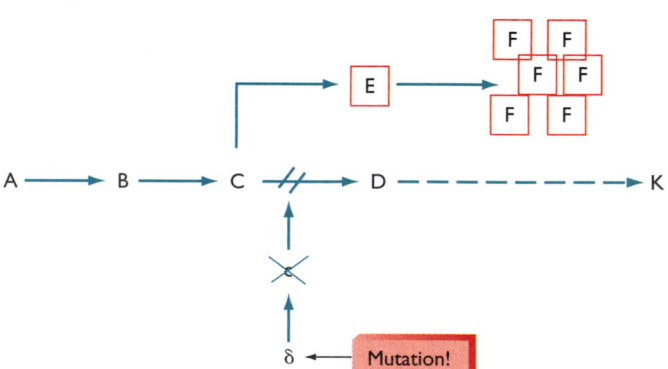

Figure 13-9 Consequences of a mutation in gene δ, resulting in lack of enzyme c, interruption of the metabolic pathway, and opening of an alternate pathway. The outcome is accumulation of byproduct F. Prototype gene dysfunction in phenylketonuria (PKU).

SINGLE GENE (MENDELIAN) INHERITANCE

The concept of gene, by definition, does not determine the expression of that gene. A gene is defined as a segment of nucleic acid that contains genetic information necessary to control a certain function, such as the synthesis of a polypeptide. For example, the gene for Tay-Sachs disease is a site on a chromosome that controls the synthesis of the enzyme HexA. The possible expressions of this gene would be HexA^{+}, indicating the command for synthesis of

HexA, or HexA⁻, indicating the lack of such command, resulting in the absence of the enzyme. Such alternate forms of gene expression are termed **alleles** of the gene HexA. The genetic constitution of an individual at any given locus is called **genotype**, whereas the expression of that gene's function in terms of measurable or observable features of the individual is termed **phenotype**. Whether or not a gene is expressed in the phenotype depends on the arrangement of its alleles and on the concepts of dominance and recessivity. A mutation in the original, or "wild-type" allele, in this case HexA⁺, may result in a different allele, such as HexA⁻.

Dominant Gene Inheritance Pattern

Consider a gene with two alleles, the normal ("wild-type") represented by **(+)**, and the mutant allele represented by **(−)**. Figure 13-11 illustrates the three possible arrangements for the alleles in persons carrying that gene. Represented here are pairs of somatic **homologous chromosomes** (chromosomes with matching genes) where that gene is located. The model may also be used to illustrate the X chromosome pair in women. The first individual (A) received from each parent a copy of the normal allele (+/+). The second person (B) received from one parent one copy of the normal allele and from the other, one copy of the mutated allele (+/−). The third person (C) received from each parent a copy of the mutated allele (−/−). These are the only possible mathematical combinations, given one gene with two alleles. Persons (A) and (C) are **homozygous** for either allele (+/+) or (−/−). A homozygous person, or homozygote, is an individual possessing a pair of identical alleles of a given gene. Person (B) is termed a **heterozygote**, that is, an individual who has two different alleles at a given locus (+/−).

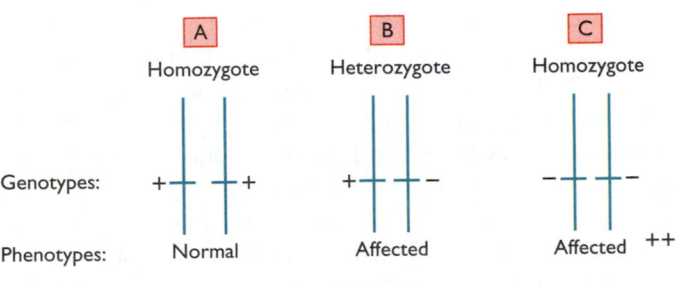

	A	B	C
	Homozygote	Heterozygote	Homozygote
Genotypes:	+ +	+ −	− −
Phenotypes:	Normal	Affected	Affected ++

+   Normal ("wild-type") allele
−   Mutant allele

Figure 13-11 Dominant inheritance pattern. Schematic of the three possible allelic arrangements of a dominant gene: genotypes and possible phenotypes. Note absence of carrier state.

Now, imagine determining by physical examination the phenotypes of these three individuals. Person (A) carries normal alleles and displays a normal phenotype. Person (C) has only mutant alleles and exhibits an affected phenotype. Person (B), the heterozygote, also displays an affected phenotype, but the clinical manifestations in person (C), the homozygote for the mutant alleles, are more severe. When this type of correlation between genotypes and observed phenotypes is obtained, the mode of inheritance is termed **dominant**. This term implies that in the heterozygote (person B) the expression of the mutant allele dominates over the expression of the normal allele. In other words, in the case of dominant genes, the presence of one copy of the mutant allele is sufficient to express the phenotype. And by extension, two copies of the mutant allele bring about a more accentuated expression of that characteristic. In summary, a dominant allele is one that is phenotypically expressed in single copy (heterozygote) and in double copy (homozygote).

In addition to the patterns of phenotypic expression described above, conditions exist that may cause a variation of expression. These include incomplete penetrance and variable expressivity.

A gene is said to have reduced or incomplete penetrance in a population when a proportion of persons who possess that gene do not express the phenotype. Usually, those who do express the affected phenotype have a complete expression of the phenotype, with all features of the syndrome present. A gene is said to have variable expressivity when individuals possessing that gene display the features of the syndrome in various degrees of expression, from mild to severe.

Vertical Transmission of Dominant Genes

A clear understanding of transmission patterns requires a few general guidelines. First of all, most genetic diseases are rare. The probability that two affected persons will produce offspring is very low for most diseases (exceptions to this rule are discussed later). Second, depending on the disease, if one parent is affected, he or she is much more likely to be heterozygous (+/−) than homozygous (−/−) for the mutant allele. Usually, an individual homozygous for the mutant allele experiences physical or mental abnormalities at a much more severe level. Those assumptions being accepted, two questions remain:

1. What are the chances for transmitting the mutant allele to the offspring?

2. What are the risks for the offspring being affected?

The outcomes of these matings are best expressed by the use of Punnett squares (Figure 13-12).

Dominant Inheritance: Punnett Squares

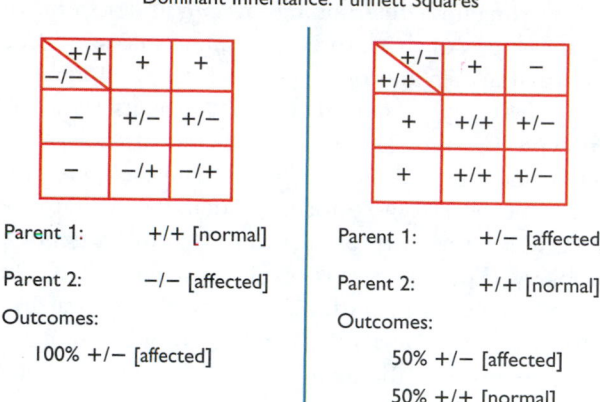

Parent 1: +/+ [normal]

Parent 2: −/− [affected]

Outcomes:

100% +/− [affected]

Parent 1: +/− [affected]

Parent 2: +/+ [normal]

Outcomes:

50% +/− [affected]

50% +/+ [normal]

Figure 13-12 Punnett squares depicting transmission of a dominant gene and resulting offspring's genotypes and phenotypes. Genotypes of the parents (top left cell), the possible gametes produced by each parent (single symbols), and the result of their random combination at fertilization. Possible outcomes in each pregnancy.

An individual who is homozygous for the mutant allele of a dominant gene (−/−) may contribute that allele (−) to all of his or her offspring. Since a single copy of the mutant allele is sufficient for the expression of the phenotype, all children will be affected, regardless of the genotype of the other parent. Panel 1 of Figure 13-12 illustrates the mating of such an affected homozygote with an unaffected partner. However, because of the often severe physical and mental manifestations found in an affected homozygote, the mating represented in panel 2 is more often encountered. Here, an affected heterozygote (+/−) will have equal chances of contributing the mutant allele (−) or the normal allele (+) to the offspring. (Random chromosome segregation during meiosis results in half of all gametes carrying the mutant allele and half carrying the normal allele.) Any time the mutant allele (−) of a dominant gene is transmitted to the offspring, the phenotype is expressed, regardless of the genotype of the other partner. Since most genetic disorders are rare, the mating illustrated in panel 2 of Figure 13-12, in which the other parent is unaffected (+/+), is representative of the majority of cases. In such mating, each pregnancy carries a 50% chance of being affected (+/−) and a 50% chance of being unaffected (+/+). These probability figures are fixed for each time conception occurs in the same set of parents, because each pregnancy is a statistically independent event.

However rare dominant diseases may be, in some circumstances the manifestations brought about by the condition serve to approximate affected individuals and increase their social interaction. One such example is achondroplasia. Because of their short stature, achondroplastic dwarfs tend to associate with persons who have the same syndrome. Here again the homozygote for the mutant allele (−/−) is often not carried to term or is born with severe malformations (e.g., hydrocephaly). Therefore,

even in the absence of genotype determination, it is more likely that two socially adept achondroplastic dwarfs are both heterozygotes (+/−). In such cases, each pregnancy produced by this couple has a 25% chance of being genotypically and phenotypically unaffected (+/+), a 50% chance of being affected with dwarfism like the parents (+/−), and a 25% chance of carrying the severe stigmata of the homozygote for the mutant allele (−/−).

As previously mentioned, the conceptual model for transmission of dominant genes applies to homologous autosome pairs and to the X chromosome pair in women (Box 13-1). The situation for sex chromosomes in men is different, since the X and the Y chromosomes contain extremely small areas of homology, so that they do not exhibit the side-by-side meiotic pairing observed with the autosomes and the X chromosome. Because of this, men are **hemizygous** for all genes on the X chromosome that do not have a homologous site on the Y, and their alleles are represented as single copies. Therefore, in the inheritance of an X-linked dominant gene, the single-copy presence of its normal or mutant allele results in the expression of the normal or mutant phenotype, respectively.

Recessive Gene Inheritance Pattern

The term **recessive** suggests the idea of "hidden" or "occult." In a genetic connotation, it reflects the behavior (expression) of the mutant allele in the heterozygote. A recessive allele is one whose phenotypic expression occurs in a homozygous or hemizygous condition; in the heterozygote, a recessive allele is masked by its dominant homologous counterpart. For example, Figure 13-13 illustrates the relationships between genotypic and phenotypic expression of a recessive gene with two alleles, (+) representing the normal or "wild-type" allele and (−) representing the mutated allele. Here again, the concepts apply to autosome pairs and the X chromosome pair in females. In the expression of a recessive gene, individuals (A) and (B) display both a normal (unaffected) phenotype, and only (C), who inherited two mutant alleles from both parents, is affected. This means that a recessive disease can only be phenotypically expressed when two copies of the mutant allele are present, and therefore, both parents must equally contribute to this outcome. In other words, in the heterozygote, the mutant allele is recessive (hidden), and the effect of the normal allele predominates (dominates), causing a normal phenotype to express. The difference between (A) and (B), however, is significant; whereas (A) can produce only gametes (ova or spermatozoa) with normal alleles, (B) carries the mutant allele and thus 50% of the gametes produced transmit this allele. This situation illustrates the concept of carriers for a genetic disease, that is, individuals who are clinically normal (or nearly normal), but who are potential transmitters of the disease.

Identification of such carriers is of paramount importance for genetic counseling. In the case of an unaffected couple who produce a child with a recessive disease, identification is easy. Because they each must contribute a mutant allele, they must be considered obligate carriers, even in the absence of specific carrier testing for that gene. Specific tests to detect heterozygous carriers of a variety of genetic diseases are available, but it would be impractical and certainly not cost-effective to screen all prospective parents without specific risk factors with all available tests. Genetic screening for carriers is usually limited to populations at risk, either because they belong to a high-risk group for a certain disorder (e.g., Ashkenazi Jews and Tay-Sachs disease), or because of a family history. Carriers for certain specific disorders can be identified by tests before conception (e.g., sickle cell disease), by means of routine screening, or after conception by means of prenatal diagnosis (e.g., Tay-Sachs disease).

Vertical Transmission of Recessive Genes

One of the most common situations in clinical practice is that of an asymptomatic couple who produce a child with a recessive disorder. Most people who seek genetic counseling fall into this category. The surprise element of this scenario is understandable if the following factors are considered:

1. Genetic disorders are rare, and therefore the chances that both parents will be heterozygous for the same gene are remote.

2. Many people remain childless for years, or they may have produced healthy children before the one affected and are unaware that they carry a deleterious gene.

3. Even when both parents are carriers, the transmission by each parent of the mutant allele (which results in an affected child) does not always occur.

Box 13-2 summarizes characteristics of recessive inheritance.

As with dominant inheritance, the best visualization of transmission of recessive genes is obtained through Punnett squares. Panel 1 of Figure 13-14 illustrates the example described previously. Both parents are asymptomatic heterozygous carriers (+/−) for a recessive gene. On forming gametes, each parent has a 50% chance of passing on the mutant allele (−). Random combination of these alleles during conception results, in each pregnancy, in a 25% chance of producing a child with a normal phenotype (+/+), a 50% chance of producing an asymptomatic carrier like themselves (+/−), and only a 25% chance of producing an affected child (−/−). Panel 2 of Figure 13-14 demonstrates that even when one of the parents is affected

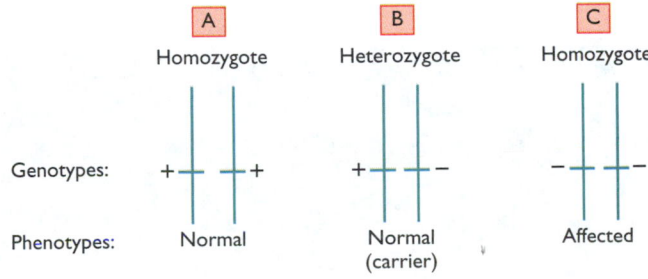

A	B	C
Homozygote	Heterozygote	Homozygote

Genotypes: + +   + −   − −

Phenotypes: Normal   Normal (carrier)   Affected

+   Normal ("wild-type") allele
−   Mutant allele

Figure 13-13 Recessive Inheritance Pattern. Schematic of the three possible allelic arrangements of a recessive gene. Genotypes and possible phenotypes. Note the introduction of a heterozygous carrier (B).

Box 13-2 Characteristics of Recessive Inheritance

Autosomal Recessive Pattern*

1. A carrier state exists; both males and females can be carriers.

2. Both males and females are equally likely to be affected.

3. The disease appears to "skip a generation." Members of that generation who have affected children are asymptomatic carriers.

4. Carrier parents have a 25% chance to produce an affected child in each pregnancy.

5. Parent consanguinity (mating between blood relatives) may be a factor when a child is affected with a *rare* recessive disease.

X-Linked Recessive Pattern*

1. Most affected persons are male; affected females are extremely rare.

2. Male-to-male transmission of the X-linked mutant allele does not occur. Males transmit their X chromosomes to their daughters.

3. All daughters of an affected male are (heterozygous) **carriers**, none are **affected** (homozygotes).

4. Sons of carrier females have a 50% chance of inheriting the mutant allele and being **affected** (hemizygotes). Daughters have a 50% risk of inheriting the mutant allele and being (heterozygous) **carriers**.

———————

*Unless otherwise specified, all affected or carrier persons' partners are normal.

Recessive Inheritance: Punnett Squares

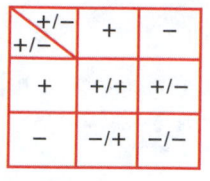

Parents: +/− [carriers]

Outcomes per pregnancy:

   25% +/+ [normal]

   50% +/− [carriers]

   25% −/− [affected]

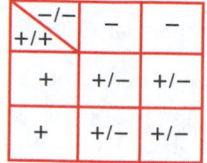

Parent 1:   −/− [affected]

Parent 2:   +/+ [normal]

Outcomes per pregnancy:

   100% +/− [carrier]

Figure 13-14 Punnett squares depicting transmission of a recessive gene and resulting offspring's genotypes and phenotypes. The genotypes of the parents (top left cell), the possible gametes produced by each parent (single symbols), and the result of their random combination at fertilization. Results are possible outcomes in each pregnancy.

pletely controlled by the action of a single gene. The majority of traits in the human body are controlled by several genes working in cooperation to produce the final effect: these are **polygenic** traits. When environmental factors also contribute to the expression of the phenotype, these are **multifactorial** traits. One of the primary characteristics of polygenic and multifactorial inheritance is the existence of a *continuous variation* in the trait, as opposed to an all-or-nothing distribution: for example, distribution of height in or the distribution of various body shapes. Box 13-3 summarizes characteristics of multifactorial inheritance.

Included in the many pathologic conditions that are polygenic and multifactorial in nature are coronary artery disease, diabetes mellitus, hypertension, obesity, and common psychiatric illnesses, such as schizophrenia and bipolar disorder. Even though an undeniable genetic predisposition to these conditions exists, they are heavily influenced by environmental factors, such as lifestyle, dietary habits, and stressful events.

(−/−), the other parent's genotypically normal (+/+) contribution ensures that they cannot produce an affected child (−/−). All their children will be carriers (+/−). However, in very common diseases, such as sickle cell disease among African Americans, it is possible that an affected person (−/−) and a heterozygous carrier (+/−) will produce an affected child (−/−). The risk for this event in every pregnancy is 50%, with another 50% probability of producing a carrier (+/−) i.e, 50% carrier/50% affected.

POLYGENIC AND MULTIFACTORIAL INHERITANCE

Risk calculation with single gene disorders, as discussed previously, follows strict Mendelian rules and is fairly straightforward. However, very few phenotypes are com-

Box 13-3 Characteristics of Multifactorial Inheritance

1. No clearly defined pattern of inheritance within a single family.

2. The recurrence risk increases when more than one family member has the trait.

3. The recurrence risk increases with increasing severity of the malformation.

4. The recurrence risk increases with consanguinous parents (mating between blood relatives).

Risk determination in polygenic and multifactorial inheritance is made on the basis of *empirical observation* of a large number of cases, followed by a specific statistical analysis for each trait. For several disorders, risk prediction and determination tables exist that take into consideration family history, number of cases in the family, and extent or severity of the malformations. By consulting these tables, the nurse and other clinicians can help clients understand the likelihood of genetic disorders occurring in future pregnancies.

SINGLE-GENE DISORDERS

By comparison with multifactorial inheritance, single-gene disorders are in the minority. However, precise molecular information has been developed using monogenic disorders as a framework. The work of Ingram (1956) on sickle cell disease is a clear example. McKusick's latest (2000) on-line cataloguing of *Mendelian Inheritance in Man* (OMIM) lists 11,807 single-gene disorders, of which 11,072 are autosomal, 637 are X-linked, 38 are Y-linked, and the remaining 60 result from mitochondrial gene action (see Resources). Table 13-1 lists some examples of monogenic disorders, their mode of inheritance, and frequency of occurence.

Autosomal Dominant Disorders

Selected autosomal dominant disorders are discussed in this section, including achondroplasia, Ehlers-Danlos syndrome, familial hypercholesterolemia, Marfan syndrome, neurofibromatosis (type 1), osteogenesis imperfecta, and polycystic kidney disease.

Achondroplasia

The most common form of dwarfism (adult stature, 48 to 52 inches) is achondroplasia, characterized by shortened limbs, especially proximally (rhizomelia), and a normal length torso. Common features include lordosis, prominent forehead with flattened nasal bridge, and short hands with stubby fingers. Life span and IQ are within normal limits among heterozygotes. One of the common complaints is backaches and there is an increased risk of spinal cord compression. Gynecologic problems include premature menarche, enlarged breasts, and premature menopause. Pregnancy often results in increased mechanical and locomotive burden. Skeletal malformations also affect the normal progress of pregnancy and delivery: because of a small chest cavity, adverse cardiorespiratory conditions

Table 13-1 Selected Single-Gene Disorders

Disorder	Classification	Frequency
Achondroplasia	Autosomal dominant	1:26,000
Albinism (occulocutaneous)	Autosomal recessive	1:10,000 to 1:12,000
Cystic fibrosis	Autosomal recessive	1:2,000 to 1:2,500 (all persons) 1:17,000 (African Americans)
Cystinuria	Autosomal recessive	1:10,000
Duchenne muscular dystrophy	X-linked recessive	1:3,000–5,000 (males)
Ehlers-Danlos syndrome	Autosomal dominant	1:150,000
Familial hypercholesterolemia	Autosomal dominant	1:200 to 1:500
G6PD deficiency	X-linked recessive	1:10 (African American males) 1:50 (African American females)
Hemophilia A (classic)	X-linked recessive	1:2,500 to 1:5,000 males
Hemophilia B (Christmas)	X-linked recessive	1:30,000 males
Huntington disease	Autosomal dominant	1:18,000 to 1:25,000 (US and UK) 1:333,000 (Japan)
Hypophosphatemic vitamin D–resistant rickets	X-linked dominant	1:20,000
Marfan syndrome	Autosomal dominant	1:10,000 to 1:20,000
Mucopolysaccharidoses	Autosomal recessive	1:20,000 (type III most common)
Neurofibromatosis type I	Autosomal dominant	1:4,000 to 1:5,000
Osteogenesis imperfecta	Autosomal dominant	1:20,000 (all types combined)
Phenylketonuria	Autosomal recessive	1:15,000
Polycystic kidney disease	Autosomal dominant	1:200 to 1:1,250
Sickle cell disease	Autosomal recessive	1:400 to 1:600 (African Americans)
Tay-Sachs disease	Autosomal recessive	1:3,600 (Ashkenazi Jews) 1:360,000 (all other groups)

may develop, and because of a contracted pelvis, delivery by cesarean section is often recommended. Increased paternal age may be a factor in producing a child with achondroplasia.

Ehlers-Danlos Syndrome

This genetic disease is an umbrella term for a group (with nine sub-types) of disorders of connective tissue that result in hyperelasticity of skin, hyperflexible joints, vascular fragility, and poor wound healing. Common complications include a tendency for bruising, hernias, and varicose veins, all of which are aggravated during pregnancy. Poor wound healing and a predisposition to hemorrhaging are risk factors during and after delivery (e.g., an episiotomy may be complicated by these factors). The life span may be limited by vascular events, such as aneurysms and rupture of large vessels. Even though the three most common variants are inherited as autosomal dominant traits, autosomal recessive and X-linked inheritance patterns have been reported. Prenatal diagnosis is possible in type V, since enzyme (lysyl oxidase) activity is present in normal amniotic cells.

Familial Hypercholesterolemia

Also called hyperlipoproteinemia IIa, this is one of various disorders of lipoproteins, along with abetalipoproteinemia and familial combined lipoproteinemia. Familial hypercholesterolemia (FH) is one of the most common single-gene disorders, in which the manifestations are sensitive to environmental (dietary) variations, to the point of being classified at times as a multifactorial disorder. However, individuals who are homozygous for this gene tend to develop severe and life-threatening conditions, such as early onset of atherosclerotic disease that affects the coronary, cerebral, and peripheral circulation. Postmortem examination of young children (ages 3 and 4) and young adults has revealed early arterial changes with lipid deposition and some plaque formation. Variants of the FH gene have been described, increasing the genetic complexity of this disease. Prenatal diagnosis has been accomplished by measurement of the hydroxymethylglutaryl coenzyme A (HMG CoA) reductase.

Marfan Syndrome

Marfan syndrome is another disorder of connective tissue, involving a triad of ocular, skeletal, and cardiovascular alterations. The most common ocular abnormality is a subluxation of the lens. Common skeletal findings include: tall stature, arachnodactylic ("spider-like") hands and feet, and scoliosis. Severe scoliosis may compromise respiratory function in pregnant women with Marfan syndrome. The major life-threatening risk, however, is the frequent occurrence of aortic fusiform or dissecting aneurysms. Fifty percent of aortic aneurysms in affected women under age 40 occur during pregnancy, with rupture most likely to occur in the third trimester (Godfrey, 1993). Aortic valve abnormalities found in Marfan syndrome also contribute to an increased mortality rate during pregnancy. As a point of curiosity, historians have suggested that President Abraham Lincoln had Marfan syndrome and may have died from a dissecting aneurysm if he had not been felled by the assassin's bullet. Average life span with Marfan syndrome is 40 to 50 years.

Neurofibromatosis

The hallmark of type I multiple neurofibromatosis (MNF I), or von Recklinghausen disease, is the development of multiple soft tumors of peripheral nerves, or neurofibromas, and an abnormal skin pigmentation. In early childhood, the disease presents with multiple brown (or café-au-lait) spots, usually on the torso, and then progresses, from adolescence onwards, in the form of neurofibromas. This progression has also been reported in association with pregnancy, with the possibility of some regression after delivery. An important finding is that apparently, affected infants born to affected mothers have a worse prognosis than those who had affected fathers and those without a family history (fresh mutations) (Simpson & Golbus, 1992). This fact emphasizes the importance of genetic and reproductive counseling for clients with MNF I. As many as 75% of patients with MNF I go through life without developing some of the complications of this disease: scoliosis, moderate to severe mental retardation, learning difficulties, hypertension, seizures, spinal cord or root compression, optic gliomas, pheochromocytomas, and malignant changes in the neurofibromas (Seashore & Wappner, 1996).

Osteogenesis Imperfecta Type I

All four types of osteogenesis imperfecta (OI) involve osteoporosis and recurrent fractures of long bones with minimal trauma. Type I disease is also characterized by blue sclera, conductive deafness (secondary to otosclerosis), and discolored teeth resulting from dentinogenesis defects. (Type II results in perinatal lethality with multiple fractures during gestation and birth). Life span of type I OI is usually normal in spite of the multiple fractures throughout life. Pregnancy in women with OI type I is complicated by respiratory difficulties among those with kyphoscoliosis and by cephalopelvic disproportions among those with previous pelvic fractures. Special precautions during delivery must also be observed for the safeguard of both mother and child (who may also have OI). In some cases, OI has been identified prenatally via sulfate incorporation test.

Polycystic Kidney Disease

This is a fairly common disorder that causes cysts in the kidneys, liver, pancreas, and spleen. Renal cysts may remain asymptomatic until the third or fourth decade of life, when the onset of renal failure or hypertension prompts a diagnosis of polycystic disease. Occasionally, an enlarged kidney is detected on X-ray studies before the onset of other manifestations, such as hematuria and proteinuria. Polycystic renal disease accounts for approximately 10% of all adult cases of chronic renal failure (Gabow, 1993). Since asymptomatic women have no related complications during pregnancy and the risk for an adverse outcome increases with progressing renal disease, it is important that reproductive counseling be provided to women with a family history of polycystic renal disease who want to have children. Prenatal diagnosis has been accomplished through linked polymorphism genetic tests.

Autosomal Recessive Disorders

The most common autosomal recessive disorders include cystic fibrosis, mucopolysaccharidoses, phenylketonuria, sickle-cell disease, and Tay-Sachs disease.

Cystic Fibrosis

Cystic fibrosis (CF) is the most common lethal genetic disease affecting Caucasians. Clinical manifestations include abnormal exocrine gland function with pancreatic insufficiency and malabsorption, chronic pulmonary disease, and excessive salt in sweat (sodium in excess of 60 mmol/L and chloride exceeding 70 mmol/L) (Pagana & Pagana, 1999). The pancreatic insufficiency results in pancreatic juice that lacks trypsin, an enzyme that must be exogenously replaced throughout life. Chronic lung disease is secondary to recurrent infections resulting from the inability of the ciliated epithelium to secrete excessive mucus. Pulmonary function progressively deteriorates and a large number of affected children die before age 10. Presently, over 50% of children with cystic fibrosis live beyond age 20, and survival depends on the extent of the disease and on additional involvement of body systems (Ferri, 1999). Other manifestations include: rectal prolapse, neonatal meconium ileus, cirrhosis of the liver, gall stones, and salivary gland obstruction. Pregnancy for women with cystic fibrosis obviously presents serious risks of increased morbidity and mortality. A classic national survey of cystic fibrosis reported the outcome of 97 pregnancies in women with cystic fibrosis (Cystic Fibrosis "GAP" Conference Report, 1975). According to this survey, the most detrimental factor to the success of a pregnancy was a decreasing vital lung capacity secondary to pulmonary disease. Prenatal diagnosis is available.

Mucopolysaccharidoses

This diverse group of mucopolysaccharide accumulation disorders (MPS) encompasses 6 different syndromes, whose primary types are: Hurler syndrome (type I), Hunter syndrome (type II), Sanfilippo's syndrome (type III), and Morquio syndrome (type IV). All but type II are inherited as autosomal recessive traits. Hunter syndrome is an X-linked recessive disorder.

Individuals with type I disease exhibit coarse facies in infancy, short stature, skeletal and joint deformities, deafness, corneal clouding, umbilical hernia, progressive mental retardation, and death in the second decade of life. Type II (X-linked) is similar to type I, except for later onset, clear corneas, and death in the third decade. Type III is the most common type, with normal facies, stature, and corneas, progressive mental retardation in early childhood, and death in the second decade. Type IV results in normal intelligence, facies, and corneas; short stature with scoliosis; and death in the third decade. Some types of mucopolysaccharidosis can be detected prenatally, since their defective enzymes (listed here in parentheses) have been identified: Hurler syndrome (α-L-iduronidase); Hunter syndrome (α-L-iduronic acid-2-sulfatase); Sanfilippo syndrome (type A: heparin sulfatase; type B: N-acetyl-α-D-glucosaminidase); Morquio's syndrome (chondroitin sulfate-N-acetylhexosamine sulfate sulfatase).

Phenylketonuria

One of the most fascinating genetic diseases, phenylketonuria (PKU) represents a success story in the management of a genetic disorder. As previously mentioned, PKU results from an enzyme (phenylalanine hydroxylase) deficiency, and the consequent accumulation of the amino acid phenylalanine and its byproducts cause mental retardation and other manifestations. Management for PKU consists of removing phenylalanine from the newborn's diet and maintaining a low dietary phenylalanine intake throughout life. If initiated within the first days of life, a low-phenylalanine diet ensures a normal development and life span. However, the offspring of "rescued" (treated) women with PKU are at risk for mental retardation, microcephaly, congenital heart disease, and intrauterine growth retardation. This is not a result of their genetic makeup, since children of homozygous mothers ($-/-$), except in the rare case of the father being a heterozygous carrier ($+/-$) for PKU, are unlikely to be homozygous for the mutant allele. Fetal damage is the result of intrauterine exposure to high levels of maternal phenylalanine and its metabolites, and the degree of damage is proportional to the maternal phenylalanine blood level. Placing a rescued woman with PKU on a

REFLECTIONS FROM A NURSE

"J.X. and S.T., a married couple, had just delivered their first child, after an uncomplicated pregnancy. The newborn girl weighed 3500 g at birth and began feeding well. However, 10 days after the delivery, results of biochemical tests indicated that the child had phenylketonuria (PKU). The baby's serum phenylalanine level was 30 mg/dL, the normal level is less than 2 mg/dL. On a subsequent office visit, I informed the parents that PKU is an inborn error of metabolism that prevents the use of an amino acid, phenylalanine, found in most foods. The disorder is inherited as an autosomal recessive trait, which indicates that both parents are heterozygous carriers for the PKU gene. I recommended that the baby be placed on a low-phenylalanine diet to prevent mental retardation and ensure a healthy life. I also told the parents that a low-phenylalanine diet must be observed throughout the child's life span, because an increase in dietary phenylalanine during childhood or adolescence may result in loss of cognitive function and in emotional disorders. While ac-

knowledging the difficulty of maintaining a child on such a strict diet, I also stressed the need for adherence and suggested referrals to counseling and support group activities. In addition, I told the parents that, on reaching child-bearing age, their 'PKU-rescued' daughter would need to be aware that increases in dietary phenylalanine may increase her chances of producing children with mental retardation.

As a nurse working with this family, I found that my ability to provide nursing care was greatly enhanced by a strong procedural knowledge and understanding of the condition and its implications. This prepared me to answer the parents' questions regarding:

- *Their risks for transmitting this condition to future offspring*
- *The consequences of this condition for normal life activities of this child*
- *The chances of this child passing on the condition to her offspring."*

---

low-phenylalanine diet before a pregnancy to maintain her blood levels at 120 to 480 μmol/L produces good outcome. Unfortunately, the treatment is often initiated after conception, at times too late to prevent microcephaly and cardiac damage to the fetus. The possibility of preventing malformations and mental retardation among the offspring of rescued mothers with PKU is a strong argument in favor of early identification or disclosure of those women at risk. Initiated in the 1960s and now a legal requirement in all states, screening for PKU in newborns has made early initiation of treatment and the prevention of mental retardation possible in most cases. Prenatal diagnosis by means of measuring fetal phenylalanine hydroxylase has been accomplished.

Sickle Cell Disease

Sickle cell disease (SCD) is a serious, chronic hemolytic anemia that results from homozygosity for the mutant allele (−/−) of the *HbS* gene. As a consequence of this genetic imbalance, hemoglobin S (HbS), an abnormal hemoglobin, replaces the normal adult hemoglobin A. HbS has reduced oxygen-carrying capacity and red blood cells have a decreased life span. The affected red blood cells acquire a sickle-shaped appearance, a morphologic change that greatly contributes to obstruction of small vessels and further ischemia. Infarctions of the lungs, kidneys, spleen, and bones are common. The result is a lifelong series of sickle cell crises, with recurrent pneumoccocal infections and salmonellal osteomyelitis, painful leg ulcers, dactylitis, priapism, and other manifestations. Renal failure is a common serious complication. The life span is significantly shortened, even with aggressive management.

The gynecologic and obstetric management of the woman with SCD requires special attention. Complications during pregnancy include aggravation of sickle cell crises and infections, development of other anemias, and toxemia. The prevalence of SCD is extremely high among African Americans and significant among people of Mediterranean extraction. The prevalence of homozygotes (−/−) among African Americans is approximately 1 in 400, with a heterozygote carrier frequency of 1 in 10.

Tay-Sachs Disease

Tay-Sachs disease (TSD) is a lipid storage disorder, with accumulation of GM$_2$ ganglioside in cells of the nervous system, resulting in a progressive neurologic disorder. The genetic defect results in decreased production of the enzyme β-hexosaminidase A (HexA), from a significant reduction in the heterozygote carrier (+/−) to total absence in the homozygote (−/−). During their short life, children with TSD experience a progressive and steady neurologic deterioration in a series of mental and motor deficits, which begin at approximately 6 months of age. Manifestations at various ages include loss of the developmental milestones acquired before the onset of the disease, along with deafness, blindness, seizure activity, and death by age 3 to 5. TSD is highly prevalent among the Ashkenazi Jews (Jews of Central and Eastern European origin), with a frequency of approximately 1:3,600 for homozygotes (−/−), 1:25 to 30 for heterozygote carriers (Jorde, Carey, Bamshad, & White, 1998). By comparison, among Sephardic Jews (Jews of Southern European, North African, and Middle-Eastern origin) and gentiles, the gene is 100 times rarer (1:360,000). Prenatal diagnosis by determination of fetal HexA levels is commonly performed.

X-Linked Disorders

Genetic disorders whose causative gene is located on the X chromosome include Duchenne muscular dystrophy, glucose-6-phosphate dehydrogenase deficiency, the hemophilias, and Lesch-Nyhan syndrome.

Duchenne's Muscular Dystrophy

One of two types of X-linked recessive muscular dystrophies (the other being Becker's muscular dystrophy), Duchenne muscular dystrophy (DMD) results in progressive muscle weakening, atrophy, and contractures, beginning in early childhood. In the majority of cases, the age of onset is less than 5 years and the disease is characterized by delayed walking. A pseudo-hypertrophy of the calf (in which muscle is replaced by adipose tissue) may mask the disease to the inexperienced clinician. Affected children are usually unable to run, and 95% of affected children are using a wheelchair by age 12 (Korf, 1996). Mild mental retardation occurs in about 1 of 4 cases. Death, often from respiratory insufficiency, usually occurs in the second decade. Prenatal diagnosis is done by assessing for various mutations that lead to the deficiency of dystrophin, the deficient protein in various muscular dystrophies.

Glucose-6-Phosphate Dehydrogenase Deficiency

This common, self-limiting hemolytic anemia is often used as a prototype for genetic environmental interaction. Glucose-6-phosphate dehydrogenase (G6PD) deficiency is usually asymptomatic until the affected male is exposed to one of many environmental triggers, such as certain drugs (antimalarial agents, aspirin, sulphonamides) or certain foods (especially fava beans, from which the popular name "favism" originates). The hemolytic episode may also be precipitated by infections. In one disease subtype (B variant), affected males suffer from a chronic hemolytic anemia in the absence of environmental triggers. Carrier females (+/−) remain asymptomatic even when exposed to a trigger agent. Homozygote females (−/−) do exist, as progeny of a carrier female (+/−) and an affected hemizygous (−/−) male. Pregnancy in women with G6PD deficiency (homozygotes) presents several complications. Hemolytic episodes are more frequent; urinary infections, common in pregnancy, cannot be treated with sulpha-based drugs; and exposure of a fetus with G6PD deficiency to maternally ingested trigger substances may result in fetal hemolysis, hydrops fetalis, and death. The incidence of anemia, hyperbilirubinemia, and kernicterus is also increased among newborns with G6PD deficiency.

Hemophilia A

Classic, or type A, hemophilia is a fairly common X-linked recessive disorder of coagulation, resulting from deficiency or defect in clotting factor VIIIc. In 10% of clients, the factor VIIIc level is normal, but its activity is reduced (Jorde, et al., 1998). Variable degrees of deficiencies are probably caused by genetic heterogeneity (different mutations). In the presence of severe factor VIIIc deficiency, massive hemorrhages after trauma and surgical procedures (including dental procedures) can occur. "Spontaneous" bleeding frequently occurs in areas subject to trauma (e.g., joints, resulting in hemarthroses). Petechiae and echymoses are usually absent. Prenatal diagnosis by measurement of factor VIII is possible.

Lesch-Nyhan Syndrome

Also known as HGPRT deficiency, Lesch-Nyhan syndrome is a rare X-linked recessive disease characterized by a tendency toward self-mutilation, mental retardation, choreoathetosis, spasticity, and hyperuricemia. Prenatal diagnosis is made by determination of fetal levels of HGPRT.

CHROMOSOME ABNORMALITIES

Both the autosomes and the sex chromosomes can experience numerical and structural chromosomal abnormalities that have clinical consequences. Table 13-2 shows the prevalence of chromosomal abnormalities in newborns. Structural chromosomal abnormalities do not alter the total chromosome number, but in some cases, they can cause

Table 13-2 Incidence of Selected Chromosomal Abnormalities in Newborns

Chromosome Abnormality	Incidence
Numerical, Autosomes	
Trisomy 21 (Down syndrome)	1 : 650 to 700 live births
Trisomy 16–18 (Edward syndrome)	1 : 8,000 live births
Trisomy 13–15 (Patau syndrome)	1 : 20,000 live births
Other autosomal anomalies	1 : 50,000 live births
Numerical, Sex Chromosomes	
47, XXY (Klinefelter syndrome)	1 : 1,000 male births
47, XYY (Jacobs syndrome)	1 : 1,000 male births
Other male anomalies	1 : 1,350 male births
45, X0 (Turner syndrome)	1 : 10,000 female births
47, XXX (triple-X female)	1 : 1,000 female births
Other female anomalies	1 : 2,700 female births
Structural, Autosomes	
Balanced robertsonian, t(Dq/Dq)	1 : 1,500 live births
Balanced robertsonian, t(Dq/Gq)	1 : 5,000 live births
Reciprocal translocations	1 : 7,000 live births
46, XX or XY, B(5)p⁻ cri du chat syndrome	1 : 20,000 live births
Total Chromosome Abnormalities	**1:160 live births**

Data adapted from Simpson and Golbus, 1992

clinical consequences as devastating as those resulting from numerical changes. As previously mentioned, numerical alterations resulting in hyperploidy (3n, 4n, and so on) produce a wide spectrum of malformations that render them incompatible with life. However, small variations around the normal diploid number (46), such as occurs in trisomies (total chromosome number 47), are often found in clinical practice. The only monosomy compatible with life is a missing X chromosome in persons with Turner's syndrome.

Numerical Abnormalities of the Autosomes

Numerical alterations of the autosomes include some of the most common trisomies found in humans: trisomy 21 (Down syndrome), trisomy 18 (Edwards' syndrome), and trisomy 13 (Patau syndrome).

Trisomy 21

Down syndrome is the most common aneuploidy compatible with development to full term with a reasonable quality of postnatal life. Physical and mental abnormalities vary enormously in spectrum (Jorde, et al., 1998). Mean IQ is 50, with a range of 25 to 70. Multiple physical anomalies include craniofacial abnormalities (brachycephaly, flat occiput, low-set ears, oblique palpebral fissures, epicanthal folds, Brushfield spots (on the iris), broad nasal bones and flattened profile, and open mouth with protruding tongue); skeletal abnormalities (broad, short fingers, clinodactyly of fifth finger); cardiac malformations (ventricular and atrial septal defects, patent ductus arteriosus); and various other abnormalities (hypotonia; increased susceptibility to respiratory infections and to acute leukemia; palmar simian crease; and abnormal dermatoglyphics, or fingerprint pattern). In spite of modern medical developments, life expectancy is still shortened, with 22% dying in the first decade and 50% by age 60, mostly from hematologic malignancies and cardiac defects. Males with Down syndrome are usually sterile, but a few females have reproduced. About one third of their offspring are also trisomic for chromosome 21.

The chromosomal constitution of Down syndrome is variable, with three possible configurations:

1. Free trisomy, 47, XX or XY, $G(21)^+$, is the pattern in 95% of all cases of Down syndrome; the extra chromosome 21 is unattached and segregates freely during meiosis. This type of Down syndrome increases linearly in frequency with increasing maternal age (from 1:1,500 live births for mothers age 20, to 1:30 live births by age 45) (Korf, 1996).

2. Translocation Down syndrome, 46, XX or XY, t(Gq/Dq)$^+$ or t(Gq/Gq)$^+$, accounts for approximately 4% of all Down syndrome cases. The majority of cases are sporadic (without family history), but about 40% have one balanced-translocation carrier parent. When one such carrier and a normal partner reproduce, their chances of producing a child with Down syndrome range from 33% (for carriers of t(Gq/Dq) and t(21q/22q)) to 100% (for carriers of t(21q/21q)). This latter situation is one of the rare examples in genetics in which an abnormality is passed on to *all* living progeny. The incidence of translocation Down syndrome is slightly elevated (9%) among mothers who are older than age 30 at conception (compare with 2% for mothers younger than age 30) (Gelehrter, Collins, & Ginsburg, 1998).

3. Mosaic Down syndrome, 46, XX or XY/47, XX or XY, G(21)$^+$. This rarer type of Down syndrome (about 1% of all cases) results from mitotic nondisjunction that occurs during early embryonic development of a normal zygote. Persons with this type have mixed cell populations, some with the normal karyotype, others with the extra chromosome. Contrary to what might be expected, children with Down syndrome mosaicism do not necessarily have a better developmental outcome than those with the free trisomy syndrome.

Trisomy 18

Edwards' syndrome is a fairly common trisomy affecting mostly chromosome 18. In addition to severe mental retardation, children with this defect present with severe craniofacial abnormalities (dolichocephaly with a prominent occiput, low-set and malformed ears, and micrognathia), skeletal abnormalities (clenched fist with overlapping fingers, flexion deformities, adducted hips, "rocker-bottom" feet), cardiac anomalies (ventricular and atrial septal defects, patent ductus arteriosus), and urogenital malformations ("horse-shoe" kidneys, hydronephrosis, cryptorchidism, prominent genitals). Hypotonia is also common. Although the life span is longer for females (10 months, average), females are more often affected. Mean survival for males is about 3 months. Overall, 30% of these children die in the first month, 50% die in the second month, and few survive 1 year (Simpson & Golbus, 1992).

Trisomy 13

Patau syndrome causes more severe malformations than the previous two trisomies discussed, which is consistent with the increased size of the extra chromosome and a greater gene imbalance. Craniofacial anomalies are much more pronounced: microcephaly, low-set and malformed ears, microphthalmia or anophthalmia, coloboma of the iris, and cleft lip and palate. Skeletal abnormalities include polydactyly and syndactyly; overlapping, flexed fingers; and hypoplasia of the pelvis. Systemic anomalies include cardiac defects (ventricular and atrial septal defects, patent ductus arteriosus) and urogenital malformations (malformed kidneys, hydronephros, polycystic kidneys, cryptorchidism, bicornuate uterus). Mean life expectancy is 4 months, with 45% dying in the first month and fewer than 5% surviving 3 years (Simpson & Golbus, 1992).

Numerical Abnormalities of the Sex Chromosomes

Alterations in number may also involve the sex chromosomes. Some of the most common genetic disorders caused by sex chromosome aneuploidies are Klinefelter, Jacobs, Turner, and the triple-X female syndromes.

47, XXY

Klinefelter syndrome is characterized by multiple X chromosomes and one Y chromosome. The greater the total chromosome number, the more severe the anomalies that result from increased gene imbalance. Physical abnormalities include elements of decreased masculinization, such as gynecomastia; hypogonadism (with sterility caused by degeneration of seminiferous tubules); and increased pubis-to-sole length, reflecting elongated lower limbs. Mental development is normal in most cases; mental retardation, if it occurs, is in the IQ range of 50 to 85. Delayed language skills, however, are common. Chromosome mosaicism (46,XY/47,XXY) rarely occurs; when it does, it results in individuals with milder manifestations than their trisomic counterparts.

47, XYY

Jacobs syndrome was reported in the early 1960s by Patricia Jacobs, a Scottish cytogeneticist who detected a higher-than-expected frequency of double-Y males among inmates of penal institutions in Britain. In early reports, an extra Y chromosome was seen as responsible for an individual's increased tendency toward aggression against property (as opposed to aggression against humans). A detailed statistical analysis by Borgaonkar and Shah (1974), of more than 200 cases later revealed that the only correlates with an extra Y chromosome were tall stature (more than 6 feet) and skin disorders, such as persistent adult acne. Mental retardation and aggressive tendency correlations with XYY were not found to be significant in that large study, and the syndrome remains a scientific curiosity. A majority of children produced by XYY fathers have normal chromosomal constitution, probably reflecting a selective advantage of normal haploid gametes over aneuploid ones.

45, XO

Turner syndrome, originally described clinically as ovarian dysgenesis (with gonads consisting of streaks of connective tissue and devoid of germ cells), is an example of a monosomy that is compatible with quasi-normal life. Clinical manifestations include: low birth weight and short adult stature (4'6″ to 4'8″); low posterior hair line and webbing of the neck; shield-shaped chest with divergent nipples; short fourth metacarpals; cubitus valgus; coarctation of the aorta; urinary tract abnormalities; lymphedema of hands and feet in the newborn; and fetal cystic hygroma and hydrops. Intellectual development is normal, with verbal IQ exceeding performance IQ. Due to decreased secondary sexual characteristics, administration of female hormones at puberty is a common practice. However, it tends to further stunt growth and must be judiciously considered. Treatment for the reduced growth with growth hormone and anabolic steroids is also in practice. Mosaicism also occurs in Turner syndrome (46, XX/45, X0), resulting in milder expression of the phenotype.

47, XXX

Occasionally, triple-X females have been reported in textbooks under the unfortunate term "super females." Whereas this nomenclature is valid in fruit flies, where the extra X chromosome causes an exacerbation of female characteristics, the term is totally unjustified in humans. A relatively common condition (1:1000 live female births), triple-X females display a normal phenotype, with perhaps a slight decrease in mental capacity, when compared to their euploid sisters. Gynecologic complications include a delayed menarche and a premature menopause. As with XXY males, the offspring of XXX females are largely normal, indicative of a selective advantage of euploid gametes.

Structural Chromosomal Abnormalities

Structural abnormalities include a variety of chromosome defects (e.g., deletions, translocations) that do not alter the total chromosome number. They include the cri du chat (cat's cry) syndrome, fragile X syndrome, and several chromosome instability syndromes, in which the hallmark is chromosome breakage or rearrangement.

46, XX or XY, B(5)p

Cri du chat, or cat's cry, syndrome is a rare (1 in 50,000 live births) (Jorde et al., 1998) chromosome deletion syndrome resulting from loss of the small arm of chromosome B(5). In early infancy, this syndrome presents with a typical but nondistinctive facial appearance, often a "moon-shaped" face, with wide-spaced eyes (hypertelorism). As the child grows, this feature is progressively diluted, and by age 2, the child is undistinguishable from age-matched controls. Profound mental retardation persists throughout a short life; most affected children die in infancy from multiple genetic imbalances. Typical of this disease is a crying pattern that is abnormal and cat-like. At times, it sounds like an angry cat; at others, like a soft mewling sound. This is a result of laryngeal atrophy, which improves with age. By age 3, the crying pattern is still abnormal, but it acquires a normal pitch and loses its cat-like quality.

Fragile X Syndrome

Although listed here as a structural abnormality, fragile X syndrome acquired its name from the fact that in *in vitro* conditions, the X chromosome frequently displays breaks and gaps in its terminal portions. However, this is an X-linked dominant condition with increased prevalence among males (approximately 1 in 1,250 males and 1 in 2,500 females are affected). Clinical features include mental retardation and a typical facial appearance, including an elongated face and long, elf-like ears (Jorde et al., 1998).

Chromosome Instability Syndromes

This is a heterogeneous group of genetic disorders characterized by a high frequency of chromosome breakage that is observed *in vitro*. They include ataxia-telangiectasia (or Louis-Bar's syndrome), Fanconi anemia, and xeroderma pigmentosum. These syndromes are associated with decreased immune function and an increased incidence of cancer, mostly lymphomas and leukemias.

GENETIC SCREENING

Because of the complexity and magnitude of genetic damage, treatment for genetic disorders is rarely successful. The primary weapon against increases in the prevalence of genetic disease is an aggressive program of genetic screening and counseling. The first corollaries of any such intervention must be *voluntary participation, equal access to all,* and *confidentiality* (both in conducting the tests and in handling records and results). In addition, education and counseling about tests and procedures must be an integral part of any screening program. Attention must be paid to ensure quality control of all aspects of testing and laboratory procedures.

Purposes for genetic screening are threefold:

1. To provide early recognition of a disease for which effective intervention and therapy exist, before symptoms occur. Example: PKU.

2. To provide identification of carriers of a genetic disease for the purpose of maximizing parenthood planning options. Example: Tay-Sachs disease.

3. To obtain population data on frequency, spectrum, and natural history of a genetic disease. Examples: chromosomal abnormalities in newborns.

Screening for genetic disorders can occur during various times in a person's life:

- Screening of selected populations for heterozygous carriers (e.g., mass screening of African Americans for sickle cell disease, as it occurred in the 1970s in clinics sponsored by the Black Panther Party)

- Screening of relatives of a known carrier or affected individuals within a family, for the purpose of reproductive decision making

- Preconception screening for carriers (e.g., screening for Tay-Sachs disease among couples contemplating parenthood, as it occurred in synagogues in the U.S. after development of testing methods)

- Postconception (prenatal) testing (e.g., screening for Tay-Sachs disease in the product of a pregnancy by two heterozygous carriers)

- Newborn testing (e.g., testing for PKU in all newborns, as mandated by law in all U.S. states). The benefits of early detection of PKU and treatment initiation warrant mandatory testing.

An ideal genetic screening test must have high sensitivity (ability to detect true-positive results) and specificity (ability to detect false-negative results); it must yield rapid results and be safe and cost-effective; and it should cause minimum physical and emotional discomfort to all involved. Geneticists and other members of the genetics team must be prepared to weigh all favorable and unfavorable consequences of genetic screening before implementing a program or conducting a screening activity.

Among the potential benefits of screening for carriers is the removal of a stigma and restoration of self-esteem when the results do not reveal a carrier status. It also facilitates genetic counseling, and reproductive planning, and provides useful information to other potentially affected family members. Testing newborns for genetic defects provides for early detection and treatment initiation, maximizing quality of life.

Risks incurred in genetic screening include the potential for stigmatization of those identified as carriers or affected individuals and for the development of feelings of inadequacy and guilt often seen in conjunction with genetic disease. A positive test result for one family member may result in the disclosure of genetic risks to other family members who did not seek or want to know the outcome of the tests.

GENETIC COUNSELING

In its narrower sense, genetic counseling consists of one or more encounters with the probands and their families with the objective of providing information about their genetic disease. A **proband** is a clinically identified person who displays the characteristics or features of the disease in question. This information includes risk figures, options, and provides a framework for a course of action to be taken by the individual or family. It should also include an assessment of psychosocial family dynamics, which are an integral part of a genetic disease, and an exploration of feelings and perceptions often elicited by the newly obtained knowledge. **Genetic counseling**, in its broader definition, refers to a series of procedures that include processing the initial referral, assessing the needs, deciding on the appropriate tests, interpreting the results, and finally, communicating these findings to the proband and family.

In the majority of families that request genetic counseling, the precipitating event is the birth of an affected child. In the case of dominant diseases, usually one of the parents is affected, and there is some degree of preparation for the possibility of an affected child. In recessive disorders, however, the parents are usually clinically normal, which precludes any warning of a potentially negative outcome.

The counseling process has been referred to as a specialized form of family counseling. However, two factors make genetic counseling a unique process. First, there is the total lack of preparation and anticipatory grief. Even with the knowledge of a potentially negative outcome, a certain amount of hope and denial usually prevails until the birth of the affected child brings the family back to reality. Second, the parents' knowledge that they are biologically responsible for their child's condition is a burden often too heavy to carry without emotional damage. The physical contact with that person, sometimes for a lifetime, is a constant reminder of what may be perceived as "reproductive failure" and "bad seed."

For these reasons, a strong medical-psychological-spiritual support system is essential. These forms of support are usually available to the client through diverse sources. Medical and client care issues are covered by the health care professionals, such as nurses and physicians. The nurse is often in a position to offer initial and ongoing support. Emotional support is provided by family members, counselors, social workers, or even through question-and-answer columns in daily newspapers and on the Internet. Spiritual, religious, and ethical support may be received from a hospital chaplain or family clergy. Unfortunately, in many instances, the helping efforts of these three areas function independently from one another and in an uncoordinated manner. Efforts should be made to ensure effective communication among the services provided by professionals in these three areas. Since no health care provider alone can provide all needed services, the best approach to genetic counseling is a team approach. Members of the team should include a generalist

Critical Thinking

So You Want to be Part of a Genetic Team?

Until the mid-70s, the field of medical genetics was exclusively in the hands of physicians who did not have a formal education in genetics. Most medical geneticists of the time were self-taught and came from a medical specialty: most were pediatricians (who saw several cases of the same genetic disorder and became interested experts), obstetricians (after observing a recurrent birth defect or fetal loss), endocrinologists (who may have been repeatedly consulted for delayed puberty), and family physicians. Medical genetics was taught in the medical curricula not in comprehensive courses, but as part of specific body systems.

In 1981, the American Society of Human Genetics instituted a Medical Genetics Board with certification in several specialties: M.D. clinical geneticist, Ph.D. medical geneticist, clinical cytogeneticist, or biochemical geneticist, all required clinical or research doctorates. Genetic counselor was the only entry point for a master's-degree prepared genetic counselor. Nurses, at first hesitant in undertaking an activity for which they were not originally trained, soon became invaluable members of medical genetics teams. Several programs in genetic counseling soon followed the pioneer efforts at Sarah Lawrence University.

If you want to know more about applying nursing skills and technology to medical genetics and genetic counseling, visit the Genetics Society of America/American Association for Human Genetics WebPage or the University of Kansas Medical Center WebPage. Another excellent resource is the Creighton University's International Society of Nurses in Genetics (ISONG) website, which contains useful genetics-related hyperlinks (see Resources).

physician, geneticist, medical specialist, nurse, psychologist (psychiatrist, clinical social worker, or therapist), and clergy.

Typically, the genetic counseling process begins when a clinician refers a family in which a genetic disease has been identified. It is important at this point to have a conclusive diagnosis of the condition, as many errors in genetics counseling are a result of mistaken or incomplete diagnoses. Provided with this information, a member of the genetic counseling team (GCT) contacts the family and describes the process that is about to begin. The parents should be informed that they need to collect data about their family, such as previous disease cases, causes of death, degree of closeness of relationships (e.g., consanguinity), and how to secure medical records. In small communities, especially in traditional rural cultures, a family Bible is often a good source of information.

In the first personal interview, the GCT gathers pertinent information from family members. Once a detailed **pedigree chart** is generated, the GCT identifies the mode of inheritance and confirms the initial diagnosis. Testing of other family members, if recommended, is initiated at this time, and a second appointment is made. It is important in the first contact that the family members be made to feel at ease, and that ample time be allotted for answering all questions. In the second interview, with all the previous information processed, the GCT discusses with the family all the implications of the findings, presents options, and clarifies possible outcomes. Team members should be prepared to handle ethical and religious issues that often surface, such as the possibility of therapeutic abortion or sterilization, in a sensitive and caring manner. It is of paramount importance that genetic counseling remain a nondirective process, with the GCT members refraining from pressuring family members in any possible direction and remaining supportive but neutral about decisions that must be made. At times, this may present a challenge to a health care provider who feels that he or she has the correct answers and that the family is mistaken about the decision they have made. It must be remembered that the family members are the ones who will have to live with their decision, and therefore their decision, once made, must be respected and supported by all health care team members.

Prenatal Diagnosis

One of the commonly used tools in genetic counseling is prenatal diagnosis of genetic disorders. Several approaches for prenatal diagnosis have been developed: screening procedures include a trisomy profile test and a ultrasound-assisted nuchal translucence test. The two main diagnostic procedures are midtrimester amniocentesis and chorionic villi sampling (CVS). In addition, routine ultra-

Critical Thinking

Genetic Counseling Situation

Mrs. B. presents to the emergency service with a broken tibia, the result of a fall. While taking a medical history, the nurse discovers that Mrs. B. is 12 weeks into her fifth pregnancy. The nurse finds out further that, of the previous children, three have osteogenesis imperfecta (OI), as has Mr. B. The nurse calls for an obstetric consult and places the hospital chaplain on alert. The obstetric resident discovers that Mrs. B. is well-informed about OI, its mode of inheritance, and the risk for this pregnancy. Apparently all of the children are in good shape, as is Mr. B., and the disease seems to present no major concerns to them. However, the resident feels that it is his duty to offer to Mrs. B. a therapeutic abortion and tubal ligation. Mrs. B. refuses both suggestions on the basis of her religious beliefs. The resident is convinced that Mrs. B. is making the wrong decision and presents forceful arguments, accompanied by color photographs of people with severe OI. Mrs. B. is unmoved. The hospital chaplain is called into consultation and, after a long interview, concurs that Mrs. B. is making a well-informed decision that is based on her strong religious convictions. Mrs. B. returns to her small rural community. The obstetrics department is later informed in a follow-up letter from the local physician that Mrs. B. has delivered her fifth child, the fourth to be born with OI.

Do you think that the obstetric resident should have been more forceful and tried to convince Mrs. B. to have an abortion and a tubal ligation? Would you be able to accept Mrs. B.'s decision, given the severity of this disease?

sonography provides invaluable information in a noninvasive manner.

Trisomy Profile Test

It has been known since 1984 that maternal serum **alpha-fetoprotein** (MSAFP) levels are, on the average, lower in pregnancies affected by Down syndrome compared with levels in a normal pregnancy. The accuracy of the test was later increased by taking into consideration maternal age. In 1987, it was discovered that maternal serum levels of human chorionic gonadotropin (hCG) were twice as high in Down syndrome pregnancies during the second trimester. In addition, unconjugated estrogen (uE_3) levels

in maternal serum were found to be 25% lower in the presence of a Down syndrome pregnancy. The trisomy profile maternal serum test presently includes maternal age, MSAFP, hCG, and uE_3 and has a high rate of identification of common chromosome disorders.

Nuchal Translucency on Intravaginal Ultrasonography

This high-resolution ultrasonography is being used more and more often to detect increased nuchal translucency, as an indicator of Down syndrome. An increased nuchal translucency or the presence of cystic hygromas (septated, fluid-filled sacs in the nuchal region) are common features of several fetal aneuploidy conditions, including the common trisomies 13, 18, and 21. The sensitivity of this test for these trisomies combined is approximately 62%, and for trisomy 21 alone, 54%. (Taipale, Hiilesmaa, Salonen, & Ylostalo, 1997) The procedure can be performed earlier in the pregnancy than serum screening, and it may decrease the need for future CVS or amniocentesis.

Midtrimester Amniocentesis

This method was applied for the first time for diagnosis of genetic disorders in the early 1960s and has been widely used since then. The procedure is commonly performed between the 14th and 16th weeks of gestation, under ultrasound guidance, and consists of transabdominally withdrawing approximately 20 mL of amniotic fluid for analysis of cells sloughed off by the developing embryo. The material obtained is then cultured to obtain a large number of cells. Two basic sets of tests are performed: chromosome analysis and biochemical analysis of the fluid (e.g., alpha-fetoprotein measurements for the assessment of neural tube defects) or cell products (e.g., hexosaminidase A determinations for the diagnosis of Tay-Sachs disease). The high accuracy of amniocentesis in detecting chromosomal and biochemical defects has been well-established. However, one serious concern still remains: since the test is run as late as the 16th (and sometimes the 17th) week of pregnancy, the results are often returned at a quite advanced phase of pregnancy, making the possibility of a late therapeutic abortion an issue of ethical and medical concern. Potential sources of error include the mistaken analysis of maternal cells (but only if the embryo is female) or when mosaicism masks the presence of aneuploid cells. However, if a sufficient number of cells is studied, the abnormal cells eventually are detected. The risks involved in this procedure are small but measurable, at approximately 0.5%, and include risks for the developing embryo (needle perforations and scratches), for the continuation of the pregnancy ("spontaneous" abortions), and for the mother (immunologic cross-reactions) (Jorde et al., 1998). However small the risk, this is an invasive procedure that should be used only after careful consideration. Indications for amniocentesis include: maternal age above 35; previous history of chromosomal abnormalities; family history of genetic disorders that can be diagnosed by amniocentesis; and an increased risk of neural tube defect.

Chorionic Villi Sampling (CVS)

This recently developed prenatal diagnosis technique is rapidly replacing the traditional midtrimester amniocentesis, mostly because it can be performed at an earlier time (usually 9th to 12th week), yields results sooner, and its safety approaches that of the midtrimester test. The test is accurate in 99% of the cases, provided true chorionic villi material is obtained. One major disadvantage of CVS is that alpha-fetoprotein determination for detection of neural tube defects cannot be obtained and must be attempted at a later date, when the concentration of this substance increases.

NURSING IMPLICATIONS

One of the most important advances in biomedical science is the mapping of the human genome. This project has the potential to make dramatic changes in all health care and certainly will affect the care of women and infants. Apart from a few genetic disorders that have a direct expression in disease, the majority of genetic information is more complex and, in many cases, a genetic predisposition to a disease interacts with environmental conditions for expression. The latter has the most implications for nurses because of the need to teach environmental modification through lifestyle modification, risk avoidance, and health management.

The nurse is likely to interact with the client and family in a number of ways related to genetics. The involvement can vary depending on setting and level of education.

Web Activities

- Visit the University of Indiana biotechnology website at http://biotech.chem.indiana.edu for an excellent basic review of general principles of genetics and molecular biology.

- Visit the March of Dimes website at http://modimes.org and explore the various resources available to families and health care professionals about birth defects.

- Visit the Cytogenetics Gallery at the University of Washington (Seattle) website at http://www.pathology.washington.edu/Cytogallery and explore different karyotypes and their association with disease processes and clinical manifestations.

- Visit the Genetic Alliance website at http://www.geneticalliance.org and use this resource to guide a family with a genetic disorder.

- Visit the National Institutes of Health, Office of Rare Diseases, at http://rarediseases.info.nih.gov/ord/patient-support.html to connect with various resources that assist you in understanding the management of genetic disorders.

- Visit the National Human Genome Research Institute home page at http://www.nhgri.nih.gov and engage in a discussion on "How to Conquer a Genetic Disease."

- Visit the Human Genome Project Information website at http://ornl.gov/hgmis and participate in ethical, legal and social debates on applications of the Human Genome Project. Communicate with experts and peers in a chat room.

- Visit the Med Help International website at http://medhelp.org to retrieve a list of support organizations to assist families with genetic disorders.

- Visit the Journal of Gene Therapy website (England) at http://www.wiley.co.uk/genetherapy/ for the latest information on various approaches to the treatment of genetic disease using gene therapy technology.

- Visit the Center for Bioethics, University of Pennsylvania website at http://med.upenn.edu/~bioethic to review articles on discrimination, privacy, and other ethical issues in genetic screening.

The staff nurse should have a general knowledge of genetics and genetic terminology to answer client questions and direct them to resources. There are major implications in supporting couples in reproductive decision making and in coping with potential genetic risks. Additionally, nurses may be in the position to provide education and support for risk management for clients who have their own genetic risk factors, such as breast cancer.

Nurses in advanced practice may function as genetic counselors, provided they have appropriate education in genetics and counseling. They may also work in birth-defect clinics and provide risk screening for normal prenatal or high-risk populations. Advanced practice nurses also are in a position to screen their clients for genetic conditions, even if the appropriate management would include referral to another member of the health care team.

All nurses need to have read and learned from current literature related to genetic information and to be able to provide information to clients about rapidly changing information and technology related to this field. Nurses in any area of practice are likely to be faced with ethical issues regarding the advancing knowledge of genetics. Each new discovery in genetics raises questions about who should have genetic information about individuals and families. Who should be treated for genetic conditions? When should treatment be given and what should be treated? What treatment is appropriate? These questions must be answered. As new treatments evolve, the cost concerns regarding distribution of scarce resources becomes an issue that must be addressed.

Key Concepts

- An alteration in a single gene may cause multiple physical and mental derangements without changing the gross structure of a chromosome, or altering the total chromosome number of an individual. Therefore, genetic disorders may be classified under gene disorders and chromosome abnormalities.

- Structural genes encode genetic information for the synthesis of enzymes. A mutation in one gene may result in the synthesis of an abnormal enzyme, thus interrupting a metabolic pathway and causing a genetic syndrome. Many genetic syndromes are single-gene (Mendelian) disorders.

- Many genes often cooperate to create or modify a given phenotype. Many human characteristics follow this polygenic inheritance pattern.

- Chromosomal abnormalities may result from alterations in individual chromosomes (structural abnormalities) or from alterations in the total number of chromosomes (numerical abnormalities). Either situation may cause significant phenotypic alterations and pathologic conditions.

- Genetic screening is the process by which individuals or populations can be assessed for various genetic disorders to detect the presence of a gene before it expresses as a genetic disease or to identify the carrier of a recessive trait.

- Many genetic disorders are not treatable with conventional techniques. In many instances, the prevention of a genetic disease is only possible through genetic counseling of persons at risk.

Review Questions and Activities

1. The parents of a newborn with Down syndrome (DS) inquire about what could have caused this abnormality. One of the following responses is *not* appropriate:
   a. DS was caused by an accidental chromosomal nondisjunction.
   b. DS is an inborn error of metabolism.
   c. DS is a rare event for the age group of these parents.
   d. DS in this child could have been identified by prenatal chromosome analysis.

   The correct answer is b.

2. The same parents are concerned about the possibility of having other children with DS. What correct information can be conveyed to them?
   a. Free trisomy 21 is not inheritable and therefore is unlikely to recur.
   b. Future pregnancies may be tested prenatally.
   c. Free trisomy is hereditary, and the recurrence risk for future pregnancies is high.
   d. Both *a* and *b* are correct.
   e. Both *b* and *c* are correct.

   The correct answer is d.

3. The parents of a newborn with phenylketonuria (PKU) ask what PKU means. One of the following is *not* a correct response to their question:
   a. PKU is an enzyme deficiency resulting in the inability to metabolize phenylalanine.
   b. PKU is an inborn error of metabolism.
   c. PKU results from a chromosomal abnormality called nondisjunction.
   d. PKU is transmitted as an autosomal recessive disorder.

   The correct answer is c.

4. What information should the same parents be given about the consequences of PKU?
   a. High dietary levels of phenylalanine may help induce enzyme production.
   b. PKU is commonly associated with other congenital anomalies.
   c. Failure to avoid dietary phenylalanine results in progressive mental retardation.
   d. Mental retardation is inevitable.

   The correct answer is c.

5. A woman is heterozygous for an *autosomal dominant* disease. If she mates with a normal man, what are the chances of the coupling producing an affected child in any pregnancy?
   a. 1:4
   b. 1:2
   c. 1:400 (1/10 × 1/10 × 1/4 = 1/400)
   d. No risk, since she is a carrier and he is not.

   The correct answer is b.

6. Three siblings have a *rare autosomal recessive* disease. Both parents are clinically normal. Which of the following statements apply?
   a. Both parents are homozygous for the normal allele.
   b. Both parents are homozygous for the defective allele.
   c. All three children are homozygous for the defective allele.
   d. All three children are heterozygous.

   The correct answer is c.

7. The term "autosomal recessive" refers to the mode of inheritance of a disorder:
   a. That is always expressed in heterozygotes.
   b. Whose causative gene is located on an autosome.
   c. That is always present at birth.
   d. That cannot be transmitted from mother to son.

   The correct answer is b.

8. Choose the correct statement about the carrier state:
   a. The son of a mother with hemophilia has a 50% chance of being a carrier.
   b. The son of a woman with achondroplasia has a 50% chance of being a carrier.
   c. The son of a man with achondroplasia has a 50% chance of being a carrier.
   d. None of the above statements is correct.

   The correct answer is d.

9. The son of a man with Y-linked hairy ears marries the daughter of a man with the same condition.
   a. All their children will have hairy ears.
   b. All their boys will have hairy ears.
   c. None of their children will have hairy ears.
   d. Half of their boys will have hairy ears.

   The correct answer is b.

10. If a man who is affected with an X-linked recessive disorder marries a woman who is phenotypically and genotypically normal,
   a. All his sons will be carriers.
   b. All his daughters will be carriers.
   c. Half his sons will be carriers.
   d. Half his daughters will be carriers.

   The correct answer is b.

References

Beadle, G. W., and Tatum, E. L. (1941). Genetic control of biochemical reactions in *Neurospora. Proc Natl Acad Sci U.S., 27,* 499–506.

Borgaonkar, D. S., and Shah, S. A. (1974). The XYY chromosome male or syndrome? In, A. G. Steinberg and A. G. Bearn (eds), *Progress in medical genetics,* vol X, pp 135–222, New York; Grune & Stratton.

Cox, T. M., & Sinclair, J. (Eds.) (1997) *Molecular biology in medicine.* Boston: Blackwell Scientific.

Cystic Fibrosis "GAP" Conference Report. (1975). *Problems in reproductive physiology and anatomy in young adults with cystic fibrosis.* Atlanta: Cystic Fibrosis Foundation.

Ferri, F. F. (1999). *Ferri's clinical advisor: Instant diagnosis and treatment.* St. Louis: Mosby.

Gabow, P. (1993). Medical progress: Autosomal dominant polycystic kidney disease. *New England Journal of Medicine, 329,* 332–342.

Garrod, A. E. (1902). The incidence of alkaptonuria: A study in chemical individuality. *Lancet, 2,* 1616.

Gelehrter, T. D., Collins, F. S., & Ginsburg, D. (1998). *Principles of medical genetics.* (2nd ed.). Philadelphia: Lippincott, Williams & Wilkins.

Godfry, M. (1993). The Marfan Syndrome. In, P. Beighton (ed.) *McKusick's Heritable Disorders of Connective Tissue,* 5th ed. pp. 51–123, St. Louis; Mosby-Yearbook.

Ingram, V. M. (1956). A specific chemical difference between the globins of normal and sickle-cell anemia hemoglobins. *Nature* 178, 792–794.

Jorde, L. B., Carey, J. C., Bamshad, M. J., & White, R. L. (1998). *Medical genetics.* (2nd ed.) St. Louis: Mosby.

Korf, B. R. (1996). *Human genetics: A problem-based approach.* Cambridge, MA: Blackwell Science.

Online Mendelian inheritance in man, OMIM. McKusick-Nathans Institute for Genetic Medicine, Johns Hopkins University, Baltimore, MD, and National Center for Biotechnology Information, National Library of Medicine, Bethesda, MD, 2000.

Pagana, K. D., & Pagana, T. J. (1999). *Diagnostic testing and nursing implications: A case study approach.* St. Louis: Mosby-Year Book.

Pauling, L., Itano, H., Singer, S. J., & Wells, I. C. (1949). Sickle cell anemia, a molecular disease. *Science,* 110, 543–548.

Seashore, M. R., & Wappner, R. S. (1996). *Genetics in primary care and clinical medicine.* Stamford, CT: Appleton & Lange.

Simpson, J. L., & Golbus, M. S. (1992). *Genetics in obstetrics and gynecology* (2nd ed.). Philadelphia: W. B. Saunders.

Taipale, P., Hiilesmaa, V., Salonen, R., & Ylostalo, P. (1997). Increased nuchal translucency as a marker for fetal chromosomal defects. *New England Journal of Medicine,* 337, 1654–1658.

Suggested Readings

Clarke, A. (Ed). (1994). *Genetic counselling practice and principles.* New York: Rutledge.

Clarke, J. T. R. (1996). *A clinical guide to inherited metabolic diseases.* New York: Cambridge University Press.

Connor, J. M., & Ferguson-Smith, M. A. (1997). *Essential medical genetics* (5th ed.). Boston: Blackwell Science.

Drilica, K. (1997). *Understanding DNA and gene cloning: A guide for the curious* (3rd ed.). New York: John Wiley & Sons.

Fuller, G. M. & Shields, D. (1998). *Molecular basis of medical cell biology.* Stamford, CT: Appleton & Lange.

Godfrey, M. (1993). The Marfan syndrome. In P. Beighton (ed.), *McKusick's heritable disorders of connective tissue* (5th ed.). St. Louis: Mosby-Year Book.

Jones, K. L. (1997). *Smith's recognizable patterns of human malformation* (5th ed.). Philadelphia: Saunders.

King, R. A., Rotter, J. I., & Motulsky, A. G. (Eds.). (1992). *The genetic basis of common diseases.* New York: Oxford.

King, R. C., & Stansfield, W. D. (1997). *A dictionary of genetics* (5th ed.). New York: Oxford University Press.

McKusic, V. A. (2000). *Mendelian inheritance in man. Catalogs of human genes and genetic disorders* (12th ed.). Baltimore: Johns Hopkins University Press.

Pawlowitzki, I.-H., Edwards, J. H., & Thompson, E. A. (Eds.). (1997). *Genetic mapping of disease genes.* New York: Academic Press.

Robertson, J. A. (1994). *Children of choice: Freedom and the new reproductive technologies.* Princeton, MA: Princeton University Press.

Schardein, J. L. (2000). *Chemically induced birth defects* (3rd ed.). New York: Marcel Dekker.

Scriver, A. L. (Ed.). (2000). *The metabolic basis of inherited human diseases* (8th ed.). New York: McGraw-Hill.

Simpson, J. L., & Elias, S. (1993). *Essentials of prenatal diagnosis.* New York: Churchill Livingstone.

Snustad, D. P., Simmons, M. J., & Jenkins, J. B. (1997). *Principles of genetics.* New York: John Wiley & Sons.

Strachan, T., & Read, A. P. (1996). *Human molecular genetics.* New York: John Wiley & Sons.

Trent, R.J. (1997). *Molecular medicine: An introductory text.* New York: Churchill & Livingstone.

Resources

Classic papers in genetics, articles by Mendel, Garrod, Hardy, and others: http://www.gdb.org/rjr/history.html

Creighton University, International Society of Nurses in Genetics (ISONG): http://nursing.creighton.edu/isong/

Genetics Society of America/American Association for Human Genetics: http://www.faseb.org/genetics/gsa/careeres/bro-menu/htm

Glossary of genetic terms: http://helios.bto.ed.ac.uk/bto/glossary/

Human Genome Project (general information): http://www.ornl.gov/TechResources/Human Genome/home.html

Mendelian (after Gregor Mendel) inheritance rules and facts http://www.netspace.org/MendelWeb/MWolby.intro.html

McKusick's *Online Mendelian Inheritance in Man (OMIM),* a catalog of single-gene disorders (2000), http://www.ncbi.nlm.nih.gov/omim/

OMIM, Updated Statistics, http://www.ncbi.nlm.nih.gov/Omim/Stats/mimstats.html

Online Mendelian Inheritance in Man, OMIM (TM). McKusick-Nathans Institute for Genetic Medicine, Johns Hopkins University (Baltimore, MD) and National Center for Biotechnology Information, National Library of Medicine (Bethesda, MD), 2000, http://www.ncbi.nlm.nih.gov/omim/

Online Mendelian Inheritance in Man (OMIM), http://www3.ncbi.nlm.nih.gov/Omim/searchomim.html

National Institutes of Health gene sequencing databases, http://www.ncbi.nlm.nih.gov/BLAST/

The University of Kansas Medical Center, http://www.kumc.edy/GEC/

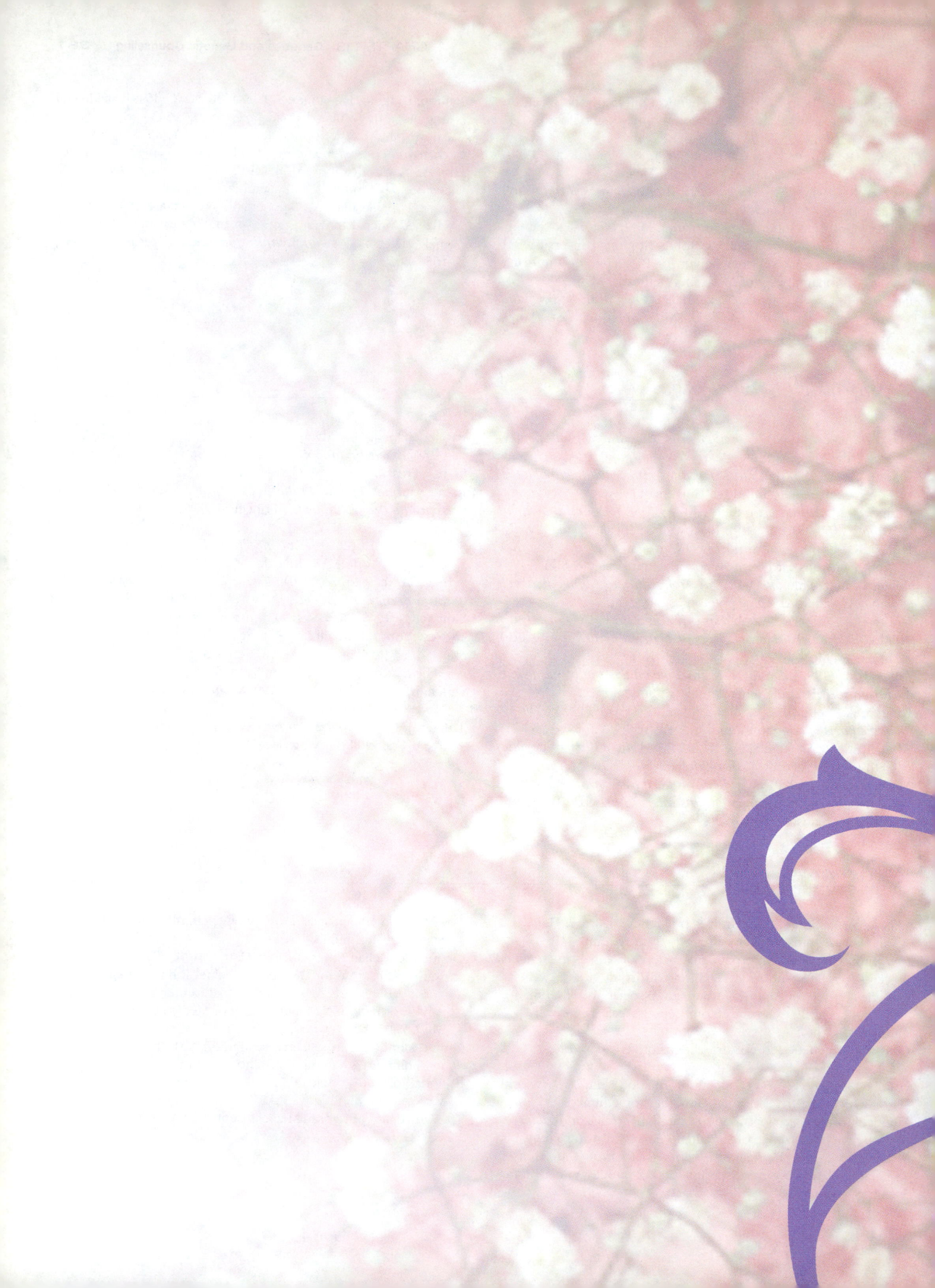

CHAPTER 14

Family Planning

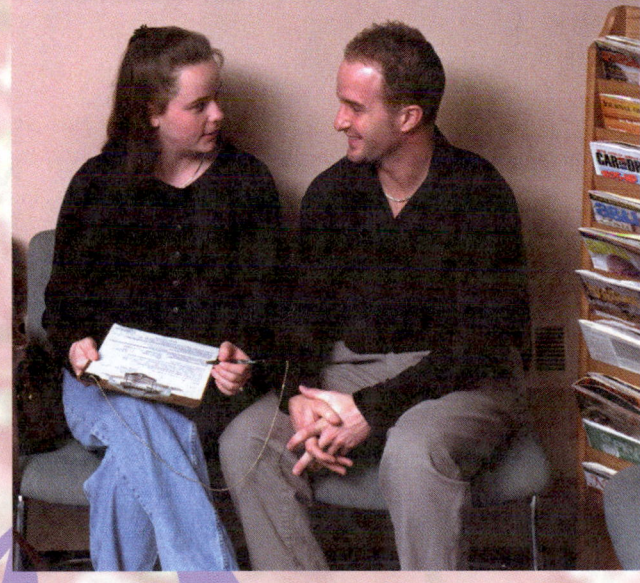

he nurse often is viewed by the public as a person who has vast medical knowledge and is capable of communicating that knowledge in lay terms that are easily understood. Questions that arise vary from simple to complex. How would you answer the following questions?

- *What is the difference in action of combined oral contraceptives and progestin-only contraceptives?*

- *How would you counsel an adolescent about contraception who is sexually active but insists that her parents must not know of her decision to be sexually active or to use contraceptives?*

- *What would you say to the 50-year-old woman who asks if she needs to use a contraceptive method?*

Key Terms

Abortion	Emergency	Injectable contraception	Tubal ligation
Cervical cap	contraception	Ovulation prediction	Vaginal ring
Coitus interruptus	Family planning	Sperm capacitation	Vasectomy
Contraception	Implantable	Spermicide	
Diaphragm	contraception	Sterilization	

Competencies

Upon completion of this chapter, the reader should be able to:

1. Discuss the currently available methods of contraception.
2. Identify the risks and benefits of each form of contraceptive device.
3. Discuss the mechanism of action of each form of contraception.
4. Describe the steps in successful reproductive decision-making.
5. Describe some of the implications of an unplanned and unwanted pregnancy.
6. Use the nursing process to determine a client's need for contraception.

amily **planning** involves cognitive decisions and behavioral practices that enable a woman to conceive a wanted pregnancy and avoid an unwanted or a badly timed pregnancy. Family planning decisions are complex and may be made by the woman, her partner, or the couple in cooperation. These decisions are made in a number of ways.

Each year in the United States, 49% of pregnancies are unintended (Dailard, 2000). The unintended pregnancy rate is approximately 3.5 million pregnancies per year in the United States (La Valleur, 2000). A pregnancy may occur at a time in a woman's life that she recognizes is inappropriate for having a child. Many of these unplanned and badly timed pregnancies involve women under aged 20 years. This chapter prepares the nurse to assist women of childbearing age in many different settings to adapt and identify their health care needs regarding how many children they will have and the timing of having children.

In this chapter, reproductive decision-making is discussed as are currently available methods of contraception and nursing care to meet the health care needs of women of childbearing age. For the nurse, an understanding of reproductive decision-making is important because many times women do not recognize choices they have. Understanding there is a choice is necessary before the woman can determine if she wants a method of contraception and which method is best for her.

REPRODUCTIVE DECISION-MAKING

In nearly every situation in life, one has choices about the actions one takes. Many of the choices have such obvious negative consequences that they are quickly eliminated and thus it may appear as if there are no choices. For example, every student has a choice to refuse to turn in required course work, take examinations, or attend classes. Most students do not consider these options viable choices because the consequences generally are undesirable.

In reproductive decision-making, **contraception**, or prevention of pregnancy, often is the topic for which couples will seek information. Interestingly, despite the fact that choosing a contraception method often is a decision made jointly by couples, little is known about how men and women differ in this regard. Grady, Klepinger, and Nelson-Wally (1999) found that women ranked pregnancy prevention as the most important factor and ranked the health risks associated with the method and protection from sexually transmitted diseases (STDs) second. By contrast, men considered protection from STDs as the most important factor. It is likely that women make most decisions regarding reproduction because the direct consequences of pregnancy have the greatest impact on women.

Ideally, reproductive decision-making is a rational process based on the premise that human beings are agents with free will. Nurses need to honor the choices of

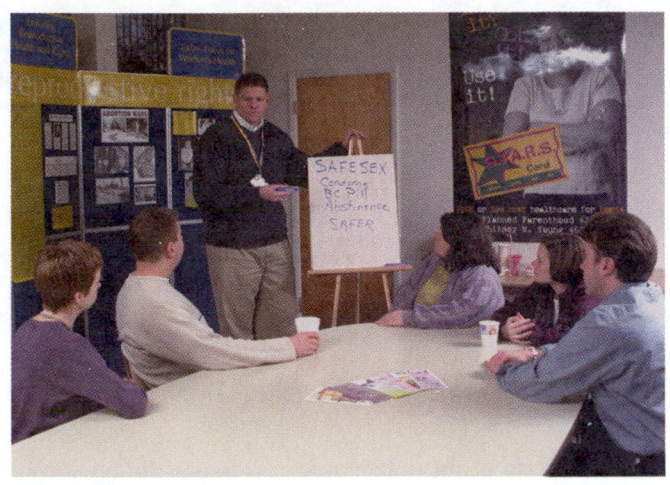

Figure 14-1 Rational decision-making in family planning is based on having accurate information about various options and their associated risks and benefits.

their clients and become aware of their personal values. This awareness is helpful so that the nurse does not impose personal values on clients. Rational decision-making is a logical process based on accurate information. A rational approach allows for an active rather than a passive approach to decision-making. An active approach involves projective planning in which individuals assess the situation; consider available options; and examine the risks, benefits, and consequences of various options (Figure 14-1). Box 14-1 identifies the steps in this process.

Factors Affecting Reproductive Choices

Although the rational process appears straightforward, in reality, decision-making is complex. In a study of 800 women, 75% changed methods at least once and reported

Box 14-1 Steps in Rational Decision-Making

- Recognize that there is a decision to be made and identify the problem.
- Seek information about options for problem resolution.
- Evaluate the options based on risks, benefits, and feasibility.
- Select the most acceptable option.
- Develop a realistic plan to implement the option.
- Implement the option.
- Evaluate the plan and make revisions or adaptations to resolve obstacles.

1,889 method choices and gave 1,036 reasons for changing (Matteson & Hawkins, 1997). In another study that examined prenatal contraceptive decision-making with postpartum behavior, only 54% of women planning to use oral contraceptives actually used them and 31% of women planning to use condoms used them (Miller et al., 2000). Psychological factors, sociocultural factors, and spiritual and religious beliefs and values influence choices. Many women find themselves with unintended pregnancies because they were passive and made no decision. Reproductive decision-making can be life altering and is an area in which nurses often are engaged with clients in helping to make these decisions.

Psychological Influences

Reproductive decisions often are influenced by feelings about one's self. For example, a young man may feel his self-concept is enhanced by performance in sexual activity. A young woman may feel that achieving pregnancy enhances her self-esteem. Sometimes women may agree to sexual activity to satisfy a sense of belonging, to feel needed, or to feel important. The accompanying emotional issues involving sexuality and relationships may cloud a logical process.

In their study of female psychology, Gilligan, Ward, & Taylor (1988) found that girls make decisions based on relationships rather than by using an objective, purely rational process. The importance of the role of attachment and connection in young girl's decision-making is reiterated over multiple studies, which may help to understand the gender differences in reproductive decision-making. Ironically, the use of contraception is lower in couples who have just met than in couples with an established relationship. In a study of sexually active females under 18 years of age, 52% who had just met their sexual partner used no method compared with 24% who were going steady (Manning, Longmore, & Giordano, 2000). Adolescent girls who first had sex with a man 6 or more years older than they had an even greater decreased rate of practicing contraception.

Pender's (1996) Health Promotion model specifies personal and experiential factors as strong predictors for health-promoting behaviors. Pender also identifies a client's perceptions about the benefits and barriers to a health-related behavior as core areas of intervention. A sense of *self-efficacy,* or judgment about personal capability to execute actions, is another psychological aspect of health behaviors.

Sociocultural Influences

The immediate social situation or social group greatly influences reproductive decision-making. Decisions often reflect the patterns of one's immediate social group. Pender

(1996) identified family, peers, providers, norms, support and models, and the situational influences as important contributors to client behavior. Cultural values regarding sexuality and gender roles, the power dimensions of adolescent's lives, and economic disadvantage exert powerful influences on decision-making (Gage, 1998). Adolescents, in particular, are influenced by peer pressure and may subject themselves to unprotected intercourse through the belief that everyone does it. The peer group also may influence the adolescent girl if the group regards the use of contraception as a label of sexual activity, thus dissuading the use of planned contraception. With these pressures, she may not consider the consequences, weigh the options, or consider her own needs and aspirations. Oddens (1997) found that contraceptive use was principally determined by social influences, attitudes, and self-efficacy.

Social circumstances are significant in making decisions regarding reproductive actions. For example, a woman with little money may not be able to afford to purchase contraceptives. A homeless woman may not use contraceptives because it is inconvenient and she has nowhere to keep them to have available when needed. A woman also may agree to sexual intercourse through the influence of romantic surroundings and a persuasive partner.

Cultural beliefs, values, and customs structure gender roles and reproductive behavior. It is important for nurses to understand the client's cultural beliefs about the acceptable age of childbearing, marriage requirements, how the father is chosen, spacing of pregnancies, and health behaviors during pregnancy. The general culture influences behavior through movies, music, and other media. Exposure of young children to explicit sexual activity has resulted in increasingly younger children acting and dressing as adults. Some have speculated that this exposure contributes to early sexual activity in adolescents.

Spiritual and Religious Influences

Spiritual and religious beliefs impact reproductive decision-making. Many belief systems condone sexual activity only within marriage, and some view sexual activity only for the express purpose of procreation. In other systems, sexual intimacy between a couple may be viewed as being sacred. The Roman Catholic Church, for example, does not condone the use of most contraceptives or abortion. The only acceptable method is natural family planning. For Muslims, although contraception is acceptable, there may be religious objections to abortion.

Readiness for Decision-Making

Honoring the client's need to make the best decision for herself, while providing the best information and facilitat-

CLINICAL ASSESSMENT OF REPRODUCTIVE DECISION-MAKING

- Is the client free to make a choice?
- Is the client competent to make a choice?
- Does the client recognize situations in which she has a choice?
- Does the client have adequate knowledge to make an informed choice?
- Can the client reasonably implement the choice? What are the barriers or obstacles to using this contraceptive method?

ing the rational decision-making process, is best achieved through a process of shared decision-making. This process is increasingly advocated as the ideal model for the medical encounter and has the following characteristics: client and provider are 1) both involved, 2) share information, 3) build consensus regarding the plan, and 4) reach an agreement on implementation (Charles, Gafini, & Whelan, 1997).

Freedom to Make Choices

Rational decision-making is based on the premise that clients are agents with free will to make choices; however, in reality, not all clients are free to make choices. Women who are victims of rape or sexual violence have had their freedom compromised. In some states, minors are not free to obtain contraceptive methods or abortion without parental consent. In other states, minors seeking medical care, including contraceptive information, methods, and in some cases abortions, are considered emancipated minors. Thus, health care providers can legally provide services without parental notification, approval, or consent. Nurses need to be aware of institutional policies and state practice regulations.

Many health care providers assume that the woman is free to make reproductive decisions independently; however, in many cultures this is not the case. The decisions regarding children and contraception reside with the husband, are shared between husband and wife, or involve the entire extended family.

Competence to Make Choices

Cognitive skills of abstract thinking are necessary to contemplate the risks, benefits, and consequences of various options. Persons without these skills need special consideration, and the health care provider may need to take more responsibility in the decision-making process to find a responsible party to make decisions. Young adolescents may not have developed abstract thinking and the ability to project into the future to process the potential consequences of sexual intimacy. In these cases, nursing interventions may need to facilitate the development of these skills and the processing of projecting the consequences of choices.

Recognition of Decision Points

Decisions are more likely to be reactive or passive, and therefore not reasoned, when the client is unaware that she is at a decision point or that options are possible. One nursing intervention may be simply to make the client aware that she has an opportunity for choices. For example, a young girl may not recognize that she can refuse to have intercourse unless her boyfriend uses a condom. Closely related to the recognition of choice is being aware of options. For example, a woman cannot make a decision to use an emergency method of contraception after intercourse if she is unaware of that option.

Three decision points are relevant to contraceptive use: 1) sexual activity, 2) preventive contraception, and 3) emergency contraception. Differentiating these decision points may be useful in recognizing opportunities for choices.

Sexual Activity

Some women make generalized decisions about sexual activity. For example, a woman may decide to be abstinent until after marriage, or after finishing school, or until she gets a job. Another may feel that if she has a sexual encounter with a particular individual, then she has made a decision related to that relationship and no longer has choices as to whether she will have sexual relations with that person in the future. '

Choices about sexual activity often are not made proactively. Many women think that proactive decisions inhibit spontaneity. Women should recognize that they have choices regarding if, with whom, when, and where intercourse should occur. Each opportunity for intercourse is a decision point.

Preventative Contraception

Most contraceptive decisions are made to avoid or postpone pregnancy. In contrast, making a decision to have a baby is the most proactive approach. Some women do not use contraceptives because they feel they are not vulnerable to pregnancy because they are too old or too young. Many women fail to use contraception when they have sporadic sexual encounters or are not in a stable relationship. This is not a good rational decision because pregnancy can result from one sexual encounter and the chances for partner support are decreased.

Emergency Contraception

Postcoital contraception, also known as **emergency contraception**, is now available and includes pregnancy termination, morning-after contraception, and RU 486. Many women however are not aware of this availability. Because a postcoital method may be inconsistent with some belief systems, preventive contraception may be more appropriate.

Knowledge Level

Informed reproductive decision-making involves more than awareness of options; it requires accurate information regarding the risks, benefits, and consequences of each option. Informed reproductive decision-making includes weighing the risks, benefits, and consequences of not using contraception. This process allows the client to make a choice regarding the risk-benefit ratio with which she is comfortable. Knowledge of how to effectively use the contraceptive method also is important and needs to be considered (Figure 14-2). A survey by Fuchs, Prinz, & Koch (1996) found that most women are poorly informed about oral contraceptive use and are largely unaware of the important long-term noncontraceptive benefits.

Implementation of the Choice

The nurse also must be aware of contraindications and obstacles to use. In this process of information sharing, the

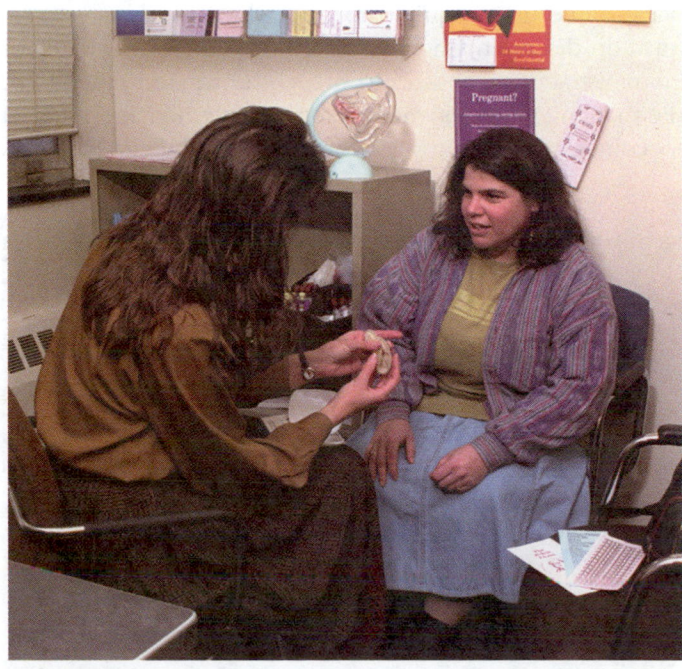

Figure 14-2 Clients must understand and return-demonstrate proper use of contraceptive devices to ensure their effectiveness.

nurse might share her knowledge of medical contraindications. For example, a woman with a history of thromboembolism should not take certain oral contraceptives. The client also might share her knowledge of potential obstacles to use. For example, an adolescent may be uncomfortable touching herself and thus would be a poor candidate for the female condom or many of the barrier methods.

Possible barriers and obstacles should be explored: Which actions on the part of the client are necessary to effectively use the chosen method? An adolescent without transportation may not be able to come to the clinic to get a monthly injection. When a teenager is living at home and believes her parents will not approve of contraception, a method that provides evidence for her parents to detect is not a good choice. A woman may choose condoms as her preferred method; however, if her partner refuses to use them, she needs to have an alternative plan. A woman may choose oral contraceptives but, in reality, cannot remember to take them regularly.

By assessing the decision-making process and the client's knowledge, the nurse can be more effective in facilitating satisfactory use of contraceptives. This interactive approach involving the client and family members as appropriate may promote greater effectiveness of contraceptive strategies.

CONTRACEPTIVE METHODS

Contraceptive methods currently available are either reversible or permanent (Figure 14-3). Reversible methods vary in the time required for reproductive capacity to return on discontinuance, and they vary in the frequency of administration necessary to prevent unwanted pregnancy. Permanent methods vary in regard to when the method becomes permanent. For example, oral contraceptives

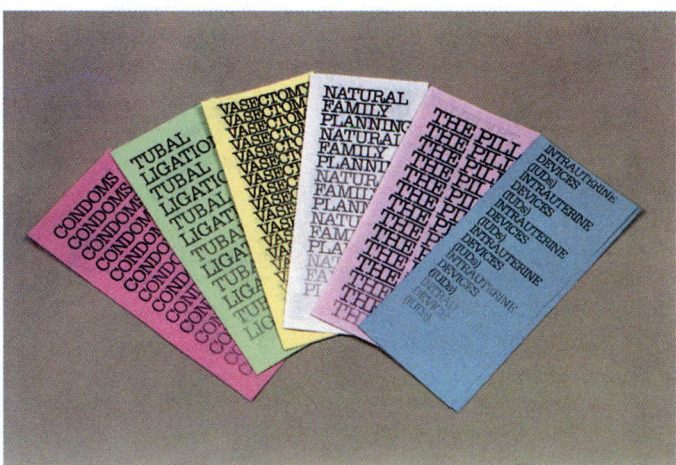

Figure 14-3 In addition to face-to-face teaching, clients should be offered printed information on family planning choices.

must be taken daily, whereas injectible methods may require monthly administration or action of the medication may last as long as 3 months, depending on the method chosen. An excellent example with regard to permanent methods is that the vasectomy is not considered permanent until follow-up sperm counts show that the count has approached or reached zero.

Reversible Methods

The numbers and kinds of reversible contraceptive methods is ever expanding. Each year several new products are marketed that are designed to refine those products already available or meet the needs of women who experience side effects.

Oral Methods

Oral methods of contraception include combined oral contraceptives and progestin-only contraceptives.

Combined Oral Contraceptives

Combined oral contraceptives have been available to women since the 1960s. The Food and Drug Administration approved this type of contraception in 1960 (Speroff & Darney, 1992). Approximately 60 million women worldwide have used combined oral contraceptives as a method of choice (Speroff & Darney, 1992).

There are three basic types of combined oral contraceptives (COC): monophasic, biphasic, and multiphasic pills. Monophasic COCs contain estrogen and progestin in the same dosage for 21 days of the menstrual cycle. If 28 pills are in the package, the remaining 7 pills may be inert or iron pills. Biphasic pills may have a stable dose of estrogen throughout the cycle and an increase in progesterone in the second half of the cycle, or the dosage of both hormones may change in the second half of the cycle. This type of COC was designed to alleviate problems some women have with breakthrough bleeding. Multiphasic COCs have three different dosages of estrogen and progesterone during the monthly cycle. This type of COC also was designed to alleviate the side effects and breakthrough bleeding some women experience with monophasic or biphasic COCs.

Pharmacology

Combined oral contraceptives are composed of steroids of the hormones estrogen and progesterone. Two types of estrogens have been used in the formulation of COCs. Mestranol was used in the pills having a higher dose when COCs initially were developed. It was determined, however, that mestranol was broken down to ethinyl estradiol before its use. In contemporary COCs, ethinyl estradiol is the only estrogen available in these preparations.

The net affect is that estrogen prevents breakthrough bleeding by potentiating the action of progestin, and enabling lower doses of progestin to be used for the same effect.

By contrast, progestin diminishes the release of leuteinizing hormone (LH) by the anterior pituitary gland. LH ordinarily is released in pulses, with a sharp increase in pulsatile action immediately before ovulation. In fact, a surge of LH is responsible for release of the mature ovum at the time of ovulation. Progestins make cervical mucous less receptive, making it impervious to sperm passage. Progestins make the endometrium less receptive to implantation. Progestins also influence secretions and peristalsis of the fallopian tubes, impeding mobility of the sperm and ovum.

Types of Combined Oral Contraceptives

Numerous preparations of COCs are sold by various pharmaceutical companies (Figure 14-4). Each year there are additional kinds of preparations added to the list. The wide variety of preparations meets individual needs and reduces undesired side effects or management problems. Table 14-1 contains some of the currently available preparations.

Efficacy

The combined oral contraceptive is the most effective reversible method available to women today. The failure rate is less than 1% (Jensen & Speroff, 2000).

Benefits and Risks

Combined oral contraceptives offer contraceptive benefits and noncontraceptive benefits. Both kinds of benefit make it to a woman's advantage to choose oral contraception. COCs are relatively inexpensive, safe, effective, and easy to use. Return to fertility is almost immediate on discontinuance of this method.

Contraceptive Benefits

Over the past 30 years, no drug has been as well studied as has the COC. Most women who use COCs do so for contraception. COCs are highly reliable. When used appropriately, COCs are more than 99% effective (Jensen & Speroff, 2000). Successful use of COCs is highly related to the woman's understanding about how the preparation works and compliance with certain practices. These practices are summarized in the Client Education Box.

Noncontraceptive Benefits

Combined oral contraceptives offer several important non-contraceptive benefits that reduce morbidity and mortality in women. The number of these recognized benefits has increased with data gathered from many women who have used COCs over many years (Burkman, 2001).

 Protection Against Ovarian Cancer Ovarian cancer is the fourth leading cause of cancer death in American women and has the highest mortality rate of any gynecologic cancer. Its onset is insidious. By the time of detection, ovarian cancer has metastasized in 60% of cases. There is a survival rate of 40% at 5 years for women treated for ovarian cancer.

When a woman has ever used them, COCs offer a 40% to 80% reduction in the risk for ovarian cancer (Burkman, 2001). The degree of protection increases with the length of use. A minimally protective effect is present with 3 to 6 months of use. The protective effects of COCs last at least 15 years after discontinuance. This reduction in risk is present in all four subtypes of ovarian cancer.

 Protection Against Endometrial Cancer The incidence of endometrial cancer is reduced by the use of COCs. Overall, studies suggest that there is a reduction in risk of 50% beginning approximately 1 year after initiation of use (Burkman, 2001). The reduction is apparent in all

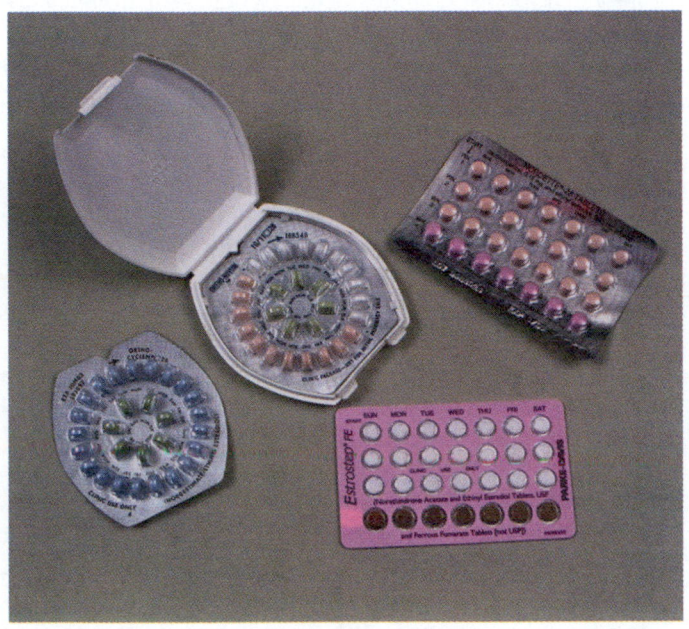

Figure 14-4 Birth control pills.

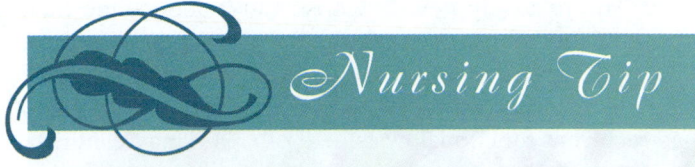

UNDERSTANDING COCs

Clients who are considering the use of combined oral contraceptives should have the benefit of information about mechanism of actions, benefits, risks, adverse effects, and contraindications to assist them in making their decision.

Table 14-1 Currently Available Combined Oral Contraceptives

Monophasic Preparations		Biphasic Preparations	Multiphasic Preparations
Brevicon	Norethin 1/35 E	Ortho-Novum 10/11	Jenest
Demulen	Norethin 1/50 M	Gracial	Ortho-Novum 7/7/7
Demulen 1/35	Norinyl 1 + 35	Jenest	Ortho Tri-Cyclen
Desogen	Norinyl 1 + 50		Tri-Levlen
Genora 1/35	Norlestrin 1/50		Tri-Norinyl
Genora 1/50	Ortho-Cept		Triphasil
Levlen	Ortho-Cyclen		Estrostep
Loestrin Fe 1.5/30	Ortho-Novum 1/35		Tricylcen
Loestrin Fe 1/20	Ortho-Novum 1/50		
Lo Ovral	Ovcon-35		
Modicon	Ovcon-50		
Nelova 1/35E	Ovral		
Nelova 0.5/35	Alesse		
Nordette	Mircette		

histologic subtypes of endometrial cancer. Protection lasts up to 15 years after discontinuance of the medication.

❧ *Reduction in Incidence of Salpingitis* Salpingitis has been reduced with the use of COCs. The mechanism of action is thought to be a chemical reaction in the woman's body that changes the cervical mucous and impedes ascent of infectious organisms. It has been estimated that a 50% reduction in hospital admissions for salpingitis can be attributed to COCs (Burkman, 2001).

❧ *Reduction in Incidence of Ectopic Pregnancy* Combined oral contraceptives have been given credit for reducing the rate of ectopic pregnancy by approximately 90% (Burkman, 2001). The mechanism of action is thought to be through inhibition of ovulation. This is a secondary benefit to preventing salpingitis.

❧ *Prevention and Treatment of Functional Ovarian Cysts* The relatively new low-dose COCs reduce the incidence of functional ovarian cysts by preventing ovulation. Preparations containing 50 µg of ethinyl estradiol have been associated with reducing cyst formation. If a woman has recurrent functional cysts, use of COCs may eliminate recurrence (Hatcher et al., 1998).

❧ *Reduction in Incidence of Anemia* Combined oral contraceptives reduce the incidence of anemia in two ways. Women who use these preparations are likely to have lighter menses, resulting in less blood loss. The 28-day formulations also supply iron replacement. This protection lasts beyond the treatment period with COCs.

❧ *Menstrual Cycle Benefits* Women who have heavy menses and those with painful menses benefit from the use of COCs. The resulting increase in progestin is likely to decrease flow and reduce or eliminate cramping some women experience during menstruation.

❧ *Reduction in Incidence of Benign Breast Disease* The reduction of benign breast disease is thought to be due to inhibition of ovulation. When a woman ovulates, certain proliferative breast changes occur. When ovulation ceases, these changes typically do not occur. The decrease in benign breast changes occurs even at the lowest dose of oral contraceptive.

❧ *Reduction in Acne* Acne can vary from person to person and can be worse at certain times in the same person. Certain COCs can be very effective in reducing or eliminating the incidence of acne. In the very young woman who has acne the benefits increase if she also has menstrual cramping or functional ovarian cysts.

❧ *Improvement in Bone Mineral Density* Bone mineral density peaks in women between the ages of 20 and 25 years, stays constant for approximately 10 years, and progressively decreases during the later reproductive years (Burkman, 2001). Estrogens act on bone by increasing absorption of calcium and directly decreasing reabsorption of calcium through inhibition of osteoclasts. One case control study indicates that there is a 25% reduction in hip fracture risk among women who use COCs.

Client Education Box

Oral Contraceptives

Women who are going to use combined oral contraceptives (COCs) should understand several important points about their successful use.

1. COCs, especially low-dose preparations, are more likely to be effective when taken the same time every day.

2. COCs may be begun on the Sunday after the first day of the woman's menses. If she begins the pill immediately it should be effective in 7 to 10 days. If she wants to be really safe, she may want to consider using a backup method with the pill for the first month.

3. The woman should know that COCs do not offer protection against exposure to the human immunodeficiency virus (HIV). She or her partner should use a condom in combination with the pill for this type of protection.

4. The woman needs to know that there are various types and dosages of COCs, and they are not necessarily interchangeable.

5. When a woman forgets to take one pill, it should be taken when she remembers; the next pill should be taken at the regularly scheduled time.

6. When a woman misses more than one pill, there is the possibility of escape ovulation. She should use a backup method along with the pill for 7 days or refrain from intercourse for the remainder of the cycle (Hatcher et al., 1998).

7. When starting a new preparation, the woman should know it might take 3 months for hormone levels to stabilize. Breakthrough bleeding may diminish after the third cycle is completed (Lynch, 2000).

8. The woman should be aware of signs and symptoms that should warn her to discontinue the pill immediately, including the following:

   Visual loss, diplopia, or blurred vision

   Unilateral numbness, weakness, or tingling

   Severe pains in the chest, left arm, or neck

   Hemoptysis

   Severe pain, tenderness, swelling, warmth, or palpable cords in the legs

   Slurring of speech

   Hepatic mass or tenderness

   If any of these signs or symptoms occurs, the woman should stop taking her pills immediately and contact a health care provider immediately.

9. The woman should know about less serious conditions that may occur and do not require immediate discontinuance of the pill but do require evaluation by a health care provider. Many of these symptoms and conditions can be easily alleviated or treated so that the woman may continue to use combined oral contraceptives. The use of COCs in the presence of relative contraindications requires clinical judgment on the part of the health care provider (Speroff & Darney, 2001). Relative contraindications include migraine headaches, hypertension, uterine fibroids, gestational diabetes, elective surgery, epilepsy, sickle cell disease, diabetes, and gall bladder disease.

Reduction in Risk for Colorectal Cancer There is growing epidemiologic evidence that oral contraceptives protect women against colorectal cancer. Although the exact mechanism of action for this protection is unknown, it has been hypothesized that reduction in bile acid concentration may explain the protective effect (Burkman, 2001). The reduction in risk may be from 40% to 50%.

Reduction in Risk for Uterine Fibroids Uterine fibroids are benign uterine tumors that increase in size and cause heavy menses. Research has shown a 70% reduction in risk for developing fibroids among women using oral contraceptives (Jensen & Speroff, 2000).

Indications

Combined oral contraceptives are used specifically for family planning but also may be used to treat certain gynecologic conditions. Young women often have problems with cycle control. These women may benefit from the use of COCs to regulate irregular cycles, reduce flow, and control dysmenorrhea. Women with polycystic ovarian syndrome may benefit from COCs because they reduce circulating androgens. Premenstrual symptoms may be improved with the use of COCs. Older women often experience anovulatory cycles with heavy bleeding owing to unopposed estrogen and also can benefit from COCs. This type of bleeding often is associated with perimenopause. COCs also can help alleviate other perimenopausal symptoms as well in women who do not have contraindications up to age 50 (Long, 1998).

Contraindications

Absolute and relative contraindications have been described related to oral contraceptives. If the woman has an absolute contraindication to the pill, she should not be given oral contraceptives under any circumstances. If she has a relative contraindication to the pill, she may take the pill under certain circumstances with direct supervision of her physician. Box 14-2 describes the absolute contraindications to oral contraception, and Box 14-3 describes the relative contraindications.

Side Effects

Most women experience relatively few side effects of the pill. Many times, side effects may be eliminated by changing pill formulation or dosage. Some side effects that have been reported are weight gain, breast tenderness, breakthrough bleeding, depression, decreased libido, and nausea. Table 14-2 describes the side effects and their relationship to hormones in the pills.

Another common concern is the effect of COCs on the lipid profile (Long, 1998). The concern was that the pill had adverse effects on the lipid profile by causing elevated triglycerides, which have been associated with cardiovascular disease and stroke. It appears that low-dose pills and the new progestins have moderated this risk for users.

Progestin-Only Contraceptives

A progestin-only contraceptive also is referred to as a minipill. This type of preparation is especially attractive for women who want oral contraception and cannot take COCs. This would include women who cannot take or do not tolerate estrogen, lactating women, and women with chronic medical conditions.

Three brands of progestin-only pills currently are available in the United States. The trade names are Nor-Q.D., Micronor, and Ovrette. Nor-Q.D. and Micronor contain norethindrone, 0.35 mg; Ovrette contains norgestrel, 0.075 mg.

Pharmacology

Unlike the COC, the minipill does not act by preventing ovulation. Instead, its mechanism of action is that the progestin acts to make the endometrium hostile to implantation and the cervical mucus becomes thick and impermeable

Box 14-2 Absolute Contraindications to the Use of Combined Oral Contraceptives

- Presence or a history of deep venous thrombosis or pulmonary embolism.
- Cerebrovascular accident or a history.
- Coronary artery or ischemic heart disease, or a history of either.
- Structural heart disease complicated by pulmonary hypertension, atrial fibrillation, or subacute bacterial endocarditis, or a history of any of these conditions.
- Diabetes with nephropathy, retinopathy, or neuropathy, or other vascular disease.
- Diabetes of over 20 years duration.
- Breast cancer.
- Pregnancy.
- Lactation.
- Liver problems.
- Headaches.
- Major surgery.
- Cigarette smoker over the age of 35 years.
- Blood pressure levels over 160/100.

Data adapted from Hatcher, R.A., Trussell, J., Stewart, F., Cates, W., Stewart, G., Guest, F., & Kowal, D. (1998). *Contraceptive Technology* (17th ed.). New York, NY: Ardent Media, Inc.

Box 14-3 Relative Contraindications to the Use of Combined Oral Contraceptives

- Absence of menses.
- Spotting or breakthrough bleeding.
- Right upper quadrant pain.
- Midepigastric pain.
- Migraine headaches.
- Severe, nonvascular headaches.
- Galactorrhea.
- Jaundice and pruritis.
- Depression.

Data adapted from Hatcher, R.A., Trussell, J., Stewart, F., Cates, W., Stewart, G., Guest, F., & Kowal, D. (1998). *Contraceptive Technology* (17th ed.). New York, NY: Ardent Media, Inc.

Table 14-2 Side Effects of Combined Oral Contraceptive Related to Hormones and Dosage

General Side Effects

Estrogen Excess
Chloasma
Chronic nasopharyngitis
Gastric influenza
Hay fever and allergic rhinitis
Urinary tract infection

Progestin Excess
Appetite increase
Depression
Fatigue
Hypoglycemia
Decreased libido
Neurodermatitis
Weight gain

Estrogen Deficiency
Nervousness
Vasomotor symptoms

Androgen Excess
Acne
Cholestatic jaundice
Hirsutism
increased libido
Oily skin and scalp
Rash and pruritis
Edema

Reproductive Side Effects

Estrogen Excess
Breast changes
Cervical extrophy
Dysmenorrhea
Hypermenorrhea
Menorrhagia
Clotting with menses
Increased breast size
Mucorrhea (mucus discharge)
Uterine enlargement
Uterine fibroid growth

Progestin Excess
Cervicitis
Decreased flow
Moniliasis

Estrogen Deficiency
Absence of withdrawal bleeding
Continuous bleeding
Hypomenorrhea
Pelvic relaxation
Atropic vaginitis

Progestin Deficiency
Breakthrough bleeding
Delayed withdrawal bleeding
Dysmenorrhea
Heavy flow with clots

Cardiovascular Side Effects

Estrogen Excess
Capillary fragility
Cerebrovascular accident
Deep venous thrombosis
Telangiectasis
Thromboembolic disease

Progestin Excess
Hypertension
Leg vein dilation

Premenstraul Side Effects

Estrogen Excess or Progestin Deficiency
Bloating
Dizziness
Edema
Headache
Irritability
Leg cramps
Nausea and vomiting
Visual changes
Weight gain

Data adapted from Dickey, R.P. (2001). *Managing contraceptive pill patients.* Durant, OK: Essential Medical Information Systems, Inc.

Nursing Alert

COC CONTRAINDICATIONS

Be sure to tell your clients that certain drugs interact with COCs to reduce their efficacy, including:

- Carbamazepine (Tegretol)
- Griseofulvin
- Phenobarbital
- Phenytoin (Dilantin)
- Rifabutin
- Rifampin
- Topiramate

Data Adapted from Hatcher, R. A., Trussell, J., Stewart, F., Cates, W., Stewart, G., Guest, F., & Kowal, D. (1998). *Contraceptive Technology* (17th ed.). New York, NY: Ardent Media, Inc.

(Speroff & Darney, 1992). Approximately 40% of women will ovulate while taking the minipill.

Efficacy

The minipill is considered to be more than 99% effective when used properly. It must be taken at the same time each day because there is a higher potential for ovulation and pregnancy than with the COC when a dose is late or missed. There is no significant metabolic effect, and fertility returns to normal almost immediately after discontinuance (Speroff & Darney, 1992).

Benefits and Risks

Minipills are of benefit to women who are unable to take COCs. In lactating women and women over the age of 40 years, the protection approaches 100% with proper use (Speroff & Darney, 1992). This high rate of efficacy in these groups may be due to the decreased fertility in this client population. The World Health Organization states that progestin-only pills have no adverse effects on lactation and can be started as early as 6 weeks postpartum (Adams, 2000). The minipill also is useful for women who experience decreased libido with COCs. The minipill offers many of the same noncontraceptive benefits as do COCs; however, these benefits may be at a reduced level. Because it is thought that the minipill produces no metabolic effect, it should be safe for use in women who have diabetes and those over the age of 35 years. Return to fertility is almost immediate on discontinuance.

In the first year of use, there typically is a 5% failure rate among the general population. This rate is slightly higher than that of COCs but better than use of no contra-ceptive, which has a pregnancy rate of 80% within 1 year of unprotected intercourse.

Women who use the minipill will develop more functional ovarian cysts, which usually will resolve without treatment. The major problem with use of the minipill is that of breakthrough bleeding.

Indications

As is the combined oral contraceptive, the minipill is designed to be used as a contraceptive. It also may be used to decrease bleeding related to unopposed estrogen. Some minipills can be used for emergency contraception, which is discussed later in this chapter.

Contraindications

Minipills should not be used in the presence of pregnancy. Progestin is considered a teratogen to the unborn fetus. The minipill also is contraindicated in women who have breast cancer, women taking certain medications, and women who have liver disease.

Side Effects

The major side effect of the minipill is irregular bleeding. Women who use this method may not have regular menses for the duration of its use. They may have irregular periods of spotting. Because the bleeding is light, however, this side effect is not bothersome for some women.

Intrauterine Methods

The intrauterine device has been available in the United States for more than 70 years, although it has been accepted widely as a contraceptive device only for the past 40 years (Figure 14-5). Present perceptions of this method are strongly influenced by some problems that arose with one particular IUD in the 1970s. That IUD was called the Dalkon Shield. Some women using Dalkon Shields developed pelvic inflammatory disease (PID). At the time, there was much discussion about safety, resulting in all but one type of IUD being removed from the market. Today, there is some discussion that the major contributing factors to removal from the market were ignorance of the facts, fear of medical liability, inadequate medical training in insertion, and confusion about the mechanism of action. As a result, physicians stopped recommending this method (Department of Health and Human Services [DHHS] & The National Institute of Child Health and Human Development [NICHHD], 1996). The IUD has been re-released for use but is not as widely used as it was before removal from the market.

Two types of intrauterine devices currently are available in the United States. Paragard T 380A is a T-shaped device made of polyethylene, and Progestasert is a T-shaped device made of ethylene vinyl acetate copolymer.

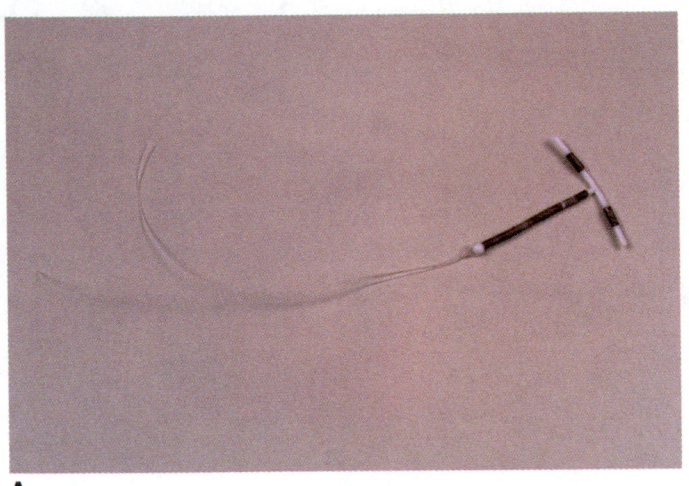

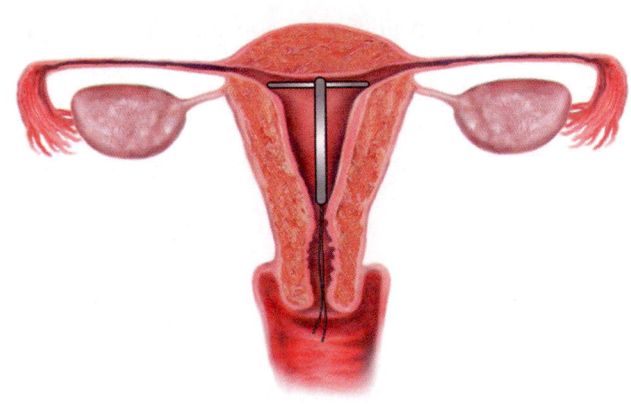

A.   **B.**

Figure 14-5 A. Intrauterine device (IUD). B. Proper insertion of an IUD.

Composition

The Paragard has a 380-mm² exposed surface of copper on its arms and stem. The Progestasert contains a reservoir of 38 mg of progesterone that is released at a rate of 65 µg/d (Nelson, 2000). Some other types of IUD from previous years with an unlimited life span may remain in use even though they are not available on the market today.

Mechanism of Action

It is thought that the IUD works by interfering with sperm transport from the cervix to the fallopian tubes. This interference makes viable sperm scarce in the fallopian tube. It is also thought that the IUD inhibits sperm capacitation and survival. **Sperm capacitation** is the process by which the sperm becomes hypermobile and there is a breakdown of the plasma membrane and merging with the aerosmal membrane which allows the sperm to bind with the zona pellucida of the ovum (Speroff, Glass, & Kass, 1999). It is thought to inhibit implantation. It also is thought that the IUD alters the biochemical or cellular composition of uterine fluid, or both, causing impairment of the viability of gametes (DHHS & NICHHD, 1996).

The copper IUD is a functional spermicide. The copper ions released from the device interfere with sperm motility and create a reaction to the foreign body that results in a spermicidal endometrium (Nelson, 2000). Progestasert is believed to act through thickening the cervical mucus and rendering it impermeable to sperm.

Efficacy

The copper IUD has a first-year failure rate of 0.7% with typical use. The copper T has a 10-year failure rate of 2.1% to 2.7% (Nelson, 2000). Progestasert has a first year failure rate of 2% with typical use. The median time from removal of the IUD to planned pregnancy is 3 months (Nelson, 2000).

Benefits and Risks

In properly selected women, the IUD can offer a method of contraception for those who cannot or do not want to take oral contraceptives. The woman should be in a mutually monogamous relationship with her partner. The IUD is ideally suited to women that have chronic medical problems that restrict their use of hormones (Kjos, 1997). Unlike pills that must be taken daily, the IUD provides prolonged protection. Paragard is approved for 10 years of use before replacement; Progestasert is approved for 1 year of use before replacement (Stewart, 1998).

The IUD requires little maintenance. The woman should check the length of the tail string in her vagina after each menses. If the string is not found, she should notify her health care provider immediately.

Insertion issues are related to IUDs. The two most serious problems are vasovagal response and uterine perforation. A vasovagal response involves rapid decrease in blood pressure on insertion of a probe or IUD into the uterus. It occurs in approximately 1% of women on manipulation of the cervix. This response usually is mild and transient; however, occasionally, the woman will require resuscitation. Therefore, resuscitation equipment should be immediately available.

Perforation of the uterus occurs in approximately 1 in 770 to 1,600 insertions (Nelson, 2000). Most perforations occur when the uterine sound is inserted to determine the depth of the intrauterine cavity. Using current techniques that do not require the use of uterine sound has reduced this risk.

Indications

Client selection is an important consideration when using the IUD. The woman should have had a previous pregnancy, must not have a history of PID, and must be in a monogamous relationship. The woman who has never been pregnant has a smaller uterine cavity and thus is at risk for expulsion.

Mishell (1996) indicated four misconceptions that prevent more women from choosing IUDs. The first reason is the fallacy that IUDs work as an abortifacient, resulting in failure of implantation of a fertilized egg. The second is that IUDs cause pelvic infections or PID. The third fallacy is that IUDs cause ectopic pregnancies. The fourth reason is the belief that the problems encountered in the past with the Dalkon Shield are common to all IUDs.

Contraindications

Nelson (2000) enumerates contraindications for IUD insertion. General contraindications include pregnancy, acute cervicitis, a distorted uterine cavity, uterine or cervical carcinoma, unexplained vaginal bleeding, severe immunocompromise, and multiple sexual partners.

Specific contraindications for IUD insertion include issues specific to copper or progesterone (Nelson, 2000). Contraindications to copper devices include uterine cavity size of less than 6 or greater than 9 cm, copper allergy, Wilson disease, severe anemia, heavy menses, and severe dysmenorrhea. Contraindications for the progesterone device are uterine cavity size of less than 6 or greater than 9 cm, a history of ectopic pregnancy, and diabetes.

Side Effects

Bleeding and cramping are the two most common side effects encountered after insertion of the IUD. These symptoms usually are minimal and temporary; however, occasionally, they occur to the extreme, necessitating removal of the device.

Other adverse effects include infection, accidental pregnancy, and expulsion of the device (Nelson, 1995). Infection is related to insertion and STD. These side effects make client selection a very important factor.

Intravaginal Methods

The **vaginal ring** (which delivers steroids through the vaginal mucosa) is a contraceptive device that had its beginnings in the 1970s (Ballagh, 2001). It became apparent that drug absorption could occur in the vaginal mucosa. Duncan at Upjohn first patented vaginal delivery of sex steroids through a polysiloxane tube or disk in 1970. Since that time, more than a dozen patents for contraceptive rings have been filed.

Various ring designs have been used. Modifications have been made to ensure sustained, even steroid release over a period of time. The result has been a highly effective product.

Composition

Vaginal rings are available that contain progestins alone or a combination of estrogen and progestin.

Mechanism of Action

The steroids are absorbed through the upper vaginal mucosa. In the combination form of the intravaginal ring, ethinyl estradiol is released at 20 μg/d and norethindrone at 1 mg/d. These dosages are equivalent to those in oral contraceptives. The mechanism of action is through prevention of ovulation, increased viscosity of cervical mucus, and endometrial atrophy.

Types of Intravaginal Devices

Ballagh (2001) described various types of vaginal rings. The progestin-only rings may include progesterone, etonogestrel, levonorgestrel-norgestrel, megestrol, nestorone, or norgestrienone. Combined estrogen-progestin devices can contain the previously mentioned progestins in combination with ethinyl estradiol.

Benefits and Risks

One of the benefits of the vaginal ring is that it does not require the rigor necessary to use oral contraceptives. The vaginal ring allows a sustained release of steroids over a 3-week period. The method is reversible by the woman. The only requirement for discontinuance is nonreplacement of the device at the end of the use-free week. Acceptance of the ring is high among women, except those who find placing a foreign object in their vagina unacceptable (Grow & Ahmed, 2000).

Indications

The vaginal ring is designed for women who do not want to use a method that must be administered daily, for example, women who travel or who do not have a perma-

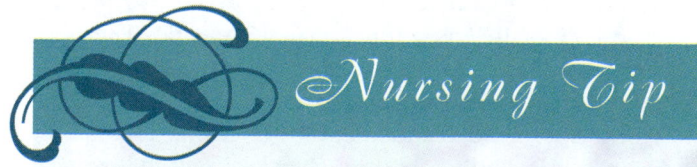

VAGINAL RING

The vaginal ring is designed to be left in the vagina for 3 weeks and removed for 1 week to allow menses. The ring may be removed or remain in place during intercourse.

nent place to store pills. The woman who uses the vaginal ring must be comfortable inserting and removing an object from her vagina. Vaginal rings also are useful in relieving menopausal symptoms.

Contraindications

Because the steroids from the ring are absorbed directly from the vaginal mucosa into the bloodstream, use of the vaginal ring is contraindicated in women who cannot use oral estrogen or progestins.

Adverse Effects

Occasionally, the vaginal ring can be expelled when straining to have a bowel movement or on tampon removal. Some women experience discomfort with intercourse when the vaginal ring is in place. Some women have an odor that they attribute to the ring. Some women also complain of vaginal discharge they attribute to the vaginal ring.

Barrier Methods

Barrier methods of contraception include condoms, diaphragms, and cervical caps. Spermicide is a chemical barrier method.

Condoms

Condoms are available for men and women. Condoms are the most frequently used barrier method of contraception. Six billion condoms were sold worldwide in 1990 (Speroff & Darney, 1992). They are sold without a prescription at most drug stores and in other public places. Condoms are available in various colors and textures and with a lubricant inside that contains a spermicide (Figure 14-6). Condoms have a typical effectiveness rate of 88% and a theoretical ef-

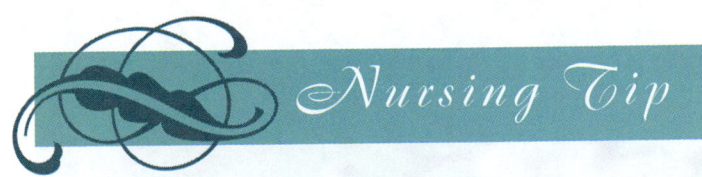

Nursing Tip

CONDOM USE

Care must be taken to leave space at the end of the male condom when it is applied. If this space is not allowed, there is a tendency for the condom to break. The condom must be removed before the penis becomes flaccid. The condom also must be secured at the base of the penis as it is removed to avoid having the condom remain in the vagina when the penis is withdrawn.

fectiveness rate of 98%. The difference in the two rates has to do with improper use, lack of use, and breakage.

The female condom has been available since the 1990s (Figure 14-7). It is inserted into the vagina and covers the perineum. It is a polyurethane sheath 7.8 cm in diameter and 17 cm long. It contains two polyurethane rings. One ring is at the closed end of the sheath and is designed to be placed into the vagina. The ring at the open end remains outside the vagina after insertion. The outside portion of the female condom provides some protection for the external genitalia of the woman and the base of the penis of the man during intercourse. Unlike the lubricant in the male condom, the female condom does not contain spermicide.

Male condoms have been available for centuries and have been made of sheepskin and other materials. Currently, the most prevalent material is latex. Latex condoms have pores small enough to protect against the HIV virus and herpes simplex viruses.

Mechanism of Action

The condom acts as a barrier to prevent sperm from entering the vagina during intercourse. Both types of condom are designed for single use. Because the mechanism of action is as a barrier, a worn or torn condom negates its action.

Benefits and Risks

Condoms are inexpensive, readily available, require no contact with the health care system, and when used properly are quite effective as a method of contraception. When applied properly, condoms are almost as reliable as the oral contraceptive. The major risks of contraceptive failure with the condom involve use failure caused by breakage, accidental removal, or partner dissatisfaction with its use.

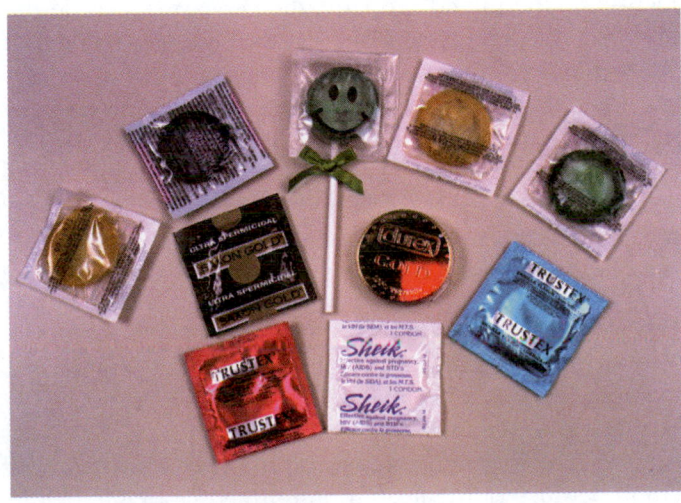

Figure 14-6 Male condoms.

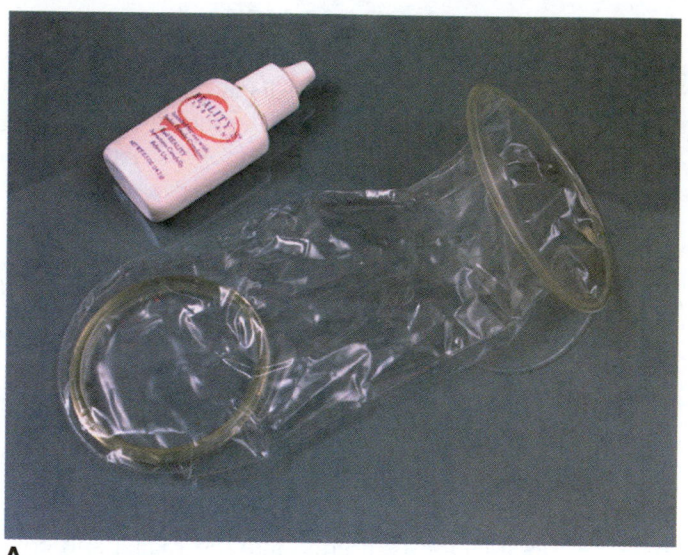

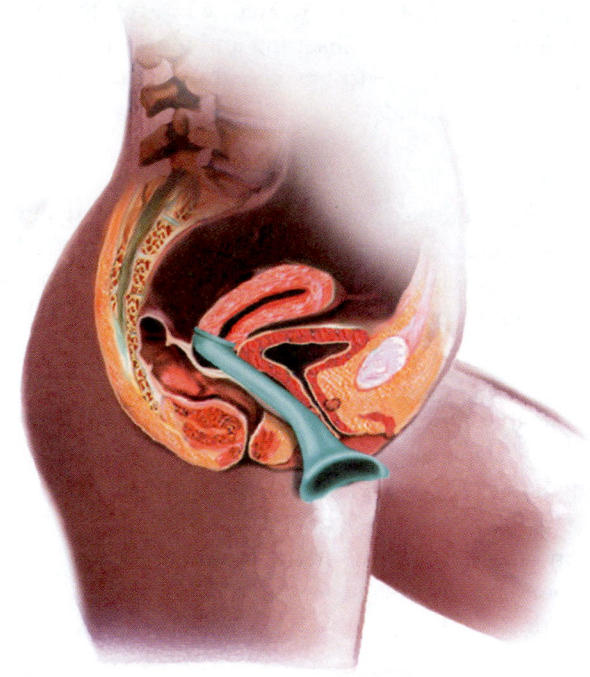

A. B.

Figure 14-7 A. Female condom. B. Proper insertion of a female condom.

Indications

Both male and female condoms are indicated for use as a contraceptive device and as a method to prevent STDs. There are a number of reasons a couple may decide to use the condom as the primary form of contraception.

Contraindications

Condoms should not be used by the person with an allergy to latex.

Side Effects

If a person is sensitive to latex or spermicide, hypersensitivity reactions to the male condom may develop. Hypersensitivity is less likely to develop with use of the female condom because it is not made of latex.

Diaphragm

The **diaphragm** is a latex device available by prescription from a health care provider. The woman must be meas-

Nursing Alert

EXTRA PRECAUTION

Cautious women should use a spermicide as a secondary means of contraception in case of failure of the primary mode.

ured for adequate fit. Diaphragms are measured in millimeters and come in several sizes and styles to meet the needs of nulliparous and multiparous women. Measurement is so important to effectiveness that a woman must be refitted if she delivers a child or has a substantial weight change (Figure 14-8).

Mechanism of Action

The diaphragm is designed to provide a barrier between the cervical os and semen. The diaphragm is fitted snuggly behind the symphysis pubis anteriorly. The sides of the diaphragm should extend laterally to encompass the entire cervix and rest in the lateral fornices. In the posterior dimension, when fitted properly, the cervix rests inside the diaphragm. A spermicidal gel is placed inside the dome of the diaphram and around the rim to ensure that sperm do not enter. If intercourse is undertaken more than once, additional spermicide should be applied into the vagina. The diaphragm should remain in place for 6 hours after intercourse. On removal, care should be taken to wash the diaphragm with a mild soap and water solution before it is returned to its case for storage.

Benefits and Risks

The diaphragm is a long-established contraceptive device that requires little upkeep. Its theoretical failure rate is 6%, giving it the potential as an excellent method of contraception. The failure rate in typical use is somewhat lower (18%) because of the need to insert the diaphragm before intercourse. It must be left in place for 6 hours after inter-

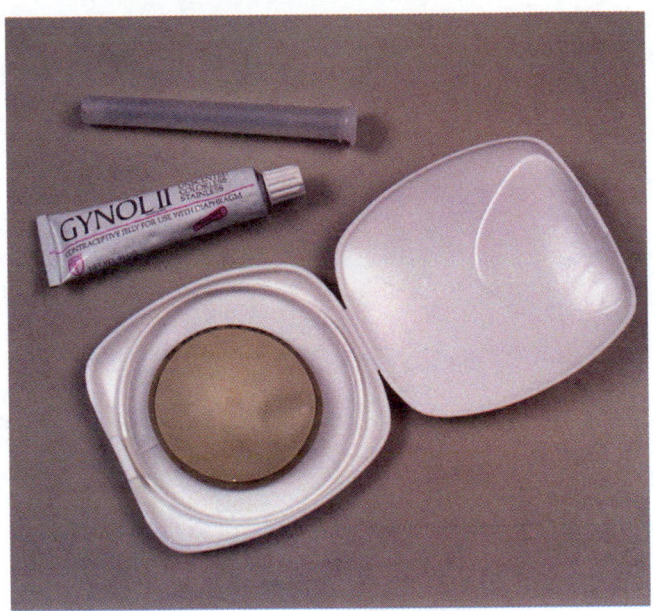

A.

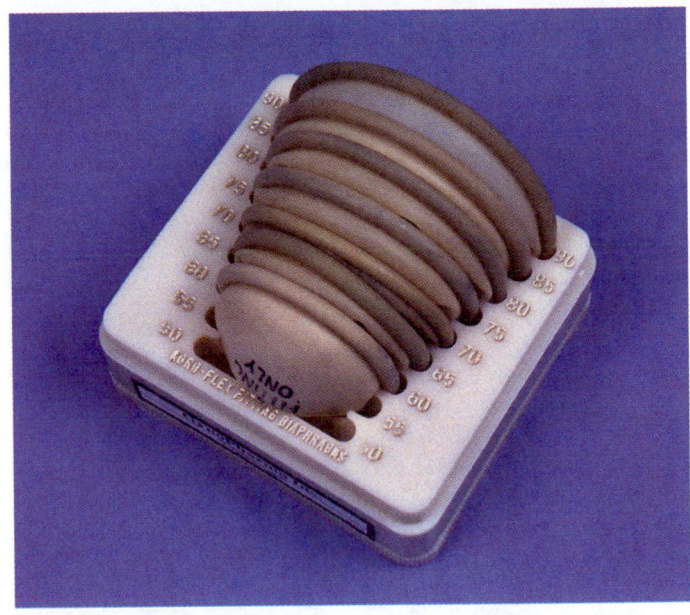

B.

Figure 14-8 A. Diaphragm with contraceptive jelly. B. Various sizes of diaphragms to be fitted by health care provider.

course and may remain in place up to 24 hours (Speroff & Darney, 1992). When properly cared for, the diaphragm can be used for many years without replacement. However, it must be inspected frequently for holes or deterioration of the latex.

Contraindications

There are no contraindications for the use of a barrier device. However, women who have allergies to latex or spermicide would probably not want to use this method. Hatcher et al. (1998) suggest that women at high risk for failure use another method. Women at risk are those who have intercourse three or more times per week; who are under aged 30 years; whose personal style or sexual patterns make consistent use difficult; who have had previous contraceptive failures, who have ambivalent feelings about the desirability of a pregnancy; and who intend to delay and not prevent pregnancy. These women are least likely to have success with this method.

Cervical Cap

The **cervical cap** is a rubber barrier device designed to be applied to the cervix (Figure 14-9). It must be fitted to the woman by the health care provider to conform to the cervix. When properly fitted, the cervical cap is a few millimeters in diameter larger than is the cervix. The device is folded for insertion and fits against the cervix with suction. Once inserted, the device must be checked to ensure it is applied to the cervix and that suction is applied. Spermicide is placed in the dome of the cup and remains in placed until the cervical cap is removed.

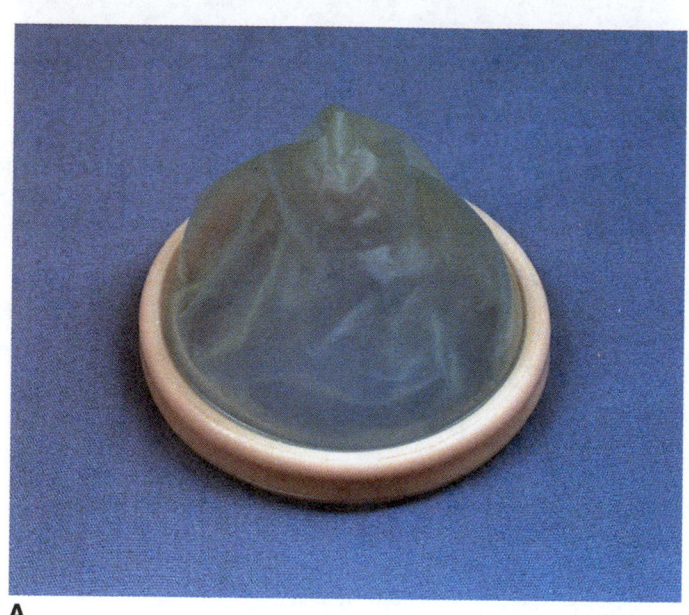

A.

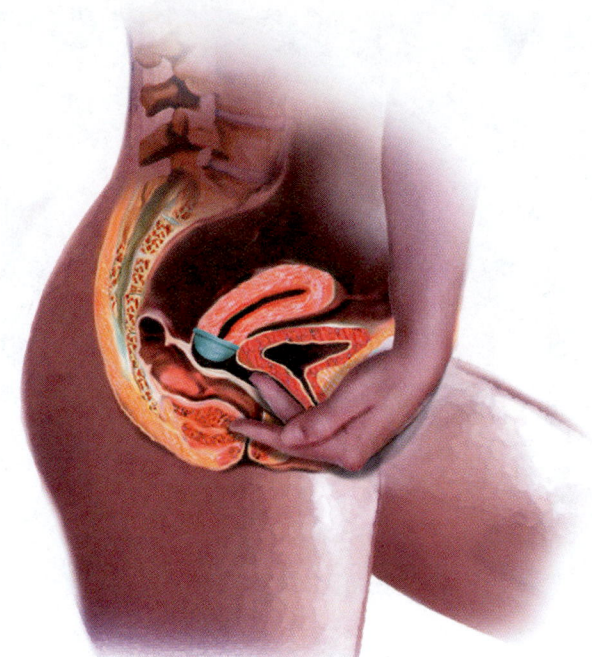

B.

Figure 14-9 A. Cervical cap. B. Proper insertion of a cervical cap.

Benefits and Risks

The cervical cap is similar to but has an advantage over the diaphragm. Additional spermicide does not need to be applied with each act of intercourse. The cervical cap can be left in place for 36 to 48 hours after intercourse but should not remain inserted for prolonged periods of time. After a few days women may complain of a foul-smelling discharge.

Some women cannot wear the cervical cap because of irregularity of the cervical contour or other reasons. The cap must be left in place for 6 hours after intercourse because there may still be motile sperm in the vagina. Because the efficacy of the device depends on maintaining suction of the cap against the cervix and there may be dislodgement of the device during intercourse, the possibility of an accidental pregnancy exists.

Adverse Effects

When a cervical cap is left in place too long the potential for infection and cervical erosion exists. Antibiotics to treat the infection and another method of contraception may be required until the infection is healed. Cervical erosion may affect the outcome of the woman's Pap smear and also may necessitate removal of the device and use of another method.

Spermicide

Spermicide is a chemical method of contraception based on varying formulations of the chemical nonoxynol. The

delivery system for this chemical can be foam, sponge, gel, cream, suppository, or film (Figure 14-10). This type of contraceptive has a failure rate of about 20% when used alone. When used in combination with another barrier method, its rate of effectiveness increases. Hatcher et al. (1998) suggest that the combination of spermicide and a barrier method, backed up by abortion for failure, is one of the safest contraceptive options. Each spermicidal device must remain in the vagina for a period of time after intercourse that is sufficient to kill the sperm. This means the woman should not bathe or douche for 6 hours after intercourse.

Types of Spermicide

Contraceptive gel or cream is designed to be used in combination with diaphragms and cervical caps. Spermicides however can be used alone. Spermicides come with applicators, and therefore, a measured dose of the product will be used with each application. Contraceptive sponges also are designed to be used alone. Suppositories can be used alone or with a condom. The woman must allow 15 to 30 minutes before intercourse for dispersion of the medication. Contraceptive film can be used alone or in combination with a diaphragm or cervical cap. When used alone, the film should be placed high in the vagina in contact with or near the cervix. When used with the diaphragm, the film should be used inside the diaphragm near the cervix. Fifteen minutes is required for the insert to dissolve so that the spermicide is available for use.

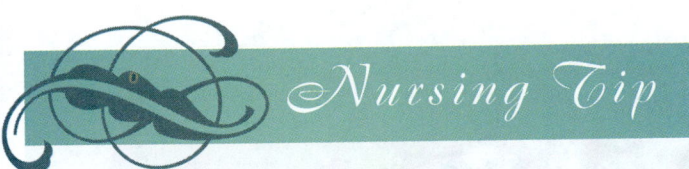

SPERMICIDE USE

When using one of the spermicides for contraception, a second application of the product is necessary when intercourse is repeated.

Mechanism of Action

Nonoxynol 9, the spermicide available in the United States, is a surfactant that destroys the sperm cell membrane. Other spermicides are used in other parts of the world.

Benefits and Risks

Spermicide may lower the risk of becoming infected with a STD by as much as 25% (Hatcher et al., 1998). Spermicides are stored easily for those who have intercourse infrequently. Another benefit may be that the male partner does not have to be involved with this type of method. It is an excellent backup method in case a woman runs out of pills or expels her IUD.

One of the disadvantages of this type of product is allergy or sensitivity to the ingredients. This sensitivity will result in skin irritation. Frequent use results in a greater likelihood of irritation. Some of the products effervesce and some women dislike this feeling. Use of the sponge or diaphragm may result in frequent yeast infections.

Implantable Methods

When **implantable contraception** (contraceptive device surgically implanted) is discussed, Norplant comes to mind (Figure 14-11). This device has been available in the United States for approximately 10 years. Several types of implantable devices are available. Over 6 million women worldwide have used Norplant (Meckstroth & Darney, 2000).

Meckstroth & Darney (2000) discussed the new types of implantable devices that are becoming available. Norplant is still available in the standard six-capsule form; a new device that contains two rods of levonorgestrel is available, which is called Jadelle. A second type of implant called Implanon is available in a single rod for implantation. Uniplant is a silastic capsule containing nomegestrol acetate that can be implanted as a single silastic capsule. Biodegradable implants include Capronor and Anuelle, which are under investigation. Capronor is a single biodegradable capsule, and Anuelle is marketed in the form of biodegradable pellets.

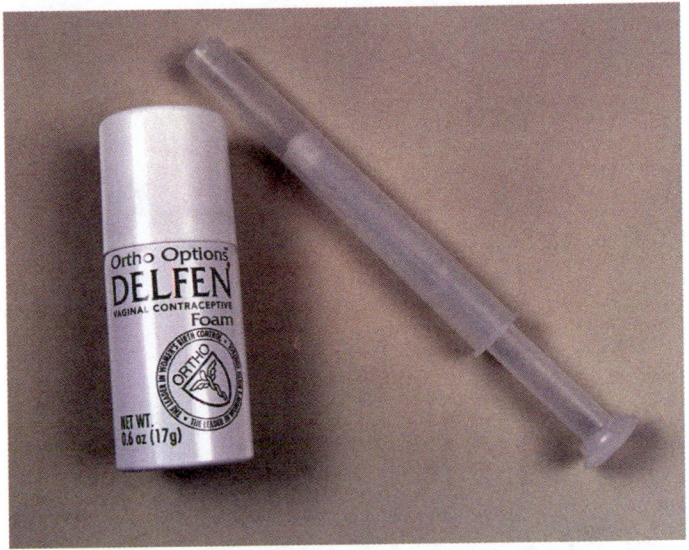

A.

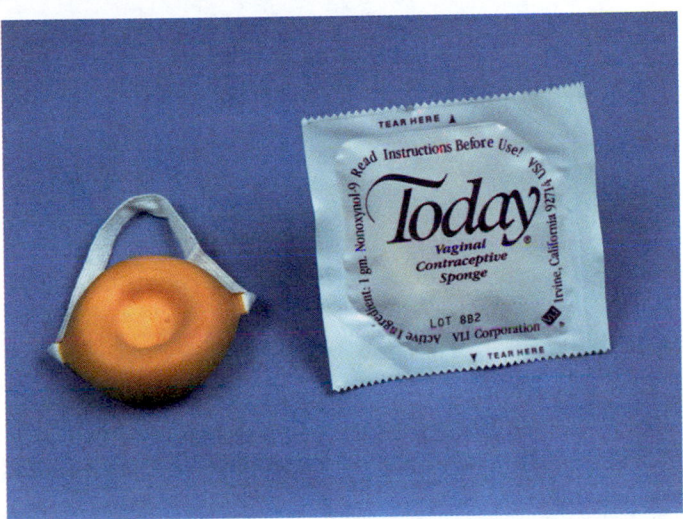

B.

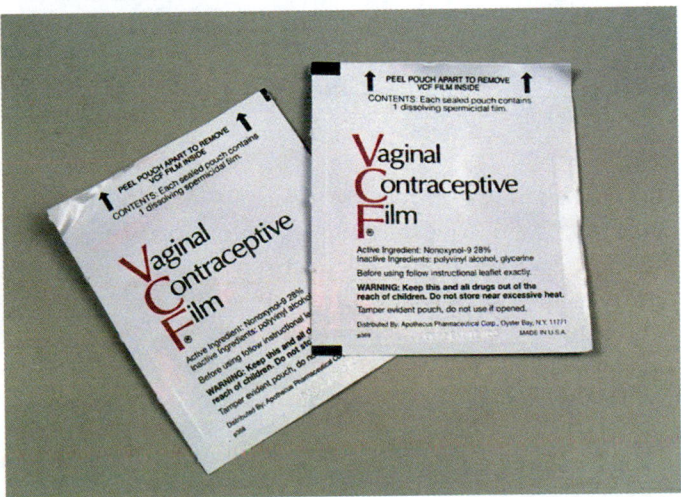

C.

Figure 14-10 Spermicides. A. Foam. B. Sponge. C. Film.

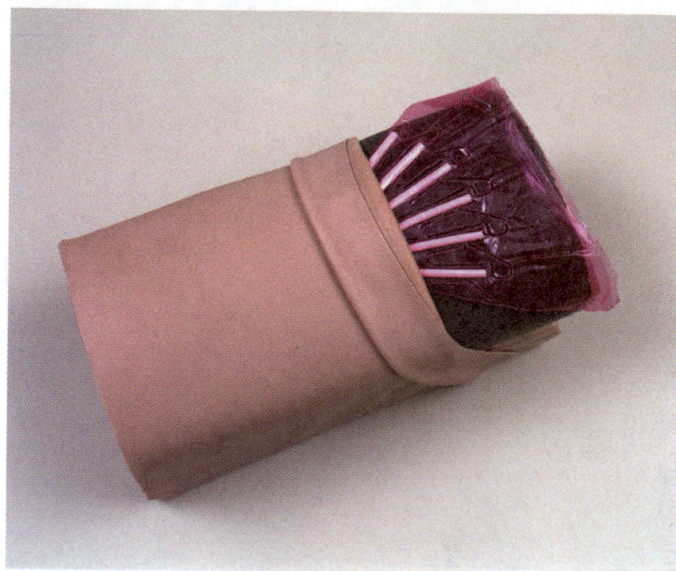

Figure 14-11 Implantable contraceptive.

Composition

Each of these implantable devices contains a progestin. Norplant contains 6 levonorgestrel capsules. Jadelle contains 2 levonorgestrel capsules. Implanon contains a single rod of the progestin etonogestrel, which is a metabolite of desogestrel. Uniplant contains nomegestrol acetate, which is a 19-nor-progesterone derivative. Nestorone is a potent progestin. Capronor contains levonorgestrel and Anuelle contains norethindrone (Meckstroth & Darney, 2000).

Mechanism of Action

Pregnancy is prevented in several ways. Inhibition of ovulation is one mechanism of action but not the primary one. Some women continue to ovulate infrequently. Changes in the cervical mucus and endometrium is the primary mechanism of action.

Efficacy

Several factors that affect the efficacy of this method include progestin concentration, the woman's weight, and her age. Another factor in effectiveness is the period of time that has passed since insertion. Implantable devices are thought to be more effective initially when inserted in the first 5 to 7 days of the menstrual cycle. A backup method is used for 1 week after insertion.

Benefits and Risks

A benefit of this type of contraceptive method is that once implanted, the woman has long-term contraception. Norplant is effective for 5 to 7 years' use, although it has been approved for 5 years' use. Norplant II/Jadelle has been approved for 3 to 5 years' use before replacement is re-

quired. Implanon has been approved for 3 years' use before replacement is required. Uniplant has been approved for 1 year of use; Nestorone has been approved for 2 years' use; Capronor is approved for 1 year of use; and Anuelle is approved for 2 years' use.

Implants require a minor surgical procedure for insertion and removal. Removal sometimes can be complicated by broken or deeply placed implants or bleeding. Scar tissue around the implants may also contribute to difficulty in removal.

Indications

Implantable devices are designed to be used only for contraception.

Contraindications

Absolute contraindications for this type of product include active thrombophlebitis or thromboembolic disease, undiagnosed genital bleeding, acute liver disease, benign or malignant liver tumors, and known or suspected breast cancer. Refer to Box 14-4 for additional contraindications.

Side Effects

These implants are thought to have little metabolic effect. Menstrual changes occur in about 75% of users (Meckstroth & Darney, 2000). Alterations in the pattern of menstrual bleeding may occur. In the first 3 months of use, menses are likely to be prolonged, with spotting between menses. Other side effects that occur less frequently include headaches, weight change, acne, ovarian cysts, and mood changes.

Some women have a local foreign body reaction producing inflammation and occasionally infection of the insertion site. There are no data suggesting the products used in implants can potentiate autoimmune disease (Meckstroth & Darney, 2000).

Injectable Methods

Two types of injectable contraceptives currently are available in the United States. Depo-Provera (depot medroxyprogesterone acetate, or DMPA) is a progestin-only formulation administered intramuscularly (IM) every 3 months (Figure 14-12). Lunelle is a combination of medroxyprogesterone and estradiol cypionate (MPA/E2C). This combination injection is designed to be given IM monthly.

Mechanism of Action

Depot medroxyprogesterone acts by inhibiting ovulation. The 150-mg dose inhibits ovulation for 3 months. The mechanism of action for Lunelle also is through inhibition of ovulation, and a dose of 0.5 mL provides contraception for 1 month.

Benefits and Risks

Depot medroxyprogesterone allows for 3 months' contraception without any effort on the part of the woman. DMPA is effective and well tolerated by most women and is safe for use by women who are lactating.

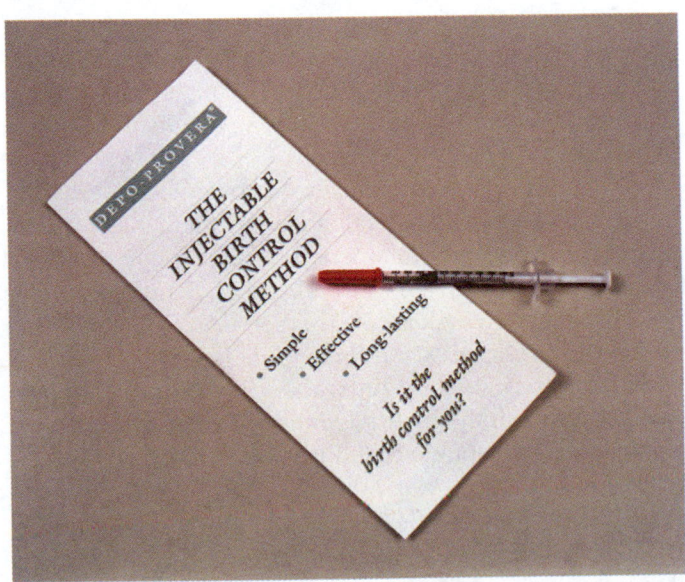

Figure 14-12 Injectible contraceptive.

If subsequent DMPA injections do not occur within 14 weeks, there is real potential for method failure and an unplanned pregnancy. Clients should be instructed to come in for re-injection immediately at 12 weeks to avoid an unplanned pregnancy.

Lunelle has a very high efficacy. Its failure rate is estimated at 0.1 per 100 women-years (Kaunitz, 2000). Return to fertility is rapid after discontinuance of the injection.

In contrast with DMPA, Lunelle must be administered monthly. This regimen requires more frequent reproductive decision-making. The safety and adverse event profile are similar to that of combined oral contraceptives.

Indications

Depot medroxyprogesterone and Lunelle are used for contraception.

Contraindications

Contraindications for DMPA include known or suspected pregnancy, undiagnosed vaginal bleeding, active thrombophlebitis, history of thromboembolic disorder, current or past history of cerebrovascular accident, liver dysfunction, known or suspected malignancy of the breast, and known hypersensitivity to DMPA.

Contraindications for Lunelle include known or suspected pregnancy, undiagnosed vaginal bleeding, thrombophlebitis or a history of thrombophlebitis or thromboembolic disease, cerebrovascular disease, coronary artery disease, cholestatic jaundice, and carcinoma of the endometrium. Known hypersensitivity to the medication also is an absolute contraindication.

Side Effects

The side effects of DMPA can include menstrual, weight, and mood changes. Menstrual changes are very common in women who use DMPA. In the first 3 months of use, heavy and irregular bleeding is most common. After 3 months, amenorrhea becomes more common. Menstrual

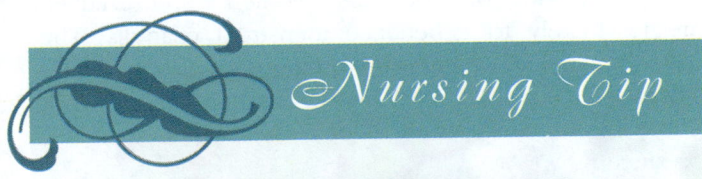

Nursing Tip

TIMING OF INJECTABLE CONTRACEPTION

It is best to administer either injectable product, DMPA or Lunelle, within the first 5 days of the menstrual cycle to ensure that the woman is not pregnant and allow time to prevent ovulation.

Research Highlight

DMPA and Weight Changes

Purpose

To determine the effects of DMPA on weight.

Method

This observational study was undertaken in Thailand, where DMPA is a prevalent means of contraception. Two groups of women, with 50 women receiving depot medroxyprogesterone (DMPA) and 50 women receiving intrauterine devices, were compared on age, parity, income, body weight, and blood pressure at the onset of contraception and at 120 months.

Findings

The mean body weight at 120 months for the group receiving DMPA was 60.5 kg ±7.5 kg; the mean body weight for the group receiving the IUD was 62.1 kg ±9.3 kg. No statistically significant difference was seen in the two groups based on body weight or blood pressure.

Nursing Implications

Nurses are in the position to answer client's questions about weight gain with various contraceptives. Despite anecdotal information, research has not been able to validate significant weight gain with DMPA (Depo-Provera).

Taneepanichskul, S., Reinprayoon, D., & Jaisamrarm, U. (1999). Effects of DMPA on weight and blood pressure in long-term acceptors. *Contraception, 59,* (3), 301–303.

---

disturbances are likely to be the reason women discontinue this form of contraception.

Weight gain is a problem encountered by many women and is a factor involved in discontinuance of contraception. Some women who use DMPA complain of weight gain. This weight gain however has not been validated by controlled studies.

The overall incidence of depression in women who use DMPA is low but does exist. Women who use Lunelle are less likely to experience menstrual changes. They may experience weight gain similar to that with DMPA. There are no reports of mood change with Lunelle. There have been reports of decreased libido with both products.

Natural Family Planning Methods

Two methods are available as natural family planning devices. Coitus interruptus is primarily controlled by the man, and ovulation prediction is primarily controlled by the woman.

Composition

Coitus interruptus involves removal of the male penis from the vagina before ejaculation. It is probably one of the least effective methods of contraception, with a failure rate of 19% (Hatcher et al., 1998). This method however is much preferable to using no contraceptive method with a failure rate of 85%.

Ovulation prediction, also known as the rhythm method, is the female natural family planning method. The woman predicts her fertile period through the use of basal body temperature charts, cervical mucus changes, or both. She abstains from intercourse for the period of time during which she is fertile. When timing intercourse, the woman must determine the day on which she ovulates and take into account that the male sperm is active for 48 hours and the ovum is susceptible to fertilization for 24 hours.

Mechanism of Action

Both of these methods, in fact, are barrier devices because they place time or distance between the sperm and ovum to prevent conception.

Benefits and Risks

These methods are inexpensive and, when used properly, can be effective. Caution must be used with coitus interruptus because seminal fluid may escape before ejaculation and before removal of the penis from the vagina. The result can be an unwanted pregnancy.

With ovulation prediction methods, it is not safe to assume that because ovulation occurred on day 14 of one cycle that it will do so each month. Ovulation at another time can result in an unplanned pregnancy.

Indications

Natural family planning methods are for those persons who do not believe in or cannot use other methods. These methods are vastly more reliable that is intercourse without the use of any method.

Contraindications

There are no known contraindications to natural family planning.

Emergency Contraception

Emergency contraception is available to prevent unintended pregnancy. This type of contraception has been available in the United States for approximately 20 years but it is not widely used or known by women. In the United Kingdom, however, the method has been used over 4 million times with few reported side effects (Grow & Ahmed, 2000).

Several types of postcoital contraception are available. Hormonal methods include administration of the COC, progestins, gonadotropin-releasing hormone (Gn-RH) agonists, antiprogestins, and high-dose estrogen Gn-RH agonists. The copper IUD also may be used for these purposes. Surgical abortion is also an option.

Combined Oral Contraceptives

In 1974, Yuzpe published the first results of successfully using 100 μg of ethinyl estradiol and 1 mg/dL norgestrel in combination as a single dose for emergency contraception. The current standard is to give the equivalent of 100 μg of ethinyl estradiol and 1 mg of levonorgestrel in combination for this purpose (Hatcher et al, 1998). The medication must be initiated within 72 hours of unprotected intercourse, and a second dose of the medication is given 12 hours after the initial dose. Table 14-3 summarizes some of the protocols used in contemporary health care.

Mechanism of Action

If COCs are administered before ovulation, ovulation may be delayed or suppressed for that menstrual cycle. The suppression is through action on the anterior pituitary. If administered after ovulation, the action is thought to be

Table 14-3 Emergency Contraception with Combined Oral Contraceptives	
Trade Name	**Dosage**
Ovral	2 pills immediately and 2 pills in 12 hours
Lo/Ovral	4 pills immediately and 4 pills in 12 hours
Nordette	4 orange pills immediately and 4 orange pills in 12 hours
Levlen	4 orange pills immediately and 4 orange pills in 12 hours
Alesse	5 pink pills immediately and 5 pink pills in 4 hours
Tri-Levlen	4 yellow pills immediately and 4 yellow pills in 4 hours
Triphasil	4 yellow pills immediately and 4 yellow pills in 4 hours
Prevens	2 pills immediately and 2 pills in 12 hours

Adapted from Hatcher et al., 1998.

through suppression of endometrial hormone receptors, possibly leading to inadequate maturation of the endometrium and thus preventing implantation (La Valleur, 2000).

Efficacy

After treatment, the pregnancy rate ranges from 0.5% to 2.5%. The variation has to do with when in the menstrual cycle the woman had unprotected sex, how soon she received treatment, and whether the woman develops side effects such as vomiting.

Benefits and Risks

Emergency contraception with COCs offers women a chance to prevent an unwanted pregnancy for a number of reasons. There are no noncontraceptive benefits to be had because of the short-term nature of this regimen.

Risks with this method include failure of the method to prevent pregnancy. Failure will result in the woman having to decide whether to seek pregnancy termination or continue the pregnancy.

Indications

Postcoital contraception is designed as a secondary method of contraception, not as a first choice. Women who repeatedly find themselves in need of this type of contraception are not being proactive in their reproductive decision-making and require counseling.

Contraindications

The only absolute contraindication to emergency contraception with COCs is pregnancy. Use of progestin-only emergency contraception may be best for the woman with a history of thromboembolism.

Side Effects

The major side effects of emergency contraception using COCs are nausea and vomiting. Providing an antinauseant medication before taking the COCs can reduce this side effect. There may be an increased incidence of ectopic pregnancy if conception does occur. There may be menstrual disturbance even in the absence of pregnancy because of the high doses of hormones involved in emergency contraception regimens. Other side effects can include headache, fatigue, and mood swings (La Valleur, 2000).

Progestin-Only Pills

Levonorgestrel has been used in Europe and China for emergency contraception. It is given in a dose of 0.75 mg within 72 hours of unprotected intercourse, and the dose is repeated in 12 hours (La Valleur, 2000). Hatcher et al. (1998) determined that this dose could be obtained by taking 20 yellow tablets of Ovrette immediately and 20 additional tablets in 12 hours. Currently, one 0.75-mg formulation is available that is marketed solely for emergency contraception. The trade name is Plan B. Each of these packets contains two levonorgestrel tablets. One tablet is for immediate use, and the other is for use in 12 hours. This medication must be used within 72 hours of unprotected intercourse (Speroff, 2000).

Antiprogestins

Mifepristone (RU 486) is a synthetic steroid that prevents progesterone from binding to its receptors. Mifepristone has been used extensively in Europe as an abortifacient and as an emergency contraceptive method (Thomas, 2001).

Benefits and Risks

A benefit of this type of emergency contraception is that it is a medical rather than a surgical approach to pregnancy termination. This method is less invasive and has fewer complications than does surgery. Pills are easier to obtain than is a surgical procedure and are very effective. Despite the many benefits, this drug has been very controversial in this country because of questions about when life begins.

Indications

Mifepristone has been investigated for use as an abortifacient and as an emergency contraceptive method. Mifepristone is more effective the earlier in the pregnancy it is used (Cates & Ellertson, 1998).

Contraindications

Contraindications to administering this drug are known or suspected pregnancy unless there is commitment to preg-

nancy termination. Mifepristone also is not used with known or suspected ectopic pregnancy or if there is an undiagnosed adnexal mass. Mifepristone should not be used in clients who have adrenal failure and clients who use long-term steroid therapy, It should not be used in clients who have hemorrhagic disorders or who are using anticoagulants. Clients who have an allergy to the product should not use it.

Side Effects

The major side effects are cramping and vaginal bleeding. Cramping usually can be managed with Tylenol with codeine. Aspirin and ibuprofen are avoided because they are antiprostaglandins and would tend to negate the actions of mifepristone. Bleeding usually is mild but occasionally can be heavy, depending on the age of gestation. When heavy bleeding is a problem, dilatation and curettage may be required.

Intrauterine Devices

Intrauterine devices can be used for emergency contraception. The device should be inserted within 5 to 10 days after unprotected intercourse. In addition to the usual mechanism of action, an IUD inserted for emergency contraception acts as a toxin to the blastocyst (La Valleur, 2000). The IUD is extremely effective as an emergency contraceptive in selected clients.

Surgical Methods

Abortion can be a medical or a surgical procedure. Discussion about the medical method is in the emergency contraception section of this chapter. The purpose of abortion is to terminate a pregnancy. It is not designed to be used as a primary method of contraception but is more appropriate as a backup method in case of failure of the primary method.

Although this surgical procedure has been legally available in the United States since 1973, abortion is still very controversial. Many Americans do not approve of pregnancy termination in any form. The result of this division of thought has been observable in numerous attempts to reverse legalization of abortion. Zealots have tried to prevent women from entering clinics where abortions are performed, picketed clinics, and even have bombed abortion clinics.

Several methods are used for abortion. The choice of methods depends on factors such as the gestational age of the pregnancy. Vacuum extraction can be used only early in the pregnancy. Dilatation and evacuation have been used to abort pregnancies that have progressed beyond the time at which vacuum extraction or aspiration is possible.

Permanent Methods

Sterilization refers to the use of a surgical procedure to produce permanent loss of reproductive capability. Surgical sterilization has become very common for married couples who have decided to permanently limit the size of their family. More women have surgical sterilization than do men.

Female Methods

Worldwide more than 190 million couples use sterilization as their contraceptive method (Pati & Cullins, 2000). Sterilization is the most prevalent method used by married couples in the United States and is used by 39% of couples. Female tubal sterilization, also called **tubal ligation**, accounts for 72% of the sterilization procedures performed in the United States. Female sterilization can be done by tubal ligation or hysterectomy. Hysterectomy usually is used when a gynecologic problem exists at the same time the woman wants permanent sterilization. When a woman has no gynecologic problem, tubal ligation can be performed immediately after delivery by minilaparotomy. A small abdominal incision is made through which the fallopian tubes are grasped and a segment of each is removed. Tubal ligation at any other time usually is a laparoscopic procedure in which a small periumbilical incision and a small lower quadrant incision are made. The tubes may be cauterized, or a clip may be placed on the tube to allow for later removal (Figure 14-13). The woman considering tubal ligation should know that it is a permanent sterilization method. Reversal of this procedure has been done; however, such attempts are not always successful and can be expensive.

Some health care providers believe the appropriate time for a woman to have a tubal ligation is early in the menstrual cycle so there is no possibility for pregnancy. Many times the woman is using birth control pills as a method of contraception, which lessens the importance of when the procedure is done because the woman is not ovulating. If the woman is taking birth control pills, the remainder of the cycle of pills should be taken after the procedure to prevent hormonal problems associated with stopping the pills before the cycle is completed.

Benefits and Risks

Tubal ligation is effective immediately and is considered permanent. These are two very great benefits for women and couples who have finished childbearing. There are no devices to use or details to remember. Laparoscopic tubal ligation can be performed easily on an outpatient basis. It is quite common for a woman to have the surgery on Friday and return to work on Monday.

Although the tubal procedure is considered permanent, there is a small failure rate. Occasionally, the tube will reopen. When this occurs, an unwanted pregnancy may result. In this case, some women have had the procedure a second time. Others decide they want their partner to undergo the next procedure.

Indications

Permanent female sterilization should be reserved for those women who have completed their family. A common discussion with these women includes directions by the health care provider for the woman to consider what her thoughts would be if something would happen to her existing family. If the woman thinks she might want to have more children under those circumstances, she may be encouraged to use a different method of birth control.

Contraindications

Contraindications for this method include women whose health condition is not good enough to withstand the procedure. This contraindication is uncommon.

Adverse Effects

Tubal ligation is a common procedure but is not without complications. The woman has a risk of death from anesthesia or infection. The mortality rate of tubal ligation has been reported to be 1 to 2 deaths per 100,000 procedures. This mortality rate compares favorably with that of hysterectomy, which is 5 to 25 deaths per 100,000 procedures, and childbirth, which is 8 deaths per 100,000 live births in the United States (Pati & Cullins, 2000). Other potential injuries include hemorrhage and damage to the bladder or bowel. Another long-term potential adverse effect is that the woman may regret having had the procedure. The final adverse effect would be failure of the procedure to provide contraception.

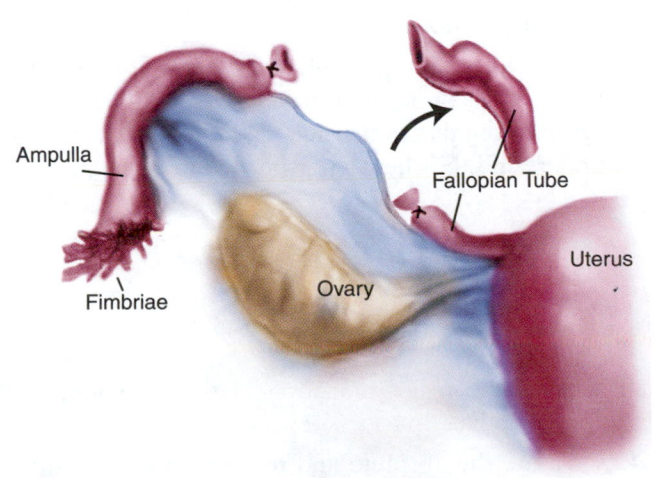

Figure 14-13 Tubal ligation.

Male Methods

The male sterilization procedure is called vasectomy. The vas deferens transport sperm from the epididymis to the seminal vesicle for mixture with other seminal fluids before ejaculation. **Vasectomy** ligates the vas deferens, thus interrupting sperm transport (Figure 14-14). The procedure can be done in an outpatient setting under local anesthesia.

As is sterilization in women, vasectomy is considered permanent. Reversal of the procedure has been done but is not always successful. Postoperative follow-up is important in vasectomy because the sperm count does not immediately decrease to zero. Vasectomy is not considered effective until the man has two negative sperm counts.

NURSING IMPLICATIONS

Nurses often are in a position to teach about contraception and counsel women who are undecided about the method

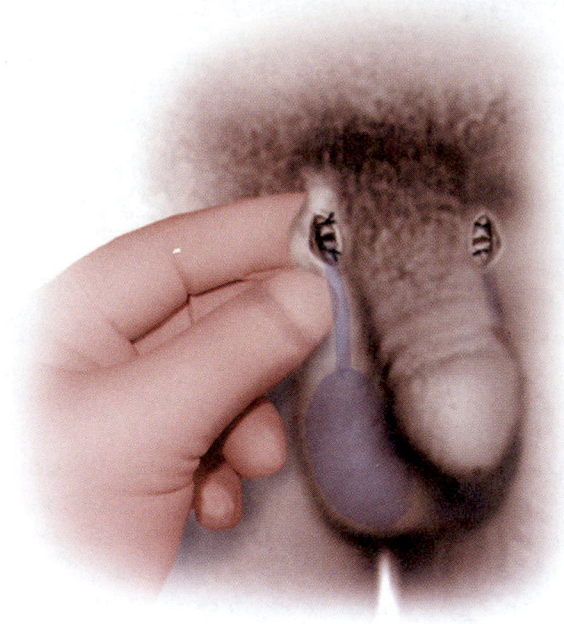

Figure 14-14 Vasectomy.

of contraception they want to use. The nurse must stay informed about the new technologies that are being developed because many times these methods may be preferable for the woman for a number of reasons.

Advanced practice nurses in many settings are able to prescribe contraceptive devices. It becomes even more important for this group of nurss to be informed about currently available contraceptive devices and methods.

Web Activities

1. Go to the NARAL homepage at www.naral.com. What are the issues of interest to this group?

2. Go to nlrc.org. What is the agenda for this group?

Key Concepts

- To use a contraceptive effectively requires the use of a rational decision-making process.

- To use the least effective contraceptive method will prevent unwanted pregnancy significantly better than will unprotected intercourse.

- Complex factors influence a couple's choice and use of contraception.

- To assist couples in family planning, the nurse must realize the couple may have a very different value system from that of the nurse. The nurse will need to understand the client's perspective to be helpful.

Review Questions and Activities

1. What is the difference in the mechanism of action between combined oral contraceptives and the minipill?

2. Which factors are involved in the reproductive decision-making process?

3. What is the major limitation of the combined oral contraceptive?

4. What are the absolute and relative contraindications of COCs?

5. What is the difference between monophasic, biphasic, and triphasic birth control pills?

6. What time limitations are involved with emergency contraception?

7. What are the reasons the IUD is not used more widely?

References

Adams, D. M. (2000). Breastfeeding and oral contraceptives: Exploring opinions and options. *AWHONN Lifelines, 4,* (3), 45–47.

Ballagh, S. A. (2001). Vaginal ring hormone delivery systems in contraception and menopause. *Clinical Obstetrics and Gynecology, 44,* (1), 106–113.

Burkman, R.T. (2001). Oral contraceptive: Current status. *Clinical Obstetrics and Gynecology, 44,* (1), 62–72.

Cates, W. & Ellertson, C. (1998). Abortion. In *Contraceptive Technology* (17th ed.). New York: Ardent Media, Inc.

Charles, C., Gafini, A., & Whelan, T. (1997). Shared decision-making in the medical encounter: What does it mean? (Or it takes at least two to tango). *Social Science and Medicine, 44,* (5) 681–692.

Dailard, C. (2000). Issues in brief: Abortion in context in the United States: Alan Guttmacher Institute. *www.agi-usa.org.* Accessed 3-3-01.

Department of Health and Human Services (DHHS) & The National Institute of Child Health and Human Development (NICHHD). (1996). IUD's: State-of-the-art conference. *Clinical Courier, 14,* (12), 1–7.

Dickey, R.P. (2001). *Managing contraceptive pill patients.* Durant, OK: Essential Medical Information Systems, Inc.

Fuchs, N., Prinz, H., & Koch, U. (1996). Attitudes to current oral contraceptive use and future developments: the women's perspective. *European Journal of Contraceptive and Reproductive Health Care, 1,* (3) 275–284.

Gage, A.J. (1998). Sexual activity and contraceptive use: the components of the decision making process. *Studies in Family Planning, 29,* (2) 154–166.

Gilligan, C., Ward, V., & Taylor, J. (1988). *Mapping the moral domain.* Cambridge, MA: Harvard University Press.

Grady, W.R., Klepinger, D.H., & Nelson-Wally, A. (1999). Contraceptive characteristics: The perceptions and priorities of men and women. *Family Planning Perspectives, 31,* (4), 168–175.

Hatcher, R.A., Trussell, J., Stewart, F., Cates, W., Stewart, G., Guest, F. & Kowal, D. (1998). *Contraceptive Technology* (17th ed.). New York: Ardent Media, Inc.

Grow, D.R., & Almed, S. (2000). New contraceptive methods. *Obstetrics and Gynecology Clinics of North America, 27,* (4), 901–916.

Jensen, J.T., & Speroff, L. (2000). Health benefits of oral contraceptives. *Obstetrics and Gynecology Clinics of North America, 27,* (4), 705–721.

Kaunitz, A.M. (2001). Injectible long-acting contraceptives. *Clinical Obstetrics and Gynecology, 44,* (1), 73–91.

Kjos, S.L. (1997). Contraception for women at risk: A case for the intrauterine device. *Contemporary Ob/Gyn, 42,* (11), 105–121.

La Valleur, J. (2000). Emergency contraception. *Obstetrics and Gynecology Clinics of North America, 27,* (4), 817–839.

Long, V.E. (1998). Between childbearing and menopause: Contraceptive options for women over 40. *Advance for Nurse Practitioners, 6,* (12), 52–58.

Lynch, C. M. (2000). Breakthrough bleeding with ocs: Practical management considerations. *Contemporary Ob/Gyn,* 12 (Suppl.), 3–19.

Manning, W.D., Longmore, M.A., & Giordano, P.C. (2000). The relationship context of contraceptive use at first intercourse. *Family Planning Perspectives. 32,* (3), 104–110.

Matteson, P.S., & Hawkins, J.W. (1997). Women's patterns of contraceptive use. *Health Care of Women International, 18,* (5), 455–466.

Meckstroth, K.R., & Darney, P.D. (2000). Implantable contraception. *Obstetrics and Gynecology Clinics of North America, 27,* (4), 781–815.

Miller, V.L., Laken, M.A., Ager, J., & Essenmacher, L. (2000). Contraceptive decision making among Medicaid-eligible women. *Journal of Community Health, 25,* (6), 473–480.

Mishell, D.R. (1996). IUDs: Historical perspective and mechanisms of action. In *Intrauterine Contraception in the U.S.: A Current Perspective.* Little Falls, NJ: Health Learning Systems, Inc.

Nelson, A. L. (2000). The intrauterine contraceptive device. *Obstetrics & Gynecology Clinics of North America, 27,* (4), 723–740.

Nelson, A. (1995). Patient selection is the key to IUD success. *Contemporary Ob/Gyn, 40,* (10), 49–62.

Oddens, B.J. (1997). Determinants of contraceptive use among women of reproductive age in Great Britain and Germany. II: Psychological factors. *Journal of Biosocial Science, 29,* (4), 437–470.

Pender, N. (1996). Health promotion in nursing practice. Stamford, CT: Appleton & Lange.

Pati, S., & Cullins, V. (2000). Female sterilization: Evidence. *Obstetrics and Gynecology Clinics of North America, 27,* (4), 859–899.

Speroff, L. & Darney, P.D. (2001). A Clinical Guide for Contraception. 3rd ed. Baltimore, MD: Williams & Wilkins.

Speroff, L. (2000). Oral contraceptives and carbohydrate metabolism. *Dialogues in Contraception, 6,* (4), 18.

Speroff L. & Darney P.D. (1992). *A clinical guide to contraception.* Baltimore, MD: William & Wilkins.

Taneepanichskul, S., Reinprayoon, D, & Jaisamrarm, U. (1999). Effects of DMPA on weight and blood pressure in long-term acceptors. *Contraception, 59,* (3), 301–303.

Suggested Readings

Speroff, L., Glass, R. H. & Kase, N. G. (1999). *Cervical Endocrinology Infertility* (6th ed.). Baltimore, MD: Williams & Wilkins.

Stewart, G. K. (1998). Intrauterine devices. In *Contraceptive Technology*. (17th ed.). New York: Ardent Media, Inc.

Thomas, MA (2001). Postcoital contraception. *Clinical Obstetrics and Gynecology, 44,* (1), 101–105.

Resources

Alan Guttmacher Institute this or provides a broad range of information about www.agi-usa.org

Family Planning Network, www.familyplanning.net

Planned Parenthood Federation, www.plannedparenthood.org

UNIT IV

Pregnancy

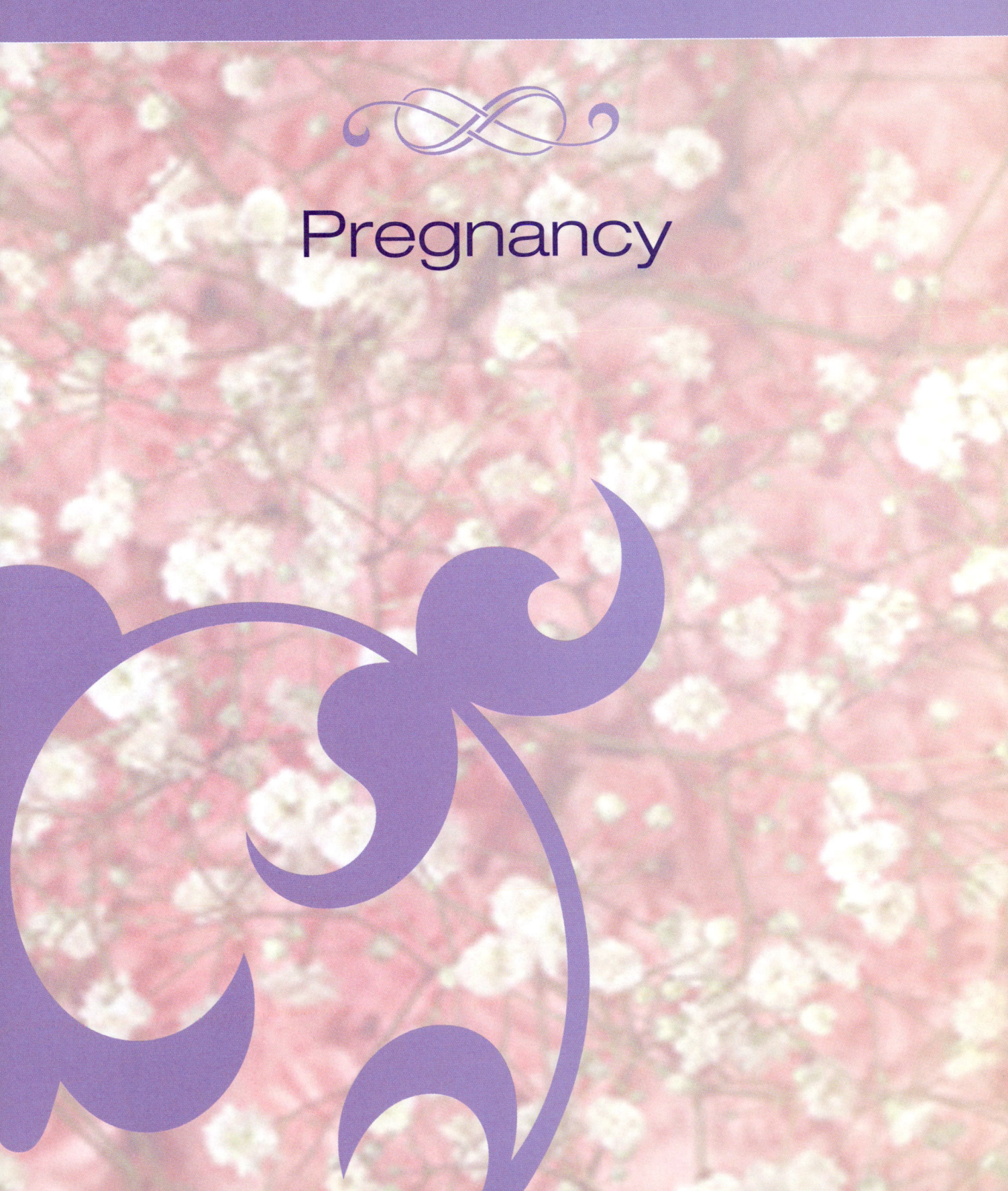

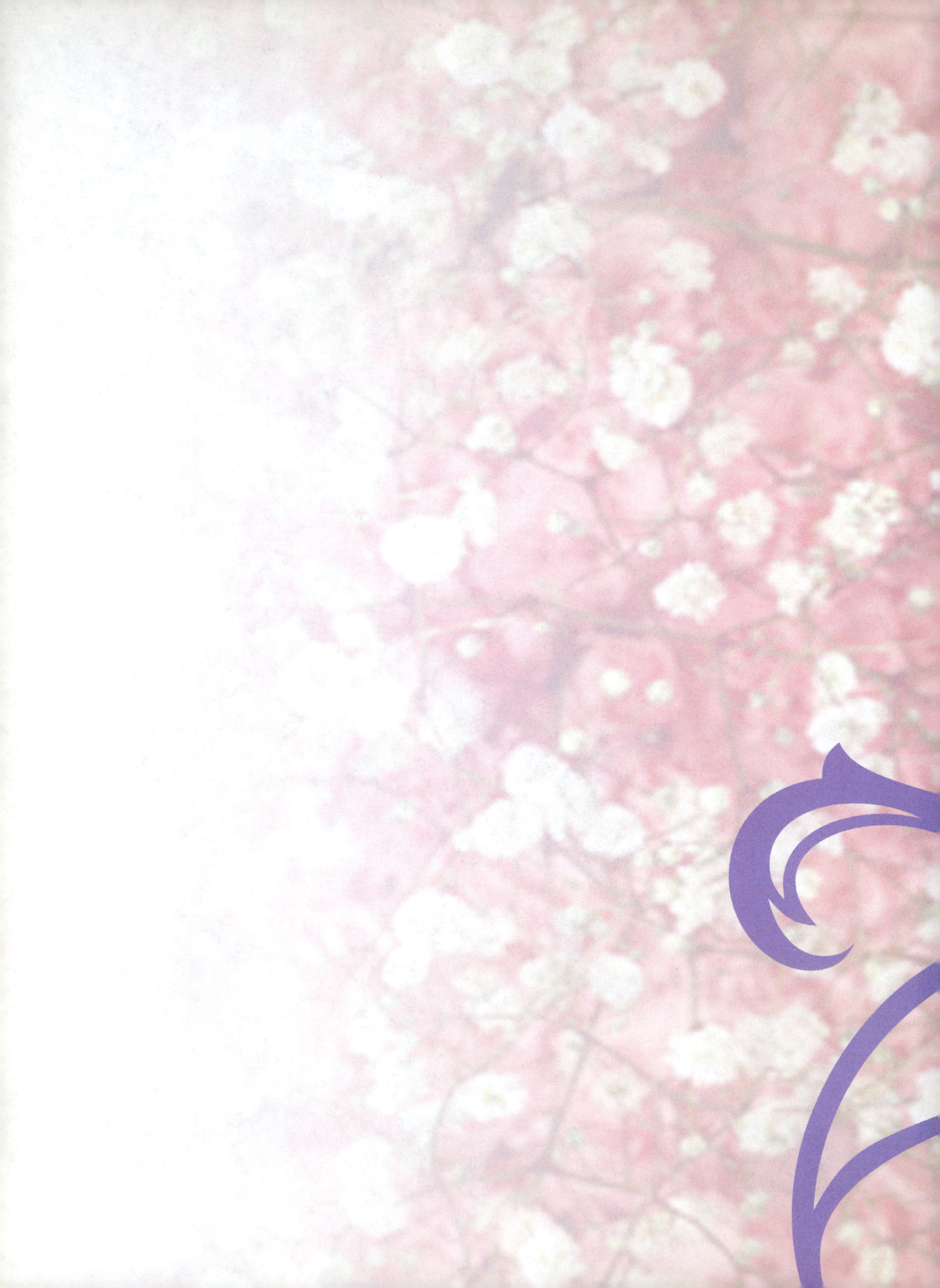

CHAPTER 15

Normal Pregnancy

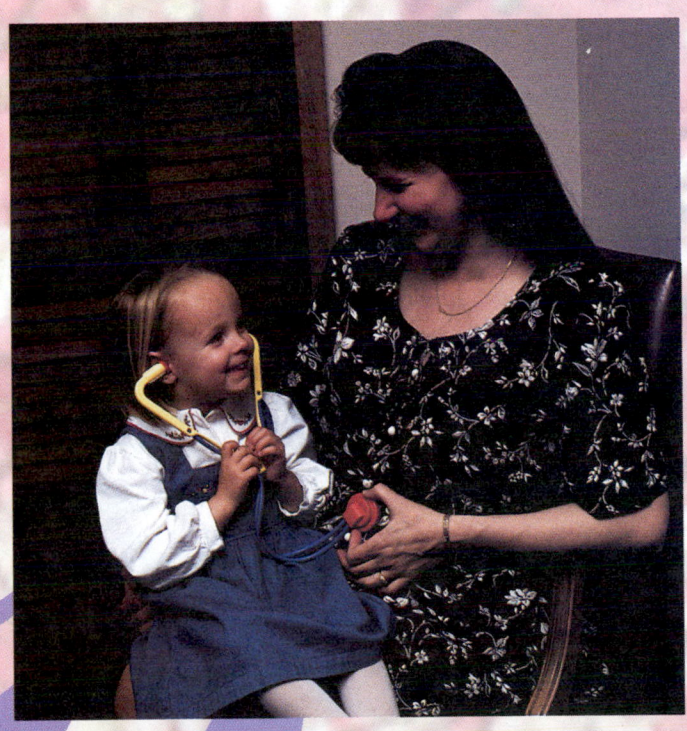

For a woman, pregnancy is a time of great change and adaptation. Many times, women proceed through the process unaware of the total picture. Nurses can play a vital role in helping a woman achieve a healthy, successful pregnancy by supporting, nurturing, educating, and caring for the pregnant woman and her family. Small gestures, such as always remembering her name, inquiring about family happenings, and being supportive and nonjudgmental, aid the nurse in rendering accurate, effective, and sensitive care. To be a nurse and provide care to a woman during this special life transition and to provide that care with compassion and respect is a great privilege.

Amenorrhea
Chadwick's sign
Chloasma

Colostrum
Goodell's sign
Hegar's sign

Linea nigra
Physiologic anemia of
    pregnancy

Quickening
Striae gravidarum

Competencies

Upon completion of this chapter, the reader should be able to:

1. List the presumptive, probable, and positive signs of pregnancy.
2. Describe the anatomic and physiologic adaptations to pregnancy.
3. Explain how the anatomic and physiologic adaptations to pregnancy relate to the common discomforts of pregnancy.
4. Outline self-help tips to assist the client in relieving the discomforts of pregnancy.
5. Describe methods of teaching health topics to the pregnant woman.
6. List the developmental tasks that successfully integrate the motherhood role into the woman's personality.
7. Explain how understanding a client's culture can affect her plan of care.

Pregnancy is a time of enormous change in a woman's body and mind. These changes affect her physical well-being, self-esteem, interactions with others, daily activities, and future plans. She looks for answers to questions that arise during her pregnancy from many different sources. The nurse's role is uniquely suited to forming a professional bond with the pregnant client and to offering impartial and accurate information that will guide her 9-month journey.

The nurse-client relationship can serve as a "safe haven" for the pregnant woman to ask questions and discuss concerns. Initially, the questions are related to how the pregnancy and birth of the newborn will affect her activities of daily living, her relationship with others, and her interaction with her health care providers. The information may not always be sought by direct questions; therefore, the nurse must be skilled in interviewing and physical assessment techniques with which to meet the woman's needs.

A woman's body changes dramatically to maintain a viable pregnancy. The knowledge and understanding of how these changes occur gives the nurse the ability to assess, make diagnoses, plan, intervene, and evaluate to ensure that the expected outcomes are achieved.

SIGNS OF PREGNANCY

There are many signs of pregnancy. Some signs are suggestive of pregnancy and are referred to as *presumptive* (subjective) signs; these signs could be caused by other conditions, so they do not establish a diagnosis of pregnancy. *Probable* (objective) signs of pregnancy can be documented by physical examination and are signs that are most often only characteristic of pregnancy; these findings could also be caused by other conditions, however, and therefore do not establish a diagnosis of pregnancy. Only three physical findings can establish a diagnosis of pregnancy; these are referred to as *positive* signs. In today's fast-paced world, women are more likely to use an over-the-counter home pregnancy test at the first hint of pregnancy and later seek final confirmation from their healthcare provider.

Presumptive Signs

Amenorrhea, absence of menses for 3 or more months, is usually the first sign to alert a woman to a possible pregnancy. Other factors, such as excessive exercise, emotional stress, chronic disease states, the onset of menopause, and the use of oral contraceptives, can stop regular periods. The cause of amenorrhea should be assessed and validated.

Nausea and vomiting is another subjective sign that can appear after the first missed period and continue into the fourth month of pregnancy. Women most often report feeling sick in the morning, hence the phrase "morning sickness," but nausea and vomiting may occur at any time of the day. The cause is not clear; it may be the increased levels of hormones. Many women report that emotional factors, noxious smells, irregular eating schedules, and fatigue contribute.

The fatigue of pregnancy is an overwhelming need for rest and sleep and is distressing. The client may voice concerns that she is more tired or drowsy after a normal day during pregnancy than she was after a normal day before she became pregnant.

In the first few weeks of pregnancy, the pressure exerted on the bladder by the enlarging uterus causes urinary frequency. In the second trimester, the uterus grows into the abdomen, somewhat relieving the pressure. Late in pregnancy, as the fetus grows and descends into the pelvis, urinary frequency returns. Do not assume urinary frequency is caused by the changes of pregnancy; assess for signs of infection.

Changes in the breasts are another presumptive sign of pregnancy. Increased amounts of estrogen and progesterone cause the breasts to swell and become tender. The initial changes in the breasts are similar to the changes that occur in the menstrual cycle. As the pregnancy progresses, the tenderness subsides, but growth of breast tissue continues.

A woman's first awareness of fetal movement is called **quickening**. The movement is usually described as a fluttery feeling, similar to being excited and having "butterflies." Quickening is initially felt between 18 and 20 weeks of gestation, but may be felt by the multigravida as early as 16 weeks. The documented date of the first fetal movement can be used in conjunction with other data in determining the expected date of delivery.

Probable Signs

At 8 to 10 weeks' gestation the bimanual pelvic examination will document an enlarged and softened uterine body. Uterine enlargement is more definitive if the growth is progressive. The fundus should be just above the symphysis pubis at 10 to 12 weeks and at the umbilicus at 20 weeks. Abdominal enlargement mirrors the uterine growth and is especially evident earlier in the pregnancy of the multigravida. A woman may hear comments from well-meaning friends and family about the way she is carrying the baby. The nurse can alleviate her concerns by telling the client about the individuality of each pregnancy.

There are other changes that may be noted on physical examination. Softening of the cervix is called **Goodell's sign**; normally the cervix is firm. The color change from pink to bluish-purplish in the mucous membranes of the cervix, vagina, and vulva is identified as **Chadwick's sign**. The increased vascularization in this area causes the color change and is attributed to the increase in the estrogen hormone. **Hegar's sign**, usually evident at 6 to 8

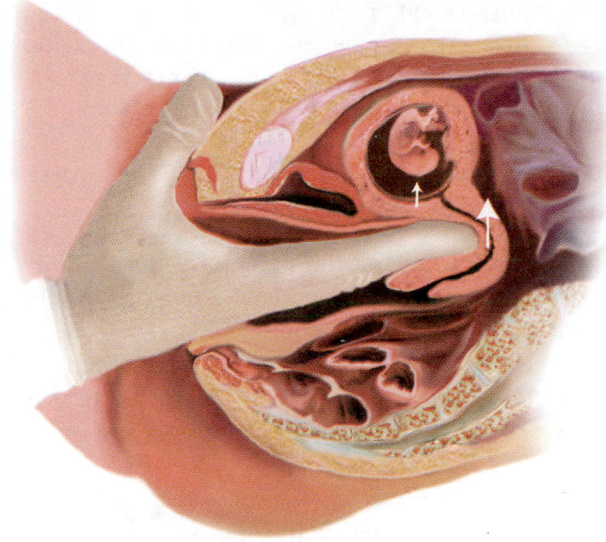

Figure 15-1 Ballottement.

weeks' gestation, is the softening of the isthmus of the uterus, often referred to as the lower uterine segment.

During the fourth or fifth month, if the fetus is pushed upward through the vagina or abdomen, the floating fetus rebounds against the examiner's fingers; this is known as **ballottement** (Figure 15-1). This occurs only while the fetus is small in comparison to the amount of amniotic fluid.

Today, pregnancy tests are available in inexpensive commercial kits that can be done quickly. Tests that are performed by trained personnel are highly accurate and, with correct technique, precise. Most pregnancy tests work on the same premise: they identify human chorionic gonadotropin (hCG) hormone, or a subunit, by detecting an antibody to the hCG molecule in urine or serum. Commercial laboratory tests that measure hCG in the urine are accurate close to 100% of the time and can detect a pregnancy as early as 10 days after conception. The hormone hCG can be detected in maternal blood at 7 days after conception with sensitive assays; the exact level of hCG can assist in dating the pregnancy. Most sensitive commercial test kits can detect a pregnancy with precision after the first missed period.

Home pregnancy test kits are readily available and relatively inexpensive. Similar to the urine test done in the physician's office or laboratory, the test is sensitive for the presence of hCG in urine. Although the tests have become simpler to use, the number-one concern is operator error. A false-negative result can mislead the woman, who may ignore the presumptive signs of pregnancy and cause a delay in seeking prenatal care. A positive test result may cause a delay in seeking follow-up care, because many women feel the first visit to a practitioner is only for diagnosis of pregnancy. Preconception counseling is crucial for educating women on caring for their body before pregnancy. At that time, it is beneficial to share information on the appropriate management of pregnancy diagnosis and the initiation of prenatal care.

Positive Signs

Positive signs (noted by the examiner) that confirm the pregnancy are fetal heart sounds and fetal movement and visualization of the fetus during ultrasound.

The fetal heartbeat can be auscultated with a fetoscope at 18–20 weeks. The heartbeat can be detected at 10–12 weeks with an electronic doppler. Normal fetal heart rate is 120 to 160 beats/min.

The earlier the fetal heart beat is detected, the more likely it may be confused with other sounds that can be detected in pregnancy. The uterine souffle is the sound made by the increased amount of blood perfusing the uterus and mimics the maternal pulse. The sound heard as the blood flows through the umbilical cord is called the funic souffle.

Fetal movement detected by a qualified examiner is another sign that is diagnostic of pregnancy. At 18 to 20 weeks' gestation, the movement is felt as a faint fluttering and progresses to rolling and kicking in the late second and third trimester. The movement in later gestation can often be seen on visual inspection of the abdomen.

The use of ultrasound is very common in today's obstetric practice. The ultrasound examination is accomplished by placing a transducer on the abdomen above the symphysis pubis (Figure 15-2). A normal pregnancy can be detected at as early as 4 weeks' gestation, using the last menstrual period for dating. Thus, confirmation of the pregnancy is possible before some common tests for hCG in the urine show positive results. The fetal brain and heartbeat can be visualized by 8 weeks' gestation.

ACCURATE DETECTION OF THE FETAL HEART RATE

To ensure an accurate diagnosis of the fetal heart beat, it must be distinguished from the maternal pulse. To do this, the fetal heartbeat should be auscultated, while simultaneously assessing the maternal radial pulse.

The use of a transvaginal transducer placed into the vagina is helpful when using ultrasound to confirm a pregnancy or seek pathology in the obese woman or to detect a pregnancy in a complicated case. The fetal heart rate can be detected via transvaginal ultrasound as early as 4 weeks after conception. A transvaginal ultrasound examination produces better visualization than abdominal ultrasound, and cannot only detect an early pregnancy but also extrauterine structures, such as an ectopic pregnancy or ovarian mass (Gabbe, Niebyl, & Simpson, 1996).

EXPECTED DATE OF DELIVERY

The mean duration of pregnancy can differ between groups of women by ethnicity, geographical location, or age, but the most common period used as the mean is 280 days, or 40 weeks from the first day of the last period. Naegele's rule is the most commonly used calculation for date of expected delivery. To calculate the gestational or menstrual age, add 7 days to the date of the first day of

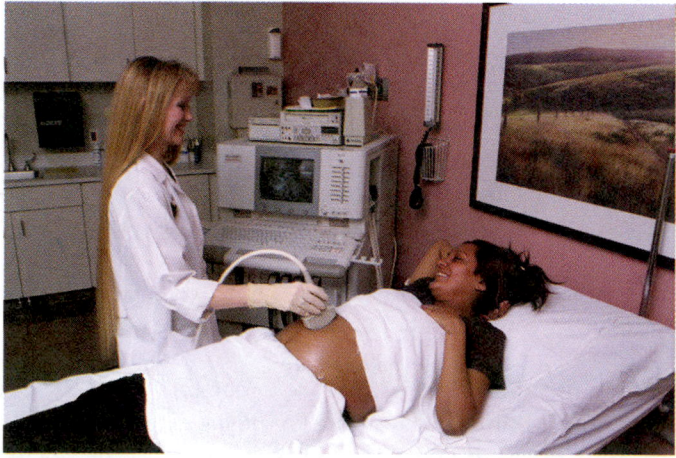

A.

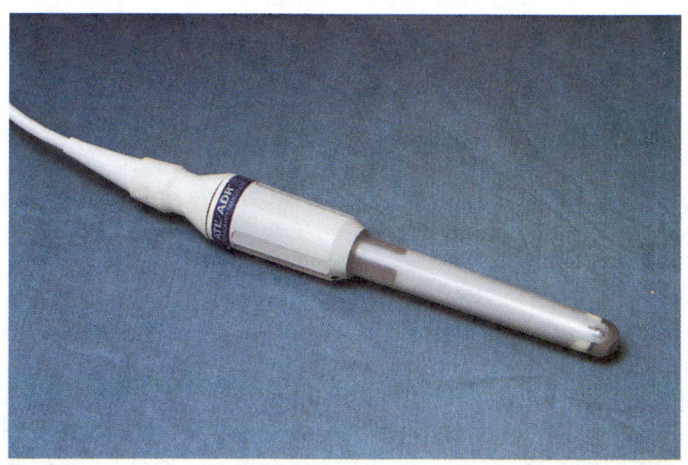

B.

Figure 15-2 A. Abdominal ultrasound; B. Transducer for transvaginal ultrasound.

EXAMPLE OF NAEGELE'S RULE

First day of last period was January 12, 2001.
Calculate: 1/12/2001 + 7 days = 1/19/2001
Count back 3 months to October. The expected delivery date is 10/19/2002.

PHYSIOLOGIC ADAPTATION TO PREGNANCY

Many physiologic changes take place in a woman's body when she is pregnant. The nurse and client must be able to distinguish between those changes that are normal adaptations and responses to the pregnant state and those changes that are outside the realm of normal and require intervention.

Reproductive System

Each organ of the reproductive system undergoes dramatic changes during pregnancy.

Uterus

Although every system in a woman's body changes to adapt to the growing fetus, the uterus undergoes the most dramatic transformation (Figure 15-4). Beginning as an almost solid organ the size of a human fist, the uterus enlarges to a thin-walled, hollow organ that can hold a volume of 15 to 20 liters. The initial changes in the structure of the uterus are caused by hypertrophy, the enlargement of existing myometrial cells, with only a small percentage of the growth attributed to hyperplasia, the increase in the number of myometrial cells. The increased production of estrogen and progesterone is thought to initiate the process of uterine growth, but the exact trigger mechanism is unclear. This hypothesis is based on the observation that uterine hypertrophy occurs even if the

the last normal menstrual period and count back 3 months.

This date is an estimated date of delivery and it can be inaccurate by 2 weeks. Because gestation, measured in weeks, is so important for the management of the pregnancy, other clinical indicators should be monitored. During the first physical examination, the size of the uterus can be determined; the fetal heart rate can be heard at 10 to 12 weeks by electronic Doppler ultrasound; the first fetal movement can be felt at about 20 weeks; and the measurement of fundal (top of the uterus) height with each prenatal visit can track gestational age (Figure 15-3). If the results of the physical examination do not correspond with the estimated weeks of pregnancy, as determined by calculating the delivery date, an ultrasound examination may be performed between 12 and 18 weeks to obtain fetal measurements that result in a more accurate delivery date.

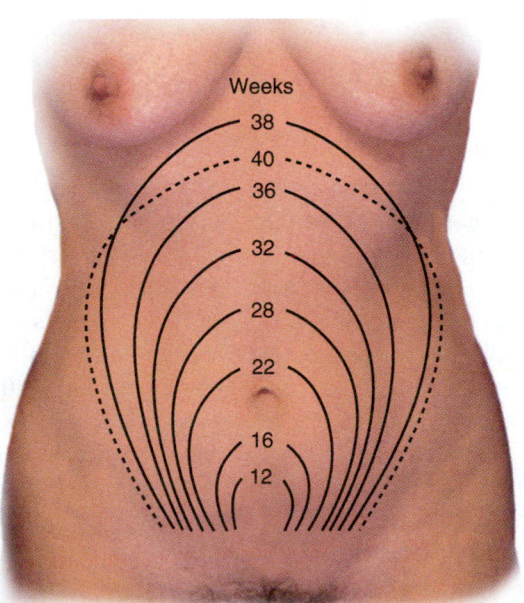

Figure 15-3 Approximate height of the fundus as the uterus enlarges.

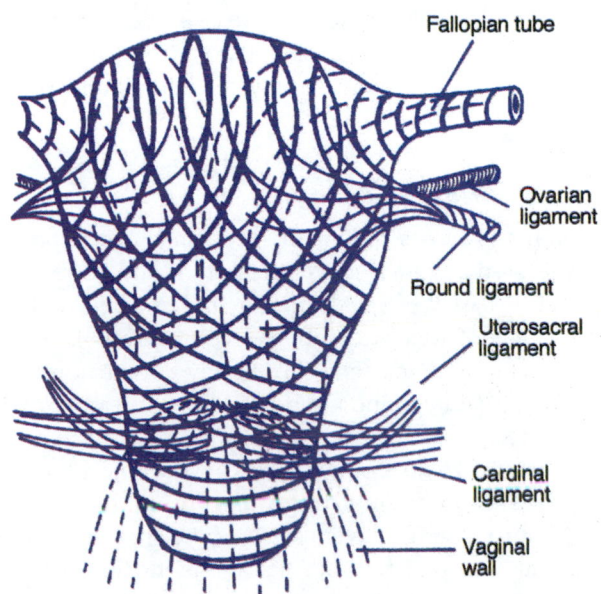

Figure 15-4 The configuration of muscle layers allows the uterus to expand evenly in all directions during pregnancy.

embryo has implanted outside the uterus (Blackburn and Loper, 1992).

It is not until the twelfth week of gestation, when the fetus reaches a crown-to-rump length of 8 to 9 centimeters, that the growth of the uterus can be attributed to mechanical distention. The increase in intrauterine pressure results from the growing fetus, placenta, and increase in volume of amniotic fluid. Growth of the uterus is not symmetrical and occurs predominantly in the fundus. The walls of the uterus become thin but are strengthened by the accumulation of fibrous tissue in the muscle layers and an increase in elastic tissue. At twelve weeks, the fundus rises above the symphysis and begins to displace the intestines. It will continue to grow upward and slightly rotate to the right. When the pregnant woman is upright, the broad and round ligaments anchor the gravid uterus and the anterior abdominal wall provides support. The weight of the uterus may produce tension on these ligaments that causes inflammation and discomfort. In the supine position, the uterus of the pregnant woman falls backward and puts pressure on the vertebral column and the great blood vessels.

Uteroplacental Blood Flow

Although not visibly evident to the pregnant woman, the changes that begin at conception progress rapidly. The placenta is mature at 8 to 10 weeks and remains larger than the fetus until 15 to 16 weeks. To achieve adequate exchange of nutrients and waste, there is an increase in the supply of blood to the uteroplacental unit. The body is able to accommodate the necessary volume by increasing the number and diameter of the vessels feeding the uterus. The proportion of the blood volume needed to perfuse the uterus and intervillous space increases over the weeks of gestation. By term, a total of 20% to 25% of the maternal cardiac output is used to supply the uterus and placenta (Haun, 1991).

Uterine Contractility

The uterus is never quiescent; even in the non-pregnant state the uterus will contract (Blackburn and Loper, 1992). Contractions in the first trimester are undetected by the maternal client, but she can feel contractions late in the second trimester. Normally these early contractions are irregular and painless and are referred to as **Braxton Hicks contractions**. As the pregnancy progresses toward full term, Braxton Hicks contractions can become more regular, occur at more frequent intervals, and cause discomfort. The client may make several visits to her practitioner or to the hospital only to be told that she is in "false labor." At this point, the woman may become embarrassed and doubt her ability to recognize the symptoms of true labor. One component of prenatal education is to communicate

to the client the symptoms of preterm and term labor and the importance of notifying her health practitioner if she has any questions.

Cervix

Although the cervix does not undergo the same dramatic changes as the uterus, it plays an instrumental role in the maintenance of the pregnancy and the delivery of the infant. In the prepregnant state, the cervix is firm and feels similar to the top of the ear. As early as 4 weeks after conception, biochemical changes occur and cause the connective tissue of the cervix to become swollen with water (edematous) and congested with blood (hyperemic). These changes, in conjunction with the hypertrophy and hyperplasia of the cervical glands, demonstrate the characteristic cervical softening of Goodell's sign and cervical cyanosis of Chadwick's sign. At this time, a digital examination of the cervix demonstrates a softened consistency, similar to the feel of the ear lobe.

The changes that occur in the cervix demonstrate the amazing adaptability of the body. The cervix provides support to maintain an intact pregnancy and, as delivery approaches, it softens and opens to allow delivery of the infant.

A mucus plug forms within the cervix and serves to protect the fetus and the membranes from bacteria that may ascend through the vagina during pregnancy. As labor becomes imminent, the mucus plug is expelled (sometimes over a period of time) as the cervix begins to dilate. As the cervix dilates, small arteries may burst and the blood mixes with the normal mucus, producing what is known as bloody show.

Vagina, Perineum, and Vulva

In preparation for the delivery of the neonate, there is increased vascularization, softening of the connective tissue and hypertrophy of the smooth muscle in the vagina, perineum, and vulva. The vagina turns the characteristic purplish color of Chadwick's sign and vaginal secretions increase as a result of increased vascular engorgement. The walls of the vagina must expand without trauma during the delivery, therefore the mucosa thicken and the rugae (vaginal folds) become pronounced. Upon vaginal examination, the caregiver may note that the rugae that line the lower portion of the anterior wall of the vagina are so enlarged that they protrude through the vulva.

As the physiologic changes progress, the cells of the vagina contain increasing amounts of glycogen. The cells slough off the walls of the vagina and contribute to the increase in discharge. The *Lactobacillus acidophilus* found in normal vaginal secretions breaks down the glycogen into lactic acid (Cunningham, MacDonald, Gant, et al., 1997). The environment of the vagina is acidic and prevents the growth of many bacterial infections. If the client complains of increased vaginal discharge, the amount, color, consistency, and odor of discharge must be assessed so that an appropriate diagnosis can be made. One of the most frequent infections in pregnancy is a vaginal yeast infection (candidiasis), which grows readily in the normal acidic discharge.

Ovaries

Once conception has occurred, the production and release of follicles from the ovaries ceases. The corpus luteum is formed within the ovary and secretes progesterone, with production peaking at 8 days. Progesterone is necessary for the maintenance of the pregnancy, so that if implantation occurs, the trophoblast secretes hCG to stimulate the corpus luteum to continue with the production of progesterone (Tucker and Loper, 1992). The placenta begins manufacturing progesterone at 6–7 weeks gestation. At this time the placenta assumes this function and the involution of the corpus luteum begins.

Breasts

The changes in the physical characteristics of the breasts are caused by the increased production of estrogen and progesterone. Early in pregnancy, the breasts become full and tender. In preparation for feeding the infant, the number of mammary alveoli increase and the breasts become physically larger. As the breasts enlarge, a web of veins may become visible under the skin. The pregnant woman may question the slightly reddened or darkened, depressed streaks that appear on the skin of the breasts. These striations (stretch marks) occur most often on breasts that enlarge significantly. The striae eventually fade to a soft silver color, but do not disappear completely. The areolae broaden and become darker in color as a result of increased pigmentation. The tubercles of Montgomery are sebaceous glands located on the areolae that become more visible through hypertrophic changes. In preparation for lactation, the glands secrete a substance that helps maintain the suppleness of the areolae. Increased sensitivity of the now larger and more erect nipple contributes to the later establishment of lactation. The pregnant woman may notice leaking of colostrum, a protein-rich yellowish fluid, from her breasts after the first few months of pregnancy.

Women with small breasts may welcome the increase in size, but women with large breasts may find it difficult to tolerate. Wearing a properly fitted bra that supports the breasts should be emphasized in early prenatal visits.

Hematologic System

The changes in the hematologic system occur to maintain homeostasis during the pregnancy and the postpartum period. Blood volume increases to nourish the fetus and to protect the mother from excessive blood loss during and after delivery and placental separation. Being aware of these changes and how they affect normal hematologic values helps the nurse in identifying the difference in expected adaptations and pathologic alterations (Table 15-1).

Blood Volume

The blood volume of the pregnant woman is 40% to 50% more than the prepregnant state. Obese women and women who have multiple fetuses or a fetus that is large for gestation age may attain a blood volume that is double their usual blood volume. Progesterone causes the tone of the vasculature to relax and enables the body to accommodate the massive increase in blood volume that is necessary to meet the increased needs of the pregnancy. Hypervolemia of pregnancy is an expected and necessary change and affects the plan of client care.

Table 15-1 Normal Changes in Maternal Laboratory Values

Test	Normal Value	Change during Pregnancy
Hematocrit	37%–47%	Decreased
Hemoglobin level	12–16 g/dL	Decreased
Platelet count	150,000–350,000/mm^3	Increased after delivery
Partial thromboplastin time (PTT)	12–14 sec	Slightly decreased
Leukocyte	6.0(4.5–11) $\times$ 10^3/mm^3	9.2(6–16) $\times$ 10^3/mm^3
Fibrinogen level	250 mg/dL	Increased

Burraw & Duffy (1999).

Plasma volume begins to increase at 6 to 8 weeks' gestation, increases rapidly until about 32 to 34 weeks, and then reaches a plateau until term. The increase in the plasma volume is 40% to 45% and measures 1200 to 1600 mL above prepregnant volume. As in most changes that occur during pregnancy, the exact mechanism that triggers this change is not well understood. One influencing factor may be increased hormone production. Another close link may be the changes that take place in the fluid balance in the renal and cardiovascular systems.

Blackburn and Loper (1992) noted that placental mass and birth weight are positively correlated with plasma volume, demonstrating the close relationship of fetal weight to plasma volume. In pathologic states, such as pregnancy-induced hypertension, there is a decrease in plasma volume related to the changes that occur in the vasculature. A common risk factor for the fetus of the woman with pregnancy-induced hypertension is fetal intrauterine growth retardation. The knowledge of this risk factor enables the caregiver to individualize the client's plan of care to obtain the best outcome.

Red Blood Cells

An increase in the number of red blood cells is another significant adaptation to pregnancy. The red blood cell mass increases up to 33% (450 mL) with iron supplementation and increases up to 18% (200 mL) without supplementation (Blackburn and Loper, 1992). The volume increase is progressive without the plateau at term that is observed in the plasma volume.

During the pregnancy, the plasma begins to expand earlier and to a volume three times greater than the red blood cell mass. The disproportion of these volumes causes a dilution of the red blood cell mass, thus lowering the hemoglobin of the pregnant woman and resulting in a phenomenon called **physiologic anemia of pregnancy**. Because this anemia is caused by normal physiologic changes in blood volume during pregnancy, it is not considered a true anemia. The average hemoglobin level of

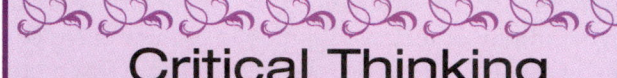

Critical Thinking

Physiologic Anemia of Pregnancy

Joan is a 16-year-old African American with a pregnancy at 28 weeks' gestation. She is attending high school and plans on living at home when the baby comes. She is feeling more tired than usual. Laboratory samples are drawn and analyzed; her hemoglobin level is 8.5 mg/dL and hematocrit is 30%.

What are the mainstays of Joan's diet? Has iron supplementation been prescribed? Is she taking the supplement? Is Joan well hydrated? What fluids is she drinking?

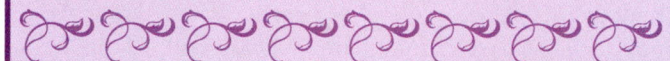

the pregnant woman at term is 12 mg/dL, with a mean hematocrit of 33.8%. Although the normal hemoglobin level can drop up to 2 mg/dL with the normal dilution of the red blood cell mass, Blackburn and Loper (1992) state that true iron deficiency anemia should always be considered, especially when the hemoglobin level drops to 10.5 mg/dL or less.

Blood Coagulation

Neither bleeding time or clotting time change in the normal pregnant woman, but there is still a popular belief in the hypercoagulability of pregnancy. Gabbe, Niebyl, and Simpson (1996) noted that although there are increases in some of the clotting factors, especially fibrinogen, the hypercoagulability of pregnancy is more likely attributable to the higher incidence of thrombus formation and coagulopathies during pregnancy. When evaluating the pregnant woman, remember that the highest incidence of thromboembolism is in the postpartum period.

Cardiovascular System

To maintain a viable pregnancy, the cardiovascular system undergoes major but reversible changes in cardiac function and hemodynamics. These changes are triggered by the increase in circulating hormones: estrogen, progesterone, and prostaglandin.

Heart

The position of the heart is changed by the inability of the diaphragm to fully expand, increasing intra-abdominal pressure. The heart is pushed upward and to the left and rotated slightly, as shown in Figure 15-5. On radiographic film, the heart may appear enlarged. The position is influenced by other anatomic changes, and the varying degrees of these changes in individual pregnancies make it difficult to diagnose cardiomegaly by X-ray studies alone.

There are no significant changes in the electrocardiogram (ECG) of the pregnant woman. In 90% of pregnant women, a systolic heart murmur can be heard at 20 weeks' gestation and disappears shortly after delivery. Also, in the majority of pregnant women, a third heart sound, or gallop, can be easily detected. Diastolic murmurs are rare in normal pregnant women and the cause of these sounds should be investigated. A murmur known as the "mammary souffle" can be heard in the left and right side between the first, second, and third intercostal spaces. The increased blood flow to the breasts is believed to be the cause of this continuous murmur.

Cardiac Output

During pregnancy, there is an increase in cardiac output beginning as early as 10 weeks and peaking at 20 at 24 weeks. Cardiac output is calculated by the heart rate times the *stroke volume,* the amount of blood leaving the heart. Early in pregnancy the increase in cardiac output is caused by an increase in the stroke volume, and the heart rate remains at the prepregnant rate. As the pregnancy progresses, the heart rate increases by up to 20 beats/min and the stroke volume declines to prepregnant rates. By means of the increase in the heart rate, the blood volume needed to adequately provide blood flow to the fetus and the maternal vital organs can be maintained. In the nonpregnant woman, average cardiac output is 4.5 L/min with the uterus receiving 2%; at term in the pregnant woman, cardiac output is about 6 L/min with about 20% going to the uterus. The percentage of the cardiac output that is mapped to the other organs remains relatively the same in the nonpregnant and pregnant woman. Because of the overall increase in blood volume, the amount of blood available to most vital organs increases.

Blood Pressure

It would seem logical to assume that the increases in the blood volume and cardiac output of the pregnant woman would lead to elevated blood pressure, but other adaptations take place to prevent this from occurring. Both systolic and diastolic blood pressure actually decrease in the first trimester by 5 to 10 mm Hg and 10 to 15 mm Hg, respectively, and begin to rise at 22 to 24 weeks, returning to normal prepregnant readings at term. The decrease in the blood pressure is probably a result of the effect of increased circulating hormones, which, in turn, decrease the peripheral vascular resistance. This adaptation must be

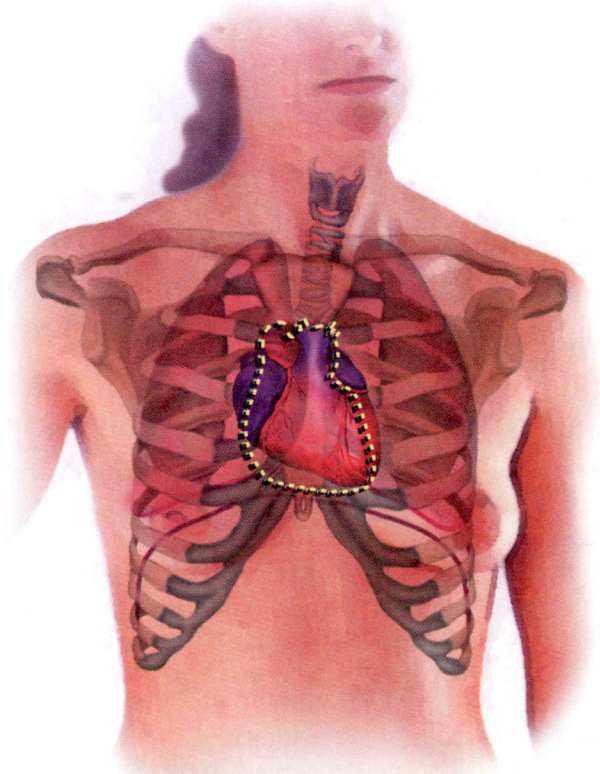

Figure 15-5 The position of the heart is changed during pregnancy. The solid line demonstrates how the heart is pushed upward and to the left and rotated slightly.

Nursing Tip

ASSESSING BLOOD PRESSURE
Prepregnant blood pressure measurements, instead of first trimester readings, should be used as the baseline when ruling out pregnancy-induced hypertension.

understood when assessing the blood pressure late in the second and into the third trimester.

The ability of the pregnant body to compensate for the increased blood volume results from the increased capacity and compliance of the vascular system. Venous pressure in the upper extremities is unchanged. In the lower extremities, the pressure may gradually increase as the uterus enlarges and begins to exert pressure on the inferior vena cava and pelvic veins. The increase in pressure below the level of the uterus can result in the development of varicose veins in the legs and perineum. When the pregnant woman is in the upright position, the uterus can interfere with the blood return to the heart. Blood pools in the lower extremities and may contribute to the dependent edema that may occur in the last half of the pregnancy. The lower extremity blood congestion seen in pregnancy can be alleviated by lying in a lateral recumbent position (Figure 15-6). Prenatal education should include teaching pregnant women to avoid prolonged standing, use support hose, and take frequent rest breaks.

Systemic Vascular Resistance

In pregnancy the increase in cardiac output and the slight decrease in mean arterial pressure results in a decrease in the *systemic vascular resistance,* or total circulatory resistance. Increased hormonal activity relaxes smooth muscle, causing vessels to dilate and thus allowing the body to accommodate the increased blood volume without pressure changes. The uteroplacental circulation provides a new and large capacity organ that diverts a portion of the increased cardiac output. Finally, increased circulating levels of prostaglandin during pregnancy serve to buffer the effects of certain vasoconstrictors. These adaptations allow the pregnant woman to accommodate the larger volume of cardiac output without the injurious side effects expected in a nonpregnant woman.

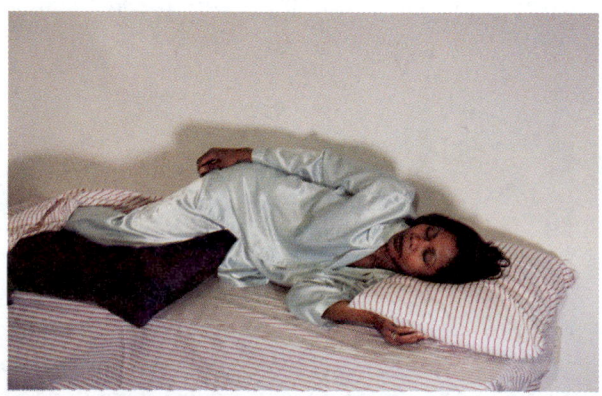

Figure 15-6 Resting in the lateral position helps to alleviate pooling of blood in the lower extremities.

The Effect of Positioning during Pregnancy

As the pregnant woman approaches term, she may report that lying on her back (supine) causes her to feel lightheaded, dizzy, or faint. The symptoms are a result of the hypotension that occurs when the weight of the gravid uterus partially occludes the vena cava and descending aorta. The occlusion of these vessels may cause a decrease in the blood return from the lower extremities to the heart, therefore causing a decrease in cardiac output and a decrease in blood pressure. If the decrease in cardiac output is prolonged, blood flow to the placenta can be affected and fetal hypoxia may occur.

Supine hypotension, also known as vena cava syndrome, occurs when the pregnant woman is supine. The enlarged, heavy uterus presses on the inferior vena cava causing a reduced blood flow back to the right atrium (Figure 15-7). The pregnant woman experiences dizziness; clammy, pale skin; and lowered blood pressure. The situation is relieved when the pregnant woman lies on her side.

The effect of positioning on the ability of the heart to pump adequate amounts of blood should be included in prenatal education sessions. When women want to lie on their backs, instruct them on the hazards of the supine position and the necessity of using a wedge under their hip to laterally tilt the uterus, alleviating vessel compression. Instruct the woman to turn to her side if she experiences the symptoms of hypotension and to use the side-lying position when resting.

Respiratory System

Changes that occur in the respiratory system are necessary to meet the increased demand for oxygen by both the pregnant woman and her fetus. These changes are both mechanical and biochemical and improve the efficiency of the maternal respiratory function.

Changes in Mechanical Function

The thoracic cavity changes early in pregnancy, contradicting the idea that anatomic changes that occur in the respiratory system result solely from the enlarged uterus and the increase in intra-abdominal pressure. The growing uterus does change the size and shape of the abdomen, causing the diaphragm to rise 4 centimeters above the normal nonpregnant resting position. Diaphragmatic excursion is increased, rather than decreased. The chest circumference increases 5 to 7 centimeters, and the transverse diameter increases approximately 2 centimeters (Gabbe, et al., 1996). Blackburn and Loper (1992) state that the flaring of the lower ribs increases the subcostal angle from 68 to 103 degrees at term. Changes in the structure of the respiratory organs takes place to prepare the body for the enlarging uterus and increased lung volume.

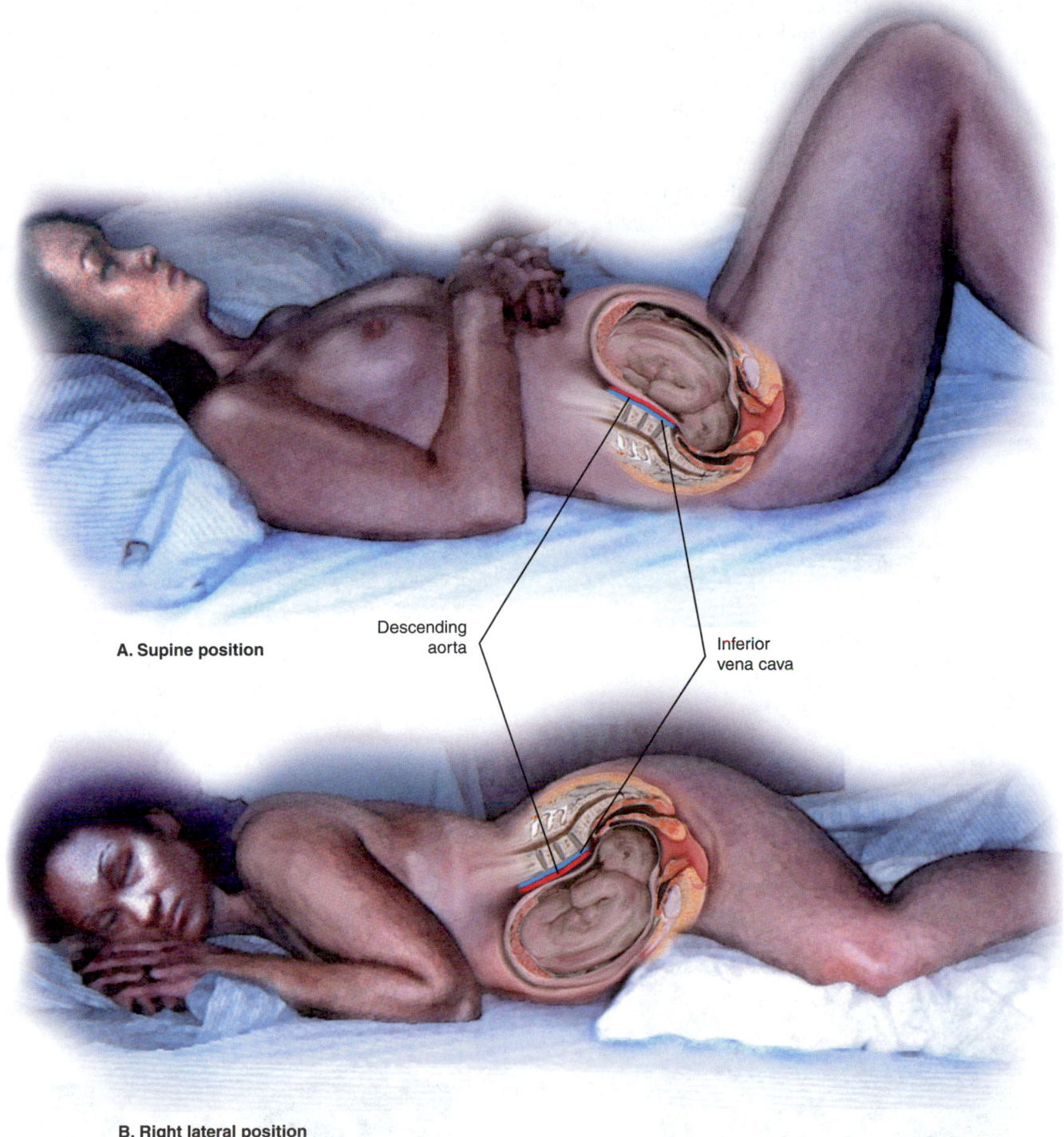

A. Supine position

Descending
aorta

Inferior
vena cava

B. Right lateral position

Figure 15-7 A. Supine hypotension can occur when the woman is in the supine position. The weight of the gravid uterus may partially occlude the descending aorta and vena cava. B. Maintaining a lateral position alleviates the compression.

Effects of Progesterone

The level of circulating progesterone increases as the pregnancy progresses. Progesterone works by direct stimulation of the central respiratory system to increase tidal volume and decrease blood PCO_2. The increased awareness of breathing or dyspnea experienced in pregnancy may be related to this change. Progesterone also plays a role in decreasing airway resistance by relaxation of smooth muscle, thus improving the efficiency of breathing.

Lung Volumes and Gas Exchange

Respiratory rate does not change significantly, so lung volume changes are based on mechanical and hormonal or biochemical influences. The greatest change is the 30% to

40% increase in tidal volume, which is the amount of air inspired and expired with each breath. The functional residual capacity, the volume of gas that remains in the lungs at the end of a normal expiration, is decreased by 20% because of the elevated position of the diaphragm. The volume changes help maintain a better mix of air and a more efficient method of gas exchange.

Lung volume changes and the effect of progesterone cause a state of compensated respiratory alkalosis. The purpose of the increased PaO_2 and the decreased PCO_2 of maternal circulation is to facilitate the removal of carbon dioxide from the fetus. The decreased maternal PCO_2 level is compensated by increased renal secretion of bicarbonate, allowing the maternal arterial pH to remain within normal limits.

Gastrointestinal System

There are anatomic and physiologic changes that occur in the gastrointestinal and hepatic system. These changes are necessary to support maternal and fetal nutrition but are also the changes most often associated with the common discomforts of pregnancy. As shown in Figure 15-8, many organs of the gastrointestinal system are displaced or compressed by the gravid uterus.

Mouth

Estrogen causes increased proliferation of blood vessels and connective tissue in the gums, causing them to become soft and edematous. The tissue is friable and may bleed easily. Chewing can cause discomfort and make meeting nutritional demands more difficult. Poor oral hygiene, periodontal disease, and increased maternal age may increase the incidence of gingivitis. Contrary to folk beliefs, there is no evidence that pregnancy increases the incidence of dental caries or tooth loss.

The saliva becomes more acidic, but an increase in the amount of saliva is not a normal change in pregnancy. There is an unusual condition called ptyalism, or an increase in saliva, that usually occurs in pregnant women who are experiencing nausea. Gabbe and colleagues (1996) state that many experts believe ptyalism is the inability to swallow the saliva normally during periods of nausea and vomiting. Pytalism can begin as early as 2 to 3 weeks and occurs most frequently in the daytime and disappears after delivery.

Some women develop pregnancy tumors in their mouths (Figure 15-9). These growths are usually benign.

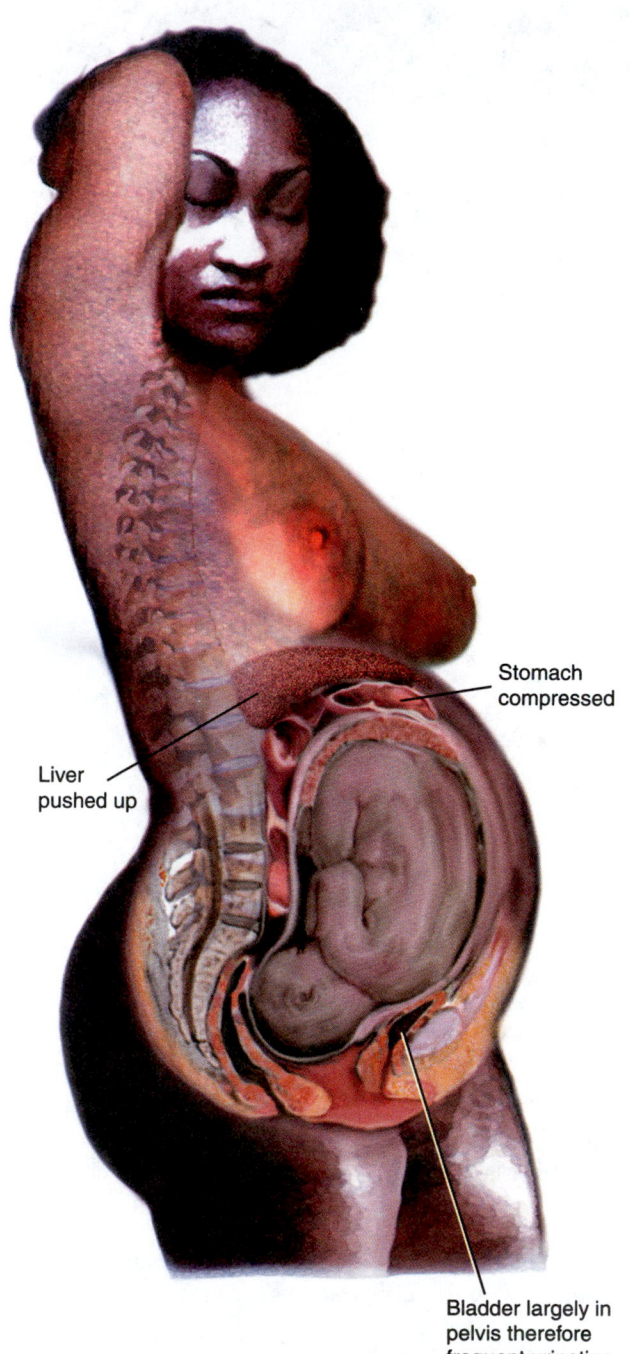

Figure 15-8 Crowding of abdominal contents by gravid uterus.

Stomach compressed

Liver pushed up

Bladder largely in pelvis therefore frequent urination

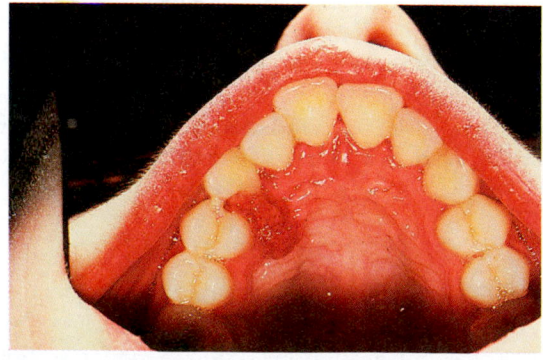

Figure 15-9 Pregnancy tumor. (Courtesy of Dr. Joseph L. Konzelman, School of Dentistry, Medical College of Georgia.)

The vascular proliferation occurs secondary to hormonal changes. These changes may not resolve at the end of pregnancy.

Esophagus

Changes in the esophagus are caused by the effects of progesterone on smooth muscle. Peristalsis of the esophagus decreases and relaxes the lower esophageal sphincter. These changes and the increase in the stomach pressure of the pregnant woman can potentiate acid reflux from the stomach into the lower portion of the esophagus. The burning sensation in the middle of the chest is called pyrosis, or heartburn.

Stomach and Intestines

When assessing the stomach and intestines, some physical findings may be changed because of the displacement of these organs by the enlarging uterus. Bowel sounds may not be evident in the four normal quadrants of the abdomen, and the appendix may be found as high as the right flank. Changes in the tone of the stomach and delayed stomach emptying may contribute to the early nausea and vomiting that sometimes accompany pregnancy.

Acid production in the stomach is decreased in the first and second trimester, gradually returning to normal prepregnant levels at term. Because normal acid production returns at term and stomach emptying is slowed during labor, the oral intake of the pregnant woman must be assessed for 6 to 8 hours before labor, because vomiting and aspiration are major risks during the administration of general anesthesia.

The progressive slowing of intestinal motility correlates with the increase in the production of progesterone as pregnancy moves to term. The slowing progression of the intestinal contents allows more efficient absorption of nutrients and fluids but also contributes to constipation. Another annoying problem, flatulence, results from the slowing of contents through the intestinal tract and the bowel compressed by the gravid uterus.

Gallbladder

The effect of progesterone on smooth muscle also decreases the tone and motility of the gallbladder. The cholesterol in the bile of the pregnant woman is more likely to crystallize, resulting in gallstones being more frequently retained.

Liver

The liver is physically displaced by the enlarging uterus, which can make the diagnosis of hepatomegaly difficult. Blood flow to the liver is not markedly changed, although the proportion of the cardiac output sent to the liver is decreased.

The most remarkable changes are in the laboratory and clinical signs that stem from the changes in the liver of the pregnant woman. These findings are commonly seen in clients who have liver disease, but in pregnancy these changes are normal. Findings include spider angiomata and palmar erythema, found in 70% to 90% of normal pregnant women. These physical findings disappear after delivery. Although liver function remains unchanged, the normal changes seen in laboratory findings of the pregnant woman are also seen in clients with liver disease. These changes include a serum albumin concentration that is decreased by 30% at term; a serum alkaline phosphatase level that is increased to two to three times normal levels; and a serum cholesterol level that is twice the level of the nonpregnant woman (Gabbe, et al., 1996).

Endocrine System

Changes in the endocrine system are manifested in many ways.

Thyroid

The thyroid gland enlarges slightly from increased vascularity and hyperplasia of the tissue. The gland does not enlarge to the extent that was once thought, and therefore any extraordinary growth should be assessed. The normal relationship of the hypothalmus, pituitary, and thyroid glands is believed to remain intact and the pregnant woman remains euthyroid. Cunningham and colleagues (1997) state that the changes that occur in the regulation of thyroid hormone production are related to high estrogen levels, effects of the placenta on function, and decreased availability of iodide resulting from increased renal clearance. These complex alterations in thyroid regulation do not dramatically change laboratory analysis but do cause a progressive increase in the *basal metabolic rate* (BMR). There is a 25% increase in the BMR, which is defined as the amount of oxygen consumed by the body over a unit of time (mL/min). The increase may be characterized by an increased pulse rate, heat intolerance, and elevated level of cardiac output.

Parathyroid

The parathyroid glands secrete parathyroid hormone, which is responsible for calcium and phosphorus metabolism. In pregnancy, the secretion of parathyroid hormone increases to meet the demands of the growing fetus for calcium. Total circulating calcium levels are decreased in pregnancy, probably resulting from fetal demands, the increase in glomerular filtration rate (GFR), and increased plasma volume.

Pituitary

The pituitary gland enlarges, with the most significant growth in the anterior pituitary. During pregnancy, the production of hormones responsible for ovulation is suppressed in the anterior pituitary; the production of prolactin is increased. Prolactin works in conjunction with other hormones for breast development in preparation for lactation. Oxytocin is produced in the hypothalmus, and the posterior pituitary stores and secretes the hormone. Oxytocin produces the uterine contractions during labor and is necessary for the ejection of breast milk. There is increased sensitivity by the myometrium to the effects of oxytocin as the pregnancy advances, probably a result of the increasing levels of estrogen.

Adrenal Glands

The adrenal glands do not change appreciably in size during pregnancy. Cortisol and aldosterone are two hormones secreted from the adrenal cortex that are important in pregnancy.

Cortisol

Cortisol works at multiple sites in the body to promote the metabolism of carbohydrate, protein, and fat. When the body needs more energy, cortisol activates gluconeogenesis to increase blood levels of glucose. Although the secretion of cortisol is decreased in pregnancy, it is hypothesized that the metabolic clearance of the hormone is slowed, thus maintaining higher than normal levels of circulating cortisol.

Aldosterone

During pregnancy the secretion of aldosterone increases, as does that of renin and angiotensin II. Renin is released from the kidneys in response to decreased perfusion pressure in the kidney. At this time, angiotensin II levels rise and act upon the maternal adrenal glands to secrete higher levels of aldosterone. It has been hypothesized that the increased circulating levels of aldosterone may protect the pregnant woman from the excessive sodium loss that is attributed to elevated progesterone levels during pregnancy.

Pancreas

The pancreas, an endocrine gland, secretes insulin from the beta cells of the islets of Langerhans. During pregnancy these beta cells increase in number and enlarge in size and cause the changes that occur in carbohydrate metabolism during pregnancy.

Placenta

Endocrine activities of the placenta are important to preserving a viable pregnancy and to the metabolic adaptations that must take place for the fetus to develop.

Human Chorionic Gonadotropin

Human chorionic gonadotropin (hCG) is secreted by a mass of trophoblastic tissue surrounding the embryo. The detection of hCG is used to confirm pregnancy. In early pregnancy, the corpus luteum increases progesterone and estrogen levels that are necessary to maintain the pregnancy. The function of hCG is to maintain the corpus luteum until the placenta is sufficiently developed to produce the needed hormones. As the pregnancy advances, hCG is involved in the suppression of the immunologic response of the maternal body to the fetus.

Human Placental Lactogen

Production of human placental lactogen (hPL) begins soon after implantation; levels gradually rise and peak at about 36 weeks. This hormone is involved in the process of making adequate glucose available for fetal growth, through the alteration of the maternal carbohydrate, fat, and protein metabolism. The hPL lowers the sensitivity of maternal cells to the action of insulin and then improves the ability of the body to metabolize and use fatty acids for energy. Therefore, as glucose levels decrease, the levels of hPL increase to allow the available glucose to be used for fetal development and growth.

Estrogen

Estrogen levels increase rapidly early in pregnancy, slow between 24 and 32 weeks' gestation, and increase again toward term. The production of estrogen is dependent on the interaction between the maternal and fetal components of the placenta. Estrogen plays an integral role in:

- Increasing blood flow to the uterus by promoting vasodilation
- Changing the sensitivity of the respiratory system to carbon dioxide
- Softening of the cervix, initiating uterine activity, and maintaining labor
- Developing the breasts in preparation for lactation and secretion of prolactin by the pituitary gland

Progesterone

Progesterone is produced by the corpus luteum in the first 5 weeks of pregnancy and then by the placenta until term. Elevated levels of progesterone ready the uterus for implantation, relax the smooth muscle of the uterus to prevent spontaneous abortion, and work to prevent a maternal immunologic response to the fetus. This hormone also relaxes smooth muscle of the gastrointestinal tract to decrease motility and improve absorption of nutrients. Relaxation of the smooth muscle of the urinary tract enlarges the ureters and bladder to increase capacity. Progesterone also plays a role in development of the alveoli and ductal system to prepare the breasts for lactation.

Changes in Metabolism

The metabolic changes that occur in pregnancy are all directed at providing the needs of the developing fetus, meeting the increased physiologic demands of the pregnancy, and providing energy for the woman throughout her pregnancy, labor, and delivery.

The metabolism of carbohydrates in the pregnant woman adapts to provide a constant source of glucose for the growing and developing fetus. In a fasting state, the pregnant woman experiences hypoglycemia, and a state of ketosis develops more quickly than in the nonpregnant woman. The speed at which this maternal response occurs is probably a result of the constant need of the fetus for glucose and the ability of the pregnant woman to more quickly utilize fat for energy. In contrast, a pregnant woman who eats a normal meal produces more glucose, insulin, and triglycerides than a nonpregnant woman does. The increased amounts of glucose and the decreased sensitivity to insulin by the cells therefore produces high amounts of circulating available glucose for the fetus. This adaptation is sometimes called the diabetogenic effect of pregnancy.

Gestational diabetes results from the inability of the pancreas of the pregnant woman to produce enough insulin to move the necessary glucose into the cells for energy production. When this happens, hyperglycemia may need to be regulated by changes in diet. Ketoacidosis may occur in a pregnant woman in whom diabetes has just been detected. Gabbe and colleagues (1996) state that because the pregnant woman is naturally in a state of insulin resistance with lipolysis and ketogenesis, ketoacidosis can occur in pregnant women with a blood glucose level as low as 200 mg/dL. To treat this disorder, the quick return of metabolic and fluid levels to normal values is necessary.

In the first two trimesters, there is an increase in triglyceride synthesis and the storage of fat at central sites. Later in the third trimester, there are more nutritional demands, both for glucose and fatty acids, by the fetus, and fat stores begin to decrease. The ability to more readily use fat as an energy source is a way to conserve glucose for the fetus and high-priority maternal needs.

Iron is necessary for the formation of hemoglobin, the oxygen-carrying component of the red blood cell. With red blood cell volume increasing by 30%, there is an increased need for iron. The intestinal tract increases its ability to absorb iron, but dietary intake and maternal stores are usually not adequate to meet all of the needs. The transport of iron across the placenta to the fetus, especially in the third trimester, takes place at the expense of maternal iron stores. Iron supplements are usually prescribed to maintain the maternal iron stores and decrease the chance of iron deficiency anemia.

Retention of water is a natural and expected part of pregnancy, resulting from changes in water metabolism. According to Cunningham and colleagues (1997), it occurs as a result of several factors:

1. The plasma osmolality is lowered in pregnancy, mainly because of the reduced serum levels of sodium and protein.

2. The intravascular pressure and permeability increase.

3. The fetus, placenta, and amniotic fluid increase the demand for fluid.

The total average volume retained can be as much as 6.5 liters. Normal water retention causes the dependent edema seen in the lower legs and ankles, most often at the end of the day. Edema that is not relieved by the elevation of the legs or excessive edema in the face, hands, or sacral area deserves further assessment (Figure 15-10).

Weight Gain

Weight gain in pregnancy is variable and recommendations should be individualized. The prepregnant weight and the pattern of weight gain that occurs over time are important factors. Tulman, Moren, and Fawcett (1998) note women with extreme prepregnancy body weights, either low or high, plus pregnancy weight gain have an increased

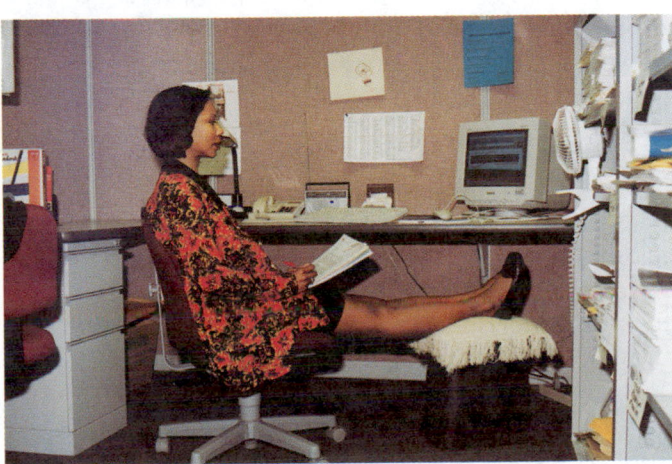

Figure 15-10 Elevating the feet while seated can help relieve edema of the ankles and feet.

Nursing Alert

SIGNS OF DIABETIC KETOACIDOSIS

- Elevated blood glucose level >200
- Polydipsia and polyuria
- Nausea and vomiting
- Headache and malaise

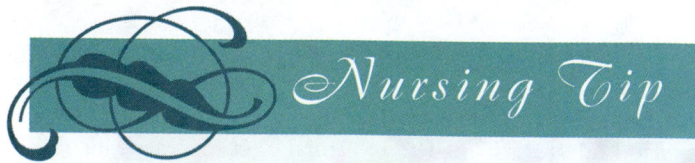

Nursing Tip

GRADING DEPENDENT EDEMA

The severity of edema is documented by grading and noticing trends in the changes.

1+   Slight pitting

2+   A somewhat deeper pit than in 1+

3+   The pit is noticeably deep; the dependent extremity is swollen and full

4+   The pit is deeper yet and lasts when the finger is removed; the dependent extremity is shiny, with extremely taut skin

risk for maternal and neonatal complications. Except at the extreme ends of the scale, a good clinical outcome is possible within a wide range weight gain. The average weight gain for healthy primigravidae is 12.5 kg (27.5 lb). Of this, the fetus, placenta, amniotic fluid, uterus, increase in maternal blood volume, breasts and the retention of water account for 9 kg (Figure 15-11). The National Academy of Science (1990) recommends the following: 12.5 to 18.0 kg (27.5 to 39.6 lb) for underweight women, 11.5 to 16.0 kg (25.3 to 35.2 lb) for normal-weight women, and 7.0 to 11.4 kg (15.4 to 25 lb) for overweight women.

In a research study, Tulman and associates (1998) examined the relationship of prepregnant weight and pregnancy weight gain as it relates to functional status, number of physical discomforts, and energy level. The results showed that the women who gained the most weight in their third trimester had a greater decrease in their functional status. The results of this nursing research suggest that nurses should be cognizant of their clients' pattern of weight gain and its effect on the woman's ability to perform her activities of daily living. Nutritional counseling is an important intervention, not only for the pregnant woman, but also for the postpartum period.

Urinary System

Changes in the urinary system, both anatomic and physiologic, are necessary for the synchronous functioning of adaptations that occur in other body systems. The key to assessing the renal system is remembering that the parameters of normal renal function are changed and that an awareness of these changes is necessary to make appropriate clinical judgments.

Anatomic Changes

As early as 16 weeks, the kidneys change in size and shape, resulting from the dilation of the renal ureters and

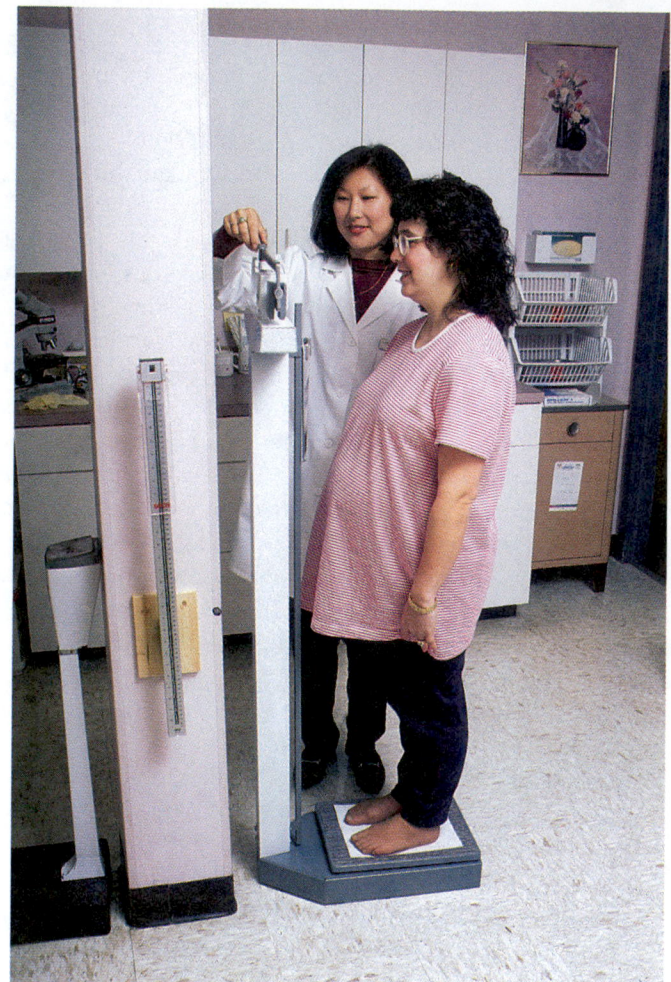

Figure 15-11 Monitoring weight gain at each prenatal visit helps the client to maintain a healthy pregnancy.

pelvices. The right kidney and ureter are larger than the left, probably because of the structural changes in other organs. Early in pregnancy, the enlargement may be caused by the effect of hormones that cause increased tone and decreased motility of the smooth muscle. After 20 weeks' gestation, the ureters are compressed at the pelvic brim by the growing uterus. Above the pelvic brim, the ureters are elongated and twisted, with a capacity to increase urine volume as much as 25-fold. Pooling of the increased volume of urine can lead to: 1) an increased incidence of pyelonephritis, 2) difficulty in the interpretation of radiographic studies of the renal system, and 3) interference with the accuracy of diagnostic studies, such as a 24-hour urine sample analysis.

By the end of the second trimester, the bladder is displaced upward and forward by the gravid uterus. The structural changes that occur with this displacement can lead to urinary frequency and incontinence. In most women, this is the first experience with incontinence, or involuntary loss of urine, and many will mistake it for the rupture of placental membranes late in pregnancy. The

Research Highlight

Prepregnant Weight and Weight Gain during Pregnancy: Relationship to Functional Status, Symptoms, and Energy Level

Purpose

To examine the relationship of prepregnancy weight and pregnancy weight gain to functional status, physical symptoms, and physical energy.

Methods

A longitudinal panel, with data, collected at the end of each trimester for 222 women whose pregnancies were low-risk, drawn from another study. The Inventory of Functional Status: Antepartum Period was the instrument used to measure functional status. To assess the physical symptoms a 21-item symptoms checklist was used. A one-item question was given to elicit the client's energy level. To calculate the body mass index (BMI) the formula (weight [kg]/height [m^2]) was used. Weight and height were self-reported.

Findings

Pregnant women who gain weight above the recommended levels in their third trimester have a decrease in their functional status. There were no significant differences in physical symptoms and energy level. The researchers speculated that excessive weight gain can contribute to an increase in energy expenditure and that this may contribute to the difficulty in completing daily activities.

Nursing Implications

The findings confirm the need for nutrition and exercise counseling during pregnancy to help the woman understand the benefits that can be achieved. Interventions to assist a woman in maintaining her functional status may help her continue to participate in social and family activities throughout her pregnancy.

Tulman, L., Morin, K. H. & Fawcett, J. (1998). Prepregnant Weight and Weight Gain During Pregnancy: Relationship to Functional Status, Symptoms, and Energy. *Journal of Obstetric, Gynecology, and Neonatal Nursing.* 27 (6), 629–634.

tone of the bladder is relaxed and capacity and the pressure within the bladder increases. These changes, along with the edema of the bladder mucosa, make this area susceptible to infection and trauma.

Physiologic Changes

Blood flow to the kidneys increases by 35% to 60%, as a result of the increase in cardiac output. In turn, this leads to an increase in the GFR, or the rate that water and solutes filter through the glomeruli, as much as 50% by 12 weeks' gestation. The increase in the GFR leads to the following changes:

1. Increased urine flow and volume
2. Decreased serum blood urea nitrogen (BUN), creatinine, and uric acid levels
3. Increased nutrients delivered to the kidneys

4. Increased filtration and excretion of water and solutes
5. Altered renal excretion of drugs, resulting, at times, in subtherapeutic blood levels

Urinalysis

The alterations that occur in tubular function increase the reabsorption of sodium, chloride, glucose, potassium, and water to prevent the depletion of these solutes. Because of the increased perfusion rate, at times reabsorption is not complete and there is a loss of glucose in the urine. Levels of glucose in the urine vary day to day and slightly elevated levels are not uncommon, but an assessment for gestational diabetes should be considered if glycosuria is recurrent. In normal pregnancy, small amounts of protein may occasionally spill into the urine. Proteinuria levels above 300 mg in 24 hours warrant further investigation, especially when accompanied by hypertension.

Glucose and protein in the urine lead to a higher susceptibility to urinary tract infections.

Integumentary System

The skin undergoes many changes that rarely cause significant physiologic problems. It is the emotional distress caused by the cosmetic alterations (that may persist until after delivery) that are problematic. Most of these skin changes disappear or lessen after the delivery of the newborn. Some of these changes are also seen in women who are taking birth control pills, which leads experts to think that the changes are related to the increase in circulating estrogen.

The vascular changes that occur may lead to changes in the integumentary system. Spider angiomas and palmar erythema, which can be found in pathologic disorders such as liver disease, are also found in pregnant women and they usually occur together. Spider angiomas or nevi usually appear between 8 and 20 weeks' gestation in about 75% of pregnant women. The nevi are central dilated arterioles that are visible or raised, with radiating branches. Appearing most often on the face, neck, throat and arms, they may be distressing to the pregnant woman. Most often the nevi fade or disappear after delivery. There is a familial tendency for palmar erythema, which appears during the first half of the pregnancy. This skin change, which causes a mottling of the fleshy portion of the palm and redness of the fingers, may be caused by an increase in estrogen level, because it disappears after delivery.

Hyperpigmentation, caused by elevated hormones, is usually visible primarily on the nipples, areolae, umbilicus, perineum, and axillae. The dark line in the midline of the abdomen caused by hyperpigmentation is called **linea nigra** (Figure 15-12). Women may also experience dark blotching on the face (Figure 15-13), similar to that seen in women who take birth control pills. This condi-

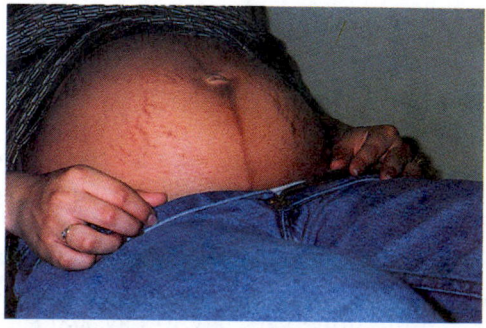

Figure 15-12 Dark line of pigmentation called linea nigra, may appear in midline of abdomen, from symphysis pubis to umbilicus.

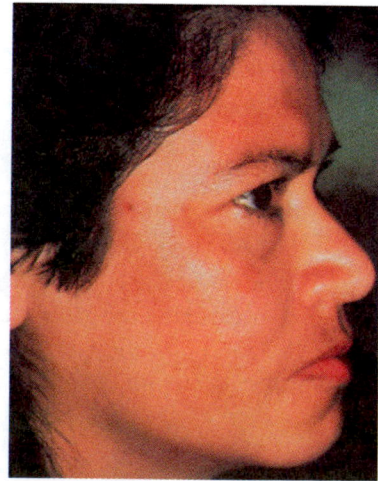

Figure 15-13 Blotches on face during pregnancy are known as chloasma. (Courtesy of Timothy Berger, MD, Chief, Department of Dermatology at San Francisco General Hospital)

tion **chloasma**, is commonly called the "mask of pregnancy." The condition may be a concern to the pregnant woman because of the cosmetic effect. Chloasma may disappear after pregnancy but often only fades. Preexisting nevi may also be affected and become darker during pregnancy. The management of these nevi should include close observation and the removal of nevi that change rapidly.

Changes that occur in the connective tissue during pregnancy can lead to the formation of **striae gravidarum**, which occurs in approximately 50% of all pregnant women. Women who have a genetic disposition may develop pink-to-purple lines on the skin from the stretching that occurs during growth of the fetus. These lines, as seen in Figure 15-14, usually appear on the breasts, lower abdomen, and upper thighs and fade to a silver color with time. "Stretch marks" do not ever completely disappear, and there is no prophylactic skin treatment to prevent them.

Musculoskeletal System

To maintain balance with the shift in weight from the growing uterus, the lumbar spine forms an exaggerated forward, convex curve (lordosis) (Figure 15-15). The body adjusts the center of gravity over the lower extremities and, unfortunately, this adjustment is often the cause of low back pain in later pregnancy. Ligaments in the pubic symphysis and sacroiliac joints soften from the effects of the hormone relaxin. This adaptation is necessary to ready the body for vaginal delivery but can also cause pelvic discomfort and an unsteady gait as the pregnancy nears term. Falls are a common occurrence; women should be instructed to wear flat, well-fitting shoes.

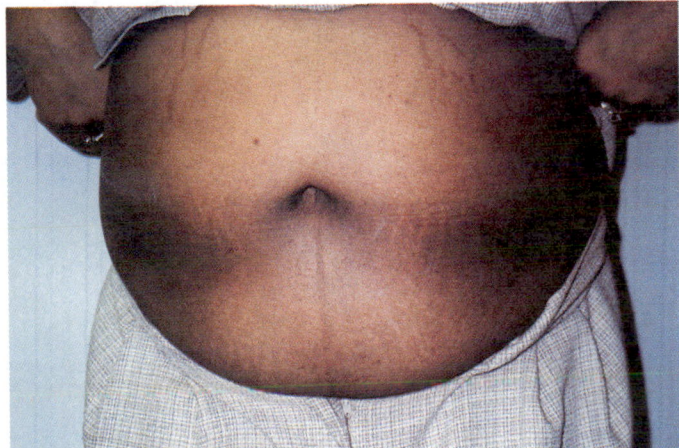

Figure 15-14 Striae gravidarum (stretch marks) are pink to purple streaks on skin. Marks are a result of linear tears in connective tissue of skin as body enlarges.

Eyes

Changes that occur in the eye normally do not affect vision, other than the transient loss of accommodation (the power of the eye to alter the convexity of the lens according to the nearness or distance of an object) that has been reported (Blackburn & Laper 1992). Ocular pressure, which is slightly decreased, is thought to change from the increased outflow of vitreous. The cornea becomes thicker, probably caused by edema. If the woman wears contact lenses, she may notice that her normally comfortable lenses are now bothersome.

DISCOMFORTS OF PREGNANCY

An important nursing responsibility during the prenatal period is educating the client regarding the discomforts that occur during pregnancy and how to remedy these, or feel better. These discomforts are usually related to the changes necessary to adapt to the growing fetus that are occurring in the body systems. Information on why the woman feels the way she does and self-help remedies usually assist in making this time more comfortable. Another

Nursing Alert

SIGNS OF POTENTIAL PROBLEMS IN PREGNANCY

Immediate assessment is required for:

Problem	Possible Cause
Persistent vomiting	Hyperemesis gravidarum
Bright red vaginal bleeding	Abruptio placenta, placenta previa
Edema of the hands and face	Preeclampsia, hypertension
Body temperature above 101°F (38.3°C)	Infection
Persistent abdominal pain, with or without a rigidity	Abruptio placenta
Epigastric pain, unrelieved by comfort measures	Preeclampsia
Dysuria	Urinary tract infection
Intermittent back pain, pelvic pressure, or abdominal pain or pressure	Preterm labor
Visual disturbances	Preeclampsia, hypertension
Changes in fetal movement	Potential fetal stress

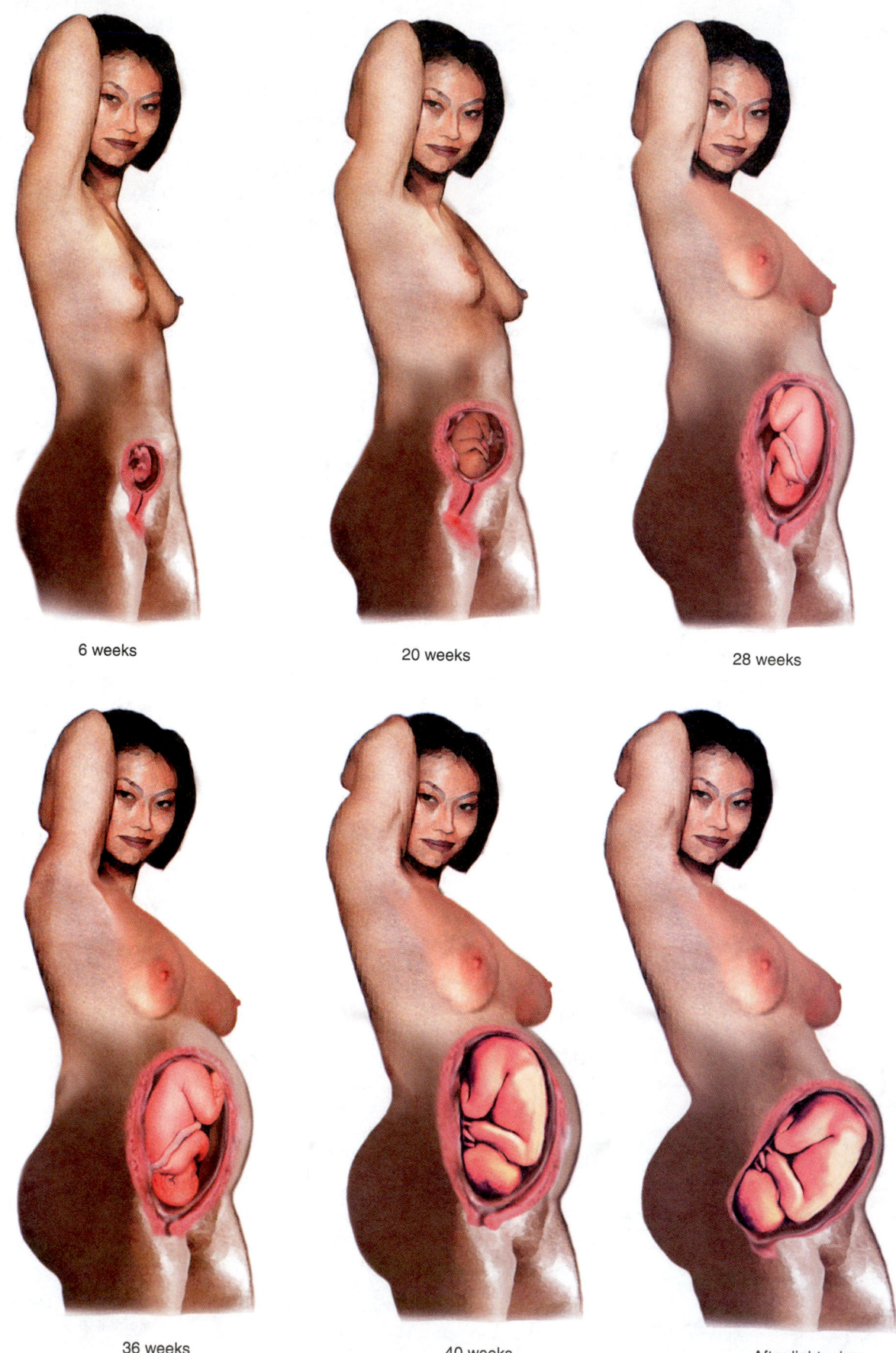

6 weeks

20 weeks

28 weeks

36 weeks

40 weeks

After lightening

Figure 15-15 As pregnancy advances, changes in posture are obvious. Exaggerated curve in the back is called lordosis.

important aspect of counseling on the discomforts of pregnancy is to help the pregnant woman distinguish between a normal discomfort and a sign that may signal a real problem in the pregnancy.

Nausea and Vomiting of Pregnancy

The discomfort of nausea and vomiting of pregnancy (NVP) can range from mild nausea (with or without vomiting) to severe vomiting (**hyperemesis gravidarum**) that occurs throughout the day. Although NVP is referred to as morning sickness, episodes can occur throughout the day. The cause of NVP is not known, but it is speculated to be related to increased levels of hCG and estrogen. Emotional factors and irregular eating habits have also been cited as possible contributors to this discomfort. The discomfort of NVP cannot be completely eliminated, but can be minimized by self-help measures. Recent research suggests that there may be a protective benefit of NVP in that it shields the fetus from potentially harmful pathogens, such as those found in undercooked meat.

Hyperemesis gravidarum is a serious complication of pregnancy and must be managed under the close observation of a health care provider. Dangerous sequelae of hyperememsis gravidarum can include weight loss, dehydration, electrolyte imbalance, and starvation.

Heartburn

Heartburn is a frequent complaint throughout pregnancy and results from the reflux of gastric acid contents into the esophagus and sometimes into the mouth. The changes that occur in the gastrointestinal system, such as decreased stomach and intestinal motility, softening of the cardiac

Critical Thinking

Nausea and Vomiting of Pregnancy

Two weeks ago Mehalia purchased a home pregnancy test, which gave positive results after she missed one of her regular periods. She has called the clinic and is experiencing nausea and vomiting.

Formulate questions for Mehalia that will help you determine the severity of her NVP and the potential for hyperemesis gravidarum, centering on:

- Frequency of vomiting
- Pain or fever
- Tolerance for food and fluids

Client Education

Nausea and Vomiting in Pregnancy

- Drink plenty of fluids, 6 to 8 glasses of water daily, to maintain hydration.
- Avoid fluids that contain caffeine or carbonation.
- Eat a diet that is high in protein and carbohydrates, in 5 to 6 small meals daily.
- Eat crackers throughout the day to avoid an empty stomach.
- Pay attention to your senses; avoid noxious odors, such as tobacco smoke, and tastes that may nauseate you.
- Limit stressful events and get plenty of rest; avoid being in a hurry, especially in the morning.
- Consider acupuncture or acupressure to assist in relieving nausea.

Client Education

Heartburn in Pregnancy

- Monitor your diet for foods that cause upset. Keep a list.
- Avoid drinking large amounts of liquid with meals; instead, spread fluid intake throughout the day.
- Remain sitting upright for at least 30 minutes after a meal and sleep with an extra pillow at night to keep the head elevated.
- Don't bend at the waist, always bend at the knees, maintaining a more upright abdominal posture.
- Try lying on your right side and using relaxation techniques to calm your stomach and promote digestion.
- Take commercial calcium-containing low-sodium antacids just before meals; check with your practitioner for brand preferences.

sphincter and esophagus, and displacement of the stomach by the uterus, seem to contribute to the burning sensation that is felt behind the sternum and in the epigastric area. Instruct the client to call her health care provider if self-help measures or antacids do not relieve persistent heartburn. Epigastric pain or right upper quadrant pain, especially when associated with edema of the hands and face, proteinuria, and elevated blood pressure, could indicate a problem in the liver.

Constipation

Constipation is another discomfort related to the changes that occur in the gastrointestinal tract. Increased levels of progesterone cause the relaxation of intestinal smooth muscle, which leads to decreased motility and increased capacity, allowing more time for the absorption of nutrients. Although this process benefits the nutrition of the mother and fetus, it can cause bloating, increased flatulence, and hard stools that aggravate hemorrhoids. Assess the frequency of bowel movements in women taking iron supplements, because iron supplements may cause constipation.

Fatigue

The fatigue that pregnant woman feel in the first trimester is real and sometimes distressing for the "superwoman" of today. The tiredness is legitimate and may seem over-

---

Client Education

Constipation in Pregnancy

If you are constipated and taking iron, do not stop taking your supplement. Try these self-help tips first.

- Increase the fiber in your diet by eating fruits and vegetables raw (or vegetables slightly steamed). Whole grains are also a good source of fiber.

- Drink plenty of fluids, avoiding caffeine; keep in mind that increasing your fiber without increasing your fluid can worsen constipation.

- Exercise to stay regular; walking, swimming, or cycling 3 to 4 times per week for 20 to 30 minutes is recommended.

- Try to establish a regular time for your bowel movement and never ignore your body's signals.

Client Education

Fatigue in Pregnancy

Find a comfortable and reasonably quiet place and try meditation. Close your mind to external sensation and outside stimulation. Pick one of the following five methods to achieve a single focus:

1. Meditative repetition: repeat a rhythmic chant, most commonly called a mantra, that is chanted over and over

2. Visual concentration: stare at an image, such as a candle, flower, or fruit

3. Repetitive sounds: listen to a sound, such as a drum, chimes, or a waterfall

4. Physical repetitive motion: perform motions such as rhythmic breathing or a rhythmic aerobic exercise

5. Repeated tactile motion: hold or manipulate a small object, such as a rosary or tumble stone

---

whelming but is of no special medical significance. The best advice for the busy pregnant woman is to give in and rest when she feels the need. She may need to take shortcuts in her daily life, and she should know that the fatigue usually disappears by the fourth month. Alleviating stress through meditation or relaxed breathing may assist in coping with the feeling of being tired.

Frequent Urination

Urinary frequency ranks at the top of the list of the most common complaints of pregnancy. In the first trimester, before the uterus ascends above the symphysis, the weight of the enlarging uterus irritates and puts pressure on the bladder. Frequent urination diminishes slightly in the second trimester, returning near term. When talking with clients, differentiate between urinary frequency and the symptoms of a urinary tract infection. If the woman has symptoms such as pain or burning urgency when urinating, a health care provider should be notified. Kegel exercises (contracting the muscles of the pelvic floor) help to prevent urinary stress incontinence.

Epistaxis and Nasal Congestion

The capillaries inside the nose become engorged with blood during pregnancy, leading to edema and hyperemia

Client Education

How to Perform Kegel Exercises

1. In the first 3 months of pregnancy, lie on your back with both knees bent to perform this exercise; after the third month, sitting or standing is a better position.

2. Contract the muscles that surround the vagina and anus and hold for 5 seconds, then slowly release. These are the same muscles you would use to stop urination. Isolating these muscles requires practice.

3. Do at least 25 to 50 repetitions. You may want to space them out during the day.

of the nasal passages. These changes can lead to *epistaxis,* or nosebleed, and nasal congestion, which can worsen in the winter months when conditions are dry and the use of home heaters is prevalent. The congestion and dryness of the nose may lead to more frequent blowing of the nose. With mucous membranes engorged with blood, blowing the nose gently may prevent epistaxis. The nurse can recommend that the client sleep with a cool mist humidifier and use commercially prepared saline spray. If the congestion becomes severe enough to interfere with activities of daily living, the client should consult her practitioner.

Client Education

Varicose Veins in Pregnancy

- Maintain good circulation in your legs; avoid sitting, standing, or crossing your legs for long periods, and wear maternity support hose during the day.
- Elevate your legs as often as you are able or flex your feet several times every few minutes while sitting.
- Take breaks and short frequent walks when performing intense, stationary work.
- Wear clothes that fit loosely and avoid wearing knee-high hose that may constrict the blood vessels in the legs.

Varicosities

Varicosities are dilated veins that occur most often in women who have a genetic predisposition for them. The valves in the veins can become incompetent, allowing a reverse of blood flow. In pregnancy, these veins may be more pronounced because of the increased blood volume, the changes in venous pressure that occur because of the enlarged uterus, and increased time in the standing position. On assessment, changes may be noted that range from mild discomfort after long periods of standing to severe tortuous and bulging blue veins that require long periods of rest with the legs elevated. Occurring most often in veins of the lower extremities, varicosities may also be present in the veins of the vulva and rectum (hemorrhoids).

Hemorrhoids

Hemorrhoids are varicosities of the rectum, which may occur outside the anal sphincter or inside the anal sphincter. Typically, hemorrhoids that are already present are exacerbated by the changes that occur in the body during pregnancy. Other factors that may exacerbate hemorrhoids are prolonged sitting or standing, straining at stool, and pushing in the second stage of labor. Hemorrhoids may continue to be problematic into the postpartum period.

Client Education

Hemorrhoids in Pregnancy

- Maintain healthy and regular bowel habits.
- Try a sitz bath: sit for about 20 minutes in a tub filled with warm water to which you have added a half-cup of baking soda.
- Apply cool compresses or cotton balls soaked with witch hazel to the swollen hemorrhoids. Commercial preparations that contain witch hazel or anesthetic compounds are also available.
- If hemorrhoids are protruding from the anus, gently push them back into the rectum. Using a glove and lubricant, gently press the hemorrhoid back through the anus and hold for a few seconds. This may be most comfortably achieved after a sitz bath.

Client Education

Back Pain in Pregnancy

- Be aware of your posture; be sure your neck, shoulders, and back are straight and your pelvis is tilted slightly forward.
- Bend at the knees, never at the waist.
- Wear comfortable, low-heeled shoes.
- Elevate one foot when standing for extended periods of time (Figure 15-16).
- Practice deep breathing and relaxation exercises that focus on the upper body.
- Get a massage to relax tired muscles.

Back Pain

The back pain of pregnancy usually occurs in the lumbar region and becomes more problematic as the uterus enlarges. Low back pain is a common complaint in pregnancy and results from the changes in posture as the uterus grows. Obesity and previous problems with back pain are also risk factors. The degree of pain is closely linked to the strain of bending, lifting, and walking. The use of good body mechanics when performing these activities limits the potential for severe injury.

Leg Cramps

Leg cramps are thought to be the result of an imbalance between the electrolytes calcium and phosphorus. During pregnancy, the ratio of calcium to phosphorus is difficult to maintain because of changes in renal absorption and diet. The decreased circulation to the lower extremities produced by the pressure of the uterus may also contribute to painful cramps. The woman may awaken at night with painful knots in the calf muscles. When the cramp occurs, getting out of bed and walking usually relieves the pain. If the pain is too severe to walk, the woman should be instructed to sit with her legs and knees straight, grab her toes, and flex her foot. A partner can also assist in relieving leg cramps by flexing the foot forward (Figure 15-17). Instruct the client to do flexibility or stretching exercises before going to bed.

Health Promotion

When considering health behavior changes, remember what it is like to be the individual attempting to change

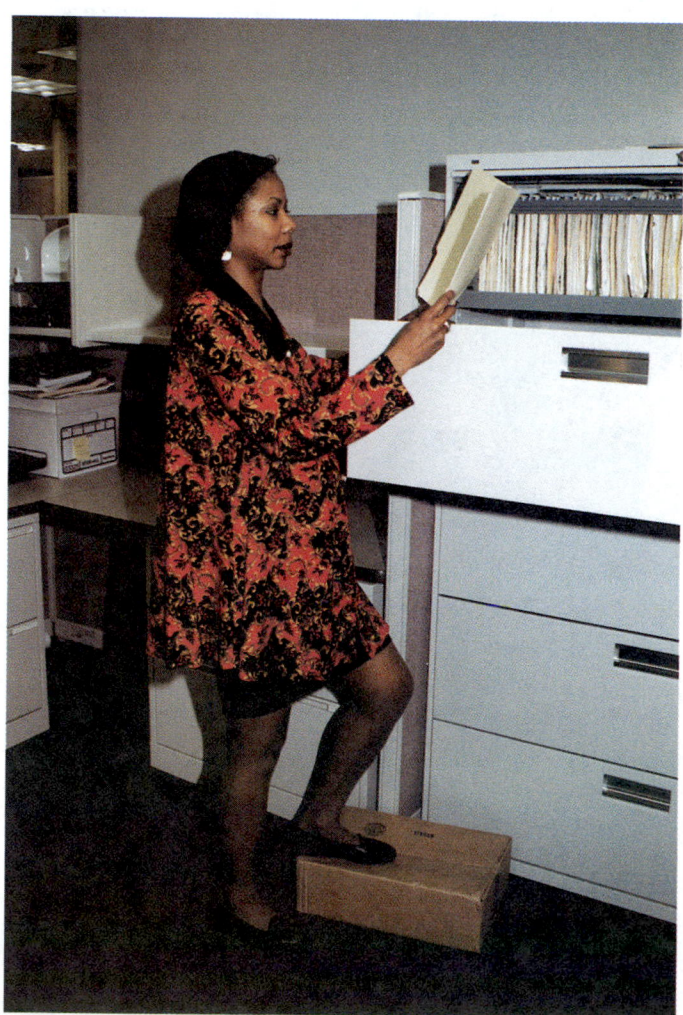

Figure 15-16 Keeping one foot elevated during prolonged periods of standing can help relieve back pain.

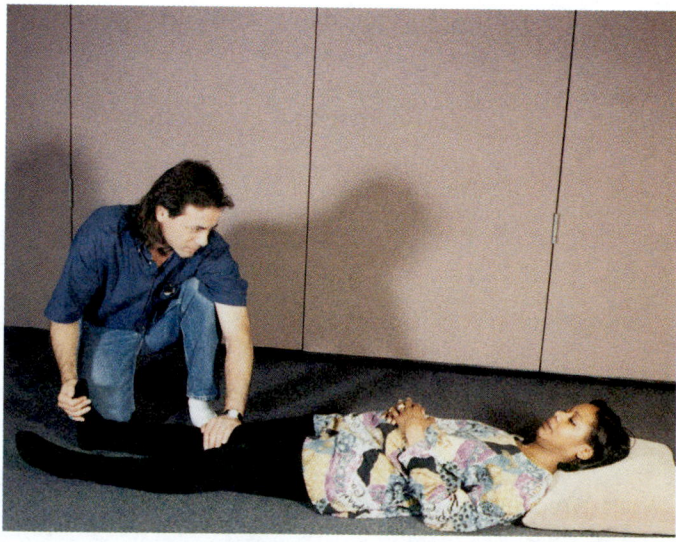

Figure 15-17 Leg cramps can be relieved by flexing foot toward knee.

Critical Thinking

Health Promotion

Formulate responses to these comments made by nurses that help nurses understand the importance of avoiding making assumptions about clients when instructing them on changing health behavior.

1. "The health change is obviously the right thing to do and everyone is motivated to change if good health is the outcome."

2. "I understand the problems concerning not changing, but why does the client not understand?"

3. "The time for change is now and if the client is not ready, then this session is over. I can only give her the advice, she has to decide to change."

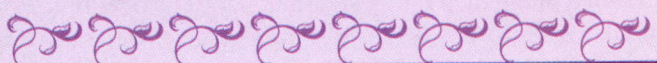

what may be long-standing habits. The nurse, as the health care provider, understands the need to change certain behaviors to achieve and maintain wellness, but the client is the person who must be ready to change.

Many women must make changes in their daily lives to achieve and maintain a healthy pregnancy. When planning education for women concerning the lifestyle changes that may need to be made, be sure to complete a physical examination, but also understand the woman's educational background, value system, and cultural beliefs. To implement change, there must be a readiness to change. If this is a new idea to the woman, she may need to complete several stages of readiness before she is able to think about changing a behavior. Relaying the importance of the change and convincing her that she can successfully make the change are also necessary. The manner in which the information is presented can either motivate the woman to change or build a wall of resistance. As a health care provider, the nurse must be sensitive to the fact that communication techniques can either make the process more difficult or can assist in the adjustments that need to be made.

Employment

At least one-half of the women of childbearing age in the United States are in the workforce. Cunningham and associates (1997) noted that women now have the legal right to work during pregnancy, and employers cannot deny any job to a woman because she is pregnant. If a job requires

excessive standing (more than 8 hours), frequent rest periods or intermittent walking should be included in the work day. Women should be instructed to avoid any work or play that may cause severe physical strain or fatigue.

Travel

Travel during pregnancy has not been shown to be harmful to the pregnant woman or her fetus. Most airlines have requirements for the woman who is traveling close to her expected date of delivery. Instruct the woman to discuss travel plans with her health care provider.

When traveling in a car, it is appropriate to use a properly positioned three-point safety restraint. The woman should be instructed to adjust the lap belt so that is positioned under her abdomen and low across her hips and the shoulder harness so that it is snug between her breasts (Figure 15-18). With any mode of travel, frequent rest periods are advantageous.

Smoking

The effect of smoking on the fetus is well-documented. Newborns born to mothers who smoke have lower birth weights, a higher incidence of sudden infant death syndrome (SIDS), a higher incidence of premature birth, and are more likely to have episodes of apnea (Cunningham, et al. 1997). The discussion concerning smoking cessation should occur in the preconception period. The nurse should assess for smoking in every client of childbearing age, review the negative effects of smoking on the fetus, and suggest ways to assist the client in quitting the smoking habit. The nurse should first understand the long-term

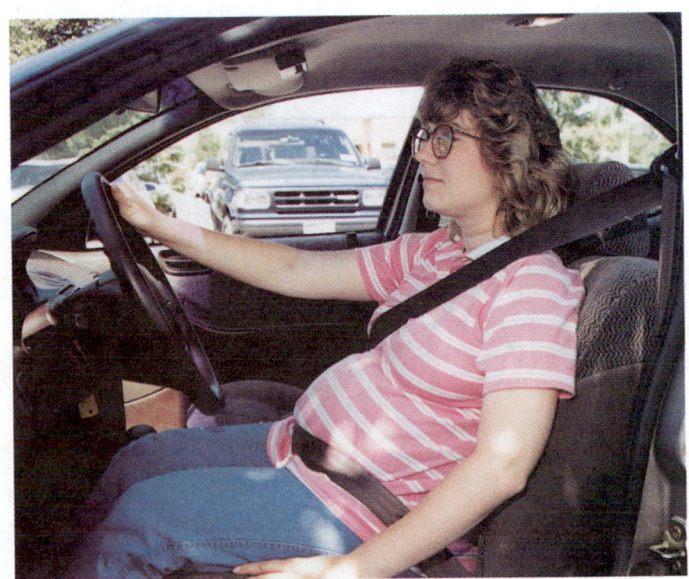

Figure 15-18 Car seatbelts should be secured low and snug under abdomen and across hips.

REFLECTIONS FROM A NURSE

"I cannot understand. I had just explained how detrimental smoking was to her baby, and in the her next breath, she wanted to go smoke a cigarette. What should my response as a concerned health care provider be?"

addiction of cigarette smoking and then work with the woman to assist in identifying her motivation to smoke. From this assessment, a plan of care can be outlined to begin the process of changing health behavior.

Alcohol Use

Women who are pregnant or are considering becoming pregnant should abstain from consuming alcohol. Experts have been unable to identify exactly how much alcohol is too much. Again, the time to identify an alcohol problem is before the woman becomes pregnant. Explaining the deleterious effects of alcohol on the developing fetus may be enough motivation for the social drinker to stop, but women who are addicted to alcohol need professional assistance and may benefit from a referral to a treatment program.

Illicit Drug Use

Large doses of illicit drugs or street drugs, such as opium derivatives, amphetamines, or barbiturates, can cause low birth weight and fetal distress (Cunningham, et al., 1997). A health care provider team that has an established program should manage the pregnant woman with a drug addiction. The newborn needs special care if the mother has remained on drugs throughout her pregnancy. If the nurse identifies a woman who has a drug addiction, quick referrals are the best avenue to obtaining a reasonably positive outcome.

Medication Use

During preconception counseling the health care provider should assess the medications that the woman may routinely consume. Almost all drugs that affect the mother systemically cross the placenta and affect the fetus. Therefore the best advice to the pregnant woman is to avoid taking any medications or herbal preparations without consulting her provider. If a drug is prescribed during pregnancy, the risk-benefit ratio should be weighed and discussed with the woman.

PSYCHOSOCIAL ADAPTATIONS TO PREGNANCY

There are developmental challenges that must be met to move to the next stage of life. Pregnancy is a maturational crisis that causes a paradigm shift for the woman and her family members. To successfully move into the new role of parenting, both the woman and her partner must complete certain tasks. The movement through this journey is affected by many variables, both internal and external. In the role of the nurse, understanding the psychological adaptations that are necessary in moving into the parenting role helps with supporting and caring for the family unit.

Psychological Responses to Pregnancy

Because pregnancy is an event that happens over time, the woman's responses are episodic in nature. Her response to certain changes may be somewhat exaggerated, while other changes are accepted with little concern. Being able to provide unbiased counsel to these women and their families is important and assists in the smooth transition from a childless couple to a family.

Acceptance of the Pregnancy

The nurse should not automatically assume that every woman has planned her pregnancy. Approximately 31% of births in the 5 years preceding 1995 were reported as unintended (Henshaw, 1998), with unintended pregnancy defined as one in which the woman did not want to have the infant or had decided not to have more children. The definition does not suggest that she will be unsuccessful in her progress through the adaptation and acceptance of her pregnancy. In fact, ambivalence to the pregnancy is a very normal initial response, and discussion concerning this topic is a productive intervention. Many women express concern over the timing of the pregnancy, wishing that planned goals or criteria had been met before becoming pregnant. Other women worry about how an infant will affect their career or their relationships with family and friends. These feelings can be confusing for the woman who feels conflict instead of elation. As her pregnancy progresses, the physical changes of an enlarging abdomen and fetal movement bring reality to her situation. As she accepts this reality, she becomes tolerant of the discomforts she may be experiencing. At this time, reassurance that what she is feeling is normal and that her conflicting feelings about the pregnancy will resolve are appropriate.

REFLECTIONS FROM A MOTHER

"In my second year of graduate school, while working part-time, I was shocked and disappointed to learn that I was pregnant. My initial reaction was, 'Oh no, not now!' I was so ashamed by the way I was feeling toward being pregnant. We had always planned to have a baby, but there were so many things we still wanted to accomplish before starting a family."

Time for Reflection

During the first trimester the woman often turns inward and reflects on what "being pregnant" means. There are few physical signs of an impending newborn, so the unstable moods that sometimes accompany early pregnancy may be unnerving to the woman and her partner. As the pregnancy advances, the focus becomes the growing fetus. Many women disengage from familiar outside activities and focus on issues that result in a safe and healthy pregnancy. At times, the plans for the newborn may completely monopolize her attention, and her partner may feel neglected or left out of the planning. The introversion that occurs is a normal psychological adaptation to the journey to motherhood. The nurse can discuss these issues with the couple and assist in providing suggestions to maintain the focus on the family.

Body Image Changes

The initial changes that occur in the woman's body validate her pregnancy, and she may demonstrate pride in her changing body. As the pregnancy progresses, her increasing size, waddling gait, and posture changes may become distressing. The discomforts of pregnancy that accompany the physical changes may add more distress to an already stressful time. Women who are experiencing difficulty adapting to the pregnancy because of real or imagined issues, such as single parenthood, marital problems, financial issues, dread of the future, or an uninterested or absent partner, typically have a more difficult time accepting the physical changes of pregnancy. The nurse and client can discuss the issues and look for solutions. It may be helpful to focus the client on the idea of pregnancy as a time-limited event.

Becoming a Mother

As the woman moves toward the maternal role, she has hopefully accomplished previous life transitions, has adequate role models, has an interpersonal support system, and the acceptance of others. During the transition, the woman is in a state of internal disequilibrium and may demonstrate disorganized behavior. The behavior may result in mood swings and changes in normal roles and relationships. Pregnancy and role changes are a life crisis. During a crisis, the woman and her family may be more open to the health care provider's expert advice and guidance. It is an important time because the change that occurs in the newly pregnant woman is integrated into her personality as her maternal identity. The incorporation of the maternal identity into the woman's life is a process that leads to the acceptance of the new infant as her child.

Development of the Maternal Role

Rubin (1984) describes the steps that must be accomplished to successfully move into the maternal role and the tools the new mother uses to accomplish this transition.

Mimicry

The pregnant woman uses mimicry in role transition when she seeks out other women who are pregnant or have been pregnant and asks to share their stories and customs. She solicits the different opinions of these experts and tries to obtain consensus before deciding which aspects of motherhood she will incorporate into her new role. Wearing maternity clothes before they are necessary, or imitating the waddling gate of other pregnant women demonstrates a trying on of the role. The role models also serve to plot a course for the expected sequence of events or changes during pregnancy. The woman finds comfort in knowing what to expect, although information that does not seem pertinent to her stage of pregnancy may be temporarily disregarded. An example of premature information would be showing a woman in her first trimester how to bathe or feed the baby. The information is stored in her memory and will be reviewed when it is more pertinent to her stage of pregnancy.

The woman's mother is the model most closely mimicked. She has an expectation that she will experience the same prenatal course and delivery as her mother experienced. When this sequence of events does not progress as anticipated, the woman may become distressed and worried. At this point, it is important to discuss with the client the differences that occur in every woman's pregnancy.

Role Play

Role play happens intermittently and is the woman's opportunity to try on the mother role. When the opportunity arises, she may offer to hold, feed, or play with a child in front of an observer. If she receives a positive response from both the infant and the observer, this encounter bolsters her confidence in successfully becoming a mother. If the infant or the observer rejects the woman, she will feel as if she has failed and will expect rejection with the next encounter. Helping the woman understand that acquiring the skills necessary for motherhood is a process that continues throughout life is a sound approach.

Fantasy

Fantasizing is common in the pregnant woman and involves imagining the infant and how she will fare as a mother. Dreams may initially focus on what the infant will look like or how the infant will look dressed in baby clothes. To test her ability to solve similar issues for her child, the mother may relive, through her dreams childhood conflicts that may have been left unresolved. As the woman moves closer to delivery, she may have dreams that question her maternal skills or her ability to cope with motherhood and a career. Fantasies are the woman's way of working through conflicts and readying herself for the motherhood role. Offering a listening ear and reassurance that dreams and fantasies are a normal adaptation to her changing role is a positive intervention.

Role Fit

After the woman has acquired a set of maternal role expectations, she matches her expectation to the actions of other mothers. As she "tries on" the different behaviors, she will either accept or reject them as agreeable to her view of the motherhood role. The investigation into the appropriate skills necessary for motherhood suggests that throughout her pregnancy the woman has successfully taken the necessary steps toward the maternal role. In sessions with new mothers, discussing ideas of motherhood and offering informational sources reinforces positive perceptions of the new role.

Maternal Tasks

In the work of Rubin (1984) a list of maternal tasks are discussed. These tasks are identified as developmental milestones that the woman must accomplish to successfully incorporate the maternal identity into her personality.

Safe Passage

The goal of safe passage is to achieve a healthy pregnancy and an intact newborn with no detrimental effects to the mother. In the first trimester, the woman will focus on herself and her pregnancy. Later in the second trimester, she becomes very aware of her responsibility to protect the fetus and does this by adhering to different aspects of her prenatal care. As she moves closer to delivery, her thoughts shift to mother and baby as a couple: what happens to one will happen to the other. The pregnant woman will seek out role models and expert advice on the best way to proceed through the pregnancy and delivery and on to parenting.

Acceptance by Others

The woman's world before pregnancy is dependent on the social interactions of the family and secondary groups, such as community activities, school, or work. Initially, the secondary groups are significant to who the woman is and how she defines her life's meaning. Throughout the pregnancy her family and especially her partner become the motivational force behind her desire to be successful as a mother. To succeed, the mother becomes aware of sacrifices that will need to be made. If she has other children, she will have to assist them in adapting to the growing family.

During this time, the most important role for the nurse is to listen to the woman's concerns and offer assistance, when applicable, in a nonjudgmental manner.

Binding in to the Child

In the first trimester, the woman focuses on herself and maintaining the pregnancy. Once fetal movement is felt, in the second trimester, the fetus becomes real and she begins to feel there is significance in working to meet the challenges of becoming a mother. At this time, the fetus becomes an independent person and all of the mother's being is directed toward the newborn's safe arrival.

Critical Thinking

Successful Role Adaptation

Rosie is a teen who is pregnant with her first baby, and she is approaching her eighth month. She is in the office for her prenatal visit and has brought her girlfriend; they are going to a party at a friend's house later that night.

1. How can you determine if Rosie has accepted her pregnancy?

2. What behaviors would you expect Rosie to report to indicate that she is successfully adapting to her impending role as mother?

3. What questions will you ask to determine if Rosie understands the changes that she will have to make in her lifestyle to care for her infant?

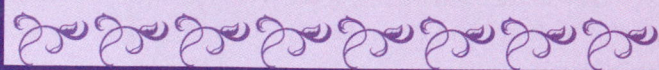

Giving of Oneself

The experience of pregnancy and childbirth could not be endured without the prospect of a healthy newborn as the outcome. Pregnancy is a time of giving gifts between couples, family, and friends. The grandmother may give the baby a family heirloom and a friend may give a baby book. The partner gives the woman a child and the woman gives the fetus a healthy diet and often eliminates unhealthy habits. The act of giving a gift is not the primary focus for the woman, but the communication of appreciative approval helps the woman to endure the changes and discomforts of the pregnant body. Health care providers who gives generously of their time to answer questions and provide guidance reinforces the importance of the sacrifices that must be made to achieve a successful pregnancy and healthy family.

Conflicting Developmental Tasks

Because pregnancy is not always a planned or intended developmental stage of the woman's or her family's life, there may be other developmental tasks that are in the process of being accomplished. These tasks may conflict with or make the accomplishment of the role transition more difficult.

An example would be the teen mother who is working on the developmental aspects of adolescence while attempting the transition to the motherhood role (Table 15-2). Many times, the tasks overlap or conflict. When this

happens, the role of the nurse is to assist in isolating the issues and to assist the teen in working through each one. The nurse may want to enlist the assistance of professionals that specialize in the care of teens or assist the teen in finding a support group for pregnant teens.

Becoming a Father

Traditionally, an assumption was made that the father of the infant was also the husband of the mother. Today, more babies are being born to single mothers, and the situation of caring for a woman without a husband is common.

The transition to fatherhood is made easier when there is a bond or relationship between the man and the woman. It is important to successful fetal attachment for both the mother and the father that the parents are united and their feelings are mutual. Wilson, White, Cobb, Curry, Greene and Popovich (2000) described mutuality as a close and emotional relationship in which each participant is secure in their own identity. In relationships that foster clear communication and the recognition that different roles are necessary to foster a healthy family, a new being can readily be accepted as a member. In families without a husband-father, the nurse can investigate how other family members may fit into the structure. A female partner, grandfather, or close friend may be the father figure in a particular family. Assisting the woman in identifying her

Table 15-2 Conflicting Development Tasks

Developmental Tasks of Adolescence	Developmental Tasks of Pregnancy	Conflicts
• Personal value system	• Seeking safe passage	• Wants the approval of others, especially peers • May conform to prenatal care only to avoid negative reaction from authority figures • May not readily express concerns about prenatal care
• Vocation or career	• Acceptance of the reality of the unborn child	• Not future-oriented • Limited means of support • Developing feminine self may assist in focusing on fetus, but role confusion may occur
• Body image and sexuality	• Acceptance of the pregnancy by self and others	• May be awkward about looking different; still struggling with own identity • Relationship with father of infant may not be as strong as she had hoped • Family may react negatively to her pregnancy
• Achievement of a stable identity	• Acceptance of the reality of parenthood	• Is attempting to develop the feminine identity; feels pregnancy may assist in her validation as a woman; may feel the conflict
• Independence from parents	• Giving of oneself	• Teen's parents may replace her as the parent figure, limiting her involvement with the newborn

emotional needs as she moves into the motherhood role helps her to adjust to any deficits that may be noted.

Transition to Fatherhood

Men have their own unique transition that must take place to incorporate the identity of father into their personality. In accepting the pregnancy, the man needs to perceive that certain goals have been accomplished before the birth of the newborn. Has he thought about becoming a father at some point in his future and has he accepted the end to his childless period? Men are concerned about the financial and emotional stability of the couple and how they will fare with this new individual entering their lives. If these questions are not positively answered, there may be some ambivalence to the pregnancy on the part of the man. The nurse's knowledge of social and community resources is helpful in assisting the couple with role adjustment.

The Stress of the Paternal Role

The adaptation of the male to the fatherhood role is a life crisis, just as it is for the woman accepting the maternal role. The woman needs her partner to be empathic, trustworthy, reliable, and available to assist in the successful completion of pregnancy and childbirth. These responsibilities, plus the change that will occur in the lifestyle of the couple, cause stress in the structure of the family. Often men note that potential financial issues, learning new routines, work conflicts, fewer hours of sleep, and caring for the infant are issues that may block the evolution of the fatherhood role. In a relationship, the woman is usually the man's emotional counselor, and in the parent role, the woman is most often focused on the needs of the newborn and not available to help the man through his challenges. The successful role adaptation of the man to fatherhood is typically closely related to the emotional health of the couple's relationship.

The custom of taking on symptoms of pregnancy and childbirth by the man is called **couvade**. There are many different theories that identify possible reasons for this condition; these include sympathy and identification with the pregnant woman, being left out, feeling guilty about putting the woman in this condition, or the stress of living in such a unpredictable situation. The symptoms may appear around the third month or at delivery and may include nausea and vomiting, abdominal pain, weight gain, food cravings, fatigue, and mood swings. Of course, these symptoms could signal illness, so a full assessment is necessary. Becoming more involved in the pregnancy, or seeking out knowledge concerning areas that the father feels insecure about, may alleviate the symptoms of couvade.

Bonding Between the Father and Infant

Fathers bond in much the same way as mothers do. Looking at and touching their infants, perceiving the infant's characteristics as unique and perfect, being attracted to the infant, and feeling happy are strong indicators of successful attachment. Early physical contact and involvement in the newborn's care are important for future positive father-child adjustment.

The Family

The family is a dynamic and complex unit that adapts to each individual's role changes and crisis resolution. The success of the family depends on the ability to continue to move forward on the developmental course while each individual moves through their own maturational and situational crises. As we enter the 21st century, the process of family life takes on a different look from the families of the early to middle 20th century. Parents may be unmarried, not living together, of the same sex, older, adoptive, or grandparents who are raising the infant.

The participation of caregivers outside the family, i.e., day care providers, is a challenge for families. The close extended family that was traditionally relied on for support and help with child care is often not geographically or financially able to assist. Nurses are finding that knowledge of community resources is necessary in assisting many of these families with the challenges of day to day living.

Duval (1985) has described developmental tasks that are necessary in the successful transition to the family role. They include adapting relationships to the realities of pregnancy; planning for the pregnancy, childbirth, and parenting; and reevaluating financial responsibilities for the impending family. The couple needs to orient themselves to their new roles and have insight into how their relationships with other family members will change. Sexual relations during pregnancy and after childbirth are different from the experience of the past. Dividing the new responsibilities that come with this change in family life, such as who takes the infant for newborn checkups or

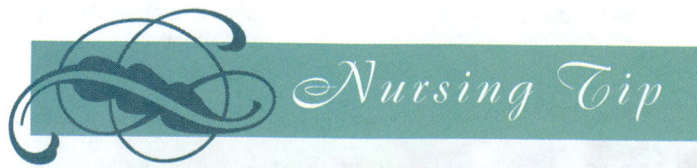

FAMILY VARIETY

In providing care to families, remember that the content of the family is the key to assisting members through a crisis and not the form that the family takes.

wakes up in the night for feedings, is a necessary task. Depending on the working status of the couple, making decisions on the physical care of the newborn will rank high on the list of tasks. In general, maintaining the morale of the family and adapting to the rapidly changing environment is most important.

Siblings

When children are already present in the family, the parents may have questions on how to handle the announcement of the expected newborn. The age of the child may dictate the timing of the announcement. If the sibling is under age 2, it may be best to wait until the fifth or sixth month to explain about a new brother or sister. A 9-month pregnancy progresses slowly for a child this age. If the mother is obviously not feeling well from the discomforts of pregnancy, it may be advantageous to tell the young child about the pregnancy. The young child may be afraid that mother is sick and that something bad will happen to her.

All children should be acquainted with the baby before it is born (Figure 15-19). There will be many questions, and these should be answered in a straightforward age-appropriate manner using the correct terminology. The nurse and the couple can discuss available age-specific books that can be used to explain the growth of the fetus as the pregnancy progresses. Children between the ages of 3 and 12 may want to track the growth of the fetus as the months progress. The older child can accompany the mother on her prenatal visits and listen for the baby's heartbeat. Also, involving siblings in preparing the home for the new baby can help them to feel that this is their baby too. Especially for the younger siblings, advance notice of the hospital stay and helping them to understand that they will be taken care of while the mother is away is extremely important. Including the child in the care of mother and baby can help with the transition once the infant is born. The nurse can assist the family in understanding that the sibling may not be immediately elated to have to share the parent's attention with this little stranger. The parents need to provide a smooth transition by keeping the sibling informed of coming events. The nurse can advise the family to monitor the attention that is showered on the new arrival and to provide a similar level of celebration for the brother or sister.

Grandparents

The grandparents' level of involvement in the pregnancy and birth of their grandchild is dependent on many variables. Today, geographic distance to the new family may not allow the level of involvement that was experienced by their grandparents. Grandparents today are typically expected to be available for the young family if an emergency arises. The new parents may call and ask advice or seek counsel from the experienced older parents. The financial situation, health, mental capacity, and working status influence the grandparents' ability to assist the new parents.

In today's family, both grandparents may be involved in careers and be focused on a retirement goal. The younger grandparent may have difficulty adjusting to the connotation of aging when they are called grandmother or grandfather. Grandparents with an active business and social life may resist being involved at the level others feel is appropriate. The conflict between reality and expectations can cause discord between family members. Nurses can discuss these issues during prenatal visits to assist the new parents in planning the involvement of the grandparents in ways that fit into everyone's lifestyle.

A growing phenomenon in the United States is the increasing number of grandparents who are raising their grandchildren. In 1997, Thomson, Minkler, and Driver (2000) reported, 3.7 million grandparents had taken their grandchildren into their homes to raise; of these, 2.3 million were single grandmothers. Many times, the parents are not living in the home with the family, which places great stress on the unprepared guardians. Grandparents are attempting to accomplish their own developmental tasks and the new role of late parenting may cause confusion and social and financial concerns.

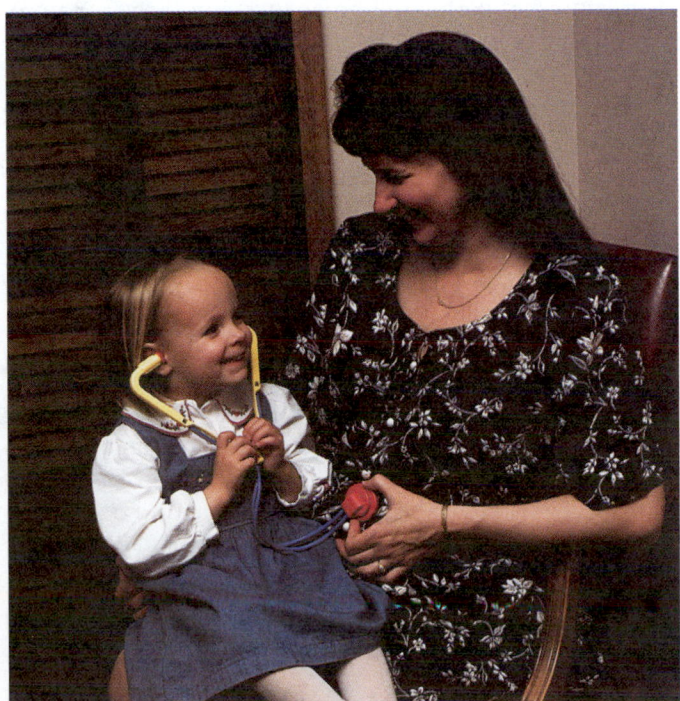

Figure 15-19 Young children can be encouraged to be involved in the pregnancy to develop a connection with the baby before birth.

CULTURAL CARING

What is a culture? The word is used to describe the intellectual, social, and artistic styles of a group of people, but for this discussion, we are referring to the customs, beliefs, and behaviors that have been learned through association with a particular group of people (Galanti, 1997). The learned behaviors of individual cultures are shared within the group and passed down to future generations. But there are factors that can dilute the culture and cause members to stray from their specific culture. When an individual has lived among people of another culture, especially since childhood, or has achieved a different social or economic class, their behaviors may deviate from their cultural heritage. The dilution or absence of the original culture is the reason why individuals should not be stereotyped. For example, the nurse assumes that because a woman appears to be from Mexico that she has or wants a large family. If the woman was born and raised in the United States in a predominantly Caucasian environment, a large family may not be a priority. It is acceptable to generalize concerning cultural behaviors, if this is used only as the beginning of an assessment to ascertain the true feelings of the individual client.

Because each person has values that are important to them, there are values that different cultures view as important. In the United States, freedom, independence, and autonomy are values that many people feel are important. In many cultures, remaining in the family home where members can assist each other with day-to-day activities is far more acceptable than obtaining independence from the family. The view of family involvement sometimes causes conflict with the American health care system's values of efficiency and self-control. Some cultures want the involvement of their family members in decision making and care and as intermediaries. Nurses must avoid ethnocentrism, i.e., the view that a certain culture's way of doing things is the only appropriate way, and attempt to be open-minded concerning the individual's values, beliefs, and behaviors, the view that is called cultural relativism (Galanti, 1997).

A person may see illness differently from the dominant health care community norms. Most medical models in the United States rely on the belief that germs, viruses, and environmental toxins cause disease and that health can be maintained through diet and exercise. Galanti (1997) states that, in some cultures, the world view is focused on the belief that these aspects of life are out of human control and in the hands of a greater being. Some cultures also relate to the natural aspect of all things and strive to obtain harmony with the earth. These individuals may prefer to treat ailments with herbal medicine or through prayer, touch, or meditation. There are cultures that do not view pregnancy as a medical condition, so the pregnant woman may not see the necessity of prenatal care. In these situations, it is necessary to explain the importance of health teaching and maintenance and not assume that everyone views healthy behaviors in the same way.

Another aspect of cultural differences that often becomes evident in pregnancy is the relationship of the father and mother. Most Americans believe that the man or partner should be involved in every aspect of the pregnancy and delivery. In some Middle Eastern families the man is present during the pregnancy and delivery to protect the woman's virtue, not to assist the woman with the birth. The woman of Mexican heritage may prefer her mother to attend her delivery, and the man may feel that his presence is inappropriate.

Nurses have an opportunity to act as advocates to the women of different cultures that make up the American population. Nurses can design and implement programs that integrate the customs and values of the culture into the care of pregnant women. Mayberry, Affonson, Shibuya and Clemmens (1999) described a health care program, *"Malama Na Wahine",* or Caring for Pregnant Women for the native Hawaiian, Filipino, and Japanese women living in Hawaii. Mayberry and associates designed the program to acknowledge the value and self-esteem of the women they served by incorporating their customs and beliefs into every aspect of their care. Examples of cultural interventions that were used in the program included:

1. Enlisting the assistance of local cultural healers to participate in the program as recruiters and caregivers.

2. Using "talk story," a form of communication that is used by the women in this culture to deliver knowledge.

Nursing Tip

PREPARATION FOR THE INFANT

A lack of preparation for the birth of the baby may indicate a problem in meeting the task of role transition. However, some cultures or families do not actually purchase any items for the baby until after birth, because purchasing gifts for the baby before birth is believed to bring bad luck. Nurses must be sensitive to cultural practices different from his or her own and not assume that the couple who has not established a nursery before the birth is not eagerly awaiting the new baby's arrival.

3. Helping women choose a name for their newborn that honors their culture.

4. Providing *lomilomi* massage, which demonstrates health promotion, as part of the care of the woman and newborn.

The nurse's role in caring for clients of different cultures is to develop an individualized plan of care for each woman that supports her beliefs and customs and, at the same time, provides healthy and safe interventions for a positive outcome.

COMPLEMENTARY THERAPIES

Consumers of health care are turning to complementary therapies in large numbers. The odds that a pregnant client is practicing some type of complementary therapy are high. Strasen (1999) defines "complementary medicine" as any practitioner or practice that is not in the realm of traditional medicine. This definition opens up a wide range of healing methods to consumers as a complement to what maybe viewed as usual health practices. Assisting clients to feel good on emotional, spiritual, and physical levels is a common goal of complementary therapists. Frequently, complementary practitioners may view their role much the same as the holistic role of the nurse, i.e., to assist the client in bringing optimal health to the body, mind, and spirit.

In pregnancy, most of the complementary therapies practiced today can be beneficial in assisting the woman with easing the discomforts of pregnancy and providing mental calm in the midst of a fast-paced world. The area in which caution may be necessary is that of herbal medicine. In 1994, the FDA passed the Dietary Supplement Health and Education Act (DSHEA), which places herbal products within the dietary supplement category and, with this act, herbal preparations became available over the counter. To date, there is no regulation of the quality of these supplements, and research into the effects of these supplements on pregnancy is just beginning. Women who request information on the use of herbs during pregnancy should be advised to avoid using them in any form during the first trimester and to seek the advice of their health care practitioner concerning the use of herbs in later pregnancy.

Because a large number of women are using complementary therapies, the nursing assessment should include questions concerning these practices. The information enables the nurse to advise the woman on the continuation of these therapies or to seek further consultation concerning the safety of the practice during pregnancy.

NURSING PROCESS

The nursing process in the care of the pregnant woman represents a map for the most direct route to wellness. The steps included in the nursing process operate in a continuum to provide a framework for individualizing the client's care.

Assessment

In performing the client assessment, there are many tools available to the nurse. Prerequisites for a thorough assessment include being nonjudgmental, open-minded, empathic, and a skilled interviewer; having a knowledge of physical assessment skills and parameters; and exhibiting the ability to communicate and to collaborate. As the assessment is continuous, every time the nurse has contact with the client, her family, her friends, or other health care professionals, a synthesizing process should take place.

Interviewing is a skill that is essential to the nurse's data collection. The data that is collected should come directly from clients and their families. An important aspect of interviewing is to listen in an unbiased manner, understanding that the client and her family are the experts in this portion of the data collection. The questions should explore biophysical, psychosocial, cultural, and spiritual aspects of the client's well-being. The interview is an opportunity to begin to develop a relationship with the client and accumulate a primary list of needs.

The setting, client complaint, and client status guide the direction of the physical assessment and at what point in the health continuum that the nurse-client interaction occurs. In a physician's office the role of the nurse may be to assist with the assessment and in the emergency room an initial focused assessment may be appropriate, but on hospital admission after stabilization, the nurse should complete a full physical assessment. The nurse caring for the pregnant woman must remember that there are two clients, the woman and her fetus; each requires an assessment that entails specific parameters. During the prenatal course, the nurse plans and organizes the care process over a period of time, documenting the outcomes clearly. The assessment data that is contained in the prenatal record provides a basis for the prenatal needs assessment and also for the intrapartum and postpartum needs assessment.

Data obtained from diagnostic studies is included in building the database. Studies that are completed in the prenatal period are used to identify client care needs throughout pregnancy, labor, and delivery. Computerized documentation that can be shared between the prenatal provider's office and hospital or birthing center is invaluable because of easy access at all hours of the day or night.

Nursing Diagnosis

Nursing diagnoses provide a uniform method of communicating the pregnant client's concerns and needs. The nursing diagnoses reflect the nurse's clinical judgment concerning actual or potential problems for the client, the family, or the community. When prioritizing needs of the pregnant women, the nurse should involve the client, family, and other disciplines to be sure the plan is correctly focused and realistic.

Outcome Identification

The pathway for nursing care is outlined in the outcomes defined for the nursing interventions. For the pregnant woman, outcomes are typically centered on nursing diagnoses relating to a healthy pregnancy, successful adaptation to new family roles, and preparation for motherhood. In identifying desired outcomes, the nurse should make every effort to involve the pregnant client's partner or family, according to client wishes, and to incorporate the client's personal goals for her pregnancy.

Planning

Once the nursing diagnoses and outcome statements have been developed, the nurse and client should plan care that will result in an achievable and desired response of the client, family, or community to the nursing interventions. Planning should take into account such factors as quality of life, acuity of medical condition, resources, time, finances, and situation. Working with the client to establish an individualized plan of care is important, because both the client and the nurse are accountable for accomplishing the planned outcomes.

Nursing Intervention

Interventions are derived from the nurses' knowledge base and through consultation with other disciplines. The interventions should be based on scientific principles and implemented with an understanding of where the pregnant client is on the continuum of wellness. Other healthcare providers may complete some of the interventions that are

SUCCESSFUL EVALUATION

Questions that the process of evaluation will answer are:

1. Were the diagnoses correct?
2. Have the outcomes been met?
3. Should the interventions be changed?
4. Have new problems occurred?
5. Should new healthcare providers be involved?
6. What interventions were most effective and should other interventions be included?
7. Are new outcome criteria required?

The evaluation process should be thought of as a flowchart of the client's care with ongoing assessment of the client's needs.

included in the plan of care for the pregnant client, and the role of the nurse may be coordination or delegation. It remains the nurse's responsibility to ensure that the plan of care is updated as the interventions are completed; this is accomplished through complete documentation at each prenatal visit.

Evaluation

The nurse must assess the pregnant client's response to the interventions, and then make adjustments to the plan of care. By interviewing the client at each prenatal visit, the nurse can ascertain the client's comfort level with the plan of care and make adjustments as new diagnoses present or other factors change.

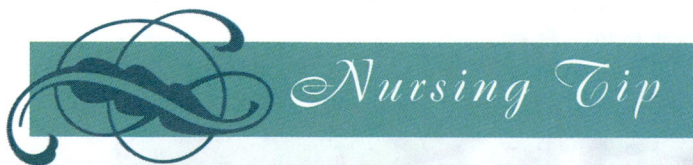

SUCCESSFUL PLANNING

Because the plan of care is a communication tool to organize and prioritize the client's care, all entries should be timed, dated, and initialed.

Critical Thinking

Additional Nursing Diagnoses

Refer to the case study of 16-year-old Rhonda. Develop a care plan that includes these additional nursing diagnoses:

Compromised family coping

Risk for impaired parenting

Deficient knowledge (infant care)

Home maintenance management, risk for impaired

Case Study/Care Plan

ADOLESCENT PREGNANCY

Rhonda is a 16-year-old female at 26 weeks' gestation. Her vital signs are within normal limits and her weight gain is at 17 pounds. She states she is still smoking because she is concerned about gaining too much weight. She presents to the clinic for only the second time, complaining of difficulty having a bowel movement. Rhonda has stopped taking her prenatal vitamins because one of her friends told her they could make her constipated. She is living with the father of her baby. She continues to wear the clothes she wore before she was pregnant, although they appear tight and uncomfortable.

Assessment

- Age 16 at 26 weeks' gestation
- Vital signs normal
- Risk for fetal injury results from maternal smoking and lack of prenatal care
- Constipation
- Body image disturbance

Nursing Diagnosis

Risk for fetal injury related to cigarette smoking and limited prenatal care

Expected Outcomes   The client will:
Verbalize understanding of the risk to the fetus from cigarette smoking
Verbalize importance of prenatal visits to maintain a healthy pregnancy
Demonstrate lifestyle changes that reduce the risk to the fetus

Planning   Collaborating with client, determine desired means of delivering necessary information, based on client's learning style and preferences.

Nursing Interventions	Rationales
1. Stress the importance of ongoing prenatal care to monitor the growth of the newborn and to prevent maternal complications.	1. Many teens feel well and do not understand the necessity of prenatal visits.
2. Explain the hazards to the fetus from maternal cigarette smoking.	2. Smoking can cause growth retardation and an increased incidence of SIDS.
3. Help client to identify her motivation to smoke and her motivation to stop smoking.	3. Teen mothers are more receptive to changing health habits if the reasons are outlined in a nonjudgmental manner. Offering the option of cutting down and then quitting may soften the request.
4. Refer her to a support group or find another teen who has successfully stopped smoking to discuss options with her.	4. Engaging Rhonda in group or peer support sessions may help her to feel less socially isolated.

Evaluation   At Rhonda's next visit, she was able to verbalize the necessity to stop or at least curtail her smoking. She had cut her smoking down to three cigarettes a day and was working to completely stop smoking. She still appeared doubtful that the prenatal visits were necessary. Refer Rhonda to the clinic's teen childbirth classes.

(continued)

Nursing Diagnosis

Constipation related to smooth muscle relaxation, slowed intestinal motility, ingestion of iron supplements, and diet.

Expected Outcome Rhonda will maintain her normal pattern of bowel function.

Planning Determine with client her usual bowel patterns and what routine would make her comfortable.

Nursing Interventions	Rationales
1. Assess for prepregnant elimination patterns.	1. With appropriate diet, usual elimination patterns should be maintained.
2. Assess for dietary history and make recommendations based on nutritional needs	2. A dietary history tells the practitioner what modifications need to be made.
3. Instruct on the benefits of increasing fiber intake. Consult the dietitian to identify high-fiber foods that are acceptable to a teen. (fruit and salads may be the most acceptable to the teen).	3. Adequate bulk and fiber assists in regulating bowel movements; a teenager's eating habits are influenced by peer pressure.
4. Advise client to increase fluid intake, avoiding drinks with caffeine. Encourage water, flavored water, fruit juices, or sports drinks.	4. An increase in fiber without an increase in fluids may compound the elimination problem.
5. Encourage mild exercise, such as brisk walking or riding a bicycle.	5. Exercise promotes peristalsis and may help to prevent constipation.
6. Encourage client to continue taking prenatal vitamins and, if constipation remains a problem after dietary adjustments, contact the healthcare provider.	6. Remind the client that prenatal vitamins are important to a healthy pregnancy and to the proper development of the baby.
7. Caution against the use of stool softeners or laxatives.	7. Never take medications that have not been approved by a healthcare provider.

Evaluation The nurse called Rhonda at home 5 days after her visit. She had increased her fluid intake to 6 to 8 glasses per day of water or a sports drink. She was eating fresh and dried fruit and salads. She continued to take her prenatal vitamins and her bowel movements had returned to her normal pattern.

Nursing Diagnosis

Disturbed body image related to pregnancy, as evidenced by wearing of prepregnancy clothing.

Expected Outcome Client will: verbalize understanding and acceptance of body image changes that are occurring

Demonstrate a positive self-image by maintaining an appropriate appearance

Planning Collaborate with client to understand her self-image and what she is or is not willing to change.

Nursing Interventions	Rationales
1. Determine Rhonda's attitude toward her pregnancy, changing body image, and her peers' and significant other's reactions. Suggest that her significant other accompany her to her next prenatal visit.	1. Her views on her pregnancy affect how she feels about her body and about becoming a mother. The father of the baby is a strong influence on health behaviors.
2. Identify Rhonda's sense of self-esteem in relationship to her pregnancy and her new role. Assess her relationship with her mother and the availability of other female role models.	2. Honest, nonjudgmental, respectful treatment facilitates interactions with the client. Female role models are helpful in the transition to the motherhood role.

(continued)

Nursing Interventions	Rationales
3. Review the physiologic changes of pregnancy and why these changes are necessary for the development of her fetus; assure her that mixed feelings are normal.	3. Show her that the changes in her body are normal and beneficial to the growth of the fetus. Talking through her feelings helps to decrease the stress she may be feeling.
4. Assess her ability to purchase or borrow comfortable maternity clothes. Make a referral to social services or targeted case management for assistance.	4. Embarrassment concerning financial issues may prevent her from purchasing or borrowing appropriate clothing.

Evaluation The case manager made a visit to Rhonda's home with several maternity outfits that were appropriate for a teenager. She discussed the role of parenthood with both Rhonda and her significant other. While in the home, she assessed the couple's plans for caring for the infant and adapting to the changes they need to make in their lifestyle. Rhonda had new questions about the changes occurring in her body and felt comfortable discussing these with the case manager.

Key Concepts

- The presumptive signs of pregnancy are the subjective signs noted by the woman and include amenorrhea, nausea and vomiting, urinary frequency, changes in the breast, and quickening. Probable signs of pregnancy are the objective signs noted by the examiner, such as uterine enlargement, Goodell's sign, Chadwick's sign, Hegar's sign, and positive results on pregnancy tests. Detecting the fetal heart rate and fetal movement and visualization of the fetus by ultrasound are the positive signs of pregnancy.

- There are anatomic and physiologic changes that occur in virtually every body system of the pregnant woman. These changes are necessary to accommodate the growing fetus.

- Plasma volume increases by 50%; red blood cell volume increases by 18% to 30%. The disproportionate increases in volume cause a dilution of the red blood cell volume that results in the physiologic anemia of pregnancy.

- Maternal cardiac output increases from 4.5 L/min to 6.0 L/min. The uteroplacental unit requires approximately 17% of this volume to achieve adequate perfusion.

- In preparation for lactation, the number of mammary alveoli increase, the breasts become physically larger, areolae broaden, nipples become firmer and more erect, and the tubercles of Montgomery, sebaceous glands, begin to secrete a substance that keeps the areolae supple.

- The position of the heart is changed; it is pushed upward to the left and rotated. These changes mimic cardiomegaly on normal radiographic films. In 90% of pregnant woman, a systolic heart murmur can be heard at 20 weeks' gestation.

- When the woman lies in the supine position, the gravid uterus may compress the vena cava and descending aorta. The compression can cause maternal hypotension and decrease the blood return to the heart.

- Many of the discomforts of pregnancy can be linked to changes that occur in the body systems to accommodate a pregnancy.

- Blood flow to the kidneys is increased, which in turn increases the glomerular filtration rate. Because of this increase, absorption is not always complete and glucose periodically spills into the urine. Protein may also be detected in the urine, but proteinuria of more than 300 mg in 24 hours warrants further investigation, especially when accompanied by hypertension and edema.

- Individuals, as well as families, are challenged to successfully accomplish developmental tasks that move them toward role adaptation.

- Siblings need assistance in dealing with the changes that occur when a new individual is brought into the family.

- An assessment to identify cultural values, customs, and beliefs should be completed for every client. The information gathered should be incorporated into the client's plan of care.

- The involvement of the client, her family, and the community is the key to planning a realistic and achievable plan of care.

Web Activities

- What resources can you locate that give mothers self-help tips on alleviating the discomforts of pregnancy? Do they offer resources to download?

- What types of organizations offer this information?

- Would you encourage your clients to use the Web? If so, what type of advice would you give concerning the use of Web resources?

Review Questions and Activities

1. All of the following are considered presumptive (subjective) signs of pregnancy except:
a. Nausea and vomiting
b. Urinary frequency
c. Fetal heart beat
d. Fatigue

The correct answer is c.

2. During pregnancy, the plasma volume increases by 50% and the red blood cell volume increases by 18% to 30%; the disproportionate increases results in the following:
a. Iron deficiency anemia
b. Sickle cell anemia
c. Thalassemia
d. Physiologic anemia of pregnancy

The correct answer is d.

3. An assessment to determine what aspects of the client's culture may affect her plan of care should include:
a. Traditional customs and behaviors related to preparation for birth
b. Beliefs related to who should be present at the birth
c. Values related to congenital defects
d. All of the above

The correct answer is d.

4. A new baby affects the family unit, especially the newborn's siblings. What measures should be avoided in helping siblings adjust to the transition?
a. Involve the sibling in planning the nursery.
b. Answer questions in a honest and straightforward manner.

c. Use age-specific books to inform the sibling of the fetus' growth.
d. Avoid telling the sibling when it is time to go to the hospital for delivery.

The correct answer is d.

5. Maternal cigarette smoking can be hazardous to the growing fetus. Which of the following is not a common risk of maternal cigarette smoking?
a. Heart defects
b. Increased incidence of SIDS
c. Low birth weight
d. Increased incidence of apnea

The correct answer is a.

6. When a pregnant woman lies in the supine position, what potentially harmful physiologic processes occur?
a. Increased edema in the hands and face
b. Maternal hypotension
c. Decreased blood return to heart
d. After a prolonged period, decreased oxygen to the fetus

The correct answer is d.

7. During adaptation to the role of motherhood, the woman must accomplish all but which of the following developmental tasks?
a. Giving of oneself
b. Binding in to the child
c. Fantasizing or dreaming
d. Shift her affections and alliance from her husband to the developing infant.

The correct answer is d.

8. Complementary therapy is becoming more accepted in the United States. Which of the following therapies would you as the nurse be cautious about suggesting to the pregnant woman?
   a. Reflexology
   b. Meditation
   c. Herbal therapy
   d. Imagery

The correct answer is c.

References

Blackburn, S. T., & Loper, D. L. (1992). *Maternal fetal and neonatal physiology: A clinical perspective*. Philadelphia: W. B. Saunders.

Burrow, G. M., S. Duffy, T. F. (1999). *Medical complications during pregnancy*. 5th ed. Philadelphia: W. B. Saunders.

Cunningham, F. G., MacDonald, P. C., Gant, N. F., Leveno, K. J., Gilstrap, L. C., Hankins, G. D. V., & Clark, S. L. (1997). *Williams' Obstetrics*. (20th ed.). Stamford, CT: Appleton & Lange.

Duvall, E. M. (1985). *Marriage and family development*. (6th ed.). New York: Harper & Row.

Gabbe, S. G., Niebyl, J. R., & Simpson, J. L. (1996). *Obstetrics: normal & problem pregnancies*. (3rd ed.). New York: Churchill Livingstone.

Galanti, G. A. (1997). *Caring for patients from different cultures*. (2nd ed.). Philadelphia: University of Pennsylvania Press.

Henshaw, S. K. (1998). Unintended pregnancy in the United States, *Family Planning Perspectives, 30* (1), 24–29, 46.

National Academy of Science, Institute of Medicine. (1990). *Nutrition during pregnancy: Weight gain and nutrients*. Washington, DC: National Academy Press.

Mayberry, L. J., Affonson, D. D., Shibuya, J. & Clemmens, D. (1999). Integrating cultural values, beliefs, and customs into pregnancy and postpartum care: Lessons learned from a Hawaiian public health nursing project. *The Journal of Perinatal and Neonatal Nursing, 13* (1), 15–26.

Rubin, R. (1984), *Maternal identity and maternal experience*. New York: Springer.

Strasen, L. (1999). The silent health care revolution: The rising demand for complementary medicine. *Nursing Economics, 17,* (5), 246–251.

Thomson, E. F., Minkler, M., & Driver, D. (2000). A profile of grandparents raising grandchildren in the United States. In C. B. Cox (Ed.). *To grandmother's house we go and stay.* (pp. 20–31). New York: Springer.

Tulman, L., Morin, K. H., & Fawcett, J. (1998). Prepregnant weight and weight gain during pregnancy: Relationship to functional status, symptoms, and energy. *Journal of Obstetric, Gynecologic, & Neonatal Nursing, 27,* (6), 629–634.

Wilson, M. E., White, M. A., Cobb, B., Curry, R., Greene, D., Popovich, D., (2000). Family dynamics, parental-fetal attachment and infant temperment. *Journal of Advanced Nursing 31,* (1), 204–210.

Suggested Readings

Allaire, A. D., Moos, M. K., & Wells, S. (2000). Complementary and alternative medicine in pregnancy: A survey of North Carolina certified nurse-midwives. *Obstetrics & Gynecology, 95,* (1), 19–23.

Acevedo, M. C. (2000). The role of acculturation in explaining ethnic differences in the prenatal health-risk behaviors, mental health, and parenting beliefs of Mexican American and European American at-risk women. *Child Abuse & Neglect, 24,* (1), 111–127.

Belew, C. (1999). Herbs and the childbearing woman: Guidelines for midwives. *Journal of Nurse-Midwifery, 44,* (3), 231–252.

Charlish, A. (1996). *Your natural pregnancy: A guide to complementary therapies*. Berkeley: Ulysses Press.

Doenges, M. E., & Moorhouse, M. F. (1999). *Maternal/newborn plans of care*. (3rd ed.). Philadelphia: F. A. Davis.

Doswell, W. M., & Erlen, J. A. (1998). Multicultural issues and ethical concerns in the delivery of nursing care interventions. *Nursing Clinics of North America, 33,* (2), 353–361.

Drake, P. (1996). Addressing developmental needs of pregnant adolescents. *Journal of Obstetric, Gynecologic, & Neonatal Nursing, 25,* (6), 518–524.

Eisenberg, A., Murkoff, H. E., & Hathaway, S. E. (1996). *What to expect when you're expecting*. (2nd ed.). New York: Workman Publishing.

Gorrie, T. M., McKinney, E. S., & Murray, S. S. (1998). *Foundations of maternal-newborn nursing*. (2nd ed.). Philadelphia: W. B. Saunders.

Lederman, R. P. (1996). *Psychosocial adaptation to pregnancy*. New York: Springer.

Malnory, M. E. (1996). Developmental care of the pregnant couple. *Journal of Obstetric, Gynecologic, & Neonatal Nursing, 25* (6), 525–532.

National Safety Council. (1995). *Stress management*. Boston: Jones & Barlett.

Sawyer, L. M. (1999). Engaged mothering: The transition to motherhood for a group of African American women. *Journal of Transcultural Nursing, 10,* (1), 14–21.

Sears, W., Sears, M., & Hole, L. H. (1997). *The pregnancy book.* Boston: Little, Brown.

Tiller, C. M. (1995). Father's parenting attitudes during a child's first year. *Journal of Obstetric, Gynecologic, & Neonatal Nursing, 24,* (6), 508–514.

Resources

American Botanical Council, P. O. Box 144345, Austin, TX 78714-4345, 1-512-926-4900, www.herbalgram.org

American College of Nurse Midwives (ACNM), 818 Connecticut Ave., NW, Suite 900, Washington, DC 20006, 1-202-728-9860, www.acnm.org

American College of Obstetrics and Gynecology (ACOG), 409 12th St. SW, P. O. Box 96920, Washington, DC 20090-6920, www.acog.com

Association of Women's Health, Obstetric and Neonatal Nurses (AWHONN), 2000 L. Street, NW, Suite 740, Washington, DC 20006, 1-800-673-8499 (USA), 1-800-245-0231 (Canada), www.awhonn.org

March of Dimes, 1275 Mamaroneck Avenue, White Plains, NY 10605, 1-888-MODIMES (663-4637), www.modimes.org

CHAPTER 16

Management and Nursing Care of the Pregnant Woman

N ursing care centered around health promotion and health maintenance during pregnancy presents an excellent opportunity for nurses to teach mothers about normal changes expected and alert them to a variety of risk factors. You may be in contact with clients who have thoughts, values, feelings, and circumstances that are different from your own. Examine your feelings and values elicited by the following questions:

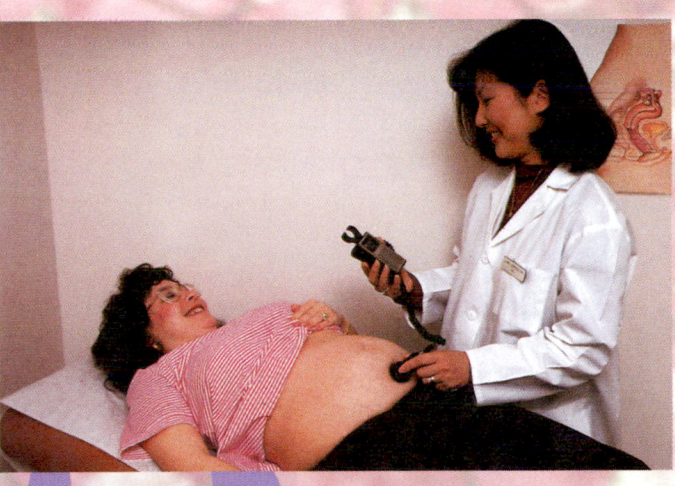

- *How do I feel about my own past or potential future experiences with pregnancy? Would my feelings be different about a planned compared with an unintentional pregnancy?*

- *How do I view all the physical changes that occur during pregnancy? How do I feel about these things happening to my body?*

- *Have I ever known a woman who did not value prenatal care as a priority in her childbearing life? How do I feel toward her and her family?*

- *What are my feelings about the varying degrees of importance attached to childbearing in my culture? In other cultures?*

- *How do I feel about families having several babies while they are receiving public assistance or welfare? What are my feelings as I see them for prenatal care?*

Key Terms

Biischial diameter	Health maintenance	Multipara	Pelvic outlet
EDB	Health promotion	Nägele's rule	Pregnancy-induced
EDC	Interspinous diameter	Obstetrical conjugate	hypertension (PIH)
EDD	LMP	Para	Preconception care
F.P.A.L.	Midpelvis	Pelvic inlet	Primipara
Gravida			

Competencies

Upon completion of this chapter, the reader should be able to:

1. Discuss the advantages of preconception care and counseling for a woman and her partner who are planning a pregnancy.

2. Discuss factors related to accessing prenatal care.

3. Describe areas of physical and psychosocial assessment that are covered in an initial prenatal visit and in subsequent visits.

4. Summarize normal physiologic changes encountered during each of the three trimesters of pregnancy.

5. Explain nursing interventions and teaching points used to assist clients in dealing with the commonly occurring discomforts of pregnancy.

6. Describe risk-assessment measures recommended for routine prenatal visits in uncomplicated pregnancies.

7. List eight danger signs for which clients should be taught to seek immediate medical attention.

8. Discuss the teaching materials and aids available to nurses and clients.

Most health professionals who provide perinatal care can readily and easily explain the goal of prenatal care. They report, very succinctly, that the goal is the delivery of a healthy infant by a healthy mother at the end of a healthy pregnancy. Indeed, this is the ideal outcome that, if achieved with each pregnancy in the United States, would be very impressive in light of the goals listed in *Healthy People 2000* and *Healthy People 2010*.

Pregnancy and childbirth are normal physiologic processes that traverse dynamic, but still normal, changes from conception to delivery. The nurse has a unique opportunity to reinforce the normalcy of these processes and, at the same time, assess clients for possible deviations that require intervention. Additionally, the nurse can interpret for clients the changes that are taking place and provide valuable guidance for clients and their families, thereby facilitating their progression through the process with understanding and confidence.

Early contact between the health care team and the pregnant client provides the opportunity to address the complementary yet separate concepts of health promotion and health maintenance. **Health promotion** consists of education and counseling activities that help enhance and maintain health and healthy behaviors. The focus is on increasing knowledge to foster deliberate, active participation in achieving or attaining an optimal state of well-being. **Health maintenance** is the concept of prevention or early detection of particular health deviations through routine periodic examinations and screenings. Prevention is the primary goal; earliest possible detection and eradication or alleviation is the secondary goal. Part of this process is the identification of risk factors, particularly in vulnerable populations.

BENEFITS OF EARLY CARE

For many years health care professionals have supported the idea that the general health, and particularly the nutritional status of a woman before pregnancy, is the best predictor of her pregnancy outcome. Generally stated, the healthier the client before pregnancy and the better her nutritional state, the better the pregnancy outcomes, especially in terms of the baby's health. Although this may be accepted as an accurate statement, the nurse must not overlook the elements involved here. It is unlikely that a state of good health "just happened" for those particular women. Closer examination usually reveals that a conscientious self-help effort took place to produce this healthy state. These efforts encompassed good nutrition patterns, regular exercise, and avoidance of known deterrents to good health. Additionally, these women were probably diligent in seeking routine periodic health examinations and in maintaining the recommended immunization status.

PRECONCEPTION CARE

With the empirical evidence available suggesting that healthy infants are born to mothers who were in optimal health before pregnancy, researchers have undertaken an examination of factors of importance before pregnancy and, thus, even before early prenatal care. This approach is **preconception care**, or consultation with health care professionals by a client before pregnancy to facilitate optimal pregnancy outcomes (Figure 16-1). Proponents of preconception care emphasize that the most critical and vulnerable time for a developing fetus is the interval of days 17 to 56 after fertilization of the ovum. These earliest days usually have passed before even the most conscientious client seeks prenatal care. Therefore, in order to avoid known potentially damaging agents to the embryo, preconception care can be even more valuable than early prenatal care (Perry, 1996). Hazards encountered during this time frequently translate into high infant morbidity or mortality rates.

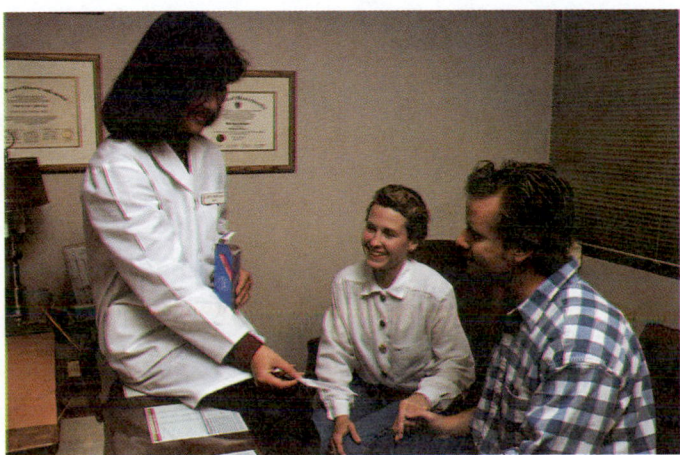

Figure 16-1 Many couples visit their health care provider for preconception counseling.

Researchers have carefully examined maternal and perinatal morbidity and mortality rates for many years. The elements of these statistics, such as incidences of stillbirths, preterm births, congenital defects, and spontaneous abortions, have been categorized and classified in many different ways. Data are available relative to total numbers of incidences from year to year, incidence by socioeconomic group, by race or ethnic group, by maternal education level, and by early compared with late entry into the health care system for prenatal care. Despite all that is known about the statistical correlations and relationships between and among these factors and pregnancy outcomes, little progress has been made in decreasing the negative outcomes. In other words, knowledge of factors associated with poor pregnancy outcomes does not automatically translate into lowering of subsequent morbidity and mortality rates.

Two problems for the neonate, low birth weight and congenital anomalies, have remained a challenge for health care professionals (Cefalo & Moos, 1995). Obstetrical care procedures and practices are not proving to be the answer to these two persistent problems in the United States. As Cefalo and Moos pointed out, the incidence of low-birth-weight neonates is not significantly different from that in the mid 1960s; more striking is the fact that the incidence of congenital anomalies has only minimally decreased in the last century. According to the Centers for Disease Control and Prevention, the most favorable data reflected only a 2% per year decrease in the incidence of neural tube defects, congenital rubella syndrome, and Rh hemolytic disease.

Early prenatal care is acknowledged as an important factor in achieving positive pregnancy outcomes, even though documentation of the cost savings (by decreasing the number of low-birth-weight and premature babies) is elusive (Huntington & Connell, 1994). Stated another way, the cost of care for premature and low-birth-weight infants is known; however, what is unknown is the numbers of these at-risk births that are remedied by early prenatal care. In many instances of early prenatal care, low birth weight and congenital anomalies (with varying degrees of severity) continue to occur in infants.

Preconception Assessment

Preconception care is ideally managed by specialists in gynecology and perinatology and involves a team approach. The team leader may be a physician, nurse practitioner, Certified Nurse Midwife, or other comparably trained professional. Findings during the initial session may indicate the need for inclusion of other personnel on the team. For example, an endocrinologist can provide valuable input for a client who has diabetes or a geneticist may clarify risk factors for a client with a family history of genetically transmitted disorders.

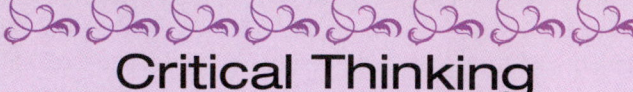

Critical Thinking

Congenital Anomalies as a Major Cause of Infant Deaths in the United States

You often work with clients who give birth to infants who have congenital anomalies with known causes. Examine your feelings about the client's responsibilities for a birth anomaly.

- Did they knowingly risk exposure to any teratogens?
- Were they innocent victims of exposure?
- Are your feelings toward these clients different?
- Is the quality of your care influenced when you feel a client has been careless in taking care of herself and her developing fetus?

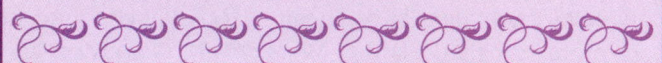

Many of the elements of preconception care can be introduced in a variety of health care settings. In the absence of an available specialized team, nurses in primary care settings (particularly in the community) can initiate care and distribute literature during routine health screenings or during group classes for health promotion (Perry, 1996). Clients interested in having children "some day" should have access to all information pertaining to factors associated with healthy pregnancy outcomes.

Early Interventions

Cefalo and Moos (1995) have summarized the components of preconception care into three general categories. The first category is systematic identification of risks from the comprehensive histories of the client and her partner, such as social factors, medical concerns, nutritional status, family structure, reproductive issues, medication use, and history of infectious disease. Next is the provision of educational materials that are indicated for each individual client and her partner. These should be factually accurate and culturally sensitive materials. Third, access to complementary and supplementary services such as special nutritional counseling or smoking cessation programs should be facilitated.

PRENATAL CARE

Early prenatal care presents benefits to the client, her partner, her family, and the health care team assuming responsibility for her care. Numerous teaching opportunities arise, especially regarding interpretation of normal physio-

logic changes that occur as the pregnancy progresses. In addition, psychological concerns can be addressed early on, thus avoiding stress and undue concern for clients. In summary, early prenatal care allows psychological, physiologic, cultural, and social concerns to be addressed while maternal and fetal well-being and the overall pregnancy status are monitored simultaneously.

Availability and Accessibility of Care

Many clients have reported that a major factor in seeking early prenatal care is access to care. Location of facilities and ease of getting into the "system" frequently are cited as factors that determine when a client goes in for her first visit. Whereas many clients seek care from physicians with offices in medical complexes or corporate-type buildings, many others prefer a neighborhood clinic where they have more convenient access. Nurse practitioners and nurse midwives practice in a variety of settings but generally are found in community clinic settings. When the work setting is in the community, nurses can glean a clearer understanding of their clientele, possible environmental concerns, and available resources. Additionally, the nurse can develop a deeper cultural sensitivity to clients and their families.

The report of The Pew Health Professions Commission (1991), Healthy America: Practitioners for 2005, presented an agenda for action as a guide for schools and professionals themselves. The focus was twofold: present competencies expected of health care practitioners, and present strategies for achieving changes that must occur in the education of health care professionals. The report is replete with emphasis on delivery of primary care that is community-based, teaching oriented, and involves clients and families in decision-making. The emphasis of this report reinforces what nurses have known for years: community-based health care by well-educated professionals that involves client and family involvement in mutual decision-making is ideal for the childbearing family.

Facilitation of Client Access to Care

Approaching the health care system can provoke fear in many clients, especially those with language or cultural differences. Additionally, concerns about costs and lack of knowledge regarding affordable resources can be deterrents for clients needing prenatal care. A very helpful model has been presented by McFarlane (1996) that uses a grass-roots approach for facilitating entry into the health care system for primary care. This particular program, called De Madres a Madres, or "Mothers to Mothers," is truly community-based. It is centered around training selected women in the community and increasing their knowledge of community resources and the health care system. These women, in turn, assist other women in their community by sharing resource information and facilitating entry into the primary care setting. Empowerment of community residents is the basis for the success of such programs (McFarlane & Fehir, 1994).

Public education programs can be very effective in facilitating early and consistent use of prenatal care. The nurse can make a valuable contribution to these programs by participating in public service announcements or becoming active in organizations, such as the March of Dimes, whose efforts are directed toward formal educational programs and development of professional and lay literature.

Barriers and perceived barriers to adequate prenatal care have been studied for many years. Through the years, as poor pregnancy outcomes have become associated with late or limited prenatal care, more research has emerged related to the reasons for limited care. The Institute of Medicine (Brown, 1998) published a compilation of such studies and an in-depth review of numerous programs throughout the United States developed to enhance use of prenatal care. Numerous studies report typical, predictable barriers: finances; transportation; inconveniences of language, clinic hours, and location; and work schedule problems. More recently, clients have reported concerns about the possibility of being asked to have an abortion, having their baby taken away, or facing deportation because of their lack of citizenship.

Many communities have programs or plans to assist clients with the specific concerns listed previously. Barriers can be viewed as challenges awaiting creative or innovative solutions. The nurse should be tuned in to self-imposed barriers of clients that reflect a poor understanding of or attaching little value to prenatal care. Situations of this nature require a sensitive approach to fact-finding regarding the client's and family's beliefs and values. This information can then be incorporated into a teaching plan that encourages early and consistent prenatal care. As an example, most clients and their partners value the health of their children, even in the absence of concern about their own immediate health state. The value of prenatal care can then be presented in terms of a healthy start for their baby at birth.

Components of Prenatal Care

Once the client and her partner have entered the health care system for prenatal care, several areas of assessment and monitoring will be covered at each visit. Depending on the findings for each individual case, the monitoring may vary slightly at each visit. For example, a client with prepregnancy diabetes may receive more frequent or closer monitoring for complications associated with diabetes. Other clients would receive routine (prescriptive) monitoring for glucose in the urine.

Based on assessments, specific client education or anticipatory management usually is indicated. Regardless of individual conditions or circumstances, all prenatal care covers assessment of maternal and fetal well-being from all aspects: physiologic, psychologic, economic, and sociocultural.

The Initial Prenatal Visit

The initial prenatal visit, especially in the absence of preconception care and counseling, can be rather lengthy. At this time a detailed medical history and physical examination are completed for baseline data. Accuracy of this baseline data is particularly important because health care providers will be referring back to it throughout the pregnancy. Nurses can assist clients through this time-consuming process by pointing out the importance of each step and by emphasizing that subsequent visits should be briefer.

As appropriate, nurses should congratulate clients for seeking early prenatal care and encourage early prenatal care for subsequent pregnancies. Aside from the logical benefits of early care, the physical examination for pregnancy confirmation, determination of uterus size, and measurements of the pelvis can be done more easily and with more comfort for the client in early pregnancy than later in the pregnancy. The practitioner also can make a

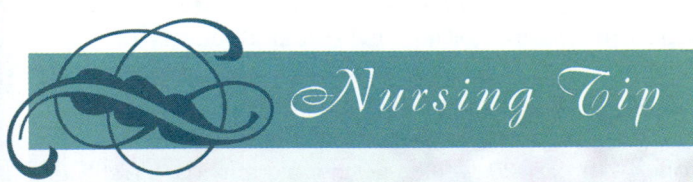

Nursing Tip

ENCOURAGE THE CLIENT TO KEEP ALL APPOINTMENTS FOR PRENATAL CARE

- Provide the client with a schedule of frequency of visits by trimester.

- Emphasize the timing of various screening and monitoring activities at each visit. Explain why the time of the monitoring is so important.

- Point out the importance of all screening and monitoring activities scheduled. Indicate which tests are for the mother's benefit and which are for the baby's benefit.

more accurate physical assessment when the client is not in an advanced state of pregnancy.

Pregnancy Confirmation

Many times clients and partners appear at a prenatal clinic for one distinctive purpose: to find out for sure if they are pregnant or not. Some clients may have already conducted an at-home pregnancy test and are seeking validation of the results. The availability and affordability of over-the-counter test kits have made them increasingly popular. However, the accuracy of the results is highly dependent on proper use of the kits, a point emphasized in the manufacturers' instruction sheets. Confirmation of pregnancy in the office or clinic setting usually is by means of a urine test for the presence of human chorionic gonadotropin (hCG). If necessary, a blood test for the same placental hormone can be performed (Cunningham, MacDonald, Gant, Leveno, Gilstrap, Haulcius & Clark, 1997).

Estimation of Due Date

After confirmation of a pregnancy, the next logical query from prospective parents is to estimate the date the baby is due to be born. This is commonly and historically referred to as the **EDC**, or expected date of confinement, reflecting the notion of the mother being confined to a specific area for the delivery. Other terms in common use are **EDD** for expected date of delivery, or **EDB** for expected date of birth. Clients usually refer to the EDB as their due date.

The EDC usually is calculated from the menstrual history, using a method called **Nägele's rule**. The calculation begins with the *first* day of the last menstrual period (or **LMP**); from this date, 3 months are subtracted and then 7 days are added. For example, if the first day of the LMP was September 15: LMP − 3 months + 7 days = EDC 9/15 (− 3 months) = 6/15 (+ 7 days) = 6/22.

The resulting calculated EDC is based on the presumption of ovulation occurring 14 days *before* the next anticipated period rather than 14 days *after* the last period began. This calculation usually is confirmed by a second method, measurement of uterine size, particularly as the pregnancy progresses. Neither method alone is deemed to be exact; however, the correlation of the findings of the two methods is fairly reliable. In clients with irregular menses, uterine size can be helpful in either confirming or redating the duration of the pregnancy.

Pregnancy wheels (Figure 16-2) are used to determine the EDC by aligning the arrow of the first day of the LMP and then reading off the date that corresponds with the 40-week mark. Aside from the dates, pregnancy wheels usually contain other information, such as corresponding weight and length of the fetus and height of the fundus at various weeks' gestation.

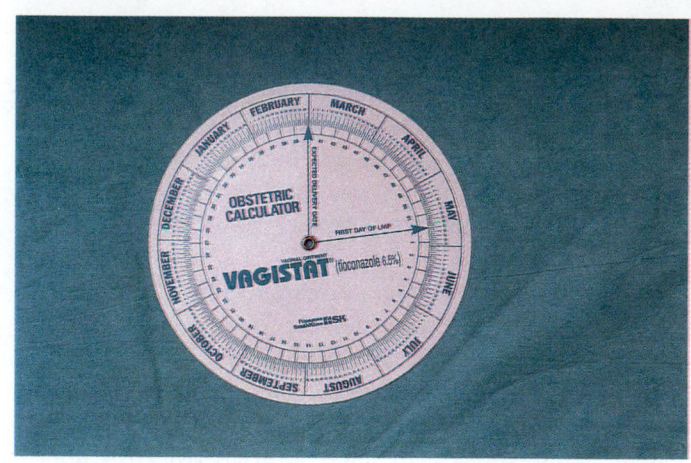

Figure 16-2 Gestation wheel. Place arrow labeled *first day of LMP* on date of LMP. Read date at arrow labeled *expected delivery date.*

Determination of Gravidity and Parity

Gravidity and parity are elements of an obstetric history that reflect number(s) of pregnancies and number of births, respectively. Gravidity and parity are used much like a shorthand way of recording these aspects without using lengthy phrases. **Gravida** is the term reflecting the number of pregnancies, regardless of duration or outcomes. A client who is pregnant for the first time thus is a gravida 1, a client experiencing her second pregnancy is a gravida 2, and so on. Sometime the gravida 1 client is referred to as a *primigravida,* meaning, literally, that this is her first pregnancy. Accompanying the gravida number is **para**, which is the number of births after 20 weeks' gestation, whether live births or stillbirths. Additionally, the term para, when expressed as a single number, does not reflect the number of infants born at a delivery but rather the number of pregnancies that have gone past 20 weeks' gestation. Thus, a client who has had only one pregnancy and gave birth to term twins would be considered a para 1 (one birth past 20 weeks' gestation), gravida 1 (reflecting her only pregnancy to date). If this same client experiences a second pregnancy, she would, at that time, be considered a para 1 (birth of her twins), gravida 2 (second pregnancy), using the para-gravida system of classification for obstetrical status.

Para also can be used in a four-digit system that gives more detailed information about past deliveries. This system refers only to past pregnancies and their outcomes; it does not reflect a current pregnancy. The four digits **(F.P.A.L.)** indicate the following in this order: the number of full-term deliveries (usually considered to be 37 to 40 weeks' gestation), the number of premature or preterm deliveries (between 20 and 36 weeks' gestation), the number of abortions (induced or spontaneous terminations of pregnancy before 20 weeks' gestation), and the number of living children born to the client who are alive at the time of data collection. This number does not include adopted children or infants born alive who later (at any age) died. As an example, a woman who has had three term pregnancies, delivered three live infants, but suffered the loss of her 6-year-old son in an accident would be considered a para 3-0-0-2.

This system of classifying deliveries may seem even more confusing than the para-gravida system; however, it provides more comprehensive information. Until this system becomes thoroughly familiar, the nurse may prefer to use a mnemonic device such as "Florida Power And Light" to remember the terms. (Students in the 60s and 70s used "Flower Power And Love".) The nurse is encouraged to remember that the first three digits are in order of time in utero, from longest to shortest. Doing so may assist in remembering the digits and their representations.

Other commonly used terms to describe the parity status of clients are **primipara**, a woman who has experienced only one birth after 20 weeks' gestation, and **multipara**, a woman who has had two or more births after 20 weeks' gestation.

Medical History and Family Medical History

Comprehensive medical histories for the client and her partner should be obtained. Information is gathered and recorded in such a manner that critical elements and risk factors pertinent to the pregnancy can be identified. Sometimes even the simplest data may give rise to early identification of risk factors or the need to monitor the pregnancy more closely. For example, age, race, ethnic background, and even address may not be viewed as crucial information, yet each can provide the health care professional with a wealth of information for monitoring. The age group identifies at-risk clients, such as teens and women of advanced age. Race and ethnic background can direct the need for monitoring for certain genetic conditions, such as the sickle cell trait or anemia or inborn errors of metabolism (see Chapter 13). Similarly, ethnic background can direct attention to potential associated problems such as Tay-Sachs disease. The client's or partner's work and residence addresses may be important factors in relation to known contaminants or pollution, ranging from allergens to toxic industrial materials responsible for disease and birth defects.

All entries in a client's records are purposeful and should be explored accordingly with the client and her partner. The medical history provides an excellent starting point for the nursing process, particularly the sharing of expert knowledge and analysis and interpretation of information. The mutuality of data exploration cannot be

Nursing Alert

IMMUNIZATIONS CONTRAINDICATED IN PREGNANCY

- Immunizations with live (attenuated) viruses should not be given during pregnancy because of potential damage to the fetus.
- Preconception care encompasses assessment of immunization status with the opportunity to update immunizations, assuming avoidance of pregnancy in the near future.

Immunizations may be given in the postpartum period with emphasis on the use of contraception (for at least 3 months) to avoid an immediate pregnancy with possible fetal harm.

overemphasized. Clients and their partners often have information readily available but are unaware of its significance to their health status without interpretation by caregivers.

Information gathered for the medical histories is the same as for any client, with a few exceptions. The elements of the medical history provide an excellent database to identify risk factors that may or may not affect the pregnancy outcomes. Additionally, the medical history flags some items to be monitored as the pregnancy progresses. The gynecologic and obstetrical histories become more important with a pregnancy because factors may require special attention not required if, for example, the client is seeking medical care for a broken ankle.

A psychosocial history can be helpful in making an assessment of readiness for parenting. This history identifies a pregnancy as an intended compared with an unintended or a wanted compared with an unwanted pregnancy and the client's attitude toward the pregnancy. Intervention and referral as indicated at this time may prevent a situation of child abuse in the future. Other areas to be assessed from this history are the client's expectations from the pregnancy and the baby, that is, whether they are realistic.

Also included in the social history of the client and her partner is the use of alcohol, tobacco, or drugs. Positive findings provide health maintenance and health promotion teaching opportunities for the prospective parents and their infant.

The Physical Examination

The initial prenatal visit includes a physical examination that, with some exceptions, follows the systematic approach seen in routine physical assessments. A complete physical examination usually is performed only at the time

Client Education

Prenatal Visits

For a client to understand her time commitment and plan ahead for prenatal visits, she should know how often her return visits will be scheduled:

- Up to 28 weeks' gestation (covers first and second trimesters), every 4 weeks.
- 29 to 36 weeks' gestation, every 2 weeks.
- 37 to 40 weeks' gestation, every week.

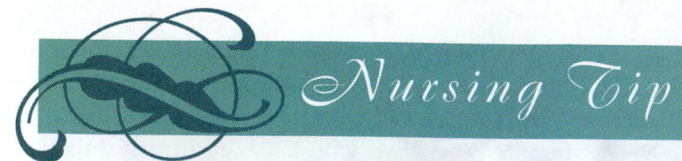

Nursing Tip

LABORATORY TESTS AT THE INITIAL VISIT

1. Blood work: complete blood count, hemoglobin, hematocrit, Rh status, and blood type. Screening for sickle cell trait, as indicated. Serology for syphilis; rubella titer, human immunodeficiency virus (HIV), and hepatitis screening, as indicated or as per department policy or client request. Glucose screening if the first visit is at 24 to 28 weeks' gestation. Alpha-fetoprotein screening if the first visit is at 16 to 18 weeks' gestation.

2. Urinalysis (with culture, if indicated): examine for glucose, protein, erythrocytes, leukocytes, and bacteria.

3. Pelvic laboratory tests: Pap smear, cultures for gonorrhea, Chlamydia, and group B *Streptococcus* if the first visit is after 24 weeks' gestation.

of the first visit. Thereafter, the elements of the repeat visits are very much abbreviated, yet specific to the progress of the pregnancy and the well-being of the mother and fetus. As the nurse explains the routine of subsequent visits, she can once again explain that future visits will be briefer.

Several physical findings in pregnancy are abnormal in nonpregnant clients. In addition, changes occur from trimester to trimester that vary from the baseline but still are normal anticipated findings. An example of the latter are the hemoglobin and hematocrit values. Assuming a normal baseline of 12 to 15 g/dL and 35% to 45%, respectively, the nurse would not be alarmed to see these values (especially hemoglobin) decrease slightly in the third trimester. As the circulating blood and fluid volume increases with the progression of the pregnancy (see Chapter 15), the appearance of a true decrease in hematocrit is given. In reality, the number of erythrocytes is essentially the same; however, the erythrocytes are suspended in a larger amount of fluid, thereby yielding a smaller percentage value. This effect is sometimes referred to as physiologic anemia of pregnancy.

Laboratory Tests

Comprehensive prenatal care indicates specific laboratory tests that need to be performed at the initial visit and periodically throughout the pregnancy. The timing of some laboratory testing is crucial for an accurate assessment. If blood is collected too early or too late in the pregnancy, the values will not be very reliable. For example, initial hemoglobin and hematocrit testing at 30 weeks' gestation certainly provides information to the nurse; however, without an early baseline for comparison, assessment of normal compared with abnormal changes is difficult. In addition, some laboratory testing is time-sensitive within a tighter timeframe. An example is the glucose testing in which the glucose level is measured from a blood sam-

ple drawn 1 hour after the client drinks a glucola preparation.

Ultrasonography

In addition to a urine or blood test for pregnancy confirmation, ultrasonography is often used, depending on the length of gestation. This technology has been refined throughout the years to a very high level of sophistication. It can be used to identify a yolk sac, a fetal heart before it is audible with Doppler ultrasonography, the sex of the fetus, and internal structures of the developing fetus. Routine use usually is limited to pregnancy confirmation; assessment of fetal development and well-being, as indicated; sex determination, if indicated or desired; and overall fetal size as term approaches.

Further use of ultrasonography is indicated in cases of unusual findings that suggest deviations from a normal prenatal course. Examples of these situations include a fundal height inconsistent with calculated dates of pregnancy (larger, often with multiple gestation or some known fetal anomalies, or smaller, which may indicate poor fetal growth), or inability to find the fetal heart beat using routine methods.

Pelvic Examination

The pelvic examination, including collection of pelvic cultures and smears and the performance of the bimanual examination usually is the last part of the initial physical examination. The pelvic laboratory specimens are collected first. Some of these (e.g., for chlamydia and gonorrhea) may be by DNA probe or culture. The bimanual examination is done to determine the uterine size and to assess for deviations in expected shape or size. Normal cervical and uterine changes expected in pregnancy (see Chapter 15) also are noted.

Assessment of the Bony Pelvis

Assessment of the bony pelvis is necessary to determine the probability of a fetus of normal size being delivered vaginally. A client who has already delivered an infant of 7 pounds or larger is said to have a "tried" pelvis, one with large enough measurements for delivery of another infant of normal size. True measurement of the pelvic structure usually is done using X-ray films; however, a reliable indirect measurement is possible with a pelvic examination by a skilled nurse or physician. Borderline or questionable measurements are cause for either further evaluation or careful monitoring for labor progression.

The pelvis consists of four bones: two os innominate (or os cocci), the sacrum, and the coccyx. The ischium, ilium, and symphysis pubis are anatomic regions of the bones and should not be confused with actual bones. The joints formed by the four bones are the symphysis pubis, two sacroiliac joints (junction of the sacrum and each os innominate), and the sacrococcygeal joint (connection of the sacrum and coccyx). The status of these joints takes on greater significance as the pregnancy progresses and these joints "soften."

The pelvis is visually divided into three planes. The first plane is the **pelvic inlet**, with the transverse segment being corresponding points on the brim of the true pelvis and the anterior-posterior points being the back side of the symphysis pubis and the sacral promontory. This anterior-posterior diameter of the pelvic inlet is the smallest diameter. This is called the **obstetrical conjugate**; it is measured indirectly by the diagonal conjugate (Figure 16-3). The examiner inserts the middle and index fingers of the examining hand and touches the tip of the middle finger to the sacral promontory. At this point, notation is made of where the examining hand touches the symphysis pubis. The measurement of this distance on the examiner's hand can be done with an obstetrical caliper (Figure 16-4).

From this diagonal conjugate, the obstetrical conjugate (smallest diameter) can be estimated fairly accurately by subtracting 1.5 or 2 cm. The resulting measure should be at least 10.5 cm, assuming normal thickness and tilt of the symphysis pubis. A smaller measurement requires further evaluation.

The second pelvis plane is known as the **midpelvis**. The smallest diameter of the midpelvis or midplane is the transverse or **interspinous diameter** (between the two ischial spines). The ischial spines are evaluated by palpation for their prominence or flatness (Figure 16-5).

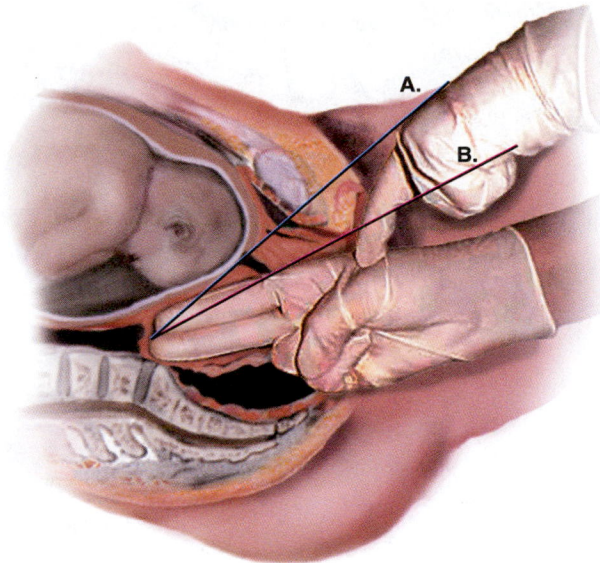

Figure 16-3 Diameters of the pelvic inlet and outlet.

Prominent converging spines can compromise this diameter or, in the least, cause a "tight fit" for the fetal head, with possible tissue damage to the mother during delivery. The sacral curvature (or flatness) is evaluated. A curved sacrum allows more room in the midpelvis than does a flat sacrum, thus becoming somewhat of a compensatory mechanism for a marginal interspinous measurement.

The third plane, the **pelvic outlet**, is the plane of greatest compensation. The smallest measurement is the distance between the two ischial tuberosities; this measurement usually is called the intertuberous or **biischial diameter**. The size is estimated by the knuckles of the examiner's fist being placed across the perineum at the level

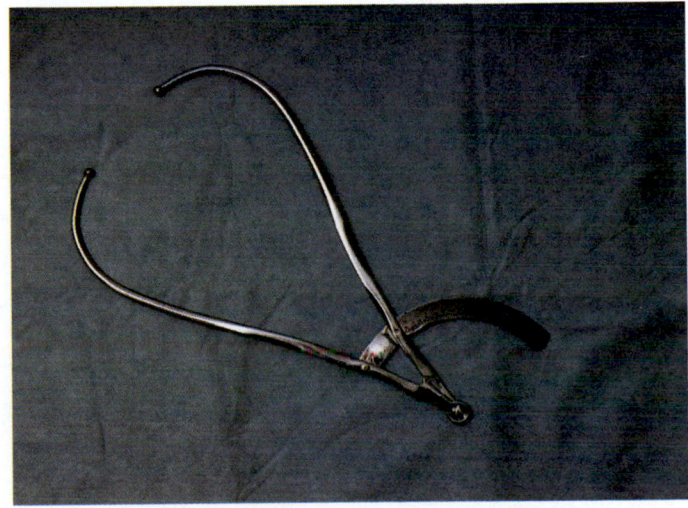

Figure 16-4 Obstetrical caliper.

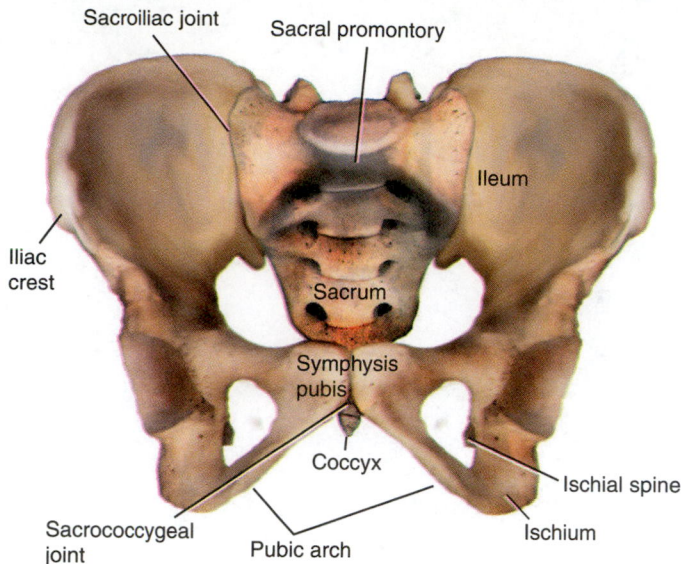

Figure 16-5 Anterior view of the female pelvis.

of the tuberosities (Figure 16-6). Assuming a fist size of at least 8 cm, the knuckles usually do not touch both tuberosities simultaneously, indicating a diameter of 8 cm or greater. The anterior-posterior measurement is from the bottom of the symphysis pubis to the tip of the sacrum, at the sacrococcygeal joint, which usually is about 10 to 11.5 cm. The coccyx is evaluated for mobility by examination finger touch. A mobile nonprominent coccyx allows for some flexibility in the pelvic outlet plane. The angle of the subpubic arch is evaluated as part of the pelvic outlet. In the normal female pelvis, this angle is about 90 degrees

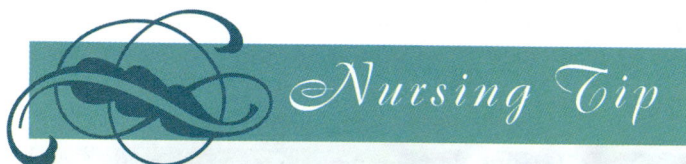

Nursing Tip

TEACHING PARTNERS HOW TO HELP PREVENT CLIENT ACCIDENTS AND FALLS

If the client's partner is made aware of pregnancy changes such as a shift in her center of balance and the softening of pelvic joints that result in "wobbly" ambulation, he can identify opportunities to be of assistance to her, particularly in avoiding falls or near-falls that easily can happen. He can do stooping and lifting for her, assist her with ambulation, particularly over irregular surfaces, help her in and out of the car, and assist her with stair steps. His attention to accident prevention is likely to be enhanced if he has an understanding of the physiologic changes that produce the risks.

and allows room for the upward extension of the fetal head at delivery (see Chapter 23).

Subsequent Visits

A schedule of future visits is given to each client. This time is an excellent opportunity to explain what is done at each visit, to give printed instructions and educational materials,

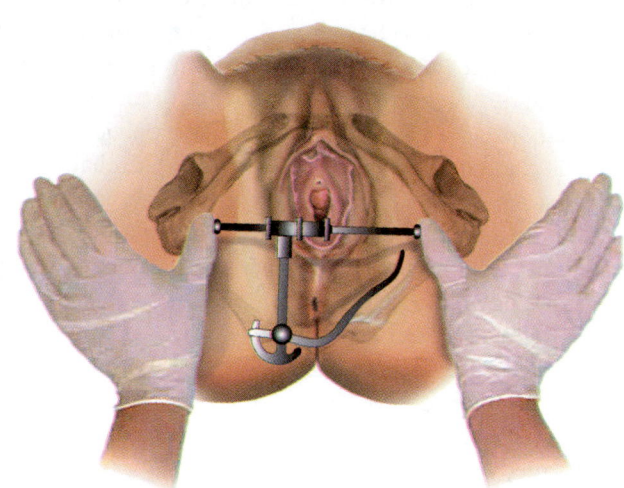

A.

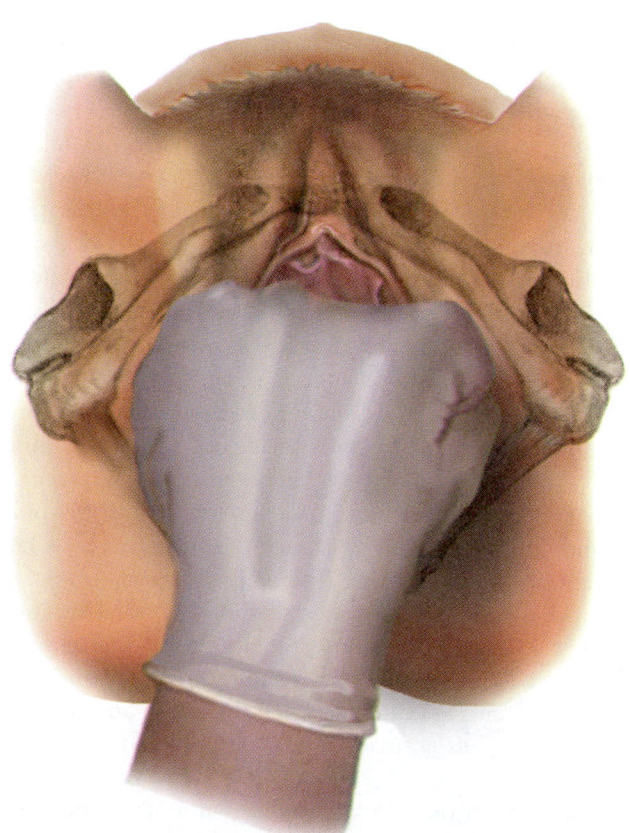

B.

Figure 16-6 Measurement of the biischial diameter with (A) ruler or (B) clenched fist.

and to anticipate client concerns during the intervening time before her next appointment. The client should be given thorough instructions regarding nutrition and fluid intake (at least eight glasses of water a day plus other fluids), the normal changes of pregnancy, recommendations regarding exercise and general hygiene, and recommended treatment of various discomforts she may encounter as the pregnancy progresses. This is also an appropriate time to give the client printed materials about designated danger signs for which she should seek immediate assistance (Figure 16-7). Although these signs usually are not seen until the last trimester, it is still not too early to give clients these materials.

Subsequent Visits

To assist in proper monitoring of the pregnancy, the following are evaluated in each visit.

- Blood pressure. Blood pressure is evaluated for any increase from baseline (Figure 16-8). An increase may be an alert to the onset of **pregnancy-induced hypertension (PIH)**, also referred to as preeclampsia or toxemia of pregnancy. Typically, PIH is characterized by elevated blood pressure, persistent edema, and proteinuria. Guidelines for signs and symptoms that should be reported to the nurse or physician are included in the danger signs listed below.

- Weight. Weight is assessed for appropriate weight gain (Figure 16-9). Too little or too much gain requires further assessment and counseling. Either may be indicative of a high-risk pregnancy.

- Fundal height. Fundal height should be consistent with dates. The uterus is palpable above the symphysis at about 12 weeks' gestation; is midway

Nursing Alert

ATTENTION TO BASELINE BLOOD PRESSURE

At each prenatal visit the blood pressure finding should be compared with the baseline value. A client may have a blood pressure reading that seems to be within normal limits but is actually a significant increase for her. This is especially true for very young clients whose normal blood pressure values are around 90–92/58–60 mm Hg. In these cases, a seemingly normal blood pressure value of of 120/82 mm Hg may be a caution flag for the need to monitor for further signs of PIH.

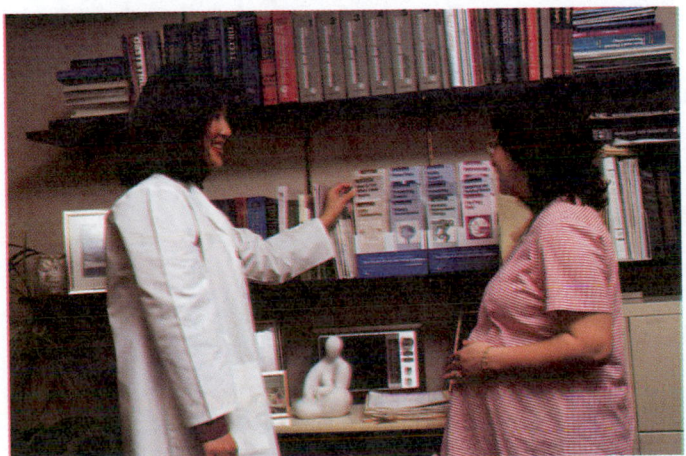

Figure 16-7 Supplying clients with information on a healthy pregnancy and potential risks and danger signs is an important nursing responsibility.

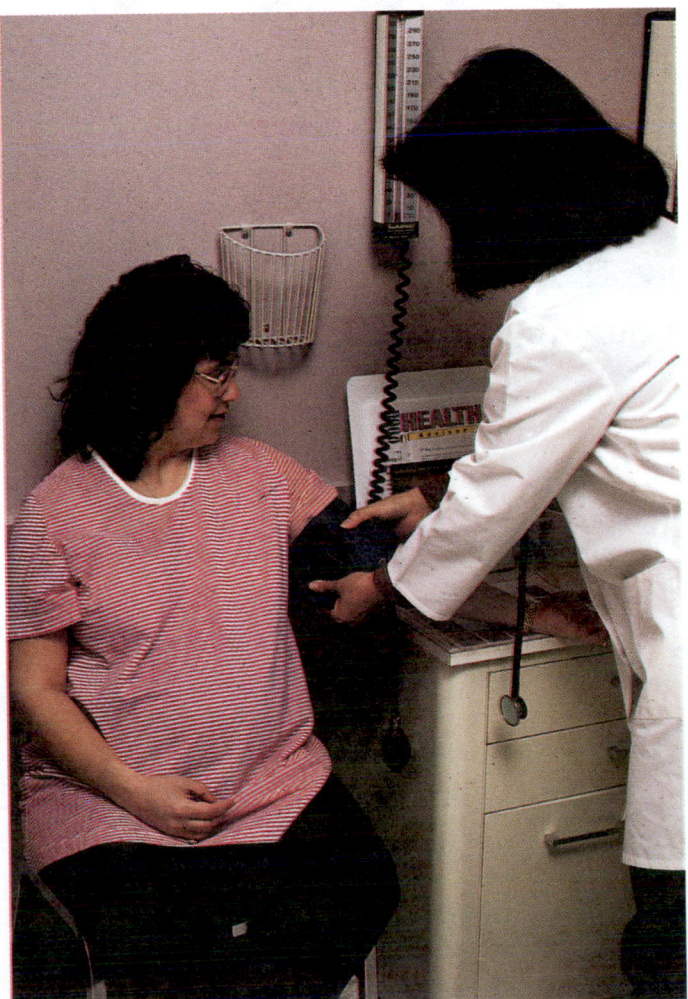

Figure 16-8 Blood pressure is measured at each prenatal visit.

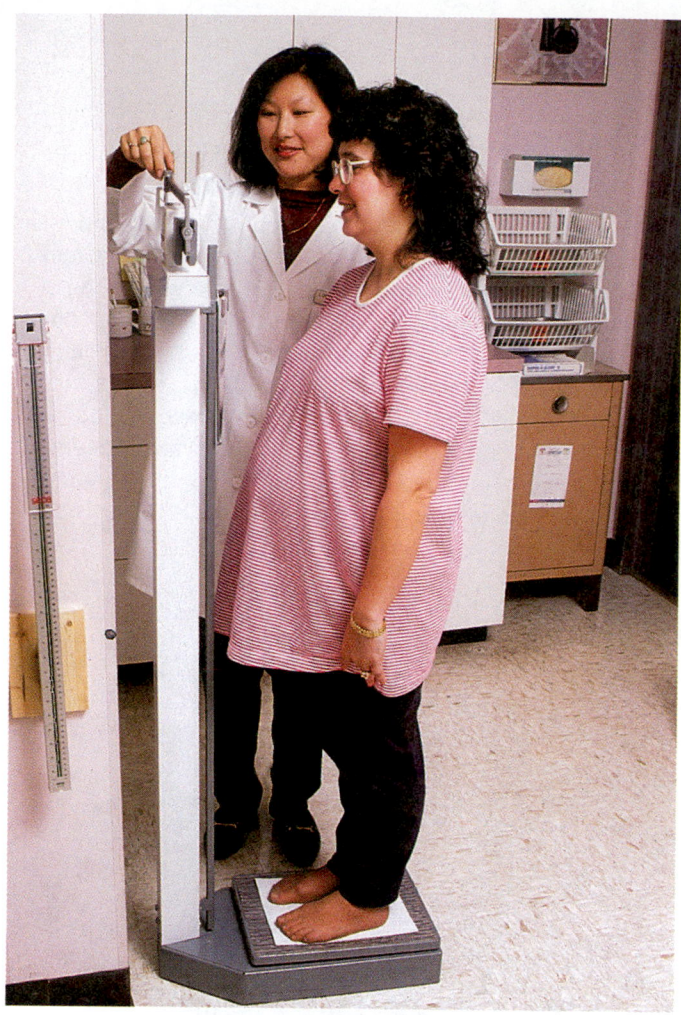

Figure 16-9 Weight gain is tracked throughout the pregnancy.

Client Education

Weight Gain

Clients should be instructed in the importance of and necessity for a recommended weight gain of about 25 to 35 lb in a pattern similar to the following:

● First trimester: approximately 3 to 5 lb.

● Second trimester: approximately 12 to 15 lb.

● Third trimester: approximately 12 to 15 lb.

Remind clients that pregnancy is not a time for weight loss.

between the symphysis pubis and umbilicus at 16 weeks' gestation; and at the umbilicus at 20 weeks' gestation (now measuring 20 cm). Overall fundal height changes generally are reflective of fetal growth. Small uterine size for dates may indicate a fetus that is not growing appropriately; large uterine size for dates may be associated with a multiple pregnancy (more than one fetus), congenital anomaly, or another complication to be assessed. Measurement is by flexible tape measure (McDonald's method; Figure 16-10A,B) held by the examiner at either a curved pattern from the symphysis pubis to the fundus (top of the uterus), or a straight pattern from the symphysis pubis to the point where the examiner's hand is directly above the fundus at a 90-degree angle. Either method is acceptable but should not be interchanged because slightly different readings are obtained. Fundal height in centimeters correlates very closely with the number of weeks of pregnancy

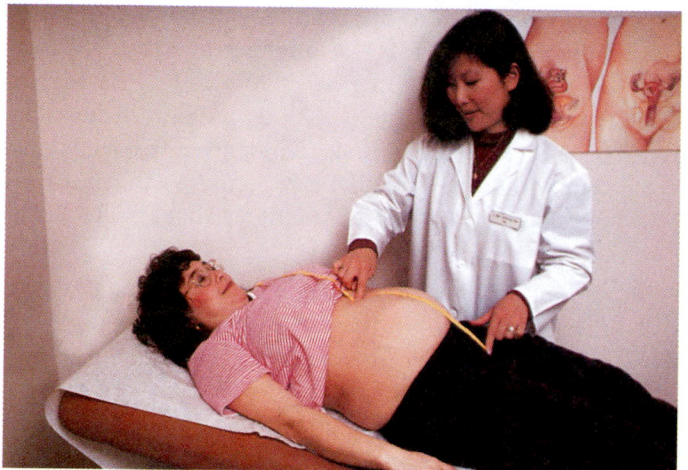

A.

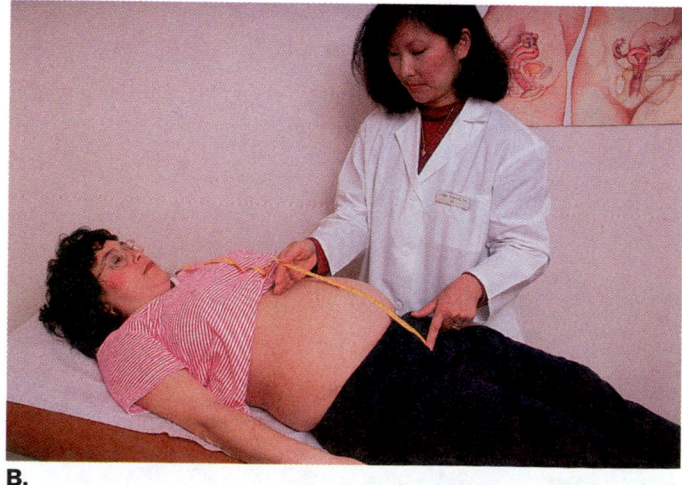

B.

Figure 16-10 Fundal height is measured by placing the end of the tape measure at the symphysis pubis and extending it in either a curved (A) or straight (B) pattern to the fundus.

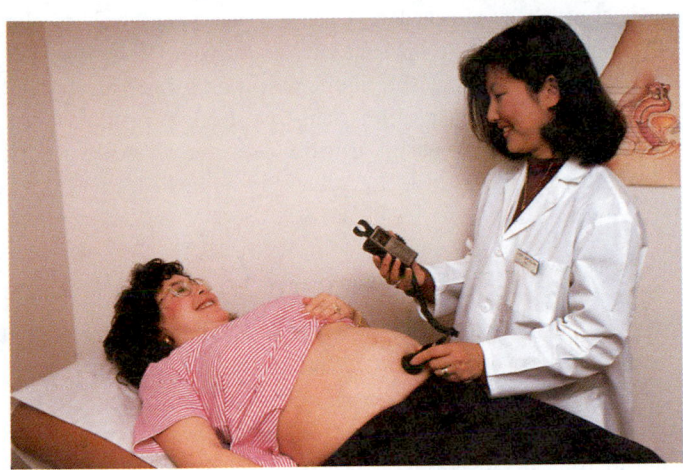

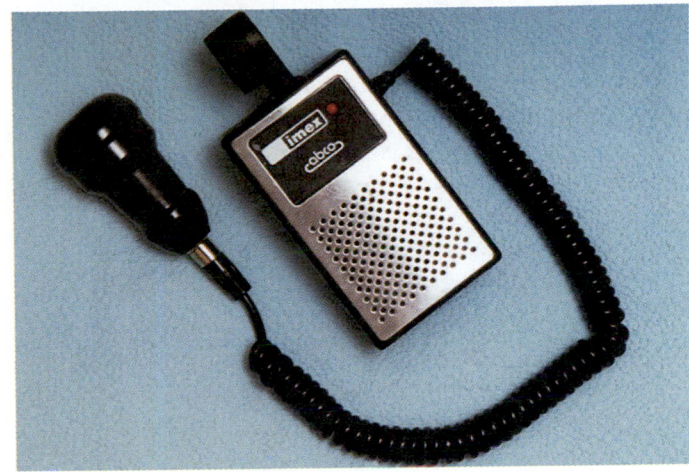

Figure 16-11 Fetal heart tones are measured with a hand-held Doppler.

after 18 weeks' gestation. Discrepancies call for further evaluation.

- Fetal heart tones. Fetal heart tones are assessed for rate and rhythm (Figure 16-11). Normal rate is 120 to 160 beats per minute.

- Urine. Urine is tested for the presence of glucose or protein (albumin) (Figure 16-12). Clients should be instructed in obtaining a clean-catch urine specimen to avoid a positive protein caused by mucoid vaginal secretions in the specimen. Proteinuria may be in-

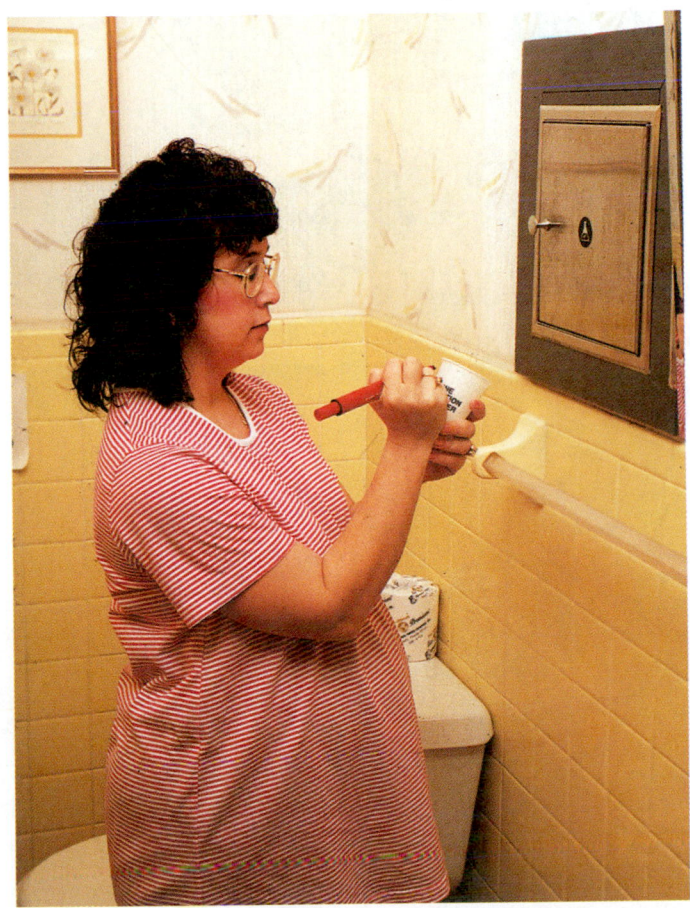

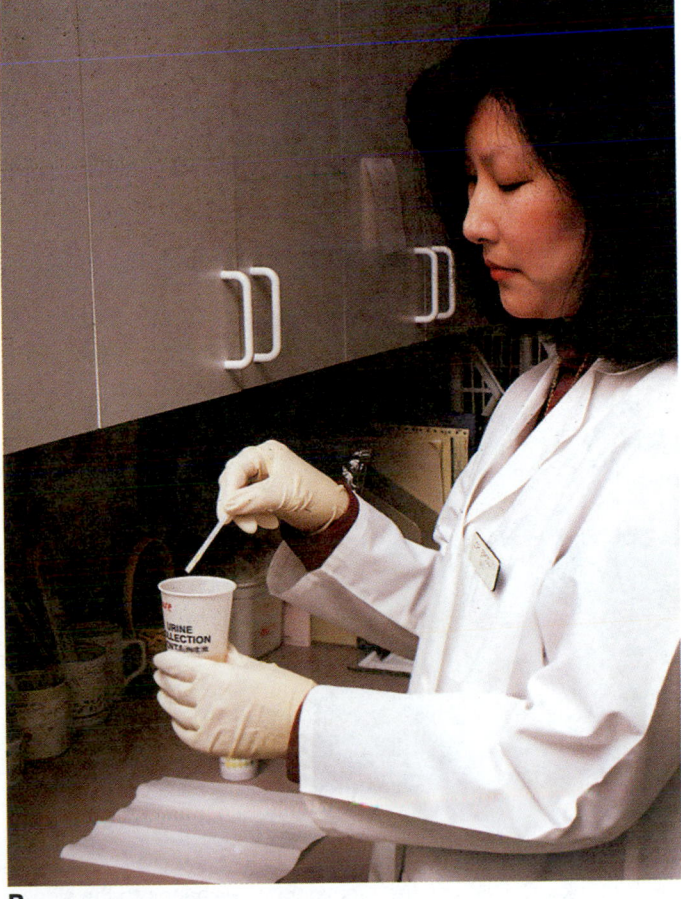

A.   B.

Figure 16-12 Urine is tested at each visit for glucose and protein. A. Client provides a clean catch urine sample. B. Nurse uses urine dipstick to measure glucose and protein.

dicative of PIH, especially if seen in the presence of elevated blood pressure and edema. Glucose in the urine may reflect the relatively normal change in glomerular filtration that allows the larger glucose molecule to be excreted. Further evaluation is still needed. Glucose screening usually is done between 24 and 28 weeks' gestation. If blood glucose is elevated, a glucose tolerance test usually is scheduled.

🔊 Edema. Edema is evaluated at each visit. Dependent edema of the feet and legs is not unusual toward the end of pregnancy. A ring sizer can be used to screen for edema in the fingers. Edema of the face is more ominous; when this is noted, the client should be evaluated for other signs and symptoms of PIH. All edema should be assessed for pitting.

🔊 Other. Each visit should include an opportunity for the client to ask questions and share concerns. Time should be allotted to explore her adaptation to the pregnancy as well that of her partner. It should not be assumed that the client who has a history of alcohol, tobacco, or other drug use before pregnancy is not using that drug during pregnancy. Assessment and referral should be provided as indicated.

Selected Subsequent Visits

As previously noted, the first prenatal visit usually is the most detailed. Monitoring activities continue throughout the pregnancy, with some less frequent than others. In the absence of abnormal findings or the identification of risk factors that necessitate closer scrutiny, other evaluations are done only at selected visits or at particular times during the pregnancy. Some examples of periodic evaluations are as follows:

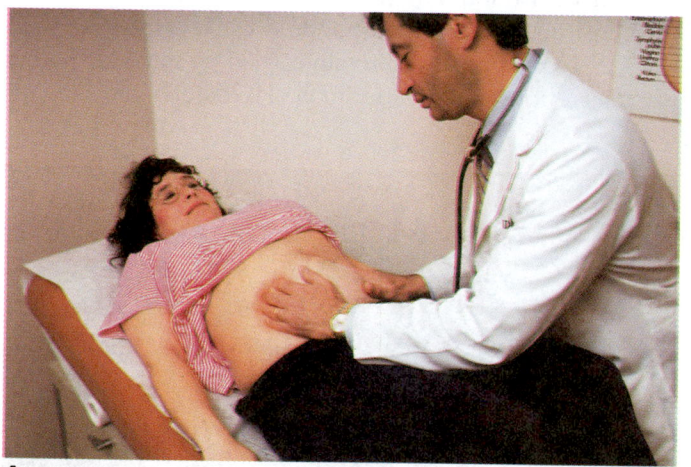

A.

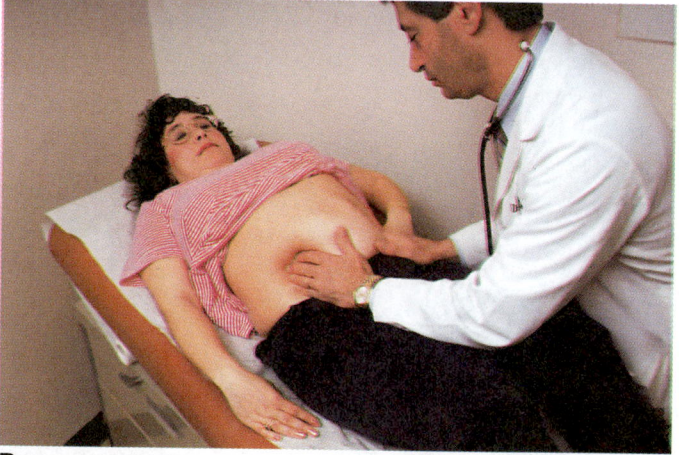

B.

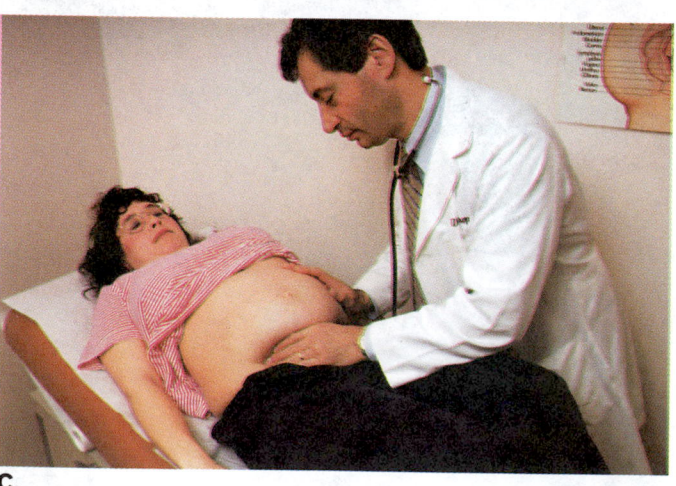

C.

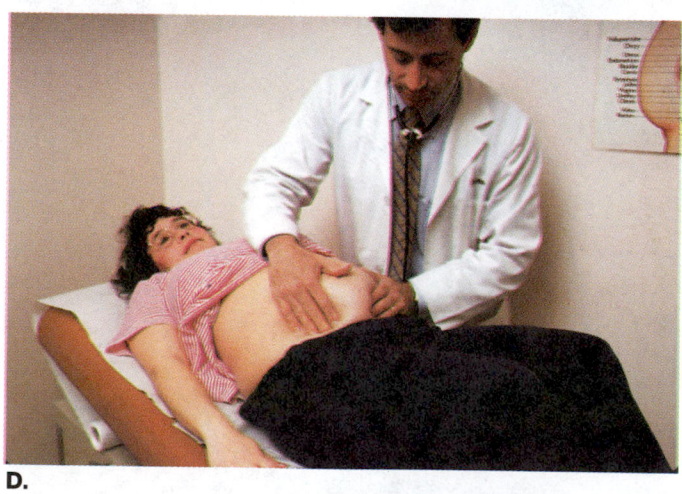

D.

Figure 16-13 Leopold's maneuvers. A. First, the examiner palpates to determine which fetal part is in the fundus. Generally, it is the buttocks. B. Second, the examiner moves hands to the sides of the uterus and determines on which side of the mother the fetal back is located. C. Third, the examiner's hand is placed above the symphysis pubis to note whether the head or breech is near the pubic symphysis (this should correlate with the first maneuver). D. Fourth, the examiner changes position to face the client's feet, and palpates the sides of the abdomen to determine on which side the cephalic prominence presents.

🌸 Additional pelvic examinations usually are not necessary until the time of weekly visits, which usually occurs in the last 3 to 4 weeks of an uncomplicated pregnancy. The cervix can be evaluated for softening, thinning, and dilation. An assessment can be made of the fetal presenting part and status of descent after lightening (see Chapter 15). Prior to this time, Leopold's maneuvers can be used to evaluate the size and position of the fetus (Figure 16-13).

🌸 Laboratory tests. In the absence of anemia at the initial screening or development of signs and symptoms subsequently, hemoglobin and hematocrit screenings usually are not repeated until 28 to 34 weeks' gestation (third trimester) and again immediately before delivery. Alpha-fetoprotein screening is done at 16 to 18 weeks' gestation, glucose screening at 24 to 28 weeks' gestation, and culture for group B *Streptococcus* (GBS) at 35 to 37 weeks' gestation. Antibody titer for clients who are Rh negative is done at 22 weeks' gestation and as indicated. Triple screening (maternal serum alpha-fetoprotein, hCG, and estriol) sometimes is done at 16 to 18 weeks' gestation or 16 to 20 weeks' gestation as a combined evaluation of fetal well-being and for predictors of genetic or congenital anomalies (see Chapters 13 and 22). In some areas of the United States, triple screenings are used routinely; in other areas, they are used more on an as indicated basis (Table 16-1).

Table 16-1 Screening Tests in Pregnancy

Test	Results
Complete Blood Count RBC WBC	3.75 million/mm^3 due to hemodilution. Rises to 18,000/mm^3 by late pregnancy. Mostly an increase in neutrophils.
Hemoglobin (Hgb)	May decrease to 11.5g/dL later in pregnancy due to hemodilution. Repeat at 28 and 36 weeks.
Hematocrit (Hct)	33% lowest acceptable, due to hemodilution.
Blood Type	A, B, AB, or O
Rh factor	Positive or negative. If negative, do indirect Coomb's test. Check father's Rh.
Coomb's Test	Should remain negative. Retest Rh negative woman at 28 weeks.
Rubella Titer (HAI)	> 1 : 10 indicates immunity. < 1 : 10, immunize after birth of infant.
Blood Glucose	Should be 60–110 mg/dL. Retest at 24 and 32 weeks.
VDRL or RPR (Syphilis)	Should be negative.
Cervical/Vaginal Culture Gonorrhea Chlamydia Group B *Streptococcus*	Should be negative.
Hepatitis B Surface Antigen (HB$_s$Ag)	Positive indicates either active hepatitis or carrier state.
Antibody Titer HB$_s$Ag	Positive indicates immunity to hepatitis.
HIV (many states mandate that it be offered)	Should be negative.
Tuberculosis Skin tests: Mantoux or Tine	Should be negative. If positive, do chest x-ray.
Urinalysis Color, specific Gravity, pH, ketones, albumin, glucose	Same as nonpregnant. Repeat at 28 weeks. Trace of glycosuria may occur in pregnancy.
Alpha-fetoprotein (AFP)	Check with laboratory for normal range for each week of gestation. If elevated, may have neural tube defects. If decreased, may have Down syndrome.

Research Highlight

Collection of Specimens for Group B Streptococcus *Screening*

Purpose

To determine how well patients did in collecting group B *Streptococcus* (GBS) samples compared with physician collection and to determine patient preference for self-collection compared with physician-collected swabs.

Methods

Women receiving prenatal care from five family physicians and eight obstetricians in Toronto, Canada, constituted the sample. All 163 women were seen during a regular visit at 26 to 28 weeks' gestation. Each woman was given a questionnaire (survey) and instructions and directions for collecting her own vaginal-anorectal swab for GBS screening. After the woman completed the survey and obtained her own swab for culture, the physician then collected the GBS specimen in the usual manner.

Findings

Of the 163 matched pairs of GBS swabs, the researchers used any positive results as the gold standard and found the prevalence to be 24% (39 of 163). Patients detected 38 cases, whereas physicians detected a smaller number of 32. The sensitivities of these detections were 97% and 82%, respectively. The 161 surveys returned showed that 25% of the women preferred that their physician take the swab, and 75% were indifferent or preferred self-collection of the specimen.

Nursing Implications

Clients can be taught GBS collection that is at least as reliable as physician-collected swabs. Self-swabbing is an excellent opportunity for women to actively participate in their own care with confidence.

Molnar, P., Biringer, A., McGeer, A., & McIsaac, W. (1997). Can pregnant women obtain their own specimens for group B *Streptococcus*? A comparison of maternal versus physician screening. *Family Practice, 14,* (5), 403–406.

DISCOMFORTS OF PREGNANCY

The normal progression of a pregnancy to produce a healthy infant requires, by necessity, a variety of physiologic changes within the mother. Several of these changes have a cascading effect and subsequently produce conditions of discomfort. Whereas some clients view these as annoyances to be dealt with, others perceive them to be interferences that are sometimes intolerable. In most cases, a detailed explanation of what is happening and suggestions for alleviation are sufficient, especially when clients have a social support system in place. For the other category of clients, further exploration of their feeling about and attitude toward the pregnancy is warranted.

Recommendations to clients should be made with sensitivity to the client's cultural background. The nurse should listen when clients want to discuss home remedies or alternative interventions for various problems. A sensible approach calls for ruling out known harmful practices (with careful explanations) and exploring all options that are within the realm of the client's social, cultural, or spiritual preferences and background. When clients are taught to blend cultural mores and self-care practices with specific basics of routine prenatal considerations (e.g., avoidance of alcohol, caffeine, and certain medications), they will be empowered to make wise choices for themselves. Furthermore, clients can share their new knowledge with others in their community. In doing so they foster the idea that clients can be proactive in their care, using health care professionals for joint decision-making and establishing mutual goals.

The following are some commonly encountered discomforts, their causes, and some recommended interventions. Nurses are encouraged to review resources (such as the Internet) that are available and to assess information for accuracy and advisability, especially before referring clients to a particular website. All information should be consistent with normal, routine, and mainstream prenatal care protocols.

Urinary Frequency

The physical sensation of needing to void frequently, and sometimes accompanied by a feeling of urgency, is encountered primarily in the first and last trimester. The gravid, growing uterus presses on the bladder, and the fetus puts direct pressure on the bladder. In addition to these mechanical factors, the pregnant client also experiences an increase in circulating fluid volume, especially in the third trimester, and frequently an increased glomerular filtration rate, which further adds to frequency. The good news for clients is that they will experience some relief from this problem during the second trimester when the uterus is higher in the abdomen and the combined weight of the fetus and uterus is not as great as it is in late pregnancy. Clients should be cautioned not to decrease their fluid intake in an attempt to control urinary frequency. Doing so is appropriate only for short periods of time, such as a car trip for an hour or so, or in anticipation of a meeting of a similar time frame. Fluid intake for any 24-hour period should not be less than the recommended amount, or 8 glasses of water plus other fluids.

Nausea and Vomiting

Nausea and vomiting are problems usually associated with the first trimester. Although sometimes referred to as morning sickness, the nausea and vomiting may occur at any time of the day. A variety of stimuli, such as certain smells and, the sight of some foods, can produce the sensations. Nausea seems to be more of a problem than does vomiting. Many clients experience nausea, with minimal vomiting. The hormones of pregnancy are the generally acknowledged basis for morning sickness. General guidelines for prevention call for eating dry toast or crackers without liquids before getting out of bed. Avoidance of known offenders, such as spicy foods and acidic citrus fruit on an empty stomach, is recommended. Other measures may include favorite decaffeinated teas. Peppermint tea is preferred by many clients because it tends to calm a queasy stomach.

Indigestion

Indigestion is a common annoyance that shares some common causes with nausea. Also, the hormones progesterone and relaxin are implicated because they relax the cardiac sphincter and allow reflux to occur. Many clients have identified specific offending foods and beverages that caused them problems, even before pregnancy. Obviously, these foods should be avoided as much as possible. If reflux is a problem at bedtime, the use of an extra pillow may be helpful in overcoming the gravity factor that can enhance reflux. Caution clients about the use of antacids, especially those with a high sodium content. Mild herbal teas of the client's preference should be encouraged.

Constipation and Hemorrhoids

Constipation and hemorrhoids are closely related and often contribute to each other. Constipation and subsequent straining with defecation contribute to the formation of hemorrhoids. As with edema, the sluggish circulation and venous return combined with the direct pressure of the uterus and fetus all make avoidance of hemorrhoids a challenge. Gentle evacuation is encouraged by ample fluid intake, a diet high in fiber, use of certain stool softeners, and walking (preferably at a brisk rate, if tolerated). High-fiber foods that also are good sources of iron include prunes and apricots.

Edema of Lower Extremities

Swelling of the feet and lower legs is most commonly seen later in pregnancy, with several factors coming together to cause it. The increased circulating fluid volume, relaxed blood vessels, sluggish venous return, and mechanical obstructive nature of the heavy uterus and fetus on vessels of the lower extremities all contribute to the problem. Avoidance of long periods of standing without walking around helps to prevent edema. Clients should be advised to have their feet and legs elevated as much as possible while sitting. Clients also should be cautioned to avoid sitting with the hips at a sharp angle when the feet are elevated because doing so will further impede venous return and aggravate the original problem. Moderate walking is of great help in controlling edema (contracting muscles facilitate venous return) and preventing constipation (walking increases peristalsis). Walking is also an excellent exercise for pregnant women, especially when done at a sensible pace, avoiding fatigue and extreme weather conditions. For clients fortunate enough to live near a seashore, wading in the surf is very therapeutic. Not only does this improve venous return from lower extremities but it does so at pressures that are ideal; that is, the pressure of the water is greatest at the bottom (feet) and decreases toward the surface (farther up the legs). Also, the psychological benefits of reflective thinking and clearing the mind contribute to the client's overall well-being.

Danger Signs to be Reported

With the availability of so much educational materials from a variety of sources, many clients are very knowledgeable about pregnancy and the various changes that occur. Even though information sources caution clients about the need for medical care and supervision, it remains the responsibility of the nurse to provide certain information without the assumption that clients have access to it elsewhere.

There are a number of possible events in pregnancy that reflect one or more complications, at best, these require assessment to rule out a problem. Whereas it may sound overreactive to refer to these as danger signs, and the policy of a clinic or facility may be to avoid use of the term danger for fear of alarming clients, it is imperative that clients be made aware of events that require immediate reporting to their health care provider. The nurse must reinforce the importance of reporting any of these things immediately, rather than making a note to report them at the next scheduled visit. A detailed explanation of the physiology and implications is not necessary for the client unless she requests it; however, she should know that immediate assessment is for the good of her health and her baby's health. Signs and symptoms that require immediate attention are the following:

- Any vaginal bleeding. The only exception to this is if a vaginal examination has been done within the past 24 hours and the examiner has told the client to expect some slight spotting of old blood. This phrase should be carefully explained, complete with a pencil drawing of how much spotting is acceptable. Some practitioners and physicians do not even mention the exception; they want to be notified of any spotting so they can assess it at that time.

- Swelling of the face and fingers. As a general rule, the higher the edema above the feet and ankles, especially in the face, coupled with suddenness of onset, the more ominous. This finding is usually associated with PIH.

- Severe headache that is continuous. Headache may be caused by a dangerously elevated blood pressure and associated with the onset of PIH. Other causes are possible.

- Vision changes, such as blurring or dimming of vision, or spots or flashes of light before the eyes. These changes also may be associated with PIH.

- Abdominal pain. There is no need to differentiate the epigastric pain of PIH from the onset of labor for the client; both require evaluation.

- Chills and fever. Instruct the client to report these and not to wait for other "flu" symptoms to appear.

- Persistent vomiting. Even though client may have read "somewhere" that nausea and vomiting are common in pregnancy, she should not dismiss persistent vomiting as normal.

- Sudden gush of fluid from the vagina. This usually signals spontaneous rupture of membranes and requires assessment for possible cord prolapse, prevention of infection, and evaluation for the onset of labor.

In instances in which the client, after receiving these instructions, reports events or symptoms that are subsequently evaluated as nonemergencies or not indicative of a

REFLECTIONS FROM FAMILIES

"During my last pregnancy the nurse gave me a list of things called 'Topics to Report Right Away.' One of the things listed was 'Rupture of membranes or escape of fluid from the vagina.' My neighbor, Rhonda, and I were out shopping. I was in my last month, with delivery about 3 weeks away. Just as we went back to the car and I reached to open the door, it happened. Fluid ran down my leg to about my knees. It wasn't a lot, but it was there. I just wanted to go home and clean myself up. Rhonda asked me if this wasn't one of the things I was supposed to report right away to my doctor. I called the office from her car phone. The nurse told me to come straight to the doctor's office, which was about 2 miles from the mall. So we went. They checked me out right away and tested the fluid. It turned out to be urine! Can you imagine? I was so embarrassed. I told the nurse I'd never be back for that again. She told me that this happens a lot, and that I shouldn't be embarrassed. She said I did the right thing. I felt better. And Rhonda didn't laugh at me. Thank goodness she didn't call my husband to meet us at the hospital!"

Case Study/Care Plan

Susan M. is a 30-year-old gravida 3, para 1, who is 20 weeks pregnant with a 5-year-old daughter at home. She experienced an early spontaneous abortion before her daughter was born. Her F.P.A.L. status is 1-0-1-1. She works full-time in a large downtown investment firm.

Susan and her husband bought a house in an adjacent rural area. They discussed the length of the daily commute for each of them, but decided it was worth it to live in their dream house.

This pregnancy was planned and has thus far progressed uneventfully. During her last prenatal visit she expressed a strong desire to avoid constipation with this pregnancy and to prevent hemorrhoids. She has been told by some co-workers that the more constipation she had, the more certain she was to develop hemorrhoids. Constipation had been a problem for her with the last pregnancy. Her nutritional status is good. She is taking a daily prenatal vitamin with iron, primarily because of her irregular eating habits at lunch. Weight is normal for height. Weight gain has been minimal. Immunizations are complete and current. She has no difficulty getting time off from work for prenatal appointments.

Assessment

Healthy 30-year-old with a 20-week intrauterine pregnancy. She has had no difficulties with this pregnancy. She is concerned about the health of herself and her family. She has strong family support from her husband and extended family. She works at a desk job 40 hours a week.

Nursing Diagnosis

Health-seeking behaviors: self-care of pregnancy related to the desire to prevent constipation and development of hemorrhoids, as evidenced by her expressed wish to avoid a previous experience with constipation.

Expected Outcome   After nursing interventions Susan will:

- Recall examples of foods and fluids recommended for their properties of constipation prevention.
- Report a pattern of regular bowel movements that do not require straining.
- Remain free of the signs and symptoms of hemorrhoids for the remainder of the pregnancy.

Planning   Because Susan has had a previous experience with constipation in pregnancy, it is important to explore with her those approaches that worked in resolving the problem. These approaches should be incorporated with any new recommendations. With her previous pregnancy, Susan did not understand the role of walking in preventing constipation; this intervention should be explored with this pregnancy.

Nursing Interventions	Rationales
1. Review with Susan the major areas involved in prevention and resolution of constipation: diet, exercise, and fluid consumption.	1. An accurate knowledge base is essential for clients to make informed decisions in caring for themselves.
2. Discuss things Susan did to alleviate constipation with her last pregnancy.	2. Healthy self-care practices should be encouraged; others should be modified as indicated. Clients can be empowered in self-care with sensitive guidance and instructions.
3. Encourage fluid intake of eight glasses of water daily, above other fluid intake.	3. Water is essential to prevent dry, hard stools. Fluids containing sugars and caffeine usually are excreted by the kidney without contributing to fluid content of the lower intestine.

(continued)

Nursing Interventions	Rationales
4. Review and encourage intake of high-fiber foods (see Chapter 8). Focus on Susan's favorite foods as well as those she found helpful in her last pregnancy.	4. High-fiber foods, when combined with adequate fluid intake, form sufficient bulk in the stool to stimulate peristalsis. High-fiber dry foods, such as cereals, in the absence of adequate fluid intake can cause or contribute to constipation.
5. Encourage walking as a daily exercise.	5. Walking helps to stimulate peristalsis and to stimulate the general circulation. Hemorrhoids are prevented by avoidance of constipation and prevention of sluggish pelvic circulation.
6. Explore Susan's perception of iron supplement relative to constipation in the past pregnancy.	6. Whereas iron tends to contribute to constipation in some clients, it may be responsible for loose stools or diarrhea in others.
7. Review the list of stool softeners recommended for use as needed by Susan's physician and nurse practitioner.	7. Some laxatives and oil-based stimulants can interfere with nutrient absorption and may cause harsh evacuations. The potential for dependence also exists.

Evaluation   Susan was able to verbalize the role of fluids, diet, and exercise in preventing constipation and hemorrhoids. She had tried the recommended dried prunes with her last pregnancy but found that they worked better for her if she cooked them instead. Walking, particularly during her lunch hour was convenient. She and her friend opted for daily walks around the perimeter of an enclosed ice skating rink located in a building adjacent to her office; this is a safe area where they can walk during any weather conditions. Susan reports having regular soft bowel movements with no straining. No signs of hemorrhoids.

complication, the nurse must be very tactful with and sensitive to the client. The nurse must not allow the client, or the client's family, to feel as though she has acted inappropriately. She should not be intimidated by thoughts of future false alarms.

NURSING PROCESS

Care of the pregnant woman is unique in that nursing care must be planned for two individuals, the mother and the fetus, with consideration for the family. The dynamic relationship between the mother and fetus must be the basis for all planning and interventions.

Assessment

Assessment is designed for early detection to facilitate prevention of complications. Assessment is done on the initial visit and includes a thorough maternal history and physical examination. This examination incorporates an assessment of the condition of the fetus and the maternal progress of the pregnancy. During this assessment, the nurse should pay attention to the family's preparation for pregnancy, labor, and parenting. Actual and potential risk factors are identified. The objective of planning nursing care for the maternal-infant dyad is to minimize morbidity and facilitate the most positive birth experience for the mother and family.

Nursing Diagnoses

Nursing diagnoses common to women receiving prenatal care are likely to include the following:

- Knowledge deficit related to inexperience with the physiologic changes of pregnancy.
- Alterations in comfort related to the physiologic changes in pregnancy.
- Alterations in nutritional status (greater than ideal body weight) of excessive caloric intake.
- Knowledge deficit related to the importance of prenatal care.

Outcome Identification

Outcomes planned for women experiencing an uncomplicated pregnancy may include the following:

- The client is able to remain free from the common discomforts of pregnancy.
- The client incorporates strategies to increase her comfort as the pregnancy progresses.
- Weight gain does not exceed 1 lb/wk in the first 36 weeks of pregnancy and 0.5 lb/wk the last month.
- The client comes regularly to her prenatal visits.

Planning

Planning should focus on the physical and emotional needs of the woman in relation to the changes she will experience in each trimester. The client's partner, family, or support system should be included in the planning, as desired by the client.

Nursing Intervention

The client should be taught strategies to deal with the common discomforts of pregnancy, because many of these can be prevented or minimized by lifestyle modifications. Many times it is difficult for a client to discriminate between a benign cause of discomfort and a serious complication; if discomfort does occur, the client should not hesitate to call the health care provider.

The client should also be taught expected weight gain parameters and common dietary pitfalls. The more weight a woman gains above 35 to 40 lb, the greater the risk of maternal-fetal morbidity, as well as health risks related to obesity for the mother after delivery.

The nurse should also be sure to teach the client the importance of early detection and treatment of abnormalities as well as the health-promoting benefits to herself and her baby. During the course of prenatal care, the mother will obtain information about lifestyle choices that ensure better health for her and her infant. Regular prenatal care allows for early detection and intervention for many pregnancy complications.

Evaluation

Each expected outcome must be evaluated with each client-nurse interaction to determine if the current goals have been accomplished or need to be modified.

Critical Thinking

Refer to the Case Study

Assessment: Do you think that her job (sitting at a desk, with very little walking) may contribute to Susan's possibly experiencing constipation?

Nursing Diagnosis: What are some other possible nursing diagnoses pertaining to health-seeking behaviors in women who are eager to be in control of their care?

Expected Outcomes: Is there a single outcome listed that is more important than the others? Or, are they all equally important in meeting the goal?

Planning: Which approaches might you take to be sure the planning phase is actually joint decision-making?

Interventions and Rationales: Examine these to see if you can identify any that may be unacceptable to a client who wants to be in control of her self-care activities.

Evaluation: If Susan developed constipation at a later point in her pregnancy, how would you revise the planning? What information would you need or which questions would you ask to say that a revised plan was necessary?

Web Activities

- Visit the web sites of some nursing organizations, such as the Association of Women's Health Obstetric and Neonatal Nurses (AWHONN) and the American Nurses Association (ANA). What information do they offer regarding nursing care of the women during an uncomplicated pregnancy? Do they also include any information targeted for the client?

- Find the sites listed in the Resources for this chapter. Read the information that will be most useful to you as you begin working with pregnant clients and their families.

Key Concepts

- Preconception care is the ideal approach to child-bearing. Many risk factors can be identified and dealt with before pregnancy begins.

- Health care communities must develop plans for availability and accessibility of prenatal care for their citizens. Barriers should be minimized.

- Early and consistent prenatal care is essential for proper monitoring of any pregnancy. Prevention of potential complications is possible with monitoring.

- The pregnancy experience can be enhanced when clients are aware of changes taking place in their bodies.

- Clients can be empowered with involvement in decision-making about their care.

- Nurses have a responsibility to review all materials recommended for client information.

- Danger signs in pregnancy may affect the health of the mother, baby, or both. Special attention is needed.

Review Questions and Activities

1. Low birth weight and congenital anomalies remain two problems on which prenatal care has had litle impact in the past 40 years. Explain how preconception care can decrease the incidences of these problems.

2. Becky S. is seeing the nurse midwife with her fifth pregnancy. Her first two babies were born prematurely but are healthy youngsters now. Her third pregnancy resulted in a miscarriage at 18 weeks' gestation, and her fourth went to term with delivery of an 8 lb, 6 oz boy. How is her F.P.A.L. status correctly noted?

3. Diane's last normal menstrual period began on May 10th, and her pregnancy test (7 weeks later) was positive. Calculate her EDC. Give the month, date, and year.

4. Explain the physiologic anemia usually seen in pregnancy.

5. List one commonly encountered discomfort of pregnancy for each of the three trimesters. Explain why each is likely to occur in that particular trimester.

6. Discuss comfort measures for each of the three identified common discomforts.

7. What are some examples of pregnancy risk factors that can be identified from a client's psychosocial history? From her partner's medical history?

8. Your neighbor thinks she is pregnant and has made an appointment with her family doctor. How would you respond to her inquiry about what to expect during the visit?

References

Cefalo, R. C., & Moos, M. K. (1995). *Preconceptional health care: A practical guide* (2nd ed.). St. Louis, MO: Mosby.

Cunningham, F. G., MacDonald, P. C., Gant, N. E., Leveno, K. J., Gilstrap, L. C. III, Hankins, G. D. V., & Clark, S. L., (1997) *Williams Obstetrics* (20th ed) Stamford, CT: Appleton-Lange.

Huntington, J., & Connell, F. A. (1994). For every dollar spent: The cost savings argument for prenatal care. *New England Journal of Medicine, 331,* (19), 1303–1307.

McFarlane, J. (1996). De madres a madres: An access model for primary care. *American Journal of Public Health, 86,* (6), 879–880.

McFarlane, J., & Fehir, J. (1994). De Madres a Madres: A community, primary health care program based on empowerment. *Health Education Quarterly, 21,* (3), 381–394.

Molnar, P., Biringer, A., McGeer, A., & McIsaac, W. (1997). Can pregnant women obtain their own specimens for group B *Streptococcus?* A comparison of maternal versus physician screening. *Family Practice, 14,* (5), 403–406.

Perry, L. E. (1996). Preconception care: A health promotion opportunity. *Nurse Practitioner, 2,* (11), 24–26.

Pew Health Professions (1991). *Healthy America. Practitioners for 2005.* San Francisco. Pew Health Professions Commission.

Suggested Readings

American Academy of Pediatrics and The American College of Obstetricians and Gynecologists. (1997). *Guidelines for perinatal care* (4th ed.). Washington, DC: American Academy of Pediatrics and The American College of Obstetricians and Gynecologists.

Association of Women's Health, Obstetrical and Neonatal Nurses (AWHONN). (1999). *Clinical competencies and education guidelines: Limited ultrasound examinations in obstetrics and gynecology/infertility settings.* Chicago, IL: AWHONN.

Brown, S. (Ed.). (1988). *Prenatal care: Researching mothers, reaching infants.* Institute of Medicine: Washington, DC: National Academy Press.

Expert Panel on the Content of Prenatal Care. (1989). *Caring for our future: The content of prenatal care.* Washington, DC: U.S. Department of Health and Human Services.

Jakobi, P., Goldstick, O., Sajov, P., & Itskovitz-Eldor, J. (1996). New CDC guidelines for prevention of perinatal group B streptococcal disease. *Lancet, 348,* (9032), 969.

Knuppel, R. A., & Drukker, J. E. (1993). *High risk pregnancy: A team approach.* Philadelphia, PA: W.B. Saunders.

Kogan, M. D., Martin, J. A., Alexandar, G. R., Kotelchuck, M., & Frigolette, F. (1998). The changing pattern of prenatal care utilization in the United States, 1981–1995, using different prenatal care indices. *Journal of the American Medical Association, 279,* 1623–1628.

LaVeist, T. A., Keith, V. M., & Gutierrez, M. L. (1995). African American/Caucasian differences in prenatal care utilization: An assessment of predisposing and enabling factors. *Health Services Research, 30,* (1), 43–58.

Lin, G. G. (1998). Birth outcomes and the effectiveness of prenatal care. *Health Services Research, 32,* (6), 805–807.

Murray, M. (1997). *Antepartal and intrapartal fetal monitoring.* Albuquerque, NM: Learning Resources International.

Rosenstein, N. E., & Schuchat, A. (1997). Opportunities for prevention of perinatal group B *Streptococcal* disease: A multistate surveillance analysis. The neonatal Group B *Streptococcal* Disease Study Group. *Obstetrics & Gynecology* 90, (6), 901–906.

Simpson, K. R., & Creehan, P. A. (1996). *Perinatal nursing.* Philadelphia, PA: Lippincott-Raven.

Taylor, M. C., Mercer, B. M., Engelhardt, K. F., & Fricke, J. L. (1997). Patient preference for self-collected cultures for group B *Streptococcus* in pregnancy. *Journal of Nurse Midwifery, 42,* (5), 410–413.

U.S. Department of Health and Human Services. (1989). *Caring for our future: The content of prenatal care.* National Institutes of Health: Washington, DC.

U.S. Department of Health and Human Services. *Healthy People (2010)* (Conference Edition, in Two Volumes). Washington, DC: January 2000.

For more information about *Healthy People 2010* or to access *Healthy People 2010* documents online, visit: http://www.health.gov/healthypeople/ or call 1-800-367-4725.

Youngkin, E. Q., & Davis, M. S. (1994). *Women's health: A primary care clinical guide.* Norwalk, CT: Appleton & Lange.

Resources

www.fetal.com
www.medphys.ucl.ac.uk/mgi/fetal
www.amnionet.com
www.med.upenn.edu/meded

www.public/berp/overview
www.cpdz.com/cpdx
www.docboard.org

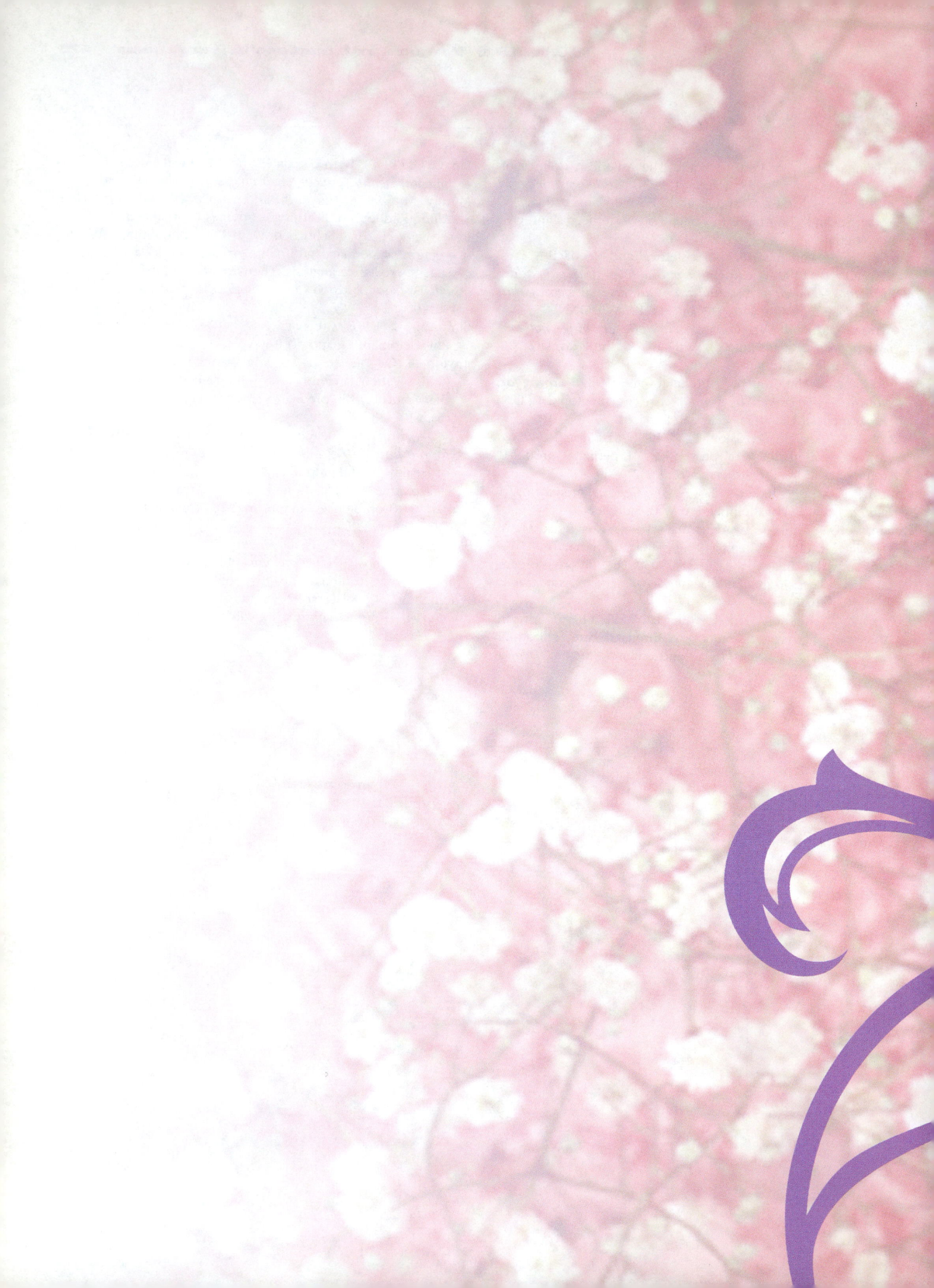

CHAPTER 17

Childbirth Preparation and Perinatal Education

*I*magine you are pregnant with your first child. How might you answer the following questions to examine your personal beliefs regarding childbirth preparation:

- *What do I fear most about child-birth?*

- *What are my expectations?*

- *What would I need to know about how to manage the pregnancy?*

- *What would help me prepare for the birth experience?*

- *Which types of things would I like to know about caring for an infant?*

- *Who is qualified to teach prenatal classes, and how will I find a legitimate class?*

- *Which types of preparatory classes and activities are available to other family members?*

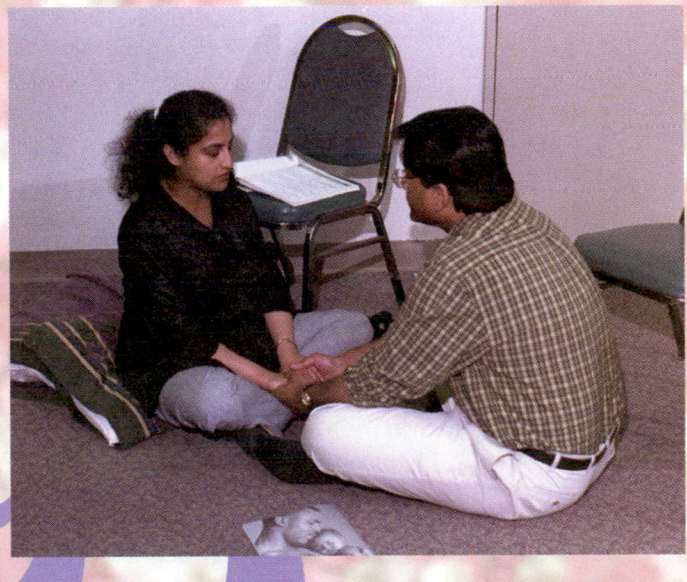

Key Terms

Childbirth education
Cleansing breath
Focal point

Medicalization of
   childbirth

Modified-paced
   breathing
Paced breathing

Patterned-paced
   breathing
Perinatal education

Competencies

Upon completion of this chapter, the reader should be able to:

1. Discuss the history of childbirth preparation classes and current trends in perinatal education.

2. Discuss the educational principles of adult learning and the group process as they relate to perinatal education.

3. Describe the major approaches to childbirth education.

4. Apply the strategies of paced breathing to enhance relaxation.

5. Discuss different strategies to enhance relaxation, such as biofeedback, imagery, touch, meditation, and music.

6. Identify options regarding labor and birth attendants, childbirth classes, and birth settings.

Childbirth education, more recently referred to as **perinatal education**, began as a consumer movement to humanize the birth experience and promote an active role by women in the birth process. Preparation for the birth and subsequent parenting responsibilities has expanded beyond learning breathing techniques for labor. The increasing involvement of the expectant woman's partner or supportive friends also has given rise to educational programs. The movement toward perinatal education has changed the hospital environment and now is an integral part of health care for childbearing women.

The movement toward perinatal education historically has involved nurses, both as consumers and educators. The Nurses Association of the American College of Obstetrics and Gynecologists (NAACOG), forerunner of the Association of Women's Health, Obstetrics, and Neonatal Nurses (AWHONN), developed guidelines for childbirth education in 1981, which were revised in 1987 and again in 1993 (AWHONN, 1993). These guidelines provide recommendations for improving the quality of perinatal education to promote healthy birth outcomes and emotionally satisfying birth experiences (AWHONN, 1993). Partnerships between health care providers and community resources provide a mechanism for offering educational preparation for childbirth and a link to support systems after the birth.

Many expectant women consider childbirth a significant challenge. Health care providers and systems have been responsive to changes suggested and, at times, demanded by childbearing families. Currently, expectant families have choices regarding care providers, birth attendants, delivery settings, and educational preparation formats. Nurses play a pivotal role in providing information and assistance to clients and their families and thus can foster active participation in and preparation for the upcoming birth. Many couples are motivated to learn and attend classes because they want strategies to cope with impending labor and ensure a healthy baby. Expectant parents often have a heightened interest in health-promoting behaviors during pregnancy. Thus, nurses have a golden opportunity to promote healthy lifestyles and meet the educational needs of the parents. Health education offered to families during pregnancy may form the foundation for lifelong health practices. Couples or persons who participate in group classes also often form continuing friendships. In both clinic and hospital settings, nurses also are in a position to use some of the techniques that have been developed to help women relax during labor and to teach clients who have not taken prenatal classes. Application of the nursing process assists the nurse to identify and meet the needs of expectant families. Evaluation of family outcomes leads to continued improvement in the approaches nurses use to prepare families for childbirth.

FROM CHILDBIRTH EDUCATION TO PERINATAL EDUCATION

The birth event often has been the focus of medicine and nursing. Early childbirth education classes were focused entirely on developing and practicing techniques for use in managing pain and facilitating the progress of labor. More recent developments in perinatal education have broadened the focus to incorporate family adaptation to the pregnancy and parental roles for the newborn. The relationship of the couple during pregnancy and incorporation of the infant into the family constellation now are included in perinatal education. The process of moving the parents into the roles of mothers and fathers is included, especially in the case of a first child. For families with children, with each subsequent pregnancy the family needs to re-establish these parenting roles. Family adaptation also includes the adaptation of siblings and the entire family unit. Additional content has been added to childbirth education curricula that includes breastfeeding, infant care, transition to parenthood, relationship skills, family health promotion, marital intimacy, and sexuality; some curricula have added the role of perinatal bereavement counselor (Humenick, 1999; 2000).

The childbirth education movement has had a significant impact on the delivery of perinatal health care. As consumers became more knowledgeable and active in decision-making, changes were made in hospital policies in regard to allowing nonmedical persons to be present at the birth, working in partnership with the laboring woman and her partner and providing more family-oriented maternity care. In 1996, the Coalition for Improved Maternity Services (CIMS) ratified a document called the Mother-Friendly Childbirth Initiative. This document was based on up-to-date research and the beliefs that childbirth is a natural process and that a wellness model of maternity services reduces interventions and provides cost-effective and improved care for all women (CIMS, 1996). Hospitals may receive mother-friendly designation by carrying out the philosophic principles and following the 10 steps outlined in the document.

History of Childbirth Education

Childbirth education is not an innovation of the last half of the 20th Century. Throughout history women have been providing informal education to other women about childbirth. Even with formalized childbirth preparation classes, many women are taught about childbearing and childrearing by their mothers and other family and friends. Childbirth education became very popular in the United States

and Europe over the past 50 years as a response to the **medicalization of childbirth** and the emergence of the woman's movement. This social movement did much to change the approach of the health care industry to childbirth. The woman's movement has helped give women more power in decision-making and the labor process, foster development of more family-centered care, foster the use of strategies to control stress and pain, and change the delivery of health care to a more holistic and humanistic model. In these areas the philosophy of childbirth education parallels that of nursing.

Early Childbirth Preparation

Across cultures, women have been assisting other women in preparing for childbirth and the role of mother and have been informally handing down these traditions. In many cultures, women attend the birth and support the mother whereas men are prohibited from attending the birth. Female midwives in Europe attended births until the 17th Century (Wertz & Wertz, 1989). During the 20th Century, childbirth moved into hospitals. As medical care became more oriented to specific diseases and as more technology began to be used, childbirth also became medicalized. This medicalization resulted in women being separated from family and, in many cases, a supportive environment. Childbirth began to be treated as are other medical or, more often, surgical events. The primary goal was a mechanically safe passage through the birth process for mother and infant. Many women and infants benefited from some of the medical interventions and methods of assessing the labor progress; however, the social, cultural, psychological, and spiritual aspects of childbirth often were ignored and replaced with an environment of surgical asepsis and technology (Davis-Floyd, 1992).

By the mid-1900s, most births occurred in hospitals and midwives were used only in remote areas. In the 1960s the prepared childbirth movement began. Through education of the public, hospital care changed to permitting support persons (often the husband) in the delivery room, allowing more time for mother and infant to stay together (e.g., by rooming-in, mother-baby care, or couplet care), and increasing support for breast-feeding. The emphasis on preparation and a more natural approach to birth has decreased many of the risks from unnecessary medical interventions and allowed a birth experience that better addresses the psychological, cultural, social, and spiritual aspects of the experience.

METHODS OF CHILDBIRTH PREPARATION

Early childbirth classes were held by the Red Cross and the Maternity Center Association in the early 1900s to teach hygiene to women who were poor or immigrants and to provide information to cope with the stresses of birth (Zwelling, 1996). In Europe, a movement was beginning that spread from Russia to France (Lamaze method), with a parallel movement in Great Britain (Dick-Read method). In Russia, the concept of behavioral reconditioning was successfully applied to labor pains. This technique provided an excellent alternative to chemical means of reducing pain. The notion that pain could be controlled by psychological preparation became the foundation for childbirth education and preparation.

Lamaze Method of Psychoprophylaxis

Fernand Lamaze, a French physician, developed a version of psychoprophylaxis that became very popular throughout Western Europe. Lamaze pioneered this educational approach to childbirth preparation using body conditioning exercises, education, and relaxation techniques (Lamaze, 1972). Lamaze found that mental and physical conditioning were extremely effective in his own practice. These conditioned responses were acquired through training and repetition whereby the client learns to respond to pain with breathing and relaxation. American society was introduced to the Lamaze approach to childbirth though the publication of the book *Thank you, Dr. Lamaze* by Marjorie Karmel (1959), a client of Lamaze. Elizabeth Bing, author of *The Lamaze Method: Six Practical Lessons for an Easier Childbirth* (1967), along with Karmel formed the American Society of Psychoprophylaxis in Obstetrics (ASPO/Lamaze, later changed to Lamaze International, Inc.). This organization has certified programs and childbirth educators in the Lamaze method since 1965.

Most childbirth preparation classes offered in North America today provide content and instruction based on the Lamaze method. The fundamental techniques for instruction are conditioning, discipline, and concentration (Figure 17-1). Conditioning teaches the mother to adapt her responses to the physical and emotional demands of labor by becoming skillful in tuning into her body. Discipline enables the person to stick to the program or regimen because she has specific goals and is committed to accomplishing them. Concentration provides the essential mental edge so the woman can stay focused on the task at hand. Concentration breaks the flight or fight response by substituting muscle release and deep oxygenation for tension and breath holding.

Early Lamaze classes focused on getting the laboring woman into a comfortable position. Use of a **focal point** allowed the woman to concentrate on something other than the pain of labor. This focal point could be a picture, sound, or mental image. Practice during pregnancy allowed the woman to build up a discipline of concentra-

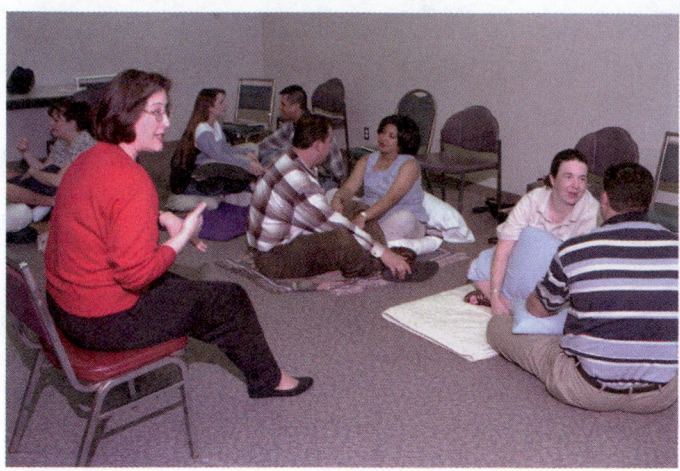

Figure 17-1 Couples practice conditioning and concentration techniques during childbirth preparation classes.

tion. The couple practiced using verbal and other cues to recondition the tension response to pain. For example, the partner might touch her on her neck and, through practice, she would develop a conditioned response of relaxation to that stimulus. Thereby the usual response to pain, which is tension, would be replaced by relaxation. Basic breathing patterns were taught to class attendees and practiced frequently in preparation for labor. The more time devoted to practice of the patterns the more automatic they will become and the more likely they will be used during childbirth. Originally, very specific breathing techniques were taught for different periods of labor. These techniques had many different names. As research advanced regarding the physiology of breathing and the understanding of relaxation during labor, paced breathing became more individualized and the centrality of relaxation became more important than were the specific breathing techniques. The most widely offered classes use this approach.

Dick-Read Method

Around the same time Lamaze was developing his psychoprophylactic method, British obstetrician Dr. Grantly Dick Read (1979) incorporated into his practice an educational program for the expectant mother. His goal was to decrease the amount of pain experienced during childbirth. He promoted the belief that the degree of fear could be diminished with increased understanding of the normal physiologic response to labor. Dick-Read's book entitled, *Childbirth without Fear,* (1979) advocated childbirth education from the first prenatal visit. Since the 1950s, the British National Childbirth Trust has trained childbirth educators and breast-feeding and postpartum counselors (Ondeck, 2000). Select physical conditioning exercises were included in the program to strengthen the muscles used in

Research Highlight

Waterbirths: A Comparative Study on More than 2,000 Waterbirths

Purpose

To compare the safety and outcomes of three types of births: waterbirths, use of the Maia-birthing stool, and bedbirths.

Method

A prospective study of 7,508 spontaneous births in a large university clinic in Switzerland was conducted. Three types of birth methods were compared and described. The three groups were comparable in parity, age, and newborn birth weight. Vacuum extractions were excluded.

Findings

In this study, 2,014 were waterbirths, 1,108 were Maia-birthing stool births, and 2,362 were bedbirths. Episiotomies were performed in 12.8% of waterbirths, 27.7% of birthing stool births, and 35.4% of bedbirths (bedbirths also showed the highest third- and fourth-degree lacerations at 4.1%). These findings were statistically significant. Maternal blood loss was lowest, fewer painkillers were used, and the birth was rated more satisfying among the women experiencing waterbirths. Average arterial blood pH of the umbilical cord as well as Apgar scores at 5 and 10 minutes were significantly higher after waterbirths. Infections in neonates did not occur more often after waterbirth than after the other methods, and no cases of aspiration or water-related complications were reported.

Nursing Implications

Waterbirth and alternative forms of birthing, such as the Maia-birthing stool, do not demonstrate increased birth risks for mothers or infants with similar medical monitoring of birth.

Geissbuhler, V., & Eberhard, J. (2000). Waterbirths: A comparative study. A prospective study on more than 2,000 waterbirths. *Fetal Diagnosis and Therapy, 15*, (5), 291–300.

childbirth and assist in lowering the tension level during labor. Relaxation techniques were taught that interrupt the circular pattern of fear, tension, and pain (Figure 17-2). Breathing and relaxation techniques during labor are the key features of the Dick-Read approach to childbirth. Dick-Read also argued against "unnatural aids," such as analgesics and anesthesia. Classes are available that follow the Dick-Read method.

Bradley Method

In 1965, Robert Bradley, a Denver-based obstetrician and follower of Dick-Read, wrote a popular book entitled *Husband-Coached Childbirth*. The key feature to this method is the involvement of the husband or significant other as a primary coach during the childbearing experience (Bradley, 1965). Use of conditioning, breathing, and

relaxation exercises are commonalties shared with the Dick-Read approach. The source of strength and support during childbirth is the partner or coach (Figure 17-3). Extensive preparation of the mother and coach is emphasized in the classes. A quiet environment for labor and delivery also is advocated. Classes are available that follow the Bradley method.

Expectant parents should be encouraged to carefully review the variety of classes available. Comparison of basic principles, theoretical foundations, and educator preparation and philosophy will assist the expectant parents in selecting a class best suited to meet their needs. Perinatal nurses often are asked to offer opinions regarding the types of childbirth preparations.

Women have increased their role as decision-makers regarding childbirth. Childbirth preparation classes provide information that allow families to be partners with

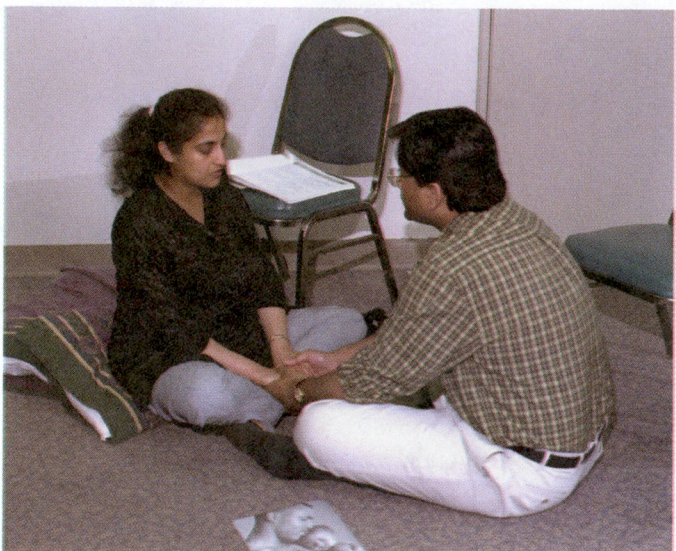

Figure 17-2 Breathing and relaxation techniques are practiced in anticipation of labor.

the health care team in their choice of anesthesia and analgesia and in making decisions about the birth setting and process. Perinatal education also includes support for breast-feeding, from education for decision-making early in pregnancy to support during the early postpartum period. Perinatal education also covers women's concerns in preparing for childbirth, starting before conception and lasting until the postpartum period. The focus is to prepare the woman and her family for the birth and care of an infant and for the impact the child will have on the family.

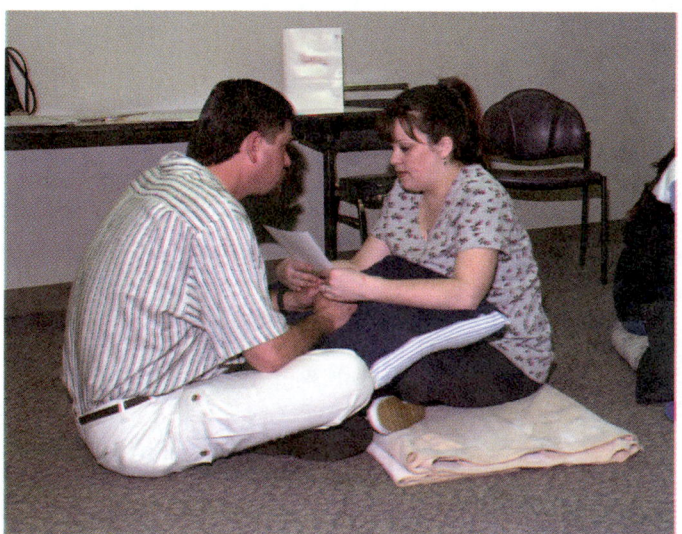

Figure 17-3 Partner support is a critical component of childbirth education courses.

Kitzinger's Psychosexual Method

Sheila Kitzinger developed a method of preparation for couples that focuses not only on the birth but on the relationship of the couple. Birth is seen as a mutual endeavor of the couple and an extension of their relationship of love. Her book entitled, *The Experience of Childbirth* (1981), promoted a reconceptualization of childbirth from a mechanical process of the fetus through the birth canal to a holistic experience that the husband and wife share as part of their intimate relationship. She advocated for political change in the way health care is delivered to birthing families.

Water Immersion

The healing powers of water have been heralded since ancient times and are associated with both ritual healing and general healing properties. The use of water during labor (Figure 17-4) and birth recently has become popular, albeit

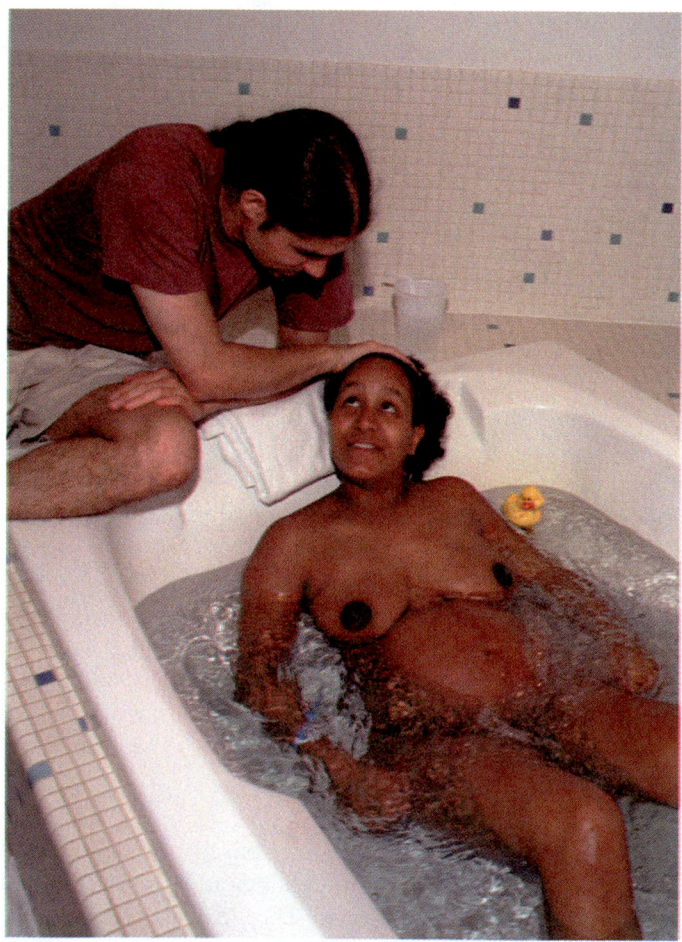

Figure 17-4 Water therapy can be extremely relaxing to the woman in labor.

controversial (Koehn, 2000). A more contemporary movement centered in Moscow and France (Odent, 1984; 1990). Tcharkovsky, a Moscow swimming instructor, became interested in the ability of infants to adapt to water and promoted underwater birthing. In France, Leboyer promoted water immersion of the neonate immediately after birth. His book entitled, *Birth without Violence* (1975) and book and film *Loving Hands* became popular in the 1970s. In Pithiviers, France, Odent pioneered waterbirth and a method of working with families and providing an environment to allow the woman and her husband to instinctively find the right position and way of birth (Odent, 1984).

THEORETICAL BASIS FOR CHILDBIRTH PREPARATION

Strategies of prepared childbirth are based on the theories about pain management and personal mastery discussed subsequently.

Relaxation Theories

Relaxation is the central concept in preparation for childbirth (Humenick, Shrock, & Libresco, 2000). Relaxation is the antithesis of the stress response. Relaxation can assist in the cognitive skills of focusing and receptivity and in the acquisition of new skills. Stress or fear signal the fight or flight mechanism, which activates the sympathetic branch of the autonomic nervous system and thus increases the heart rate, blood pressure, and breathing. Fear and tension during labor result in tense muscles that use oxygen, making it less available to the uterus and fetus. Tense striated muscles contribute to an increased lactic acid buildup that impinges on pain receptors, increasing pain perception and fatigue. Resistance from a tense abdominal wall decreases the efficiency of uterine contractions. A tense pelvic floor creates unnecessary pain in the second stage of labor.

Relaxation strategies influence the cognitive thoughts that in turn influence fear and stress, thus reducing the perception of stressful stimuli. Conscious relaxation of other muscles allows the uterus and cervix to do their work unimpeded and more efficiently. When a woman can consciously control stress, her sense of mastery and self-confidence are increased. Right brain stimulation, such as imagery, color, music, rhythm, odors, and so on, can foster activation of the parasympathetic system and facilitate childbirth (Humenick, Shrock, & Libresco, 2000). During pregnancy a state of low sympathetic arousal increases oxygen and decreases the levels of stress hormones reaching the fetus. During labor this state of low sympathetic arousal reduces pain and increases oxygen and energy for the work of labor. Relaxation aids in breast-feeding and the stresses of parenthood. The skills of evoking a relaxation response are useful throughout life. Often, childbirth preparation is the first time women and their partners learn about and practice relaxation techniques. Relaxation now is being taught in many other areas of health care as a treatment adjunct for many disorders.

Pain Management Theories

Several theories of pain management are used in childbirth preparation. Cognitive control works by modulating pain by focusing on mental activities rather than the pain. A laboring woman might focus on the motion of uterine contractions or the work of dilation of the cervix to dissociate the painful aspects from the source of stimulation (Jimenez, 2000). She also may use distraction techniques, such as watching TV, using paced breathing, and using visualization to interfere with the transfer of the pain message. These techniques are learned through cognitive rehearsal in preparation for labor. Desensitization also is used to help the person overcome fears.

Some physiologic theories have been proposed to explain how these techniques may reduce the pain of labor. Levels of endorphins or endogenous opiates have been found to be high during pregnancy and higher still during labor; these levels remain elevated in the postpartum period. Endorphins are natural pain inhibitors and are suppressed with use of exogenous opiates, such as meperidine (Demerol) (Jimenez, 2000). Research is being conducted on the effects of other endogenous substances, such as serotonin, oxytocin, and melatonin.

Melzak and Wall proposed the gate-control theory of pain in 1965 (Melzak & Wall, 1965). This theory states that

---

Nursing Alert

EFFLEURAGE

Light touch, such as effleurage, travels along the same small-fiber pathways as do pain stimuli and therefore can increase pain perception. Many women prefer a harder massage as labor progresses.

Relaxation and stress reduction are beneficial for many physical conditions and pain control. Positive effects also may be related to the special attention and support the laboring woman receives from the nurse, her labor partner, or a doula. This positive effect can reduce fear and pain. Other mechanisms may be related to the benefits of spiritual connection with the supportive presence of others who have intent to help.

pain stimuli can be modified as they travel on small-diameter nerve fibers along the ascending pathway through the spinal cord. A gating mechanism can be activated by sensations traveling through large-diameter fibers, which transmit messages more quickly than do the small fibers. This gating mechanism is activated by massage and by heat and cold. Habituation may occur in 15 to 20 minutes and may be mistaken for an increase in actual pain rather than in perception. Changing the site or type of stimulus can reactivate the "gate" (Jimenez, 2000).

RESEARCH RELATED TO CHILDBIRTH PREPARATION

Much of the focus in childbirth has been on pain reduction. However, research has repeatedly shown that maternal satisfaction with childbirth is more strongly related to the woman's ability to participate actively in decisions related to the childbirth experience (Humenick, 1997). The focus of the media and many providers continues to be pain reduction. The first randomized controlled trial of epidural anesthesia in 1993 was stopped because ethical conflicts arose owing to an increase in the cesarean birth rate among women in the group receiving epidural anesthesia (Ondeck, 2000). Research is inconclusive regarding the physiologic effects of catecholamines and the use of anesthesia and analgesia during labor. These subjects currently are being debated among researchers and practitioners.

Some researchers believe that maternal stress levels contribute to the release of catecholamines, thus causing vasoconstriction of uterine blood vessels and resulting in lower levels of oxygen reaching the placenta and thus the fetus (Steiner, 2000). Concerns exist that this decreased oxygenation could contribute to fetal distress. The use of analgesia and anesthesia is supported because it reduces maternal stress, making birth less stressful for the mother and infant. In contrast, a body of research exists that suggests the presence of catecholamines is important to fetal survival and that the surge during labor is protective (Steiner, 2000).

The response of the fetus to catecholamines could be misinterpreted as fetal distress, because when fetal scalp blood pH levels were drawn, true asphyxia was present only in those with levels of catacholamines in excess of normal labor. These researchers concluded that the high levels of catecholamines found in normal deliveries protected the infant during the stress of the birth experience and also facilitated normal breathing in the first hours of life by increasing the metabolic rate and enhancing blood flow to vital organs. The risk of interfering with this healthy response should be considered in decisions of managing labor (Steiner, 2000). Childbirth educators are

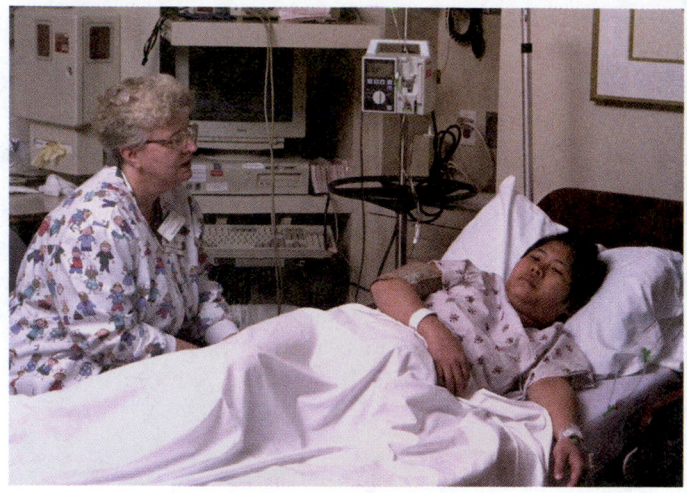

Figure 17-5 The nurse knows that her encouraging words and soothing voice will help this first-time mother to relax as her labor progresses.

encouraged to employ evidence-based practice (Figure 17-5). This approach integrates research from various areas: education for the most effective methods and strategies, medicine related to the physiology of labor and fetal development, medical management of pregnancy and labor, and social sciences related to physiologic, social, cultural, and spiritual aspects of childbearing.

The strategies for labor have been strongly influenced by research. In 1993, Lamaze International, Inc., revised its guidelines related to breathing strategies based on the scientific literature (Nichols, 2000). Research into the various relaxation strategies, such as touch, music, and so on, also is increasing. As more nurses become aware of evidence-based practice and use of research results, perinatal education will be impacted.

STRATEGIES FOR LABOR MANAGEMENT

Prenatal or childbirth education may be with individuals, families, or groups. Nurses can design educational content using trimesters as guidelines, allowing for standardized content. Many agencies have designed specific classes for various topics and stages of pregnancy. Adaptations always must be made to accommodate individual family needs.

Relaxation Techniques

Relaxation is central to many of the techniques for coping with labor. Relaxation is a systemic response that reduces fear and tension during labor. Reduction in fear and ten-

RELAXATION

"Relaxation is the foundation of all childbirth preparation techniques" (Nichols, 2000).

sion facilitates the body's efficient use of energy for labor, thereby reducing fatigue and thus making labor more effective. Tense abdominal muscles form resistance to uterine contractions and use oxygen, resulting in less oxygen available to the fetus. Tension increases lactic acid build-up, which increases pain. Relaxation during pregnancy results in increased oxygen to tissues and organs and fewer stress hormones reaching the fetus. Relaxation skills also are helpful after delivery in coping with the demands of a new baby and helping establish breast-feeding. Developing relaxation skills promotes the health of the entire family (Humenick, Shrock, & Libresco, 2000). The authors reviewed research studies on relaxation techniques for birth. Benefits extended into the postpartal period and included lower anxiety, less depression, increased self-esteem, and improved immune function. Several techniques are employed to promote relaxation. Some of the more popular techniques are described subsequently. Many of these techniques also are discussed in Chapter 4 on complementary and alternative therapies. The use of these techniques specifically for pregnancy and childbirth also is discussed subsequently.

Paced Breathing

Current scientifically based breathing techniques are flexible, individualized, and focused on using a slow-paced breathing rate throughout labor. Breathing strategies for labor now are understood to be a relaxation-enhancing strategy (Nichols, 2000). Breathing strategies are based on scientific understanding of respiration and changes during pregnancy and labor. Normal respiratory rates range from 12 to 16 breaths per minute. In pregnancy, the respiratory rate increases slightly, respiratory effort increases owing to uterine enlargement and resultant pressure on the diaphragm, and oxygenation requirements increase. The increased need for oxygen generally is accommodated by an increased depth of respiration and a slight increase in rate.

Paced breathing decreases stress and pain and increases relaxation. The term paced breathing now is used to describe the research-based breathing techniques used to decrease stress responses and thus decrease pain. Paced breathing has been shown to promote relaxation through reducing the sympathetic response of the autonomic nervous system and to stimulate the parasympathetic branch.

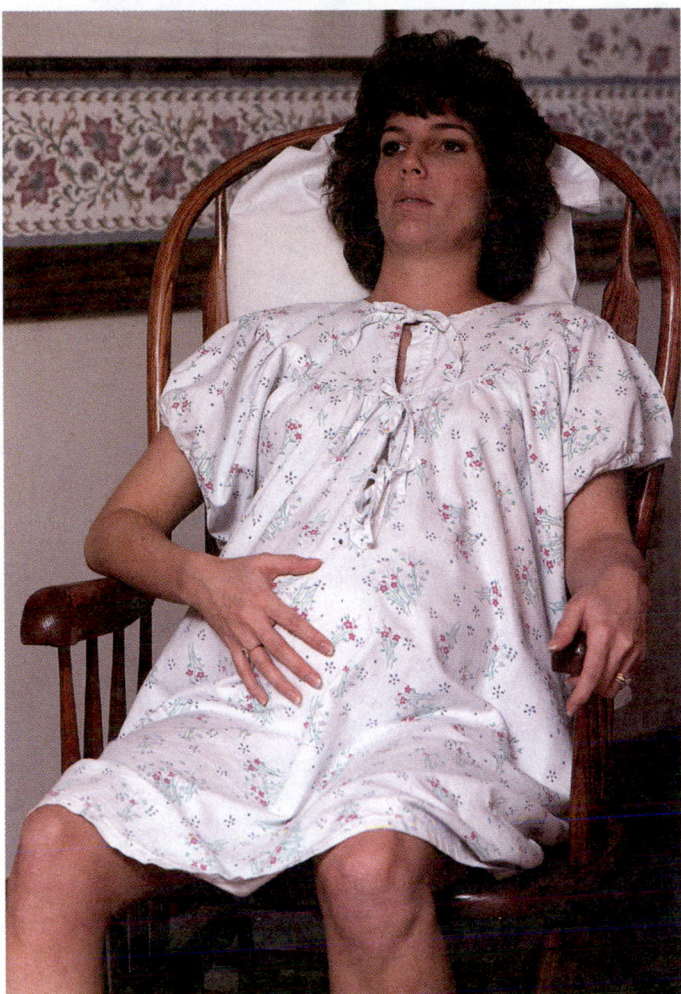

Figure 17-6 Using paced breathing, the laboring woman controls and regulates her breathing patterns.

This type of breathing also implies self-regulation. In 1983, Lamaze International adopted the standards for prepared childbirth based on the paced breathing patterns discussed subsequently (Nichols, 2000). Paced breathing techniques use a slow rate and individualized and flexible approaches to promote relaxation of the laboring woman (Figure 17-6).

Cleansing Breath

A **cleansing breath** is a deep relaxed breath, such as a sigh, designed to signal relaxation and provide deep ventilation. This breath often is used to signal the beginning of a contraction and separates the stimulus of the contraction that usually has a response of alarm and tension. Cleansing breaths often have been used along with a focal point to help the woman in labor concentrate and focus on relaxation. Contractions of the uterus or other muscles contracted during stress use additional oxygen and result in aerobic work. Cleansing breaths also help provide additional oxygen for the aerobic work of a contraction or can

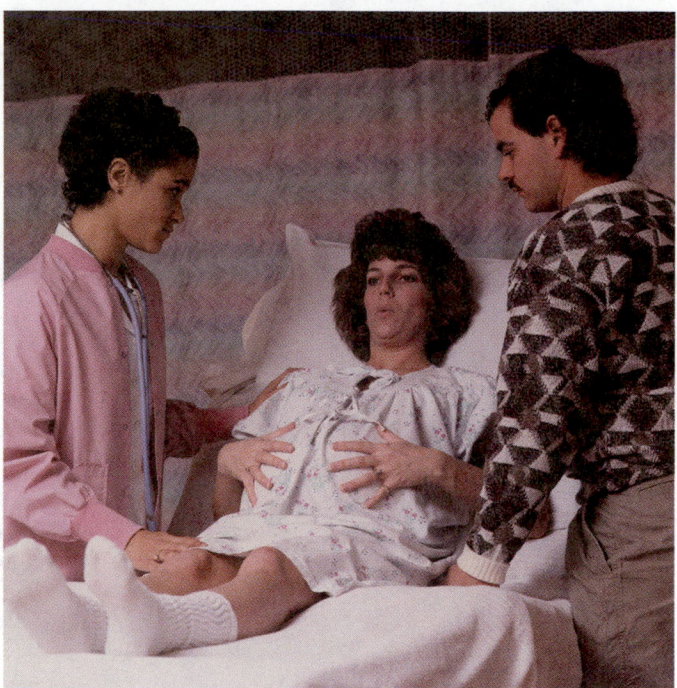

Figure 17-7 Slow-paced breathing provides comfort to the mother and adequate ventilation to both mother and fetus during labor.

serve to repay the oxygen debt from previous work. Cleansing breaths should be effortless and as deep as is comfortable.

Slow-Paced Breathing

Slow deep breathing is associated with relaxation. Research had shown that slow-paced breathing is associated with increased relaxation and decreased anxiety, pain, psychological response to threats, and stress (Nichols, 2000). Early childbirth instruction differentiated between abdominal and chest breathing; current classes emphasize a more flexible approach.

The rate of breathing should be comfortable for the woman and provide adequate ventilation for the mother, fetus, and work of labor. A rate of half the woman's normal rate is appropriate during the early part of labor.

EFFECTIVE BREATHING

Always work with the woman to help her breathe at her comfort level. Avoid complicated breathing techniques that interfere with relaxation. Remember that relaxation is the key.

Often, couples will learn the woman's normal rate and practice slowing breathing in preparation for labor (Figure 17-7). Abdominal or chest breathing may be used; however, confining the breathing to either area may interfere with relaxation, which is the main goal. Nose or mouth breathing may be used, whichever is more comfortable. If mouth breathing is used, moisture in the woman's mucous membranes will need to be replenished during labor. The woman should be encouraged to use the slow-paced breathing pattern for as long as possible. As labor progresses and habituation occurs, however, she may need to modify her breathing.

Modified-Paced Breathing

During increased work or stress, the respiratory rate increases. **Modified-paced breathing** paces this increase at a controlled rate. Patterned-paced breathing is a more rhythmic pattern and requires increased attention by the laboring woman. These techniques are learned and are best practiced during pregnancy for optimal use during labor. The rhythm aids the woman in concentrating and therefore increases her ability to relax. Respiratory physiology requires that the lungs adequately empty to result in good ventilation. Respiratory rates that are too fast decrease the tidal volume. It is recommended that the respiratory rate not exceed twice the woman's normal rate and that there be a balance of breathing deeply enough to cause alveolar ventilation but not so shallow as to stop air movement. When the woman feels as if she needs to catch her breath, she should deepen her breathing.

Nursing Alert

SLOW-PACED BREATHING

The rate of slow-paced breathing should be no less than half of the woman's normal respiratory rate. Less than this rate may not provide adequate ventilation.

MAINTAINING MOUTH MOISTURE

Offer a laboring woman sips of water, clear liquids, or crushed ice to help keep her mouth moist, per physician or institution policy.

Patterned-Paced Breathing

Patterned-paced breathing is similar to modified-paced breathing but with the addition of a rhythmic pattern. One of the rhythms that frequently is taught in childbirth classes is 4—1, which means four light breaths plus one similar inspiration followed by an exhalation, such as that used when blowing out a candle. Different patterns may be used, such as 4—1, 6—1, 4—1. Many couples use pyramids or other patterns. The patterns sometimes help the woman to focus. Any pattern is encouraged as long as the basic principles of rate and relaxation are met.

Progressive Muscle Relaxation or Neuromuscular Relaxation

The technique of progressive muscle relaxation or neuromuscular relaxation uses the client's ability to recognize muscle tension and relaxation in her own body. The client thus learns to release muscle tension and relax through systematic contraction and relaxation of specific muscle groups. This technique generally is done with a partner who observes the tension in the muscle groups and cues the woman into achieving overall relaxation. This focused relaxation increases oxygenation to muscles, especially the uterus, and decreases the perception of pain. As couples practice this technique, some eventually are able to relax a muscle by applying a specific stimulus, such as touch.

Neuromuscular Dissociation

Neuromuscular dissociation focuses on differentiating tension from relaxation. The woman practices by tensing some muscles while simultaneously relaxing other muscle groups. This technique often is taught to couples. The partner checks muscle groups and coaches the client on relaxing and tensing various muscles. Eventually, couples may practice substituting a relaxation response rather than tension to painful stimuli.

Autogenic Training

Autogenic training is a form of passive concentration whereby the woman acquires control over autonomic processes through concentration on visual, auditory, or somatic imagery. The training often employs commands such as "My hands are warm" or "My arm is heavy."

Meditation

Meditation has been used for centuries in Eastern religious and health practices. The meditative state is attained through quiet concentration on a mantra or a repetitious sound. The purpose is to empty the mind of thoughts and concerns, thereby quieting the mind and therefore the body. This discipline requires practice and may produce excellent reduction in anxiety.

Biofeedback

Biofeedback is the use of instruments to detect select physical status, making clients more aware of their physical state and thus enabling them to bring the physical state under voluntary control. Most biofeedback equipment monitors muscle tension, skin temperature, blood pressure, and brain activity. Clients increase their sensitivity to internal events and can learn to regulate heart rate and blood pressure, control symptoms, and stimulate a relaxed state. Humenick and Marchbanks (1981) indicate that some childbirth educators have the potential to be as accurate as is biofeedback equipment in determining the degree of relaxation.

Touch

Touch has been associated with comfort and caring across cultures and over time. Human touch is vital to the well-being of infants and has been used by midwives to support women in birthing for centuries. Various techniques of touch are used with women in labor that range from gentle comforting touch to massage and acupressure (Figure 17-8). Infant massage historically has been used in India and recently has gained popularity in the United States. Therapeutic touch and healing touch are discussed in more detail in Chapter 4.

Imagery

Athletes may imagine a physical activity and public speakers and performers may prepare for a performance by visualizing the desired actions. Imagery also has been used in health care to prepare people for surgery, resulting in

Nursing Alert

IMAGERY

Although using imagery may seem harmless, psychological clinicians warn that it should not be used in clients who have psychoses or are mentally unstable. When using this technique with a group, the lights may be kept on and participants instructed to open their eyes if they are more comfortable. No more than 20 minutes should be spent in deep relaxation states because excessive use of imagery may be associated with withdrawal from everyday life, insomnia, and hallucinations. Unless they are experienced counselors, educators should never probe memories of past trauma that may be elicited or interpret images that clients may have. Clients taking medications for metabolic disorders should be monitored.

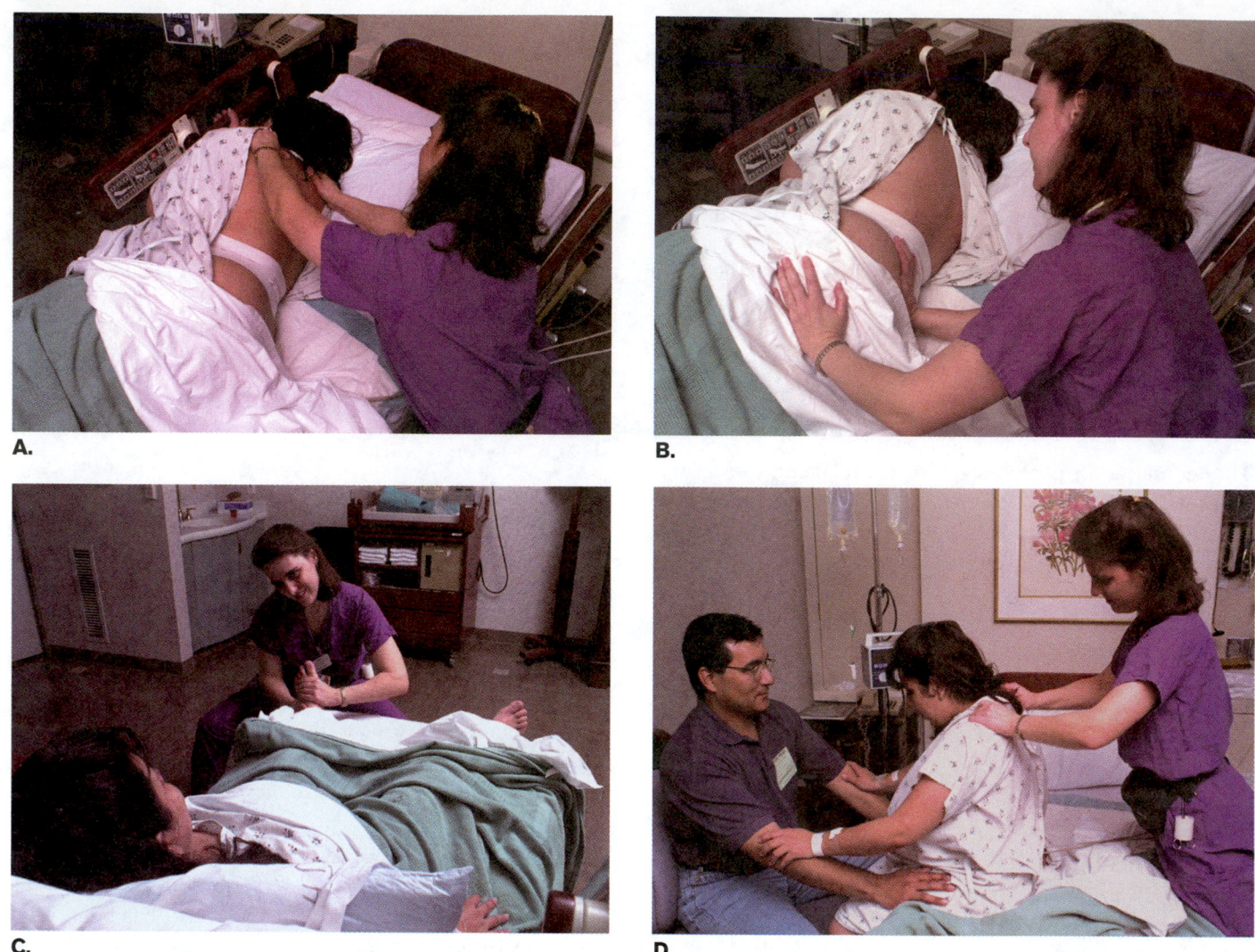

Figure 17-8 Touch therapy for the woman in labor may include the following. A. Shoulder massage. B. Low back pressure to relieve the pain of back labor. C. Foot massage. D. Partner-supported touch.

the need for less pain medication and decreasing complications. Imagery has been used to decrease headaches and lower blood pressure; it has been used in patients with cancer and those undergoing skin grafts (Achterberg, 1985; Achterberg et al., 1994). Although the scientific understanding of how imagery works is unclear, it appears that the brain does not differentiate between an image of reality and a visualized image (Steffes, 2000). Imagery has been used in childbirth, starting with the focal point for concentration and using pleasant images for relaxation training. Use of these images involves multiple senses, including vision, sound, and smell to transform pain into a less stressful sensation. Imagery in childbirth is used alone or in combination with other relaxation techniques. For example, Lamaze (1972) suggested that the laboring woman visualize contractions like waves in the rising tide and waning of contractions as the ebbing tide. Some childbirth educators encourage woman to visualize their cervix dilat-

ing during labor. Most people self-select and use the type of relaxation technique most comfortable for them. The Academy for Guided Imagery reported no adverse effects from the professional or lay community when imagery was used (Steffes, 2000).

Music Therapy

Music has been used as a therapeutic agent throughout history and across cultures. Early studies of the therapeutic properties of music were conducted in dentistry as a method to reduce pain (DiFranco, 2000). A meta-analysis of music in medical and dental literature indicates that music enhanced medical objectives in psychological, self-evaluative, physiologic, and behavioral observations (Standley, 1986). Music appears to have effects on the autonomic nervous system, immune system, and psychological system. In childbirth preparation, music is used alone or in combination with imagery to induce relaxation and reduce pain. Halpren & Savary (1986) believe that the human biologic rhythm corresponds with a 4:4 musical beat and when exposed to a new rhythm, tries to balance by adapting to the new rhythm. Thus, some rhythms are soothing, others are rousing, and others are antagonistic to biologic rhythms. Repetition is a feature of music that, in combination with rhythm, may be calming (DiFranco, 2000). Low-pitched tones have a more relaxing effect than do high-pitched tones; intensity also is an important feature, with loud music increasing respiratory activity. Loud music increases the fetal heart rate. The effect of fetal intrauterine exposure to loud music or noise is unknown. Music has been used to facilitate calming in newborns. Personal preference also is important in selecting music.

Acupressure

Acupuncture and acupressure have been used for pain relief and anxiety reduction for thousands of years. A consensus panel of the National Institutes of Health (NIH) on the use of acupuncture and acupressure has concluded that these treatments may be effective for many pain-related conditions and the nausea related to chemotherapy and pregnancy (NIH, 1997). Data on the use of acupuncture and acupressure in childbirth is sparse; however, empirical evidence supports its use for the discomforts of pregnancy, labor, birth, and the postpartum period. Acupressure is similar to acupuncture but is not invasive and applies manual pressure to the acupuncture sites. Acupuncture requires administration by a trained professional; however, some acupressure techniques can be incorporated into childbirth preparation. The acupressure point may be tender to the touch and feels less resistant to the touch than do other points on the body. Generally, the thumb or finger is used to apply pressure. A point on the wrist is used for nausea in pregnancy (Figure 17-9). Points around the sacrum are used for labor pain and back pain. Before using or teaching clients the acupressure technique, the nurse should become familiar with the various points because some may induce labor contractions (Koehn, 2000).

SUPPORT DURING LABOR

One of the most significant elements of the childbirth education movement has been to legitimize the importance of the presence of a supportive person who stays with the woman throughout labor. Around the world, women support other women in childbirth. Since the 1970s in the United States, husbands or partners have moved into this role as a result of the childbirth movement. Since that time, many childbirth classes have described the father's role as coach and he was instructed to coach his partner through the various breathing techniques. This role has been challenged because many men feel the role is inappropriate. Currently, the father's role is more flexible but men are encouraged to accompany their partners through labor if the couple wishes.

Currently, health care professionals and doulas are employed more frequently by health care institutions or contracted by the family to provide support during labor. Whereas the role of support person seems ideal for the nurse, the greater the medical needs of the women the less available is the nurse to provide emotional support (Simkin & Fredrick, 2000). In addition to midwives and nurse midwives, a new group of health providers has emerged as labor companions. They have many names. Some are called birth assistants or labor assistants who often are laypersons with some midwifery skills. Doulas are labor companions trained and experienced in childbirth. They provide continuous emotional support, physical comfort, and informational support. The labor support person may be an untrained, inexperienced friend who accompanies the woman during labor. A montrice is a nurse who can provide nursing care and assessment in addition to labor support.

Studies have demonstrated that women who were accompanied by doulas or montrices had better outcomes, including a lower rate of epidural use; fewer episiotomies; and in one study, a lower cesarean rate and less need for forceps (Klaus, Kennell, & Klaus, 1993; Hodnett and Osborn, 1989). Doulas and montrices generally work with mothers and fathers to help the couple work closely together and to support a positive experience for the family.

The support person works with the laboring woman to make sure she understands the physical changes of labor, encourages distracting activities and relaxation activities, and assists in finding comfortable positions throughout labor. (Some of these positions are illustrated in Figure 17-10.) Often, the nurse, nurse midwife, doula, or montrice works with the family before delivery and thus

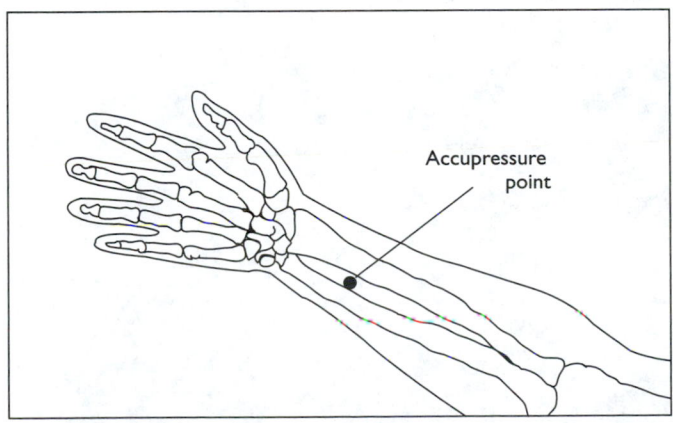

Figure 17-9 Acupressure to the wrist often alleviates the feeling of nausea in pregnancy.

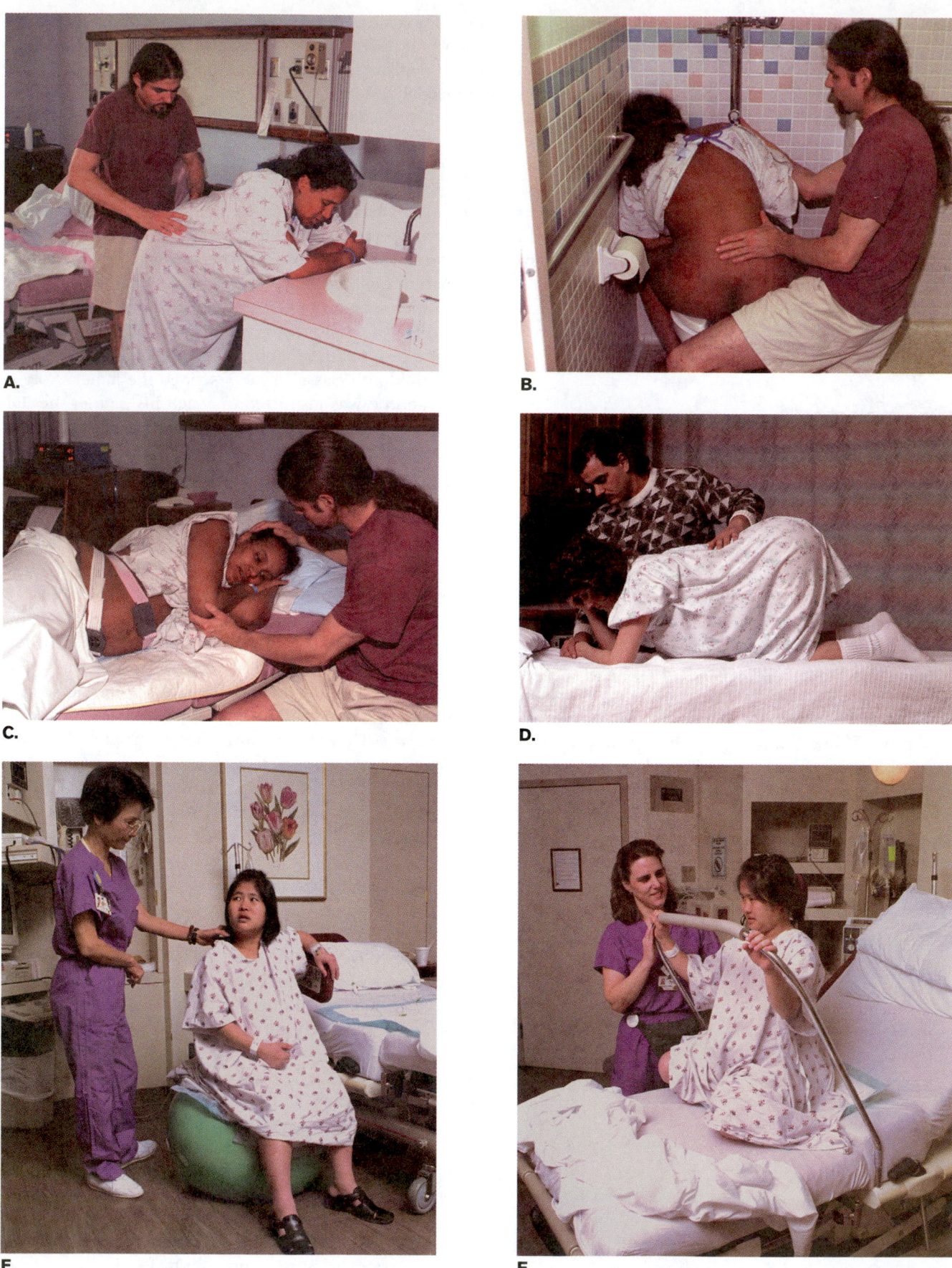

Figure 17-10 Various positions can ease the discomforts of and assist in the progress of labor. A. Standing. B. Sitting on toilet. C. Side-lying position. D. Hands and knees position. E. Sitting on birthing ball. F. Squatting with birthing bar.

applies the types of relaxation techniques the couple has been practicing.

Labor often has been regarded by health care providers as a high-risk medical event, using an active model of aggressively managing the labor process; alternatively, many childbirth educators and nurses view labor as a normal physiologic process (Wooley & Nelsson-Ryan, 2000). Some, echoing Odent's philosophy of intuitive birth—or the physiologic model—believe that labor can evoke a basic intuitive response that allows the woman the best experience.

Active Model

The active model of labor assumes that the second stage of labor is a singular event from the full dilation of the cervix to the expulsion of the fetus (Wooley & Nelsson-Ryan, 2000). Full dilation is assessed by vaginal examinations, and the woman is encouraged to bear down and push when complete cervical dilation and effacement has occurred. She often is instructed to take a deep breath, hold it, and push. She may be given anesthesia and analgesia. The fetus is carefully monitored and medical interventions are initiated if the process is prolonged.

Physiologic Model

The physiologic model supports the woman's natural process of labor and attempts to use interventions that enhance or replace the physiologic process (Wooley & Nelsson-Ryan, 2000). This model divides the second stage of labor into two phases: (1) the interval between full dilation and active and spontaneous bearing down; and (2) the press period, or the bearing-down phase, which extends from the time of active spontaneous pushing to the birth of the baby. Thus, the second stage may extend to 3 hours. The active model encourages the woman to actively and consciously push to shorten this stage. The longer stage of the physiologic model encourages the woman to follow the natural impulses of her body (Roberts, 1996). Following the natural impulses avoids involuntary pushing that may unnecessarily exhaust the woman and evoke a Valsalva maneuver, in which the intrathoracic pressure from straining impedes venous return to the heart and causes decreased cardiac output and disrupted blood to the uterus. The physiologic approach also encourages the woman to make whatever sounds are spontaneous. Many women will use an open glottis while pushing, which sounds more like grunting than straining when bearing down.

In a review of literature on the second stage of labor, Minato (2000) concludes that laboring down should be incorporated whenever possible in caring for laboring women. *Laboring down* refers to allowing the mother to rest while contractions produce the descent of the fetal head through the birth canal, until rectal pressure or other physical sensations of the urge to push occur. The mother is not encouraged to push until after this rest period. This technique reduces maternal exhaustion, produces less perineal edema, and appears to have no adverse effects on fetal or newborn well-being.

Positioning during the second stage of labor can increase uterine efficiency and protects the perineum. In studies of nonmedicalized births, an upright position often is used. The upright position is described as an active position achieved by standing, sitting, squatting, or kneeling (Wooley & Nelsson-Ryan, 2000). These positions allow gravity to assist the work of the uterus, and they reduce back pain and the length of the second stage of labor. Many birthing beds or chairs have been designed to put the woman in a more upright position, which facilitates labor. Good evidence exists to support that the dorsal position for birth, which fails to use the forces of gravity, is unfavorable because it lengthens the labor and may cause fetal hypoxia and maternal hypotension. A birthing bed that allows the mother freedom of movement and a variety of active positions seems to be the optimal choice.

In the physiologic model, interventions follow the form of enhancing the physiologic process. For example, breast stimulation is used before administering oxytocin (Pitocin) to stimulate uterine contractions. Perineal massage during pregnancy and labor also is used to reduce lacerations. Extensive research supports the fact that routine episiotomies are not justified and carry additional unnecessary risks.

Families, either through their childbirth preparation classes or exposure to friends and the media, also develop a philosophy about labor. A supportive physical and emotional environment for the second stage of labor is important in any case. Health care providers are encouraged to work with the family regarding their philosophy of birth.

Parenting, Role Transition, and Family Adaptation

The perinatal educator approaches childbearing in a broader sense than the focus on the birth, incorporating education about family adjustment to the pregnancy and the new infant. Infant feeding and infant care are major components of client education.

ADDITIONAL CLASSES OFFERED TO CHILDBEARING FAMILIES

Special classes may need to be adapted for families. The following may need to be taken into consideration: cesarean birth, vaginal birth, vaginal birth after cesarean section, parents, grandparents, siblings, single parents, specific cultural groups, high-risk pregnancies, pregnant adolescents, parents with handicaps, parents with medical problems, communication barriers, and preconceptual classes (AWHONN, 1993). Some of these classes are discussed.

First Trimester–Early Pregnancy Class

Early pregnancy classes are offered by hospitals that provide women's health care services. This introductory course focuses on the physiologic and psychological changes that occur during the first 3 months of pregnancy. Educators are able to respond to questions and, perhaps, decrease anxiety for clients through frank discussion and exploration of feelings during this initial stage of attachment to the growing baby. Hospitals also may view this class as a mechanism for marketing the services they provide; therefore, a tour of labor and delivery, nursery, neonatal, and postpartum units often is included in the class. The importance of continued prenatal care, education, and preparation is promoted. Additional classes or prepared childbirth and infant care programs may be introduced.

An important benefit of this type of class is education. An increased level of knowledge regarding changes that occur throughout the pregnancy is gained by the significant others of the expectant mother. Optimally, childbirth education is started before conception and includes ensuring the mother has appropriate treatment for minor health problems and begins good health habits. These health habits include good nutrition; avoiding alcohol, cigarette smoking, and other drugs; and avoiding exposure to toxic substances that could cause harm to the developing fetus. Ideally, childbirth education builds throughout the pregnancy, which allows for specific content to be covered in each trimester. Other material is introduced early and expanded or reinforced throughout the pregnancy. When the nurse has not been able to begin the education early in the pregnancy, the material should be covered whenever the client is available for teaching. Many facilities provide classes on specific topics that can augment formal childbirth preparation classes and individual teaching.

Content appropriate for teaching childbearing families is outlined for each trimester in Box 17-1.

Pregnancy Exercise Classes

The pregnant woman's desire to maintain or improve her physical conditioning in preparation for birth has resulted in the development of exercise classes designed specifically for pregnant women. The American College of Obstetricians and Gynecologists (ACOG, 1994) published guidelines for exercise during pregnancy that have become the standards for the content, exercise selection, and maternal parameters of these classes. Classes may be coordinated through sports medicine or hospital wellness departments that use or rely on the expertise of exercise physiologists. Commonly, a physician's approval is required before acceptance into the program. Postpartum conditioning also has been included in some exercise programs that also serves to unite new mothers, resulting in the formation of informal support networks.

Mild exercise for strengthening muscles taxed by pregnancy or giving birth has been a standard part of perinatal education. Concerns have been raised about vigorous exercise during pregnancy, such as the risks for hyperthermia, fetal distress miscarriage, and maternal injury. The risks of vigorous exercise are low; in contrast, vigorous exercise has many benefits, including weight control, physical fitness, and positive mental health (Hammer, Perkins, & Parr, 2000). The first ACOG standards regarding exercise in pregnancy were published in 1985 (ACOG, 1985) and contained specific guidelines related to heart rate and duration. These standards were revised to be more flexible, indicating that continuing or beginning an exercise program during pregnancy is now viewed as safe (ACOG, 1994). The benefits of exercise during pregnancy include healthy weight maintenance, cardiovascular fitness, improved posture, positive psychological benefits, and fewer miscarriages; other benefits are relief of minor discomforts, easing of labor, prevention or treatment of pregnancy-induced complications of gestational diabetes, and possible prevention of pregnancy-induced hypertension (PIH) (Hammer, Perkins, & Parr, 2000). The benefits are weighed against the risks that include trauma, strains, and sprains. The risk of fetal hypoxia occurred only in women who were not physically fit and who engaged in sporadic vigorous exercise and, in some cases, high-altitude activities (above 9,000 ft) or scuba diving (exceeding depths of 12 to 16 ft). Fetal risks related to hyperthermia are greatest in the first trimester; core temperature of 102°F to 104°F may be related to neural tube developmental defects and teratogenesis. Pregnant women are advised to avoid vigorous exercise in hot ambient conditions (Hammer, Perkins, & Parr, 2000). Hypoglycemia can be avoided by consumption of a sports drink or fruit during (every 30 minutes) or after exercise. Women should maintain adequate hydration during exercise. Differences in health status, physical fitness, and previous exercise require that recommendations be individualized; monitoring may be advised (Figure 17-11).

Breast-Feeding Classes

Breast-feeding classes provide information and assist the mother in making a decision regarding breast-feeding. Participants are encouraged to attend these informational and supportive classes before delivery because they provide the knowledge related to the benefits, mechanisms, and skills of breast-feeding. Classes are commonly conducted by breast-feeding educators or, when possible, certified

Box 17-1 Specific Educational Content for Each Trimester

First Trimester

Knowledge of the Pregnancy

- Anatomy and physiology of pregnancy
- Physical and emotional changes related to pregnancy
- Fetal development
- Importance of prenatal care
- Diagnostic tests, such as chorionic villus sampling, amniocentesis, and ultrasonography
- Warning signs of complications
- Dangers of substance abuse and exposure to toxins and teratogenic hazards

Management of Pregnancy

- Morning sickness
- Sleep disturbances
- Libido changes
- Urinary frequency
- Fatigue
- Emotional liability

Relaxation Techniques

Introduction to stress management:
- Awareness of the stress response: breathing patterns, muscle-tension, and other physical symptoms of stress in contrast with relaxation
- Awareness of stimuli for tension and relaxation
- Introduction to relaxation techniques
- Slow-paced breathing
- Body awareness

Exercise and Nutrition

- Nutritional needs
- Vitamin supplements
- Exercise
- Body mechanics
- Stretching
- Kregel's exercises
- Pelvic tilt exercises
- Toning and aerobic exercises

Family Adaptation

- Choices of provider and birth setting
- Response to emotional and physical changes of pregnancy
- Sexuality
- Infant feeding method
- Exploring maternal and paternal roles
- Communication skills to discuss adaptive changes in the family
- Introduction of discussion of financial and spatial family adaptation to the expanding family

Second Trimester

Builds on previous teaching or incorporates previous trimester teaching if necessary

Knowledge of Pregnancy

- Physiologic changes of pregnancy
- Fetal development and characteristics
- Fetal movement
- Review of warning signs and complications

Management of Pregnancy

- Management of heartburn, back pain, and so on
- Changes in body and body image
- Comfort and hygiene measures

Relaxation Techniques

- Explore and identify techniques, such as imagery, massage, music, touch, visualization, and so on
- Work together as a couple (client and support person) to elicit relaxation to stimuli
- Practice slow-paced breathing, modified-paced breathing, and patterned-paced breathing

Exercise and Nutrition

- Continue good nutrition, and monitor weight gain
- Increase repetitions of exercise
- Modify activity related to physical changes

Family Adaptation

- Identity of the fetus as a separate individual and building maternal-fetal attachment

(continued)

Box 17-1 Continued

- Financial considerations; may include a discussion of working or career in relation to the pregnancy
- Paternal concerns: role in labor, role as father, financial concerns, and provision of safety for the mother and fetus
- Sibling preparation
- Preparation of the home for the infant
- Discussion of feeding choices for the infant
- Selection of a pediatric provider

Third Trimester

Often the time for formal classes and need to include all of the above if not already covered

Knowledge of Pregnancy

- Anatomy and physiology of late pregnancy
- Mechanisms and signs of labor
- Additional testing or medical information related to specific conditions
- Medications and anesthesia
- Policies and practices of the facility chosen for delivery
- Postdelivery physical and emotional changes
- Signs and symptoms of labor
- Warning signs of complications
- Progress of labor

Management of Pregnancy

- Preparation for labor
- Comfort measures
- Sleep patterns

Relaxation Techniques

- Practice relaxation techniques
- Practice all methods of breathing for labor
- Practice additional relaxation techniques

Exercise and Nutrition

- Continue good eating patterns
- Monitor appropriate weight gain
- Watch body mechanics, safety, and comfort
- Prepare for delivery: tailor sitting, pelvic tilt, and Kregel's exercises
- Perform walking and other conditioning exercises
- Introduce postpartum exercise

Family Adaptation

- Rehearse preparation for delivery and role of support person
- Evaluate family and extended family's preparation for birth
- Discuss normal appearance, care, and feeding of the infant
- Discuss breast-feeding techniques and preparation
- Discuss parental roles
- Discuss sexual adjustment

lactation consultants. Many health care organization and insurance plans also provide breast-feeding support classes and information for parents postpartally, which may gradually have an impact on the length of time an infant is breast-fed. Partners often gain a great deal of understanding and knowledge from attending these classes, and they can provide emotional support for the new mother.

Sibling Classes

The focus on family-centered maternity care has led to the inclusion of all family members in the preparation for the upcoming birth. Classes for siblings are conducted in a relaxed atmosphere that allows family members to ask questions, practice infant care skills, and tour the facility where the mother and neonate will stay. Classes often target specific age groups, allowing for development of age-appropriate content. The use of slide presentations, coloring books, stuffed animals, and treats, such as cookies and punch, can prove very effective in familiarizing the child with the hospital environment. Sibling preparation is intended to decrease the anxiety experienced by both child and parent when a new family member is added.

Grandparent Classes

Many times grandparents are very active in the preparation for childbirth. Many changes in maternal and newborn care have occurred over the past several decades, especially in including extended family members in the preparation and care of the new infant. Grandparents can become familiar with changes in approaches to infant care, such as sleep position recommendations; infant feeding; and new products, equipment, or services available to the new family.

Vaginal Birth after Cesarean Preparation

Classes have been formed to accommodate the specific educational needs of women who have elected to attempt a vaginal delivery after a previous cesarean section birth. Class participants often spend the first part of the program discussing factors that contributed to the operative delivery. These factors may detract from the confidence the couple may have regarding labor. The program covers techniques and strategies for expectant mothers and support partners to use during labor that increase the likelihood of a successful vaginal delivery.

Infant Care Classes

The desire to prepare for parenthood is a concern of mothers and fathers. At times, care of the newborn can seem overwhelming to new parents. In many areas of the country classes are held that provide instruction on the safe and responsible approach to infant care. These programs typically include an American Heart Association infant cardiopulmonary resuscitation course and demonstrations covering basic newborn care concerns such as bathing and diapering. This course is an excellent way for parents and child care providers to acquire knowledge related to newborns and to discuss topics such as stimulation, feeding choices, safety concerns in the home environment, and adjustment to the parenting role.

PREPARATION FOR THE EDUCATOR ROLE

Nurses and laypersons may be certified as perinatal educators. The position statement of the International Childbirth Education Association (ICEA) states that no single training or academic background is necessary to become a childbirth educator (ICEA, 1999). AWHONN (1993) guidelines for nurses specify that perinatal educators are expected to have completed appropriate previous education and training and have experience in both general nursing practice

and teaching techniques. For nurses, some experience working in obstetrics or woman's health serves is a good background for the educator role. The guidelines describe teaching and content competencies.

Formal preparation for the perinatal educator role is available from several professional organizations, including the International Childbirth Education Association (ICEA), the Bradley method, ASPO/Lamaze, Prepared Childbirth Educators, Inc., and other organizations. Perinatal educators must be able to clearly communicate the following: scientific bases of pregnancy and the birth process, psychosocial and cultural aspects of childbearing, and most current information for promoting health throughout the pregnancy and preparation for birth. According to AWHONN (1993) guidelines, the educator should work as a team member and demonstrate a philosophy of perinatal education that honors pregnancy as a state of wellness and respects the beliefs and attitudes of families. Specific content includes health education regarding pregnancy and childbirth, specific coping and relaxation strategies for childbirth, preparation of support persons, and provision of anticipatory guidance for the family in the postpartum period.

Families are encouraged to be active participants in the education process, and one of the goals of the classes is to encourage the woman and her partner to take an active role in their health care and the birth of their child. Perinatal education is founded on the premise of freedom of choice based on information about the process and knowledge of options.

The nursing process can be useful in determining and meeting individual educational needs in addition to the anticipatory guidance that may be provided to groups or clients as part of standard care. Assessment of needs should occur during the first prenatal visit. Some of these anticipated needs may be based on trimesters and progression of the pregnancy.

Prenatal education must respond to changes in technology, consumer demands, and trends in health care services provided to expectant parents. The perinatal educator must be knowledgeable about the risks and medical management of pregnancy and birth and be able to prepare and interpret these to the client. The educator needs to be aware of the many educational products, such as literature, films, and other materials, that can be used effectively for family preparation for childbirth. Prepared materials should be assessed for accuracy of information, literacy level, and cultural appropriateness. Clients also are exposed to information about pregnancy and birth through the popular media. The educator should assist clients in interpretation of this information for accuracy and relevance to their situation.

Perinatal education can be in formal groups or with individual clients. Participation in formal prenatal education

Client Education

Good Posture during Pregnancy

- Standing: head should be held erect with chin tucked, shoulders relaxed, and knees slightly bent (Figure 17-11A).

- Sitting: knees should be level with or higher than hips; a pillow may be placed behind the lower back for comfort (Figure 17-11B).

- Lying on your side: a pillow should be placed under the upper leg, keeping the leg slightly flexed. A pillow also may be placed under the abdomen for support (Figure 17-11C).

- Lying on your back: A pillow should be placed under the knees to elevate the legs (Figure 17-11D); a pillow under the right hip displaces the uterus and prevents vena cava syndrome. This position should not be used after the fourth month of pregnancy.

Exercises for Pregnancy

Specific exercises can be taught to clients to help strengthen muscle tone in preparation for birth.

- The pelvic tilt reduces back strain and strengthens the abdominal muscles. Figure 17-11E illustrates how to perform the pelvic tilt in both a standing and kneeling position. Exhale, roll the hips and buttocks forward, hold for a count of five, then inhale and relax.

- Abdominal muscle tightening with every breath increases abdominal muscle tone. This exercise can be done anywhere in any position. While slowly taking in a deep breath, expand the abdomen. Then exhale slowly while pulling the abdomen in until the muscles are completely contracted. Relax a few seconds and repeat the exercise.

- Kegel's exercises strengthen and tighten the perineal muscles. Tighten these muscles and pull them up toward the vagina as if trying to stop urination midstream. This exercise also can be done anytime, anyplace.

- The tailor sit (cross-legged sit) stretches the inner thigh muscles; adding arm reaches stretches the sides and upper body and helps relieve upper backache. Sit cross-legged and stretch one arm high over your head, then release and exhale. Repeat on the other side. Figure 17-11F illustrates the tailor sit and arm reaches.

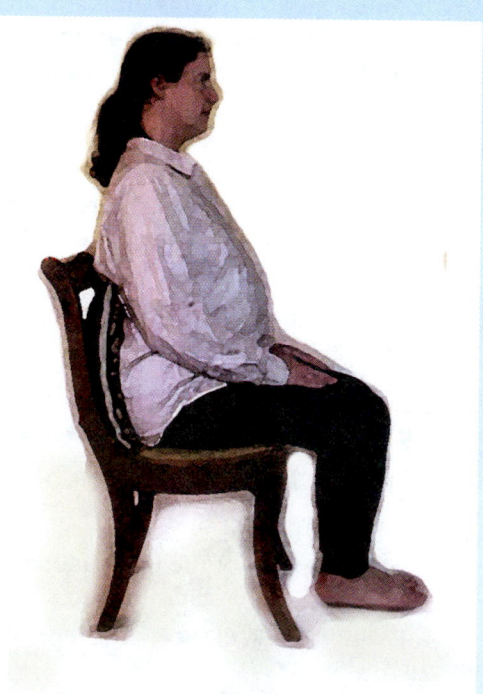

A.   **B.**

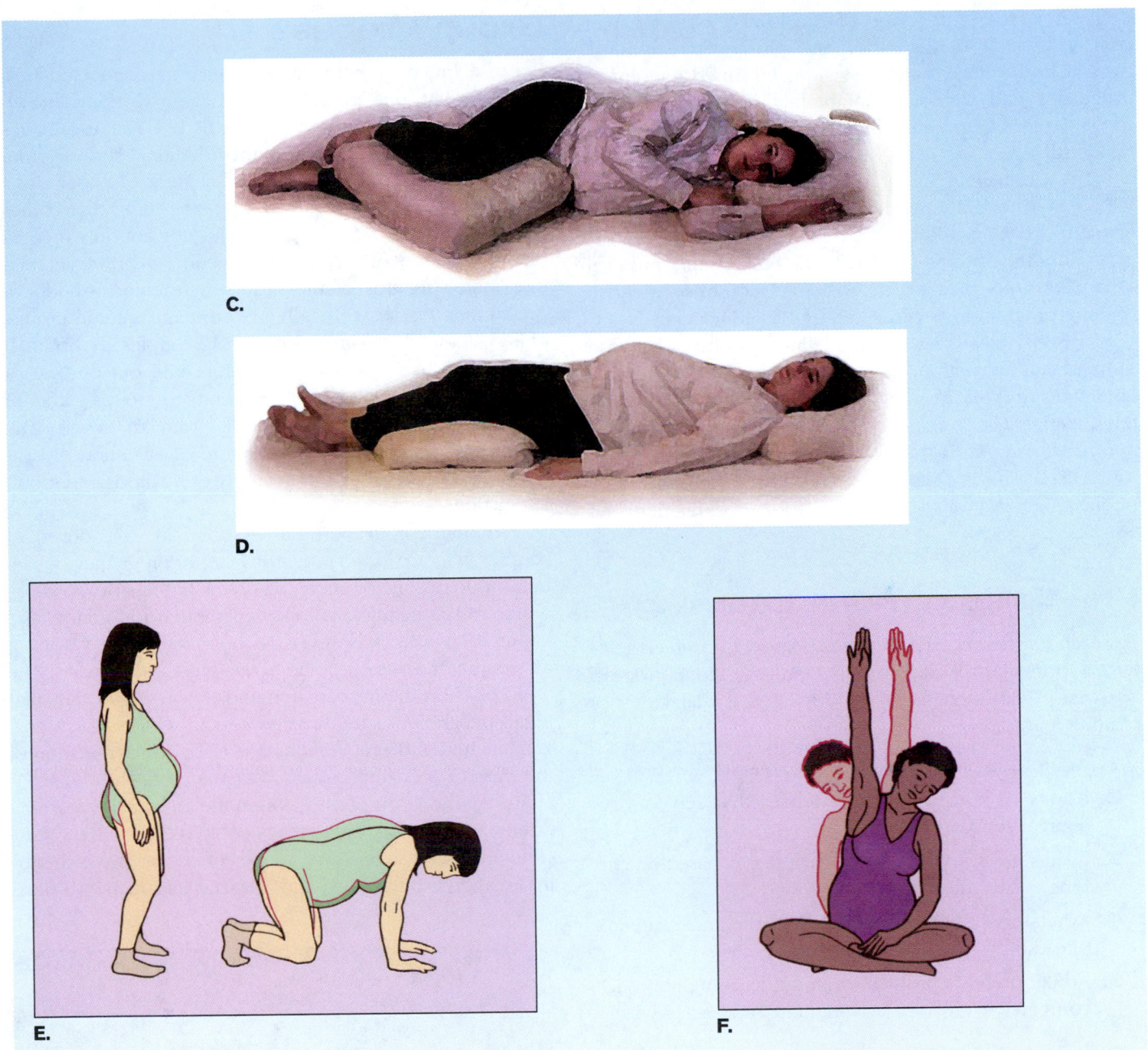

C.

D.

E.

F.

classes frequently is included in the plan of care for clients. It is important that an evaluation be conducted regarding how well the educational needs of the client are being met. Individualized teaching often is necessary to augment formal classes.

Organizations that Support and Certify Childbirth Educators

In addition to the organizations that support the various childbirth methods, such as the Bradley method and Lamaze method, the following organizations have formed to provide information, publish journals, direct policy, and certify educators.

The International Childbirth Education Association (ICEA) was formed in 1960 by consumer groups (Ondeck, 2000). It certifies educators, holds regular conferences, and publishes the *International Journal of Childbirth Education*. The ICEA requires continuing education for recertification and supports workshops, conferences, and publications. The organization has issued several position statements that can be obtained through its website or from its headquarters. The ICEA has issued position statements on the following topics: substance abuse during pregnancy, role and scope of the doula, assessment of fetal well-being during labor and birth, cesarean birth, vaginal birth after cesarean section, informed consent in pregnancy and childbirth, infant feeding, epidural anesthesia, role of the childbirth educator, and scope of childbirth.

The Council of Childbirth Education Specialists, Inc. (CCES), is an independent not-for-profit organization formed in 1972 to address the need for formal preparation of childbirth educators. Registered nurses and physical therapists who practice in obstetrics complete a 3-day training program to become certified as educators.

The AWHONN provides guidelines for nurses engaged in perinatal education. This organization also provides guidelines and information across the spectrum of perinatal nursing. *The Journal of Obstetric, Gynecologic, and Neonatal Nursing* (JOGNN) is the official journal of AWHONN. The AWHONN website also contains many publications related to guidelines for nurses in perinatal education.

Principles of Adult Learning

To teach effectively, nurses need to know the subject matter, the principles of adult learning, and the group process. Knowles (1980) identified the following five characteristics of adult learners:

1. Adult learners are independent and self-directed.
2. Adults have previous experiences that serve as resources for learning.
3. Adults have a readiness to learn that is based on current social roles and tasks.
4. Adults prefer to learn things that have immediate application.
5. Adults prefer a problem-oriented learning approach compared with a subject-oriented approach.

Nurses can incorporate these principles while developing an education plan for clients. Pregnancy is an ideal time to provide education because the family is approaching new or expanded social roles and tasks. The timing of the classes reflects a subject-oriented approach to an impending application, that is, the birth of the infant. Many prenatal education classes engage the participants in discussing their past experience and knowledge related to childbirth. These classes allow for much self-direction as the partners work out their own birth plan and rehearse strategies for labor.

Nurses can use these principles to direct group and individual client education, especially education of clients who do not participate in formal classes. The education of adolescents may require modification of content and presentation style.

Group Process

Because much of perinatal education is conducted in a group format, the educator must have a working knowledge of the group process (Figure 17-12). The advantages of working in a group include the additional support from the members, broader insight and sharing of experiences that members contribute, and subtle learning that comes from social interactions. A good educator not only focuses on presentation of material but incorporates the interactions and strengths of the group in teaching. Childbirth preparation classes generally are content-centered groups of 2 to 30 members (groups of 5 to 12 couples are optimal) who are focused on specific content and outcomes (Edwards & Nichols, 2000). Content-centered groups gather to acquire information about a topic from an expert. The group process includes presentation of scientific or academic information through a variety of methods and group interactions.

Childbirth education classes often are composed of couples who are in the same trimester of pregnancy, which helps to focus on common content. A process of warm-up, work, and integration is followed though the course and within each class (Edwards & Nichols, 2000). The warm-up allows the group to become acquainted and focused. The work phase is the introduction and processing of new material. Integration is the final process in which the material is integrated and preparations are made for termination of the class or group meetings. After the group has been established, the work phase is when the most active learning of new information and practice of skills take place. Often, childbirth classes consist of a series of classes at which new information is introduced and previous information is prac-

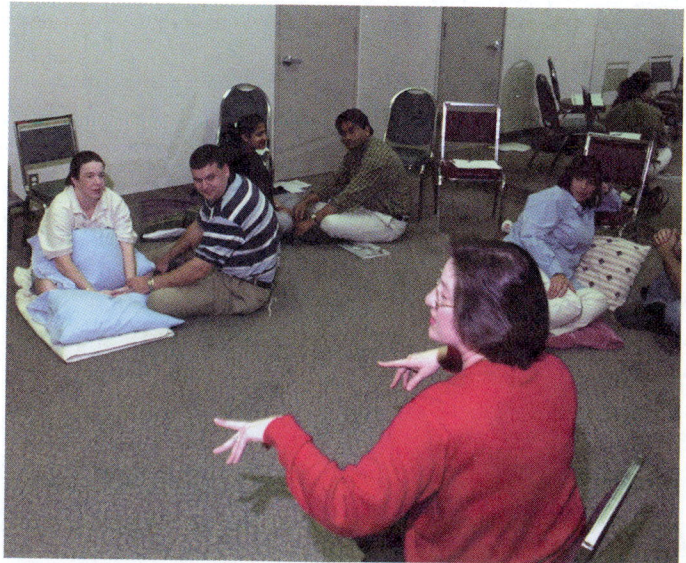

Figure 17-12 Many childbirth preparation classes are done in a group format.

ticed. Some classes invite previous class members who have delivered their infants to come to the group and discuss how they used the techniques during labor; this helps the class integrate the information. An important part of group process is planning the termination of the group. Often in the last class, little new information is introduced. Instead, rehearsals and integration of previous materials are the focus. Many groups will exchange information, and some will plan reunion meetings.

One technique in these classes is to divide into smaller groups for specific tasks. Often, small group activities are introduced during the first class to allow the group to become acquainted and to establish the group as a working unit. The first class also is the time to set out some of the expectations and instructions, such as type of clothing to wear if the group will be practicing exercises. The group process allows the members to feel there is consensus about problems and concerns addressed in the classes. For example, one educator asks the class what they would want to know if they went into labor (Edwards & Nichols, 2000). This information allows the educator to incorporate the concerns of the class into the class content.

According to AWHONN guidelines (AWHONN, 1993), the perinatal educator should be able to conduct a needs assessment, write goals and objectives, and use a variety of strategies in teaching. The perinatal educator should be able to create a flexible learning environment that fosters self-efficacy in the learner and uses principles of group process. The educator also needs to evaluate and refine the teaching accordingly.

CULTURAL CONSIDERATIONS IN CHILDBIRTH PREPARATION

Childbirth is enmeshed in cultural beliefs and values. These beliefs direct behaviors from conception through childrearing. Spiritual meanings pervade issues regarding when a soul enters the body and the vulnerabilities of the mother, fetus, and family during pregnancy and the birth processes. Cultural beliefs and traditions also dictate a great deal of maternal behavior during pregnancy, especially about activities that might have a negative effect on the baby. Many women will use amulets, charms, chanting, prayers, or special ceremonies to ensure the safety of their infant and themselves throughout the pregnancy and birth. Cultural practices also determine the place or setting for birth; who should be present at the birth; and in many cases, much of the process of birth and ceremonies surrounding the birth. For example, among Palestinians, men, pregnant women, and menstruating women should not be present at a birth (Shilling, 2000). Among Orthodox Jews, the husband may not touch his wife during

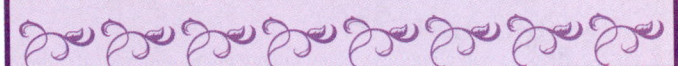

Critical Thinking

Considerations in Childbirth

Examine your own cultural beliefs about birth. Imagine that you or your partner are pregnant and in an unfamiliar culture.

- Which things would you feel are necessary for a safe pregnancy?
- Who would you want to be present at the birth?
- Where and with whom would you want to give birth?

labor and cannot view the genital area during labor or delivery; childbirth classes are held with couples sitting around a table because men are not allowed to view another's wife performing exercises (Lutwak, Ney, & White, 1988). Many African American's will choose to have their mother or another close female as a support person during labor.

Many symbolic practices are associated with preparing for labor, such as undoing knots, opening windows, and avoiding ideas of getting stuck. Some childbirth educators incorporate visual exercises of "opening up" or cervical dilation. In many cultures, specific procedures, reflecting symbolic meanings, exist for cutting of the cord or disposal of the placenta and umbilical cord. Many traditions also exist related to particular foods that should or should not be eaten during pregnancy or when approaching labor. One example of a culturally adaptive way of delivering health care occurred in Chiapas, Mexico. When the Indian women in the town would not give birth in the newly built hospital, a local medicine woman was hired to set up an altar in a birthing room and deliver babies in the hospital (Shilling, 2000).

Expression of pain during labor reflects culturally appropriate ways of managing pain and the meaning of pain related to childbirth. Culture affects women's behavior during the postpartum period, for instance, the amount of activity she should engage in, her personal hygiene, and her relationship to other family members. For example, in some parts of India the mother of the husband may have the most authority regarding the care of the newborn. Some families may not want the mother or infant to wear white because it is the color of mourning. In some cultures, a woman who does not appear to pay much attention to her infant is protecting it from bad luck; whereas in others, it may be important for the mother to take the infant to bed with her (Shilling, 2000).

Research Highlight

Collaborative Research Project: Effectiveness of Birth Preparation Classes at a Community Hospital

Purpose

To explore the content and effectiveness of birth preparation classes at a community hospital. The questions included the following: Which aspects of the classes did the mothers perceive as most effective in coping with the birth experience? Was there a relationship between the selected coping strategies and the mother's overall childbirth satisfaction?

Methods

An exploratory descriptive design was employed. Using a convenience sample from women attending the childbirth preparation classes, 127 participants were tracked through the childbirth experience. Within 1 week after the birth, these participants were surveyed using the coping with childbirth questionnaire and the childbirth satisfaction scale. The return rate of surveys was 66%, or 75 participants. Descriptive statistics were used in the analysis. Content analysis was used for the questions on most helpful strategies used.

Findings

The participants were primarily Caucasian (98%), married (91%), college educated (84%), and having their first child (93%). All had a labor support person with them, and most (64%) planned to use anesthesia. Actual use of anesthesia was 74%, and 85% delivered vaginally. Most (85%) were satisfied with the overall experience. The presence of the support person, information about the hospital, process of labor and birth, medications, birth choices, complications of labor were identified as helpful elements of the classes. Slow-paced breathing was the most frequently used breathing technique (64%). The only significant correlation was related to information and satisfaction.

Nursing Implications

Similar with other research on childbirth education this study supports the importance of information, breathing techniques, and a support person as being helpful to mothers during childbirth. Variations among clients and labor and delivery experiences necessitates, including information about and practicing various pain control options to allow the couple to individualize methods.

Slaninka, S. D., Galbraith, A. M., Strzelecki, S., & Cockroft, M. (1996). Collaboration research project: Effectiveness of Birth Preparation Classes at a community hospital. *Journal of Perinatal Education, 5,* (4), 29–36.

Nurses should continually develop their cultural awareness and understand that much variation exists within cultural groups and between ethnic groups. Open-minded approaches to diverse ways of thinking and acting to accommodate their clients are the first steps in developing cultural competence. Astute nurses will incorporate cultural awareness into their assessments of individual families and endeavor to adapt their nursing care according to the family's cultural beliefs and practices.

VARIABLES INFLUENCING THE NEED FOR CHILDBIRTH PREPARATION

The mother's orientation to pregnancy and birth are important considerations. Some women see pregnancy and birth as a time of enjoyment, greater marital closeness, and eagerness to engage in prenatal classes for childbirth preparation; other women are extremely fearful and have a more negative orientation. A woman's expectations and orientations about pain during labor will influence her decision regarding use of anesthesia and analgesia during labor. Several studies have been cited that mothers who received epidurals were less satisfied with the birth experience despite having less pain (Nichols & Gennaro, 2000). Nurses can be instrumental in helping pregnant women make informed choices regarding use of medications during labor.

Pain is influenced by many factors: fatigue, anxiety, presence of a support person, confidence in the ability to cope with labor, age, education, socioeconomic status, personal history, parity, and spiritual and cultural beliefs. In general, women from the middle and upper middle classes, women with a high level of education, multigravidas, and women with strong social support and a sense of mastery had the highest levels of satisfaction with the birth experience (Nichols & Gennaro, 2000).

Nurses can be instrumental in educating the client and family to prepare for childbirth, thus reducing some of the fears and anxieties about the birth process. Nurses also can help create an environment for birth that reduces stress and promotes comfort. Childbirth preparation has been found to have positive effects on the birth experience by stimulating a positive attitude and by reducing pain, the need for medications, and the use of forceps (Nichols & Gennaro, 2000). Reducing the need for medical interventions has significant benefits and reduction of risks for both mother and infant.

CHOICE OF PROVIDER

Ideally, selection of a health care provider before conception would result in the establishment of a strong client-provider relationship throughout pregnancy and childbirth. Realistically, often it is only after conception that many women begin the search for a provider. Women have many choices available in selecting a provider, including obstetricians, family practice physicians, certified nurse midwives, women's health care practitioners, and lay midwives. Before meeting with providers, expectant families should be encouraged to identify specific desires relating to prenatal, intrapartal, newborn, and postpartal care. Questions should be formulated to obtain information about approaches to obstetric care and practice standards to identify a provider most compatible with issues important to the client. The provider's educational background and preparation, specialty certification, and affiliation with birth settings are additional factors that may influence the client's selection. Economic considerations are increasingly important, because the development of health maintenance organizations and physician provider networks that are aligned with selected insurance carriers may limit the selection of providers and settings from which clients may choose.

Client Education

Health Care Providers

A number of health care providers are available to clients who are pregnant. Nurses may be asked to provide information about the credentials of various providers.

- Obstetricians: Licensed medical doctors who have specialty preparation in obstetrics.
- Family practice physicians: Medical doctors who are generalists and provide prenatal care and delivery services for uncomplicated pregnancies and referrals to specialists for high-risk pregnancies.
- Nurse practitioners: Nurses who specialize in women's health and provide prenatal and postpartal care. They generally work in collaboration with obstetricians who supervise the delivery.
- Certified nurse midwives: Licensed nurses certified to provide prenatal and postpartal care and perform uncomplicated deliveries. They also generally collaborate with physicians for high-risk care.
- Lay midwives: Unlicensed women who see clients and deliver infants in the home or community setting. In some states they are required to register with the health department.

CHOICE OF DELIVERY SETTING

Nurses frequently are a source of information used by families to reach a decision regarding the choice of a setting in which to give birth. Clients may choose from among five settings:

Home Birth

Home births represent a return to a common practice of the past. Certified nurse midwives are the most common providers of these services, with medical backup provided by a physician. Extensive preparation of the home environment and the expectant family is the underlying requirement for the home to be a safe alternative to hospitalization for childbearing. Active participation in decision-making in the comfort of a familiar environment is an important advantage to a home delivery.

Free-Standing Birth Center

Free-standing birth centers are located in relatively large urban cities and frequently are owned and staffed by nurse midwives and occasionally physicians. These centers offer the atmosphere and comfort of a homelike environment and often are located close to a hospital that provides obstetric services. Expectant parents come to the center at the beginning of the labor process and are able to deliver, recover, and complete a postpartum period in a home-type room. The care provider and family work closely together during the childbirth experience to balance individual desires and safety. Empowerment related to decision-making and active participation in the birth process frequently are cited as positive family outcomes from this delivery setting. A disadvantage that bears consideration is the fact that should significant obstetric complications arise, the client may require emergency transport to a hospital.

Birth Center in a Hospital

Available as an alternative to traditional labor and delivery units, birth centers in hospitals offer services to low-risk obstetric clients in a relaxing homelike environment. Providers in this setting primarily are nurse midwives who work collaboratively with obstetricians in developing a plan of care for clients. The opportunity to blend a midwifery approach to childbearing with the availability of surgical services, a pediatrician, and a neonatal unit is very appealing to many clients.

Labor, Delivery, and Recovery Unit

Labor, delivery and recovery (LDR) units are available in hospitals providing obstetric services to both low- and high-risk clients. Attractively decorated rooms are the settings in which the client completes the labor and delivery and then begins the recovery process. The length of the postpartum stay in this type of setting may be up to 4 hours followed by transfer of the client to a traditional postpartum unit (Figure 17-13).

Labor, Delivery, Recovery, and Postpartum Unit

Labor, delivery, recovery, and postpartum (LDRP) units in hospitals are designed to enhance provision of family-centered care. Clients are admitted to a suite for the birth of the child followed by a seamless transition to mother and infant care for the entire postpartum stay. The opportunity for increased continuity of care for all family members is a strong advantage of this setting.

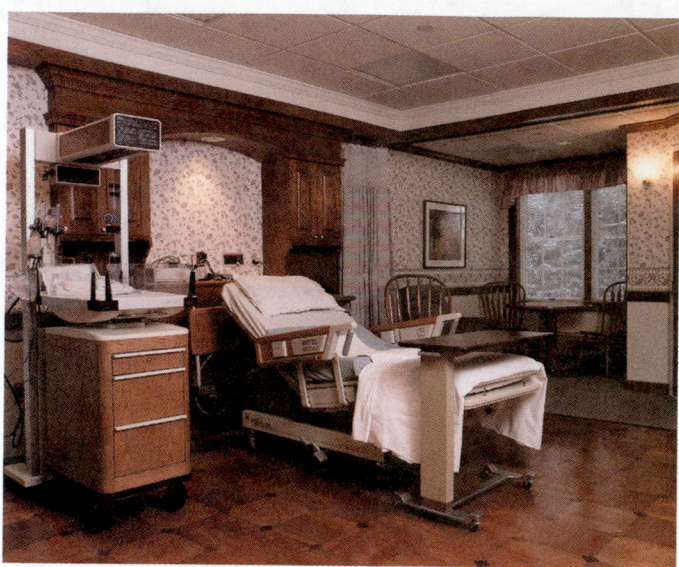

Figure 17-13 Comfortable labor, delivery, recovery units and labor, delivery, recovery, and postpartum units are the norm in many hospitals today.

NURSING IMPLICATIONS

Nurses can help clients make informed choices regarding the most appropriate model of care and preparation for the birth. Nurses can assist clients to find and connect with a particular childbirth course that matches their needs and cultual beliefs. Techniques that have been developed in various childbirth preparation courses can be used with any client. It is helpful for the nurse to know a variety of techniques for client comfort because one technique will not work with all women. The techniques and philosophies regarding childbirth can be applied to make the hospital birth environment more family-centered and provide a more satisfying experience for the mother, infant, and entire family.

Web Activities

- Acorn Accords is a coalition that fosters optimal early parenting. It is forming an initiative for prenatal parent preparation. To view the working draft of their philosophy statement, contact the website at www.thewellspring.com/coalitionprinciplePts.html.

- Go to a local bookstore and examine the books and journals for expectant parents.

- Read women's magazines and critique articles related to childbearing women.

- Search the Internet for information for expectant parents and critique the information available.

Key Concepts

- The popularity of prepared childbirth classes coincided with the woman's movement and involved both nurses and lay educators.

- Nurses who are engaged in childbirth preparation have used an expanded approach: that of perinatal educator and can obtain additional certification.

- Childbirth education employed cognitive preparation and relaxation techniques to break the fear-tension-pain cycle.

- The leading methods of childbirth education were Lamaze, Dick-Read, Bradley, and Kitzinger.

- The theoretical basis for childbirth preparation were based on relaxation theories, and pain management theories.

- Although paced breathing is the most commonly used technique to decrease stress and increase relaxation, other strategies are also used. These include neuromuscular dissociation, autogenic training, medication, biofeedback, touch, imagery, music, acupressure, labor support.

- Many perinatal educators advocate a physiological model for second stage labor. This model encourages the woman to follow her natural impulses for pushing.

- Perinatal education has included classes on early pregnancy, exercise, breastfeeding, sibling preparation, grandparent preparation, vaginal birth after a cesarean (VBAC), and infant care classes.

- One of the main purposes of perinatal education is to facilitate the woman's decision making and preparation for childbearing.

Review Questions and Activities

1. How was the psychoprophlactic method of childbirth preparation introduced in the United States?
   a. Through recommendations by the American College of Obstetricians and Gynecologists to hospitals
   b. Through recommendations by the American College of Obstetricians
   c. Through a consumer movement that began in the popular press
   d. Through an official alliance with the French Obstetric Council

   The correct answer is c.

2. Which principle of adult education by Knowles often is applied to childbirth education?
   a. Women respond best to science-based techniques
   b. Repetition of facts helps change behavior
   c. Women respond to their social networks and learn best in groups
   d. Adults learn best when there is immediate application

   The correct answer is d.

3. What are some of the unique needs that might best be accommodated by a specialized perinatal education class?

4. Which childbirth preparation method specifically involves the husband with an active role in labor?

   a. Bradley method
   b. Kitzinger's psychosexual method
   c. Lamaze method
   d. Dick-Read method

   The correct answer is a.

5. Which techniques are important in paced breathing during labor?
   a. The mother should use patterned breathing as soon as she is in labor
   b. The breathing technique needs to be individualized to the mother and her normal breathing pattern
   c. Exaggerated blowing and vocalization in patterned-paced breathing are necessary for optimal benefit
   d. Cleansing breaths should be avoided because hyperventilation may occur

   The correct answer is b.

6. Which complementary therapies are useful in preparing for childbirth?
   a. Herbal remedies
   b. Trauma release
   c. Visual imagery
   d. Rebirthing

   The correct answer is c.

References

Achterberg, J. (1985). *Imagery in healing: Shamanism and modern medicine.* Boston, MA: New Science Library.

Achterberg, J., Dossey, L., Gordon, J. S., Hegedus, C., Herrmann, M. W., & Nelson, R. (1994). *Mind-body intervention, alternative medicine: Expanding medical horizons, a report to the National Institutes of Health on alternative medical systems and practices in the United States.* Washington, DC: U.S. Government Printing Office.

American College of Obstetricians and Gynecologists (ACOG). (1985). *Exercise during pregnancy and the postnatal period.* Washington, DC: American College of Obstetricians and Gynecologists.

American College of Obstetricians and Gynecologists (ACOG). (1994). *Exercise during pregnancy and the postpartum period* (ACOG Technical Bulletin 189). Washington, DC: American College of Obstetricians and Gynecologists.

American Society for Psychoprophylaxis in Obstetrics, Inc. (ASPO/Lamaze). (1992). *National prepared childbirth statistics.* Washington, DC: ASPO/Lamaze.

Association of Women's Health, Obstetric, and Neonatal Nurses (AWHONN). (1993). *Competencies and program guidelines for nurse providers of perinatal education.* Washington, DC: Association of Women's Health, Obstetric, and Neonatal Nurses.

Bing, E. (1967). *The Lamaze method: Six practical lessons for an easier childbirth.* New York: Grosset & Dunlap.

Bradley, R. (1965). *Husband-coached childbirth.* New York: Harper & Row.

Coalition for Improving Maternity Services (CIMS). (1996). The mother-friendly childbirth initiative, Washington, DC: ASPO/Lamaze. (Also www.cims@healthy.net.)

Davis-Floyd, R. B. (1992). *Birth as an American rite of passage.* Berkeley, CA: University of California Press.

Dick-Read, G. (1979). *Childbirth without fear.* New York: Harper & Row.

DiFranco, J. T. (2000). Relaxation: Music. In F. H. Nichols & S. S. Humenick (Eds.). *Childbirth education: Practice, theory and research* (2nd ed). Philadelphia, PA: W. B. Saunders.

Edwards, M. R., & Nichols, F. H. (2000). Group process. In F. H. Nichols & S. S. Humenick (Eds.). *Childbirth education: Practice, theory and research* (2nd ed.). Philadelphia, PA: W. B. Saunders.

Geissbuhler, V., & Eberhard, J. (2000). Waterbirths: A comparative study. A prospective study on more than 2,000 waterbirths. *Fetal Diagnosis and Therapy, 15,* (5), 291–300.

Halpern, S., & Savary, L. (1986). *Sound health.* Philadelphia, PA: Harper & Row.

Hammer, R. L., Perkins, J., & Parr, R. (2000). Exercise during the childbearing year. *Journal of Perinatal Education, 9,* (1), 1–13.

Hodnet, T. E. and Osborn, R. W. (1989). Effects of continuous intrapartum support on childbirth outcomes. *Research in Nursing and Health, 12,* 289–297.

Humenick, S. S. (1981). Mastery: The key to childbirth satisfaction? A review. *Birth and the Family Journal, 8,* (2), 79–83.

Humenick, S. S. (1997). The normalcy of birth. *Journal of Perinatal Education, 6,* (4), v–vi.

Humenick, S. S. (1999). The versatility of the perinatal educator. *Journal of Perinatal Education, 8,* (2), vi–vii.

Humenick, S. S. (2000). The evolution of childbirth educator to perinatal educator. *Journal of Perinatal Education, 9,* (1), vi–vii.

Humenick, S. S., & Marchbanks, P. (1981). Validation of a scale to measure relaxation in childbirth education classes. *Birth and the Family Journal, 8,* 145.

Humenick, S. S., Shrock P., & Libresco, M. M. (2000). Relaxation. In F. H. Nichols & S. S. Humenick, (Eds.). *Childbirth education: Practice, theory and research* (2nd ed.). Philadelphia, PA: W. B. Saunders.

International Childbirth Education Association (ICEA). (1999). ICEA position paper: The role of the childbirth educator and the scope of childbirth education. *International Journal of Childbirth Education, 14,* (4), 33–41.

Jimenez, S. L. M. (2000). Comfort and pain management. In F. H. Nichols & S. S. Humenick (Eds.). *Childbirth education: Practice, theory and research* (2nd ed.). Philadelphia, PA: W. B. Saunders.

Karmel, M. (1959). *Thank you, Dr. Lamaze.* Philadelphia, PA: J. B. Lippincott.

Kitzinger, S. (1981). *The experience of childbirth.* Middlesex, England: Penguin Books.

Klaus, M., Kennell, J., & Klaus, P. (1993). *Mothering the mother: How a doula can help you have a shorter, easier and healthier birth.* Reading, MA: Addison-Wesley.

Koehn, M. L. (2000). Acupuncture and acupressure. In F. H. Nichols & S. S. Humenick (Eds.). *Childbirth education: Practice, theory and research* (2nd ed.). Philadelphia, PA: W. B. Saunders.

Knowles, M. (1980). *The modern practice of adult education.* Chicago, IL: Associated Press.

Lamaze, F. (1972). *Painless childbirth: The Lamaze method.* New York: Pocketbooks.

Leboyer, F. (1975). *Birth without violence.* Wildwood House: Aldershot.

Lutwak, R., Ney, A., & White, J. (1988). Maternity nursing and Jewish law. *MCN, 13,* (1), 44–46.

Melzak, R., & Wall, P. (1965).*Science, 150,* 971–979. *Pain mechanisms: A new theory.*

Minato, J. F. (2000). Is it time to push? Examining rest in second-stage labor. *Lifelines, 4,* (6) 20–23.

National Institutes of Health (NIH). (1997). NIH panel issues consensus statement on acupuncture, http://www.nih.gov.

Nichols, F. (2000). Paced breathing techniques. In F. H. Nichols & S. S. Humenick (Eds.). *Childbirth education: Practice, theory and research* (2nd ed.).Philadelphia, PA: W. B. Saunders.

Nichols, F., & Gennaro, S. (2000). The childbirth experience. In F. H. Nichols & S. S. Humenick (Eds.). *Childbirth education: Practice, theory and research* (2nd ed.). Philadelphia, PA: W. B. Saunders.

Odent, M. (1984). *Birth reborn.* New York: Pantheon.

Odent, M. (1990). *Water and sexuality.* London, England: Arkana.

Ondeck, M. (2000). Historical development. In F. H. Nichols & S. S. Humenick (Eds.). *Childbirth education: Practice, theory and research* (2nd ed.). Philadelphia, PA: W. B. Saunders.

Roberts. (1996). A second look at the second stage of labor. *JOGNN, 25,* (5), 415–423.

Shilling, T. (2000). Cultural perspectives on childbearing. In F. H. Nichols & S. S. Humenick (Eds.). *Childbirth education: Practice, theory and research* (2nd ed.). Philadelphia, PA: W. B. Saunders.

Simkin, P., & Frederick, E. (2000). Labor support. In F. H. Nichols & S. S. Humenick, (Eds.). *Childbirth education: Practice, theory and research* (2nd ed.). Philadelphia, PA: W. B. Saunders.

Slaninka, S. D., Galbraith, A. M., Strzelecki, S & Cockroft, M. (1996) *Journal of Perinatal Education, 5* (4), 29–36. Collaborative research projects. Effectiveness of birth preparation classes at a community hospital.

Standley, J. (1986). Music research in medical/dental treatment: Meta-analysis and clinical applications. *Journal of Music Therapy, 23,* 56.

Steffes, S. A. (2000). Relaxation: Imagery. In F. H. Nichols & S. S. Humenick (Eds.). *Childbirth education: Practice, theory and research* (2nd ed.). Philadelphia, PA: W. B. Saunders.

Steiner, S. (2000). Medication/anesthesia. In F. H. Nichols & S. S. Humenick (Eds.). *Childbirth education: Practice, theory and research* (2nd ed.). Philadelphia, PA: W. B. Saunders.

Wertz, R., & Wertz, D. (1989). Lying-in: A history of childbirth in America. New Haven, CT: Yale University Press.

Wooley, D., & Nelsson-Ryan, S. (2000). Second-stage labor. In F. H. Nichols & S. S. Humenick (Eds.). *Childbirth education: Practice, theory and research* (2nd ed.). Philadelphia, PA: W. B. Saunders.

Zwelling, E. (1996). Childbirth education in the 1990's and beyond. *Journal of Obstetric, Gynecologic, and Neonatal Nursing, 25,* (5), 425–432.

Suggested Readings

Castor, R. C. (1997). The Council of Childbirth Education Specialists, Inc. www.councilces.org

DiFranco, J. T. (2000). Biofeedback. In F. H. Nichols & S. S. Humenick (Eds.) *Childbirth education: Practice, theory and research* (2nd ed.). Philadelphia, PA: W. B. Saunders.

Enkin, M. (1995). *A guide to effective care in pregnancy and childbirth* (2nd ed.). Oxford: Oxford University Press.

Hodnett, E. (1997). *Commentary: Are nurses effective providers of labor support? Should they be? Can they be? Birth, 24,* 78–80.

Koehn, M. L. (1993). The psychoeducational model of prepared childbirth education. *AWHONN Clinical Issues, 4,* (1). Perinatal and Women's Health nursing. Philadelphia: J. B. Lippincott.

Lothian, J. A. (1999). Does Lamaze "Work"? *Journal of Perinatal Education, 8,* (3), x–xii.

Maloney, R. (1985). Childbirth education classes: Expectant parents' expectations. *Journal of Obstetric, Gynecologic, and Neonatal Nursing, 14,* 245.

Nichols, F. H. (1993). Issues in perinatal education. *AWHONN Clinical Issues, 4,* In perinatal & woman's health nursing. Philadelphia: J. B. Lippincott.

Zwelling, E. (2000). The pregnancy experience. In F. H. Nichols & S. S. Humenick (Eds.). *Childbirth education: Practice, theory and research.* (2nd ed.). Philadelphia, PA: W. B. Saunders.

Resources

Association of Women's Health, Obstetric, and Neonatal Nurses (AWHONN). (1993). *Competencies and program guidelines for nurse providers of perinatal education.* Washington, DC: Association of Women's Health, Obstetric, and Neonatal Nurses.

Beginnings: www.PrenatalEd.com

Growing Family: www.GrowingFamily.com

International Childbirth Education Association: www.icea.org

International Journal of Childbirth Education

March of Dimes (storks_nest): www.modimes.org

Mayo Clinic (click on pregnancy center): www. mayoclinic.org

National Center for Education in Maternal and Child Health: www.ncemch.org

Neonatology Information (for professionals): www.neonatology.org

Prepared childbirth education, inc: www.childbirtheducation.org

Websites for expectant parents

Baby Center (information for parents): www.babycenter.com

Fit Pregnancy: www.fitpregnancy.com

Life serve: www.Babyserv.com

Parent books: www.parentbookstore.com

Pregnancy Weekly: www.PregnancyWeekly.com

Rose Baby (products for baby care): www.rosebaby.com

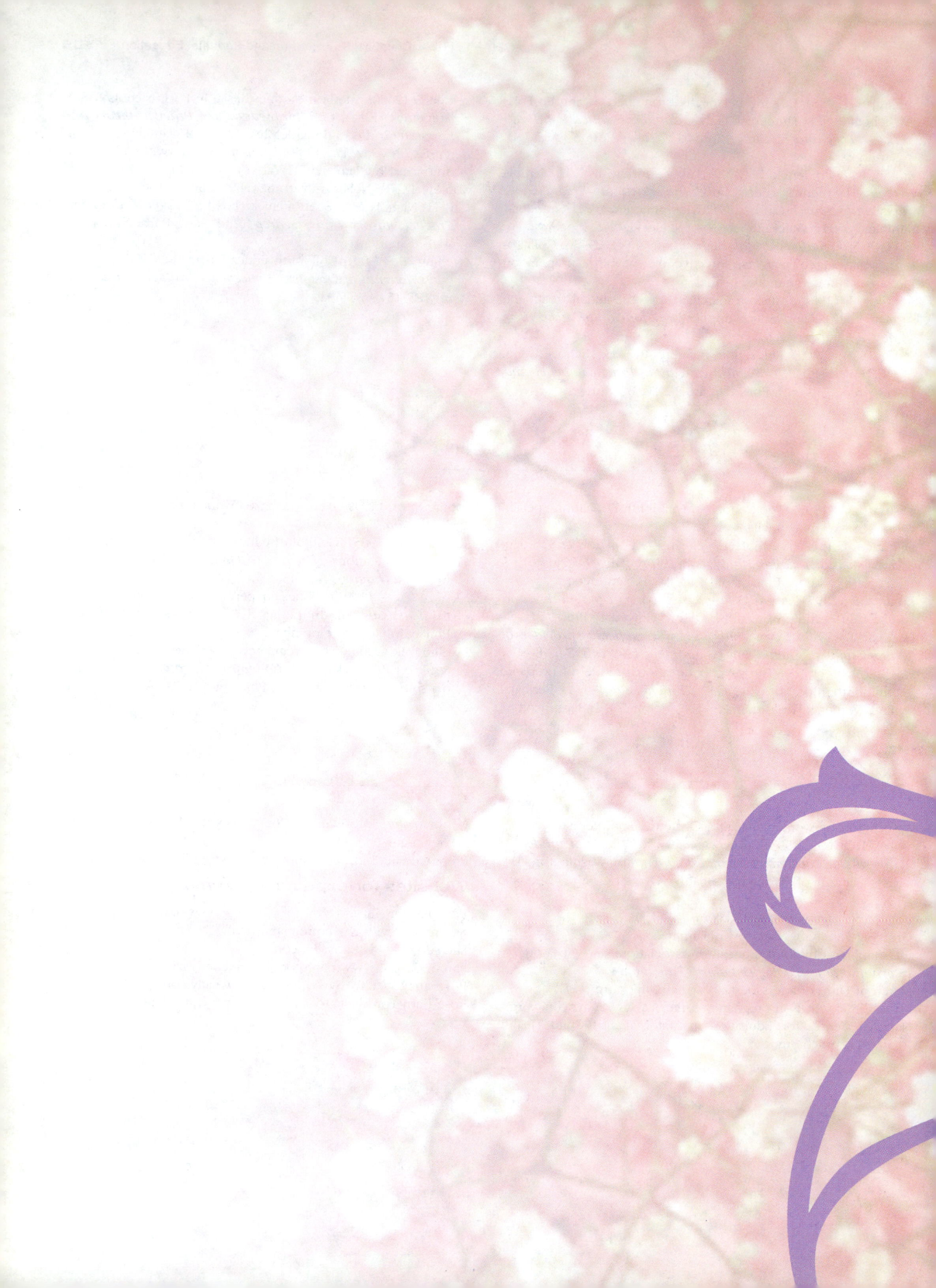

CHAPTER 18

Management and Nursing Care of the High-Risk Client

he birth of a child generally is thought of as a joyous occasion for families. Whereas many women experience an uncomplicated pregnancy and childbirth, complications can develop at any point in the pregnancy, labor and delivery, or postpartum period. These complications can lead to serious illness, injury, and even death for the pregnant woman and her baby and place tremendous stress on the family.

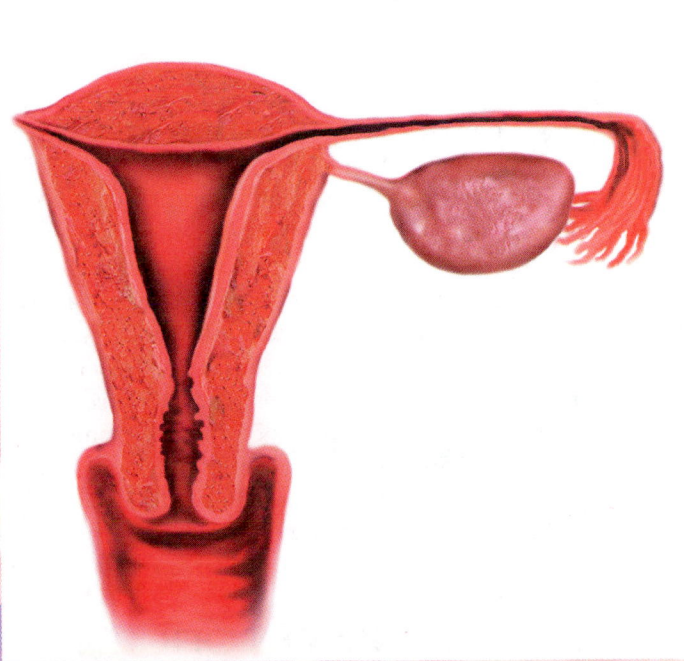

Key Terms

ABO incompatibility
Abortion
Abruptio placentae
Amniocentesis
Amnioinfusion
Cerclage ·
Chronic hypertension
Disseminated
   intravascular
   coagulation (DIC)
Dizygotic
Eclampsia

Ectopic pregnancy
Elective abortion
Gestational diabetes
HELLP syndrome
Hydramnios
Hydrops fetalis
Incompetent cervix
Induced abortion
Ketoacidosis
Low-lying placenta
Marginal placenta previa
Monozygotic

Nonimmune hydrops
   fetalis (NIHF)
Oligohydramnios
Percutaneous umbilical
   blood sampling
   (PUBS)
Placenta previa
Polyhydramnios
Postterm pregnancy
Preeclampsia
Premature rupture of
   membranes (PROM)

Preterm labor
Preterm premature
   rupture of membranes
   (PPROM)
Spontaneous abortion
Therapeutic abortion
Thrombocytopenia
Thyrotoxicosis
Type I diabetes mellitus
Type II diabetes mellitus

Competencies

Upon completion of this chapter, the reader should be able to:

1. Discuss potential complications of pregnancy-induced hypertension.
2. Apply the nursing process to plan and implement care for the woman with diabetes in pregnancy.
3. Discuss nursing interventions for the pregnant client who is experiencing vaginal bleeding.
4. Outline common risk factors for preterm labor.

The maternal mortality rate in the United States was reported to be 7.5 deaths per 100,000 live births from 1982 to 1996 (Centers for Disease Control and Prevention, 1998). Identification of common medical and obstetric conditions that place the client and fetus at increased risk for morbidity and mortality is essential in developing a nursing plan of care and achieving optimal outcomes for both. Assessment of family values, available resources, and learning needs also is a critical part of nursing care for these families who are at risk for serious health problems or even loss of a family member.

This chapter provides a broad overview of some common conditions that place mother and fetus at risk and provides guidelines for nursing assessments and interventions.

HEMORRHAGIC DISORDERS

Obstetric hemorrhage is a common cause of maternal mortality occurring in 1.4 per 100,000 live births (Chichakli et al., 1999). In this section some common causes of obstetric hemorrhage are discussed. The most common obstetric hemorrhagic event, postpartum hemorrhage, is discussed in detail in Chapter 28.

Abortion

Abortion is termination of pregnancy before fetal viability. This term usually is applied to pregnancy termination before 20 weeks' gestation. **Spontaneous abortion** refers to pregnancy termination that occurs naturally and commonly is referred to as miscarriage. Box 18-1 lists categories of spontaneous abortion.

Induced abortion is termination of pregnancy before fetal viability by medical or surgical intervention. Induced abortions may be **therapeutic**, in which case the pregnancy is terminated because of health risks to the mother in continuation of the pregnancy or for fetal disease. The terms **elective abortion** and voluntary abortion are used to describe termination of pregnancy before fetal viability at the request of the client.

Incidence

Most spontaneous abortions occur in the first trimester of pregnancy, possibly before the woman realizes she is pregnant. The exact cause of spontaneous abortion is not always identified. Approximately half of these losses are attributed to chromosomal abnormalities (Cunningham et al., 1997).

Box 18-1 Categories of Abortion

Complete

All products of conception are expelled, and uterine bleeding and cramping cease.

Incomplete

A portion of the products of conception is expelled, and a portion is retained. Bleeding and cramping continue until the uterus is evacuated.

Threatened

Uterine bleeding and cramping occur; however the products of conception have not be expelled. Cervical dilation may occur.

Missed

A pregnancy becomes nonviable; no uterine bleeding, cramping, or passage of tissue has occurred.

Habitual

Term used to describe a woman who has three or more successive spontaneous abortions.

Clinical Presentation

Vaginal bleeding or bloody discharge in the first trimester of pregnancy with or without cramping is a sign of threatened abortion, although other causes of vaginal bleeding are possible. The amount of vaginal bleeding may be minimal but may persist for days or weeks. The presence of pain along with vaginal bleeding usually is a poor prognostic indicator for continuation of the pregnancy (Cunningham et al., 1997).

Management

Clients presenting with vaginal bleeding are examined to determine if cervical dilation has occurred, making abortion inevitable. Other potential causes of vaginal bleeding to be considered are cervical lesions and physiologic bleeding at the time normal menses would occur.

The woman with a threatened abortion may be managed expectantly, which may include bed rest and serial laboratory tests to assess for decreasing hemoglobin and hematocrit levels and the presence of infection. Pain medication may be necessary in some cases.

The client who experiences a spontaneous abortion is observed closely for hemorrhage after delivery. The physician will assess the client, fetus, and placenta to determine if all products of conception have been expelled. In the

Nursing Tip

FACTORS THAT MAY PREDISPOSE WOMEN TO POSTPARTUM UTERINE ATONY

- Overdistended uterus (e.g., from multiple gestation or polyhydramnios)
- Intrapartum oxytocin administration
- High parity
- Intrapartum administration of magnesium sulfate
- History of previous postpartum hemorrhage
- Distended urinary bladder

event of retained tissue or postpartum hemorrhage, curettage may be performed.

Nursing Care

Nursing care of the client experiencing an abortion or threatened abortion includes assessing for amount and character of blood loss, assessing for signs and symptoms of shock or infection, and responding promptly to complications. Resuscitative measures may be necessary, such as volume and blood replacement, oxygen therapy, and medical and surgical interventions. All procedures and the plan of care should be communicated clearly to the client. The nurse should provide emotional support to the client and family during this difficult experience. Spiritual support,

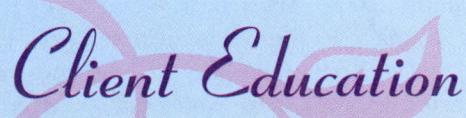

Client Education

Clients as Resources

Pregnant women are a very valuable resource in assisting with prenatal care. They are only able to help if they know what to expect. For example, some women can have spotting early in a pregnancy, and it is not serious. In other cases, spotting may suggest a missed abortion or ectopic pregnancy. You should teach clients that even if they think their spotting is not serious, they should notify their health care provider immediately so that the cause can be identified.

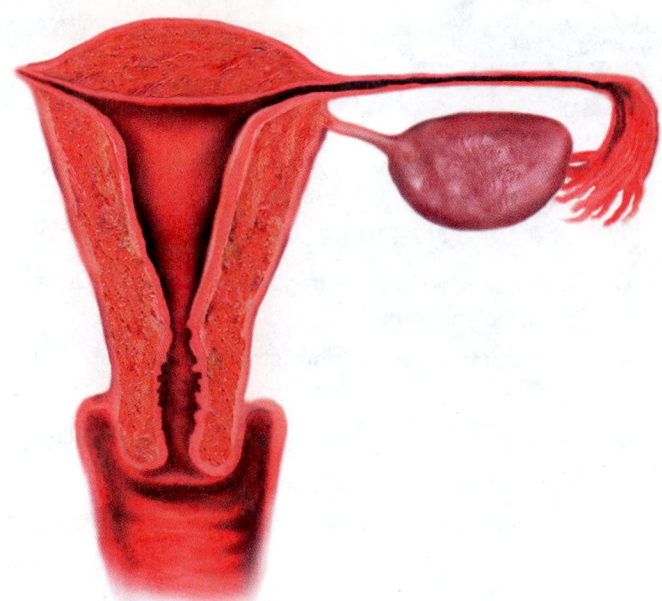

Figure 18-1 Sites of implantation in ectopic pregnancy.

client literature for education, and information about support groups where available may be offered.

Ectopic Pregnancy

Ectopic pregnancy is the implantation of the fertilized ovum in a location other than the endometrial lining (Figure 18-1). The most common implantation site is the fallopian tube; however, implantation may occur in numerous locations, including the ovaries, cervix, and abdomen (Hankins et al., 1995).

Incidence

In the United States, the rate of ectopic pregnancy in women 15 to 45 years of age is about 19.7 per 1,000 pregnancies (Tenore, 2000). Many factors contribute to ectopic pregnancy. Damage to the fallopian tubes from pelvic inflammatory disease (PID) is sited as the most common cause of ectopic pregnancy. *Neisseria gonorrhoeae* is a common causative organism implicated in the development of PID (Kamwendo et al., 2000). A previous surgery, chromosomal abnormalities of the embryo, the use of intrauterine contraceptive devices, ovarian hyperstimulation as the result of assisted reproductive technology, and peritoneal dialysis also have been implicated as causes of ectopic pregnancy (Hankins et al., 1995; Davison & Lindheimer, 1999). Ectopic pregnancy can be a life-threatening event because hemorrhage may occur with rupture if this complication is not diagnosed and treated promptly. Ectopic pregnancy is the leading cause of pregnancy-related deaths during the first trimester in the United States (American College of Obstetricians and Gynecologists [ACOG], 1999).

Clinical Presentation

The client with an ectopic pregnancy often presents with vaginal bleeding, severe abdominal and pelvic pain, tenderness of the abdomen on palpation, and severe pain on movement of the cervix on pelvic examination.

Management

Once an ectopic pregnancy is confirmed, medical management of the client may include surgery; administration of methotrexate, a drug used to resolve the pregnancy; or expectant management. Laboratory assessments include a complete blood count (CBC) to evaluate for blood loss and infection and a serum pregnancy test. The client also may undergo vaginal or abdominal ultrasonography to determine the location of the pregnancy. The site of implantation helps determine the medical management. A culdocentesis also may be performed to assess for the presence of nonclotting blood in the peritoneum (Hankins et al., 1995).

Nursing Care

Nursing care for the client experiencing an ectopic pregnancy includes assessment for the amount and character of vaginal bleeding and for signs and symptoms of shock. The nurse obtains laboratory tests and procedures, such as ultrasonography, and reports the findings to the physician promptly. The woman with an ectopic pregnancy often will experience a great deal of pain, and pain medication should be administered as ordered. The nurse prepares the client for the surgical procedure, including a clear explanation of the planned procedure. The woman who has an ectopic pregnancy may experience grief as a result of pregnancy loss. The nurse should offer emotional support, spiritual care, client literature for education, and information about support groups when appropriate.

PLACENTAL ABNORMALITIES

Abnormalities in placental form and function include placenta previa and abruptio placentae.

Placenta Previa

In placenta previa the placenta lies over or near the cervical os (Figure 18-2). There are three classes of placenta previa (Clark, 1999):

1. **Placenta previa** in which the cervical os is covered by the placenta in the third trimester of pregnancy.
2. **Marginal placenta previa** in which the placenta lies within 2 to 3 cm of the cervical os but does not cover it.

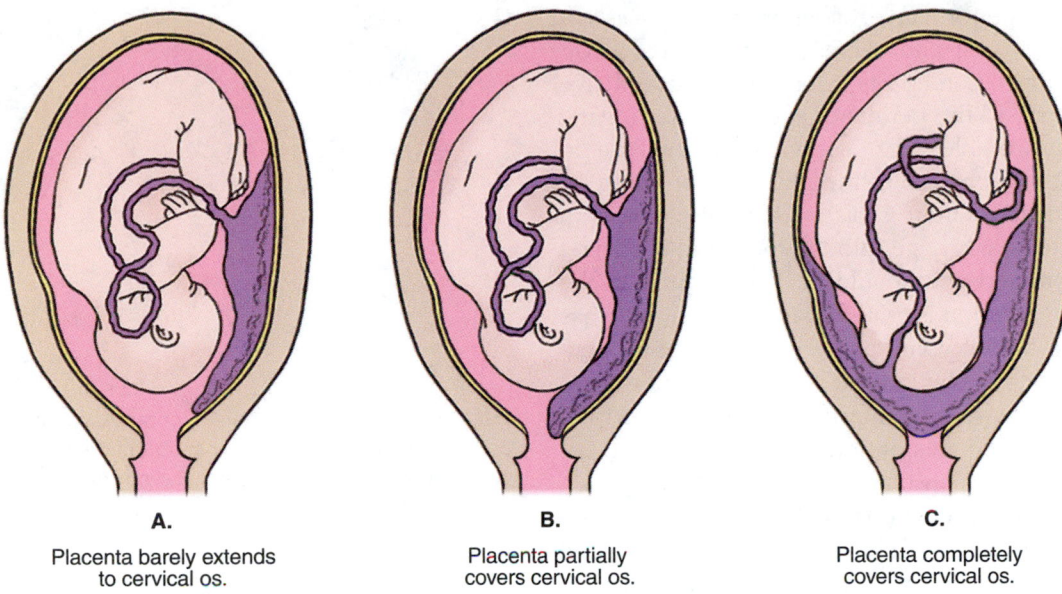

A.
Placenta barely extends
to cervical os.

B.
Placenta partially
covers cervical os.

C.
Placenta completely
covers cervical os.

Figure 18-2 Placenta previa. A. Low implantation (marginal). B. Partial placenta previa. C. Total placenta previa.

3. **Low-lying placenta** in which the exact relationship of the placenta to the cervical os is not determined, or in the case that an apparent placenta previa occurs before the third trimester of pregnancy.

Incidence

Placenta previa is a fairly uncommon complication of pregnancy; however, the consequences can be very serious for the mother and fetus. The incidence of placenta previa is reported to be from 0.3% to 2.0%, or 1 in 200 deliveries (Hendricks et al., 1999).

Previous cesarean section and induced abortion increase the risk for occurrence of placenta previa. The risk increases as the number of previous cesarean sections increases (Castles et al., 1999; Ananth, Smulian, & Vintzieleos, 1997). Multiparity and advancing age of the woman also are associated with placenta previa, as is maternal smoking (Cunningham et al., 1997; Castles et al., 1999; Ananth, Smulian, & Vintzieleos, 1999). Cocaine use by the mother is an independent risk factor for the development of placenta previa (Macones et al., 1997).

Clinical Presentation

The diagnosis of placenta previa frequently is made after onset of sudden, painless vaginal bleeding in the second or third trimester of pregnancy. The amount of bleeding varies and may stop spontaneously; however, in some cases, bleeding can be so perfuse as to life-threatening. The diagnosis of placenta previa is made after ultrasonographic examination.

Management

Management of the woman with placenta previa is determined by the degree of placenta previa present, gestational age of the fetus, and presence and amount of vaginal bleeding.

In cases of severe hemorrhage, delivery is undertaken despite the gestational age of the fetus. Volume resuscitation and transfusion of blood products frequently are required. An emergency cesarean section delivery is performed to prevent further blood loss that could occur with disruption of the placenta during vaginal delivery.

Laboring patients who present with a diagnosed placenta previa generally are delivered by cesarean section even in the absence of active bleeding. This decision is determined by the degree of placenta previa present. In the case of a marginal placenta previa, some clients are allowed to labor as long as facilities for an emergency are immediately available (Clark, 1999).

In the woman who is preterm and nonlaboring, delivery may be delayed if the bleeding has stopped or is minimal and the mother and fetus are in stable condition. The physician may order hospitalization until the time of delivery or may allow select clients to remain at home. The decision is individualized according to placental location, physician preference, and the condition of the mother and fetus (Maloni, Cohen, & Kane, 1998).

Nursing Care

Nursing care specific to the client diagnosed with placenta previa includes assessment for signs and symptoms of vaginal bleeding, performance of laboratory tests as ordered, supportive care, and client education. A peripad count is kept and recorded for clients who have active vaginal bleeding, and the perineum is checked frequently for the presence of bleeding. A significant increase in bleeding should be reported to the physician promptly. A large-bore IV catheter often is placed for quick access in the case of acute hemorrhage. Blood typing and screening generally are ordered and should be kept current in the event a blood transfusion is required. In the client who has active bleeding, blood typing and crossmatching for several units of blood may be indicated.

Occupational or recreational therapy may be helpful to the woman who requires prolonged hospitalization. Social services should be consulted for client and family concerns, financial assistance, and travel and lodging arrangements. Thorough skin assessment and attention to hygiene are important aspects of nursing care when the woman is placed on bed rest with very limited physical activity. A mattress protective to skin and tissues may be useful to prevent skin break down and to help alleviate client discomfort.

Information should be given to the client and family regarding the proposed plan of care and the potential complications that may arise from this condition. On occasion, vaginal bleeding may begin with no warning and may be hemorrhagic in nature. This emergency situation is very alarming to the woman and family members. The nurse should make an effort to prepare them for this possibility, explain the series of events that would follow in preparation for an emergency cesarean section, and provide reassurance if this should occur. Women who are discharged with placenta previa should receive instructions to return immediately in the event of uterine contractions or vaginal bleeding.

Abruptio Placentae

Abruptio placentae (abruption) is separation of the placenta from its implantation site before delivery of the fetus (Figure 18-3). Bleeding associated with a placental abruption may be concealed in a space between the now detached placenta and uterus. More often, external vaginal bleeding is present. Placental abruptions can be total, with ensuing fetal death likely, or partial, in which case a portion of the placenta remains intact and perfusion to the fetus is possible (Cunningham et al., 1997).

Incidence

Abruption occurs in about 1 in 150 deliveries (Cunningham et al., 1997). According to Chichakli et al. (1999), abruptio placentae was the leading cause of pregnancy-related deaths in the United States from 1979 to 1992.

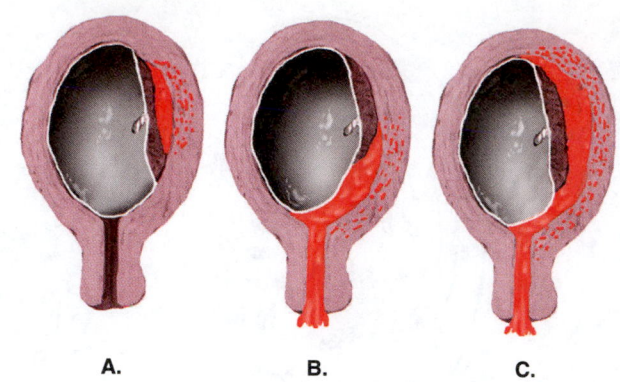

Figure 18-3 Abruptio placentae A. Central abruption, concealed hemorrhage. B. Marginal abruption, external hemorrhage. C. Complete abruption, external hemorrhage (could also be concealed).

African American women in this study had a three-fold increased risk for death compared with Caucasian women.

The condition most commonly associated with placental abruption is hypertension in pregnancy (Hauth et al., 2000). Preterm premature rupture of membranes and maternal trauma, especially associated with high-speed automobile accidents also have been associated with abruption (Reis, Sander, & Pearlman, 2000). Cocaine use during pregnancy and cigarette smoking also have been associated with a large number of placental abruptions (Cunningham, et al., 1997; Castles et al., 1999; Ananth et al., 1999).

Clinical Presentation

The diagnosis of abruptio placentae may be difficult to make and often is made only after excluding other potential causes of the presenting symptoms. Common presenting symptoms are vaginal bleeding and abdominal pain, tenderness, or rigidity. On admission assessment, fetal heart sounds may be absent or there may be a nonreassuring fetal heart pattern and high-frequency uterine contractions on electronic fetal monitoring.

The amount of vaginal bleeding present does not necessarily reflect the extent of abruption. Up to 10% of women who have an abruption present with concealed bleeding. Ultrasonographic examination to assess the presence of an abruption often is not helpful in establishing this diagnosis (Cunningham et al., 1997; Clark, 1999).

Maternal morbidity in abruption is common and can be serious. In a review of pregnancy-related mortality in the United States, placental abruption was the leading overall cause of death as a result of hemorrhage (Chichakli et al., 1999). Acute blood loss from both placenta previa and abruptio placentae can lead to shock in the mother. Decreased perfusion to the kidneys during massive blood loss may cause oliguria, which usually responds to volume resuscitation with intravenous (IV) fluids and blood. Acute

Research Highlight

Purpose

To develop a scale to measure perinatal grief intensity (PGIS) to predict the intensity of grief response to early pregnancy loss.

Method

A sample of 186 women who experienced a miscarriage before 16 weeks' gestation completed a Likert type–scale questionnaire. Factor analysis was performed.

Findings

Fourteen items were retained. Three factors were found to influence the intensity of grieving: (1) reality of the pregnancy and baby, (2) congruence between the actual miscarriage and the woman's standard of the desirable, and (3) confrontation of others, which is the ability of parents to make decisions or act in ways to increase the congruence. The most intense grief experiences were associated with parents for whom the pregnancy and baby were perceived as real, whose miscarriage experience was incongruent with the desired standard, and who perceived themselves unable to do anything about this incongruence.

Nursing Implications

The PGIS establishes beginning reliability and validity in predicting grief intensity. Although further testing will determine the usefulness with other types of pregnancy loss and establish levels of the predictive value of scores, a method of measuring perinatal grief may be helpful to nurses to determine the type of follow-up appropriate for families.

Hutti, M. H., dePacheco, M., & Smith, M. (1998). A study of miscarriage: Development and validation of the perinatal grief intensity scale. *Journal of Obstetric, Gynecologic, and Neonatal Nursing, 27,* (5), 547–555.

tubular necrosis and renal failure are serious complications that can occur when there is a delay in or inadequate treatment for blood loss and hypovolemic shock (Clark et al., 1997; Cunningham et al., 1997).

Abruption is the most common obstetric cause of **disseminated intravascular coagulation (DIC)**. This process occurs as a result of excess consumption of some components of coagulation. With the massive consumption of circulating clotting factors and activation of the fibrinolytic system the client experiences hemorrhage, end-organ ischemia, vascular permeability, and hypotension (Sisson & Ruth, 1999; Clark et al., 1997; Cunningham et al., 1997).

Neonatal complications of placenta abruptio include preterm birth, anemia, and respiratory distress syndrome (RSD) (Crane et al., 1999). The perinatal mortality rate for abruptio placentae is reported to be from 20% to 35%, accounting for a large percentage of third-trimester fetal deaths. Even when infants survive, they may be seriously affected by the decreased perfusion to the placenta and may develop neurologic sequelae (Cunningham et al., 1997).

Management

The treatment for abruptio placentae depends on the condition of the mother and fetus. When bleeding is not severe and the mother is stable, fetal status and gestational age often determine the plan of care. The physician may choose to manage the woman who is stable with a preterm fetus expectantly under close observation and may employ the use of tocolytic agents to stop uterine contractions (Clark, 1999). The viable fetus that is near full term often is electively delivered to avoid a larger abruption that could seriously compromise the fetus or result in fetal death (Cunningham et al., 1997).

In the case of acute hemorrhage, resuscitation with blood transfusion and IV fluids and immediate delivery are indicated. This life-threatening complication usually requires aggressive volume resuscitation with IV fluids, blood pressure support, oxygen therapy, and evacuation of the uterus (Clark et al., 1997).

In the event of an abruption in which there is an intrauterine fetal death, delivery will be induced once maternal stability is achieved, and the woman will be closely observed for complications.

Nursing Care

Nursing care of the client with an abruption includes an assessment of the amount and nature of vaginal bleeding. A peripad count may be indicated in the presence of ongoing bleeding. The nurse should palpate the uterus to assess for tenderness and rigidity and for the location and nature of pain. It is sometimes difficult for the client to describe the pain associated with an abruption when she also is experiencing painful uterine contractions.

In an acute bleeding episode, vital signs are monitored closely for signs of hypovolemic shock. The fetus may be compromised as a result uteroplacental insufficiency, and therefore, continuous electronic fetal monitoring usually is employed for assessment of the viable fetus. In the event of hemodynamic changes in the client or a nonreassuring fetal heart rate, resuscitative measures should be initiated by the nurse and the physician should be notified immediately.

In the case of acute blood loss, a large-bore IV catheter is indicated for fluid and possibly blood replacement. The nurse obtains ordered laboratory tests that usually include blood typing and screening or blood typing and cross-matching, a CBC, and clotting studies. A Foley catheter is indicated, with hourly intake and output measured and recorded. The nurse may prepare the client for an emergency cesarean section, as indicated.

When induction of labor is ordered as a result of intrauterine fetal loss, the nurse should ensure adequate pain relief according to the client's wishes. The nurse should be familiar with the medications used to induce labor and their potential side effects.

Once stabilized, the client should receive a thorough explanation of her condition and that of the fetus. The potential complications and proposed plan of care should be discussed with the client and family. Grief support and spiritual care should be offered to the woman and family in the event of fetal or neonatal death.

LABOR DISORDERS

Disorders that fall into this category include incompetent cervix, preterm labor, and postterm pregnancy.

Incompetent Cervix

Incompetent cervix describes the often painless dilation of the cervix in which the pregnancy is lost and may result from a congenital cause such as diethylstilbestrol (DES) exposure, or an acquired cause, such as trauma to the cervix from previous gynecologic or obstetric procedures (Iams, 1999).

Incidence

The reported incidence of cervical incompetence varies greatly but may account for 8% to 15% of spontaneous pregnancy losses (Hankins et al., 1995).

Clinical Presentation

The diagnosis of an incompetent cervix may be made after repetitive spontaneous second-trimester pregnancy losses, incidentally on an ultrasonographic examination, or acutely with the advanced cervical dilation and effacement (Iams, 1999). The client may present with complaints, such as lower abdominal pressure, bloody show, or urinary frequency. As the bag of water protrudes through the cervix, small frequent contractions may occur.

Management

Management of cervical incompetence is achieved primarily through a surgical procedure, a **cerclage**, to suture the cervix. The suture usually removed in the late third trimester of pregnancy. Contraindications to this procedure include active vaginal bleeding, rupture of membranes, active labor, chorioamnionitis, and major congenital abnormalities of the fetus (Iams, 1999). Complications such as rupture of the membranes and ensuing intrauterine infection may occur with surgical intervention (Hankins et al., 1995).

Nursing Care

Nursing care for the client with an incompetent cervix includes obtaining a complete history of the events of current and past pregnancies. The client should be observed for signs of impending delivery, such as rupture of membranes, active bleeding, and regular painful uterine contractions. Emotional support is a key element of nursing care because these clients and families often are very anxious about the well-being of the fetus. The nurse should explain the plan of care and all procedures to the client and family.

Preterm Labor and Premature Rupture of Membranes

Preterm labor is defined as labor that occurs before 37 completed weeks' gestation. **Premature rupture of membranes (PROM)** is defined as spontaneous rupture of membranes before the onset of labor. **Preterm premature rupture of membranes (PPROM)** is PROM before 37 weeks' gestation.

Incidence

Preterm births account for approximately 8% to 15% of births in the United States; worldwide, 13 million prema-

Client Education
Preterm Labor

All pregnant women should recognize the signs and symptoms of preterm labor that can be stimulated by

- Urinary tract infection
- Diarrhea
- Dehydration
- Laxatives

Nursing Alert

COMMON TOCOLYTIC MEDICATIONS AND POTENTIAL COMPLICATIONS

Magnesium sulfate:

- Respiratory depression or arrest
- Pulmonary edema
- Hypotension
- Cardiac arrest
- Profound hypotension

Beta-adrenergics (ritodrine, terbutaline):

- Hyperglycemia
- Hypokalemia
- Hypotension
- Arrhythmias
- Pulmonary edema
- Myocardial ischemia

Indomethacin:

- Gastrointestinal bleeding
- Renal failure
- Hepatitis
- Premature closure of the ductus arteriosus, necrotizing enterocolitis, and intracranial hemorrhage in the fetus or neonate

Nifedipine:

- Profound hypotension
- Possible decrease in uteroplacental perfusion

ture infants are born, accounting for the overwhelming majority of perinatal morbidity and mortality (Althabe et al., 1999; Cunningham et al., 1997; Shellhaas & Iams, 1998).

Clinical Presentation

Despite vast improvements in obstetric care the ability to predict which clients will develop preterm labor, and therefore to have an impact on its prevention, has been unsuccessful (Althabe et al., 1999). Numerous risk factors for preterm labor have been cited, including the following: multiple gestation; previous preterm labor; exposure to DES; more than one second-trimester abortion; infectious causes, such as bacterial vaginosis; pyelonephritis; cigarette smoking; poor maternal weight gain; history of cervical conization; maternal age; and maternal parity (Schieve et al., 2000; McGregor & French, 2000; Kyrklund-Blomberg & Cnattingius, 1998). The most frequently cited risk factor is a history of a previous spontaneous preterm delivery. These clients have an increased risk for preterm delivery in their current pregnancy of about 2.5 times that of a normal pregnancy. A previous preterm delivery caused by PPROM and preterm labor are significantly associated with a similar event in the current pregnancy (Mercer et al., 1999).

The client who has preterm labor may present with a variety of complaints. Common sign and symptoms of preterm labor include uterine contractions, menstrual-like

Nursing Alert

TOCOLYTIC AGENTS

Tocolytic medications can have serious adverse effects. You must be knowledgeable about the tocolytic agent and carefully monitor clients receiving these medications.

cramps, dull backache, diarrhea or intestinal cramps, increased vaginal discharge, and vaginal bleeding.

Complications of preterm labor to the mother are related largely to the tocolytic agents used in treatment. See the Nursing Alert for common medications, side effects, and complications.

Infants with birth weights of less than 1,500 g or gestational age under 34 weeks have greatly increased risks for RDS, intraventricular hemorrhage, and necrotizing enterocolitis (NEC). Long-term complications of preterm birth include bronchopulmonary dysplasia, cerebral palsy, developmental delays, blindness, and deafness (Cunningham et al., 1997). Whereas the incidence of these major complications decreases in babies born after 32 weeks' gestation, other complications, such as feeding difficulties and hypothermia, occur frequently until 35 weeks' gestation and can prolong hospitalization (Seubert et al., 1999). The preterm low-birth-weight infant generally is not discharged from the hospital until 35 to 37 postconceptional weeks, or approximately the time of the infant's original due date (Rawlings & Scott, 1996).

The economic impact of preterm births in the United States is enormous. Extended stays in the neonatal intensive care unit can cost hundreds of thousands of dollars. Estimated cost per first year of survival for premature infants ranges from $74,000 to $280,000 and is highly dependent on birth weight. The cost of hospitalization for infants having very low birth weight (less than 750 g) is approximately four times that for neonates weighing from 1,000 to 1,499 g (Rogowski, 1998). Compare this with the total birth costs of less than $10,000 for term infants at 39 to 42 weeks' gestation (Luke et al., 1996).

Management

The treatment for preterm labor is intended to improve outcomes for neonates by prolonging the pregnancy or by affecting their adaptation to the extrauterine environment. Treatment options are highly individualized and depend on physician and client preference, gestational age of the fetus, and additional medical or obstetric complications.

The medical therapies for preterm labor range from nonintervention to the use of tocolytic agents to stop preterm contractions. IV hydration and sedation may be ordered when the client initially presents with signs and symptoms of preterm labor. When labor does not progress the client may be admitted to the hospital for a period of observation. Once discharged, she most likely will be placed on bed rest or asked to modify physical activities.

The physician may order antibiotics to treat presumed or confirmed infections that can be causative factors in preterm labor. Corticosteroids may be given to the client to enhance fetal lung maturity. In the case of ongoing preterm labor, the client may receive tocolytic medication given in an attempt to stop uterine contractions.

Nursing Care

Nursing care for the woman experiencing preterm labor includes prompt and thorough assessment of the client on presentation to the hospital, obtaining or assisting in collection of laboratory specimens, administration of prescribed medications and therapies, and client education. Nursing assessment should include taking vital signs, including temperature; assessing the fetal heart rate, evaluating uterine activity, and obtaining a history of the pregnancy and events associated with the onset of the current symptoms. The client should be asked about the presence of vaginal bleeding and rupture of membranes. Common laboratory tests specific for assessment of the client who has preterm labor include urinalysis, urine culture and sensitivity, cervical cultures, and CBC. The nurse must be familiar with the actions, contraindications, and potential side effects of common medications administered in the treatment of preterm labor. The tocolytic agents frequently ordered may have serious side effects (Table 18-1).

The client who is at risk for delivering a preterm infant often is very anxious about the risks to the infant and herself and about the medical therapies ordered. Coincidental concerns often exist about separation from family and loss of income during prolonged hospitalization.

Occupational or recreational therapy often is helpful in providing diversional activities during prolonged hospi-

Table 18-1 Side Effects and Complications of Tocolytic Medications

Medication	Side Effect	Complications
Magnesium sulfate	Flushing, drowsiness, muscle weakness, blurred vision, nausea and vomiting	Pulmonary edema, respiratory depression or arrest, cardiac arrest, profound hypotension **Neonate:** hypermagnesemia
Beta-adrenergics (ritodrine, terbutaline)	Tachycardia, shortness of breath, chest pain, nausea and vomiting, diarrhea, anxiety	Pulmonary edema, arrhythmias, hyperglycemia, hypokalemia, hypotension, myocardial ischemia
Prostaglandin inhibitors	Epigastric pain, nausea and vomiting	Gastrointestinal bleeding, renal failure **Fetus or neonate:** premature closure of the ductus arteriosus, necrotizing enterocolitis, intracranial hemorrhage
Calcium channel blockers	Flushing, tachycardia	Profound hypotension, possible decrease in uteroplacental perfusion

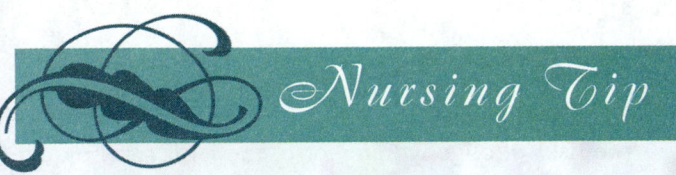

talization. Social services can be of assistance in financial, housing, and transportation concerns for the client and family.

The nurse should provide information for the client regarding the plan of care for both mother and infant to enable decision-making and reduce anxiety. It may be helpful for the client and family to speak to a health care provider from the nursery about the care planned for the neonate in the event of delivery.

Postterm Pregnancy

Postterm pregnancy is defined as a pregnancy that is greater than 42 postmenstrual weeks' gestation (Resnik & Calder, 1999).

Incidence

Approximately 4% to 14% of pregnancies are postterm and are associated with increased fetal morbidity and mortality (Resnik & Calder 1999). Some risks to the fetus include umbilical cord compression because of decreased amniotic fluid (oligohydramnios), meconium aspiration, large for gestational age fetus (macrosomia), and shoulder dystocia. The frequency of labor induction and cesarean section delivery is increased in this group of postterm clients (Cunningham et al., 1997).

Management

The postterm pregnancy may be managed initially with antepartum fetal testing beginning at 41 to 42 weeks' gestation (Resnik & Calder, 1999). Antepartum fetal surveillance tests include a nonstress test, an oxytocin challenge test, and a biophysical profile and may be scheduled weekly or twice weekly. Clients also are asked to monitor fetal movement and to notify the health care provider if they note a significant decrease in fetal activity. Induction of labor often is ordered when antepartum testing is not reassuring or the pregnancy exceeds 42 weeks' gestation.

Nursing Care

Nursing care specific to the postterm pregnant client usually includes assessing fetal well-being by performance of

fetal surveillance testing as ordered and performing induction of labor as ordered by the provider.

Antepartum surveillance tests should be carried out according to unit protocol or physician's order and the results should be reported to the physician.

Induction of labor should be performed according to unit protocol or physician's order. As with administration of any medication, the nurse must be knowledgeable about the actions, contraindications, and potential side effects of the medications that are ordered.

The posterm client and family often are anxious. Client education is a key aspect of nursing care and can provide some reassurance. The plan of care, including tests, procedures, and ordered medications, should be thoroughly explained to the client and family.

DISORDERS OF AMNIOTIC FLUID VOLUME

Disorders of amniotic fluid volume include polyhydramnios and oligohydramnios. Each condition can be a sign of negative fetal outcomes.

Polyhydramnios

The average amount of amniotic fluid at term is approximately 800 mL. **Polyhydramnios**, also referred to as **hydramnios**, is diagnosed when more than 1,500 to 2,000 mL of amniotic fluid has accumulated (Brace & Resnik, 1999).

Clinical Presentation

Amniotic fluid volume may be affected by a number of factors. During the second trimester of pregnancy the fetus swallows and urinates amniotic fluid. In most cases of severe polyhydramnios a fetal anomaly is present. These anomalies are generally those of the gastrointestinal (GI) system, inhibiting the ability of the fetus to swallow fluid, or the central nervous system (CNS), wherein increased volumes of amniotic fluid can be transferred from the spinal defect into the amniotic cavity (Cunningham et al., 1997). Idiopathic hydramnios is not associated with increased rates of poor outcomes that may be found in fetal anomalies or maternal diabetes mellitus (Panting-Kemp et al., 1999). Yancy and Richards (1994) described the effect of altitude on amniotic fluid volume and found that the average amniotic fluid volume is increased at altitudes of 6,000 feet.

The largely overdistended uterus may put pressure on the surrounding organs. In cases of excessive polyhydramnios the pregnant woman may experience dyspnea secondary to pressure on the lungs and edema of the lower extremities and vulva because of decreased venous return.

The client with polyhydramnios is at increased risk for preterm delivery secondary to contractions occurring with uterine distension.

Management

The client who has mild to moderate polyhydramnios usually does not require treatment. In severe cases of polyhydramnios that causes dyspnea or pain the client may be hospitalized. In these cases an amniocentesis may be performed to relieve these symptoms. In this procedure a catheter is placed through the maternal abdomen into the amniotic cavity and is attached to a IV tubing set, which drains amniotic fluid into a container placed at floor level. The rate of fluid drainage is controlled to avoid rapid decompression (Cunningham et al., 1997). This procedure can provide immediate symptomatic relief for the client.

Nursing Care

Nurse caring for the client with polyhydramnios includes monitoring the client for symptoms of dyspnea, abdominal pain, uterine contractions, and severe edema of the lower extremities and vulva. When a therapeutic amniocentesis is performed, the nurse assists the physician in the procedure by positioning the client and helping with the mechanism of the drainage apparatus. The nurse monitors the rate of fluid drainage, amount and characteristics of the fluid, and response of mother and fetus. The nurse ensures that the client has an opportunity to ask questions and understands the procedure.

Oligohydramnios

Oligohydramnios can occur as a result of premature rupture of membranes or may not have a clear cause. Regardless of the cause, the condition may require a decision regarding whether the fetus should remain in utero.

Clinical Presentation

When the amniotic fluid volume decreases to as little as 500 mL, the condition is termed **oligohydramnios** (Brace & Resnik, 1999). The cause of oligohydramnios is not always apparent. Any condition that prevents the fetus from making urine or that blocks the entry of urine into the amniotic sac can cause oligohydramnios. Leaking of the bag of water or frank rupture of membranes also may cause oligohydramnios. Hypertension in pregnancy, uteroplacental insufficiency, and diabetes also are factors associated with oligohydramnios in late pregnancy (Cunningham et al., 1997). The diagnosis of oligohydramnios is made by ultrasonographic examination because as the client will have no presenting symptoms.

Oligohydramnios more frequently develops late in pregnancy. The volume of fluid normally is diminished after 35 weeks' gestation. The development of oligohydramnios in early pregnancy may be an ominous sign (Cunningham et al, 1997; Brace & Resnik, 1999).

The risks of oligohydramnios to the fetus can be quite serious. Umbilical cord compression may occur, diminishing perfusion to the fetus. Adhesions can develop between the fetus and the amnion, which can cause serious fetal deformities and possibly amputation of fetal parts. The fetus also may suffer from musculoskeletal deformities as it is compressed in utero (Cunningham et al., 1997). Pulmonary hypoplasia possibly related to mechanical restriction of the fetal chest can occur in the presence of very low amniotic fluid levels (Brace & Resnik, 1999).

Management

The client who has oligohydramnios may be managed outside the hospital setting, with serial ultrasonographic evaluations and fetal surveillance testing. Once delivery is inevitable and the membranes have ruptured, an **amnioinfusion** may be performed to replace fluid in the amniotic cavity (Brace & Resnik, 1999). In this procedure crystalloid fluid is infused through an intrauterine catheter placed through the cervix into the uterine cavity. The infusion is administered in a controlled manner to prevent overdistension of the uterus.

Nursing Care

The client who has oligohydramnios and a viable fetus and is not hospitalized will require periodic evaluation of fetal well-being. Nursing care may include fetal surveillance testing, such as a nonstress test or contraction stress test. In the intrapartum period the nurse observes for fetal intolerance of labor and may assist in the performance of amnioinfusion. When amnioinfusion is ordered the nurse infuses fluid into the client's uterus by way of an intrauterine catheter at a prescribed rate. The return of amniotic fluid onto the bed linen and maternal and fetal tolerance of the procedure should be observed and documented. The nurse should provide an explanation of the plan of care to the client and family.

HIGH-RISK FETAL CONDITIONS

Fetal conditions that increase the risk for negative fetal outcomes include multiple gestation, Rh isoimmunization and ABO incompatibility, and nonimmune hydrops fetalis.

Multiple Gestation

Multiple gestation increases pregnancy risks because of the high risks for preterm labor and delivery and conditions related to prematurity.

Incidence

The incidence of multiple births in the United States is relatively infrequent yet represents a large proportion of poor pregnancy outcomes. Multiple gestation pregnancies are at increased risk for preterm delivery and intrauterine fetal demise. Maternal morbidity is significantly increased in these pregnancies (Malone & D'Alton, 1999).

The incidence of twins, triplets, and higher-order multiples has dramatically increased because of the widespread use of fertility drugs and advanced reproductive techniques (ACOG, 1998b). Twins frequently are the result of two separate ova, called **dizygotic** or "fraternal" twins. The incidence of this type of twinning is highly variable according to maternal age, race, parity, and heredity. Twins resulting from a single fertilized ovum that then divides are called **monozygotic** or "identical" twins; the incidence of identical twins is about 1 in 250 births (Cunningham et al., 1997). The process is the same in higher-order multiples, with quadruplets being the result of either one or four fertilized ova.

Clinical Presentation

In the second trimester a discrepancy between the measured fundal height and gestational age of the fetus often is the first clue that there may be a multifetal pregnancy. The diagnosis of a multiple gestation pregnancy generally is made or confirmed by ultrasonographic examination.

Multiple gestation pregnancies are at increased risk for many complications. Early pregnancy loss is more common in a multifetal pregnancy. Multiple gestations also have a greater incidence of low birth weight secondary to intrauterine growth restriction or preterm delivery (ACOG, 1998b).

Maternal complications in a multiple gestation pregnancy can be significant. The incidence of pregnancy-induced hypertension (PIH), gestational diabetes, postpartum hemorrhage, anemia, urinary tract infections (UTIs), endometritis, and need for cesarean delivery are increased in multifetal pregnancies. Among parous women, multiple gestation is associated with a two-fold increase in risk of death compared with a singleton pregnancy (Conde-Agudelo, Belizan, & Lindmark, 2000; Myatt & Miodovnik, 1999).

The incidence of spontaneous abortion is higher for monozygotic than for dizygotic twins (Cunningham et al., 1997). A further complicating condition referred to as twin-to-twin transfusion describes the process in which blood is shunted from one twin to the other. The twin who is underperfused becomes anemic, and the other, the overperfused twin, becomes polycythemic (Malone & D'Alton, 1999).

Significant weight differences can develop in twins in the second or third trimester of pregnancy, with one twin being growth restricted. The incidence of fetal death in these discordant twin pregnancies is greatly increased (Cunningham et al., 1997).

Management

The client with a multifetal pregnancy likely will be followed throughout her pregnancy with serial ultrasonographic examinations to assess for fetal growth and development. Fetal surveillance testing often is initiated late in the second trimester. The client who develops signs and symptoms of preterm labor and whose fetus develops complications often will be managed in the hospital setting, which allows for closer and more frequent observation.

The intrapartum period can be a particularly risk-filled time in the multifetal pregnancy. These pregnancies are at increased risk for complications, such as fetal malpresentation, dysfunctional labor, PIH, abruptio placentae, umbilical cord prolapse, cesarean delivery, and endometritis (Conde-Agudelo, Belizan, & Lindmark, 2000; Myatt & Miodovnik, 1999). In the intrapartum period, electronic fetal monitoring is employed to evaluate for fetal tolerance to labor or evidence of cord prolapse. After vaginal delivery of the first twin the client is reassessed to determine if vaginal delivery of the second twin is possible and imminent. Vaginal delivery of the second twin may be minutes to hours after the first delivery. The client may require cesarean section for the second twin if it is in a nonvertex position (Malone & D'Alton, 1999).

Nursing Care

Outpatient nursing care for the client with multifetal pregnancy focuses on assessment of the client at each visit for signs and symptoms of possible complications, such as threatened abortion, PIH, and preterm labor. Once the decision is made to initiate fetal surveillance testing, the nurse performs nonstress tests or contraction stress tests.

Clients who are admitted to the hospital for complications such as PIH or preterm labor receive care as discussed in the applicable sections of this chapter. The client admitted for labor and planned vaginal delivery usually receives continuous electronic fetal monitoring to provide assessment data for both uterine activity and fetal tolerance to labor. Adequate personnel to attend to the mother and to each neonate should be available at the time of delivery. The client and family should be informed of the potential for cesarean delivery and all questions should be answered.

Rh Isoimmunization and ABO Incompatibility

Immunization, or sensitization, occurs when fetal blood enters the maternal circulation causing antibodies to be formed in the maternal blood. Once formed, these antibodies are able to cross the placenta into the fetal circulation and attack fetal erythrocytes, with resulting hemolysis. **Rh sensitization** is the most common and most significant cause of maternal immunization and hemolysis in the fetus or newborn (Bowman, 1999). In this process an Rh-negative mother, or a mother with absent $Rh_o(D)$ antigen, who is carrying an Rh-positive fetus forms anti-D antibodies whenever fetal erythrocytes enter the maternal bloodstream. A very small amount of Rh-positive fetal blood in the maternal bloodstream can result in the formation of antibodies (Duffy, 1999). The amount of hemolysis that results varies, with severe hemolysis causing fetal anemia. The severely affected fetus develops **hydrops fetalis** in which the fetus and placenta have severe edema; the fetus also may develop pleural and cardiac effusions, cardiac enlargement, hepatomegaly, and splenomegaly (Cunningham et al., 1997).

Clinical Presentation

The injection of fetal blood into the maternal circulation occurs most commonly at the time of delivery but may occur during the course of the pregnancy. A significant number of women who become Rh immunized do so at about 28 weeks' gestation or within 3 days after delivery. Approximately 75% of women have some evidence of a transplacental hemorrhage during the pregnancy or in the immediate postpartum period (Bowman, 1999). Sensitization may occur in the antepartum period after abortion; after an invasive procedure, such as amniocentesis; or in the disruption of the placenta with abruption or placenta previa (Cunningham et al., 1997). Once antibodies are formed, subsequent pregnancies are at risk for hemolytic disease of the fetus and newborn.

ABO incompatibility is a less serious form of isoimmunization that may occur when a mother who has type O blood is pregnant with a fetus who has type A or B blood. The mother may form antibodies that can lead to hemolysis in the fetus and neonate. These infants may develop hyperbilirubinemia, requiring phototherapy. The development of hydrops in ABO incompatibility is rare (Bowman, 1999).

Management

Pregnant women undergo routine screening for sensitization at the first prenatal visit when blood is drawn for blood typing, determination of Rh factor, an antibody titer test, or indirect Coombs test (ACOG, 1996b). The presence of anti-$Rh_o(D)$ antibodies on the laboratory test results indicates sensitization has occurred and alerts the clinician to the possibility of an affected fetus. The fetus is monitored throughout the pregnancy, and the mother has repeated titer tests. A titer of 1:8 or higher usually indicates the

need for further testing and evaluation (Cunningham et al., 1997).

The client who has titer values that are increasing will undergo repeated ultrasonography to evaluate fetal growth, amniocentesis, or percutaneous blood sampling to evaluate fetal condition. In an **amniocentesis** fluid is withdrawn from the uterus with a needle to evaluate for the presence and amount of bilirubin, which is evidence of hemolysis. Amniotic fluid with high levels of bilirubin may indicate a fetus who needs immediate treatment to survive. **Percutaneous umbilical blood sampling (PUBS)** is a direct sampling of fetal blood from the umbilical cord guided by ultrasonography. The severely affected fetus may undergo intrauterine fetal transfusion. This is accomplished by transfusion of blood into the fetal peritoneal cavity or directly into the umbilical vein (ACOG, 1996b). Intravascular transfusion into the umbilical vessels is associated with good long-term outcomes (Grab et al., 1999).

Preterm delivery may be necessary for the severely affected fetus. The neonate is evaluated at birth for severity of hemolytic disease of the newborn and may require treatment ranging from phototherapy to exchange transfusion.

The client with negative indirect antibody test results on entry into prenatal care usually is retested at 28 weeks' gestation. If the test results remain negative, at that time the mother is given a prophylactic dose of $Rh_o(D)$ immune globulin (RhoGAM) (ACOG, 1999a). Administration of this Rh antibody can prevent an active antibody response by providing passive immunity to the mother (Bowman, 1999).

In the postpartum period, clients who are Rh-negative are considered for postpartum administration of RhoGAM. Mothers of infants who are Rh-positive will receive RhoGAM as prophylaxis within 72 hours after delivery. Women experiencing a first-trimester pregnancy loss or those undergoing invasive procedures, such as amniocentesis or fetal blood sampling, also should receive RhoGAM (ACOG, 1999).

Nursing Care

In the antepartum period the nurse should evaluate routine maternal laboratory tests and alert the primary care provider of the maternal blood type in the $Rh_o(D)$-negative client. It is very important that RhoGAM be administered as ordered at approximately 28 weeks' gestation. The administration of RhoGAM should be documented in the client's medical records.

Clients who are determined to be sensitized will need thorough explanation of the implications of Rh isoimmunization and the plan of care for the pregnancy. The invasive procedures described previously that may be performed in the severely affected fetus are very anxiety-provoking for most clients. The nurse should provide support to the mother and family as the mother undergoes these procedures.

In the postpartum period the nurse obtains maternal and neonatal laboratory values, assesses the need for RhoGAM, and administers the prophylactic dose as ordered by the primary care provider.

Nonimmune Hydrops Fetalis

Nonimmune hydrops fetalis (NIHF) is severe edema of the fetus that is not the result of isoimmunization. This syndrome has many different causes, including fetal cardiac anomalies; fetal heart rate abnormalities; chromosomal abnormalities; fetal malformations; twin-to-twin transfusion; and viral infections, such as parvovirus or herpes infection (Wilkins, 1999).

Clinical Presentation

The diagnosis of NIHF initially is made by ultrasonographic examination. Further testing is performed in an attempt to determine the cause of NIHF. Maternal blood tests are performed to assess for maternofetal hemorrhage and infection. PUBS is performed to evaluate the fetus for hematologic, genetic, or infectious causes. Many cases of NIHF ultimately will result in intrauterine fetal demise, with a reported mortality rate of greater than 50% (Wilkins, 1999). As reported by Rodis et al. (1998), NIHF occurring early in pregnancy may spontaneously resolve before term; otherwise treatment largely is based on the cause.

Management

Once a determination of the cause of NIHF is made, treatment is directed toward resolution of the cause if possible. When disturbances of fetal heart rate are determined to be a causative factor, medications (such as digoxin or an antidysrhythmic agent) may be administered to the mother to improve fetal cardiac function (Cunningham et al., 1997). Anemia may result from hematologic or infectious causes and is treated much the same as is anemia caused by Rh isoimmunization, which has been discussed previously.

Nursing Care

Once the diagnosis of hydrops is made the nurse may assist in obtaining a detailed medical history from the client in an effort to identify potential causative factors. Nurses caring for the pregnant client whose fetus has NIHF should provide explanations for the disease process and the proposed plan of care and allow the client and family an opportunity to ask questions. The prognosis for the fetus often is poor. The nurse should offer emotional support to the client and family. In the event of fetal or neona-

tal death the client should be offered additional support, such as client educational materials, spiritual support, and information on support groups if available.

HYPERTENSION

Over 20 large clinical trials involving more than 50,000 participants have established that antihypertensive treatment in adults with mild to moderate hypertension reduces mortality and morbidity (Murrow et al., 2000). Few randomized trials have been undertaken to examine issues related to pregnancy and hypertension.

Terminology used in describing hypertension in pregnancy has changed over many years of studying this disease process. The National High Blood Pressure Education Program Working Group on High Blood Pressure in Pregnancy (2000) recently published a report that includes classification, pathophysiology, and management of the hypertensive disorders of pregnancy. Hypertension as defined by this group is a blood pressure 140 mm Hg systolic or higher or 90 mm Hg diastolic or higher. The classifications developed by the group are as follows:

- Chronic hypertension is defined as hypertension that occurs before pregnancy or is diagnosed before 20 weeks' gestation. Hypertension diagnosed for the first time during pregnancy that persists beyond the postpartum period also is classified as chronic hypertension.

- Preeclampsia-eclampsia is a pregnancy-specific syndrome usually occurring after 20 weeks' gestation. The diagnosis is determined by (1) increased blood pressure, over 140 mm Hg systolic or over 90 mm Hg diastolic in a woman who has had normal blood pressure before 20 weeks' gestation; and (2) proteinuria, which is defined as more than 0.3 g of protein in a 24-hour urine collection. **Eclampsia** is the occurrence of seizures in a pregnant woman who has preeclampsia that cannot be attributed to another cause. The presence of edema has long been included as one of the classic signs of preeclampsia but has been excluded as a marker by this Working Group because it is a common finding in normal pregnancies.

- Preeclampsia superimposed on chronic hypertension is "highly likely" with the findings of (1) women with hypertension and no proteinuria before 20 weeks' gestation that have new onset of proteinuria; and (2) women who have hypertension and proteinuria before 20 weeks' gestation who develop any of the following: (a) sudden increase in proteinuria, (b) sudden increase in blood pressure, (c) thrombocytopenia, (d) increase in alanine aminotransferase or asparate aminotransferase.

REFLECTIONS FROM A FAMILY

"I was really excited to find out I was pregnant. My husband and I had planned a family for a long time. Then my wonderful pregnancy turned into a horror show when I developed preeclampsia. The doctor was not able to control my condition at home. I was admitted to the hospital at 32 weeks' gestation, and was told I would need to stay in the hospital on bed rest until my due date. I cannot explain how that changed my life. I went from being happy and excited to being full of dread and fear. Luckily, the nurses on the unit where I was hospitalized were able to teach me what to expect. It reduced my fear tremendously."

❧ Gestational hypertension is used to describe blood pressure elevation occurring for the first time after midpregnancy and without proteinuria. This diagnosis may change to that of preeclampsia if other symptoms develop. The definitive diagnosis of gestational hypertension can only be made if the hypertension has resolved after 12 weeks postpartum.

Incidence

Hypertension occurs in 6% to 8% of pregnancies and is the second leading cause of maternal mortality in the United States, accounting for 15% to 18% of deaths (ACOG, 1996a; Berg et al., 1996). Complications of PIH are outlined in Table 18-2.

Clinical Presentation

Many theories regarding the cause of PIH have been proposed but none proven. PIH has been shown to occur more commonly in the primipara, in women with pregestational diabetes mellitus, in multiple gestation pregnancies, and in older women who have an increased incidence of chronic hypertension (Myatt & Miodovnik, 1999; Sibai et al., 2000a; Sibai et al., 2000b; Abu-Heija, Jallad, & Abukteish, 2000). The only known "cure" for PIH is delivery of both fetus and placenta.

Preeclampsia is a disease characterized by generalized vasospasm, a significant decrease in circulating blood volume, and an activation of the coagulation system. The end

Table 18-2 Potential Complications of Pregnancy-Induced Hypertension

Organ or System	Potential Complications
Cardiopulmonary	Pulmonary edema, hypertensive crisis, stroke
Renal	Decreased glomerular filtration, increased plasma uric acid and creatinine, necrosis (rarely)
Neurologic	Retinal detachment (rarely), cerebral edema, seizures, cerebral hemorrhage, coma
Hematologic	Thrombocytopenia, hemorrhage, disseminated intravascular coagulation
Hepatic	Hematoma, rupture
Fetus	Intrauterine growth restriction, hypoxia, intrauterine death, prematurity

result of these changes is hypertension, decreased perfusion, and resultant ischemia particularly to the placenta, kidneys, liver, and brain (National High Blood Pressure Working Group, 2000).

The fetus may be significantly impacted by decreased uteroplacental perfusion. In cases of long-standing hypertension the fetus is at increased risk for mortality and morbidity, such as intrauterine growth retardation. The additional complication of superimposed preeclampsia significantly increases the risk to the fetus (National High Blood Pressure Working Group, 2000). Delivery of the fetus may be indicated by worsening maternal or fetal condition, placing the fetus of the client who has preeclampsia at increased risk for low birth weight and prematurity.

Renal blood flow and the glomerular filtration rate are decreased in preeclampsia. Proteinuria is a common finding in preeclampsia but is highly variable from hour to hour, and thus, is not a sensitive marker for severity of the disease process. Oliguria may occur in severe disease. Renal insufficiency is rarely severe enough to cause permanent damage, and the client usually will have complete recovery of renal function after delivery (Cunningham et al., 1997; Roberts, 1999).

The coagulation effects of preeclampsia may include **thrombocytopenia,** a decrease in platelets to less than 100,000, placing the client at increased risk for hemorrhage. This coagulation problem may occur at any time during pregnancy. Symptoms may antecede blood pressure elevation.

HELLP Syndrome is a complication of pre-eclampsia/eclampsia. In 1982, Weinstein first described 29 cases of severe preeclampsia/eclampsia complicated by hemolytic anemia, elevated liver enzymes, and low platelet counts.

This syndrome was given the acronym HELLP to describe its clinical presentation of Hemolysis of red blood cells, Elevated Liver enzymes, and low Platelet count. Since 1982, numerous cases of this syndrome have been reported.

Boston and Sibai (2001) discuss a classification system for HELLP syndrome. Class 1 is the most severe and occurs when the platelet count reaches a low of <50,000 per mm^3. Class 2 occurs when the platelet count reaches a low between 51,000 and 100,000 per mm^3. Class 3 occurs when the platelet count reaches a low of 101,000 to 150,000 per mm^3. These classes are used to predict postpartum disease recovery, risk of recurrence of HELLP syndrome, perinatal outcome, and the need for plasmaphoresis.

At University of Tennessee in Memphis, where much research has been done related to PIH and its complications, they have developed the following criteria for the diagnosis of HELLP syndrome. The criteria for hemolysis are abnormal peripheral blood smear; a total bilirubin of 1.2 mg.d/L or greater; and LDH (lactic dehydrogenase) of 600 U/L. To meet the criteria for elevated liver enzymes requires serum aspartate aminotransferase of ≥ 70 U/L; and a LDH of >600 U/L (Barton & Sibai, 2001).

The incidence of HELLP syndrome is significantly higher in the Caucasian population and multiparous women as well as among pre-eclamptics who are being managed conservatively (Barton & Sibai, 2001).

Clinical manifestations of HELLP syndrome include remoteness from term with right upper quadrant pain, some have nausea and vomiting, and others have nonspecific flu-like symptoms. Clients with HELLP syndrome usually exhibit significant weight gain and generalized edema. They usually have severe hypertension.

Pathophysiology of HELLP syndrome involves hemolytic anemia, this type of anemia can occur in other conditions besides HELLP syndrome and may confuse the diagnosis. The elevated liver enzymes are a result of liver involvement. The most common liver lesion is liver necrosis. Periportal hemorrhage is associated with fibrin deposition. Steatosis or fat degradations is associated significantly with abnormalities in platelet count Barton & Sibai, 2001).

Management of HELLP syndrome involves stabilization of the maternal condition, evaluation of fetal well being, and estimation of fetal lung maturity. Management may be aggressive or conservative. Aggressive management includes delivery of the infant by Cesarean Section as quickly as the maternal condition is stabilized.

Conservative management includes use of antihypertensives and MgSO4. The predominate reason for terminating the pregnancy is fetal distress or fetal demise. Usually the pregnancy is not terminated due to maternal conditions. Potential risks associated with conservative management are abruption of the placenta, pulmonary edema, acute renal failure, eclampsia, perinatal death, and maternal death (Barton & Sibai, 2001).

Complications of HELLP syndrome may include delayed wound closure, eclampsia, and hematoma or infarction of the liver. If a hepatic hematoma occurs, there is potential for liver rupture. Other severe complications include DIC, acute renal failure, severe ascites, pulmonary edema, pulmonary effusions, cerebral edema, retinal detachment, and laryngeal edema (Barton & Sibai, 2001).

HELLP syndrome can occur in the antepartum or postpartum period. If the woman survives this complicated pregnancy, there is a 19-27% risk of developing recurrent HELLP syndrome in future pregnancies (Barton and Sibai, 2001).

Management

Clients who develop mild elevation of blood pressure in pregnancy may be managed conservatively by the physician and placed on bed rest at home, with increased frequency of office visits and laboratory evaluations (National Heart, Lung and Blood Institute, 2000). Once the client is admitted to the hospital for evaluation and management of preeclampsia, the course of treatment is highly individualized and based on disease severity. A client with mild preeclampsia may be managed on an antepartum unit, with evaluation for signs and symptoms of worsening disease, fetal evaluation, and laboratory testing. In the case of worsening or severe preeclampsia the client often is managed with administration of magnesium sulfate, frequent targeted assessments, laboratory tests, electronic fetal monitoring if indicated by the gestational age, and possibly the induction of labor. Those clients who are more severely affected are likely to be found on the labor and

Nursing Tip

TARGETED ASSESSMENTS IN CLIENTS WITH PREECLAMPSIA

- Blood pressure measurement
- Urine dipstick evaluation for protein
- Intake and output measurements
- Physical assessments for:
  presence and location of edema
  Deep tendon reflexes
  Presence of headache and visual changes
  Presence of nausea, vomiting, and epigastic or right upper quadrant pain
- Fetal evaluation appropriate for gestational age and fetal well-being

delivery unit where they can receive more intensive nursing care.

Nursing Care

Skilled nursing assessments are necessary for the pregnant woman with preeclampsia. A thorough physical assessment should be performed at the start of each shift, followed by frequent targeted assessments. Magnesium sulfate, antihypertensive agents, and medications for cervical ripening and induction of labor are administered as ordered. The nurse must be familiar with the actions of, side effects of, and complications that may arise from the use of these medications. Laboratory tests should be obtained as ordered, and abnormal results should be reported to the physician promptly. Significant findings from nursing assessments also should be reported promptly (see the Nursing Alert).

Client and family education should begin as soon as the diagnosis is made. Education should include an explanation of the disease process; signs and symptoms of worsening disease; proposed course of treatment, including physical and laboratory assessments; medications; potential complications for the client and fetus; and the plan for delivery, as indicated. If the infant is to be delivered preterm, it is very important for the client and family to be made aware of the proposed plan of care for the baby.

ENDOCRINE DISORDERS

Endocrine disorders may predate pregnancy or be precipitated by pregnancy. Either way, these disorders can have profound effects on the pregnant woman and her fetus.

Diabetes

Diabetes has serious implications for the mother and fetus even though survival rates for both have improved dramatically over the past few decades.

Incidence

Diabetes results in complications in 2% to 3% of all pregnancies in the United States and is the most common medical complication in pregnancy (ACOG, 1994; Cunningham et al., 1997). Pregnancy outcomes for women with diabetes have improved dramatically since the beginning of the 20th Century, when perinatal survival was approximately 40% and maternal death was common (Cunningham et al., 1997). The use of insulin in the 1920s greatly impacted maternal survival but had little impact on perinatal survival (Inzucchi, 1999). In the late 1940s the development of the Caucasian classification of diabetes, which is based on age of onset, duration, and vascular complications of diabetes, demonstrated fetal risk proportional to severity of the disease. Prediction of pregnancy outcome

and timing of the delivery on an individual basis improved perinatal survival rates to about 85% by the late 1950s (Cunningham et al., 1997). The improvement in survival rates has now reached mortality rates similar to those in normal pregnancy after accounting for fetal malformations, which occur approximately four times more often in women with pregestational diabetes (ACOG, 1994). Although death in the pregnant woman with diabetes is rare, the mortality rate is greatly increased compared with that of the general population. Death often is the result of diabetic ketoacidosis, concomitant hypertension or PIH, and complications associated with pyelonephritis (Cunningham et al., 1997).

Clinical Presentation

Diabetes is classified into three categories: **Type I diabetes mellitus**, or insulin-dependent diabetes; **Type II diabetes mellitus**, or non–insulin-dependent diabetes; and **gestational diabetes**, or diabetes diagnosed during pregnancy. Type I diabetes, is an immune disorder in which the beta cells of the pancreas are destroyed, resulting in a lack of insulin secretion. This type of diabetes is most often diagnosed before the age of 30 years and requires lifelong insulin therapy and dietary management. Type II diabetes, is characterized by abnormal insulin secretion and insulin resistance and most often is found in persons over the age of 40 years and in overweight individuals. This type of diabetes may be managed by diet alone or with oral hypoglycemic agents, although oral hypoglycemic agents are contraindicated during pregnancy. Gestational diabetes is the onset of abnormal carbohydrate metabolism diagnosed during pregnancy. Approximately 90% of clients with diabetes treated during pregnancy have gestational diabetes (Inzucchi, 1999; Kendrick, 1999; ACOG, 1994).

In general, pregnant women with any form of diabetes are at increased risk for additional maternal, fetal, and neonatal complications. Women with pregestational Type I diabetes are at increased risk for the development of preeclampsia and adverse neonatal outcomes, and the rates of these complications increase with disease severity (Sibai, 2000). Hypoglycemia generally occurs with greater frequency and severity in early pregnancy (Inzucchi, 1999). This increase in hypoglycemia may be related to the strict glycemic control attempted in this population but also may be induced by nausea and vomiting associated with pregnancy and an increased sensitivity to insulin in the first trimester (Kendrick, 1999).

The pregnant woman who has diabetes has an increased incidence of UTIs. Screening for asymptomatic bacteriuria may reduce the impact of this complication. The incidence of hydramnios also is more common in women who have diabetes (Moore, 1999).

Approximately 1% of diabetic pregnancies are affected by ketoacidosis. This complication is more common in the pregnant woman who has diabetes (Inzucchi, 1999). **Ketoacidosis** is diagnosed when glucose levels are greater than 300 mg/100 mL, positive serum ketones are at a level of 1:4, and metabolic acidosis is present (Moore, 1999). This life-threatening condition may result from poor compliance, hyperemesis gravidarum, infection, or use of beta-sympathomimetic drugs or corticosteroids (Moore, 1999). Diabetic ketoacidosis caries a perinatal mortality rate of approximately 20%, making prompt recognition and treatment critical (Cunningham et al., 1997).

The major causes of fetal death are congenital malformations, RDS, extreme prematurity, and unexplained stillbirth during the antepartum period (Cunningham et al., 1997; Moore, 1999). Perinatal mortality, especially late fetal death, is significantly increased for the fetus of the woman with Type II diabetes (Cundy et al., 2000).

From 15% to 45% of infants of mothers who have diabetes may be at increased risk for *macrosomia,* defined as a fetal weight of 4,000 g or higher, and therefore may be at increased risk of a difficult delivery (Moore, 1999).

Hypoglycemia occurs in approximately 30% to 50% of neonates and may be manifested immediately after delivery and for the next 24 hours of life. The incidence of hypoglycemia is increased significantly in infants of mothers with poor glucose control in the antepartum period and elevated glucose levels during labor (Inzucchi, 1999). Infants of mothers who have diabetes also may develop significant hypocalcemia in the first few days of life, the cause of which has not yet been clearly determined (Moore, 1999). Hyperbilirubinemia is common, occurring in 20% to 25% of infants born to mothers who have diabetes.

Infants of mothers who have diabetes are at increased risk for RDS because of physiologic pulmonary immaturity (Inzucchi, 1999). This risk is taken into account in the determination of planned deliveries and care is taken to avoid delivery of a premature infant.

Management

Screening for gestational diabetes is a routine test in pregnancy that usually is performed at 26 to 28 weeks' gestation. A serum glucose measurement is obtained 1 hour after administration of 50 g of glucola. A serum glucose level of 140 mg/dL is considered abnormal and is followed up with a 3-hour glucose tolerance test with administration of 100 g of glucola (ACOG, 1994) (Box 18-2).

Management of the pregnant woman who has diabetes is focused on tight glycemic control and evaluation of fetal well-being throughout the pregnancy. Prenatal visits are scheduled with greater frequency than in a normal pregnancy. Control of diet is an essential aspect of client management, and nutritional counseling regarding a dia-

Box 18-2 Diagnostic Criteria for the 3-Hour Glucose Tolerance Test

	Fasting	1-Hour	2-Hour	3-Hour
Results (mg/dL)	105	190	165	145

For results to be considered abnormal, two of the values must exceed the normal values listed here.

betic diet is critical in this effort. The goals for glycemic control include fasting blood glucose levels consistently less than 105 mg/dL and 2-hour postprandial levels of less than 120 mg/dL (ACOG, 1994). The woman is asked to monitor her blood glucose levels several times daily and to record her dietary intake. Insulin therapy usually is begun when the prescribed diabetic diet does not result in a consistent fasting glucose level of less than 105 mg/dL or a 2-hour postprandial glucose of less than 120 mg/dL (ACOG, 1994). Women with poorly controlled diabetes or concomitant hypertension usually are hospitalized.

In the antepartum period the pregnant woman who has diabetes typically receives serial ultrasonographic evaluations of fetal growth and additional fetal surveillance testing, such as a nonstress test, an oxytocin challenge test, or a biophysical profile, beginning at about 28 to 34 weeks' gestation (Moore, 1999). Fetal surveillance may be ordered earlier than 26 weeks' gestation for clients with uncontrolled diabetes or those with additional complications (ACOG, 1994).

Delivery timing is individualized and ideally occurs around term. Maintaining maternal glucose levels within the normal range during the intrapartum period is important to avoid stimulation of the fetal pancreas, with resulting fetal or neonatal hypoglycemia. In the client who has Type I diabetes, long-acting insulin is avoided during labor and an infusion of regular insulin along with an IV glucose infusion may be ordered to be administered by way of infusion pump (Moore, 1999). Blood glucose is checked frequently during this period, and adjustments are made to the infusion. Additional boluses of insulin may be ordered as needed.

The increased insulin resistance occurring in the pregnant woman who has diabetes often resolves in a matter of a few hours after delivery. The insulin infusion generally is discontinued at the time of delivery, and many women will not require insulin during the first 24 hours. Because clients with type I diabetes can have sharp decreases in insulin requirements during the first 24 hours after delivery, the insulin dose is titrated to measured blood glucose levels in the immediate postpartum period (Inzucchi, 1999).

Pregnant women who develop gestational diabetes may be counseled about the strong possibility of developing overt diabetes in the next 20 years (Buchanan & Kjos,

1999). It is important that a 1-hour glucose tolerance test be performed 6 to 8 weeks postpartally to ensure return to normoglycemia.

Nursing Care

Antepartum nursing care of the pregnant woman who has diabetes may include reviewing blood glucose values obtained between prenatal visits and obtaining blood glucose values at the time of the visit. All pregnant women should have routine screening of blood glucose levels. Nursing care also often will include performance of fetal surveillance testing, such as a nonstress test or an oxytocin challenge test, as ordered. Nonreassuring test results should be reported to the physician promptly.

In the intrapartum period the frequency of vital sign and fetal assessments is individualized based on the client's condition and the stage of labor. The nurse should be alert for signs of fetal intolerance to labor and report these to the physician promptly. A continuous insulin infusion may be ordered and serum or capillary blood glucose levels are monitored as ordered by the physician during labor. The nurse should assess the client frequently for signs and symptoms of hypoglycemia and institute prompt administration of glucose according to unit protocol or physician's order. Hourly intake and output monitoring usually is initiated during the intrapartum period.

Education of the diabetic gravida and her family members is critical for the successful management of diabetes. The diagnosis of diabetes can be very frightening, and the volume of information needed to be imparted to the woman and family can be overwhelming. The plan of care for antepartum management should be reviewed carefully. Teaching regarding a culturally appropriate diabetic diet is very important and may need to be reinforced periodically. The dietician is a valuable member of the health care team and can assist in tailoring the diet for the client's preferences. Clients and family members also will need thorough instruction on blood glucose testing, goals for blood glucose values, insulin administration, and common signs and symptoms of hypoglycemia and hyperglycemia. In addition to these self-management principles the potential maternal, fetal, and neonatal complications should be addressed.

Hypothyroidism

Hypothyroidism is a condition frequently encountered in women of childbearing age. This condition has been associated with difficulty in conception and other negative outcomes.

Incidence

Thyroid disease occurs more commonly in women than in men (Burrow, 1999). Hypothyroidism occurs in about 1 of every 1,600 to 2,000 pregnancies (Montoro, 1997). Clients with severe hypothyroidism often have difficulty conceiving, and women with hypothyroidism are at increased risk for pregnancy loss (Burrow, 1999).

Clinical Presentation

Hormonal and metabolic changes that occur in pregnancy may stress thyroid function. Clients who have mild or moderate hypothyroidism generally are able to achieve pregnancy, and the disease does not significantly impact the pregnancy in most cases (Glinoer, 1999).

In general, the client who has hypothyroidism may present with complaints of cold intolerance, coarse hair, and dry skin. Hypothyroidism rarely is first diagnosed during pregnancy. Women who are pregnant and have hypothyroidism may complain of increased fatigue in addition to the above-mentioned complaints. Laboratory assessments may reveal an elevated level of serum thyroid-stimulating hormone (TSH) and a low serum level of free thyroxine, or T_4 (Seely & Burrow, 1999).

Congenital hypothyroidism is difficult to diagnose clinically and is found in about 1 in 4,000 to 7,000 infants (Cunningham et al., 1997). Because of the risk of severe neurologic deficits as a result of a deficiency of thyroid hormone, screening of neonates is strongly recommended (Seely & Burrow, 1999).

In regions where there is dietary deficiency of iodine, fetal brain damage may result. The severe manifestation of this damage is referred to as cretinism, which is characterized by marked developmental retardation, deaf mutism, spasticity, strabismus, and abnormal sexual development (Haddow et al., 1999; Seely & Burrow, 1999).

Management

Replacement thyroxine is given to the pregnant woman, with dosages titrated until thyroid function tests are within the normal range. The dosage usually is increased approximately every 4 weeks until TSH levels are within the normal range (Seely & Burrow, 1999). Clients who have received thyroxine replacement therapy before pregnancy often require higher dosages during pregnancy (Brent, 1999).

Nursing Care

Antepartum nursing care for the client with hypothyroidism includes monitoring for signs and symptoms of worsening disease, such as increased fatigue, dry skin, and coarse hair. The nurse should provide education to the client regarding the disease process and the medical management plan. There are no specific nursing care issues in the intrapartum period. In the postpartum period, clients may not have thyroid hormone replacement therapy until thyroid function studies can be evaluated several weeks after delivery.

Hyperthyroidism

Hyperthyroidism can cause menstrual irregularities but usually does not affect fertility, and pregnancy does not alter the disease (Major & Nageotte, 1999). The primary maternal concern is uncontrolled disease called thyroid storm, which is a medical emergency. Heart failure also is of concern. Hyperthyroidism has been associated with adverse fetal outcomes.

Incidence

Hyperthyroidism, or **thyrotoxicosis**, is common in the general population, affecting approximately 2% of women and 0.02% of men (Gittoes & Franklyn, 1998). Similar to hypothyroidism the diagnosis of hyperthyroidism rarely is made during pregnancy, and the disease causes complications in about 0.2% of pregnancies (Mestman, 1997).

Clinical Presentation

The classic signs of hyperthyroidism include heat intolerance, diaphoresis, warm skin, fatigue, anxiety, emotional lability, tachycardia, and vomiting, which also are found frequently in a normal pregnancy. A lack of weight gain, unanticipated weight loss, and increased heart rate above the norm for pregnancy may be signs that would help differentiate hyperthyroidism from the symptoms of a normal pregnancy. Laboratory values in the diagnosis of hyperthyroidism indicate an elevated serum level of free thyroxine and a low TSH level (Cunningham et al., 1997; Seely & Burrow, 1999).

Approximately 95% of cases of hyperthyroidism are caused by Graves disease, which is an autoimmune process (Seely & Burrow, 1999). Perinatal outcomes in hyperthyroidism are largely dependent on control of the disease state in pregnancy. Adverse outcomes associated with hyperthyroidism include an increased risk for PIH, preterm labor, congestive heart failure, and intrauterine fetal demise (ACOG, 1993; Burrow, 1999). Rarely, clients will undergo thyroid storm, which is a potentially life-threatening complication resulting in cardiac failure (Cunningham et al., 1997).

Rarely, fetal and neonatal hyperthyroidism may result from transplacental passage of thyroid-stimulating immunoglobulins. Fetal hyperthyroidism may increase the risk for intrauterine growth retardation, nonimmune hydrops, and intrauterine fetal death (Zimmerman, 1999). The neonate born to a client who has hyperthyroidism also may have hyperthyroidism that may require medical treatment. These infants may demonstrate hyperkinesis, irritability, poor feeding, vomiting, diarrhea, poor weight gain, jaundice, ophthalmopathy, cardiac failure, hypertension, and thrombocytopenia up to 5 to 10 days after delivery (Zimmerman, 1999; Seely & Burrow, 1999). A neonate who has been exposed to antithyroid medication in utero also may develop hypothyroidism, with development of a goiter and exophthalmos.

Management

Hyperthyroidism usually is managed with thionamide drugs, such as propylthiouracil (PTU). The dosage of this medication is titrated until the free thyroxine levels are within the normal range for pregnancy and the clinical symptoms appear to be improved. The drug is administered at the lowest possible dosage to maintain normal serum levels. In many cases, PTU can be discontinued at about 32 to 36 weeks' gestation (Seely & Burrow, 1999). In rare cases during pregnancy, a thyroidectomy may be performed when medical management fails (Cunningham et al., 1997).

Nursing Care

The nursing care of the client with hyperthyroidism includes monitoring for signs and symptoms of worsening disease and client education regarding the disease process and medical plan of management. The nurse also may perform fetal surveillance testing as ordered. The client with thyroid storm or cardiac failure will need intensive nursing care, the discussion of which is beyond the scope of this chapter.

CARDIOVASCULAR DISORDERS

Cardiovascular disease in pregnant women is either congenital or acquired. The consequences of heart diseases for the mother and fetus depend on disease type and severity.

Clinical Presentation

In the recent past, many women with congenital or acquired heart disease were counseled to avoid pregnancy and in some cases did not survive to childbearing age themselves. Advances in health care have allowed for surgical repair of structural defects and have vastly improved outcomes for this group of women. Women with existing heart disease can present a challenge to the health care team because many significant cardiovascular changes occur during pregnancy.

Most pregnant women with significant cardiovascular disease are diagnosed before pregnancy. Some cases of heart disease are first detected during pregnancy when the hemodynamic changes of pregnancy begin to place stress on the heart. Normal symptoms found in pregnancy, such as palpitations, tachypnea, fatigue, edema, and syncope, are similar to symptoms of cardiovascular disease. A careful evaluation of existing symptoms is needed for the pregnant woman and any new or additional symptoms, or an increase in symptoms with exertion, should be cause for further evaluation. Symptoms that should prompt further evaluation include severe dyspnea, syncope with exertion, hemoptysis, paroxysmal nocturnal tachycardia, and chest pain on exertion (Shabetai, 1999).

Many specific cardiovascular structural defects may be affected by pregnancy. The discussion of these defects is beyond the scope of this chapter because each one would require a discussion of the specific defect and a detailed discussion of the medical management. Cardiovascular conditions that are specific to or common in pregnancy or that need special consideration include peripartum cardiomyopathy, cardiac arrhythmias, and myocardial infarction (MI).

Peripartum cardiomyopathy is a rare form of heart failure occurring during pregnancy or in the first 5 months postpartum (Hibbard, Lindheimer, & Lang, 1999). Approximately 1,000 women in the United States are expected to develop this complication each year (Brown & Bertolet, 1998). The mortality rate for this complication is significant at 25% to 60% (Aziz et al., 1999; Hibbard, Lindheimer, & Lang, 1999). The cause of peripartum cardiomyopathy is unknown; however, viral and autoimmune causes often are associated with this type of heart failure (Heider et al., 1999; Brown & Bertolet, 1998).

The woman with peripartum cardiomyopathy presents in a way similar to clients with other types of congestive heart failure, that is, with edema, fatigue, and dyspnea. Weight gain, jugular vein distension, and an enlarged heart may be present on examination (Shabetai, 1999). The management of cardiomyopathy is primarily supportive (Heider et al., 1999). Approximately 30% of women who develop peripartum cardiomyopathy will recover to their baseline ventricular function within 6 months of delivery (Lampert, Wernwor, Thippert, Korcarz, Lindheimer, & Lang, 1997).

Cardiac arrhythmias appear to increase in frequency during pregnancy, often are benign, and do not require treatment (Wolbrette & Patel, 1999; Shabetai, 1999). Sustained and symptomatic arrhythmias may jeopardize the health of the mother and fetus and may be life-threatening (Shabetai, 1999).

Myocardial infarction is a rare event in pregnancy, occurring in 1 per 10,000 to 30,000 deliveries (Samuels et al., 1998; Webber, Halligan, & Schumacher, 1997). The mortality rate from this complication is high, reportedly from 37% to 50%. Mortality increases in clients experiencing MIs in the third trimester of pregnancy, when delivery occurs within 2 weeks of the event, in clients less than 35 years of age, and in clients who deliver by cesarean section (Webber et al., 1997).

Pregnancy generally is contraindicated in clients who have experienced an MI before becoming pregnant and who have severe left ventricular damage and heart failure (Shabetai, 1999). When pregnancy occurs accidentally, the woman may be asked to consider terminating the pregnancy if her condition is severe.

Management

Each client with cardiovascular complications should have an individualized plan of care determined by a multidisciplinary team and based on her underlying disease process or structural defect. Certain principles in the management of the pregnant women with cardiovascular disease can be applied to most all types of disease. These clients generally should have frequent prenatal visits and consultation with a specialist. They also may need to be placed on bed rest at any point in the pregnancy as they become symptomatic or as cardiac function is impaired (Shabetai, 1999). The physician may choose conservative management of clients who are stable and not hemodynamically compromised, including observation and bed rest.

The pregnant woman with peripartum cardiomyopathy usually is treated similarly to clients with congestive heart failure, with bed rest, digitalization, diuretics, and sodium restriction (Clark et al., 1997). Clients who do not exhibit improved ventricular function may be considered for heart transplantation (Heider et al., 1999; Aziz et al., 1999).

Women who have certain tachyarrhythmias may first be instructed to use vagal maneuvers to alleviate the dysrhythmia (Cunningham et al., 1997). If these maneuvers fail and the client is symptomatic, she is frequently managed with antiarrhythmic drugs. These drugs usually are well tolerated by clients and pose relatively low risk in pregnancy (Cunningham et al., 1997; Joglar & Page, 1999). Beta-blockers frequently are prescribed in the treatment of tachyarrhythmias. These medications may cause neonatal hypoglycemia and bradycardia; however these conditions usually are not serious. Beta-blockers are excreted in the breast milk and may cause bradycardia and hypotension in the neonate (Clark et al., 1997).

A pacemaker may be used to treat certain arrhythmias, and these devices should not impact the pregnancy (Shabetai, 1999). Cardioversion has also been effectively used to treat maternal dysrhythmias and is well tolerated by the client and fetus (Joglar & Page, 1999; Shabetai, 1999).

The woman who has experienced a MI previously is counseled to wait 1 year before becoming pregnant (Shabetai, 1999). Once pregnant, women often will be placed on bed rest during pregnancy. The client whose delivery occurs within 2 weeks of the MI has an increased risk for death, and therefore, adequate rest during this time is very important (Clark et al., 1997; Shabetai, 1999). In the intrapartum period, efforts are made to minimize hemodynamic changes and optimize perfusion. The client is labored in a lateral position, provided with adequate pain relief, and given oxygen (Clark et al., 1997). Invasive hemodynamic monitoring may be necessary (Clark et al., 1997; Shabetai, 1999).

The specific cardiovascular complications and the condition of the client will help determine the method of delivery. In general, the mode of delivery usually is decided based on obstetric indications. The second stage of labor may be shortened by the use of forceps or vacuum extraction to avoid the prolonged Valsalva maneuver in pushing (Cunningham et al., 1997). In some specific cardiac complications, to avoid the strain of labor an elective cesarean section may be performed. The stress of major surgery, the potential for infection, and increased blood loss as compared with vaginal delivery is taken into consideration in planning the method of delivery (Clark et al., 1997).

Clients with cardiovascular complications who will undergo labor and anticipated vaginal delivery often need special considerations. During the intrapartum period attempts are made to minimize changes in blood pressure and pulse, including placing the client in a lateral position, adequate pain management, and the avoidance of hemorrhage. The avoidance of infection is an important consideration because an infection can have a detrimental effect on the client's overall condition. Supplemental oxygen and antibiotics frequently are prescribed (Clark et al., 1997).

Nursing Care

Nursing care of clients who have cardiovascular disease can be very challenging. In some cases, nurses from the obstetric, cardiovascular, or critical care service may need to collaborate in the care. Thorough physical assessments should be performed, and any change in cardiopulmonary status should be reported to the physician promptly. Meticulous care should be given to aseptic technique to avoid an infection because infection could have a serious impact on the client's overall condition. Intake and output should be monitored closely in most clients with cardiovascular disease to avoid volume overload. The nurse should have a thorough understanding of the pathophysiology of the specific cardiovascular disease and be familiar with any vasoactive drugs that may be used.

Clients and families are often very anxious and need thorough explanations regarding the plan of care. Emotional support is an essential piece in the care of these clients, and spiritual needs should be considered.

PULMONARY DISORDERS

Pulmonary disorders that can complicate pregnancy include asthma and tuberculosis (TB). The impact this disease has on the mother and fetus is related to the severity of the disease process.

Asthma

Asthma is considered to be an obstructive pulmonary disease.

Incidence

Asthma affects about 1% to 4% of pregnancies, which is a lower incidence than in the general population in which the reported incidence is 3% to 5% (Kurinczuk et al., 1999; Weinberger & Weiss, 1999).

Clinical Presentation

Bronchospasm and increased mucous production cause air flow to be limited, especially during expiration. Exacerbation of asthma may be related to specific events or "triggers," such as dust, animal dander, exercise, and respiratory infection; in contrast, there may be no obvious precipitating event. Symptoms of exacerbation of asthma, or an "attack," include coughing, wheezing, and dyspnea. Maternal and perinatal outcomes in clients with asthma depend on disease severity and treatment adequacy throughout pregnancy (Weinberger & Weiss, 1999).

Asthma usually begins in childhood but can occur at any age. The course of asthma in pregnancy is unpredictable; some clients experience worsening of the disease, some improve, and an equal number remain unchanged (Weinberger & Weiss, 1999). Pregnant clients rarely will experience an asthma attack during pregnancy, although the reason for this is not clear (Swiet, 1999).

Management

Treatment for women with asthma who are pregnant compared with that for those who are not pregnant varies little. Treatment is aimed at preventing and relieving bronchospasm. Undertreatment of pregnant women with asthma is common and based on fears about the effects medications used to treat asthma may have on the fetus. A study by Cydulka et al. (1999) found that pregnant women who presented to the emergency room for acute asthma attacks were less likely to receive appropriate treatment with corticosteroids. Most medications used for treatment of asthma in the general population are safe for use in pregnancy (Swiet, 1999). The risks to the patient of leaving severe asthma untreated are greater than are the risks of using medication to control asthma during pregnancy (Schatz, 1999). Poorly controlled asthma in the pregnant client places the fetus at greater risk than do most medical therapies used in the treatment of asthma (Weinberger & Weiss, 1999; Schatz, 1999).

Clients with mild or occasional asthma attacks are generally managed outside the hospital setting with inhaled beta-agonist agents, such as albuterol. Clients experiencing several attacks a week may be placed on scheduled doses of inhaled anti-inflammatory medications as a preventive measure. Inhaled corticosteroids also are used to prevent airway inflammation in clients who have moderate or severe asthma (Swiet, 1999; Cunningham et al., 1997). In very severe cases of asthma, parenteral or oral steroids may become necessary. The treatment is usually converted to inhaled steroids over time (Cunningham et al., 1997).

The Working Group on Asthma and Pregnancy, National Institutes of Health, National Heart, Lung, and Blood Institute, was established in 1993 by the National Asthma Education and Prevention Program to address the problems of asthma management in pregnancy. Key concepts from the recommendations of this Working Group include aggressive asthma management principles integrated with obstetric care. This Working Group suggests that management be as aggressive for the pregnant patient as for the nonpregnant patient and that medications used to treat asthma should include a short-acting beta-agonist and a long-term daily medication to reduce inflammation (Clark, 1993; Luskin, 1999).

In a severe asthma attack the goals are to correct maternal hypoxia, relieve bronchospasm, ensure adequate ventilation, and support uteroplacental perfusion. Intubation and mechanical ventilation may be necessary for clients who are unresponsive to medical therapy (Clark et al., 1997).

Nursing Care

Client education is a key part of nursing care for the pregnant woman who has asthma. The client should be counseled that her asthma might possibly improve, worsen, or remain unchanged during pregnancy. The importance of using inhalers and other prescribed medications as ordered by the primary care provider should be stressed. Many pregnant women are fearful of taking any type of drug during pregnancy and should be reassured about the safety of these medications.

The technique of inhaler use should be evaluated because proper dosing depends on adequate use of the device. Clients who have difficulty with traditional inhalers can be offered the use of a spacer, an additional device that helps deliver accurate doses.

A severe asthma attack is a medical emergency. A pregnant woman who is experiencing a severe asthma attack should be observed closely and receive a thorough physical assessment. The client should be placed in a lateral recumbent position to optimize ventilation and uteroplacental circulation. The client's response or lack of response to medications should be noted and reported to the physician.

The client experiencing an asthma attack will exhibit anxiety and often will be anxious about the fetal condition and her own. Reassurance should be offered to the client and family as should thorough explanations about procedures, medications, and the medical plan of management.

Tuberculosis

Tuberculosis is a worldwide health concern and a major cause of illness and death. The prevalence of TB is increasing worldwide. Many causes have been implicated in the resurgence of TB in recent years in the United States: presence of the human immunodeficiency virus (HIV), development of drug-resistant strains of TB, an increase in the number of immigrants, difficulty accessing medical care in the population with TB, and lack of adequate resources to handle the increasing number of cases (Saade, 1997; Hageman, 1997; Anderson, 1997).

Clinical Presentation

The lung is the major site of involvement. Some clients, however, will have extrapulmonary disease, including endometrial, lymphatic, intestinal, skeletal, renal, meningeal, and genital TB (Jana et al., 1999; Soussis et al., 1998). The diagnosis of TB generally is made by isolation of the organism *Mycobacterium tuberculosis* from involved sites. The organism is cultured from a sputum specimen in the case of pulmonary TB. Infection is caused by inhalation of the *M. tuberculosis* organism. Clients can be asymptomatic at the time of primary infection. TB may lie dormant for long periods of time before reactivating. Clinical manifestations include symptoms of pneumonia, such as fever and a cough that may be nonproductive, pleuritic chest pain, hemoptysis, and weight loss. Outcomes for clients who have TB during pregnancy are related to disease severity and treatment adequacy.

Management

The tuberculin skin test is a routine but important screening test for TB that may be performed in high-risk women during pregnancy (Nolan, Espinosa, & Pastorek, 1997; Riley, 1997). Clients at high risk include those who have HIV, those with close contact with persons known to have TB, persons who recently have immigrated to the United States, and clients who are incarcerated or in long-term care facilities (Cunningham et al., 1997). A chest radiograph may be performed in the client who has a positive result on a skin test and who previously has had a negative test result, or in the client whose medical history or physical examination is suggestive of TB. When a chest radiograph is indicated, it should be delayed until after the first trimester if possible to avoid exposing the rapidly developing fetus to radiation. Shielding also can be used to reduce fetal exposure.

Pregnant women who test positive for TB but do not have clinical evidence of active disease may delay treatment until after delivery (Cunningham et al., 1997). Treatment of pulmonary TB in pregnant women is similar to that in women who are not pregnant (Saade, 1997). Treatment consists of daily doses of isoniazid (INH), rifampin, pyrazinamide, and ethambuton over a 6-month period. These first-line agents appear to have minimal risks for the development of congenital anomalies and may be started as soon as the diagnosis of TB is made (Brost & Newman, 1997). Clients who have HIV and TB are placed on extended regimens. Hepatitis is a major side effect of INH; therefore, clients may require serial liver enzyme testing (Cunningham et al., 1997).

Neonatal infection is uncommon if the mother has received adequate treatment for at least 2 weeks before delivery. The neonate is at greatest risk for the development of TB shortly after birth because the newborn is susceptible to TB infection (Starke, 1997). The newborn is isolated from the mother for up to 2 weeks if she has active disease (Swiet, 1999).

Nursing Care

Clients who are in high-risk groups should be screened for TB in pregnancy. A thorough medical history will include information on potential exposure to TB and any signs and symptoms of the disease. The client will often need education about the disease process, potential complications, and management plan. Compliance to the medication regimen, if prescribed, is key to optimal outcome in the mother and fetus and should be stressed.

The pregnant client who has TB will need emotional support in dealing with the implications of the disease. The client who must be isolated from her newborn may be very distraught. She should be made aware of the rationale for isolation and offered the opportunity to verbalize her concern and grief.

AUTOIMMUNE DISEASE

Autoimmune disease is a condition in which a person demonstrates an immune response to constituents of one's self. It is thought to be caused by a combination of factors, including environment, genetics, and host factors (Branch & Porter, 1999).

Systemic Lupus Erythematosus

Systemic lupus erythematosus is an inflammatory autoimmune disease that affects multiple organ systems. Autoimmune diseases occur most commonly in women of childbearing age and with greater frequency in African American and Hispanic women than in Caucasian women (Silver & Branch, 1997).

Clinical Presentation

The diagnosis of lupus generally is based on the presence of clinical signs and symptoms. The most common complaints are a low-grade fever that comes and goes, extreme fatigue, muscle and joint pain, and weight loss (Clark et al., 1997; Swiet, 1999). Other symptoms used as criteria for the diagnosis of lupus include malar or discoid rash; photosensitivity; arthritis; and specific renal, neurologic, and hematolgic manifestations. The client who has lupus undergoes periods of remission and may improve, worsen, or remain unchanged during pregnancy. Confirmation of the diagnosis is made by the presence of autoantibodies on antinuclear antibody tests (Swiet, 1999).

The development of PIH in the client who has lupus is common and reported to occur in 20% to 30% of pregnancies (Clark et al., 1997). The differentiation between a lupus flare-up and PIH is difficult because of the similarity in clinical presentation, each one having common findings of hypertension and proteinuria. There are no tests that are helpful in distinguishing between the two diseases, and in some cases the client may actually be experiencing a flare-up of lupus (Clark et al., 1997).

The rate of pregnancy loss in women with lupus is increased related primarily to hypertension, renal complications, and premature rupture of membranes (Swiet, 1999; Meng & Lockshin, 1999; Rahman, Gladman, & Urowitz, 1998; Reichlin, 1998). Most pregnancy losses are intrauterine fetal deaths occurring in the second and third trimesters of pregnancy (Clark et al., 1997). Lupus also is associated with an increased risk of intrauterine growth retardation, and premature delivery. Premature delivery may be medically induced because of maternal or fetal complications. Clients who have active disease, who have had established lupus rather than late onset, and who have uncontrolled disease have higher rates of abortion and premature birth. The remission of lupus in the 6 to 12 months before pregnancy most likely decreases the chance for a flare-up during pregnancy and the postpartum period (Silver & Branch, 1997).

Neonatal lupus erythematosus is rare and is characterized by skin lesions; cardiac abnormalities, such as heart block; and hematologic abnormalities, such as thrombocytopenia and anemia (Meng & Lockshin, 1999; Reichlin, 1998; Rabinerson et al., 1997). Skin lesions are the most common finding, appearing in the first few weeks after delivery; they usually resolve at about 6 months of age.

Management

Glucocorticoids, such as prednisone, are used in the treatment of lupus in the general population and are continued during pregnancy (Silver & Branch, 1997). Patients are monitored closely for an increase in the symptoms of lupus. Mild to moderate exacerbations of lupus symptoms generally are treated with an increased oral dose of prednisone for several days to weeks (Cunningham et al., 1997; Swiet, 1999). Tapering of the drug is initiated after an improvement in symptoms (Cunningham et al., 1997). Severe exacerbations, including renal or CNS involvement, require large doses of IV glucocorticoids over several days. The client is then placed on oral therapy and weaned over approximately 1 month. Clients who have been on continuous administration of glucocorticoids will require a supplemental IV dose, or "stress dose," during labor or surgical procedures (Clark et al., 1997; Gladman & Urowitz, 1999).

Nursing Care

The client who has lupus can be counseled to postpone pregnancy until she has had a period of 6 to 12 months without a flare-up of the disease. These women will have frequent prenatal visits, and at each visit should be asked about an increase in symptoms or new symptoms of lupus. Clients who are newly diagnosed will require extensive education about the disease process, the implications for pregnancy, and the long-term prognosis. Clients and families should receive emotional support in dealing with the diagnosis of lupus and with the prospects for perinatal complications.

In the intrapartum period clients should be closely monitored for signs of worsening disease, such as the presence of hypertension, CNS involvement, or renal involvement.

HEMATOLOGIC DISORDERS

Hematologic disorders in pregnancy range from iron deficiency anemia to idiopathic thrombocytopenic purpura. Some of these disorders are a mere annoyance, whereas others are life-threatening.

Immunological Idiopathic Thrombocytopenic Purpura

Immunologic thrombocytopenic purpura (ITP), also referred to as idiopathic thrombocytopenic purpura, is a process in which antibodies are directed against platelets and usually is an immune response to drugs or viral infections (Duffy, 1999).

Clinical Presentation

Acute cases of thrombocytopenia often follow a viral infection and usually resolve spontaneously (Cunningham et al., 1997). Chronic cases of ITP are most common in young

women and occur in about 7% to 8% of pregnancies. The initial diagnosis of ITP sometimes is made during pregnancy when a routine CBC reveals a decreased platelet count (ACOG, 1999b). It is unclear what impact pregnancy could have on chronic ITP.

Antibodies are able to cross the placenta and cause thrombocytopenia in the fetus and neonate. Concern exists that the fetus with thrombocytopenia is at risk for intracranial hemorrhage during labor and delivery, prompting direct measurement of fetal platelet count by PUBS or fetal scalp sampling (Cunningham et al., 1997). The actual incidence of moderate to severe neonatal thrombocytopenia and intracranial hemorrhage is low (Payne et al., 1997; Song et al., 1999; Burrows & Kelton, 1993). It is estimated that significant neonatal thrombocytopenia occurs in 10% of babies born to patients with ITP (Bussel, 1997).

Management

Once thrombocytopenia is diagnosed, secondary causative factors are investigated, such as lupus, leukemia, and lymphoma. Clients whose very low platelet counts persist (less than 50,000) are usually treated with steroids. The goal of therapy is to decrease the incidence of hemorrhage. Improvement usually occurs within 2 to 3 weeks. More than 70% of clients will have an increase in platelet count, and the steroid dose is tapered as the platelet count is normalized (Kilpatrick & Laros, 1999). Clients who continue to have persistent severe thrombocytopenia and who are bleeding despite steroid therapy may require a splenectomy; however, this is rarely required in pregnancy (Bussel, 1997; Duffy, 1999). Women who are asymptomatic and have ITP and a platelet count greater than 50,000 usually do not require treatment (Duffy, 1999).

Clinicians have attempted to predict fetal and neonatal thrombocytopenia based on maternal characteristics without much success (Cunningham et al., 1997; Payne et al., 1997). Some clinicians will opt to deliver the baby by cesarean section if the fetus has thrombocytopenia (Duffy, 1999; Cunningham et al., 1997). Laboratory tests used to determine fetal platelet count are expensive, and there is a significant risk to the fetus from the procedures (Burrows & Kelton, a 1993; Song et al., 1999; Payne et al., 1997). Studies have been performed that have found that neither the determination of fetal platelet count nor performance of a cesarean section significantly impact neonatal outcomes. Although this remains a controversial issue, many clinicians determine the route of delivery based strictly on obstetric indications. (Payne et al., 1997; Song et al., 1999; Burrows & Kelton, 1993b; Silver, Branch, & Scott, 1995).

Nursing Care

Clients diagnosed with ITP will need thorough explanations of the disease process and of possible maternal and fetal implications. The medical plan of management, including considerations for the route of delivery, should be discussed with the client and family.

Sickle Cell Disease

Sickle cell disease encompasses several inherited disorders of hemoglobin synthesis, with sickle cell anemia (SS disease), sickle cell–hemoglobin C disease (SC disease), and sickle cell–β-thalassemia (S-β-thalassemia) being the most common forms.

Clinical Presentation

Sickle cell anemia (SS disease) occurs when the gene for S hemoglobin is inherited from both parents. Sickle cell trait, which is the inheritance of one gene for the production of S hemoglobin and one for normal hemoglobin, occurs in 1 of 12 African Americans. SC disease, in which there is a gene for the production of hemoglobin C, occurs in approximately 1 in 2,000 African American women (Cunningham et al., 1997). S-β-thalassemia occurs with the inheritance of an S gene and a β-thalassemia gene. S-β-thalassemia occurs in approximately 1 of every 2,000 women (Cunningham et al., 1997). Pregnancy places a strain on women with sickle hemoglobinopathies and, accordingly, they have significant maternal and perinatal morbidity and mortality.

The diagnosis of hemoglobinopathies is made by hemoglobin electrophoresis, which identifies the type and percentage of abnormal hemoglobin.

Most of the signs and symptoms of SS disease are a result of hemolysis, vaso-occlusive disease, or increased susceptibility to infection (Kilpatrick & Laros, 1999). Patients with SS disease experience sickling of erythrocytes and resulting occlusion of the microvasculature precipitated by hypoxemia. Chronic anemia and episodes of "crises" in which there is vaso-occlusion causing ischemia, acute pain, and possible organ failure are characteristic of the disease. These painful episodes of sickle cell crisis may occur in the long bones, abdomen, chest, or back; these episodes are potentially life-threatening and often increase in frequency during pregnancy (Clark et al., 1997; Kilpatrick & Laros, 1999).

In general, clients who have SS disease are more susceptible to infection. Infections and pulmonary complications are major causes of morbidity and mortality in women who have SS disease and are more common in pregnancy (Cunningham et al., 1997).

During pregnancy women who have SC disease may have an increased incidence of severe bone pain and additional serious complications, even though they often are asymptomatic before pregnancy. Maternal and perinatal mortality rates are higher than in the general population but much lower than in SS disease (Duffy, 1999).

Pregnancy outcomes for clients who have β-thalassemia usually are good. These women may experience mild to moderate anemia during pregnancy (Duffy, 1999).

Management

Hemoglobin electrophoresis may be ordered prenatally as a screening test for African American women. The pregnant woman with a sickle hemoglobinopathy generally will have chronic hemolytic anemia and requires increased folic acid supplementation throughout pregnancy. Disease treatment mainly consists relieving symptoms, with the objective being to end painful crisis and fight infection (Kilpatrick & Laros, 1999).

Transfusions of erythrocytes are used in cases of chronic anemia to prevent acute or chronic complications based on the client's symptoms (Simon et al., 1998).

Clients are monitored throughout pregnancy for asymptomatic bacteriuria because women with sickle cell hemoglobin have a greatly increased risk for bacteriuria (Pastore, Savitz, & Thorp, 1999). Infections are poorly tolerated and are managed aggressively to avoid precipitation of a crisis.

The management of sickle cell crisis usually involves hospitalization, evaluation for sources of potential infection, rest, hydration, and pain management. IV therapy to correct dehydration is a key aspect of therapy because it can lower the blood viscosity and may help alleviate vaso-occlusion (Kilpatrick & Laros, 1999). Oxygen therapy is reserved for clients who are experiencing hypoxia, those with a pulmonary infection, and those in labor (Clark et al., 1997). The pain of sickle cell crisis can last for up to a week and is managed according to severity; some clients require narcotic analgesia.

Nursing Care

Clients who have sickle hemoglobinopathies require education about the impact of pregnancy on their disease. Avoidance of infection is an important consideration and should be stressed. Pregnant women are more susceptible to UTIs than are women in the general population, and clients should be instructed to alert their health care provider as soon as the first symptoms of UTI appear. In fact, routine screening is likely to be included in prenatal care because of asymptomatic bacteriuria.

Clients experiencing crisis will require supportive care: a warm restful environment, adequate pain control, IV hydration, and oxygen therapy as ordered. Intake and output should be recorded; however, catheterization should be avoided because of risk of infection. Crisis is an extremely anxiety-provoking event, with the very real threat of death. Clients require emotional support and reassurance from family and health care providers.

NEUROLOGIC DISORDERS

Neurologic disorders, namely epilepsy, can affect the health of the mother and baby.

Seizure Disorders

Seizure disorders may be acquired as a result of trauma, tumors, or metabolic disorders.

Incidence

Most frequently the seizure activity is idiopathic and is known as epilepsy (ACOG, 1996d). Epilepsy is common in the general population and affects an estimated 1 million women of childbearing age (Chang & McAuely, 1998). Seizure disorders are the most common major neurologic complication seen in pregnancy, affecting approximately 0.5% of all pregnancies (Nulman, Laslo, & Koren, 1999; ACOG, 1996d). This section focuses on epilepsy.

Clinical Presentation

Preconceptual counseling for women of childbearing age who have epilepsy is very important. The outcome of the pregnancy is greatly determined by control of the seizure disorder, achieving therapeutic blood levels of the prescribed anticonvulsant, compliance with the medication regimen, and vitamin supplementation.

During pregnancy psychological, hormonal, and pharmokinetic changes can cause an increase in seizure activity. As many as half of women with epilepsy will experience an increase in seizure activity during pregnancy (Cunningham et al., 1997). Status epilepticus is a rare condition in which recurrent generalized seizures occur. This condition is an emergency because the mother and fetus are at risk for hypoxia. This complication seems to occur more frequently in the third trimester (Licht & Sankar, 1999; ACOG, 1996d).

Serum levels of anticonvulsant drugs can change dramatically during pregnancy, usually decreasing as the pregnancy progresses. These changes may be related to nausea and vomiting, delayed gastric emptying, increased plasma volume, and altered protein binding. Serum levels fluctuations may cause a nontherapeutic level of the anticonvulsant drug or, in some cases, maternal toxicity (Nulman, Laslo, & Koren, 1999; ACOG, 1996d). Therefore, close monitoring is required during pregnancy.

Most anticonvulsant drugs interfere with metabolism of the essential vitamins folic acid and vitamin K. Folic acid deficiency is associated with an increased incidence of neural tube defects and other major malformations. Interference with vitamin K metabolism places the neonate at increased risk for bleeding because certain clotting factors are dependent on vitamin K (Chang & McAuely, 1998; ACOG, 1996d).

Children born to women without seizure disorders have a 0.5% to 1% risk of developing epilepsy. Children born to a woman with epilepsy are four times more likely to develop epilepsy (ACOG, 1996d). Children exposed to phenytoin in utero are at risk for cleft lip and fetal hydantoin syndrome.

Management

Women of childbearing age who have epilepsy may be started on folic acid supplementation even before conception. Once pregnant, the woman should receive folic acid supplementation throughout the first trimester (Nulman, Laslo, & Koren, 1999; Lewis et al., 1998; Morrell, 1998; Chang & McAuely, 1998; ACOG, 1996d). Some clinicians prescribe vitamin K supplementation during the last month of pregnancy. The infant also receives a vitamin K injection at birth (Nulman, Laslo, & Koren, 1999; ACOG, 1996d).

The woman with epilepsy should be counseled regarding possible teratogenic effects of uncontrolled seizures and the increased risk for major congenital malformations associated with the anticonvulsant medications (Nulman, Laslo, & Koren, 1999; Samren et al., 1999; Holmes et al., 2000). There is about a two to three times increased risk for birth defects in infants with mothers who have epilepsy compared with the general population (ACOG, 1996d). Seizure control is preferably achieved at least 6 months before conception.

Medical therapy during pregnancy is ideally accomplished with the lowest possible effective dose of a single antiseizure medication (Morrell, 1998; Chang & McAuely, 1998; Ellers, Patterson, & Webb, 1997; ACOG, 1996d). Because serum levels of drugs considered therapeutic in patients who are not pregnant are not reliable during pregnancy and because of the fluctuations, drug levels are checked periodically as the pregnancy progresses. Clients should be educated regarding the signs and symptoms of drug toxicity (ACOG, 1996d).

Some clients are reluctant to take the prescribed anticonvulsant medications because of fear of fetal effects (ACOG, 1996d). Patients should be strongly advised to adhere to the medical regimen and report increase in seizure activity. Because lack of sleep and stress may cause an increase in seizure activity, the pregnant client should be encouraged to get adequate rest.

During the early antepartum period clients are offered screening for potential neural tube defects using a maternal serum alpha-fetoprotein determination and ultrasonography. If these tests are inconclusive the woman may be offered an amniocentesis for a definitive diagnosis. Frequently, a comprehensive ultrasonography to assess for congenital malformations is performed at approximately 18 to 22 weeks' gestation. Further antepartum surveillance is not always necessary and is determined based on the individual client's condition (ACOG, 1996d).

In the event of status epilepticus the physician may order IV phenytoin, which must be administered slowly to avoid significant cardiac dysrhythmias. Phenobarbital or diazepam may be ordered alternatively; however, both these drugs may cause respiratory depression. Emergency supplies for endotracheal intubation, oxygen, and suction equipment should be readily available (ACOG, 1996d).

During labor the client may be unable to take prescribed oral medications. Serum drug levels may be evaluated and the client may receive an anticonvulsant parenterally.

In the postpartum period serum levels of anticonvulsants may increase rapidly. When the drug dosage is increased during pregnancy, it frequently needs to be decreased in the postpartum period (Aminoff, 1999). Serum levels are checked frequently to avoid toxic drug levels (ACOG, 1996d). Antiepilectic drugs interact with oral contraceptives, making them less effective. Clients should be counseled on the need for increased dosage or a second method of birth control to avoid an unplanned pregnancy (Chang & McAuely, 1998; ACOG, 1996d).

Infants born to mothers with epilepsy who are receiving barbiturates may experience withdrawal symptoms beginning about 1 week after birth and lasting 1 to 2 weeks. A breast-fed infant may develop withdrawal with abrupt cessation of breast-feeding and may require low-dose phenobarbital with gradual withdrawal (ACOG, 1996d).

Nursing Care

In the antepartum period most clients will need education regarding the effect their pregnancy might have on their disease, medical therapy prescribed, potential complications for the fetus and neonate, and the medical plan of care. Clients diagnosed with epilepsy and their families may be fearful of the effects their disease can have on their babies and will need accurate information about their disease and emotional support throughout the pregnancy.

NURSING IMPLICATIONS

Few events over the course of a lifetime have such a momentous impact on women and their families as do a pregnancy and the eventual birth of the baby. Pregnancy can be a time of great hope and joy or, when complications arise, a time of great concern and even despair. Major advances in obstetric care have been made in the last half of the 20th Century that have allowed women with serious medical and obstetric complications to achieve positive pregnancy outcomes. The availability of adequate prenatal care, early identification of risk factors, and an interdisciplinary approach to the management of the high-risk pregnancy is critical to optimize outcomes for the family.

The role of the nurse in caring for the high-risk obstetric client will vary depending on the condition and setting. For the client being managed in the community, your role may be one of counseling, teaching, and case management. It is very important that the client and family understand the pathophysiology of the condition and which self-help measures can be taken. It also is important to teach danger signs and the procedure that should be followed in the event of a change in the woman's condition. The intervention depends not only on the condition but the severity of the condition, with home care used for milder cases in which client compliance is not likely to be an issue.

Nurses working with pregnant women and families must be familiar with common complications that can arise during the course of pregnancy. Nurses should be prepared to function as an integral part of the health care team, performing thorough nursing assessments, administering medications and treatments, and providing clients and families with education and support.

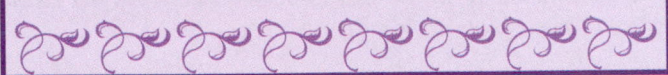

Critical Thinking

Significant Findings from Nursing Assessment

Nurses are in a position to detect early signs of obstetric risks. What might be the significance of the following findings from a nursing assessment?

- Oliguria of less than 30 mL/h
- Significant change in vital signs
- Diastolic blood pressure of 110 mmHg or higher
- Nonreassuring fetal status
- Seizure activity
- Vaginal bleeding
- Severe epigastric or upper right quadrant pain
- Altered mental status
- Signs and symptoms of pulmonary edema
- Abnormal laboratory results

Web Activities

- Use a search engine such as PubMed or Ovid to search a specific condition discussed in this chapter.

- Visit the website of the American College of Obstetricians and Gynecologists for clinical guidelines on managing pregnant clients with hypertensive and cardiovascular disorders.

Key Concepts

❧ Pregnancy is considered a normal process with minimal risks. However, the potential exists for development of risks.

❧ The best practice is to anticipate and attempt to reduce risks or prevent the occurrence of complications.

❧ A pregnant woman has the potential for changing from being normal to being high risk very quickly.

Review Questions and Activities

1. Why is it important for you to differentiate the following: complete abortion, threatened abortion, and missed abortion?

2. Which signs and symptoms would alert you to a potential ectopic pregnancy?

3. When providing care for a woman who is in the third trimester of pregnancy and bleeding, what should you include in emergency preparations?

4. When magnesium sulfate is given to the pregnant woman, which complications or adverse effects will you need to monitor?

5. Why is it important to identify the blood type and Rh factor of all pregnant women?

6. Why is gestational diabetes a health problem for the pregnant woman? For the neonate?

7. What are the differences between chronic hypertension, pregnancy-induced hypertension, and superimposed hypertension?

8. What is peripartum cardiomyopathy, and why is this complication significant?

9. What is the HELLP syndrome and how does it affect the pregnant women?

References

Abu-Heija, A., Jallad, M., & Abukteish, F. (2000). Maternal and perinatal outcomes after the age of 45. *Journal of Obstetrics and Gynaecology Research, 26,* (1), 27–30.

Althabe, F., Carroli, G., Lede, R., Belizan, J., & Althabe, O. (1999). Preterm delivery: Detection of risks and preventative treatment. *Pan American Journal of Public Health, 5,* (6), 373–385.

American College of Obstetricians and Gynecologists (ACOG). (1993). *Thyroid disease in pregnancy* (ACOG Technical Bulletin Number 181). Washington, DC:

American College of Obstetricians and Gynecologists. (1994). *Diabetes and pregnancy* (ACOG Technical Bulletin Number 200). Washington DC:

American College of Obstetricians and Gynecologists. (1996a). *Hypertension in pregnancy* (Technical Bulletin Number 219). Washington, DC:

American College of Obstetricians and Gynecologists. (1996b). *Management of isoimmunization in pregnancy* (ACOG Educational Bulletin Number 227). Washington, DC:

American College of Obstetricians and Gynecologists. (1996d). *Seizure disorders in pregnancy* (ACOG Technical Bulletin Number 231). Washington, DC:

American College of Obstetricians and Gynecologists. (1998b). *Special problems of multiple gestation.* (ACOG Educational Bulletin Number 253). Washington, DC:

American College of Obstetricians and Gynecologists. (1999a). *Prevention of Rh D alloimmunization* (ACOG Practice Bulletin Number 4). Washington, DC:

American College of Obstetricians and Gynecologists. (1999b). *Thrombocytopenia in pregnancy* (ACOG Practice Bulletin Number 6). Washington, DC:

Aminoff, M. (1999). Neurologic disorders. In R. Creasy & R. Resnik (Eds.). *Maternal fetal medicine* (pp. 1091–1119). Philadelphia, PA: W. B. Saunders.

Ananth, C., Smulian, J., & Vintzileos, A. (1997). The association of placenta previa with history of cesarean delivery and abortion: A metaanalysis. *American Journal of Obstetrics and Gynecology, 177,* (5), 1071–1078.

Ananth, C., Smulian, J., & Vintzileos, A. (1999). Incidence of placental abruption in relation to cigarette smoking and hypertensive disorders during pregnancy: A meta-analysis of observational studies. *Obstetrics and Gynecology, 93,* (4), 622–628.

Anderson, G. (1997). Tuberculosis in pregnancy. *Seminars in Perinatology, 21,* (4), 328–335.

Aziz, T., Burgess, M., Acladious, N., Campbell, C., Rahman, A., Yonon, N., & Deiraniya, A. (1999). Heart transplantation for peripartum cardiomyopathy: A report of 3 cases and a literature review. *Cardiovascular Surgery, 7,* (5), 565–567.

Barton, J. B., & Sibai, B. M. (2001). HELLP syndrome. *In Hypertensive Disorders in Women* (B. M. Sibai Ed.) Philadelphia, PA: W. B. Saunders.

Berg, C., Atrash, H., Koonin, L., & Tucker, M. (1996). Pregnancy-related mortality in the United States, 1987–1990. *Obstetrics and Gynecology, 88,* 161.

Bowman, J. (1999). Hemolytic disease (erythroblastosis fetalis). In R. Creasy & R. Resnik (Eds.). *Maternal fetal medicine* (pp. 736–767). Philadelphia, PA: W. B. Saunders.

Brace, R., & Resnik, R. (1999). Dynamics and disorders of amniotic fluid volume. In R. Creasy & R. Resnik (Eds.). *Maternal fetal medicine* (pp. 632–643). Philadelphia, PA: W. B. Saunders.

Brauch, D. W., & Porter, T. F. (1999). Autoimmune disease. In (D. K. James, P. J. Steer, C. P. Weiner & B. Gonik (Eds.). *High risk pregnancy: Management options.* Philadelphia, PA: W. B. Saunders.

Brent, G. (1999). Maternal hypothyroidism: Recognition and management. *Thyroid, 9,* (7), 661–665.

Brost, B., & Newman, R. (1997). The maternal and fetal effects of tuberculosis therapy. *Obstetrics and Gynecology Clinics of North America, 24,* (3), 659–673.

Brown, C., & Bertolet, B. (1998). Peripartum cardiomyopathy: A comprehensive review. *American Journal of Obstetrics and Gynecology, 178,* (2), 409–414.

Buchanan, T., & Kjos, S. (1999). Gestational diabetes: Risk or myth? *Journal of Clinical Endocrinology, 84,* (6),1854–1857.

Burrow, G. (1999). Thyroid diseases. In G. Burrow & T. Duffy (Eds.). *Medical complications during pregnancy* (pp. 135–161). Philadelphia, PA: W. B. Saunders.

Burrows, R., & Kelton, J. (1993a). Fetal thrombocytopenia and its relation to maternal thrombocytopenia. *New England Journal of Medicine, 329,* (20), 1463–1466.

Burrows, R., & Kelton, J. (1993b). Pregnancy in patients with idiopathic thrombocytopenic purpura: Assessing the risks for the infant at delivery. *Obstetrical and Gynecological Survey, 48,* (12), 781–788.

Bussel, J. (1997). Immune thrombocytopenia in pregnancy: Autoimmune and alloimmune. *Journal of Reproductive Immunology, 37,* (1), 35–61.

Castles, A., Adams, E., Melvin, C., Kelsch, C., & Boulton, M. (1999). Effects of smoking during pregnancy: Five meta-analyses. *American Journal of Preventative Medicine, 16,* (3), 208–215.

Centers for Disease Control and Prevention. (1998). *Morbidity and Mortality Weekly, 47,* (34), 705–707. Maternal Mortality, United States, 1982–1996.

Chang, S., & McAuely, J. (1998). Pharmacotherapeutic issues for women of childbearing age with epilepsy. *Annals of Pharmacotherapy, 32,* (7-8), 794–801.

Chichakli, L., Atrash, H., Mackay, A., Musani, A., & Berg, C. (1999). Pregnancy-related mortality in the United States due to hemorrhage: 1979–1992. *Obstetrics and Gynecology, 94,* (5, Pt. 1), 721–725.

Clark, S. (1993). Asthma in pregnancy. National Asthma Education Program Working Group on Asthma and Pregnancy. National Institutes of Health, National Heart, Lung, and Blood Institute. *Obstetrics and Gynecology, 82,* (6), 1036–1040.

Clark, S. (1999). Placenta previa and abruptio placentae. In R. Creasy & R. Resnik (Eds.). *Maternal fetal medicine* (pp. 616–631). Philadelphia, PA: W. B. Saunders.

Clark, S., Cotton, D., Hankins, G., & Phelan, J. (Eds). (1997). *Critical care obstetrics,* (3rd ed.). Malden, MA: Blackwell Science.

Conde-Agudelo, A., Belizan, J., & Lindmark, G. (2000). Maternal morbidity and mortality associated with multiple gestation. *Obstetrics and Gynecology, 95,* (6, Pt. 1), 899–904.

Crane, J., van den Hof, M., Dodds, L., Armson, B., & Liston, R. (1999). Neonatal outcomes with placenta previa. *Obstetrics and Gynecology, 93,* (4), 541–544.

Cunningham, F., MacDonald, P., Gant, N., Leveno, K., Gilstrap, L., Hankins, G., & Clark, S. (Eds.). (1997). *Williams obstetrics* (20th ed.). Stamford, CT: Appleton and Lange.

Cydulka, R., Emerman, C., Schreiber, D., Molander, K., Woodruff, P., & Camargo, C. (1999). Acute asthma among pregnant women presenting to the emergency department. *American Journal of Respiratory and Critical Care Medicine, 160,* (3), 887–892.

Davison, J., & Lindheimer, M. (1999). Renal disorders. In R. Creasy & R. Resnik (Eds.). *Maternal fetal medicine* (pp. 873–894). Philadelphia, PA: W. B. Saunders.

Duffy, T. (1999). Hematologic aspects of pregnancy. In G. Burrow & T. Duffy (Eds.). *Medical complications during pregnancy* (pp. 79–95). Philadelphia, PA: W. B. Saunders.

Ellers, D., Patterson, C., & Webb, G. (1997). Maternal and fetal implications of anticonvulsant therapy during pregnancy. *Obstetrics and Gynecology Clinics of North America, 24,* (3), 523–524.

Friedman, S. A., Lubarsky, S. L., and Lim, K. H. (2001). Mild gestational hypertension and pre-eclampsia. In *Hypertensive Disorders in Women* (B. M. Sibai, Philadelphia, PA: W. B. Saunders.

Gittoes, N., & Franklyn, J. (1998). Hypothyroidism. Current treatment guidelines. *Drugs, 55,* (4), 543–553.

Gladman, D., & Urowitz, M. (1999). Rheumatic disease in pregnancy. In G. Burrow & T. Duffy (Eds.). *Medical complications during pregnancy* (pp. 415–438). Philadelphia, PA: W. B. Saunders.

Glinoer, D. (1999). What happens to the normal thyroid during pregnancy? *Thyroid, 9,* (7), 631–635.

Grab, D., Paulus, W., Bommer, A., Buck, G., & Terinde, R. (1999). Treatment of fetal erythroblastosis by intravascular transfusion: Outcome at 6 years. *Obstetrics and Gynecology, 93,* (2), 165–168.

Haddow, J., Palomaki, G., Allen, W., Williams, J., Knight, G., Gagnon, J., O'Heir, C., Mitchell, M., Hermos, R., Waisbren, S., Faix, J., & Klein, R. (1999). Maternal thyroid deficiency during pregnancy and subsequent neuropsychological development of the child. *New England Journal of Medicine, 341,* (8), 549–555.

Hageman, J. (1997). Congenital and perinatal tuberculosis: Discussion of difficult issues in diagnosis and management. *Journal of Perinatology, 18,* (5), 389–394.

Hankins, G., Clark, S., Cunningham, G., & Gilstrap, G. (Eds.). (1995). *Operative obstetrics.* Stamford, CT: Appleton Lange.

Hauth, J., Ewell, M., Levine, R., Esterlitz, J., Sibai, B., Curet, L., Catalano, P., & Morris, C. (2000). Pregnancy outcomes in healthy nulliparas who developed hypertension. Calcium for Preeclampsia Prevention Study Group. *Obstetrics and Gynecology, 95,* (1), 24–28.

Heider, A., Kuller, J., Strauss, R., & Wells, S. (1999). Peripartum cardiomyopathy: A review of the literature. *Obstetrical and Gynecological Survey, 54,* (8), 526–531.

Hendricks, M., Chow, Y., Bhagavath, B., & Singh, K. (1999). Previous cesarean section and abortion as risk factors for developing placenta previa. *Journal of Obstetrics and Gynaecology Research, 25,* (2), 137–142.

Hibbard, J., Lindheimer, M., & Lang, R. (1999). A modified definition for peripartum cardiomyopathy and prognosis based on echocardiography. *Obstetrics and Gynecology, 94,* (2), 311–316.

Hutti, M. H., dePacheco, M., & Smith, M. (1998). A study of miscarriage: Development and validation of the perinatal grief intensity scale. *Journal of Obstetric, Gynecologic, and Neonatal Nursing, 27,* (5), 547–555.

Iams, J. (1999). Cervical incompetence. In R. Creasy & R. Resnik (Eds.). *Maternal fetal medicine* (pp. 445–464). Philadelphia, PA: W. B. Saunders.

Inzucchi, S. (1999). Diabetes in pregnancy. In G. Burrow & T. Duffy (Eds.). *Medical complications during pregnancy* (pp. 25–51). Philadelphia, PA: W. B. Saunders.

Jana, N., Vasishta, K., Saha, S., & Ghosh, K. (1999). Obstetrical outcomes among women with extrapulmonary tuberculosis. *New England Journal of Medicine, 341,* (9), 645–649.

Joglar, J., & Page, R. (1999). Treatment of cardiac arrhythmias during pregnancy: Safety considerations. *Drug Safety, 20,* (1), 85–94.

Kamwendo, F., Forslin, L., Bodin, L., & Danielsson, D. (2000). Epidemiology of ectopic pregnancy during a 28 year period and the role of pelvic inflammatory disease. *Sexually Transmitted Infections, 76,* (1), 28–32.

Kendrick, J. (1999). Diabetes in pregnancy. In L. Mandeville & N. Troiano (Eds.). *High-risk and critical care intrapartum nursing* (pp. 224–255). Philadelphia, PA: J. B. Lippincott.

Kilpatrick, S., & Laros, R. (1999). Maternal hematologic disorders. In R. Creasy & R. Resnik (Eds.). *Maternal fetal medicine* (pp. 935–963). Philadelphia, PA: W. B. Saunders.

Kurinczuk, J., Parsons, D., Dawes, V., & Burton, P. (1999). The relationship between asthma and smoking during pregnancy. *Women & Health, 29,* (3), 31–47.

Kyrklund-Blomberg, N., & Cnattingius, S. (1998). Preterm birth and maternal smoking: Risks related to gestational age and onset of delivery. *American Journal of Obstetrics and Gynecology, 179,* (4), 1051–1055.

Lewis, D., Van Dyke, D., Stumbo, P., & Berg, M. (1998). Drug and environmental factors associated with adverse pregnancy outcomes. Part I: Antiepileptic drugs, contraceptives, smoking, and folate. *Annals of Pharmacotherapy, 32,* (7-8), 802–817.

Licht, E., & Sankar, R. (1999). Status epilepticus during pregnancy. A case report. *Journal of Reproductive Medicine, 44,* (4), 370–372.

Luke, B., Bigger, H., Leurgans, S., & Sietsema, D. (1996). The cost of prematurity: A case-control study of twins vs singletons. *American Journal of Public Health, 86,* (6), 809–814.

Luskin, A. (1999). An overview of the recommendations of the Working Group on Asthma and Pregnancy. *Journal of Allergy and Clinical Immunology, 103,* (2 Pt. 2), s350–s353.

Macones, G., Sehdev, H., Parry, S., Morgan, M., & Berlin, J. (1997). The association between maternal cocaine use and placenta previa. *American Journal of Obstetrics and Gynecology, 177,* (5), 1097–1100.

Major, C. A., & Nageotte, M. P. (1999). Thyroid disease. In D. K. James, P. J. Steer, C. P. Weiver, & B. Gonik (Eds.). *High-risk pregnancy: Management options.* Philadelphia, PA: W. B. Saunders.

Malone, F., & D'Alton, M. (1999). Multiple gestation: Clinical characteristics and management. In R. Creasy & R. Resnik (Eds.). *Maternal fetal medicine* (pp. 598–615). Philadelphia, PA: W. B. Saunders.

Maloni, J., Cohen, A., & Kane, J. (1998). Prescription of activity restriction to treat high-risk pregnancies. *Journal of Women's Health, 7,* (3), 351–358.

McGregor, J., & French, J. (2000). Bacterial vaginosis in pregnancy. *Obstetrical and Gynecological Survey, 55,* (suppl. 1), s1–s19.

Meng, C., & Lockshin, M. (1999). Pregnancy in lupus. *Current Opinion in Rheumatology, 11,* (5), 348–351.

Mercer, B., Goldenberg, R., Moawad, A., Meis, P., Iams, J., Das, A., Caritis, S., Miodovnik, M., Menard, M., Thurnau, G., Dombrowski, M., Roberts, J., & McNellis, D. (1999). The preterm prediction study: Effect of gestational age and cause of preterm birth on subsequent obstetric outcome. *American Journal of Obstetrics and Gynecology, 181,* (5 Pt. 1), 1216–1221.

Mestouan, J. H. (1997) Perinatal thyroid dysfunction: Prenatal diagnosis and treatment. *Medscape Womens Health 2,* (7), 2.

Montoro, M. (1997). Management of hypothyroidism during pregnancy. *Clinical Obstetrics and Gynecology, 40,* (1), 65–80.

Moore, T. (1999). Diabetes in pregnancy. In R. Creasy & R. Resnik (Eds.). *Maternal fetal medicine* (pp. 964–995). Philadelphia, PA: W. B. Saunders.

Morrell, M. (1998). Guidelines for the care of women with epilepsy. *Neurology, 51,* (5 suppl 4), S21–S27.

Mucrow, C. D., Chiquette, E., Ferree, R. C., Sibai, B. M., Stevens, K. R., Harris, M., Montgomery, K. A. & Starum, K. (2000). *Management of chronic hypertension during pregnancy.* Bethesda: Agency for Healthcare Research and Policy.

Myatt, L., & Miodovnik, M. (1999). Prediction of preeclampsia. *Seminars in Perinatology, 23,* (1), 45–57.

National Heart, Lung, and Blood Institute. (2000). *Working group report on high blood pressure in pregnancy.* Washington, D.C.: National Institutes of Health.

National High Blood Pressure Education Program Working Group on High Blood Pressure in Pregnancy Report. (2000). *American Journal of Obstetrics and Gynecology, 183,* (1), S1–S22.

Nolan, T., Espinosa, T., & Pastorek, J. (1997). Tuberculosis skin testing in pregnancy: Trends in a population. *Journal of Perinatology, 17,* (3), 199–201.

Nulman, I., Laslo, D., & Koren, G. (1999). Treatment of epilepsy in pregnancy. *Drugs, 57,* (4), 535–544.

Panting-Kemp, A., Nguyen, T., Chang, E., Quillen, E., & Castro, L. (1999). Idiopathic polyhydramnios and perinatal outcome. *American Journal of Obstetrics and Gynecology, 181,* (5 Pt. 1), 1079–1082.

Pastore, L., Savitz, D., & Thorp, J. (1999). Predictors of urinary tract infections at the first prenatal visit. *Epidemiology, 10,* (3), 282–287.

Payne, S., Resnik, R., Moore, T., Hedriana, H., & Kelly, T. (1997). Maternal characteristics and risk of severe neonatal thrombocytopenia and intracranial hemorrhage in pregnancies complicated by autoimmune thrombocytopenia. *American Journal of Obstetrics and Gynecology, 177,* (1), 149–155.

Rabinerson, D., Gruber, A., Kaplan, B., Lurie, S., Peled, Y., & Neri, A. (1997). Isolated persistent fetal bradycardia in complete A-V block: A conservative approach is appropriate. A case report and review of the literature. *American Journal of Perinatology, 14,* (6), 317–320.

Rahman, P., Gladman, D., & Urowitz, M. (1998). Clinical predictors of fetal outcome in systemic lupus erythematosus. *Journal of Rheumatology, 25,* (8), 1526–1530.

Rawlings, J., & Scott, J. (1996). Postconceptual age of surviving preterm low-birth-weight infants at hospital discharge. *Archives of Pediatrics and Adolescent Medicine, 150,* (3), 260–262.

Reichlin, M. (1998). Systemic lupus erythematosus and pregnancy. *Journal of Reproductive Medicine, 43,* (4), 355–360.

Reis, P., Sander, C., & Pearlman, M. (2000). Abruptio placentae after auto accidents. A case control study. *Journal of Reproductive Medicine, 45,* (1), 6–10.

Resnik, R., & Calder, A. (1999). Post-term pregnancy. In R. Creasy & R. Resnik (Eds.). *Maternal fetal medicine* (pp. 532–540). Philadelphia, PA: W. B. Saunders.

Riley, L. (1997). Pneumonia and tuberculosis in pregnancy. *Infectious Disease Clinics of North America, 11,* (1), 119–133.

Roberts, J. (1999). Pregnancy-related hypertension. In R. Creasy & R. Resnik (Eds.). *Maternal fetal medicine* (pp. 833–872). Philadelphia, PA: W. B. Saunders.

Rodis, J., Borgida, A., Wilson, M., Egan, J., Leo, M., Odibo, A., & Campbell, W. (1998). Management of parvovirus infection in pregnancy and outcomes of hydrops: A survey of members of the Society of Perinatal Obstetricians. *American Journal of Obstetrics and Gynecology, 179,* (4), 985–958.

Rogowski, J. (1998). Cost-effectiveness of care for very low birth weight infants. *Pediatrics, 102,* (1), 35–43.

Saade, G. (1997). Human immunodeficiency virus (HIV)-related pulmonary complications in pregnancy. *Seminars in Perinatology, 21,* (4), 336–350.

Samren, E., van Duijn, C., Christiaens, G., Hofman, A., & Lindhout, D. (1999). Antiepileptic drug regimens and major congenital abnormalities in the offspring. *Annals of Neurology, 46,* (5), 739–746.

Samuels, L., Kaufman, M., Morris, R., & Brockman, S. (1998). Postpartum coronary artery dissection: Emergency coronary bypass with ventricular assist device support. *Coronary Artery Disease, 9,* (7), 457–460.

Schatz, M. (1999). Interrelationships between asthma and pregnancy: A literature review. *Journal of Allergy and Clinical Immunology, 103,* (2 Pt. 2) s330–s336.

Schieve, L., Cogswell, M., Scanlon, K., Perry, G., Ferre, C., Blackmore-Prince, C., Yu, S., & Rosenberg, D. (2000). Prepregnancy body mass index and pregnancy weight gain: Associations with preterm delivery. *Obstetrics and Gynecology, 96,* (2), 94–200.

Seely, B., & Burrow, G. (1999). Thyroid disease and pregnancy. In R. Creasy & R. Resnik (Eds.). *Maternal fetal medicine* (pp. 996–1014). Philadelphia, PA: W. B. Saunders.

Seubert, D., Stetzer, B., Wolfe, H., & Treadwell, M. (1999). Delivery of the marginally preterm infant: What are the minor morbidities? *American Journal of Obstetrics and Gynecology, 181,* (5 Pt. 1), 1087–1091.

Shabetai, R. (1999). Cardiac diseases. In R. Creasy & R. Resnik (Eds.). *Maternal fetal medicine* (pp. 793–820). Philadelphia, PA: W. B. Saunders.

Shellhaas, C., & Iams, J. (1998). Ambulatory management of preterm labor. *Clinical Obstetrics and Gynecology. Ambulatory Obstetric Management, 41,* (3), 491–502.

Sibai, B. (2000). Risk factors, pregnancy complications, and prevention of hypertensive disorders in women with pregravid diabetes mellitus. *Journal of Maternal-Fetal Medicine, 9,* (1), 62–65.

Sibai, B., Caritis, S., Hauth, J., Lindheimer, M., VanDorsten, J., MacPherson, C., Klebanoff, M., Landon, M., Moidovnik, M., Thurnau, G., Roberts, J., & McNellis, D. (2000a). Risks of preeclampsia and adverse neonatal outcomes among women with pregestational diabetes mellitus. *American Journal of Obstetrics and Gynecology, 182,* (2), 364–369.

Sibai, B., Hauth, J., Caritis, S., Lindheimer, M., MacPherson, C., Klebanoff, M., VanDorsten, J., Landon, M., Miodovnik, M., Paul, R., Meis, P., Thurnau, G., Dumbrowski, M., Roberts, J., & McNellis, D. (2000b). Hypertensive disorders in twins versus singleton gestation. National Institute of Child Health and Human Development Network of Maternal-Fetal Medicine Units. *American Journal of Obstetrics and Gynecology, 182,* (4), 938–942.

Silver, R., & Branch, D. (1997). Autoimmune disease in pregnancy. Systemic lupus erythematosus and antiphospholipid syndrome. *Clinics in Perinatology, 24,* (2), 291–320.

Silver, R., Branch, D., & Scott, J. (1995). Maternal thrombocytopenia in pregnancy: Time for a reassessment. *American Journal of Obstetrics and Gynecology, 173,* (2), 479–482.

Simon, T., Alverson, D., AuBuchon, J., Cooper, E., DeChristopher, P., Glenn, G., Gould, S., Harrison, C., Milam, J., Moise, K., Rodwig, F., Sherman, L., Shulman, I., & Stehling, L. (1998). Practice parameters for the use of red blood cell transfusions: Developed by the Red Blood Cell Administration Practice Guideline Development Task Force of the College of American Pathologists. *Archives of Pathology and Laboratory Medicine, 122,* (2), 130–138.

Sisson, M., & Ruth, D. (1999). Disseminated intravascular coagulation. In L. Mandeville & N. Troiano (Eds.). *High-risk and critical care intrapartum nursing* (pp. 214–223). Philadelphia, PA: J. B. Lippincott.

Song, T., Lee, J., Kim, Y., & Choi, Y. (1999). Low neonatal risk of thrombocytopenia in pregnancy associated with immune thrombocytopenic purpura. *Fetal Diagnosis and Therapy, 14,* (4), 216–219.

Soussis, I., Trew, G., Matalliotakis, I., Margara, R., & Winston, R. (1998). In vitro fertilization treatment in genital tuberculosis. *Journal of Assisted Reproduction and Genetics, 15,* (6), 378–380.

Starke, J. (1997). Tuberculosis: An old disease but a new threat to the mother, fetus, and neonate. *Clinics in Perinatology, 24,* (1), 107–127.

Swiet, M. (1999). Rheumatologic and connective tissue disorders. In R. Creasy & R. Resnik (Eds.). *Maternal fetal medicine* (pp. 1082–1090). Philadelphia, PA: W. B. Saunders.

Tenore, J. (2000). Ectopic pregnancy. *American Family Physician, 61,* (4), 1080–1088.

Webber, M., Halligan, R., & Schumacher, J. (1997). Acute infarction, intracoronary thrombosis, and primary PTCA in pregnancy. *Catheterization and Cardiovascular Disease, 42,* (1), 38–43.

Weinberger, S., & Weiss, S. (1999). Pulmonary diseases. In G. Burrow & T. Duffy (Eds.). *Medical complications during pregnancy* (pp. 363–400). Philadelphia, PA: W. B. Saunders.

Wilkins, I. (1999). Nonimmune hydrops. In R. Creasy & R. Resnik (Eds.). *Maternal fetal medicine* (pp. 769–782). Philadelphia, PA: W. B. Saunders.

Wolbrette, D., & Patel, H. (1999). Arrhythmias and women. *Current Opinion in Cardiology, 14,* (1), 36–43.

Yancy, M., & Richards, D. (1994). Effect of altitude on the amniotic fluid index. *Journal of Reproductive Medicine, 39,* (2), 101–104.

Zimmerman, D. (1999). Fetal and neonatal hyperthyroidism. *Thyroid, 9,* (7), 727–733.

Suggested Readings

American College of Obstetricians and Gynecologists. (1996c). *Pulmonary disease in pregnancy*. (Technical Bulletin Number 224). Washington, DC:

American College of Obstetricians and Gynecologists. (1998a). *ACOG practice bulletin. Medical management of tubal pregnancy* (ACOG Practice Bulletin Number 3). Washington, DC:

Bowman, J. (1997). The management of hemolytic disease of the fetus and newborn. *Seminars in Perinatology, 21,* (1) 39–44.

Creasy, R., & Iams, J. (1999). Preterm labor and delivery. In R. Creasy & R. Resnik (Eds.). *Maternal fetal medicine* (pp. 498–531). Philadelphia, PA: W. B. Saunders.

Cundy, T., Gamble, G., Townend, K., Henley, P., MacPherson, P., & Roberts, A. (2000). *Diabetic Medicine, 17,* (1), 33–39.

Gordon, C. (1998). Use of intravenous immunoglobulin therapy in pregnancy in systemic lupus erythematosus and antiphospholipid antibody syndrome. *Lupus, 7,* (7),429–433.

Holmes, L., Rosenberger, P., Harvey, E., Khoshbin, S., & Ryan, L. (2000). Intelligence and physical features of children of women with epilepsy. *Teratology, 61,* (3), 196–202.

Joffe, G., Esterlitz, J., Levine, R., Clemens, J., Ewell, M., Sibai, S., & Catalanes, P. (1998). The relationship between abnormal glucose tolerance and hypertensive disorders of pregnancy in healthy nulliparous women. *American Journal of Obstetrics and Gynecology, 179,* (4), 1032–1037.

Katz, V., Farmer, R., & Kuller, J. (2000). Preeclampsia into eclampsia: Towards a new paradigm. *American Journal of Obstetrics and Gynecology, 182,* (6), 1389–1396.

Lampert, M., Weinert, L., Hibbard, J., Korcarz, C., Lindheimer, M., & Lang, R. (1997). Contractile reserve in patients with peripartum cardiomyopathy and recovered left ventricular function. *American Journal of Obstetrics and Gynecology, 176,* (1 Pt. 1), 189–195.

Lu, J., & Nightengale, C. (2000). Magnesium sulfate in eclampsia and preeclampsia: Pharmokinetic principles. *Clinical Pharmokinetics, 38,* (4), 305–314.

Malone, F., & D'Alton, M. (1997). Drugs in pregnancy: Anticonvulsants. *Seminars in Perinatology, 21,* (2), 114–123.

Moore, S., Turnpenny, P., Quinn, A., Glover, S., Lloyd, D., Montgomery, T., & Dean, J. (2000). A clinical study of 57 children with fetal anticonvulsant syndromes. *Journal of Medical Genetics, 37,* (7), 489–497.

Norris, T. (1997). Management of postpartum hemorrhage. *American Family Physician, 56,* (3), 737–738.

Roach, V., Hin, L., Tam, W., Ng, K., & Rogers, M. (2000). The incidence of pregnancy-induced hypertension among patients with carbohydrate intolerance. *Hypertension in Pregnancy, 19,* (2), 183–189.

Santolaya, J., Alley, D., Jaffe, R., & Warsof, S. (1992). Antenatal classification of hydrops fetalis. *Obstetrics and Gynecology, 79,* (2), 256–259.

Silver, R., & Branch, D. (1999). Immunologic disorders. In R. Creasy & R. Resnik (Eds.). *Maternal fetal medicine* (pp. 465–483). Philadelphia, PA: W. B. Saunders.

Szal, S., Croughan-Minihane, M., & Kilpatrick, S. (1999). Effect of magnesium prophylaxis and preeclampsia on the duration of labor. *American Journal of Obstetrics and Gynecology, 180,* (6 Pt. 1), 1475–1479.

CHAPTER 19

Pregnancy in Special Populations

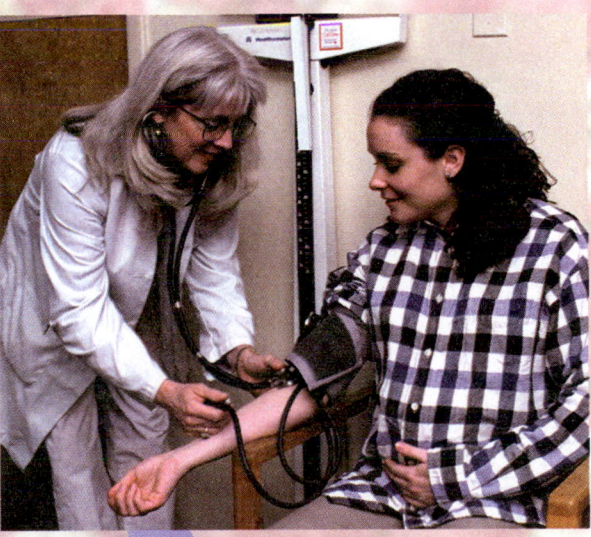

*W*orking with young, HIV-positive, or older pregnant clients can be a challenging and rewarding nursing experience. Understanding the complex psychosocial factors that lead these women to become pregnant is essential in providing supportive care to them and to their families. You may need to explore your own feelings relative to adolescent sexuality, AIDS, and pregnancy after age 35 to facilitate a therapeutic relationship with these clients. Consider the following:

- *How do I feel about teens who are sexually active?*

- *How do I feel about unmarried teens who become pregnant?*

- *What role do I think unmarried teen fathers should play in their partners' pregnancy and delivery?*

- *How can I relate to an HIV-positive woman who chooses to complete a pregnancy? Can I offer sensitive care to this client and her newborn?*

- *Do I know the risks of pregnancy after age 35? What is my opinion of pregnancy resulting from use of fertility drugs?*

Key Terms

Acquired
  immunodeficiency
  syndrome (AIDS)
Adolescence
Adolescent pregnancy

Advanced reproductive
  age
Antiretroviral therapy
Cognitive development
Developmental tasks

Elderly primagravida
Embryo transfer (ET)
Human
  immunodeficiency
  virus (HIV)

Seroconversion
Sexual maturation
Vertical transmission

Competencies

Upon completion of this chapter, the reader should be able to:

1. Describe the scope and significance of adolescent pregnancy.

2. Analyze the reasons that adolescents become pregnant.

3. Describe the psychosocial and physical risks for pregnant adolescents and their children.

4. Discuss adolescent sexuality and appropriate contraceptive methods.

5. Formulate a nursing care plan for pregnant adolescents.

6. Describe the significance of HIV infection in pregnant adolescents and young adults.

7. Discuss the importance of prevention of vertical and perinatal transmission of HIV infection.

8. Discuss the clinical manifestations and medical management of HIV-infected pregnant women and neonates.

9. Identify the effects of aging on reproductive function.

10. Discuss the medical risks for older women during pregnancy.

11. Discuss the issues concerning artificial conception in postmenopausal women.

12. Provide anticipatory guidance for older first-time pregnant couples.

Pregnancy in special populations refers to those populations that have unique issues related to the physical and psychosocial aspects of pregnancy. The populations discussed in this chapter include the pregnant adolescent; the pregnant HIV-infected woman; and the pregnant middle-aged and post-menopausal woman. Each of these special populations provides a unique challenge to nurses in providing holistic and age-appropriate nursing care during pregnancy and delivery. Advances in medical technology account for the following: (1) effective low-dose hormonal methods of contraception that should significantly decrease the teen birth rate, although statistics remain remarkably high; (2) improved outcomes for pregnant women with HIV infection, using new multi-drug antiretroviral therapy; and (3) innovative methods for fostering conception and full-term births in older women. Along with the advances in technol-

ogy come many controversial ethical and social issues related to pregnancy outcomes, most of which have been highly debated in professional and lay literature and have received widespread media attention. This chapter discusses issues relevant to pregnancy in special populations.

PREGNANCY IN ADOLESCENCE

The period known as **adolescence** spans ages 11 to 19 and is defined as the biologic and psychologic transition from childhood to adulthood. Pregnancy in adolescence is not a new phenomenon but is of increasing concern because childbearing during the teenage years has profound socioeconomic and physical consequences for both the teen mother and her offspring. **Adolescent pregnancy** (the state of pregnancy in young females ages 11 to 19) is a complex, multifaceted problem with no easy or obvious solutions. The burden of an unintended pregnancy is especially heavy for young teens who are still in high school and are trying to juggle their education, their own identity formation, and the physical and emotional changes occurring with pregnancy (Stevens-Simon, 1997).

Incidence and Significance

Approximately 1,000,000 teen pregnancies occur in the United States annually (Alan Guttmacher Institute, 1997). The majority (about 82%) of teen pregnancies are unplanned (Stevens-Simon, 1997) and most teens (about 79%) who had a baby in 1998 were unmarried (National Center for Health Statistics, 1999).

According to the 1999 data from the National Center for Health Statistics (NCHS), the worldwide rate of adolescent pregnancy is declining, although the adolescent pregnancy rate in the United States remains among the highest in the industrialized world. When compared to other developed countries, such as Canada, France, Sweden, and Great Britain, the United States has higher rates of adolescent pregnancies, births, and elective abortions, despite comparable levels of sexual activity among adolescents. Overall, teen pregnancy rates have declined in the past decade from a peak in 1992 to a low in 1996 (Ventura, Mosher, Curtain, Abma, & Henshaw, 1999) (Figure 19-1). In 1998, the number of births to teenage girls ages 15 to 19 increased slightly but was still less than the record highs in 1990 and 1991 (NCHS, 1999). Reasons for the decline in teen pregnancy rates include decreased sexual activity, increased condom use, and the use of injectable and implant contraceptives (Ventura et al., 1999). While these statistics may initially appear encouraging, the facts suggest that teen birth rates have remained relatively stable over

the past decade (Figure 19-2). Reasons for the stability in birth rates are the decrease in spontaneous abortions (miscarriages) and elective abortions among adolescents.

Because poor, unmarried teens are more likely to become parents than their more affluent peers, some believe that welfare in the form of Aid to Families with Dependent Children (AFDC) contributes to early and out-of-wedlock births. Others argue that poverty, the loosening of social mores, and the decline of the family structure are the driving forces behind adolescent pregnancy; the adolescent's poverty predates her pregnancy. Although unintended pregnancies among Caucasian, unmarried teens have increased, "the African American teenage mother has come to personify the social, economic, and sexual trends that in one way or another have affected almost everyone in America" (Luker, 1996, p. 83). Ethnicity appears to play a part in teen pregnancy. The pregnancy rates for non–Hispanic African American and Hispanic teenagers are about twice that of non–Hispanic Caucasian teens (Ventura et al., 1999).

The cost of adolescent pregnancy is staggering; the estimate is $25.1 billion for 1992 and up to $29 billion for 1996 (Maynard, 1996). Cost estimates in 1996 included AFDC, food stamps, Medicaid, loss of productivity, foster care, and the entire web of social problems that confront adolescent parents and lead to poor outcomes for their children. Estimates suggest that a cost savings of $10 billion could be achieved if adolescents delayed giving birth until after the age of 20 and focused on completing their basic education and initiating employment (Burnhill, 1994). Approximately two-thirds of adolescent mothers are high school dropouts and obtain less work experience, receive lower wages, and earn less over a lifetime than young women who delay childbearing (Greene & Cromer, 1991). Others argue that because poverty is often an antecedent to pregnancy among adolescents, pregnancy only compounds a pre-existing condition in which

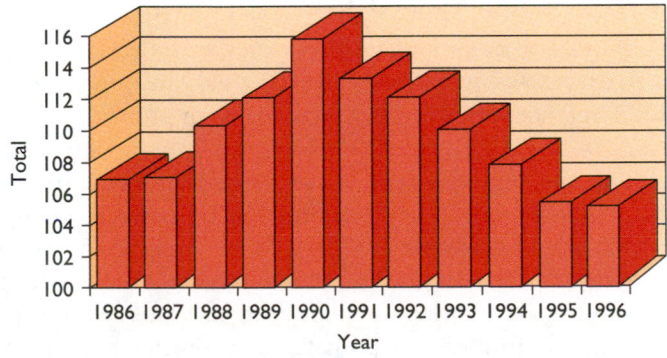

Figure 19-1 Birthrates Per Thousand Women Ages 15–19, 1986–1996. (Note: Data from Highlights of trends in pregnancies and pregnancy rates by outcome: Estimates for the United States, 1976–1996, by Ventura, S., Mosher, W., Curtain, S., Abma, J., & Henshaw, S. (1999) *National Vital Statistics Reports* 47, (29), 1–10.)

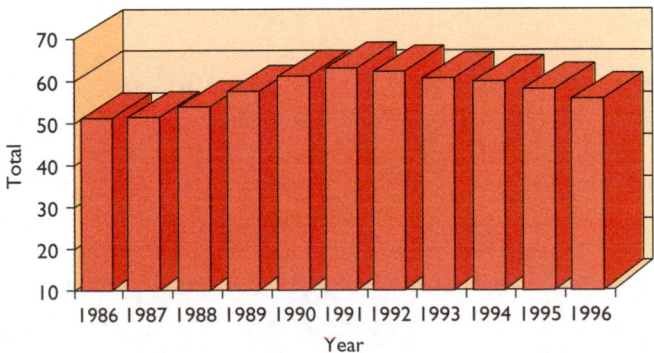

Figure 19-2 Birthrates per thousand women, ages 15–19, 1986–1996. (Note: Data from Highlights of trends in pregnancies and pregnancy rates by outcome: Estimates for the United States, 1976–1996, by Ventura, S., Mosher, W., Curtain, S., Abma, J., & Henshaw, S. (1999) *National Vital Statistics Reports* 47, (29), 1–10.)

poverty is the established standard (Luker, 1996). In a synthesis of the literature on adolescent pregnancy over the past decade, investigators concluded that "adolescent childbearing is a means of adapting to urban poverty" (Stevens-Simon & Lowy, 1995, p. 912). Childbearing is viewed as a personal accomplishment and is recognized by others as a transition to adulthood. Many of the studies suggest that adolescent parents often drop out of high school before they become pregnant. Therefore, school attendance and achievement before pregnancy is the best predictor of academic success after pregnancy. The completion of high school is a basic educational achievement, but the lack of a high school diploma prevents young people from entering the military, obtaining a postsecondary degree, and participating in many of the vocational training programs that enhance employment opportunities.

Adolescent Abortion

The number of induced abortions among adolescents has declined for all age groups in the past two decades. However, induced abortions among older adolescent women (ages 18 to 19) remain significantly higher than for younger adolescents (under age 17) (Ventura et al., 1999). Adolescents who elect abortion differ from those who do not in that they are more likely to remain in or complete high school, have higher educational aspirations, and come from families of higher socioeconomic status. Impoverished teens from minority backgrounds who do not seek birth control are more vulnerable to unplanned pregnancies and most often keep their babies after delivery. Approximately 2% to 3% of adolescent mothers put their babies up for adoption (Stevens-Simon & McAnarney, 1992). Making the decision to relinquish a baby is a complex and multifaceted task that requires a degree of maturity lacking in many teen parents. Those mothers who are older and more educated are more likely to offer a child for adoption. More female babies are relinquished than males; some researchers believe that male infants are less likely to be given up for adoption because of the greater interest shown by the baby's father (Bachrach, Stolley, & London, 1992).

With the legalization of abortion in the 1970s, the rate of abortion among pregnant adolescents initially increased and then leveled off in the mid-1980s. Racial differences in abortion rates explained higher pregnancy rates among African American adolescents; yet proportionately, abortion among ethnic or racial groups is comparable during the teen years (U.S. Bureau of the Census, 1993). However, these statistics may change as state and federal dollars decline for elective abortions among indigent women, and the controversy continues as to whether parents of minors should be informed when their adolescent children

under the age of 18 seek pregnancy termination. Proponents of parental notification or consent for adolescent abortion believe that this legislation would discourage sexual activity. Those opposed to such legislation believe that teens would be more inclined to (1) hide their pregnancy from adults and parents; (2) not obtain prenatal health care, thus increasing perinatal morbidity and mortality rates; (3) delay action beyond the gestational age limits of legal abortion; (4) seek illegal or self-induced abortions; or (5) try to deliver the fetus alone with no medical assistance. Recent cases of criminal charges against adolescents, who delivered and then hid or discarded newborns in trash cans, increase concerns about limiting abortion options for teens (Reuters News Service, 1997).

Adolescent Fathers

Although adolescent mothers have been studied extensively, there is little data on adolescent fathers. However, adolescent mothers are known to fare better in terms of maternal satisfaction when they have the emotional and financial support of their family and the baby's father. In one study that examined the characteristics of adolescent fathers, the investigators found that those who were teen fathers or those older than 20 who fathered babies born to teen mothers, were severely educationally disadvantaged (Hardy & Duggan, 1988). More than 50% of fathers are over the age of 20, but they have disproportionately more problems with academics, behavior, and substance abuse than their childless peers (Stevens-Simon & McAnarney, 1992). The relationships between teen parenting (by either sex) and inadequate education and low-paying occupations appear well-established, regardless of whether adolescent pregnancy is the cause or the consequence of poverty.

Infant and Child Outcomes

Costs related to adolescent pregnancy can also be measured in terms of negative infant and child outcomes (Table 19-1). Infants born to adolescents are often premature (less than 37 weeks' gestation) or low-birth-weight (less than 2500 grams), constituting the two most common and serious risks associated with adolescent pregnancy. Infants born to adolescents under the age of 16 are twice as likely to be of low weight at birth, which is largely the result of the adolescent mother's smaller body and the lack of appropriate nutrition and prenatal care during pregnancy (Stevens-Simon & McAnarney, 1992).

In addition, untreated sexually transmitted diseases (STDs), smoking, and substance abuse are factors that contribute to preterm labor, prematurity, intrauterine growth retardation (IUGR), and low-birth-weight infants. Cigarette smoking among pregnant women of all ages has been shown to have a significant relationship to delivery of low-birth-weight infants. It is estimated that 25% of low-birth-weight infants are born to teen mothers and that these infants are 50 times more likely to die than normal-weight infants (Tsang, 1993). Premature infants born to teen mothers are more likely to experience infant death and to suffer from serious respiratory complications, cerebral palsy, and chronic cognitive deficits.

In the postneonatal period, the mortality rate of infants born to adolescent mothers, age 17 and younger, is twice as high as that of infants born to more mature women. The lack of knowledge about child development, appropriate discipline, supervision, and adequate health care are thought to contribute to the increased incidence of illness, injury, and mortality among infants and young children of teenage parents (Stevens-Simon & McAnarney, 1991).

Adolescents under age 18 who become pregnant are more likely to engage in other risk-taking behaviors than young women who are not pregnant. Cigarette smoking has increased among teens in recent years; 64% of high school seniors report smoking and 41% report using marijuana (Bragg, 1997). The likelihood of smoking among pregnant teens is high. However, a recent study found that, although drug use is common among pregnant teens, with education, these young women substantially decreased drug use during pregnancy for the benefit of the fetus (Gilchrist, Hussey, Gillmore, Lohr, & Morrison, 1996). The investigators did note that a steady increase in substance abuse occurred during the first 6 months postpartum, suggesting that substance abuse among adolescent mothers is significant and potentially harmful to infants and young children. Maternal drug use may adversely affect parenting capabilities and the safety of the environment in which children are raised.

Client Education
Teen Pregnancy and Smoking

You may wish to provide and discuss information with expectant teen mothers on the adverse effects of cigarette smoking during pregnancy, including the following points.

- There is a clear association between maternal smoking and perinatal loss.
- Smokers have three and one-half to four times more risk for small-for-gestational-age babies than nonsmokers.
- The average weight of infants born to smokers is 170 to 200 grams less than infants born to nonsmokers.
- Studies have shown increased premature rupture of membranes in smokers.
- Newborns of smokers are smaller at every gestational age.
- Infants who are born to women who have stopped smoking early in their pregnancy are of normal weight at birth.
- There may be an increase in sudden infant death syndrome (SIDS) among infants born to mothers who smoke.

Note: Data from *Smoking and women's health* by American College of Obstetricians and Gynecologists, 1997. *ACOG Educational Bulletin,* No. 240, copyright 1997 by American College of Obstetricians and Gynecologists.

Table 19-1 Negative Infant/Child Outcomes Indirectly Related to Adolescent Pregnancy

Infant	Child
Prematurity	Neglect and abuse
Low-birth-weight	Chronic cognitive defects
Infant death	Developmental delays
Serious respiratory problems	Chronic behavioral problems
Blindness/deafness	School failure/withdrawal
Cerebral palsy	Chronic runaway
Mental retardation	Foster/alternative placement

Note: Data from *Kids having kids: A Robin Hood foundation special report on the costs of adolescent childbearing* by Maynard, R. (1996). New York: The Robin Hood Foundation; and Teenage childbearing, by Stevens-Simon, C. & Lowry, R. (1995). *Archives of Pediatric and Adolescent Medicine, 149,* 912–915.

Clearly, the psychosocial consequences for children born to adolescent mothers appear to be less than optimal. Children of adolescent mothers exhibit greater cognitive and behavioral problems and more frequently repeat school grades because of low academic achievement; it is estimated that only 77% earn a high school diploma by adulthood. Such children are also more frequently abused or neglected and are recipients of harsh discipline, which may contribute to chronic runaway behavior and the use of alternative living placements, such as shelters or group homes. Daughters of adolescent mothers are at a significantly higher risk of becoming adolescent parents themselves, and the sons of adolescent mothers are almost three times more likely to become incarcerated (Maynard, 1996). Because the typical profile of the adolescent mother is unmarried and poor, there is a strong association between the effects of poverty, single parenting, and negative child outcomes.

Adolescent Psychosocial Development

The physical and psychosocial consequences for adolescent mothers and their offspring are substantial. To understand the context of adolescent pregnancy, a knowledge of adolescent psychosocial development and acquisition of developmental tasks is necessary. **Developmental tasks** of adolescence include the competencies in psychosexual development related to identity formation, sexual and vocational identity, and independence. Adolescence overlaps with the younger, school-age child in the developmental tasks of early adolescence at one end of the age continuum and with the young adult in the developmental tasks of young adulthood at the other end. Although the adolescent years have been described as a period of turmoil, many adolescents experience a smooth transition into adulthood. In the search for their personal identity, adolescents try on many new roles, until they discover a role that fits and an identity is formed. Having completed identity formation, the adolescent is emancipated from the family and becomes independent. According to Erikson (1968), the major developmental tasks of adolescence are the development of identity and the establishment of autonomy, or the ability to be self-governing. The adolescent achieves autonomy by the use of abstract reasoning, which allows analytical thinking, problem solving, and planning for the future. Other developmental tasks include the formation of a sexual and vocational identity (see Box 19-1).

Cognitive development, or the age-related development of intellectual reasoning and perception, influences every aspect of adolescent psychosocial development. According to Piaget (1969), cognition moves from concrete to abstract thinking during the three phases of adolescent development (i.e., early, middle, and late adolescence). Concrete thinking focuses on the present, with little thought to later consequences; abstract thinking in early adolescence encompasses inductive and deductive reasoning and the ability to connect separate events and to understand later consequences; and abstract thinking, in late adolescence, is increasingly logical and complex. Some older adolescents remain concrete thinkers because of low intellect, lack of education, or chronic substance abuse.

Critical Thinking

Counseling and Cognition

You need to consider the adolescent's cognitive capacity when doing any counseling or education. Counseling a group of teens about birth control may be ineffective if the consequences of their behavior are tied to the future, when their thinking focuses only on the present. What other aspects of adolescent's behavior would you need to consider in relation to cognitive capacity?

The acquisition of cognitive abilities and the resolution of developmental tasks occur over time. While age parameters are suggested for the completion of developmental tasks, they are somewhat variable and adolescents may move back and forth on the developmental continuum, depending on their personal circumstances. For example, it is not unusual for teens to regress in their level of independence during the uncertainty of pregnancy, labor, and delivery and to become more reliant on their parents, usually mothers, in this period.

The adolescent is described as being egocentric or self-absorbed. Frustrated parents often describe teenagers as self-centered, lazy, or irresponsible because they spend their time and energy concentrating on themselves. The

Box 19-1 Adolescent Developmental Tasks
- Formation of identity/self-perception
- Acquisition of education/vocation
- Emancipation from family/independence
- Formation of sexual identity
- Development of social network of peers

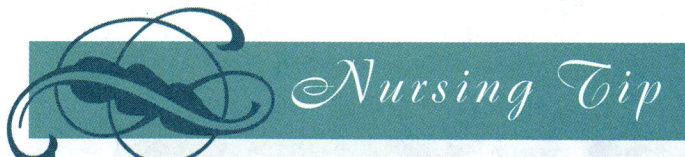

Nursing Tip

NEGOTIATING WITH TEENS

Whenever possible, you should negotiate choices with teens and always consider how teens are judged by their peers. Knowledge of specific peer group norms is essential and limits should appear reasonable and acceptable to teens. For example, when educating pregnant teens about the importance of prenatal nutrition, you should be sensitive to food preferences and develop a diet plan that is realistic for teens to follow. Adequate intake of calcium can be obtained by a variety of products, such as yogurt, ice cream, and cheese. Diet planning also should include meals consumed outside the home, such as those at school and teen social events.

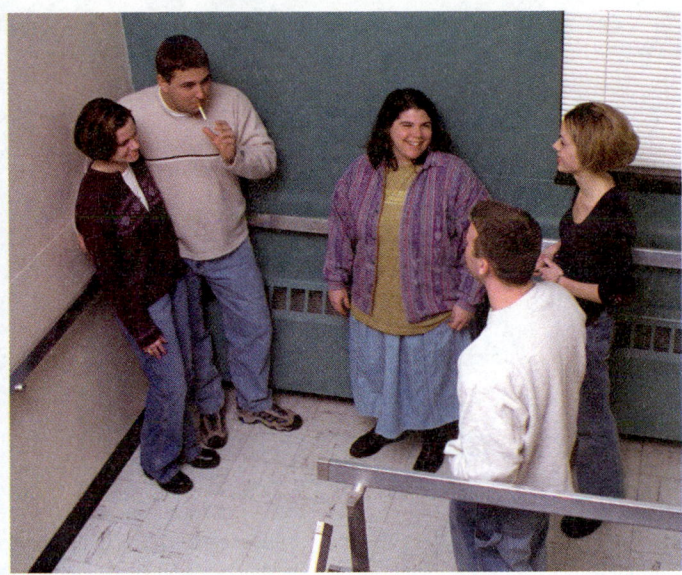

Figure 19-3 Interaction with peers is a key factor in adolescent development.

transition from childhood to adulthood is a phase of experimentation during which teens are not yet ready to make a commitment or make ones that are only tentative. The lack of commitment is illustrated by the adolescent's frequent change of interests; this has implications for the young adolescent mother. The reality of raising an infant may conflict with the adolescent's interest in trying on new roles; the role of parent is not so easily abandoned.

The peer group plays an essential role in adolescent identity formation (Figure 19-3). The peer group provides support as adolescents emotionally move away from the family and struggle with their own identity. Teenagers take their cues for appearance, social behavior, and language from the peer group; the peer group validates acceptable

behavior. In a peer group where early sexual activity, pregnancy, and parenting are the norm, it is difficult for the adolescent to break away from the accepted cycle of behavior. Changes in the adolescent's body image, psychosocial development, and peer group acceptance are closely related.

There is a wide developmental age span between early and late adolescence (ages 11 to 21). Each age group has unique reactions to the developmental tasks, which are influenced by the adolescent's cognitive thinking and are tied to the adolescent's sexuality (Table 19-2).

Early Adolescence

Early adolescents (ages 11 to 14) have intense feelings about body image and concerns about whether the changes taking place are normal. Young teens have many questions about normal body functions such as menstruation, spontaneous nocturnal ejaculation, and masturbation. The nurse is in a pivotal role to answer the teen's questions about physical changes and to use correct terminology in discussing sexual functions. Sexual fantasies involving celebrities (like rock and movie stars) and crushes on both sexes are not uncommon. Young teens are less confident with members of the opposite sex and tend to have best friends and form groups of the same sex (Figure 19-4). Sexual experimentation among early adolescents is increasing as the age of sexual maturation declines, but experimentation has not yet reached the intensity of middle adolescence (Stevens-Simon, 1998). Incest and sexual abuse

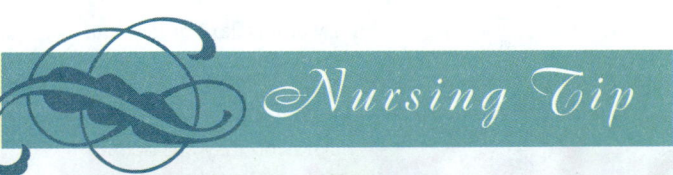

ASSESSMENT AND SEXUAL ABUSE

You should always consider aspects of sexual abuse in any health care encounter as young teens begin to reach physical and sexual maturation. Questions relative to the adolescent's sexuality should be included in the health history. For example, you may begin a discussion of the teen's sexuality by stating: "Many young people your age begin to think about sexual behavior, tell me what you think." Consider what your responsibilities are in asking teens about sexually sensitive information.

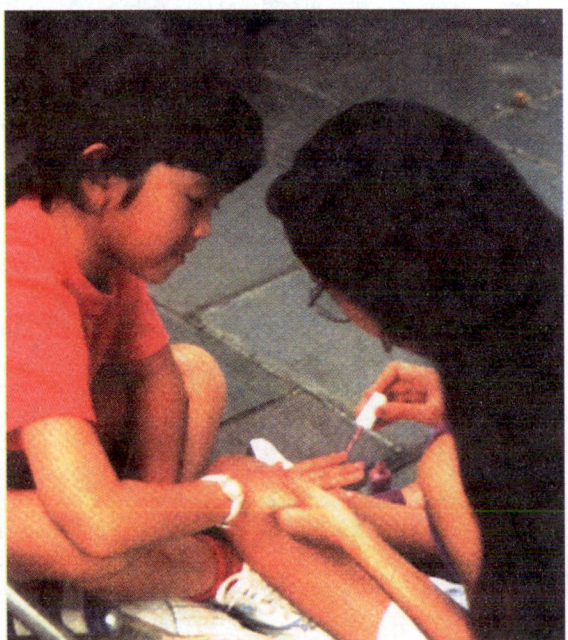

Figure 19-4 In the early years of adolescence, teens often prefer the company of friends of the same gender.

Table 19-2 Stages of Cognition and Aspects of Adolescent Sexuality and Pregnancy

	Early Adolescence (ages 11–14) Concrete Thinking	Middle Adolescence (ages 15–17) Early Abstract Thought	Late Adolescence (ages 18–21) Abstract Reasoning
Cognitive Thinking	Limited abstract thought Appreciates the here and now Little sense of later consequences	Use of inductive/deductive reasoning Ability to understand later consequences of actions Ability to connect separate events and to project into the future Introspective/narcissistic	Ability to abstract and conceptualize Ability to analyze and plan for the future Consider another's needs above their own Concern for society as a whole
Issues in Sexuality	Changing body image Sexual fantasy Sexual vocabulary Sexual abuse/incest Masturbation Menstruation Nocturnal emissions Limited sexual experimentation Same sex peers	Sexual experimentation Peer pressure for sex activity Self-esteem issues and sexuality Over-the-counter contraception Sexual abuse/incest Homosexuality/safe sex practices Sexually transmitted diseases Responsible decision-making related to sexual issues Adequate/effective contraception Sexual preference may still be in flux Short-term commitments to partners Peer acceptance at peak	Responsible sexual decision making Correct use of contraceptive Sexual preference set Greater intimacy/long-term commitments Pregnancy/parenting Some continuation of sexual experimentation More realistic expectation of partner's role Peers of less influence
Issues in Pregnancy	Failure to recognize signs of pregnancy Denial of pregnancy if recognized Fear of telling partner/parents/other adults about pregnancy Delay in seeking pregnancy diagnosis Delay in seeking prenatal care Disturbed about body changes Family upset about pregnancy Ambivalence about pregnancy Other coexisting risk-taking behaviors (drugs; etc.) Conflict in maternal role Lacks problem-solving abilities re: pregnancy Fears related to labor and delivery Lack of ability to plan for the future Partner often not involved	Same Same Same Seeks pregnancy diagnosis from over-the-counter-test kits May seek professional diagnosis of pregnancy Ambivalent about body changes Same Same or desires pregnancy May be the same Same Some problem-solving skills present re: pregnancy Able to learn about labor and delivery but still may fear experience May be able to plan for pregnancy and consider future consequences Partner sometimes involved	Recognizes signs of pregnancy Confirms pregnancy Tells partner and/or parents about pregnancy Seeks professional diagnosis of pregnancy Seeks prenatal care early Accepts body changes Family ambivalent or accepts pregnancy Realistic decisions about pregnancy Less risk-taking evident although risk-taking may still occur Accepts maternal role if pregnancy is desired Able to solve problem re: pregnancy Realistic about labor and delivery Able to plan for future Considers options to pregnancy Partner may be involved, especially for older adolescent/young adult

may occur in both sexes as the adolescent approaches sexual maturity and bodily changes become evident.

The early adolescent is very egocentric and preoccupied with appearances. A great deal of time is spent looking in the mirror and selecting clothing that is desired and sanctioned by the peer group. Self-conscious behavior is thought to be the result of the physical and emotional transition to middle adolescence. The early adolescent is losing the familiar role of the child but does not yet feel comfortable with the role of the adult. Concrete thinking limits the young adolescent to the here and now, and ambivalence towards the future is not uncommon. When early adolescents become pregnant and give birth, they may be ambivalent about caring for the baby and may see child care responsibilities as their parent's concern rather than their own. Caring for the baby and planning for even basic needs, such as child and medical care, may prove challenging for the young adolescent mother who is most preoccupied with herself.

Middle Adolescence

Middle adolescence (ages 15 to 17) is described by parents as the most frustrating period of adolescent development because teens become even more introspective and narcissistic. Conformity to peer group norms becomes even more important, and conflicts between teenagers and parents often escalate (Figure 19-5). The testing of limits and outright rebellion may occur in relation to just about anything; activities related to sex, drugs, alcohol, and violence may have negative outcomes that can last a lifetime. Parental expectations become clear when discipline and structure are consistent. Parental involvement actually makes adolescents feel more secure; decision making can be shared between parent and teen. However, parents must be aware that middle-stage adolescents are impulsive, impatient, and egocentric. Because of their egocentrism, adolescents see themselves as invulnerable; negative consequences (such as HIV infection) "can't happen to me." Concern by parents may be viewed by teens as interference and may be met with resistance and resentment.

Feelings about self-image and social relationships with the opposite sex are intense. Dating in couples occurs and sexual experimentation becomes common. Sexual activity, peer pressure, and self-esteem issues are frequently linked, and adolescents with the poorest self-esteem are most vulnerable to engaging in risky behaviors. Relationships are generally short-term and sexual activity is often unplanned, with little regard to later consequences. Over-the-counter contraception may be used: condoms have become more popular because the public has become more educated about HIV and AIDS. Long-term methods of contraception have proven less effective among teens, because relationships are short-term and contraceptive practices are inconsistent (Stevens-Simon, 1998).

Nurses may help by providing accurate information to assist adolescents in making appropriate choices related to sexuality and by encouraging parents to maintain open communication and guide teenagers in sexual decision making (Figure 19-6). Parental guidance regarding sexual behavior is not an easy task during middle adolescence, when privacy is of extreme importance and communication tends to decrease with parents and increase with peers. Guided peer-group discussion has been shown to

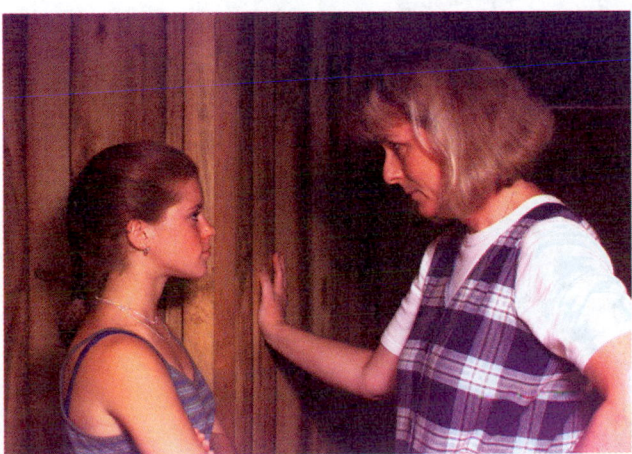

Figure 19-5 Making adjustments in family power configurations is necessary to provide opportunities for teenagers to develop their own identities.

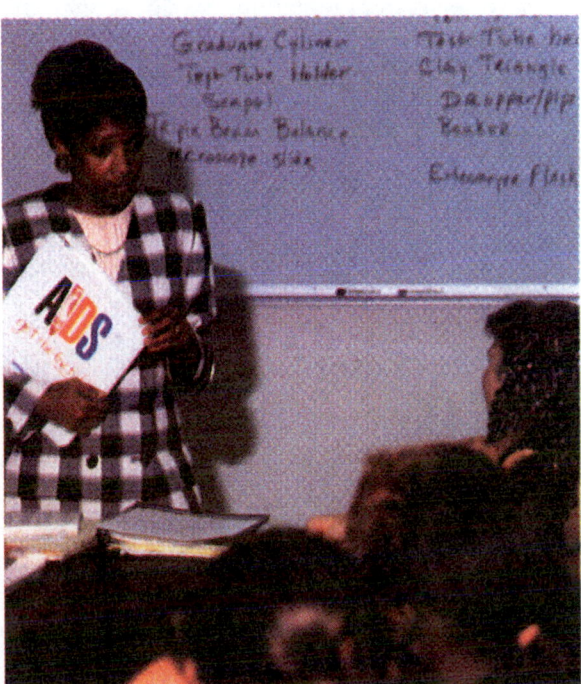

Figure 19-6 Wellness promotion for the adolescent may include in-school seminars by school nurses, such as this one on AIDs prevention.

be beneficial in providing information on sexually related issues and allowing teens to express their feelings about their own sexuality. As adolescents move from concrete to abstract reasoning, the consequences of their sexual decisions become more real to them.

Late Adolescence

Late adolescence (age 18 to 19) is characterized by abstract thinking, verbal conceptualization, and anticipation of the consequences of actions. Teens in late adolescence tend to be idealistic about love, social issues, ethics, and lifestyles, until their experiences modify their beliefs. Conformity becomes less important as teens become more confident of their personal identity. Parent-teen relationships may become more respectful, unless values clash, and relationships with both family and friends become important. Intimate relationships become more mutual, and expectations of partners become more realistic. Although some degree of sexual experimentation may continue, older adolescents typically have a greater capacity for long-term commitment.

Emancipation is a major issue. Teens in late adolescence prepare themselves to meet this challenge by education or vocational training. Older adolescents and young adults are generally better suited to parenthood by virtue of their greater education, greater earning power, and more sustained relationships than younger teens. However, emancipation may become difficult if the adolescent is single, unmarried, and impoverished. Dependence on welfare payments and the existing family is often the end result, and the developmental tasks of adolescence may never be fully achieved.

Issues Related to Adolescent Sexuality, Pregnancy, and Parenting

Adolescence is a period of transition: Pregnancy at any stage of adolescent development, but particularly in early and middle adolescence, poses an additional transition that makes identity formation more difficult. Sadler and Catrone (1983) describe adolescent pregnancy as a "dual developmental crisis" and describe major areas of potential conflict (Table 19-3).

The change in body image is particularly distressing to young adolescents who may find labor, delivery, and lactation not only frightening but unpleasant and undesirable. The father-to-be may also find his partner's body changes unattractive, throwing the young expectant mother into despair over her rapidly changing appearance. Because relationships are relatively short during early and middle adolescence, partners may terminate the relationship before the baby's birth (Figure 19-7). Approximately two-thirds of teen relationships in which pregnancy occurs end

Table 19-3 Dual Developmental Tasks of Adolescent Mothers

Adolescence	Versus	Parenthood

Adolescence	Parenthood
• Narcissistic and egocentrist/introspective, self-absorbed; focus on own needs	• Empathy with the child; place child's needs before own
• Ambivalent attachment to child	• Mutuality between mother and child; mother's needs met through parenting
• Identity formation through role experimentation; no firm commitment to a specific role	• Maternal role identification and definition
• Sexual identity formation/body image development	• Body image changes of pregnancy, delivery, and postpartum
• Emancipation from family	• Family role reassignments: from child to mother
• Cognitive development: transition from concrete to abstract thinking	• Problem solving and decision making skills necessary for raising child

Adapted with permission from The adolescent parent: A dual developmental crisis, by Sadler, L., & Catrone, C. (1983). *Journal of Adolescent Health Care. 4,* 102.

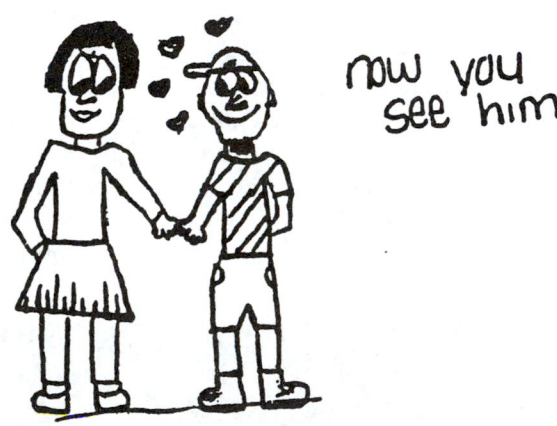

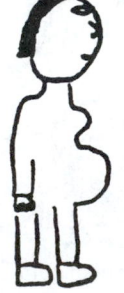

Figure 19-7 Teen pregnancy: now you see him, now you don't.

before delivery. A recent study showed that fathers who attend prenatal care sessions, visit the infant in the hospital after birth, and have an established relationship with the young mother's family are more likely to still be involved when their children are 24 months old (Cox & Bithoney, 1995). Programs that acknowledge and promote a more active participation by young fathers are needed to encourage the formulation of paternal roles and responsibilities.

Adolescents who give birth may actually have little understanding of their own body functions or their own sexuality. Nurses are in an excellent position, in both the prenatal and postpartum periods, to explore these areas with teen mothers. Pregnancy and subsequent parenthood limit the teen's time, mobility, and ability to experiment with new roles because the responsibilities of child care must be assumed. Conflicts may arise regarding whose needs are being met as the adolescent mother attempts to differentiate her needs from her infant's needs during the normal adolescent transition period. Emancipation issues may become an area of conflict for the teen mother and her family. Developmentally, the teen mother needs to move away from the family and become autonomous, but realistically, she may be dependent on the family for financial and child care assistance.

Who's in charge and how the infant is raised is a likely area for disagreement. It is not uncommon to see the young adolescent mother step aside as her own mother takes over decisions related to the child's health and welfare. Finally, all aspects of parenting are influenced by the mother's cognitive development. Adolescent parents who lack the cognitive skills to understand their child's behavior and development may have unrealistically high expectations for their infants and young children and may be harsh disciplinarians who use physical punishment frequently. A young mother who does not realize that a toddler has a limited memory may become easily frustrated and angry when the child fails to follow her commands. The mother's ability to understand the principles of child development and to project and plan for the future has a definitive effect on the child's well-being (see Table 19-2).

Adolescent Sexual Activity

The scenario in the "Reflections" box is not uncommon among teen mothers, and yet, after over 30 years of effective and available birth control measures, adults often ask, why. The path to teen pregnancy is influenced by many factors. Experimentation with sexual relationships, the need to love and be loved, peer pressure, promotion of self-esteem, partner pressure, and the need to feel grown up are reasons cited by teens as motivation for early sexual activity (Moore, 1996). Furthermore, teens state that loneliness, lack of understanding child care responsibilities, poor self-respect, lack of knowledge about their bod-

REFLECTIONS FROM A TEEN MOTHER

"I never expected to get pregnant," says 15-year-old Alyce, "It just sort of happened. Now I'm struggling with school, and I have to get up a lot earlier just so I can get the baby ready, take him to daycare, and make it to class. It's getting harder to stay in school as he gets older; he wants my attention all the time. I wish my mother would just take care of him so I could get on with my life."

ies and birth control, drinking and drug use, and a general dissatisfaction with their lives contribute to an early, unplanned pregnancy (Chassler, 1997).

On a national level, the use of drugs and alcohol among adolescents has risen steadily, the family structure and social mores that discouraged unwed motherhood have diminished, and religious affiliations have declined. Responsible sexual behavior and the consequences of sexual risk-taking are not taught consistently. Some adolescents view having a child as their only real accomplishment, when even a high school diploma doesn't guarantee a job. One young man, who had fathered several children by different women, described his children as "something I can leave to the world, sort of like art work." The fact that he was unemployed and did not support any of his children appeared to be of little concern to him.

The age at which adolescents initiate sexual activity has declined as the age of **sexual maturation** (the establishment of menstruation and ovulation in females and the development of spermatogenesis in males) has declined. Unfortunately, emotional maturity develops later than physical maturity, and many adolescents who engage in sexual relations to meet their biologic needs do not think of future consequences. Young people are confronted with sexual feelings and opportunities for sexual activity for which they may be cognitively and emotionally unprepared. This lack of preparation undoubtedly predisposes American teenagers to the negative consequences of sexual experimentation, among which are unintended pregnancy and STDs. Approximately 50% of all adolescent pregnancies occur within the first 6 months of initiating sexual intercourse, but only about 40% of teens seek contraceptive services within the first year of initiating sexual activity; two-thirds do not use birth control routinely (The Contraception Report, 1995). Contraceptive practices are often influenced by the adolescent's limited cognitive ability or lack of ability to think abstractly.

Taking an accurate sexual history from adolescents during routine health care visits is an opportunity to discuss the adolescent's sexuality and to assist her or him in selecting a method of contraception or help prepare for the initiation of sexual intercourse (Figure 19-8). Adolescents respond best to direct, open questions that are stated clearly and in terms they understand. It is necessary to be sincere and to demonstrate empathy, support, and understanding when questioning the adolescent about such sensitive issues (Box 19-2).

The average age of first-time sexual experience in girls is age 17 and in boys, age 15 to 16 (Centers for Disease Control and Prevention [CDC], 1994b). Approximately 24% of American youth report first intercourse before age 15 (Haffner, 1995). Variation in the age of first-time sexual intercourse is often culturally driven. African American adolescents are shown to engage in sexual intercourse earlier than Caucasian and Hispanic adolescents, African American males are the youngest to initiate sexual activity (CDC, 1996). According to the 1995 Youth Risk Behavior Surveillance System (YRBSS), which surveyed over 10,000 high school students nationally in grades 9 through 12,

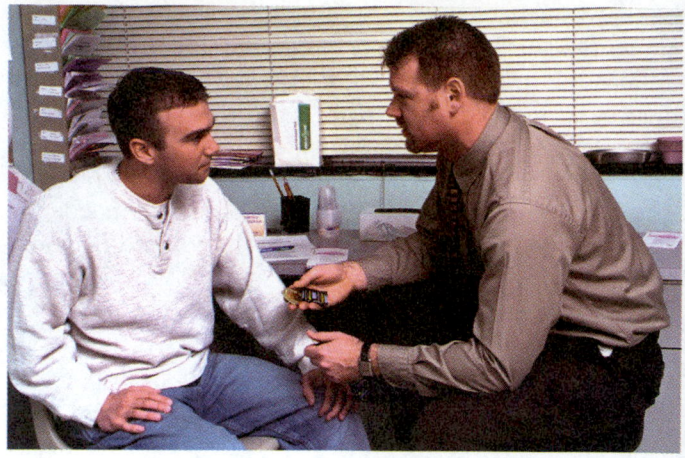

Figure 19-8 A straightforward, friendly approach when taking a health history from a teen facilitates a discussion about sexuality and birth control.

African American males were significantly more likely to initiate sexual intercourse before age 13, have sexual intercourse with multiple partners, use alcohol or drugs at the time of sexual intercourse, and to impregnate a partner. On a more positive note, African American males were

---

Box 19-2 Taking the Adolescent Sexual History

- Many young people your age begin to have sexual thoughts and feeling. Tell me about yours.

- What age did you start menstruation/ejaculation? Tell me how you are feeling about this development.

- You do have a choice about whether or not you want to have sex. Do you feel that you have a choice? Tell me something about what choices you have made.

- Are you having sex now? *(If yes)* With females/males/both? Oral or anal sex? With the same partner or different partners? At what age did you have your first sexual experience? Is having sex pleasurable for you? Tell me about the last time you had sex. Are you or your partner using anything to prevent pregnancy or sexually transmitted diseases STDs? What methods do you use?

- Have you ever been pregnant? Tell me about it.

- Have you ever had a sexually transmitted disease? How was this treated? Was your partner(s) treated also? What do you understand about this disease?

- What would you do if you (or your partner) became pregnant?

- Would you like to know about methods to prevent pregnancy?

- Tell me what you know about HIV/AIDS. Do you know what it means to have "safe sex"? Have you ever used (or practiced using) a condom? What would you like to know about condoms?
  (If no to sex now) Have you had sex in the past? Tell me how you felt about it.

- Are your friends having sex? having babies?

- Before having sex, would you talk to your parent(s) about making that decision? Perhaps to a friend or another adult? How do you feel about using condoms? Have you considered what method of birth control you would use? How do you feel about becoming pregnant now?

- Have you ever been sexually assaulted? Sexually abused? Touched in a private way that you did not want? *(If yes)* Tell me about what happened to you. How did you feel about this? Who supported you after this happened? Did you have any counseling? *(If yes)* Describe how you felt about the counseling. *(If no)* Would you consider counseling now?

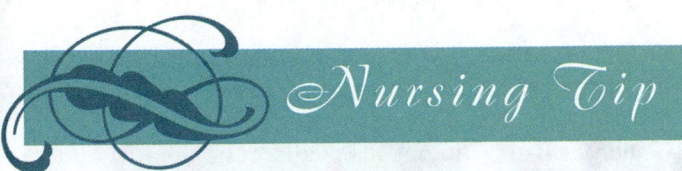

CONFIDENTIALITY AND REFERRAL

You should know the laws of confidentiality in your state for providing care to adolescents and have resources available for all adolescents, including minors, who are pregnant or are engaging in high-risk sexual behaviors.

significantly more likely to have used a condom at last intercourse and to have discussed HIV infection and AIDS with a parent or another adult.

Adolescent Attitudes Toward Contraception

While it is commonly believed that adolescents do not use contraception because sexual relations are impulsive and unplanned, there are other factors that also contribute to lack of contraceptive use. Many unplanned and untimely pregnancies are suspected to really be planned and wanted. For some teens, a pregnancy, which was neither planned or unplanned, is an occurrence that validates their level of maturity through fertility. In some cultural groups, the state of pregnancy confers adult status. In a recent study, investigators examined the reasons for lack of contraceptive use among indigent adolescent women, ages 13 to 18 (Stevens-Simon, Kelly, Singer, & Cox, 1996). The findings of this study suggest that indigent adolescent females have positive or ambivalent feelings about becoming pregnant that interfere with consistent, effective contraceptive use. Young people may view parenting as a means to escape a current living situation, maintain a tenuous relationship, or please an older sexual partner. Still other reasons for lack of contraceptive use include: lack of knowledge about and access to birth control, defiance of parental authority, fear of being discovered as sexually active by parents, denial of participating in sexual activity that requires birth control, fear of contraceptives or a pelvic examination, contraceptive failure, and feelings of invulnerability, i.e., "it can't happen to me" (Stevens-Simon, 1997). Clearly nurses, especially those in schools or adolescent specialty clinics, are in a key position to educate young people about risk-taking behaviors related to sexual activity.

Adolescent Contraceptive Methods

"Just say no," or abstinence-only, programs aimed at sexually mature teens have proven to be unrealistic and largely ineffective in significantly delaying the initiation or slow-

ing the frequency of sexual activity (Stout & Kirby, 1993). Abstinence-focused pregnancy prevention programs given in combination with reproductive and contraceptive information are more effective in reducing early sexual involvement but their efficacy in preventing adolescent pregnancy is questionable. Programs that stress knowledge content, values clarification, decision-making, and communication skills between partners and parents are thought to improve decision-making skills of teens with regard to sexual behavior. However, a review of these intervention programs demonstrated little effect on sexual or contraceptive behavior past the immediate period after the programs (Stout & Kirby, 1993).

Because of the high rate of pregnancy and STDs among all adolescents, nurses and other health care providers should not shy away from suggesting abstinence as a means of contraception. Teens need to consider abstinence as an option and to know that they have a choice about becoming sexually active. Abstinence not only prevents pregnancy but offers the greatest protection against STDs. Some adolescents, in the face of peer pressure, may need continued support to maintain abstinence. Whatever contraceptive method is chosen, the most effective contraceptives for teens are those that are acceptable to teens and match their needs; obviously, contraceptives that are not used will not be effective. Chapter 14 discusses contraceptives in greater detail.

Choosing an appropriate contraceptive is a decision that should ideally be made by couples. Nurses working with adolescents should emphasize that contraception is a shared responsibility (Figure 19-9). Studies suggest that teens agree that contraception should be a shared responsibility (Sheehan, Ostwald, and Rothenberger, 1988), but clinical evidence suggests that often nobody takes responsibility. A contraceptive method that is not acceptable to both partners is likely to be unused. Factors that should be

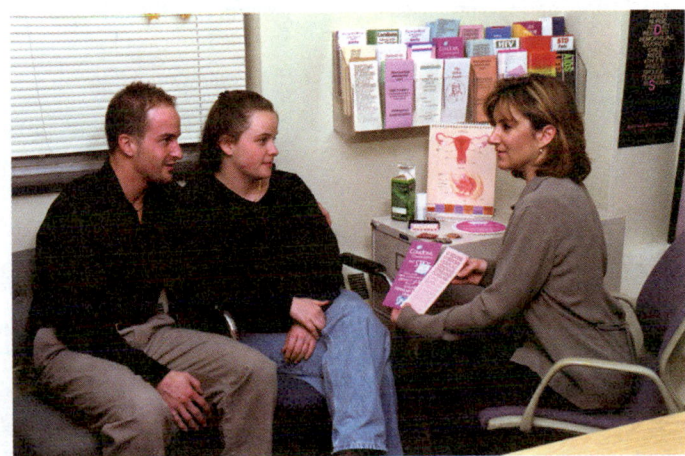

Figure 19-9 Learning about contraceptive choices as a couple helps teens learn that birth control is a shared responsibility.

considered in selecting contraceptive methods are described in Table 19-4.

Adolescents use withdrawal, condoms, and oral contraceptive pills (OCPs) as the most frequent methods of contraception (Stevens-Simon, 1997). Most adolescents rarely maintain consistent compliance, and failure rates are much higher than those described for adults. Cost and easy accessibility are two of the most important factors in selecting contraceptive methods. For these reasons, condoms and withdrawal are methods likely to be selected first by sexually active teens. Methods such as diaphragms or injections, which are expensive or require contact with health care services, are less likely to be used. School-based clinics and free or sliding scale primary care clinics marketed for teens increase the availability of all methods of contraception.

The withdrawal method of contraception is the removal of the penis from the vagina before ejaculation. Withdrawal is relatively ineffective (18% failure rate) and requires a great deal of control. Seminal fluid is often deposited into the vagina before ejaculation, and pregnancy can and does occur. However, withdrawal does not cost money and may be the only option when sexual intercourse is spontaneous and unplanned.

Condoms are becoming more popular as awareness of AIDS has increased among adolescents. According to the 1995 YRBSS study, 54% of high school males and 48.6% of high school females reported condom use at last intercourse (CDC, 1996). Condoms are available at a relatively low cost but are only moderately effective (9% to 12% failure, rate if used consistently and properly). Condoms made out of latex provide the best protection from pregnancy and disease. Latex helps prevent the passage of HIV, herpes virus, and hepatitis virus, although no condom is 100% effective. Adolescents should be encouraged to read labels and select condoms that are made in the United States. The U.S. Food and Drug Administration (FDA) has strict requirements regarding permeability, strength, and shelf life (expiration date). Lubricated condoms that contain the spermicide nonoxynol-9 are the most effective against disease and pregnancy. In addition to killing sperm, nonoxynol-9 is known to be somewhat effective as an antibacterial and antiviral agent.

Adolescent couples need explicit instruction on condom use and should be able to demonstrate how to safely put on and remove a condom (Figure 19-10). Teens should be encouraged to use condoms along with spermicides containing nonoxynol-9, such as contraceptive foam, cream, or suppositories, for greater protection. When used consistently and correctly, the efficacy of condoms plus spermicides approaches that of oral contraceptives. Of the spermicides on the market, contraceptive foam is most preferred by adolescents because it provides additional lubrication, yet leaves little residue after intercourse. Spermicidal jelly, KY Jelly, or other water-based products can be used for additional lubrication. A lack of sufficient lubrication in adolescent females can account for condoms slipping when being used by teen couples. Products containing oil, such as petroleum jelly or baby lotion, can cause latex to deteriorate and make condoms ineffective. Misuse

Table 19-4 Factors to Consider in the Selection of Adolescent Contraception

- Cognitive development (concrete vs abstract thinking)
- Clarification of attitudes and values
- Sexual maturity rating (SMR)
- Communication with partner
- Use of more than one Method
- Frequency of intercourse
- Appropriate Information (3 messages per visit)
- Knowledge of back-up methods
- Problem solving abilities (appeal to logic and feelings of power over body)
- Communication with parents or other adults
- Physical/mental health
- Motivation of both partners
- Concrete, graphic instruction on all methods
- Number and gender of partners
- Encouragement that abstinence is OK
- Availability of resources

Note: Adapted with permission from The adolescent, Busen, N. (1997). In J. Ashwill & S. Droske (Eds.), *Nursing Care of Children: Principles and Practice* (p. 168). Philadelphia: W.B. Saunders Co.

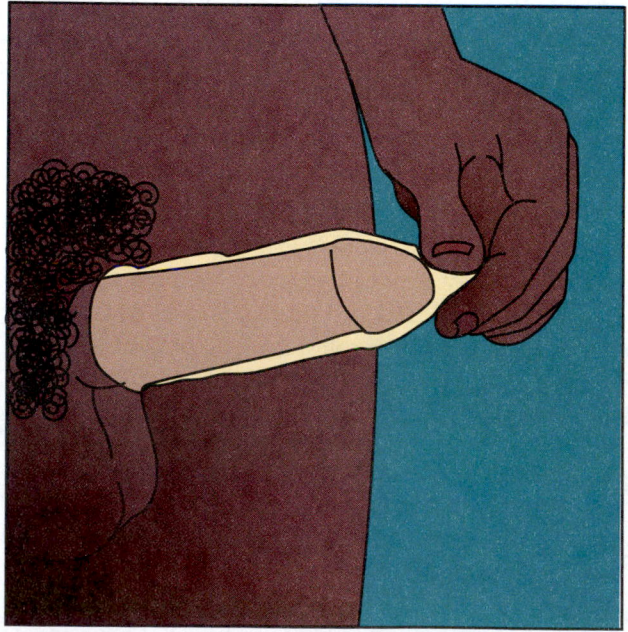

Figure 19-10 The condom should be unrolled on an erect penis, all the way to the base, having about a half-inch of space at the end for a semen reservoir.

of condoms accounts for the higher failure rate of condoms among teens. Other barrier methods, such as diaphragms, are relatively unpopular or ineffective. Adolescent females must be comfortable with their bodies and highly motivated to use the cervical cap or diaphragm (Figure 19-11), and the use of spermicidals alone has a high failure rate (21%) (Hatcher et al., 1998).

The most effective method of birth control for adolescent females is OCPs, if used correctly. According to Hatcher et al. (1998) combination OCPs (those containing estrogen and progestin) have a failure rate of 0.1%. The actual failure rate for teens using OCPs for the first time is 5%. Teens are doubly vulnerable to birth control failures in that they have intercourse frequently and are often less experienced and less motivated to use a method consistently. OCPs are stopped when relationships end and not necessarily restarted appropriately with a new sexual partner. Combined OCPs work by suppressing ovulation, increasing the thickness of the cervical mucosa (preventing penetration by sperm), and decresing the thickness of the uterine lining (preventing implantation of the egg). Side effects of combined OCPs include weight gain, breast tenderness, headaches, and breakthrough bleeding. Teens experienc-

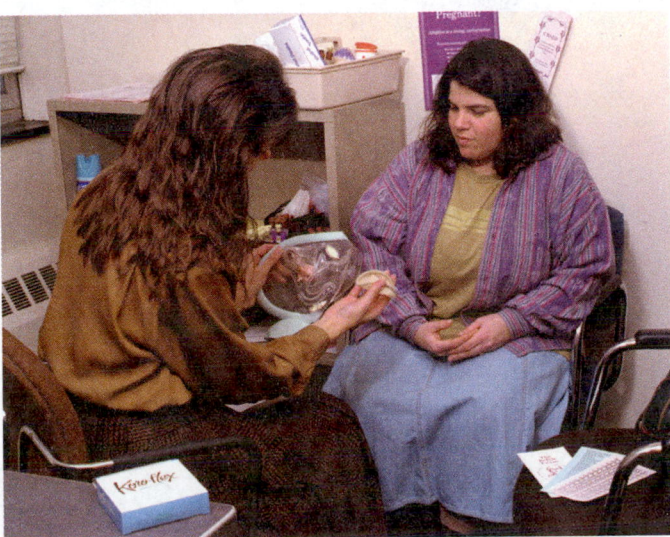

Figure 19-11 Demonstration with an anatomical model helps this teen understand correct diaphragm use.

ing OCP side effects should not discontinue pills but contact their health care provider. Side effects are generally from the amount of estrogen and progestin contained in the pill. With numerous OCPs on the market, changing pills can usually minimize undesirable side effects. In addition to preventing pregnancy, OCPs are known to confer protection against ovarian and endometrial cancers, pelvic inflammatory disease, ectopic pregnancy, and toxic shock syndrome (Stevens-Simon, 1997).

Relatively new to the U.S. market are injectable medroxyprogesterone, Depo-Provera, and a subdermal progestin, Norplant. Neither of these methods of birth control contains estrogen, which makes them particularly suitable for women with cardiovascular conditions or who are lactating. The progestin-only methods work in a similar manner to combined OCPs but have the added advantage of long-acting contraception not tied to sexual activity. Depo-Provera is an injection that is received every 3 months and is effective for approximately 16 weeks. Norplant, a set of capsules containing progestin that is placed under the skin in the hip or upper arm, is visible if inserted correctly. The visibility of the Norplant may be an issue with teens who desire the utmost privacy about their sexual activity. The set of capsules releases a continuous dose of progestin for 5 years.

The injectable and implantable devices are highly effective methods of birth control, but can cause side effects that include amenorrhea, irregular periods, heavy bleeding, and weight gain. Headaches, hair loss, and depression are less common side effects but warrant consideration. The long-term methods of birth control are appealing to young women who do not plan pregnancy any time in the near future. However, problems with the frequency of progestin-related side effects and the visibility and necessity for removal of the capsules in the Norplant system have made use of long-acting progestin methods of contraception controversial (Mashburn, 1994).

In 1997, the FDA gave approval for the use of certain oral contraceptives to be used as a postcoital, or "morning-after," method of birth control. Although these have been used for years in the U.S. and other countries, drug companies were not allowed to advertise combined pills as a postcoital method of contraception because such use had not yet been approved by the FDA. The use of the OCPs as a postcoital method of contraception is commonly recommended after rape, and the method has also become popular among college students. Controversy has surrounded the use of morning-after pills as an abortifacient; the method of action prevents fertilization of an egg or stops a fertilized egg from implanting in the uterus.

Two combined oral contraceptive pills containing 200 μg of ethinyl estradiol and 2 mg of levonorgestrel are taken within 72 hours of intercourse (preferably within 12 to 24 hours); then two more pills are taken 12 hours later.

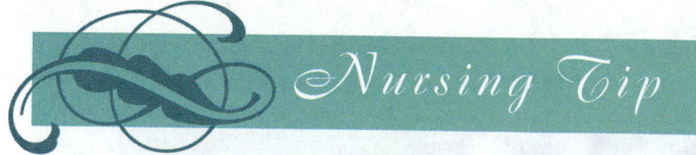

CONTRACEPTIVE METHODS

Whatever method of contraception is used by teens, it should *always* be accompanied by condom use to decrease the likelihood of transmission of STDs.

The morning-after method is known to be effective, with few side effects other than nausea and cramping. The pills are most often given with an antiemetic to minimize nausea and vomiting. Bleeding generally occurs between 14 to 21 days after taking the pills and lowers the risk of pregnancy to less than 8%. It is essential to determine if the teenager is already pregnant; if pregnancy is confirmed, the morning-after pills should not be given. If used correctly, postcoital contraception is highly effective in preventing an unwanted pregnancy but should not serve as a substitute for a consistent, effective method of birth control.

Adolescents should be encouraged to discuss their sexuality, sexual behavior, contraception, and pregnancy with their parents or another trusted adult whenever possible, but nurses must guarantee the confidentiality of such communication. The nurse's professional role is to assist adolescents in making knowledgeable and responsible decisions regarding their sexual behavior (Figure 19-12). Primary prevention must emphasize assisting adolescents to develop coping strategies to meet their needs in ways other than through sexual behavior. Life skills training programs, organized sports, and church activities can help point the adolescent's time and energy in a positive direction. On a national level, social welfare policies should promote educational and vocational experiences that are meaningful and accessible to adolescents as a means of encouraging future planning and discouraging early parenting.

Adolescents can be educated to consider the negative outcomes of risky sexual behavior and weigh the consequences of their actions. In a school-based or primary care clinic, the nurse's role may be one of "gatekeeper" or case manager in facilitating access to intervention programs and

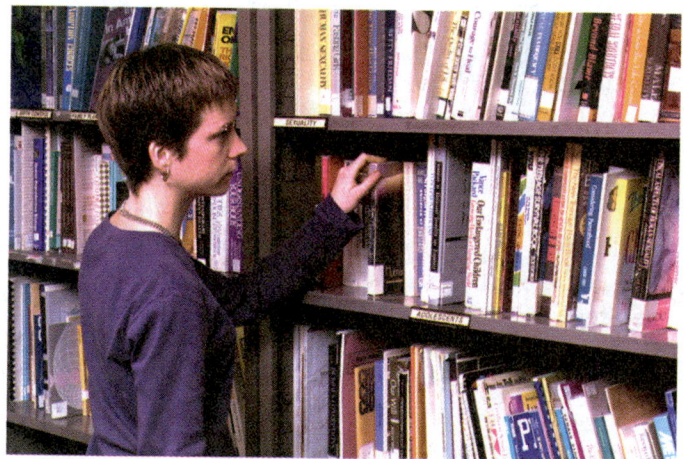

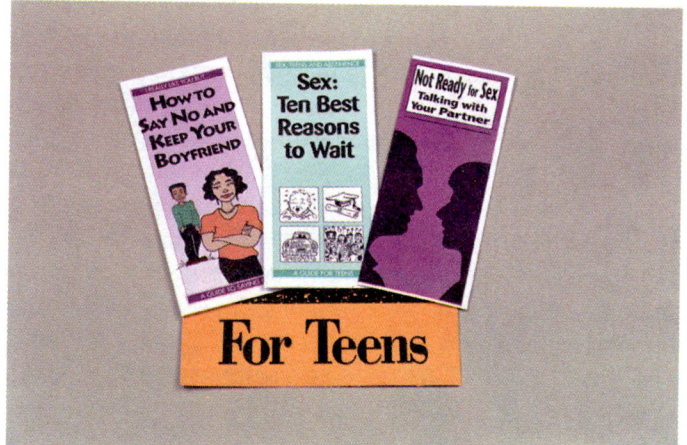

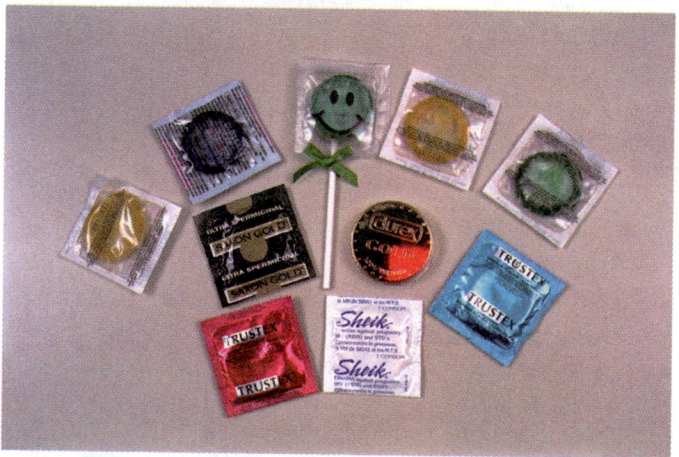

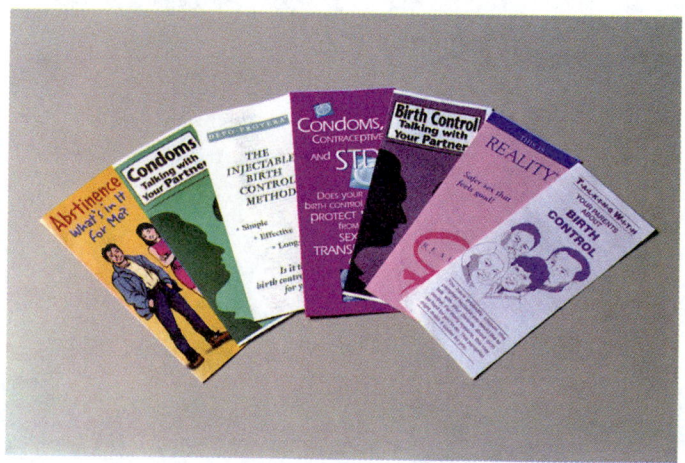

Figure 19-12 Adolescents may wish to look up information on sexual behaviors as they make decisions about their own sexuality. Nurses can also counsel teens and offer information and devices designed specifically for the adolescent population.

Critical Thinking

The Nurse and Sexuality

Nurses who are open, honest, and comfortable with their own sexuality are the most likely to gain the adolescent's trust and confidence, and to interact with adolescents in a confidential atmosphere. How comfortable are you with your own sexuality and discussing sexual issues with teens? How do you feel about maintaining confidentiality with information that you think an involved parent might want to know?

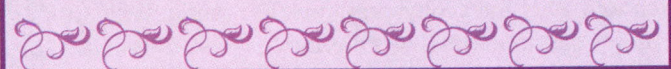

other community resources. Dealing with the unwanted consequences of adolescent pregnancy can be complicated and collaboration with other health care providers is essential in meeting the needs of sexually active youth.

Repeat Adolescent Pregnancy

Without effective contraception and intensive postpartum support and follow-up to maintain contraception, repeat adolescent pregnancy is common. The repeat pregnancy rate is estimated to be 30% in the first year after delivery and 25% to 50% during the second postpartum year. Young women at highest risk for a second pregnancy are those who (1) are under 16 years of age at conception of the first pregnancy, (2) have a boyfriend older than age 20, (3) are high school drop-outs, (4) are below appropriate grade level for age, (5) are dependent on welfare compensation after the first birth, (6) had complications with the first pregnancy (such as prematurity), and (7) had no established method of birth control after hospital discharge (Stevens-Simon & McAnarney, 1992). Multigravidity, which has its roots in adolescence, is consistently linked to educational disadvantage and poverty. The risk of a preterm delivery increases with each successive adolescent pregnancy and positive neonatal outcomes decline.

Nursing Implications

Early diagnosis of an adolescent pregnancy is important for counseling purposes and for early entry into prenatal care. Many adolescents delay diagnosis and have no prenatal care in the first trimester of pregnancy. Early and consistent prenatal care is known to decrease the negative outcomes to the fetus, especially those born to women under the age of 16 (Stevens-Simon & White, 1991). Pregnant adolescents may initially present for confirmation or diagnosis of pregnancy with a variety of complaints. Some present with typical signs and symptoms of pregnancy, others present with vague complaints that may or may not be helpful in establishing a diagnosis of pregnancy. Teens who are in denial may be vague with respect to their last menses and complain of fatigue, headache, or abdominal pain. Because adolescents often do not know when they became pregnant, pelvic ultrasound is helpful in estimating gestational age. Approximately one-third of adolescents have vaginal bleeding during the first trimester and may mistake this for regular menses, denying the possibility of a pregnancy. The adolescent's sense of invulnerability may be in full operation and denial is common. "I thought I was too young to get pregnant" and "I had sex a lot and I didn't get pregnant so I thought I couldn't" are frequent comments when pregnancy is confirmed.

The use of a good sexual history is essential in obtaining information that leads to the confirmation of pregnancy. Once the pregnancy is confirmed, the adolescent should be counseled regarding her options and appropriate referrals should be made. Pregnant adolescents may have difficulty in solving problems and making decisions related to the pregnancy. Because adolescents need a great deal of support they should be strongly encouraged to share their pregnancy with their parents or another adult who can help them solve problems. Young women should also be encouraged to share confirmation of their pregnancy with the father of the baby. Teens who have short-lived relationships are often reluctant to share pregnancy information with the father of their child. Roles for the adolescent father can include taking responsibility for the pregnancy, participating in the decision-making process related to the pregnancy, and offering financial and emotional support if possible (Figure 19-13).

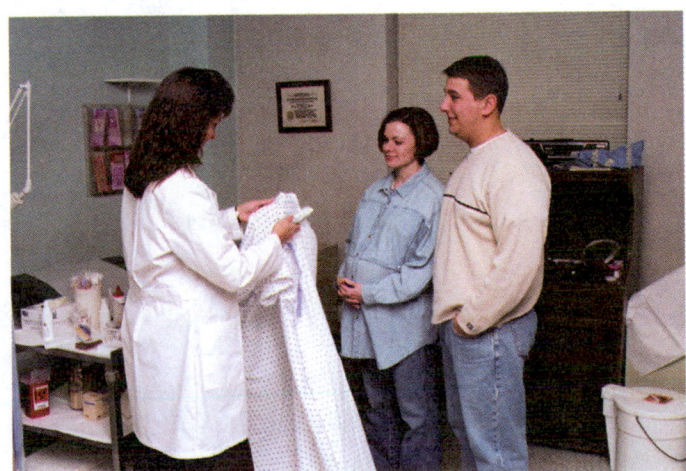

Figure 19-13 Expectant fathers who participate in prenatal visits gain a better understanding of pregnancy and the imminent responsibilities of parenthood.

Prenatal Care, Labor and Delivery, and Postpartum Care

If the adolescent decides to continue the pregnancy, she should be referred to a comprehensive adolescent maternity program. Such programs are best at providing age-appropriate care and for offering prenatal education that is developmentally appropriate. Young teens who are concrete thinkers are best taught by simple, graphic instruction and demonstration. Videotapes, role modeling, interacting with other teen mothers, parenting exercises, and a hands-on approach to prenatal care are methods of instruction that are more effective than just providing verbal and written materials to pregnant teens. Being in a similar peer group assists the pregnant adolescent in adjusting to the pregnancy and becoming engaged in the activities necessary for a successful outcome. School-based clinics and programs, such as Communities in Schools (CIS), that provide prenatal education for pregnant couples are effective in preparing young teens for pregnancy, labor, delivery, and parenting. Prenatal education should include anatomy and physiology of the mother's body, the developing fetus, and the physiologic aspects of labor and delivery. Young women are particularly interested in seeing pictures of the developing fetus and graphic illustration (such as videotapes) of labor and delivery. Graphic illustrations provide the adolescent with a visual experience and help to decrease the misconceptions about body changes and what to expect during labor and delivery.

Other aspects of prenatal care should include the importance and frequency of:

- Prenatal visits
- Prenatal diet and exercises
- Treatment of STDs
- Immunizations
- Use of medications and abstinence from cigarettes, alcohol and other drugs
- Preparation for labor and delivery
- Recognition of signs of labor, who to call, and where to go
- Discharge planning and postpartum follow-up

Prenatal education involving the infant would include:

- Information on breast feeding, formulas, and infant nutrition
- Identification and acquisition of the necessary clothing and equipment for the newborn
- The need for and identification of appropriate resources for well child care
- Basic skills, such as bathing, diapering, and feeding newborns
- How to take a temperature

- Recognition of urgent and emergent conditions in newborns
- Identification of emergency resources
- Automobile and child safety
- Infant and child development with particular emphasis on age-appropriate discipline

Ideally, comprehensive maternity programs include the baby's father and offer classes with other young expectant couples over a series of weeks or months in preparation for the baby's birth. Adolescents should be strongly encouraged to remain in school during the pregnancy, and school-based maternity programs are particularly supportive to that outcome. Community- or school-based programs designed especially for teens also emphasize issues in the transition to parenting and offer guidance for couples in maintaining relationships and dealing with conflicts related to their change in lifestyle. Negotiating an intimate relationship is often difficult enough for teen couples; the additional stress of finances and childrearing can be devastating given the tenuous nature of many adolescent relationships. More children of teen mothers grow up in a single-parent household than any other group in the U.S. (Maynard, 1996).

Pregnant teens under the age of 16 years are at greatest risk for obstetric complications. These complications are thought to be less causally related to physiologic factors but strongly linked to factors associated with teen pregnancy, such as poverty, poor nutritional habits, and inadequate and late prenatal care. Pregnant teens are at greater risk for iron-deficiency anemia that is secondary to poor nutritional intake. Teens need help in selecting iron-rich foods that are palatable and acceptable; most maternity services refer to a nutritionist to assist teens in developing diet plans that are nutritionally sound but include "fast foods" that are popular with teens. For low-income families with a pregnant adolescent, federal- and community-supported food resources are generally available. Body changes may be disturbing, and pregnant teens may restrict their caloric intake to maintain a pre-pregnant figure. Information on the increased nutritional needs of the body and the developing fetus is important. Assurances that diet and exercise after birth will return the teen to her pre-pregnant weight are encouraging.

Pregnancy-induced hypertension appears to be related to parity and weight gain. In multiparous adolescents, blood pressure and weight gain should be monitored frequently after baseline data have been established (Figure 19-14). Cephalopelvic disproportion (CPD) is common only in very young adolescents (ages 11 to 13) who have not established complete pelvic growth and is more causally related to body type than to maternal age. STDs and substance abuse are known to be common co-existing factors in adolescents who exhibit other high-risk behav-

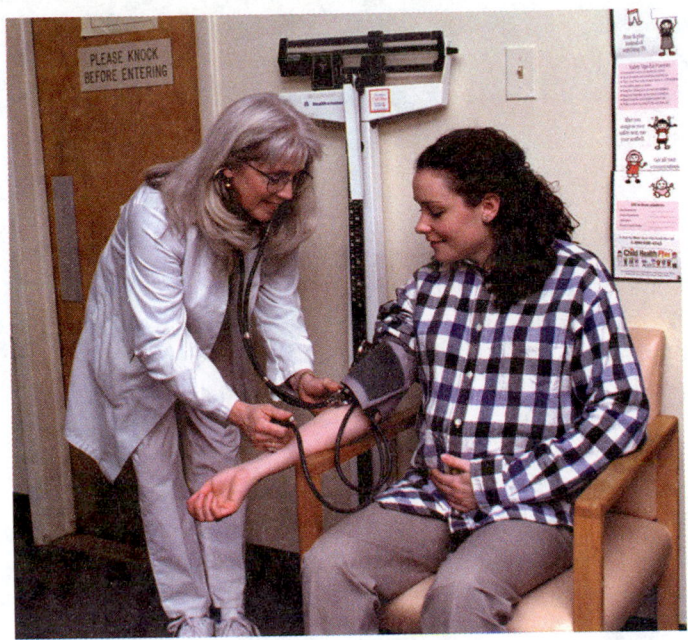

Figure 19-14 The adolescent's blood pressure should be carefully monitored throughout a pregnancy.

iors. Therefore, STDs and substance abuse must be considered in any adolescent pregnancy. Adolescents with a history of multiple partners and drug abuse should be counseled and tested for HIV infection. Specific and consistent follow-up is extremely important in decreasing the **vertical transmission** of HIV from the mother to the fetus during pregnancy or delivery and to the neonate during breastfeeding. STDs should be treated appropriately for both partners. Pregnant teens should also receive education regarding the effects of smoking, alcohol, and drugs on themselves and the developing fetus. Teens with a casual drug habit are more inclined to discontinue or decrease drug use during pregnancy. Teens who are addicted are more likely to remain addicted during pregnancy; crack cocaine is frequently the drug of choice. Referral to substance abuse treatment may be a viable option.

Although the postpartum period most often focuses on maternal identity and infant care, ongoing primary care for the mother and the baby should be identified early and become well-established. Adolescent mothers often seek care for their baby but lack care for themselves. Clinics that offer health care for both the mother and child are more successful in delivering services that support child health and consistent contraceptive practices, thus decreasing repeat pregnancy and encouraging education and vocation (Figure 19-15). Young couples with multiple social problems are best referred to comprehensive

Client Education

Home Visit Guidelines for Adolescent Parents

- Assess the social support system (parents, relatives, friends, neighbors, community agencies) for the adolescent parents

- Encourage ongoing contact with the health care system for parents and infant, including community agencies such as the Visiting Nurse Service (VNS)

- Review the parents's knowledge of child development and expectations for their child

- Identify school- and community-based services that would encourage continuing education for the parents and enhance infant development

- Provide support to adolescent couples who may experience stress in the parenting role

- Include the baby's father in all aspects of infant care, when possible

- Identify referral sources for social, educational, and vocational needs

- Provide information on reproductive physiology and family planning

- Provide support for future plans, if adolescent parents choose to stay together

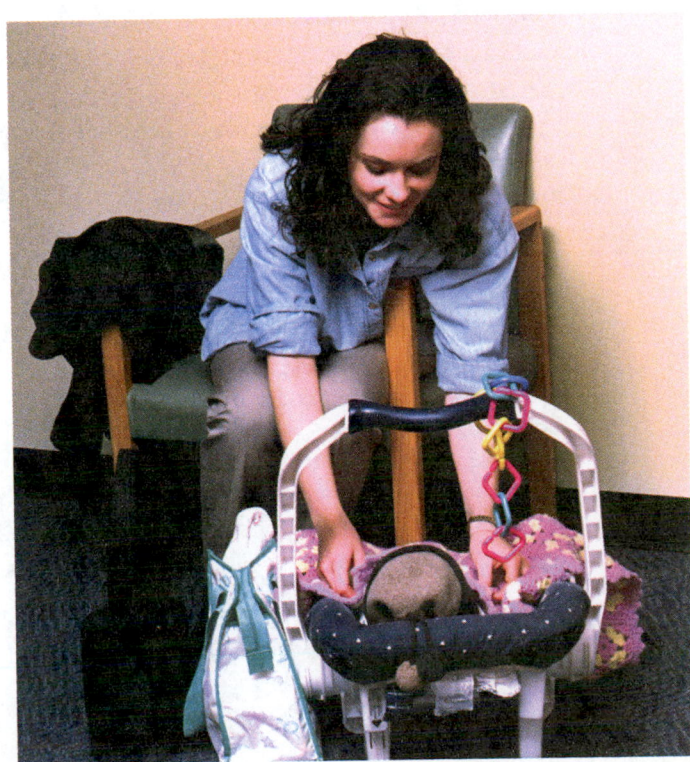

Figure 19-15 Postpartum and infant health check-ups are especially important for new teenage mothers who are learning to care for themselves and their new babies.

Case Study/Care Plan

ADOLESCENT PREGNANCY

Shannon, a 10th grader, is an average student, yet outgoing and popular. It seems that she always has a new boyfriend and is hopelessly romantic. She talks on the phone to her friends for hours about boys and dreams that someday she will become an actress. Shannon is 15 years old and presents to the school-based clinic complaining of nausea and a headache. Shannon's symptoms are vague, but she says that she has had nausea and some vomiting in the morning off and on for the past couple of months. After doing a complete health history and a brief physical examination, the nurse asks Shannon if she thinks she might be pregnant. Shannon denies being pregnant and tells the nurse that she can't possibly be pregnant because she broke up with her boyfriend over 6 weeks ago and she is having regular periods. On further questioning, Shannon admits the couple only used condoms "sometimes." She further adds that her periods are a little different, and she hasn't had as much bleeding as she usually does. She's also noticed that her breasts are tender and somewhat enlarged. After a positive result on a urine pregnancy test and a pelvic examination, she is estimated to be approximately 10 to 12 weeks pregnant. Shannon begins to cry and says, "What am I going to do? My parents will kill me! They were so glad when I broke up with my boyfriend and now this! Please, don't tell my mother," she sobs.

Assessment

- Single, pregnant adolescent
- High school student
- Lives with parents
- Unplanned pregnancy

- Unknown date of conception
- Concrete thinker
- Emotionally upset at confirmation of pregnancy
- Inadequate support at present

Nursing Diagnosis

Ineffective individual coping related to confirmation of unplanned pregnancy and parental notification.

Expected Outcome Shannon will receive support and assistance from the health care staff and her family in problem solving, planning, and decision making regarding the current pregnancy.

Planning Encourage Shannon and help her to outline the steps she feels are necessary to come to terms with this pregnancy.

Nursing Interventions	Rationales
1. Encourage Shannon to verbalize her fears related to the pregnancy and notification of her parents and the baby's father.	1. Decreases anxiety level and encourages beginning to solve problems.
2. Encourage Shannon to tell her parents immediately about the pregnancy and also encourage her to tell the baby's father.	2. Adolescent mothers need family support and also support from the baby's father, if possible. If the baby's father cannot support Shannon, he should be encouraged to assume some responsibilities related to the pregnancy.
3. Offer to assist Shannon in parental notification of the pregnancy but assure her of confidentiality if she refuses.	3. In developing a therapeutic relationship with adolescents, confidentiality is of utmost importance. Some teens welcome assistance in notifying their parents of an unplanned pregnancy and others prefer to tell them on their own. Nurses and other health care staff can assist adolescents with decisions about notification and provide support in this process.

(continued)

Nursing Interventions	Rationales
4. Have Shannon identify who will be her immediate support person regarding the pregnancy today.	4. An immediate support person can decrease Shannon's anxiety about the pregnancy confirmation and parent and partner notification and assist her in immediate decision making.

Evaluation Shannon identified her best friend as an immediate support person and, with her assistance, notified her parents of her pregnancy. She chose not to notify the baby's father at this time. Shannon's anxiety decreased and she is considering her options regarding the pregnancy.

Nursing Diagnosis

Knowledge deficit related to lack of experience with the normal signs and symptoms of pregnancy.

Expected Outcome Shannon will demonstrate a basic understanding of the signs and symptoms of pregnancy.

Planning Gather materials for Shannon that outline the normal indicators of pregnancy.

Nursing Interventions	Rationales
1. Discuss the signs and symptoms of pregnancy in the first trimester.	1. Providing information related to the normal physiologic and emotional changes of pregnancy allows Shannon to adjust to the pregnancy and decrease her anxiety about what is normal. Simple graphic instruction, in terms Shannon understands, will not overwhelm her in this time of crisis.
2. Encourage Shannon to ask any questions related to the pregnancy and provide anticipatory guidance. Provide written information for Shannon about the signs and symptoms of pregnancy during the first trimester.	2. Adequate knowledge about the pregnancy will assist Shannon to set immediate expectations and decrease her anxiety about the pregnancy.

Evaluation After discussion with the nurse, Shannon understood how she got pregnant, approximately when, and why she still had minimal monthly bleeding and other signs of pregnancy.

Nursing Diagnosis

Knowledge deficit regarding decisions about pregnancy alternatives.

Expected Outcome Shannon will make an informed decision about the alternatives regarding her pregnancy.

Planning Gather materials and information appropriate to her level of understanding to share with Shannon the different pregnancy options.

Nursing Interventions	Rationales
1. Discuss all the possible alternatives relative to the pregnancy: termination, adoption, and keeping the baby.	1. Although many adolescents know of alternatives to pregnancy, they are often unaware of the timing of pregnancy termination, available resources, how to access resources, and costs. Health care providers can assist the adolescent and their support persons through this decision-making process in a nonjudgmental manner.

(continued)

Nursing Interventions	Rationales
2. Encourage Shannon to discuss her feelings, values, and needs related to each alternative presented.	2. It is important to allow Shannon to discuss the consequences of all possible outcomes of the pregnancy and to support her in the decision she makes.
3. Encourage Shannon to discuss her decision regarding pregnancy alternatives with her parents.	3. Shannon needs support from her parents in whatever decision she makes. Cultural mores and family and religious values often play a part in the decision to terminate or retain a pregnancy.

Evaluation   After an ultrasound examination which established an estimate 10-week pregnancy, Shannon elected to undergo pregnancy termination. Shannon's ex-boyfriend was not consulted about this decision, and Shannon has continued with school. She is currently unattached and is not sexually active, but she says that she will seek a birth control method before becoming sexually active in the future. Shannon's parents have remained supportive and have encouraged Shannon to concentrate on school and set realistic expectations for the future.

adolescent parenting classes that are designed to meet their social, psychological, and health care needs. Such programs are generally available through state and federal maternal-child health services at low cost or free to the participants. More comprehensive information on normal pregnancy, prenatal care, labor and delivery, and postpartum care is covered in Chapters 15, 16, 23, and 29.

PREGNANCY IN HIV-INFECTED WOMEN

AIDS is a debilitating and life-threatening condition caused by HIV, a retrovirus. HIV is transmitted by exposure to an infected person's body secretions, including blood, vaginal fluid, semen, breast milk, and saliva.

Incidence and Significance

Women of reproductive age are increasingly affected by HIV infection; many women become HIV-infected during the adolescent years and manifest the symptoms of AIDS as young adults. One in five of all reported cases of AIDS occurs in the persons ages 20 to 29, and adolescent minority females are more proportionately represented than adolescent males (King, 1996). Given that the mean time from viral infection to the development of AIDS is approximately 10 years, many of those in the 20 to 29 age category were infected with HIV as adolescents.

The statistics on women with HIV infection and AIDS are alarming. HIV infection is a major cause of morbidity and mortality among women and children in the U.S. In 1995, women accounted for approximately 19% of all reported AIDS cases compared with 12.8% in 1991. Infection

by HIV and the subsequent development of AIDS is reported as the third leading cause of death for all women ages 25 to 44 and is the leading cause of death among African American women in this age group (CDC, 1996). The racial distribution of AIDS has changed dramatically over the past decade. During the first part of the AIDS epidemic, Caucasians were overwhelmingly affected. By 1991, however, 46% of all men with AIDS and 75% of all women with AIDS were African American or Hispanic; transmission in these populations was largely the result of heterosexual contact or infection by contaminated needles (CDC, 1993a).

Over 90% of the reported cases of pediatric AIDS in the U.S. are acquired by transmission from an HIV-infected mother. An estimated 7000 infants are born annually to HIV-infected women and approximately 15% to 30% of these infants would become HIV-infected if no treatment with **antiretroviral therapy** (medications used to suppress HIV replication and reduce viral load) were instituted (CDC, 1996). Approximately 25% to 50% of children with perinatally acquired HIV infection manifest AIDS in the first year of life, and about 80% have clinical symptoms of the disease within 3 to 5 years (Mauskopf, Paul, Wichman, White, & Tilson, 1996). Recognizing the devastating effects of HIV infection on children and their caregivers, it is clear that, from an economic and a humanitarian perspective, prevention of vertical and perinatal transmission is essential.

The most effective way to reduce vertical and perinatal transmission of HIV infection is through prevention of infection of women during their reproductive years. However, despite adequate screening, detection, and educational efforts, the HIV-infection rate among heterosexual women of reproductive age continues to rise. In 1996, the overall incidence of AIDS-related opportunistic infections declined for the first time since 1985, except among African American and Hispanic males and African American females who had heterosexual risk or exposures (CDC, 1997c). The number of deaths attributed to AIDS also declined among all ethnic groups and men but increased 3% among women. With grave implications for perinatal transmission, the infection rate by heterosexual contact among young females between ages 13 and 24 is significantly higher in comparison to adolescent males, through 1996 (Figure 19-16).

The young heterosexual female population accounts for an increase in new HIV **seroconversions** (i.e., conversion of the blood serum from negative to positive for HIV infection), primarily from transmission by HIV-infected intravenous drug users to their heterosexual partners (CDC, 1997a). For many young women, the only identifiable risk factor is their male sexual partner. During the 1980s, the proportion of adolescents who reported being sexually active increased significantly, yet many young women remain naive about their partner's history of sexual activity or of intravenous drug use (IVDU). Because

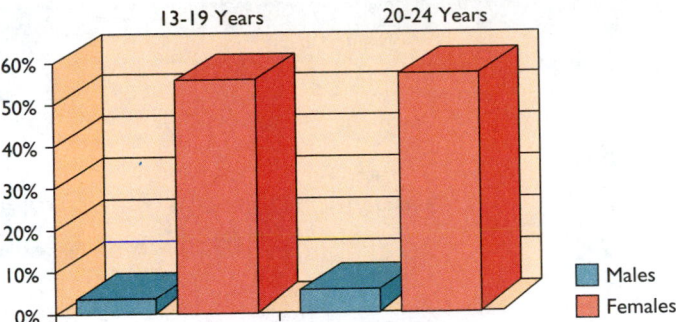

Figure 19-16 AIDS cases in male and female adolescents and young adults by heterosexual contact through 1996, United States. (Note: Adapted from *AIDS Surveillance in Adolescents. L265 Slide Series,* by Centers for Disease Control and Prevention (1997). http://www.edc.gov/nchstph/hiv_aids/graphics/adolescent.htm)

adolescents and young adults have proportionately higher rates of STDs, they are more vulnerable to HIV infection. HIV transmission during sexual contact may be facilitated by STDs that cause open genital lesions, such as herpes, syphilis, and chancroid. A break in the skin and mucous membranes of the perianal and genital areas is thought to increase the risk of transmission of HIV during intercourse, and male-to-female transmission is significantly greater than female-to-male (Padian, Shiboski, & Jewell, 1991).

Screening, Testing, and Diagnosis

Although the cure for AIDS is yet undetermined, the statistics on longevity among women and their children appear promising, if antiretroviral therapy is initiated in a timely manner. Until an effective vaccine is developed, early detection and treatment, behavioral risk reduction, and other preventative strategies targeted toward high-risk populations remain the most effective methods of reducing the spread of HIV to noninfected persons and delaying the onset of full-blown AIDS in those who are infected. However, many HIV-infected women are not tested for the virus until symptoms of AIDS are apparent or they deliver a child who has an AIDS-related condition.

Controversy continues about who should be screened for HIV. Because of the availability and efficacy of early antiretroviral treatment and the problems associated with selecting who should be screened, many authorities advocate voluntary prenatal testing of all pregnant women, regardless of their actual or perceived risk of infection. Young women, especially teenagers, often believe AIDS to be a disease that occurs only among homosexual men or IVDUs, and therefore feel invulnerable to the disease. Because many women do not receive any prenatal care or receive prenatal care only in the last trimester of pregnancy, counseling and testing are recommended for all adoles-

REFLECTIONS FROM A NEW MOTHER

"I always wanted to have children," states 22-year-old Janice. "I never dreamed that it would end up being like this. Our baby developed pneumonia in the newborn nursery and didn't respond well to treatment, so they tested him for HIV. We thought this was just routine and we were shocked when he was HIV-positive. How could that be? Where could he get HIV? My doctor looked at me and said, 'He got it from you, and both you and your husband need to be tested as soon as possible.' We were stunned. I had sex with different partners in high school and college and my biggest fear was getting pregnant, not getting HIV. I didn't think that anyone I knew could be HIV-positive. I admit I wasn't always as careful as I should have been. I just didn't think this could happen to me. Now my baby is sick, my husband is in shock, and I am so afraid. What will happen to us?"

Research Highlight

Economic Impact of Zidovudine Treatment for HIV-Infected Pregnant Women and Newborns

Purpose

The purpose of this study was to examine the number of pediatric HIV cases and the costs of screening and prophylactic ZDV treatment in pregnant women compared with the long-term costs of treatment of HIV infection in pediatric clients.

1. To estimate the economic impact of treating pregnant women who are HIV-positive with ZDV during pregnancy.

2. To estimate the economic impact of voluntary screening programs for pregnant women and of offering antiretroviral treatment with ZDV for those women who are HIV-positive.

Methods

Cost estimates were based on a study of 100 HIV-positive women who were treated with ZDV compared with 100 HIV-positive women who received no antiretroviral treatment during pregnancy. Cost estimates were then projected for treatment and care of offspring of the infected women, based on a number of reported parameters. Cost and health effects were also estimated for voluntary screening of a hypothetical 1000 pregnant women, whose HIV status was unknown, and for treatment of those who were found to be infected. A cost-threshold analysis was performed relative to HIV infection prevalence rates and the impact of ZDV on disease transmission.

Findings

Using ZDV according to the ACTG 076 Protocol, treatment costs of $104,502 for 100 HIV-positive pregnant women and their offspring were offset by a reduction in costs of $1,701,333 because of the lower number of cases of pediatric HIV infection in the treated group, which resulted in a net savings of $1,596,831.

Nursing Implications

Providing ZDV treatment to HIV-positive pregnant women has the potential to decrease the number of pediatric HIV infections by vertical transmission and to significantly reduce health care costs. Voluntary screening programs for pregnant women further reduce perinatal transmission of HIV because HIV-positive women are identified early in pregnancy and treatment is offered in a timely manner.

Note: From Economic impact of treatment of HIV-positive pregnant women and their newborns with zidovudine, by Mauskopf J, Paul J, Wichman D, White A and Tilson H, (1996), *JAMA*. 132–138;276:(2).

cents and young adults who use drugs or engage in unprotected sexual intercourse, especially those with multiple partners and those diagnosed with STDs. Broadening the scope of screening and testing may identify those who are infected with HIV before pregnancy or early in an existing pregnancy (CDC, 1999). The economic impact of a significant cost-saving through screening, early intervention, and the prevention of vertical transmission to neonates is considerable (see Research Highlight box). Additionally, any persons who consider themselves at risk and request testing should be offered that option. Box 19-3 identifies women who are considered to be at risk for HIV infection and for whom screening and testing services should be made available. Mandatory pre- and post-test counseling should always be available in a confidential setting.

HIV infection (seroconversion) is identified by the use of the enzyme-linked immunosorbent assay (ELISA), which detects serum antibodies to HIV and is confirmed by the Western blot test. Results of these diagnostic tests are highly reliable; false-positives and false-negatives rarely occur. Seroconversion among adolescents and adults generally occurs from 6 to 12 weeks after transmission of the virus. The diagnosis of HIV infection in infants born to HIV-positive mothers is confounded by the presence of maternal immunoglobulin G (IgG) antibodies to HIV. Detection of HIV DNA and RNA by polymerase chain reaction (PCR), detection of the serum p24 antigen, and viral cultures for the virus are the tests used to confirm HIV in the neonate (Barrett & Sleasman, 1997). A presumptive diagnosis of HIV infection is confirmed by two positive results on PCR tests or viral cultures. Because some HIV-infected neonates have undetectable virus levels, diagnostic tests should be repeated at 1 and 4 months. The HIV ELISA should be used to test for HIV in these infants from 6 months to 18 months of age. In uninfected neonates, the maternal antibodies disappear by approximately 18 months of age, and the child remains asymptomatic.

After HIV is confirmed by screening tests, the level of immunocompetence is measured by counting the CD4+ T-lymphocyte cells and, in research settings, by measuring plasma RNA levels of HIV. Progressive depletion of CD4+ T-lymphocytes and rising plasma levels of HIV RNA are associated with an increased likelihood of clinical disease and opportunistic infections (CDC, 1997b; Carpenter et al., 1997). The average CD4+ T-lymphocyte cell count in healthy individuals is approximately 1000 cells/μL. HIV-infected persons lose approximately 200 to 300 CD4+ T-lymphocyte cells per microliter of blood in the first year of infection, followed by a subsequent decline of 50 to 80 CD4+ T-lymphocyte cells per microliter yearly thereafter (Stein, Korvick, & Vermund, 1992). Opportunistic infec-

---

Client Education

Pre-Test Counseling for HIV Infection

- Explain that testing is confidential
- Assess the client's understanding of HIV risk
- Obtain a careful sexual history
- Explain the modes of HIV transmission
- Explain the relationship between infection and transmission
- Discuss the prevention of transmission to others, including methods of safe sex
- Provide age-appropriate reading materials on HIV transmission, detection, and treatment
- Describe and explain the serologic tests used to confirm HIV infection
- Discuss what test results mean, including false-negative and false-positive results
- Make a plan for the client to receive test results and post-test counseling

Note: Adapted from *HIV Counseling, Testing, and Referral Standards and Guidelines,* Centers for Disease and Control, 1994a. Washington, DC: U.S. Department of Health & Human Services.

Box 19-3 Characteristics of Women at Risk for HIV Infection

- Current or past history of drug use, especially intravenous drug use
- History of prostitution
- Frequent sexual intercourse with multiple partners
- Sexual intercourse under the influence of drugs
- Sexual intercourse with men who also have sex with men
- Residence in an area of the country with high prevalence of HIV infection, particularly in the northeast and southeast areas of the United States
- Received a blood transfusion or blood products before 1985, when HIV screening became available for blood donors
- Current or past history of sexual intercourse with any persons with any of these characteristics

---

tions and clinical symptoms of AIDS generally occur when the CD4+ T-lymphocyte cell count declines to 200/μL or less. While many factors influence the progression of HIV disease, time remains the most significant prognostic indicator of mortality in clients with HIV infection. In 1993, the CDC expanded the AIDS surveillance case definition to include persons with CD4+ T-lymphocyte cell counts of less than 200 cells/μL along with HIV-related wasting syndrome, HIV-related dementia, disseminated tuberculosis (TB); or one of the following conditions: pulmonary TB, recurrent bacterial pneumonia within 12 months, or invasive cervical carcinoma (CDC, 1993b).

Clinical Manifestations of HIV Infection in Pregnant Women

While there is no conclusive data that nongynecologic opportunistic infections of HIV differ in men and women, it has been suggested that women present with higher rates of candidal esophagitis as an AIDS-defining condition (Carpenter et al., 1997). HIV-infected women may initially present with complicated gynecologic conditions rather than the traditional AIDS-defining diagnoses. The most frequent manifestation of HIV infection in females is recur-

Client Education

Post-Test Counseling and Education for HIV Infection

HIV-Negative Results

- Inform client of negative results and the need for future testing related to exposure

- Review pre-testing educational materials, the need to screen partners, and avoidance of other risk behaviors

- Offer contraception information

- Offer counseling and education to partners

- Review safe sex practices

- Identify community resources for health care and substance abuse if necessary

- Advise client not to donate blood, plasma, or organs until HIV status is firmly established

HIV-Positive Results

- Offer immediate psychological support

- Help the client understand what the test result means

- Review methods of transmission and assess the client's risk of transmitting HIV to others

- Explain that treatment is available

- Identify immediate health care resources

- Identify immediate psychiatric services, as appropriate

- Assist the client in developing a plan to notify all sexual partners of exposure

- Help the client develop a plan to notify all others who may need to know about their HIV status

- Offer counseling and education to partners

- Offer contraception information

- Review safe sex practices and other risk reduction strategies

- Advise client not to donate blood, plasma, or organs

Note: Adapted from *HIV Counseling, Testing, and Referral Standards and Guidelines,* Centers for Disease and Control, 1994a. Washington, DC: U.S. Department of Health & Human Services.

rent vaginal candidiasis in otherwise healthy women. As the number of CD4+ T-lymphocyte cells decline, women exhibit: (1) candidal vaginitis; (2) pelvic inflammatory disease (PID), which may lead to abscess formation and resistant to antibiotic therapy; (3) genital herpes infections, which are frequent, persistent, and progress to severe ulcerating disease; (4) human papillomavirus (HPV) infection, with an accelerated progression to cervical neoplasia; (5) rapidly progressing cervical neoplasia; and (6) co-infection with syphilis, which has an aggressive progression to neurosyphilis (Eldred and Chaisson, 1996). Women rarely exhibit Kaposi's sarcoma, but do present with *Pneumocystis carinii* pneumonia (PCP), wasting syndrome, and HIV-related dementia (McDonnell & Kessenich, 2000).

There is no conclusive evidence that maternal HIV infection has an adverse effect on the fetal outcome in pregnancy. Studies conducted in the U.S. that have been controlled for substance abuse factors have not shown significant obstetrical or perinatal complications. Limited studies identified low birth weight, preterm deliveries, and fetal deaths as complications to HIV-related pregnancy (Koonin et al., 1989; Temmerman et al., 1994). However, poverty, lack of prenatal care, drug abuse, and HIV infection are often concomitant, and the combination is costly in terms of obstetrical and perinatal complications and adverse neonatal outcomes.

Clinical Manifestations of HIV in Neonates

Although studies are inconclusive, it appears that HIV can be transferred from mother to the baby during pregnancy or birth and while breastfeeding and that most perinatal transmission occurs at the time of labor and delivery (Riley and Green, 1999). Many attempts have been made at identifying predictors of HIV transmission, but the results are inconclusive. In a study of twins born to HIV-infected mothers, it was found that the first twin to pass through the birth canal had a significantly greater chance of becoming HIV-infected (Goedert, Duliege, Amos, Felton, & Biggar, 1991). It was speculated that the first twin experiences more trauma during birth and may be exposed longer to potentially infectious blood, mucus, and vaginal secretions. However, cesarean delivery alone has not significantly reduced transmission of the virus. It has also been hypothesized that HIV viral load, severity of illness at delivery, and fetal membranes ruptured more than 4 hours before delivery have some predictive value related to fetal and neonatal transmission (Mofenson, 1998).

Clinical signs of HIV infection in the neonatal period are difficult to identify. In approximately 20% of vertically infected infants, high levels of plasma viral load in the first year of life appear to predict rapid progression of disease (Barrett and Sleasman, 1997). These infants are likely to manifest signs of opportunistic infections such as PCP, interstitial lymphocytic pneumonia (ILP), candidal diaper rash, thrush, diarrhea, and other recurrent bacterial infections. Growth failure, neurologic problems, and developmental delays are also common.

Nursing Implications

Pregnant women who are HIV-positive or who have clinical AIDS should be identified as soon as possible during pregnancy for early intervention (Figure 19-17). Early identification of either pregnancy or HIV status assumes contact with the health care system. However, poor minority women, who are either IVDUs or have unprotected sex with infected persons, are more vulnerable to HIV infection and are less likely to seek health care early. In a recent study of inner-city pregnant women, investigators found that drug users were less likely than non–drug users to initiate early prenatal care, more likely to abort if HIV-positive, and uninformed about HIV transmission and

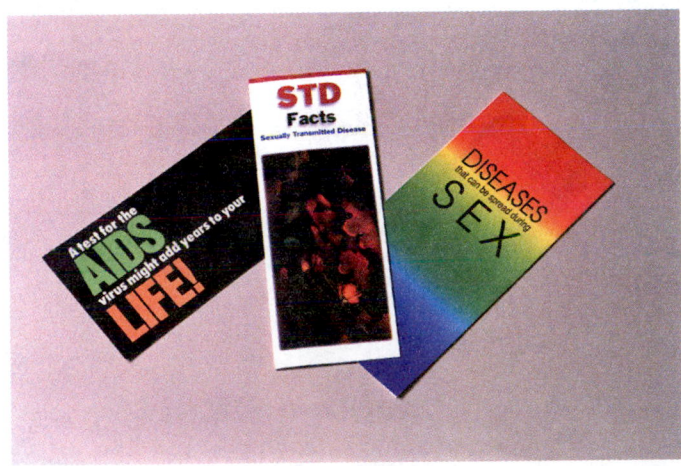

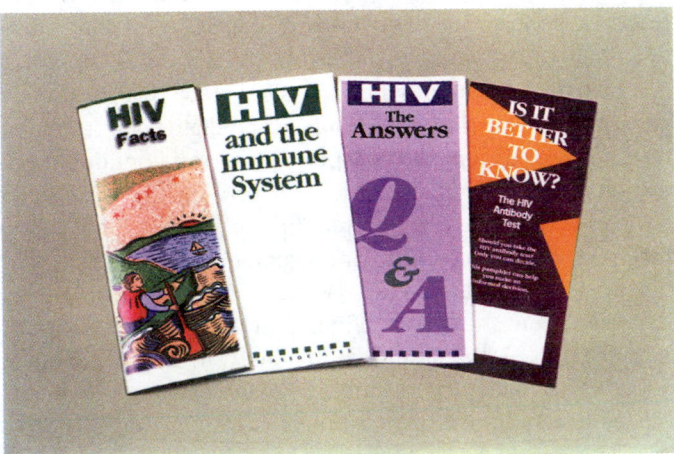

Figure 19-17 Pregnant woman at risk for AIDS or other sexually-transmitted diseases should be tested immediately, and information on health promotion and treatment options should be provided.

Box 19-4 ACTG-076 Protocol for Administration of Zidovudine During Pregnancy

Client Eligibility Criteria

- Confirmed pregnancy of 14–34 weeks' gestation
- No antiretroviral drug treatment during current pregnancy
- No clinical indication for antiretroviral drug therapy during the antenatal period
- CD4+ T-lymphocyte count ≥ 200 μL at initial assessment

Zidovudine Regimen for Mother and Baby

- Zidovudine (ZDV), 100 mg orally, 5 times daily, begun at 14–34 weeks' gestation and continued throughout pregnancy
- During labor, an intravenous loading dose of ZDV of 2 mg/kg over 1 hour, followed by continuous infusion of 1 mg/kg/hr until delivery
- For the neonate, ZDV syrup orally 2 mg/kg, every 6 hours for 6 weeks, beginning 8–12 hours after delivery

Note: Adapted from, Zidovudine for the prevention of HIV transmission from mother to infant. Centers for Disease Control and Prevention, (1994c). Morbidity and Mortality Weekly Report, 43, (16), 286.

---

treatment for HIV during pregnancy. Over half the sample thought HIV transmission to the fetus occurred most of the time or always, and only 20% had heard of a drug to treat HIV during pregnancy but 95% would take such therapy if it was offered (Silverman, Rohner, & Turner, 1997).

In 1994, the AIDS Clinical Trials Group Protocol #076 (ACTG 076) demonstrated that zidovudine (ZDV), given to HIV-infected women during pregnancy and labor and delivery plus 6 weeks of oral ZDV therapy for the neonate decreased vertical transmission from 25.5% to 8.3% (Connor, Sperling, & Gelber, 1994). The ACTG 076 protocol showed such promising results that the clinical trials using a placebo group were terminated prematurely once the effectiveness of ZDV was demonstrated and all participants were offered the drug. The efficacy of ZDV in decreasing vertical transmission of HIV was a major breakthrough in treatment. Box 19-4 describes the ACTG 076 protocol for administration of ZDV in pregnancy. Table 19-5 identifies various clinical situations of women during pregnancy and ZDV therapy currently recommended to prevent vertical transmission. In all drug treatment regimens offered to pregnant women with HIV infection, the known and unknown risks and benefits to mother and fetus should be

Table 19-5 Recommended Zidovudine Therapy for Prevention of Vertical HIV Transmission

Clinical Status	Recommendations
HIV-infected pregnant women, no previous antiretroviral therapy	Clinical, immunologic, viral evaluation. Risk/benefits of therapy discussed. Three-part ZDV chemoprophylaxis (ACTG Protocol) initiated at 10–12 weeks' gestation.*
HIV-infected pregnant women receiving antiretroviral therapy during pregnancy	Continue antiretroviral therapy if identified after first trimester. If identified during first trimester, risks/benefits of therapy should be discussed and continuation of therapy should be considered. If drug therapy is discontinued during first trimester, drugs should be simultaneously reintroduced to avoid development of drug resistance. If current drug regimen does not contain ZDV, it should be added after 14 weeks' gestation. ZDV is recommended for the pregnant woman during the intrapartum period and for the newborn according to the ACTG Protocol.
HIV-infected pregnant women in labor with no previous antiretroviraltherapy	ACTG Protocol 076 for intrapartum and postpartum period along period along with the 6-week regimen for the newborn. Woman should be evaluated to determine if antiretroviral therapy should be recommended.
Infants born to HIV-infected women who received no antiretroviral therapy during pregnancy or delivery	The ACTG Protocol for neonates should be discussed with the mother and offered for the newborn. ZDV should be initiated as soon as possible after delivery—preferably within 12–24 hours after birth. Woman should be evaluated to determine if antiretroviral therapy should be recommended.

*Dosing of ZDV has changed from the original ACTG Protocol, which recommended 100 mg five times daily, to 200 mg three times daily, or 300 mg twice daily.
Note: Adapted from Public Health Service task force recommendations for the use of antiretroviral drugs in pregnant women infected with HIV-1 for maternal health and for reducing perinatal HIV-1 transmission in the United States. Centers for Disease Control. (1998). *Morbidity and Mortality Weekly Report. 47*, (No. RR-2), 1–31.

considered and discussed before drug treatment is instituted during pregnancy or at delivery.

In 1996, the final results of the ACTG 076 protocol reported mother-to-baby transmission rates of less than 8% (CDC, 1998). Research continues on the use of ZDV in the treatment of pregnant women, with the emphasis on decreasing the frequency of dosing to increase drug compliance among clients and the use of combination therapy (i.e., ZDV and other antiretroviral agents). In 1998, the U.S. Public Health Service Task Force on antiretroviral medications during pregnancy recommended the use of combination therapy for HIV-positive pregnant women. The long-term effects of the ACTG 076 protocol ZDV regimen on women and children is currently unknown, although there appears to be no immediate adverse consequences to the mother or infant or to child development during the first 2 years after therapy (CDC, 1998).

The most promising strategy for reducing perinatal transmission is the combination of elective cesarean section and ZDV therapy. The combined approach reduces the transmission rate to 2% (Read, 1999). However, elective cesarean section is not financially possible for all women, and women undergoing a cesarean section have more complications than those delivering vaginally (Mofenson, 1998).

Pregnant women who are HIV-infected and already on antiretroviral therapy should immediately inform their health care provider of their pregnancy and continue medications as directed. Treatment of HIV-infected pregnant women should be considered in the context of optimal health care for the mother and pregnancy termination may be considered as an option. Because ZDV is the only drug that has been shown to significantly reduce vertical HIV transmission, ZDV should be included in any regimen of antiretroviral therapy during pregnancy whenever possible. Currently, if pregnant women are taking combinations of antiretroviral drugs that have reduced their plasma levels of HIV to undetectable levels, these women should be encouraged to continue the drug regimen, especially if treatment with ZDV alone has failed (Carpenter et al.,

1997). More research is needed on combination antiretroviral therapy in pregnancy before recommendations can be made relative to efficacy (CDC, 1998).

Multidrug regimens include the use of three types of antiretroviral agents, as described in Table 19-6. Combination therapy, or the "triple-drug cocktail," has been successful in suppressing HIV to undetectable levels when measured by standard tests and improving the health, length, and quality of life for individuals with HIV. However, the eradication of HIV has remained elusive, and individuals with HIV should continue the expensive ($15,000/year) triple-drug cocktails indefinitely. While combined therapy is promising, approximately one-third of HIV-infected clients are unresponsive to the drugs, particularly if they have been on previous ZDV therapy. Side effects can include intense nausea, diarrhea, oral ulcers, anemia, peripheral neuropathy, and pancreatitis, and clients must be sufficiently motivated to take more than 20 pills a day at specific times. Failure to follow specific regimens can lead to viral mutations that are resistant to the drug's effects.

In addition to antiretroviral therapy, pregnant women with HIV infection may also be taking prescribed drugs for treatment or prophylaxis for opportunistic infections or clinical symptoms of AIDS. The management of pregnancy in HIV-infected women can be complex and referral to special health care providers is usually indicated. There is little data available on HIV-infected women who use multidrug therapy during pregnancy, and safety data on the drug effects on the developing fetus are currently unknown. Therefore, it is essential that initiation or continuation of multidrug treatment regimens for HIV-infected pregnant women occur only after a full discussion of the risk/benefit ratio of combined antiretroviral therapy. Carpenter and colleagues (1997) state that "because

ASSESSMENT OF THE HIV-POSITIVE CLIENT

- Client history
  Age
  Parity
  Complete health history
  Risk level for HIV infection
    Drug history (particularly injected-drug use)
    Sexual exposure
    Environmental or occupational exposure
  Subjective symptoms of HIV infection
  Perceptions of HIV status and anxiety level
  Social support system

- Physical examination
  Review results of complete physical examination, especially any physical findings related to HIV infection

- Diagnostic studies
  Enzyme-linked immunosorbent assay (ELISA) and confirmatory Western blot test
  CD4+ T-lymphocyte cell count, if the client HIV-positive

of the dearth of information on use of antiretroviral drugs other than ZDV during pregnancy, all women who choose to take antiretroviral drugs during pregnancy should be encouraged to enroll in the Antiretroviral Pregnancy Registry managed by several pharmaceutical companies in conjunction with the CDC and the National Institute of Health." (p. 1967 and see "Resources" at end of chapter).

Contraception for HIV-infected pregnant women should always be addressed in the antepartum period. All methods of contraception should be discussed and selection should focus on methods that are highly effective and fit into the client's lifestyle. Effective contraception, including the concepts of potential sterilization and abstinence, is of great importance, because women who are HIV-infected are often at high risk for unplanned pregnancies. In addition to contraception, HIV-infected women should use latex condoms with every episode of sexual intercourse to prevent transmission of the virus to others. Nurses are in an excellent position to counsel women regarding effective contraception and safe sexual practices. Additional information on HIV infection, AIDS, and contraception is addressed in Chapters 9, 10, and 14.

Table 19-6 Antiretroviral Drug Therapy	
Type	**Drugs**
Nucleoside reverse transcriptase inhibitors	• Zidovudine (ZDV, AZT) • Didanosine (ddl) • Zalcitabine (ddC) • Lamivudine (3TC) • Stavudine
Non–nucleoside reverse transcriptase inhibitors	• Nevirapine • Delaviridine • Lovridine
Protease inhibitors	• Saquinavir • Indinivir • Ritonavir • Nelfinavir

Case Study/Care Plan

HIV TESTING AND COUNSELING

Because Janice and her husband have recently learned that their newborn has HIV-related pneumonia, they are referred for testing, for HIV and counseling before and after testing. Refer back to "Reflections from a New Mother."

Nursing Diagnosis

Anxiety related to unknown HIV status and fear of a positive result.

Expected Outcome Client will identify support systems and experience a reduction in anxiety.

Planning With clients, make a list of potential support persons with whom they can share their news.

Nursing Interventions	Rationales
1. Assure Janice that test results and any information she shares is confidential.	1. Clients are more likely to share sensitive information if confidentiality is assured.
2. Encourage Janice to vent her feelings related to a possible HIV-positive test result.	2. Allowing Janice to express her fears will assist her in coping with the testing process.
3. Provide Janice with information about the HIV testing process and what the laboratory test results mean.	3. Providing Janice with factual information will allow her to set her expectations relative to the testing procedure and assist her in understanding what a positive result means for herself and her family.
4. Assist the client in appropriate disclosure of HIV status with others who need to know.	4. Disclosing HIV status is a difficult and sensitive matter. Discrimination against HIV-positive individuals does exist. However, disclosure is important in obtaining appropriate medical and psychosocial support.
5. Encourage Janice to identify immediate support systems within her family and community.	5. Social support increases coping and assists the client in initial problem solving.

Evaluation After discussing her feelings of fear with the nurse, Janice identified her parents, her family physician, and the pastor at her church as a support system for herself and her family. The nurse encouraged Janice to role-play to help decide how and what she would disclose about her HIV status with others, and Janice felt more prepared to share her uncertainty at this difficult time. Factual knowledge of the testing procedure assisted Janice in making an appointment for learning the test results and identifying a support person when obtaining the test results. Although still fearful of a positive result, Janice has identified an initial plan for coping with the test results.

Nursing Diagnosis

Knowledge deficit related to HIV disease process.

Expected Outcome Client will increase understanding of disease process and treatment.

Planning Gather materials, resources, and referrals to ensure that the couple can react to the news from a base of knowledge.

(continued)

Nursing Interventions	Rationales
1. Assess the client's understanding of HIV risk.	1. Before the nurse can begin client education about HIV, it is important to identify what is known.
2. Provide information on HIV transmission and effective measures to decrease transmission.	2. If the client understands the basis for transmission of HIV, appropriate precautions can be taken to prevent the spread of the disease.
3. Encourage the client to avoid breastfeeding.	3. Current literature suggests that HIV can be transmitted in breast milk. If the infant is HIV-positive, repeated exposure to the virus can increase viral load.
4. Discuss sexual abstinence and the use of latex condoms if the client sexually active.	4. Female-to-male transmission is less common than male-to-female transmission. Latex condoms help to decrease viral transmission to either HIV-positive or HIV-negative partners. Repeated exposure to the HIV virus can increase viral load.
5. Encourage the client to refrain from the use of drugs and alcohol.	5. Because of a compromised immune system in HIV-positive individuals, drugs and alcohol should be used in limited quantities or not at all.
6. Advise client not to donate blood, plasma, or organs.	6. Blood, blood products, and body organs may contain HIV and thus be transmitted to others.
7. Assure client that if test results are positive, treatment and counseling are available.	7. Although there is currently no cure for HIV infection, effective treatment can decrease viral load to undetectable levels in the blood. If viral load remains low, opportunistic infections are less likely to occur. Because a diagnosis of HIV can be psychologically devastating, counseling should be made available for the family.

Evaluation Janice has expressed understanding of the disease process and is encouraged that effective treatment is available. She denies other risky behaviors, such as drug and alcohol use and recent exposure to partners other than her husband. If she is HIV-infected, she will seek the nurse's assistance in identifying a plan to notify partners before her marriage. Janice is open to referral to an HIV specialist if her test result is positive.

PREGNANCY IN WOMEN OVER AGE 35

In the past decade, the number of American women over the age of 35 who are giving birth has increased dramatically.

Incidence and Significance

According to the National Center for Health Statistics, in 1993, the number of births among women ages 35 to 39 was higher than in any year since 1960, and the number of births for women over age 40 was the highest since 1968 (Ventura, Martin, Taftel, Mathews, & Clarke, 1995). From 1976 to 1986, the number of first-time births doubled among women age 40 or older. This trend continues as the disproportionately large number of women in today's childbearing age group (the result of the "baby boom" between 1946 and 1964) reach the end of reproductive maturity. There are numerous explanations for the shift in childbearing among older women, including a longer life expectancy; effective, available contraception; enhanced roles for women; increased female participation in the work force; delayed first marriage; frequency of divorce and remarriage; advanced technology in the treatment of infertility; and other various lifestyle decisions related to career and educational opportunities. Women who delay childbearing are known to have greater educational and economic status (Aldous & Edmonson, 1993).

The Effects of Age on Reproduction

Fertility decreases proportionately as women age, with the maximum potential for conception at ages 20 to 25, declining to very low levels after age 40. A 95% decrease in fertility occurs in women ages 40 to 45 (Maroulis, 1993). Several factors contribute to the decline in fertility among older women:

- The reproductive system's decreased efficiency
- The increased frequency of infectious diseases, diabetes, hypertension, and obesity that may occur with aging
- The number of pack-years that have accumulated among women who smoke
- Years of delaying childbearing, during which couples postpone pregnancy until reproductive capability is markedly decreased (Maroulis).

Spermatogenesis declines in males as they age and oocyte depletion in females is an ongoing process from birth to menopause. Oocyte aging is thought to be the most frequent cause of chromosomal abnormalities, decreased fertility, and increased spontaneous abortions in older pregnant women (Aldous & Edmonson, 1993; Maroulis, 1993; Sauer, Paulson, & Lobo, 1995). Fertilized ova in older women do not implant as well as in younger women, which may be caused by aging of the uterus. The blood supply to the uterus may be compromised by calcification of the uterine vessels. In fertility studies, it has been demonstrated that fertilized ova from young donors implant more often than in women under the age of 35. However, adequate implantation with donor ova has occurred in older women who have been receiving progesterone supplementation after **embryo transfer** (ET), which is the transfer of an externally fertilized egg in embryonic stages by transcervical or other methods. Despite the effects of aging, successful pregnancy and delivery of viable neonates has occurred with ET and exogenous hormone supplementation, even in women who are postmenopausal (Sauer et al, 1995.)

As women age, the endocervix changes with varying levels of estrogen and progesterone. Because of declining estrogen in older women, the cervical mucus becomes dense, making penetration by sperm very difficult. Ovum transport through the fallopian tubes is influenced by normal hormonal functioning. Tubal motility is affected by age and a subsequent decline in estrogen and progesterone levels. Motility of the egg through the fallopian tube decreases, making fertilization less likely. The frequency of ectopic pregnancy increases with age, but the exact causal mechanism is unknown. The changes in transport with the decreased motility of the fallopian tubes may affect the location of ovum fertilization.

REFLECTIONS FROM A MOTHER

"This is a second marriage for us both," says 42-year-old Claire. "We both wanted a large family, even though we realized that we were starting late. We tried for 5 years and I miscarried once during that time. I tried fertility drugs but I felt bloated and irritable, so I didn't stick with them for very long. I also worried about getting pregnant with multiple babies. I kept thinking that I would get pregnant the natural way, but when nothing happened, we saw a fertility specialist who put me on a low-potency fertility drug that didn't make me sick. We were nearly ready to give up when I missed a period. Later, I had an amniocentesis done, and we were told we had a healthy baby girl. I think that was the happiest day of my life."

Medical Risks for Older Pregnant Women and Their Neonates

Although there is no precise age at which women become more susceptible to the complications related to childbearing, age 35 most commonly serves as a reference point, especially when referring to women who are pregnant for the first time. The term **elderly primagravida** was first adopted by the International Federation of Obstetricians and Gynecologists to describe women who were pregnant for the first time and were over age 35. The incidence of maternal complications, including trisomy 21 or Down syndrome, in women over age 35 compared with women in the "ideal" childbearing age range of 20 to 25 received increased attention (Cunningham & Leveno, 1995). Medical evidence suggests that the risk of Down syndrome increases steadily with age, although approximately 70% to 80% of children with Down syndrome are born to women under age 35 (Pauker & Pauker, 1994).

For the past 20 years, amniocentesis and, more recently, chorionic villus sampling (CVS) have been routinely recommended for pregnant women over age 35 to screen for Down syndrome and other chromosomal abnormalities. In the 1980s, it was found that serum levels of alpha fetoprotein were lower in the presence of Down syndrome and two additional serum markers, human chorionic gonadotropin (hCG) and unconjugated estriol, were elevated (Haddow, Palomaki, Knight, Cunningham, Lustig, & Boyd, 1994). Amniocentesis cannot be performed until 14 to 16 weeks' gestation, although CVS may be done at 8 to 10 weeks and the results are available in the first trimester of pregnancy. Prenatal screening is very useful in detecting chromosomal defects and for providing information to assist couples in decision making relative to pregnancy termination. Nurses are in an excellent position to refer couples for genetic counseling and to support couples who may experience difficult decisions related to pregnancy and abortion (see Chapters 13 and 37).

Medical conditions, such as infections, diabetes, hypertension, and obesity, are more common and thus present a challenge in management of pregnant women over age 35. The incidence of type II (insulin-dependent) diabetes mellitus increases with age, and gestational diabetes is more common in older pregnant women, who are also at substantially greater risk for pregnancy-induced hypertension (PIH) or pre-eclampsia than their younger counterparts. Diabetes and PIH account for numerous complications during pregnancy and adverse fetal outcomes. Pregnancies complicated by hypertension are associated with lower gestational age and lower weight at birth and an increased risk of placental abruption and fetal death. Premature separation of the placenta (placenta previa) is thought to be related to aging uterine vessels and chronic hypertensive conditions. Fibroid tumors (leiomyomas) are also more common among older women as a result of the increased secretion of estrogen during pregnancy and may contribute to miscarriage. Large fibroid tumors may contribute to postpartum bleeding because of an inability for adequate contraction after delivery. Because of the potentially serious bleeding complications characteristic of placenta previa, placental abruption, and fibroid tumors, cesarean sections are more common in women over age 35.

The results of the most recent studies related to fetal and maternal mortality vary, although most studies support advanced maternal age as a significant risk factor. In 1995, Fretts and colleagues demonstrated that, even when controlling for coexisting medical conditions, women of age 35 or older had a risk of fetal death twice as high as younger women, a finding that is supported by earlier studies. The relationship between advanced maternal age and fetal death twice as high as younger women, a finding that is supported by earlier studies. The relationship between advanced maternal age and fetal death remains unexplained.

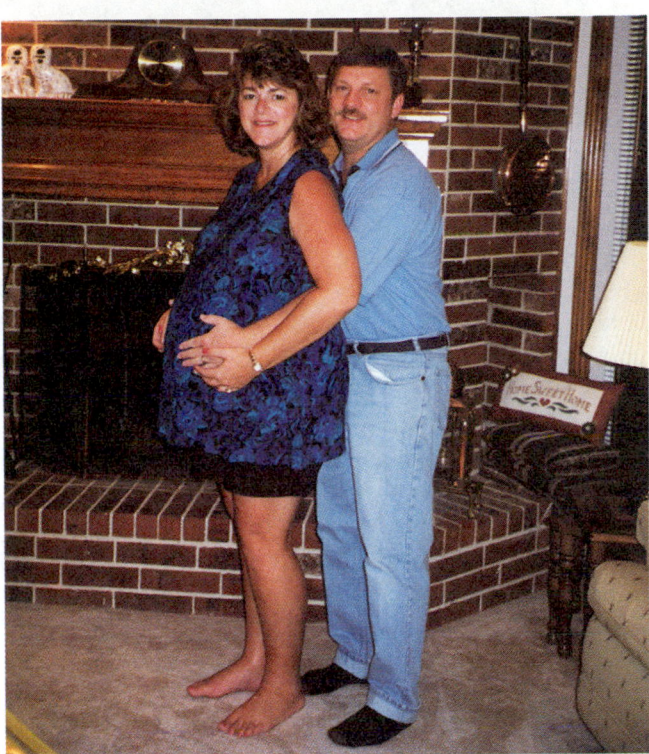

Figure 19-18 The older expectant couple before delivery.

In addition to maternal complications, neonates born to older women have increased perinatal morbidity and mortality. Spontaneous abortions, preterm delivery, low birth weight, fetal anomalies, and antepartum stillbirths occur more commonly in older women (Aldous & Edmonson, 1993; Cunningham & Leveno, 1995). However, because the rate of pregnancy among older women is increasing, studies directed to this population have found that older pregnant women tend to be more likely to be economically secure, carry health insurance, seek early and continuous prenatal care, and be motivated to achieve the best pregnancy outcome. Many of the chronic disorders that go along with aging can be treated and are well controlled during pregnancy. With advanced technology, good counseling, and good medical and nursing care, the outlook for older pregnant women remains optimistic and obstetric and perinatal outcomes appear good (Figure 19-18).

Achieving Pregnancy in Postmenopausal Women

Oocyte donation and embryo transfer (ET) has been used for over 10 years to establish pregnancy in women who were unable to become pregnant as a result of ovarian failure or other structural and functional problems. However, the extension of these services to women of **advanced reproductive age,** who are ages 45 to 50 and are perimenopausal or postmenopausal, remains controversial.

While studies on postmenopausal pregnancies are scarce, preliminary data are positive, and oocyte donation, in vitro fertilization (IVF), and ET for women of advanced reproductive age are gaining in worldwide popularity.

To assist older women in achieving pregnancy, hormone replacement, in the form of sequential estrogen and progesterone, is given to stimulate the secretory response of the endometrium, followed by endometrial biopsy during several cycles to determine if the endometrium is adequate for implantation. Oocyte donors are generally anonymous, although in some cases, relatives act as donors. Sperm is sometimes obtained from husbands or from anonymous donors. The use of semen from men over age 55 is discouraged because of the increased risk of genetic disorders (Sauer, Paulson, & Lobo, 1995). In most procedures, five embryos are transferred transcervically, potentially leading to multiple gestations. Once the pregnancy is confirmed by measurement of serum β-human chorionic gonadotropin (β-hCG) levels and pelvic ultrasonography, a selective reduction is performed on excess embryos. The selective reduction process also remains controversial, particularly when multiple gestations receive popular media attention. From a medical perspective, selective reduction is performed to give a single or twin gestation the best environment in which to develop. Multiple gestations often result in adverse fetal outcomes and fetal death.

Women seeking pregnancy at an advanced reproductive age are generally screened extensively for physical and psychological problems before ET. However, in a 1995 study of the largest series of delivered pregnancies in women over age 50, the incidence of multiple gestations, gestational hypertension, gestational diabetes, preterm labor, and pre-eclampsia were significant (Sauer, Paulson, & Lobo, 1995). The investigators concluded that pregnancy, especially with multiple gestations, precipitated underlying medical problems, yet the perinatal and maternal outcomes in this study were excellent.

Despite the many personal reasons for desiring pregnancy beyond the normal reproductive age, controversy exists in the public domain regarding artificial conception in postmenopausal women. Concerns about treating women beyond reproductive capability focus on the well-being of the child, the potential complications for the mother, and the longevity of the parents in providing for their children.

Nursing Implications

Nursing care for pregnant women over age 35 is much the same as that for other pregnant women. However, several issues are germane to older pregnant women, and older first-time mothers may experience unique stressors in their role transition. Older women becoming pregnant for the first time may have concerns about their ability to carry a pregnancy to term and their ability to manage labor and delivery. Peer groups of like individuals are helpful in supporting the expectant mother through the pregnancy and delivery process and in the immediate postpartum period. The nurse may assist the older pregnant woman to identify such support groups or help her contact other women in similar circumstances. Because preterm labor is common among older primiparas, bedrest may become necessary at some point during the pregnancy. The nurse could serve as a facilitator for a bedrest support group or inform the pregnant woman of support groups that are available either independently or in association with fetal monitoring equipment companies.

Women over age 35 receive genetic counseling and learning about the increased incidence of medical complications and genetic abnormalities may be stressful for both parents. If genetic screening is performed, waiting for the results is a difficult time for most older expectant couples. If abortion is an option for the couple, the decision may still be stressful: couples need a great deal of support during this period. Nurses working with this population may function in a supportive capacity to individuals or groups or may refer couples to support groups that deal with these issues.

Couples who delay childbearing are generally well-educated. The woman, while having made a conscious decision to have a child, may still be uncomfortable with the role transition from career woman to mother and have doubts about her ability to "keep up" with an active small child. The support of those in the immediate work setting is often perceived as a loss when the new mother is no longer working and has less contact with professional colleagues. Some older mothers may find themselves interacting primarily with new mothers many years younger than themselves. While their concerns for their children may be similar, their life experiences may differ significantly. The need for social interaction with similar individuals is considerable. Also, older women often have higher expectations for themselves as mothers because they have already

Critical Thinking

Counseling and Postmenopausal Conception

Nurses need to consider their own values and feelings when counseling individuals about sensitive or controversial issues. How do your own values about parenting influence your beliefs about postmenopausal conception by oocyte donation and embryo transfer? What are the issues that come to mind?

Early identification of older primiparas with special needs would allow for appropriate nursing interventions, which can begin in the first trimester. Such interventions might include guidance and counseling services related to the pregnancy and delivery, providing parenting classes to address the older couple's special needs, and the development of or referral to parent support groups appropriate for older couples.

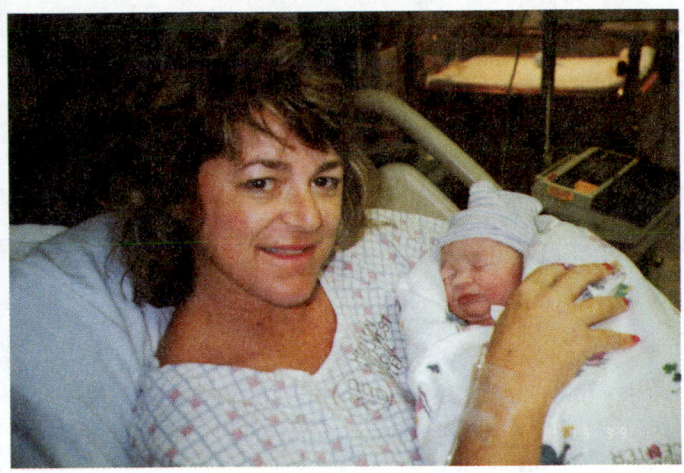

Figure 19-19 The elderly primipara after delivery.

achieved a measure of success in their careers. Because of their high expectations and the lack of role models, older mothers may experience lower levels of satisfaction with parenting, especially in the first several months postpartum (Reece, 1993). On a positive note, older mothers may feel more financially secure, be devoted to childrearing, and bring a level of maturity to parenting (Figure 19–19).

Web Activities

- Visit the websites listed above. What types of information do they provide? Is the material targeted to the client or the health care provider?

- What other Internet resources can you find for pregnant teens (i.e., chat rooms, adoption services)?

- Visit nursing and government websites to find their guidelines on optimum ages for pregnancy.

- What does the CDC's site say about pregnancy HIV infection, and AIDS?

Key Concepts

- Adolescent pregnancy is of increasing concern because childbearing during the teenage years has profound socioeconomic and health consequences for teen mothers and their children. The burden of an unintended pregnancy is especially heavy for young teens who are still in high school and are trying to manage their education, develop their own identity, and adapt to the physical and emotional changes occurring with pregnancy.

- The factors contributing to adolescent pregnancy are multifaceted and complex; they are influenced by the adolescent's cognitive and psychosocial development as well as cultural mores and socioeconomic status.

- The psychosocial and physical risks of pregnancy in adolescence are closely related to the adolescent's health and psychosocial well-being and the achievement of normal adolescent developmental tasks. Age, degree of substance abuse, level of nutrition, use of prenatal care, level of family support, and socioeconomic factors greatly influence maternal and neonatal outcomes.

- Adolescence is a period of sexual experimentation for many teens. Appropriate contraceptive methods

for them are ones that are effective, acceptable, and will be consistently used by adolescents. Ideal contraception for adolescents are those methods that are highly effective in prevention of pregnancy and transmission of STDs.

- HIV infection has a significant physical and emotional impact on pregnant adolescents and young adults. Early detection and treatment of HIV infection is essential. With current antiretroviral therapy, vertical and perinatal transmission of HIV can be dramatically reduced and the outlook for greater longevity for mothers and children is promising.

- Childbearing among women over age 35 is becoming increasingly common. With advanced medical technology and appropriate prenatal care, maternal and fetal outcomes are good.

- Older first-time expectant couples experience unique stressors in their transition to parenthood. Anticipatory guidance includes counseling related to prenatal genetic testing, such as amniocentesis and chorionic villus sampling, identification of appropriate social support, and adaptation to parenting.

Review Questions and Activities

1. Which of the following socioeconomic factors contributes to the high incidence of adolescent pregnancy in the United States?
   a. The lack of adequate birth control
   b. Poverty
   c. The lack of information on safe sex
   d. The availability of public assistance for unmarried mothers
   The correct answer is b.

2. Which of the following is the most effective contraceptive method for adolescents?
   a. Condoms and contraceptive foam
   b. Norplant implants
   c. OCPs and condoms
   d. DMPA injection
   The correct answer is c.

3. Which of the developmental tasks listed is most affected by an unplanned pregnancy in early to middle adolescence?
   a. Identity formation
   b. Sexual identity
   c. Vocational identity
   d. Emancipation
   The correct answer is a.

4. When is HIV passed from mother to infant?
   a. Prenatal period
   b. Intrapartum period
   c. Postpartum period via breast feeding
   d. All of the above
   The correct answer is d.

5. Which of the following is the drug used to decrease the vertical transmission of HIV from mother to baby?
   a. Saquinivir
   b. Ritonivir
   c. Zidovudine
   d. Stavudine
   The correct answer is c.

6. Which of the following groups in the United States is experiencing an increase in the rate of HIV infection?
   a. Homosexual men
   b. Heterosexual men
   c. Intravenous drug users
   d. Heterosexual female adolescents and young adults
   The correct answer is d.

7. What age defines the elderly primigravida?
   a. Over age 30
   b. Over age 35
   c. Over age 40
   d. Ages 45 to 50
   The correct answer is b.

8. Which genetic screening test for chromosomal abnormalities provides an older expectant couple with information within the first trimester?
   a. Chorionic-villus sampling (CVS)
   b. Amniocentesis
   c. Genetic karyotyping
   d. Ultrasonography
   The correct answer is a.

References

Alan Guttmacher Institute. (1997). *Contraception counts: State-by-state information*. New York: Alan Guttmacher Institute.

Aldous, M., & Edmonson, B. (1993). Maternal age at first childbirth and risk of low birth weight and preterm delivery in Washington state. *Journal of the American Medical Association. 270,* (21), 2574–2577.

American College of Obstetricians and Gynecologists. (1997). Smoking and women's health. *ACOG Educational Bulletin. No. 240.* Washington, DC: American College of Obstetricians and Gynecologists.

Bachrach, C., Stolley, K., & London, K. (1992). Relinquishment of premarital births: Evidence from national survey data. *Family Planning Perspectives. 24,* 27.

Barrett, D., & Sleasman, J. (1997). Pediatric AIDS: So now what do we do? *Contemporary Pediatrics, 14,* (6), 111–124.

Bragg, E.J. (1997). Pregnant adolescents with addictions. *Journal of Obstetrical and Neonatal Nursing. 26,* (5), 577–584.

Carpenter, C. et al. (1997). Antiretroviral therapy for HIV infection in 1997. *Journal of the American Medical Association. 277,* (24), 1962–1969.

Centers for Disease Control and Prevention. (1993a). *HIV/AIDS surveillance report*. Atlanta, Georgia: CDC. January, 1–23.

Centers for Disease Control and Prevention. (1993b). 1993 revised classification system for HIV infection and expanded surveillance case definition for AIDS among adolescents and adults. *Morbidity and Mortality Weekly Report. 41,* 1–19.

Centers for Disease Control and Prevention. (1994a). *HIV counseling, testing, and referral standards and guidelines*. U.S. Department of Health & Human Services.

Centers for Disease Control and Prevention. (1994b). Pregnancy, sexually transmitted diseases, and related risk behaviors among U.S. adolescents. Atlanta, Georgia: Centers for Disease Control and Prevention.

Centers for Disease Control and Prevention. (1994c). Zidovudine for the prevention of HIV transmission from mother to infant. *Morbidity and Mortality Weekly Report. 43,* (16), 286.

Centers for Disease Control and Prevention. (1996). HIV testing among women aged 18–44 years—United States, 1991 and 1993. *Morbidity and Mortality Weekly Report. 45,* (34), 733–736.

Centers for Disease Control and Prevention. (1997a). Aids cases in male and female adolescents and young adults by heterosexual contact through 1996, United States. *AIDS Surveillance in Adolescents.* L265 Slide Series. http://www.edc.gov/nchstph/hiv__aids/graphics/adolesnt.htm

Centers for Disease Control and Prevention. (1997b). 1997 revised guidelines for performing CD4+ T-cell determinations in persons infected with human immunodeficiency virus (HIV). *Morbidity and Mortality Weekly Report. 46,* (RR-2), 1–3.

Centers for Disease Control and Prevention. (1997c). Update: Trends in AIDS incidence, deaths, and prevalence—United States, 1996. *Morbidity and Mortality Weekly Report. 46,* (8), 165–173.

Centers for Disease Control and Prevention. (1998). US Public Health Service Task Force recommendations for the use of antiretroviral drugs in pregnant women infected with HIV-1 for maternal health and for reducing perinatal HIV-1 transmission in the United States. *Morbidity and Mortality Weekly Report. 47,* (No. RR-2), 1–31.

Centers for Disease Control and Prevention. (1999). Status of perinatal HIV prevention: U.S. declines continue. *National Center for HIV, STD, and TB Prevention-Divisions of HIV/AIDS Prevention.* http://www.cdc.gov/nchstp/hiv__aids/pubs/facts/perinatl.htm

Chassler, S. (1997, February 2). What teenage girls say about pregnancy. *Parade Magazine,* 4–5.

Connor, E., Sperling, R., & Gelber, R. (1994). Reduction of maternal-infant transmission of human immunodeficiency virus type 1 from mother to infant. *New England Journal of Medicine. 331,* 1173.

The Contraception Report Contraception and adolescents. (1995). *July,* 5–12.

Cox, J., & Bithoney, W. (1995). Father of children born to adolescent mothers. *Archives of Pediatric and Adolescent Medicine. 149,* 962–966.

Cunningham, F.G. & Leveno, K. (1995). Childbearing among older women: The message is cautiously optimistic. *New England Journal of Medicine. 333,* (15), 1002–1003.

Eldred, L., & Chaisson, R. (1996). The clinical course of HIV infection in women. In R. Faden & N. Kass (Eds.), *HIV, AIDS, and childbearing.* (pp. 15–25). New York: Oxford Press.

Erikson, E. (1968). *Identity: Youth and crisis.* New York: W.W. Norton.

Gilchrist, L., Hussey, J., Gillmore, M., Lohr, M., & Morrison, D. (1996). Drug use among adolescent mothers: Prepregnancy to 18 months postpartum. *Journal of Adolescent Health. 19,* 337–344.

Goedert, J., Duliege, A., Amos, C., Felton, S., & Biggar, R. (1991). International registry of HIV-exposed twins. *Lancet. 338,* 1471–1475.

Greene, E., & Cromer, S. (1991). Adolescent pregnancy. *North Carolina Medical Journal. 52,* (10), 494–495.

Haddow, J., Palomaki, G., Knight, G., Cunningham, G., Lustig, L., & Boyd, P. (1994). Reducing the need for amniocentesis in women 35 years or older with serum markers for screening. *New England Journal of Medicine. 330,* (16), 1114–1118.

Haffner, D.W. (1995). *Facing facts: Sexual health for America's adolescents: The report of the national commission on adolescent sexual health.* New York: SIECUS.

Hardy, J., & Duggan, A. (1988). Teenage fathers and the fathers of infants of urban teenage mothers. *American Journal of Public Health. 78,* (8), 919–922.

Hatcher, R., Stewart, F, Trussell, J., Kowal, D., Guest, F., Stewart, G., Cates, W., & Policar, M. (1998). *Contraceptive technology.* (17th ed.) New York: Irvington.

King, P. (1996). Reproductive choices of adolescent females with HIV/AIDS. In R. Faden & N. Kass (Eds.), *HIV, AIDS, & childbearing.* (pp. 345–363). New York: Oxford Press.

Koonin, L., et al. (1989). Pregnancy-associated deaths due to AIDS in the United States. *Journal of the American Medical Association, 261,* 1306–1309.

Luker, K. (1996). *Dubious conceptions: The politics of teenage pregnancy.* Cambridge, MA: Harvard University Press.

Maroulis, G. (1993). Fertility, pregnancy, and the older woman. *Contemporary OB/GYN. 5,* 101–123.

Mashburn, M. (1994). Levonorgestrel implant use among adolescents. *Journal of Pediatric Health Care. 8,* (6), 255–260.

Mauskopf, J., Paul, J., Wichman, D., White, A., & Tilson, H. (1996). Economic impact of treatment of HIV-positive pregnant women and their newborns with zidovudine. *Journal of the American Medical Association. 276,* (2), 132–138.

Maynard, R. (1996). *Kids having kids: A Robin Hood foundation special report on the costs of adolescent childbearing.* New York: The Robin Hood Foundation.

Mofenson, L. (1998). Simplified ZDV prophylaxis against mother-to-child transmission. *Medscape Conference News Online.* http://www.medscape.com/Medscape/CNO/1998/AIDS/06.29/p11/aids.p11.html

McDonnell, M., & Kessenich, C. (2000). HIV/AIDS and women. *Primary Care Practice: HIV-Related Illness. 4,* (1), 66–73.

Moore, R. (1996). Overview of developmental physical milestones and psychosocial issues. *Current Practice Issues in Adolescent Gynecology,* 4–7.

National Center for Health Statistics. (1999). Declines in teenage birth rates, 1991–98: Update of national and state trends. *Monthly Vital Statistics Report. 47,* (26), 1–12.

Padian, N., Shiboski, S., & Jewell, N. (1991). Female to male transmission of the human immunodeficiency virus. *Journal of the American Medical Association. 266,* 1664–1667.

Pauker, S., & Pauker, S. (1994). Prenatal diagnosis—why is 35 a magic number? *New England Journal of Medicine. 330,* (16), 1151–1152.

Piaget, J. (1969). *The theory of stages in cognitive development.* New York: McGraw-Hill.

Read, J. (1999). The mode of delivery and the risk of vertical transmission of human immunodeficiency virus, type 1. *New England Journal of Medicine. 340,* (13), 977–987.

Reece, S. (1993). Social support and the early maternal experience of primiparas over 35. *Maternal-Child Nursing. 21,* (3), 91–98.

Reuters News Service. (1997, October, 28). Teen pleads not guilty in prom baby case. *The Houston Chronicle,* 7A.

Riley, L.E., & Greene, M.F. (1999). Elective cesarean delivery to reduce transmission of HIV. (Editorial). *The New England Journal of Medicine. 13,* 1032–1033.

Sadler, L., & Catrone, C. (1983). The adolescent parent: A dual developmental crisis. *Journal of Adolescent Health Care. 4,* (2), 100–105.

Sauer, M., Paulson, R., & Lobo, R. (1995). Pregnancy in women 50 or more years of age: Outcomes of 22 consecutively established pregnancies from oocyte donation. *Fertility and Sterility. 64,* (1), 111–115.

Silverman, N., Rohner, D., & Turner, B. (1997). Attitudes toward health-care, HIV infection, and perinatal transmission interventions in a cohort of inner-city, pregnant women. *American Journal of Perinatology. 14,* (6), 341–346.

Stein, D., Korvick, J., & Vermund, S. (1992). CD4+ lymphocyte cell enumeration for prediction of clinical course of human immunodeficiency virus disease: A review. *Journal of Infectious Diseases, 165,* 352–363.

Stevens-Simon, C. (1998). Providing reproductive health care and prescribing contraceptives for adolescents. *Pediatrics in Review, 19,* (12), 409–417.

Stevens-Simon, C. (1997). Reproductive health care for your adolescent female patients. *Contemporary Pediatrics, 14,* (2), 35–69.

Stevens-Simon, C., Kelly, L., Singer, D., & Cox, A. (1996). Why pregnant adolescents say they did not use contraceptive prior to conception. *Journal of Adolescent Health. 19,* 48–53.

Stevens-Simon, C., & Lowy, R. (1995). Teenage childbearing. *Archives of Pediatric and Adolescent Medicine. 149,* 912–915.

Stevens-Simon, C., & McAnarney, E. (1992). Adolescent pregnancy. In W. McAnarney, R. Kreipe, D. Orr & G. Comerci (Eds.), *Textbook of Adolescent Medicine* (pp. 689–695). Philadelphia: W.B. Saunders.

Stevens-Simon, C., & McAnarney, E. (1991). Adolescent pregnancy: Continuing challenges. In D. Greydanus & M. Wolraich (Eds.), *Behavioral Pediatrics.* New York: Springer-Verlag.

Stevens-Simon, C., & White, M. (1991). Adolescent pregnancy. *Pediatric Annals, 20,* (6), 322–331.

Stout, J. & Kirby, D. (1993). The effects of sexuality education on adolescent sexual activity. *Pediatric Annals, 22,* (2), 120–126.

Temmerman, M. et al. (1994). Maternal human immunodeficiency virus-1 infection and pregnancy outcome. *Obstetrics and Gynecology, 83,* (4), 495.

Tsang, R. (1993). Teenage pregnancy is preventable—a challenge to our society. *Pediatric Annals, 22,* (2), 133–135.

U.S. Bureau of the Census. *Statistical abstract for the United States* (1993), (13th ed.) Washington, DC: U.S. Bureau of the Census.

Ventura, S., Martin, J., Taftel, S., Mathews, T., & Clarke, S. (1995). Advance report of final natality statistics, 1993. *Monthly Vital Statistics Report, 44,* (Suppl), 1–88.

Ventura, S., Mosher, W., Curtain, S., Abma, J., & Henshaw, S. (1999). Highlights of trends in pregnancies and pregnancy rates by outcome: Estimates of the United States, 1976–96. *Monthly Vital Statistics Report, 47,* (29), 1–10.

Suggested Readings

Becker, K., & Walton-Moss, B. (2000). Young women with recurrent yeast infections. *Primary Care Practice. 4,* (1), 125–131.

Bode, J. (1999). *Kids still having kids: Talking about teen pregnancy.* Boston, Mass.: Horn Book, Inc.

Burnhill, M. (1994). Adolescent pregnancy rates in the U.S. *Contemporary Pediatrics, 11,* 43–50.

Busen, N. (1997). The adolescent. In J. Ashwill & S. Droske (Eds.), *Nursing care of children: Principles and practice* (p. 168). Philadelphia: W.B. Saunders.

Castro, W., Mayden, B., & Annitto, M. (1999). *First talk: A teen pregnancy prevention dialogue among Latinos.* Washington, DC: Child Welfare League of America.

Endersbe, J. (2000). *Teen fathers: Getting involved.* Mankato, MN: Capstone Press.

Fretts, R., Schmittdiel, J., McLean, F., Usher, R., & Goldman, M. (1995). Increased maternal age and the risk of fetal death. *New England Journal of Medicine. 333,* (15), 953–957.

Hershberger, P. (1998). Smoking and pregnant teens. *Association of Women's Health, Obstetric, and Neonatal Nurses Lifelines, 2,* (4), 27–31.

Jamiolkowski, R. (1997). *A baby doesn't make the man: Alternative sources of power and manhood for young men.* New York: Rosen.

Jones, M. (1998). Motherhood after 35: Choices, decisions, options. Tucson, AZ: Fisher Books.

Lavin, E.R., Wood, S. (1998). *The essential over 35 pregnancy guide: Everything you need to know about becoming a mother later in life.* New York: Avon Books.

Lindsay, J., Schilling, M., & Enright, S. (1997). *Books, babies and school-aged parents: How to teach pregnant and parenting teens to succeed.* Buena Park, California: Morning Glory Press.

Lindsay, J.W. (1997). *Pregnant? Adoption an option.* Buena Park, CA: Morning Glory Press.

Lynch, M., & Pugh, K. (2000). Uneven ground: HIV in women of color. *Advance for Nurse Practitioners, January,* 45–48.

Maloni, J. (1998). Averting the bed rest controversy. *Association of Women's Health, Obstetric, and Neonatal Nurses Lifelines. 2,* (4), 64, 61–63.

Passero, V., Wellman, L., Damas, K., & com Freda, M. (1995). *The mature gravida: Pregnancy at age 35 and older.* Wilkes-Barre, PA: March of Dimes Birth Defects Foundation.

Prysak, M., Lorenz, R., & Kisly, A. (1995). Pregnancy outcome in nulliparous women 35 years and older. *Obstetrics and Gynecology. 85,* (1), 65–70.

Putnik, J. (1996). Welfare bill: Legislating morality? *New York Times,* August 19, B1.

Raines, C. (2000). Antiretroviral treatment in HIV infection. *Primary Care Practice, 4,* (1), 83–100.

Trapani, M. (1997). *Listen up!: Teenage mothers speak out.* New York: Rosen.

Resources

Antiretroviral Pregnancy Registry, phone (800) 722-9292, extension 38465

American Academy of Pediatrics: www.aap.org/

First-time mothers over age 35: www.midlifemommies.com/

International Childbirth Education Association: www.icea.org

Interactive teen website: www.cyberisle.org

Sidelines National Support Network for pregnant women on bed rest: www.sidelines.org

Society for Adolescent Medicine: www3.uchc.edu/~sam/introduction-low.shtml.com

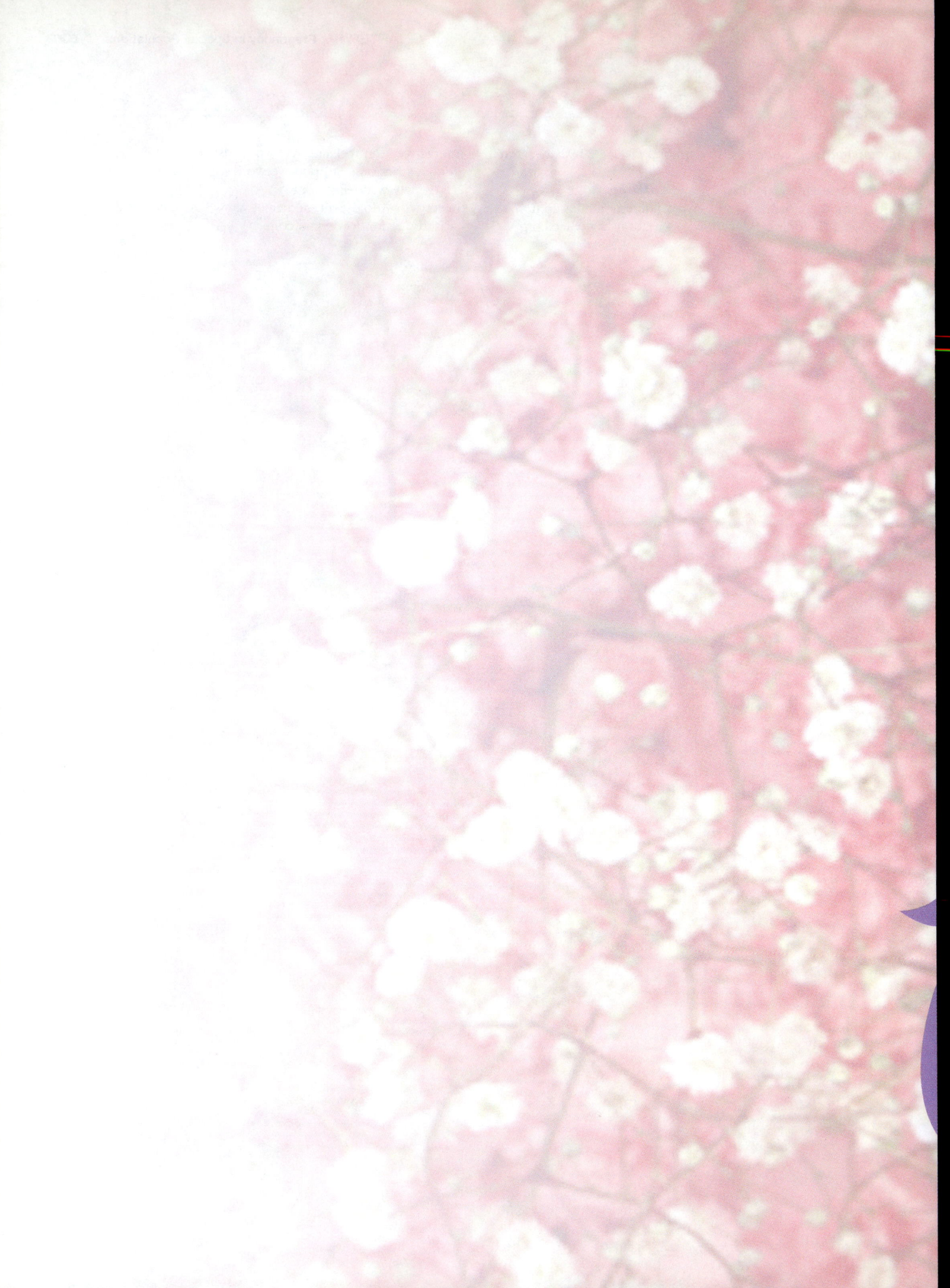

UNIT V

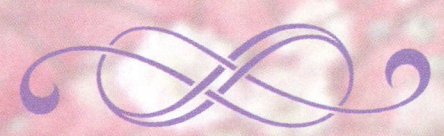

Assessment
of Fetal Well-Being

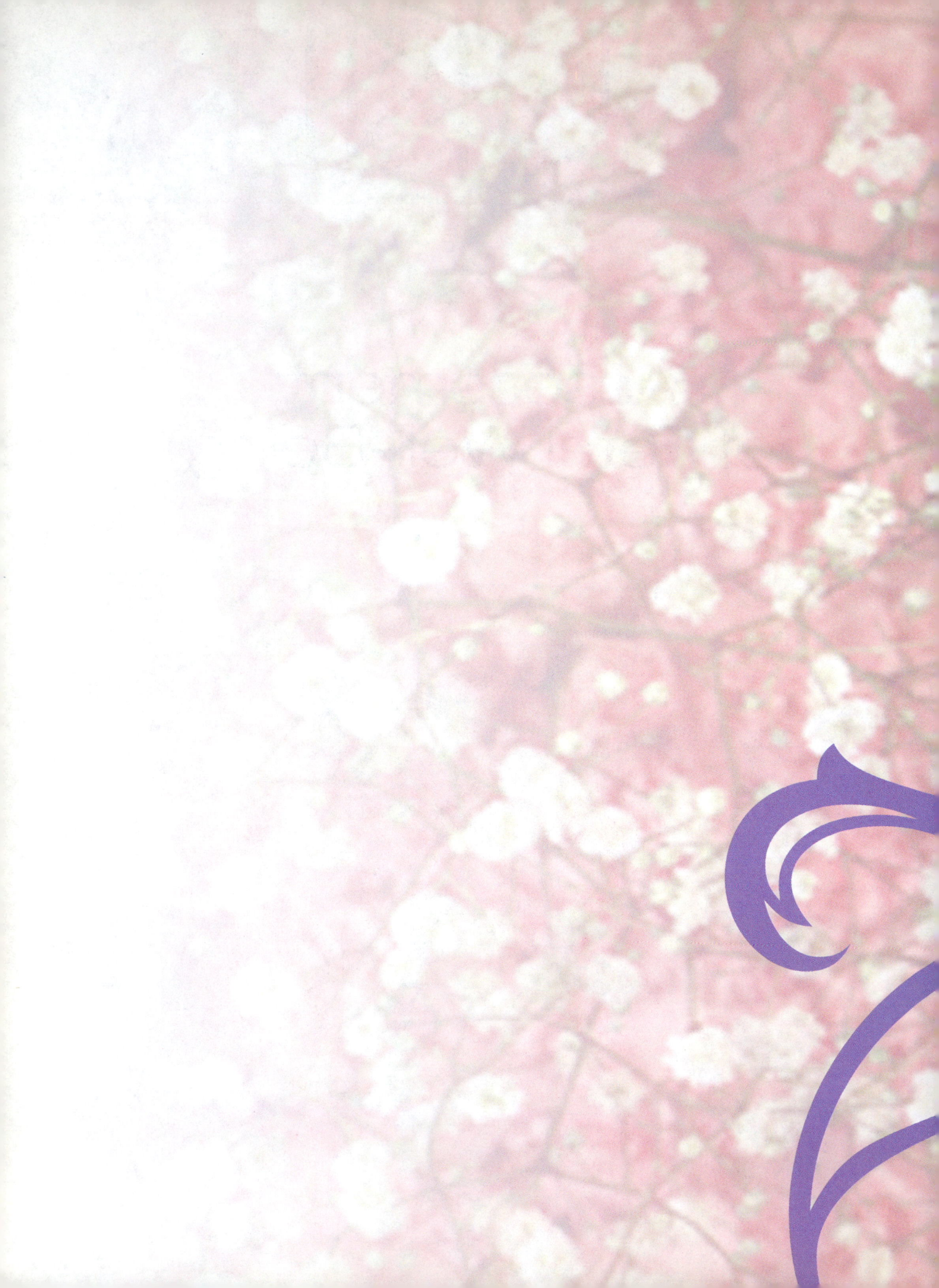

CHAPTER 20

Fetal Development

*H*ave you ever considered what a baby looks like at various stages of fetal development? Organs and systems are almost totally complete at the end of the first trimester of pregnancy. Other systems, such as the nervous system, are not fully developed. What implications does fetal development have for your nursing practice?

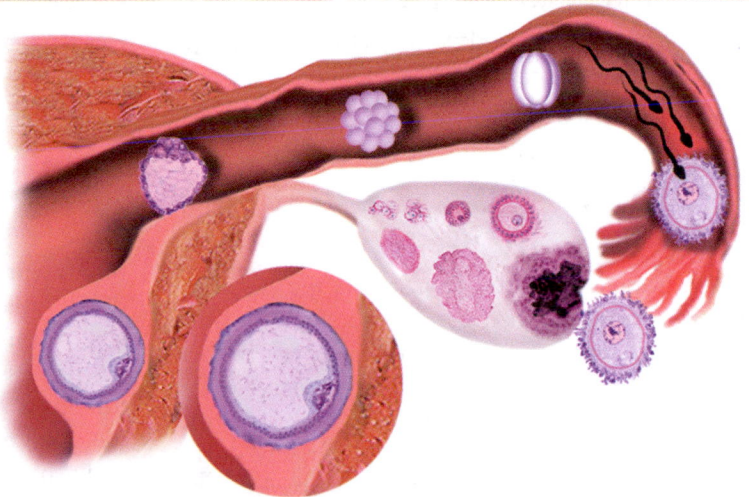

Key Terms

Allantois	Decidua	Implantation	Somite
Amnion	Decidua basalis	Langhan's layer	Spermatozoon
Amniotic fluid	Decidua capsularis	Lanugo	Syncytiotrophoblast
Blastocyst	Decidua vera	Meconium	Teratogen
Capacitation	Embryo	Meiosis	Trophoblast cells
Chorion	Fertilization	Mesenchyme	Wharton's jelly
Chorionic villi	Fimbriae	Mitosis	Zona pellucida
Corona radiata	Graafian follicle	Morula	Zygote
Cotyledons	Human chorionic	Nuchal cord	
Cytotrophoblast	gonadotropin (hCG)	Organogenesis	

Competencies

Upon completion of this chapter, the reader should be able to:

1. Describe the process of fertilization, implantation, and cell differentiation.
2. Delineate the structure and function of the placenta, amniotic fluid, and umbilical cord.
3. Identify the major stages of fetal development.
4. Identify the critical developmental stages of organogenesis that may be affected by environmental hazards.
5. Apply the knowledge of fetal growth and development to create high-quality nursing care and teaching plans for the expectant mother and her developing fetus.

There is no process as amazing as the development of a human being from two single cells. In about 40 weeks, a fertilized egg grows from a single cell to a fully developed fetus able to survive the birthing process. Fetal development is an incredible and multifaceted event. This chapter gives an overview of the developmental stages, starting with early cell division, and then reviews fetal development. The organizing framework for this chapter is chronological development of the fetus. Throughout the chapter, concepts that relate to the educational needs and concerns of clients are highlighted.

CELL DIVISION

This chapter presents an overview of fertilization through embryonic and fetal development. A fertilized egg grows from a single cell carrying all the required genetic material, to a fully developed fetus, eventually growing into an adult.

Human development occurs through two cell division processes: mitosis and meiosis. **Mitosis** refers to the process in which body cells duplicate themselves and then separate into two new daughter cells. This is how the human body grows and increases in size. Mitosis is a con-

tinuous process whereby the cell material duplicates and divides and enables the growth of the fetus. The distinct stages of mitosis are illustrated in Figure 20-1. **Meiosis** is the process by which the ovum and sperm divide and mature. In contrast to mitosis, meiosis results in a reduction in the number of human chromosomes. All human cells normally have 46 chromosomes, except the sex cells (ovum and sperm). These chromosomes are paired, thus each cell contains 22 pairs of autosomes and one pair of sex chromosomes. The ovum and sperm undergo the process of meiosis (reduction in total number of chromosomes). In the meiotic process (Figure 20-1) each gamete receives only one chromosome from each pair. Thus each mature ovum and spermatozoon has 23 chromosomes.

IMPLANTATION AND FERTILIZATION

Human development begins before **implantation**, which is the embedding of the fertilized ovum into the endometrium. During ovulation in the female, the ovum is expelled from the **graafian follicle** in the ovary and swept up into the fallopian tube (Figure 20-2). The ovum is surrounded by a layer of cells (**zona pellucida**) and a

Cell Division

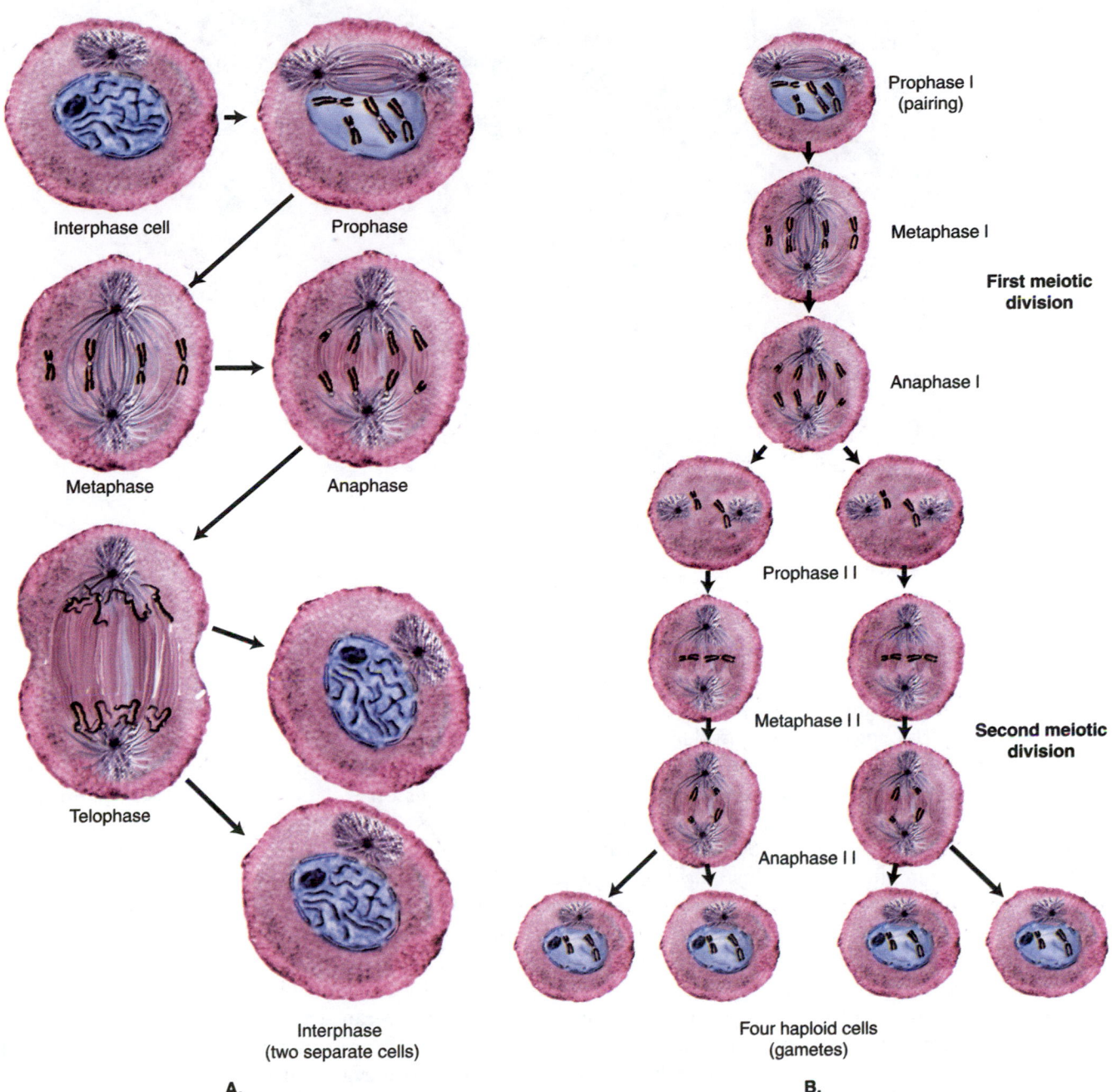

Interphase cell

Prophase

Metaphase

Anaphase

Telophase

Interphase
(two separate cells)

A.

Prophase I
(pairing)

Metaphase I

**First meiotic
division**

Anaphase I

Prophase I I

Metaphase I I

**Second meiotic
division**

Anaphase I I

Four haploid cells
(gametes)

B.

Figure 20-1 Cell division. A, mitosis; B, meiosis.

band of cells, known as the **corona radiata**. These layers of cells facilitate the migration of the ovum along the fallopian tube to the uterus. The ovum is propelled through the fallopian tube by waves of fine hair-like structures **(fimbriae)**, that line the fallopian tubes. **Fertilization** (Figure 20-3) of the ovum occurs within the first 24 to 48 hours after the release of the ovum into the fallopian tube. If the ovum is not fertilized within this time, the ovum wastes away and becomes nonfunctional. Since the life of

spermatozoa is approximately 48 to 72 hours, the total time span during which fertilization may occur depends on ovulation occurring during the life of the deposited sperm.

At ejaculation during coitus, 200 to 600 million spermatozoa are deposited in the vagina. The spermatozoa propel themselves into the uterus and eventually into the fallopian tube. Only a few sperm survive to reach the ovum. The surviving sperm cluster around the ovum. To penetrate the

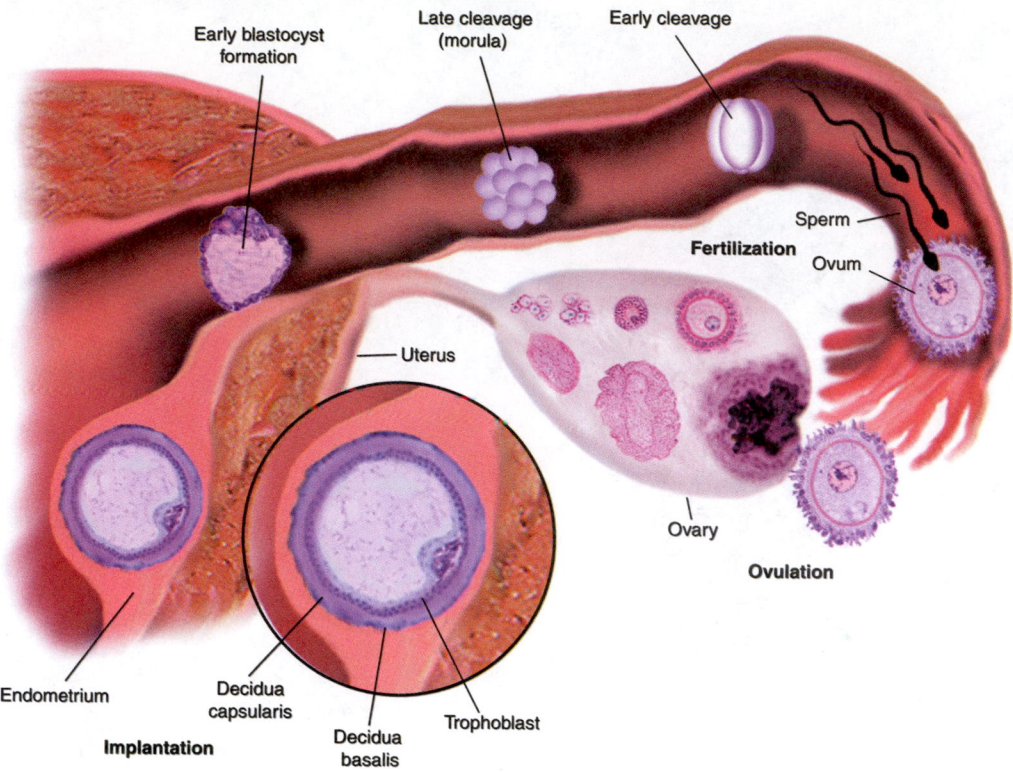

Figure 20-2 Ovulation, fertilization, and implantation.

ovum, the head of the sperm must undergo **capacitation**. This process consists of changes in the plasma membrane of the sperm head. The sperm releases hyaluronidase (a proteolytic enzyme) that dissolves the layer of cells protecting the ovum. When a single sperm penetrates the zona pellucida of the ovum, a chemical reaction occurs that prevents other sperm from entering the ovum. Immediately upon entering the ovum, the chromosomal material of the ovum and spermatozoa fuse, resulting in a **zygote**. The fertilized ovum not only forms the fetus but also the accessory structures (placenta and yolk sac) that the fetus will need to support itself during intrauterine life.

Once fertilization is complete, the zygote travels along the fallopian tube toward the uterus. This journey takes approximately 3 to 4 days. During this time, mitotic cell division, or cleavage, occurs. The first cleavage is complete at about 24 hours after fertilization, and this process continues once every 22 to 23 hours. By the time the zygote reaches the uterus, it should consist of 16 to 64 cells. This mass of cells is referred to as a **morula** because of its resemblance to a mulberry. The morula continues to multiply for about 4 more days. During this time, large cells **(trophoblast cells)** cluster on the perimeter of the morula, resulting in a fluid-filled space surrounding the inner cluster of cells, called a **blastocyst**. The outer layer of cells (trophoblast) is part of the structure that forms the placenta, while the inner cluster of cells (blastocyst) develops into the embryo.

On the seventh day after fertilization, the corona and zona pellucida dissolve and disappear. This permits the trophoblast to deeply embed into to the endometrium of the uterine wall. The trophoblastic cells produce an enzyme that dissolves the endometrial tissue, permitting the blastocyst to tunnel into the endometrium. As the invasion continues, the cell mass establishes a communication network with the circulatory system of the endometrium.

Implantation generally occurs high in the uterus. If the implantation occurs lower in the uterus, the growing placenta may obstruct the cervix (a situation referred to as placenta previa). Probably one-third of fertilized eggs never implant because there is a major defect in the zygote or the endometrium is not receptive to the invading blastocyst. Of those zygotes that do implant, fewer than one-third progress to establish a productive pregnancy (Moore & Persaud, 1998).

The corpus luteum in the ovary continues to function producing estrogen and progestin, because of the influence of **human chorionic gonadotropin** (hCG), produced by the trophoblast cells. This allows the endometrium to continue to grow and sustain the pregnancy. At this stage, the endometrium is called the **decidua**. The decidua has three regions: (1) the part resting directly between the embryo and the uterine wall under the **embryo (decidua basalis)**, (2) the portion of the endometrium that surrounds the surface of the trophoblast **(decidua capsularis)**, and (3) the remaining

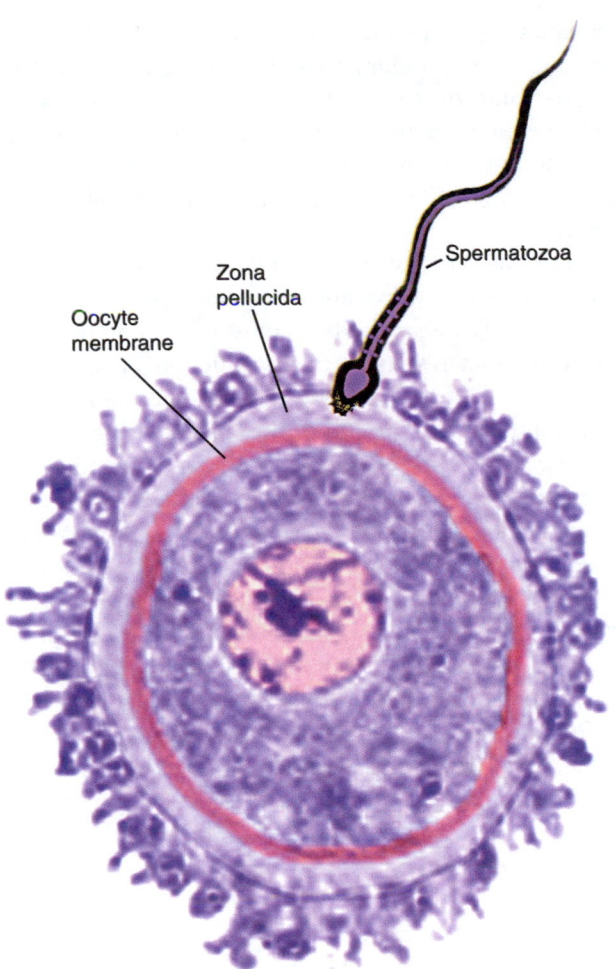

Figure 20-3 Fertilization.

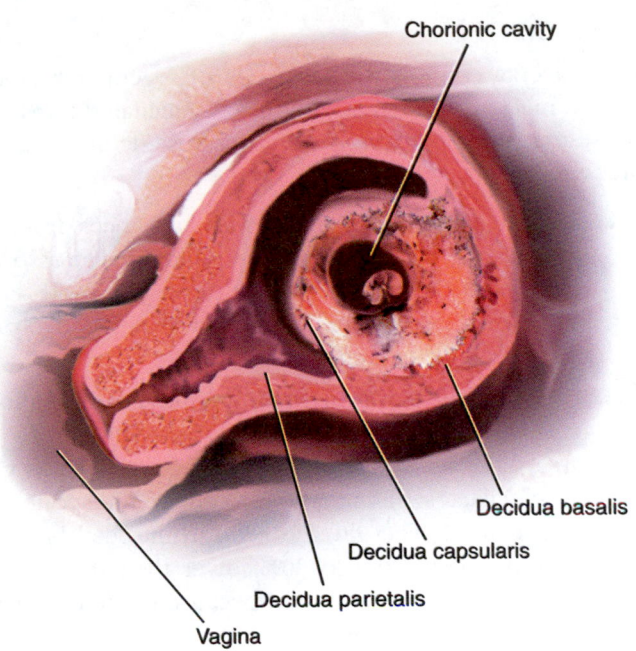

Figure 20-4 Decidua.

portion of the uterine lining **(decidua parietalis)** (Figure 20-4) (Larsen, 1997).

Once implantation occurs, the trophoblastic layer of cells begins to mature. By the 12th day, **chorionic villi** form and begin to expand into the uterine endometrium. The chorionic villi have a central core of connective tissue that contains fetal capillaries and is covered by two layers of trophoblast cells. The **syncytiotrophoblast** is the outer layer, which facilitates the production of several placental hormones (hCG, human placental lactogen HPL, estrogen, and progesterone). The inner layer **(cytotrophoblast, or Langhan's layer)** is present as early as 12 days after fertilization but it disappears between the 20th and 24th weeks of gestation (Larsen, 1997). This layer of cells protects the growing embryo from certain infectious organisms, such as syphilis; however, it does not provide protection against many other viral agents.

PLACENTA

After implantation, the placenta begins to develop. The placenta develops from the trophoblast cells at the site where the developing embryo attaches to the uterine wall. The placenta eventually serves as the lungs, kidneys, endocrine system, and gastrointestinal tract for the fetus. Placental development and circulation begins around the third week of embryonic development. The placenta continues to grow in size until the 20th week of gestation, at which time it covers nearly one-half of the uterine wall. After the 20th week, the placenta becomes thicker but not larger in diameter. At term, the placenta is about 6 to 8 inches (15 to 20 cm) in diameter, with walls 1 to 1.5 inches (2.5 to 3.0 cm) in thickness, and weighs approximately 14 to 21 ounces (400 to 600 g).

The placenta has two parts: the maternal portion and the fetal portion. The maternal portion consists of the decidua basalis and its circulation. Its surface is red, rough, and segmented into irregular convex areas, referred to as **cotyledons**. The fetal portion consists of the chorionic villi and the surface is covered by the amnion, which gives it a shiny, gray appearance.

Functions of the Placenta

The placenta begins to function shortly after implantation and is involved in the metabolic, endocrine, and transport activities necessary for fetal development (Carlson, 1999).

Metabolic

The placenta produces glycogen, cholesterol, and fatty acids for fetal use and hormone production and numerous enzymes required for fetoplacental transfer. It also stores glycogen and iron.

Transport

The placenta controls the exchange of several substances by five mechanisms: simple diffusion, facilitated transport, active transport, pinocytosis, and hydrostatic and osmotic pressure.

1. Simple diffusion occurs when substances from an area of higher concentration pass to an area of lower concentration. Substances that move by simple diffusion are water, oxygen, carbon dioxide, electrolytes, anesthetic gases, and certain drugs.

2. Facilitated transport involves the movement of molecules from an area of greater concentration to an area of lower concentration. Molecules such as glucose, galactose, and some oxygen are transported by this method. The glucose level in the fetal blood is approximately 20% to 30% lower than the glucose level in the maternal blood because the fetus metabolizes glucose rapidly.

3. Active transport can work against a concentration gradient, allowing molecules to move from areas of lower concentration to areas of higher concentration. Amino acids, calcium, iron, iodine, water-soluble vitamins, and glucose are transferred in this manner.

4. Pinocytosis is the process of cellular ingestion by engulfing the cell. Pinocytosis is important for transferring large molecules, such as albumin and gamma globulin. Amoeba-like cells, forming plasma droplets, engulf materials.

5. Hydrostatic and osmotic pressure allow the bulk flow of water and some solutes to the fetus.

Other mechanisms of transfer also exist, for example, fetal red blood cells may pass into the maternal circulation through breaks in the placental membrane. Maternal leukocytes and certain microorganisms can cross the placental membrane under their own power. There is no mixing of maternal blood with fetal blood. As the maternal blood picks up waste products and carbon dioxide from the fetus, it drains back into the maternal circulation. The transfer of substances, the ratio of blood on either side of the placenta, and the binding abilities of certain molecules in the blood affect changes in blood flow between the fetus and the maternal intervillous spaces.

Endocrine

The placenta produces hormones that are vital to the survival of the fetus. These include hCG, human placental lactogen (hPL), and two steroid hormones, estrogen and progesterone.

The hormone hCG prevents the normal involution of the corpus luteum at the end of the menstrual cycle. If the corpus luteum stops functioning before the 11th week of pregnancy, spontaneous abortion occurs. The hCG stimulates the corpus luteum to secrete increased amounts of estrogen and progesterone. hCG reaches its maximum level around the 60th day and then decreases, as placental hormone production increases. hCG and hPL play a role in preventing the rejection of the placenta and embryo by the mother's body.

After the 11th week, the placenta produces enough progesterone and estrogen to maintain pregnancy. In the male fetus, hCG also exerts a cell-stimulating effect on the fetal testes that results in the production of testosterone. The secretion of testosterone during embryonic development stimulates the growth of the male sex organs.

Progesterone is essential for the maintenance of the pregnancy because it increases the secretions of the fallopian tubes and uterus. These secretions provide appropriate nutritive elements for the developing morula and blastocyst. Progesterone also assists in the transport of the ovum through the fallopian tube. Progesterone causes decidual cells to develop in the uterine endometrium, and it must be present in high levels for implantation to be successful. Progesterone also decreases the contractility of the uterus, thus preventing uterine contractions, which may result in spontaneous abortion. The production of progesterone by the corpus luteum peaks between the seventh and 10th day after ovulation, and implantation occurs at this time. After the 10th week, the placenta takes over the production of progesterone.

By the seventh week, the placenta produces more than 50% of the estrogen in the maternal circulation. Estrogen has a generating function on the uterus, the breasts, and the breast glandular tissue.

Placental Circulation

After the blastocyst implants, the cells differentiate into fetal cells and trophoblastic cells. The trophoblast invades the decidua basalis of the endometrium, resulting in the opening of the uterine capillaries and eventually the larger uterine vessels (Figure 20-5). At the same time, the chorionic villi continue to grow and eventually form the fetal vessels. On about the 12th day, maternal blood pools in the intervillous spaces surrounding the chorionic villi. By the end of the 21st day, oxygen, glucose, and other nutrients diffuse from the maternal blood to the chorionic villi and are transported to the developing embryo.

By the 12th week of gestation, the placenta develops into a discrete organ. The cotyledons on the maternal surface contain branches of the placental villi, allowing for some compartmentalization of the uteroplacental circulation. Each cotyledon contains branching vessels that are distributed throughout the lobules.

The capillaries of the villi are lined with thin endothelium and are surrounded by a layer of connective tissue

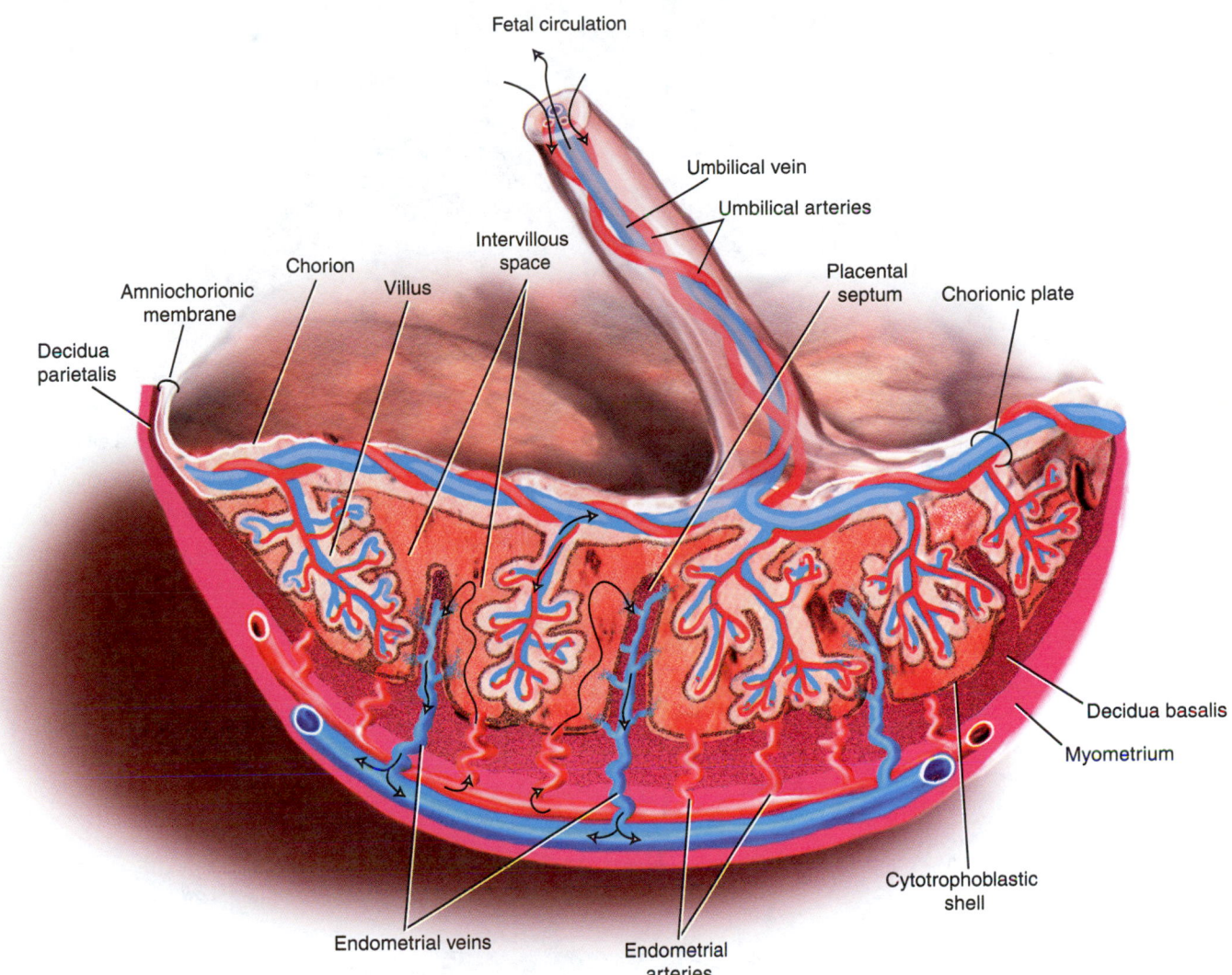

Figure 20-5 Placental circulation.

(mesenchyme). In the fully developed umbilical cord, fetal blood flows through two umbilical arteries to the capillaries of the villi and oxygen-enriched blood flows back through the umbilical vein to the fetus.

Maternal blood, rich in oxygen and nutrients, spurts from the uterine arteries into the intervillous spaces. The blood is directed toward the chorionic plate and, as the pressure decreases, it spreads out. Fresh maternal blood enters and exerts pressure on the intervillous spaces, thus pushing blood toward the basal plate. Blood is then drained through the uterine and pelvic veins.

Circulation within the intervillous spaces depends on maternal blood pressure. The lumen of the uterine artery is narrow when it pierces the chorionic plate and enters the intervillous space, resulting in an increase in blood pressure locally. The pressure in the arteries forces the blood into the intervillous space and bathes the villi in oxygenated blood. As the pressure decreases, the blood flows back from the chorionic plate toward the decidua, where it enters the endometrial veins. Placental exchange functions occur only in fetal vessels that are in intimate contact with the covering syncytial membrane. The syncytium villi have borders containing many microvilli, which greatly increase the exchange rate between maternal and fetal circulation.

Fetal Circulation

The blood circulation after birth is much different from that of the fetus. During fetal development, the lungs are collapsed and do not function. The placenta performs the role of supplying oxygen to the blood and removing carbon dioxide. This requires that there be unique structures (i.e., foramen ovale, ductus venosus, and ductus arteriosus) that play major roles in fetal circulation and disappear after birth.

The blood from the placenta flows through the umbilical vein, which penetrates the abdominal wall of the fetus

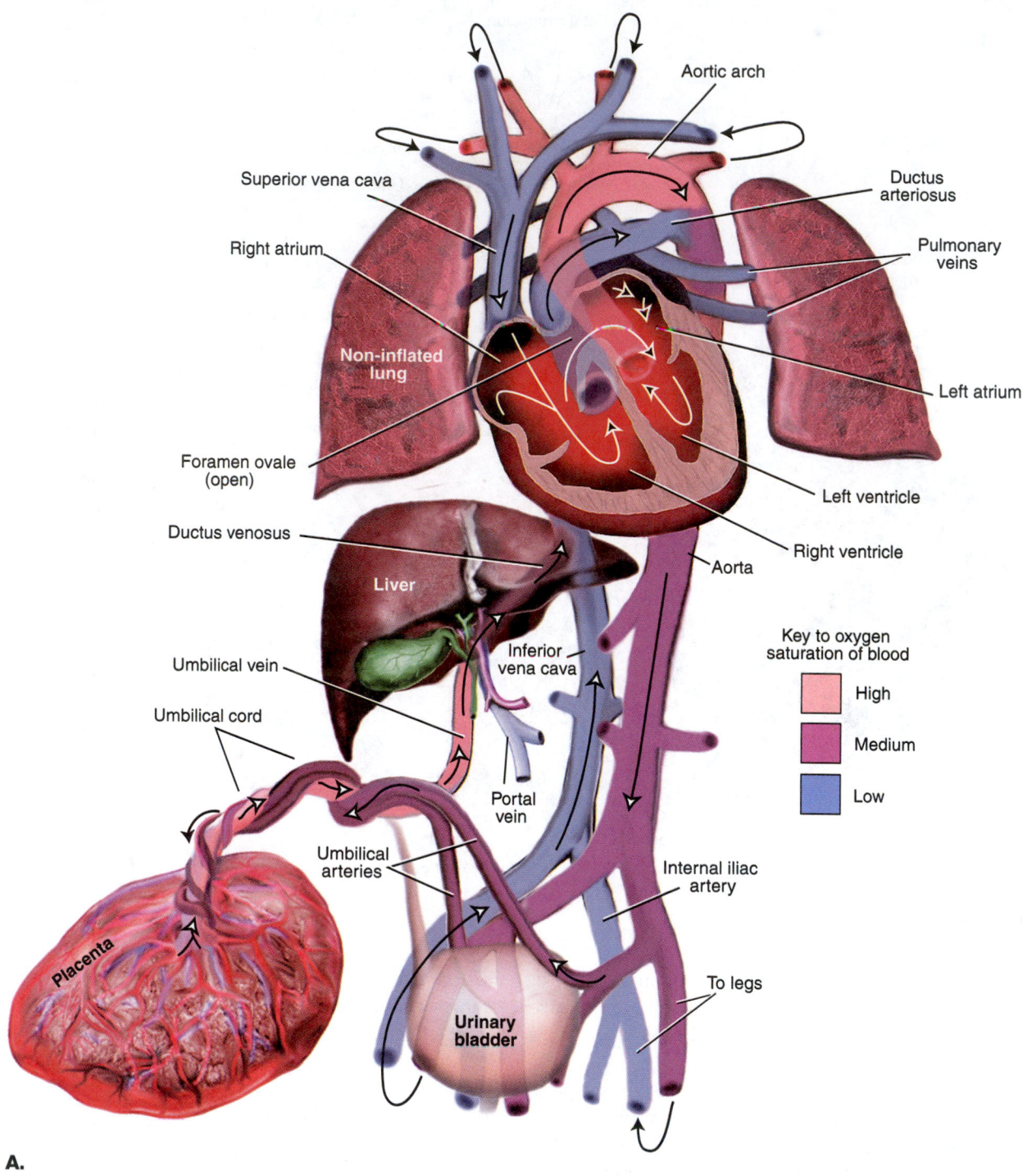

Key to oxygen saturation of blood

High	
Medium	
Low	

Figure 20-6 A. Fetal circulation.

at the site of the umbilicus (Figure 20-6A). It divides into two branches, one of which circulates a small amount of blood through the fetal liver and empties into the inferior vena cava through the hepatic vein. The second and larger branch, called the ductus venosus, empties directly into the fetal vena cava. This blood then enters the right atrium, passes through the foramen ovale into the left atrium, and pours into the left ventricle, which pumps it into the aorta. Some blood returning from the head and upper extremi-

ties by way of the superior vena cava is emptied into the right atrium and passes through the tricuspid valve into the right ventricle. This blood is pumped into the pulmonary artery, and a small amount passes to the lungs and provides nourishment only. The larger portion of blood passes from the pulmonary artery through the ductus arteriosus and into the descending aorta, bypassing the lungs. Finally, blood returns to the placenta through the two umbilical arteries, and the process is repeated.

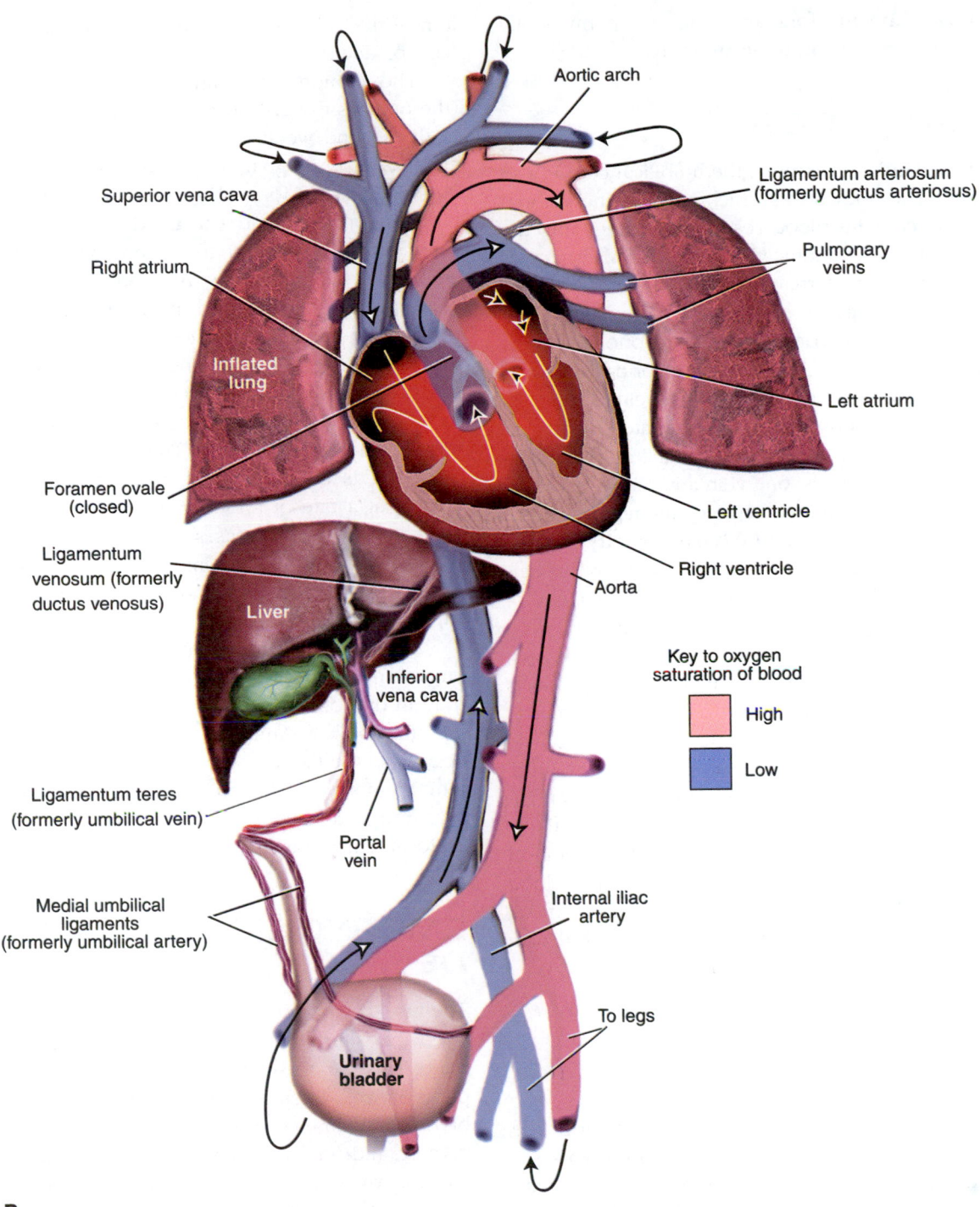

B.

Figure 20-6 *(continued)* B. Newborn circulation.

The fetus receives oxygen via diffusion from the maternal circulation. Fetal hemoglobin facilitates obtaining oxygen, since it carries as much as 20% to 30% more oxygen than adult hemoglobin. Fetal circulation delivers the highest available oxygen concentrations to the head, neck, brain, and heart and a lesser amount of oxygenated blood to the abdominal organs and the lower body. This circulatory pattern leads to cephalocaudal (head-to-tail) development of the fetus.

Newborn Circulation

Fetal circulatory shunts are not necessary after birth because the baby is able to oxygenate the blood through the lungs rather than the placenta (Figure 20-6B). As the newborn breathes, the foramen ovale closes as a result of the increased blood flow to the lungs and the decreased pressure in the right side of the heart. The ductus venosus closes when the blood from the umbilical cord stops. The ductus venosus and the foramen ovale are permanently closed as tissue develops in these structures.

UMBILICAL CORD

While the placenta is developing, the umbilical cord is also being formed. The body stalk, which attaches the embryo to the yolk sac, contains blood vessels that extend into the chorionic villi. As the chorionic villi initiate circulatory communication with the maternal circulatory system, the villi begin to fuse into large vessels. As the body stalk elongates, the vessels in the cord contract into one large vein and two smaller arteries. The larger vein brings the oxygenated blood from the placenta to the fetal circulatory system. The two small arteries carry deoxygenated blood and waste products back to the placenta. About 1% of umbilical cords have only two vessels: one vein and one artery. This may be seen in conjunction with congenital malformations. A specialized connective tissue **(Wharton's jelly)**, which is an extension of the amnion, surrounds the blood vessels in the umbilical cord. This tissue, plus the high volume of blood in the vessels, prevents compression of the umbilical cord. The major function of the cord is to transport oxygen and nutrients to the fetus and to return waste products from the fetus to the placenta. At term, the cord is almost 1 inch (2 cm) across and about 22 inches (55 cm) long. The cord can attach itself to the placenta at various sites. Central insertion into the placenta is considered the norm. Umbilical cords can look twisted or spiraled; this is most likely caused by fetal movement. A true knot in the umbilical cord is rare, because of the high pressure and rapid blood flow in the cord. More common are so-called false knots, caused by the folding of the cord vessels. A **nuchal umbilical cord** is one that encircles the fetal neck.

MEMBRANES AND AMNIOTIC FLUID

The fetal membranes include the **amnion** and the chorion; both surround the fetus, along with the yolk sac and the **allantois**. The yolk sac develops in the second week and serves several functions for the embryo in its early stage of development. The yolk sac transfers nutrients to the embryo while the placental circulation is being developed. The yolk sac is important in blood development in the first few weeks of the embryo's life. Blood forms on its walls until the fetal liver takes over the function of blood formation. During the fourth week, the yolk sac becomes incorporated into the embryo and serves as the foundation for the primitive gut. The remaining portion of the yolk sac decreases in size and eventually becomes detached from the embryo. The allantois appears in the third week. It is a small diverticu-

lum of the yolk sac and eventually develops into the urinary bladder.

The amnion is the inner of the two fetal membranes (the outer is the **chorion**). The amnion begins to appear in the second week of gestation. It envelops the embryo and, as the pregnancy progresses, it adheres to the chorion. The sac formed by the amnion and chorion contains an opaque fluid **(amniotic fluid)**. The fluid surrounds the embryo and, as the pregnancy progresses, the amount of fluid increases. Amniotic fluid consists of 98% water and 2% organic and inorganic materials. The composition of the fluid changes as pregnancy advances. In the early stages of pregnancy, the amniotic fluid has a composition similar to maternal plasma; later in pregnancy, the amniotic fluid becomes hypotonic as a result of the presence of fetal urine. The volume of amniotic fluid increases as the pregnancy progresses. The volume increases at a rate of about 25 ml per week until the 15th week, and then it increases 50 ml per week until the 28th week. Amniotic fluid volume reaches a peak of approximately 1 L at 38 weeks and then stabilizes or decreases slightly until delivery.

Amniotic fluid's main function is to provide an optimal environment for the fetus. The fetus begins to swallow the fluid in the fourth month and thus it may be important to fetal metabolism. Amniotic fluid helps to dispose of secretions from the kidneys and the respiratory tract, allows the fetus to move with ease in the uterus, equalizes the pressure from sudden external forces, and keeps the fetus at a uniform temperature.

EMBRYONIC AND FETAL DEVELOPMENT

The first days of human development, starting on the day the ovum is fertilized, are referred to as the pre-embryonic stage. This period is characterized by rapid cellular multiplication, cell differentiation, and establishment of the embryonic membranes and primary germ layers. Specific embryonic and fetal assessments to determine the status of the embryo or fetus are described here. The pattern of development is cephalocaudal, proximal to distal, and general to specific.

Embryonic Stage

The stage of the embryo begins about the 14th day and continues until approximately the eighth week of development. The embryonic stage is a period of tissue differentiation, forming of essential organs, and development of external features. During this period, the embryo is vulnerable to **teratogens** (Table 20-1). Teratogens are environmental substances that may cause adverse effects on

Table 20-1 Stages of Fetal Development

	Stage	Fetal Development
	Embryonic or Germinal Stage	
	Weeks 1 and 2	Rapid cell division and differentiation. Germinal layers form.
	Embryonic Stage	
	Week 3*	Primitive nervous system, eyes, ears, and RBCs present. Heart begins to beat on day 21.
 4 weeks	Week 4* Wt 0.4 g L 4–6 mm (crown–rump, C–R)	Half the size of a pea. Brain differentiates. GI tract begins to form. Limb buds appear.
	Week 5* L 6–8 mm (C–R)	Cranial nerves present. Muscles innervated.
	Week 6* L 10–14 mm (C–R)	Fetal circulation established. Liver produces RBCs. Central autonomic nervous system forms. Primitive kidneys form. Lung buds present. Cartilage forms. Primitive skeleton forms. Muscles differentiate.
	Week 7* L 22–28 mm (C–R)	Eyelids form. Palate and tongue form. Stomach formed. Diaphragm formed. Arms and legs move.
 8 weeks	Week 8* Wt 2 g L 3 cm (1.5 in) (C–R)	Resembles human being. Eyes moved to face front. Heart development complete. Hands and feet well formed. Bone cells begin replacing cartilage. All body organs have begun forming.
	Fetal Stage	
	Week 9	Finger and toenails form. Eyelids fuse shut.
	Week 10 Wt 14 g (½ oz) L 5–6 cm (2 in) crown–heel (C–H)	Head growth slows. Islets of Langerhans differentiated. Bone marrow forms, RBCs produced. Bladder sac forms. Kidneys make urine.
	Week 11	Tooth buds appear. Liver secretes bile. Urinary system functions. Insulin forms in pancreas.

(continued)

Table 20-1 Stages of Fetal Development (continued)

	Stage	Fetal Development
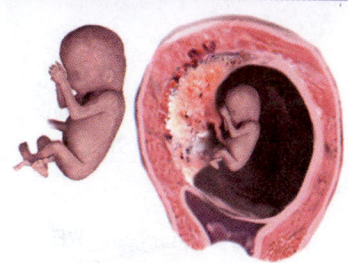 12 weeks	Week 12 Wt 45 g (1.5 oz) L 9 cm (3.5 in) (C–R) 11.5 cm (4.5 in) (C–H)	Lungs take shape. Palate fuses. Heart beat heard with Doppler ultrasound. Ossification established. Swallowing reflex present. External genitalia. Male or female distinguished.
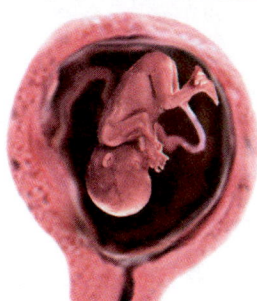 16 weeks	**Second Trimester** Week 16 Wt 200 g (7 oz) L 13.5 cm (5.5 in) (C–R) 15 cm (6 in) (C–H)	Meconium forms in bowels. Scalp hair appears. Frequent fetal movement. Skin thin, pink. Sensitive to light. 200 mL amniotic fluid. (Amniocentesis possible.)
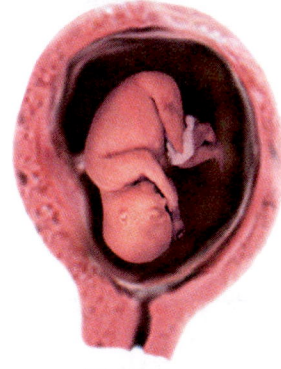 20 weeks	Week 20 Wt 435 g (15 oz) L 19 cm (7.5 in) (C–R) 25 cm (10 in) (C–H)	Myelination of spinal cord begins. Peristalsis begins. Lanugo covers body. Vernix caseosa covers body. Brown fat deposits begun. Sucks and swallows amniotic fluid. Heartbeat heard with fetoscope. Hands can grasp. Regular schedule of sucking, kicking, and sleeping.
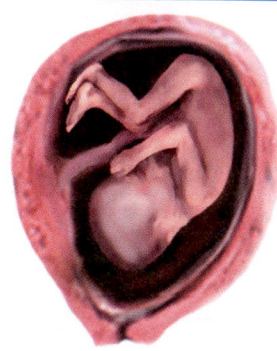 24 weeks	Week 24 Wt 780 g (1 lb, 12 oz) L 23 cm (9 in) (C–R) 28 cm (11 in) (C–H)	Alveoli present in lungs, begin producing surfactant. Eyes completely formed. Eyelashes and eyebrows appear. Many reflexes appear. Chance of survival if born now.

Table 20-1 Stages of Fetal Development (continued)

	Stage	Fetal Development
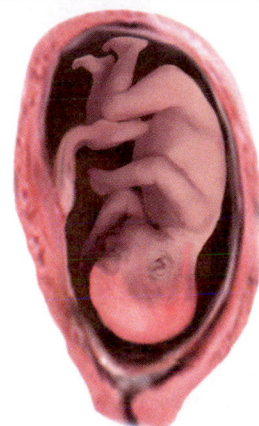 28 weeks	**Third Trimester** Week 28 Wt 1200 g (2 lb. 10 oz) L 28 cm (11 in) (C–R) 35 cm (14 in) (C–H)	Subcutaneous fat deposits begun. Lanugo begins to disappear. Nails appear. Eyelids open and close. Testes begin to descend.
	Week 32 Wt 2,000 g (4 lb, 6.5 oz) L 31 cm (12 in) (C–R) 41 cm (16 in) (C–H)	More reflexes present. CNS directs rhythmic breathing movements. CNS partially controls body temperature. Begins storing iron, calcium, phosphorus. Ratio of the lung surfactants lecithin and sphingomyelin (L/S) is 1.2:2.
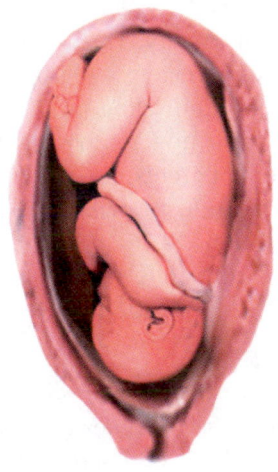 32 weeks		
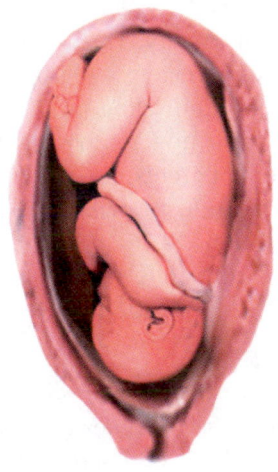 36 weeks	Week 36 Wt 2,500–2.750 g (5 lb, 8 oz) L 35 cm (14 in) (C–R) 48 cm (19 in) (C–H)	A few creases on soles of feet. Skin less wrinkled. Fingernails reach fingertips. Sleep-wake cycle fairly definite. Transfer of maternal antibodies.
	Week 38	L/S ratio 2:1

(continued)

Table 20-1 Stages of Fetal Development *(continued)*

	Stage	Fetal Development
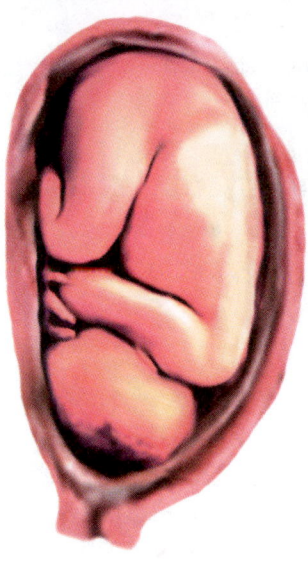 40 weeks	Week 40 Wt 3,000–3,600 g (6 lb, 10 oz–7 lb, 15 oz) L 50 cm (20 in) (C–H)	Lanugo only on shoulders and upper back. Creases cover sole. Vernix mainly in folds of skin. Ear cartilage firm. Less active, limited space. Ready to be born.

*Vulnerable to teratogenic effects.

the developing fetus. A teratogen has the greatest effect on an organ during that organ's period of differentiation and development. Brain development occurs throughout the pregnancy, and teratogens can affect mental development throughout gestation.

Embryonic Assessment

Continual improvements in the area of prenatal diagnosis are making the availability of testing relatively safer, more acceptable, reliable, and accessible. Transvaginal sonography is one diagnostic procedure that can be used for early evaluation of the embryo. This procedure gives fairly accurate estimates of gestational age by measuring the biparietal diameter of the head, head circumference, and ab-

dominal circumference. This procedure is considered safe and is not invasive.

Embryoscopy can be used in early pregnancy (around 6 weeks). This procedure requires the insertion of a minute viewing scope into the mother's abdomen through a canula about the size of a needle used to draw blood. This procedure is gaining acceptance for use in embryonic diagnosis and, in some cases, fetal surgery. This is an invasive procedure; the mother requires extensive support in preparation for the procedure and counseling on the possible risks and benefits gained from undergoing this test. The ultimate decision rests with the parents; however, they need current and accurate information to make the most appropriate decision for their family. The nurse should maintain a nonjudgmental and emotionally supportive approach to families who undergo embryoscopy.

3 Weeks

In the third week, the embryonic disk becomes elongated and pear-shaped, with a broad cephalic end and a narrow caudal end. The ectoderm forms a long cylindrical tube called the notochord, from which brain and spinal cord develop. The most advanced organ is the heart, which appears as a single tube outside the embryo's body cavity. The heart muscle is able to contract, and peristaltic waves pass along the heart tube. The cardiovascular system begins to form and blood begins circulating in the primitive heart. The gastrointestinal tract, created from the endo-

Critical Thinking

Medical History

Review obstetric and medical history for risk factors (detrimental lifestyle, abusive relationship, inappropriate use of medications, and potential teratogens, such as alcohol or nicotine). Which of these factors is most likely to produce birth defects, and why?

derm, appears as a tube-like structure that communicates with the yolk sac.

4 Weeks

During the fourth week, **somites** form on either side of the embryo's midline. Somites are formed by the division of the mesoderm next to the midplane and eventually form the vertebrae and the spinal column. The main divisions of the central nervous system (CNS) are established. The pharyngeal arches, which will form the lower jaw, hyoid bone and cartilage of the larynx, develop at this time. The pharyngeal pouches appear; they will form the eustachian tube and cavity of the middle ear, the tonsils, and the parathyroid and thymus glands. The primordia of the ear and eye are also present. By the end of 28 days, the tubular heart is beating at a regular rhythm, and the contractions are efficient enough to produce circulation

through the main fetal blood vessels. The stomach begins as a spindle-shaped bulge in the lower part of the foregut, and the pancreas begins as two small buds of endodermal cells growing out of the foregut. The liver starts as a small bud, forming at the lower end of the foregut. Before the fourth week, arm and leg buds are not visible, but the tail bud is present.

5 Weeks

By this time, the brain has differentiated into five areas, and ten pairs of cranial nerves are recognizable. During the fifth week, the optic cups and lens vesicles of the eye form and the nasal pits develop. Partitioning in the heart begins with the dividing of the atriam. The heart, circulatory system, and brain show the most advanced development. The embryo has a marked C-shaped body, accentuated by the rudimentary tail and the large head that is folded over a protuberant trunk. By day 35, the arm and leg buds are well-developed, with paddle-shaped hand and foot plates.

6 Weeks

At six weeks, the head structures are more developed, and the trunk is straighter than in earlier stages. The upper and lower jaws are recognizable, and the external nares are formed. The trachea has developed, and its caudal end is bifurcated, heralding the beginning of lung formation. The lung buds extend into the abdomen. The upper lip is present and the palate is developing. The ears continue to develop. The heart now has most of its definitive characteristics, and fetal circulation begins. The liver starts to produce blood cells. The arms have begun to extend ventrally across the chest, and both arms and legs have digits, although they may be webbed. There is a slight bend in the arms, which are more advanced in development than the legs. At this stage of development, the prominent tail begins to recede.

7 Weeks

During the seventh week, the head of the embryo is rounded and nearly erect. The eyes have shifted from their original lateral position to a forward location, in which they are closer together, and the eyelids are beginning to form. The palate is almost complete, and the tongue is developing in the formed mouth. The diaphragm begins to divide the thoracic cavity from the abdomen. The lung buds migrate up into the chest cavity. If the diaphragm fails to close, the fetus is born with a diaphragmatic hernia. The gastrointestinal and genitourinary tracts undergo significant changes during the seventh week. Before this time, the rectal and urogenital passages formed one tube that ended in a blind pouch; now they begin to separate into two tubular structures. The intestines enter the extraembryonic coelom in the area of the umbilical cord (called umbilical herniation). At this point the beginnings of all essential external and internal structures are present.

8 Weeks

At eight weeks, the embryo is approximately 1.2 inches (3 cm) long and resembles a human being. **Organogenesis** is complete. The facial features continue to develop. The eyelids begin to fuse. Auricles of the external ears begin to assume their final shape, but they are still set low. The circulatory system through the umbilical cord is well-established. External genitals appear, but the embryo's sex cannot be determined visually. The rectal passage opens with the perforation of the anal membrane. Long bones are beginning to form, and the large muscles are now capable of contracting.

Fetal Stage

By the end of the eighth week, the embryo is sufficiently developed to be called a fetus. Every organ system and external structure that is found in the full-term newborn is

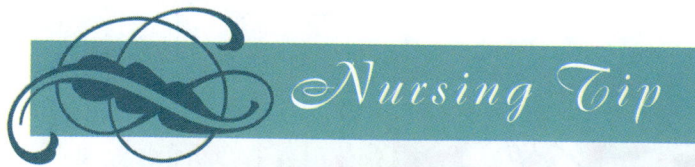

FETAL TESTS

Be aware of available fetal tests and support the family in preparing for the tests (ultrasound, amniocentesis, triple-marker screening [analysis of maternal serum for abnormal levels of alpha-fetoprotein, hCG, and estriols]) that may predict chromosomal and neural tube defects.

COMMUNITY RESOURCES

Inform the clients of the resources in the community that assist clients who need further support and information regarding problems identified through antepartal testing.

present (England, 1996). The remainder of gestation is devoted to refining structures and perfecting function.

Fetal Assessment

There are several tests that can be used to assess fetal well-being. These tests may provide information about the fetus's development, fetal lung maturity, and the location of the placenta in the uterus. Some of the tests that can be used to determine fetal status are diagnostic ultrasound (intermittent high-frequency sound waves used to create an image of the fetus), fetal stress tests, chorionic villus sampling (CVS) for chromosome analysis, and amniocentesis for lung maturity.

9 to 12 Weeks

By 10 weeks, the fetus reaches 2 inches (5 cm) in length and weighs about ½ ounce (14 g). The head is large and comprises almost half of the fetus. The neck is distinct from the head and body, and both the head and neck are straighter than in previous stages of development.

By 12 weeks, the fetus reaches 3.2 inches (8 cm) in length and weighs about 1.6 ounces (45 g). The face is well-formed: the nose protrudes, the chin is small and recedes, and the ears are acquiring a more adult shape. The eyelids close at about the 10th week and do not reopen until about 28 weeks. Some reflex movements of the lips, suggestive of the sucking reflex, have been observed as early as 12 weeks. Tooth buds now appear for all 20 of the

REFLECTIONS FROM A CLIENT

"I really didn't even realize I was pregnant until I heard my baby's heartbeat. Then I saw her heart beating on ultrasound and found out it was a girl. I'm amazed to think my baby has all her systems developed and functioning so early."

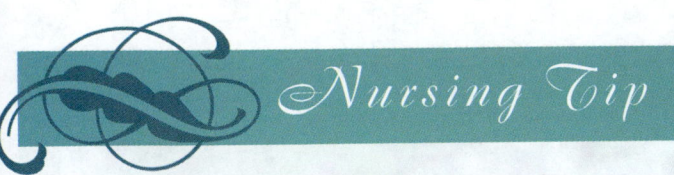

child's first teeth (baby teeth). The liver primarily produces red blood cells. The heart rate is 120 to 160 beats/min. The urogenital tract completes its development, well-differentiated genitals appear, and the kidneys begin to produce urine. The limbs are long and slender, with well-formed digits. The fetus can curl the fingers toward the palm and make a tiny fist. Ossification centers begin to form in the bones. The legs are still shorter and less developed than the arms. Ultrasonographic devices can easily ascertain spontaneous movements between 6 and 12 weeks.

13 to 16 Weeks

At 13 weeks, the fetus weighs 2 to 2½ ounces (55 to 60 g) and is about 3.6 inches (9 cm) in length. Fine hair (**lanugo**) begins to appear, especially on the head. The skin is transparent and the blood vessels are clearly visible. Active movements are present; the fetus stretches and exercises its arms and legs. The fetus begins making sucking motions, swallowing amniotic fluid, and producing meconium in the intestinal tract. Bronchial tubes are branching out in the primitive lungs, and sweat glands are developing. Fetal heart tones may be heard for the first time with a doppler device. The liver and pancreas begin to function. By the beginning of week 16, skeletal ossification is clearly identifiable. Muscle tissue and the body skeleton are developed, resulting in the fetus being straighter in body position.

17 to 19 Weeks

This is a period of somewhat slower growth, but the fetus becomes more active. The mother may feel fetal movements. Rapid brain growth occurs during this time, and myelination of the spinal cord is initiated. The fetal heart tones may be heard through a stethoscope. The fetus actively sucks and swallows amniotic fluid. The kidneys continue to secret urine into the amniotic fluid.

20 to 23 Weeks

The fetus now measures about 8 inches (19 cm). Fetal weight is between 15.2 to 16.3 ounces (435 and 465 g).

The head is covered with fine hair, and the eyebrows and eyelashes are beginning to form. Lanugo covers the entire body and is especially prominent on the shoulders. Subcutaneous deposits of brown fat, which has a rich blood supply, makes the skin less transparent. Nipples appear over the mammary glands. The fetus has nails on both fingers and toes. The fetus begins to produce antibodies, and passive antibody transfer between the mother and fetus is established. **Meconium** is present in the upper intestines. Muscles are well-developed, and the fetus is active. Fetal movement is now strong enough to be felt by the mother.

24 Weeks

The fetus at 24 weeks reaches a length of 11 inches (28 cm) and weighs about 1 lb, 10 oz (780 g). The hair on the head is longer, and the eyebrows and eyelashes are formed. The eye is structurally complete and soon opens. The alveoli of the lungs are just beginning to form, and surfactant is present. The fetus has a reflex handgrip and, by the end of 6 months, a startle reflex. Skin covering the body is reddish and wrinkled, with little subcutaneous fat. Skin on the hands and feet has thickened, with skin ridges on the palms and soles, forming distinct footprints and fingerprints. The skin over the entire body is covered with a protective cheese-like, fatty substance secreted by the sebaceous glands, called vernix caseosa. Meconium is present in the rectum.

25 to 28 Weeks

At 6 months, the fetal skin is red, wrinkled, and covered with vernix caseosa. The fetus at 28 weeks is about 14 to 15 inches long (35 to 38 cm) and weighs 2 lb, 10 oz to 2 lb, 12 oz (1200 to 1250 g). During this time, the brain is developing rapidly, and the CNS is complete enough to provide some degree of regulation of body functions. The eyelids open and close under neural control. The alveoli of the lungs mature, and surfactant is present in the amniotic fluid. Even though the lungs are still physiologically immature, they are sufficiently developed to provide gas exchange. A fetus born at this time requires immediate and prolonged intensive care to survive. If the fetus is a male, the testes begin to descend into the scrotal sac.

29 to 32 Weeks

The fetus is gaining weight from an increase in body muscle and fat and weighs about 4 lb, 6 oz (2000 g) with a length of about 15 to 17 inches (38 to 43 cm). The CNS has matured enough to direct rhythmic breathing movements and has partial control of body temperature. At 30 weeks, the pupillary light reflex is present. The fetus responds to sounds outside of the mother's body. The fetus begins storing iron, calcium, and phosphorus. Bones are now

Research Highlight

Fetal Hemodynamic Changes

Purpose

To assess the relationship between the pressure pulses and flow velocity in the fetal descending aorta in fetuses with intrauterine growth retardation compared with fetuses with normal growth development.

Method

A serial study done between the 21st and 40th weeks of gestation was conducted on 22 pregnant women who had normal fetal growth, 25 pregnant women with fetuses who were small for gestational age (SGA), and six women with fetuses that were large for gestational age (LGA). Echocardiographic tracking was used to measure resistance and changes in fetal blood pressure.

Findings

Normal fetal growth was associated with an increase in systolic and diastolic diameters in the fetal descending aorta and advancing gestational age. SGA fetuses also had the similar pattern; however, there was a definite increase in both the systolic and diastolic pressures with increasing fetal weight.

Nursing Implications

It may be possible to measure the pressure pulse in relationship to velocity, thus identifying potential circulatory abnormalities. Ultrasound technology can be used to measure fetal blood circulation and systolic and diastolic pressure and velocity. This may help in identifying fetuses who are at risk.

Mori, A., Iwabuchi, M., & Makino, T. (2000). Fetal haemodynamic changes during fetal development evaluated by arterial pressure, pulse, and blood flow velocity. *British Journal of Obstetrics and Gynecology, 107*, (5), 669–677.

fully developed but are soft and flexible. In males, the testicles may be located in the scrotal sac but are often still high in the inguinal canal.

33 to 36 Weeks

The fetus is less wrinkled because of increasing deposits of subcutaneous fat. At 36 weeks, the fetal weight is usually 5 lb, 12 oz to 6 lb, 11.5 oz (2500 to 2750 g), and the crown-heel length of the fetus is about 16 to 19 inches (42 to 48 cm). Lanugo is beginning to disappear, and the nails reach the edge of the fingertips. By 35 weeks, the fetus has a firm grasp and exhibits spontaneous orientation to light. An infant born at this time has a good chance of surviving but may require some special care.

38 to 40 Weeks

The fetus is considered full-term at 38 weeks after conception. The length can vary from 19 to 21 inches (48 to 52 cm). The weight at term is approximately 6 lb, 10 oz to 7 lb, 15 oz (3000 to 3600 g) (Figure 20-7). The skin is pinkish immediately after birth. African American infants' skin color darkens within 1 to 2 hours after birth. There is a small amount of lanugo left on the upper arms and shoulders. Vernix caseosa is present, with heavier deposits remaining in creases and folds of the skin. The body and extremities are plump, with good skin turgor, and the fingernails extend beyond the fingertips. The chest is prominent but still a little smaller than the head, and mammary glands protrude in both genders. As the fetus enlarges, amniotic fluid diminishes to about 500 ml or less, and the fetal body mass fills the uterine cavity. The fetus assumes what is referred to as its position of comfort. The head is generally pointed downward, following the shape of the uterus (and also possibly because the head is heavier than the feet). The extremities and often the head are flexed. After 5 months, feeding patterns, sleeping patterns, and activity patterns became established, so the fetus at term has its own body rhythms and individual style of response. The testes are in the scrotum or are palpable in the inguinal canals.

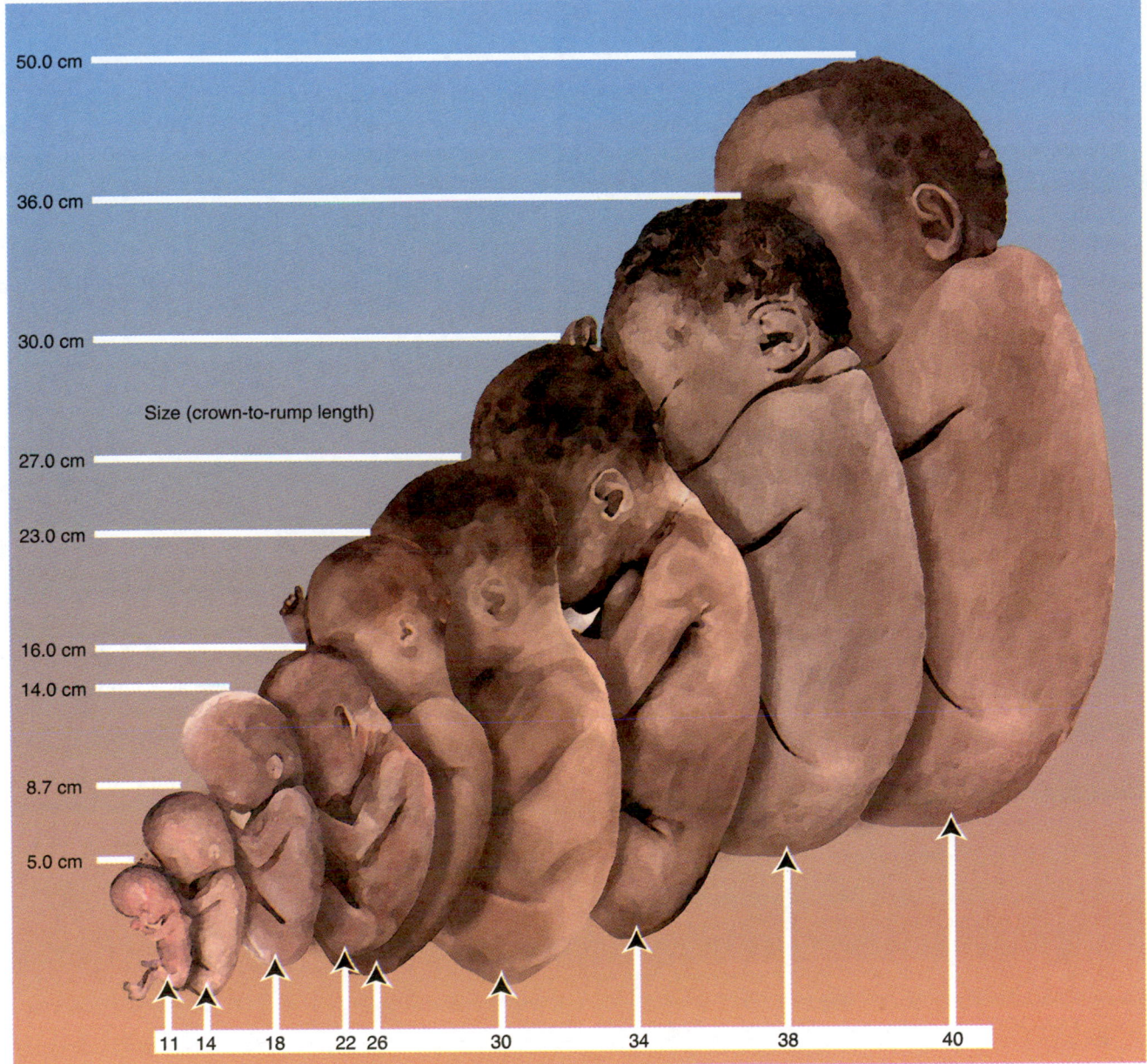

50.0 cm
36.0 cm
30.0 cm
Size (crown-to-rump length)
27.0 cm
23.0 cm
16.0 cm
14.0 cm
8.7 cm
5.0 cm

11 14   18   22 26   30   34   38   40

Gestational age in weeks

Figure 20-7 Fetal size by gestational age.

Web Activities

- Visit the March of Dimes website to review fetal growth and development: http://www.noah.cuny.edu/pregnancy/march-of-dimes/pre-preg.plan/babygrow.html

- Identify two ways that you could incorporate the information provided at this site into your nursing care plan for mothers who are in the first trimester, second trimester, and third trimester.

- Identify two websites that can provide information on maintaining a healthy lifestyle during pregnancy. Evaluate the sites for their reliability and the scientific accuracy of data. Do the sites provide additional resources for individuals seeking more information?

Key Concepts

- Fertilization occurs in the uterine tube within 24 hours after ovulation, and implantation occurs approximately 6 days after fertilization.

- Organ systems and external features develop during the embryonic period (between third to eighth week after fertilization). The embryo is now most vulnerable to teratogenic exposure.

- Refinement of organ structures and function occurs from 10th week to the time of birth.

- The placenta carries out two major functions: transport and exchange of products between the fetus and the mother and hormone production.

- Fetal circulation is supported by the umbilical cord, ductus venosus, placenta, foramen ovale, and ductus arteriosus, and it is dependent on maternal placental circulation.

- Fetal development proceeds cephalocaudal and proximal to distal.

- Fetal development proceeds from generalization to differentiation.

Review Questions and Activities

1. When does implantation occur?

2. How is the embryo nourished before the placenta develops? After the placenta is developed?

3. When is the embryo susceptible to damage from teratogens?

4. What is the difference between the time of fertilization and implantation? Which time is used in calculating gestational age?

5. How does fetal development progress? Describe the sequence.

6. What is the function of amniotic fluid?

7. Attend an antepartal testing clinic: interview personnel that conduct antepartal testing and identify the preparation, purpose, process, and risks for each test. Ascertain what follow-up is routinely done for clients with abnormal test results.

8. Find a research article on fetal development and determine how the study results can be applied to your nursing practice.

9. View the film "Miracle of Life," produced by WGBH for "NOVA."

References

Moore, K. I., & Persaud, T. V. (1998). *Before we are born: Essentials of embryology and birth defects,* (5th ed.). Philadelphia: W. B. Saunders.

Mori, A., Iwabuchi, M., & Makino, T. (2000). Fetal haemodynamic changes in fetuses during fetal development evaluated by arterial pressure pulse and blood flow velocity. *British Journal of Obstetrics and Gynecology, 107,* (5), 669–677.

Suggested Readings

American College of Obstetricians and Gynecologists (ACOG). (1996). *Nutrition in women.* (ACOG Educational Bulletin No. 229). Washington, DC: Author.

Carlson, B. M. (1999). *Human Embryology and Developmental Biology.* 2nd Ed. St. Louis, MO: Mosby.

England, M. A. (1996). *Life before birth,* (2nd ed.). London: Mosby-Wolfe.

Kellogg, B. (2000). Fetal development. In Mattson, S., & Smith, J., eds. *Core curriculum for maternal-newborn nursing,* (2nd ed.). Philadelphia: Saunders.

Kellogg, B. (2000). Placental development and functioning. In Mattson, S., & Smith, J., eds. *Core curriculum for maternal-newborn nursing,* (2nd ed.). Philadelphia: Saunders.

Larsen, D. J. (1997). *Human Embryology.* 2nd Ed. New York: Churchill-Livingstone.

Lavery, J. P. (1987). *The human placenta: Clinical perspectives.* Rockville, MD: Aspen.

Spears, G. (1999). Ultrasound in obstetric triage. *Journal of Nurse-Midwifery, 44,* (5), 480–492.

Resources

March of Dimes: www.noah.cuny.edu/pregnancy/march_of_dimes/"Miracle of Life" NOVA film produced by PBS (WGBH in Boston) available from PBS or in some video stores.

The National Center for Human Genome Research: www.nchgr.nih.gov

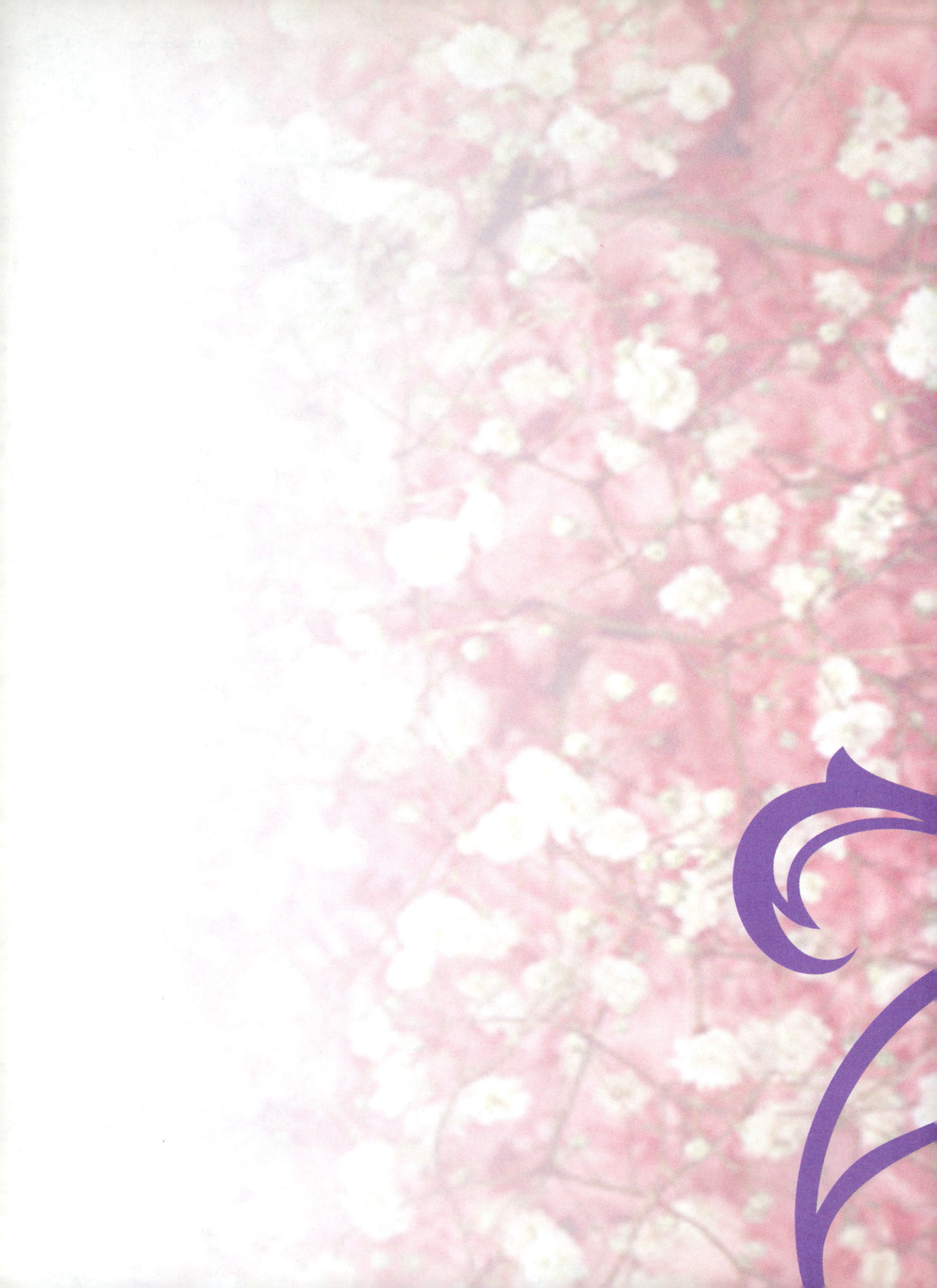

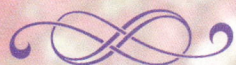

CHAPTER 21

Environmental Risks Affecting Fetal Well-Being

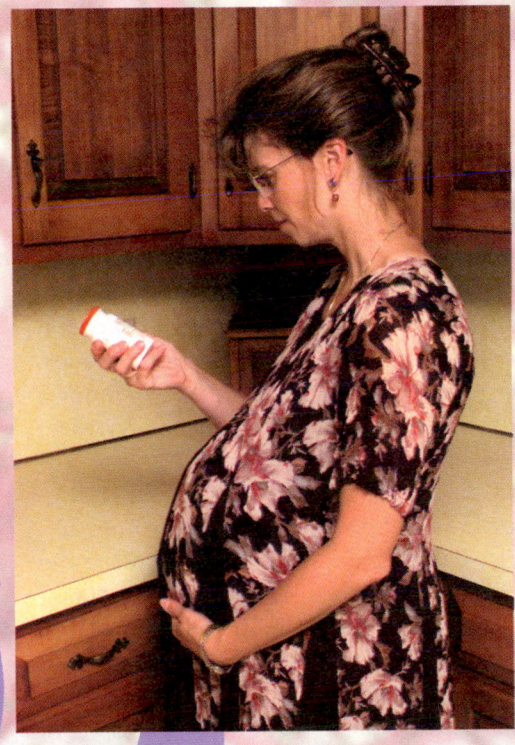

Sometimes it is difficult to determine how much choice a woman has regarding her environment and lifestyle. Consider these questions as you reflect on your own feelings about reducing risks in pregnancy:

- *Have I ever tried to break an unhealthy habit, such as smoking or overeating? How difficult was it?*

- *Do I feel angry or disgusted when I hear about pregnant women using illegal drugs that may harm their fetuses? What would it be like for me to provide nursing care for a pregnant woman who uses drugs?*

- *How do I feel about making home visits to pregnant women in neighborhoods where violence occurs or where tuberculosis has been reported?*

- *If I were pregnant and my job increased my risk of miscarriage, would I stop working even if I were the only wage earner in my family?*

- *Is my home neighborhood at risk for a nuclear or chemical accident? How could I find out whether the soil or air has dangerous pollutants?*

Key Terms

Agonists
Chorioretinitis
Fetal alcohol
   syndrome
Heavy metal

Hemolytic disease of
   the newborn
Herbicide
Hyperthermia
Ionizing radiation

Neonatal abstinence
   syndrome
PCBs and PBBs
Pesticide

Solvent
Sympathomimetic
Teratogen
TORCH

Competencies

Upon completion of this chapter, the reader should be able to:

1. Describe contaminants found in air, water, food, and soil that may increase the risks to pregnant women.

2. Discuss threats to fetal well-being found in some workplaces and job requirements.

3. Explain how stress and strain may increase the risks to pregnant women.

4. Teach the client which food products and common medications to avoid during pregnancy.

5. Identify several types of resources that may assist a woman who has a chemical dependency to change her behavior.

Early physicians and scientists believed that the mother's body protected her fetus from harm and that the womb was a peaceful and safe setting for new life to begin. They believed that the mother's skeleton and integumentary system shielded the fetus from injuries. The placenta was considered a filter that would remove any dangerous substance before it diffused into the fetal bloodstream.

Although most pregnancies proceed normally and result in healthy newborns, we now know that some substances and events in the environment can increase the risk of death or injury to the developing fetus. Many chemicals diffuse readily from the maternal bloodstream into that of the fetus. Radiation and heat reach fetal tissue and can affect fetal development. Violent injury to a mother also may injure her fetus. Fetal growth and development are intimately affected by the mother's geographic location; chemical exposures; stresses at work and at home; use of medications and other substances, some of which are illegal; and infections, some of which may have been acquired by risky behavior.

Approximately 3% to 5% of newborns have some form of congenital anomaly. More than half of congenital malformations have an unknown cause. Genetic defects and inherited tendencies brought on by environmental risks taken together explain about a third of all defects.

The role of the registered nurse in caring for pregnant women is to:

- Assess clients for environmental and behavioral risks.
- Design individualized plans of care that support women in reducing risks in their lifestyles.
- Intervene using teaching, support, observations, and referrals to minimize environmental risks in pregnancy.
- Provide ongoing evaluation of maternal and fetal well-being so that care can be tailored to each client's changing needs.

This chapter begins by examining the larger picture of how regional geography and political environments can create risks for pregnant women. The focus then narrows to the workplace environment, centering on how a woman's job, which may be a means of economic survival, can increase risks to fetal survival. Last, home environment, personal lifestyle, and behavior are considered to determine how these factors can be modified through nursing interventions to reduce fetal risk.

RISKS RELATED TO GEOGRAPHIC LOCATION

A woman may be at risk for a poor pregnancy outcome simply as a result of the geographic location of her home or neighborhood. Conditions and substances in a woman's environment affect her health and that of her fetus. Many women may be unaware of the risks faced from the environment. Nurses can identify women whose surroundings hold threats to well-being and intervene to promote safety during pregnancy.

Nuclear and Chemical Accidents

Residents in modern nations of the Western hemisphere are exposed daily to small amounts of **ionizing radiation** (energy in wave or particle form, such as X-rays) that is capable of releasing ions from irradiated tissue. Background radiation in the atmosphere has no measurable effect on health. In catastrophic industrial or warfare-related accidents, however, pregnant women can be exposed to large amounts of chemicals or radiation. Fortunately, these events are rare.

The fetal central nervous system (CNS) is vulnerable to high-dose radiation, particularly between 7 and 15 weeks' gestation when neurons are developing rapidly and the cerebral cortex is being formed. In the 1920s it was noted that women who received radiation to the pelvic area as part of medical treatment and later were found to be pregnant had increased risks of delivering newborns with microcephaly and CNS disturbances. Infants born to Japanese mothers in Hiroshima and Nagasaki after the atomic bombings of 1945 also had increased rates of microcephaly and mental retardation, with the risk of retardation increasing with the dose of radiation to which mothers were exposed. Children exposed to radiation also experienced retardation of growth and mental development after birth (Persaud, 1990).

In the late 1980s, a catastrophic nuclear power plant accident in Chernobyl, in the former Soviet Union, released large amounts of radioactive cesium, resulting in an unusually high incidence of neural tube defects and other malformations in infants born in the months after the accident (Persaud, 1990). Women living in the wider region surrounding the area of the accident also experienced greater than normal risks of spontaneous abortions and fetal growth retardation (Muratova et al., 1994).

Industrial chemicals also pose a danger to developing fetuses when released into the environment in large quantities. In 1984, at Bhopal, India, nearly 40 metric tons of methylisocyanate were released from a U.S.-owned pesticide plant. Among many other serious health consequences to residents was a spontaneous abortion rate in women in the region nearly four times above normal; perinatal and neonatal mortality rates also were higher, although the rate of birth defects did not increase (Bajaj, Misra, Rajalakshmi, & Madan, 1993).

Another chemical once produced for agricultural use in treating seed to prevent the growth of fungi is methyl-

mercury. In Iraq, in 1971 and 1972, the government distributed treated seed to farmers for planting the next spring. A severe drought had limited that year's harvest, however, and many families used the grain to bake bread. They soon showed signs of mercury poisoning, including paresthesias and other CNS disturbances. Close to 5,000 people died. Mothers who survived delivered children with severe CNS damage, including cerebral palsy and reduced brain growth.

Mercury played a role in another environmental disaster, in Minamata Bay off the coast of Japan in the early 1950s. An inorganic form of mercury used in chemical production had been released into the ocean, where microorganisms converted it to the deadly methylmercury. Fish became heavily contaminated. Japanese who ate these fish experienced the same health problems and fetal CNS damage as did the Iraqi victims of mercury poisoning. Since these two disasters, use of mercury in industry and agriculture has been more carefully controlled.

Pesticides

Pesticides are chemicals designed to kill insects, rodents, or other unwanted lower life forms harmful to crops or human habitation. **Herbicides**, chemicals designed to kill unwanted plant life, such as weeds, are often classified as pesticides. Humans are exposed to these chemicals through contact with contaminated air, soil, and water, and through consumption of foods treated during planting and cultivation. Humans also may eat fish or livestock that have ingested the chemicals from contaminated environments. Pesticides and herbicides are widely used not only in the agricultural industry but in homes, lawns, and gardens to destroy insects and weeds.

Over fifty pesticides have been identified as **teratogens**, substances that in doses of one thousand times or less the usual human exposure have been found to interfere with the formation or normal development of the human fetus. Some of the more commonly known harmful pesticides include Captan, copper sulfate, dichlorodiphenyltrichloroethane (DDT), and diethylmetatoluamide, the active ingredient in OFF. Herbicides include 2,4,5-trichlorophenoxyacetic acid (2,4,5-T), used until 1970 along roadsides to control weeds; Agent Orange, used by U.S. military forces to destroy crops and remove leaves from trees in the Vietnam conflict; and dioxin, not an herbicide in itself but a long-lasting byproduct of the manufacture of other herbicides. Pesticides and herbicides appear to increase the risks of spontaneous abortion and fetal death and also can result in more subtle malformations, such as cleft lip or extra fingers (Needleman & Bellinger, 1994).

One group of women at particular risk of pesticide exposure during pregnancy is migrant workers and female members of agricultural laborer families. By living near fields, vineyards, or orchards where pesticides are used, women may absorb high doses over time. The chemicals can accumulate in the liver and other body tissues, including fetal tissue. Women who are malnourished may face even greater maternal and fetal risks, if the maternal or fetal liver is not functioning well enough to detoxify the chemicals in the bloodstream (Needleman & Bellinger, 1994).

Another group of women at risk are those whose partners work with these dangerous chemicals. Either through the effects of the chemicals on male gametes or exposure of pregnant women to substances on their partner's clothing, paternal pesticide and herbicide exposure has been linked to spontaneous abortion and birth defects (Sever, Arbuckle, & Sweeney, 1997).

Although many dangerous pesticides have been banned by industrialized nations, risks still exist for women in agricultural regions of developing countries. As new pesticides are invented, their risks may emerge over time. All new products used in the United States must be tested for safety and approved by the Environmental Protection Agency. The human effects of chemicals are difficult to isolate because many substances are present in the environment, including residues from harmful products used in past years. Most products are tested on animals before being approved for human use; however, the effects on animal fetuses may be different from those on human fetuses. Testing must be adequate to ensure that these compounds are safe for human exposure. Nurses can advocate for complete safety testing of these products before they are released for public use.

Industrial Contaminants

Factories, machines, furnaces, and automobiles are among the many sources of pollution of soil, water, and air. Waste products or accidental spills of harmful products into the environment are a major complication of industrialization. Some of the effects of these products on human reproduction have been studied. Other substances have been studied only in animals.

Heavy Metals

Heavy metals, chemical substances such as lead or mercury, are byproducts of industry that may be found in the environment. Methylmercury, already discussed as a hazard when released accidentally, can be present in low levels in lakes. These low levels of mercury in lake water can accumulate in the tissues of fish. In some areas of the Great Lakes, the Adirondacks, Canada, and Florida, fish flesh has been found to contain 3 ppm of mercury, whereas 1 ppm is considered the level at which safety concerns should be raised. Women may consume large amounts of these fish throughout pregnancy. In two studies, one of Cree Indians in northern Quebec and the other in New Zealand, the hair of mothers who consumed fish in large amounts during pregnancy showed evidence of mercury exposure. Their children were more likely than were other children to show delayed motor development or abnormal muscle tone and reflexes (Needleman & Bellinger, 1994).

Lead has been known to cause reproductive problems since the early twentieth century. Lead exposure can occur as a result of water or air pollution; from exhausts of cars using leaded gasoline; and in workplace exposure in industries such as smelting, battery and paint manufacturing, and typesetting. Exposures to high levels of lead during pregnancy can cause miscarriage, fetal demise, and prematurity and can lead to later developmental and growth delays in children (Needleman & Bellinger, 1994). Women whose male partners are exposed to lead also face increased risks of fetal malformations (Sever, 1994). Arsenic, lead, and mercury in mothers' drinking water have been linked to increased risks of cardiac defects and other adverse outcomes in newborns (Aschengrau, Zierler, & Cohen, 1993).

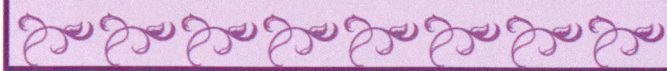

Critical Thinking

Activism to Reduce Harmful Substances in the Environment

Nurses have been active in advocating for public health since the profession was first recognized. Continuing in that tradition, the American Nurses Association (1996) issued a position statement on lead poisoning and screening in 1994. The Association stated its support of:

- Screening and intervention for lead poisoning in children.
- Efforts to make lead poisoning a reportable disease.
- Community outreach and funding to identify and clean up high-risk residences and neighborhoods.
- Legislation restricting the amount of lead in manufactured products.

Are you aware of activism taking place in the community of your home or college?

Are nurses among those in your state who are calling for a safer environment?

Polychlorinated and Polybromated Biphenyls

Polychlorinated biphenyls **(PCBs)** and polybromated biphenyls **(PBBs)**, chemicals now banned but once produced in industry, are halogenated aromatic hydrocarbons used in the production of flame retardants, coolants, and sealants. These chemicals are highly stable and thus last for long periods of time in the environment and the human body. Exposure to PCBs and PBBs in pregnancy is hazardous, causing spontaneous abortion, growth deficits, and other fetal problems. In addition, there is some evidence that abnormal genetic syndromes may result from the father's exposure to vinyl chloride (Colie, 1993).

Although manufacture has been banned in the United States since 1979, these compounds still contaminate air, soil, water, and foods in some regions, including fish from the Great Lakes. These chemicals are present in electrical equipment manufactured before the 1979 ban and in landfills (Needleman & Bellinger, 1994). PCBs and PBBs are extremely fat-soluble, which results in concentrations in fatty tissue and breast milk of up to one hundred times those of maternal serum levels. In one incident in Japan, mothers who consumed PCB-contaminated cooking oil delivered infants with dark-pigmented skin, gum hyperplasia, and low birth weights (Office of Technology Assessment, 1985). Breast-fed infants whose mothers were exposed to PCBs and infants whose cord blood showed PCB exposure during pregnancy had lower cognitive performance and increased risk of developing attention and learning difficulties later in childhood (Needleman & Bellinger, 1994).

Solvents

Solvents, organic compounds widely used in industry to clean and manufacture mechanical or electronic components, are hazardous to fetal well-being. Solvents are found in dry-cleaning products, spray adhesives, paints, nail polish removers, felt-tipped pens, and many other products. Solvents may be used as mind-altering drugs by inhaling the agent. Either maternal or paternal exposure to toluene in the workplace has been associated with cardiovascular malformations (Sever, 1994), and paternal exposure to toluene has been linked to increased rates of miscarriage and anencephaly (Colie, 1993).

Carbon Monoxide

Carbon monoxide is a colorless, odorless, and extremely toxic gas. It is produced when burning occurs, including in internal combustion engines. The fetus may be exposed when a pregnant woman is exposed to automobile or furnace exhaust, or to cigarette smoke. Studies in animals have shown that maternal carbon monoxide exposure has

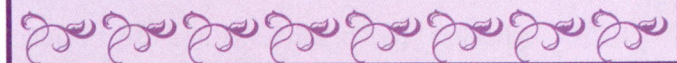

Critical Thinking

Environmental Racism?

Since the 1980s, Americans have been concerned that polluting industrial plants, toxic waste dumps, sewage discharge areas, and incinerators have been situated in communities whose residents are least able to speak out against these dangers—in low-income urban and rural areas populated by people of color and immigrants, and on Native American lands (Bullard, 1994; Szasz, 1994). In 1991, the First People of Color Environmental Summit gathered and put forth principles of environmental justice, and in 1994 then-President Clinton formed an Interagency Working Group charged with identifying and addressing disproportionately adverse human health or environmental effects of policies and programs on minority and low-income populations.

Can you identify areas of high pollution or environmental risks in your community that are located in low-income, minority-populated areas?

Is there any community resistance to the dangers?

Does the need for jobs and tax revenue from these industries outweigh the harms to the environment and human health?

What can nurses do to help educate people about the health effects of environmental hazards?

led to fetal death, neurologic abnormalities, and low birth weights (Needleman & Bellinger, 1994). The effects of cigarette smoke are discussed later in this chapter.

Rural or Urban Residence

Living in a rural or urban area may increase a woman's risks of pregnancy and birth complications. Women living in isolated rural areas may be hindered by distance or terrain from obtaining prenatal care or seeking help for problems that develop during pregnancy. These women also may have limited education and have received little assistance in improving hygiene and preventing disease. In contrast, urban living has its own unique stresses and dangers that create different types of pregnancy risks. Women living in urban areas who have low incomes are especially vulnerable to the harmful effects of poor living conditions, poor nutrition, and lack of health care.

Obstetrical care by family doctors and general practitioners in some rural areas is declining. For example, in

Mississippi, a 1993 survey revealed that although the number of obstetricians had remained steady over 8 years, a significant proportion of general and family practitioners either had stopped providing pregnancy care or were planning to stop. Doctors cited costs of malpractice insurance, concerns about litigation, and lack of time as reasons for terminating prenatal care services (Copeland et al., 1993). In many rural areas, women must travel long distances to obtain preventive care, including prenatal care and well-baby care.

Living in a rural area, however, does not always lead to poor pregnancy and birth outcomes. For example, although women in rural areas of Wisconsin were found to receive less prenatal care overall than did women in urban areas of the state, the urbanites with inadequate prenatal care were most likely to deliver low-birth-weight infants (Hueston, 1995). This study suggests that other problems in the urban environment had an especially harmful influence on these women.

Nurse researchers have determined that health behaviors and demographic risk factors such as low income and limited education were more important in predicting low birth weight than was urban or rural residence. Rural women were more likely than were urban women to be single, poorly educated, and of African American descent. They had lower incomes, lower pregnancy weight gain, and poorer nutrition than did the urban group. However, urban women were more likely to smoke and use illicit drugs. These factors rather than location alone created the risk of low birth weight (Alexy, Nichols, Heverly, & Garzon, 1997).

Health behaviors and health care use can be influenced by nurses who design and run outreach services and innovative health care agencies serving both urban and rural women. When nurses and others have developed comprehensive outreach programs to underserved rural areas, birth outcomes have improved (Boettcher, 1993; Carcillo et al., 1995). One well-known example of a nursing effort to bring safe maternity care to a very remote area is the Frontier Nursing Service, founded by Mary Breckinridge in Kentucky in 1925 (Figure 21-1). Nurse-midwives lived in remote mountain areas and provided comprehensive public health care to whole districts of poor families. Not only birth outcomes but the health of whole families was improved by this important service, which continues today (Frontier Nursing Service, 1997).

Warfare and Political Violence

Living in a frightening environment under threat of injury or death creates extreme risks for pregnant women. Both the injuries pregnant women have suffered as bystanders

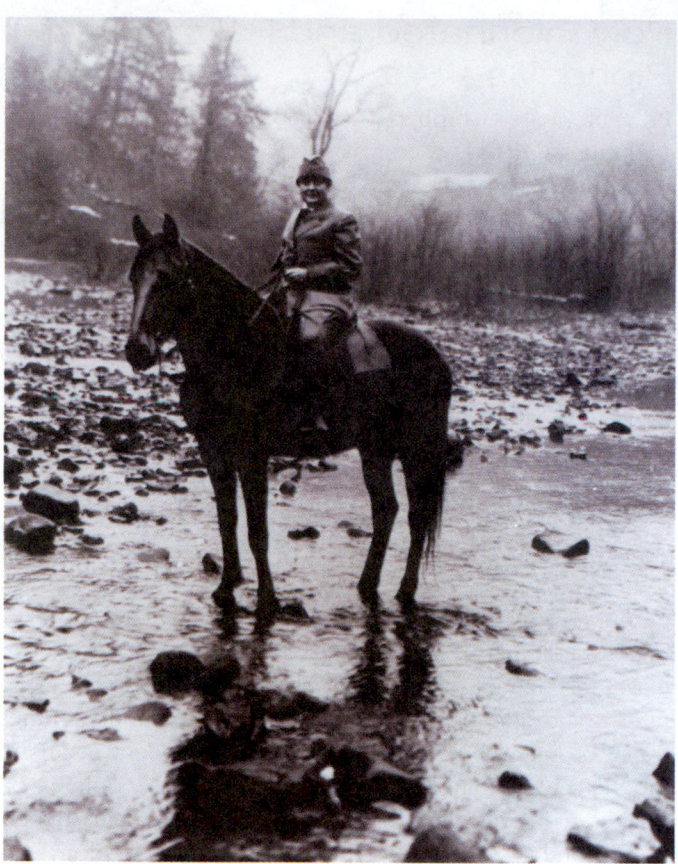

Figure 21-1 Under the leadership of Mary Breckenridge, nurse-midwives of the Frontier Nursing Service have reduced the risks of geographic isolation and poverty for rural Kentucky families. (Courtesy of Frontier Nursing Service, Hyden, KY)

in armed conflicts and the deprivation and the extreme stress they have endured during war have been found to harm fetal development.

During World War II, women in Norway, the Netherlands, and other regions experiencing extreme food shortages and harsh conditions, along with women who received inadequate food in the third trimester of pregnancy, were at high risk for fetal growth retardation. Moreover, their daughters' pregnancies are now showing the long-term effects of malnutrition. Women who themselves were exposed to famine during the first and second trimesters of their mothers' pregnancies, although their own birth weights were normal, are more likely to deliver low-birth-weight and preterm infants (Lumey, Stein, & Ravelli, 1995).

The stress of living in a war zone affects prenatal health and newborn outcomes of otherwise healthy and well-nourished women. Maternal blood pressure was found to be increased by war stress during the Israeli Yom Kippur war, especially in young women whose husbands may have been serving in the front lines (Rofe & Goldberg, 1983). During civil war in Chile, women who lived in neighborhoods with high rates of bomb threats, political demonstrations, military presence, and undercover surveillance were significantly more likely than were women from neighborhoods with low violence to experience pregnancy complications (Zapata et al., 1992).

In war-torn regions of Croatia, a slight overall increase in prematurity was seen. The greatest risk, however, was suffered by women who were expatriated or exiled from their native regions as a result of the conflict. Women refugees were twice as likely to deliver prematurely, probably due to fear, deprivation, and loss of prenatal services (Kuvacic et al., 1996). In babies born in a Sarajevo hospital during that war, perinatal mortality increased from 15.8 deaths per 1,000 to 36 per 1,000, and the rate of malformations increased from 0.4% before the war to 3.0% during the war (Simic et al., 1995).

The Persian Gulf conflict in 1990 and 1991 also revealed risks to pregnant women. In Kuwait, significant increases in the rates of spontaneous abortions, low birth weights, and major anomalies were observed in 1991 and 1992, and stillbirth and perinatal mortality increased in 1991 (Makhseed et al., 1996). In the neighboring country of Israel, which suffered Iraqi missile attacks during the Gulf War, transient fetal bradycardia was associated with air-raid sirens (Yoles et al., 1993). However, birth outcomes were not affected (Schenker & Mor-Yosef, 1993).

Effects on newborns of their fathers' exposures to chemicals during military activities has been a concern (Figure 21-2); however, no definite harmful effects have been observed. Men exposed to Agent Orange and dioxin during the Vietnam war had changes in sperm formation (Colie, 1993) but they could not be definitely linked to increased risks of delivering newborns with malformations or illnesses. However, these chemicals have been shown to cause reproductive problems in animals (Wolfe et al., 1995).

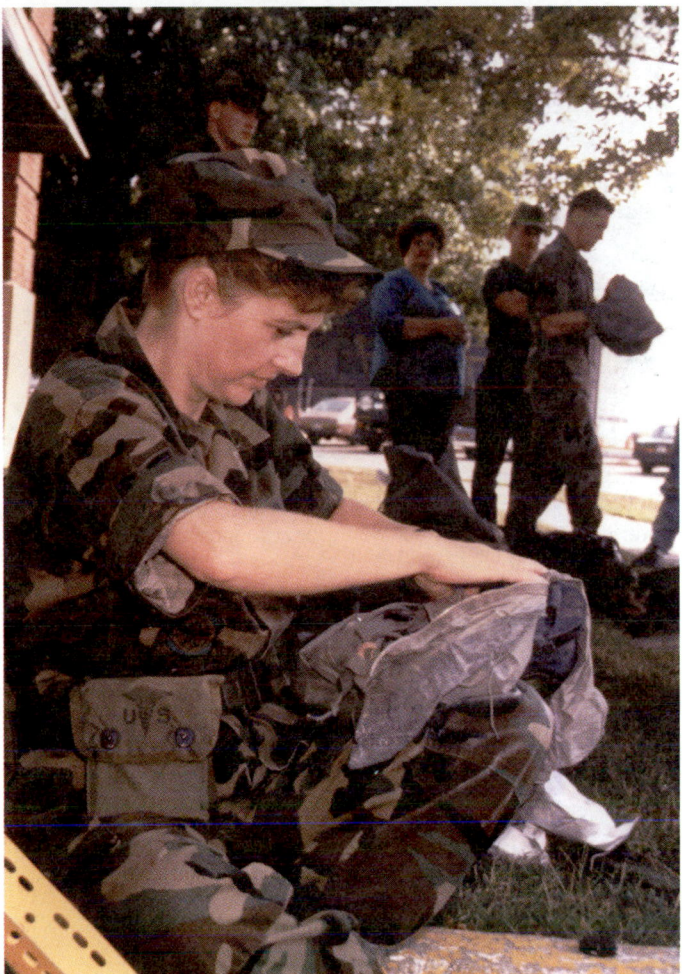

Figure 21-2 Exposure of either the male or female parent to harmful chemicals during war can increase pregnancy complications. This Persian Gulf War soldier is packing her gas mask before being deployed to Saudi Arabia for Operation Desert Storm. (Courtesy of Defense Visual Information Center)

RISKS RELATED TO EMPLOYMENT

Most pregnant women are employed outside the home. Work itself does not appear to increase pregnancy risks; in fact, in one California county, employed African American women at all income levels were less likely than were unemployed African American women to deliver low-birth-weight infants (Poerksen & Petitti, 1991). Work may increase women's access to health care, sense of well-being, physical fitness, and financial autonomy and may have other healthy effects. However, work also may bring women into contact with harmful substances and physical dangers. Unfortunately, very few of the thousands of chemicals and other risks in modern workplaces have been studied for their effects during pregnancy. Predictions of possible risks often are based on assumed exposures, anecdotal evidence, and animal studies.

Heat and Radiation

Work environments that include the presence of ovens or furnaces and outdoor work in hot climates expose the pregnant woman to excessive heat. As yet, no definite evidence exists of pregnancy harm specifically caused by exposure to heat, or cold, in the workplace (Gold & Tomich, 1994).

Radiation in the workplace comes from a variety of sources. Ionizing radiation is used in diagnostic and therapeutic x-rays studies. Radiation is also used during chemical processing, food and chemical preservation, and sterilization. Because some of these industrial processes are relatively new, the hazards to developing fetuses of women workers are not yet fully understood.

Diagnostic x-ray procedures are considered safe by some scientists when they involve less than 0.05 Gy of radiation; however, complete avoidance of X-ray exposure during the first 15 weeks of pregnancy is recommended.

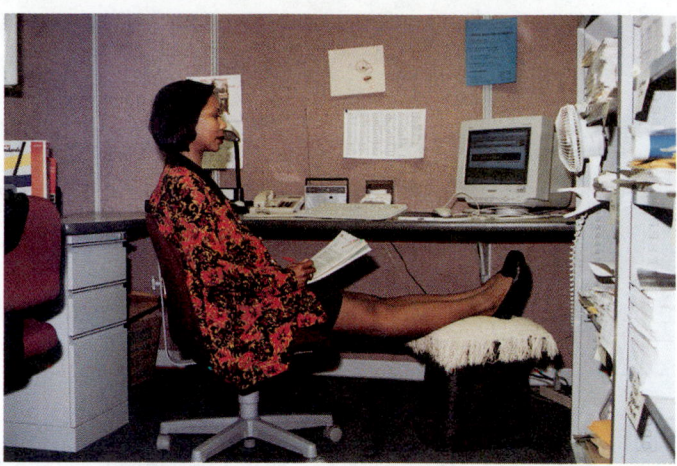

Figure 21-3 Despite early concerns, radiation from computer monitor screens does not appear to increase the risk of pregnancy complications.

Exposure to greater than 0.2 Gy of radiation during pregnancy is known to cause birth defects, and lower-level exposures of 0.01 to 0.10 Gy have been linked to leukemia and mental retardation in children. Employers have been advised by federal agencies that exposure during any potential pregnancy should be limited to no more than 0.005 Gy (Office of Technology Assessment, 1985). Radiology workers in health care agencies and nurses working in areas where x-rays are frequently used should wear meters to detect cumulative radiation exposure.

Video display terminals, or computer monitor screens, are a potential source of exposure to low-level electromagnetic radiation for many employed women (Figure 21-3). Some clusters of spontaneous abortions and birth defects were reported in women computer workers in the early years of computerization; however, many subsequent studies using careful measurements and controls have shown no increase in the risk to pregnancy (Gold & Tomich, 1994).

Chemical Exposure

Heavy metals, solvents, pesticides, and other harmful chemicals are present in the workplaces where these products are manufactured or used in producing other products. Many chemicals are so new that their effects on pregnancy are not fully understood, although animal evidence is used to estimate human risks in pregnancy. In the United States, each workplace is required by law to maintain Material Safety Data Sheets (MSDS) listing all chemical substances to which workers may be exposed, their components, any toxic effect, and protective measures being taken; each workplace also must have in place a Hazard Communication Program that educates workers about these substances (Stanhope & Lancaster, 1996).

As described earlier, exposure to metals such as lead and mercury is hazardous in pregnancy, and these metals are present in some manufacturing plants. Other substances with potential risks include arsenic, which is produced as a byproduct of copper and lead smelting and is present in ceramics, paints and dyes, wood preservatives, and rat poison. In addition, pesticides and chemicals that are hazardous to women working in agricultural jobs are equally hazardous to women who work where these substances are manufactured.

When analyzed by occupation, certain job categories appear to have increased reproductive risks. Pulp and paper workers, laboratory workers, textile workers, and agricultural workers have been found to be at some increased risk, as have women exposed to solvents in factory work. Solvents include toluene, which was noted earlier as a hazardous substance in the environment and in some home products such as glues. Exposure to toluene and other solvents in the workplace has been linked to increased risk of spontaneous abortion along with fetal oral, renal-urinary, and gastrointestinal (GI) defects (Gold & Tomich, 1994). Solvents are used in many modern industries, including microchip manufacturing. Women may also be exposed in industrial settings where metal parts are cleaned or painted. Solvents also are present in some anesthetic gases such as tricholoroethylene and ether.

Although it is difficult to measure women's exposures to these common chemicals, and not all studies have shown poor outcomes, animal studies have shown problems with development of the fetal nervous system. Infants of women exposed in workplaces (including operating rooms) and of women who used spray adhesives have had greater than normal incidences of fetal death and congenital defects. Nurses should advocate for extreme caution by employers using toluene and insist that manufacturers monitor worker exposure and minimize risks.

Anesthetic agents, including nitrous oxide, halothane, and cyclopropane, have been blamed for increased rates of spontaneous abortion and birth defects among operating room workers; however, the quantity of exposure is difficult to measure, and the effect is not consistent. Safety measures in the operating room that reduce leakage of gases and volatile liquids are important to minimize risks. Another area of risk in hospitals is where instruments are sterilized. Ethylene oxide is a gas used in sterilization as well as in the manufacture of antifreeze. This chemical is known to cause genetic mutations in laboratory experiments, and an increase in spontaneous abortion in sterilization workers has been found in several studies (Gold & Tomich, 1994).

Women who are employed in agriculture, spreading pesticides on crops or working in fields during crop-dusting, are at high risk. For example, in a study of infants born to over 34,000 licensed pesticide appliers in Min-

Critical Thinking

The Case of The Johnson Controls Company

The Johnson Controls Company manufactures lead-acid batteries. In 1982, the company adopted a policy to prevent exposure of pregnant women to lead. This policy barred all fertile women from jobs in which lead exposure was likely. One woman had a tubal ligation to keep her job; however, no fertile women, even those not planning to or likely to become pregnant, were permitted to continue to work. A male employee requested transfer out of the high-lead area to protect his ability to father a healthy child; however, his request was denied.

The U.S. Supreme Court ruled that The Johnson Controls Company policy constituted discrimination in employment based on sex, and that fetal protection, although a worthwhile goal, could not be pursued by discriminatory means. The Court stated that decisions about welfare of future children must be left to the parents, rather than to employers (Bertin, 1994). Women now have the choice to pursue an economic role even if it creates a threat to their reproductive role.

Do you think this decision solved the problem of employment risk?

Should companies protect all their workers from harmful chemicals, regardless of the possibility of pregnancy?

What is your role as a nurse in promoting healthy work policies in industry, and in educating workers?

---

cause significant fatigue. Strenuous activity also results in increased body temperature and thus creates concerns about **hyperthermia**, which is a dangerous elevation in body temperature resulting from fever or external heat sources.

For many women, and particularly for those in urban areas, getting to work involves long commutes on buses and trains, which also can be extremely tiring. Many women are not formally employed but still must engage in

Client Education

Reducing the Risks of Work in Pregnancy

Women who are employed outside the home during pregnancy or who have strenuous responsibilities within the home or family farm can reduce the risks of having infants with birth defects, and preterm infants, or low birth-weight infants by:

- Becoming aware of hazardous chemicals in the workplace and obtaining protective clothing or a work reassignment if exposure is unavoidable. At most companies, the Human Resources Department keeps a listing of hazardous substances information.

- Limiting heavy lifting and carrying at work and home after 20 weeks' gestation, including avoiding carrying children and heavy grocery bags up several flights of stairs. Request work reassignment and use family or home health aid assistance in the home.

- Reducing prolonged standing or sitting. A pregnant woman should take breaks in which she can change position, get up, and walk around if her job involves sitting, or rest with her feet up if her job involves standing. Women who stand at factory assembly lines or cash registers can request a high stool to sit on and a low stool to rest one foot on while standing. If this is not possible, work reassignment should be requested.

- Maintaining adequate food and fluid intake. Pregnant women should have access to drinking water in the workplace and should have at least one meal break and two snack breaks during an 8-hour shift.

---

nesota, the rate of birth defects between 1989 and 1992 was significantly greater than that in infants born to other Minnesota women during that time period. Circulatory, respiratory, urogenital, and musculoskeletal defects were increased, especially in regions where chlorphenoxy herbicides were used, and especially among fetuses conceived in the spring. Women living in these farming areas who were not employed as pesticide appliers also had a lesser but still increased risk of delivering infants with birth defects (Garry et al., 1996).

Fatigue and Physical Risks

Many jobs require women to stand for long periods, lift heavy objects, climb stairs, bend over for long periods (as in picking vegetables), and perform other physical exertion. Simply standing or sitting for an 8-hour workday can

Research Highlight

Reproductive Risks for Nurses

Purpose

To determine whether nurses face increased risks to their fetuses during pregnancy. The work environments of nurses may include hazards such as viruses, bacteria, anesthetic and sterilizing gases, antineoplastic drugs, and X-ray films.

Methods

Using data from 1968 to 1980, researchers in Atlanta, GA, analyzed the records of 4,915 babies born with congenital defects and 3,027 babies born without defects. The researchers compared the infants of nurses with infants whose parents had other occupations to determine whether having a nurse as a parent increased the likelihood of a defect.

Findings

Regardless of maternal age, education, and alcohol consumption, children whose mothers worked in nursing during early pregnancy were twice as likely as were those of nonnurses to be born with anencephaly, spina bifida, or coarctation of the aorta, and were more than three times as likely to have urinary system defects. There was no increase in defects among babies whose fathers worked in health care.

Nursing Implications

Because birth defects are quite rare in the general population (3%–5% of births), even if these findings hold true for nurses today, the risk of defects still is quite low. In addition, employers and nurses are better educated than they were in the 1970s about preventing hazardous exposures during pregnancy. Nonetheless, nurses should pay attention to hazards in their environments and alert their employers to potential risks.

Matte, T., Mulinare, J., & Erickson, J. (1993). Case-control study of congenital defects and parental employment in health care. *American Journal of Industrial Medicine, 24,* 11–23.

---

hard physical work to maintain a family farm, care for children, seek out financial assistance, and perform other activities. Therefore studies of formally employed women also may be relevant to other women.

The activities most likely to cause preterm birth and low birth weight are prolonged standing, long working hours, and lifting heavy objects (Simpson, 1993). Extreme physical effort at work was linked to fetal growth retardation in one study, although standing and walking were not (Spinillo et al., 1996). In another study, physical exertion did not increase miscarriage risks, except for women with a history of two or more previous spontaneous abortions. For these women, standing at work more than 7 hours a day greatly increased their risk of additional spontaneous abortion (Fenster et al., 1997).

In response to studies such as these, the American Medical Association has published guidelines for work limitations during pregnancy (AMA Council on Scientific Affairs, 1984) that suggest prolonged standing (for more than 4 hours), repeated stooping and bending (more than twice an hour), climbing ladders, climbing stairs more than 4 times per shift, and repeated lifting of over 25 pounds should be restricted after 20 to 28 weeks' gestation. Nurses should make an individualized assessment of each pregnant woman's work-related risks as well as the personal beneficial factors related to work.

Stress

Job-related psychological stress may be as much of a burden to employed pregnant women as is physical exertion. Just as the stress and fear of living in a war zone may cause pregnancy risks, the pressure of a job with low rewards, high demands, low decision-making power, or other causes of worry and pressure may also place fetuses at risk. Some studies have suggested that pregnancy-induced hypertension is more common in women with low-status jobs with limited decision-making, high job pressures, and little control over their work environment (Landisbergis & Hatch, 1996); for most pregnant women, however, job stress does not seem to lead to preterm delivery (Brett, Strogatz, & Savitz, 1997; Hickey et al., 1995). Clearly, more research is needed before nurses will be able to advise pregnant women on their stress-related pregnancy risks. In the meantime, however, nurses can provide emotional and practical support to employed pregnant women and facilitate support from others.

RISKS RELATED TO HOME ENVIRONMENT AND LIFESTYLE

Although industrial workplaces probably have the most intense concentrations of hazardous substances, the products produced in industry are used in the home. Foods are another source of harmful exposures. Medications and illicit drugs used in the home also can place the fetus at risk. Nurses can reduce some of the pregnancy risks related to home and lifestyle through teaching, home visiting, and ongoing support.

Food Additives and Contaminants

Food preparation and processing involve many chemical substances that serve as stabilizers, colorings, preservatives, leaveners, flavorings, sweeteners, and so forth. Some additives come from natural sources, such as red dye made from beets, and others are produced artificially. Whether an additive is natural or artificial has no bearing on its safety. In fact, artificial additives are often purer and more consistent than are natural ingredients (Food and Drug Administration, 1992).

In addition to compounds added directly to foods, indirect additives occur when a substance used in packaging, storage, or other handling becomes a part of the food in trace amounts. The Food and Drug Administration (FDA) must approve both direct and indirect food additives for marketing in the United States. The manufacturer must provide convincing evidence to the FDA in the form of animal or human studies to prove that based on the best scientific information available, this product is safe for human use. Evidence of safety in pregnancy must also be provided.

Pregnant women often are concerned about additives such as artificial sweeteners and preservatives. Preservatives have not been found to cause birth defects or other problems in pregnancy; however, the nutritional value of processed foods may be less than that of raw or home-cooked foods. "Diet" soft drinks are a popular beverage for young women. Aspartame, the artificial sweetener in diet drinks, has not been found to cause harm in pregnancy (Briggs, 1995). Saccharin, another artificial sweetener, also is considered safe. Women who are concerned that consumption of these additives early in pregnancy may have caused harm to their fetuses can be reassured that the risk of harm is very low. However, sugar-free and artificially sweetened soft drinks have no beneficial nutritional value.

Caffeine, found in high concentrations in coffee, tea, and some soft drinks, has been linked to risk of spontaneous abortion in the past; however, recent studies indicate that caffeine consumption alone does not increase the risk of prematurity or low birth weight in infants. Many smokers consume more caffeine than do nonsmokers, however, and smokers who drink large amounts of coffee have an even greater risk of having an infant of low birth weight than do smokers who do not drink coffee (Cook et al., 1996; Peacock, Bland, & Anderson, 1995; Shu, et al., 1995).

Food contaminants are bacteria or chemicals that are present in foods in unsafe amounts. The U.S. Department of Agriculture and the FDA regulate and supervise foods for purity and safe processing. Occasionally, however, an accidental contamination occurs. Imported fruits such as raspberries may not undergo the same testing as do U.S.-grown fruit products and may be contaminated by viruses or bacteria. Poorly processed or stored meats also occasionally are found to have harmful levels of illness-causing bacteria, such as *Escherichia coli*. Pregnant women are subject to the same health risks as are nonpregnant women when contaminated food is ingested. Fortunately, there are no known direct risks to fetal development from food contaminated with bacteria.

Lead and mercury contamination of food may pose a greater risk to pregnant women than to the general population. Pregnant women should be advised not to drink hot acidic beverages on a regular basis from mugs that have been glazed improperly with high-lead glazes. The heat combined with the acid in coffee or tea speed the leaching of lead from the glaze into the liquid. Cracked or chipped ceramicware should be disgarded. All ceramicware manufactured on a large scale in the United States is tested for safety. Pottery workers and craft groups in the United States currently are being educated about the importance of using safe glazes on all products made of clay that will contain food or drink (Foulke, 1997).

Mercury contamination occurs through consumption of fish from waters with a high mercury content, as noted in an earlier section of this chapter. All fresh, canned, and frozen fish processed and sold commercially, including tuna, is regulated and must meet safety standards. However, some pregnant women may consume fish caught by sports fishing and thus not subject to testing. Nurses should advise pregnant women to contact local environmental protection or water safety agencies to determine whether high mercury levels have been found in specific fishing locations before consuming fish caught by friends or family (Foulke, 1994).

Medications

Medications are one of the many possible forms in which pregnant women may be exposed to teratogens. It was once thought that the placenta served as a barrier between the fetus and harmful substances in the mother's system. Now it is known that most medications pass to the fetus to some degree. Of the many thousands of medications available today, only a few drugs or certain drugs classes have been proven to be teratogens: aminopterin; androgens; angiotensin-converting enzyme (ACE) inhibitors; busulfan, cocaine, when abused; coumarin derivatives; cyclophosphamide; diethylstilbestrol (DES); etretinate; isotretinoin; lithium; methotrexate; tetracycline; thalidomide; the antiseizure medications carbamazepine, paramethadione, trimethadione, phenytoin, and valproic acid; and dosages of vitamin A over 18,000 IU/day (Briggs, 1995). Other drugs and drug classes have been linked only anecdotally to fetal problems. (Ethanol, also called grain or ethyl alcohol, also is a teratogen.)

Although it is wise to be cautious about taking medications, some pregnant women may require over-the-counter or prescription medications for chronic medical conditions, complications of pregnancy, or discomforts and common illnesses. In addition, women may take potentially harmful medications in the early weeks of gestation, before they realize they are pregnant. In order to provide preconceptual counseling for women who take medications on a regular basis for chronic illness such as diabetes, cardiovascular disease, or seizure disorders, and to provide current and accurate information for women who are pregnant, nurses must be aware of the many factors that affect how chemicals are metabolized during pregnancy.

The nature of the drug itself affects the rate at which it is diffused into the fetal circulation. Medications with high molecular weights, which are highly ionized, that are not readily fat-soluble, or that readily bind to proteins are less likely to diffuse across the capillary membranes between the maternal circulation and the placenta. The stage of pregnancy also affects fetal exposure. Early in pregnancy the membranes between fetal and maternal circulation are thick, making transport difficult; whereas at term the membranes are very thin, making transport easier. The volume of blood circulating through the placenta also greatly increases during pregnancy, which would increase the rate at which drugs are transferred to the fetus.

These factors would suggest that early in pregnancy the fetus is better protected from harm. To the contrary, however, the most vulnerable period for fetal malformations is in the first trimester, particularly weeks 3 through 8 after conception. Even a small amount of a harmful substance can cause damage during this time. Moreover, the blood-brain barrier, which protects the adult CNS from certain harmful substances, does not form until 20 weeks' gestation. Therefore, the CNS is more vulnerable early in pregnancy than it is later, although different periods of pregnancy have factors that increase fetal vulnerability.

Most medications are quite safe during pregnancy. Even during critical periods of organ formation, most drugs present less than 10% risk of fetal damage, compared with the 3% risk of birth defects in the general population. Although the risk of injury is low, nurses must use available information to minimize these risks whenever possible. Nurses should be aware of the major teratogens but also must consult up-to-date reference books and other resources before giving advice about medications to pregnant women. As shown in Table 21-1, prescription medications are rated for safety by the FDA based on available research to date. The ratings are included in all product information and in drug reference materials for physicians and nurses.

Vitamins

Most care providers advise pregnant women to take prenatal multivitamins, which contain the recommended daily allowances of many vitamins and minerals important for the pregnancy. The two minerals most essential to fetal development are calcium and iron. One B vitamin essential to normal CNS development is folic acid, or folate. Pregnant women should receive 0.4 mg/day or more of folic acid, most importantly during the early first trimester when the neural tube forms (Rose & Mennuti, 1994). Some medications, such as anticonvulsants and trimethoprim, increase the need for folic acid. Many health care providers advise nonpregnant women of childbearing age to take a multivitamin tablet daily, because the critical period for neural tube closure is soon after conception, when women may not realize they are pregnant.

Another vitamin, vitamin A, is healthy in therapeutic doses but is teratogenic in certain forms. When pregnant women took vitamin A for acne, in the isomer form of isotretinoin (Accutane®), a high rate of severe defects and spontaneous abortions occurred. In the topical form of the oral medication isotretinoin, tretinoin (Retin-A®), the dose is lower; however, some risk still may exist (Briggs, 1995).

Pain and Fever Relievers

Acetaminophen has been widely used in pregnancy to relieve minor pain and fever, and no fetal harm has been ob-

Table 21-1 Teratogenic Risks of Drugs: FDA Categories

Category	Risk
A	Controlled studies in women fail to demonstrate a risk to the fetus in the first trimester or later trimesters. Possibility of fetal harm appears remote.
B	Animal reproduction studies have not demonstrated a fetal risk, but there are no controlled studies in pregnant women. *Or* Animal studies have shown an adverse effect but the risk is not confirmed in human studies in the first trimester (and there is no evidence of risk in later trimesters).
C	Studies in animals have revealed adverse effects on the fetus, and there are no controlled studies in pregnant women. *Or* Studies in women and animals are not available. Drugs should be given only if the potential benefit justifies the potential risk to the fetus.
D	There is positive evidence of human fetal risk, but the benefits from use may be acceptable despite the risk.
X	Studies in animals or humans have demonstrated fetal abnormalities. *And/or* There is evidence of fetal risk based on human experience. The risk of use in pregnant women clearly outweighs any possible benefit. The drug is contraindicated in women who are or may become pregnant.

Adapted from Spratto, G., & Woods, A. (2002). *PDR nurses' handbook.* Albany, NY: Delmar.

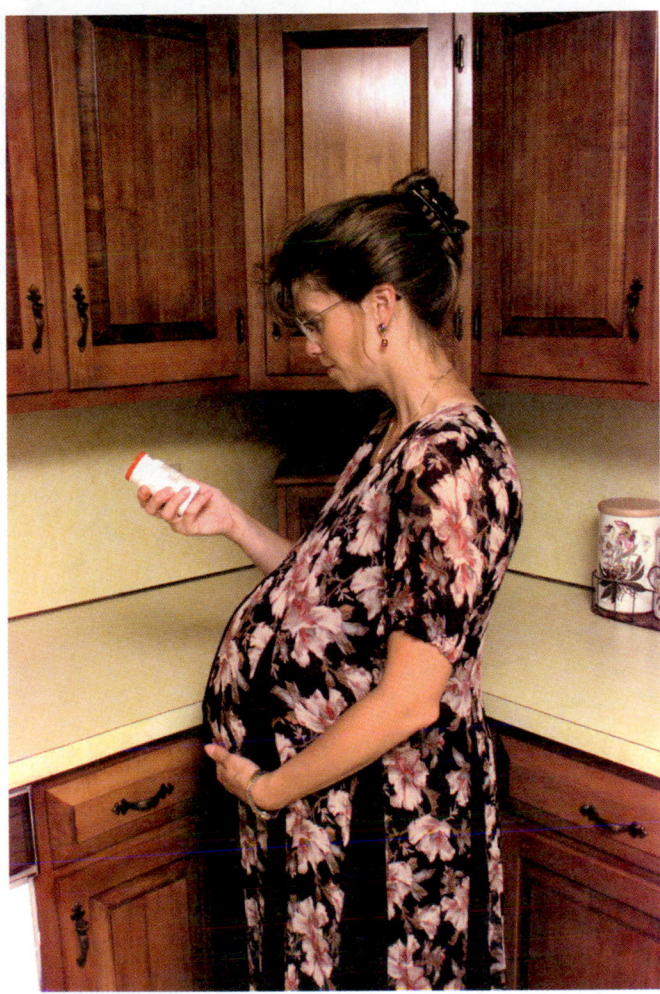

Figure 21-4 Nurses can help pregnant women recognize which over-the-counter medications are safe for use in pregnancy.

served (Figure 21-4). Aspirin, on the contrary, although consumed inadvertently by many pregnant women, is less safe. Aspirin has been known to cause bleeding problems and premature closure of the fetal ductus arteriosus when taken daily in late pregnancy for chronic illnesses such as arthritis (Rayburn & Conover, 1993). In some special cases, however, it may be used to reduce the inflammatory process blamed for some forms of pregnancy-induced hypertension. Nonsteroidal anti-inflammatory drugs, or NSAIDs, such as ibuprofen (Motrin®) have not been linked to fetal harm; however, because of their similarity to aspirin, most practitioners do not recommend the use of NSAIDs during pregnancy. Narcotic pain relievers such as meperidine or morphine are safe in therapeutic doses but can cause problems when taken chronically or abused. When used in high doses late in pregnancy, fetal sedation, neonatal respiratory depression, and neonatal withdrawal may result (Briggs, 1995).

Antihistamines, Decongestants, and Cough Medications

Diphenhydramine (Benadryl®), an antihistamine sometimes taken for nausea, has been linked to malformations in a few cases; however, the evidence is not conclusive, and it may be safely used after the first trimester. Pseudoephedrine (Sudafed®) is considered relatively safe and is the best option for antihistamine use in pregnancy (Conover, 1994). Some decongestants have been linked to anomalies. Chlorpheniramine (Chlor-Trimeton®) has been taken without problems; however, some studies indicate an increased risk of anomalies when used in the first trimester (Briggs, 1995).

Cough medicines (such as Robitussin DM®) containing dextromethorphan and guaifenesin are considered safe when used in therapeutic doses. Medicines containing codeine, however, carry the risks noted previously for narcotics. Codeine also may increase the risk of respiratory tract malformations after first-trimester exposure. It is important to note that cough syrups containing potassium iodine should be avoided because iodine can severely damage the fetal thyroid.

Gastrointestinal Medications

Constipation can be a major discomfort for many pregnant women. Increased fluid and fiber intake should be tried before medications are added. Stool softeners and laxatives, if needed, are not known to cause fetal harm. Laxative dependence generally is not a problem, because after childbirth the sluggish bowel usually returns to normal function.

Heartburn is another GI discomfort that affects many pregnant women. Antacid preparations containing calcium compounds as the main ingredient are considered safe. Those containing aluminum or magnesium are less well studied, and although no problems have been reported, a calcium-containing preparation is probably a better choice during pregnancy (Conover, 1994). Cimetidine (Tagamet®) and other systemic medications that reduce gastric acid production are fairly new but appear safe for use in pregnancy. Several types are available over the counter.

Sleep Medications

Sedatives such as secobarbital (Seconal®) and pentobarbital (Nembutal®) have been used in all trimesters of pregnancy without problems. Amobarbital has been linked to defects after first-trimester use, however, and neonatal respiratory depression can occur if the drug is given a short time before birth. Over-the-counter sleep aids such as

doxylamine (Unisom®) should be used with caution; however, no definite link to fetal malformations has been established (Briggs, 1995).

Antinausea Medications

Bendectin®, an antinausea medication containing pyridoxine (vitamin B_6) and doxylamine (now found in an over-the-counter sleep aid), was removed from the U.S. market after litigation about possible birth defects. Subsequent research could not prove this association. This medication still is available over the counter in England. Some women experience relief from nausea after taking oral or parenteral doses of B_6 and B_{12}.

Metochlopramide (Reglan®), an autonomic nervous system agent that works by speeding up GI motility to aid stomach emptying, is considered safe in pregnancy. Most other prescription antiemetics (such as perchlorperazine [Compazine®]) are from the phenothiazine group. In modest doses, they are considered safe for use during pregnancy.

Antibiotics

Most antibiotics are safe for use during pregnancy. Indeed, their use may be important because infection can cause serious complications, including preterm labor and fetal death. The penicillins, erythromycin, and many cephalosporins can be safely used in pregnancy. Several types of antibiotics are known or suspected teratogens, however, and their use should be carefully avoided.

Tetracycline and doxycycline can cause malformations early in pregnancy and produce tooth and bone discoloration after 20 weeks' gestation. They are considered teratogens. Drugs in the quinolone group, including ciprofloxacin (Cipro®) and norfloxacin (Noroxin®), should not be used because they may cause joint and bone problems in the fetus, as they have been found to do in infants and young children. Streptomycin, kanamycin, and gentamycin have been known to cause damage to the 8th cranial nerve, including hearing loss, in fetuses exposed during pregnancy. Chloramphenicol has been linked to a "gray baby syndrome" involving cardiovascular collapse in a newborn whose mother had taken it late in pregnancy, and therefore, this drug also should be avoided (Briggs, 1995).

Therapy for tuberculosis should be continued during pregnancy. Isoniazid and rifampin, common treatments, have been linked to isolated defects but overall are considered relatively safe. Women with resistant forms of tuberculosis who need other medications should be referred to a specialist in infectious diseases for treatment planning. Isoniazid and rifampin reduce the amount of vitamin K in the body. Therefore, vitamin K supplementation during labor for the woman and at delivery for the newborn is

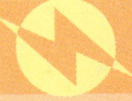

tion should receive intramuscular vitamin K during labor, and newborns should receive an increased dose of vitamin K after delivery (Briggs, 1995).

Another common antiseizure medication is carbamazepine (Tegretol®). Although some consider this to be the best choice of an anticonvulsant during pregnancy, like phenytoin, it has been linked to a syndrome of malformations. A third type of antiseizure medication is valproic acid (Depakene®). This medication is considered especially harmful during pregnancy, and women who take this drug should seek consultation immediately with their neurologists to switch to another medication. A fourth drug is diazepam (Valium®), used to treat severe seizures. This drug should be avoided during pregnancy because it has been linked to many fetal problems, including anomalies and neonatal jaundice. Diazepam and related compounds also are used to treat anxiety disorders. They should be replaced with other less dangerous drugs.

All the anticonvulsants are believed to be potent folate **agonists**, drugs that block or reduce the action of this vitamin in the human body. Therefore folic acid supplementation is important, ideally beginning before conception. It is important to remember, however, that seizures are far

recommended to reduce the risk of **hemolytic disease of the newborn**. This disease results in destruction of the neonate's erythrocytes owing to either isoimmunization (Rh or ABO incompatibility) or an inadequate amount of vitamin K, which leads to an inability to produce clotting factors and consequent risk of hemorrhage (Briggs, 1995).

Anticonvulsants

Pregnant women with seizure disorders face an increased risk of birth defects, although it is unclear how much of these are linked to medications and how much to the disease being treated (Conover, 1994). In addition, to avoid injury during seizures, it is especially important for women with seizure disorders who take anticonvulsant medications to use effective forms of contraception and receive preconceptual counseling to minimize the risks to their fetuses. A change in drug type or dosage may be considered if pregnancy is planned. Folic acid supplementation also will be advised because antiseizure medications interfere with absorption of this vitamin, which is important to reduce the risk of neural tube defects.

Phenytoin (Dilantin®) is the most common antiseizure medication and is associated with a 10% risk of a definite syndrome of malformations. These malformations include growth retardation, hypoplasia of the fingers and toes, and craniofacial changes, such as a broad nasal bridge, a low hairline, epicanthal folds, and a short neck. Mental retardation sometimes is present. Phenytoin also causes a deficiency in vitamin K–dependent clotting factors in about half of exposed newborns. Mothers who take this medica-

more harmful to the fetus than is the risk of minor malformations, and women should be counseled about the benefits and risks of taking their medications.

Antianxiety and Antidepressant Medications

Medications used for mental health conditions have differing levels of safety during pregnancy. As already mentioned, antianxiety medications from the diazepam group should be avoided. Alprazolam (Xanax®), a related compound that is one of the most common drugs used to treat anxiety, has been linked to isolated cases of birth defects and neonatal withdrawal (Briggs, 1995) but when used very sparingly may be relatively safe.

Tricyclic antidepressants also have been associated with isolated defects and withdrawal symptoms in newborns but overall are considered fairly safe. The selective serotonin reuptake inhibitor, or SSRI, antidepressants such as fluoxetine (Prozac®), although fairly new, have not been reported to cause adverse effects and appear to be a good choice during pregnancy (Briggs, 1995; Conover, 1994). Lithium, used for bipolar disorder, has caused cardiac defects and neonatal problems for exposed fetuses (Briggs, 1995); however, the incidence of problems appears to be decreased when serum levels are monitored closely and the lowest therapeutic dose is maintained.

Cardiovascular Medications

Drugs used to treat cardiac function and hypertension on an outpatient basis generally are safe in pregnancy. These include digoxin, quinidine, nifedipine (Procardia®), and other calcium channel blockers. When used in therapeutic doses they have not been found to be harmful, and in fact, vasodilation may be important for hypertensive women to enable placental perfusion and fetal oxygenation. There is one exception, however. ACE-inhibitors, such as captopril (Capoten®), have caused severe fetal toxicity in the second and third trimesters of pregnancy, and should be avoided. Diuretics are not advised during pregnancy. By removing water from the plasma, they also reduce the circulating volume to the placenta, and thus place the fetus at risk.

Hypertension that arises during pregnancy or that is present before pregnancy can be treated safely with methyldopa (Aldomet®), labetalol (Normodyne®), or atenolol (Tenormin®); hydralazine (Apresoline®) also may be used. Bedrest is an important first step to manage high blood pressure and reduce edema. Fetal surveillance with regular nonstress tests and periodic biophysical profiles should be initiated for all pregnant women with hypertension regardless of medication use, to observe for

fetal compromise. The mother's renal and liver status also should be carefully monitored.

Anticoagulants

Warfarin (Coumadin®) should not be used in pregnancy because it is known to cause serious fetal defects. Women who need anticoagulation medication, such as those with artificial heart valves or clotting disorders, must be switched to heparin before pregnancy, if possible. This change must be made carefully while observing laboratory clotting values, because thrombosis may occur when drug levels are subtherapeutic. Heparin is a very large molecule and does not cross the placenta. Because heparin can cause bone demineralization when used in high doses, calcitriol should be added to a pregnant woman's medication regimen if heparin therapy will be needed throughout the pregnancy (Briggs, 1995).

Hormones and Steroids

Sex hormones in large dosages can be harmful in pregnancy. Diethylstilbestrol (DES), a potent estrogen given until the early 1970s to prevent miscarriage, is known to cause malformations and epithelial changes in the genital tracts of female offspring and altered semen, epididymal cysts, and other genital problems in male offspring. Estrogens therefore are contraindicated in pregnancy (Briggs, 1995). In very low doses, however, such as with accidental exposure to low-dose oral contraceptives, harm has not been observed (Raman-Wilms et al., 1995). Androgens such as danazol (Danocrine®) may cause masculinization of female fetuses.

Thyroid hormone is safe during pregnancy, and in fact, it is important that mothers with hypothyroidism take adequate thyroid replacement to avoid impaired motor and mental development in their newborns. Drug therapy can be monitored using laboratory values, and doses will need to be increased during pregnancy because thyroid hormone binding increases during pregnancy. The most common antithyroid treatment to reduce hyperthyroidism, propylthiouracil, is safe during pregnancy. Thyroid diagnostic or therapeutic agents containing iodides should not be used, however, because the iodide can destroy the fetal thyroid.

Steroid use during pregnancy generally is safe when needed to treat serious maternal conditions. For example, steroids can be used to control the inflammatory process in bowel disease, asthma, and systemic lupus erythematosus. Topical steroids for dermatologic inflammation can be used safely, as can hemorrhoid treatments containing cortisone. Some steroids cross the placenta more readily than do others. Betamethasone (Celestone®), used to enhance fetal lung maturity, crosses the placenta readily, whereas prednisone does not. When the desired target is not the

The oral vaccine, now most commonly used, has no known harmful effects to the fetus. Tetanus toxoid has been linked to a slight increased risk of malformations (Briggs, 1995).

The rubella vaccine has not caused fetal rubella syndrome when given accidentally during pregnancy. Because it is a live vaccine, however, its use is avoided in pregnancy, and it is given in the postpartum period instead. Influenza vaccines from live viruses should be avoided; however, newer inactivated virus forms may be safe and should be offered to pregnant women who are immunocompromised and others who may receive important benefits (Briggs, 1995). Likewise, the hepatitis vaccine may be given during pregnancy when a mother is at high risk of exposure to the disease, although immunization during the first trimester should be avoided whenever possible. Vaccines given for travel to tropical countries may be risky during pregnancy; the pregnant woman should consult a specialist in tropical medicine.

In general, few problems are reported with immunizations. However, they should be administered during pregnancy only when the benefits outweigh the risks. For example, for a pregnant woman at high risk of contracting varicella (chickenpox) from her young child who has the disease, the benefit of giving the varicella vaccine is prevention of stillbirth or preterm delivery if she were to develop varicella later in her pregnancy. In this case, the small risk of a reaction to the vaccination outweighs the risks to the fetus.

Alcohol Use

Although public concern tends to focus on illegal drug use during pregnancy, alcohol and tobacco use are much more common and are more common causes of harm to the fetus. Many women who use illicit drugs also use alcohol and tobacco, making it difficult to separate the effects caused by illegal drugs from those caused by the more commonly ingested legal substances. In the 1980s and 1990s, nurses and other health care professionals began to take seriously the risks of alcohol and tobacco use in pregnancy and to become involved in helping their clients to stop using these substances.

Women who use illegal drugs have been found to be much less likely than nonusers to obtain prompt and adequate prenatal care. These women may be afraid of being reported or stigmatized for their drug use, or of losing custody of their newborns. In addition, women involved in illegal drug use are more likely to have chaotic, violent, and risky livestyles and be ambivalent about continuing their pregnancies (Kearney, 1995). Reaching and gaining the trust of pregnant women who use illicit drugs present special challenges for nurses employed in community health and prenatal care.

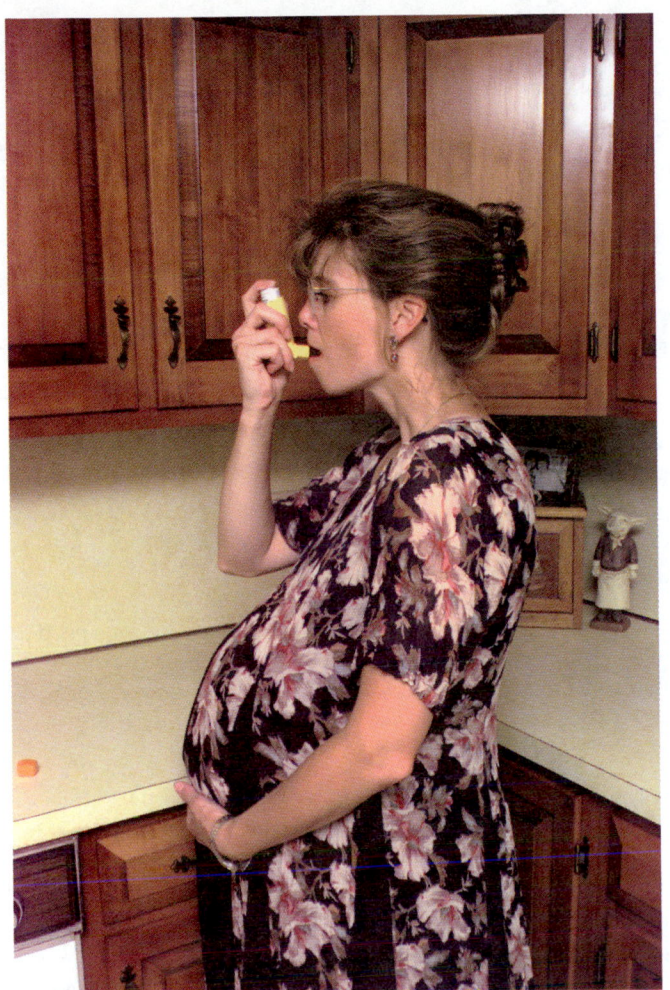

Figure 21-5 Pregnant women with asthma should continue to take their medications to prevent respiratory distress, which may also reduce oxygen to the fetus. Most asthma medications are safe in pregnancy.

fetus, the forms that cross the placenta less readily should be used.

Asthma treatments generally are safe in pregnancy. Bronchodilators, such as theophylline, can be used. **Sympathomimetic** agents, such as terbutaline (Brethine®) and isoproterenol (Isuprel®), that stimulate the sympathetic nervous system also are safe. Drugs that can be taken by inhaler are preferable to oral agents; however, oral or IV drugs should be used when needed. It is important to treat asthma promptly and effectively to maintain fetal and maternal oxygenation (Figure 21-5).

Immunizations

Pregnant women may need immunizations to protect against viral infections that threaten health during pregnancy. The inactivated polio vaccine, at one time given routinely in pregnancy, did not cause fetal malformations but did increase the risk of childhood cancers in offspring.

Prenatal alcohol use is the leading cause of childhood mental retardation, surpassing Down syndrome (Streissguth, Barr, Sampson, & Bookstein, 1997). Yet prenatal care providers probably spend more time counseling and testing women for fetal abnormalities such as Down syndrome than they do in assessing for and intervening in alcohol use. The National Institute for Drug Abuse has estimated that 18% of newborns are exposed to some alcohol during gestation (Young, 1997).

Heavy alcohol use throughout pregnancy (two or more drinks per day) has a 10% risk of producing **fetal alcohol syndrome** (FAS), which is a collection of physical and behavioral problems seen in children of women who drink heavily during pregnancy. Alcohol-related birth defects may include physical defects such as growth retardation; microcephaly; facial malformations, such as a flat midface, thin upper lip, and low or wide nasal bridge; malformations of joints and organs, such as the heart and kidney; and eye anomalies. FAS may also cause mental retardation, which is associated with microcephaly, and seizure disorders. Behavioral problems such as learning and attention difficulties and hyperactivity also have been associated with FAS. Fetal alcohol effect is a less severe form of alcohol-related problems.

A newborn exposed to alcohol during gestation with normal appearance and weight at birth still may have suffered brain damage. Newborns with low birth weight from maternal alcohol intake usually reach normal size by 8 months of age; however, CNS damage does not improve over time. Large amounts of alcohol cause physical malformations. Even small amounts consumed during pregnancy—so-called social drinking—can cause problems that persist into the teenage years and beyond: CNS damage; subtle cognitive delays; and motor, attention, and learning deficits (Streissguth, Barr, Sampson, & Bookstein, 1997). Thus, pregnant women and those planning pregnancy should be strongly advised to abstain from all alcohol use, because there is no known safe amount of alcohol consumption during pregnancy.

Tobacco Smoking and Passive Smoke

Approximately 20% to 30% of pregnant women report they smoke cigarettes with an average intake of about 14 cigarettes per day (Lawrance & Gruchow, 1996) (Figure 21-6). Tobacco use of over five cigarettes per day in pregnancy doubles a woman's risk of delivering a low-birth-weight infant (Lieberman, Gremy, Lang, & Cohen, 1994) (Figure 21-7). From 21% to 39% of low birth weights in infants are believed to be related to maternal smoking, and the effect on birth weight is proportional to the amount of tobacco used. The greatest effect is an in-

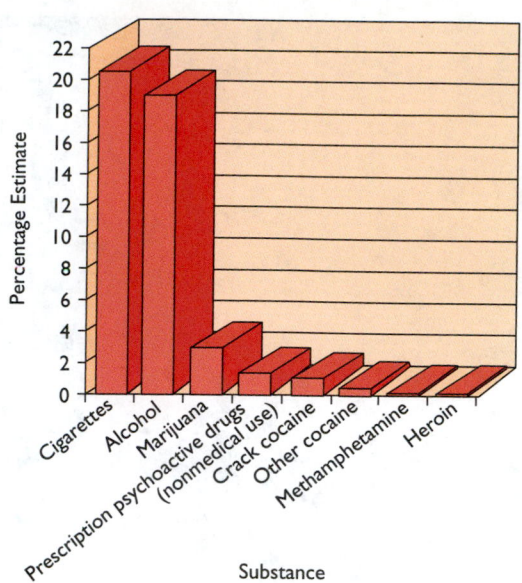

Figure 21-6 Estimated percentage of women who used selected substances in pregnancy, 1992. (Data from National Institute on Drug Abuse 1996. *National Pregnancy and Health Survey: Drug use among women delivering live births: 1992.* Rockville, MD: Author. NIH Pub. No 96-381 9, p. 36.)

creased risk of newborns who are small for gestational age; however, prematurity, infant mortality, and other pregnancy complications (such as spontaneous abortion, placenta previa, placental abruption, and premature rupture of fetal membranes) also are increased (Lieberman, Gremy, Lang, & Cohen, 1994). There is some evidence that prenatal tobacco exposure causes learning and atten-

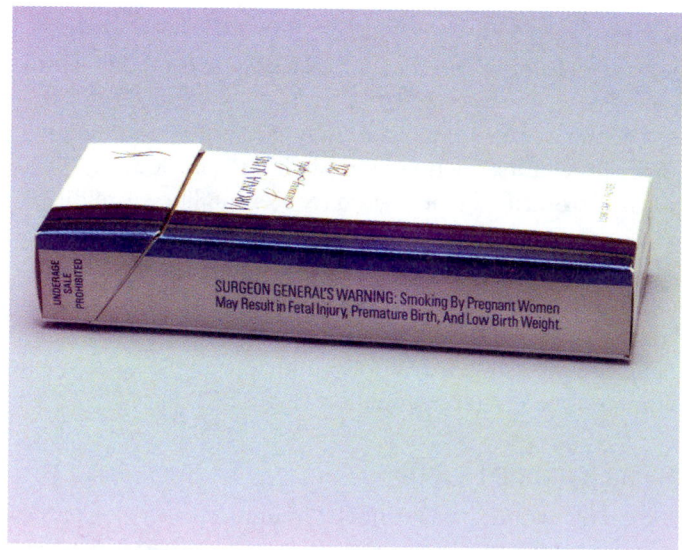

Figure 21-7 Warnings of risk to pregnant women on packages of cigarettes and alcoholic beverages must be supplemented by nursing advice and support.

tion problems in children but less consistently than does alcohol exposure (Streissguth, Barr, Sampson, and Bookstein, 1997).

Both nicotine and carbon monoxide are thought to cause the problems resulting from cigarette smoking in pregnancy. Nicotine constricts blood vessels and reduces perfusion to the fetus. Carbon monoxide binds to hemoglobin, reducing its oxygen-carrying capacity. Some women may be at special risk from cigarette smoking. Although more Caucasion than non-Caucasion women smoke cigarettes during pregnancy, the harm may be greater to African American women than to other groups. Cotinine, a metabolite of nicotine, is found in higher amounts in the urine of African American than of Caucasion smokers, even when their tobacco intake is the same (English, Eskenazi, & Christianson, 1994). Also, the older the woman, the more likely smoking will result in her having a low birth weight infant (Fox, Koepsell, & Daling, 1994).

Nursing Tip

ASKING CLIENTS ABOUT SUBSTANCE USE IN PREGNANCY

The most important point to remember is to ask *all* pregnant women about substance use. Do not make assumptions about which women are likely to be smokers or to use illicit drugs. Practice asking these kinds of questions and use them in assessment of all pregnant clients.

Keep these ideas in mind as you assess substance use:

1. Create a private setting to do a social assessment. The presence of other clients or family members may restrict the woman's willingness to discuss stigmatizing conditions such as substance use or domestic violence.

2. Ask about substance use in the part of the assessment that covers family, home life, and social environment. Linking these behaviors to the environment reduces the implication that they are personal failings of the woman. Ideally, ask them after you have established rapport with the client.

3. Consider asking, "Are you exposed to cigarette smoke in your home?" Then ask, "Who are the smokers in your home? Are you a smoker?" Inquire how many cigarettes the woman and her family members smoke each day and whether they have made any changes since the pregnancy began.

4. Use the same calm, warm tone of voice to inquire about alcohol use and then other drug use. Do not simply ask, "Do you use any other drugs?" Be specific: name illicit drugs, including heroin, cocaine, and marijuana.

5. Watch your body language. If you hurry through the questions, shake your head "No," or look away when asking these questions, the woman may assume you do not want to hear the answer.

6. If the woman admits substance use during pregnancy, do not give in to the urge to immediately explain all the risks of these substances and advise her to quit, which may alienate her. Unless she indicates a desire to continue to discuss it, simply say, "Thank you for sharing this, it is important to the health of you and your baby. We'll talk about this more later."

7. Complete the assessment, and then inquire, "You mentioned (substance use) earlier. I would like to review some of the effects of (this substance) during pregnancy and perhaps make some suggestions. Are you interested in discussing this?" If she declines, reply, "I will be happy to go over this information at any time." Offer printed literature on the topic.

8. Continue to treat her warmly and offer support and encouragement so that she develops trust in you. Over time, your positive relationship may enable you to revisit the topic. Your goal is to build her confidence and self-esteem, which will aid in her willingness to try to change her behavior.

9. Remember that she may be focusing on other personal priorities that seem much more urgent to her, such as surviving a violent relationship or keeping a job that her family depends on. She may value the stress reduction and sense of autonomy she gets from smoking more than protecting her fetus from a risk that seems small. Nurses are most effective when they work within the client's personal goals, helping the client see how improving health behaviors will help them meet their other goals as well.

One of the concerns of health care providers is whether pregnant women are reliable in their reports of how much alcohol and tobacco they use. In one study, only about half the women whose newborns had nicotine in their urine admitted to being smokers (Walsh, Redman, & Adamson, 1996). Nurses who conduct prenatal screening interviews must work to establish a secure, confidential environment for these assessments and develop rapport with their clients before asking potentially stigmatizing questions about alcohol, tobacco, and drug use in pregnancy.

When a woman's partner or work colleagues smoke cigarettes during her pregnancy, she is exposed to passive smoke. Passive smoke also causes low birth weight, although its effects may not be as severe as active cigarette smoking by the pregnant woman (Ellard et al., 1996). When a partner smokes cigarettes, it makes it more difficult for the woman to abstain from doing so during and after the pregnancy.

A woman who acknowledges cigarette smoking on an early prenatal visit may be encouraged to learn that it is not too late to avoid pregnancy risk. If she is able to stop by the third trimester, her risk of delivering a low-birth-weight infant decreases to normal levels (Lieberman, Gremy, Lang, & Cohen, 1994). However, many women who reduce or quit cigarette smoking during pregnancy resume their habit after giving birth, increasing the risk to the health of their newborns (Stotts, DiClemente, Carbonari, & Mullen, 1996). Nursing teaching and support are important to help women remain abstinent from cigarette smoking in the postpartum period.

Illicit Drug Use

Pregnant women who use illicit drugs often feel unwelcome in nursing care settings such as prenatal clinics. They fear they will be shamed or reported to legal or child protective authorities (Kearney, 1995). In order to provide nonjudgmental care and support for women who use illicit drugs, nurses must understand not only the effects of illicit drugs in pregnancy but how addiction affects a woman's lifestyle and self-concept. Nurses must conduct a complete and nonjudgmental assessment of each pregnant woman's use of all forms of legal and illegal drugs and provide accurate and unbiased teaching to pregnant women and their families. Ongoing support will be needed to help women use treatment resources, remain abstinent from substances, and continue and commit to avoiding relapse after giving birth.

Marijuana

Marijuana, also known as cannabis, is the illegal drug most commonly used in pregnancy. From 3% to 12% of pregnant women have traces of cannabis in their urine, with the higher rates found in women living in urban areas (Buchi, Varner, & Chase, 1993; Vaughn et al., 1993). Marijuana causes relaxation, euphoria, and sleepiness; may enhance appetite; and may reduce nausea and vomiting. Marijuana is not believed to be physically addictive or to cause withdrawal symptoms during periods of abstinence. Psychological dependence is possible, however.

The effects of marijuana smoking on pregnancy are not yet fully understood. There is some evidence that marijuana may cause decreased birth weight, birth length, and gestational age, as well as changes in infant sleep electroencephalograms and neurologic status; however, other studies do not support this evidence (Richardson, Day, & Goldschmidt, 1995). There are very few studies on the long-term effects of prenatal marijuana use on child development. Other factors in the lives of pregnant women who use marijuana, such as other substance use and poor nurturing from the home environment, seem to have as much impact on newborn and child health as does the drug itself.

Cocaine and Other Stimulants

Cocaine, a stimulant manufactured from the coca plant, is used by 0% to 12% of pregnant women, with the higher rates found in women living in urban areas (Vaughn et at., 1993; Young, 1997). Cocaine causes excitement, euphoria, and anorexia. Cocaine can be inhaled in powder form, injected, or smoked. The rates of perinatal cocaine use were highest in the late 1980s and early 1990s and declined in the late 1990s. Amphetamines, also known as "speed," "crank," or "ice," are other stimulants that can be injected, smoked, or taken orally. Their effects are believed to be similar to those of cocaine.

Cocaine is not physically addictive, meaning that use can be stopped without the risks of seizures or other life-threatening physical problems associated with withdrawal. Long-term use reduces the level of neurotransmitters produced in the body, however, resulting in intense behavioral dependence and producing psychological effects (such as depression) when cocaine use stops. Cocaine causes vasoconstriction, increased blood pressure, and tachycardia. Cocaine reduces placental blood flow. Chronic use in the second and third trimesters can lead to low birth weight, the most common effect of cocaine use in pregnancy (Bateman, Ng, Hansen, & Heagarty, 1993). Sudden decreases in placental blood flow may result in placental abruption. Scattered, rare reports link cocaine to congenital anomalies. Some infants exposed to cocaine in utero show increased irritability, difficulty in soothing, and changes in orientation and motor processes. These symptoms are not a result of physiologic withdrawal but of the effect of cocaine on the nervous system. These neurologic effects are temporary in full-term infants (Richardson, Conroy, & Day, 1996).

Long-term effects of cocaine on development and cognition also have been found in some studies (Azuma & Chasnoff, 1993). Other studies, however, have not found differences between children who were exposed to cocaine in utero and those who were not who come from similarly deprived backgrounds, suggesting that the home environment may have an important influence on whether children outgrow the effects of cocaine (Richardson, Conroy, & Day, 1996; Weathers, Crane, Sauvain, & Blackhurst, 1993). Alcohol and tobacco are used heavily by many users of cocaine (Richardson, Day, & Goldschmidt, 1995), making it difficult to separate the effects of cocaine use from those of alcohol and tobacco use.

Heroin

Heroin is a narcotic related to morphine that causes sedation, relaxation, and euphoria. Less than 1% of pregnant women use heroin, its prescribed substitute methadone, or other opiates. Heroin can be inhaled or injected. It is physically addictive, and withdrawal in either mother or newborn can cause vomiting, diarrhea, diaphoresis, respiratory distress, seizures, or death. When pregnant women who are addicted to heroin withdraw use suddenly or sharply reduce their use, intrauterine fetal demise can occur.

The most common harmful effect of heroin on newborns is withdrawal, or **neonatal abstinence syndrome**. This collection of symptoms may include sneezing, vomiting, diarrhea, irritability, and seizures and is seen in newborns withdrawing from prenatal exposure to narcotics. In a few studies, heroin has been linked to anomalies and low birth weight. In some cases, children who are exposed to heroin or methadone in utero have shown deficits in developmental and cognitive testing; however, poor maternal-child interaction and other factors of the home environment probably contributed to this effect (Richardson et al., 1996).

Injection drug use—whether of cocaine, heroin, amphetamines, or other drugs—increases a woman's risk of exposure to the human immunodeficiency virus (HIV) through contaminated needles. Illegal drug use also carries the risk of acquiring a sexually transmitted disease (STD) because women may trade sex for drugs, provide sexual favors to earn money for drugs, or maintain relationships with drug users (Henderson, Boyd, & Mieczkowski, 1994). Prescribed oral methadone maintenance, given to reduce heroin withdrawal symptoms, can reduce exposure to HIV and other STDs if it helps the woman to stop injecting other drugs. However, methadone has the same withdrawal consequences for women and newborns as does heroin.

Critical Thinking

Caring for Pregnant Women who Abuse Substances

When caring for clients who abuse substances in prenatal or perinatal care, you may be faced with conflicting emotions. As a nurse, you spend your career working for healthy mothers and babies. When a mother places a child at risk, you may feel anger, dislike, or impatience. You may even wish the court system would place the mother under surveillance to prevent substance use. This is not currently legal in any state in the United States because a fetus does not have full legal status as a person with rights of its own.

You are facing a conflict among three ethical principles important in providing health care: *beneficence,* doing good; *paternalism,* taking care of those who are unable to use good judgment for themselves; and *autonomy* (self-determination), the right of an adult to make personal decisions about her own behavior even when it places a fetus at risk. Forcibly controlling a woman's behavior may further diminish her ability to make good decisions on her own.

To promote the health of the fetus while building the mother's confidence and self-esteem, think about how you could form a respectful and interested professional relationship with her. This will help her feel worthwhile and competent, and she may be more likely to continue in prenatal care and seek alternatives to substance abuse.

Infections

Infections during pregnancy can be acquired from humans, animals, or the natural environment. They fall into two broad categories: STDs, acquired through intimate sexual contact; and other infections, including rubella, *E. coli,* and hepatitis, that may be acquired through casual exposure to infected persons or animals or through food or water. Maternal infections, mainly rubella, toxoplasmosis, and cytomegalovirus, account for approximately 2% of major congenital malformations occurring during pregnancy (Briggs, 1995).

Sexually Transmitted Diseases

One potent route of infection during pregnancy is sexual exposure, which introduces harmful organisms into the maternal system by way of the genital tract (Figure 21-8).

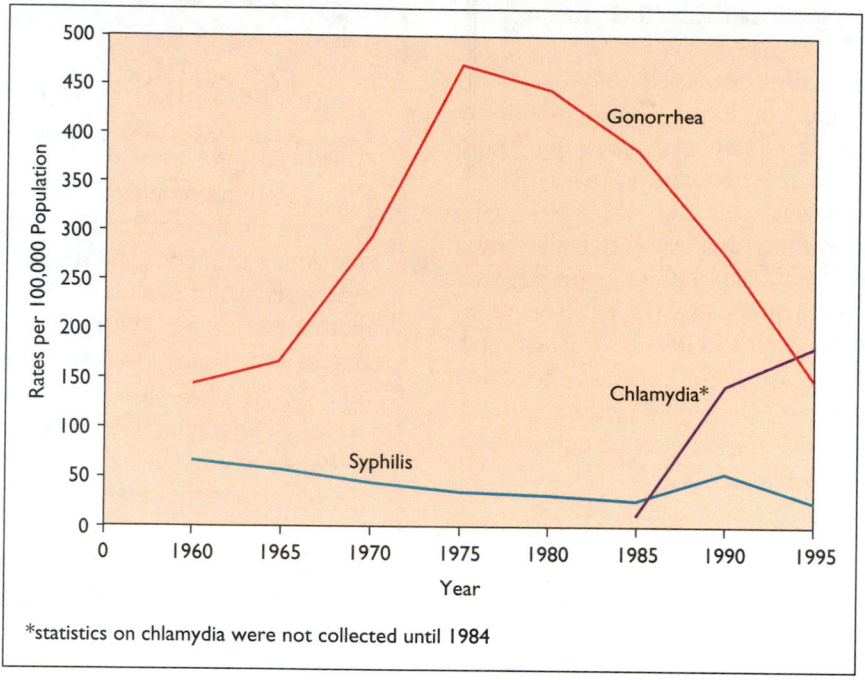

Figure 21-8 Estimated rates of sexually transmitted diseases per hundred thousand population, 1960–1995. (Data from Centers for Disease Control and Prevention. 1996. *Sexually transmitted disease surveillance, 1995*. Atlanta, GA: CDC, U.S. Department of Health and Human Services, Public Health Service.)

Many diseases are known to be transmitted sexually. Although many cause discomfort or pose a risk to the mother, not all cause harm to the fetus. Examples of infections that do not seem to place the fetus at risk include trichomoniasis and candidiasis. Figure 21-8 displays incidence data concerning STDs.

Syphilis

Syphilis infection, caused by the spirochete *Treponema pallidum,* increases the risks of spontaneous abortion, stillbirth, and live birth with congenital syphilis. Congenital syphilis affects about 250 infants annually in the United States (Sweet & Gibbs, 1995). The longer the mother has been infected, the greater the risk to the fetus.

In the mother, a new case of syphilis causes a painless lesion in the area of contact, which soon disappears while the progress of the infection continues. In the newborn, congenital syphilis may have no symptoms. A distinctive rash on the palms and soles of the feet and around the mouth and anus usually appears 2 to 6 weeks after birth, along with rhinitis. By 4 months of age, bone problems can be detected, sometimes accompanied by meningitis and enlarged liver and spleen. Later in childhood, other changes are found, including perforated nasal septum, pointed or notched teeth, and facial abnormalities. Bone and joint problems, deafness, and CNS damage can occur.

All pregnant women should receive a blood serology test for syphilis as early as possible in pregnancy. Women with evidence of active infection should have repeat VDRL (Venereal Disease Research Laboratory) testing during antibiotic treatment until the titer level decreases to a negligible one. Syphilis can be effectively treated during pregnancy using penicillin. Other substitute antibiotics (such as doxycycline or erythromycin) used for women who are allergic to penicillin and are not pregnant do not work as well during pregnancy. Pregnant women who have syphilis and are allergic to penicillin usually should undergo desensitization to be able to receive penicillin treatment (Sweet & Gibbs, 1995).

Gonorrhea and Chlamydia

Gonorrhea, caused by *Neisseria gonorrhoeae,* and chlamydia, caused by *Chlamydia trachomatis,* are transmitted sexually and cause no symptoms in 85% of infected women. If symptoms are present, they usually consist of vaginal discharge and dysuria (painful urination). Each disease affects about a half million women annually in the United States. The rate of chlamydia infection is increasing, and the rate of gonorrhea infection is slowly decreasing. Adolescent women and women of color are disproportionately affected by these infections (CDC, 1996).

If left untreated, these STDs can lead to pelvic inflammatory disease (PID) in up to 40% of women. In turn, PID leads to scarring of the reproductive tract that causes infertility in 20%, ectopic pregnancy in 9%, and chronic pelvic pain in 18%. Gonorrhea and chlamydia infections can cause neonatal conjunctivitis and blindness, and chlamydia infection can cause neonatal pneumonia. Blindness can be prevented by prophylactic treatment of the newborn with ointment applied to the eyes at birth; however, prevention of pneumonia requires that chlamydia infection be treated during pregnancy (CDC, 1996).

Although not universally practiced, some health professionals recommend screening of all pregnant women for these infections, just as all women are screened for syphilis. The test for syphilis shows current and past infection. Therefore, tests for other STDs such as gonorrhea and chlamydia should be considered because unprotected sexual encounters also may have caused multiple infections. Women with chlamydia or gonorrhea infection should receive antibiotic treatment with a medication safe for use in pregnancy. Oral erythromycin is used to treat chlamydia, and intramuscular injection of cephtriaxone plus oral erythromycin is used to treat gonorrhea. Nurses should discuss with clients the likelihood of GI irritation with erythromycin therapy and the importance of contacting a health professional for an alternative plan if they are unable to complete the prescribed regimen. A reduced dosage for a longer treatment period may be prescribed.

Human Papilloma Virus

The human papilloma virus (HPV) is a common one that produces warts in the anogenital area known as the condyloma acuminatum. Because several subtypes of this virus have been implicated in cancer of the cervix, women with a history of this infection should have more frequent Pap smears, ideally every 6 months. Although the warts themselves are not harmful, when large they may block the passage of the fetus through the vagina or bleed excessively. In these cases, cesarean birth may be recommended. Exposure of the fetus to HPV during labor and birth has been linked to later development of laryngeal papillomas; however, the risk is less than 1 in 100. Although no treatment has been proved effective in permanently eradicating the HPV virus, the warts may be removed using laser, cryocautery, or topical chemicals that are safe during pregnancy. Maintaining a healthy immune system may help a pregnant woman fight off the infection (Sweet & Gibbs, 1995).

Herpes Simplex Virus

The herpes simplex virus (HSV) is a common one that causes painful, pruritic blisterlike lesions and is carried by 0.1% to 4% of pregnant women. Herpes is a chronic recurrent infection. The virus is shed heavily during the primary infection as well as during recurrences (Sweet & Gibbs, 1995). Fetal and neonatal risks from HSV occur mainly when a primary infection occurs in pregnancy. Rarely, the fetus may become infected through transplacental trans-

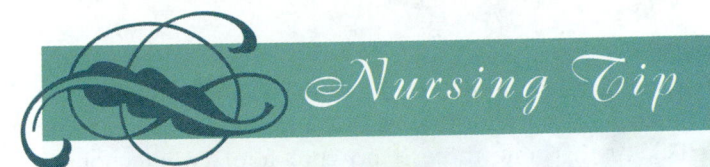

REDUCING RISKS RELATED TO THE HERPES SIMPLEX VIRUS

Isolation in a private room is no longer considered necessary for mothers and full-term newborns when the mother has HSV. Practicing and teaching good hand-washing technique are very important. The mother, all family members, and all visitors should wash their hands thoroughly before handling the newborn. The infant should be protected from exposure to herpes lesions. This includes advising the family not to kiss the infant if they have orofacial HSV lesions. Face masks may be worn by persons with orofacial herpes lesions to reduce the risk of spreading the virus in droplet form.

Protecting the newborn and other clients is important, as is treating the family with respect and understanding. The family will feel stigmatized if nurses avoid them or demonstrate a lack of enthusiasm in caring for them.

When the nurse has an orofacial herpes lesion, scrupulous handwashing and coverage of the lesion with a dressing is essential. Lesions are less contagious when crusted over, about 5 to 7 days after onset. Some institutions temporarily reassign nurses with herpes lesions to an area of the unit away from newborns.

mission or infection of the membranes, which can cause spontaneous abortion, preterm delivery, or intrauterine growth retardation. The most common route of transmission to the fetus is genital contact during vaginal delivery when the mother has a primary genital HSV infection. In this situation, neonatal HSV infection may occur in 25% to 50% of newborns; 40% to 60% of these newborns are at risk for death, and the remainder are likely to suffer CNS damage.

During a primary infection when the membranes are intact or have been ruptured for less than 4 hours, cesarean delivery may be recommended to reduce the exposure of the neonate to the virus. During a recurrent infection, the risk of transmission to the neonate is estimated at 0% to 4%; however, cesarean delivery may be performed as a precaution. Neonates also can be infected by hospital personnel or visitors with HSV lesions, and occasionally a newborn will develop an infection when the mother has no history of lesions but has a positive result on culture for HSV (Sweet & Gibbs, 1995).

Human Immunodeficiency Virus

Approximately 1 in 600 births in the United States are to women infected with the human immunodeficiency virus (HIV). At this time there is no cure for HIV infection. It leads to cancers and opportunistic infections, and ultimately death results as a result of depletion of the immune system. For childbearing women, a major concern is transmission of HIV to the fetus. Without antiviral therapy, approximately 25% of newborns of women infected with HIV will become infected with HIV. HIV in these infants causes growth retardation, repeated infections, and early death. Transmission risk is increased by advanced maternal disease and prolonged ruptured membranes. With zidovudine therapy during the second and third trimesters and treatment of the newborn for the first 6 weeks of life, infection of the newborn is reduced by as much as two thirds, to a rate of 8% to 11% (CDC Fact Sheet, 1996).

During pregnancy, nurses must focus on outreach to pregnant women who are HIV-positive to encourage them to obtain early and comprehensive prenatal care, including treatment with antiviral medications to maintain their own health and minimize the risk of perinatal transmission of the infection. Nutritional support, preventive care to avoid opportunistic infection, and other wellness promotion may reduce the risk of low birth weight and preterm delivery. Women who became infected with HIV through illicit drug use or unprotected sex should be offered referrals to treatment sources and teaching on prevention of sexual exposures.

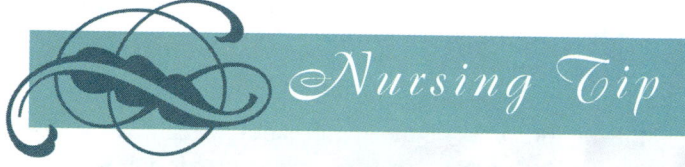

HIV TESTING IN PREGNANCY

Although some practitioners believe that all pregnant women should be tested for HIV, regardless of consent, this practice would be contrary to the ethical principle of autonomy for health care clients. Voluntary counseling and testing has resulted in increased use of zidovudine therapy during pregnancy and reduced transmission of HIV to newborns (CDC Fact Sheet, 1996).

You must provide information and counseling on voluntary testing for HIV to all pregnant women. Explain that this testing will enable the detection of infection early enough to provide zidovudine and other important treatment. Advise women diagnosed with other STDs that they may also have been exposed to HIV. Repeated testing over 6 to 12 months is necessary to detect recent infection.

Nursing Alert

PREVENTING THE SPREAD OF HIV AND OTHER INFECTIONS

You must maintain standard infection control precautions during prenatal and perinatal procedures to minimize the risk of contamination of the environment with blood or body fluids containing the HIV virus and other pathogens. These precautions apply to all pregnant and postpartum women, not only those known to be infected with HIV.

You must remember that HIV and other infections may be present in any woman, including those whose HIV status was negative at the last test. If the infection is recent, antibodies may not have yet developed that can be detected with testing. Some women may have refused testing because of fear of stigma or loss of employment or insurance coverage if they are found to be HIV-positive. Others may never have been offered the HIV test. You should refrain from making judgments about which women are likely to be infected with HIV and use standard precautions for all clients.

During labor and birth, women known to be infected with HIV should receive the same consideration and level of support and care as do other mothers. These mothers may suffer fear and depression as they await the results of laboratory testing of their newborns for HIV infection. Because all newborns exposed to HIV will be born with maternal HIV antibodies, virologic tests must be performed to determine whether the virus itself is present in the neonatal system. Mothers with HIV should be counseled not to breast-feed their infants, because HIV can be transmitted to infants through breast milk.

Other Infections

Pregnant women may acquire infections from contaminated food, water, or nonsexual contact with infected persons. Although many kinds of infections may be contracted from these sources, some are known to have harmful effects on the fetus and newborn.

Hepatitis B

This viral infection is transmitted through blood and body fluids and predominantly affects the liver. The acute infection can be fatal or cause permanent liver damage or carcinoma. Infection in pregnancy may cause spontaneous abortion and has been linked to preterm labor. Maternal-infant transmission can occur transplacentally, through intrapartum or postpartum contact with

STANDARD PRECAUTIONS

When following Standard Precautions, you must:

1. Wear gloves to prevent transmission of blood-borne infections, such as HBV and HIV, when you are at risk of coming into contact with any bodily fluids that contain blood or amniotic fluid from the client, bedding, or instruments. You must also change gloves between clients. Do not reuse gloves.

2. Wear a mask, eye protection, a face shield, and a fluid-resistant gown in all situations in which bodily fluids are likely to be splashed or propelled onto you.

3. Wear a gown and gloves when handling newborns until all blood and amniotic fluid have been removed by bathing.

4. Do not recap, bend, or break needles. Do not remove needles from syringes. Store all sharps safely for disposal.

5. Perform resuscitation and suctioning using protective equipment rather than by mouth-to-mouth contact or use of a DeLee catheter.

contaminated surfaces, or through breast milk or colostrum. Approximately 5% to 10% of newborns of infected mothers will become infected unless they receive treatment in the neonatal period, and the rate is much higher if the mother carries a virulent form of the disease caused by the hepatitis B e (HBeAg) antigen (Sweet & Gibbs, 1995).

All pregnant women should be tested for hepatitis B surface antigen (HBsAg), the surface antigen indicating infectivity with hepatitis B. Women who are HBsAg-positive should receive careful instruction as to blood and body fluid precaution to prevent infection of family members. Public health service referrals may be used to assist in notifying all sexual contacts of a pregnant woman infected with hepatitis B and providing immunoglobulin and immunization therapy to family members to reduce the risk of infection. The neonate of a mother with hepatitis B should receive hepatitis B immune globulin and the first of three injections of hepatitis B vaccine before being discharged from the hospital. Most states require that all parents be offered the opportunity to have their newborns receive the first hepatitis B immunization injection during the nursery stay.

Varicella Zoster

The varicella virus causes the chickenpox infection. Chickenpox is a common childhood disease causing fever, malaise, and pruritic pustules. It is highly contagious, and more than 90% of adults show evidence of past infection and are immune. For this reason, infection during pregnancy is rare, only about 5 cases per 10,000 pregnancies. The most severe complication for adults with chickenpox is varicella pneumonia, which can be fatal. In most cases, however, adult chickenpox is a fairly low-risk disease.

In pregnancy, however, varicella can be extremely harmful. Varicella infection in the first trimester of pregnancy has approximately a 10% risk of causing congenital varicella syndrome, which includes limb and digit hypoplasia, eye anomalies, mental retardation, and growth retardation. Infection of the mother late in pregnancy can cause preterm labor and stillbirth and places the newborn at risk for life-threatening neonatal varicella infection. The risk of death can be averted by giving exposed newborns varicella-zoster immune globulin (VZIG), although some may still show signs of infection (Sweet & Gibbs, 1995).

When a women who does not believe she has had chickenpox is exposed during pregnancy, blood for a varicella antibody titer should be drawn. If the results are negative, VZIG may be given to prevent or minimize infection. If the titer level is moderate, the woman is immune. If the titer level is high, current infection probably is present. Varicella vaccine is now available and can be given to pregnant women with negative results on varicella titer tests before exposure occurs. Immunization will prevent the serious sequelae of infection during pregnancy.

Cytomegalovirus

Cytomegalovirus (CMV) has been linked to serious neonatal infection and malformations. CMV causes mild flulike symptoms in the healthy adult or no symptoms at all, and as many as 75% of adult women have antibodies to CMV. Primary infection occurs in 1% to 2% of susceptible women during pregnancy and may be completely asymptomatic for the mother. The virus can be detected for long periods after infection and may be shed intermittently through body fluids. CMV can be transmitted to the fetus transplacentally and at the time of birth. Pregnancy may reactivate CMV infection in women who carry the virus. When CMV is present on the cervix at birth, 30% to 50% of neonates acquire the virus (Sweet & Gibbs, 1995).

Newborns infected with CMV have a 10% risk of symptomatic disease at birth. The infection can cause hepatosplenomegaly, jaundice, deafness, and eye problems. Mental retardation, chorioretinitis, cerebral calcifications, and microcephaly or hydrocephaly are long-term effects. Unfortunately, although antiviral treatments are used to

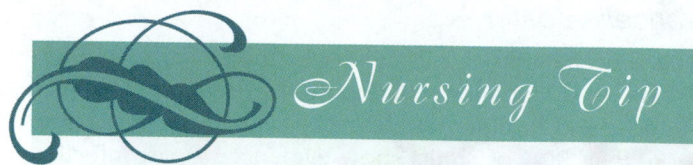

limit the extent of disease, no fully effective treatments are available.

Pregnant women can be tested for immunity or current infection using the **TORCH** serum screening panel (see Nursing Tip). For an asymptomatic disease such as CMV, expensive serial titer testing would be needed to detect the presence of primary infection; however, no effective treatments are known for women diagnosed with primary CMV. Nurses should be prepared to counsel pregnant women about this difficult situation and provide support. Some women who have CMV infection may choose to terminate the pregnancy even though the likelihood of a healthy outcome is 90% (Sweet & Gibbs, 1995).

Parvovirus

Also known as Fifth disease, parvovirus causes erythema infectiosum in childhood, a disease involving low-grade fever and erythema of the cheeks. Parvovirus can have more serious effects in adults, including pneumonia and hemolytic anemia. One strain, human parvovirus B19, has been found to cause severe fetal anemia, cardiac failure, nonimmune hydrops fetalis, and intrauterine fetal death. Approximately 1% of pregnant women are infected with B19, which can be diagnosed with antibody testing. Fetal damage is believed to occur in 30% to 40% of pregnancies. Treatment is limited at the present time. Serial ultrasonography can detect early signs of heart failure and hydrops, and intrauterine transfusion may be used to treat fetal anemia (Sweet & Gibbs, 1995). Some women infected with B19 may choose therapeutic abortion.

Toxoplasmosis

Toxoplasma is an intracellular parasite that is found in animals, including sheep and mice. It is transmitted in the feces of cats who have consumed infected mice and in meat from infected animals. The disease in humans may have no symptoms or may cause lymphadenopathy, fever, fatigue, sore throat, eye pain, and rash. It may be mistaken for influenza or mononucleosis.

At least half of all pregnant women in the United States have antibodies to toxoplasma. The rate of infection in pregnancy is fewer than 1 in 1,000 births. When infection does occur, spontaneous abortion, preterm delivery, and intrauterine growth retardation may result. At least half of all neonates born to mothers infected with toxoplasma during pregnancy show laboratory evidence of infection. The most severe effects occur when the mother is infected in the first trimester. These effects can include **chorioretinitis** (inflammation of the membrane of the retina of the eye), anemia, liver damage, CNS abnormalities, and perinatal death. Toxoplasmosis can be treated with antibiotics if infection is diagnosed early; however, some neonatal disease may still occur. Nurses play an important role in home assessment and prenatal teaching to prevent this infection.

This preventive advice has significantly reduced the incidence of toxoplasmosis in areas where it has been used systematically (Sweet & Gibbs, 1995).

Other Parasitic Diseases

Pregnant women in underdeveloped countries and tropical areas may be exposed to a variety of parasites in the environment. Many parasites have primarily GI effects, and some cause systemic infection.

Protozoans are the cause of amebiasis, giardiasis, leishmaniasis, trypanosomiasis, and malaria. Amebiasis causes ulcerative disease of the colon, giardiasis affects

Box 21-1 Home Visit Guidelines

1. Before the visit, gather information about environmental hazards present in the neighborhood of your client, such as toxic waste dumps, incinerators, factories with dangerous emissions, unsafe water supply, and other risks.

2. As you approach the residence, observe for potential pregnancy risks (and hazards to your own safety) in the social environment, such as street violence, drug dealing, and unsafe housing.

3. During your visit, observe the home for hazards such as peeling paint, toxic chemicals such as bug killers or lawn chemicals, or homemade ceramic mugs that may contain lead glaze.

4. During your nutritional assessment, ask to see the contents of cupboards and the refrigerator. Inquire about imported fruits and any fish or game that may not have been inspected.

5. Ask permission to look in the medicine cabinet. Point out over-the-counter medications that are unsafe for use in pregnancy.

6. Observe for the odor of tobacco, cigarette butts, and ashtrays. If a family member smokes, inform the pregnant woman about the risks of passive smoke to herself and her baby both before and after birth. Help the woman to problem-solve to reduce her exposure to tobacco smoke. Provide information for her and her family on stop-smoking classes and other resources.

While completing a nursing assessment of a client's medical and obstetrical history and risk factors, you should explore these other important areas through nursing observations and questioning the client on the following topics.

1. Geographic risks:
   a. Are you or have you been exposed to violence, urban poverty, or chemical or nuclear accidents?
   b. Are pesticides and herbicides used in agriculture present in your residential area?
   c. Are there industrial wastes such as heavy metals, solvents, PCBs, or PBBs in the food and water where you live?
   d. Is geographic isolation an obstacle that prevents you from obtaining prenatal care?

2. Employment-related risks
   a. Are you exposed to extreme heat, radiation, chemical, or gas exposures at work?
   b. Are you an agricultural worker exposed to pesticides or herbicides?
   c. Does your job entail long hours of standing, heavy lifting, extreme physical exertion, or psychological stress?

3. Risks in the home environment
   a. Do you frequently drink hot beverages from ceramic mugs that may contain lead?
   b. Do you eat fish caught by sports fishermen that may contain high levels of lead or mercury?
   c. Do you live in an area where waterborne or insectborne parasites are a threat, or have an untested well as your source of drinking water?
   d. Do you have cats as pets?
   e. Have you traveled to or emigrated from an area in which parasitic infections are common, such as a tropical climate?

4. Medication risks
   a. What prescribed medications do you take for chronic or intermittent medical conditions?
   b. What over-the-counter medications do you use on a regular basis, and what have you taken since the time of conception of the current pregnancy?

5. Recreational drug and tobacco risks
   a. Do you smoke cigarettes, and if so, how many per day? Do other household members smoke?
   b. Do you drink alcohol recreationally or regularly? How much and how often? How much since conceiving this pregnancy?
   c. Have you ever tried cocaine, marijuana, heroin, or other drugs? How recently? How much have you used since conceiving this pregnancy?

6. Risks from STDs
   a. Do you have one sexual partner or more than one? Do you practice safe sex?
   b. Do you or your partner have any symptoms of vaginal or perineal infection, such as itching, discharge, burning, sores, or growths on the perineal area?

(continued)

Box 21-1 continued

    c. Have you or your partner ever been diagnosed with an STD?

    d. Have you ever experienced PID? If so, do you have any symptoms of ectopic pregnancy, such as pelvic pain, vaginal bleeding, or shoulder pain that may be caused by internal bleeding?

    e. Does your prenatal laboratory tests indicate infection with syphilis, parvovirus, toxoplasmosis, HIV, hepatitis B, gonorrhea, or chlamydia?

    f. Have you been immunized against or have a history of past infection with rubella and varicella (chickenpox)?

7. Knowledge level, behavior, and social conditions

    a. Are you aware of the more common risks to the fetus, including those from over-the-counter medications, tobacco, and alcohol?

    b. Are you motivated to change your behavior if you are a habitual user of substances that are dangerous in pregnancy? Have you made changes since your pregnancy was diagnosed, such as quitting smoking or avoiding alcohol?

    c. What resources such as support and treatment are available to you? What is the level of family support present for behavior change such as stopping tobacco, drug, or alcohol use?

    d. What is your overall nutritional and physical health status, which reflects your body's resistance to infections and ability to provide nourishment to a fetus?

    e. What are your financial constraints that might affect your ability to change your employment setting if hazards are present?

    f. What are your home responsibilities that may affect your ability to rest and care for yourself if you must continue to do strenuous work?

the duodenum, and leishmaniasis causes ulcers of skin and mucous membranes. Trypanosomiasis has two forms: Chagas' disease, which causes cardiac disease and intestinal problems and can be transmitted prenatally and through breast milk; and African sleeping sickness, which has rapidly progressive, fatal CNS effects and usually causes death of the woman before the pregnancy reaches full term. Malaria, the most common protozoan worldwide, is spread by mosquitoes and causes recurrent fever and chills, nausea, vomiting, liver damage, and sometimes rupture of the spleen. In pregnancy, malaria can cause spontaneous abortion, intrauterine growth restriction, and preterm delivery, as well as congenital infection of the newborn (Sweet & Gibbs, 1995). Protozoan infections can be treated with antibiotics during pregnancy.

Helminths are worms capable of parasitizing humans. Helminths include GI nematodes (roundworms), such as ascariasis, pinworms, and hookworms. Helminths also include tissue nematodes, such as filariasis, transmitted by mosquitoes, and trichinosis, spread by consuming infected meat. Trematodes, or flatworms, include schistosomiasis, a bloodborne infection that can penetrate skin in contact with infected water. Schistosomiasis can be fatal, and the drugs used for treatment are not advised during pregnancy. Cestodes, or tapeworms, inhabit the GI tract and are acquired by eating infected meat. Although cestodes cause unpleasant symptoms and treatment is available, it

usually is delayed until after delivery to avoid exposure to harmful medications (Sweet & Gibbs, 1995). Although the fetus is not harmed directly by these parasites, nutritional deficits and loss of body fluids in the mother may produce intrauterine growth restriction.

Nurses should counsel pregnant women who travel to tropical and undeveloped areas to avoid exposure to insects, bodies of water, water that has not been treated for drinking, and meat that is not fully cooked. Women who come to prenatal care from these areas should be assessed for signs of parasitic disease and treatment provided when appropriate. Blood and stool cultures can be used to detect many parasites. It is important for the nurse to teach women about the low risk to the fetus of many parasitic conditions and to provide emotional support and instructions on hygiene if treatment must be delayed until after childbirth.

NURSING PROCESS

Nurses are the ideal health care provider to identify and intervene with women exposed to environmental risks during pregnancy. Nursing's holistic focus on clients within the context of their families and environments promotes sensitivity to factors in addition to medical and obstetrical risks that may threaten the well-being of pregnant women and their fetuses.

Assessment

When providing care for pregnant women in acute, ambulatory, or home care settings, you must be aware of and assess for environmental and lifestyle risks that may endanger the mother and fetus. These assessments can take place in a health care setting or during a home visit.

Nursing Diagnoses and Outcome Identification

Nursing diagnoses along with expected outcomes are listed in Table 21-2.

Table 21-2 Common Nursing Diagnoses, Causes, and Outcomes

Nursing Diagnosis	Cause	Expected Outcomes
Risk for (or present) infection	Unsafe sexual practices, preexisting sexually transmitted disease, lack of immunity to childhood diseases that place the fetus at risk, environmental hazards such as parasites	Fetus is protected from infection by immunization, maternal antibiotic treatment, maternal safer sex practices and lifestyle precautions, and safe food handling and preparation.
Risk for injury (fetal)	Industrial waste, employment conditions that expose pregnant woman to dangerous chemicals or activities	Fetus is protected from injury by removing hazards from environment, protecting pregnant woman from exposure, and modification of employment or household conditions.
Ineffective tissue perfusion (placental)	Cigarette smoking, cocaine use, stress	Placental perfusion is adequate, as demonstrated by appropriate fetal growth and reassuring fetal assessments.
Impaired gas exchange (placental-fetal)	Cigarette smoking, carbon monoxide exposure, maternal anoxia from seizures	Fetus demonstrates adequate oxygenation by reactive nonstress tests and other assessments. Risk is reduced by reduction in maternal cigarette smoking and maintenance of therapeutic level of anticonvulsants.
Delayed growth and development (fetal)	Inadequate nutrition or malformations from chemical or drug exposure	Alterations are diagnosed promptly. Chemical exposures are minimized or eliminated. Pregnant woman and family are informed of risks and supported in decision-making. Pregnant woman and family have adequate support and preparation for birth of an infant with possible altered development.
Imbalanced nutrition, less than body requirements	Substance abuse and consequent anorexia, cognitive alterations, lifestyle disruption	Pregnant woman who abuses substances demonstrates adequate weight gain and fetal growth. Adequate support and teaching are provided to reduce substance abuse and promote healthful lifestyle.
Fatigue	Strenuous employment demands	Pregnant woman demonstrates moderation in physical activity and adequate rest periods.
Ineffective role performance	Role burdens (work and home) changing roles	Employment conditions and role expectations are modified to promote prenatal health.
Fear	Possible birth of damaged infant from exposure to a hazardous substance or infection	Pregnant woman and family report reduction in fear, and demonstrate knowledge of likelihood of fetal harm and measures to minimize fetal damage.
Deficient knowledge	Lack of information about pregnancy, hazards, risk reduction strategies	Pregnant woman and family can state potential risks of their environmental conditions for fetal health, and describe and demonstrate risk reduction strategies.
Ineffective individual and family coping	Substance abuse	Pregnant woman and family demonstrate improved safety in behavior and home management and increased motivation toward healthful behaviors.

Planning

For each nursing and medical diagnosis that applies to a pregnant woman and her family, you should work with the client to develop a plan of care that addresses health needs within the goals, capabilities, and context of the family. In planning to address each health issue, you should:

1. Consider the values behind the health goal, and clarify that the values are compatible with the client's choices. For example, a pregnant woman who smokes a pack of cigarettes per day may not value prevention of low birth weight as much as she values the autonomy and stress reduction of smoking.

2. Provide the education needed to convey the benefits of behavior or lifestyle changes. For example, if a pregnant woman works in an agricultural environment, explain the relative risks of harm from pesticide exposure and heavy lifting, and the reduction in risk that would be achieved if she were able to eliminate these exposures and activities.

3. Select interventions to reduce risks that are feasible within the client's unique situation and context. These may be client-initiated or nurse-initiated, or initiated by referral to another helping professional. Client-initiated interventions might include preparing meats at home in a different way to reduce the risk of trichinosis or other parasites. Nurse-initiated interventions might include weekly supportive phone calls to help a woman maintain abstinence from alcohol, or performing nonstress tests weekly to monitor reactivity in the fetus of a woman who uses cocaine. Referral-initiated interventions include actions such as providing information about Alcoholics Anonymous (AA) meetings, helping the woman make an appointment with a family counselor if a partner's substance abuse is placing her at risk, or sending a pregnant woman with a chronic illness to her specialist medical provider to have type and dosage of medications adjusted to maintain safety during pregnancy.

Nursing Intervention

Nurses should focus on the whole pregnancy, not just the present time, as they intervene to help pregnant women reduce environmental risks. Many actions may be initiated as a result of the initial assessment; however, follow-up is extremely important. Behavioral changes such as stopping smoking are extremely difficult to sustain, reducing activities at work may not be permitted over the entire course of pregnancy, and other conditions may increase the chance of reverting to the prior risk status. The nurse must maintain an active problem list and through telephone, home visits, and scheduled ambulatory care appointments, let the pregnant woman know that support is always available as she maintains these difficult changes.

One way of monitoring successful behavioral change is through voluntary testing. A pregnant woman may appreciate the motivating influence of regular testing of urine for alcohol, drugs, or cotinine. Testing should not be initiated without her knowledge or against her will, because doing so would constitute criminal assault and violate the principle of informed consent and client autonomy. Another type of periodic testing is monitoring of blood levels of prescribed medications to ensure adequate dosages and avoid excessive fetal exposure. A third type of continual monitoring is fetal assessments initiated in the third trimester to ensure fetal growth, oxygenation, and normal development.

Evaluation

Interim evaluations should be made of client knowledge, behavior, environmental conditions at work and at home, and maternal and fetal physical and psychosocial well-being. The ultimate outcome of nursing care to reduce risks during pregnancy is the birth of a healthy infant. Parents must be counseled that some exposures do not reveal their effects until later in childhood. For example, alcohol exposure may cause subtle learning and attention difficulties that are not detected until school age. Parents should also be advised that a nurturing, interactive, and educationally stimulating home environment can minimize the developmental effects of many prenatal exposures.

FUTURE DIRECTIONS: IMPROVING PUBLIC AWARENESS AND POLICIES FOR PREGNANCY SAFETY

Much more research is needed to fully understand the effects of many environmental influences during pregnancy. Because experimental studies cannot ethically be conducted on humans, information will continue to be gathered retrospectively from human experiences of exposures to newly identified hazards. Sadly, it is only after damage has occurred that many substances are labeled as harmful. With rapid development of new chemicals and forms of radiation for use in industry and health care, research on pregnancy safety must keep pace.

Yet, we do know a great deal about the impact of many environmental influences. Nurses have an important role to play in educating clients and families about reducing environmental risks during pregnancy and in advocating for clients with their employers, landlords, other social service providers, and families. In addition, much more

Case Study/Care Plan

SUBSTANCE USE IN PREGNANCY

Janice Lord is a 31-year-old (gravida 3, para 2) single Caucasian woman who arrives for her first prenatal visit. She is 16 weeks pregnant. Her first pregnancy ended with delivery of a healthy full-term male infant who is now 3 years old. Her second pregnancy ended in a spontaneous abortion at 18 weeks owing to placental abruption. She has no chronic diseases or known exposures to industrial chemicals or radiation. She lives with her son in a public housing project where gang fighting and public intoxication is common. She is employed full-time as a house cleaner.

Janice smokes 20 cigarettes per day, drinks two or three 12-ounce beers each night to relax after work, and smokes crack cocaine on weekends with her boyfriend. Her mother, also a cigarette smoker, watches Janice's son during the day. Her boyfriend does not live with her but spends most of each weekend in her apartment.

Janice was originally ambivalent about continuing the present pregnancy and also was delayed in seeking prenatal care because she did not have health insurance. She tells you that she believes the previous pregnancy loss was due to a cocaine binge, and she wants to do her best to protect the present fetus from harm. She hopes to move out of public housing sometime soon and relocate to a suburban area with less street violence.

Janice's initial physical examination is within normal limits, with the exception of a foul-smelling vaginal discharge and mild hypertension (140/90 mm Hg). Wet prep slide of discharge reveals Trichomonas infection; other culture results are negative. Fetal heart tones are normal, and fetal activity is palpated.

Assessment

Based on nursing knowledge of obstetrical, public health, and psychosocial risks, the nurse determined that the following assessments indicated need for nursing intervention:

1. History of late spontaneous abortion, violent home area, smoking by both Janice and her mother, cocaine use, and hypertension, all of which may increase the risk of vasoconstriction and inadequate blood supply to the placenta and fetus.

2. Reported alcohol and cocaine use in early pregnancy, suggesting an increased risk of fetal injury from these substances.

3. Trichomonas infection, suggesting unsafe sex practices and risks of other STDs and HIV.

4. Self-reported substance use, indicating ineffective coping strategies.

Nursing Diagnosis

Ineffective tissue perfusion (placenta) related to vasoconstriction from cigarette smoking, cocaine use, hypertension, and chronic stress.

Expected Outcomes   Maintain adequate fetal-placental perfusion, as demonstrated by appropriate fetal activity and growth; absence of drugs in maternal urine; and self-reported reduction in cigarette smoking.

Planning   Adequate perfusion demonstrated by stable activity counts and reactive non-stress tests.
Normal fetal growth demonstrated by fundal height and ultrasonography.
Reduced risk, as measured by absence of substance in urine screening sample and self-reported reduction in substance use.
Pregnancy continues to term without evidence of preterm labor or placental abruption.

(continued)

Nursing Interventions	Rationales
1. Educate about effects of nicotine, carbon monoxide from cigarettes, and neurologic and vasoconstrictive effects of cocaine in pregnancy, as well as effects of passive smoking on her and her son's health. Offer referrals to stop-smoking and substance abuse treatment programs. Provide ongoing emotional support to maintain behavior change. Engage mother and boyfriend in educational and stop-smoking programs.	1. Information about health risks along with a referral to resources are important to begin change.
2. Monitor placental function with activity counts, nonstress tests. Monitor blood pressure.	2. Monitoring the pregnancy is part of prenatal care.
3. Provide letter to employer requesting activity limitations as recommended by the American Medical Association, and follow-up with phone call, if needed.	3. Interventions may need to be taken at the workplace to facilitate a healthy environment.

Evaluation   Janice describes reduction in smoking to 5 cigarettes per day, and abstinence from alcohol and cocaine. Her partner and mother attend stop-smoking classes sporadically. Janice expresses appreciation for support from the nurse as she continues to work on making changes at home and work. Activity counts and nonstress tests are within normal limits. Blood pressure decreases to normal levels as smoking decreases. Janice denies preterm contractions, uterine pain, and vaginal bleeding.

Nursing Diagnosis

Risk for fetal injury; risk factors include prenatal alcohol and cocaine exposure.

Expected Outcomes   Minimize risk to fetus of further substance exposure, as demonstrated by Janice's understanding of the risks of drugs and alcohol use in pregnancy, her reports of abstinence from alcohol and drugs, and negative urine screening.

Planning   Client will be able to state risks to fetus of alcohol and cocaine use in pregnancy.

Alcohol and cocaine intake will stop for remainder of pregnancy, as demonstrated by negative urine screening results and client self-reporting.

Nursing Interventions	Rationales
1. Educate client and family about effects of cocaine and alcohol, as well as impairment of parenting interactions when intoxicated.	1. Knowledge of effects of substance abuse on family and parenting abilities may motivate client to modify behaviors.
2. Refer to AA or Narcotics Anonymous for peer support; refer to formal drug and alcohol treatment, if desired.	2. Education and referral provide the client the tools to make lifestyle changes.
3. Provide ongoing support and encouragement.	3. Client may be more inclined to adopt healthy behaviors if nurse is a strong supporter and change agent.
4. Discuss advantages of regular screening for substances.	4. Knowledge of the benefits of regular screening may encourage client to have frequent contact with a health care provider, resulting in better and more consistent prenatal care.
5. Provide assessment and intervention for newborn alcohol and cocaine effects, if present.	5. Continued assessment and monitoring of newborn risks allows for early intervention and treatment.

(continued)

Evaluation   Janice reports abstinence from alcohol and cocaine since the time of committing to continue the pregnancy. She attends AA meetings weekly where she has met another pregnant woman who has become a friend. Janice's boyfriend continues to drink and use drugs but not in her apartment. Ultrasonography shows no apparent anomalies.

Nursing Diagnosis

Risk for fetal and maternal infection; risk factors include maternal exposure to STDs.

Expected Outcomes   Complete treatment for current infection, consider HIV testing for self and partner, and use safer sex to prevent future infection.

Planning   Client will complete treatment for documented infection.
Client will report safer sex practices to prevent future infection.
Client will report her decision regarding HIV testing in pregnancy.

Nursing Interventions	Rationales
1. Educate client about implications of Trichomonas infection—not harmful in itself but a sign of other possible STD exposure.	1. Client needs to understand the risks and implications of STDs on her health and that of her developing fetus.
2. Provide treatment with metronidazole (safe after first trimester), and recheck for cure after completion of treatment.	2. Complete course of medication is effective in fighting the infections.
3. Discuss with client and partner importance of safer sex practices and merits of testing for HIV and other STDs. Advise partner to be treated.	3. Treatments will be most effective if involved partner also undergoes treatment and therapy.

Evaluation   Janice reports she took all medication. Repeat testing is negative for Trichomonas infection. Boyfriend obtained medication, but Janice is unsure about his completion of therapy. Janice reports she has insisted on condom use since learning of risks of STDs in pregnancy. Other STD tests and HIV test are negative. Boyfriend has not yet agreed to HIV testing.

Nursing Diagnosis

Ineffective coping related to lack of alternatives to harmful substances, environmental prevalence of substance use, fatigue, and lack of social support.

Expected Outcomes   Replace ineffective coping strategies (substance use) with alternative activities.

Planning   Client will demonstrate abstinence from substance use or progress toward abstinence and can describe alternative methods of coping with fatigue and stress.

Nursing Interventions	Rationales
1. Provide reading materials and refer for counseling to uncover alternative means of recreation and relaxation such as walking, movies, games, playing with her son, and naps in late afternoon while grandmother watches her son.	1. Client may need help in identifying alternatives to substance use as a means of recreation; activities that involve her son and family may help strengthen family bonds.
2. Discuss new sources of social support such as women's groups, religious groups, family, or clubs.	2. Offering client an array of choices will allow her to choose those options most appealing to her, thereby increasing the likelihood of compliance.

(continued)

Evaluation Janice remains abstinent from all substances except cigarettes. She has found a friend at a local AA meeting held in a church. She and her son have discovered friends at a playground of a local public library and have begun to go there in the evenings. She describes some distance between herself and her boyfriend but hopes that he will see the benefit of this healthier lifestyle.

can be done on a large scale to improve public health. More stringent federal and state policies for industrial waste emission and cleanup of toxic waste hazards are needed. Public education about safe food products and food preparation should be promoted by nurses. Nurses can advocate for safe housing for even the poorest residents of their communities to reduce stress from neighborhood violence and drug commerce, the risk of lead poisoning from unsafe paint, and the risk of infection from substandard water supplies.

A major area for nursing advocacy is that of federal policies for family work leave and work modification for pregnant and parenting women. Paid leave for the last 2 months of pregnancy and first 6 months postpartum is common in other industrialized nations, as is subsidized or free child care. Pregnant women should be able to change their job responsibilities during pregnancy to reduce risk without loss of income or fear of losing their jobs completely. Such family-friendly policies promote the health of mothers and children, reduce the risk of low birth weight, and foster strong and nurturing family bonds while maintaining financial stability.

Web Activities

• Visit some of the government web sites listed in this chapter. Can you locate specific information regarding avoiding hazards in pregnancy? Do these sites also contain guidelines for health professionals who counsel pregnant women and their families?

• Choose a specific toxin discussed in this chapter and search the web for information on its effects on a developing fetus.

Key Concepts

• Many substances found in air, soil, food, and water, as well as prescribed and over-the-counter medications, have potential effects on fetal development.

• A pregnant woman's living conditions, geographic location, work environment, and neighborhood activities can increase fetal risks. Neighborhood violence, proximity to chemical wastes, or isolation from adequate health care can create hazards and stressors while reducing a woman's ability to obtain help.

• Behaviors such as substance abuse may be hazardous to the developing fetus. Alcohol and tobacco use are responsible for widespread fetal risks.

• Nursing assessment of the pregnant woman must include careful and sensitive history-taking to reveal potential pregnancy risk in her neighborhood,

home, work environment and activity, and personal behavior.

• Pregnant women must be educated to avoid all medications until advised by a health professional. They also can be reassured that most food additives are not harmful. Preconceptual counseling is important for women who must take medications to control chronic illnesses.

• Ongoing support and monitoring by the nurse will help pregnant women maintain a low-risk environment for fetal development. Lifestyle changes for substance users are difficult to make; outside support from counselors, social service workers, substance abuse treatment professionals, and others can assist the pregnant woman.

Review Questions and Activities

1. Contact the Environmental Protection Agency and the Centers for Disease Control and Prevention. Obtain information about potential hazards in your geographic area, including industrial wastes currently being discharged into the environment, toxic waste storage areas or contaminated land, and infection sources. Create a poster for a prenatal clinic to educate women and their families about local risk and how to protect themselves.

2. Visit a local factory or hospital. Ask for information on hazardous substances in that work environment. Prepare an educational pamphlet for pregnant woman in that work setting.

3. Visit an AA meeting. (Some are specified as open, and others may be limited to clients who abuse substances or restricted to specific members.) Note the personal circumstances and family histories of persons who disclose their past experiences. Analyze the difficulties and obstacles to substance abuse recovery. Explore other local resources for pregnant women who want to begin recovery from substance abuse.

4. Research the safety of use during pregnancy of medications commonly prescribed for chronic illnesses such as hypertension, asthma, epilepsy, diabetes, or multiple sclerosis. Use local teratology hotlines. Develop a guideline for nurses caring for this group of patients to advise them of which medications are safe and which may need alteration or substitution during pregnancy.

5. Prepare a travel advisory for pregnant women who plan to go to a particular tropical nation. Explore the tropical diseases prevalent in that area. Using reference materials, list the safe vaccinations and other recommendations for pregnant women to avoid infection.

References

Alexy, B., Nichols, B., Heverly, M., & Garzon, L. (1997). Prenatal factors and birth outcomes in the public health service: A rural/urban comparison. *Research in Nursing & Health, 20,* 61–70.

AMA Council on Scientific Affairs. (1984). Effects of pregnancy on work performance. *Journal of the American Medical Association, 251,* 1995–1997.

American Nurses Association. (1996). *Compendium of ANA position statements.* Washington, DC: American Nurses Association.

Aschengrau, A., Zierler, S., & Cohen, A. (1993). Quality of maternal drinking water and the occurrence of late adverse pregnancy outcomes. *Archives of Environmental Health, 48,* 105–113.

Azuma, S., & Chasnoff, I. (1993). Outcome of children prenatally exposed to cocaine and other drugs: A path analysis of three-year data. *Pediatrics, 92,* 396–402.

Bajaj, J., Misra, A., Rajalakshmi, M., & Madan, R. (1993). Environmental release of chemicals and reproductive ecology. *Environmental Health Perspectives, 101 suppl. 2,* 125–130.

Bateman, D., Ng, S., Hansen, C., & Heagarty, M. (1993). The effects of intrauterine cocaine exposure in newborns. *American Journal of Public Health, 83,* 190–193.

Bertin, J. (1994). Reproductive hazards in the workplace: Lessons from UAW vs. Johnson Controls. In H. Needleman & D. Bellinger, Eds. *Prenatal exposure to toxicants: Developmental consequences* (pp. 297–316). Baltimore: Johns Hopkins University Press.

Boettcher, J. (1993). Promoting maternal-infant health in rural communities: The Rural Health Outreach Program. *Nursing Clinics of North America, 28,* 199–209.

Brett, K., Strogatz, F., & Savitz, F. (1997). Employment, job strain, and preterm delivery among women in North Carolina. *American Journal of Public Health, 87,* 199–204.

Briggs, G. (1995). Teratogenicity and drugs in breast milk. In L. Y. Young & M. Koda-Kimble, Eds., *Applied therapeutics: The clinical use of drugs* (6th ed.) (pp. 45/1–45/39). Vancouver, WA: Applied Therapeutics.

Buchi, K., Varner, M., & Chase, R. (1993). The prevalence of substance abuse among pregnant women in Utah. *Obstetrics and Gynecology, 81,* 239–242.

Bullard, R. (1994). *Unequal protection: Environmental justice and communities of color,* New York: Random House.

Carcillo, J., Diegel, J., Bartman, B., Guyer, F., & Kramer, S. (1995). Improved maternal and child health access in a rural community. *Journal of Health Care for the Poor and Underserved, 6,* 23–40.

CDC (Centers for Disease Control and Prevention). (1996, September). *Sexually transmitted disease surveillance 1995.* Atlanta, GA: Division of STD Prevention, CDC, U.S. Department of Health and Human Services, Public Health Service. Also available online at www.cdc.gov.

CDC Fact Sheet. (1996). *Mother-to-child HIV transmission decreases in the US but challenges remain for perinatal prevention.* Online at www.cdc.gov.

Colie, C. (1993). Male-mediated teratogenesis. *Reproductive Toxicology, 7,* 30–9.

Conover, E. (1994). Hazardous exposures during pregnancy. *Journal of Obstetric, Gynecologic, and Neonatal Nursing, 23,* 524–532.

Cook, D., Peacock, J., Feyerabend, C., Carey, I., Jarvis, M., Anderson, H., & Bland, J. (1996). Relation of caffeine intake and blood caffeine concentrations during pregnancy to fetal growth: Prospective population-based study. *British Medical Journal, 313,* 1358–1362.

Copeland, D., Replogle, W., Meeks, G., Morrison, J., Pittman, K., & Crane, S. (1993). An assessment of obstetric services in Mississippi. *Journal of the Mississippi State Medical Association, 34 (5),* 143–146.

Ellard, G., Johnstone, F., Prescott, R., Ji-Xian, W., Jian-Hua, M. (1996). Smoking during pregnancy: The dose dependence of birth weight deficits. *British Medical Journal, 103,* 806–813.

English, P., Eskenazi, B., & Christianson, R. (1994). African American-Caucasian differences in serum cotinine levels among pregnant women and subsequent effects on infant birthweight. *American Journal of Public Health, 84,* 1439–1443.

Fenster, L., Hubbard, A., Windham, G., Waller, K., & Swan, S. (1997). A prospective study of work-related physical exertion and spontaneous abortion. *Epidemiology, 8,* 66–74.

Food and Drug Administration [FDA]. (1992). Food additives. Washington, DC: International Food Information Council Brochure. Also online at www.fda.gov.

Foulke, J. (1994). Mercury in fish: Cause for concern? *FDA Consumer,* online at www.fda.gov.

Foulke, J. (1997). Lead threat lessens, but mugs pose problem. *FDA Consumer,* online at www.fda.gov.

Fox, S., Koepsell, T., & Daling, J. (1994). Birth weight and smoking during pregnancy: Effects modification by maternal age. *American Journal of Epidemiology, 139,* 1008–1015.

Frontier Nursing Service. (1997). At website www.barefoot.com/fns/.

Garry, V., Schreinemachers, D., Harkins, M., & Griffith, J. (1996). Pesticide appliers, biocides, and birth defects in rural Minnesota. *Environmental Health Perspectives, 104,* 394–399.

Gold, E., & Tomich, E. (1994). Occupational hazards to fertility and pregnancy outcome. *Occupational Medicine: State of the Art Reviews, 9,* 435–469.

Henderson, D., Boyd, C., & Mieczkowski, T. (1994). Gender, relationships, and crack cocaine: A content analysis. *Research in Nursing & Health, 17,* 265–272.

Hickey, C., Cliver, S., Mulvihill, F., McNeal, S., Hoffman, H., & Goldenberg, R. (1995). Employment-related stress and preterm delivery: A contextual examination. *Public Health Reports, 11,* 410–418.

Hueston, W. (1995). Prenatal care and low birth weight rates in urban and rural Wisconsin. *Journal of the American Board of Family Practice, 8,* 17–21.

Kearney, M. (1995). Damned if you do, damned if you don't: Crack cocaine users and prenatal care. *Contemporary Drug Problems, 22,* 639–662.

Kuvacic, I., Skrablin, S., Hodzic, D., & Milkovic, G. (1996). Possible influence of expatriation on perinatal outcome. *Acta Obstetricia et Gynecologica Scandinavica, 75,* 367–371.

Landisbergis, P., & Hatch, M. (1996). Psychosocial work stress and pregnancy-induced hypertension. *Epidemiology, 7,* 346–351.

Lawrance, L., & Gruchow, H. (1996). Adequacy of prenatal care and pregnancy outcomes in cigarette smoking and nonsmoking mothers. *Journal of Women's Health, 5,* 609–614.

Lieberman, E., Gremy, I., Lang, J., & Cohen, A. (1994). Low birthweight at term and the timing of fetal exposure to maternal smoking. *American Journal of Public Health, 84,* 1127–1131.

Lumey, L., Stein, A., & Ravelli, A. (1995). Timing of prenatal starvation in women and birthweight in their first and second born offspring: The Dutch Famine Birth Cohort Study. *European Journal of Obstetrics, Gynecology, and Reproductive Biology, 61,* 23–30.

Makhseed, M., el-Tomi, N., Moussa, M., & Musini, V. (1996). Postwar changes in the outcome of pregnancy in Maternity Hospital, Kuwait. *Medicine, Conflict, and Survival, 12,* 154–167.

Matte, T., Mulinare, J., & Erickson, J. (1993). Case-control study of congenital defects and parental employment in health care. *American Journal of Industrial Medicine, 24,* 11–23.

Muratova, R., Zhilenko, M., Iakovlevna, N., Aleksandrova, A., Tsvetaeva, T., Karlin, N., & Sukhov, V. (1994). Perinatal care for the fetus is women exposed to ionizing radiation after the Chernobyl nuclear plant accident. *Meditsina Truda I Promyshlennaia Ekologiia, 10,* 25–27 (English abstract).

Needleman, H., & Bellinger, D., Eds. (1994). *Prenatal exposure to toxicants; Developmental consequences.* Baltimore: Johns Hopkins University Press.

Office of Technology Assessment (1985). *Reproductive hazards in the workplace.* Washington, DC: Government Printing Office.

Peacock, J., Bland, J., & Anderson, H. (1995). Preterm delivery: Effects of socioeconomic factors, psychological stress, smoking, alcohol, and caffeine. *British Medical Journal, 311,* 531–535.

Persaud, T. (1990). *Environmental causes of human birth defects.* Springfield, IL: Charles C. Thomas.

Poerksen, A., & Petitti, D. (1991). Employment and low birth weight in African American women. *Social Science & Medicine, 33,* 1281–1286.

Raman-Wilms, L., Tseng, A., Wighart, S., Einarson, T., & Koren, G. (1995). Fetal genital effects of first-trimester sex hormone exposure: A meta-analysis. *Obstetrics and Gynecology, 85,* 141–149.

Rayburn, F., & Conover, E. (1993). Non-prescription drugs and pregnancy. In J. Studd (Ed.). *Progress in obstetrics and gynecology, vol. 10* (pp 101–109). Edinburgh: Churchill Livingstone.

Richardson, G., Conroy, M., & Day, N. (1996). Prenatal cocaine exposure: Effects on the development of school-age children. *Neurotoxicology and Teratology, 18,* 627–634.

Richardson, G., Day, N., & Goldschmidt, L. (1995). Prenatal alcohol, marijuana, and tobacco use: Infant mental and motor development. *Neurotoxicology and Teratology, 17,* 479–487.

Rofe, Y., & Goldberg, J. (1983). Prolonged exposure to a war environment and its effects on the blood pressure of pregnant women. *British Journal of Medical Psychology, 56 (pt. 4),* 305–311.

Rose, N., & Mennuti, M. (1994). Periconceptual folate supplementation and neural tube defects. *Clinical Obstetrics and Gynecology, 37,* 605–620.

Schenker, E., & Mor-Yosef, S. (1993). Did anxiety during the Gulf War cause premature delivery? *Military Medicine, 158,* 789–791.

Sever, L. (1994). Congenital malformations related to occupational reproductive hazards. *Occupational Medicine: State of the Art Reviews, 9,* 471–494.

Sever, L., Arbuckle, T., & Sweeney, A. (1997). Reproductive and developmental effects of occupational pesticide exposure: The epidemiological evidence. *Occupational Medicine: State of the Art Reviews, 12,* 305–325.

Shu, X., Hatch, M., Mills, J., Clemens, J., & Susser, M. (1995). Maternal smoking, alcohol drinking, caffeine consumption, and fetal growth: Results from a prospective study. *Epidemiology, 6,* 115–120.

Simic, S., Idrizbegovic, S., Jaganjac, N., Boloban, H., Puvacic, J., Gallic, A., & Dekovic, S. (1995). Nutritional effects of the siege on newborn babies in Sarajevo. *European Journal of Clinical Nutrition, 49 (suppl 2),* S33–S36.

Simpson, J. (1993). Are physical activity and employment related to preterm birth and low birth weight? *American Journal of Obstetrics and Gynecology, 168,* 1231–1238.

Spinillo, A., Capuzzo, E., Baltaro, F., Paizza, G., Nicola, S., & Iasci, A. (1996). The effect of work activity in pregnancy on the risk of fetal growth retardation. *Acta Obstetricia et Gynecologica Scandinavica, 75,* 531–536.

Stanhope, M., & Lancaster, J. (1996). *Community health nursing: Promoting health of aggregates, families, and individuals* (4th e). St. Louis: Mosby.

Stotts, A., DiClemente, C., Carbonari, J., & Mullen, P. (1996). Pregnancy smoking cessation: a case of mistaken identity. *Addictive Behaviors, 21,* 459–471.

Streissguth, A., Barr, H., Sampson, P., & Bookstein, F. (1997). Prenatal alcohol and offspring development: The first fourteen years. *Drug and Alcohol Dependence, 36,* 89–99.

Sweet, R., & Gibbs, R. (1995). *Infectious diseases of the female genital tract.* Baltimore: Williams & Wilkins.

Szasz, A. (1994). *Ecopopulism: Toxic waste and the movement for environmental justice.* Minneapolis: University of Minnesota Press.

Vaughn, A., Carzoli, R., Sanchez-Ramos, L., Murphy, S., Khan, N., & Chiu, T. (1993). Community-wide estimation of illicit drug use in delivering women: Prevalence, demographics, and associated risk factors. *Obstetrics & Gynecology, 82,* 92–96.

Walsh, R., Redman, S., & Adamson, L. (1996). The accuracy of self-report of smoking status in pregnant women. *Addictive Behaviors, 5,* 675–679.

Weathers, W., Crane, M., Sauvain, K., Blackhurst, D. (1993). Cocaine use in women from a defined population: Prevalence at delivery and effects on growth of infants. *Pediatrics, 91,* 350–354.

Wolfe, W., Michalek, J., Miner, J., Rahe, A., Moore, C., Needham, L., & Patterson, D. (1995). Paternal serum dioxin and reproductive outcomes among veterans of Operation Ranch Hand. *Epidemiology, 6,* 17–22.

Yoles, I., Hod, M., Kaplan, B., & Ovadia, J. (1993). Fetal "fright-bradycardia" brought on by air-raid alarm in Israel. *International Journal of Gynaecology and Obstetrics, 40,* 157–160.

Young, N. (1997). Effects of alcohol and other drugs on children. *Journal of Psychoactive Drugs, 29,* 23–42.

Zapata, C., Rebolledo, A., Atalah, E., Newman, B., & King, M. (1992). The influence of social and political violence on the risk of pregnancy complications. *American Journal of Public Health, 82,*685–690.

Suggested Readings

Briggs, G., Ed. (1994). *Drugs in pregnancy and lactation: A guide to fetal and neonatal risk.* Baltimore: Williams & Wilkins. (A comprehensive reference on drug safety in pregnancy and breastfeeding)

Dorris, M. (1989). *The broken cord.* New York: Harper and Row. (A nonfiction account of an adopted child with fetal alcohol syndrome)

Lipson, A., Collins, F., & Webster, W. (1993). Multiple congenital defects associated with maternal use of topical tretinoin. *Lancet, 341,* 1352–1353.

Paul, M. (1992). *Occupational and environmental hazards: A guide for clinicians.* Baltimore: Williams & Wilkins. (A review of known risks in workplace and environment)

Reinarman, C., & Levine, H. (1989). Crack in context: Politics and media in the making of a drug scare. *Contemporary Drug Problems, 16,* 535–577. (A thought-provoking analysis of the influence of politics on public awareness of drug use)

Resources

Videotape:

"A Challenge to Care: Strategies to Help Chemically Dependent Women and their Children." Association for Women's Health, Obstetric, and Neonatal Nursing (AWHONN), 1990.

Accessible on the Worldwide Web:

Association for Women's Health, Obstetric, and Neonatal Nursing (AWHONN), www.awhonn.org

Centers for Disease Control and Prevention (CDC), www.cac.gov

Food and Drug Administration (FDA), www.fda.gov

Environmental Protection Agency (EPA), www.epa.gov

National Institute for Occupational Safety and Health (NIOSH), www.ede.gov/niosh

TOXNET: National Library of Medicine database of toxicology research, www.nlm.nih.gov/databases/

Telephone Resources:

Teratology Information Services: Hotlines for clinicians are available in each geographic area.

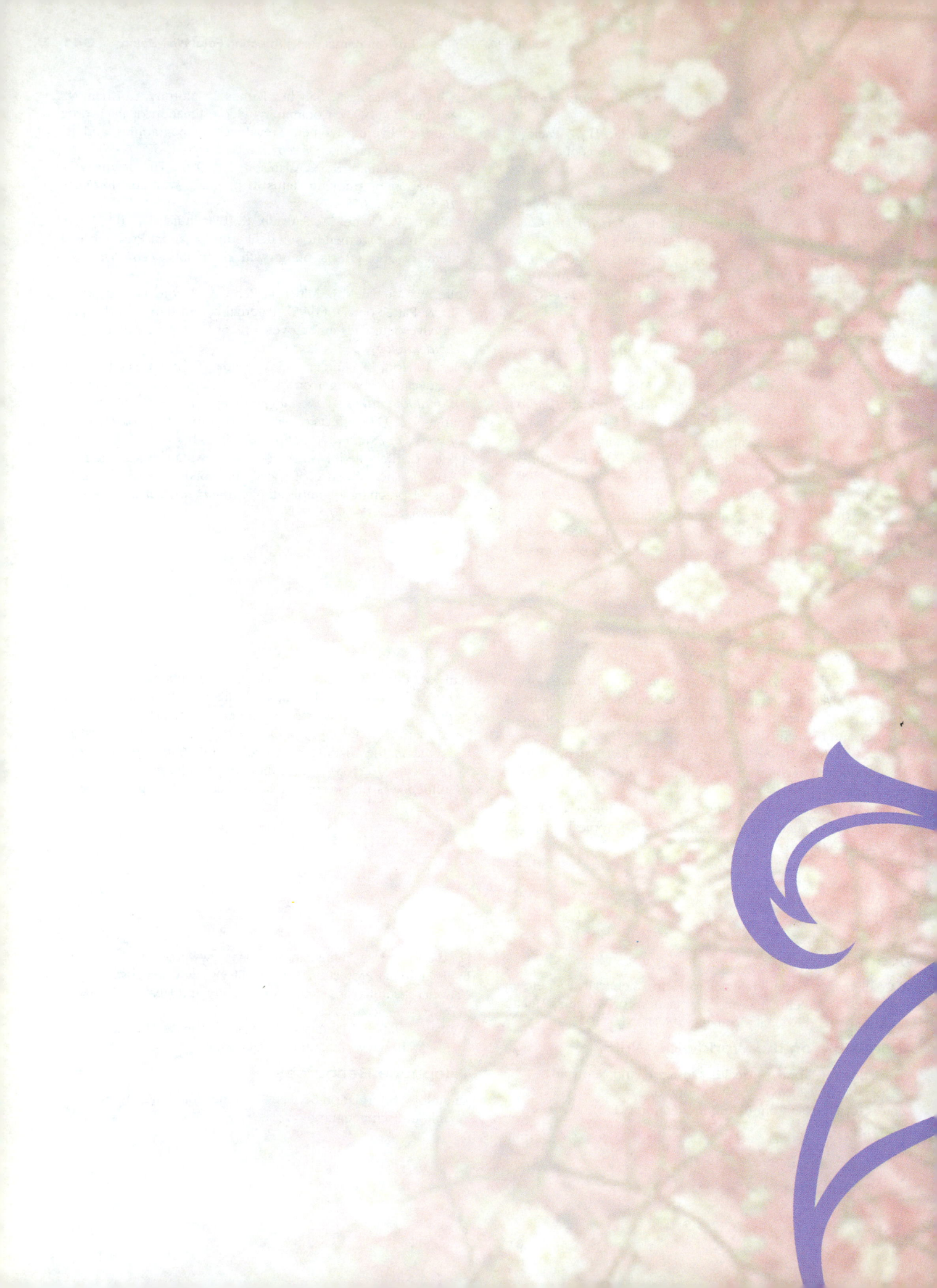

CHAPTER 22

Evaluation of Fetal Well-Being

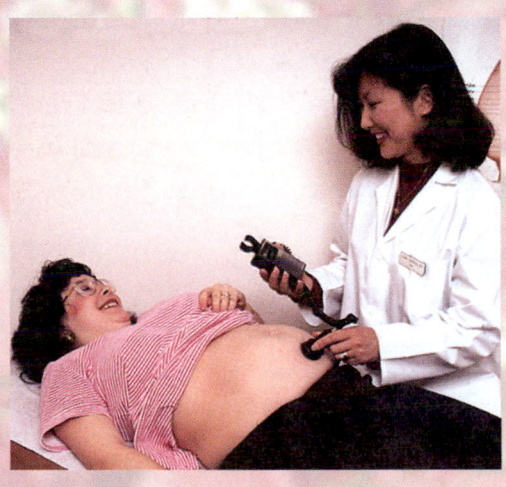

Kristen is a 40-year-old woman who has been married to Jack for 6 months. This is a second marriage for both Kristen and Jack. Kristen has three children (aged 14, 11, and 8 years) from her previous marriage, and Jack has two teenagers with his first wife. Kristen was diagnosed with Crohn's disease five years ago. She has been experiencing irregular and infrequent menstrual cycles for the past 3 years. She was advised that in view of her chronic bowel disease and family history she was most probably experiencing premature menopause.

Kristen began to experience extreme fatigue and urinary frequency. She visited her primary care physician and, much to her surprise, discovered she was approximately 14 weeks pregnant. After the initial shock, Kristen and Jack were very happy. They viewed this pregnancy as a gift and a sign of their everlasting love and life together.

As part of her prenatal laboratory testing, maternal serum–α-fetoprotein (MS-AFP) and estriol levels were measured. When the results were returned, the MS-AFP level was low. Kristen was informed that this finding indicated that she was at greater than average risk for carrying a fetus with Down syndrome. Kristen was advised to have an amniocentesis for karyotyping of the fetus and a definitive diagnosis of whether or not the fetus had an extra chromosome 21.

Kristen and Jack were greatly distressed. Kristen states she could never have her pregnancy terminated, no matter what the test indicates, and Jack is supportive of her position. The physician is strongly advocating for an amniocentesis stating, "We need to know what we are dealing with." Finally, Kristen tearfully says, "I wish I never had that blood test!"

Key Terms

Amniocentesis
Biophysical profile (BPP)
Chorionic villus sampling (CVS)
Contraction stress test (CST)
Doppler blood studies

Fetal fibronectin (fFN) testing
Fetal movement counting (FMC)
Fetal tissue sampling
Human chorionic gonadotropin (hCG)

Human placental lactogen (hPL)
Magnetic resonance imaging (MRI)
Maternal serum–alpha-fetoprotein (MS-AFP)
Nonstress test (NST)

Percutaneous umbilical blood sampling (PUBS)
Ultrasonography

Competencies

Upon completion of this chapter, the reader should be able to:

1. Discuss the clinical applications of ultrasonography.
2. Identify the role of the nurse in the evaluation of fetal well-being.
3. Identify the criteria for interpreting a nonstress test.
4. Explain fetal diagnostic techniques to families.
5. Differentiate between screening and diagnostic procedures.
6. Describe three procedures used to identify genetic alterations during pregnancy.
7. Teach the client how to perform fetal movement counts.
8. Describe a method to evaluate fetal maturity.

Technology and science have become prominent components of obstetrical care. Technology can provide useful information about the status of the pregnancy and condition of the fetus; however, it is imperative to balance technologic capabilities with responsiveness to the human needs of the woman and her family. Many of the fetal evaluation techniques described in this chapter are performed in outpatient settings. In addition, many of these procedures, especially those performed during the first half of pregnancy, are technically oriented and have minimal direct care responsibilities for the nurse during the procedure itself. However, the nurse does have a major role in identifying, preparing, counseling, supporting, and educating clients regarding the implementation and understanding of fetal evaluation throughout the period of gestation. Fetal evaluation is an interdisciplinary endeavor involving physicians, sonographers, laboratory technicians, and nurses. However, the nurse often is the only care provider who can establish a therapeutic and holistic relationship with the client and who has the opportunity to interact with the client before, during, and after the procedure. Consequently, nurses need to have a complete knowledge base of fetal diagnostic and screening technologies; the disease processes that warrant fetal evaluation; and the meaning of the findings of these procedures to the woman, the pregnancy, and the family. The counseling, support, and education provided by the nurse are vital interventions to assist the woman during the experience of fetal evaluation.

EVALUATION OF FETAL WELL-BEING

A variety of diagnostic techniques and monitoring parameters are used to evaluate *fetal well-being,* that is, the growth and health of the developing fetus as well as its ability to tolerate the physiologic stresses of pregnancy, labor, and birth. Fetal development is a complex and, at times, mysterious process. The introduction of fetal evaluation technologies has allowed health care providers to peer into the intrauterine environment and gather data related to some of the mysteries of fetal growth and development. Fetal surveillance techniques have dramatically affected the understanding of fetal anatomy, physiology, and behavior. In addition, technologic advances have facilitated the ability to diagnose anatomic abnormalities, growth failure, and the potential for fetal hypoxia and neonatal sequelae. The rapid growth of technologic advances in evaluating fetal conditions, however, has introduced the possibility of the use of such technology without a comparable level of knowledge of its effects and implications.

The average duration of human pregnancy is 40 weeks, or 280 days after the first day of the last menstrual period. The gestational period typically is divided into the period of the embryo (the first 8 weeks) and the period of the fetus (9 weeks to birth). The embryonic period is a time of growth, differentiation, and organization of the cellular components of the developing being. During the embryonic period, evaluation is done primarily to assess for normal implantation, viability, and abnormalities with a genetic base. By the end of the 8th week of gestation, all body systems are present in at least a rudimentary form. During the remainder of the gestational period, the fetal period, these rudimentary body systems grow, change, and evolve into specialized tissues and organs in preparation for existence outside the uterus. During this period of pregnancy fetal well-being can be assessed and monitored using a number of biochemical, physical, and physiologic surveillance techniques.

Routine assessment of fetal well-being has included intermittent auscultation of fetal heart rate, measurement of fundal height, and maternal perception of fetal movement. These parameters provide indirect measures of fetal condition (Figure 22-1). As knowledge about the causes of fetal compromise has grown and technology has progressed, however, three areas of particular concern to

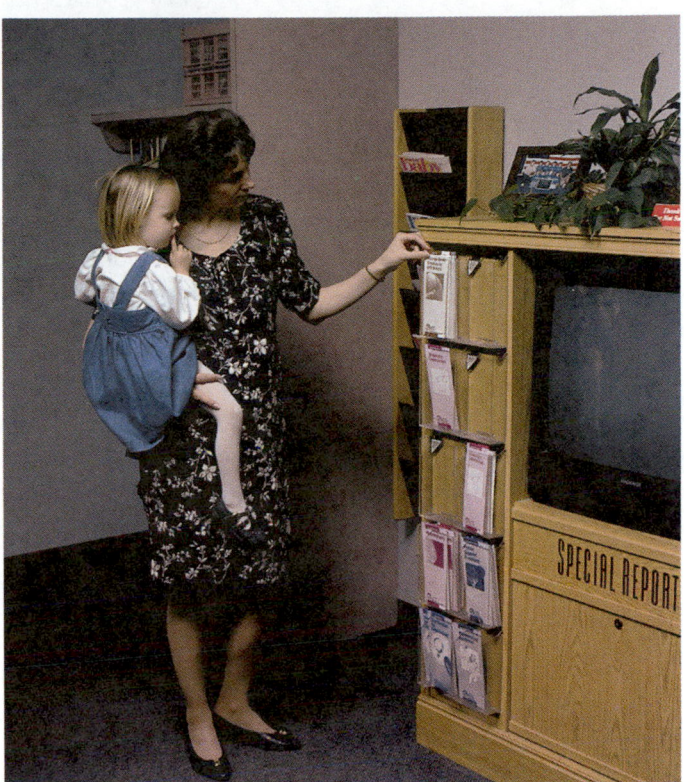

Figure 22-1 Literature should be made available to the expectant parents who will be undergoing fetal evaluation testing. The nurse should also help the client understand and interpret information and be ready to answer questions.

nurses regarding fetal surveillance techniques have emerged: purpose, process, and consequences.

Purpose

We examine the purposes of the proposed fetal evaluation technologies: for use as diagnostic testing, screening procedures, and reassurance procedures. Some of the testing modalities described in this chapter are diagnostic, for example, amniocentesis and chorionic villus sampling for determination of chromosomal complement. Diagnostic testing modalities confirm the presence or absence of a specific condition. Other testing modalities are screening procedures to identify clients at greater risk of having a condition than the general population. These screening procedures identify a fetus as being at greater risk than other fetuses but do not confirm or rule out the condition in either group. Examples of screening procedures used during the prenatal period are MS-AFP and fetal fibronectin measurements. Thus, a positive finding that results from one of the screening technologies opens the door to further use of fetal evaluation technologies in attempts to obtain diagnostic data. A third group of evaluation technologies is reassurance procedures. These procedures

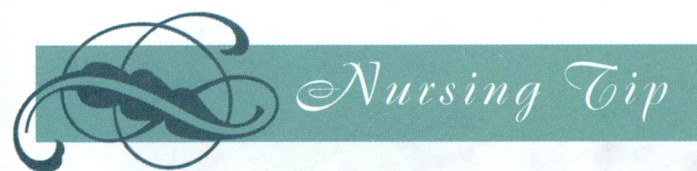

PRENATAL SCREENING

When considering whether prenatal screening should be done, ask the following questions:

1. Is the screening procedure justified in this population?

2. What is the risk to the pregnancy?

3. What is the risk to the woman?

4. What will the results reveal about the status of the pregnancy?

5. Which options are available to the woman and her family if the results indicate increased risk?

6. Which resources are available to support the woman and her family?

include the nonstress test. This test provides data predictive of fetal health and well-being; however, when the results are abnormal, no concrete evidence of danger to the fetus is provided. The client must understand the purpose or goal of a particular fetal evaluation technology in order to provide consent to undergo the procedure.

Fetal surveillance procedures should be considered for women with one or more of the following risk factors: maternal age over 35 years; a family history of chromosomal anomaly; carrier status, including a balanced translocation; and an X-linked disorder or an autosomal recessive trait. Table 22-1 outlines certain risk factors and the related recommended assessment techniques. Prenatal determination of fetal gender is a valid indication for prenatal surveillance only when the possibility exists of the presence of an X-linked disorder.

Process

We discuss the process of implementing the chosen fetal evaluation technology. The overriding goal of fetal evaluation is to obtain information about the growth, development, and well-being of the fetus; however, it is impossible to do so without invading the woman's bodily

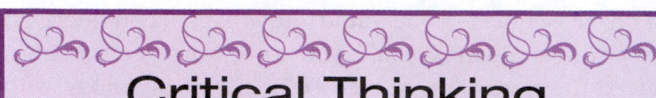

Critical Thinking

Gender Selection

How do you respond to a 36-year-old client (gravida 6, para 5) (all boys) who tells you she wants genetic testing done because if this baby is not a girl, she wants to terminate the pregnancy.

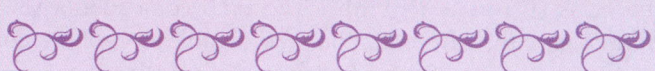

integrity. Whether it is drawing blood, obtaining amniotic fluid, or placing a transducer on the abdomen, the woman is physically impacted during the implementation of fetal evaluation. Consequently, the rights and autonomy of the woman as an individual are potentially in opposition to the rights and well-being of the fetus. Therefore, the decision by the client to undergo prenatal surveillance procedures requires careful consideration of the prevalence and severity of the condition under investigation, the sensitivity and specificity of the testing modality, and the economic

Table 22-1 Assessment for Increased Risk of a Genetic Disorder

Risk Factors	Related Risks	Assessment Techniques
Maternal age	At the age of 35, the risk of fetal loss from invasive prenatal testing equals the risk of having a child with a chromosomal anomaly.	Collection of demographic data Interview and general survey
Ethnic background	Certain genetic diseases are found in populations with a specific ethnic background, e.g., • Tay-Sachs disease: Eastern European Jews • Thalassemia: Mediterranean descent • Sickle cell trait: African Americans	Interview Pedigree or genogram to analyze patterns
Family history	The presence of certain diseases (hemophilia, Huntington's chorea, and cystic fibrosis), birth defects (neural tube defects and abdominal wall defects), or mental retardation in the family history increases the risk for future offspring.	Careful family history Pedigree or genogram to analyze patterns
Reproductive history	Previous poor perinatal outcomes, e.g., • Stillbirths • Repeated spontaneous abortions • Children with birth defects or disorders	Careful family history Medical record review
Maternal disease	Some diseases have the increased risk of transmission from mother to fetus.	Careful review of past medical history, current health status, and medication ingestion
Environmental hazards	Exposure to chemicals, radiation, hot tubs, nutrition, or other potential teratogens	Behavior evaluation Preconception education about hazard exposure

Table 22-2 Types of Fetal Surveillance Procedures		
Screening	**Diagnostic**	**Reassurance**
Estriol	Amniocentesis	Nonstress test
Human chorionic gonadatropin	Chorionic villus sampling	Contraction stress test
Maternal serum–alpha-fetoprotein	Percutaneous umbilical blood sampling	Biophysical profile
Human placental lactogen	Fetal tissue sampling	Fetal movement counting
Fetal fibronectin screening	Fetal cell isolation	

and emotional costs. Table 22-2 provides an overview of the types of fetal surveillance procedures available.

Providing an explanation of the procedure and its risks, benefits, and implications from the perspective of the woman as well as from that of the fetus is important. The nurse needs to be a nondirective counselor, committed to helping the client make a well-informed decision. It is the client who should decide if she wants to have the pregnancy screened or the fetus tested. It is also the client who should decide which actions should be taken based on the results of these tests. The woman and her family need a clear and thorough explanation of all the problems and potential outcomes of the current pregnancy. They then need to examine the information in view of their

personal, social, religious, cultural, and familial beliefs and values. The client needs time to think carefully about the potentially serious implications of pregnancy screening and fetal testing, without feeling pressured to make a decision.

Attention to maternal physical and emotional well-being is equally important in evaluating fetal or uterine response to evaluation technologies. For example, the following should be considered in deciding to initiate fetal evaluation procedures and in selecting specific evaluation modalities:

- Comparison of the specific differential procedures and risks of termination of a first- versus a second-trimester pregnancy.
- The impact of a procedure-induced loss of pregnancy compared with the risk of having a child that is not affected by a specific condition.
- The risk of maternal physical or psychological injury from the procedure.
- The resources available to provide support to the client and family who may experience a loss.

The nurse often is in the position of being the client's advocate and is a key person in assisting the client in

REFLECTIONS FROM A NURSE

"My client, Svetlana, received early and consistent prenatal care. She had no complications during her pregnancy. She had a CVS and two ultrasound examinations, and she performed daily fetal movement counts from 28 weeks on. All test results were within normal parameters. When her infant was born, however, he had a rare congenital anomaly. Svetlana and her family were devastated, and as her primary nurse, I was surprised and saddened. She and her family asked again and again, 'How can this happen?'"

Critical Thinking

Client Preparation for Fetal Evaluation

When preparing a client for fetal evaluation procedures, be sure you are prepared to respond to all of the following questions:

- Why is the procedure being done?
- Is the procedure safe?
- How accurate is the test?
- What information will the test provide?
- Who will preform the procedure?
- Is any physical preparation necessary?
- What does the procedure involve?
- How much time will the test take?
- What will I feel?
- What is the recovery time after the procedure?
- Who will interpret the results?
- When will I be informed of the results?
- Who will talk with me about the results?
- Who will answer my questions and address my concerns about the test and the results?
- What other options are available?

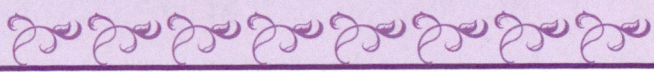

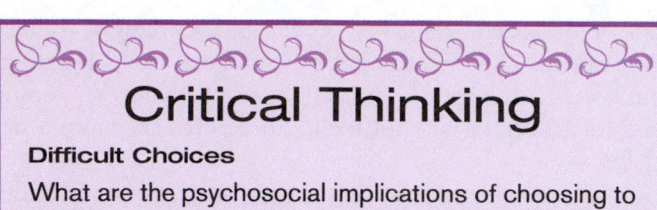

Critical Thinking

Difficult Choices

What are the psychosocial implications of choosing to have prenatal diagnosis and the implied consideration of pregnancy termination on the development of family bonds and trusting relationships?

accessing and synthesizing the information necessary to make decisions. Also, as with any technical procedure, it is incumbent on the nurse to ensure that the appropriate equipment and resources are available in the event a complication necessitating emergency intervention arises.

Consequences

We discuss the consequences of fetal evaluation technologies. As with any procedure that generates information, one must think about how that information will be used. Information can have both positive and negative implications. Information obtained from fetal evaluation technologies may significantly alter the course of a pregnancy. Based on the information obtained from fetal evaluation technologies, women are faced with choices about terminating the pregnancy, pursuing fetal therapy or intrauterine surgical procedures, waiting and accepting the test results, or hoping the test was wrong. There are no right answers, and even more questions will arise as technology continues to advance. These questions and the consequences of each option need to be explored in a knowledgeable and supportive environment.

Considering the consequences of fetal evaluation when a problem is detected is as important as considering the impact of fetal evaluation when the postulate condition is not confirmed. A "good" result from fetal evaluation technologies can result in a false sense of security. Fetal evaluation technologies do provide data about a wide variety of fetal conditions; however, many other conditions and factors exist that can impact pregnancy outcome. Fetal evaluation does not guarantee a perfect baby; it only provides data that confirm the presence or absence of a specific condition for which the testing modality was searching (Raines, 1996).

GENETIC AND BIOCHEMICAL EVALUATION

Prenatal evaluation has become increasingly important since the development of amniocentesis in the 1950s. The concept underlying genetic and biochemical testing is the application of biochemical techniques to fetal tissue or cells as a means of detecting potentially harmful alterations. These alterations may be genetic, such as alterations in chromosomal number, change in molecular structure, metabolic deviation, and hematologic variation (Table 22-3). Biochemical analysis also can provide information related to fetal maturity and placental function that, in turn, can provide the critical data needed to develop a therapeutic treatment plan for managing a high-risk pregnancy. Genetic and biochemical evaluation of pregnancy status can be grouped into invasive fetal diagnostic studies and maternal serum studies.

Invasive Fetal Diagnostic Studies

Invasive fetal procedures involve violating the integrity of the fetal-placental-uterine environment and include amniocentesis, chorionic villus sampling, percutaneous umbilical blood sampling, and other tests. These studies facilitate direct testing of fetal tissues and byproducts. Invasive fetal diagnostic studies can identify a number of fetal conditions. These diagnostic tests are the first steps in the development of fetal intrauterine surgical interventions and the implementation of gene therapy to correct potentially life-threatening or life-altering conditions detected during the gestational period.

Specific concerns, both maternal and fetal, related to the possible risks and complications are discussed for each testing modality. However, a general concern relevant to all invasive fetal procedures is the risk of maternal-fetal hemorrhage. Therefore, blood type should be obtained for all pregnant women undergoing invasive fetal testing

Table 22-3 Areas of Genetic and Biochemical Evaluation

Type of Condition	Example
Alteration in chromosomal number	Trisomy 21, Down syndrome Trisomy 18, Edwards' syndrome Trisomy 3, Petau syndrome Klinefelter's syndrome Monosomy: Turner's (or Noonan's) syndrome
Molecular structure	Cystic fibrosis Hemophilia Duchenne muscular dystrophy
Metabolic	Tay-Sachs disease Gaucher's disease
Hematologic	Sickle cell disease β-Thalassemia

procedures. Women who are Rh-negative are candidates for Rh$_o$(D) Immune globulin (RhoGAM®). Prophylactic RhoGAM minimizes the potential for maternal sensitization and prevents antibody formation in the event of a minor maternal-fetal bleeding.

Amniocentesis

Amniocentesis is one of the oldest invasive methods of fetal evaluation. Use of amniocentesis was first documented in the 19th century as a treatment for polyhydramniosis (Romero et al., 1991). The first documented use of amniocentesis for prenatal diagnosis was in 1966 when Steel and Breg cultured amniotic cells and identified the karyotype of the resulting cells (Steel & Breg, 1966). Today, with the increased knowledge of molecular genetics, am-

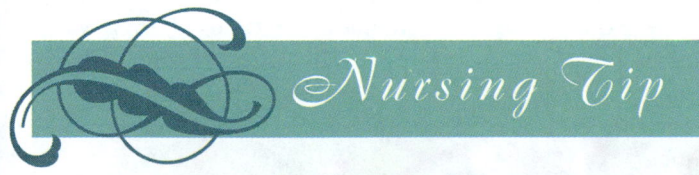

Nursing Tip

INDICATIONS FOR AMNIOCENTESIS IN THE FIRST HALF OF PREGNANCY

1. Maternal age over 35 years.
2. Previous offspring with abnormal chromosomal pattern.
3. Altered chromosomal pattern, including a balanced translocation, aneuploidy, or mosaicism in either parent.
4. Trisomy 21 (Down syndrome) or other chromosomal abnormality in close family members.
5. Pregnancy after three or more spontaneous abortions.
6. Elevated MS-AFP level.
7. Personal or family history leading to increased risk for a neural tube defect.

niocentesis is used to obtain amniotic fluid for the diagnosis of a variety of disorders through enzymatic analysis and DNA testing (Reece, 1997). In addition, the fluid obtained by amniocentesis can be used to evaluate fetal hemolytic disease by measuring bilirubin levels and fetal lung maturity by analyzing phospholipid ratios later in pregnancy.

Description

Amniocentesis is the removal, collection, and analysis of a sample of amniotic fluid from the amniotic sac. Amniotic fluid has long been established as a commonly used medium for prenatal diagnosis. Amniotic fluid is fetal in origin. It contains a variety of chemical substances and electrolytes. Amniotic fluid also contains a mixture of cells shed by the fetus from its skin and the linings of its gastrointestinal, respiratory, and genitourinary tracts. The cellular and biochemical components of amniotic fluid change with gestational age and fetal maturation. Consequently, amniotic fluid analysis is useful to determine chromosomal disorders early in pregnancy and to evaluate fetal health and maturity later in pregnancy.

Timing and Indications

Amniocentesis can be performed at different times during pregnancy for a variety of indications. Amniocentesis was originally used and continues to be most commonly performed between 15 and 17 weeks' gestation. During this stage of the pregnancy the amniotic sac is more accessible because the uterus has migrated from the pelvis to the abdomen; the volume and continuous replacement of amniotic fluid are adequate for sampling and fetal protection; and the ratio of viable to nonviable cells is greatest (Reece, 1997). Amniocentesis performed at this time usually is referred to as a mid-trimester procedure. Multicenter studies have demonstrated the procedure to be relatively safe, with an estimated pregnancy loss of 1 in 400 (0.25%) (Davis 1993). Studies also have demonstrated that mid-trimester amniocentesis is not associated with problems related to birth weight, gestational age, or maternal-fetal complications (Davis, 1993). One of the major disadvantages of mid-trimester amniocentesis is the need to wait until 15 weeks' postmenstrual gestational age to perform the procedure. Combined with the time necessary to culture and grow cells, test results may not be available until the pregnancy is physically evident to others and the woman has felt fetal movement. In addition, when the decision for pregnancy termination is made, the client must accept the increased risk of morbidity associated with second-trimester termination procedures. As a result, early amniocentesis involving the aspiration of fluid at or before 14 weeks' gestation has been explored (Davis, 1993). Early amniocentesis is technically more difficult because the uterus is still positioned within the pelvis and a smaller volume of amniotic fluid is present. The procedure-related loss rate for early amniocentesis is 2.0% to 3.0%, which is greater than the loss rate for mid-trimester procedures (Reece, 1997).

Throughout pregnancy, but most significantly before 18 weeks' gestation, analysis of amniotic fluid samples can provide information about fetal karyotype, metabolic disorders, DNA pattern, and other biochemical components. Because the desquamated cells found in amniotic fluid are fetal in origin, they contain genetic information identical to the fetus (Callen, 2001). The list of conditions identifiable through amniotic fluid analysis includes chromosomal disorders, such as translocation, aneuploidy, and trisomy; autosomal recessive disorders; X-linked disorders; metabolic diseases; enzyme defects; hematopoietic diseases; and immunodeficiencies. As the number of genes identified by the Human Genome Project continues to grow, the list of conditions identifiable through amniotic fluid analysis also will continue to grow and may include individual traits and attributes as well as medical conditions or syndromes.

In the second half of pregnancy, amniotic fluid analysis can be used to identify fetal hemolytic disease caused by maternal red blood cell (RBC) antigens. Isoimmune hemolytic disease of the fetus culminates in hemolysis and phagocytosis of fetal RBCs. As the fetus becomes increasingly anemic, the bilirubin level in the amniotic fluid increases. On spectrophotometry, bilirubin levels produce an optical density peak at 450 nm. Therefore, titers of bilirubin in the amniotic fluid can be measured and evaluated. Increased levels of ocular density indicate advanced hemolysis. The degree of fetal involvement is evaluated by graphing the ocular density measure of bilirubin correlated with gestational age to identify the severity of fetal hemolytic disease.

Amniotic fluid values also can be used to evaluate fetal well-being through the use of gram-staining techniques to identify intraamniotic infections and measurement of creatinine levels reflective of fetal kidney development and fetal muscle mass.

A common use of amniotic fluid analysis in late pregnancy is to evaluate fetal surfactant production and respiratory system maturity in anticipation of the transition to extrauterine existence. Evaluation of the lecithin-to-sphingomyelin ratio is the most widely used method of fetal lung maturity assessment. Sphingomyelin levels remain relatively constant throughout pregnancy, whereas lecithin levels increase dramatically with the production of mature surfactant. Consequently, pulmonary maturity is established when the lecithin-to-sphingomyelin ratio is 2:1 or greater. A specific phospholipid, phosphatidylglycerol (PG), found in the amniotic fluid also is an indicator of fetal lung maturity. The presence of PG takes on added significance in women with conditions such as gestational diabetes, blood incompatibilities, and methadone use. In these conditions, the mature pathway for surfactant production is delayed and the lactase/sucrase ratio may be borderline, but the presence of PG almost ensures pulmonary maturity.

A newer technique for evaluating lung maturity by amniotic fluid analysis is counts of lamellar bodies. Lamellar bodies are excreted by type II alveolar cells, and the concentration of lamellar bodies increases exponentially with gestation (Greenspoon et al., 1995). Fetal pulmonary maturity is associated with counts of lamellar bodies of over 30,000 particles/μL (Fakhoury, Daikoku, Benser, & Dubin, 1994).

Client Preparation

Amniocentesis usually is performed as an outpatient procedure. Informed consent procedures include a dialogue outlining the risks, benefits, and limitations of the procedure as needed. When amniocentesis is done in early pregnancy, the bladder may be filled to elevate the uterus and increase visualization of a fluid pocket. In the second half of pregnancy, the bladder is emptied to prevent confusion between it and the uterine sac. Maternal vital signs and fetal heart tones are evaluated before the procedure. During the procedure, the client is placed in a supine position. In late pregnancy, a hip roll may be used to prevent supine hypotensive syndrome. The client needs to know that some women experience a sensation of pressure, cramping, or both during the procedure.

Before and during amniocentesis, the nurse is a support person and patient advocate. The need for the procedure and the potential outcome are sources of anxiety and uncertainty for most women. Anticipating the client's anxieties and feelings and responding verbally and nonverbally are critical components of client preparation by the nurse.

Procedure

Amniocentesis is performed after ultrasound examination to identify an adequate pocket of amniotic fluid free of fetal parts, umbilical cord, or placental mass (Figure 22-2). The maternal abdominal wall is cleansed with an antiseptic solution and prepared and draped as a sterile field. In some situations, a local anesthetic may be used before amniocentesis is performed. Using an ultrasound probe with a sterile cover, the physician introduces a 20- or 22-gauge spinal needle through the abdominal wall and uterus and into the pocket of amniotic fluid. As the needle stylet is removed, amniotic fluid should freely flow from the needle. The initial fluid sample may be contaminated by maternal blood or cells and usually is discarded. In amniocentesis done early in the pregnancy, approximately 1 mL of fluid for each gestational week is collected. In amniocentesis performed at mid-trimester, approximately 20 to 30 mL of

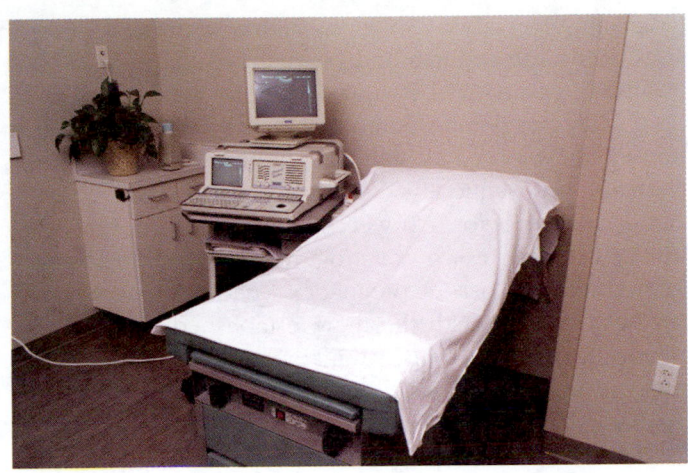

A.

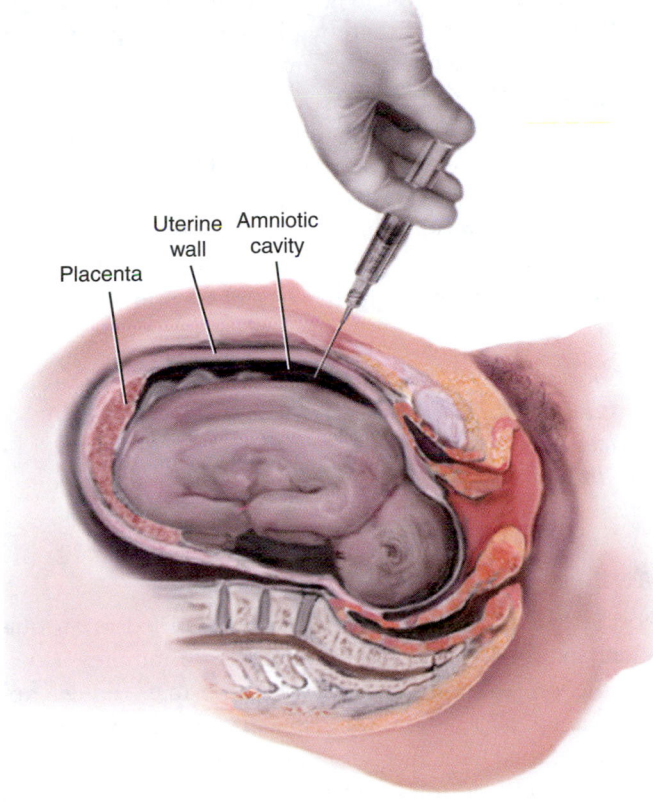

Placenta

Uterine wall

Amniotic cavity

B.

Figure 22-2 A. An amniocentesis setup. B. During amniocentesis, a sample of amniotic fluid is aspirated for evaluation.

for analysis. Culture tubes sometimes require special handling to protect the specimen. For example, specimens for bilirubin analysis must be placed in tubes covered with an opaque material to prevent breakdown of the bilirubin by light rays. After fluid collection the needle is withdrawn, pressure is applied to the site, and the site is dressed.

Follow-up

Maternal vital signs and fetal cardiac activity are documented at the conclusion of the procedure. When amniocentesis is performed before the age of viability, cardiac activity is an indicator of fetal survival. As gestational age of the pregnancy advances, monitoring of fetal tolerance to the procedure is increased and may incorporate other modalities to evaluate fetal well-being, such as a nonstress test.

Many women experience mild cramping for a few hours after the procedure. Women should be instructed to rest until the cramping subsides and then resume normal activity. However, women should refrain from sexual intercourse, heavy lifting, and strenuous physical activity for 24 hours. The abdominal puncture site should be kept clean, and no special skin care is required.

Maternal complications after amniocentesis, including vaginal spotting, fluid leaking, and uterine contractions, are uncommon and usually self-limiting (Tabor et al., 1986; Reece, 1997). Women need to report any vaginal discharge, severe or persistent uterine cramping, and increased temperature to the health care provider.

Women need emotional support and education during the interval between the procedure and availability of the results, especially when the purpose of the testing is for identification of a condition that may threaten the well-being and continuation of the pregnancy. The client needs to be informed of when the results will be available, who will contact her, and how she will learn the outcome. Ongoing support during this period of uncertainty is a critical role for the nurse.

Chorionic Villus Sampling

Chorionic villus sampling (CVS) is an alternative to amniocentesis. The primary stimulus for the development of CVS

fluid is collected. In amniocentesis performed in the third trimester, the volume of fluid collected will vary based on the number and types of tests being performed. If the attempt to obtain amniotic fluid is unsuccessful, a second needle may be inserted at a different site. However, studies have indicated that fetal loss rates increase in proportion to the number of needle insertions. Therefore, no more than two attempts should be performed on any given occasion (Reece, 1997). After withdrawal the fluid is placed in culture tubes, labeled, and sent to the laboratory

technology was its use in earlier diagnosis, during the first trimester when the pregnancy is not yet physically visible to others. The major disadvantages of CVS are inability to diagnose the presence of a neural tube defect and higher rate of pregnancy loss.

Description

Chorionic villus sampling is a procedure to obtain fetal cells in the first trimester of the developing pregnancy. Chorionic villi cells are living cells fetal in origin, thereby reflecting the chromosomes, enzymology, and DNA content of the fetus. However, unlike amniocentesis, CVS cannot determine the presence of a neural tube defect because the level of α-fetoprotein can only be tested using serum or amniotic fluid.

Timing and Indications

Chorionic villus sampling is usually performed between 10 and 12 weeks' menstrual age of gestation (American College of Obstetricians and Gynecologists, 1995). At this gestational age, the amniotic sac does not fill the uterine cavity, thereby facilitating the passage of the sampling instrument into the uterus to remove a tissue specimen. A small tissue aspiration device is inserted into the developing placenta, allowing the chorion frondosum (which ultimately will form the placenta) to be biopsied. The chorion frondosum are mitotically active cells that provide tissue for karyotype determination and tissue cultures as well as fetal RBCs for identifying RBC antigens (Wapner, 1997). Because the chorionic villi are composed of spontaneously dividing cells, it is not necessary to grow cell cultures in the laboratory.

The chorion frondosum eventually will develop into the placenta, and can be visualized on ultrasonography. Only a small amount (10 to 20 mg) of villi is required for most diagnoses. This quantity of cells represents less than 1% of the villi destined to become the functioning placenta.

The greatest benefit of CVS is earlier diagnosis of fetal disorders and a shorter interval between test performance and availability of the results. CVS is performed in the first trimester of pregnancy, before the obvious changes in maternal physical appearance and before the experience of quickening. If the woman chooses to end the pregnancy based on the diagnosis, a first-trimester termination procedure, with a lower risk of complications and lower cost, is an option. The waiting time between obtaining the specimen of chorionic villi and test results also is decreased because the specimen consists of actively dividing fetal cells as opposed to the cells shed by the fetus that are grown in culture medium after amniocentesis.

The risks associated with CVS include spontaneous pregnancy loss. One confounding factor in calculating

pregnancy loss after CVS is the differentiation of loss related to the procedures and pregnancies that would have naturally terminated between 9 and 20 weeks' gestation. One study has demonstrated that 2% to 5% of pregnancies shown to be viable by ultrasonography at 7 to 12 weeks' gestation subsequently become nonviable or spontaneously abort before 20 weeks' gestation (Rodesch et al., 1987). Data from two collaborative studies have demonstrated that the risk of pregnancy loss is not significantly greater than that with the more established mid-trimester amniocentesis procedure (Canadian Collaborative Study, 1989; Rhoads et al., 1989). Concern has been voiced about the increased risk of fetal structural anomalies after CVS. Froster-Iskenius and Baird (1989) reported a greater than 1% incidence of oromandibular-limb hypogenesis in CVS sampled pregnancies. This syndrome has a prevalence of 0.057 per 10,000 births, thereby providing strong suspicion of an association between the procedure and the presence of anomalies (Froster-Iskenius & Baird, 1989). While the cause of this malformation is not clear, it appears that the association is related to the timing of the CVS procedure, between 55 and 65 days' gestation (Hsieh et al., 1995). While the association is unclear, the American College of Obstetricians and Gynecologists (1995) has made the following statement related to the use of CVS in the clinical setting.

> *Chorionic villus sampling is a relatively safe procedure when performed at 10–12 weeks and is an acceptable alternative to amniocentesis. Chorionic villus sampling is not recommended prior to nine weeks' gestation.*

Client Preparation

Chorionic villus sampling usually is performed in an outpatient setting and takes approximately 20 minutes. However, the preparation and recovery time may require approximately 2 hours in the clinical setting. Before the procedure, the client and her family should receive genetic counseling and be informed about its benefits, risks, and limitations. Informed consent must be obtained. The client needs thorough education about what to expect during the procedure, and a comprehensive assessment of maternal-fetal status is completed. A full bladder is used to serve as an acoustic window. Some women experience discomfort during the procedure as a result of bladder fullness and pressure from the ultrasound transducer.

Procedure

Two techniques currently are in widespread use for performing CVS: the transcervical catheter aspiration technique and the transabdominal needle aspiration technique (Figure 22-3). The choice of a transvaginal or transabdominal approach usually is based on client preference

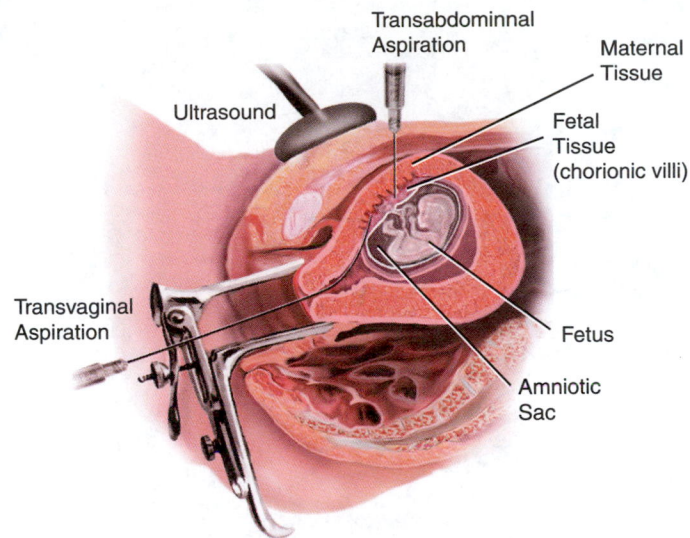

Figure 22-3 During chorionic villus sampling, a small tissue sample is aspirated from the fetal side of the placenta. Needle insertion is made either transabdominally or transvaginally.

and provider skill. In some situations, however, client-specific factors such as the presence of cervical polyps, uterine position and placental location, or active cervical or vaginal herpes infection determine the procedural approach. Both approaches require two practitioners, one performing the sampling and one providing the ultrasound guidance.

If the transcervical technique is selected, an ultrasound examination is completed to confirm fetal viability and to locate the chorion frondosum. The woman is placed in lithotomy position, and a sterile speculum is inserted to visualize the cervix. A transcervical catheter with a malleable obturator, capable of negotiating the cervicouterine angle and being directed to the biopsy site is selected. Under real-time ultrasound guidance, the physician passes the catheter through the cervix and into the chorion frondosum. Once at the selected site, the obturator is removed, a 20-mL syringe is attached to the catheter, and negative pressure is applied to aspirate the villi into the syringe. The catheter is removed with continuous negative pressure being applied to prevent leakage into the amniotic sac. If an inadequate sample is obtained, the procedure is repeated with a new sterile catheter. In general, no more than three attempts are made. The presence of fetal cardiac activity, appearance of the amniotic sac, and the chorion frondosum are verified after each attempt.

Ultrasound verification of fetal viability, gestational age, and location of the chorion frondosum is the first step in transabdominal CVS. After ultrasound examination, the maternal abdomen is draped and prepared with an antiseptic solution in a way similar to that of the amniocentesis procedure. Under ultrasound guidance, an 18- or 20-gauge needle is inserted through the abdominal and uterine wall and guided into the chorion frondosum. A 20-mL syringe is attached to the hub of the needle, and negative suction is applied to aspirate the sample of villi. The tip of the needle is kept under ultrasound visualization at all times. If an inadequate sample is obtained, the procedure is repeated using a new sterile setup.

The specimen from either technique is inspected visually for the presence of villi, which have a distinctive frondlike appearance with budlike projections. The specimen is placed in a sterile medium for transport and cytogenic analysis.

Follow-up

After the procedure the woman's vital signs are evaluated and assessment of uterine status is completed. Uterine cramping should not occur. Vaginal spotting may occur after the transcervical approach, and usually resolves within 3 days. Heavy bleeding or passage of clots, tissue, or amniotic fluid is abnormal and should be reported to the health care provider. After the CVS procedure, the client is advised to avoid sexual activity and strenuous physical activity until all vaginal spotting has resolved. The client also needs to be informed to contact the physician if cramping, vaginal bleeding, or flulike symptoms are experienced within the week. Women usually have follow-up ultrasonography a week after the procedure and at 16 weeks' gestation to reconfirm integrity of the products of conception.

Percutaneous Umbilical Blood Sampling

Percutaneous umbilical blood sampling (PUBS), also known as cordocentesis, has expanded the possibilities for fetal surveillance and treatment. Improved ultrasound guidance techniques have enhanced the safety of this highly invasive technique. A major consideration in the decision to perform PUBS is whether premature birth and neonatal care would be more effective or associated with lower risk than this highly invasive prebirth procedure.

Description

PUBS is an evaluation technique that provides direct access to the fetal circulation and involves direct aspiration of fetal blood. The most common site for needle placement is the umbilical cord, within 2 cm of the placental insertion site. This site is preferred because it provides a relatively fixed target for puncture as opposed to a free-floating loop of cord. Conditions such as maternal obesity, marked hydramnios or oligohydramnios, or unfavorable fetal position may make the cord-placenta junction inaccessible. Thus, alternative sites include the fetal intrahepatic vein and the cardiac ventricle.

Timing and Indications

Percutaneous umbilical blood sampling can be performed any time after 17 weeks' gestation. Because the medium assayed is fetal blood, PUBS is useful in conducting a wide variety of blood studies and in diagnosing a variety of conditions including the following: chromosomal alterations; intrauterine infections; coagulopathy; hemoglobinopathies and RBC disorders; immunodeficiency states; and platelet disorders, including RBC counts for identifying isoimmune disease and fetal thrombocytis levels. In cases of suspected intrauterine growth retardation, PUBS can be used to evaluate fetal hypoxia and determine fetal acid-base status. PUBS also can be used for intrauterine transfusion and fetal drug therapy.

Client Preparation

Percutaneous umbilical blood sampling can be performed in either an outpatient or inpatient setting. The actual sampling procedure takes approximately 10 minutes for specimen collection. Women must give informed consent because of the invasive nature of the procedure. The client needs to understand the reason, risks, benefits, and nature of the follow-up of the PUBS procedure. Depending on uterine size, a full bladder may be necessary. The client can be informed that physical discomfort during the procedure is minimal and similar to the pressure and cramping sensations experienced during other intrauterine procedures such as amniocentesis. Physical care of the woman includes documenting baseline vital signs and fetal cardiac activity. When PUBs is performed after the fetus is viable, preparation for a cesarean birth in the event of fetal distress must be discussed and considered by the client before the procedure is implemented. Preparation also involves ensuring that emergency equipment and personnel are available.

Procedure

Percutaneous umbilical blood sampling is performed under ultrasound guidance to identify the target sampling site. Antiseptic preparation of the maternal abdomen is completed and a local anesthetic may be used. A 20- or 22-gauge spinal needle is inserted through the abdominal and uterine walls and is directed into the umbilical vessel, most commonly the umbilical vein (Figure 22-4). A site approximately 1 to 2 cm from the insertion of the cord into the placental is desirable. This site minimizes the risk of cord injury and the chance of obtaining maternal blood from the placenta. If fetal movement interferes with the procedure, a sedative can be administered intravenously to the mother, or intravenously or intramuscularly to the fetus. Once the umbilical vein is accessed, the blood sample can be aspirated and placed in the appropriate microtube for the desired testing. Confirmation that the blood

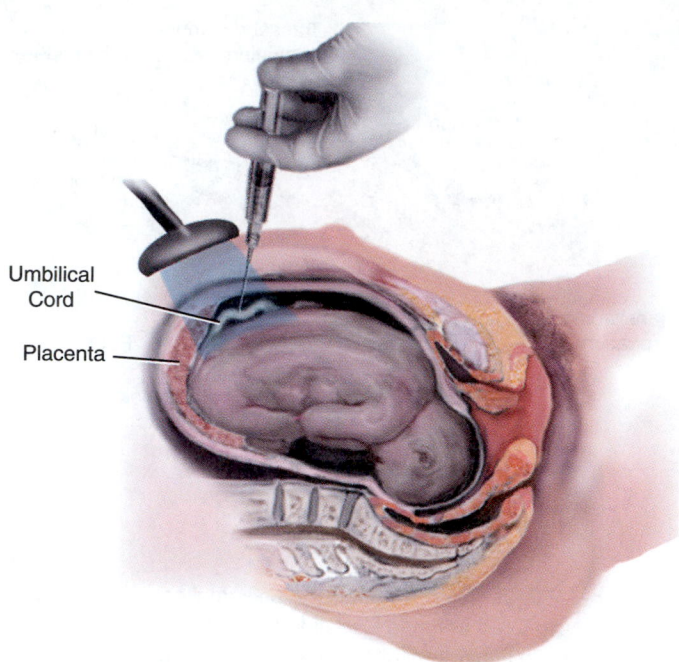

Umbilical Cord

Placenta

Figure 22-4 The percutaneous umbilical blood sampling technique is performed using ultrasound guidance and transabdominal aspiration of a sample from the fetal umbilical vessel.

sample is fetal in origin can be accomplished by assessing the mean corpuscular volume (MCV), which is greater in the fetus than in the adult.

Percutaneous umbilical blood sampling, or cordocentesis, also provides an access site for administration of medications or blood transfusion to the fetus. After the blood specimen is obtained or the infusion completed, the needle is removed, the site is inspected for bleeding, and fetal cardiac activity is confirmed by ultrasonography.

Follow-up

Postprocedure care includes monitoring maternal vital signs, fetal heart rate, and uterine activity. The fetal heart rate is evaluated for signs of reactivity and the absence of distress. PUBS is associated with a 2% risk of complications that include bleeding from the puncture site, fetal bradycardia, infection, thrombosis, and hematoma formation (Scott et al., 1994). Because of the increased risk of infection, some providers prescribe prophylactic antibiotics. The client also should be instructed to monitor her temperature twice a day to detect temperature elevation.

Other Genetic and Biochemical Evaluations

Fetal tissue sampling and fetal fibronectin are two of the lesser used modalities for evaluation of the status of a pregnancy.

Fetal tissue sampling involves a direct biopsy of fetal tissue. Collection of fetal tissue is accomplished using biopsy forceps through an angiocatheter or a double-needle system under ultrasound guidance. Tissue samples of fetal skin can be used to diagnose severe skin disorders such as epidermolysis bullosa, Harlequin ichthyosis, and oculocutaneous albinism; liver biopsies can identify inborn errors of metabolism such as glucose-6-phosphate dehydrogenase deficiency and alanine–glyoxalate aminotransferase deficiency; and lung biopsy can provide data about masses detected with ultrasonography (Chitty and Bobrow, 1994). Fetal tissue sampling is a highly invasive procedure and is not widely used in the clinical setting.

Fetal fibronectin (fFN) testing is a screening procedure for the prediction of preterm labor. Fetal fibronectin is a protein substance that helps connect the amniotic sac to the inside wall of the uterus. The FDA (Food and Drug Administration) has approved a test for fFN detection between 22 and 31 weeks' gestation. Determination of cervicovaginal fetal fibronectin as a marker for risk of preterm birth has been proposed for two uses: to test women identified as being at high risk and thus leading to reassurance that early birth is unlikely and to screen low-risk populations to identify women at higher than normal risk. The test for fFN involves obtaining a swab of vaginal and cervical secretions. It is believed that fetal fibronectin leaks into the cervix when the interaction between the fetal membranes and the uterine wall weakens. Consequently, a positive finding may predict the onset of labor. The more useful finding may be a negative result, which is correlated with a low incidence of labor onset in the next 7 to 14 days (Weismiller, 1999).

Maternal Serum Studies

The interaction of the maternal-placental-fetal unit, present from the earliest point of the pregnancy, forms the basis for genetic and biochemical screening through maternal serum studies. Maternal serum testing technologies examine byproducts of the gestational state found in the maternal system but do not invade the integrity of the uterine-placental-fetal unit. Before the technologic advances that now facilitate direct examination of uterine-placental-fetal cells, maternal serum analysis was the primary method of fetal surveillance in early pregnancy. Although more direct ways of examining the fetus have made some maternal serum studies less widely used today, this method is recognized as a valuable tool in screening women for high-risk pregnancies. Maternal serum studies measure maternal hormone levels, MS-AFP levels, and fetal cell isolation, with MS-AFP measurement being the most widely used prenatal screening modality today. Maternal serum studies are primarily screening procedures to identify pregnancies that are at high-risk for complications or negative out-

comes. In contrast, many of the invasive fetal studies described previously are diagnostic of specific conditions. Screening procedures simply identify pregnancies at risk for complications or alterations, whereas diagnostic procedures confirm the presence or absence of specific conditions. Therefore maternal serum screening techniques, if the results are altered, lead to more invasive diagnostic techniques.

Maternal Hormone Levels

Human chorionic gonadotropin, estrogen and estriol, and human placental lactogen are hormones associated with the state of pregnancy. Levels of these hormones can be measured in a sample of maternal venous blood. Maternal serum hormones are used in the diagnosis of pregnancy, differential diagnosis of intrauterine and ectopic pregnancies, and prediction of poor perinatal outcomes. With more accurate and more direct modalities to evaluate the status of a pregnancy, maternal hormone levels are not routinely used in the management of high-risk pregnancies. Follow-up includes referral for the appropriate diagnostic testing based on the results of maternal serum studies.

Human Chorionic Gonadotropin

Human chorionic gonadotropin (hCG) is a protein hormone secreted by the syncytiotrophoblast early in pregnancy. hCG is detectable in maternal serum 8 days after conception. hCG is exclusively produced during pregnancy and therefore is the basis for many pregnancy tests. Maternal plasma levels of hCG increase rapidly, doubling approximately every 1.5 to 2.5 days after conception, and then rapidly decline. Values that deviate from the expected pattern suggest an abnormally developing pregnancy: low or slowly increasing levels are associated with threatened abortion and ectopic pregnancies, and highly elevated levels are associated with hydatidiform moles. hCG levels that persist into the mid-trimester of pregnancy may be predictive of Down syndrome, when considered in conjunction with maternal age and MS-AFP and estriol levels (Palomaki et al., 1992).

Estrogen and Estriol

Maternal estrogen levels increase progressively over the course of pregnancy. The increased estrogen level is due primarily to estriol, which increases a thousand times over nonpregnant levels and accounts for 90% of total estrogen levels (Cunningham et al., 1997). Estriol precursors are secreted from the fetal adrenal cortex, and the conversion to estriol is accomplished in the placenta. Thus, compromise in either the fetus or placenta can result in decreased estriol production (Martin & Cowan, 1990). In the past, serum estriol levels were used as an indicator of fetal condition in high-risk pregnancies. Decreased levels of estriol suggest fetal jeopardy. In multiple gestation pregnancies or pregnancies complicated by erythroblastosis, estriol levels may be elevated.

Human Placental Lactogen

Human placental lactogen (hPL) levels also increase progressively over the course of pregnancy. hPL is produced by the syncytiotrophoblast cell as early as the third week after ovulation and is detectable in the maternal serum 4 weeks after fertilization. The level of hPL is continually increasing throughout the gestational period and peaks at 35 weeks' gestation. hPL promotes fetal and placental growth. The level of hPL in the maternal circulation is directly related to fetal and placental weight. Therefore, alteration in maternal serum levels of hPL may indicate altered placental function, providing a basis for screening for complications.

Maternal Serum–alpha-Fetoprotein Screening

Maternal serum–alpha-fetoprotein (MS-AFP) testing is the basis for screening for neural tube defects (elevated levels) and trisomy 21 (decreased levels) during the second trimester of pregnancy. MS-AFP testing screens maternal blood for the presence and volume of AFP, which is the major serum protein of early fetal life. AFP is present as early as 6 weeks' gestation and initially is produced by the yolk sac and later by the fetal liver. Levels increase rapidly, with peak concentrations found at the end of the first trimester. The absolute level of AFP produced and secreted by the fetus remains constant throughout the remainder of the gestational period; however, the circulating concentration of AFP is diluted as the fetal blood volume increases. The presence of AFP in the amniotic fluid is largely maintained by fetal urination. Another source contributing to AFP in the amniotic fluid is leakage from fetal capillaries in the absence of keratinization of the skin (Ruoslahti, Engvalli, Pekkpola, & Seppala, 1978). AFP enters the maternal circulation by way of diffusion across the amnion. MS-AFP concentrations increase geometrically until 30 weeks' gestation and then decline. Normal ranges have been identified for each week of pregnancy. The optimal time for testing is 16 to 18 weeks' gestation (Cunningham et al., 1997). The American College of Obstetricians and Gynecologists (1996) recommends that all pregnant women be offered MS-AFP screening. Significant variations in the serum levels of AFP have been reported among different laboratories. Thus, to increase standardization, results are reported as multiples of the laboratory's median level (multiples of the median [MoM]) in unaffected pregnancies adjusted for gestational age. MS-AFP testing has high sensitivity but low specificity. Therefore, when al-

tered levels of MS-AFP are obtained, the first course of action is to repeat the screening. When abnormal levels persist, the client is referred for both ultrasonography to examine for structural anomalies and amniocentesis to further quantify AFP levels and obtain chromosomal analysis.

Several variables can affect the level of AFP in the maternal circulatory system: large women have lower levels, whereas African American women have higher levels than do Caucasion or Asian women. Other factors that can alter AFP levels include inaccurate gestational dating; multiple pregnancy; and maternal disease states such as diabetes, lupus, and blood group sensitization. High levels of AFP suggest an increased risk of an open neural tube defect, and low levels suggest an increased risk of Down syndrome. The specificity of MS-AFP in the diagnosis of Down syndrome is increased when serum levels of hCG and unconjugated estriol also are measured. This procedure is known as the triple Marker Serum Screen and detects 2.3 times more cases of Down syndrome than does MS-AFP testing alone (Haddow & Palomaki, 1993).

Before obtaining a specimen for MS-AFP analysis, informed consent needs to be obtained. Clients need to understand the nature of this procedure (a screening test, not a diagnostic test), the potential outcomes of the test, and the procedures that will be followed if the results are altered. Because of the wide variation of "normal levels" among healthy women, fetuses, and pregnancies, the possibility of a false-positive result should be discussed.

Fetal Cell Isolation

A promising development in prenatal genetic diagnosis is the retrieval of fetal cells from the maternal peripheral blood. Fetal cells that "leak" into the maternal circulation include trophoblasts, lymphocytes, and RBCs. Fetal nucleated RBCs appear to be a useful source for fetal diagnostic studies because they are unique to the adult circulation, express several unique antigens, produce fetal hemoglobin, have a short life span, and do not persist from one pregnancy to another (Steele & Berg, 1996). Fetal cell isolation is an attractive concept and the outlook for clinical application is promising; however, this method currently is in the investigational phase.

PHYSICAL AND PHYSIOLOGICAL SURVEILLANCE

Visualization of the physical size, structure, and movement of the fetus is possible with the use of ultrasonography, Doppler flow studies, and magnetic resonance imaging (MRI). Physiologic integrity of the placenta and of fetal compensatory mechanisms can be measured with electronic fetal monitoring and biophysical profile evaluation. Through the use of these technologies, practitioners can gather information about the physical status and structural anatomy and about the physiologic status and functional behavior of the fetus, respectively. Physical and physiologic surveillance of the fetus includes imaging, heart rate monitoring, and behavior studies.

Fetal Imaging

Fetal imaging is based on the belief that the ability to "see" the fetus and its environment profoundly shifts the factual and psychologic basis of the management of pregnancy (Manning, 1995). The primary means of fetal imaging include ultrasonography, Doppler studies, and MRI. Before the introduction of high-resolution imaging procedures, visualization of the fetus and intrauterine environment was limited to indirect measures such as fundal height assessments and manual palpation for fetal size. The introduction of fetal imaging has transformed the fetus from a hidden and mysterious being to a "patient" to be viewed, examined, evaluated, and in some situations treated.

Ultrasonography

Ultrasound technology has made possible direct noninvasive visualization of the fetus. Ultrasonography is the imagery modality most widely used to assess the pregnant client and developing fetus. In obstetrical settings, both the transabdominal and transvaginal approaches to ultrasound examination are used.

Description

Ultrasonography is the use of high-frequency (>20,000 Hz) sound waves to detect differences in tissue density and visualize outlines of structures within the body. Ultrasonography used in obstetrical settings to generate images operates on the pulse-echo principle. According to this principle, a short pulse is emitted by the transducer, the pulse is reflected from underlying fetal structures as an echo, and the rebounding echo is detected by the transducer and displayed as an image. The pulse or sound wave passes through various tissues at different speeds based on tissue density and elasticity. The pulse travels through tissue until it comes to a tissue interface or another tissue with a different density. The change in density causes a small proportion of the pulse to be echoed back to the transducer. The echo is converted into electrical signals and displayed as an image on the monitor. The time interval from emission of the impulse to detection of the echo determines the physical position of an underlying structure. Dense tissues produce a higher velocity of sound transmission, which translates to brightness of the image on the monitor. Most state-of-the-art ultrasound equipment displays 128 shades of gray correlated with differences in signal strength. Differences among signals result in color gradient changes that indicate structure density:

- Bright white areas: strong echoes from high-density structures such as bone tissue.
- Gray areas: small echoes from intermediate density tissues, such as brain, renal, or cardiac tissue.
- Black areas: no echo related to a fluid-filled areas, such as a pocket of amniotic fluid or a filled bladder.

Therefore, ultrasonography provides physical measures of tissue density, size, and location. The translation of these physical measures into estimates of gestational age or fetal weight is based on data from clinical research (Docker, 1992). Real time or B-scan ultrasonography uses a multiple-pulse system of sound waves to note fetal movements, whereas conventional or M-mode scan ultrasonography uses a single pulse that produces a static image. Real-time ultrasonography is most commonly used in obstetrical practice because of its capability to display motion-picture-like two-dimensional sectional images. However, M-mode scan ultrasonography, or static images, is valuable in gaining information about individual structures, such as the dynamic changes occurring in the fetal heart.

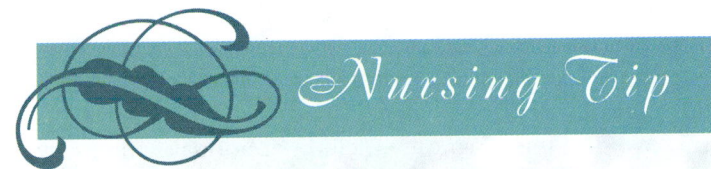

Nursing Tip

INDICATIONS FOR ULTRASOUND DIAGNOSIS IN THE SECOND TRIMESTER

1. Estimation of gestational age for women with uncertain clinical dates.
2. Evaluation of fetal growth.
3. Estimation of fetal weight.
4. Vaginal bleeding of unknown cause.
5. Suspected multiple gestation.
6. Adjunct to amniocentesis or PUBS.
7. Adjunct to cervical cerclage placement.
8. Significant uterine size or clinical dates discrepancies.
9. Suspected uterine abnormality.
10. Suspected alteration in amniotic fluid volume.
11. Premature labor.
12. Abnormal AFP level.
13. Serial evaluation of fetal growth in multiple gestation.

Timing and Indications

Ultrasonography is used progressively throughout the gestational period for a variety of indications. According to the American College of Obstetricians and Gynecologists (1993) the ultrasound examination may take one of three forms: basic, or level I, examination; comprehensive, or level II, examination; and limited, or targeted, examination.

Level I, or basic, ultrasonography is used to:

- Detect the gestational sac as early as 5 weeks after the last menstrual period.
- Identify the number of fetuses.
- Document fetal life.
- Detect gross fetal structural anomalies.
- Estimate gestational age.
- Determine fetal position.
- Locate the placenta.
- Estimate amniotic fluid volume.
- Evaluate maternal pelvic masses.

The basic examination takes approximately 20 minutes and is a component of the obstetrical standard of care. The basic examination is the most common use of ultrasonography in obstetrical practice (Tucker, 2000).

A level II, or comprehensive, ultrasound examination is done when the provider suspects a client is carrying an anatomically or physiologically abnormal fetus. Indications for level-II ultrasonography include abnormal findings on clinical examination, history of an abnormal fetus, and validation of information obtained in the level-I examination. The focus of a comprehensive examination is to survey fetal anatomy for specific malformations. A level II, or comprehensive, ultrasound examination is used to:

- Evaluate gestational age.
- Measure fetal growth.
- Perform specific examinations of the brain, heart, kidney, and cord insertion.
- Quantify amniotic fluid volume.
- Determine placental location.

A level II examination usually is performed after 18 weeks' gestation and is done by a perinatologist.

The third type of examination, limited or targeted, is performed when specific information is needed but a complete survey of the fetus and intrauterine environment is not needed. Limited examination usually is performed in conjunction with another procedure or event. Limited ultrasound examinations are performed during amniocentesis, PUBS, or a biophysical profile to confirm fetal cardiac activity as a result of decreased fetal movement, and iden-

tify fetal presentation or locate the placenta after the onset of spontaneous bleeding or labor.

Client Preparation

As with any procedure the client needs to be informed about its purpose, content, and limitations. Before transabdominal examination, the client will need to fill her bladder. To establish adequate bladder filling the client should drink 1 to 2 quarts of water 1 hour before the procedure. Maintaining a full bladder can be a source of discomfort for many clients, especially in late pregnancy. When a transvaginal examination is planned, the client will be asked to empty her bladder before the procedure to minimize obscuring the view into the pelvic cavity.

Procedure

Obstetrical ultrasonography can be performed using either a transabdominal or transvaginal scanning approach (Figure 22-5). Transabdominal scanning is the more traditional approach and can be used throughout gestation but is most useful in the second and third trimesters. Transabdominal ultrasonography provides a clear view of the fetus and placenta. When this approach is used a filled bladder or an acoustic window is necessary to displace the gas-filled bowel, which obstructs pelvic structures, and to lift the uterus higher into the abdominal cavity. During transabdominal ultrasonography, a lubricating gel is applied to the abdomen and the probe is moved over the abdominal surface. The lubricating reduces friction and enhances transmission and reception of the sound waves by the probe.

Transvaginal ultrasonography is most useful in the first trimester of pregnancy. During this procedure, a handheld probe is inserted into the vagina, allowing detailed examination of the pelvic anatomy and earlier diagnosis of intrauterine pregnancy (Cunningham et al., 1997). Using a transvaginal approach an acoustic window is not necessary. Another advantage of transvaginal scanning is the closer proximity to the pelvic structures, facilitating clearer visualization and reducing interference by thick abdominal tissue. Therefore, this method is especially useful in clients who are obese. Transvaginal scanning has limited usefulness in visualizing fetal anatomy and obtaining fetal measurements after 16 weeks' gestation because the enlarging uterus moves into the abdominal cavity and away from the vaginal vault. Guzman and coauthors (1998), however, have used transvaginal ultrasonography as an adjunct to abdominal scanning in the second half of pregnancy to evaluate preterm labor.

The findings of an obstetrical ultrasound examination can provide valuable data to influence the management plan during the course of gestation. In addition to data about the physical status of the fetus (e.g., number of

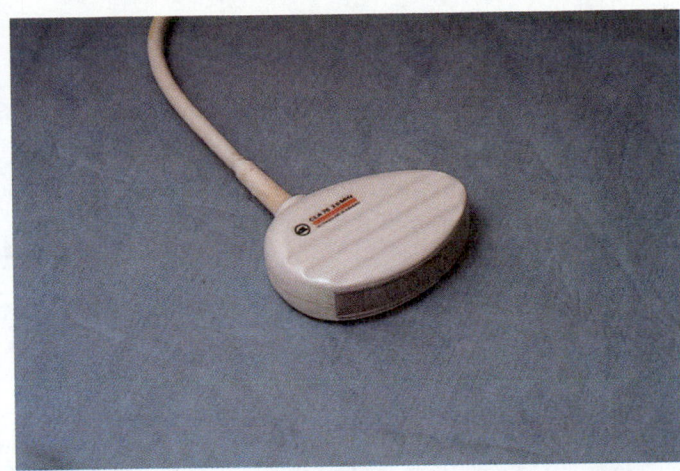

A.

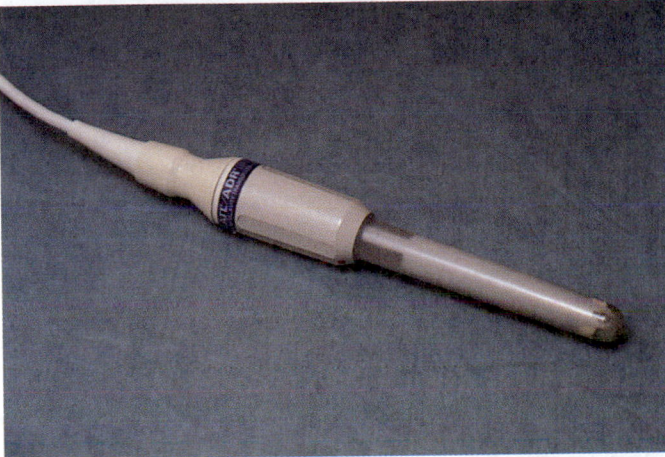

B.

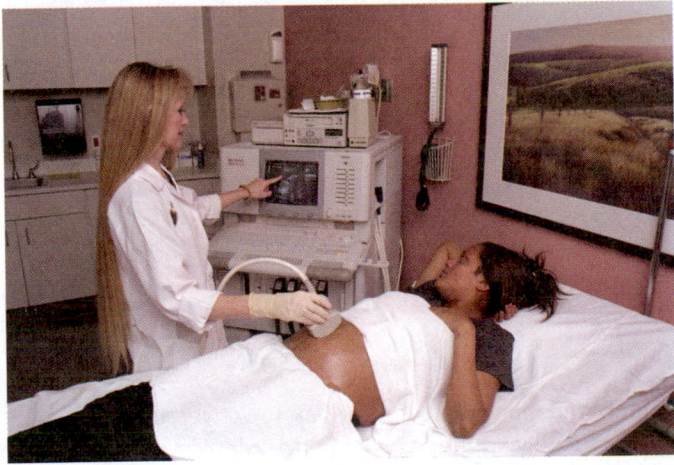

C.

Figure 22-5 A. Transabdominal scanner. B. Transvaginal scanner. C. The nurse and client look at the features of the fetus, as shown on the monitor during transabdominal ultrasonography.

fetuses, presentation, and anatomical survey), data obtainable from an ultrasound examination includes fetal cardiac activity, gestational dating and fetal growth, placental position and function, and amniotic fluid volume.

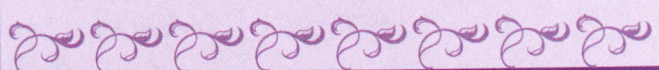

Critical Thinking

Is Ultrasonography a Routine Procedure?

A study by Berkowitz (1993) concluded that routine ultrasound screening for low-risk women did not improve pregnancy outcome. The author suggested that savings for prenatal care could total about $1 billion if there was a decrease in the number of screening ultrasound examinations in routine pregnancy.

- Do you agree with this position?
- In your opinion, what are the risks of discontinuing routine ultrasounds?

Using an echo scanner, cardiac activity can be documented as early as 6 to 7 weeks' gestation. The lack of cardiac activity, in association with fetal scalp edema, and maceration are signs of fetal death. By 9 to 10 weeks' gestation, the lack of fetal cardiac activity and the proliferation of trophoblastic tissue are diagnostic of gestational trophoblastic disease.

Ultrasonography can be used to obtain gestational dating of a pregnancy. During the first 20 weeks' gestation, normal fetuses grow at approximately the same rate. The four methods use to determine gestational age are

- Determination of gestation sac dimensions at about 8 weeks' gestation.
- Measurement of crown-rump length between 7 and 14 weeks' gestation.
- Measurement of biparietal diameter (BPD) after 12 weeks' gestation.
- Measurement of femur length after 12 weeks' gestation.

In the second half of pregnancy, accurate determination of fetal age is enhanced by serial measurements. When three composite measures are obtained at least 2 weeks apart, between 24 and 32 weeks' gestation, a highly accurate estimate of actual age is achievable (Manning, 1999). These measurements can also be used to evaluate fetal growth. Serial evaluations of BPD and femur length can identify reduced fetal growth. Intrauterine growth restriction (IUGR) can be symmetric, reflecting a chronic insult to fetal growth, or asymmetric, indicating an acute state of deprivation impacting fetal growth.

Differentiation between placental and endometrial tissue is evident by about 14 to 16 weeks' gestation. However, determining the exact relationship of the placenta to the internal cervical os is difficult before the end of the second trimester. Therefore, the diagnosis of placenta previa before 27 weeks' gestation is questionable because of the elongation and stretching of the lower uterine segment in late pregnancy.

Placental grading and classification of placental maturity are accomplished by ultrasound scanning. Grading of the placenta is based on the identification and distribution of calcium deposits on the fetal surface of the placenta (Manning, 1999). A relationship has been established between placental grade and fetal pulmonary maturity (Manning, 1999).

Amniotic fluid volume (AFV) can be objectively quantified using ultrasound technology. The AFV is calculated by measuring the depth of the amniotic fluid pocket in the

Research Highlight

Effects of Symmetric and Asymmetric Fetal Growth on Pregnancy Outcome

Purpose

Obstetrical ultrasonography was used in a study to assess the prevalence of head-abdomen circumference (HC/AC) asymmetry among small for gestational age (SGA) infants and to determine adverse fetal outcomes among symmetric versus asymmetric SGA infants when compared with their average gestational age (AGA) counterparts.

Methods

A retrospective cohort study was undertaken in which antepartum sonography was completed on women within 4 weeks of delivery. Data were collected between January 1, 1989, and September 30, 1996, on 33,740 women who delivered live singleton infants without anomalies. A HC/AC normogram was derived from this database. Fetuses were considered to have HC/AC asymmetry if the normogram value was greater than or equal to the 95th percentile for gestational age. Neonatal morbidity and outcome data were based on diagnosis by neonatal intensive care faculty.

Findings

Of infants in the study, 16% (1,364) were at or below the 10th percentile (SGA). Among those, 80% (1,090) were symmetric and 20% (274) were asymmetric. Major anomalies were detected among asymmetric SGA infants. The mean birth weight was significantly lower in SGA infants. Preterm induction of labor was more common among asymmetric SGA fetuses. Intrapartum hypertension requiring delivery at or before 32 weeks' gestation was significantly more common in the asymmetric SGA group. Finally, cesarean delivery owing to nonreassuring fetal heart rate tracings was significantly more common in SGA than in AGA fetuses and was nearly twice as frequent among pregnancies complicated by asymmetric versus symmetric growth restriction.

Nursing Implications

A third trimester ultrasound can be a valuable diagnostic tool in identifying infants at risk for adverse outcomes related to birth weight and growth symmetry of HC/AC. Identifying those clients at risk for delivering SGA infants with asymmetrical growth patterns will afford the nurse the opportunity to educate the clients about their likelihood of delivering an infant with an anomaly. The nurse can also help prepare the clients mentally and emotionally for a change in birth plan, which might include the need for preterm induction of labor, an early delivery to control intrapartum hypertension, or a c-section delivery in the event of nonreassuring fetal heart rate tracings.

Dashe, J. S., McIntire, D. D., Lucas, M. J., & Leveno, K. J. (2000). Effects of symmetric and asymmetric fetal growth on pregnancy outcomes. *Obstetrics and Gynecology, 96,* 321–327.

four quadrants surrounding the maternal umbilicus. The measurements obtained from each quadrant are totaled to provide the amniotic fluid index. Values of 5 to 19 cm are considered normal, whereas values under 5 cm indicate oligohydramnios and over 20 cm indicate hydramnios (Chervenak & Gabbe, 1996). Altered AFV is a marker of a chronic fetal condition.

Follow-up

Ultrasonography is a noninvasive procedure. Follow-up care is primarily education, counseling, and support as referral for additional testing or treatment based on ultrasound findings is implemented.

Since its introduction more than 30 years ago the safety of ultrasonography, especially during critical periods of embryonic development, has been questioned. Although the use of ultrasonography is apparently free from physical danger to the mother and fetus when pulse intensity is within predetermined safety zones, no conclusive empirical findings or longitudinal data are available to support this claim (Sabbagha, 1994; Anthony, 1996).

Doppler Studies

An addition to ultrasound imaging technology is color-enhanced Doppler flow studies, also called umbilical vessel velocimetry. Based on recent data, The American College of Obstetricians and Gynecologists (ACOG, 1997) has endorsed the use and clinical value of umbilical vessel Doppler studies in high-risk pregnancies.

Description

Doppler blood studies, or umbilical vessel velocimetry, is the measurement of blood flow velocity and direction in major fetal and uterine structures. The Doppler effect provides information about blood flow in supplying vessels and reflects changes in the connecting fetal-uterine vascular system. The Doppler effect, or Doppler shift, occurs when a sound wave is reflected from a moving object, and there is a change in the frequency of the reflected wave relative to that of the transmitted wave. This principle can be applied to fetal RBCs moving through the umbilical vessels. The velocity of the RBC can be determined by measuring the change in the frequency of the sound wave reflected off the cell. Therefore, Doppler ultrasonography detects the movement of RBCs in vessels and is used to measure blood flow velocity.

Timing and Indications

Velocity waveforms can be detected as early as 15 weeks' gestation. With advancing gestation there is a progressive decrease in resistance in the umbilical vessels. Consequently, a high-velocity umbilical artery flow or a lower systolic-to-diastolic ratio is found in normally growing fetuses. Decreased umbilical vessel flow is found in fetuses with intrauterine growth retardation (IUGR) and in pregnancies complicated by pregnancy-induced hypertension (PIH) or postdates, when a pregnancy exceeds its edc, usually 42 weeks. In addition, exposure to nicotine from maternal smoking has been shown to decrease blood flow velocity (Schulman, 1990).

Client Preparation

From the client's perspective, physical preparation is similar to the preparation for imaging ultrasonography. Additional counseling and education are needed specific to the indications for the addition of Doppler velocity.

Procedure

The technique of transabdominal ultrasound is used to obtain blood flow velocity measurements. A Doppler waveform of a vessel represents the systolic and diastolic flow velocities within the vessel. Doppler measurements include the systolic-to-diastolic ratio (systolic/diastolic measure), pulsatility index (systolic-diastolic/mean value of the maximum frequencies) and resistance or Pourcelot's index (systolic-diastolic/systolic). High values (>3) in the second half of pregnancy may indicate increased resistance of the placental vascular bed and decreased diastolic flow (Reed, 1995; Cundiff, Haubrick & Hinzman, 1990). Doppler waveforms can measure the blood flow velocity in several vessels, including the intracerebral, renal, femoral, and umbilical arteries. The most common application is measurement of blood flow velocity from the fetus to the placenta or in the umbilical artery. Doppler flow studies therefore primarily measure placental and not fetal health (Whittle, 1992). However, Doppler studies have been considered a valuable screening tool because abnormalities in the placental vascular status are theoretically associated with fetal problems or compromise. An abnormal flow is either an absent end-diastolic flow or a flow index greater than 2 standard deviations above the mean for gestational age.

Color-enhanced flow imaging is an extension of Doppler velocimetry. With color-flow instrumentation, multiple samples of blood flow velocity are obtained. A mean velocity is calculated and assigned a color by the instrument. An image of the vessel is displayed in color, and the direction and velocity of blood flow are represented by color changes coinciding with the cardiac cycle (Hung et al., 1997).

Follow-up

Follow-up care includes providing information and support to the client and her family, explaining the management plan, and making referrals as needed.

Magnetic Resonance Imaging

The newest imagery modality in pregnancy is magnetic resonance imaging (MRI). MRI generates excellent pictures of soft tissue, similar to those of computerized tomography (CT). Unlike CT, however, ionizing radiation is not used, thus eliminating any known biological risk.

Description

Magnetic resonance imaging (MRI) is a noninvasive diagnostic tool that provides high-resolution cross-sectional images of fluid-filled soft tissues. MRI produces a magnetic field that causes the hydrogen nuclei of the body to align and emit a signal, which is converted to a computer image (Fishbach, 2000). Similar to ultrasonography, MRI can provide images in a variety of planes. Unlike sonography, however, with MRI there is no interference from skeletal, fatty, or gas-filled structures and a full bladder is not necessary for imaging structures deep in the pelvis.

Timing and Indications

In pregnancy, MRI has been used as early as 10 weeks' gestation to demonstrate placental location and biparietal diameter, and the results are comparable with ultrasound imaging. However, MRI is specifically suited for the detection of soft-tissue abnormalities not easily identifiable on ultrasonography, such as hydatiform mole and fetal anomalies (e.g., cystic hygroma, urethral obstruction, and hydronephrosis) (Fishbach, 2000). The uses of MRI technology during pregnancy include evaluation of fetal structure, placental tissue, amniotic fluid quantity, maternal structures, biochemical status of tissue and organs, and soft tissue or functional anomalies.

Client Preparation

During the procedure, which can take 20 to 60 minutes, the client must lie completely still.

Procedure

The client is placed in a supine position on a table that is then moved into the bore of the main magnet. Because it takes a significant amount of time to produce magnetic resonance images, the probability of fetal movement during image generation is high. Movement leads to image distortion. Consequently, the major drawbacks of MRI imagery during pregnancy are the following: inability to select the plane of imaging, making true measurement of fetal structures impossible; and the relatively long time period needed to produce a single image, resulting in distortion secondary to fetal movement. MRI is advantageous in situations that are not conducive to ultrasound examination, such as maternal obesity and oligohydramnios. Thus, the utility of MRI during pregnancy may be increased in conditions such as oligiohydramnios where fetal movement is limited and in which ultrasound examination of

the fetus and uterine contents is inhibited by the lack of amniotic fluid (Johnson, 1992). The overall cost and length of time required to complete imaging has reserved the use of MRI in pregnant women to situations in which the results of other imaging modalities are unacceptable.

The client will be given a follow-up appointment for results.

Fetal Heart Rate Monitoring

Fetal heart rate monitoring is integral to fetal surveillance. Intermittent auscultation of the fetal heart rate has been a basic component of fetal physiologic surveillance for many years and is a standard component of each prenatal visit (Figure 22-6). The introduction and widespread acceptance of electronic fetal monitoring techniques have allowed the development of testing modalities to evaluate fetal condition over time and in response to intrauterine events. The goal of fetal evaluation with electronic fetal monitoring in late pregnancy is to determine whether the intrauterine environment continues to be supportive of the fetus. Antenatal electronic fetal monitoring can identify the gradual deterioration of placental function, ultimately resulting in fetal hypoxia. As the fetus experiences sustained hypoxemia, cardiac output, arterial blood pressure, and cerebral and cardiac blood flow are decreased (Parer, 1999). These physiologic alterations are manifested as characteristic changes in fetal heart rate patterns.

Fetal heart rate variability or rhythmic change in baseline heart rate values is a reassuring indicator of a supportive intrauterine environment. Variability is designated as a nonperiodic fetal heart rate change because it is not related to changes in fetal or uterine activity. Periodic fetal heart rate changes are defined as alterations in the fetal heart rate pattern in response to fetal movement or uterine contraction. The major designations of periodic changes

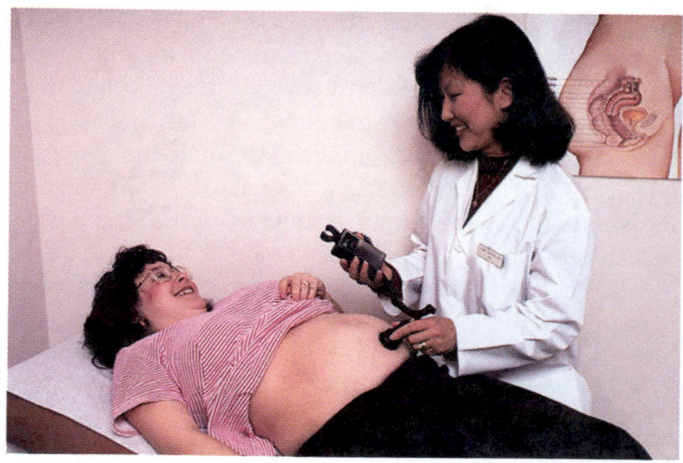

Figure 22-6 Fetal heart rate monitoring is a routine factor in each prenatal visit.

are accelerations and decelerations. An acceleration is a responsive or stimulated increase of fetal heart rate by a minimum of 15 bpm with a duration of at least 15 seconds. A deceleration is a decrease in fetal heart rate in response to fetal or uterine activity. Decelerations in response to uterine contractions are further differentiated by their relationship to the onset, peak, and resolution of the contraction. Analysis and classification of the fetal heart rate pattern are the foundation of antenatal fetal heart monitoring evaluation. The methods of electronic fetal monitoring used for fetal evaluation include nonstress tests with or without the addition of fetal acoustic stimulation (FAS) and contraction stress tests (CST).

Nonstress Test

A nonstress test (NST) is a noninvasive method that combines detection of fetal heart rate accelerations and presence of spontaneous or evoked fetal movement. A NST is a relatively inexpensive procedure and has no known contraindications. NSTs are performed by nurses in a variety of settings including outpatient, inpatient, and home environments.

Description

A **nonstress test (NST)** is the evaluation of fetal heart rate in response to an increase in either spontaneous or stimulated fetal activity.

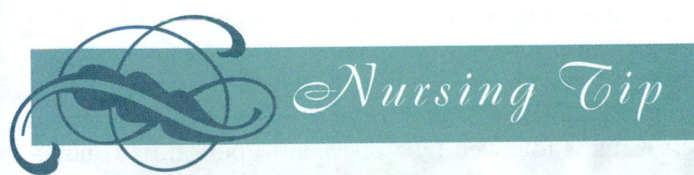

INDICATIONS FOR THE NST

1. Suspected postmaturity
2. Maternal diabetes mellitus
3. Maternal hypertension: chronic and pregnancy-related disorders
4. Suspected or documented intrauterine growth restriction (IUGR)
5. Sickle cell disease
6. History of previous stillbirth
7. Isoimmunization
8. Older gravida
9. Chronic renal disease
10. Decreasing fetal movement
11. Severe maternal anemia
12. Multiple gestation
13. High-risk antepartal conditions: premature rupture of fetal membranes, preterm labor, bleeding

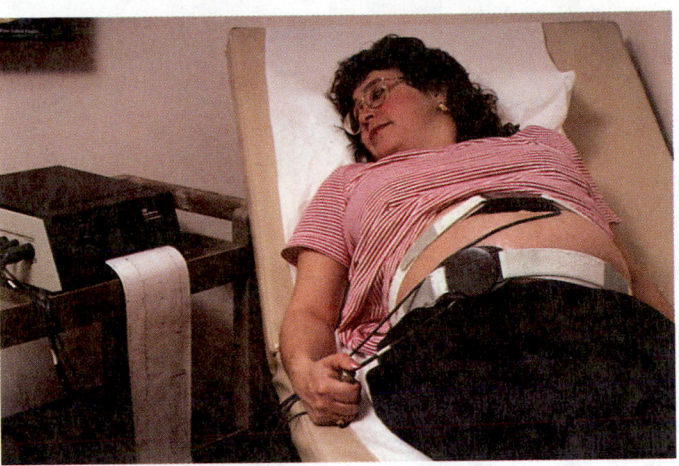

Figure 22-7 A client undergoing a nonstress test is asked to depress a button when fetal movements are felt.

Timing and indications

Nonstress testing can be reliably performed after 28 weeks' gestation, when maturity of the fetal autonomic nervous system is achieved. A positive relationship between fetal heart rate acceleration and fetal movement is dependent on the integration of peripheral receptors, the autonomic nervous system, and myocardial function (Paul & Miller, 1995). In the healthy fetus with a functional central nervous system (CNS), 90% of fetal body movements are associated with accelerations in fetal heart rate (Tucker, 2000).

Client Preparation

The NST is a noninvasive procedure that can be performed in an outpatient setting. The client's blood pressure is taken and documented. The woman is placed in a reclining position or a Semi-Fowler position with a lateral tilt to avoid supine hypotension. An external mode of fetal monitoring is placed on the abdomen. The woman may be instructed to depress an event button to mark episodes of fetal movement on the monitoring strip (Figure 22-7).

Procedure

The fetal heart rate is detected and recorded by the Doppler transducer. Fetal movement is documented either by the event button or use of the tocotransducer to document fetal movements as intermittent changes in uterine pressure. The test usually is completed in 20 minutes but may take longer if the fetus is in a sleep state.

The criteria for a reactive NST are two accelerations in a 20-minute test period and a normal baseline fetal heart rate. Failure to fulfill the criteria as a reactive pattern over a total of a 40-minute test period is deemed a nonreactive NST. A nonreactive result is the absence of accelerations during the test period (Figure 22-8). The 40-minute time frame for observation accounts for fetal sleep-wake cycles. A third result is an inconclusive, or equivocal, test

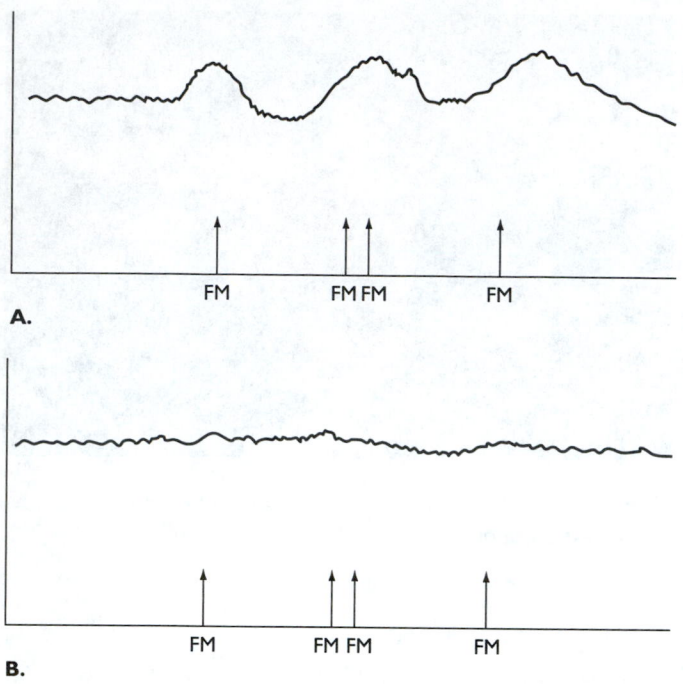

A.

B.

Figure 22-8 A. A reactive nonstress test pattern shows fetal heart acceleration with movement. B. The nonreactive pattern shows absence of accelerations during the test period.

result. An inconclusive test result is the finding of less than two accelerations in the 20-minute test window, accelerations that do not meet the criteria of an amplitude increase of 15 bpm for a duration of 15 seconds, or a poor-quality recording that is inadequate for interpretation.

When the NST is reactive, it is highly predictive of fetal health and well-being. However, the use of the NST in identifying the fetus at risk for a poor perinatal outcome is less reliable. NSTs have a significantly high false-positive rate of over 75%; in other words, more than 75% of fetuses with nonreactive NSTs are in fact healthy (Gauthier, 1979; Smith, 1995).

In an attempt to reduce the incidence of false-positive results on NSTs and to differentiate a healthy fetus at rest from one who is sick or asphyxiated, vibroacoustic stimulation has been used. An artificial larynx that provides acoustic and vibratory stimuli has received FDA approval for prenatal use between 28 and 42 weeks' gestation. Vibroacoustic stimulation usually is initiated after 10 minutes of nonreactivity during the NST. To provoke fetal activity, the stimulation is applied to the maternal abdomen for 1 second. The stimulus startles the fetus, causing a behavioral state change, and generates a state of reactivity. If the fetus does not respond, the stimuli can be repeated twice. After stimulation, the fetus is observed until a reactive pattern is attained or until 40 minutes have elapsed. Fetuses exposed to vibroacoustic stimulation exhibit more movements and therefore are more likely to have a reactive test pattern (Marsden et al., 1997).

REFLECTIONS FROM A NURSE

"I recently worked with a woman who was 33 weeks pregnant and eager to see the end of a rough pregnancy marked by daily nausea, a great deal of back pain, and swollen feet. After a nonreactive NST, the woman emphatically stated: 'I want to have a cesarean birth right now, so the nursery can take care of my baby!' Being a mother of three myself, I empathized with her plight, but took it upon myself to gently remind her of the benefits of seeing a pregnancy through to at least 38 weeks. I also made some suggestions for exercise and diet changes, which I thought could help relieve some of her discomforts"

Follow-up

When the NST is reactive, most practitioners will repeat the examination twice weekly. The pregnancy is continued if the results remain reassuring. When the results are inconclusive or equivocal, either the NST is repeated within 12 to 24 hours or further testing is scheduled, based on the evaluation of the clinical situation. A nonreactive test result is followed by a decision to perform a contraction stress test or a biophysical profile to further evaluate fetal well-being.

Contraction Stress Test

The contraction stress test (CST) is one of the original forms of fetal testing. It is a graded fetal stress test based on the principle that a stage of fetal compromise can be identified by exposing the fetus to gradual stress. Stress is applied by uterine contractions that cause intermittent interruption of oxygenated blood into the villus spaces, resulting in a transient decrease in the partial pressure of oxygen to the fetus. If the fetus has a baseline oxygen deficit, it will be manifested as a change in the fetal heart rate pattern.

Description

A **contraction stress test (CST)** stimulates uterine contractions for the purpose of assessing fetal response. It evaluates the presence or absence of fetal heart rate de-

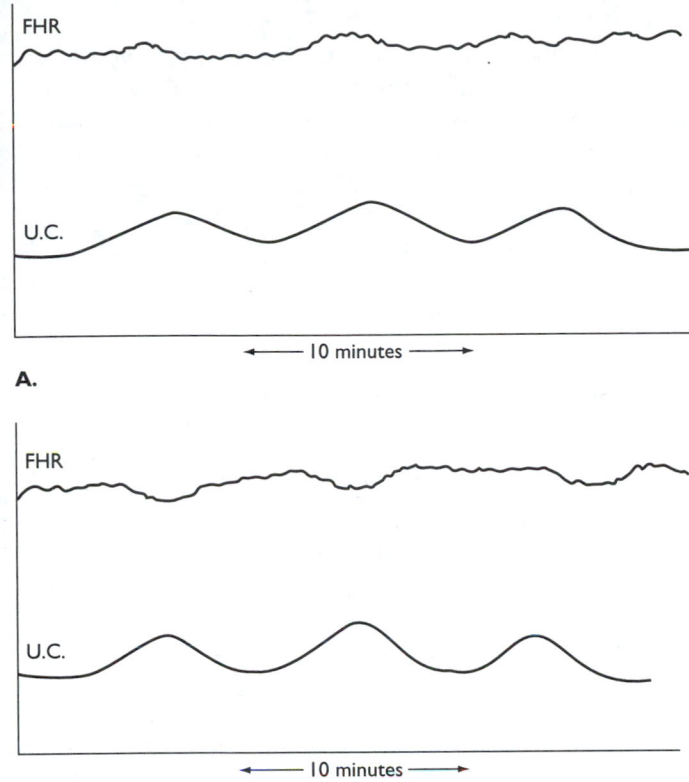

Figure 22-9 A. Negative contraction stress test. B. Positive contraction stress test.

celerations in the presence of uterine contractions (Figure 22-9). The presence of a late deceleration pattern of the fetal heart rate during a uterine contraction is indicative of uteroplacental insufficiency and altered fetal cardiorespiratory reserves. In a healthy fetus, cardiorespiratory reserves are adequate to tolerate the decreased or interrupted intravillous blood flow associated with uterine contraction whereas inadequate fetal cardiorespiratory reserves lead to decreased tolerance of altered uteroplacental blood flow that is manifested as late decelerations.

Timing and Indications

A CST usually is performed after a nonreactive finding on a NST. Although a NST is noninvasive, with no known contraindications, the CST is not. The potential for preterm labor after a CST has led to it being contraindicated in clients with a predisposition to preterm labor or a gestation age at which the risk for preterm birth is greater that is the benefit of the information provided.

Client Preparation

Because the CST is an invasive procedure, informed consent must be documented. A discussion of potential risks should include the possibility of the need for preterm vaginal or abdominal birth.

Procedure

A CST is an invasive procedure because it stimulates uterine contractions. To perform a CST, the client is placed in a Semi-Fowler position and baseline maternal vital signs and fetal heart rate tracings are obtained. Uterine contractions can be induced by either nipple stimulation or administration of exogenous oxytocin. The results of a CST are documented as follows:

- Negative: no late decelerations with three adequate uterine contractions in a 10-minute window, normal baseline fetal heart rate, and accelerations with fetal movement.
- Positive: Late decelerations with more than half the uterine contractions.
- Suspicious: Late decelerations with fewer than half the uterine contractions.
- Unsatisfactory: Inadequate fetal heart rate recording or less than three uterine contractions in 10 minutes.

A CST is a lengthy procedure, averaging 90 minutes. It also is an invasive surveillance measure that carries the risks of labor and premature delivery of the pregnancy as a result of stimulation of the uterus. Consequently, these risks must be considered in the decision to undertake a CST. Similar to the NST, the CST also has a high false-positive rate of 50% to 75% (Gauthier, 1979, Paul & Miller, 1997). Therefore, external fetal monitoring as a surveillance technique identifies the healthy well-oxygenated fetus but is of limited use in identifying the at-risk or compromised fetus.

Follow-up

If the CST is negative, the oxytocin source is discontinued. Intravenous fluids are continued until uterine activity has returned to preprocedure status. A negative CST is reassuring that the fetus is likely to survive labor should it occur within 1 week if there are no other changes in either maternal or fetal condition. Immediate retesting is needed if any change in maternal condition occurs. If the CST is positive, continued monitoring and assessment of fetal well-being are needed. A positive result may lead to a decision to end the pregnancy and care for the newborn in the nursery.

Fetal Behavior Studies

Documenting the woman's perception of fetal movement is the traditional method for evaluating fetal behavior. Whereas maternal perception of fetal activity provides valuable data, the addition of ultrasound technology has provided direct measurements of fetal behavior.

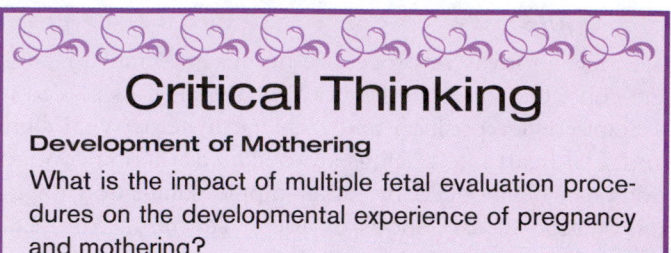

Critical Thinking

Development of Mothering

What is the impact of multiple fetal evaluation procedures on the developmental experience of pregnancy and mothering?

Fetal Movement Count

Fetal movement counting, also known as kick counting, is a simple noninvasive form of surveillance that can be done anywhere.

Description

Fetal movement counting (FMC) is the daily maternal assessment of fetal activity by counting the number of movements within a specified time period. The pregnant woman's observation of fetal movement has been validated through an 80% to 90% correlation of maternal perception of movement with movement detected on real-time ultrasonography (Moore & Piacquadio, 1989).

Timing and Indications

The American College of Obstetricians and Gynecologists ACOG (1994) recommends daily fetal movement counting beginning at 28 weeks' gestation for pregnant women at increased risk for antepartal fetal death. Because of the simplicity of this surveillance, however, all pregnant women could benefit from instruction in fetal movement counting.

Maternal perception of fetal movement usually is related to motion of the trunk or limbs and total body movements, such as flips. During the second half of pregnancy, fetal movement becomes more organized and movements become stronger. The frequency of fetal movement peaks at 32 weeks' gestation and gradually decreases as the pregnancy approaches 40 weeks' gestation (Rayburn, 1995). A number of other factors can influence fetal movement: time of day, glucose loading, and maternal smoking, alcohol, or medication consumption.

Maternal perception of fetal movement correlates with fetal well-being. Decreased fetal movements may be associated with chronic as opposed to acute states of fetal distress (Rayburn, 1995). As the fetus experiences intrauterine compromise, the decreased activity leads to decreased oxygen requirements manifested as altered growth and oxygenation patterns.

Client Preparation

Fetal movement counting is a no-cost noninvasive method used to heighten the pregnant woman's awareness of fetal activity and behavior. Fetal movement counting can be initiated with all pregnant women after 28 weeks' gestation. Pregnant women should be taught the significance of fetal movement, the procedure for counting, how to record the findings, and when to report changes to the health care provider.

Procedure

A variety of counting methods exist. Two of the most widely used are the following:

- Record a start time. Place the hands over the abdomen to palpate fetal movement. Count until 10 movements are palpated, and record the time.

- Select a predetermined time interval. Place the hands on the abdomen to palpate fetal activity. Count the number of movements within the selected time period.

To perform fetal movement counts, the woman should be in a relaxing environment and a comfortable position, that is, semi-Fowler, reclining, or side-lying. A side-lying position promotes placental circulation and increases detection of fetal movements. Fetal movement counting should be done at the same time each day, preferably after a meal or when the fetus is most active.

Follow-up

Neither an ideal number of fetal movements nor an ideal interval for fetal movement counting has been established. A trend toward decreasing motion should be reported. In general, a count of less than three fetal movements within 1 hour necessitates further evaluation, usually with a NST or biophysical profile.

Biophysical Profile

The biophysical profile (BPP) is a dynamic noninvasive surveillance technique that combines the strong points of ultrasound imagery and external fetal monitoring technologies.

Description

The **biophysical profile** is a noninvasive dynamic assessment of the fetus and fetal environment. The BPP is based on the premise that the predictive accuracy of observing a number of biophysical variables is greater than the predictive value of a single observation. The BPP consists of five parameters: fetal heart rate reactivity, fetal breathing movements, gross body movement, fetal tone, and amniotic

Table 22-4 Biophysical Profile Variables and Scoring Criteria

Variable	Normal (Score = 2)	Abnormal (Score = 0)
Fetal breathing movements	One or more episodes of 30 seconds' duration during the 30-minute test period	Absent or breathing movement is <30 seconds' duration
Gross body movement	A minimum of three discrete body or limb movements during the 30-minute test period (active continuous movement is considered one movement)	Less than three fetal movements during the test period
Fetal tone	One or more episode of active extension with return to flexion of fetal limbs or trunk, or opening and closing of the hand	Slow extension with return to flexion, movement of limb in full extension, or absence of fetal movement
Amniotic fluid volume index	One or more pockets of amniotic fluid measuring ≥1 cm in two perpendicular planes	Pockets of amniotic fluid are <1 cm or absent
Nonstress test	Reactive	Nonreactive

Adapted from: Manning, F. A. (1995). Dynamic ultrasound-based fetal assessment: The fetal biophysical profile score. *Clinical Obstetrics and Gynecology, 38,* 26–44.

fluid volume (Manning, 1995). Each area receives a score of 0 (absent) or 2 (present) based on established criteria (Table 22-4). Therefore, BPP evaluates fetal status using a methodology modeled after the *Apgar score,* a numerical expression of the condition of a newborn.

Timing and Indications

The decision to perform a BPP usually is the sequella of a nonreassuring finding on a NST. BPP scoring is based on the assessment of both acute and chronic markers of fetal compromise. In response to systemic hypoxia the fetus demonstrates alterations in movement, muscular tone, breathing, and heart rate pattern. Therefore, normal biophysical activities are a proxy measure of a functional CNS (Manning 1995).

Client Preparation

The BPP is indicated as a result of a nonreassuring finding from a previous fetal surveillance technique. Therefore, a primary area of client preparation is emotional support, education, and counseling in the face of a potential pregnancy crisis.

Procedure

Level II, or comprehensive, ultrasonography is used to examine the variables of fetal breathing movements, gross body movements, fetal tone, and amniotic fluid volume. A NST is completed before the ultrasound examination.

A BPP score of 8 to 10 is normal, a score of 6 is equivocal, and a score of 4 or less indicates fetal compromise. The biophysical activities of the fetus provide a reflection of CNS activity because the CNS is among the tissues most sensitive to altered oxygen supply. Based on the gradual hypoxia principle, therefore, progressive fetal hypoxia is manifested as loss of biophysical function. The multiple-variable input of the BPP scoring system improves the specificity and sensitivity of the technique compared with the use of a single surveillance variable. BPP has a low false-negative rate of less than 1 infant per 1,000 (0.726 per 1,000) pregnancies with adequate BPP scores. Therefore, the incidence of fetal compromise is not underestimated with BPP testing. Thus, the BPP is an accurate indicator of impending fetal crisis and should be acted on (Manning, 1995).

Follow-up

The BPP is an accurate indicator of impending fetal demise. When the BPP score is low, induced labor is considered. When the BPP score is normal, intervention is indicated only for specific obstetrical or maternal factors.

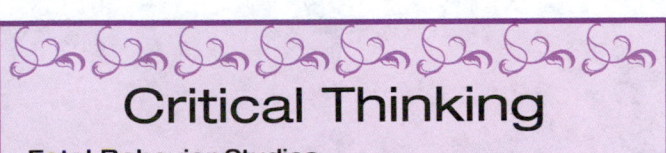

Critical Thinking

Fetal Behavior Studies

How do you respond to a client who has a nonreactive NST and BPP score of 4, but is refusing a cesarean birth because she is afraid of having surgery?

NURSING PROCESS

In the area of fetal evluation interdisciplinary collaboration and coordination of the client's care is a significant component of nursing care. Some of the fetal evaluation technologies discussed in this chapter are not within the scope of nursing practice; however, the nurse's role in the care of the client surrounding the procedure is essential and needs to be a component of the nursing management plan for the woman's pregnancy.

Assessment

A comprehensive nursing assessment is completed during the initial prenatal contact to identify risk factors or indications of the need for fetal evaluation. An interrelationship among biophysical, psychosocial, sociodemographic, and environmental variables can impact maternal response to the pregnant state, fetal development and well-being, desirability of the intrauterine environment, and the ultimate pregnancy outcome. The initial comprehensive assessment may reveal indicators for immediate testing or may uncover indicators for testing at some future point in the pregnancy.

The nursing assessment needs to include physical and physiologic factors as well as cultural and emotional ones that influence the woman's need for and perception of fetal evaluation technologies. Nurses must be aware and knowledgeable about predisposing conditions along with procedures and resources available for prenatal fetal surveillance. The assessment process should result in collection of an individualized database that facilitates selection of fetal evaluation modalities within the context of the client's situation.

Once the need for a fetal evaluation procedure has been identified, the nurse often is the primary liaison between the pregnant client, testing facility, and associated specialist and staff. At the time of the procedure, a focused assessment of both maternal and fetal status is completed. The purpose of this assessment is to identify factors that may alter or contraindicate the performance of a fetal evaluation procedure. For example, the presence of a vaginal infection would contraindicate transvaginal CVS, the inability to auscultate the fetal heat tone would lead to additional assessment to confirm fetal viability before amniocentesis, and the presence of uterine irritability or cervical change would necessitate an evaluation of the decision to perform a CST.

A significant component of the nursing assessment is to evaluate the client's psychosocial status to identify the levels of stress and anxiety being experienced. Stress and anxiety can interfere with the client's ability to make decisions and cope with test procedures and outcomes.

Stress and anxiety also can impact the client's level of understanding. The client's ability to take, assimilate, and process information about the need, risks, benefits, and limitations of the procedure and its outcomes must be assessed. When faced with the crisis of a problem pregnancy, clients may be unable to absorb information about the procedure, diagnosis, follow-up, and options for alternative modes of evaluation and interventions. Consequently, in addition to a complete physical and psychosocial assessment, the nurse needs to assess the client's ability to participate in the informed decision-making process (Figure 22-10).

Client Education

Fetal Evaluation

To encourage critical thinking by the client, the nurse may ask the following questions:

- What do you know about the status of your pregnancy and fetus?

- How did you learn this information?

- How do you explain this concern to yourself?

- What do you think will help you to deal with your concern?

- How does this situation affect your daily life?

- If you could have one question answered, what would it be?

- How much control do you think you have over this situation?

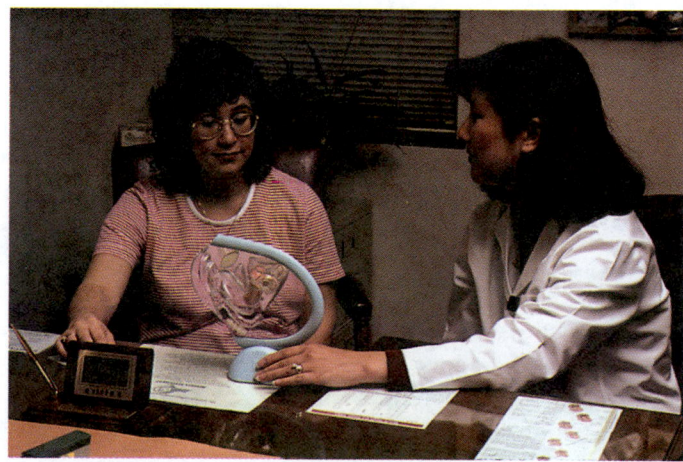

Figure 22-10 Part of the nurse's responsibilities during fetal evaluation procedures is to ensure the client is fully informed and able to participate in the decision-making process.

The woman's individual belief system also is an integral component of the assessment. Racial, ethnic, and cultural differences are particularly important in assessing clients. A recent study has revealed that African American and Hispanic women are less likely to use fetal diagnostic testing compared with Caucasion and Asian women, suggesting that the meaning of testing, pregnancy termination, and raising a disabled child may be unique within cultural groups (Kuppermann, Gates, & Washington, 1996). The meaning of pregnancy, the status ascribed to the fetus, beliefs about disability and disease, attitudes about pregnancy termination, family dynamics, and decision-making patterns must be analyzed within the context of the client's dominant cultural paradigm. The cultural role of women, the perception of childbearing as a developmental process or a role-gender responsibility, a choice versus a fate, and the choice of being an active participant and decision-maker or a follower and producer of offspring have profound influences on the client's perception and use of fetal evaluation technologies. It is important to avoid cultural stereotyping however; that is, the nurse must recognize that not all clients of a specific cultural origin will hold the same values and beliefs. Therefore, assessing the client's cultural perspective is essential in developing a plan of care that is culturally sensitive and congruent.

A comprehensive holistic assessment is essential to identifying the client's need for fetal evaluation and to developing an individualized plan of care. Because the fetal environment can change quickly and the woman's physiologic response to the pregnant state can vary from adaptive to maladaptive, assessment needs to be an ongoing process throughout the duration of the gestational period.

Nursing Diagnoses

Appropriate nursing diagnoses are based on clustering, interpretating, and validating client-specific assessment data to determine mutually agreed on client needs. Consequently, a thorough assessment and knowledge base about fetal evaluation procedures are essential in formulating reliable and valid nursing diagnoses. A list of nursing diagnoses is provided to give some insight into the types of health care needs typically associated with fetal evaluation testing. The following nursing diagnostic labels can be applied to most of the procedures discussed in this chapter. The cause and supporting data components of the diagnostic statement, however, must be individualized based on the context of the testing situation and client-specific assessment data.

- Risk for injury of the invasive diagnostic technique.
- Powerlessness related to feeling inadequate to properly care for the fetus, inability to control events impacting fetal well-being, and inability to protect the fetus.

- Pain related to manipulation during the diagnostic procedure.
- Anxiety related to the possibility of an abnormal test result and uncertainty.
- Fear related to possible complications of the procedure and possible pregnancy loss.
- Ineffective coping related to stress and the inability to control or influence events.
- Spiritual distress related to the possibility of a negative outcome of the testing procedure and association of the outcome with pregnancy termination.
- Anticipatory grieving related to the loss of a "perfect" pregnancy.

Outcome Identification

The outcomes reflect the needs and desired goals for the woman, fetus, and family. Consistent with a variety of theoretic frameworks, goals are initially prioritized to reflect physiologic needs followed by psychosocial and emotional needs. However, pregnancy is a developmental episode in the client's life. Therefore outcome identification specific to fetal evaluation technologies needs to be formulated within the context of the pregnancy experience and the individualized client database. Consequently, because the priority outcome may be related to a psychosocial or emotional state, the risk of physical complications may be considered a secondary outcome by the woman. The important point is that the rationale for the designated priority be based on scientific principles yet be consistent with the values and beliefs of the client and mutually agreeable to all involved in the care-giving situation. Because of the amount of time required by some fetal evaluation procedures, the expected outcomes for each proposed group of nursing interventions should be documented in the client's medical record to allow for continuity of care. Possible outcomes for the client experiencing fetal evaluation include the following:

- The woman and fetus experience no injury or complication from the procedure
  - The fetal heart rate is audible and within normal parameters based on gestational age.
  - The client has no uterine cramping, or uterine cramping resolves within 24 hours.
- The fetus maintains a state of well-being.
  - Fetal movement level is unchanged.
  - Fetal heart rate is consistent with the norms for gestational age, and accelerations are present.
- The compromised fetus is identified, and timely referral for follow-up is made.
- The woman participates in the decision-making process related to the selection and use of fetal evaluation procedures.

– She verbalizes concerns and questions related to fetal evaluation technologies.

– She verbalizes the meaning of the fetal evaluation testing results.

– She states her options based on the testing results.

🐦 The woman and family psychologically adapt to the process and results of fetal evaluation procedures.

Planning

The nurse is responsible for planning client care in accordance with established standards of care as defined by state nursing practice acts, professional scope of practice statements, professional education, and employer policies and guidelines. Some fetal evaluation procedures such as CVS, amniocentesis, PUBS, and BPPs are performed by sonographers, laboratory specialists, and physicians. In these situations, the planning component of the nursing process involves facilitating communication and coordination among activities, settings, and practitioners.

RECOMMENDATIONS OF THE U.S. PREVENTIVE SERVICES TASK FORCE: STRATEGIES IN HEALTH EDUCATION AND COUNSELING

1. Frame the teaching to match the client's perception.

2. Fully inform clients of the purpose and expected effects of the intervention and when to expect these effects.

3. Be specific.

4. Use a combination of strategies.

5. Involve others.

6. Refer.

7. Monitor progress through follow-up contacts.

Ask yourself:

● How do you feel about women who come for prenatal care but refuse to undergo fetal evaluation testing?

● How do your personal values and beliefs about pregnancy, children, and disability influence your interactions with these clients?

U.S. Preventive Services Task Force. (1996). *Guidelines to clinical preventive services* (2 ed.). Philadelphia: Williams & Wilkins.

Other fetal evaluation technologies, such as NSTs and CSTs, are performed by the nurse. Not only does the nurse need the competencies to carry out the procedure but the skill to recognize nonreassuring patterns and to initiate interventions and notification of appropriate personnel.

An important component of planning is ensuring that the persons significant to the client are included in the procedure and decision-making process, as desired by the client. An assessment of family dynamics and communication patterns consistent with the client's cultural values and beliefs will assist the nurse to empower the client to include those persons important to her.

A growing number of nurses are performing ultrasound scans, BPPs, and other fetal evaluation procedures. Nurses who have training and competence, usually in the form of additional education, can perform these procedures if it is within the scope of practice as defined in the practice act of their state (Treanor, 1998).

Nursing Intervention

Nursing interventions are concentrated primarily in the area of counseling, support, and education. Before the procedure, nursing interventions encompass explaining the indications, risks, accuracy, technical aspects, rationale, and limitations of the specific evaluation modality. Performance of fetal evaluation procedures such as CVS, amniocentesis, PUBs, and MRI are not within the scope of nursing practice. The nurse is integrally involved in preparing the client, however, and may be present during the procedure. In these situations the nurse plays a vital role in explaining the technical and sensory aspects of the procedure. When the nurse is present during the performance of the procedure, her role is twofold: assisting the physician and supporting the client. During the procedure, the nursing activities may include assisting with skin preparations, positioning the woman, and specimen collection and labeling. The more significant role of the nurse, however, is as client advocate and a source of support. During the procedure, the nurse should be in continuous contact, verbal or nonverbal as appropriate, with the client. The nurse can provide anticipatory guidance about what will happen next, provide comfort measures, use anxiety reduction techniques, and monitor for potential and real problems.

After the procedure, nursing interventions include monitoring the pregnancy for complications that include amniotic fluid leakage; bleeding; uterine irritability; fetal distress, including changes in fetal cardiac activity; and maternal physiologic parameters of distress, such as fever, pain, and changes in baseline vital signs. Facilitating the client's verbalization of her perception of the experience, her concerns, and her coping strategies and support systems while awaiting the results are vital interventions.

Case Study/Care Plan

CLIENT IN A SECOND PREGNANCY

Maria presents for her first prenatal visit. Maria, who is 40 years old, is accompanied by her husband of 14 years, Alex. Maria is a loan officer and Alex is a 43-year-old stockbroker. Both Maria and Alex are very religious. They have not used contraceptive methods during their marriage. They had begun to explore adoption during the past year, with the belief that pregnancy was not in God's plan for their lives.

This is Maria's second pregnancy. Her first pregnancy was at aged 16 and produced a 3-pound male infant at 39 weeks' gestation. The infant was placed for adoption, and Maria has had no contact with him.

Assessment

The client reports she has missed two menstrual periods and has had a positive home pregnancy test.

Both Maria and Alex are excited about this pregnancy and the prospect of being parents. They state that they desire this baby and are certain everything will be okay since they have waited so long.

Family history is significant because Maria's older sister gave birth to a stillborn infant with an "open sore on her back" 20 years ago. Alex's family history is without evidence of genetic or birth-related conditions.

Maternal vital signs and prepregnancy weight are within normal limits.

Maria is referred for an amniocentesis for karyotyping and evaluation of AFP level. Maria and Alex tearfully agree to the procedure stating, "We love this baby. There can't be anything wrong. Please tell us everything will be okay."

Nursing Diagnosis

Deficient knowledge related to unfamiliarity with the testing procedures and lack of understanding of genetic predisposition.

Expected Outcome   Client will understand importance of family history related to risk factors.
Client will understand general parameters of the procedure.
Client will feel empowered during the procedure.

Planning   Referral for comprehensive ultrasonography specifically to examine for neural tube closure, movement of lower extremities, and bladder filling. In later pregnancy, Maria will need to be monitored for IUGR based on a previous history of a low-birth-weight infant and a family history of a stillbirth.

Nursing Interventions	Rationales
1. Teach the client about the indications, risks, benefits, and limitation of amniocentesis for fetal karyotype and AFP analysis.	1. Client acceptance of the procedure is based partly on an understanding of how it works and what it does.
2. Provide emotional support during the procedure.	2. The client's fears and feelings of loss of power can be kept in check with thoughtful and sensitive nursing care.
3. Encourage consultation with clergy or presence of religious article, as desired by the client.	3. Show respect for the client's preferences by considering factors that are important to her during the decision-making process.

Evaluation

1. The client is able to state the purpose, process, and alternatives to the chosen procedure.
2. The client's spiritual needs are met consistent with her beliefs and values.

Some fetal evaluation procedures, such as fetal movement counts, are completely within the scope of nursing practice. Nurses can initiate the procedure by teaching the client the purpose and process of fetal movement counting. When a decrease in fetal movement is detected, the nurse collaborates with and refers to the physician or certified nurse-midwife for further evaluation and testing.

Evaluation

The woman, pregnancy, and family unit need to be reevaluated in the context of the results of fetal evaluative procedures and the individual client's values and choices. Depending on the results of the testing procedure, evaluation of nursing interventions and achievement of nursing care goals may lead to formulation of a new nursing care plan focused on promoting a healthy pregnancy or adapting to and coping with an affected fetus, a high-risk pregnancy, or perinatal loss.

FUTURE DIRECTIONS

Support for the continued use and further dissemination of fetal surveillance technologies was identified in the objectives of Healthy People 2000, which stated, "increase to at least 90% the proportion of women enrolled in prenatal care who are offered screening and counseling on prenatal detection of fetal anomalies" (U.S. Department of Health and Human Services, 1991). Prenatal fetal testing is becoming increasingly recommended during pregnancy. Combined with continued technologic advances in genetics and instrumentation, this trend is not likely to be reversed. In addition, the wide dissemination of information about fetal evaluation modalities has resulted in consumers who request procedures, sometimes based on incomplete knowledge or information. Another practice that can influence the use of fetal surveillance procedures is the practice of defensive medicine. The use of fetal evaluation technologies to prevent a potential legal action as opposed to using it to promote maternal well-being

should be a point of concern. Much of the literature related to emerging technologies is focused on safety, accuracy, and financial costs of different procedures and not on the broader implications of the use of that knowledge within the context of society. As patient advocates, nurses must ensure that decisions are made consistent with the client's values and not directed solely by technology or the dominant values of the health care system.

Fetal surveillance technologies can produce a sense of anxiety and a feeling of powerlessness in women and their families. Decisions related to the use of fetal surveillance can alter family dynamics and can impact the bond between mother and the fetus or infant (Raines, 1996). Simply because the technology is available does not mean that every procedure is right for every pregnancy. Questions about the purpose, process, and consequences of fetal evaluation are critical to holistic nursing practice and individualized, quality nursing care. Sometimes a little mystery is a good thing.

Web Activities

The following web sites have information concerning assessment of fetal status. Visit these sites for additional information.

- www.fetal.com
- www.medphys.ucl.ac.uk/mgi/fetal
- www.amnionet.com
- www.med.upenn.edu/meded
- www.public/berp/overview
- www.cpdx.com/cpdx
- www.virtualbirth.com
- www.sgvp.com
- www.docboard.org

Key Concepts

Most fetal evaluation procedures have benefits and risks to both mother and fetus. There are limitations to the amount of information provided from these testing modalities.

- Reactive NST and negative CST are reassuring signs of fetal well-being.
- A BPP is an evaluation of fetal well-being and condition of the intrauterine environment.

- Ultrasonography is a commonly used imaging modality during pregnancy with no known side effects.
- Amniocentesis is performed throughout pregnancy for differing indications: from 15 to 18 weeks' gestation for identification of chromosomal alteration or altered AFP level, in the second trimester for elevated bilirubin levels, and in the third trimester for a lung maturity profile.

❧ Alterations in AFP levels are not detectable by CVS.

❧ MS-AFP is a screening procedure that identifies pregnancies at increased risk for a neural tube defect.

❧ The nurse's role in fetal surveillance includes teaching, counseling, and supporting the client and family.

Review Questions and Activities

1. Identify nonreassuring fetal heart rate patterns using electronic fetal monitoring and discuss the physiology and nursing interventions for each pattern.

2. What are the characteristics of a reassuring fetal heart rate pattern?

3. What is the difference between a screening test and a diagnostic test? Provide examples of each type of test used in the care of the pregnant woman.

4. What are the indications for a NST and how are the results interpreted?

5. Compare and contrast the NST with the BPP.

6. What is the purpose of a CST?

References

American College of Obstetricians and Gynecologists. (1993). Ultrasound in Pregnancy (Technical Bulletin 187). Washington, D.C.: *American College of Obstetricians & Gynecologists*.

American College of Obstetricians and Gynecologists: Committee on Genetics. (1995). Chorionic Villus Sampling (Committee Opinion No. 169). Washington, D.C.: *American College of Obstetricians & Gynecologists*.

American College of Obstetricians and Gynecologists: Committee on Educational Bulletins. (1996). Maternal serum screening. *ACOG Educational Bulletin, 28,* 1–9.

Anthony, A. (1996). Biological effects and safety. In T. Dubose (Ed.). *Fetal sonography.* Philadelphia: W. B. Saunders.

Berkowitz, R. L. (1993). Should every pregnant woman undergo ultrasonography? *New England Journal of Medicine, 329,* 874–880.

Callen, P. W. (Eds.). (2001). *Ultrasound in obstetrics and gynecology* (4th ed.). Philadelphia: W. B. Saunders.

Canadian Collaborative CVS-Amniocentesis Clinical Trial Group. (1989). Multicentre randomized clinical trial of chorion villus sampling and amniocentesis. *Lancet, 1,* 1–6.

Chervenak, F., & Gabbe, S. (1996). Obstetrical ultrasound: Assessment of fetal growth and anatomy. In S. Gabbe, J. Niebyl, & J. Simpson (Eds.). *Obstetrics: Normal and problem pregnancies* (3rd ed.). New York: Churchill Livingstone.

Chitty, L. S., & Bobrow, M. (1994). Techniques in current use in prenatal diagnosis. *International Journal of Technology Assessment in Health Care, 104,* 604–627.

Cundiff, J., Haubrich, K., & Hinzman, N. (1990). Umbilical artery Doppler flow studies during pregnancy. *JOGNN, 19,* 475–481.

Cunningham, F. G., MacDonald, P. C., Gant, N. F., Leveno, K. L., Gilstrap, L. C., Hankins, G. D. V., & Clark, S. L. (1997). *Williams obstetrics* (20th ed.). Stamford, CT: Appleton & Lange.

Davis, J. G. (1993). Reproductive technologies for prenatal diagnosis. *Fetal Diagnosis and Therapy,* 8 (supp 1), 29–38.

Docker, M. F. (1992). Ultrasound imaging techniques. In D. J. H. Brock, C. H. Rodeck, M. A. Ferguson-Smith, Eds. *Prenatal diagnosis and screening.* (pp. 69–81). London: Churchill Livingston.

Fakhoury, G., Daikoku, N. H. Benser, J., & Dubin, N. H. (1994). Lamellar body concentrations and the prediction of fetal pulmonary maturity. *American Journal of Obstetrics and Gynecology, 170,* 72–76.

Fishbach, F. (2000). *A manual of laboratory and diagnostic tests* (6th ed.). Philadelphia: Lippincott-Raven.

Froster-Iskenius, U., & Baird, P. (1989). Limb reduction defects in over 1,000,000 consecutive live births. *Teratology, 39,* 127–135.

Gauthier, R. J. (1979). Antepartum fetal heart rate testing II: Intrapartum fetal heart rate observations and newborn outcome following a positive contraction stress test. *American Journal of Obstetrics and Gynecology, 133,* 34–39.

Guzman, E. et al. (1998). Longitudinal assessment of endocervical length between 15-24 weeks' gestation in women at risk for pregnancy loss or preterm birth. *Obstetrics and Gynecology, 92,* 31–37.

Haddow, J. E., & Palomaki, G. E. (1993). Prenatal screening for Downs syndrome. In J. L. Simpson, S. Elias, Eds. *Essentials of prenatal diagnosis* New York: Churchill Livingstone.

Hearns-Stebbins, B. (1995). Fetal growth assessment: A literature review. *Journal of Diagnostic Medical Sonography, 11,* 176–187.

Hsieh, F. J., Shyu, M. K., Sheu, B. C., Lin, S. P., Chen, C. P., & Huang, F. Y. (1995). Limb defects after chorionic villus sampling. *Obstetrics and Gynecology, 85,* 84–88.

Hung, J. H. H., Ng, H. T., Pan, Y. P., Yang, M. J., & Shu, L. P. (1997). Color Doppler ultrasound, pregnancy-induced hypertension and small for gestational age fetuses. *International Journal of Gynecology and Obstetrics, 56,* 3–11.

Johnson, I. R. (1992). Radiologic and magnetic visualization techniques. In D. J. H. Brock, C. H. Rodeck, & M. A. Ferguson-Smith, Eds., Prenatal diagnosis and screening. London: Churchill Livingston.

Kuppermann, M., Gates, E., & Washington, E. (1996). Racial and ethnic differences in prenatal diagnostic test use and outcomes: Preferences, socioeconomic or patient knowledge? *Obstetric and Gynecology 87,* 675–682.

Manning, F. A. (1995). Dynamic ultrasound-based fetal assessment: The fetal biophysical profile. *Clinical Obstetrics and Gynecology, 38,* 26–44.

Manning F. (1999). General principles and application of ultrasound. In R. Creasy & R. Resnik, (Eds.). *Maternal-fetal medicine* (4th ed.). Philadelphia: W. B. Saunders.

Martin, J. N., & Cowan, B. D. (1990). Biochemical assessment and prediction of gestational well-being. *Obstetric and Gynecology Clinical of North America, 17,* 81–93.

Palomaki, G. E., Knight, G. J., Hadaow, J. E., Carick, J. A., Seller, D. N. Jr & Panizza, D. S. (1992). Prospective intervention trial of a screening protocol to identify fetal trisomy 18 using maternal serim AFP, UE3, and hcg. *Prenatal Diagnosis, 12,* 925–930.

Parer, J. (1999). Fetal heart rate. In R. Creasy & R. Resnik, Eds. *Maternal-fetal medicine* (4th ed). Philadelphia: W. B. Saunders.

Paul, R. H., & Miller, D. A. (1995). Nonstress test. *Clinical Obstetrics and Gynecology, 38,* 3–10.

Raines, D. A. (1996). Fetal surveillance: Issues and Implications. *JOGNN, 25,* 559–564.

Rayburn, W. (1995). Fetal movement monitoring. *Clinical Obstetrics and Gynecology, 38,* 59–67.

Reece, E. A. (1997). Early and Midtremester Genetic Amniocentesis. *Obstetric and Gynecologic Clinical of North America, 24,* 71–81.

Reed, K. (1995). Using doppler ultrasound to detect fetal problems. *Contempory Obstetrics and Gynecology, 40,* 15–28.

Rhoads, G. G., Jackson, L. G., Schlesselman, S. E., de la Cruz, F. F., Desnick, R. J., Golbus, M. S. Ledbetter, D. H., Lubs, H. A., Mahoney, M. J., & Pergament, E. (1989). The safety and efficacy of chorionic villus sampling for early prenatal diagnosis of cytogenetic abnormalities. *New England Journal of Medicine, 320,* 609–617.

Romero, R., Puplin, M., Oyarzun, E. et al. (1991). Amniocentesis. In A. C. Fleischer, R. Romero, F. A. Manning, et al., Eds. *The principles and practice of ultrasound in obstetrics and gynecology* (pp. 439–454). Norwalk, CT: Appleton & Lange.

Ruoslahti, E., Engvall, E., Pekkpola, A., & Seppala, M. M. (1978). Developmental changes in carbohydrate moiety of human alpha-fetoprotein. *International Journal of Cancer, 221,* 515–520.

Sabbagha, R. (1994). *Diagnostic ultrasound applied to obstetrics and gynecology.* (3rd ed.). Philadelphia: J. B. Lippincott.

Schulman, H. (1990). Doppler ultrasound. In R. Eden & F. Boehm, Eds. *Assessment and care of the fetus: Physiological, clinical and mediolegal principles.* Norwalk CT: Appleton & Lange.

Scott, J., DiSaia, P., Hammond, C. et al. (1994). *Danforth's obstetrics and gynecology* (7th ed). (pp. 284, 317–321, 409–411). Philadelphia: J. B. Lippincott.

Smith, C. V. (1995). Vibroacoustic Stimulation. *Clinical Obstetrics and Gynecology, 38,* 68–77.

Steele, C. D., Wapner, R. J., Smith, J. B., et al. (1995). Prenatal diagnosis using fetal cells isolated from maternal peripheral blood: a Review. *Clinical Obstetrics and Gynecology, 39,* 801–813.

Steele, M. W., & Berg, W. R. (1966). Chromosomal analysis of human amniotic cells. *Lancet, 1,* 383.

Tabor, A., Phillip, J., Madsen, M. et al. (1986). Randomized controlled trials of genetic amniocentesis in 4606 low risk women. *Lancet, 1,* 287.

Treanor, C. (1998). Exploring nurses' role in limited ultrasound. *AWHONN's Lifeline, 2,* 13–14.

Tucker, S. (2000). *Pocket guide to fetal monitoring and assessment* (4th ed). St. Louis: Mosby

U.S. Department of Health and Human Services. (1991). *Healthy People 2000: National health promotion and disease prevention objectives.* Washington D.C.: U.S. Government Printing Office.

Wapner, R. J. (1997). Chorionic Villus Sampling. *Obstetric and Gynecologic Clinics of North America, 24,* 83–109.

Whittle, M. J. (1992). Doppler. In M. L. Druzin, Eds. *Antepartal fetal assessment* (pp. 45–61). Boston: Blackwell Scientific Publications.

Suggested Readings

A.W.H.O.N.N. (1999). *Clinical competencies and education guide: Limited ultrasound examinations in obstetrics and gynecology/infertility settings.* Chicago: Association of Women's Health, Obstetrics, and Neonatal Nursing.

Feinstein, N, Sprague, A., & Trepanier, M. J. (1999). *Fetal auscultation.* Washington, D.C.: Association of Women's Health Obstetric and Neonatal Nurses.

Gilbert, E. S., & Harmon, J.S. (1998). *High risk pregnancy and delivery.* St. Louis: Mosby.

Minihan, C. A. (1998). *Limited sonography in obstetric and gynecologic triage.* Philadelphia: Lippincott.

Murray, M. (1997). *Antepartal and intrapartal fetal monitoring.* Albuquerque: Learning Resources International Inc.

Sanders, R. (1996). *Structural fetal anomalies: The total picture.* St. Louis: Mosby.

Simpson, K. R. & Creehan, P. A. (1996). *Perinatal nursing.* Philadelphia: Lippincott.

Simpson, K. R., & Creehan, P. (1996). *Perinatal nursing.* Washington, D.C.: Association of Women's Health Obstetric and Neonatal Nurses.

Rodesch, F., Lambermont, M., Donner, C., Simon, P., Romasco, F., Schwers, J., & Wybran, J. (1987). Chorionic biopsy in management of severe kell alloimmunization. *American Journal of Obstetrics and Gynecology, 156,* 124–125.

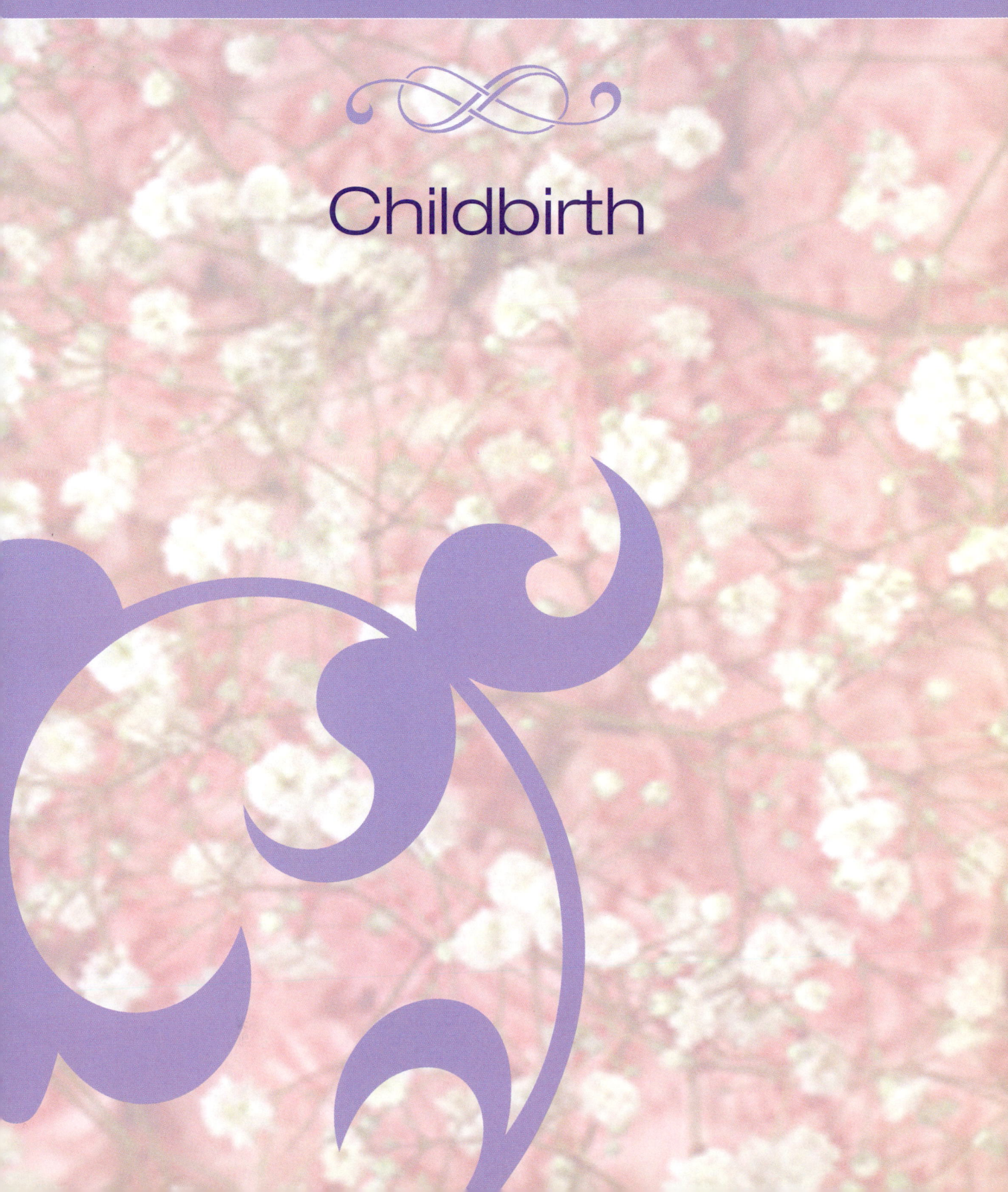

UNIT VI

Childbirth

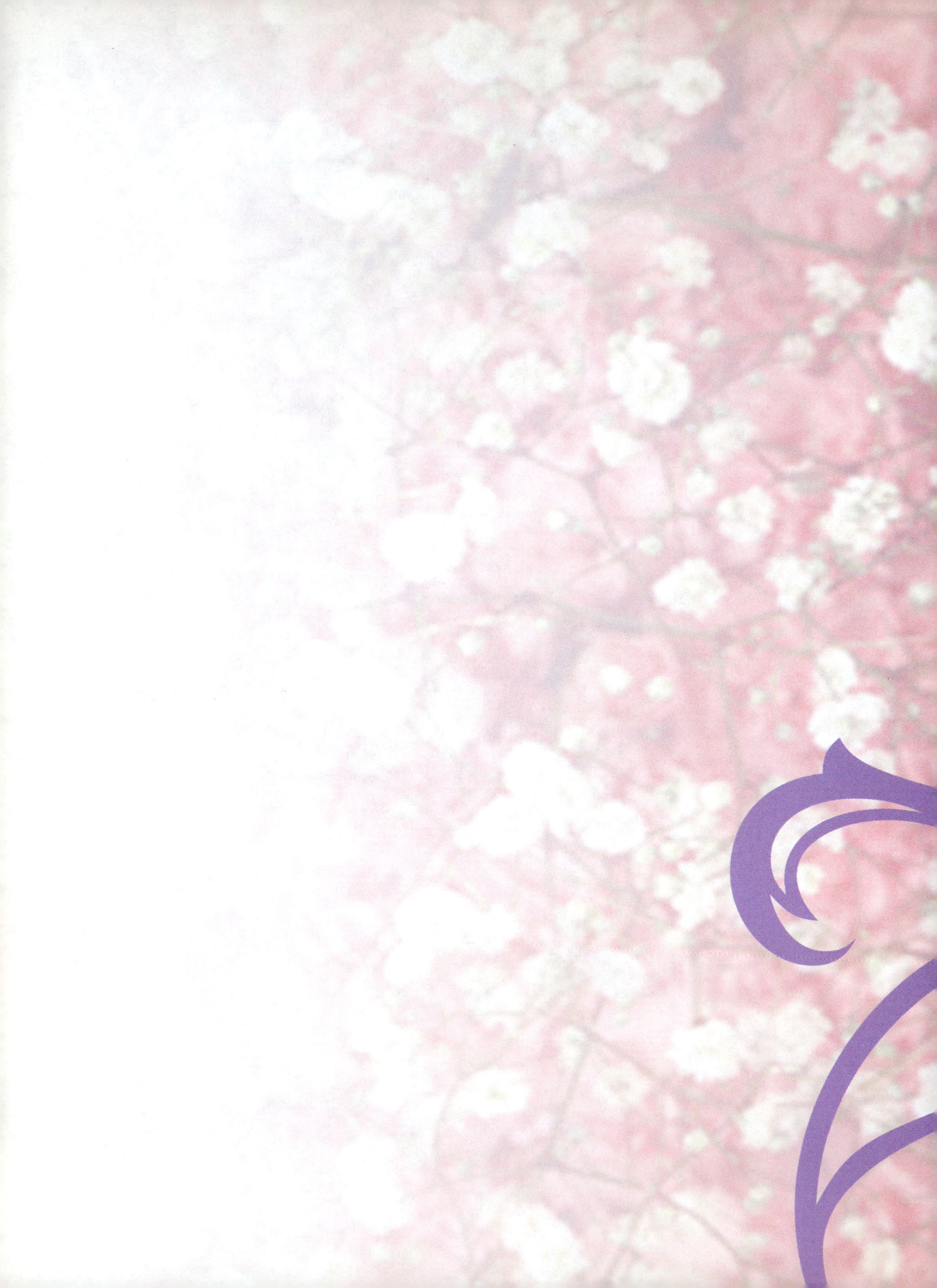

CHAPTER 23

Processes of Labor and Delivery

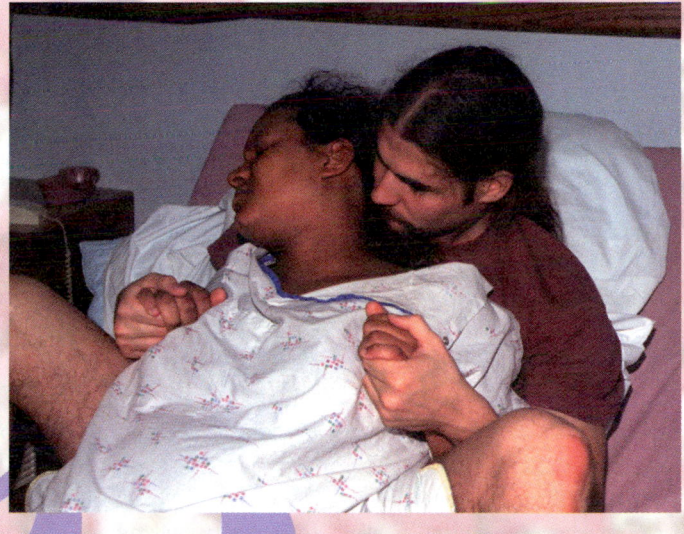

One evening, a group of women began talking about their labor experiences. Each woman could clearly remember the details. It did not matter if it was her first or her fourth child, she could recall many of the details of the labor and delivery, even when the events had occurred decades before. This fact represents how significant the process is and how important it is for the nurse to have a thorough understanding of the physiologic and psychologic changes that occur during labor. Because the labor nurse often is the person who has the most contact with the client during labor, this knowledge can help assist the nurse in making the experience a positive and safe one for both mother and baby. The labor and delivery process is a pivotal point in a woman's life, a time when she is making the transition to her role as mother. A positive experience can have major effects on the key people in the woman's life, such as her spouse or partner, other children, parents, and friends.

Key Terms

Active phase
Amniotomy
Augmentation of labor
Bloody show
Braxton Hicks contraction
Cervical dilation
Cesarean section
Crowning
Descent

Dystocia
Effacement
Fetal attitude
Fetal lie
Fetal position
Fetal presentation
First stage of labor
Flexion
Fontanels
Fourth stage of labor

Labor
Labor induction
Latent phase
Leopold's maneuvers
Lightening
Maternal role attainment
Molding
Nesting (energy spurt)
Oxytocin
Parturition

Placental stage
Primary powers
Pushing stage
Recovery stage
Second stage of labor
Secondary powers
Station
Third stage of labor
Transition

Competencies

Upon completion of this chapter, the reader should be able to:

1. Understand the theories of the onset of parturition or labor.
2. Define the signs and symptoms of impending labor.
3. Define the five Ps of labor.
4. Describe the psychologic response of the mother during labor.
5. Define the four stages of labor.
6. Explain the maternal adaptations to labor.
7. Explain the fetal adaptations to labor.

*L*abor is the bridge between pregnancy and motherhood, and for the laboring woman it often is the most intense experience of the pregnancy. Most nulliparous women can readily visualize themselves as pregnant and their future role as a mother; however, most women cannot or do not visualize what labor is or can be. Labor is both a physical process for the mother and an emotional passage. Family members and friends often are involved in the labor process, introducing additional emotional experiences for all those participating in the labor experience. Finally, the neonate is going through the transition between intrauterine and extrauterine life.

In this chapter we explore the physiologic and psychologic processes of labor, the various stages associated with childbirth, and how labor affects both mother and child. The signs and symptoms of impending labor will be examined and the maternal and fetal adaptations reviewed. The medical and surgical interventions and indications for labor induction, augmentation, and cesarean sections will be discussed.

Because the nurse often is the caregiver who spends the most time with the laboring woman, it is important for the nurse to understand fully the physiologic process of labor and how it affects both the woman and neonate. Knowing the normal process, the nurse can assist the woman and her support group through the experience, ensuring the well-being of all involved.

PHYSIOLOGY OF LABOR

The physiologic process by which the fetus, placenta, and membranes are expelled through the uterus is called **labor** or **parturition**. Labor has four stages. Stage I begins with the onset of labor and continues until full cervical dilation occurs, typically lasting 12 hours for primigravidas and 8 hours for multigravidas. Stage II begins at the point of complete dilation of the cervix and is complete when the fetus is expelled, usually lasting 50 minutes in primigravidas and 20 minutes in multigravidas. Stage III begins with the delivery of the fetus and ends with delivery of the placenta and membranes, usually within 8 to 10 minutes of delivery of the neonate. Stage IV begins when the placenta and membranes are delivered and is complete 4 hours later. When labor fails to ensue or situations arise that do not allow a spontaneous vaginal delivery, labor induction, augmentation, assisted delivery, and cesarean section must be considered.

Theories for the Onset of Labor

Blackburn and Loper (1992) emphasize that the exact cause of the onset of labor still is not completely understood but no doubt involves both maternal and fetal factors. Progesterone withdrawal or binding, increased estrogen levels, prostaglandins, and oxytocin sensitivity are believed to have a part in the onset of labor. Fetal factors such as cortisol levels also are thought to play a role in the onset of labor.

Maternal Factors

Maternal hormone levels are partly responsible for initiation of labor.

Estrogen and Progesterone

It is believed that progesterone causes relaxation of the myometrium, whereas estrogen stimulates myometrial contraction. Estrogen levels begin to increase at about 34 to 35 weeks gestation; a decrease in uterine responsiveness to progesterone also occurs, changing the effect of the estrogen-progesterone ratio. The changes in these steroid levels are responsible for the increased number of myometrial gap junctions. *Gap junctions* are proteins that connect cell membranes, facilitating coordinated uterine contractions and myometrial stretching (Ulmsten, 1996). Estrogen also stimulates the production of prostaglandin in the decidua and fetal membranes, which increases stimulation of smooth muscle contraction of the uterus.

Prostaglandins

Prostaglandins, which act as paracrine hormones, are derived from arachidonic acid and are essential for the onset of labor. Increases in prostaglandin production occur late in pregnancy and are thought to play an important role in the onset of labor. The two most important prostaglandins associated with parturition are PGE_2 and $PGF_{2\alpha}$. Prostaglandins are produced in the myometrium, cervix, fetal membranes, and placenta. $PGF_{2\alpha}$ exerts a stimulatory effect on the myometrium, whereas PGE_2 has a stimulatory effect on the cervix. The effect of PGE_2 on the cervix causes remodeling of the connective tissue in the cervix, allowing the cervix to soften, efface, and dilate during labor.

Oxytocin

Produced in the posterior pituitary, **oxytocin** is a hormone that plays a major role in the onset and maintenance of labor. Maternal oxytocin levels increase throughout pregnancy. As a gestation nears term the number of oxytocin receptors in the uterus increases, creating increased sensitivity to oxytocin. Estrogen also increases myometrial sensitivity to oxytocin. In the absence of these end-organ changes, even external administration of oxytocin will not be successful in precipitating labor. Fetal production of oxytocin also occurs, which is thought to stimulate prostaglandin production (Blackburn & Loper, 1992).

Fetal Factors

An increase in fetal adrenocorticotropic hormone levels at term is speculated to have an effect on uterine sensitivity to oxytocin and prostaglandins, thus stimulating the onset of labor (Ulmsten, 1996). Increased cortisol levels also decrease the production of progesterone by the placenta, therefore aiding in the relaxation of the myometrium.

Mechanisms of Labor

Five important factors affect the process of labor:

1. Passageway, or the birth canal.
2. Passenger, the fetus and placenta.
3. Powers, the uterine contractions.
4. Position of the mother.
5. Psychological response of the mother (Box 23-1).

Passageway

The bony pelvis is an important structure in the birthing process to accommodate the fetus as it passes through the birth canal. The bony pelvis is composed of four bones, two innominate (each consisting of the ilium, ischium, and pubis), the sacrum, and the coccyx. The effects of hormones associated with pregnancy, relaxin and estrogen, are to soften cartilage and increase the strength and elasticity of the pelvic ligaments. These changes cause the pelvic joints to separate slightly, allowing some movement of the pelvic joints. As the pregnancy progresses, the symphysis pubis separates slightly, allowing room for the fetal head.

The pelvis is divided into the false pelvis and true pelvis. The *false pelvis* is the shallow upper section of the pelvis. The *true pelvis* is the lower curved bony canal, including the inlet, cavity, and outlet, through which the fetus must pass in the birth process (Seidel et al., 1999).

Box 23-1 The Five Ps of Labor

- **P**assageway
- **P**assenger
- **P**owers
- **P**osition
- **P**sychologic response

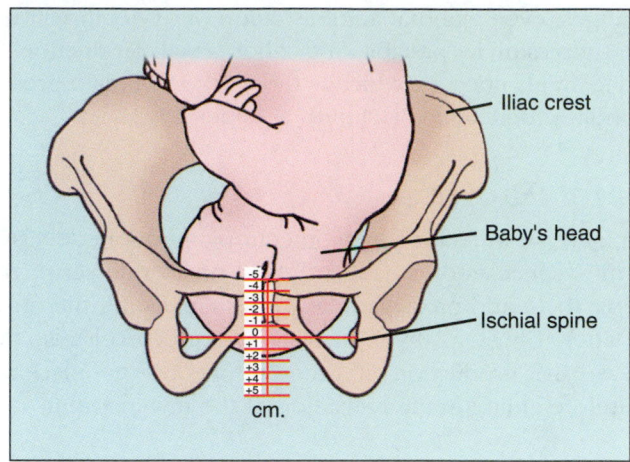

Figure 23-1 Station or relationship of the fetal presenting part to the ischial spines. The station illustrated is +2.

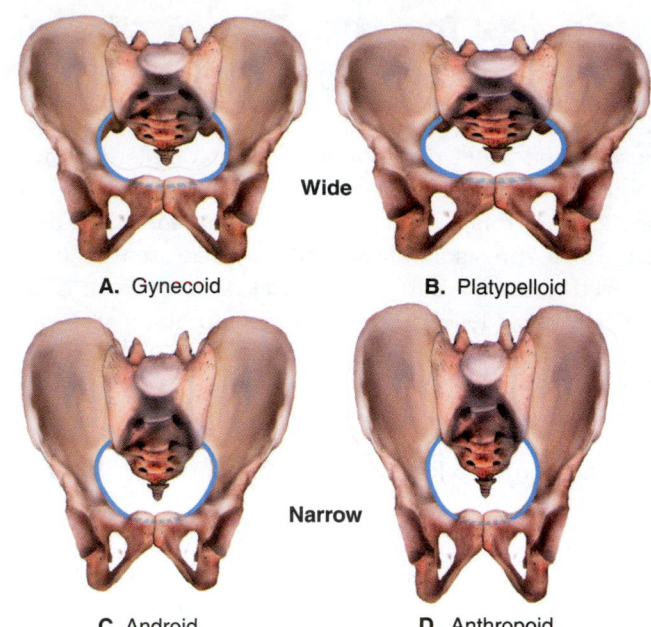

A. Gynecoid   B. Platypelloid

C. Android   D. Anthropoid

Figure 23-2 Female pelvis types.

Station refers to the relationship between the ischial spines in the passage and the presenting part of the fetus (Figure 23-1). The ischial spines are station 0 and in the normal pelvis signify the narrowest diameter the fetus encounters during a vaginal birth.

There are four types of female pelvis: gynecoid, android, anthropoid, and platypelloid. These various pelvis types can play a large role in determining the ease of a vaginal delivery. The most common type of female pelvis is the gynecoid pelvis found in about half of women. The least common type of female pelvis is the platypelloid pelvis found in about 3% of women. Figure 23-2 compares the four female pelvis types. Wide suprarpubic arches (gynecoid and platypelloid) tend to allow normal vaginal delivery, whereas narrow arches (android and anthropoid) increase the risks for forceps and cesarean deliveries.

Passenger

The ease with which the passenger goes through the pelvis is determined by many fetal factors: head size, presentation, lie, attitude, and position.

Fetal Head Size

The fetal head is composed of bony parts consisting of a frontal bone, two parietal bones, two temporal bones, and an occipital bone. The skull bones are united by membranous sutures, and the points of intersection of these are called **fontanels**. The two most important fontanels for delivery are the anterior and posterior fontanels (Figure 23-3). The diamond-shaped anterior fontanel is the largest of the two and lies at the juncture of the sagittal, coronal, and frontal sutures. This fontanel generally stays open until about 18 months of age, allowing brain growth. The posterior fontanel is trianglar shaped and is formed by the intersection of the sagittal and lambdoid sutures; it closes about 6 to 8 weeks after birth. During a vaginal examina-

tion, the fetal presentation can be determined by locating these fontanels.

The fontanels are important during the birth process because they allow molding to occur. **Molding** is the overlapping of the fetal skull that helps the fetal head to adapt to the size and shape of the maternal pelvis. Molding can be extensive, causing the fetal head to appear misshapen at birth. The effects of molding on the shape of the head usually resolve completely in 3 days.

Fetal Presentation

Fetal presentation refers to the anatomic part of the fetus that is either in or closest to the birth canal. Presentation is determined by performing a vaginal examination and feeling the part through the cervix. There are three major presentations. Cephalic or fetal head presentation is the most common, occurring in 96% of births, and is most likely to lead to a vaginal birth. Breech or buttock presentation occurs in 3% of births. Shoulder presentation occurs in the remaining 1%. These last two presentations are associated with a complicated birthing process and often require cesarean section.

Fetal Lie

The **fetal lie** describes the relationship of the fetal long (head to foot) axis to that of the maternal long axis or spinal cord (Figure 23-4). In a breech or cephalic presentation, the lie is longitudinal. With a shoulder presentation, the lie is transverse, making vaginal birth unlikely. An oblique lie indicates the fetus is at a 45-degree angle to the maternal long axis and is considered an unstable lie; the oblique lie often converts to longitudinal or transverse lie during labor.

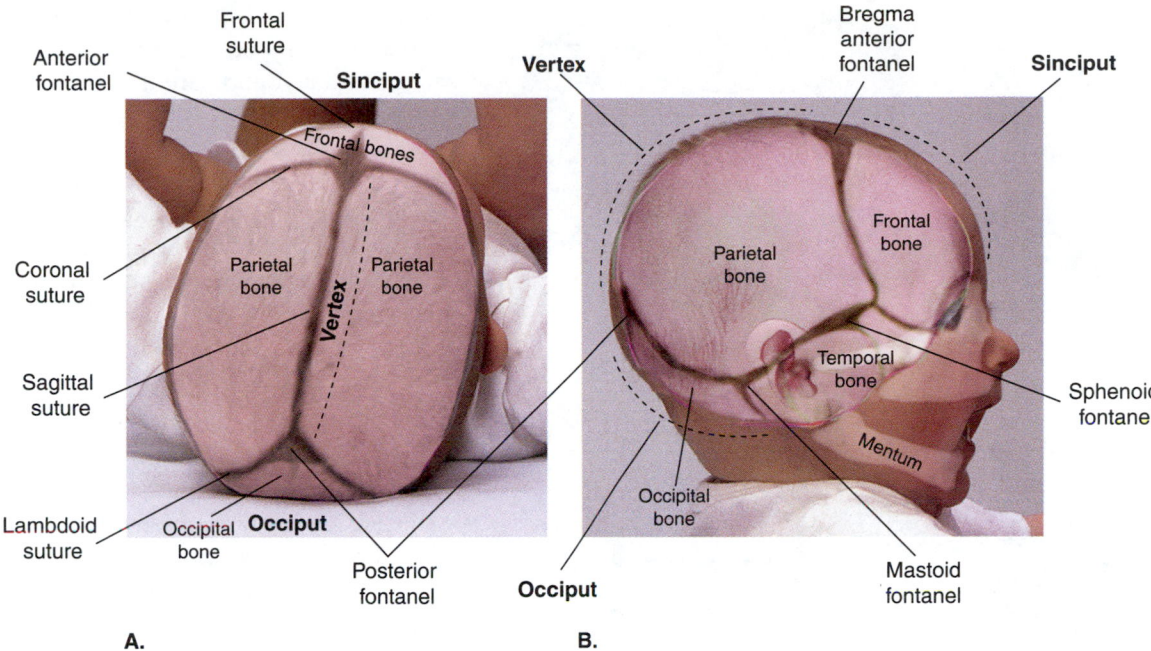

Figure 23-3 Fetal skull—sutures and fontanels. A. Superior view. B. Lateral view.

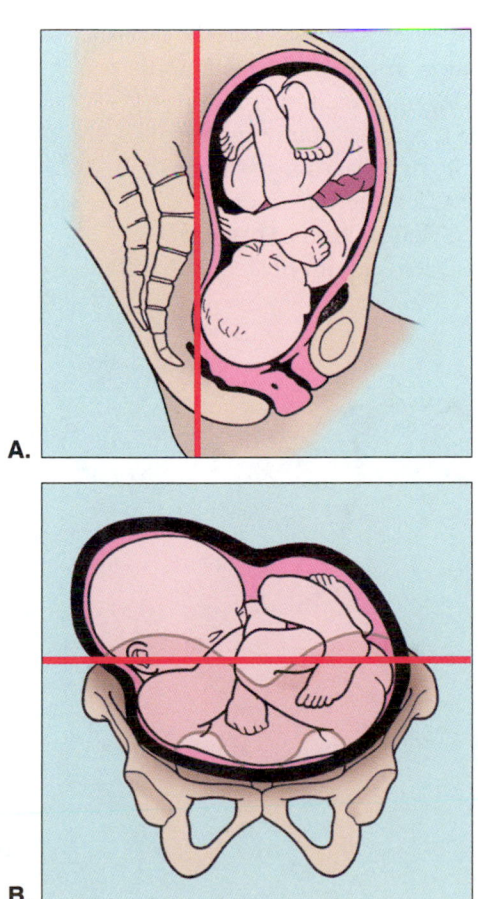

Figure 23-4 Fetal attitude and fetal lie. A. Fetal attitude flexion, fetal lie longitudinal. B. Fetal attitude flexion, fetal lie transverse.

Fetal Attitude

Fetal attitude refers to the relationship of fetal body parts to one another. The typical fetal attitude includes flexion of the head wherein the chin rests on the sternum, the arms and legs are flexed against the chest, and the back is bowed out. Throughout the pregnancy, the fetus assumes various attitudes through movement and stretching of the fetal extremities. The available space within the uterine cavity can cause changes in fetal attitude; large for gestational age infants tend to be flexed more than are normal-sized infants owing to lack of room inside the uterus.

Fetal attitude can affect the birth process. For example, when the fetal head is slightly extended (sinciput or brow presentation), it presents a larger diameter to pass through the maternal pelvis and thus increases the difficulty of labor and delivery (Figure 23-5).

The largest transverse diameter of the fetal head is the biparietal diameter, which at term is about 9.25 cm. The suboccipitobregmatic diameter is the most critical anteroposterior diameter, which is about 9.5 cm at term. If the fetal head is not fully flexed at delivery, the anterioposterior diameter increases and may prevent the head from entering the true pelvis or the deeper cavity below the inlet (Figure 23-6).

Fetal Position

Fetal position refers to the relationship of the fetal presenting part to the left or right side of the maternal pelvis. If the cephalic presentation is vertex, the position landmark is the posterior fontanel or occiput; similarly, in a

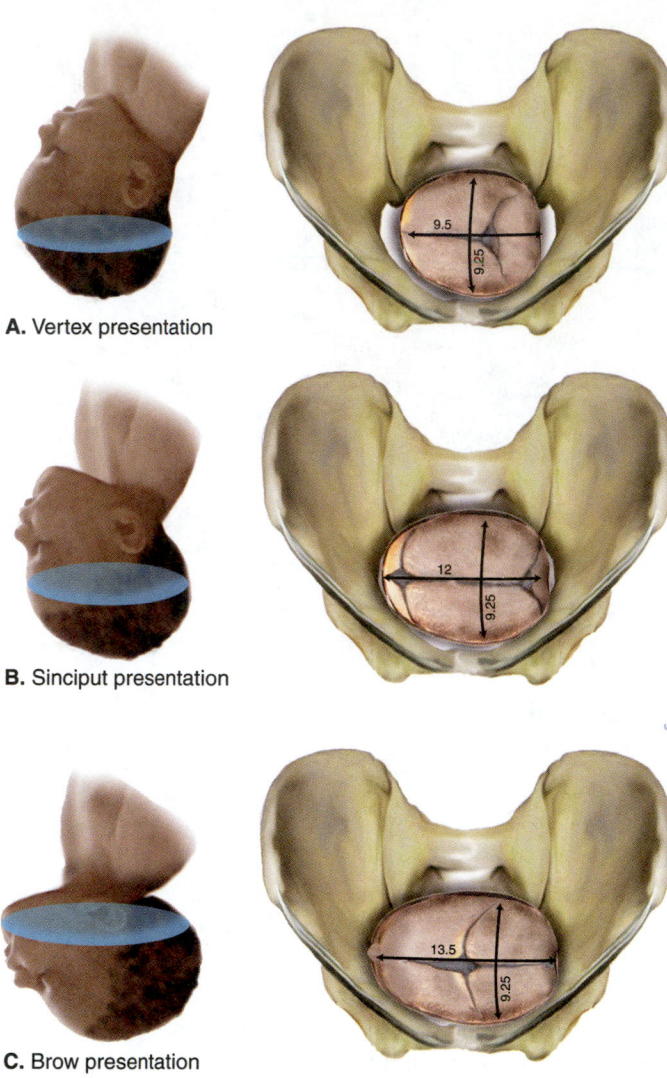

A. Vertex presentation

B. Sinciput presentation

C. Brow presentation

Figure 23-5 Diameter of presenting part in vertex, sinciput, and brow presentations.

cephalic face presentation, the mentum or chin is the presenting part. In breech and shoulder presentations, the sacrum and acromion are the landmarks, respectively. The landmark of the presenting part of the fetus is described in relation to the four quadrants of the maternal pelvis (left anterior, right anterior, left posterior, and right posterior) or the transverse portion (Figure 23-7). In a posterior position, a larger part of the head must pass through the pelvis, causing a long labor and often more back pain owing to increased pressure on the sacral nerves.

The positions for fetal presentation follow:

- Position in Vertex Presentations:
  ROA, right-occiput-anterior
  ROT, right-occiput-transverse
  ROP, right-occiput-posterior
  LOA, left-occiput-anterior
  LOT, left-occiput-transverse
  LOP, left-occiput-posterior

- Position in Face Presentations:
  RMA, right-mentum-anterior
  RMT, right-mentum-transverse
  RMP, right-mentum-posterior
  LMA, left-mentum-anterior
  LMT, left-mentum-transverse
  LMP, left-mentum-posterior

- Position in Breech Presentations:
  RSA, right-sacrum-anterior
  RST, right-sacrum-transverse
  RSP, right-sacrum-posterior
  LSA, left-sacrum-anterior
  LST, left-sacrum-transverse
  LSP, left-sacrum-posterior

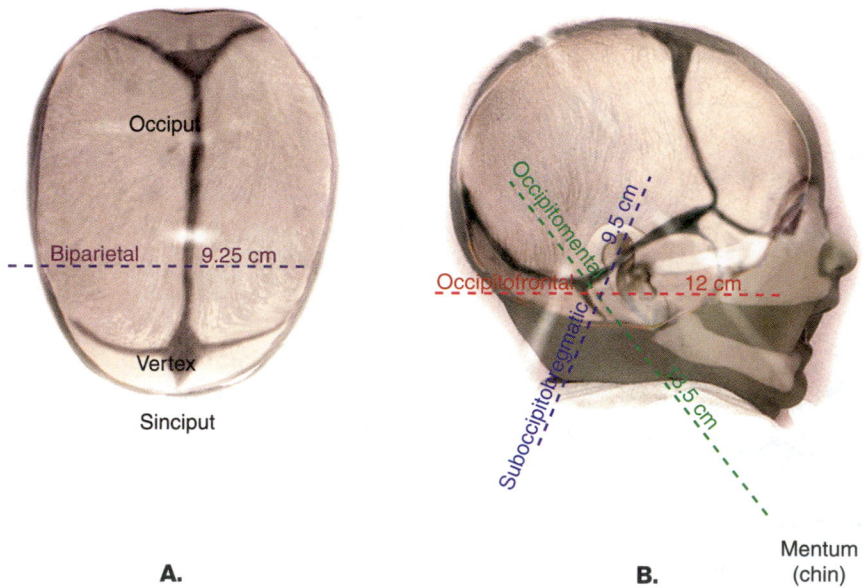

A.

B.

Figure 23-6 Fetal head measurements. A. Biparietal diameter. B. Cephalic diameters.

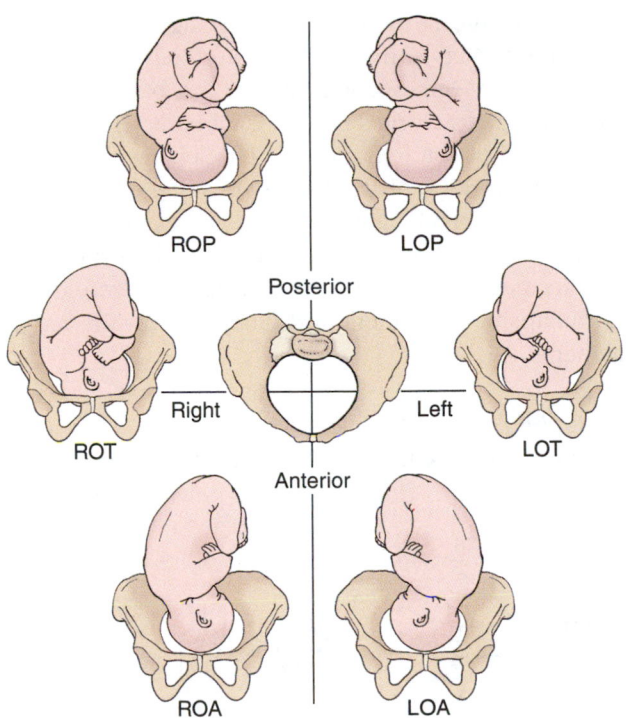

Figure 23-7 Positions of a vertex presentation.

Assessment of Fetal Presentation and Position

There are two primary means for determining the presentation and position of the fetus. The first and less invasive way is through Leopold's maneuvers; the more invasive way is through a vaginal examination.

Leopold's Maneuvers or Abdominal Palpation.

Leopold's maneuvers refer to a method of abdominal palpation to determine fetal presentation and position. These maneuvers need to be performed in a consistent and systematic fashion to be as reliable as possible. These maneuvers are a reliable method to determine position and presentation but are very limited in the obese client or the client with an anterior placenta. The examiner should stand at the side of the bed that is most convenient and face the client's head for the first three maneuvers and the client's feet for the last maneuver (Figure 23-8).

First Maneuver

With both hands, the examiner outlines the shape of the uterus, gently palpating the fundus with the fingertips to determine which fetal pole is present in the fundal area. The fetal buttocks give the sensation of a large nodular body, whereas the head is more firm, round, and ballottable.

Second Maneuver

After determining the fetal part in the fundus, the examiner's palms are placed on either side of the client's abdomen, exerting deep but gentle pressure. In a vertex or breech presentation, one side will feel smooth and firm,

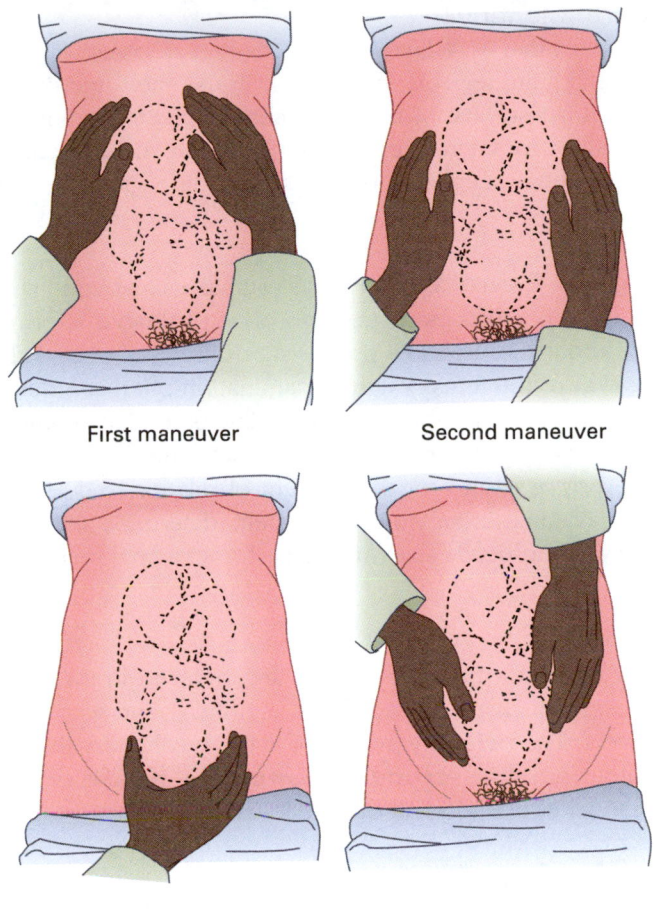

First maneuver

Second maneuver

Third maneuver

Fourth maneuver

Figure 23-8 Leopold's maneuvers.

indicating the back; whereas the other side will have numerous small irregular mobile parts, indicating the fetal extremities. Both increased amniotic fluid and maternal obesity will make feeling the individual extremities more difficult, and in some cases only the back may be palpated. Determining the location of the back more anteriorly or transversely will give the examiner a more accurate idea of the fetal lie and presentation.

Third Maneuver

The third maneuver will help determine whether the previously detected presenting part is *engaged* (deep in the pelvis), and the attitude of the fetal head is in a cephalic presentation. With the thumb and fingers of one hand, the examiner attempts to grasp the lower portion of the client's abdomen, just above the symphysis pubis. If a body part moves easily, the presenting part is not engaged. The fetal attitude can be determined in a cephalic presentation by assessing if the cephalic prominence is on the same side as are the small parts, indicating that the head is flexed and the fetus is in vertex presentation. When the cephalic prominence is on the same side as is the back, the fetal head is extended.

Fourth Maneuver

The examiner will face the client's feet to assess further the fetal attitude. This maneuver will use the fingertips of the palmar surface of the examiner's hands to outline the cephalic prominence of the fetus. When the presenting part is deeply engaged, only a small portion may be outlined.

Vaginal Examination.

The vaginal examination during the labor process is done to obtain valuable information about the mother's progression during labor and the position of the fetus. Vaginal examination often can determine the fetal station and presenting part. The mother's cervix also can be assessed vaginally for how open, thin, and short it is and for the amount of dilation and effacement. Vaginal examination can help determine the adequacy of the pelvic size and shape for a vaginal delivery.

Powers

Two important types of powers are involved in the labor process, which are characterized as primary and secondary powers. The **primary powers** are the involuntary uterine contractions. The **secondary powers** are the mother's intentional efforts to push out the fetus.

Primary Powers

Uterine contractions are involuntary and generally are independent of extrauterine control. During labor, the uterus forms what is called the physiologic retraction ring, dividing itself into two portions. The upper contractile segments become thicker as labor advances. The passive lower uterine segment and the cervix expand and thin out as labor progresses. Uterine contractions are responsible for the effacement and dilation of the cervix, allowing the descent of the fetus. Uterine contractions are measured by their frequency, from the beginning of one to the beginning of the next contraction. The length of a contraction is how long it lasts in seconds. The intensity or strength of a contraction also is evaluated by external palpation of the firmness of the uterus and the level of pain perceived by the client.

As the uterine muscle contracts, the upper uterine segment shortens and causes longitudinal traction on the cervix. This leads to **effacement**, or shortening and thinning, of the cervix. Before labor, the cervix generally is 2 to 3 cm long and about 1 cm thick. The degree of effacement is described in terms of a percentage. For example, a cervix that is halfway effaced would be described as being 50% effaced.

The widening of the cervical opening that occurs from myometrial contractions in labor is referred to as **cervical dilation**. In general, before labor the cervix is closed, progressing to 10 cm open as labor advances. Dilation accom-

modates passage of the fetal head through the birth canal. When the cervix is fully dilated and retracted into the lower uterine segment, it is no longer palpable (Figure 23-9). The uterus elongates with each contraction, causing the fetal body to straighten. This fetal change exerts pressure on the fundus of the uterus, pushing the presenting part onto the cervix and assisting in dilation; this phenomenon is called *fetal axis pressure*. In the primigravida, the effacement of the cervix usually begins before dilation. In a multipara, effacement and dilation generally progress together.

Secondary Powers

After the woman is fully dilated and effaced, the presenting part of the fetus descends to the pelvic floor. The uter-

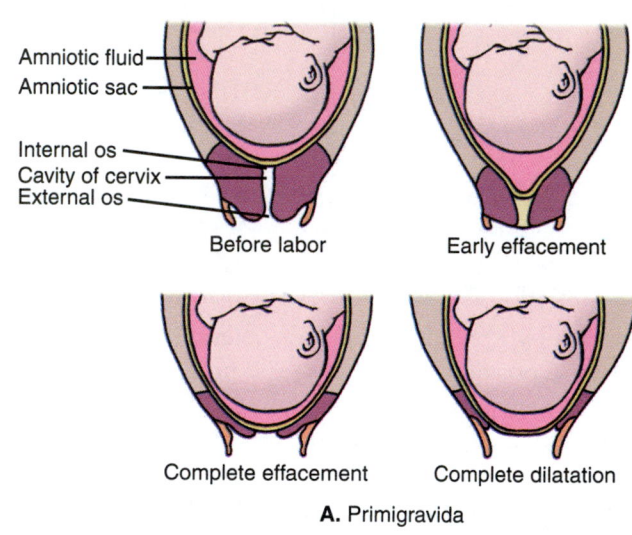

A. Primigravida

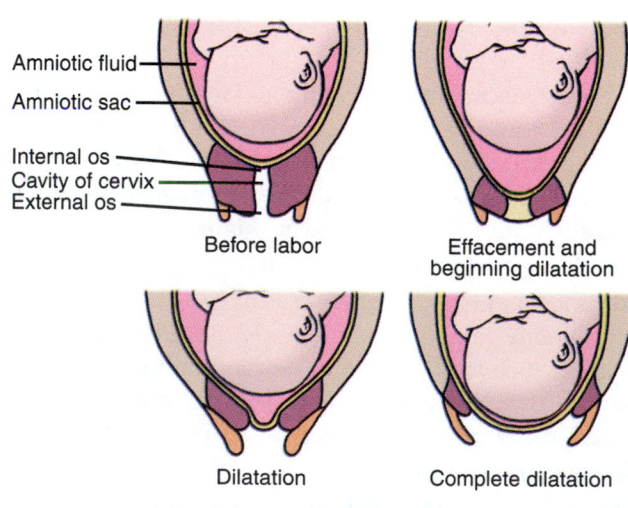

B. Multigravida

Figure 23-9 Effacement and dilation. A. Primigravida. B. Multigravida.

ine contractions begin to change and become more expulsive. The laboring woman begins to feel an involuntary urge to bear down or push. This begins the use of secondary, more voluntary efforts of labor. With each uterine contraction, the woman contracts her abdominal muscles to compress all sides of the uterus to aid in expelling the fetus. The woman's ability to push has an important role in the progression of the vaginal birth of the fetus.

Position

Maternal position in labor can have an effect on both the mother and fetus. Much disagreement exists regarding the influence of maternal position on labor progress, pain perception, and fetal well-being. During the first stage of labor, it may be psychologically beneficial for the mother not to be confined to lying supine in bed. If a client has an intravenous line in place, a movable pole should be used to allow ambulation. If a mother chooses to remain in bed, she should be encouraged to find her most comfortable position. A lateral recumbent position often is the most comfortable one and best for fetal well-being, particularly during the first stage of labor. The optimal position for an individual client, however, may range from sitting in a rocking chair to using a labor ball or being in a semi-reclined position. All positions have advantages and disadvantages. For example, although the squatting position may increase the size of the pelvic outlet, it may be difficult for a woman with an epidural to assume this position.

Many studies have examined the effects of maternal position on pain and duration of the second stage of labor. In some cultures, women give birth in an erect, kneeling, or squatting position, which has been associated with less maternal pain. A study by Gardosi, Hutson, & Lynch (1989) found that assuming a modified squatting position resulted in a shorter second stage of labor and fewer subsequent perineal lacerations.

In the absence of a clear-cut "best" position during labor, it is important to consider maternal needs, both physical and psychologic, as well as fetal well-being.

Psychological Response of the Mother

Few reports exist in the nursing literature about the psychological response to labor. Clark and Affonso (1978) identified some factors that make labor a meaningful positive event or the antithesis, a negative event for the mother. The first factor is the role of one's culture, that is, how a particular society views childbirth, which incorporates the woman's attitudes toward the labor process. Another factor that can negatively or positively affect the childbirth experience is the expectation and goals for the labor process. If the expectations about labor are realistic

and can be met, the outcome is more likely to be positive; in contrast, if the expectations are unrealistic and unattainable, the experience is more likely to be negative. Finally, feedback from other people participating in the labor and birth process can add positive or negative aspects to the experience.

It is important for the nurse to assess these factors as soon as the client arrives in the labor suite. The nurse should communicate with the client and significant others involved in the labor experience and explore cultural ideas, attitudes, expectations, and goals. For example, a specific cultural need of the client that could be explored is the role of labor coach being taken on by the laboring woman's mother instead of the husband. These needs should be met when possible, even if the nurse providing care has different cultural attitudes.

A positive labor and birth experience can help the woman more easily transition into the maternal role. **Maternal role attainment** as defined by Rubin (1984) is the process by which a woman acquires knowledge of maternal behavior that aids in transforming her maternal identity. The first developmental stage of maternal role attainment is for the mother to seek a safe passage for herself and her child during pregnancy, labor, and delivery. Many factors contribute to maternal role attainment such as age, culture, support system, childbirth preparation, and previous birth experiences. Williams, Kramma, & O'Brian (1997) describe proper childbirth preparation as a valuable tranquilizer during the birth process that can lead to decreased need for analgesics to be administered during labor.

The labor and delivery nurse should provide a supportive and caring environment for the client and should respect the client's and family's needs and attitudes. Delivery of such care is attained through therapeutic communication and assessment of client needs.

Cultural Perceptions of Childbirth

Leininger (1985) defines culture as a "particular group's values, beliefs, norms and practices that are learned and shared and that guide thinking, decisions and actions in a patterned way." In examining this definition and relating it to childbirth, culture is one of the biggest influences on childbirth perceptions and the role of motherhood. A study by Callister, Vehvilainen-Julkunen, & Lauri (1996) compared childbirth perceptions among women who were American Mormon, Canadian Orthodox Jew, and Finnish Lutheran. The results showed that Finnish Lutheran women felt that motherhood was one of many roles women would encounter in life. In contrast, Canadian Jewish women and American Mormon women felt that motherhood was their purpose in life. The author points out that family structures are different in that husbands in

Finland take a more active role in parenting. In contrast, American and Canadian fathers of these religious affiliations believe the mother's role is paramount and thus are less involved.

SIGNS AND SYMPTOMS OF IMPENDING LABOR

The signs and symptoms of impending labor are different for every woman, and an individual woman may experience all, some, or none of them. Some of the premonitory signs and symptoms of labor may include lightening, cervical changes, Braxton Hicks contractions, bloody show, an energy spurt, and gastrointestinal (GI) upset. Education of the woman and assessment of these signs and symptoms can help the nurse to provide anticipatory guidance for the onset of labor and delivery.

Lightening

Lightening is the movement of the presenting part of the fetus into the true pelvis. In primigravidas, lightening usually occurs about 2 weeks before the onset of labor. Clients often will describe a feeling of being able to breathe more easily because of less pressure on the diaphragm from the gravid uterus. Other discomforts however may become more apparent:

- Increased pelvic pressure and congestion, resulting in increased vaginal secretions and pelvic discomfort.
- Increased urinary frequency from extrinsic pressure on the bladder.
- Neuropathic pain related to the pressure of the presenting part on the nerves in the pelvis, particularly in the obturator foramen.
- Edema of the lower extremities and increased venous stasis from inhibition of blood return by the pelvic pressure of the presenting part.

Cervical Changes

As a pregnant woman approaches term, her cervix changes from being long and closed with a firm consistency to shortened (or effaced), thinned, dilated, and soft. The cervix of a multipara normally can be dilated 2 cm or more before the onset of labor. Primigravidas often will experience effacement before dilation, whereas multiparas will have concurrent effacement and dilation (Seidel et al., 1999).

Cervical changes are thought to occur from the remodeling of connective tissue secondary to the effects of prostaglandins. Braxton Hicks contractions also play a role in cervical change. Because cervical ripeness varies at the onset of labor, it does not predict when the woman will go into labor. However, cervical ripeness can help predict that a client will go into labor when contractions begin and can help in deciding who is ready for induction of labor (Varney, 1987).

Braxton Hicks Contractions

Throughout the pregnancy a woman may experience painless irregular contractions called **Braxton Hicks contractions** or false labor. These contractions produce no cervical changes. As true labor approaches, Braxton Hicks contractions may become more noticeable, frequent, painful, and difficult to differentiate from true labor without cervical examination. These contractions may be annoying and confusing to the pregnant woman, who often will come to the physician's office or hospital for evaluation. A woman experiencing false labor needs reassurance that true labor will eventually ensue.

Bloody Show

Soon after conception, thick tenacious mucus forms inside the cervical canal to act as a protective barrier. Before the onset of labor, as the cervix begins to soften and dilate, this mucous plug often is expelled. These blood-tinged secretions are referred to as **bloody show**. Labor usually ensues within 24 to 48 hours of expelling the mucous plug. It may be difficult to identify bloody show if a vaginal examination has been done within the past 24 hours, given the increased friability of the cervix near term.

Energy Spurt

Although no physiologic basis is known for this, many women experience a burst of energy, known as **nesting**, 24 to 48 hours before going into labor. Many women report having the energy to do things that they recently have not had the ability to do because of the fatigue of pregnancy, for example, cleaning the house or washing windows. In providing anticipatory guidance, the nurse should warn clients of the possible energy spurt and how they need to conserve their energy for labor.

Gastrointestinal Disturbances

Diarrhea, indigestion, nausea, and vomiting sometimes are reported just before the onset of labor. There is no known physiologic explanation for these symptoms.

STAGES OF LABOR

There are four stages of the labor process. The first and longest stage of labor occurs between the onset of true labor and the point of complete cervical dilation and effacement. The second stage of labor is expulsion of the fetus, and the third stage of labor is delivery of the placenta. The fourth stage is the first 4 hours after delivery of the placenta.

First Stage

The **first stage of labor**, which is the longest in duration, begins with regular contractions and ends when the cervix is completely dilated. This stage is divided into three phases: latent, active, and transition phases.

Latent Phase

The **latent phase** of labor begins with the onset of regular contractions, which usually are mild. During this phase, contractions may be 15 to 20 minutes apart, lasting 20 to 30 seconds. As this phase progresses, however, the contractions will occur every 5 to 7 minutes and the duration will lengthen to 30 to 40 seconds. Many women remain at home during the early parts of the latent phase. This phase usually begins with little or no cervical dilation and ends when the cervix is 3 to 4 cm dilated. For the primigravida, the latent phase lasts an average of 9 hours; whereas in the multigravida, the latent phase generally lasts an average of 6 hours. Although the woman may exhibit some anxiety during this phase, she often is comfortable enough to verbalize her concerns.

Active Phase

The **active phase** of labor begins when the women is 3 to 4 cm dilated and ends when she is 8 cm dilated. During this phase, contractions occur every 2 to 3 minutes and last up to 60 seconds. The intensity of each contraction begins as moderate and continues to increase as the woman gets closer to the transition phase. The average length of the active phase in the primagravida is 6 hours and in the multigravida is 4.5 hours. Dilation rates should be at least 1.2 to 1.5 cm/h (Troyer & Parisi, 1993). This often is the period when pain relief is requested by the laboring client.

Transition Phase

The last and shortest part of the first phase of labor is **transition**, which typically is the most intense phase for the laboring woman. In transition, contractions occur every 1.5 to 2 minutes, with a duration of 60 to 90 seconds. The intensity of the contractions is very strong in the transition phase. The woman often becomes very restless and agitated and may have difficulty focusing during contractions. Many women exhibit anger at the coach, voice a desire to leave the hospital, request a cesarean section, hyperventilate, complain of nausea and vomiting, tremble, and experience rectal pressure. The nurse plays an impor-

tant role for the client and her coach because the laboring woman often begins to withdraw from her coach's support. The coach may feel useless, and both the client and her partner will look to the nurse for reassurance and support. During this time the nurse will need to prepare the woman for the second stage of labor.

Second Stage

The **second stage of labor** begins when the cervix is completely dilated and effaced and ends when the fetus is expelled; it also is known as the **pushing stage**. The average length of the second stage of labor in a primagravida is 1.1 hours and 24 minutes in the multigravida. Many factors influence the length of the second stage of labor, including maternal parity, fetal size, uterine contractile force, presentation, position, pelvic size, method of anesthesia, and magnitude of maternal expulsive effort.

During contractions, the woman will bear down, causing the abdominal muscles to contract and helping the fetal head to descend through the birth canal. As the fetal head continues into the birth canal, the perineum begins to bulge. **Crowning** is defined as the point at which the fetal head is visible at the vulvar opening. When crowning occurs, birth is imminent.

Many women feel relief at the developing urge to push, partly because it signifies that the birth is very close. Other women, particularly those without support or child preparation classes, feel overwhelmed when it is time to push. Some women describe intense pain and burning of the perineum as the pressure increases on the vulva. Women are in various positions during the second stage of labor; the lithotomy position is the most common in the United States. Epidural anesthesia may interfere with the woman's perception of pushing and her ability to push forcefully. Nurses need to be aware of prolonged second stages of labor (Table 23-1) because intervention may be required.

Cardinal Movements or Mechanism of Labor

During the birthing process, the position of the fetal head and body must change to accommodate the maternal pelvis. These changes in fetal position are called *cardinal movements* or *mechanism of labor* (Figure 23-10). The cardinal movements are descent, flexion, internal rotation, extension, restitution, external rotation, and expulsion.

Descent

Descent is the progression of the fetal head into the pelvis, which occurs because of three forces: the pressure of the amniotic fluid, direct pressure of the contracting uterus, and effects of the contractions on the maternal

Table 23-1 Average Length of Labor Stages 1 and 2

Characteristic	First Stage			Second Stage
	Latent Phase	Active Phase	Transition Phase	
Primigravida	8–10 h	6 h	2 h	1 h
Multigravida	5 h	4 h	1 h	15 min
Cervical dilation	0–4 cm	4–8 cm	8–10 cm	
Contractions				
Frequency	10–20 progressing to 5–7 min	3–5 min	2–3 min	2–3 min
Duration	15–20 progressing to 30–40 sec	40–60 sec	60–90 sec	60–90 sec
Intensity	Mild progressing to moderate	Moderate progressing to strong	Strong	Strong

diaphragm and abdominal muscles. The head generally enters the pelvis in the transverse and oblique position. The degree of descent is measured by stations.

Flexion

Flexion occurs when the fetal head meets resistance from the pelvic floor and walls as well as the cervix, causing the head to flex with the chin against the fetal chest. This position achieves the smallest fetal diameters coming into the maternal pelvis.

Internal Rotation

The widest part of the maternal pelvis is the anteroposterior diameter because the fetal head must rotate to accommodate the pelvis. The pelvic muscles, levator ani muscle, and the fascia cause resistance to the fetal head, forcing it to rotate from the left to right and aligning the fetal head with the long axis of the maternal pelvis. This occurs mainly during the second stage of labor.

Extension

As resistance is met by the pelvic floor, the fetal head pivots beneath the symphysis pubis. The head emerges through extension, led by the occiput, then the face, and finally the chin.

Restituition

Internal rotation causes the shoulders of the fetus to enter the pelvis in an oblique position. When the head is delivered in the extended position, the neck is twisted and the head realigns with the long axis of the fetus.

External Rotation

As a continuation of the restitution, the shoulders align in the anteroposterior diameter, causing the head to continue to rotate. The trunk navigates though the pelvis with the anterior shoulders descending first.

Expulsion

As the shoulders extend under the symphysis pubis, the anterior followed by the posterior shoulders are delivered by the women's pushing effort. Once the shoulders are delivered, the trunk easily follows.

REFLECTIONS FROM A LABORING MOTHER

"During my pregnancy, my labor lasted almost 48 hours. I had an epidural and felt pretty good but was getting more and more tired. The nurses couldn't believe how long I was taking to dilate (since they saw me—unusually—on more than one rotation). Finally, after about 40 hours, a new nurse came in and reviewed my chart. She introduced herself and said, 'You are going to have this baby on my shift.' She instructed me to turn every half hour, and she came into my room to make sure I did it. She was calm yet in control. I did have my baby on her shift and I whole-heartedly believe it was because she worked with me to make it happen."

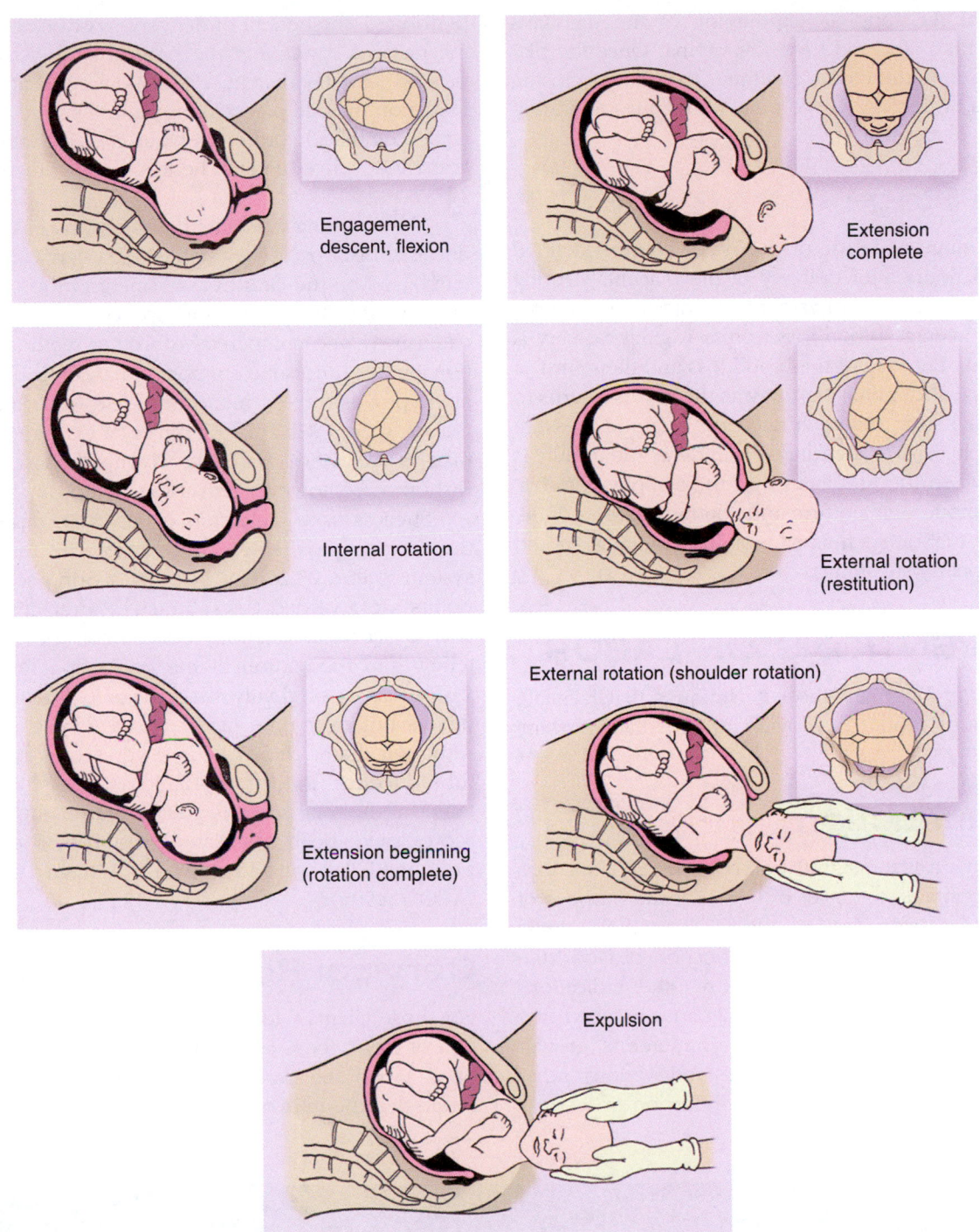

Engagement, descent, flexion

Extension complete

Internal rotation

External rotation (restitution)

Extension beginning (rotation complete)

External rotation (shoulder rotation)

Expulsion

Figure 23-10 Mechanisms of labor.

Third Stage

The **third stage of labor** or **placental stage** begins as soon as the fetus is delivered and lasts until the placenta is delivered. The mechanism of placental separation is a combination of uterine contractions and involution. After expulsion of the fetus, the uterus continues to contract every 3 to 4 minutes. As the uterus contracts and begins the process of involution, shrinkage of the site of implantation of the placenta occurs. Within 10 to 15 minutes after delivery of the infant, most of the placenta has detached from the uterine wall. At this point, vaginal bleeding from the uncovered implantation site increases, and delivery of the placenta generally soon follows. The classic signs of placental separation are rounding up of the uterus, upward movement of the fundus, lengthening of the umbilical cord, and a rush of blood from the vagina. Once the placenta is delivered, the uterus continues to contract, closing off the spiral arterioles. As the uterus continues to shrink, the bleeding decreases.

Fourth Stage

The **fourth stage of labor** or **recovery stage** is defined as the first 4 hours after delivery of the placenta. During this time, many maternal physiologic readjustments are occurring. The average blood loss from a vaginal delivery is 250 to 500 mL. Because of the blood loss and the return of a more normal abdominal anatomy as the uterus returns to a more normal size, there is a decrease in blood pressure and slight tachycardia. The fundus is midline and usually is halfway between the umbilicus and the symphysis pubis. The fundus should remain firm and contracted. Most of the discomforts of labor, such as nausea and vomiting, should be gone or clearly subsiding.

INTERVENTIONS OF LABOR

Interventions of labor are those techniques that facilitate the progress of labor or provide an alternate birthing mechanism.

Labor Induction

Labor induction is the stimulation of uterine contractions before the spontaneous onset of labor for the purpose of accomplishing delivery (ACOG, 1995). There are multiple medical and obstetric reasons for induction of labor, the most common being postterm gestation. Other indications for induction of labor include pregnancy-induced hypertension (PIH), diabetes mellitus, intrauterine growth restriction, intrauterine fetal demise, and various other maternal-fetal complications. Before induction of labor is

performed, the benefit of delivery must be compared with the risks of continuing the pregnancy and the induction process itself (Bernstein, 2000). Contraindications to labor induction include placenta previa, transverse fetal lie, prolapsed umbilical cord, a previous classical uterine incision scar, and active genital herpes virus infection (ACOG, 1995).

In attempting to ensure the safety and ease of labor induction, Bishop (1964) established a cervical scoring system based on the clinical assessment of the cervix. Developed in the 1950s, the Bishop score has been studied extensively and compared with other methods of evaluation. Some authors have reported that cervical examination alone proves to be a more predictive value than does the Bishop score (Williams, Krammer, & O'Brian, 1997; Friedman et al., 1966; Harrison, Flynn, & Craft, 1977). The Bishop score however remains standard practice.

Success with induction of labor is improved when the cervix is favorable or inducible. The Bishop scoring system (Table 23-2) is a 13-point scoring scale in which points are awarded (or subtracted) after clinical evaluation of cervical dilation, effacement, position, consistency, and the station of the presenting fetal part. The Bishop score originally was designed for use with multiparas but over time has been used with primigravids. Although many clients with lower scores have successful inductions, induction of labor is more likely to be attained if the total score is greater than eight. Low Bishop scores have been associated with failure of induction, prolonged labor, and higher cesarean section rates (ACOG, 1995).

Cervical Ripening Methods

For those clients with low Bishop scores requiring induction of labor, there are methods to enhance the readiness of or ripen the cervix. MacKenzie and Embrey (1979) found that the intravaginal administration of 0.5 mg of the

Table 23-2 Bishop Scoring System

Factor	0	1	2	3
Cervical dilation	Closed	1–2 cm	3–4 cm	5+ cm
Cervical effacement	1–30%	40–50%	60–70%	80+%
Fetal station	−3	−2	−1	+1, +2
Cervical consistency	Firm	Med	Soft	+
Cervical position	Posterior	Mid	Anterior	+

Predictive value:
Score: 0–4 45–50% induction failure rate
5–9 10% induction failure rate
10–13 0% failure rate
Bishop, E. H. (1964). Pelvic scoring for elective inductions. *Obstetrics and Gynecology* 24:266.

prostaglandin gel (PGE$_2$) dinoprostone (Prepidil) shortened the length of labor and improved the cervical condition, thus reducing the risk for cesarean section. Approved by the FDA in 1992, Prepidil gel is administered into the cervical canal through a catheter-tipped syringe or applied to a diaphragm placed next to the cervix. Doses may be applied every 6 to 12 hours, with ripening of the cervix occurring most often after two to three doses.

The vaginal insert Cervidil contains 10 mg of PGE$_2$, generic name, that is slowly released over 12 hours. One benefit of Cervidil is that the insert may be removed if hyperstimulation or active labor begins. Hyperstimulation of the uterus can be described as an inadequate rest between contractions and is a potential hazardous side effect of using any kind of PGE$_2$ for induction of labor. Maternal side effects of PGE$_2$, including vomiting, diarrhea, and fever, are avoided with local vaginal applications.

According to Keirse (1993), prostaglandin treatment can increase the spontaneous vaginal delivery rate by 33% as a result of a decrease in cesarean section and instrument-assisted delivery. Monitoring of the client after receiving PGE$_2$ includes 30 minutes to 2 hours of external fetal monitoring for uterine contractions and reassuring fetal heart tones. Bed rest should be maintained for 30 minutes to ensure proper placement of the medication. If regular uterine contractions persist, fetal heart rate (FHR) monitoring should be recorded hourly for at least the first 4 hours (ACOG, 1995).

Osmotic cervical dilators can be placed into the cervical canal under direct visualization using aseptic technique. As many dilators as possible are placed in the cervical canal and swell when left in place (usually overnight) to cause cervical dilation. Initially made of dried seaweed (*Laminaria*), there are now synthetic versions available (Dilipan). *Laminaria* has shown to be a cost-effective and safe method of cervical ripening; however, one study has shown *Laminaria* to be associated with a high incidence of increased peripartum infection (Kazzi, Bottoms, & Rosen, 1982).

Misoprostol (Cytotec) is a synthetic PGE$_1$ used for the treatment and prevention of peptic ulcer disease. Although its use for the induction of labor is not approved by the FDA, studies have been conducted using the drug intravaginally to soften the cervix. ACOG (1999) outlined strict guidelines for the use of Cytotec in labor induction stating that for cervical ripening, one quarter of a 100-μg tablet should be used for the initial dose; doses should not be given more frequently than every 3 to 4 hours; oxytocin should not be given within 4 hours of the last dose; and Cytotec should not be used in clients with a previous cesarean delivery or a previous uterine scar. Wing, Lovett, & Paul (1998) also discourage use in clients with a previous uterine scar owing to the increased incidence of uterine rupture in his randomized trial of labor.

Nursing Alert

OXYTOCIN

An accidental bolus of oxytocin can be life-threatening for both the mother and fetus. To avoid this potential hazard, oxytocin should always be administered through an infusion pump and inserted by piggyback through the main intravenous line at the port closest to the client.

Intervention for Uterine Hyperstimulation

- Turn off the pitocin.
- Change the client's position (left side-lying is best).
- Administer oxygen.

Oxytocin (Pitocin) is a hormone used to help induce labor, continue labor, or control bleeding after delivery. Pitocin is produced naturally by the posterior pituitary gland and stimulates contraction of the uterus. For those clients with low Bishop scores, cervical ripening may be initiated before using Pitocin.

Oxytocin usually is diluted with 10 U in 1 L of an isotonic electrolyte solution (ACOG, 1995), although many hospital protocols may call for 20 U of oxytocin in a 1-L

Client Education

Pitocin

Explain the following to the client:

- The medication and reasons for use: induction of labor and improvement of contractions.
- The reactions to expect: increased intensity and frequency of contractions.
- The route of administration and the rate.
- The monitoring of the fetal heart rate and contractions, including frequency, intensity, and resting tone.
- The monitoring of the maternal blood pressure, pulse, and temperature.
- The expected outcome.
- That expectations may vary according to the Bishop score and other maternal-fetal factors.

Research Highlight

Membrane Sweeping

Purpose

To determine whether cervical membrane sweeping (stripping) during labor is beneficial.

Methods

Randomized trial of labor outcomes after induction. Experimental group with membrane sweeping. Control group without membrane sweeping. Outcome measures included duration of labor, maximum dose of oxytocin used, induction-labor interval, and mode of delivery.

Findings

130 nulliparas (64 swept, 66 nonsweep); 118 multiparas (60 swept, 58 nonsweep). Among nulliparas who received intravaginal prostaglandin and oxytocin, those who had sweeping had significantly shorter induction-labor interval (P = 0.048), lower doses of oxytocin (P = 0.01), and increased normal vaginal delivery rates (P = 0.01). Sweeping also had a favorable effect on nulliparas who received oxytocin alone (P = 0.04). There were no differences on outcome measures in multiparous women.

Nursing Implications

Sweeping the membranes during induction of labor had a beneficial effect on labor and delivery of nulliparas with unfavorable cervices who required cervical priming with PGE_2. Membrane stripping is a technique physicians occasionally undertake. It is not a generally accepted practice for nurses.

Foong, L. C., Vanaja, K., Tan, G., & Chua, S. (2000). Membrane sweeping in conjunction with labor induction. *Obstetrics and Gynecology, 94,* (4), 539–542.

---

bag. Regimens for the initial dose and dose increases vary according to hospital protocols. Starting dosages of 0.5 to 2 mU/min with increases in increments of 1 to 2 mU/min every 20 to 60 minutes are acceptable dosages (ACOG, 1995).

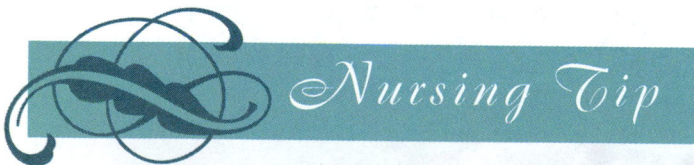

STRIPPING THE MEMBRANES

Stripping of the membranes can assist the commencement of spontaneous labor. Performed during a sterile vaginal examination, the technique entails placing the examining finger through the cervical os and sweeping in a circular motion to separate the chorioamniotic membrane from the internal surface of the lower uterus. Risks associated with the procedure include infection, bleeding, and accidental rupture of membranes. This procedure is done by physicians.

Oxytocin does not cross the placenta; therefore, no direct effects on the fetus are seen. FHR deceleration as a result of uterine hyperstimulation is the most common adverse effect (ACOG, 1995). Adverse effects for the mother include uterine rupture and hyperstimulation. Hypotension and diuresis have been shown with oxytocin use; however, these effects usually occur with a large bolus dose.

Amniotomy

Amniotomy (artificial rupture of membranes) can stimulate and reduce the duration of labor. Amniotomy may be performed early in labor for urgent inductions (e.g., for preeclampsia), or later once cervical dilation has advanced for routine inductions. The longer the membranes have been ruptured the greater the possibility of infection; therefore, amniotomy often is used in conjunction with oxytocin.

Augmentation of Labor

Augmentation of labor is the stimulation of uterine contractions after labor has begun. Indications for augmenta-

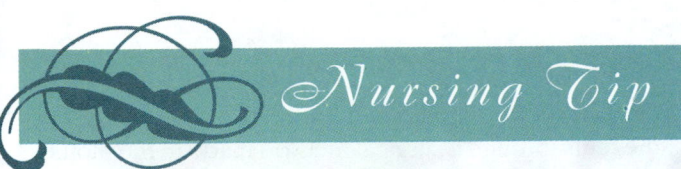

INTERVENTIONS DURING AMNIOTOMY

1. Explain the procedure to the client and family.

2. Assure the client the procedure is painless to her and her baby.

3. Assess the fluid color, odor, and consistency.

4. Note the time of rupture.

5. Note and document the fetal heart rate before and after the procedure.

6. Assess the client's temperature every 1 to 2 hours to check for infection.

7. Frequently assess the client's level of comfort.

8. Maintain adequate intake and output records.

9. Document maternal and fetal assessments in the medical record.

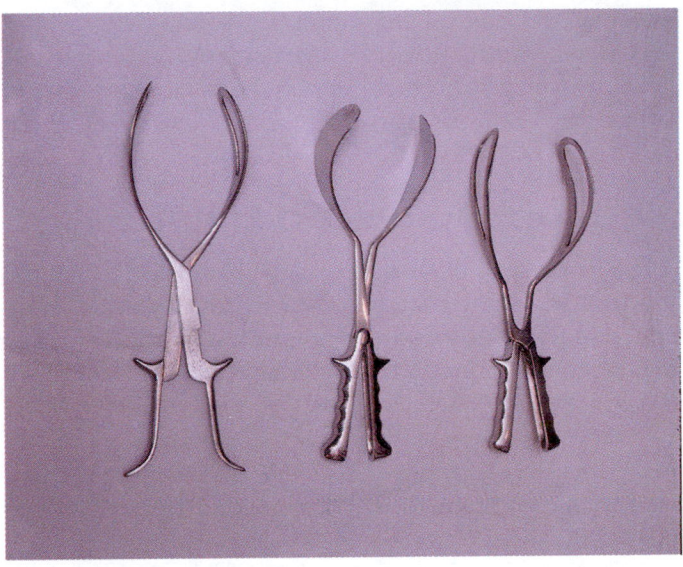

Figure 23-11 Types of forceps.

tion include prolonged labor, failure of cervical dilation to progress, or dysfunctional labor. Procedures for the augmentation of labor are the same as are those for induction. Nursing assessment and management of the client undergoing augmentation also are the same as are those for induction.

Forceps-Assisted Birth

Forceps are metal instruments used on the fetal head to provide traction or to provide a method of rotating the fetal head to an occiput-anterior position. There are several types of forceps. Some forceps have fenestrated (open) blades and some solid blades. All forceps have a locking mechanism that prevents the blades from compressing the fetal skull (Figure 23-11).

Forceps may be applied as follows:

* *Outlet forceps*—when head is crowning (Figure 23-12).

* *Low forceps*—when head is at +2 station or lower but not yet crowning.

According to Cunningham, et al (1999), the indications of forceps-assisted birth are classified as maternal and fetal. Maternal indications include; heart disease, acute pulmonary edema, intrapartum infection, certain neurological conditions; exhaustion or a prolonged second stage labor. Fetal indications are prolapse of umbilical cord, premature separation of the placenta, and worrisome FHR patterns.

Before forceps are applied, the cervix must be completely dilated, membranes must be ruptured, and position and station of the fetal head must be known. The FHR must be checked, reported, and recorded *before* forceps are applied and again *after* forceps are applied to make sure the cord is not being compressed by the forceps. It may help the mother to understand about the forceps if it is explained that the forceps blades fit around the baby's head like two teaspoons fit around an egg (Lowdermilk et al., 1999). Traction is applied to the forceps only during contractions. Rotation is performed between contractions.

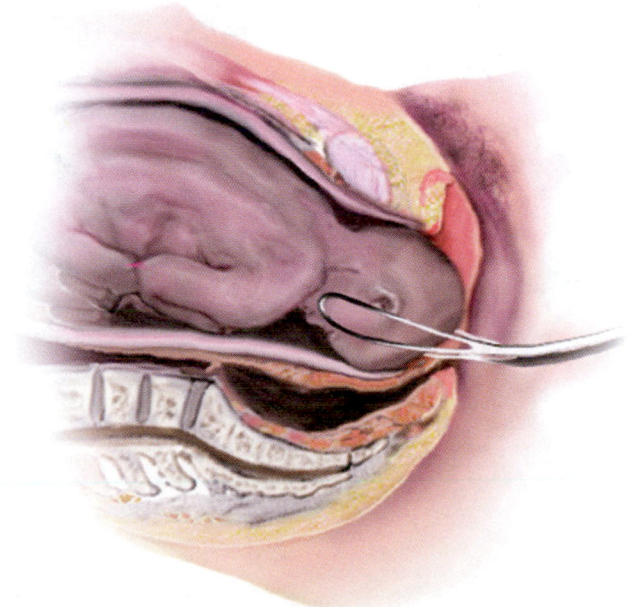

Figure 23-12 Forceps-assisted birth; traction is applied downward and outward during contractions.

After the birth of the infant, the mother must be assessed for vaginal and cervical lacerations, hematoma, and bruising. The newborn infant may have facial bruising or edema.

Vacuum-Assisted Birth

A cup connected to suction is placed over the occiput on the fetal head. After the suction (negative pressure) is attained, traction downward and outward is applied during contractions (Figure 23-13). Indications are the same as for forceps-assisted birth.

Maternal risks include vaginal and rectal lacerations. Fetal risks include cephalhematoma, brachial plexus palsy, retinal and intracranial hemorrhage, and hyperbilirubinemia (O'Brian & Cefalo, 1996).

The FDA (1998) issued a public health advisory on the need for caution in vacuum-assisted deliveries. Two life-threatening complications have been reported; subgleal hematoma (subaponeurotic hematoma) and intracranial hemorrhage. In response to the FDA report, the American College of Obstetrics and Gynecology (ACOG, 1998) recommends the continued use of vacuum-assisted deliveries when indicated. ACOG emphasizes the importance of appropriate training concerning the indications and use of all vacuum extraction deliveries.

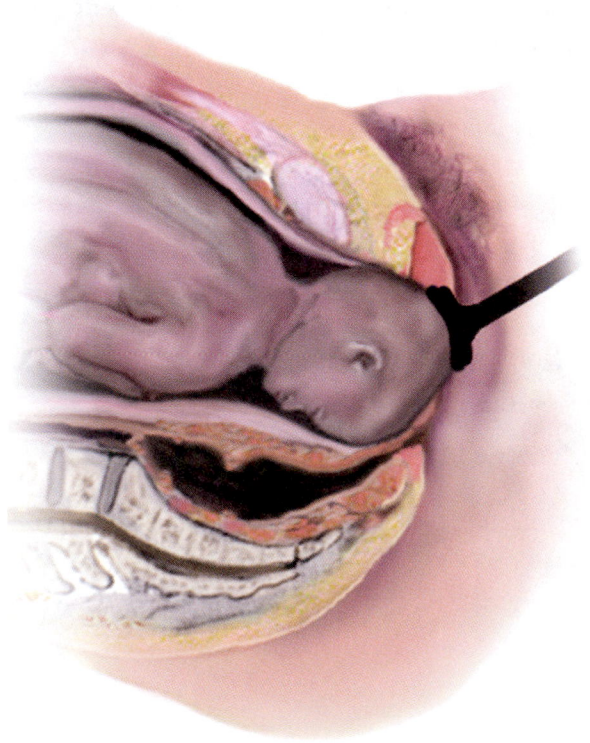

Figure 23-13 Vacuum-assisted birth.

Cesarean Section

Cesarean section, commonly called C-section, is the birth of the fetus through a surgical incision made in the mother's abdomen (Figure 23-14). The classical cesarean section involves a vertical incision through the skin and uterus and usually is performed only in cases of emergent delivery. The classical incision usually extends from the pubic hairline to the navel. The low transverse cesarean section is a horizontal (Pfannensteil) incision of the skin and uterus. The incision scar from a low transverse cesarean section is a horizontal crease under the pubic hairline. Occasionally, the physician may perform a horizontal skin incision with a vertical uterine incision. Owing to the increased risk for uterine rupture in future pregnancies associated with a vertical uterine scar, it is important to maintain adequate documentation of both the skin and uterine incisions.

Indications for cesarean section are varied. **Dystocia** (failure of labor to progress), repeat cesarean section, breech presentation, and fetal distress are among the more common indications. Other indications for cesarean section include active genital herpes infection, placenta previa, placental abruption, prolapsed umbilical cord, PIH, and other maternal-fetal complications.

Cesarean section may be performed under regional (epidural or spinal) or general anesthesia. Because most surgeons use the low transverse cesarean section, vaginal birth after cesarean section is common practice. Risk for uterine rupture increases dramatically after a vertical uterine incision and therefore is a contraindication for vaginal delivery in subsequent pregnancies.

Counseling the client in preparation for cesarean section should include information about the surgery, anesthesia, and expected course of recovery. Clients undergoing cesarean section may express feelings of loss of a natural birth. Support and emphasis on a healthy baby may enhance the client's sense of well-being. Refer to the accompanying photo story on a cesarean delivery.

MATERNAL ADAPTATIONS TO LABOR

Maternal physiologic adaptations to the process of labor are complex and change rapidly throughout labor and delivery. To assess the client's status adequately, the nurse needs to understand the changes that occur during labor in the following systems: hematologic, cardiovascular, respiratory, renal, GI, and endocrine systems.

Hematologic System

During labor, maternal hemoglobin levels increase slightly in response to the hemoconcentration. The increased hemoconcentration is related to the increases in erythro-

Skin incision   **Uterine incision**

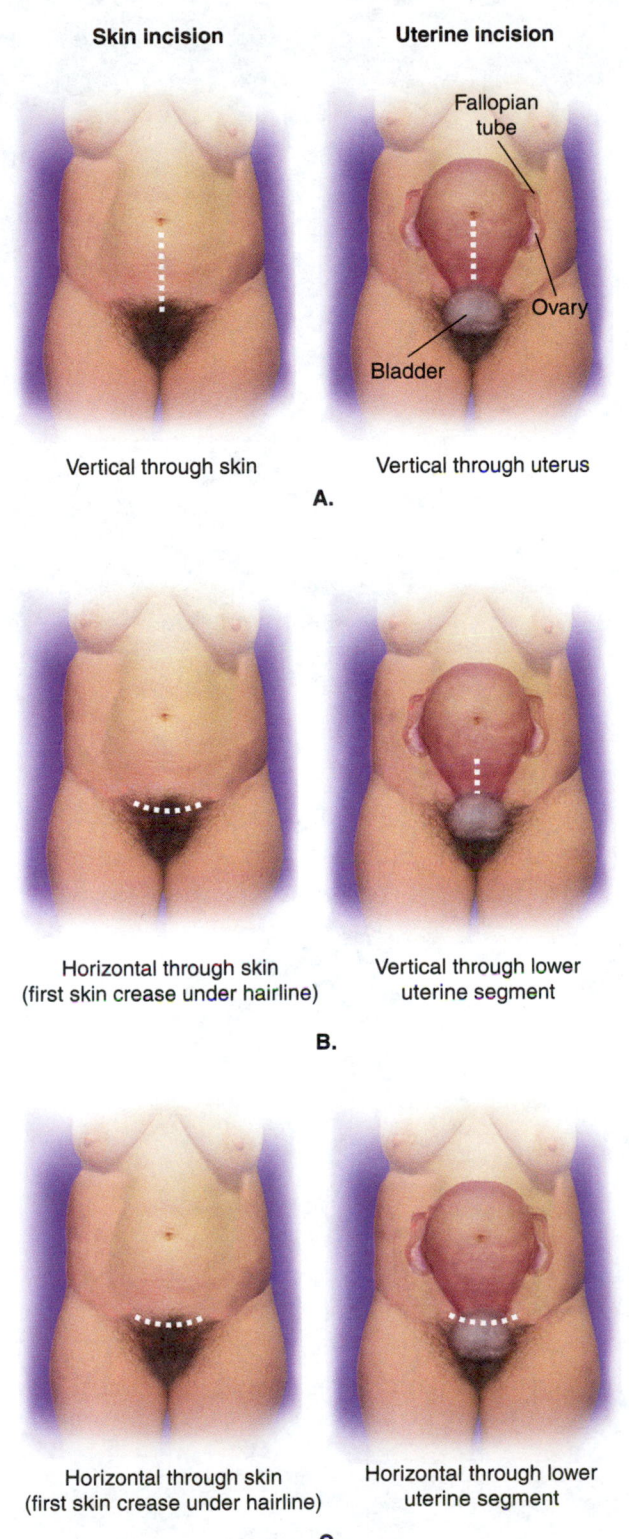

Vertical through skin   Vertical through uterus

A.

Horizontal through skin   Vertical through lower
(first skin crease under hairline)   uterine segment

B.

Horizontal through skin   Horizontal through lower
(first skin crease under hairline)   uterine segment

C.

Figure 23-14 Cesarean incisions: A. Skin and uterine incisions classic, vertical skin incision with uterine incision; seldom used except in emergency situation; B. Horizontal skin incision with low vertical uterine incision; C. Horizontal skin incision with horizontal uterine incision.

poiesis, muscular activity, and dehydration from blood and fluid loss. An increase in the leukocyte count is seen owing to an increase in neutrophils related to the stress response. It is not uncommon for a woman to have a leukocyte count from 25,000 to 30,000 mm^3 immediately after delivery, which often makes diagnosing an infection difficult.

The coagulation system is activated both before and after placental separation. The placenta and decidua are rich in thromboplastin, accounting for activation of the coagulation system. Because of all the changes in the coagulation system that occur during labor and immediately postpartum, the mother is in a hypercoaguable state. This is a compensatory mechanism to help protect the woman from postpartum hemorrhage (Blackburn & Loper, 1992).

Cardiovascular System

During labor a significant increase in maternal cardiac output occurs. Many factors contribute to this increase, including uterine contractions, pain, anxiety, and maternal position. During the first stage of labor, with each contraction approximately 400 mL of blood is emptied from the uterus into the maternal vascular system, increasing cardiac output by 10% to 15%. In the second stage of labor the increase in cardiac output is 30% to 50% (Blackburn & Loper, 1992).

An increase in blood pressure occurs during contractions, again related to the increase in blood flow to the maternal vascular system. An increase in systolic blood pressure of 10 mm Hg can be expected with contractions in the first stage of labor. In the second stage of labor, systolic blood pressure may increase by 30 mm Hg with each contraction. The diastolic pressure may increase by 25 mm Hg with each contraction. It is important to carefully assess clients with underlying hypertension. Hypotension can occur in the supine position owing to compression of the ascending vena cava and descending aorta. In addition, medications used for anesthesia in labor sometimes can cause hypotension.

During the second stage of labor, the woman often is inclined to hold her breath and tighten her abdominal muscles, called the Valsalva maneuver, when pushing. The Valsalva maneuver can cause fetal hypoxia because the maternal pulse slows and cardiac output and blood pressure increase.

Respiratory System

An increase in oxygen consumption is associated with the increase in physical activity associated with labor. In addition, mild compensatory respiratory acidosis occurs to accommodate for mild metabolic alkalosis. By the end of the second stage of labor, the respiratory system can no longer fully compensate for the metabolic acidosis. Hyperventilation, which is common in labor, can cause

One Couple's Cesarean Section Delivery and Tubal Ligation

*W*hen the operating room is set up and the client is secure on the table, anesthesia personnel monitor the client while the surgical team gathers.

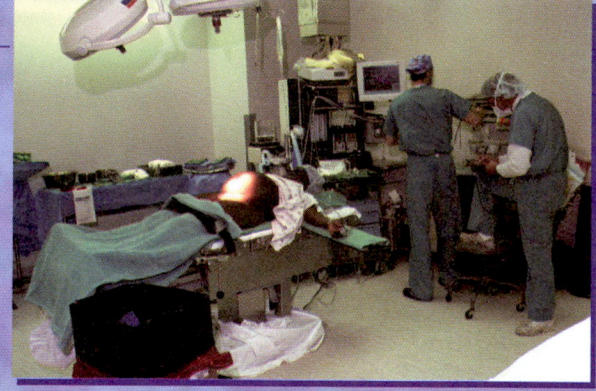

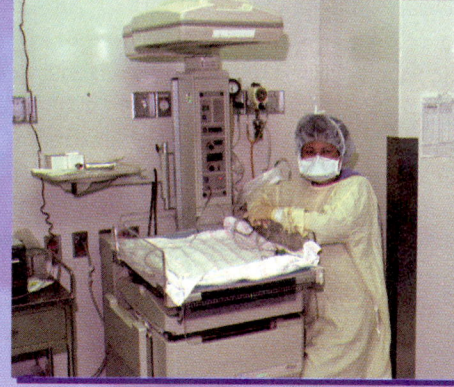

Nursery personnel arrive and check neonatal equipment and supplies in preparation to receive the newborn.

Identification bands are prepared for mother and infant.

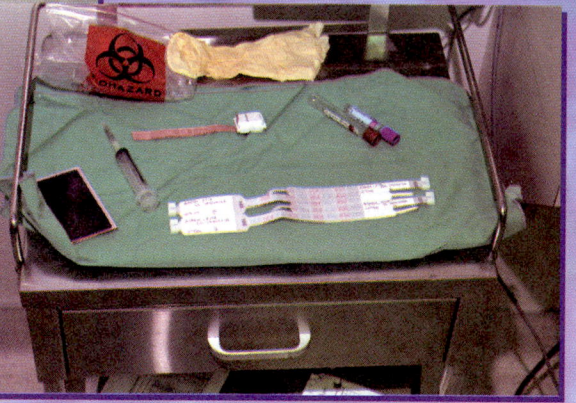

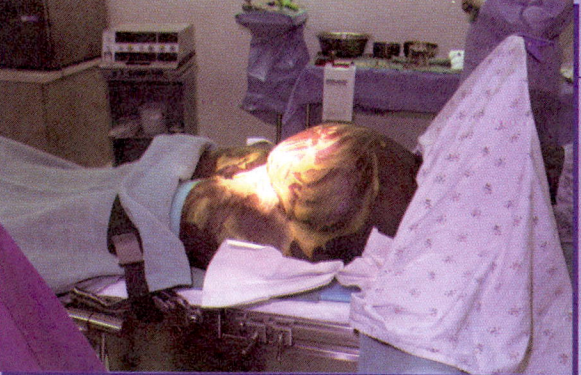

The circulating nurse performs a surgical scrub of the client's abdomen followed by a rinse with sterile water.

The client's abdomen is painted with an antiseptic solution to further reduce the risk of infection.

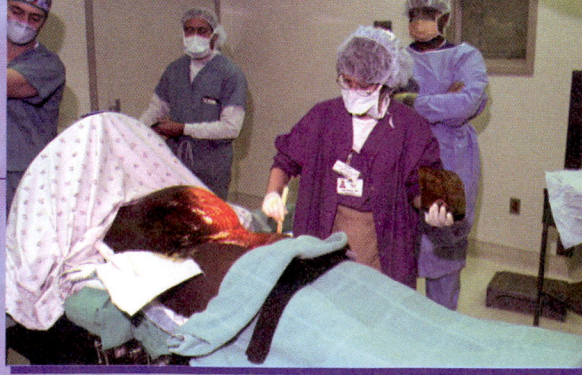

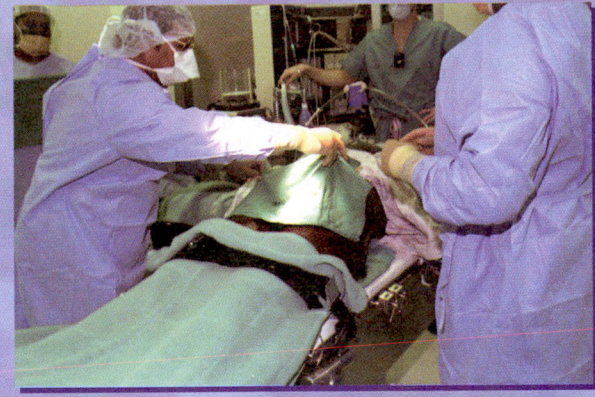

Sterile drapes are applied to provide a sterile field for the surgery.

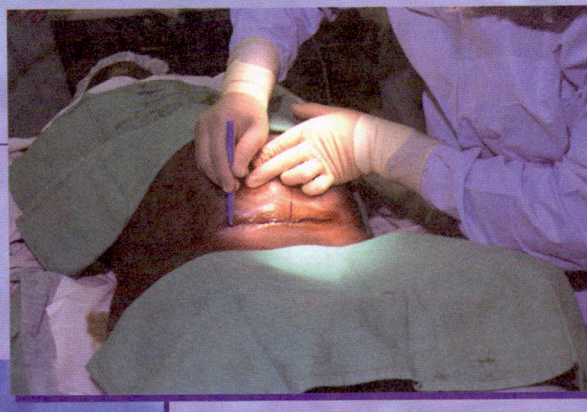

The surgeon marks the targeted incision line along the previous C-section scar.

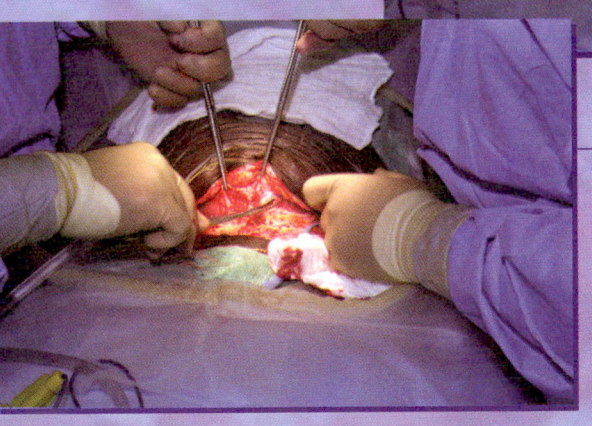

A Pfannensteil incision is made.

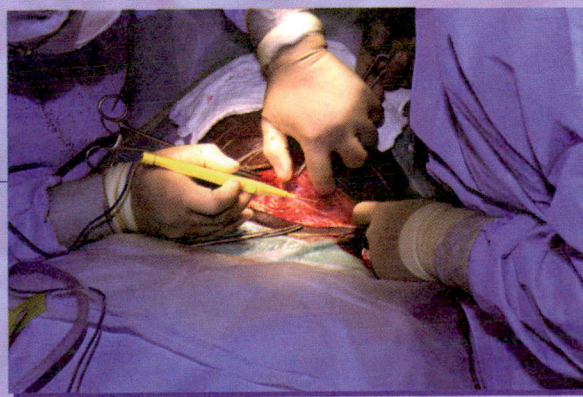

The central muscle is retracted and dissected to access the fascia.

With routine C-sections, an attempt is made to control bleeding through cauterization.

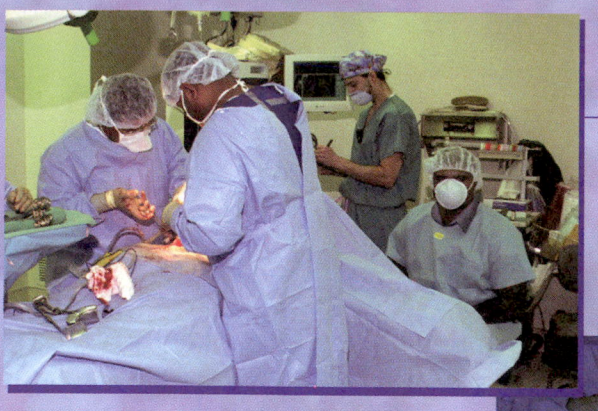

The father supports his partner and observes as the surgical team works.

Prior to incision into the uterus, the bladder must be dissected away; a bladder blade is inserted into the abdominal cavity to retract the bladder.

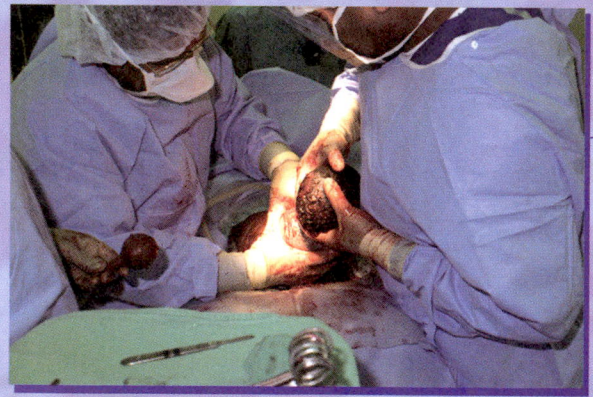

The infant's head is delivered through the incision, followed by the remainder of his body.

The infant's mouth and nose are suctioned immediately to remove amniotic fluid from the airway.

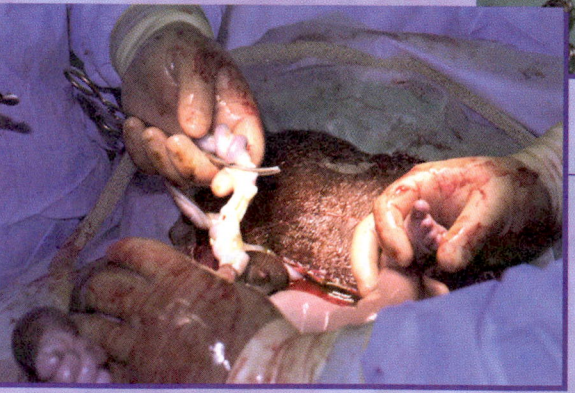

The infant's umbilical cord is cut and clamped.

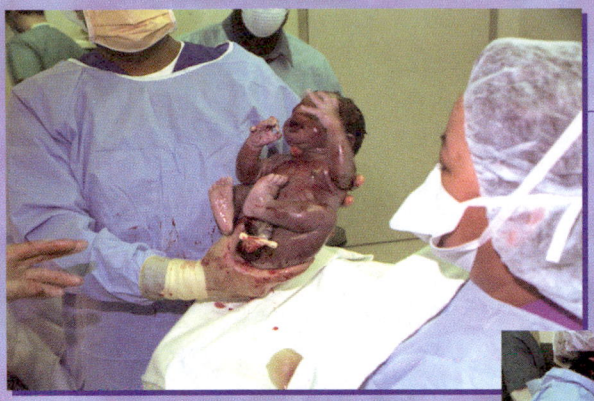

The infant is handed to the nursery personnel, who receive him in a sterile blanket.

Nursery personnel place the infant in a warmer and dry him to prevent heat loss by evaporation.

Cord blood samples are obtained.

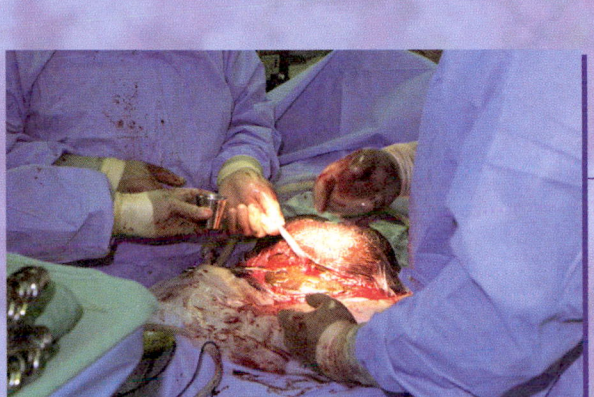

The placenta is removed and the uterine cavity is examined for fragments of retained membranes.

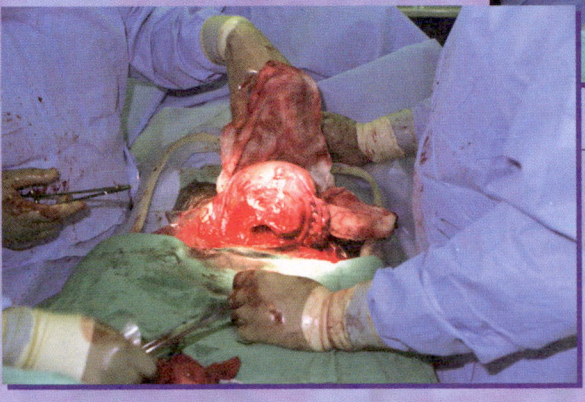

The fundus of the uterus is removed from the abdominal cavity to assist the surgeon in visualizing the lower uterine segment for closure.

The surgeon sutures the lower uterine cavity to close the incision and control the bleeding.

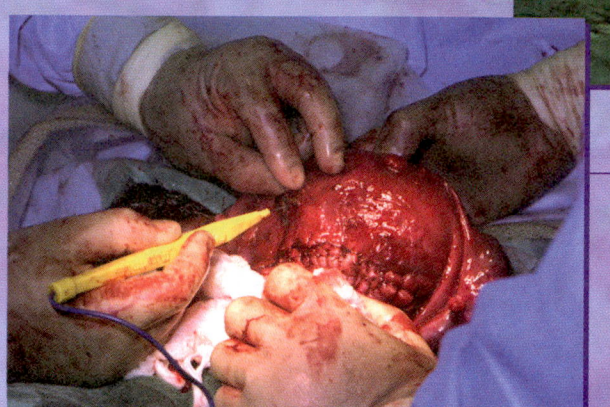

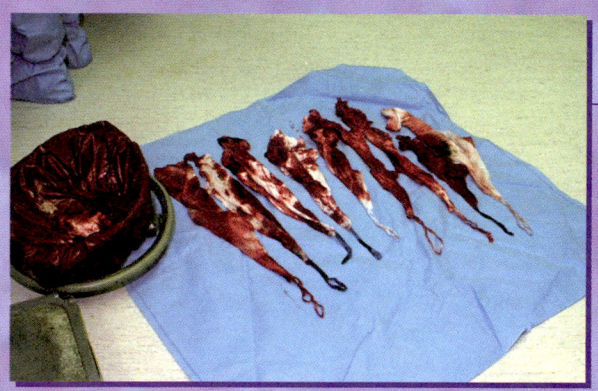

Once the major bleeding has been controlled, the smaller vessels are cauterized.

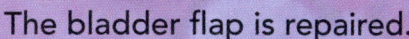

The circulating nurse and scrub nurse count lap sponges as the uterus is closed. A second sponge count occurs later, prior to closure of the peritoneum.

The bladder flap is repaired.

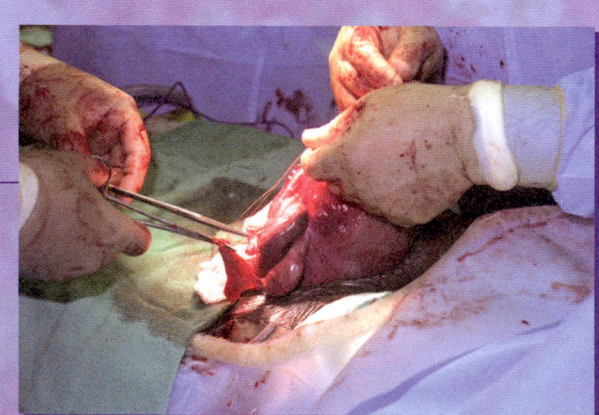

To begin the tubal ligation, the right fallopian tube is grasped with a Babcock clamp near the middle of the tube.

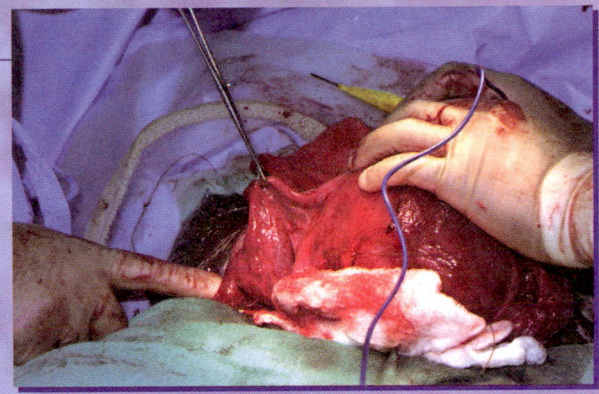

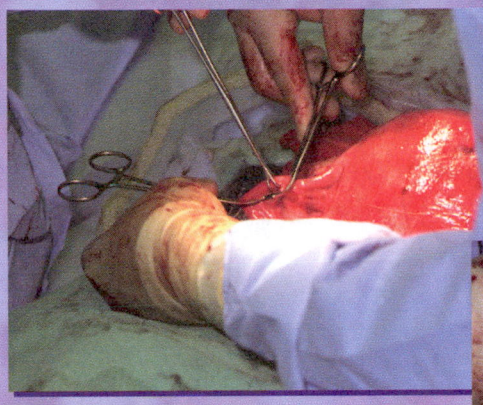

Kelley clamps are placed on each side of the Babcock.

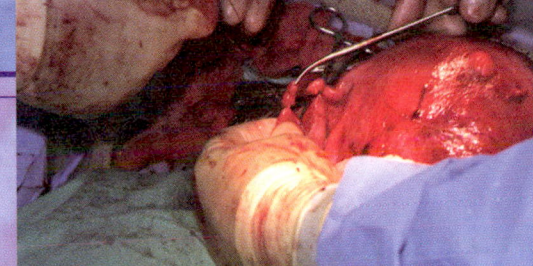

A suture is placed and tied to occlude the tube proximally and distally.

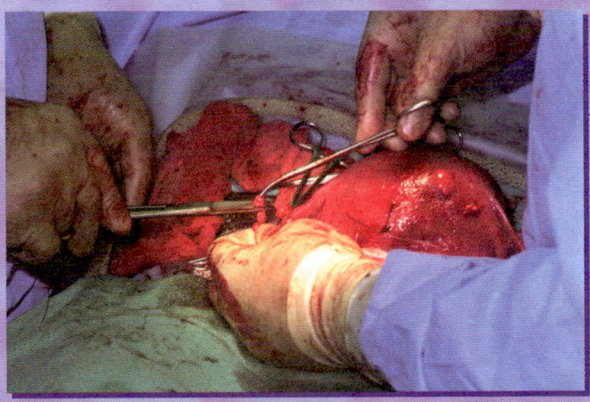

A segment of the tube between the two ligatures is removed.

After the segment of tube is removed and the ligature is placed, the proximal end of the tube may be buried as an extra precaution.

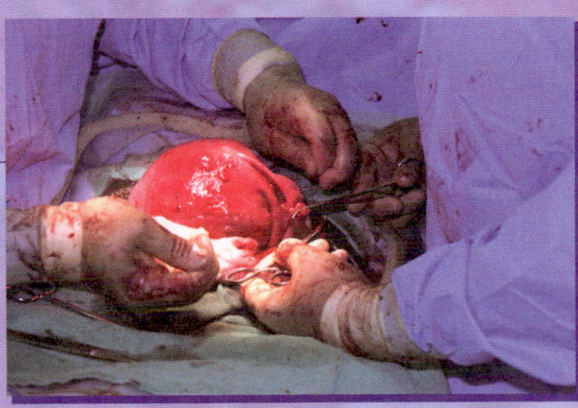

The contracted uterus is replaced into the abdominal cavity.

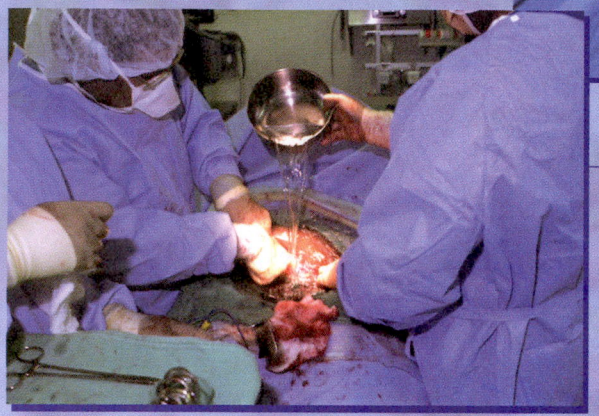

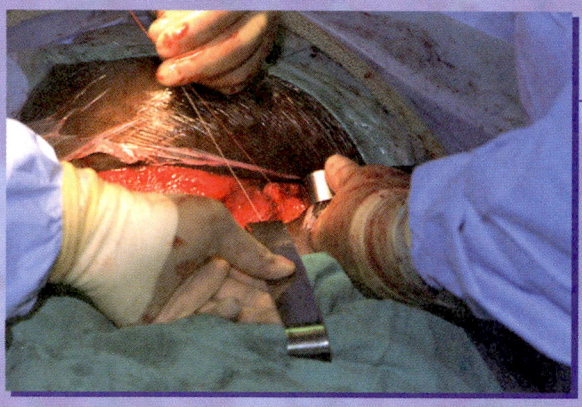

The abdominal cavity is irrigated to remove any blood clots and reduce infection.

Each layer of tissue is reapproximated and sutured.

Care is taken to cauterize small bleeders during closure.

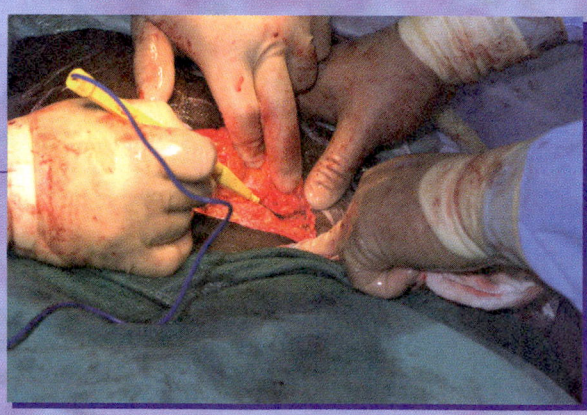

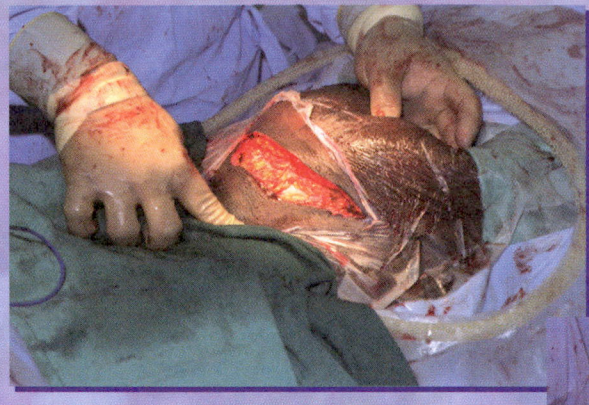

The abdominal opening is ready to be closed.

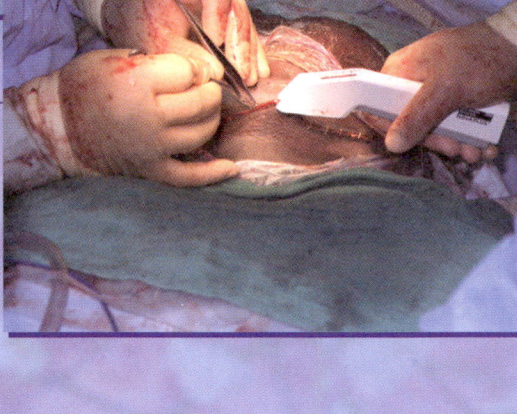

Skin staples are used to reapproximate the surface incision.

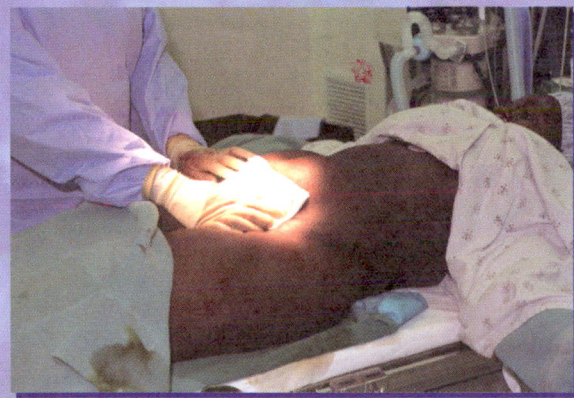

The lower abdomen is cleaned and a pressure dressing is applied.

Since the mother has been awake for this procedure, she and her husband have time to bond with their new son.

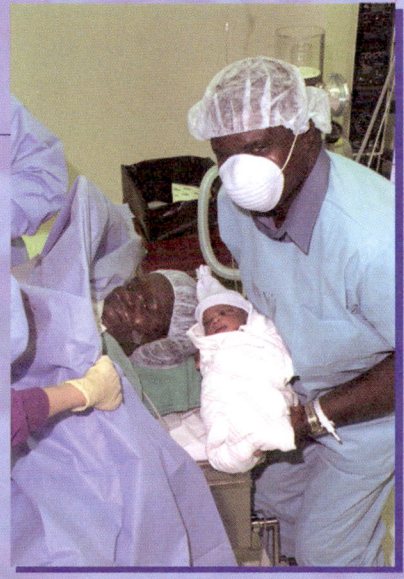

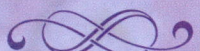

respiratory acidosis, which can result in a decrease in the partial pressure of carbon dioxide in arterial blood. Symptoms of hyperventilation include dizziness and tingling. Nursing intervention includes counting the client's respirations aloud and informing her when a contraction is ending to help her relax. The acid-base disturbance quickly resolves after delivery because the respiratory rate returns to normal.

Renal System

During pregnancy the uterus displaces the bladder anteriorly, thus making it an abdominal organ, which causes a decrease in venous return, thus making it edematous. Edema and pressure placed on the bladder during labor can make voiding during labor very difficult and can cause overdistension of the bladder, often making urinary catheterization necessary.

Increased maternal and plasma renin levels as well as increased angiotension levels are thought to be important in the control of uteroplacental blood flow (Blackburn & Loper, 1992).

Gastrointestinal System

During labor there are significant decreases in gastric emptying and gastric pH. The implication of these changes is the risk of vomiting with aspiration pneumonia. The use of narcotic pain medication can further decrease gastric emptying (Blackburn & Loper, 1992). Hyperventilation related to mouth breathing that occurs during labor can cause dehydration; however, because of the decreased gastric emptying it is important for the nurse to be cautious about the amount and type of oral fluids administered. With complete cervical dilation it is common for the client to experience nausea, belching, and sometimes vomiting. Diarrhea often is experienced at the onset of labor.

Endocrine System

As discussed previously, many changes occur within the endocrine system. In addition to the hormonal changes that occur during labor, metabolic change also occurs. An increase in the metabolic rate occurs related to the pain and work associated with labor, which is reflected by the decrease in glucose levels during labor.

FETAL ADAPTATIONS TO LABOR

Although the fetus experiences many mechanical and hemodynamic changes during parturition and birth, the full-term healthy infant can withstand these changes without adverse effects.

Fetal Heart Rate

During pregnancy the average FHR decreases from 140 to 160 beats per minute (bpm), to the normal range of 120 to 160 bpm. Although a normal fetus may have a baseline heart rate below 120 bpm, it is important to be aware that a prolonged FHR below 100 bpm during labor is likely to indicate fetal jeopardy. During labor, FHR monitoring provides a predictable and reliable measure of fetal oxygen status and well-being. Deceleration associated with fetal head compression can be as low as 40 to 50 bpm; this represents the hypoxic depression of the central nervous system, which is under vagal control. Other factors, such as movements, vaginal examinations, and contractions, can cause accelerations and decelerations of the FHR that can be normal (Figure 23-15).

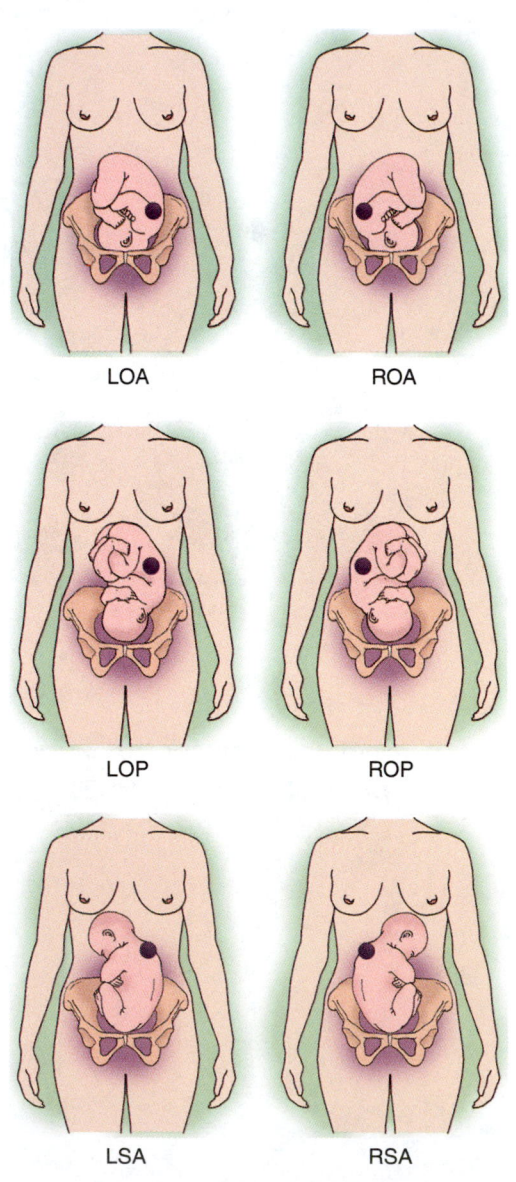

LOA   ROA

LOP   ROP

LSA   RSA

Figure 23-15 Based on Leopold's maneuvers, the fetal heart rate will best be heard in the marked areas for the various positions.

Fetal Respiratory System

The incidence of fetal breathing movements decreases before the onset of spontaneous labor. During active labor, fetal breathing movements continue to decrease. Fetal blood gases and pH change throughout the labor process. During early labor a gradual decrease in the capillary blood pH occurs; toward the end of labor this decrease is more rapid. The pH continues to decrease during the few minutes after birth. As the fetus passes through the birth canal, 7 to 42 mL of amniotic fluid is squeezed out of the fetal lungs. All of these changes help stimulate chemoreceptors in the aorta and carotids to prepare the fetus for spontaneous respirations after delivery (Manning, 1995).

Fetal Circulation

During the birth process the fetal circulation converts to that of an adult configuration within 60 seconds of the birth. The completion of this event may take up to 6 weeks. During this transition period the fetal oxygenation is transferred from the placenta to the lungs. As the placenta ceases to be the source of fetal circulation there is an increase in pulmonary blood flow and closure of the fetal cardiovascular shunts (Blackburn & Loper, 1992).

Web Activities

- Search under the Iowa Health Book: Obstetrics and Gynecology's Patient Information by Department, at www.vh.org/Patients/IHB/ObGyn.html. Create a list of client teaching tips for the primipara and multipara.
- Visit the website of the National Library of Medicine at the National Institutes of Health at www.nlm.nih.gov. What time frames are outlined for the stages and phases of labor?

Key Concepts

- The physiology of the onset of labor is a complex process involving many fetal and maternal factors.
- There are many premonitory signs and symptoms of labor, which may include lightening, Braxton Hicks contractions, cervical change, bloody show, energy spurts, ruptured membranes, and GI disturbances.
- The five Ps of labor are important factors that may affect the labor process: passageway, passenger, powers, position of the mother, and psychologic response of the mother.
- The latent phase of the first stage of labor begins with the onset of labor and lasts until the woman's cervix is 3 to 4 cm dilated.
- The active phase of labor begins when the woman's cervix is 3 to 4 cm dilated and ends when it is 8 cm dilated.
- The transition phase of the first stage of labor begins when the woman's cervix is 8 cm dilated and ends when it is fully dilated.
- The second stage of labor begins when the cervix is completely dilated and effaced and ends when the fetus is expelled.
- The third stage of labor begins when the fetus is expelled and ends when the placenta is expelled.
- The fourth stage of labor lasts for 4 hours after the placenta is expelled.
- Labor requires the adaptation of every body system of the mother.
- There are many fetal adaptations during the labor process.

Review Questions and Activities

1. How do hormones and prostaglandins affect the onset of labor?
2. Discuss the premonitory signs and symptoms of labor.
3. Name the five Ps of labor and explain how each affects the labor and delivery process.
4. Describe some aspects of the maternal attainment theory and how it is applied to labor.
5. Describe some of the maternal adaptations during the process of labor.
6. Name the different stages of labor, including the definition and the length of each.
7. Describe the fetal adaptations during the labor and delivery process.

References

American College of Obstetrics and Gynecologists (ACOG). (1998). Delivery by Vacuum Extraction (ACOG Committee on Obstetric Practice #208). Washington, DC.

American College of Obstetricians and Gynecologists (ACOG). (1995). *Induction of labor.* (ACOG Technical Bulletin #217). Washington, DC: American College of Obstetricians and Gynecologists.

American College of Obstetricians and Gynecologists (ACOG). (1999). *Induction of labor with misoprostol.* (ACOG Committee Opinion 228). Washington, DC: American College of Obstetricians and Gynecologists.

Bernstein, P. S. (2000). Predicting successful induction of labor. *The American College of Obstetricians and Gynecologists 48th Annual Clinical Meeting* [Online], Available: www.medscape.com/medscape/CNO/2000/ACOG-05.html.

Bishop, E. H. (1964). Pelvic scoring for elective induction. *Obstetrics and Gynecology, 24,* 266.

Blackburn, S. T., & Loper, D. L. (1992). *Maternal, fetal, and neonatal physiology: A clinical perspective.* Philadelphia, PA: W. B. Saunders.

Callister, L. C., Vehvilainen-Julkunen, K., & Lauri, S. (1996). Cultural perceptions of childbirth: A cross-cultural comparison of childbearing women. *Journal of Holistic Nursing, 14,* (1), 66–72.

Clark, A. L., & Affonso, D. D. (1978). *Childbearing: A nursing perspective.* Philadelphia, PA: F. A. Davis.

Foong, L. C., Vanaja, K., Tan, G., & Chua, S. (2000). Membrane sweeping in conjunction with labor induction. *Obstetrics and Gynecology, 94,* (4), 539–542.

Friedman, E. A., Niswander, K. R., Bayonet-Rivera, N. P., & Sachtleben, M. R. (1966). Relation of prelabor evaluation to inducibility and the course of labor. *Obstetrics and Gynecology, 28,* 495–501.

Gardosi, J., Hutson, N., & Lynch, C. B. (1989). Randomised controlled trial of squatting in the second stage of labour. *Lancet, 2,* (8654), 74–77.

Harrison, R. F., Flynn, M., & Craft, I. (1977). Assessment of factors constituting an "inducibility profile." *Obstetrics and Gynecology, 49,* 270–274.

Kazzi, G. M., Bottoms, S. F., & Rosen, M. G. (1982). Efficacy and safety of *Laminaria* digitata for preinduction ripening of the cervix. *Obstetricians and Gynecologists, 60,* 440.

Keirse, M. J. (1993). Prostaglandins in preinduction cervical ripening: Meta-analysis of worldwide clinical experience. *Journal of Reproductive Medicine, 38,* (Suppl.), 89.

Leininger, M. (1985). Transcultural care diversity and universality: A theory of nursing. *Nursing and Health Care, 6,* (4), 209–212.

Lowdermilk, D., Perry, S., & Bobak, I. (1999). *Maternity Nursing* (5th ed.). St. Louis, MO: Mosby Year Book.

MacKenzie, I. Z., & Embrey, M. P. (1979). A comparison of PGE_2 and $PGF_{2\alpha}$ vaginal gel for ripening the cervix before induction of labour. *British Journal of Obstetrics and Gynaecology, 86,* 167.

Manning, F. A. (1995). Fetal breathing movements. In *Fetal medicine: Principles and practices* (pp. 113–145). Norwalk, CT: Appleton and Lange.

O'Brian, W. F., & Cefalo, R. C. (1996). Labor and Delivery. In S. G. Gabbe, J. R. Niehyl, & J. L. Simpson (Eds.). *Obstetrics: Normal and problem pregnancies* (3rd ed.). New York: Churchill Livingstone.

Rubin, R. (1984). Maternal identity and the Maternity Experience. New York: Springer-Verlag.

Seidel, H. M., Ball, J. W., Dains, J. E., & Benedict, G. W. (1999). *Mosby's guide to physical examination* (4th ed.). St. Louis, MO: Mosby.

Troyer, L. R., & Parisi, V. M. (1993). Management of labor. In T. R. Moore et al. (eds.). *Gynecology & Obstetrics: A traditional approach* (pp. 575–588). New York, NY: Churchill Livingstone.

Ulmsten, U. (1996). The onset of labor. *European Journal of Obstetrics, Gynecology and Reproductive Biology,* (65), 95–98.

Varney, H. (1987). *Nurse-midwifery* (2nd ed.). Boston, MA: Blackwell Scientific Publications.

Williams, M. C., Krammer, J., & O'Brian, W. F. (1997). The value of the cervical score in predicting successful outcome of labor induction. *Obstetrics and Gynecology, 90,* (5), 784–789.

Wing, D. A., Lovett, K., & Paul, R. H. (1998). Disruption of prior uterine incision following misoprostol for labor induction in women with previous cesarean delivery. *Obstetrics and Gynecology, 91,* 828.

US Food & Drug Administration-Center for Devices and Radiological Health (1998). FDA Public Health Advisory: Need for caution when using vacuum assisted devices. http://www.fda.gov/cdrh/fetal598.html accessed 4/10/01.

Suggested Readings

American Academy of Pediatrics & American College of Obstetricians and Gynecologists (1997). *Guidelines for perinatal care* (4th ed.). American Academy of Pediatrics & American College of Obstetricians and Gynecologists. Washington, DC: Elk Grove, IL.

Moorhouse, M. F. (1999). *Maternal/newborn plans of care: Guidelines for individualizing care* (3rd ed.). Colorado Springs, CO: TNT-RN Enterprises.

Luxner, K. (1999). *Maternal infant nursing care plans.* Albany, NY: Delmar.

Gilstrap, L. C., & Hankins, G. D. V. (1997). *William's obstetrics* (20th ed.). Norwalk, CT: Appleton & Lange.

Shapiro, P. (1995). *Basic maternal/pediatric nursing.* Albany, NY: Delmar.

Rostant, D. M., Cady, R. F., & Miller, D. (1999). *Liability issues in perinatal nursing.* Philadelphia, PA: J. B. Lippincott.

Resources

American Academy of Pediatrics, National Headquarters, 141 Northwest Point Boulevard, Elk Grove Village, IL 60007-1098, Phone: 847-434-4000, Fax: 847-434-8000, www.aap.org

American College of Nurse-Midwives, Suite 900, 818 Connecticut Avenue NW, Washington, DC 20006, Phone: 202-728-9860, Fax: 202-728-9897, www.midwife.org

American College of Obstetricians and Gynecologists, 409 12th Street, S.W., P.O. Box 96920, Washington, D.C. 20090-6920, www.acog.org

Association of Women's Health, Obstetric and Neonatal Nurses, 2000 L Street, N.W., Suite 740, Washington, D.C. 20036, 800-673-8499 (U.S.), 800-245-0231 (Canada), Fax: 202-728-0575, www.awhonn.org

March of Dimes, 1275 Mamaroneck Avenue, White Plains, NY 10605, 888-MODIMES (663-4637), www.modimes.org

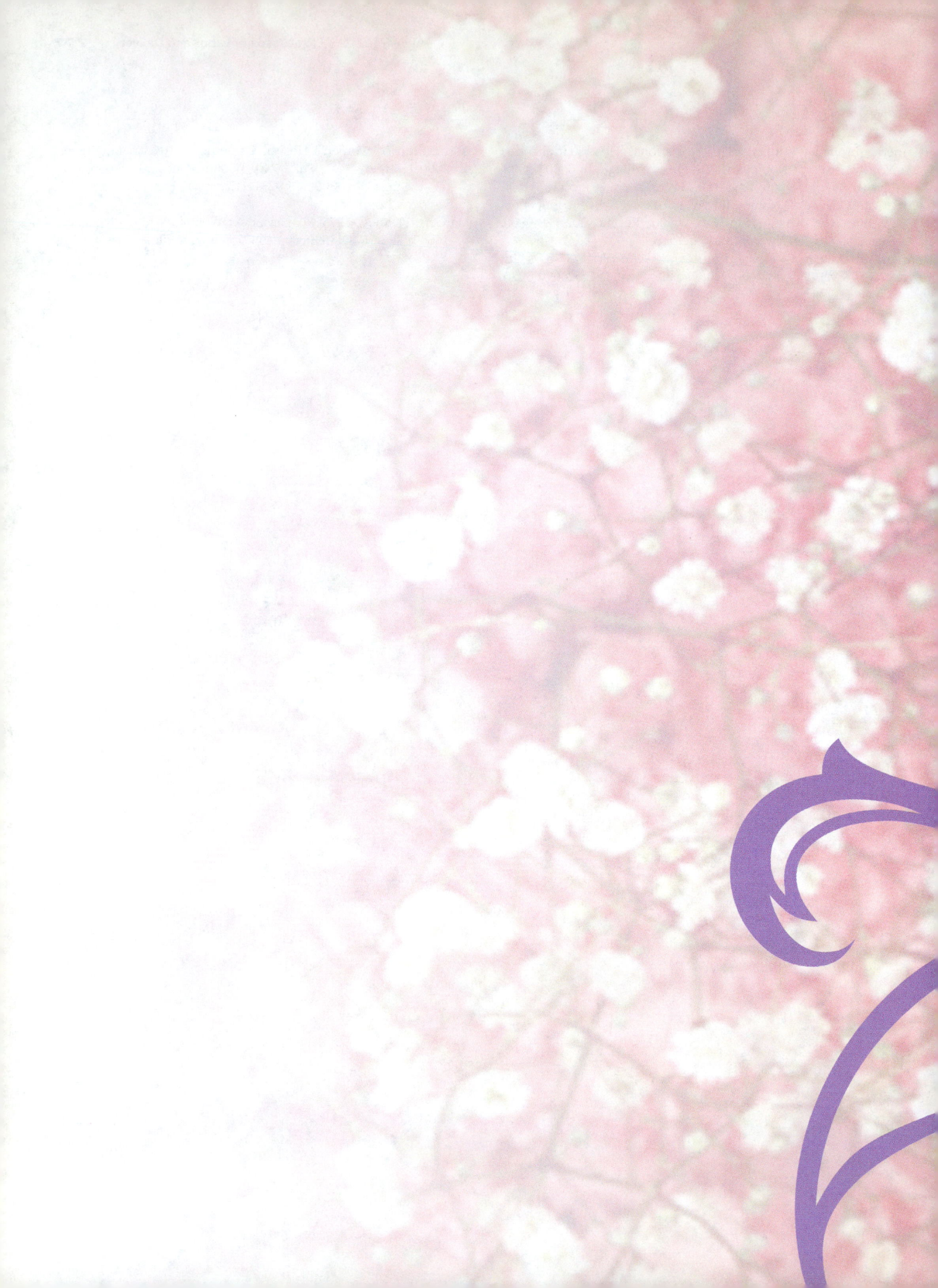

CHAPTER 24

Analgesia and Anesthesia in Labor and Delivery

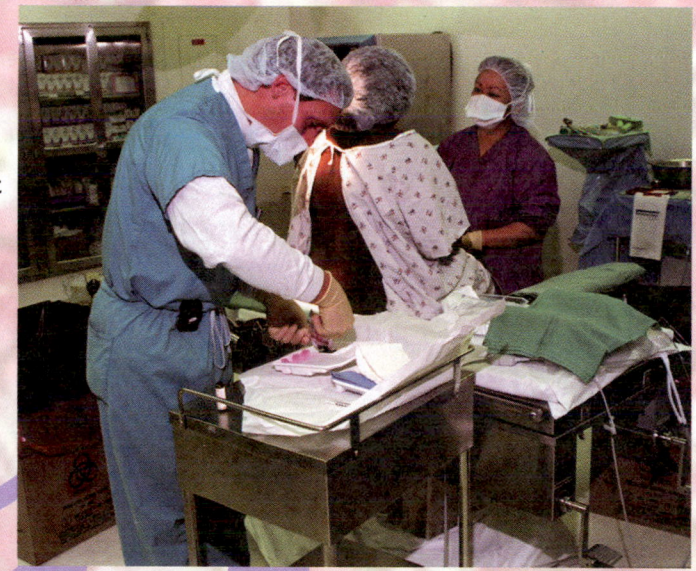

*T*here are both supporters and opponents to the use of drugs for pain relief during labor and delivery. In order to support your client during labor and delivery you must first

- *Examine your own opinions and preferences regarding the use of drugs during childbirth.*

- *Review your own knowledge of all available options for pain relief for the client in labor.*

- *Be objective regarding education of the client about all options for pain relief.*

- *Acknowledge the right of the client to choose or decline options for pain relief.*

Key Terms

Analgesia
Anesthesia
Anesthesiologist

Certified Registered
   Nurse Anesthetist
   (CRNA)
Dermatome
Epidural

General anesthesia
Intrathecal
Local anesthetic
Local infiltration
   anesthesia

Opioid
Parenteral
Pudendal block
Regional anesthesia

Competencies

Upon completion of this chapter, the reader should be able to:

1. Define and differentiate analgesia and anesthesia.
2. Describe three main types of anesthesia.
3. Explain the different options of analgesia for labor.
4. Discuss the advantages and disadvantages of specific options.
5. Describe the nursing actions necessary to prepare a client for placement of an intrathecal narcotic, epidural catheter, or both.
6. Indicate the common side effects of intrathecal and epidural analgesia.
7. Indicate the treatment of side effects of intrathecal and epidural analgesia.

The discomforts of childbirth have been acknowledged for thousands of years. For centuries it was thought that pain during childbirth was inevitable and to be endured. In comparison, the idea of pain relief during childbirth is a new concept (Morrision, Wildsmith, & Ostheimer, 1996). The advent of anesthesia in childbirth occurred in the mid-19th century in Great Britain and the United States. Dr. James Young Simpson, professor of midwifery at Edinburgh University is credited with being an early user of ether, and then chloroform, in obstetrical practice (Cohen, 1996). In 1849, the Committee on Obstetrics of the American Medical Association recommended the use of anesthesia in obstetrics, stating that pain relief in labor was justified (Morrision, Wildsmith, & Ostheimer, 1996). After the early use of anesthesia in obstetrics, debate continued. Objections included medical concerns, need for physiologic pain during childbirth, and religious reasons. Medical concerns related to the newness of the field and safety of the mother and child. Some obstetricians regarded the mother's reaction to pain as a valuable guide to the progress of labor and therefore believed pain should not be relieved (Morrision, Wildsmith, & Ostheimer, 1996). The religious objections were based on the interpretation of Genesis 3, verse 16, which was thought to imply that God had decreed that in pain would woman bring forth children (Cohen, 1996).

Rabbi Abraham De Sola, Canada's first rabbi, was asked to clarify the meaning of Genesis 3:16; in 1849, he published a three-part article detailing the interpretation. He concluded that the verse referred to the uterine contractions of labor and not the somatic sensation of pain, and therefore, the use of anesthetics for pain relief in labor was not opposed by scripture (Cohen, 1996). The controversy died in Great Britain after Dr. John Snow administered chloroform to Queen Victoria, in 1853, for the birth of her ninth child, Prince Leopold (Morrision, Wildsmith, & Ostheimer, 1996; Cohen, 1996; Kyle & Shampo, 1997; Ball, 1996). Because the Queen was the head of the Church of England and defender of the faith, her use of anesthesia led to the end of the controversy on religious grounds, at least in Great Britain. Arguments continued over the safety of the practice (Connor & Connor, 1996). By 1862, however, chloroform and ether were in general use for anesthesia in obstetrics practice (Morrision, Wildsmith, & Ostheimer, 1996).

During this same period, development proceeded in the use of parenteral opioids, first morphine and later meperidine, and the use of both parenteral and inhalation anesthesia (Morrision, Wildsmith, & Ostheimer, 1996). The early 20th Century saw an increased use of twilight sleep, a result of the addition of scopolamine to morphine, with resultant analgesia, amnesia, and maternal restlessness.

The high incidence of neonatal respiratory depression caused this technique to fall into disrepute (Morrision, Wildsmith, & Ostheimer, 1996). Although a movement known as natural childbirth began in the 1940s and 1950s, it did not become prevalent in the United States until the 1960s when the Lamaze method of prepared childbirth was introduced (Sandelowski, 1984).

The technique of epidural anesthesia was known in the first half of the 20th century; however, its use in obstetrics was limited. Refinement of the technique and improvement in the available equipment and drugs led to an increased use of epidural anesthesia (Morrision, Wildsmith, & Ostheimer, 1996). Research continues to make further refinements in techniques and medication combinations. Today, clients facing childbirth have a vast array of options for pain relief in labor and delivery.

THEORIES OF PAIN AND PAIN MANAGEMENT

Pain has been the subject of interest for centuries. By the middle of the 20th century the specificity theory of pain was prevalent. The specificity theory states that pain is a pure sensation with its own specific receptor organ and pathways for the conduction of nociceptive information to the brain, with little or no modification (Morrision, Wildsmith, & Ostheimer, 1996). Further research led to modifications of the specificity theory, yet there were still areas of pain that were not well explained by the theory. In 1965, the gate-control theory of pain was proposed by Melzak and Wall (Morrision, Wildsmith, & Ostheimer, 1996). The gate-control theory proposed that pain is a result of activity in several interacting neural systems. Each of these nervous systems, peripheral and central, has different functions. Nociception is made up of four processes: transduction, transmission, modulation, and perception. Transduction is the receiving of noxious stimuli and converting them to electrical activity at the sensory endings of peripheral nerves. Transmission is the continuation of those electrical impulses throughout the nervous systems. Modulation is the alteration of the transmissions by neural influences. Perception is the development of the sensory, subjective, and emotional experience identified by the person as pain (Fine & Ashburn, 1998). In the gate-control theory, sensory information can only pass from the peripheral nervous system to the central nervous system (CNS) when the physiologic "gate" is open. When the gate is closed due to the release of inhibitory neurotransmitters, endogenous opioids, or lock, then sensory information is blocked. This mechanism explains the effectiveness of both physical (e.g., rubbing, massage, transcutaneous electrical nerve stimulation [TENS], and water therapy) and psychological (e.g., focus points, breathing exercises, and

Nursing Alert

OVER-THE-COUNTER MEDICATIONS
Remember to ask clients about over-the-counter medications and dietary supplements, including herbal preparations. Clients often do not volunteer this information unless specifically asked. Many of these preparations can interact with analgesic and anesthetic agents.

encouragement) methods of pain relief (Nichols and Hamenck, 2000).

Pain is an individual experience. It can be influenced by a number of factors such as cultural practices, anxiety, fear, previous experiences with pain, and psychological support. These factors also are present during the experience of childbirth. It is useful for the nurse to identify in advance the most frequently seen client ethnic groups and develop profiles of culturally specific childbirth practices, including pain behaviors (Weber, 1996). However, the nurse should be concerned about stereotyping clients or failing to adapt to individual clients. The nurse must be aware of and sensitive to individual variations in a client's choices for dealing with pain in labor and delivery. The client may choose to use pharmacologic methods, nonpharmacologic methods, or both to meet her needs. The nurse must be able to teach, review, and assist the client to implement a variety of pain relief methods. The nurse also must respect the client's prerogative to choose, as long as the method chosen is safe for the mother and child at that time.

ANALGESIA AND ANESTHESIA

It is important to have a clear understanding of the concepts of analgesia and anesthesia. **Analgesia** is the relief of pain. This can be complete relief or some lesser degree of relief. Analgesia can be provided by a variety of techniques, including administration of medications. **Anesthesia** is the absence of sensation. Whereas the absence of sensation could imply complete relief of pain, the opposite is not necessarily true. Anesthesia also can be provided by a variety of techniques.

Types of Anesthesia

Anesthesia techniques fall into three categories: local, regional, and general anesthesia. The different types of anesthesia have different applications, actions, effects, and requirements. Some types of anesthesia are instituted by the obstetrician or Certified Nurse Midwife (CNM); others require the assistance of a provider whose specialty is anesthesia. The specific applications, effects, and administration of the techniques are discussed subsequently.

Local Anesthesia

Local infiltration anesthesia refers to the loss of sensation from a small area of the body after infiltration with a local anesthetic. **Local anesthetic** refers to a class of drugs that produce reversible blockade of electrical impulses along nerve fibers (Williams, 1997). Blockade is produced by preventing sodium ions from passing through selective channels in the membrane of the nerve (Stoelting & Miller, 1994). There are different types of nerve fibers, which have different functions and carry impulses that are interpreted differentially by the brain. Table 24-1 illustrates the classifications and functions of nerve fibers. Williams (1997) notes that these fibers are blocked in a specific order. B-fibers are affected first, causing autonomic blockade. Then C-fibers and A-delta fibers are affected, causing loss of superficial pain, touch, and temperature. Finally, A-alpha, A-beta, and A-gamma fibers are blocked, causing loss of motor function and proprioception. This differential blockade is very important in the technique of epidural anesthesia, which will be discussed subsequently.

Regional Anesthesia

The second category of anesthesia techniques is **regional anesthesia**, which is the loss of sensation from a large area of the body owing to blockade of neural impulses. The most common regional anesthesia techniques in obstetrics are the subarachnoid block, or spinal, and the epidural. Pudendal nerve blockade is another form of regional anesthesia found in obstetrics and also will be discussed subsequently.

General Anesthesia

The third category of anesthesia techniques is **general anesthesia**, which is the loss of sensation from the entire body secondary to the loss of consciousness produced by intravenous (IV) or inhalation anesthetic agents. Unconsciousness does not prevent the transmission of neural impulses of pain and other sensations; rather, it prevents the brain from interpreting the neural impulses into conscious awareness. Unconsciousness is not the only factor involved in general anesthesia. Other aspects—amnesia, analgesia, and muscle relaxation—also need to be provided through administration of other medications.

Types of Anesthesia Providers

Both nurses and physicians provide anesthesia services in the United States. These providers have undergone additional and extensive educational preparation in this specialty. There are institutions with only one type of provider; however, currently most anesthesia services are delivered by an anesthesia care team. This team of nurses and physicians work together to provider safe, high-quality anesthesia care to clients in a variety of situations.

Nursing anesthesia is considered the oldest nursing specialty, with a documented history of service of over 100 years (Bankert, 1989; Jordan, 1994). The **Certified Registered Nurse Anesthetist** (CRNA) is an advanced practice nurse who has completed an accredited educational program (now only at the graduate level) and passed the National Certification Examination. CRNAs administer 65% of the over 26 million anesthetics given in the United States each year. CRNAs are the sole providers of anesthesia services in 85% of America's rural hospitals (Garde, 1997). These nurses practice in a variety of arrangements, in collaboration with other legally authorized and qualified providers (Jordan, 1994). The American Association of Nurse Anesthetists (AANA) was founded in 1931. There currently are over 26,000 CRNAs nationwide, and over 96% are members of the AANA (Garde, 1997).

An **anesthesiologist** is a physician who has completed a postgraduate residency in anesthesia (and then has the option of taking the board certification examination). The American Society of Anesthesiologists was founded in 1935 and currently has over 30,000 members (Stoelting and Miller, 1994).

PAIN IN LABOR AND DELIVERY

In order to understand the requirements for analgesia or anesthesia it is necessary to briefly review the nature and transmission of pain in the process of labor. Pain is a

Table 24-1 Nerve Fibers and Functions	
Fiber Type	**Function**
A-alpha	Proprioception
	Large motor
A-beta	Small motor
	Touch
	Pressure
A-gamma	Muscle tone
A-delta	Temperature
	Sharp pain
B	Preganglionic
C	Dull pain
	Temperature
	Touch

highly individualized experience with painful stimuli interpreted within the brain (Fiedler & Shaw, 1997). The philosophy behind prepared childbirth or psychoprophylaxis is that ignorance, misinformation, fear, and anxiety appear to intensify pain (Santos, Pederson, & Finster, 1997). Education of the client regarding expectations of labor increases her ability to deal with the stress of labor. The intermittent nature of pain in labor is a primary contributor to the challenge in providing analgesia through some options. These challenges include the contrast in pain levels between the peak of a contraction and the period between contractions. What would be an appropriate blood level of medication for pain relief at the peak of contractions would be too much for the periods between contractions.

Types of Pain

The pattern of pain in labor is fairly predictable (Nichols & Humerick, 2000) (Figure 24-1). During the first stage of labor, pain results from cervical dilation and uterine contractions. These pain impulses are carried via C-fibers through the lower thoracic dermatomes T-10 to L-1 (Fiedler & Shaw, 1997). A **dermatome** is an area of the

body innervated through a specific spinal nerve (Figure 24-2). The degree of pain changes as dilation progresses, and maternal tolerance of the changes vary but often are impacted by the duration of labor. Exhaustion from loss of sleep or prolonged labor contributes to increased pain perception (Youngstrom, Baker, & Miller, 1996; Morrision, Wildsmith, & Ostheimer, 1996). When tired, a person may have less energy and a poor ability to deal with pain.

As labor progresses, with descent of the fetal head into the pelvis, another pathway appears to be the primary one (Fiedler & Shaw, 1997). The second stage of labor includes distention of the vagina and perineum by the fetal head, resulting in pain impulses being transmitted through the pudendal nerve. The pudendal nerve is composed of fibers that enter the spinal column through the sacral nerves S-2 to S-4 (Santos, Pederson, & Finster, 1997).

If the fetal head is descending in the occipitoposterior position, the force of contractions will push the fetal head into the client's sacrum and coccyx. The sacrum is in a relatively fixed position, and pressure exerted against it will result in the client perceiving pain to be in her lower back.

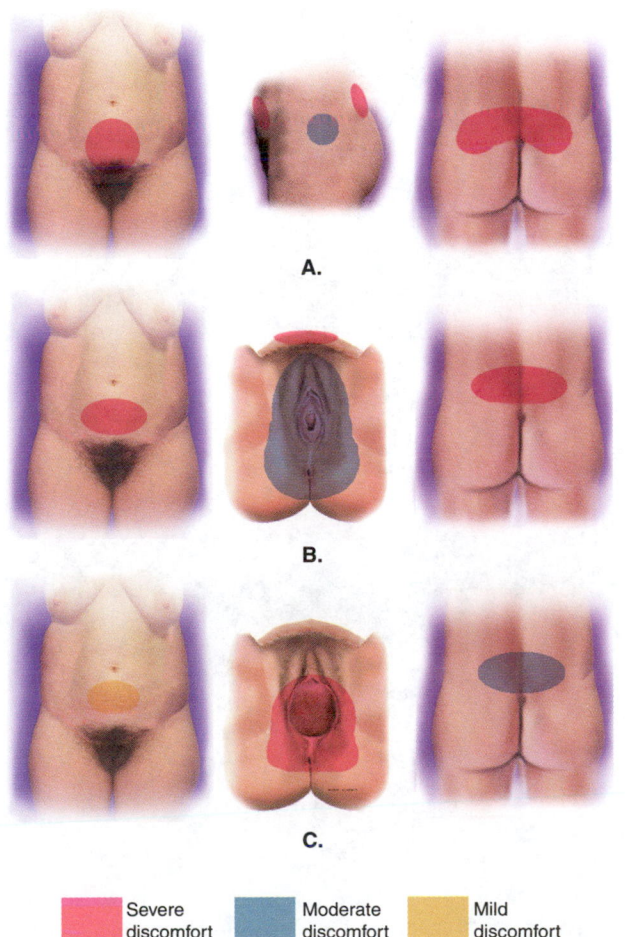

Severe discomfort / Moderate discomfort / Mild discomfort

Figure 24-1 Intensity and distribution of labor discomfort.

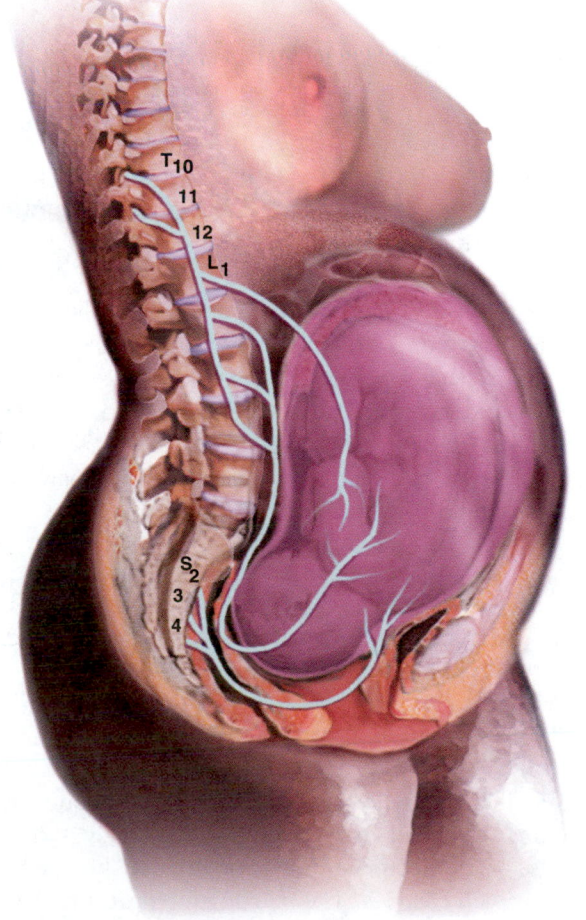

Figure 24-2 Pain pathways.

The stretching of the perineum just before delivery of the fetal head often is described by clients as an intense, burning sensation. Other specific pain sensations may be indicative of an abnormal presentation, such as an occipitoposterior position, or a different problem, such as uterine rupture (Fiedler & Shaw, 1997).

Considerations in Medication for Pain

Above all else, the first consideration regarding medication for pain in pregnancy, labor, and delivery is the safety of the mother and baby. Early in pregnancy the focal concern is the teratogenic effects of medications on the developing fetus. The critical period of fetal exposure to medications is from 4 to 10 weeks' gestation (Visconti & Rathwell, 1998). Unfortunately for many clients the critical period occurs before confirmation of a pregnancy.

In labor and delivery the focal concern is respiratory depression of either the mother or neonate and the possible complications as a result of maternal or neonatal depression. Therefore careful monitoring of clients choosing to use medications is necessary. The nurse must be vigilant and knowledgeable about the medications being used and the individual nature of the response of the client to them.

ANALGESIA IN LABOR

Clients currently have a number of options for analgesia during labor. The nurse plays an important role in client education, that is, in conveying and confirming information regarding the advantages and disadvantages of many available options to the client. The client may enter the labor process with little or no understanding of the course or expectations of labor and delivery, or the client may be highly educated and well informed but seek the opinion of those she expects to have greater knowledge and experience. An understanding of the impacts of parenteral and regional analgesia in labor will allow the nurse to anticipate problems that might, if undetected, jeopardize the safety of the mother and baby.

Nonpharmacologic Methods

Nonpharmacologic options are discussed in Chapter 17, Childbirth Preparation, and the reader is directed there for information on techniques such as focal points and controlled breathing. The reader is directed to Chapter 4, Alternative Therapies, for more information on touch therapies, visual imagery, and other relaxation techniques. Transcutaneous electrical nerve stimulation (TENS) involves transmission of electrical energy by way of skin electrodes to relieve pain (Davies, 1997). The electrical stimulation is thought to produce an inhibitory effect on transmission of

impulses that are interpreted by the brain as pain. The four electrodes are placed in pairs, with one on either side of the spine (Figure 24-3). The top pair is placed with the top edge at the level of T-10, and the lower pair is placed with the top edge at the level of S-2. The nurse should review all the information from the manufacturer before instructing the client in use of the device. TENS appears to be most helpful in the latent and early active phases of labor. Other techniques for pain management, with the exception of water therapy, may be used in conjunction with a TENS unit.

Parenteral Analgesia

Parenteral analgesia, or administration of drugs by intramuscular (IM) or IV route, has a long history of use in ob-

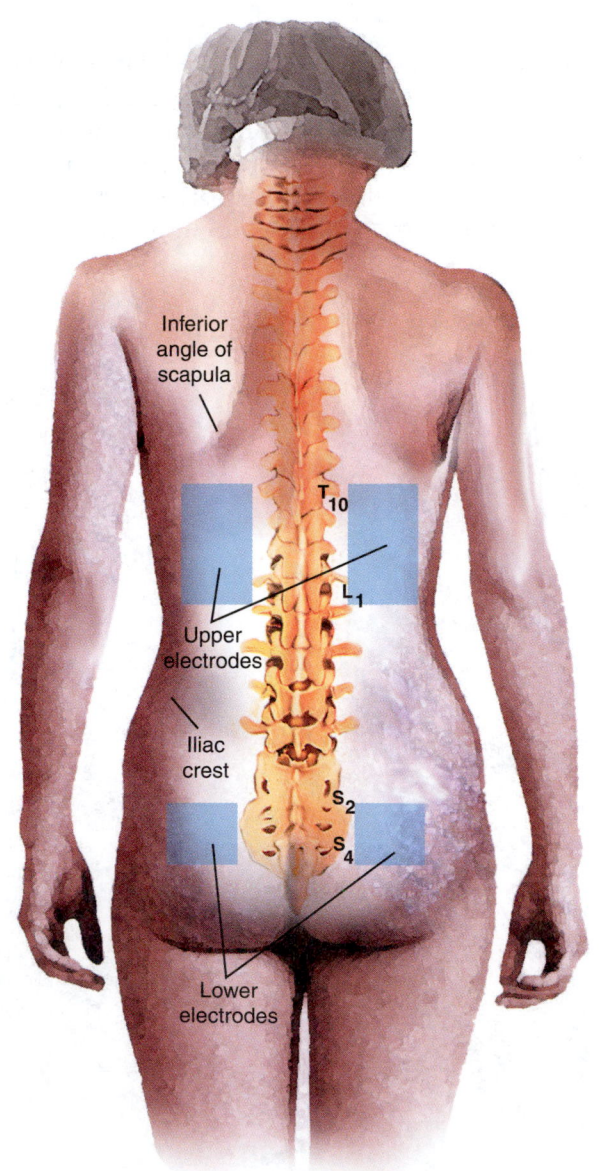

Figure 24-3 Placement of electrodes for transcutaneous electrical nerve stimulation.

stetrics to provide some degree of analgesia to the client in labor. There are two broad groups of medications administered parenterally to clients in labor: opioids and sedatives (Schnider & Levinson, 1994). Registered nurses can easily administer parenteral analgesia, which is an advantage of this method.

The disadvantages of parenteral analgesia are inadequate pain relief, neonatal CNS and respiratory depression, and maternal nausea or vomiting (Fiedler & Shaw, 1997). The route, dosage, and timing of administration are the primary factors impacting the amount of neonatal depression present at birth (Stoelting & Miller, 1994). Most drugs administered to the client will cross the placenta by simple diffusion. Molecular weight, lipid solubility, degree of protein binding, and speed of maternal metabolism will impact placental transfer of drugs (Visconti & Rathmell, 1998). Drug uptake, distribution, metabolism, and elimination by the fetus will determine the impact of medications (Schnider & Levinson, 1994). The advantages and disadvantages of parental analgesia are outlined in Table 24-2) and the factors impacting placental drug transfer are highlighted in Box 24-1.

Opioids

An **opioid**, also known as a narcotic, possesses analgesic properties because it is derived from or modeled on morphine (Hawkins, Chestnut, & Gibbs, 1996). Morphine provides excellent analgesia but its long duration of action and depressive effects in the neonate have relegated its use to the client in the prolonged latent phase of labor when delivery is not anticipated for many hours (Santos, Pederson, & Finster, 1997). Side effects include a high frequency of nausea and vomiting; possible histamine release, with resultant orthostatic hypotension; and occasional bradycardia.

Meperidine (Demerol) is probably the most frequently used opioid analgesic in labor (Santos, Pederson, & Finster, 1997). It appears to cause a lesser degree of neonatal respiratory depression than does morphine; however, its

Box 24-1 Factors Impacting Placental Drug Transfer

- Non-protein-bound amount
- Concentration gradient
- Molecular size and weight
- Lipid solubility
- Un-ionized amount
- Uterine blood flow

metabolite normeperidine has a half-life of 30 hours and may impact neonatal behavioral assessment scores (Fiedler & Shaw, 1997; Santos, Pederson, & Finster, 1997). The dosage and elapsed time from administration of meperidine can predict to some extent the degree of neonatal respiratory depression exhibited at birth.

The greatest degree of neonatal depression is seen when delivery occurs 1 to 4 hours after administration (Hawkins, Chestnut, & Gibbs, 1996). When this occurs the nurse must be prepared to carefully assess the neonate for signs of respiratory depression. The neonate with opioid-induced depression may be sleepy and not breathe properly. Appropriate care of the neonate includes stimulation, ventilation (if needed), and oxygenation. If these measures are not successful then administration of appropriate doses of an opioid antagonist naloxone (Narcan, 0.1 mg/kg) may be given IV, IM, or subcutaneously (SQ) (Hawkins, Chestnut, & Gibbs, 1996).

Naloxone should not be administered to the client just before delivery in an attempt to avoid respiratory depression in the neonate. Doing so reverses the analgesic effects when they are most needed, and there have been reported cases of maternal pulmonary edema and cardiac arrest as a

Table 24-2 Advantages and Disadvantages of Parenteral Analgesia

Advantages	Disadvantages	
Ease of administration	Maternal	Fetal
Registered nurse can administer	Inadequate pain relief	Central nervous system depression
	Nausea	Respiratory depression
	Vomiting	Decreased beat-to-beat variability
	Drowsiness	
	Possible histamine release	

Nursing Alert

NEONATAL RESPIRATORY DEPRESSION

- Opioids may cause respiratory depression in clients.
- Opioids administered to the woman cross the placenta.
- Neonates can exhibit drug-induced respiratory depression at birth. The greatest degree of drug-induced respiratory depression is seen when delivery occurs 1 to 4 hours after administration of meperidine (Demerol).

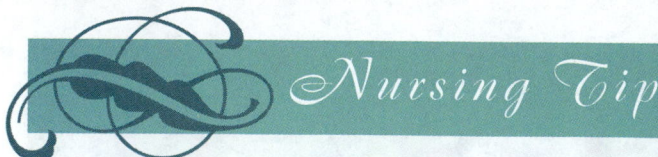

Nursing Tip

ASSESSMENT AND TREATMENT OF THE NEONATE WITH OPIOID-INDUCED RESPIRATORY DEPRESSION

1. Place infant under warmer and dry thoroughly, removing wet linen.

2. Position and open airway, if needed.

3. Suction mouth and nose.

4. Evaluate respiratory efforts.

5. Provide tactile stimulation: rub back, flick the heel, or slap the foot briefly if infant does not have adequate respirations.

6. If neonate has no respirations or only gasping respirations, begin positive-pressure ventilation with a bag and mask to deliver 100% oxygen.

7. Evaluate heart rate.

8. If heart rate is below 60, continue ventilation and begin chest compressions.

9. If heart rate is 60 to 100 and increasing, continue ventilation.

10. If heart rate is below 80 and not increasing, continue ventilation and begin chest compressions.

11. If heart rate is above 100, watch for spontaneous respirations and discontinue ventilation.

12. If heart rate remains below 80 after 30 seconds of positive-pressure ventilation with 100% oxygen, medications may be needed and additional help should be summoned.

13. Evaluate color; if blue, continue to provide 100% oxygen.

14. If pink or there is peripheral cyanosis, observe and monitor.

15. Note: Careful observation of the neonate with suspected drug-induced respiratory depression continues after this period of stimulation because the decrease in stimulation may result in hypoventilation at this point.

16. If severe respiratory depression is present or maternal opioid has been administered in the past 4 hours, naloxone (Narcan) may be needed. The dosage is 0.1 mg/kg, preferably IV, or through an endotracheal tube. IM or SQ routes are acceptable but onset of action will be delayed.

17. Note: Duration of opioid may exceed duration of naloxone. Infant will need continued observation and assessment for return of respiratory depression. Notify nursery personnel of administration.

---

result of sudden opioid reversal (Santos, Pederson, & Finster, 1997). The placental transfer is unpredictable. This affects the amount of drug delivered to the neonate and therefore its effectiveness in reversing opioid activity in the neonate (Hawkins, Chestnut, & Gibbs, 1996). It is vital to inform nursery personnel of the administration of naloxone, because its duration of action is shorter than that of some opioids. The difference in duration of opioids and naloxone results in the need for careful observation and repeated doses, if needed, for the reappearance of respiratory depression (Harmer & Rosen, 1996; Hawkins, Chestnut, & Gibbs, 1996).

Fentanyl, like meperidine, is a synthetic compound modeled on morphine (Hawkins, Chestnut, & Gibbs, 1996). Fentanyl is more potent but has a shorter duration of action than does morphine, which may limit its usefulness as a parenteral opioid except in situations where rapid onset and short duration may be advantages, such as forceps application (Santos, Pederson, & Finster, 1997). The lack of active metabolites may offer some advantage because the duration of fentanyl is not impacted by the cumulative effects of repeated doses as is the duration of other opioids (Camann, 1996).

Patient-controlled analgesia (PCA) is a method of mechanical delivery of small doses of an opioid by IV on patient demand. PCA may or may not include an underlying continuous basal rate of medication. The safety features incorporated into the PCA device include a time interval lockout and set doses that are not accessible by the client. These are safeguards against the possibility of self-administration of an overdose. The nurse should remember that these mechanical devices are not a substitute for continued vigilance and assessment. Two advantages to this method are the sense of client autonomy and the ability of clients to tailor drug administration to their perception and tolerance of pain during the course of labor. The disadvantage is the need for PCA pumps and pharmacy-prepared medications. Studies show conflicting results regarding an increase or decrease in total opioid dose used with this method (Hawkins, Chestnut, & Gibbs, 1996).

Research Highlight

A Randomized Trial of Epidural versus Patient-Controlled Meperidine Analgesia during Labor

Purpose

To assess the effects of epidural analgesia on the incidence of cesarean delivery.

Methods

In a prospective randomized trial, 715 women received either epidural analgesia or PCA IV meperidine analgesia.

Findings

Epidural analgesia was not associated with an increased incidence of cesarean delivery when compared with PCA using meperidine.

Nursing Implications

Understanding the research regarding the incidence of cesarean delivery associated with epidural analgesia is important in client education regarding this option for pain management in labor and delivery.

Sharma, S. K., Sidawi, J. E., Ramin, S. M., Lucas, M. J., Leveno, K. J., & Cunningham, F. G. (1997). A randomized trial of epidural versus patient-controlled meperidine analgesia during labor. *Anesthesiology, 87*, (3), 487–494.

Sharma et al. (1997) concluded that PCA with meperidine was a safe and effective method of analgesia during labor but noted the increased need for neonatal naloxone administration. In this study, the mean and maximum doses of meperidine were 139 ± 100 mg and 500 mg, and the authors noted that 24% of women received over 200 mg. PCA has gained in popularity in recent years but may not be in use in all hospitals (Cheek & Gutsche, 1997).

Another type of opioid drugs is known as agonist-antagonists. Two drugs of this type, butorphanol (Stadol) and nalbuphine (Nubain), are still occasionally seen in obstetrics practice. These drugs produce analgesia but also a degree of maternal sedation and dizziness (Hawkins, Chestnut, & Gibbs, 1996). The apparent ceiling effect for maternal respiratory depression (increasing doses do not appear to increase respiratory depression) is the advantage cited by some proponents (Cheek & Gutsche, 1997). These drugs appear to have a lower incidence of nausea and vomiting (Hawkins, Chestnut, & Gibbs, 1996; Santos, Pederson, & Finster, 1997). Because there is some association of fetal respiratory depression with the use of these drugs, the nurse should be prepared to assess and respond to problems at birth.

Sedatives

Sedatives or tranquilizers usually are co-administered with opioids (Cheek & Gutsche, 1997). Pentobarbital (Nembutal) occasionally is used, in combination with morphine in the prolonged latent phase of labor when delivery is not anticipated for over 12 hours (Schnider & Levinson, 1994). Promethazine (Phenergan) is the most widely used drug of this class (Hawkins, Chestnut, & Gibbs, 1996). Promethazine or hydroxyzine (Vistaril) are co-administered with meperidine to reduce narcotic requirements, decrease nausea and vomiting, and allay anxiety (Schnider & Levinson, 1994; Cheek & Gutsche, 1997). Because of the strong sedative effect of benzodiazepines such as diazepam (Valium) and midazolam (Versed), they are only used in specific situations, for example, as anticonvulsive agents in the presence of seizures (Schnider & Levinson, 1994). The nurse should be aware that benzodiazepines have amnesic properties.

Client Experience with Pain

The nurse must always recognize that pain is a very individual experience. It is subjective in nature and can only

REFLECTIONS FROM A LABORING MOTHER

"My husband and I had been to childbirth prepara-tion classes and had toured the hospital where I was planning on delivering our first baby. We were very excited and practiced the techniques we learned in the classes. Two days before my due date we had some friends over for a barbecue, and as we sat around afterward I found myself restless and kind of achy. I found that if I changed my posi-tion or rubbed my abdomen I felt better. That night I just kept feeling like I had to go to the bathroom, even if there was nothing there. I spent a couple of hours getting up and down, and finally my hus-band grumbled, 'Why don't you call the doctor?' I didn't think this was labor because it really wasn't painful. I called and was sent to the hospital. But I was only dilated to 1 cm. I thought the pain wasn't too bad. Little did I know what it would be like in the next couple of hours. The contractions got closer together and hurt more, and after awhile I couldn't walk any more. At 5 cm dilated I was ex-hausted from being up all night and ready for some pain relief. I was unprepared for the intensity of the pain, and although I had hoped for a drug-free de-livery, I was most relieved when the medications began to take effect."

be defined by the client experiencing the pain, who may communicate in many different ways that are interpreted by the nurse. Misunderstandings may arise if the nurse is not aware of the personal beliefs and biases regarding pain and pain behaviors, particularly in clients from other cultural backgrounds (Weber, 1996).

Nursing Implications

Nurses and clients should discuss plans regarding pain re-lief early in labor. Assessment of the client's understanding of different methods of pain relief can illustrate educa-tional needs. The nurse should convey information or act as the client's advocate to acquire needed information re-garding pain relief methods. If the client asks for medica-tion the nurse should inform her of what to expect regard-ing the onset, duration, and side effects of the individual medication.

Regional Analgesia

Regional techniques, alone or in combination with other techniques, are commonly used to provide analgesia for labor pain (Ellis, 1997). Regional analgesia options for labor include the use of intrathecal opioids, epidural blocks, and spinal-epidural combination. One other re-gional technique, paracervical block, is not in common use but will be reviewed for the sake of completeness.

A review of the anatomy of the spinal column and epidural space is needed to fully understand the mecha-nism by which these techniques provide analgesia or anes-thesia to the client (Figure 24-4). The spinal cord ends ap-proximately at the level of the first or second lumbar vertebrae, L-1, L-2 (Ostheimer & Leavitt, 1996). It is pro-tected by the dural sac and lies within the vertebrae.

REFLECTIONS FROM NURSES

"Before epidurals were available I gave Demerol to clients in labor. There were some things that I could watch for because they happened a lot. I al-ways put an emesis basin within reach because a fair number of the women would be nauseated or vomit. I had to really watch the multiparas when I gave them Demerol at 5 cm dilated, because after they threw up a couple of times they would look at you with eyes the size of dinner plates and say 'The baby is coming.' You had better believe them, because often they were right. The increased in-traabdominal pressure created by vomiting would push that baby down against the cervix, and they would go from 5 cm to complete in minutes. It didn't happen all the time but often enough to watch for it."

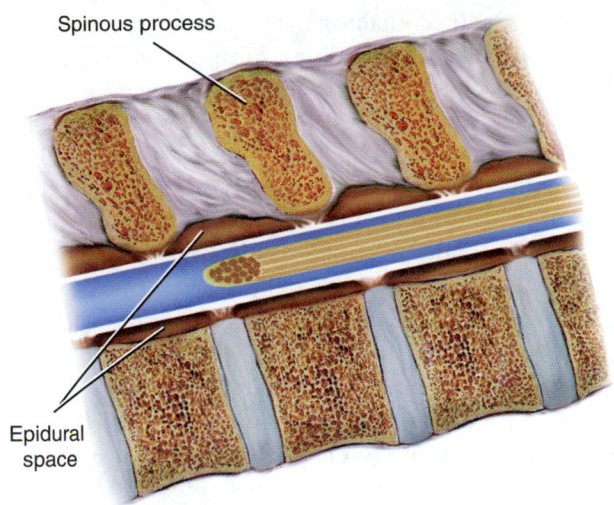

Figure 24-5 Discontinuous nature of epidural space.

Critical Thinking

Client and Partner Conflicts Regarding Analgesia and Anesthesia in Labor and Delivery

It is not unheard of for clients to change their minds regarding options for pain relief in labor and delivery, especially as pain intensifies.

- What will you do if the client requests medications or anesthesia and the partner disagrees?
- What if the client has had medications and now wants an epidural but her partner disagrees?
- Can the client give informed consent while under the influence of medication?
- What will you do?

Below L-1, L-2 the dural sac contains spinal nerve roots. The epidural space lies between the dura and vertebral canal (Benards, 1997). Nerves and blood vessels travel through the epidural space, which is occupied by fat globules (Luyendijk, 1996). The epidural spaces are discontinuous. Addition of fluid volume to the epidural space opens up the areas that appear unoccupied (Figure 24-5).

The major factors involved in analgesia or anesthesia provided by regional techniques include the types of drugs used, dosages, anatomic level and area of placement, and patient position. Individual differences in these factors impact the analgesia produced in a specific client.

Preparation of the Client

The nursing actions to prepare the client and assist the anesthesia provider during initiation of intrathecal, epidural, or combined techniques are virtually identical. When applicable, slight differences will be discussed in the sections on specific techniques.

The client's desire for regional analgesia should be confirmed and the obstetrician notified before the procedure. IV access must be obtained, if not already available, and a bolus of fluid should be given just before the procedure. The CRNA or anesthesiologist must assess the client

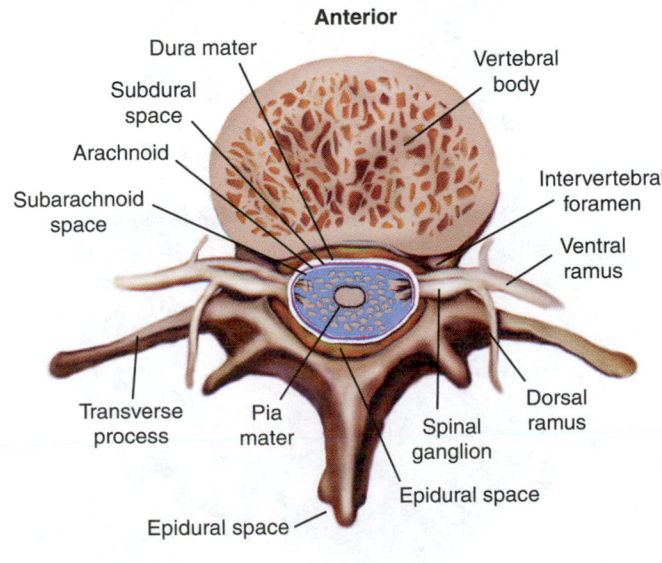

Figure 24-4 Cross-section of the spinal canal area.

Client Education

Important Information for the Anesthesia Provider

Before administration of medication, the anesthesia provider must ascertain the client's health history on the following:

- Drug or other allergies
- Smoking history
- Breathing problems
- Cardiac problems
- Other health problems
- Previous anesthetics
- Difficulties with nausea or vomiting with previous anesthetics

requesting regional analgesia. The client's medical history; physical status; understanding of the procedure, including risks and benefits; and consent for the procedure must be obtained (Fiedler & Shaw, 1997). It is very important to answer any questions the client may have regarding the risk and benefits of regional analgesia before the procedure is begun to create an atmosphere of trust and confidence and to fulfill conditions of informed consent.

After all questions of the client have been answered and informed consent has been obtained, the client is assisted to a sitting position (feet over the side of the bed, or cross-legged in front and hunched forward) or side-lying position (with knees and feet drawn up toward her chest), depending on the preference of the anesthesia provider (Figures 24-6 and 24-7). The client's gown or fetal monitor belts must be moved away from the area of the back where the needle will be placed.

The back is palpated for the appropriate landmarks and prepared with an antiseptic solution. A small wheal of local anesthetic is made, and the epidural needle is placed between the vertebrae and the epidural space identified. (When an intrathecal opioid alone or spinal anesthesia is planned, a spinal needle is used and the epidural space is not identified.) There are two methods of identification, "hanging drop" and "loss of resistance." In the hanging

drop method a drop of saline is placed in the hub of the epidural needle once the needle has entered the ligaments near the spinal canal. When the epidural needle enters the epidural space, a slight degree of negative pressure will pull the drop into the needle (Ostheimer & Leavitt, 1996). In the loss of resistance method, a 5- to 10-mL syringe filled with saline is attached to the hub and the needle slowly advanced. Keeping a steady pressure on the plunger of the syringe as the needle is advanced, resistance will be felt until the epidural space is entered, at which point the saline will be suddenly and easily injected (Ostheimer & Leavitt, 1996). Regardless of the method, the most important task of the nurse is to assist the client in not moving and remaining in an optimal position during the procedure. A knowledgeable nurse is a great asset to the anesthesia provider performing regional analgesia and anesthesia techniques (Fiedler & Shaw, 1997). The anesthesia provider will indicate when it is safe for the client to move. At this point in the administration the techniques vary slightly and will be covered in the individual sections.

Intrathecal Opioids

The technique of **intrathecal** opioid administration is a variation of the subarachnoid block, or spinal. The difference lies in the type of medication (opioid instead of local

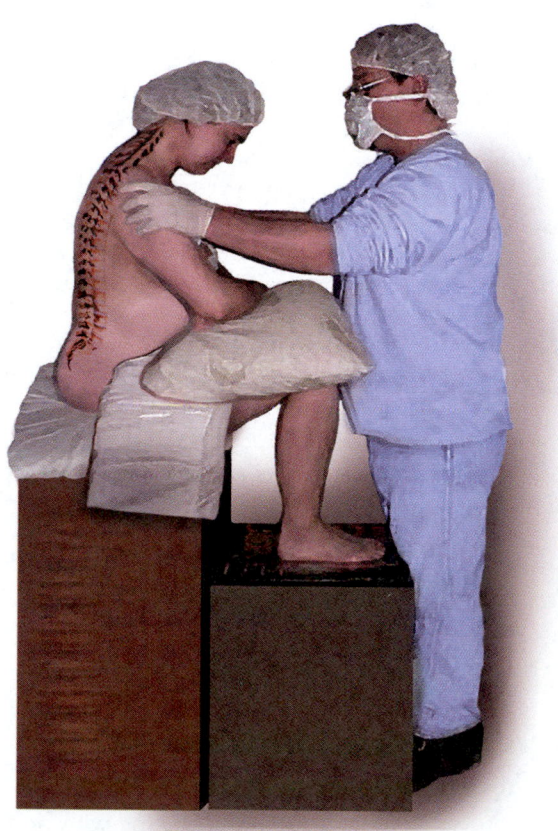
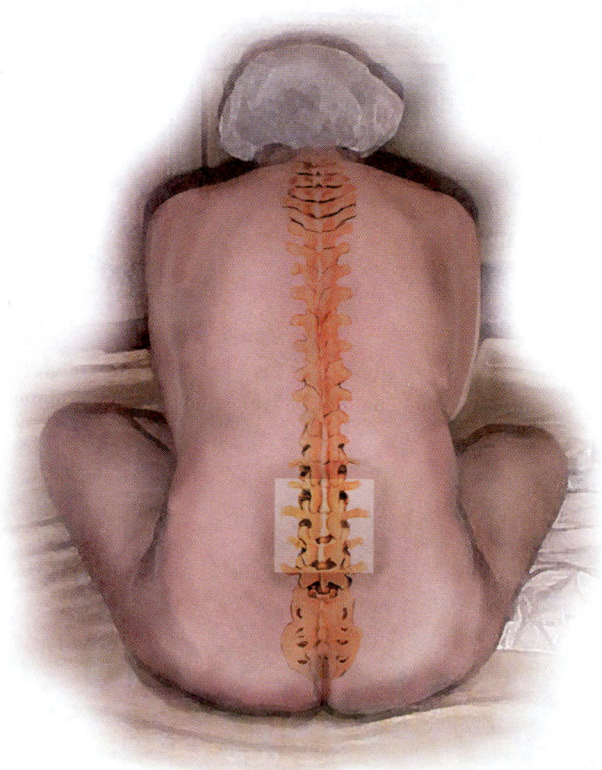

Figure 24-6 Sitting position for insertion of spinal or epidural anesthesia.

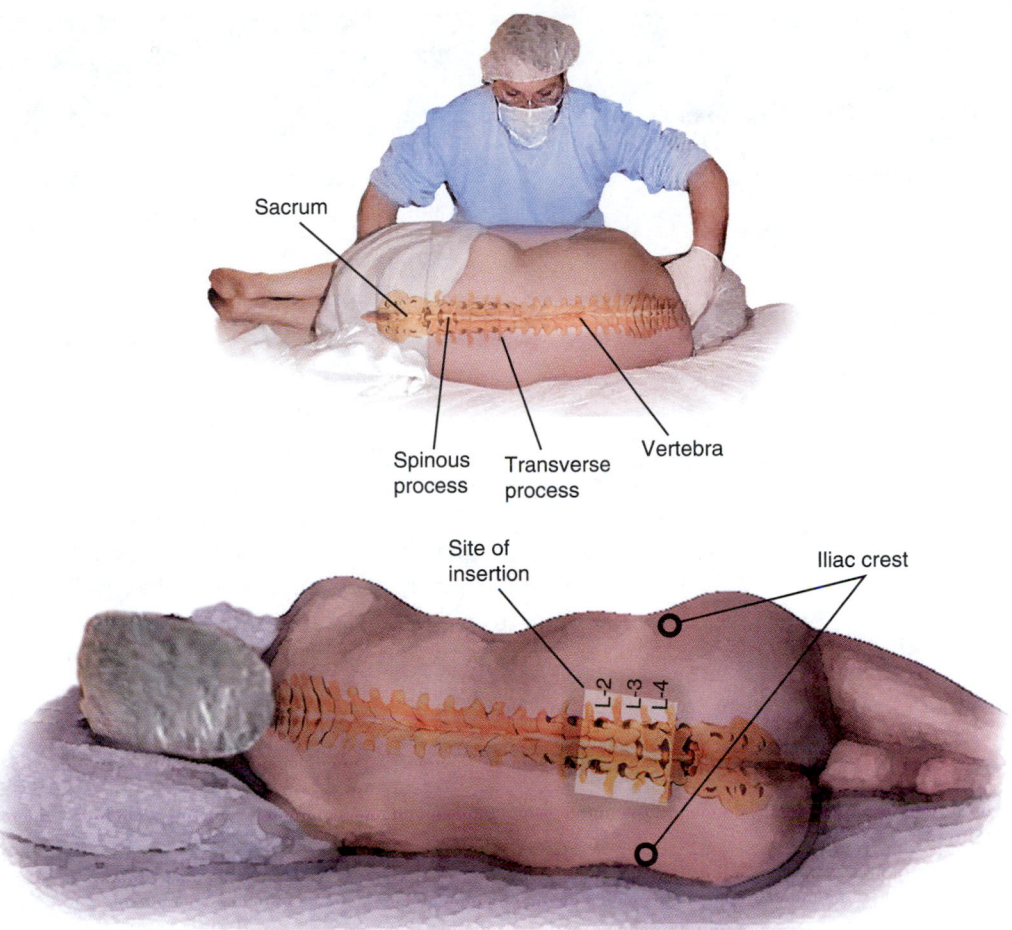

Figure 24-7 Side-lying position for insertion of spinal or epidural anesthesia.

anesthetic) deposited just inside the dural sac. This method provides analgesia through opioid activity at the receptors located in the spinal nerves. A small amount of an opioid, such as morphine, fentanyl, or sufentanil, is placed in the cerebrospinal fluid through a small-gauge spinal needle after puncture of the dural membrane. Refer to Table 24-3 for the advantages and disadvantages of this method.

The intrathecal opioid technique using fentanyl or sufentanil has the advantages of rapid onset (often less than 5 minutes) and of providing excellent analgesia without autonomic or motor blockade (Mullins & Johnson, 1996). The client's ability to ambulate without orthostatic hypotension or motor coordination is preserved (Rawal, 1996). Because there is no autonomic blockade, maternal blood pressure decreases slightly but usually not below prelabor levels. In the absence of the autonomic blockade, the IV fluid bolus requirement usually is less then 500 mL. There are drawbacks to this technique. Labor duration is highly individualized and not easily or accurately predictable and thus may outlast the duration of pain relief afforded by the dose of intrathecal opioid. Mullins and Johnson (1996) reported that 40% of clients required additional analgesia owing to duration of labor. Additional disadvantages can include sedation, nausea and vomiting, and pruritus. The incidence, duration, and severity of these symptoms are related to the drug and dosage used. Use of intrathecal morphine alone is limited due to the high incidence of side effects and the more serious occurrence of maternal respiratory depression. Fentanyl is more

Table 24-3 Advantages and Disadvantages of Intrathecal Opioids	
Advantages	**Disadvantages**
Rapid onset (fentanyl or sufentanil)	May not last as long as labor
No motor block (able to ambulate)	Pruritus
No sympathetic block (no hypotension)	Nausea (morphine)
	Vomiting (morphine)

Client Education

Intrathecal Opioids

Teach your clients what to expect after administration of an intrathecal opioid:

- Rapid (one to two contractions later) onset of relief.

- Contractions that feel more like pressure and less like pain.

- Itching that could be located anywhere but usually is mild and resolves in 30 to 40 minutes.

frequently given because of the lower incidence and decreased severity of side effects. It is beneficial to inform the client that she may experience itching shortly after administration of intrathecal fentanyl and that it usually will resolve over the next 30 to 40 minutes. Extreme cases of pruritus can be managed by the administration of naloxone; however, treatment rarely is required (Mullins & Johnson, 1996). Most clients will indicate that they prefer itching over pain.

Clients also should be educated regarding other sensations they will experience after intrathecal opioid administration. Although they still may be aware of the uterine contraction, the pain will be more like a pressure sensation, possibly rectal, than pain. Clients should be instructed to report an increase in rectal pressure sensation or a feeling of continuous pressure. Either may be an indication of progression of labor. When clients begin to feel pain again, the anesthesia provider should be notified in a timely manner because once the intrathecal opioid activity begins to diminish it may wear off quickly.

Epidural Anesthesia

The technique of lumbar **epidural** analgesia for relief of labor pain was first used during the 1940s (Ostheimer, Shea, & Van Zundert, 1996). Currently, epidural use of a dilute solution of a local anesthetic (often in combination with a small amount of opioid) is the standard against which all other modalities of pain relief in labor are measured (Vincent & Chestnut, 1996). The combination of a dilute solution of local anesthetic and an opioid appears to result in the best combination of quality analgesia and minimal side effects (Table 24-4) (Fiedler & Shaw, 1997).

An *absolute contraindication* refers to the idea that in the face of a particular condition there is no valid reason for proceeding to place an epidural. A *relative contraindi-*

Table 24-4 Advantages and Disadvantages of Epidural Analgesia

Advantages	Disadvantages
Indefinite duration	Confined to bed
Titratable	Frequent vital signs
Excellent analgesia	May interfere with pushing
	Possible postdural puncture headache

cation means that although there may be some valid reason for placing an epidural, it is not likely to offer significant benefit versus the risks involved the procedure. There are few absolute contraindications to the use of epidural analgesia and some relative contraindications (Box 24-2).

After identification of the epidural space the anesthesia provider may either give a test dose of a small amount of local anesthetic and epinephrine or pass an epidural catheter through the needle (Figure 24-8), withdraw the needle, and give the test dose through the catheter.

The combination of local anesthetic and epinephrine is designed to test for accidental placement of the needle or catheter into the subarachnoid space or into an epidural vein (Fiedler & Shaw, 1997). If the needle or catheter is in the subarachnoid space, the small amount of local anesthetic will produce a degree of spinal block. If the client indicates that her legs are heavy or feet are numb, the needle or catheter is in the subarachnoid space and will need to be withdrawn. If the needle or catheter is in an epidural vein, the small amount of epinephrine in the test dose will cause a rapid but transient increase in maternal heart rate. Continuous pulse oximetry or other assessment of mater-

Box 24-2 Contraindications to Regional Analgesia and Anesthesia

- Absolute
  - Patient refusal
  - Severe hemorrhage
  - Significant coagulopathy
  - Infection at the site
- Relative
  - Sepsis
  - Neurologic disorder
  - Heparinization
  - Spinal deformity
  - Extensive spinal surgery or hardware
  - Metastatic disease in the lumbar spine

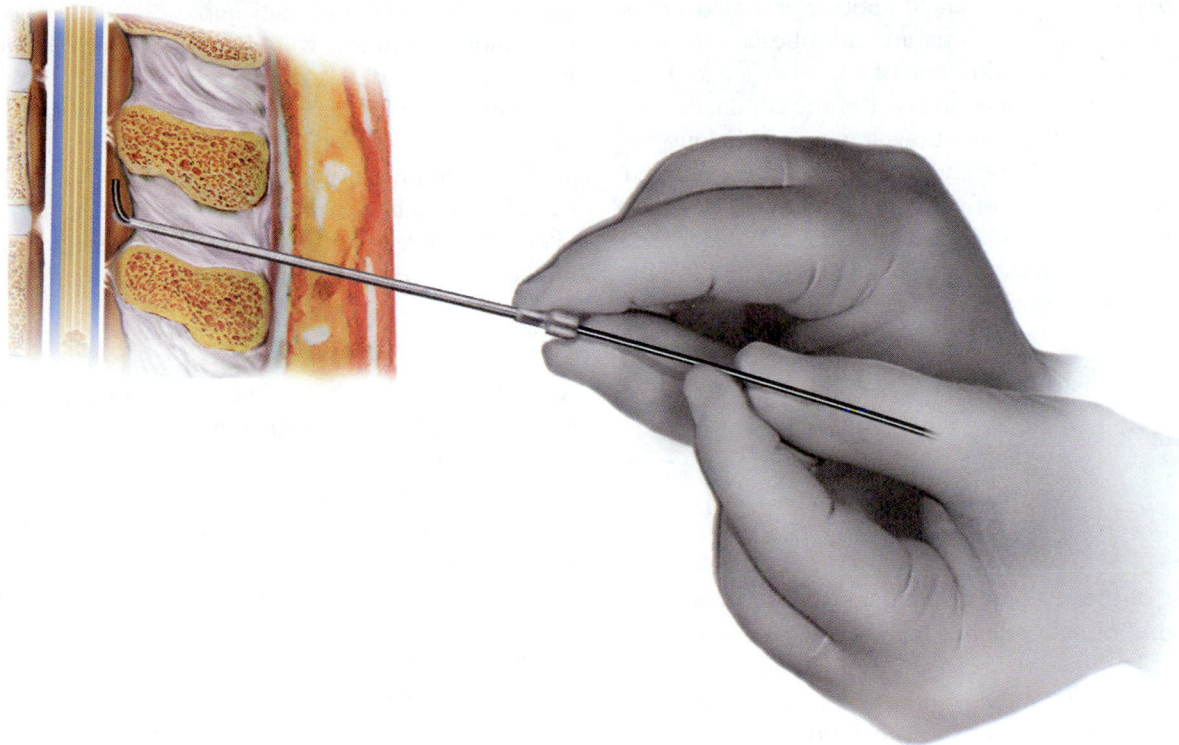

Figure 24-8 Epidural catheter passed through the needle.

nal pulse should be used to detect changes. When the results of the test dose are negative, either a bolus of medication is given through the needle or, if preferred, the catheter is passed through the epidural needle, the needle withdrawn, and the bolus administered through the catheter. The catheter is carefully passed through the epidural needle and the needle withdrawn. The anesthesia provider is careful not to move the needle forward once the catheter has been passed because doing so could result in breakage or shearing off of the catheter tip and thus

an inability to remove the catheter after use. The catheter is securely taped to the client's back, and she is assisted to a lateral position. Maternal blood pressure and fetal heart tones are assessed frequently in the initial 20- to 30-minute period after the procedure.

Local anesthetic creates a degree of autonomic blockade, which relaxes the blood vessels in the lower body and results in decreased maternal blood pressure. An adequate preload or bolus of IV fluid (500 to 1,000 mL non-dextrose–containing solution) and the judicious use of small increments of ephedrine by anesthesia providers when necessary will counteract the effects of the autonomic blockade.

Whereas epidural analgesia offers excellent analgesia and versatility for providing differing levels of analgesia for different conditions, this technique may have side effects or complications. It should be noted that complications occur very rarely. If the epidural needle accidentally punctures the dura, the larger size will make a bigger hole, which may increase the incidence of postdural puncture headache (also known as a spinal headache). The large fluid bolus needed for epidural analgesia may decrease uterine contractions; however, this side effect often is transient and responsive to oxytocin administration (Hawkins, Chestnut, & Gibbs, 1996). Epidural analgesia may contribute to prolonging the second stage of labor when the block is dense enough to obliterate the bearing-down reflex or diminish maternal ability to push (Vincent & Chestnut, 1996).

Nursing Alert

POSSIBLE SIDE EFFECTS AND COMPLICATIONS OF EPIDURAL ANALGESIA

- Hypotension
- Urinary retention
- Total spinal anesthesia
- Neurologic injury
- Unsatisfactory block
- Unintentional subarachnoid (spinal) block

It is possible to use a single shot or repeated bolus technique for epidural analgesia and anesthesia; however, uncertainty regarding the duration of labor has led to these techniques being abandoned in favor of the continuous infusion technique. In the continuous infusion technique, an infusion of dilute local anesthetic and opioid is prepared and administered by way of a syringe pump or other infusion-controlling device. As the client nears full dilation or begins to push, her motor function is assessed and the infusion rate adjusted downward, if needed (Fiedler & Shaw, 1997). Infusions may be adjusted but rarely are discontinued because doing so is likely to result in return of pain, which is unnecessary, unjustified, and counterproductive (Youngstrom, Baker, & Miller, 1996).

Combined Intrathecal-Epidural Technique

The newest of the regional techniques seeks to combine the rapid onset of pain relief of the intrathecal opioid with the ability to provide analgesia over an indeterminate period, as with a continuous epidural infusion (Cheek & Gutsche, 1997). In the combined technique the epidural space is identified and the dura punctured using a spinal needle through the epidural needle (Figure 24-9). Combination needles are available commercially. These consist of an epidural needle with an additional port and centering sleeve on the spinal needle. A small amount of fentanyl (usually 25 μg) or sufentanil (10 μg) is injected and the spinal needle withdrawn (Vincent & Chestnut, 1996).

An epidural catheter is threaded through the epidural needle and the needle is withdrawn. The catheter is securely taped to the client's back. At this point the client is monitored as described previously. After 30 minutes of monitoring and assessing for postural hypotension the client may ambulate with a support person, if desired (Cheek & Gutsche, 1997). The duration of analgesia varies from 1 to 2 hours. When the client is again uncomfortable (if ambulating, she returns to bed) the catheter is tested (as previously described) and a bolus of local anesthetic and opioid is administered and a continuous epidural infusion begun. When ambulation is not desired (or permitted) and delivery does not appear imminent, a continuous epidural infusion may be begun immediately. Thus, a seamless course of analgesia is created. By the time the analgesia

provided by the intrathecal opioid decreases, the continuous epidural infusion will have built up sufficient volume in the epidural space to provide analgesia.

The combined technique also has disadvantages. In theory, administration of a solution into the epidural space, in the presence of a dural hole, could result in accidental subarachnoid administration. Cheek and Gutsche (1997), however, argue a pressure gradient exists that is unlikely to be overcome by slow epidural injection.

Paracervical Block

A paracervical block involves submucosal injections of local anesthetic in the vaginal wall, lateral to both sides of the cervix (Figure 24-10). A blockade of the visceral sensory nerves of the uterus, cervix, and upper vagina is produced. Because a paracervical block does not block sensory nerves from the perineum, it is not effective in the second stage of labor (Schnider & Levinson, 1994). This technique is rarely used because of the high incidence of severe fetal bradycardia, fetal asphyxia, and poor neonatal outcome (Santos, Pederson, & Finster, 1997; Schnider & Levinson, 1994). It is suggested that the fetal bradycardia is a result of the proximity of the uterine artery to the area of local anesthetic administration, which causes constriction that results in decreased placental blood flow. It also has

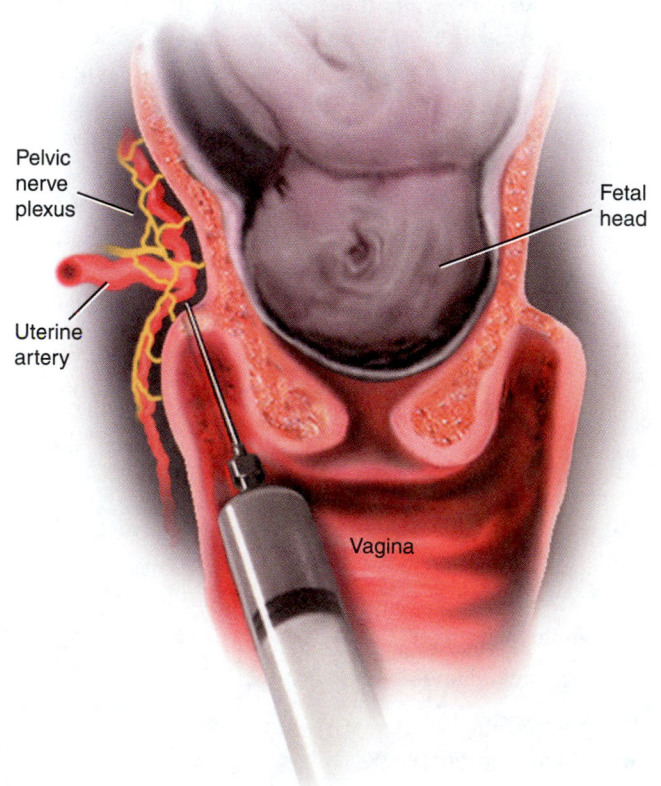

Figure 24-10 Paracervical block.

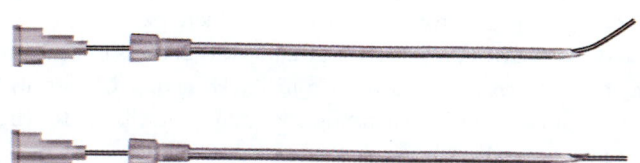

Figure 24-9 Spinal-epidural needle combinations.

been suggested that high fetal blood levels of local anesthetic, as a result of absorption into the uterine artery or fetal scalp, are the cause of the fetal bradycardia (Schnider & Levinson, 1994).

Possible Complications with Regional Anesthesia

Numerous long-term complications from regional anesthesia are possible but very rare. Knowing about such problems, however, should result in rapid recognition by the nurse. Trauma to a nerve root or spinal cord is possible. Administration of lumbar puncture below the level of L-1, L-2 decreases the risk of spinal cord trauma because the spinal cord usually ends above this level. Trauma to the nerve root is possible but extremely rare (Concepcion, 1996). An intraneural injection of local anesthetic causes immediate pain and is a signal to the anesthesia provider to stop injecting. Paresthesias or hyperalgesia in the area innervated by that nerve root indicates damage to the nerve root. Fortunately, this type of injury generally resolves within weeks to several months (Concepcion, 1996).

Drasner and Swisher (1996) indicate that risk factors for postdural puncture headache include age, body habitus, specifics of the needle, and multiple insertion attempts (Box 24-3). Postdural puncture headache occurs when the dura mater of the spinal cord is punctured. The puncture can be deliberate, such as in administration of intrathecal opioids or spinal anesthesia, or accidental, such as in the case of epidural anesthesia.

Headaches after childbirth are not uncommon; they may be due to a number of causes other than regional anesthesia. The distinguishing characteristic of a postdural puncture headache is the association between client position and headache severity. A true postdural puncture headache causes severe pain when the client is in a upright position, sitting, or standing, and is minimal or disappears completely when the client assumes a horizontal position (Chadwick & Ross, 1992). The onset usually is

within the first 5 days after the procedure. The headache may last for days and usually is not responsive to minor analgesics. The cause of the headache is tension on the meninges of the brain as a result of the loss of cerebrospinal fluid through the puncture site. The lower level of cerebrospinal fluid allows the brain to shift more than usual when the client assumes the upright position, causing more severe pain when the client is sitting or standing. Treatment of postdural puncture headache includes hydration to assist the body in replacing the cerebrospinal fluid; analgesics, which may provide some relief; and oral or IV caffeine for cerebral vasoconstriction. When these treatments are unsuccessful, the next step is an "epidural blood patch." This technique is successful in over 95% of clients. It is an invasive technique, however, and carries the risks of additional puncture of the dura, which will results in worsening of headache, and arachnoiditis (if the blood is injected into the subarachnoid space). The technique involves placement of an epidural needle, preferably in the same vertebral interspace as the original puncture, and venipuncture and withdrawal of 20 mL of the client's blood by an assistant, often the nurse. The anesthesia provider then slowly injects the blood through the epidural needle into the epidural space. The client is instructed to lie quietly for the next 30 minutes and curtail activities over the next several hours. The epidural blood patch appears to work by two different mechanisms: the blood clots and plugs the hole in the dura; and the volume of blood in the epidural space increases the pressure within the spinal canal, which increases the cerebrospinal fluid level surrounding the brain (Fiedler & Shaw, 1997).

Hematoma in the spinal canal is a rare complication but one that can result in spinal cord compression or ischemia (Drasner & Swisher, 1996). The damage may range from sensory or motor weakness to quadriplegia and death. Presenting symptoms may include lower body muscle weakness, back pain, and sensory deficit. Delays in recognition, diagnosis, and treatment have been correlated with more severe damage (Drasner & Swisher, 1996). Concern about this complication is one of the reasons that spinal and epidural anesthesia methods are contraindicated in the presence of severe coagulopathies.

Epidural analgesia may contribute to some neurologic injuries. Because of the relaxation and decreased pain sensation provided by the epidural, it is possible to excessively flex the client's legs while positioning during pushing. Overstretching of the nerves passing through the pelvis may result. Clients may report parathesias or numbness in one foot or leg that can be severe or last long enough to require the use of a cane or walker for weeks to months. Any report of numbness, parathesisa, or weakness that lasts longer that the expected duration of the regional or epidural analgesia should be referred to the anesthesia provider for further evaluation.

Box 24-3 Factors Associated with Increased Risk of Postdural Puncture Headache

- Age: younger women are at greater risk than are older women
- Body habitus: obesity carries a greater risk
- Previous postdural puncture headache
- Multiple attempts: increased number of punctures
- Needle size: large needle, more leakage
- Needle design: beveled needles, more than conical needles

The diminishment of uterine contractions after IV fluid boluses has been noted previously. Studies have indicated some diminishment in uterine activity in women receiving epidural analgesia with epinephrine-containing solutions (Chantigian & Chantigian, 1996).

An increased duration of the second stage of labor is common enough that the American College of Obstetricians and Gynecologists revised the guidelines for defining prolonged second stage of labor. In the presence of epidural analgesia, prolonged second stage of labor is defined as more than 3 hours in nulliparous women and more than 2 hours in parous women. These guidelines encourage careful assessment of the clients' motor and sensory functions as she is preparing to start pushing. It has been recommended that pushing should be delayed if the client lacks motor or sensory function (Hawkins et al., 1995).

Hawkins et al. (1995) reviewed the records of over 14,000 deliveries before and after implementation of epidural service. These authors found an increased incidence of the use of forceps for delivery in multiparous women with epidural analgesia. The nurse is reminded that association does not imply causation.

The impact of epidural analgesia on the progress of labor and modes of delivery is a topic that has been studied by numerous researchers in the past and continues to be studied today. There are multiple studies with results that support both sides of the controversy. There is no definitive answer to the questions raised; however, research continues toward improving our understanding and refin-

REFLECTIONS
FROM A LABORING MOTHER

"When I got to the hospital I was 4 cm dilated. Although I had managed pretty well so far, I knew what was coming. With my first baby, once I got to be 6 cm the contractions started to hurt a lot worse and that's when I got the epidural. Talk about the difference between day and night! I felt the contractions as pressure, but they were not as painful as they had been before the epidural. With my second baby, I asked for the epidural as soon as I just got into the labor-delivery room. I didn't want to miss getting one because my labor was moving too fast."

ing techniques. The nurse should be aware of the ongoing research to further her own knowledge and assist the client in fully understanding the risks and benefits involved in the vast array of options currently available for pain relief in labor and delivery.

Client Experience with Pain

The nurse should be sure to educate the client regarding the onset of pain relief with regional analgesia, the expected side effects, and safety concerns.

Nursing Implications

Nurses must assess the client's response to regional anesthesia; a baseline assessment of physical status is important for comparison after administration. Maternal responses can include hypotension, hypoventilation, nausea and vomiting, pruritus, and urinary retention. IV fluid boluses should be administered before an epidural with local anesthetic is performed. Evaluation of pain relief is needed to determine the level of analgesia appropriate for the stage of labor. Fetal well-being also must be assessed.

ANESTHESIA FOR DELIVERY

Anesthesia options for delivery include local anesthetic infiltration; regional techniques, such as a pudendal nerve block, a spinal, or an epidural; and general anesthesia. Without subjecting the client or fetus to unnecessary risks, the goal is to provide analgesia and anesthesia to meet the client's wishes and the requirements of the mode of delivery (Hawkins, Chestnut, & Gibbs, 1996). Modes of delivery include spontaneous vaginal, forceps (outlet, low, or mid), vacuum extraction, and cesarean section. Table 24-5 lists the specific modes of delivery and appropriate anesthesia techniques. The accompanying photo story highlights the technique of spinal anesthesia administration.

Local Infiltration

Infiltration of the perineal tissues with 10 to 20 mL of a local anesthetic (usually lidocaine) provides anesthesia during vaginal delivery to facilitate cutting or repair of the perineum and vagina. Episiotomy usually is performed by the obstetrician just before delivery of the fetal head (Schnider & Levinson, 1994). From a safety standpoint, local perineal infiltration has the least likelihood of complications (Hawkins, Chestnut, & Gibbs, 1996).

Regional Anesthesia

Regional anesthesia may be used for delivery as a continuation of the analgesia provided during labor or administered just before delivery, if required, for a specific mode of delivery.

Table 24-5 Modes of Delivery and Appropriate Anesthesia Techniques

Modes	Local Infiltration	Pudendal	Spinal	Epidural
Spontanous vaginal	X	X		X
Vacuum extraction	A	X		X
Outlet forceps		X	X	X
Low forceps		A	X	X
Cesearean section	B		X	X

A = Some clients may tolerate
B = Known technique but not used frequently

Pudendal Block

A **pudendal block** is a minor regional block that is reasonably effective and also very safe owing to its lack of fetal effects (Hawkins, Chestnut, & Gibbs, 1996). This block is administered by the obstetrician through the vagina by placing a local anesthetic in the area of the pudendal nerve, behind the sacrospinous ligament and near the right and left ischial spines (Cunningham et al., 1997; Hawkins, Chestnut, & Gibbs, 1996; Schnider & Levinson, 1994). (Figure 24-11). A pudendal nerve block can be used for spontaneous vaginal, outlet, and sometimes low forceps delivery. It also has been used effectively in some cases of vacuum extraction.

Spinal Anesthesia

Spinal anesthesia is rarely used for spontaneous vaginal delivery. It is likely to be used in low or midforceps delivery and vacuum extraction. It is often used for cesarean delivery. A list of the advantages and disadvantages of spinal anesthesia is provided in Table 24-6. Differences in the levels of spinal anesthesia for vaginal and cesarean delivery are created by the dosage of medication administered and the position of the client after placement of the local anesthetic in the dural sac (Figure 24-12).

For a vaginal delivery, the client will remain in a sitting position for a brief period (1 to 2 minutes) after the spinal anesthesia has been administered so that the hyperbaric local anesthetic solution will migrate downward toward the sacral area. *Hyperbaric* refers to the local anesthetic solution as being heavier that the cerebrospinal fluid it is placed in, and therefore, gravity pulls it downward. This block also has been referred as a "saddle block," although the term is technically incorrect because the anesthetized area is larger than that which would be in contact with a saddle (Cunningham et al., 1997).

Cesarean section requires sensory blockade to at least the level of the xiphoid process, the T-8 dermatome (Cunningham et al., 1997). To obtain these levels a greater dosage of medication is required. The client is assisted immediately to a supine position, with left lateral tilt, after administration of the spinal anesthesia. The tilt causes a more cephalad spread of anesthesia, resulting in a higher level of sensory blockade. Hazards include maternal hypotension and the possibility of complete spinal anesthesia (Hawkins, Chestnut, & Gibbs, 1996). Preloading with 1,500 to 2,000 mL of fluid may help decrease maternal hypotension (Ostheimer & Leavitt, 1996). Incremental doses of ephedrine may be administered if maternal hypotension occurs (Schnider & Levinson, 1994; Stoelting & Miller, 1994).

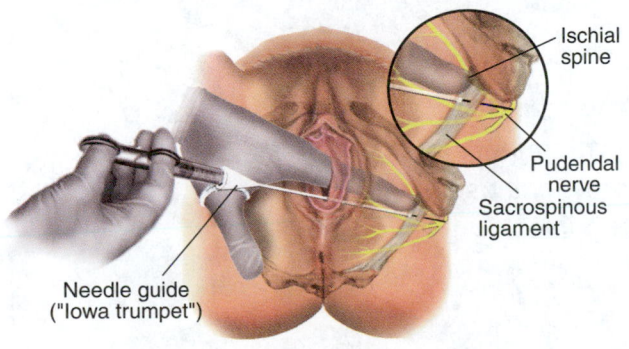

Figure 24-11 Pudendal block.

Ischial spine
Pudendal nerve
Sacrospinous ligament
Needle guide ("Iowa trumpet")

Table 24-6 Advantages and Disadvantages of Spinal Anesthesia

Advantages	Disadvantages
Rapid onset	Finite duration
Dense block	Possible severe hypotension
Less shivering	Possible total spinal
Less systemic medication	
Little placental transfer	
Awake client	

Administration of Spinal Anesthesia

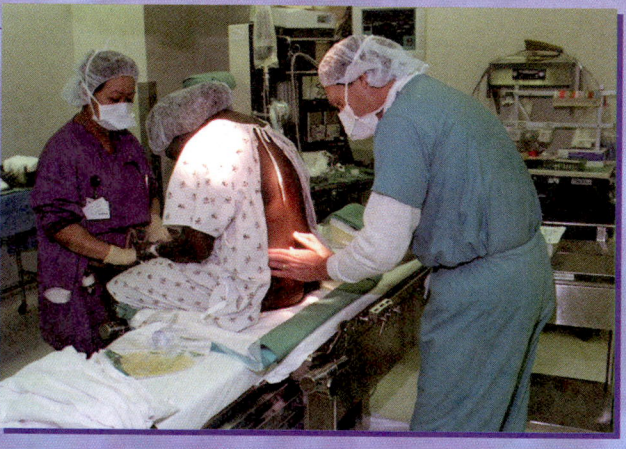

This 29-year-old female is a gravida 4, para 3 who is being prepared for a repeat C-section. She will sit on the operating table with the nurse's assistance and support while the anesthesiologist assesses physical landmarks.

Upon identification of landmarks, preparations are made to cleanse the injection site.

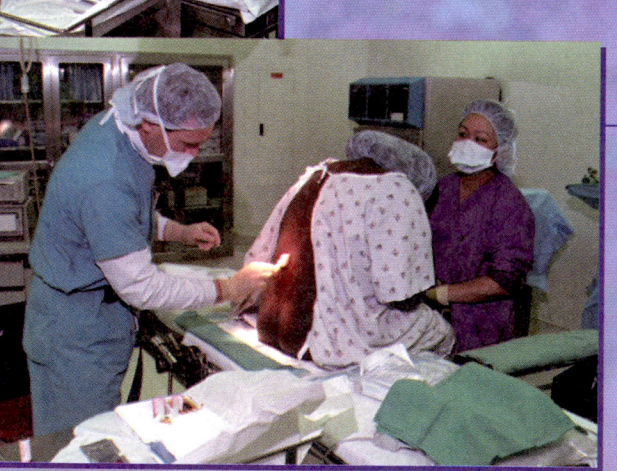

The nurse has the responsibility to promote client comfort and limit motion during the procedure.

Once the area surrounding the injection site is cleansed, a sterile sponge is used to remove Betadine from the injection site.

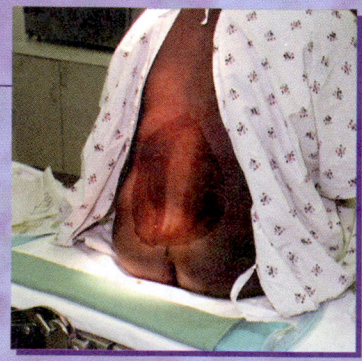

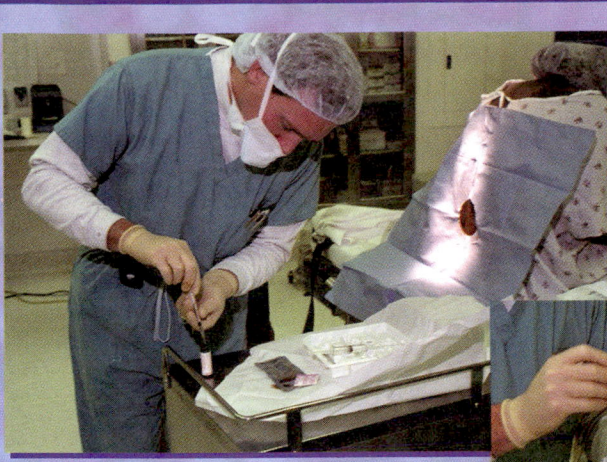

The anesthetic agent is prepared for injection using sterile technique.

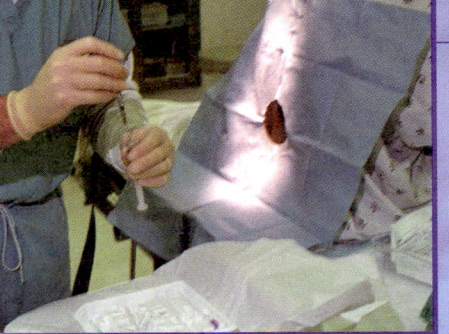

Epinephrine is added to the anesthetic agent to produce local vasoconstriction and to prolong the action of the substance.

A local anesthetic is administered prior to the spinal to increase client comfort.

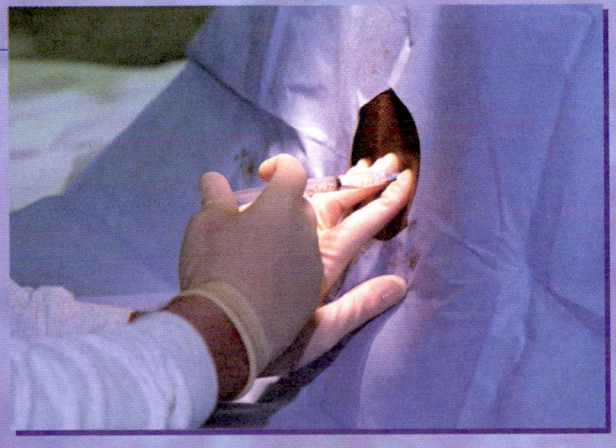

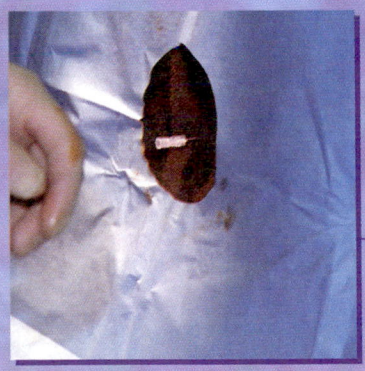

When the local anesthesia is completed, an 18-gauge introducer is inserted and the hub of the needle is left in place.

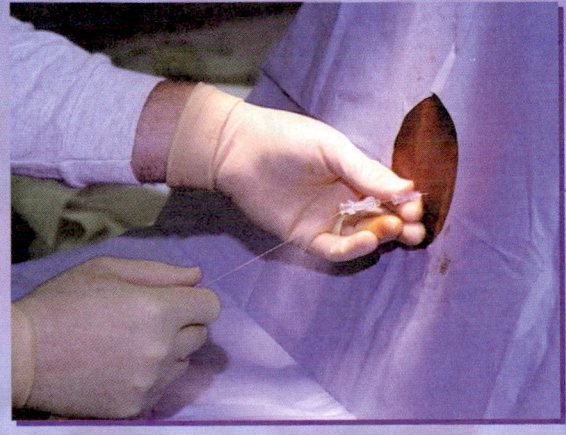

The stylus guide wire is removed from the hub of the needle and inspected for drops of spinal fluid.

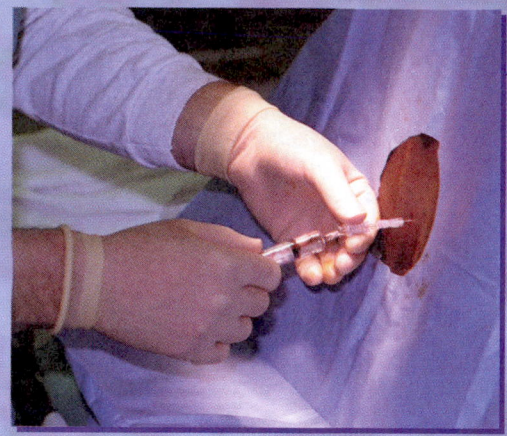

The syringe containing the anesthetic is connected to the hub of the needle.

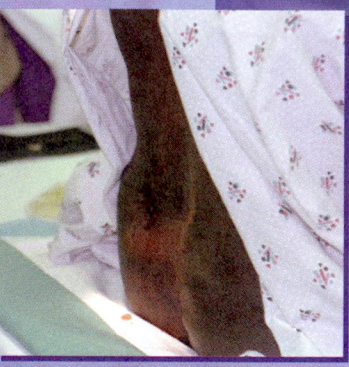

The anesthetic agent is administered.

The anesthetic equipment is removed. The nurse assists the client in remaining seated until anesthesia personnel indicate the time is appropriate for the client to lie down. It is important to avoid vena cava syndrome by inserting a wedge or pillow under the right side of her back.

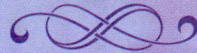

Anesthesia personnel will document the procedure and continue monitoring the client's condition.

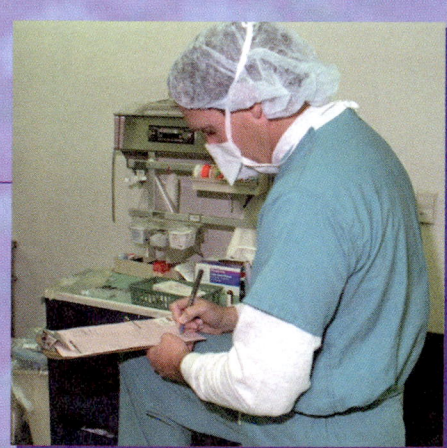

The nurse's responsibility in assisting with an epidural is the same as assisting with a spinal. The difference is the epidural needle is inserted lower (L4–L5), a larger needle is used, and a catheter remains in place for continuous dosing or reinjection.

Epidural Anesthesia

The epidural anesthesia technique provides the versatility required for all modes of delivery. This versatility is a result of differences in types, volumes, and concentrations of local anesthetics administered through a functioning epidural catheter (Figure 24-13). For a spontaneous vaginal delivery, additional local anesthesia can be administered just before delivery of the fetal head. Local anesthesia also may provide additional analgesia and anesthesia for episiotomy repair.

A slightly larger dose of local anesthetic can be administered for forceps or vacuum extraction delivery. The anesthetic should be administered 5 to 10 minutes before attempting forceps or vacuum extraction. It should be noted that the voluntary expulsive effort may be diminished with increased doses and longer elapsed time between administration and delivery. Two distinct advantages of epidural anesthesia are the ease and rapidity by which the anesthesia level can be increased to levels sufficient for cesarean delivery when forceps or vacuum extraction

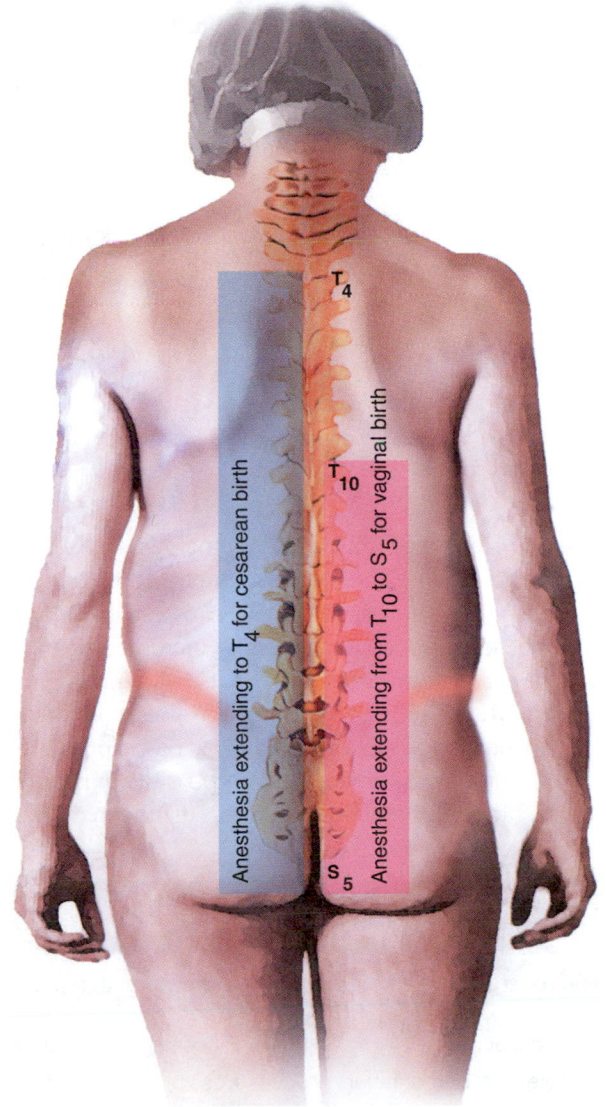

$\blacksquare$ Anesthesia extending from T_{10} to S_5 dermatomes for vaginal birth

$\blacksquare$ Anesthesia extending from T_4 to S_5 dermatomes for cesarean birth

A.

B.

Figure 24-12 Anesthesia levels for vaginal and cesarean births.

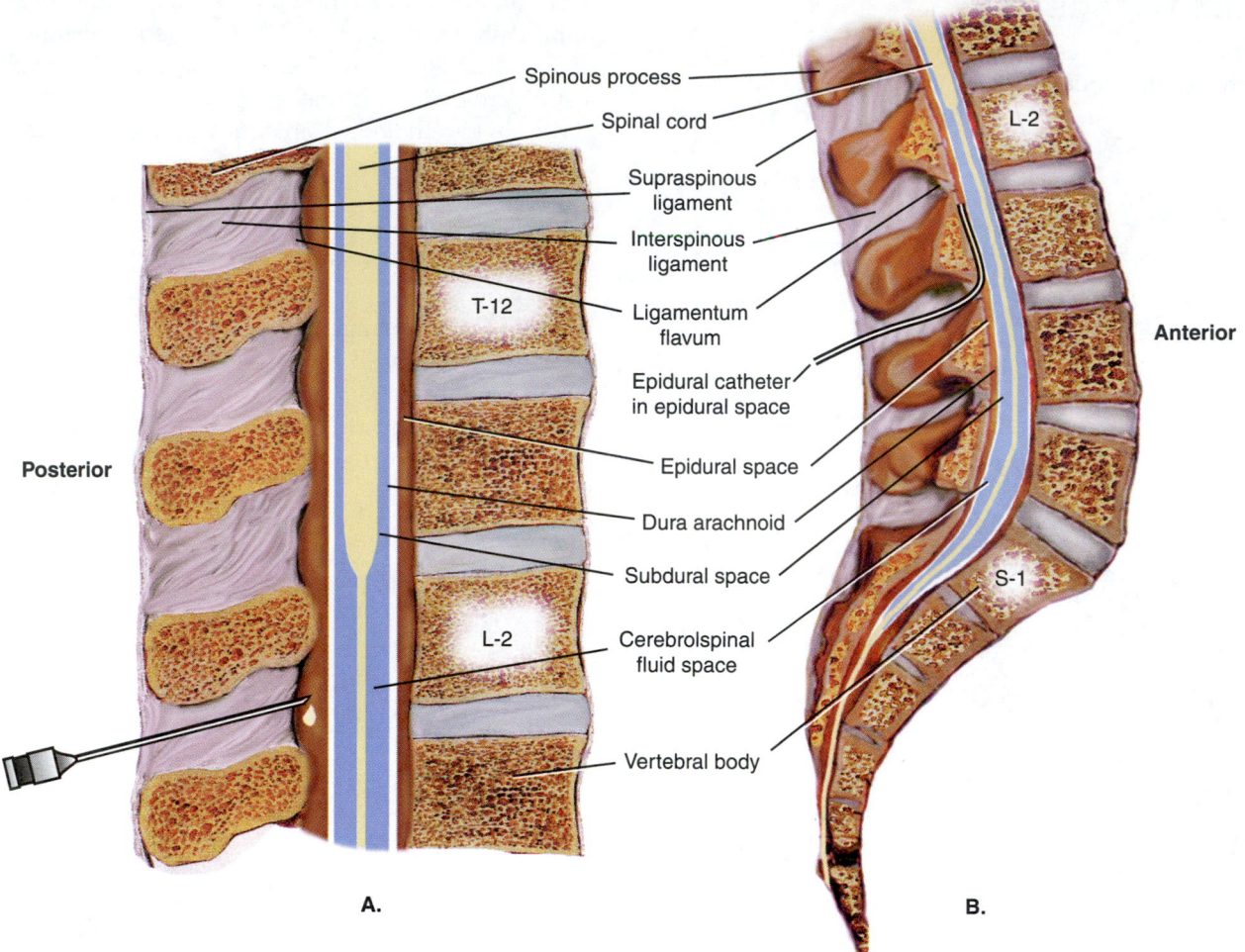

Spinous process
Spinal cord
Supraspinous ligament
Interspinous ligament
Ligamentum flavum
Epidural catheter in epidural space
Epidural space
Dura arachnoid
Subdural space
Cerebrolspinal fluid space
Vertebral body

T-12
L-2
Posterior
A.

L-2
Anterior
S-1
B.

Figure 24-13 Side view of the anatomy of the spine. A. Epidural needle placed in the epidural space. B. Epidural catheter placed in the epidural space.

attempts are unsuccessful. The advantages and disadvantages of epidural anesthesia are summarized in Table 24-7.

The fact that epidural anesthesia can be used to increase the level of sensory blockade in slow increments can be an advantage in certain cases. In clients with pregnancy-induced hypertension (PIH), epidural anesthesia offers a number of advantages: reduction of maternal blood pressure secondary to autonomic blockade, with possible improvement in uterine blood flow. Reduction in circulating maternal cat-

echolamines through relief of pain may also improve uterine blood flow. When cesarean section is needed, gradual increases in sensory blockade levels help avoid maternal hypotension and resultant decreases in placental perfusion. Use of epidural anesthesia avoids airway stimulation, owing to tracheal intubation for general anesthesia, which could precipitate hypertension and thus possibly contribute to maternal cerebral bleeding (Fiedler & Shaw, 1997).

Except in the case of severe fetal distress, an epidural usually can be used to provide sufficient surgical levels of anesthesia in a short enough period of time for urgent cesarean section. General anesthesia is the technique of choice for true emergency cesarean sections such as in cases of severe fetal distress and substantial maternal hemorrhage (Santos, Pederson, & Finster, 1997).

General Anesthesia

General anesthesia for delivery involves rendering the client unconscious and intubation of the trachea with a cuffed endotracheal tube. Afterward, ventilation, oxygena-

Table 24-7 Advantages and Disadvantages of Epidural Anesthesia	
Advantages	**Disadvantages**
Slower onset	Placement takes longer
Titratable level and duration	Possible systemic toxicity
Less hypotension	Larger placental transfer
Awake client	Higher incidence of inadequate block

Table 24-8 Advantages and Disadvantages of General Anesthesia

Advantages	Disadvantages
Total pain relief	Awareness is impossible
Optimal operating conditions	Slight risk of fetal depression

Table 24-10 Pregnancy-Induced Changes in Maternal Airway and Pulmonary System and Resultant Complications

Change	Complication
Engorgement of mucosa	Increased bleeding
Decreased upper airway size	Requires smaller endotracheal tube
Cephalad displacement of thorax	Increased difficulty of intubation
Breast enlargement	Mechanical obstruction to insertion of laryngoscope; may need short-handled scope

tion, unconsciousness, analgesia, and muscle relaxation are maintained. Emergence, or waking up the client, and extubation follow. The advantages and disadvantages of general anesthesia are given in Table 24-8). The possible maternal and fetal complications of general anesthesia are listed in Table 24-9.

All anesthetic agents, whether given by IV or inhalation, cross the placenta and affect the infant. Muscle relaxants are the exception owing to their large molecular size. Resuscitation of an infant with respiratory depression should be anticipated, with adequate equipment and personnel present at delivery.

The two major causes of maternal morbidity and mortality from general anesthesia are failure to intubate and pulmonary aspiration (Hawkins, Chestnut, & Gibbs, 1996). Pregnancy-induced changes contribute to airway management problems and are listed in Table 24-10.

Management of the airway, including tracheal intubation, is in the hands of the anesthesia provider; however, the nurse should be aware of the possible difficulties in airway management. To be able to render assistance, the nurse also must know the necessary steps to be taken by the CRNA or anesthesiologist in the case of difficult intubation. Figure 24-14 provides an algorithm for failed intubation. The nurse may be required to assist the anesthesia provider by calling for additional help, especially other anesthesia providers, if readily available because extra experienced hands can be invaluable (Johnson, Lawlor, & Weiner, 1994). The nurse also may be needed to hold cricoid pressure or hand an endotracheal tube to a solitary anesthesia provider. To maintain cricoid pressure, use the thumb and forefinger to firmly compress the cricoid ring

downward (Figure 24-15) (Chipas, 1997). The cricoid ring is the first and only tracheal cartilage ring that is a complete circle. Compression of this ring closes off the esophagus, helping to prevent passive regurgitation (Schnider & Levinson, 1994). The most important part the nurse must remember is that *cricoid pressure is not released* until after the cuff of the endotracheal tube is inflated, with proper placement confirmed or the anesthesia provider indicating it can be released (Chipas, 1997).

Table 24-9 Possible Maternal and Fetal Complications of General Anesthesia

Maternal	Fetal
Hypertension at intubation	Drug-induced depression
Difficult or failed intubation	
Aspiration of gastric contents	
Awareness	
Uterine atony	

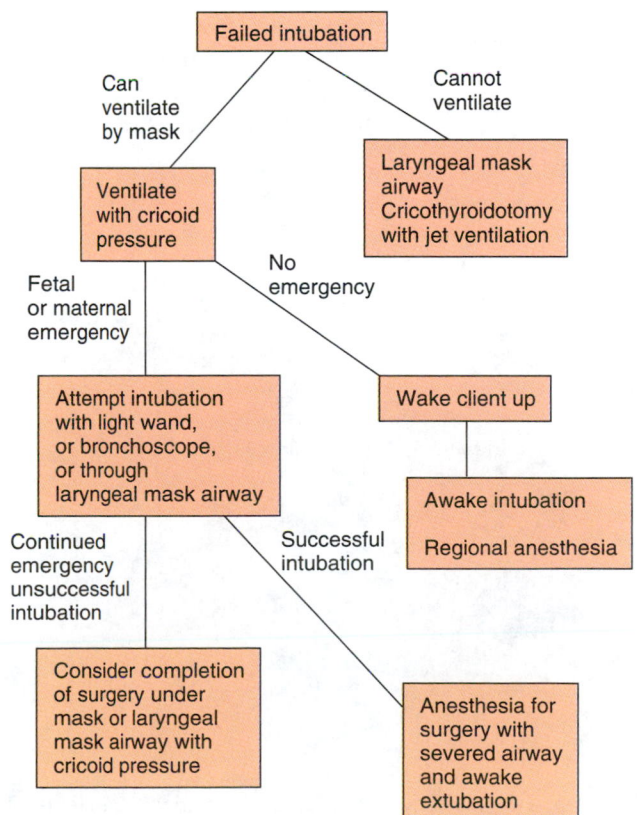

Figure 24-14 Failed intubation algorithm.

Pulmonary aspiration of gastric contents can result in obstruction of lower airways, pneumonitis, pulmonary edema, and death (Cunningham et al., 1997). Two factors impact the severity of aspiration pneumonitis: volume greater than 25 mL and pH less than 2.5 (Fiedler & Shaw, 1997). There are methods to decrease the risk of maternal aspiration or severity of a possible aspiration. The oral administration of a nonparticulate antacid (such a sodium citrate) just before induction of general anesthesia increases the gastric pH level and should be given routinely. Particulate antacids (such as Maalox) are not recommended because the particulate matter in the antacid can produce severe pulmonary reaction if aspirated (Fiedler & Shaw, 1997). Additional medications such as histamine blockers (cimetidine or ranitidine) also may be administered to decrease the gastric pH level and volume.

All pregnant clients are considered to have "full stomachs" even if they have been in labor or have not eaten for hours. The physiologic changes in the gastrointestinal system due to pregnancy that increase the likelihood of regurgitation and aspiration are shown in Table 24-11 (Bassell, 1996). The best defenses against pulmonary aspiration are use of medications, rapid sequence induction with cricoid pressure, immediate intubation and inflation of the cuff of the endotracheal tube, and extubation only after the client is awake and has regained the protective airway reflexes.

Special Considerations for Cesarean Section

After securing of the airway, the obstetrician is directed to proceed with the cesarean section. Unconsciousness of the client is maintained through the use of a volatile anesthetic agent and oxygen. After delivery of the infant, nitrous oxide is often added to enhance the anesthesia. Additional doses of muscle relaxant are given as needed to maintain surgical conditions. After the procedure the client is awakened. Once she is responsive, is spontaneously breathing with sufficient rate and tidal volume, and has the protective airway reflexes including swal-

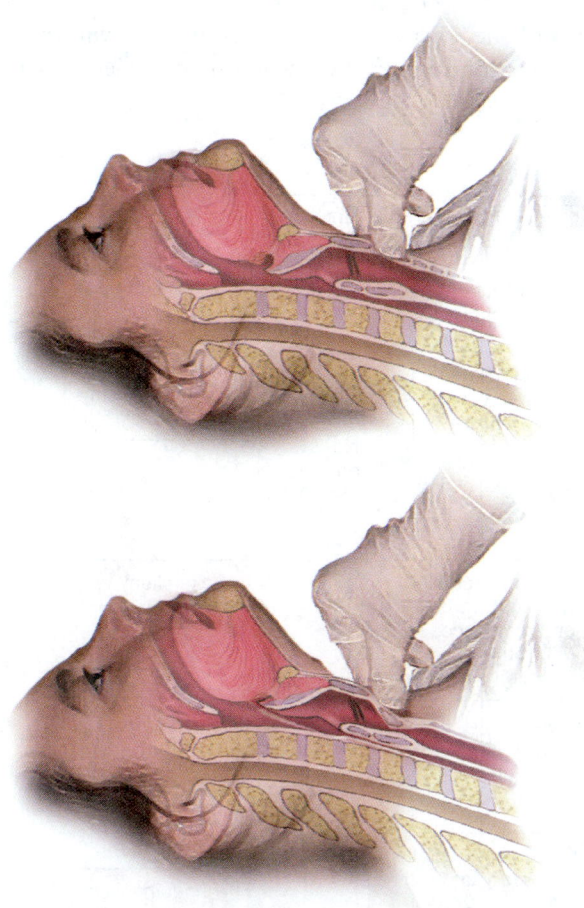

Figure 24-15 Downward force of the cricoid cartilage will compress the esophagus.

Table 24-11 Pregnancy-Induced Changes in Maternal Gastrointestinal System		
Change	**Increased**	**Decreased**
Bowel motility		X
Stomach emptying		X
Barrier pressure (at gastroesophageal junction)		X
Intraabdominal pressure	X	
Gastric acid production	X	
Pepsin production	X	

lowing, the oral cavity is suctioned, the cuff deflated, and the client extubated. At this time she is taken to the recovery room.

The two other complications listed in Table 24-9 are awareness during general anesthesia and uterine atony. It is possible for the client to have some degree of awareness under general anesthesia; this may be attributed to the attempt to minimize drug-induced depression of the neonate (Chadwick & Ross, 1992). Addition of nitrous oxide to the oxygen-volatile agent mixture can help decrease awareness but is not advocated by some practitioners until after the delivery of the fetus. Many anesthesia providers think that delivery 100% oxygen until delivery of the infant is preferred because doing so should result in the highest level of oxygen available to the fetus. After delivery of the infant, additional doses of opioids and amnesics such as midazolam (Versed) as well as increased levels of volatile agents and use of nitrous oxide can help prevent maternal awareness. If the client describes incidences of awareness the nurse should take this seriously and notify the anesthesia providers so that the client can receive further assessment and explanation of the incident.

Uterine atony is possible in all deliveries regardless of the presence of anesthesia. The volatile agents used to maintain general anesthesia can produce a degree of dose-related decrease in uterine contractility and tone (Chadwick & Ross, 1992). At the level of volatile anesthetic agents and other drugs normally used, the uterus is responsive to the administration of oxytocin to induce contractions (Schnider & Levinson, 1994).

POSTDELIVERY CARE FOR THE CLIENT RECEIVING ANESTHESIA

The care needed in the recovery period by the client who has received anesthesia varies greatly according to the type of anesthesia. The care related to the birth process itself is covered in Chapter 25. Care of the client related to analgesia and anesthesia in labor and delivery is discussed subsequently.

Local Anesthesia

The client with local infiltration anesthesia of the perineum requires little additional recovery care owing solely to the anesthetic. The nurse must be aware that the client may be unable to feel hot or cold in the area that has been anesthetized. She must ensure that ice or other sources of cold are not placed directly on the skin of the perineum because it is possible to cause cold thermal injury owing to impaired cold and pain perception in this area.

Regional Anesthesia

In the recovery of a client with regional anesthesia, the type and extent of the regional anesthesia will determine necessary care. The client with a pudendal nerve block requires the same care as does a client with local infiltration. One additional caution applies: the perineal area should be carefully assessed for swelling, which may indicate the development of vaginal wall or perineal hematoma. The impaired sensory perception may mask pain and delay the recognition of a developing hematoma.

The recovery of a client with spinal or epidural anesthesia requires careful attention to vital signs and the declining spinal level (sensory block). Monitoring of vital signs includes blood pressure, electrocardiogram, and pulse oximetry. Oxygen by nasal cannula may be needed if the client has received sedation or other depressive medications. A low spinal or saddle block has a lower sensory level and causes less maternal hypotension then does a spinal block for cesarean section. Positional changes from supine to semi-Fowler's to Fowler's position should be done incrementally, with assessment of the client for tolerance and hypotension. It is not necessary for the client to remain supine after regional anesthesia. The nurse should be aware that the sensory blockade recedes from the chest toward the feet. Analgesia for incision or episiotomy pain should be considered and administered before the block is completely gone. The client's ability to urinate may be impaired. The bladder should be assessed and catheterized if the client is unable to void.

The client with epidural anesthesia may need the care indicated above if epidural anesthesia has been used to provide sensory blockade for vaginal forceps or cesarean delivery. The type of local anesthetic used through the epidural greatly impacts the client's status in recovery. Bupivacaine is frequently used for its properties of sensory blockade with preservation of motor control. Clients who did not receive additional analgesia for delivery may not require specific care other than a warning that they will not have complete control of their legs for several hours and that full sensation does not mean full control. All clients should have assistance the first time they ambulate from the bed; however, the nurse should be even more cautious when helping to ambulate clients who have had regional anesthesia (consider additional help).

General Anesthesia

Recovery of the client from general anesthesia requires close observation and complete monitoring. Assessment of the client involves all major systems and preparations for immediate response to problems encountered. Respirations should be observed for rate and depth. Oxygen should be administered by nasal cannula or by mask (when higher concentrations are needed.) Pulse oximetry should be employed to determine changes in oxygen saturation. Continuous electrocardiogram and frequent intermittent blood pressure monitoring are done. Suction equipment should be functioning and ready in case of vomiting. The nurse should be aware that the client should not be left alone at any time and that the most dangerous time in the recovery period can be that few minutes after the initial flurry of activity involved in admission to the recovery area. After the initial stimulation of monitor placement and assessment is over, the patient may drift back to sleep and hypoventilate. Vigilance is the key word for safe recovery of the client from general anesthesia.

Web Activities

- Visit the sites listed above for both client and professional educational materials. Check out www.childbirth.org and the section Epidurals—Frequently Asked Questions. Type in the terms "childbirth" and "analgesia" in any web search engine, such as Lycos, HotBot, AltaVista, Excite, or Goto.com. You will get lists of thousands of websites. Check out a few just to see what is out there. Some information may be excellent and some may not be.

Key Concepts

- Theories of pain suggest that pain is a very individual experience influenced by cultural practices, previous experience with pain, and available support systems.
- Types of anesthesia include local (small area of the body), regional (large area of the body), and general (loss of consciousness).
- The primary consideration for use of pain medication during labor and delivery is always the health and well-being of the mother and baby.
- Sources of pain in labor and delivery include cervical dilation, uterine contractions, distension of the vagina and perineum, and pressure on the sacrum; perception of pain can be influenced by cultural expectations, exhaustion, loss of sleep, and duration of labor.
- Parenteral analgesia options during labor include opioids and sedatives. Options for regional analgesia in labor include intrathecal opioids, epidural, combined intrathecal-epidural, and paracervical analgesia.
- During delivery, pudendal, spinal, and epidural blocks are the pain relief options of choice.
- The nurse's role in caring for the client recovering from anesthesia emphasizes close observation, complete and frequent monitoring, and assessment; the nurse may also provide assistance to the client when ambulating.

Review Questions and Activities

1. Which of the following is not a process involved in nociception?
   a. Transduction
   b. Transmission
   c. Transudation
   d. Modulation

   The correct answer is c.

2. Which of the following types of anesthesia involves the loss of sensation from a large area of the body?
   a. General
   b. Regional
   c. Inhalation
   d. Local infiltration

   The correct answer is b.

3. Which of the following types of anesthesia does only a CRNA or anesthesiologist provide?
   a. General
   b. Regional
   c. Inhalation
   d. Local infiltration

   The correct answer is a.

4. In which stage of labor is the conduction of pain impulses through T-10 to L-1?
   a. Third stage
   b. Second stage
   c. First stage
   d. Fourth stage

   The correct answer is c.

5. In which stage of labor is the conduction of pain impulses through S-2 to S-4?
a. Third stage
b. Second stage
c. First stage
d. Fourth stage

The correct answer is b.

6. Which opioid is most frequently used in labor and delivery?
a. Fentanyl
b. Morphine
c. Sufentanil
d Meperidine

The correct answer is d.

7. Which of the following methods of pain management is the gold standard?
a. Intrathecal opioids
b. Parenteral analgesia
c. Epidural
d. Combined spinal and epidural

The correct answer is c.

8. Which of the following is one of the major causes of maternal morbidity and mortality from anesthesia?
a. Emergency cesarean section
b. Epidural catheter breakage
c. Pulmonary aspiration
d. Postdural puncture headache (spinal headache)

The correct answer is c.

9. Which of the following is the most dangerous period for a client after general anesthesia?
a. During transportation from the operating room to the recovery room.
b. After the initial flurry of activity on arrival to the recovery room.
c. Thirty minutes after arriving in the recovery room.
d. Just before transportation to the postpartum unit.

The correct answer is a.

References

Ball, C. (1996). James Young Simpson, 1811–1870. *Anaesthesia & Intensive Care, 24,* 639.

Bankert, M. (1989). *Watchful care: A history of America's nurse anesthetists.* New York, NY: Continuum.

Bassell, G. M. (1996). General anesthesia. In A. Van Zundert & G. W. Ostheimer (Eds.), *Pain relief and anesthesia in obstetrics* (pp. 471–484). New York, NY: Churchill Livingstone.

Benards, C. M. (1997). Epidural and spinal anesthesia. In P. G. Barash, B. F. Cullen, & R. K. Stoelting (Eds.), *Clinical anesthesia* (3rd Ed.) (pp. 645–680). Philadelphia, PA: Lippincott-Raven.

Camann, W. R. (1996). Patient-controlled analgesia. In A. Van Zundert & G. W. Ostheimer (Eds.), *Pain relief and anesthesia in obstetrics* (pp. 373–374). New York, NY: Churchill Livingstone.

Chadwick, H. S. & Ross, B. K. (1992). Causes and consequences of maternal-fetal perianesthetic complications. In J. L. Benumof & L. J. Saidman, *Anesthesia and perioperative complications* (pp. 520–547). St. Louis, MO: Mosby Year Book.

Chantigian, R. C. & Chantigian, P. D. M. (1996). Effect of lumbar epidural anesthesia on the progress of labor and the incidence of operative deliveries. In A. Van Zundert & G. W. Ostheimer (Eds.), *Pain relief and anesthesia in obstetrics* (pp. 943–954). New York, NY: Churchill Livingstone.

Cheek, T. G., & Gutsche, B. B. (1997). Analgesia for labor. In D. M. Dewan & D. D. Hood, *Practical obstetric anesthesia* (pp. 95–124). Philadelphia, PA: W. B. Saunders.

Chipas, A. (1997). Airway management. In J. J. Nagelhout & K. L. Zaglaniczny (Eds.) *Nurse anesthesia* (pp. 708–725). Philadelphia, W. B. Saunders.

Cohen, J. (1996). Doctor James Young Simpson, Rabbi Abraham De Sola, and Genesis Chapter 3, verse 16. *Obstetrics & Gynecology, 88,* (5), 895–898.

Concepcion, M. (1996). Acute complications and side effects of regional anesthesia. In D. L. Brown (Ed.), *Regional anesthesia and analgesia* (pp. 446–461). Philadelphia: W. B. Saunders.

Connor, H. & Connor, T. (1996). Did the use of chloroform by Queen Victoria influence its acceptance in obstetric practice? *Anaesthesia 51,* 955–957.

Cunningham, F. G., Gant, N. F., McDonald, P. G., Gilstrap, L. C. III, Leveno, K., Hankins, G. D. V., and Clark, S. L. (1997). *Williams Obstetrics* (20th ed.) Norwalk, Conn.: Appleton and Lange.

Davies, R. (1997). Transcutaneous electrical nerve stimulation. In S. Moore (Ed) *Understanding pain and its relief in labor.* New York: Churchill Livingstone.

Drasner, K. & Swisher, J. L. (1996). Delayed complications and side effects of regional anesthesia. In D. L. Brown (Ed.), *Regional anesthesia and analgesia* (pp. 462–476). Philadelphia, PA: W. B. Saunders.

Ellis, W. E. (1997). Regional anesthesia. In J. J. Nagelhout & K. L. Zaglaniczny (Eds.), *Nurse anesthesia* (pp. 1160–1197). Philadelphia, PA: W. B. Saunders.

Fiedler, M. A. & Shaw, B. (1997). Obstetric anesthesia. In J. J. Nagelhout & K. L. Zaglaniczny (Eds.), *Nurse anesthesia* (pp. 292–332). Philadelphia, PA: W. B. Saunders.

Fine, P. G. & Ashburn, M. A. (1998). Functional neuroanatomy and nociception. In M. A. Ashburn & L. J. Rice (Eds.), *The management of pain.* (pp. 1–16). Philadelphia, PA: Churchill Livingstone.

Garde, J. F. (1997). Specialty practice of nurse anesthesia. In J. J. Nagelhout & K. L. Zaglaniczny (Eds.), *Nurse anesthesia* (pp. 23–27). Philadelphia, PA: W. B. Saunders.

Harmer, M., & Rosen, M. (1996). Parenteral opioids. In A. Van Zundert & G. W. Ostheimer (Eds.), *Pain relief and anesthesia in obstetrics* (pp. 365–372). New York: Churchill Livingstone.

Hawkins, J. L., Chestnut D. H., & Gibbs, C. P. (1996). Obstetric anesthesia. In S. G. Gabbe, J. R. Niebyl, & J. L. Simpson, *Obstetrics: Normal and problem pregnancies* (pp. 425–468). New York: Churchill Livingstone.

Hawkins, J. L., Hess, K. R., Kubicek, M. A., Joyce III, T. H., & Morrow, D. H. (1995). A reevaluation of the association between instrument delivery and epidural analgesia. *Regional Anesthesia, 20*, (1), 50–56.

Johnson, C., Lawlor, & Weiner, M. (1994). The airway in the obstetrical patient. *AANA Journal, 62*, (2), 149–159.

Jordan, L. M. (1994). Qualifications and capabilities of the Certified Registered Nurse Anesthetist. In S. D. Foster & L. M. Jordan (Eds.), *Professional aspects of nurse anesthesia practice* (pp. 3–10). Philadelphia, PA: F. A. Davis.

Luyendijk, W. (1996). Anatomy of the lumbar and sacral spinal canal. In A. Van Zundert & G. W. Ostheimer (Eds.), *Pain relief and anesthesia in obstetrics* (pp. 167–182). New York: Churchill Livingstone.

Kyle, R. A. & Shampo, M. A., (1997). James Young Simpson and the introduction of chloroform anesthesia in obstetric practice. *Mayo Clinic Proceedings, 72*, 372.

Morrision, L. M. M., Wildsmith, J. A. W., & Ostheimer, G. W. (1996). History of pain relief in childbirth. In A. Van Zundert & G. W. Ostheimer (Eds.), *Pain relief and anesthesia in obstetrics* (pp. 3–19). New York: Churchill Livingstone.

Mullins, R. & Johnson, M. D. (1996). Epidural and subarachnoid opioids in labor and delivery: USA view. In A. Van Zundert & G. W. Ostheimer (Eds.), *Pain relief and anesthesia in obstetrics* (pp. 219–224). New York: Churchill Livingstone.

Nichols, F. H., and Humenick, S. S. (2002) *Childbirth Education: Practice, Research and Theory* (2nd ed.) Philadelphia: Saunders.

Ostheimer, G. W., & Leavitt, K. A. (1996). Epidural anesthesia: technique. In A. Van Zundert & G. W. Ostheimer (Eds.), *Pain relief and anesthesia in obstetrics* (pp. 288–295). New York: Churchill Livingstone.

Ostheimer, G. W., Shea, C., & Van Zundert, A. (1996). The development of epidural needles. In A. Van Zundert & G. W. Ostheimer (Eds.), *Pain relief and anesthesia in obstetrics* (pp. 285–287). New York: Churchill Livingstone.

Rawal, N. (1996). Combined spinal-epidural anesthesia. In A. Van Zundert & G. W. Ostheimer (Eds.), *Pain relief and anesthesia in obstetrics* (pp. 413–426). New York: Churchill Livingstone.

Sandelowski, M. (1984). *Pain, pleasure, and American childbirth: From the twilight sleep to the Read method, 1914–1960.* Westport, CT: Greenwood Press.

Santos, A. C., Pederson, H., & Finster, M. (1997). Obstetric anesthesia. In P. G. Barash, B. F. Cullen, & R. K. Stoelting (Eds.), *Clinical anesthesia* (pp. 1061–1090). Philadelphia, PA: Lippincot-Raven.

Sharma, S. K., Sidawi, J. E., Ramin, S. M., Lucas, M. J., Leveno, K. J., & Cunningham, F. G. (1997). A randomized trial of epidural versus patient-controlled meperidine analgesia during labor. *Anesthesiology, 87*, (3), 487–494.

Schnider, S. M. & Levinson, G. (1994). Anesthesia for obstetrics. In R. D. Miller (Ed.), *Anesthesia* (4th ed.). New York: Churchill Livingstone.

Stoelting, R. K. & Miller, R. D. (1994). *Basics of anesthesia* (3rd ed.). New York: Churchill Livingstone.

Vincent, R. D. Jr., & Chestnut, D. H. (1996). Analgesia during labor and delivery. In D. L. Brown (Ed.), *Regional anesthesia and analgesia* (pp. 587–608). Philadelphia, PA: W. B. Saunders.

Visconti, C. M. & Rathmell, J. P. (1998). Pain management issues in the pregnant patient. In M. A. Ashburn & L. J. Rice (Eds.), *The management of pain.* (pp. 1–16). Philadelphia, PA: Churchill Livingstone.

Weber, S. E. (1996). Cultural aspects of pain in childbearing women. *JOGNN—Journal of Obstetric, Gynecologic, & Neonatal Nursing, 25*, (1): 67–72.

Williams, J. R. (1997). Local anesthetics. In J. J. Nagelhout & K. L. Zaglaniczny (Eds.), *Nurse anesthesia*. Philadelphia, PA: W. B. Saunders.

Youngstrom, P. C., Baker, S. W., & Miller, J. L. (1996). Epidurals redefined in analgesia and anesthesia: A distinction with a difference. *JOGNN, 25*, (4), 350–354.

Suggested Readings

Dewan, D. M. & Hood, D. D. (1997). *Practical obstetric anesthesia*. Philadelphia, PA: W. B. Saunders.

Foster, S. D. & Jordan, L. M. (Eds.). (1994). *Professional aspects of nurse anesthesia practice*. Philadelphia, PA: F. A. Davis.

Resources

American Association of Nurse Anesthetists (AANA), 222 South Prospect Avenue, Park Ridge, IL 60068, www.aana.com

American College of Nurse Midwives, Suite 900, 818 Connecticut Avenue, NW, Washington, DC 20006, www.acnm.org

American College of Obstetricians and Gynecologists, 409 12th Street, SW, P.O. Box 96920, Washington, DC 20090-6920, http://acog.com

American Society of Anesthesiologists (ASA), 520 N. Northwest Highway, Park Ridge, IL 60068-2573, www.asahq.org

Association of Women's Health, Obstetric and Neonatal Nurses, Suite 740, 2000 L Street, NW, Washington, DC 20036, http://awhonn.org

Lamaze International, Suite 800, 2025 M Street, NW, Washington, DC 20036-3309, http://lamaze-childbirth.com

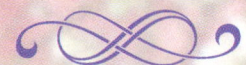

CHAPTER 25

Intrapartum Nursing Care

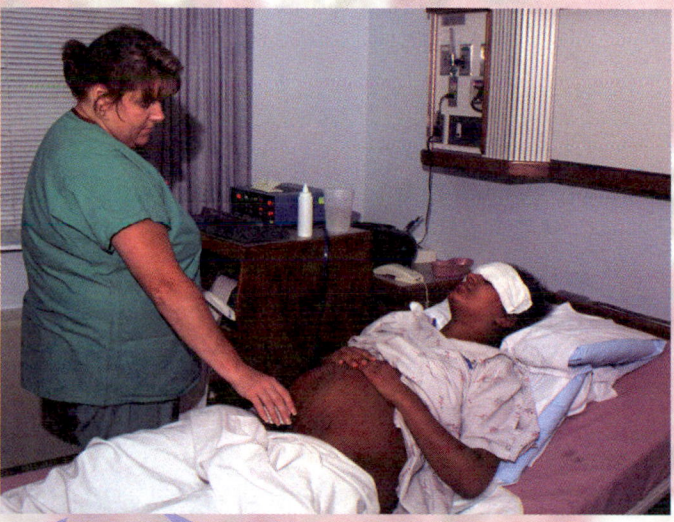

Childbirth is one of the most meaningful, unique, and exciting times for the laboring woman and her partner, yet it also can be a time of stress and anxiety. Essential components of nursing care include a comprehensive knowledge of the processes of labor and delivery, competence in providing care that conforms with current standards, and provision of support for the childbearing family through this major event. Good interpersonal skills, including listening to the client, will complement technical skills. A positive perception of the birthing experience and a feeling of empowerment are fostered by the nurse who gives sufficient information to the woman and her partner, in language they can understand, and who shows nonjudgmental support for their efforts.

A good intrapartum nurse is one who not only is skilled and knowledgeable but who deems it a privilege to provide care to a family during this momentous time. Many women remember every nuance of their labor and childbirth for many years afterward. These women especially remember the actions and demeanor of the major caregiver. Attentive and effective support, therefore, can make childbirth a satisfying experience for everyone and a treasured memory for the family.

Key Terms

Acceleration	Effacement	Meconium	Preterm premature
Acme	Emergency childbirth	Montevideo units	rupture of membranes
Acrocyanosis	Episiotomy	Multipara	(PPROM)
Active phase	Fern test	Nitrazine test	Reactive nonstress test
Amnihook	Fetal heart rate (FHR)	Nonperiodic fetal heart	Resting tone
Amnioinfusion	First stage of labor	rate changes	Saltatory pattern
Amniotomy	Frequency	Nuchal cord	Second stage of labor
Apgar score	Gravidity	Oligohydramnios	Short-term variability
Baseline fetal heart rate	Hypertonic contractions	Overshoot	Shoulder
Beat-to-beat variability	Hyperventilation	Parity	Station
Bloody show	Increment	Parturient	Striae gravidarum
Chorioamnionitis	Intensity	Periodic fetal heart rate	Third stage of labor
Contraction	Intrauterine pressure	changes	Transition phase
Crowning	catheter (IUPC)	Placenta previa	True labor
Deceleration	Inversion of the uterus	Polyhydramnios	Uterine atony
Decrement	Labor	Precipitous delivery	Uteroplacental
Dilation	Laceration	Premature rupture of	insufficiency
Doula	Late onset deceleration	membranes (PROM)	Variable deceleration
Duration	Latent stage	Presenting part	Variability
Early onset deceleration	Long-term variability	Preterm birth	Vertex

Competencies

Upon completion of this chapter, the reader should be able to:

1. Describe the initial assessment of the woman in labor.
2. Describe the subsequent maternal-fetal assessment during the four stages of labor.
3. Define the normal course of all four stages of labor.
4. Describe the primary nursing interventions in all four stages of labor.
5. Identify changes in client-fetal status that may alter the course of labor and delivery.
6. Discuss episiotomy use and subsequent nursing considerations.
7. Accurately document events and nursing interventions.

The nursing care of the woman experiencing an uncomplicated vaginal birth is discussed. All maternity clients have their individual expectations and reactions to labor and delivery. Emphasis on each of the varied roles of the nurse, as client advocate, support person, and expert caregiver, will depend on the client's particular circumstances and specific needs. For example, the young teenager who has received no childbirth preparation will need a great deal more teaching than will the client who is giving birth to her fourth child and has attended childbirth classes. A middle-class woman with a planned pregnancy, good preparation, and a supportive family is more likely to find the experience joyful and rewarding than is the single woman with an unwanted

pregnancy. The actions of the intrapartum nurse are described step-by-step through the labor and delivery process, beginning with the admission procedures and continuing with the ongoing observation and support of the client until completion of the fourth stage, or stabilization period. This is the sequence of events as the nurse encounters them. Although this chapter deals with uncomplicated vaginal delivery, every labor and delivery nurse must be able to recognize symptoms of complications that might develop and must know the appropriate nursing interventions.

Most women in the United States give birth in a hospital birthing room called a labor, delivery, and recovery room (LDR). In that setting, the woman is not transferred

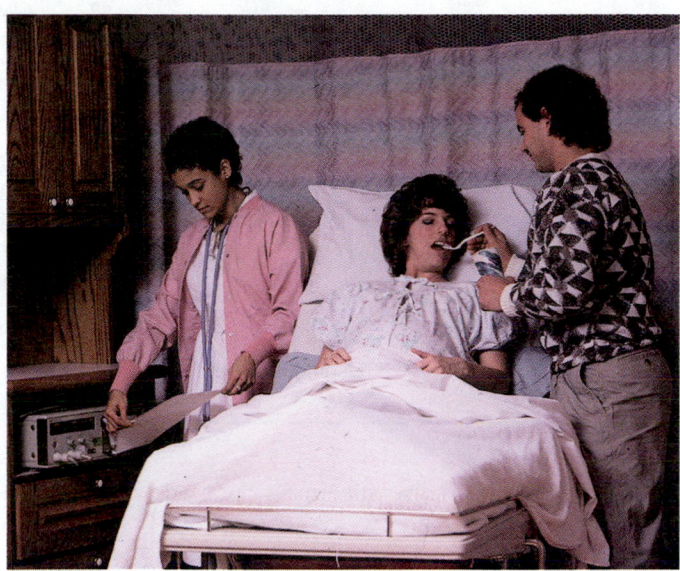

Figure 25-1 Many hospitals offer a pleasant, family-centered atmosphere for the birthing experience.

Critical Thinking

Who Delivers the Infant?

It is the woman who delivers the infant, not the physician or midwife. The laboring woman is the key player in this event. The health care team safeguards the mother and infant by providing a therapeutic environment, appropriate interventions, encouragement, reassurance, and feedback.

What do you believe is the most appropriate role for the professional nurse in providing care for the laboring woman and her fetus?

How do you think the nurse fits into the health care team?

from a labor room to a delivery room, unless the need develops for operative intervention; she remains in the LDR for at least 1 hour after delivery. During this recovery period the woman can hold and feed her infant and thus begin the bonding process. After the recovery hour, the woman is transferred to the postpartum unit. In some hospitals the woman remains in the same room (labor, delivery, recovery, and postpartum room [LDRP]) until discharge. With the introduction of LDRs, LDRPs, and birthing rooms, hospitals have attempted to create a family-centered homelike appearance that promotes an ambience of normalcy rather than a clinical atmosphere (Figure 25-1).

ASSESSMENT OF THE PHYSIOLOGIC PROCESSES OF LABOR

Most women who arrive at the labor and delivery unit are excited about the birth of their baby but also anxious that everything should progress well. A woman often is concerned about whether she really is in labor, whether she will appear foolish if sent home again, and if she is in true labor, how she will cope with the pain and stress of contractions and giving birth. The nurse can allay much of this anxiety by adopting a friendly and interested manner and by keeping the woman and her support person fully informed. Teaching plays a major role in easing anxiety and should include events of labor and what to expect in the way of procedures. Care must be taken to maintain the client's privacy and confidentiality to promote trust and avoid undue stress. The nurse is perceived as powerful but should not be controlling. The **parturient**, that is the

woman in labor, is the person of central importance in this situation, not the nurse, doctor, or nurse-midwife.

Maternal Status

Women come to the hospital or birthing center at different stages of labor and with different levels of wellness. Thorough initial and ongoing assessment by the nurse is critical to the well-being of mother and infant. Certain information is needed immediately for the nurse to establish appropriate priorities when developing the plan of care. Initial admission observations are aimed at establishing the fact that true labor has begun, ascertaining the imminence with which the birth might be expected, and alerting team members to existing or developing complications or risk factors. It is desirable for the prenatal care provider to transmit the client's health history, physical findings, and laboratory data to the hospital toward the end of the third

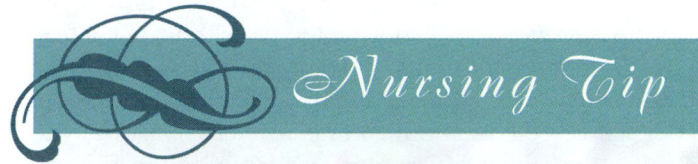

Nursing Tip

INTRODUCTIONS

When meeting a client for the first time, it is wise to bear in mind that first impressions are lasting. The nurse should introduce herself, ask the names of the client and those accompanying her, and conduct them to the triage room or the assigned labor, delivery, and recovery room.

Table 25-1 True versus False Labor

Qualifier	True Labor	False Labor
Contractions	Regular	Irregular
	Intervals shorten	Intervals do not shorten
	Intensity increases	Intensity remains unchanged
	Intensify with walking	Do not intensify with walking
Cervix	Dilates and becomes effaced	Does not dilate or efface
Sedation	Does not stop true labor	Tends to stop false labor
Show (blood-tinged mucus from the cervical canal)	Often is present	Usually is absent

trimester so that when the client is admitted to the labor and delivery unit her prenatal record can be reviewed and pertinent information recorded in the Admission Record.

Labor Onset

One of the most critical diagnoses in obstetrics is the accurate diagnosis of labor onset. The hallmark of true labor is cervical change; however, the woman at home has no way of knowing whether her cervix is dilating. Many women come to the hospital believing that they are in labor, only to be discharged home, still pregnant, after a few hours. To conserve the use of LDRs, many hospitals have a triage room in which the client's labor status is first evaluated before she is either discharged or moved to an LDR.

Although making a differential diagnosis between true and false labor sometimes is difficult, it usually can be done on the basis of certain very specific criteria (Table 25-1).

Initial Status Assessment

During the initial assessment the client is observed closely for clues to her status. Postures, facial expressions, and gestures can suggest tension, anxiety, or pain. Perspiration, varied breathing patterns, and frequent position changes also can indicate stress and discomfort. Grunting or breath-holding may signal the start of the second stage of labor. If the client is in active **labor** (the process by which the fetus is expelled from the uterus) the nurse may have to shorten the initial assessment and prioritize the questions (between contractions) to focus on her current labor status. Certain information is needed immediately to evaluate the extent of the woman's labor and to become alert to the woman with a history of rapid deliveries or problems denoting risk. The client should not have to guess the information that is important for the nurse to know; therefore, skillful interviewing is essential. Questions that the nurse should ask include the following:

1. What is your reason for coming to the hospital?
   Information Obtained: Presenting complaint (e.g., urge to push, back pain, "water" broke).

2. When is your baby due, and how many babies have you had?
   Information obtained: Expected date of delivery and parity, possibility of a rapid labor if the woman is a **multipara**, that is, a woman who has had two or more pregnancies that reached viability.

3. When did your labor begin? How far apart are the **contractions** (tightening and shortening of the uterine muscles during labor)? Have they become stronger?
   Information obtained: The length of time the woman has been in labor, and the frequency and perceived **intensity** (strength of the contraction at its peak) of the contractions.

4. Has the bag of water (membranes) broken? At what time? What color was the fluid? Have you noticed any bleeding?
   Information obtained: Possible presence of abnormal bleeding (bloody discharge without mucus) or **bloody show** (a blood-tinged mucous discharge from the vagina that occurs as the cervix starts to dilate), whether membranes have ruptured, time of rupture of membranes, possible presence of meconium-stained amniotic fluid (**meconium** is fetal stool found in the bowel of a term neonate). Presence of meconium-stained amniotic fluid indicates that the fetus has experienced an episode of hypoxia.

5. How has your pregnancy been? Have you been hospitalized during this pregnancy? Is there anything else about you or your pregnancy that I should know?
   Information obtained: Any condition or information that may have an impact on labor, delivery, and the neonate.

6. Are you allergic to any foods or medicines that you know of? Are you allergic to latex? Have you ever had a bad reaction to a blood transfusion?
   Information obtained: Any known allergies to medications, latex, or blood.

Other pertinent information can be outlined on the Obstetric Admitting Record (Figure 25-2).

Hollister™

Obstetric Admitting Record

Hollister Maternal/Newborn Record System   Page 1 of 2
To order call: **1.800.323.4060**   Re-order No. **5710**

Basic Admission Data   Date 6/23/96 Time 1020

- ☑ Ambulatory
- ☐ Stretcher
- ☑ Oriented to Unit
- ☐ Wheelchair
- ☐ Transfer From
- ☑ Safety/Security

G.	T.	Pt	A	L	LMP	EDD	Wks
III	II	0	0	II	9/28/95	7/4/96	38 3/7

EDD By Fetal Assessment 7/4/96

Race/Ethnicity Cauc.   Age 35

Advance Directives ☑ None ☐ Living Will
☐ Medical Power of Attorney

Organ Donor ☐ Yes ☑ No

Last Oral Intake
Fluids 6/23/96 Time 0630
Solids 6/22/96 Time 2200

Medications ☐ None

Type/Dose	Last Taken	With Patient No / Yes	Disposition
PNV	6/22/96	☑ / ☐	
		☐ / ☐	
		☐ / ☐	

MD/CNM	Tel No	Support Person/Relationship	Tel No
M. Brown MD	831-2467	Frank (husband)	345-9330

Allergies/Sensitivities   ☐ None
- ☑ Medication Demerol → severe N&V
- ☐ Other

Reasons for Admission
- ☑ Onset of Labor
- ☐ Induction of Labor
- ☐ Spontaneous Abortion
- ☐ Cesarean Section
  - ☐ Primary ☐ Repeat
  - (reason for primary _____)
- ☐ Tubal Ligation
- ☐ Vaginal Bleeding
- ☑ ROM ☐ Premature ☐ Prolonged
- ☐ Preterm Labor

Detail Reasons for Admission

Observation Evaluation
- ☐ Fetal Status
  - ☐ Ultrasound
  - ☐ Amniocentesis
  - ☐ NST ☐ CST
- ☐ Medical Complications
- ☐ Obstetric Complications

Personal Effects	Disposition		
Item	With Patient	With Support Person	Other (Describe)
wedding ring set	✓		
gold watch	✓		
contact lenses	✓		

Patient Triage Data   ☐ See Triage Record

Contractions ☐ None ☑ Palpation ☐ Tocotransducer
Frequency 3-4 min Duration 30-40' Intensity mild
Began on 6/23/96 Time 0930 (regular rhythm)

Membranes ☐ Intact ☐ Bulging
"leaking" ☑ Ruptured (Date 6/23/96 Time 0100)
☑ Nitrazine test (☑ pos ☐ neg) ☐ Sterile Speculum Exam
☐ Fern test (☐ pos ☐ neg) (findings _____)

Fluid ☑ Clear ☐ Bloody ☐ Meconium Stained
☐ Foul Odor ☐ No Foul Odor ☐ None Observed
Vaginal Bleeding ☑ None ☐ Normal Show
☐ Bleeding (Describe _____)
Cervical Exam By J Hall RNC
Station -2 Effacement 80% Dilatation 1 cms
Presentation ☑ Vertex ☐ Transverse Lie
☐ Face/Brow ☐ Compound
☐ Breech (type _____) ☐ Unknown

Physical Assessment

Height	Wt Pregrav/Grav	Temp	Pulse	Resp	BP
5'7"	135/160	99	84	18	112/67

Detail Abnormal Findings

System	Normal	Abnormal
HEENT	☑	☐
Neurologic	☑	☐
Skin	☑	☐
Breasts	☑	☐
Extremities	☑	☐
Cardiovascular	☑	☐
Respiratory	☑	☐
Abdomen	☑	☐
Gastrointestinal	☑	☐
Urinary	☑	☐
Genitalia	☐	☑

uterus ✓ Bicornuate uterus

Initial Problems Identified ☐ None
1. Potential for ineff UC.
2.
3.

Plan
Monitor effectiveness of UC. Oxytocin aug. if indicated. MB

Fetal Evaluation Data   Multiple Gestation ☑ No ☐ Yes

Fundal Height 40 cms
Fetal Weight (est.) 8#
FHR 130's

	Presentation	Position
1.	vertex	OP
2.		
3.		

☐ Fetoscope ☑ Fetal Monitor
☐ Doppler ☐ Other

Specimens Obtained (Check all that apply)

Urine Test	Time	Results	Blood Test	Time	Results
☐ Urinalysis			☑ Hgb	0945	
☐ C + S			☑ Hct	0945	
☐ Glucose			☐ VDRL/RPR		
☐ Albumin			☑ Type/Screen	0945	O+
☐ Ketones			☐		
☐ pH			Cervical Culture		
☐ Blood			☑ GBS	0945	
☐ Toxicology			☐		

Admitting Signature	Date/Time	Examiner Signature	Date/Time
J Hall RNC	6/23/96 1045	J Hall RNC	6/23/96 1000

Figure 25-2 Obstetric Admitting Record. Courtesy of Hollister Incorporated.

✻ Hollister™

Obstetric Admitting Record
Hollister Maternal/Newborn Record System   **Page 2 of 2**
To order call: 1.800.323.4060   Re-order No. **5710**

Significant Prenatal Data

Prenatal Records Available on Admission
☐ No ☑ Yes Source _M Brown MD_
First Visit by 13 Wks ☑ Yes ☐ No
Regular Care ☑ Yes ☐ No
Prenatal Classes ☐ Yes ☑ No _prev. exper._

Pediatric Provider _M. Smith MD_

General Health ☑ Healthy
☐ Recent Exposure to Communicable Disease
  Type/Date ___
☐ Illness (≤ 14 days prior to admission)
  Type/Treatment ___
☐ Chronic Condition
  Type ___

Nutritional Status ☑ Well-nourished ☐ Malnourished ☐ Obese
☐ Special Diet ___
Eating Disorder ☑ None ☐ Identify ___
Nutritional Problems ☑ None ☐ Identify ___

Lab Findings
☐ None
Blood Type & Rh _O+_
Rubella Titer _Immune_
Serology _NR_
HBsAg _Neg_
HIV
GBS _Neg_

Fetal Assessment Tests
☐ None

Date	Test	Result
2/14	Sono	20 6/7wk
6/6	PG LSRatio	±2.5
5/9	NST	reactive

Problems Identified ☐ None
		Active	Resolved
1.	Preterm labor	☐	☑
2.	Uterine anom.	☑	☐
3.		☐	☐
4.		☐	☐

Hospitalizations ☐ None
1. _5/9/96_ Reason _PTL_
2. ___ Reason ___

Plans for Birth and Hospital Stay ☐ Birth Plan Attached
Support Person Present in L&D ☐ No ☑ Yes _husband_
Other Family Members in L&D ☐ No ☑ Yes _parents_
Anesthesia ☐ None ☐ Local ☑ Epidural ☐ Spinal ☐ General
Delivery Site/Position _LDRP sitting-leg support_
Personal Requests _Ice chips prn_

Adoption ☑ No ☐ Yes Contact with Infant ☐ No ☐ Yes
Adoption Contact ___
Feeding Preference ☑ Breast ☐ Bottle
☐ Tubal Ligation Authorization Signed ☐ Yes ☐ No
☑ Circumcision Authorization Signed ☑ Yes ☐ No

Psychosocial Data ☑ See Prenatal Records
Emotional Status ☑ Happy ☐ Ambivalent ☐ Concerned
☐ Depressed ☐ Angry ☐ Other
Communication Barriers ☑ None
☐ Language ☐ Interpreter ___
☐ Vision ☐ Reading ☐ Writing ☐ Hearing
☐ Speech ☐ Other ___
Support System
Marital Status: S ⓜ Sep D W Father involved ☑ Yes ☐ No
Other Support ☐ None ☑ _maternal family_
Occupation _RN_ Education _16 - BSN_
Religion ☐ N/A ☑ _catholic_
Personal/Cultural/Religious Customs Affecting Care and/or Learning
☐ None ☑ Identify _Infant baptism in emergency_

Basic Needs Met Yes No If No, Explain
Food ☑ ☐
Clothing ☑ ☐
Housing ☑ ☐
Transportation ☑ ☐
Finances ☑ ☐
Life Stress No Yes If Yes, Explain
Physical Abuse ☑ ☐
Emotional Abuse ☑ ☐

Life Stress(Cont.) No Yes If Yes, Explain
Major Change ☑ ☐
Self Care Needs ☑ ☐
Serious Illness ☑ ☐
Other ☐ ☐

Substance Use No Yes If Yes, amt/day, last use
Tobacco ☑ ☐
Alcohol ☑ ☐
Prescribed Drugs ☐ ☑ _PNV ÷ daily/Terbutaline 2.5 mg po 6/7_
Illicit Drugs ☑ ☐

Educational Needs Mother Support Person Comments
Stages/Phases of Labor ☐ ☐ _Experienced_
Coping Techniques ☐ ☐
Infant Feeding ☐ ☐
Infant Care ☐ ☐
☐ ☐

Preferred Learning Methods Yes No
One-on-One Instruction ☑ ☐
Group Instruction ☐ ☑
Written Information ☑ ☐
Audio/Visual Information ☐ ☑
Demonstration/Practice ☑ ☐
Other ___

Discharge Planning Data Planned Length of Stay _one_ Days
Home Setting Yes No
Heat, running water, refrigeration ☑ ☐
Infant Care Supplies/Car Seat ☑ ☐
Phone in home ☑ ☐
Transportation available ☑ ☐
Adult assistance available ☑ ☐

Referrals
☐ RN Case Manager ☐ Utilization Review ☐ Other
☑ Home Care RN ☐ Social Service
☐ Nutritionist/Dietician ☑ Pediatric Provider

MD/CNM notified by _J Hall RNC_ Date _6/23/96_ Time _1040_
Admitting Signature _J Hall RNC_ Date _6/23/96_ Time _1045_

OBSTETRIC ADMITTING RECORD FORM #5710 (Page 2 of 2) 696

Figure 25-2 (continued)

Informed Consent

The fact that the woman comes to the birthing facility gives the implication of consent to treatment; nevertheless, informed consent should be obtained in the form of a signature before any invasive procedures are carried out. It is the physician's responsibility to give the client information and rationale for the type of interventions that may be performed, including benefits, possible risks, and available alternatives. Typically, however, it is the nurse who obtains and witnesses the client's signature on the consent form. An informed consent form should be signed before any treatment is carried out, particularly administration of medications that might impair the woman's ability to make decisions. Each hospital or birthing center may have its own variation of an informed consent form; however, all forms should cover delivery of the infant and include procedures that may be necessary in an emergency, for example, general anesthesia, cesarean delivery, blood transfusion, and hysterectomy.

Risk Factors

If the prenatal record is available, it should be reviewed before the client arrives at the unit. The nurse reviews the prenatal history and antenatal care and notes identified risk factors. To make appropriate nursing diagnoses, a comprehensive nursing database must be compiled. To achieve an optimal perinatal outcome, factors that put the woman or infant at high risk for morbidity must be recognized early so that appropriate and timely intervention can be made, including consultation with specialists in other medical departments. Early intervention can minimize fetal and maternal complications.

Many conditions in either the mother or fetus, some preexisting and others that have developed during the pregnancy, can result in a high-risk classification (Boxes 25-1 and 25-2).

Cunningham (1997) listed three major categories that can be identified antepartum that put the client at increased risk: preexisting medical illness; previous poor pregnancy outcome, such as perinatal mortality, preterm delivery, fetal growth retardation, malformations, placental accidents, and maternal hemorrhage; and inadequate maternal weight gain owing to malnutrition.

Expected Date of Delivery

The expected date of delivery (EDD) is noted in the Admission Record and the gestation calculated in weeks and days; for example, 38 weeks and 3 days would appear as 38 3/7 weeks. If the EDD is not known, the nurse may cal-

---

Box 25-1 Pregnancy Risk Factors Identified from the Mother's Medical History

- Diabetes mellitus
- Sickle cell disease
- Prior cesarean delivery
- Chronic hypertension
- Heart disease
- Anemia
- Cigarette smoking, alcohol use, substance abuse
- Renal disease
- Infection, e.g., hepatitis B, syphilis, gonorrhea human immunodeficiency virus group B *Streptococcus*, active herpes virus
- Previous perinatal loss
- Age under 16 or over 35 years

Box 25-2 Specific Risk Factors Developing During This Pregnancy

- Pregnancy-induced hypertension
- Polyhydramnios or oligohydramnios
- Preterm labor
- Bleeding in the third trimester
- Placenta abruption
- Prolonged rupture of membranes
- Gestational diabetes mellitus
- Fetal congenital anomalies
- Gestational age 42 weeks or more
- Preeclampsia
- Multiple gestation
- Placenta previa
- Abnormal presentation
- Inadequate prenatal care
- Intrauterine growth retardation
- Isoimmunization (Rh or ABO)

Critical Thinking

Noncompliance

RL has phenylketonuria. Her doctor advised her to follow a diet low in phenylalanine before becoming pregnant and throughout the pregnancy to protect the fetus. RL refused to follow the low-phenylalanine diet and gave birth to a baby boy with severe neurologic damage. You overhear another nurse say, "People like her should be put in the hospital and obliged to follow the diet so that the baby would not be harmed."

What would be your response to this nurse?

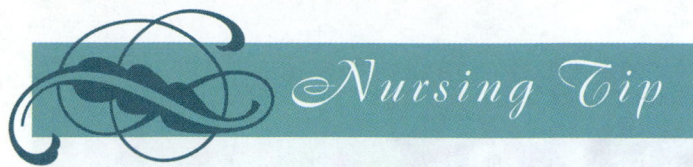

PARITY

Parity is determined by the number of *pregnancies* of viable duration, not the number of fetuses delivered. For example, a primigravida who previously delivered stillborn triplets at 29 weeks gestation is a para 1.

culate the EDD from the date of the woman's last menstrual period using Nägele's rule (see Chapter 15). **Gravidity**, the number of times the woman has been pregnant, and **parity**, the number of pregnancies that have reached viability regardless of outcome, are noted.

Two methods are used to document gravidity and parity:

5-digit method:
a. Number of times the woman has been pregnant (gravidity).
b. Number of term births (parity).
c. Number of **preterm births**, that is, births after 20 weeks' gestation and before 37 weeks' gestation.
d. Number of abortions (spontaneous or elective).
e. Number of living children.
GTPAL: G6P4014 = 5 pregnancies, 4 to term, 0 premature, 1 abortion, 4 living.

2-digit method:
a. Number of times the woman has been pregnant (gravidity).
b. Pregnancies that have reached a gestation of viability, regardless of outcome.
G_3P_2: 2 pregnancies and two live births. G includes current pregnancy prior to delivery.

Problems with Present Pregnancy

The client is asked about any problems she may have had, particularly those requiring hospitalization, pertaining to the current pregnancy. Problems such as preterm labor, vaginal infections, vaginal bleeding, gestational diabetes, and pregnancy-induced hypertension (PIH) are of particular importance.

Findings of a preliminary history and screening serve to ascertain whether the woman is, in fact, in labor and whether there are any obvious problems. Relevant information includes but is not necessarily limited to the EDD; blood pressure; temperature; pulse; respirations; pattern and amount of weight gain and present nutritional status; symptoms experienced; deep tendon reflexes; edema; and urine screening for protein, glucose, and ketones.

Health History

The nurse obtains pertinent information from the prenatal record and by interviewing the client. Risk factors that may increase morbidity or mortality are evaluated. In order to make this evaluation, the nurse must possess a knowledge of factors and chronic physical conditions that might put the pregnancy into a high-risk category. Childhood diseases, emotional problems, and genetic defects are noted in the Admission Record. Chronic illnesses, such as hypertension, diabetes, positive human immunodeficiency virus (HIV) status, cardiac disease, phlebitis, renal disease, and seizure disorders, are conditions that place an additional burden on the body; therefore, these illnesses put the client and fetus at greater than normal risk for mortality or morbidity. Surgical operations are noted, particularly uterine surgeries (e.g., cesarean delivery, myomectomy) that would leave a weakened portion of the myometrium and thus a higher than normal risk of uterine rupture.

Demographic and Psychosocial History

Demographic and psychosocial information includes age; religious and cultural factors; and use of substances such as alcohol, tobacco, and illicit drugs. If the woman smokes cigarettes, she should be asked how many are smoked per day. If the woman admits to using illicit, so-called recreational, drugs she should be asked for details such as the specific substance used and the amount taken. A drug screening should be done on any client who admits to or displays evidence that leads the caregiver to suspect substance abuse. Signs suggestive of substance abuse, such as needle marks or bruising, should be noted.

If the woman is admitted in an advanced stage of labor and is experiencing strong contractions, it may not

Critical Thinking

Cigarette Smoking During Pregnancy

Women who smoke cigarettes during pregnancy face serious health risks, including increased perinatal mortality, increased risk for placental abruption, low-birth-weight infants, small for gestational age infants, and preterm deliveries (ACOG, Sept. 1997).

If you were a nurse caring for a pregnant woman who smokes cigarettes, what would you tell her about cigarette smoking during pregnancy?

Would your advice differ if you were a cigarette smoker?

be appropriate for the nurse to make an in-depth health history record. Priority assessments, however, include the following:

Is the woman able to ask for what she needs?

Is there a language barrier?

Does she talk freely with the nurse and her partner?

Does she avoid eye contact?

How much rest has she had lately?

The woman's culture and socialization as well as her perception of previous birth experiences are likely to influence her attitude toward her current situation and her postpartum emotional adjustment (Lowe, 1996).

The woman should be encouraged to ask about practices during labor and delivery that are important to her culture, and these requests must be entertained with respect and sensitivity. When a request is made that contradicts usual practice, nurses should ask themselves the following questions: How important is this to the client? Is it safe? Is it feasible to incorporate this request into the plan of care?

Safety Screening

Estimates of the prevalence of abuse during pregnancy, developed from clinic-based studies, range from 0.9% to 20.1%, with the bulk of studies reporting a prevalence of 3.9% to 8.3% (Gazmararian et al., 1996). Many studies report that violence may begin or escalate during pregnancy (Hilliard, 1985). Thus, it is crucial for the nurse to enquire of all female clients as to the safety of their domestic situation, because hospitalization during childbirth may provide the only window of opportunity for an abused woman to seek assistance. Studies have revealed that women who are anxious during pregnancy compared with women who are not tend to have infants of lower birth weight; studies also have shown that women with high levels of stress hormones compared with those with low levels are more likely to deliver preterm (Teixeira, Fisk, & Glover, 1999; Wadhwa et al., 1998).

A client may not want to confide in the nurse about domestic violence until a relationship of trust has developed between the nurse and the client. Even then, the client may not volunteer information unless she is asked outright and is assured of confidentiality. Safety screening should always be performed in absolute privacy, when the client is alone with the nurse. Sometimes it is necessary for the nurse to ask the partner to step out into the waiting room. An Abuse Assessment Screen should be completed and placed in the client's medical record (Figure 25-3). If the client screens positive for abuse, the nurse must discuss possible options that are available, provide phone numbers of local shelters, and notify the hospital social worker. If there are overt signs of abuse, such as bruises or abrasions, the nurse should describe them and take photographs, which are than placed in the client's medical record.

Obstetric History

When this is not the woman's first pregnancy, the characteristics of previous births are noted. The number of previous deliveries and length of the client's last labor is information that might help to predict progress of the current labor. Useful details of the previous births would include birth weights, the type of anesthesia used, the kind of birth (spontaneous vaginal, forceps-assisted, vacuum-assisted, or cesarean birth), and whether there was postpartum hemorrhage.

Fetal Status

Initial assessment of fetal status gives reassurance of well-being and must be recorded appropriately. The fetal heart rate (FHR) may be evaluated by auscultation with a fetoscope or electronically by means of an ultrasound stethoscope or by electronic fetal monitoring (EFM). EFM has become routine in most labor and delivery units in the United States. The character of uterine activity and the response of the FHR to contractions are of considerable interest. Leopold's maneuvers are performed by the nurse between contractions to assess fetal presentation, lie, position, and engagement (see Chapter 23) and also to ascertain the appropriate location for auscultating the FHR. Success of external fetal monitoring depends largely on correct positioning of the transducer.

Critical Thinking

Domestic Violence During Pregnancy

Complications of pregnancy, including low weight gain, anemia, infection, preterm labor, chorioamnionitis, and first and second trimester bleeding are significantly higher in women who are abused compared with women who are not abused (Parker, McFarlane, & Soeken, 1994; Berenson et al., 1991). Also significantly higher are maternal rates of depression; suicide attempts; and use of tobacco, alcohol, and illicit drugs. Some studies report appreciably lower mean birth weights for infants born to women abused during pregnancy (McFarlane, Parker, & Soeken, 1996).

What responsibility does the nurse have in screening for domestic violence in pregnancy?

NAME _____

TODAY'S DATE _____

(Circle **YES** or **NO** for each question)

1. **IN THE YEAR BEFORE YOU WERE PREGNANT,** were you pushed, shoved, slapped, hit, kicked or otherwise physically hurt by someone? . . . . . **YES   NO**

If YES, by whom (Circle all that apply)

Husband   Ex-husband   Boyfriend   Ex-boyfriend

Total number of times _____

2. **SINCE THE PREGNANCY BEGAN** have you been pushed, shoved, slapped, hit, kicked or otherwise physically hurt by someone? . . . . . **YES   NO**

If YES, by whom (Circle all that apply)

Husband   Ex-husband   Boyfriend   Ex-boyfriend

DATE OF LAST INCIDENT _____, **SCORE** _____ (SEE BELOW)

DATE OF WORST INCIDENT _____, **SCORE** _____ (SEE BELOW)

MARK THE AREA OF INJURY ON THE BODY
SCORE THE TWO INCIDENTS according to the following scale:

1 = Threats of abuse including use of a weapon

2 = Slapping, pushing; no injuries and/or lasting pain

3 = Punching, kicking, bruises, cuts and/or continuing pain

4 = Beating up, severe contusions, burns, broken bones

5 = Head injury, internal injury, permanent injury

6 = Use of weapon; wound from weapon

(If any of the descriptions for the higher number apply, use the higher number)

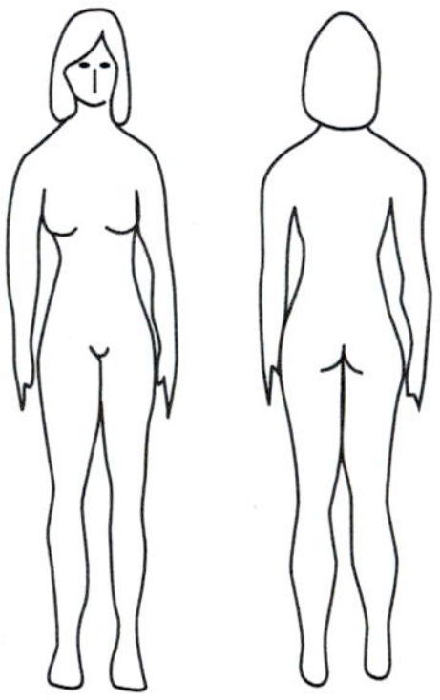

3. **IN THE YEAR BEFORE YOU WERE PREGNANT,** did anyone force you to have sexual activities? . . . . . **YES   NO**

If YES, by whom (Circle all that apply)

Husband   Ex-husband   Boyfriend   Ex-boyfriend

Total number of times _____

4. **SINCE THE PREGNANCY BEGAN,** has anyone forced you to have sexual activities? . . . . . **YES   NO**

If YES, by whom (Circle all that apply)

Husband   Ex-husband   Boyfriend   Ex-boyfriend

Total number of times _____

Figure 25-3 Abuse Assessment Screen.

CONFIDENTIALITY

The client's partner may be unaware of past pregnancies, infants given up for adoption, abortions, or a positive human immunodeficiency virus status. A client's desire for confidentiality must be respected. Therefore, some questions are best asked when the partner, all family members, and all other support persons are out of the room.

The **fetal heart rate (FHR)** is the number of times the fetal heart beats per minute (Cunningham, 1997). The Association of Women's Health, Obstetrics, and Neonatal Nurses (AWHONN) (1998) establishes guidelines for competency validation for FHR monitoring and the American College of Obstetricians and Gynecologists (ACOG) publishes technical bulletins to guide clinical practice issues such as FHR monitoring (ACOG, 1995).

Perinatal nurses are responsible for familiarizing themselves with practice guidelines regarding FHR monitoring. The FHR should be evaluated as soon as possible after the woman arrives at the labor and delivery unit (Box 25-3). The method and frequency of assessment will depend on risk factors and departmental policy. Monitoring can be continuous or intermittent.

Auscultation

Auscultation is an auditory method of monitoring the FHR. It is performed intermittently and usually with a DeLee-Hillis obstetric stethoscope or a Doppler device. Auscultation should be done during and immediately after a contraction. For the low-risk client in the active phase of the first stage of labor, auscultation should be performed at least every 30 minutes (ACOG, Dec. 1995). The Doppler ultrasound device is handheld and amplifies the sound of the FHR. The advantage of auscultation is that it allows for greater freedom of the client because she is not attached to a machine and does not have to wear belts to secure the ultrasound transducer and the tocotransducer. However, auscultation does not provide a printed record of the FHR for other medical professionals to see, nor does it provide an assessment of variability or other subtle changes in FHR.

Electronic Fetal Monitoring

Electronic fetal monitoring (EFM) is an auditory and visual monitoring method and provides a paper strip printout of

Box 25-3 Nonstress Test

1. Place the fetal monitoring device on the client.

2. A **reactive nonstress test** is:
   2 accelerations of the fetal heart rate that are at least 15 beats above the baseline and last 15 seconds or more within 10 min.

3. If unable to obtain a reactive nonstress test within 30 min:
   Change the client's position.
   Administer oral or intravenous fluid.
   Use acoustic stimulation.

4. Continue to monitor for 30 more minutes.

5. If the fetal heart rate is not reactive after this time, inform primary care giver.

FHR and variability, as well as a record of contraction frequency and duration (Figure 25-4, Box 25-4). EFM is used more frequently than is any other method; research has shown that EFM has increased the rate of surgical intervention and decreased perinatal mortality owing to fetal hypoxia (Vintzileos et al., 1995). Using EFM, the FHR can be assessed externally, or internally after the membranes have ruptured.

In external electronic monitoring, the quality of the FHR strip depends on correct placement of the transducer

Critical Thinking

Fetal Monitoring Interpretation

Intrapartum nurses are legally responsible for interpreting the fetal heart rate (FHR) pattern and initiating appropriate nursing interventions. Timely notification of the primary caregiver in the event of a nonreassuring FHR pattern and documentation of all interventions and subsequent outcomes are nursing responsibilities. Should a difference of opinion arise between the intrapartum nurse and the physician or nurse-midwife regarding the appropriate intervention, the intrapartum nurse is responsible for initiating the institutional chain of command (AWHONN, 1998).

As a labor and delivery nurse, you have a client who has what you consider to be an ominous FHR pattern. You voice your concern to the physician several times, with no response. What is your duty as a nurse to provide for the safety of your client and her infant?

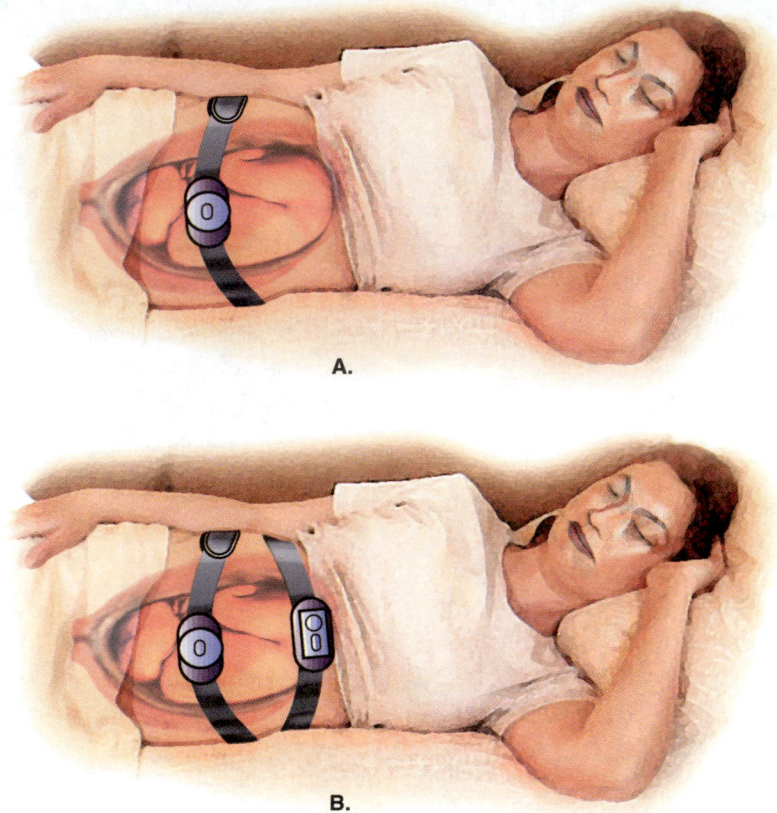

A.

B.

Figure 25-4 External fetal heart rate monitoring. A. Ultrasound transducer in place over the fetal heart. B. Tocotransducer in place over the uterine fundus.

Box 25-4 General Approach to External Fetal Monitoring

1. Explain the procedure to the client.

2. Place the client in a position in which she feels comfortable and that is a semi-Fowler's, side-lying, or semi-recumbent position, with one hip tilted to the side.

3. Perform Leopold's maneuver to ascertain the position of the fetal back.

4. Apply water-soluble gel to the underside of the transducer for conduction of the fetal heart sounds.

5. Place the Doppler transducer on the maternal abdomen over the location of the fetal back (Figure 25-5).

6. Check that the fetal heart rate (FHR) appears on the monitor screen.

7. Check that the paper strip of the FHR monitor is being printed and that the correct time appears on the strip.

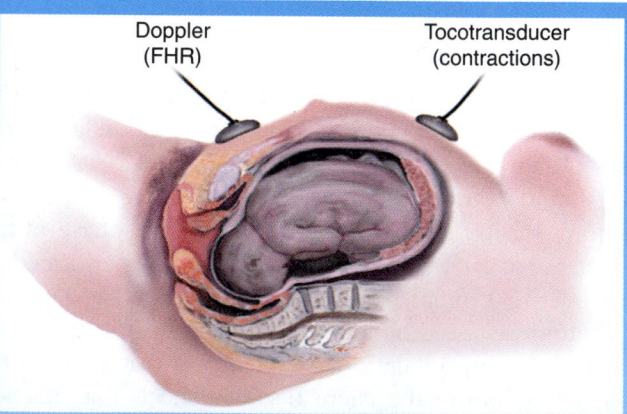

Figure 25-5 Lateral view of correct placement of Doppler and the tocotransducer on the maternal abdomen.

8. Mark the FHR monitor strip with the following information: client's name and medical record number, name of the physician or nurse-midwife, date, time, diagnosis, estimated date of delivery, and weeks of gestation.

(sometimes called a *Doppler*) on the maternal abdomen and the position of the fetus. The ultrasound waves strike the fetal heart, detecting the opening and closing of the valves, and direct a signal back to the transducer (ACOG, July 1995). The FHR can be observed from the bedside monitor or from a centrally located screen. Internal EFM requires a fetal scalp electrode (FSE) that attaches to the fetal scalp after rupture of the membranes (Figure 25-6).

The method and frequency of FHR and contraction monitoring depend on the stage of labor, maternal and fetal risk factors, and the client's preference. The nonstress test is the first line of antepartum fetal assessment (Salamalekis et al., 1997). Parameters for normal and abnormal FHR baseline in the term fetus are shown in Table 25-2 (Cunningham, 1997).

Electronic fetal monitoring gives data that are slightly more objective than does intermittent auscultation, and EFM provides a continuous graphical printout of rate pat-

Table 25-2 Classification of Fetal Heart Rates

Normal range	110–160 beats per minute (bpm)	
Tachycardia		
	Mild	161–180 bpm
	Severe	>180 bpm
Bradycardia		
	Mild	100–110 bpm
	Moderate	80–100 bpm
	Severe	<80 bpm

terns and periodic changes. If the FHR is to be monitored electronically, a 20-minute strip should be obtained on admission for evaluation.

Labor Status

The client's labor status should be assessed in terms of uterine activity, fetal membrane status, cervical status, and fetal descent.

Uterine Activity

In addition to asking the client when her contractions began and whether they are getting stronger, the nurse can evaluate the intensity of contractions by palpating the fundus. Uterine activity is assessed to identify frequency, duration, and intensity of contractions. Uterine resting tone also is evaluated. The presence of uterine irritability or strong and prolonged contractions, that is **hypertonic contractions**, is noted. Assessment of uterine contractions by palpation requires no special equipment but, rather, nursing skill and touch sensitivity. The nurse rests the palmar surface of the hand and fingertips on the fundus, where contractions start, and notes the changing firmness of the uterus as the contraction increases in intensity and then recedes. The firmness of the uterus at the **acme**, or peak, of the contraction is used to determine the intensity, which can be described as mild, moderate, or strong (Figure 25-7).

During mild contractions, the fundus can be indented easily by the fingertips. During moderate contractions, the fundus indents less easily and feels more rigid. During strong contractions, the fundus is firm and resists indenting by the slightly spread fingertips.

The **resting tone**, that is, the firmness of the uterus between contractions, should be soft. The **frequency** of contractions is measured from the beginning of one to the beginning of the next contraction. **Duration** of a contraction is the time from the beginning of a contraction until the end of the same contraction.

Electronically, contractions can be monitored by means of a tocotransducer, which is a pressure-sensing

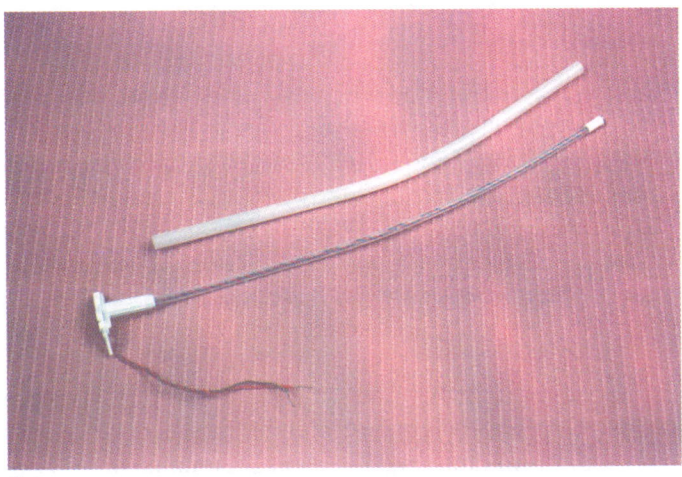

A.

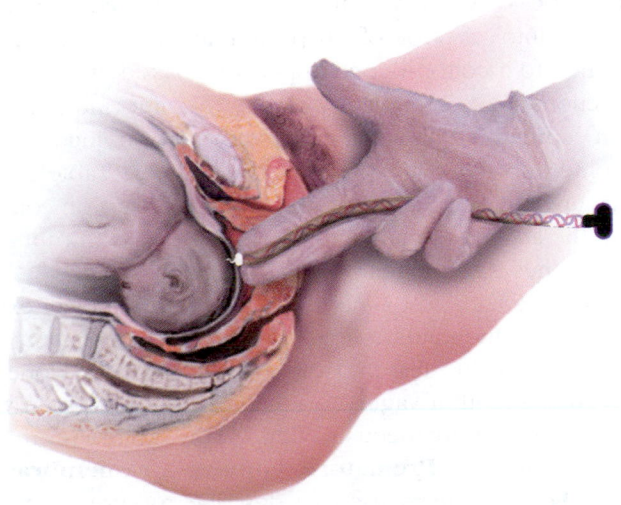

B.

Figure 25-6 A. Fetal scalp electrode. B. Placement of a fetal scalp electrode for fetal heart rate monitoring.

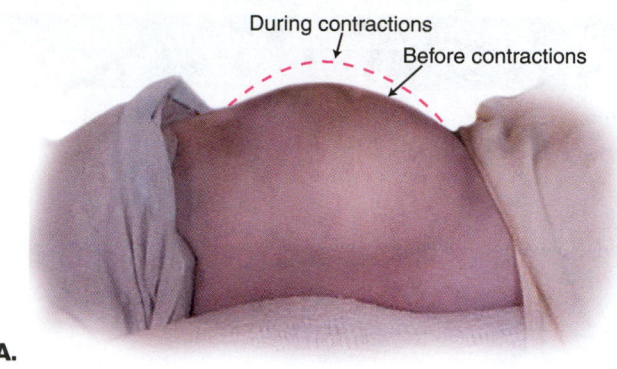

A.

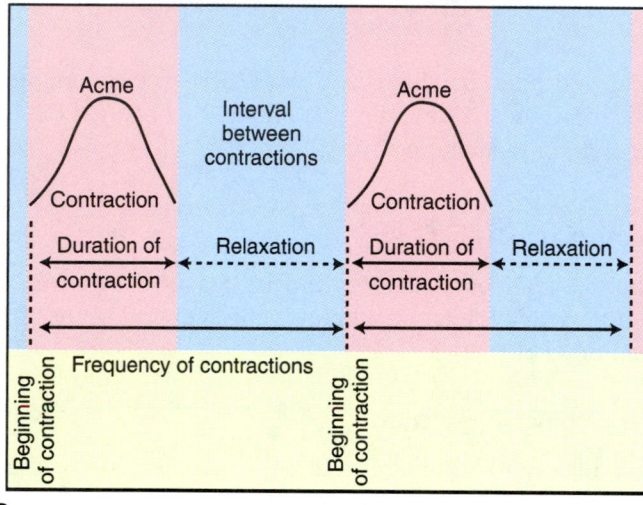

B.

Figure 25-7 A. Abdominal contour before and during a uterine contraction. B. Wavelike pattern of contractions on the fetal heart rate strip.

device placed on the fundus. The tocotransducer detects changes in the shape of the abdominal wall directly above the fundus as each contraction occurs. This noninvasive method gives the nurse information about the frequency and duration of the contractions but not the intensity. Because many women feel contraction pain in the lower back, or in the lower abdomen, they might question why the toco is placed over the fundus instead of where the pain is felt. The nurse should explain that contractions begin at the fundus even though the woman may not experience pain in that particular area.

Accurate information concerning the intensity of contractions only can be obtained internally by means of the **intrauterine pressure catheter (IUPC)**. The IUPC is a fluid-filled catheter that is inserted directly into the uterine cavity through the cervix after the membranes have ruptured (Figure 25-8). In addition to the frequency and duration of contractions, the IUPC records contraction intensity by measuring the pressure of the amniotic fluid inside the uterus in millimeters of mercury (mm Hg). Occasions that might necessitate the use of an IUPC include induction of labor, vaginal birth after cesarean section, and in the very

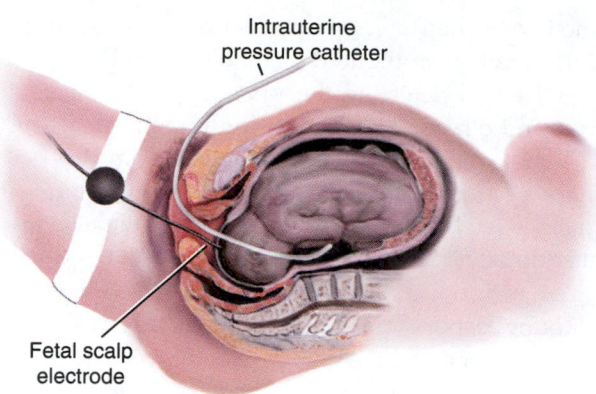

Figure 25-8 Placement of the intrauterine pressure catheter (IUPC) and fetal scalp electrode (FSE).

obese client for whom attempts at external monitoring have been unsuccessful.

Fetal Membrane Status

By the end of pregnancy the uterus contains about 1 L of amniotic fluid (Cunningham, 1997). In abnormal conditions the amount of fluid within the amniotic sac may vary from a few milliliters to several liters. The presence of more than 2 L of amniotic fluid is called **polyhydramnios** and less than 300 mL of fluid is referred to as **oligohydramnios** (Cunningham, 1997). Normal amniotic fluid is colorless and clear, and contains particles of vernix. The odor is characteristic (not foul). As the nurse observes the perineum during physical examination, there may be pooling of amniotic fluid. It is important to establish the time of membrane rupture because a delay of 24 hours or more between membrane rupture and birth, greatly increases the risk for intrauterine infection (Cunningham, 1997). Rupture of membranes may be confirmed by performing a **nitrazine test**, in which a dye-impregnated paper is dipped into a pool of suspected amniotic fluid or is touched to a cotton-tipped applicator soaked with vaginal secretions (Box 25-5). The color of the nitrazine paper is then compared with a color chart showing varying degrees of blue and the corresponding pH number (Table 25-3). Nitrazine paper that turns dark blue (pH of 6.5) on contact with the alkaline amniotic fluid is consistent with ruptured membranes (Cunningham, 1997).

If a Nitrazine test is not definitive and doubt still exists as to membrane status, a **fern test** may be done (Box 25-6).

The nitrazine test and the fern test may be done in conjunction with a vaginal examination. Most women will go into labor spontaneously within a few hours after membranes rupture. **Premature rupture of membranes (PROM)** is the term used to describe rupture of membranes before labor begins. **Preterm premature rupture of membranes (PPROM)** describes rupture of membranes in a preterm pregnancy (less than 38 weeks gesta-

Box 25-5 Procedure for Nitrazine Test for Presence of Amniotic Fluid

1. Explain the procedure to the woman and her partner.

2. Wash your hands, and put on sterile gloves. Do not use lubricating jelly.

3. Use a sterile cotton-tipped applicator to obtain fluid from the vagina. Touch the applicator to the test paper. Alternatively, a strip of nitrazine paper may be touched to the perineum when there is profuse drainage of clear fluid.

4. Compare the color of the nitrazine paper to the color chart.

5. Discard the gloves, and wash your hands.

6. Explain your findings and their implications to the client.

7. Document the numerical result.

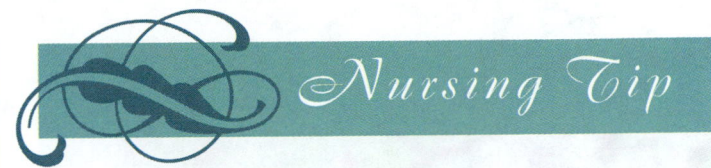

MECONIUM STAINING

Presence of meconium in the amniotic fluid can be the result of vagal stimulation from transient umbilical cord compression or can be caused by fetal hypoxia. Fresh meconium staining in the presence of a nonreassuring fetal heart rate (FHR) pattern, such as severe variables or late FHR decelerations, is an ominous sign. The primary care provider should be notified immediately and requested to come to evaluate the client.

---

tion) in the absence of contractions. Abnormal findings after rupture of membranes include meconium staining, foul odor, and dark-red fluid.

Meconium, when present in the amniotic fluid in a cephalic presentation, often is an indication that the fetus has experienced an episode of hypoxia. Meconium turns the amniotic fluid to yellow or greenish-brown, depending on the amount of meconium present in the fluid. Meconium staining in the presence of a reassuring FHR pattern may indicate that the fetus is not currently in distress. Oligohydramnios, decreased amniotic fluid, reduces the cushioning effect of the fluid. As a result, the cord is more likely to become compressed. Cord compression, and consequent shutting off of the blood flow to and from the fetus, will result in a variable FHR deceleration.

The longer the fetal membranes have been ruptured, the greater the risk of **chorioamnionitis**, which is infection of the fetal membranes.

After taking the medical history, performing FHR monitoring, and assessing the labor status, a vaginal examina-

tion is performed to ascertain whether there has been cervical dilation, that is, whether the woman is in true labor.

Cervical Status and Fetal Descent

Vaginal examination is performed to determine the degree of cervical effacement and dilation, the fetal presenting part, and station. **Effacement** refers to the taking up of the cervical canal so that the cervix changes from a long thick structure to a paper-thin layer (Cunningham, 1997); effacement is reported as a percentage.

Dilation is the term used to describe the widening of the external os of the uterine cervix from closed to a maximum of 10 cm, at which time the cervix is said to be fully

Box 25-6 Procedure for Fern Test for Presence of Amniotic Fluid

1. Explain the procedure to the woman and her partner.

2. Wash your hands, and put on sterile gloves.

3. Use a sterile cotton-tipped applicator to obtain fluid from the vagina (usually done during a sterile speculum examination).

4. Draw the fluid-soaked applicator over a glass slide, and allow it to dry.

5. Examine the glass slide under a microscope and observe for the presence of a frondlike pattern, which indicates amniotic fluid.

6. Discard the gloves, and wash your hands.

7. Explain your findings and their implications to the client.

8. Document the result, that is, a positive or negative fern test.

Table 25-3 Findings on Nitrazine Paper

Color	pH	Membranes
Yellow to olive green	5.0–6.0	Probably intact
Blue-green to deep blue	6.5–7.0	Probably ruptured

The pH values of blood, vaginal mucus, and secretions from some vaginal infections also are alkaline. Be aware of the possibility of false readings.

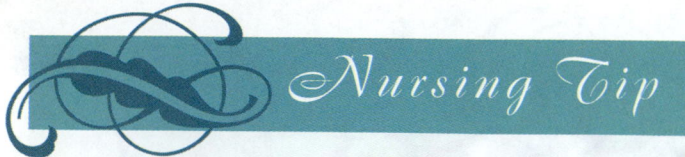

MECONIUM STAINING: BREECH PRESENTATION

In a breech presentation, meconium frequently is passed because the fetal abdomen and buttocks are under pressure. This does not necessarily mean that the fetus is in distress.

dilated (Cunningham, 1997). The **presenting part** is the body part of the fetus that is first to enter the birth canal. The most common presentation is cephalic vertex (Cunningham, 1997). **Vertex** refers to the crown of the infant's head, that is, the portion of the fetal head that is born first when the head is well flexed (Cunningham, 1997).

Station refers to the relationship of the presenting part to an imaginary line drawn between the ischial spines of the maternal pelvis (Figure 25-9), which is the narrowest diameter of the pelvis and designated as zero (0) station (Cunningham, 1997). The long axis between the pelvic inlet and the ischial spines can be divided into thirds, as described by Cunningham (1997), and labeled −3, −2, −1 accordingly; the axis between the ischial spines and the perineal outlet similarly can be divided into thirds and labeled +1, +2, and +3. When the presenting part can be seen at the woman's perineum it is said to be at +3 station.

Abdominal palpation for fetal lie and position (see Leopold's maneuvers, Chapter 23), together with a check of fetal heart tones should precede the initial vaginal examination. Situations such as PROM or preterm labor contraindicate a digital vaginal examination, unless birth appears imminent, because of the infection risk. Vaginal examination should never be done by the nurse if the woman has experienced bleeding during the last trimester of pregnancy or if placenta previa is known or suspected.

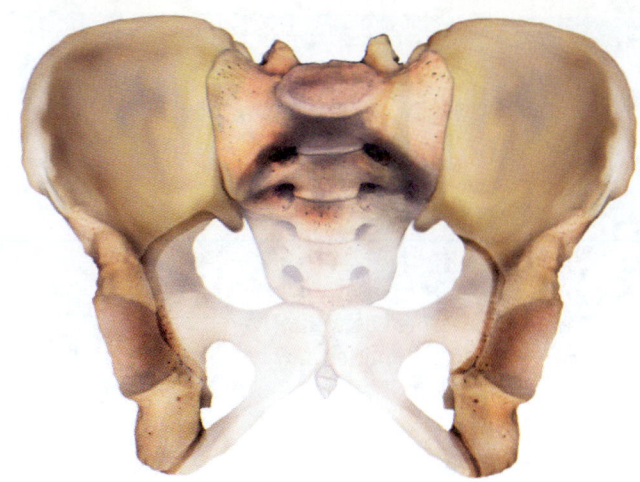

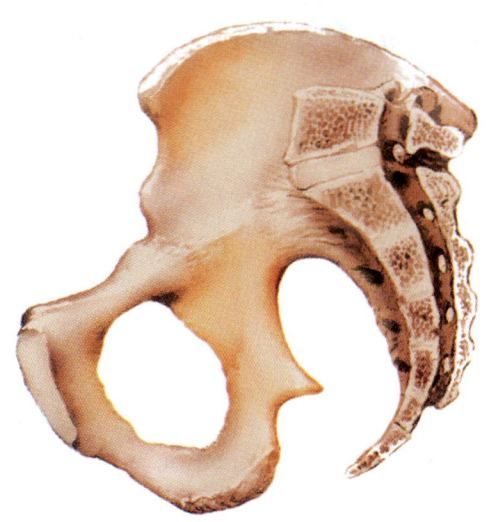

Figure 25-9 Stations of the presenting part. A. Front view. B. Lateral view.

Vaginal examination of a woman with placenta previa might cause severe bleeding.

Before vaginal examination the woman should empty her bladder; a full bladder will add to her discomfort. Vaginal examination can begin between contractions but should be continued throughout a contraction for a more accurate assessment. Examination during a contraction gives a much better picture of the fullest extent of dilation, effacement, and descent. Vaginal examination is an uncomfortable and stressful procedure for the woman. Efforts should be made to reduce stress by first giving a full explanation of the procedure and the information to be obtained from it in terms the woman can understand (Box 25-7). An informed woman is more likely to cooperate throughout

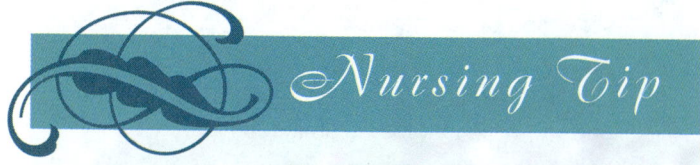

EFFACEMENT

Effacement is a measurement of cervical thickness and is measured in percentages. The uneffaced cervix is about 1-in thick (0% effaced). A cervix that is 2-in thick is 50% effaced.

Box 25-7 Performing a Vaginal Examination on a Woman in Labor

1. Explain the procedure to the client in terms she can understand. Ensure privacy.

2. Position the client on the examination bed, semi-recumbent, with knees bent and legs apart and draped.

3. Wash your hands, and apply sterile gloves.

4. Apply sterile lubricating jelly to the index and second finger of the examining hand.

5. Inspect the general area of the introitus for presence and amount of bloody show, presence and color of amniotic fluid, malodorous discharge, and presence of blisters or ulcerated areas on the labia.

6. With the hand turned sideways and the thumb pointing upward, insert the first and second fingers of the examining hand gently into the vagina, keeping the fourth and fifth fingers bent inward to the palm of the hand. Insert the fingers the length of the vagina.

Membranes

7. Palpate for a soft, bulging membrane sac through the dilating cervix. Observe for running fluid during the examination, which would indicate that the membranes have ruptured.

Effacement

8. Palpate the thickness of the cervix and estimate the degree (0 to 100%) of thinning.

Dilation

9. Dilation of the cervix is measured in centimeters. One fingerbreadth is approximately 1.5 to 2 cm in width, although this measurement will vary among practitioners. Full cervical dilation is 10 cm in diameter.

10. Palpate for the presenting part.

Station

11. Determine the station by locating the lowest portion of the presenting part, then sweeping the fingers to one side of the pelvis to feel for the ischial spines.

12. Remove the fingers, and discard the gloves.

13. Wash your hands.

Nursing Alert

VAGINAL BLEEDING

If a client presents with bright-red vaginal bleeding, particularly if it is painless, you should suspect **placenta previa**, that is, implantation of the placenta near or over the cervical os.

1. Do *not* perform sterile vaginal examination.

2. Notify the primary care provider immediately.

3. Anticipate ultrasonography to rule out placenta previa.

4. Institute continuous electronic fetal monitoring.

the examination. Privacy must be maintained and modesty respected by closing the door or screening the room or triage area and asking the client whether she would like any family members present to step into the waiting room for a few minutes. Vaginal examination should be performed without delay if the woman complains of a desire to bear down or a perception of perineal pressure (Figure 25-10).

The woman is asked to lie down on the hospital bed, with legs bent and apart. Her legs are draped to avoid unnecessary exposure. If the woman knows a relaxation technique, such as slow deep breathing, she should be asked to use it and to try to relax. If it is not certain whether the membranes have ruptured, sterile lubricating jelly is not used because it can sometimes give a false-positive result on a nitrazine test. There may be sufficient vaginal mucus or bloody show to prevent dryness, or

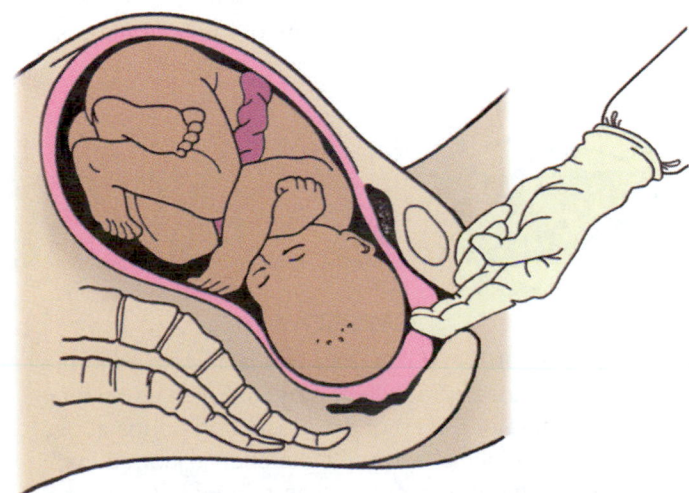

Figure 25-10 Vaginal examination to determine effacement, dilation, and fetal descent.

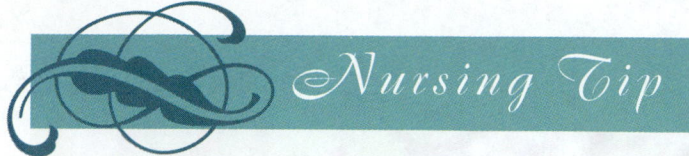

HERPES SIMPLEX VIRUS

When no lesions are visible at the onset of labor, vaginal delivery is acceptable. When primary or recurrent lesions are visible near the time of labor or when the membranes are ruptured or when there are prodromal symptoms of a recurrence (i.e., if the woman complains of herpeslike discomfort), cesarean delivery is performed (Roberts et al., 1995).

sterile water can be used instead of lubricating jelly. Presence of a large amount of bloody show indicates that labor is advanced. If raised vesicles or blisters are noted, the nurse should suspect active herpes viral infection. In the presence of active herpes infection, the examination is stopped and the primary care provider notified. Infants infected with the herpes virus during vaginal birth experience high morbidity (Kohl, 1997). Therefore, cesarean section is performed on all women who have herpes lesions at the time of delivery.

Findings of the examination are communicated to the woman and related to her progress in labor. Information about the labor status may be reassuring to the woman and her partner.

Determine the onset of **true labor** (i.e., regular, strong contractions accompanied by cervical change). When doubt exists as to whether the woman is in labor, she may be advised to ambulate for several hours, taking frequent rest periods. Walking often helps to establish a good contraction pattern. The woman should be instructed to return to her room for FHR monitoring at 30- to 40-minute intervals, or to return immediately if any of the following occur:

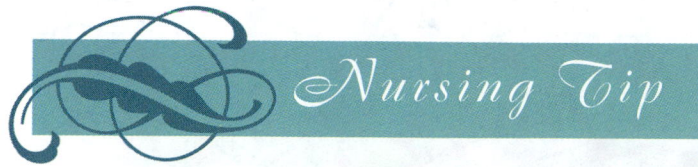

STATION

Imagine a horizontal line from one ischial spine to the other. This line represents 0 station. Estimate how far (in centimeters) the tip of the presenting part is above or below the ischial spine. If the station is judged to be beyond 0, the pelvis probably is adequate for vaginal delivery.

- Membranes rupture.
- Contractions become more frequent than 5-minutes apart.
- Bloody show increases.
- Nausea or vomiting occurs.
- An urge to push is felt.
- She requires analgesia or finds walking too tiring.

General Systems Assessment

The physical examination of the laboring woman is not as extensive as is that performed at the first prenatal visit. The initial assessment is carried out immediately to identify potential problems. Findings of the initial examination will provide a baseline for evaluation and comparison with future clinical findings. The general appearance of the woman is noted, particularly presence of edema in the face, hands, and feet as well as skin color, speech, manner, mood, state of awareness, gait, and personal hygiene. Initial information usually is recorded in the Admission Record; many facilities now have computer systems into which client information is entered directly from the bedside.

Vital Signs

Temperature, pulse, respirations, and blood pressure are assessed on admission and recorded in the Admission Record and nursing flowchart. Frequency of monitoring will depend on the risk status of the maternal-fetal dyad. Infection or dehydration will cause the client's body temperature to increase. The normal range is 97.4°F to 99.6°F, orally or tympanically. Normal heart rate range is 60 to 90 beats per minute (bpm). When auscultating the heart, the nurse will note that the point of maximal impulse is slightly more to the left than usual owing to displacement of the heart by the enlarged uterus. Increased heart rate may be due to excitement, anxiety, or contraction pain. Other possible causes of increased heart rate are cardiac problems or dehydration. Carefully taking the medical history should reveal preexisting medical problems. Dehydration should be considered as a possible reason for a rapid heart rate, in the absence of other causes, and the primary caregiver may require the administration of a 500-mL bolus of intravenous (IV) lactated Ringer's solution. The respiration rate will vary considerably, depending largely on the amount of pain being experienced. Counting of respirations should be done between contractions when the woman is not practicing a breathing technique.

Blood pressure is taken with the woman in a side-lying position, using the uppermost arm; the findings are

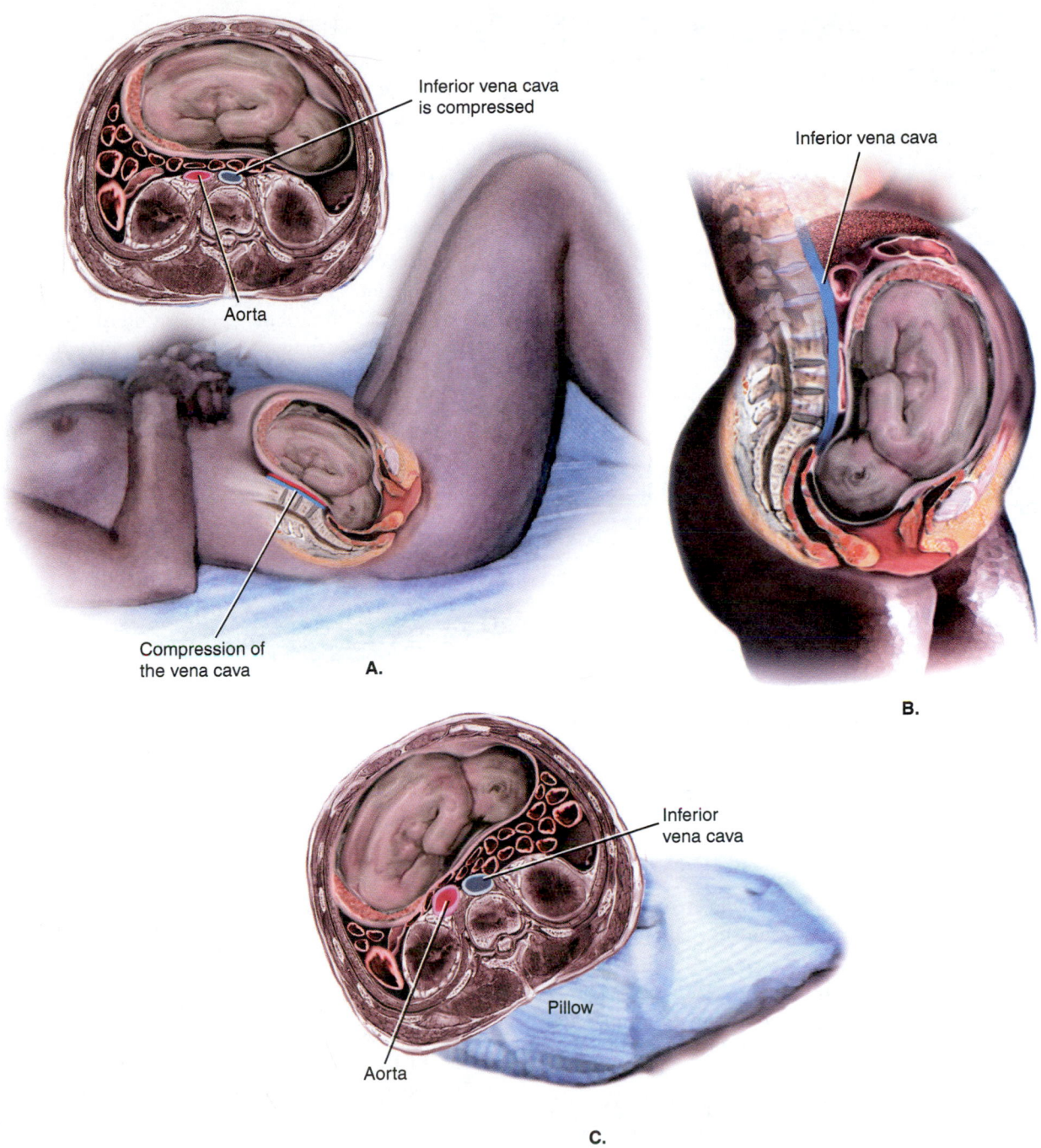

Inferior vena cava
is compressed

Aorta

Compression of
the vena cava

A.

Inferior vena cava

B.

Inferior
vena cava

Pillow

Aorta

C.

Figure 25-11 Vena caval compression (A) can be avoided by upright positioning (B) or by tilting to the side while lying supine (C).

compared with those on the prenatal record. A measurement showing an elevated systolic but normal diastolic blood pressure may indicate anxiety and should be repeated after the woman has had time to relax. To prevent supine hypotension and fetal distress caused by vena caval compression by the heavy uterus, the woman should be encouraged to lie on her side, or on her back with the uterus tilted to one side (Figure 25-11).

Abdomen

Inspect the abdomen for **striae gravidarum,** which are shiny, reddish lines that appear as a result of stretching of the skin and underlying tissue. An abnormal shape of the abdomen should alert the nurse to a possible transverse lie, which would require cesarean delivery. Transverse fetal lie can be identified using Leopold's maneuvers. Previous abdominal surgery will have been noted when the

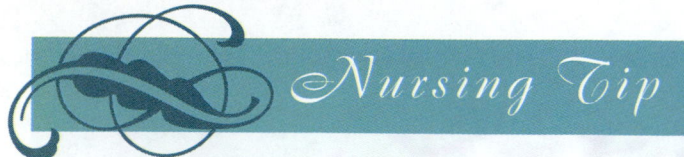

PRESENTING PART

If you feel:

- The hard skull with the sagittal suture, it is a cephalic presentation.
- The softer buttock, it is a breech presentation.
- Irregular parts such as facial features, it is a face presentation.

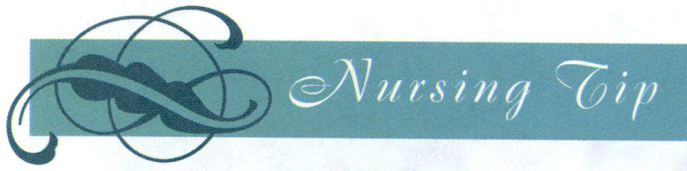

HYPERTENSION

Compare blood pressure readings with those on the prenatal record. The client has hypertension if any of the following is noted:

- Blood pressure value of 140/90 mm Hg or higher.
- A systolic increase of 30 mm Hg or higher.
- A diastolic increase of 15 mm Hg or higher.

medical history was taken, and scarring may be evident. The history of the uterine incision must be obtained. If the uterine scar is classical (not low cervical), the primary care provider should be notified immediately. If a classical incisional scar is seen on the abdomen of a woman in active labor, the primary care provider should be notified immediately because a repeat cesarean delivery will be required and the woman therefore should not be left to labor. Also, to prevent uterine rupture. Although uterine rupture occurs in only 1 of every 2,000 deliveries (ACOG, 1998), it is more of a risk for women who have had a previous transfundal cesarean delivery and can be catastrophic for both mother and fetus.

Bladder

Gently palpate above the symphysis pubis to determine bladder fullness or suprapubic tenderness. Urinary frequency is common in late pregnancy; however, when the woman also complains of burning on urination, the nurse should suspect urinary infection. The nurse should send a catheter specimen or a clean-catch urine specimen for laboratory analysis.

Lower Extremities

Inspect the legs for varicosities and palpate with both hands for tenderness or areas of particular warmth, which might indicate thrombophlebitis. Other frequent physical findings in deep venous thrombosis are swelling, redness, and a positive Homan's sign (ACOG, March 1997).

Edema

Many women experience some dependent edema of the feet during late pregnancy from constriction of blood vessels by the pressure of the pregnant uterus (Box 25-8). Dependent edema usually is less evident when the woman is in bed. Pretibial edema, however, is an abnormal finding as are edema of the hands and edema around the eyes (periorbital edema), and is one of the signs of PIH. Findings of more than 2+ edema or periorbital edema should be reported to the primary care giver along with blood pressure readings and results of dipstick analysis of urine for albumin. The three cardinal signs of PIH are edema, hypertension, and albuminuria.

Deep Tendon Reflexes

Deep tendon reflexes (DTRs) are assessed by supporting the knee in a slightly flexed and quite relaxed position. The patellar tendon is briskly tapped just below the knee cap; responses are graded as per Table 25-4.

Clonus

When the DTR is 3+ or greater (hyperactive), the nurse should be alert to the possibility of clonus, which is associated with preeclampsia. To test for clonus, the knee is supported in a partially flexed position while the nurse applies sharp dorsiflexion to the foot (Figure 25-12). As the foot is maintained in dorsiflexion it will oscillate rhythmically if clonus is present. An abnormal (positive clonus) is recorded as two or more "beats" clonus and indicates irritability of the central nervous system (CNS). The woman should be questioned about other possible indicators of

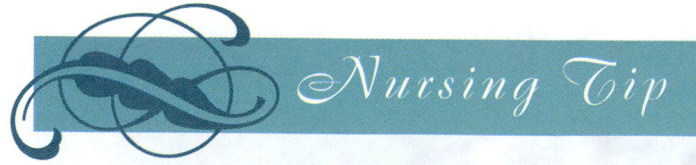

POSITIONING

Ask the client to assume a side-tilt or side-lying position. These positions allow the heavy uterus to be displaced off the ascending vena cava and descending aorta, thus preventing a decrease in cardiac output that may lead to a decrease in maternal blood pressure and subsequent fetal bradycardia.

Box 25-8 Procedure for Assessing Edema

Press firmly with the thumb for about 5 seconds over the pretibial area on both legs. Pretibial edema is assessed as follows:

1+ Small suggestion of fullness is felt.

2+ Sense of fullness.

3+ Blanching of the skin and depression seen as the thumb presses down.

4+ Indentation made by the pressure of the thumb remains for several seconds and gradually recedes.

Table 25-4 Quantifying Deep Tendon Reflexes

Response	Grading
More than normal (brisk)	3+
Normal	2+
Low or sluggish	1+
No response	0

Nursing Alert

C-SECTION INCISIONS

In assessing a woman with a history of C-section, the nurse needs to differentiate between the incision on the skin and the second incision on the uterus. The uterine incision is the determinate for repeat C-sections.

Nursing Alert

HOMAN'S SIGN

Apply dorsiflexion to the client's foot, and ask her whether this action causes calf pain. Calf pain on dorsiflexion of the foot is a positive Homan's sign and must be investigated further for deep vein thrombosis.

---

preeclampsia such as nausea, dizziness, visual disturbances such as "halos" around the lights, epigastric pain, and headache.

Setting Priorities and Making Decisions

Care is prioritized and based on information obtained from the initial prenatal record, physical assessment, and medical history. Care includes early identification and communication of conditions that might place the client in a high-risk category, educational needs, and discharge needs. A system of care is planned for the achievement of goals that are acceptable to both the client and nurse. A critical pathway of care that might be used is shown in Box 25-9. As labor progresses the plan of care is modified according to the ongoing maternal and fetal assessments as well as labor progress. Those women with critical care or high-risk conditions, or who are likely to give birth to an infant requiring neonatal intensive care, may require consultation with or transportation to a medical center with a neonatal intensive care unit.

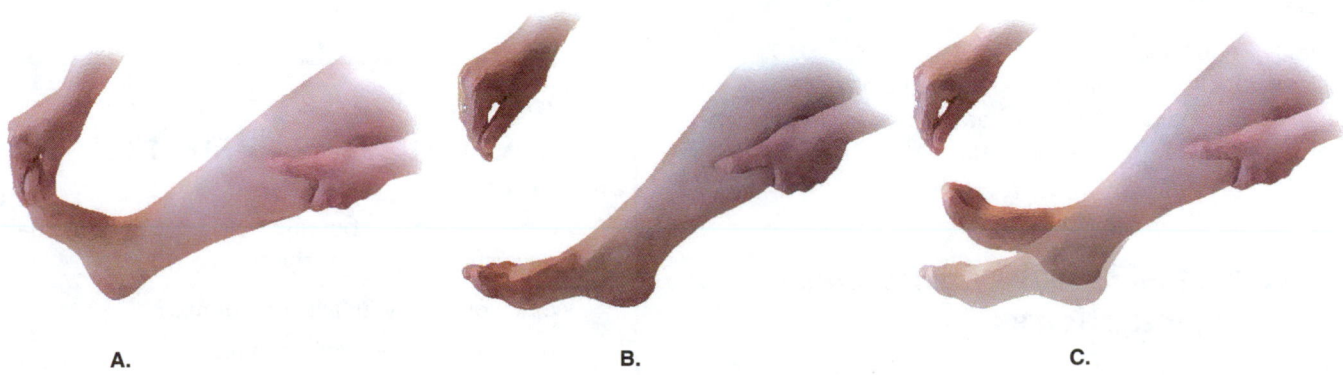

A. B. C.

Figure 25-12 Assessment for clonus. A. Dorsiflexion is applied to the foot. B. Foot returns to neutral position without pulsation. C. Foot oscillates, indicating clonus.

Box 25-9 Critical Pathway for a Client During Low-Risk Labor

Assessment

Monitor fetal heart rate and contractions as per protocol: Continuous _____   Intermittent _____

Sterile vaginal examination.

Blood pressure and pulse every hour.

Temperature every 4 h; every hour after rupture of membranes. (RDM)

Laboratory tests: Typing, Rh status, complete blood count (CBC), rapid plasma reagin (RPR), hepatitis B surface antigen (HbsAg) (unless on prenatal record); HIV test is offered.

Input and output.

Cord gases: Yes _____   No _____

Cord blood sent to laboratory if Rh-negative or blood group type O.

Placenta sent to laboratory: Yes _____   No _____

Consent form signed.

Interventions

Soapsuds enema as required.

Oxygen per non-rebreather face mask at 8–10 L/min as required.

Straight catheter as required if unable to void. If receiving epidural, may insert Foley catheter as required.

Perineal preparation and stirrups at delivery.

Nutrition

Sips of water and ice chips.

Intravenous hydration: Lactated Ringer's solution of 1 L at 125 mL/h and as required afterward.

Activity

May ambulate: Yes _____   No _____

Bathroom privileges (BRP):   Yes _____   No _____

Consultation

Notify pediatrician.

Notify anesthesiologist or Certified Registered Nurse Anesthetist as required.

Notify neonatologist as required.

Maternal-Family Support and Interactions

A woman is more likely to have positive memories of her childbirth experience when she receives kind sensitive care. Her partner, a significant family member, or friend

---

should be encouraged to stay at the bedside and support the woman in labor. The support person also will need attention and should be provided with a comfortable chair and offered opportunities to take meal breaks. The nurse can show the family member how to provide comfort to the woman and should include the support person in discussions about the plan of care. Family interaction and the support system are evaluated as labor progresses, always taking cultural beliefs into consideration. When the woman does not have a support person with her, the nurse becomes the support person.

Many women attend childbirth preparation classes and develop expectations in the form of an individualized birth plan. When presented with a birth plan the nurse should consider the safety of the plan, importance of the plan to the client, and feasibility of incorporating some or all of the woman's wishes into the nursing process. It is important for the nurse to be respectful and flexible.

Psychological Considerations During the Latent Phase of Labor

The woman who comes to the hospital in the latent phase of labor often is mildly anxious both about her well-being and that of the baby, and also about how she will react to

Critical Thinking

Prioritize!

A client is rushed to labor and delivery in a wheelchair. She says she feels like pushing.

What would be your initial response?

How would you set your priorities?

the pain of contractions. The hospital is an unfamiliar environment, and the nurse is a stranger to her. The nursing interview and interventions must be performed in a competent and respectful manner that promotes trust and facilitates relaxation. One of the most important nurse behaviors, as perceived by the patient, is that the nursing staff know what they are doing (Manogin, Bechtel, & Rami, 2000). The approach of the nurse should be accepting and supportive of the woman as an individual. Cultural practices related to childbirth also need to be considered.

To provide appropriate teaching to the client, the nurse must first evaluate the amount of preparation for childbirth she has had. Other factors to consider are the stage of labor, maturity of the client previous experience of childbirth, and educational level. During the initial orientation to the labor and delivery or triage room and the primary assessment, the nurse can make inquiries as to any childbirth classes the woman may have attended or books she has read. This also is a good time to ask whether the woman has specific concerns that may be causing anxiety. Family members also should be included in any teaching. Client teaching is an ongoing process, and it is important for the nurse to explain what is happening to the woman during each stage of labor. Examination findings also should be fully explained; some labor rooms have a chart depicting cervical dilation to which the nurse might refer.

The client participates in the plan of care. The rationale for recommended interventions, as well as risks, should be explained fully. Frequent reinforcement usually is necessary. Teaching includes an explanation of the purpose of equipment that is likely to be used, such as the electronic fetal monitor, the correct method of timing contractions, and activity that will be helpful to the woman. Many primary caregivers may allow the woman to have sips of water and ice chips during normal labor. Some women prefer to ambulate during the early phase of labor, returning to the labor and delivery room for intermittent FHR monitoring. The woman and her support person should be shown the correct method of timing contractions.

Explanations are given about the current stage of labor and available options for pain management, when and how they can be administered, and the effect they are likely to have. Although the woman may have received previous instruction about breathing and relaxation techniques, these may need to be reviewed and reinforced. Teaching and the client's response should be recorded in the flowchart.

Documentation and Communication

Admission data are documented in the medical chart and nursing flowchart and communicated to the appropriate health care team members such as the physician or nurse-midwife, social worker, pediatrician, or neonatologist. Charting of all interventions, medications, and clinical findings is done according to the accepted procedure of the facility and may involve flowcharts or computer-generated charting.

Laboratory Tests

After the initial assessment of the client, the nurse should anticipate the need for laboratory tests according to the hospital protocol.

Urine Specimen Analysis

Urinalysis can be done by the nurse, using a dipstick, to examine for the presence of protein, glucose, blood, and ketones. Urinalysis can be done using a voided specimen, as free as possible from debris. Urinalysis can alert the nurse to possible complications such as PIH (albuminuria), diabetes mellitus (glucose), or inadequate nutrition (ketones). Laboratory urinalysis can provide additional information about hydration status (specific gravity) and infection (presence of leukocytes).

Blood Tests

Blood tests vary with the hospital protocol and risk factors. Information that usually can be obtained from the prenatal record includes results of tests for the following: blood type, Rh factor, atypical antibodies, rubella, syphilis (rapid plasma reagin [RPR], or VDRL test), hepatitis B, glucose levels, and HIV.

Although sufficient information may be available from prenatal records, on hospital admission the hematocrit and hemoglobin levels should be rechecked and an RPR test performed. Many hospitals require a complete blood cell count (CBC), and confirmation of blood type and Rh factor. Blood may be saved in the laboratory for use in crossmatching should the client require a blood transfusion. A screening test for HIV is offered. The role of the nurse is to explain the purpose of drawing blood and often to draw blood and order the tests according to the hospital protocol. Only when all examinations, including laboratory review, are completed can a decision be reached about the normalcy of the pregnancy.

NURSING RESPONSIBILITIES DURING LABOR

Labor progresses through four stages, as outlined in Box 25-10. Nursing responsibilities to the laboring woman and family are tied to the stage of labor and the woman's changing needs.

> ## Box 25-10 Stages and Phases of Labor
> ### First Stage (0–10 cm dilated)
>
> Latent phase: 0–3 cm; contractions are mild every 15–30 min and last for 30 s
>
> Active phase: 4–7 cm; contractions are moderate every 3–5 min and last for 40 s
>
> Transition phase: 8–10 cm; contractions are strong every 2–3 min and last for 60 s
>
> ### Second Stage (10 cm dilated to birth)
>
> Contractions: Every 2–3 min
>
> Duration of contractions: 60–90 s
>
> Duration of second stage: 5 min–2 h
>
> ### Third Stage (birth to delivery of placenta)
>
> Duration: 5–45 min
>
> ### Fourth Stage (recovery)
>
> Duration: 1–4 h

First Stage of Labor

The **first stage of labor** begins with the initiation of regular contractions that produce cervical dilation and continues through complete dilation. The first stage is the longest one and is composed of three phases. The latent phase is followed by the active phase and then the transition phase. Nursing assessment of the mother and fetus is ongoing.

Maternal Assessment

Assessment of the woman in the first stage of labor includes evaluation of vital signs, hydration status, and elimination.

Vital Signs

Vital signs of the mother include blood pressure, temperature, pulse, and respiration. Frequency of assessment is determined by the stage of labor and risk status of the maternal-fetal dyad. Monitoring will be more frequent in high-risk situations. Vital signs are monitored between contractions and recorded on the FHR strip and the nursing flowchart.

Blood Pressure is measured between contractions every hour during active labor, if normal. During a uterine contraction approximately 500 mL of blood is shunted into the central circulation, elevating the maternal blood pressure. The normal range of blood pressure is 100 to 120 mm Hg systolic and 60 to 80 mm Hg diastolic. An increase of 30 mm Hg systolic and 15 mm Hg diastolic above the prepregnancy blood pressure level may be indicative of PIH (Cunningham, 1997). Hypertension is defined as a sustained blood pressure of 140 mm Hg systolic or 90 mm Hg diastolic, and the risk of developing PIH is increased in women with preexisting chronic hypertension (ACOG, 1996).

Temperature is an important indicator of hydration and infection and may be slightly elevated throughout labor. Temperature is taken on admission and every 4 hours until the membranes rupture, after which it is recorded every 2 hours. Once the fetal membranes are ruptured, there is an increased risk of ascending infection. For this reason all invasive procedures, such as vaginal examinations, are kept to a minimum. If the membranes are ruptured an elevated temperature could indicate chorioamnionitis, particularly if they have been ruptured for more than 12 hours. A increasing temperature should be reported to the primary caregiver. Foul odor of the amniotic fluid is a late sign of chorioamnionitis.

Meconium may support bacterial growth. For this reason, there is also a potential for chorioamnionitis when there is meconium staining.

Heart rate and respirations vary according to maternal exertion during labor, hydration, infection, and anxiety level. Respirations also are affected by the level of pain and breathing techniques used to cope with labor. **Hyperventilation**, a change in the oxygen-carbon dioxide exchange, is a consequence of breathing too rapidly and too deeply. If the woman complains of tingling sensations in the palms of her hands, she may be hyperventilating and should be urged to slow her breathing. This condition also can be corrected by having the woman rebreathe her exhaled air by breathing into a paper bag or examining glove.

Hydration and Nutrition

Gastric emptying time is prolonged during active labor, so that ingested food remains in the stomach and may be vomited. Oral fluids usually are well tolerated throughout labor but should be limited to ice chips or sips of water or clear fluids, as tolerated. The various breathing techniques used by laboring women to cope with painful contractions usually result in a dry mouth and craving for sips of water or ice chips.

The woman is asked when she last had something to eat or drink, and the times are noted in the medical record. When general anesthesia is a possibility, the woman receives nothing by mouth to prevent vomiting. Aspiration of acidic gastric contents into the lungs is life-threatening to the woman and fetus. When the primary caregiver requires the woman to be NPO, the nurse provides mouthwashes and applies petroleum jelly to the lips to alleviate dryness.

Intravenous fluids provide calories and prevent dehydration in the laboring woman. Many facilities, particularly in physician-assisted deliveries, require IV hydration as part of the routine protocol for the laboring woman. Starting an IV may be delayed for the woman in early labor who is ambulating. For hydration, an 18-gauge or 20-gauge cannula is inserted into a vein of the hand or forearm and connected to tubing attached to a 1-L bag of lactated Ringer's solution or dextrose 5% lactated Ringer's solution infusing at 125 mL/h. This constitutes the main IV line and facilitates administration of analgesics or other appropriate medications into one of the access ports. Antibiotics, oxytocics, or tocolytics can be diluted and inserted by piggyback into the main line. An accurate record of fluid intake and output should be maintained.

Elimination

Voiding every 2 hours is encouraged because a full bladder can impede descent of the presenting part. The nurse should palpate the suprapubic region to detect a distended bladder. When the bladder is readily palpated and the woman is unable to void, catheterization is indicated. If the woman wishes to get up to walk to the bathroom the nurse should assist her in doing so by lowering the bed, unplugging the FHR monitoring cables, and moving the IV pole. Urinary output is measured and dipstick testing for glucose, albumin, and ketones performed every shift. The woman who is receiving epidural anesthesia should not be permitted to get out of bed to walk to the bathroom because partial loss of muscle strength in the legs is common. A Foley catheter, attached to bedside drainage, frequently is inserted if the woman is receiving epidural anesthesia because urinary retention is a very frequent side effect of this regional anesthesia.

The use of enemas is infrequent but should be offered to the woman who is in early labor and has not had a recent bowel movement. As the fetal head descends, it exerts pressure on the lower bowel and any stool that is present will be expelled during the second stage of labor. Passage of fecal matter during the birth is embarrassing for the client and also increases the risk for infection. As the fetal head descends, the woman will experience increased pressure in the rectal area.

Fetal Assessment

The FHR is assessed as per the hospital policy, taking into consideration the phase and stage of labor and maternal and fetal risk factors. Certain abbreviations are commonly used by labor and delivery personnel when documenting baseline, variability, and periodic changes in FHR (Box 25-11).

Baseline Fetal Heart Rate

In order to determine a **baseline fetal heart rate**, that is, the FHR between contractions and accelerations, the FHR must be observed *between* contractions. Because the FHR is an inherently irregular rate, accuracy will be improved by charting it as a *range,* for example, 130 to 140 bpm. The FHR baseline during the third trimester ranges from 110 to 160 bpm, and a FHR strip of at least 10-minutes' duration should be taken before a baseline is established (ACOG, July 1995).

Fetal Heart Rate Variability

Fetal heart rate **variability** (fluctuations in the FHR) has two components: **long-term variability** (the slow rhythmic fluctuations above and below an average baseline rate, producing a wavelike pattern) and **short-term (or beat-to-beat) variability**, which are instantaneous fluctuations in the FHR. The combination of these two types of variability reflects the interaction between parasympathetic (which slows the heart) and sympathetic (which accelerates the heart) branches of the CNS.

The criteria for long-term variability (LTV) does not include accelerations or decelerations. Evaluation of the LTV helps identify changes in the fetal behavioral state

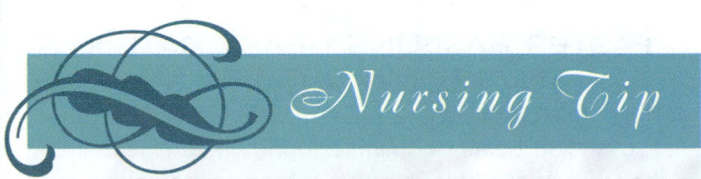

ELIMINATION

If the woman in active labor expresses the need to have a bowel movement, the nurse should perform a vaginal examination to assess cervical dilation and station. Examination may reveal significant descent of the presenting part.

Box 25-11 Common Abbreviations in Fetal Monitoring	
bpm	Beats per minute
EFM	Electronic fetal monitoring
FHR	Fetal heart rate
FSE	Fetal scalp electrode
UC	Uterine contraction
IUPC	Intrauterine pressure catheter
LTV	Long-term variability
STV	Short-term variability
TOCO	Tocodynamometer (external)
US	Ultrasonography

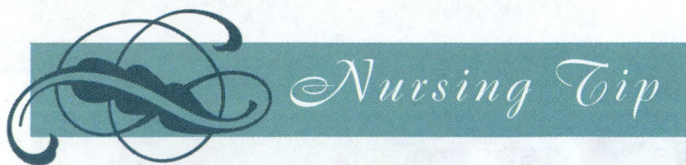

FETAL BRADYCARDIA OR MATERNAL HEART RATE?

Always make certain that the rate you are recording using the external fetal heart rate monitor is not the same rate as the woman's radical or apical pulse. When the fetus changes position, the transducer may start picking up the maternal heart rate.

and the response to labor. Absent LTV might also be described as a "flat" FHR. Marked LTV, or **saltatory pattern**, is a term that describes a baseline that is chaotic and jumps up and down multiple times each minute. The presence of two spontaneous accelerations of greater than 15 bpm for at least 15 seconds' duration in 20 minutes is a reassuring sign. When LTV is present, STV also is almost always present.

Short-term variability (STV) or beat-to-beat variability can only be realistically visualized with internal FHR monitoring and is documented as minimal, moderate, or marked. STV variability can be present in the absence of LTV.

Nursing Alert

CAUSES AND PHYSIOLOGY OF ABSENT LONG-TERM VARIABILITY

- Fetal quiescent state that may last 90 min.
- Medications, for example, central nervous system depressants.
- Hypoxia owing to placental insufficiency.
- Severe fetal anemia, for example, as a result of a fetal viral infection.
- Arrhythmia such as a supraventricular tachycardia or complete heart block.
- Fetal brain death or decerebration.
- Congenital brain anomaly, for example, anencephaly or a heart anomaly or conduction defect.
- Late sign of deterioration of the fetus having intrauterine growth retardation.
- Terminal bradycardia (low baseline and absent LTV, not related to an arrhythmia, suggesting impending intrauterine death).

Periodic and Nonperiodic Fetal Heart Rate Changes

Periodic fetal heart rate changes are transient changes in FHR in association with contractions (Cunningham, 1997). **Nonperiodic fetal heart rate changes** are transient changes in FHR not associated with contractions, although they can occur during contractions. Specific classifications are defined by ACOG (1995) as follows:

1. **Acceleration:** An increase in FHR above the baseline level, with a return to baseline within 10 minutes. An increase in FHR lasting longer than 10 minutes is classified as an increase in FHR baseline.

2. **Deceleration:** A distinct decrease below the baseline, with a return to the baseline within 10 minutes. Decelerations are classified by their shape and timing in relation to uterine contractions as follows:
   Early–U-shaped deceleration that begins and ends with the contraction. The heart rate reaches its nadir at the peak of the contraction.
   Variable–May have a V or W shape. May occur during or between contractions, on-set is usually abrupt.
   Late–Usually has a gradual onset. Nadir of the deceleration usually occurs after the peak of the contraction.

Accelerations

Accelerations are the most common type of FHR change (Figure 25-13). Periodic accelerations are not a sign of fetal distress; they are a reassuring sign that the fetus is able to increase his or her heart rate to compensate for the stress of contractions. Periodic accelerations begin with the onset of the contraction and return to the baseline at the end of

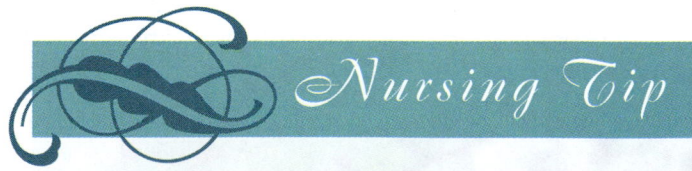

FASTER BASELINE HEART RATE IN THE PREMATURE FETUS

The normal baseline fetal heart rate (FHR) ranges from 110 to 160 beats per minute (bpm). In early fetal life the sympathetic branch of the autonomic nervous system (ANS) establishes and maintains the baseline FHR, which tends to be in the upper range (150 to 160 bpm). As the fetus matures, the parasympathetic branch of the ANS exerts a slowing effect, bringing the baseline into the lower range (110 to 140 bpm) by term.

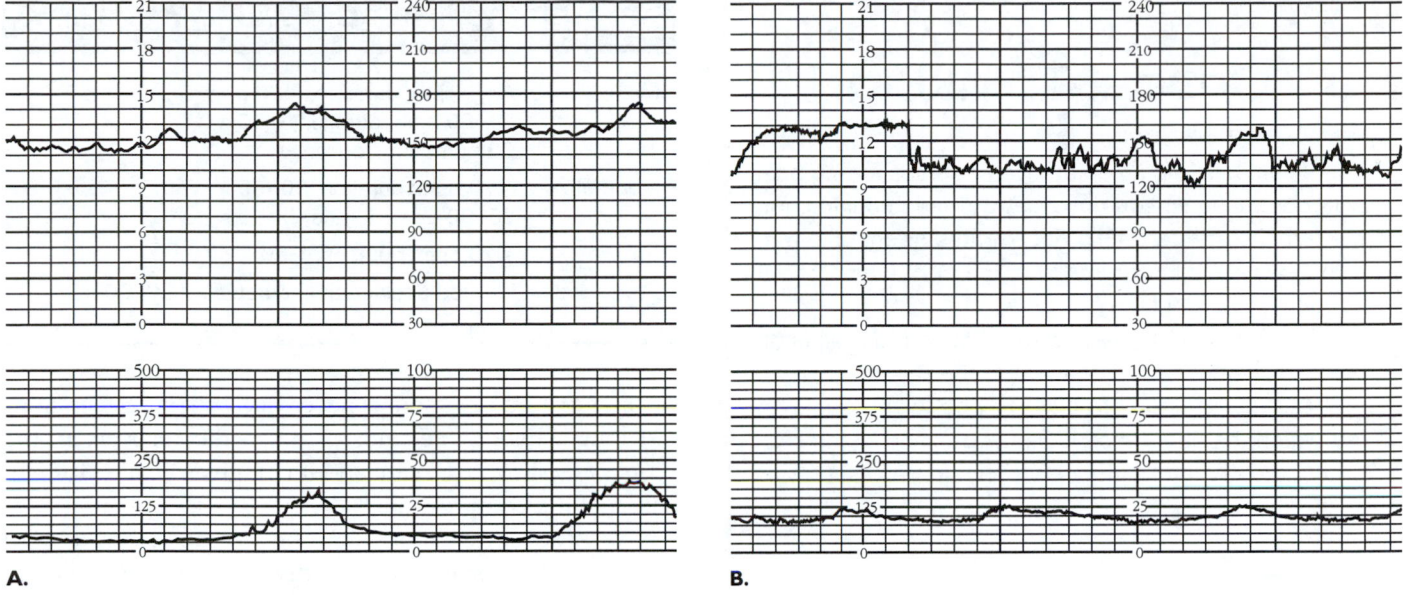

Figure 25-13 A. Periodic accelerations. B. Nonperiodic accelerations.

the contraction. Nonperiodic accelerations are not associated with contractions. Nonperiodic accelerations most often are seen with fetal activity and during pelvic examination; they are reassuring of fetal well-being. Nonperiodic accelerations have no regular pattern. The presence of spontaneous accelerations of at least 15 bpm lasting at least 15 seconds is almost always an indication of the absence of fetal acidosis (ACOG, July 1995).

Early Onset Decelerations

Early onset decelerations involve a transitory decrease in FHR caused by fetal head compression, which stimulates the vagus nerve to decrease the heart rate. Early decelerations during the second stage of labor, in the presence of adequate descent of the presenting part, usually are benign and reflect compression of the fetal head as it enters the birth canal.

An early deceleration is characterized by a gradual onset at the beginning of a contraction and a slow return to the baseline soon after the contraction ends, like a mirror image of the contraction (Figure 25-14). The slope is gradual and the depth of the deceleration reflects the intensity of the contraction. Early decelerations occur most frequently with vertex presentations in the second stage of labor, during pushing.

No treatment is necessary for early decelerations that occur in the transition phase of the first stage of labor or during pushing in the second stage, provided the vertex is descending and the FHR recovers. If, during the second stage of labor, it becomes difficult to determine the baseline owing to the frequency of early decelerations, the woman should be instructed to stop pushing until the fetus

has recovered and the FHR has returned to baseline. If early decelerations are observed while the presenting part is still above the level of the ischial spines, cephalopelvic disproportion should be ruled out.

Variable Decelerations

Variable decelerations are transitory decreases in FHR caused by umbilical cord compression. Variable decelerations are characterized by rapid onset, rapid return to baseline, and a variable relationship to the contraction (Cunningham, 1997). As long as the baseline rate remains stable

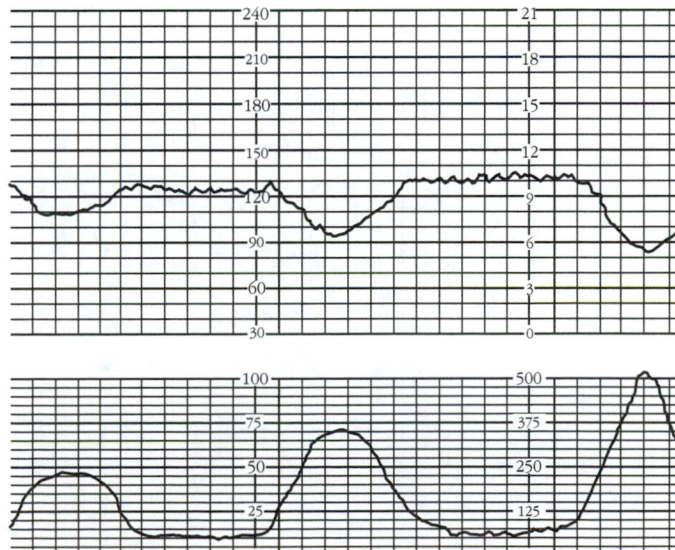

Figure 25-14 Early decelerations.

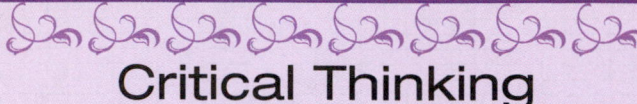

Critical Thinking

Early Decelerations

Your client has had an epidural and denies feeling pain with contractions. You note that with each contraction the fetal heart rate (FHR) decelerates so that the pattern looks like a mirror image of the contraction. What action should you take?

Perform a sterile vaginal examination to assess dilation of the cervix and descent of the presenting part.

The appearance of early FHR decelerations is an indication that labor may have progressed to the second stage; therefore, the cervix should be assessed.

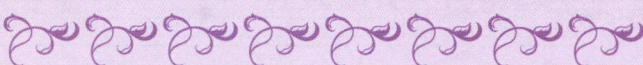

Table 25-5 Variable Decelerations Defined	
Mild	Any depth; duration, <30 s
	70–80 bpm; duration, <60 s
	80 bpm; duration, any
Moderate	<70 bpm; duration, 30–60 s
	70–80 bpm; duration, <60 s
Severe	<70 bpm; duration, >60 s
Prolonged	Isolated deceleration; duration, >60–90 s

and the variability is good, variable decelerations are not associated with poor fetal outcome. Variable decelerations have no consistent shape and may appear V-shaped, W-shaped, or U-shaped; they may begin or end at any time in relation to the contraction curve (Figure 25-15).

Variable decelerations occur most frequently after rupture of membranes, when there is less amniotic fluid to provide a protective cushion around the cord. Other circumstances that could result in compression or stretching of the cord causing variable decelerations are the following: loops of the umbilical cord around the fetal neck or shoulder, a true knot in the cord, or prolapsed cord. Variable decelerations are defined according to their depth and duration (Table 25-5). Many variable decelerations are

so brief that no treatment is necessary. When decelerations last longer than 30 seconds or when the recovery to the baseline is slow, treatment should be given to alleviate the cause of the compression.

Variable decelerations may be preceded or followed by acceleratory phases or shoulders. A **shoulder** is not an acceleration but is an acceleratory phase of a deceleration pattern. It is a compensatory sign of an intact fetal CNS. Appropriate descriptive documentation in the medical record should read as follows: "Variable decelerations with shoulders."

Occasionally a rebound increase in the FHR occurs after a variable deceleration. This is called an **overshoot** and consists of an increase of 20 or more bpm above the baseline or an increase above the baseline for more than 20 seconds. An overshoot is not an acceleration but is part of a variable deceleration pattern (Murray, 1997). An overshoot is a nonreassuring sign and could indicate significant hypoxemia or hypoxia. The primary caregiver should be notified immediately of such a FHR pattern, particularly if there is absent STV or an increasing baseline (Murray, 1997).

Late Onset Decelerations

Late onset decelerations are transitory decreases in the FHR caused by **uteroplacental insufficiency**, which is compromised blood flow from the placenta to the fetus (ACOG, July 1995). Late decelerations have the following characteristics: uniform shape similar to early onset decelerations, smooth, and U-shaped (Figure 25-16). The late

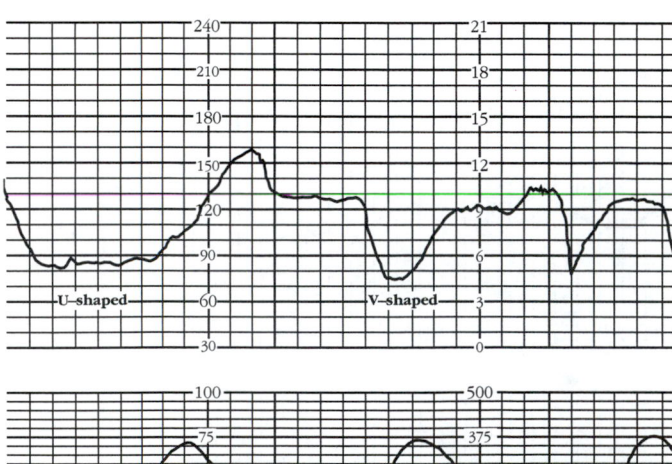

Figure 25-15 Variable decelerations.

Nursing Alert

LATE DECELERATIONS

Late decelerations are caused by uteroplacental insufficiency (low oxygen delivery) and are nonreassuring. The primary caregiver must be notified without delay of the appearance of late decelerations on the fetal heart rate monitor strip and should come to assess the client immediately.

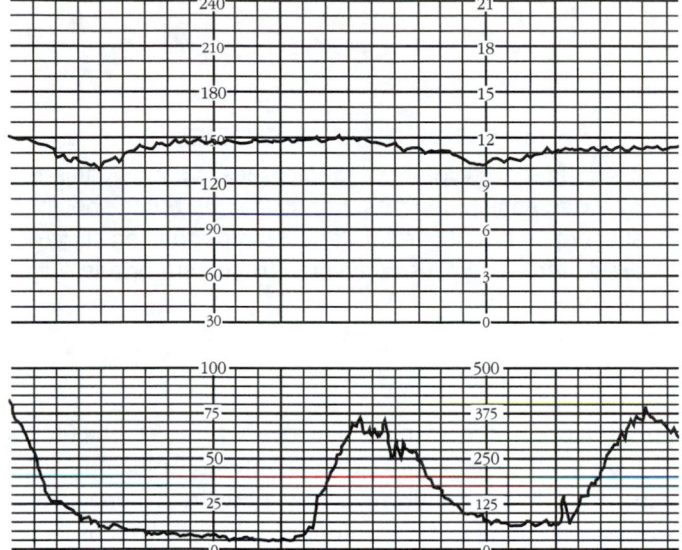

Figure 25-16 Late decelerations.

deceleration, however, starts at about the time the contraction is at its height and does not return to baseline until after the contraction has ended (ACOG, July 1995). When a pattern of late FHR deceleration occurs, the primary caregiver should be requested to review the FHR strip and assess the client without delay.

Interventions for Nonreassuring Fetal Heart Rate Pattern

Nursing interventions that should be initiated for a nonreassuring FHR pattern depend on the signs and probable cause, and include the following:

1. Change the maternal position from one side to the other side, particularly if umbilical cord compression is suspected. Changing the maternal position is almost always the first nursing intervention to consider and may be the only intervention necessary.

2. Oxygen therapy by non-rebreather face mask at 8 to 10 L/min. The theory is that oxygen therapy will saturate the mother's blood with oxygen so that when the cord compression is relieved, the fetus will have a good supply of oxygen to use in recovering a normal heart rate.

3. Increase the rate of the main IV fluid line (usually lactated Ringer's solution) to increase perfusion of the placenta, particularly if a decrease in blood pressure has occurred.

4. If moving the client from one side to the other does not relieve the problem, sterile vaginal examination should be performed to rule out prolapsed cord. If prolapsed cord is feared, move the client to the hands and knees position and have her bend her arms until she is resting on her knees and forearms (Figure 25-17). This position helps to shift the weight of the fetus off the cervix and off the umbilical cord.

5. Notify the primary care provider the time of occurrence, duration, severity, and frequency of decelerations and of nursing interventions given. The nurse also should document the rationale behind interventions provided.

6. Anticipate administration of a tocolytic such as terbutaline, 0.25 mg subcutaneously or 0.125 to 0.25 mg IV (ACOG, Dec. 1995), if the woman is experiencing hypertonic contractions, resulting in inadequate resting tone between contractions.

7. Anticipate starting an **amnioinfusion**, which is instillation of an isotonic glucose-free solution (such as

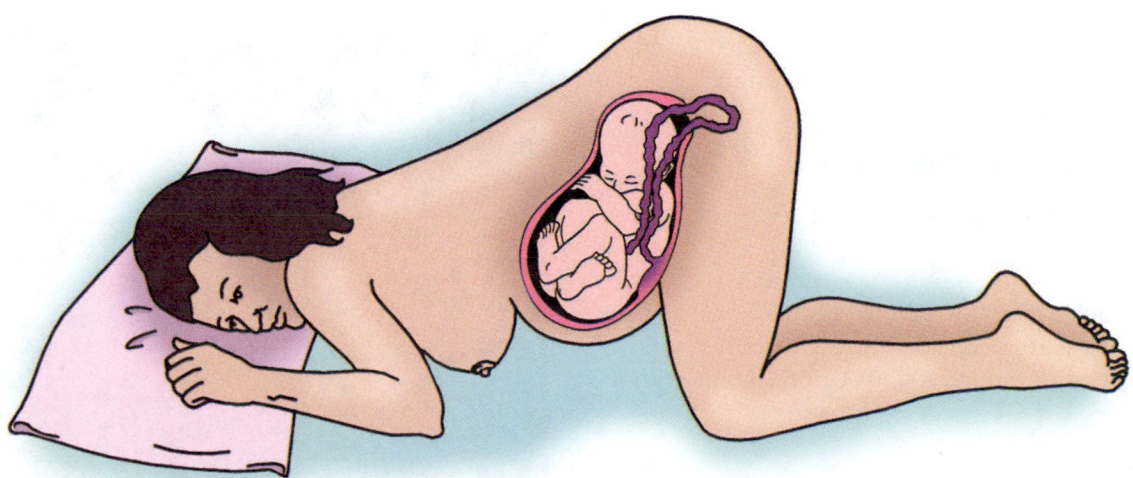

Figure 25-17 Elbows and knees position to relieve pressure on a prolapsed umbilical cord.

normal saline or lactated Ringer's solution) into the uterus to cushion the umbilical cord or to thin out meconium.

8. Chart all information, including the time the primary care giver was notified, the specific information given, and the response. It is acceptable to write, "No new orders received."

When interventions do not improve the FHR pattern, and depending on the seriousness of the deceleration and the stage of labor, the nurse should be prepared to move the client into the operating room for emergency cesarean delivery.

Labor Progress

The nurse assesses the woman throughout labor to establish normal progress during each stage and phase. The primiparous client may be expected to experience a longer labor than would the multiparous woman.

Uterine Assessment

Contraction patterns are monitored carefully, as discussed in the section on Admission Procedures. As the contractions intensify, the nurse continues to assess their frequency, duration, and intensity, and the adequacy of the resting tone. The minimal contractile pattern of 95% of women in spontaneous labor consists of three to five contractions in a 10-minute window. When the woman is having internal uterine monitoring, Montevideo Units, or MVU (a numerical method of calculating adequacy of contraction strength), can be calculated. MVU equals the total strength of contractions, in mm Hg, in a 10-minute window. The equation is as follows:

Total strength of all contractions in a 10-minute window − Total resting tone of all contractions in a 10-minute window = MVU

For example, if the woman has three contractions in 10 minutes of 90, 75, and 85 mm Hg and the resting tone is 20 mm Hg, then the MVU equals 190 mm Hg:

$$(90 + 75 + 85 \text{ mm Hg}) - (20 \text{ mm Hg} \times 3)$$

$$= 250 \text{ mm Hg} - 60 \text{ mm Hg}$$

$$= 190 \text{ mm Hg}$$

Most women achieve 200 to 225 MVU, and some achieve 300 MVU. A woman is considered to have arrested labor when she exceeds a rate of 200 MVU for 2 hours without cervical change.

Rupture of Fetal Membranes

If the fetal membranes were still intact when the woman arrived at the hospital, they may rupture spontaneously

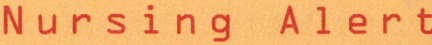

Nursing Alert

PROLAPSED CORD

If spontaneous rupture of membranes is accompanied by a decrease in the fetal heart rate, the nurse should suspect umbilical cord prolapse and perform an immediate sterile vaginal examination to confirm or rule out this emergency.

during labor. If the woman states either that she has felt a sudden gush of fluid or has inadvertently urinated in the bed, the nurse should check the bed linen beneath the woman for pooling of amniotic fluid. When membranes rupture spontaneously, the first nursing responsibility is to check the FHR, because the gush of amniotic fluid could possibly cause a segment of umbilical cord to prolapse or become pinched between the fetal head and the cervix. The first indication of such an emergency would be a variable FHR deceleration.

If fetal membranes do not spontaneously rupture, the primary caregiver may perform **amniotomy**, artificial rupture of membranes (AROM). The rationale for AROM is to slightly shorten the length of labor, although there is no research to suggest that this is beneficial to either the mother or fetus.

One benefit of AROM is the earlier detection of meconium staining of amniotic fluid. Once the membranes are ruptured, a FSE can be applied for more accurate monitoring of the FHR. Amniotomy usually is done by the use of an **amnihook**, which is a plastic implement with a blunt hook at the distal end (Figure 25-18). AROM also can be

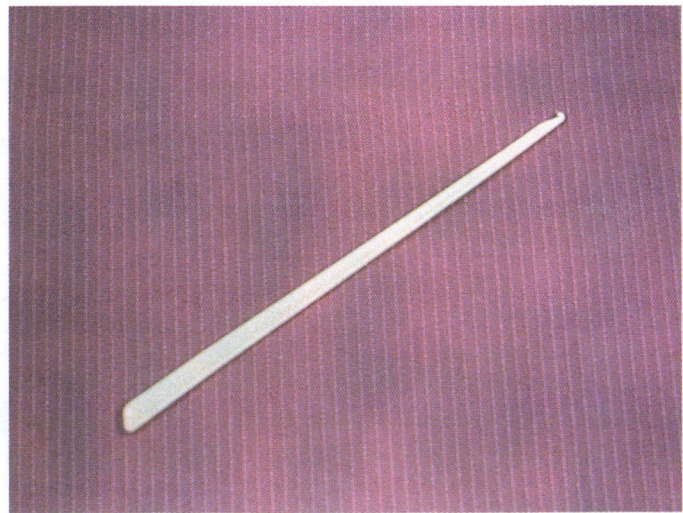

Figure 25-18 Amnihook.

Research Highlight

Amniotomy for Shortening Spontaneous Labor

Purpose

To study the effects of amniotomy on the rate of cesarean delivery on other indicators of maternal and neonatal morbidity (5-minute Apgar score of less than 7, admission to the neonatal intensive care unit [NICU]). Early amniotomy has been advocated as a component of the active management of labor.

Method

A review of all controlled trials of amniotomy during the first stage of labor. Data were extracted from published reports. Trials were assigned methodologic quality scores based on a standardized rating system. Typical odds ratios (ORs) were calculated using Peto's method.

Findings

Amniotomy was associated with a reduction in labor duration of between 60 and 120 minutes. There was a marked trend toward an increase in the risk for cesarean delivery: OR, 1.26; 95% confidence interval (CI), 0.96–1.66. The likelihood of a 5-minute Apgar score less than 7 was reduced in association with early amniotomy (OR, 0.54; 95% CI, 0.30–0.96). Groups were similar with respect to other indicators of neonatal status (arterial cord pH, NICU admissions). There was a statistically significant association of amniotomy with a decrease in the use of oxytocin: OR, 0.79; 95% CI, 0.67–0.92.

Nursing Implications

Routine early amniotomy is associated with benefits and risks. Benefits include a reduction in labor duration and a possible reduction in low 5-minute Apgar scores. The meta-analysis provides no support for the hypothesis that routine early amniotomy reduces the risk for cesarean delivery. Indeed, there is a trend toward an increased risk for cesarean delivery. An association between early amniotomy and cesarean delivery for fetal distress was noted in one large trial, suggesting that amniotomy should be reserved for women with abnormal labor progress.

Fraser, W. D., Turcot, L., Krauss, I., & Brisson-Carrol, G. (2000). Amniotomy for shortening spontaneous labour (Cochrane Review). In *The Cochrane Library, Issue 1.* Oxford: Updated Software.

effected by applying a FSE directly through the membranes, especially if there is no bulging forebag.

Nursing responsibilities during AROM are to assess the FHR both before and after amniotomy. The client usually is receiving continuous EFM. After AROM, the characteristics of the amniotic fluid are assessed and documented: color—clear, bloody, or meconium stained; odor; and amount—copious or scant. Notify the appropriate health care team members of the rupture of membranes and abnormal findings as per the hospital policy, procedure, and protocol. The primary caregiver should be notified immediately when meconium-stained amniotic fluid is first observed.

Documentation and Communication

Documentation of nursing care is made on a flowchart or entered directly into a bedside computer according to the hospital policy, procedure, and protocol and the client's clinical status communicated to other members of the health care team as appropriate (Figure 25-19). Although physicians and nurse-midwives make the obstetric management decisions, they cannot be in constant attendance at the bedside. It is the intrapartum nurse who alerts the physician or nurse-midwife when a change in the plan of care becomes necessary. Failure of the nurse to correctly interpret assessment findings is below the standard of care. Failure to communicate and document clinical findings are

Labor Progress Chart

Hollister

Labor Progress Chart
Hollister Maternal/Newborn Record System
To order call: **1.800.323.4060**   Re-order No. **5711**

Current Date: 6 23 96

Medication Allergy/Sensitivity (Identify): Demerol   ☐ None

Chart ___1___ of ___1___

1430	1445	1505	1520	1535	1550	1605	1620	1635	1658	1705	1720	1735	1750	1800	1815	1830	1845	1900	1915	1920	1945
		99.2								99											
83	80	82	81	82	84	86	84	88	84	80	84	82	81	88	91	92	87	88	85	88	83
16	16	18	16	16	16	18	18	16	16	16	16	18	16	20	20	18	16	16	18	20	18
114/91	112/68	114/70	116/71	114/72	116/70	118/70	116/78	116/78	118/72	118/72	110/76	112/72	108/76	118/76	118/76	118/73	116/70	112/72	120/72	114/70	118/76
97%																					
/	/	/	/	/	/	/	/	/	/	/	/	/	/	/	/	/	/	/	/	/	/
NS	NS	NS	NS	NS	NS	NS	NS	NS	NS	0	0	0	0	0	0	0	0	0	0	0	
2	2	2	2	2	2	2	2	2	2	2	2	2	2	3	4	4	4	5	5		
E	E	I →																			
3	3	3	3	3	2-3	2-3	3	3	2-3	2-3	2-3	2-3	4	5	5	3-4	3	3	3	3	2
40-50	40-50	40	40	40-50	50-60	60	60	60-70	60	60	80-60	60	60	60	50-60	60	60-70	70	70	70	
		40	40	40	40	40	40	40	40	40	40	50	50	60	60	60	70	pushing 100	100	100	100
		10	10	10	10	10	10	10	10	10	10	10	10	10	10	10	10	10	10	10	10
mod.	mod.	120	120	120	140	140	120	120	140	140	140	150	125	120	120	180	210	300	300	300	300
I	I	I →																			
140	144	136	136	136	136	130	130	130	132	132	128	140	144	130	130	140	144	150	152	156	90
+	+	+	+	+	+	+	+	+	+	+	+	+	+	+	+	+	+	+	+	+	
+	+	+	+	+	+	↓	↓	+	+	+	+	+	+	+	+	+	+	↓	↓	↓	
++	+	++	++	++	++	+	+	+	++	++	++	++	+	+	+	+	+	+	+	+	
V	V	E	E	E	E	E	E	E	V	V	V	V	V	V	V	V	V	V	V	V	V
C	C	C	C	MS	MS	MS	MS	MS	MS	MS	MS	scant fluid leak →									
100 ice			100			100				100											F3
								cath 400													
		2 my/M	4	6	6	8	10		12	12	12	14	14	15	16	17	DC				
CEA cont. ———																	→				
			O₂			BP 0		st. cath.										O₂↑			
LS	RS	RS	SF	SF	LS	LS	SF	LS	LS	SF	SF	LS / PC	LS	SF / MC	SF	LS	LS	SF	LS	SF	
	V/O					V			V					V - remains c̄ pt →					del 1446		
JH	JH	JH	JH	JH	JH	JH	JH	JH	JH	JH	JH	JH	LD	JH	JH	JH	JH	JH	JH	JH	JH

Acceditations
++ = 15 BPM 1 X 15 sec
+ = <15 BPM 1+/or <15 sec
0 = None
Decelerations
N = None
E = Early
V = Variable
L = Late
P = Prolonged

Membranes
I = Intact
B = Bulging
R = Ruptured
Fluid
C = Clear
M = Meconium Stained
B = Bloody
F = Foul Odor
NF = No Foul Odor

Treatments
O₂ = O₂ L/min
IVB = IV Bolus
SC = Straight Catheterization
FC = Foley Catheterization
ABD = Abdominal Hair Removal

Teaching/Support
0 = Orient to Unit
SR = Safety Review
LR = Labor Review
F = Focusing
BRT = Breathing/Relaxation Techniques
PrO = PreOp.

Touch
E = Effleurage
B = Backrub
CP = Counterpressure
M = Massage

Position/Activity
W = Walking
C = Chair
SQ = Squatting
JR = Jet Hydrotherapy
SH = Shower
K = Kneeling
LS = Left Side
RS = Right Side
KC = Knee Chest
T = Trendelenburg

Physical Care
MC = Mouth Care
SC = Superficial Cold
SH = Superficial Heat
PC = Peri Care
BP = Bedpan

Hollister Incorporated, 2000 Hollister Drive, Libertyville, Illinois 60048

LABOR PROGRESS CHART FORM #5711 696

Figure 25-19 Labor Progress Chart. Courtesy of Hollister Incorporated.

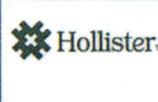

Labor Progress Chart
Hollister Maternal/Newborn Record System
To order call: **1.800.323.4060**   Re-order No. **5711**

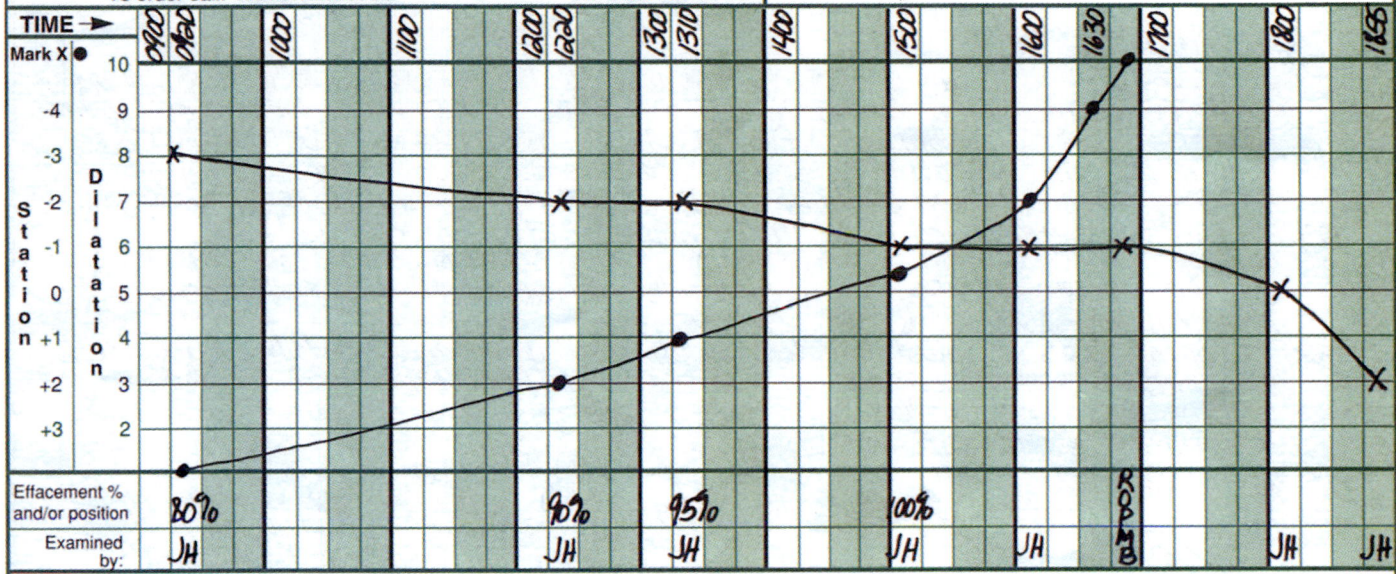

| Effacement % and/or position | 80% | | | | 80% | 95% | | 100% | | ROM MB | | 80% | |
| Examined by: | JH | | | | JH | JH | | JH | JH | MB | | JH | JH |

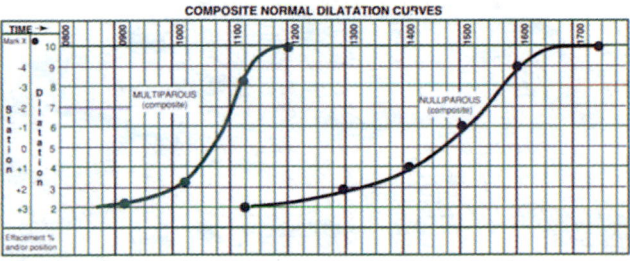

COMPOSITE NORMAL DILATATION CURVES

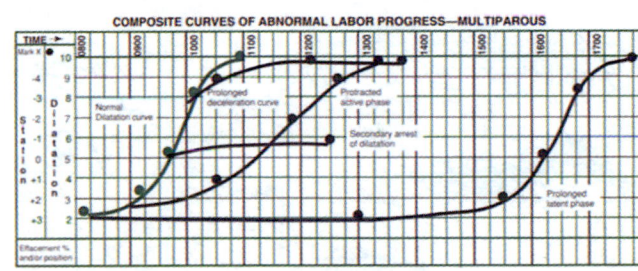

COMPOSITE CURVES OF ABNORMAL LABOR PROGRESS—MULTIPAROUS

Labor Progress Curves derived form the work of Emanual A. Friedman, M.D.

IV Record

Start Date	Time	Solution	Amount (cc's)	Medication/Dose Added	Initials	Infused Date	Time	Amount Infused
6/23/96	1130	Lact. Ringer's Sol. (F#1)	1000	—	JH	6/23	1320	1000
6/23/96	1320	Lact. Ringer's Sol. (F#2)	1000	—	JH	6/23	1940	1000
6/23/96	1510	Lact. Ringer's Sol. (F/A)	500	Oxytocin 10 mu	JH	6/24	0200	500
6/23/96	1940	Lact. Ringer's Sol. (F#3)	1000	Oxytocin 20 u p̄ del. (con't for recovery)	JH	6/23	2340	1000
				(F#IA D.C @ 1900 cont.@ 2340)				

Interval Medications

Date Time	Medication/Dose	Route	Site	Initials
6/23 1630	Bicitra 30cc	P.O	—	JH

Signature Key

Initials	Signature
JH	J. Hall RNC
MB	M. Brown MD
LD	L. Day RNC

Figure 25-19 (continued)

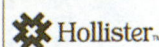

Labor Progress Chart

Hollister Maternal/Newborn Record System

To order call: **1.800.323.4060**   Re-order No. **5711**

Progress Notes

Date	Time	Year 1996
4/23	1020	A 35 yr. w/f g iii p ii c̄ EDD 7/4/96 adm. to LDRP rm. 274 c̄ c/c "leaking" small amt. clear fluid since 0100. Nitrazine ⊕ SVE = 1/80 % 1-3. Vertex firm on cx. Consents for care signed. Dr. Brown notified of status - "admit" order received. J Hall RNC
	1045	Walking in room. Tolerating U.C.'s which are becoming regular since admin. JH ———
	1100	Blood specimen drawn for lab analysis. IVLR hydration initiated pre-epidural JH
	1230	Epidural catheter placed by Dr. Miller. No medication injected yet. JH ———
	1245-1315	↓ Fetal movement - STV + LTV↓ Pt. utilizing breathing and relaxation techniques c̄ each U.C. States the UC's "are more painful in lower back". Husband massaging pt's lumbar area c̄ U.C. J Hall RNC ———
	1335	Marcaine 0.25% "bolus" injected per epidural catheter by B. Mills, MD. Catheter attached to continuous epidural infusion pump (CEA) Rate/dose documented on Anesthesia Record J. Hall RNC ———

V.S. monitored per epidural protocol:

@	1335	1337	1339	1341	1343	1345	1347	1349	1351	1353	1355
P	118/82	110/84	114/85	108/83	110/80	108/81	112/81	118/82	118/84	116/84	120/84
R	70 16	72 16	71 18	77 16	72 18	71 16	72 16	74 16	75 16	72 16	71 16

	1400	Good relief of discomf. of U.C. & the back pain. Internal scalp electrode applied. J Hall RNC
	1435	Occas. variable decels from baseline of 140's to 120 c̄ U.C. - returns to baseline by end of U.C. Repositioned side → side. Dr. Brown informed of variable U.C's. JH
	1505	Dr. Brown here - inserted IUPC to evaluate effectiveness of U.C.'s. J Hall RNC ———
	1535	IV Oxytocin 10u/500cc LR initiated by infusion pump "piggy back", main IV line. JH FH early decel 10-15 bpm c̄ each U.C. Ret'd to baseline p̄ U.C. Lt. mec. stain in amn. fluid. O₂ per mask init. 10.5 lpm JH
	1620	Dr. Brown here to evaluate labor progress and fetal status J Hall RNC ———
	1705	Bladder palpible — straight cath → 400 clear yellow urine. J Hall RNC ——— Marcaine dosage per infusion CEA reduced to promote natural vertex decent. J Hall RNC
	1705	RN in attendance to continually assess fetal monitor data and to assist in coaching pt.
	1800	FH variables contin. (approx. ↓ 10-15 bpm c̄ each U.C.) → returns to baseline p̄ U.C. J Hall RNC
	1805	Has strong urge to push. Dr. Brown present - evaluating U.C's & fetal status J Hall RNC
	1815	Using open glottis technique c̄ pushing and freq. chg. of position to assist in decent and rotation of fetal head (ROP). Variable decel. from baseline of 130 to 100 - return to baseline p̄ U.C. J Hall RNC
	1905	Dr. Brown present. FHR↓ STV + LTV - variable decel from 150's to 90-100 c̄ each U.C. O₂ per mask increased to 10 lpm Oxytocin discontinued. Caput forming - PP @ +a station JH
	1940	Prepared for forcep assistance to rotate ROP → ROA & delivery J Hall RNC ———
	1946	Male infant delivered spont. p̄ vertex rotation to ROA. Aropharynx suctioned on perineum < initial resp. J. Stone NNP present at birth to assist c̄ mgmt. of infant airway and ventilation. See L&D summary J Hall RNC ———

Hollister Incorporated, 2000 Hollister Drive, Libertyville, Illinois 60048

Figure 25-19 *(continued)*

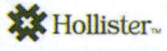
Hollister™

Labor Progress Chart
Hollister Maternal/Newborn Record System

To order call: **1.800.323.4060**   Re-order No. **5711**

Admit Date	Admit Time	Blood Type and Rh	Age	G.	T.	Pt	A.	L.	EDD / 4 96	Membranes			
6 23 96	1020	O+	35	III	II	O	O	II	LMP 9 28 95	☐ Intact ☐ Bulging	☑ Ruptured (SROM) AROM	Date 6/23/96 Time 0100	

Current Date 6 23 96	Time →	1000	1020	1045	1100	1115	1130	1145	1200	1215	1230	1245	1300	1315	1335	1345	1400	1415
Vital Signs Temperature		98⁷						98⁷					99					
Pulse		92	91		90			91	88	84	90	87	82	88	84*	82	80	82
Respiration		18	18		18			18	20	20	18	18	16	20	20	18	16	18
Blood Pressure		120/70	114/72		120/70			116/71	120/70	124/78	128/76	120/72	120/72	124/68	118/70	114/70	116/68	114/68
O₂ Saturation																		
Maternal Deep Tendon Reflexes (L/R)		/	/	/ 2+ 2+	/	/	/	/	/		2+ 2+		/	/	/	/	/	/
Urine (Protein/Sugar)		/	/	/ − −	/	/	/	/	/		− −		/	/	/	/	/	/
Vaginal Bleeding		0	0	0		0	0	0	0	0	0	0	0	0	0	NS	NS
Pain		2	2	3		4	4	4/5	4	5	6/7	9	8	3	2
Edema		H																
Uterine Activity Monitor Mode		E	E	E		E	E	E	E	E	E	E	E	E	E	E	E
Frequency		3/4 min	3 min	3 min		3 min	3	3	3/4	2-3	2-3	2-3	2	2	2	2
Duration		35 sec.	40 sec.	45 sec.		45-60	45-60	50-60	50-60	40-50	50-60	60+	60-70	60	50-60	40-50
Peak IUP																		
Resting Tone																		
Intensity / palpation		mild	mild	mild		mild	mod	mod	mod.	mod.	mod.	mod.	mod.	mod.	mod.	mod.
MVUs																		
Fetal Assessment Monitor Mode (Strip # 1996)		E	E	E		E	E	E	E	E	E	E	E	I	I	I
Baseline (FHR)		140	140	140		130	138	136	132	140	140	130	130	130	136	136
STV		+	+	+		+	+	+	+	∅	∅	+	+	+	+	+
LTV		+	+	+		+	+	+	+	↓	↓	+	+	+	+	+
Accelerations		++	++	++		++	++	++	++	+	+	++	++	++	++	++
Decelerations		N	N	N		N	N	N	N	N	N	N	N	N	N	N
Membranes/Fluid		C	C	C		C	C	C	C	C	C	C	C	C	C	C
Intake/Output (cc's/Hr) IV						Rt hand							→1500					
PO		ice chips	ice	ice		ice	ice		ice		ice							
Urine		100				75		100			125							
Emesis		∅					∅											
Cont Meds Pitocin mU/min																		
MgSO₄ gms/hr																		
Marcaine 0.25% cont. 3 pid. cath														CEA see anesth. rec.				
Intervention Treatments																		
Teaching/Support		O/LR	SR	BRT		F												
Touch									CP	CP	M							
Position/Activity		LS	W	W		C	C	C	LS	LS	RS	RS	LS	LS	SF	SF
Physical Care																		
Epid. cath. placed (P)										P								
MD visit (v) call (c) (M Brown MD) orders (o) * See prog notes for V.S.		C						C/O							C			
Initials \epid		JH	JH	JH		JH	LD	LD	JH	JH	JH	JH	JH	JH	JH	JH

Abbreviations/Key				
Deep Tendon Reflexes 0 = No Response +1 = Sluggish +2 = Normal +3 = Hyperactive +4 = Brisk + Hyperactive C = Clonus	**Vaginal Bleeding** NS = Normal Show ABN = Frank Vaginal Bleeding	**Pain** 0 = No Pain 5 = Distressing Pain 10 = Highest Intensity	**Uterine Activity Monitor Mode** P = Palpation E = External I = Internal **MVUs Montevideo Units** The sum of the peak of each uterine contraction minus its resting tone, in a 10 minute period.	**Fetal Monitor Mode** A = Auscultation (Fetoscope) D = Doppler E = External I = Internal	**STV Short Term Variability** + = Present (Roughness of Tracing Line Present) ∅ = Absent (Tracing Line is Smooth) **LTV Long Term Variability** ∅ = 0- 2 BPM = Absent ↓ = 3- 5 BPM = Minimal + = 6-25 BPM = Average ↑ = >25 BPM = Marked

LABOR PROGRESS CHART FORM #5711 696

Figure 25-19 *(continued)*

Research Highlight

Caregiver Support for Women During Childbirth

Purpose

To assess the effects of continuous support during labor (provided by the health care team or laypersons) on mothers and infants. Social support may include advice or information, tangible assistance, and emotional support.

Method

Review of 14 randomized trials involving 5,000 women. Continuous support during labor was compared with intermittent support.

Findings

The continuous presence of a support person reduced the likelihood of medication for pain relief, operative vaginal delivery, cesarean delivery, and a 5-minute Apgar score of less than 7. Continuous support also was associated with a slight reduction in the length of labor. Six trials evaluated the effects of support on mothers' views of their childbirth experiences. Although the trials used different measures (overall satisfaction, failure to cope well during labor, finding labor to be worse than expected, and level of personal control during childbirth), in each trial the results favored the group of women who had received continuous support.

Nursing Implications

Continuous support during labor from caregivers appears to have a number of benefits for mothers and their infants, and there do not appear to be any harmful effects.

Hodnett, E. D. (2000). Caregiver support for women during childbirth (Cochrane Review). In *The Cochrane Library, Issue 1.* Oxford: Updated Software.

---

two reasons that the intrapartum nurse might be named as a defendant in a malpractice claim. The Board of Nurse Examiners Rules and Regulations, Standards of Professional Practice, require nurses to "accurately and completely report and document" (Rule 217.11 (4)).

Activity

When the woman is in bed, frequent position changes allow for better comfort. During normal labor, however, the woman does not need to be confined to bed, unless analgesics are being used. Many women prefer to walk, accompanied by a support person, and return to the LDR every 30 to 45 minutes for FHR assessment according to ACOG standards (July 1995). A comfortable chair may be beneficial, allowing the woman to maintain a more upright position than being semi-recumbent in bed. Many women use a rocking chair, preferring to rock through each contraction. Continuous EFM can continue with the woman sitting in a chair at the bedside. While in bed, the laboring woman should be allowed to assume the position that af-

fords her the most comfort; additional pillows can be provided to help in positioning. The supine position should be avoided because of the danger of vena caval compression.

Comfort Measures

Anxiety levels and coping mechanisms of the client, partner, and family are assessed continually as labor progresses. Anxiety and fear tend to lower a woman's pain threshold, and the nurse should try to remain with the woman in active labor (client load permitting) to give encouragement and reassurance that normal progress is being made. Ignorance of the process and mechanism of labor can result in anxiety and fear of childbirth. Fear causes catecholamine secretion, which has the effect of decreasing peripheral blood flow. Adrenaline has a terbutaline-like effect in that it can cause labor to be prolonged as uterine contractions become less effective. The biggest factor in management of labor is nursing support and coaching. The value of having a caring skilled professional at the bedside cannot be overestimated.

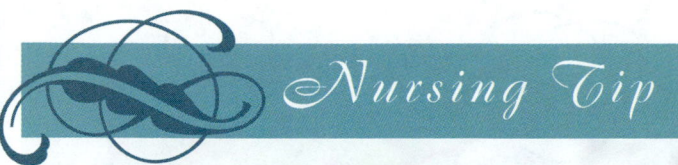

THE BOARD OF NURSE EXAMINERS

If you are named as a defendant in a malpractice suit, bear in mind that the Board of Nurse Examiners is not there to protect nurses. Its sole concern is to protect the public from incompetent nurses. It does provide the guidelines that set standards of care.

A calm, competent, and gentle manner on the part of the nurse promotes trust and goes a long way toward alleviating client anxiety. Frequent feedback should be given and the findings of each test explained in language the client can understand. It also is important to take care of the woman's partner, and this can be done by providing a comfortable chair and including the person in discussions and explanations. Support for the laboring family is individualized according to the specific needs and expectations of those concerned as well as respectfully taking into account the cultural background.

Pain Management

A common concern of the pregnant woman is whether she will be able to withstand the pain of contractions, or whether she will lose control. There are a variety of measures that will promote relaxation and assist the woman in coping as contractions intensify.

The nurse may need to instruct the woman in breathing techniques or reinforce those already learned. Some women find counterpressure massage of the sacral area helpful during contractions, particularly when contraction pain is being experienced mostly in the lower back. Some childbirth classes advise clients to bring a tennis ball to the hospital to roll in a circular fashion against the woman's lower back, while applying gentle pressure during a contraction. If the fetus is in an occipitoposterior position, the pressure of the fetal occiput on maternal spinal nerves will cause the woman to experience contraction pain mostly in the lower back. Counterpressure is helpful in lifting the occiput off these nerves, to some extent, thus providing pain relief. Changing positions frequently is helpful.

The comforting effects of a warm shower during the first stage of labor should not be underestimated. Some facilities feature a bathtub with whirlpool jets, such as a Jacuzzi, as a comfort measure to decrease muscle tension and promote relaxation (Figure 25-20). Having the client relax in a whirlpool, however, does not relieve the nurse of the responsibility of appropriate fetal assessment.

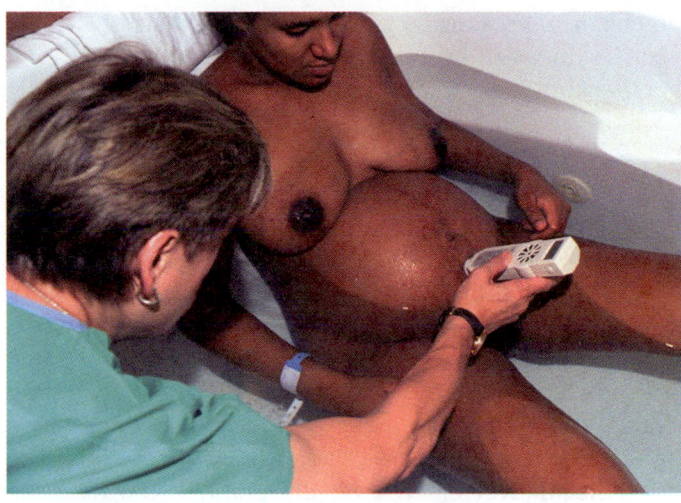

Figure 25-20 The nurse continues to monitor fetal status while the laboring woman relaxes in a whirlpool.

Bathing during labor is associated with decreased pain and increased speed of cervical dilation (Lowe, 1996).

A **doula** is a woman who is employed by the pregnant woman to assist her through labor by helping her cope with the pain. The doula has no clinical training but is able to reinforce breathing techniques, massage, and sometimes provide ice packs or warm packs. The labor partner or nurse usually is more than able to provide physical and emotional support; however, when the nurse is assigned to more than one client or if the client has no family member with her, the services of a doula are particularly valuable.

The birthing ball is a standard physiotherapy tool used in physical therapy departments worldwide. The ball provides a soft yet firm place to sit while promoting a desirable upright posture and allowing for decreased straining of the muscles. The birthing ball also is used to lie on.

Additional pain relief and pharmacologic measures are discussed in Chapter 24.

Psychologic Considerations

As labor advances, anxiety levels secondary to pain increase in the woman who has not received epidural analgesia. It is important for the nurse to be present with the woman who is in active labor and to continue to offer encouragement and reassurance to the woman and family. As the transition phase approaches, the woman experiences stronger contractions while feeling tired, irritable, and less able to cope after all the hours of labor. She may feel trapped and apprehensive because of the increasing pain and vaginal pressure and will be less interested in her appearance and outside activities. To minimize environmental change, it is advisable for the same nurse, who already has developed a trusting rapport with the laboring woman, to continue care until she gives birth. Emphasis is on enhancing coping by assuring the client that all is going well, staying with her, and coaching her as necessary with her breathing techniques through each contraction. The client needs constant support during these phases of labor.

Labor Curve

Labor progress may be plotted by use of the labor curve, which was developed by Friedman (1970) as a method of graphically plotting the relationship of time to dilation of the cervix and station of the presenting part. When preparing to plot the labor curve, the number of hours the woman labors are written across the top of the graph, the dilation in centimeters up one vertical side, and the station (in descending order) down the opposite vertical side. The first time interval entered on the graph is the time the woman reported that regular contractions began.

Role of the Support Person

The friend or relative who provides companionship and encouragement to the laboring woman may be male or female; often is the husband or father of the infant who gives emotional support at this time. Some expectant fathers see their role as coach and will actively help the woman focus on breathing through her contractions. Partners who have not attended prepared childbirth classes with their mate, though not familiar with breathing techniques, often are quite willing to give physical comfort such as sips of water and back rubs. The nurse can fill in any knowledge gaps that the support person might have.

Some expectant fathers adopt a more passive role and are content to merely be present and to witness the birth. While being available to guide and encourage the man in taking an active part in the process, the nurse should in no way impose on him any personal philosophy of what his function should be. The laboring woman may be content that her partner is present and may not require him to do more than sit in a chair and read a newspaper while she is in labor. The woman is the one who knows her partner best and probably has a fairly accurate idea of how much he will participate in her birth experience.

Second Stage of Labor

The **second stage of labor** begins when the cervix is fully dilated (10 cm) and completely effaced (100%), and ends with delivery of the baby. Inability to feel the cervix during vaginal examination confirms that the second stage has begun (Figure 25-21). When a woman has received epidural analgesia, she may not be aware that the contractions have become stronger. She will feel vaginal pressure with each contraction during the second stage of labor. Premonitory indicators that should alert the nurse that the client may have entered the second stage of labor include the following (Scott et al., 1994):

NURSING DIAGNOSES IN THE SECOND STAGE OF LABOR

Nursing diagnoses that apply to a woman during the second stage of labor might include the following:

- Disturbed sleep pattern related to the length of labor.
- Deficient knowledge related to normal labor and delivery as evidenced by client's inexperience and lack of preparation.
- Pain related to uterine contractions.

- Bearing down of her own accord.
- Complaints that her contractions have become stronger and more painful.
- Complaints of pressure on her rectum.
- Increased amount of bloody show.
- Increasing irritability and tearfulness, together with a decreased coping ability.
- Nausea or vomiting.
- Trembling limbs.

The physician or nurse-midwife should be notified when the woman has begun the second stage of labor so that he or she can be available to come to the LDR as soon as birth is imminent. The duration of the second stage varies greatly from woman to woman. A duration of more than 2 hours in a first pregnancy is considered prolonged, unless the woman is receiving epidural or other regional analgesia. In the multiparous woman, a second stage of more than 2 hours might be considered prolonged (ACOG, Dec. 1995). The nurse notifies the appropriate health care provider of progress or lack of progress.

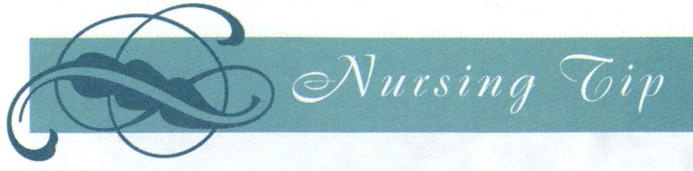

PREMATURE PUSHING

If the cervix is not fully dilated, pushing will not only tire the woman unnecessarily but will cause the cervix to become swollen and thus prolong labor. Repeated blowing or panting helps to counteract the tendency to push prematurely.

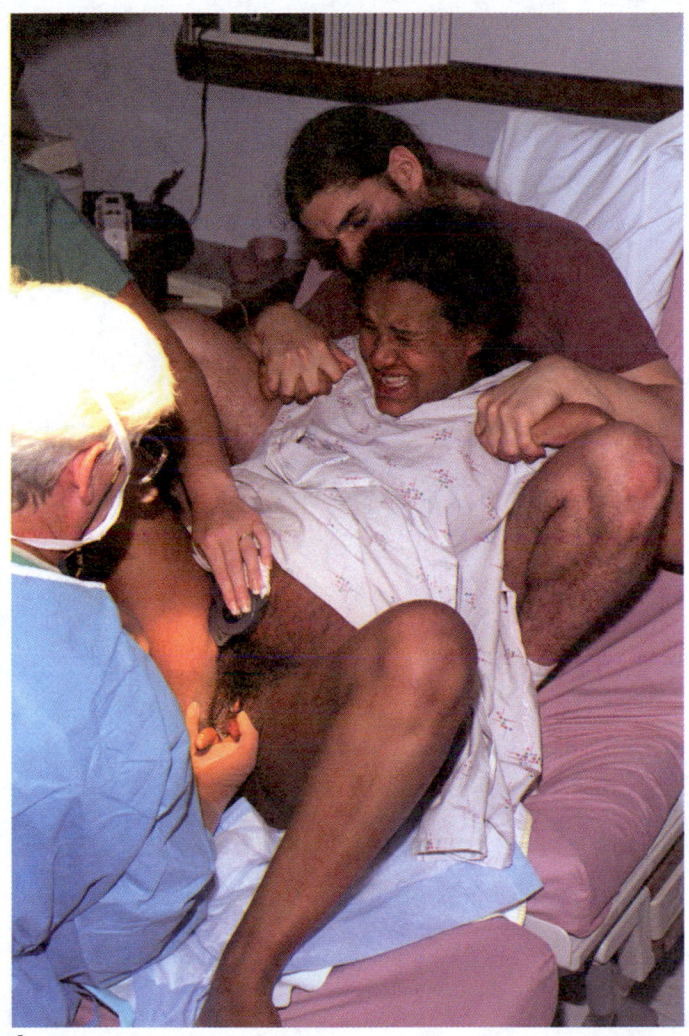

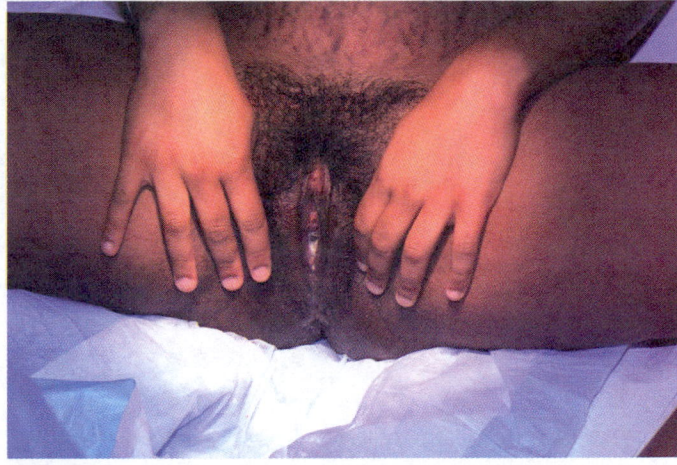

B.

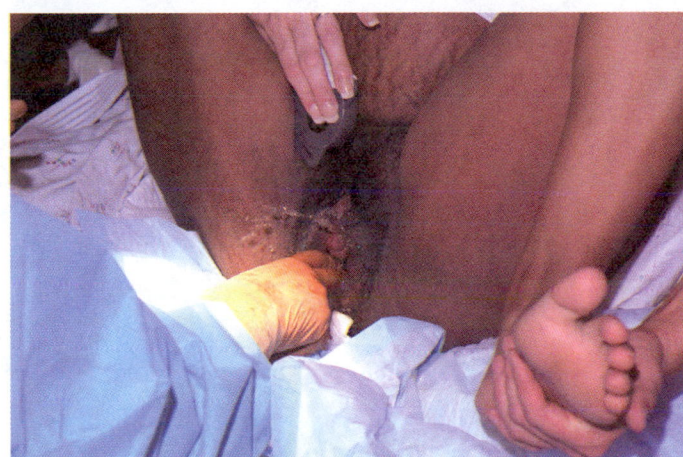

C.

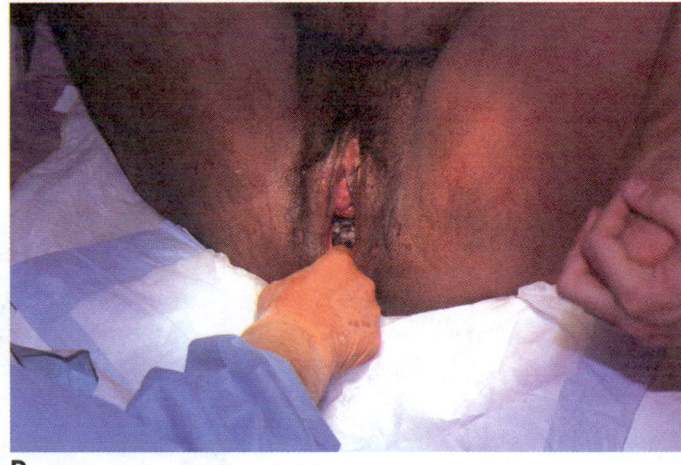

D.

A.

Figure 25-21 A. Dilation of the cervix is assessed while the woman briefly bears down. B. Many women will want to feel the perineal bulge with their fingers to be assured that labor is progressing. C. Spontaneous urination occurs during a vaginal check. D. The infant's head is clearly visible, meaning that birth is imminent.

During the second stage of labor contractions usually occur every 2 to 3 minutes, with a duration of 60 to 90 seconds, and intensity is strong by palpation or 80 to 100 mm Hg by IUPC. Uterine tone should palpate soft between contractions. Amniotic fluid is assessed for the presence of meconium, and bloody show is monitored for excessive bleeding. The FHR is assessed in accordance with institu-

tional policy. During the second stage of labor the usual protocol requires FHR and uterine activity evaluation every 15 minutes for low-risk clients and every 5 minutes for high-risk clients (ACOG, July 1995).

Refer to the accompanying photo story for a complete account of one couple's birth story.

One Couple's Birth Story

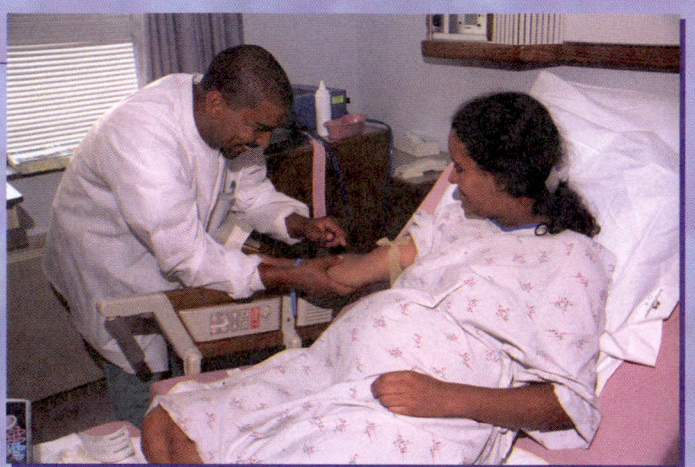

When the couple arrives at the hospital and labor is confirmed, the woman is admitted to Labor and Delivery. Certain admission procedures must be completed including gathering baseline data and lab work.

In the past, women were expected to remain NPO throughout their labor. This policy has been relaxed in most institutions and liquids are encouraged.

Many women find it more comfortable to ambulate or sit in a chair during early labor.

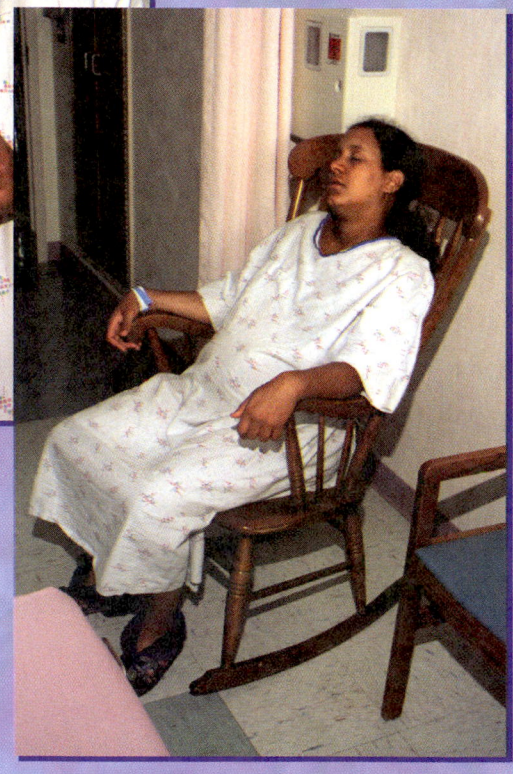

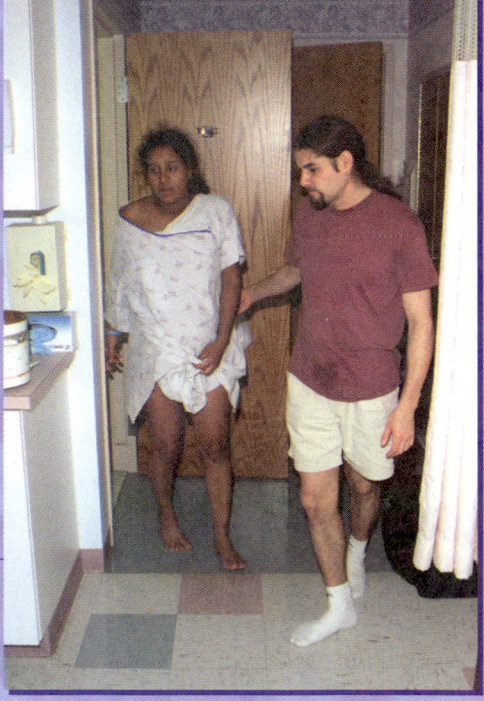

As labor progresses, the woman may want to rest in bed with the exception of trips to the bathroom.

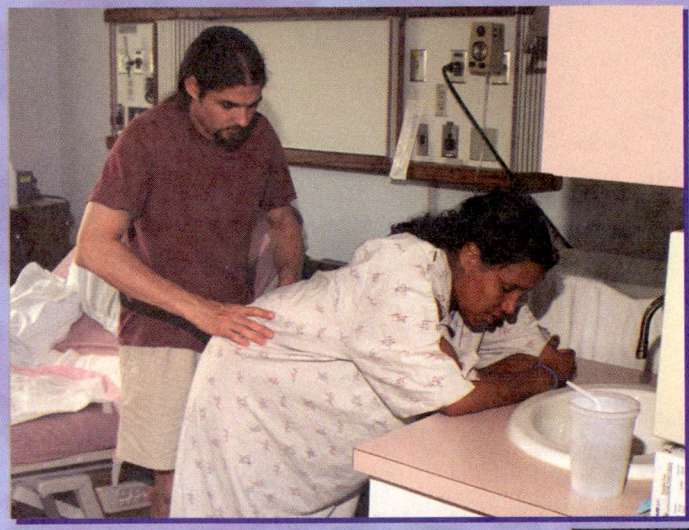

Some women find that a change of position and a backrub assists them in achieving comfort.

Most women try to rest between contractions to conserve energy.

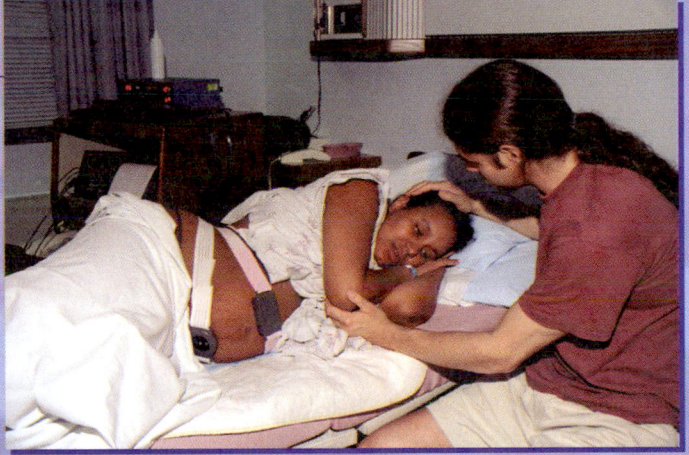

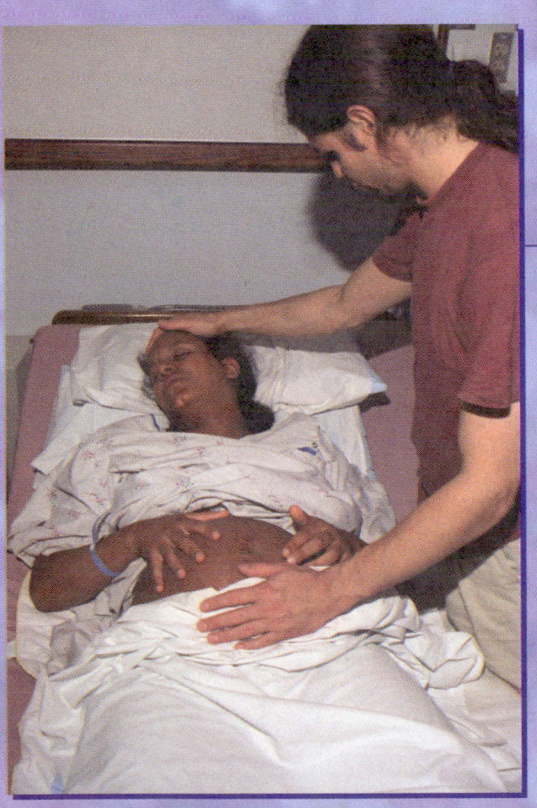

As contractions increase in frequency, duration, and intensity, the woman is less likely to be able to rest.

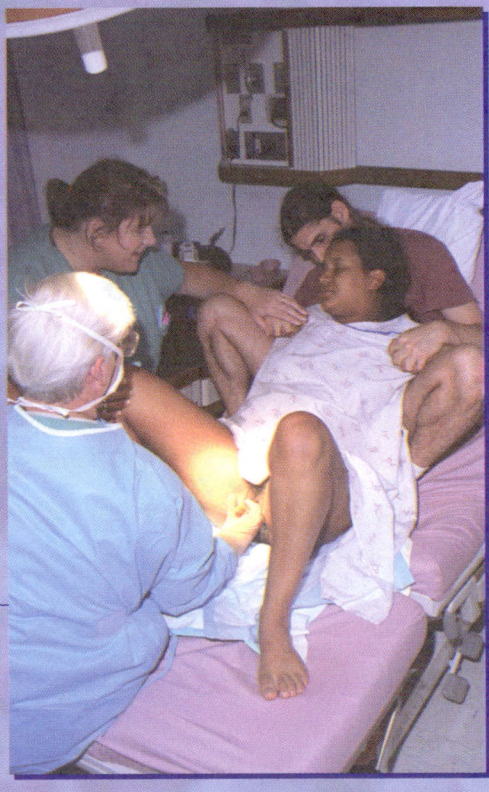

When the client becomes completely dilated, she feels an urge to push with her contractions. Her significant other is assisting her to assume a position conducive to pushing.

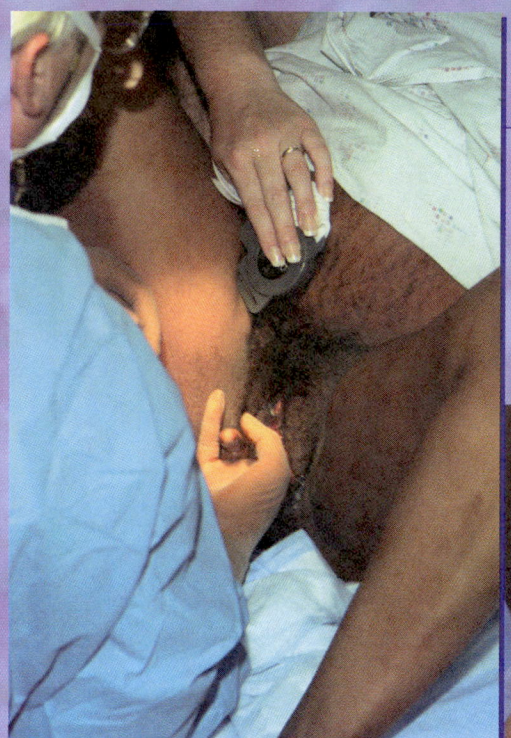

As the fetus descends through the pelvis, the nurse must monitor the fetal heart tones more frequently as well as the station of the presenting part.

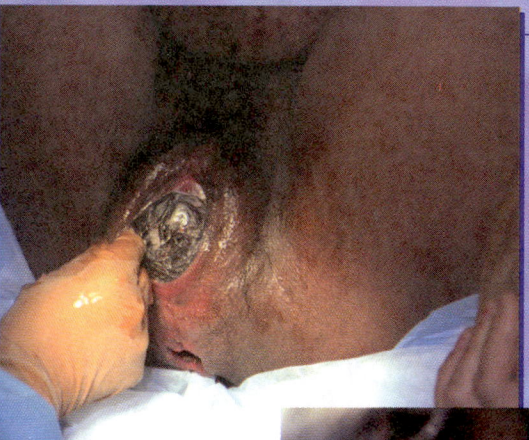

As the fetal head crowns, there is much thinning and pressure of the tissue. This pressure also involves the anus.

Finally, the baby's head is delivered between contractions to avoid perineal injury.

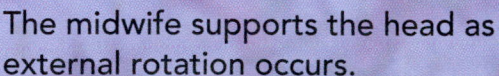

The midwife supports the head as external rotation occurs.

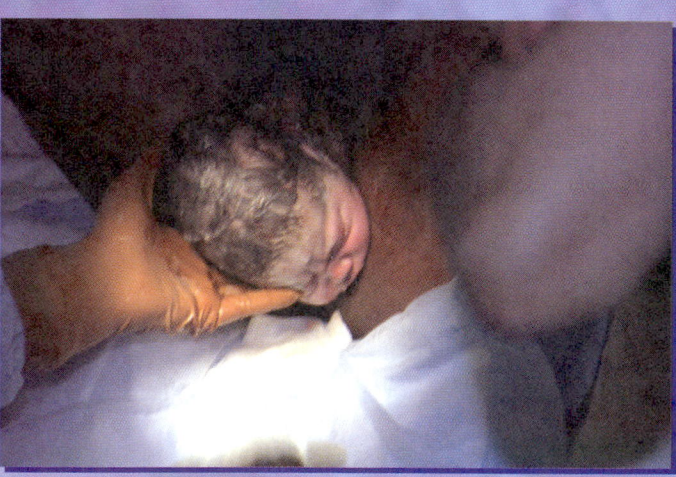

The baby's mouth and nose are suctioned immediately so the airway will be clear of amniotic fluid.

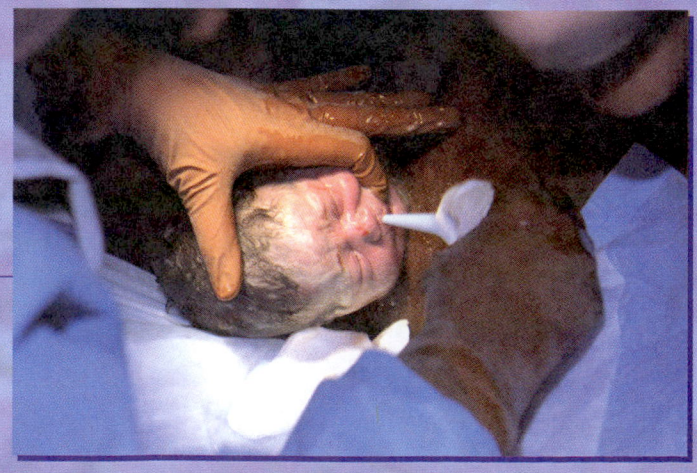

As restitution occurs, the midwife makes sure the baby's umbilical cord is not around its neck.

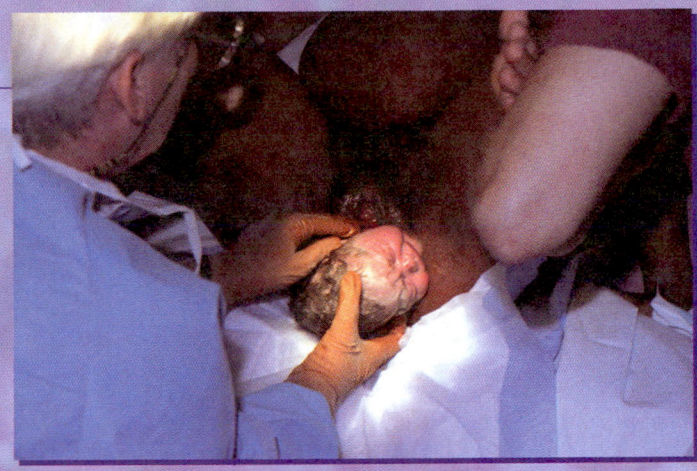

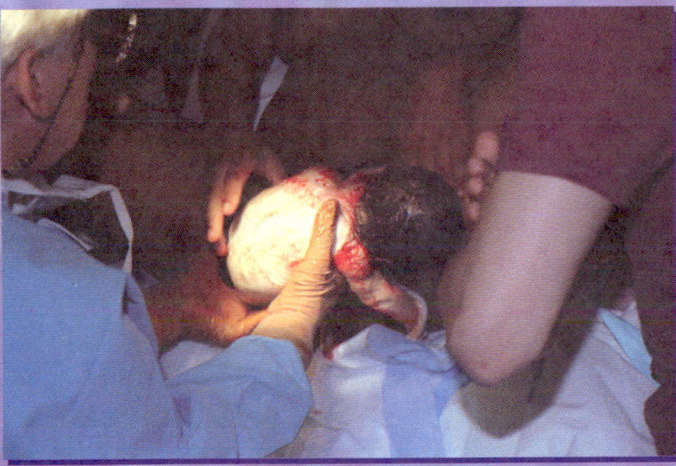

After the next contraction, the remainder of the body is delivered.

The baby is placed on the mother's abdomen while the midwife finishes the delivery.

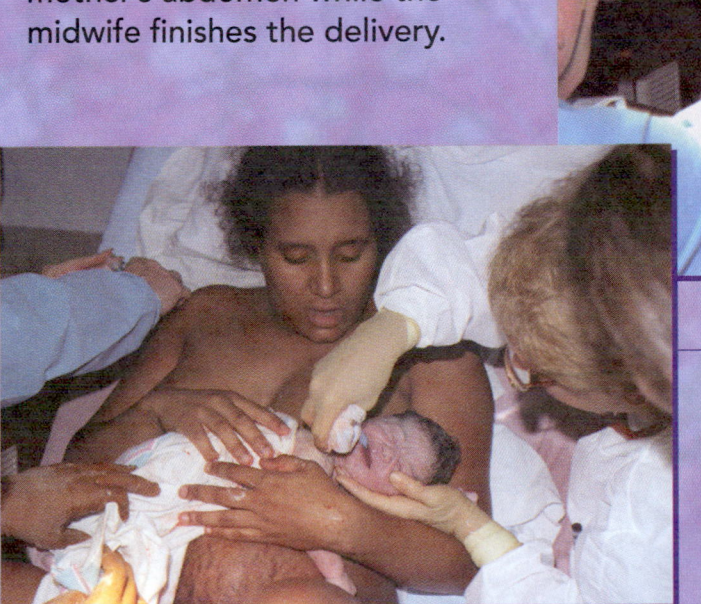

The infant is covered with a blanket and placed next to the mother's skin to prevent loss of body heat. The nurse suctions the baby's mouth again to ensure adequate air transport.

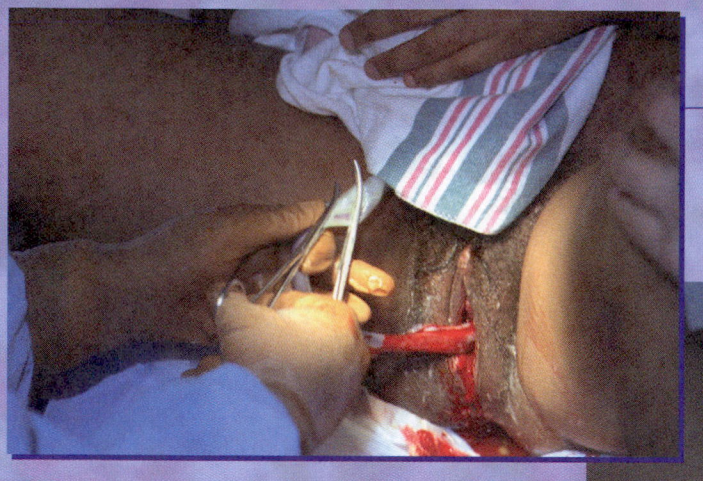

The midwife places two clamps on the umbilical cord.

The cord is cut between the two clamps by the baby's father.

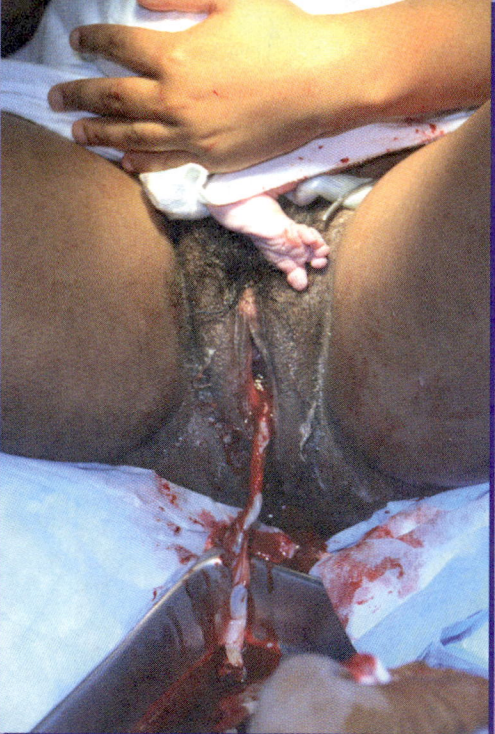

Waiting for the placenta to deliver. This usually occurs within a few minutes.

As the placenta separates, there is usually a gush of blood.

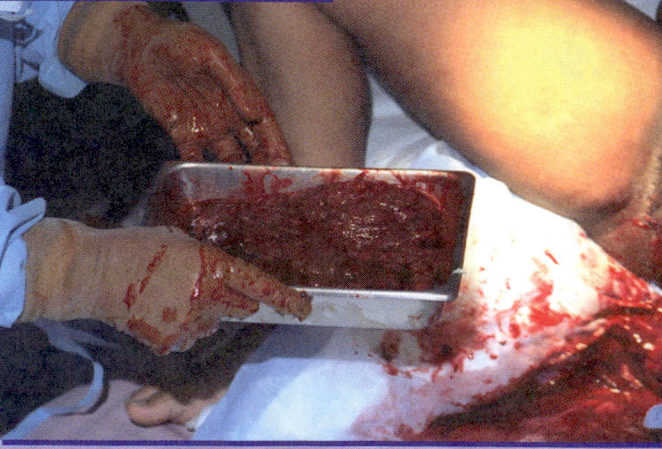

When the placenta has been delivered, it is inspected to ascertain that it is intact.

Many times women deliver without an episiotomy but may have small lacerations that need repair.

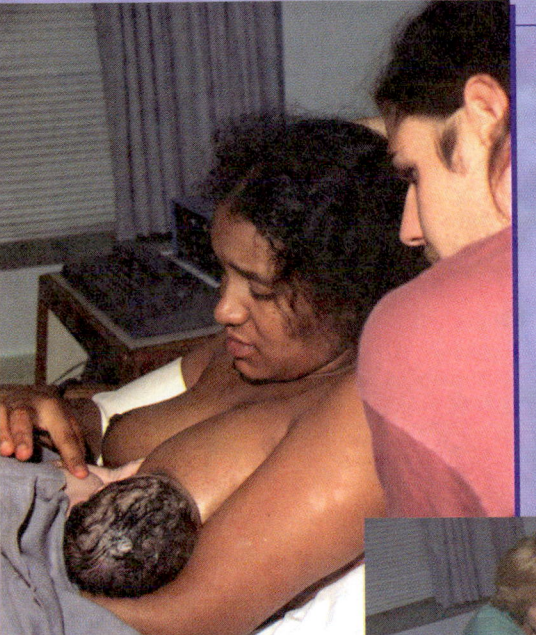

If the infant is placed at the mother's breast and sucks immediately following the delivery of the placenta, this assists in uterine involution through the release of maternal oxytocin.

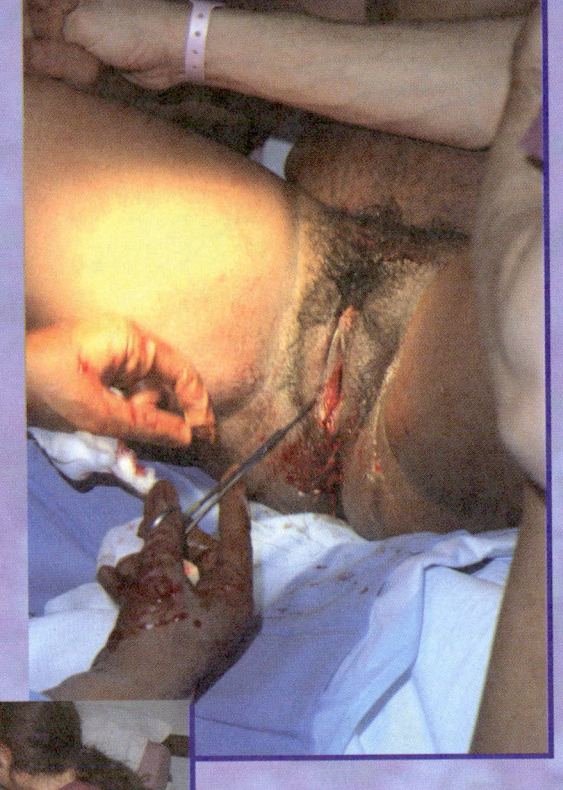

The nurse massages the fundus to assist in uterine involution while taking precautions against uterine inversion.

The baby's umbilical cord was intentionally left long at delivery. Now it is time to place a cord clamp and shorten the cord.

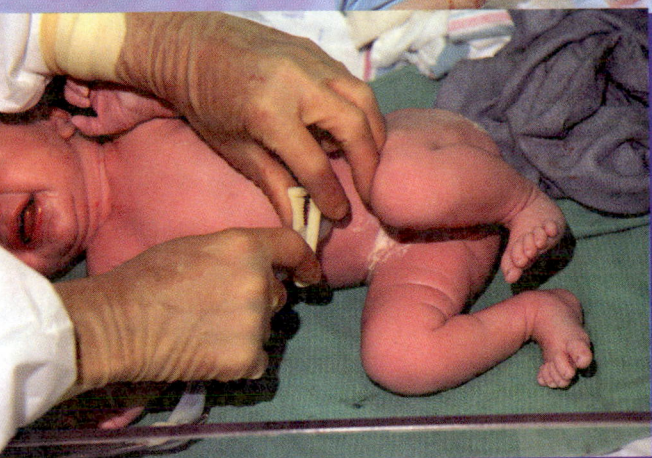

The cord is trimmed with sterile scissors.

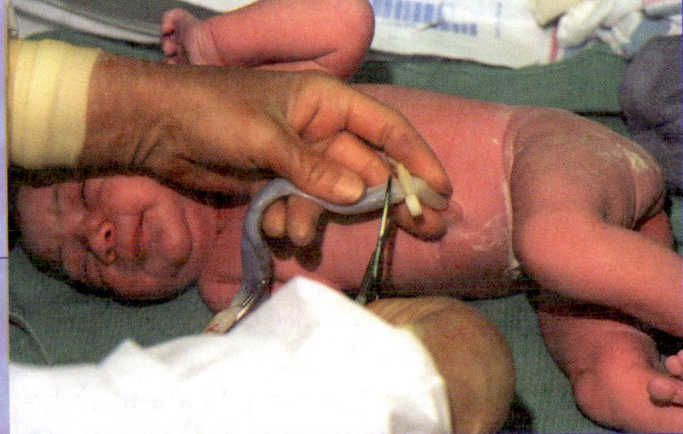

The baby has a
strong, lusty cry.

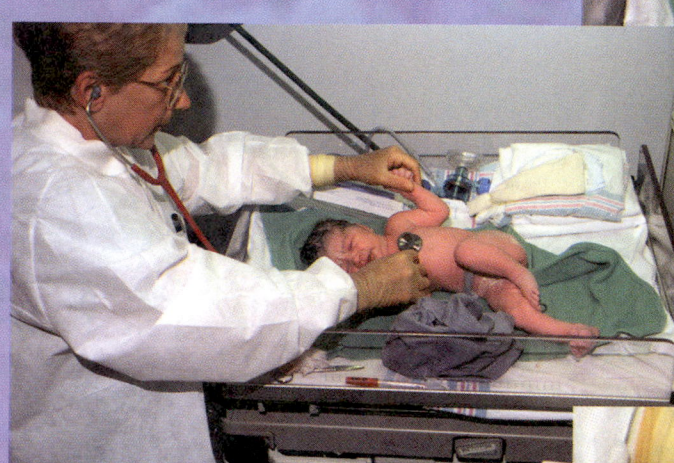

The nurse completes an
assessment of the heart rate.

Matching arm bracelets are placed on
the mother and infant for identification.

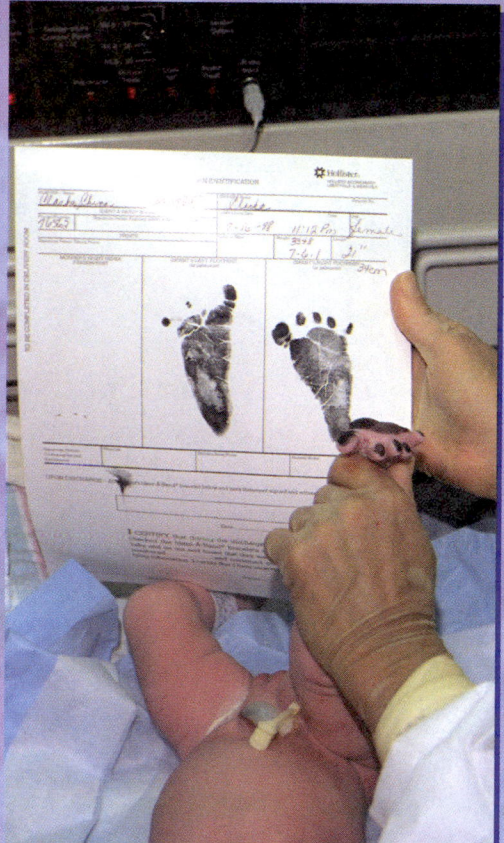

Infant footprints are obtained as a
secondary means of identification.

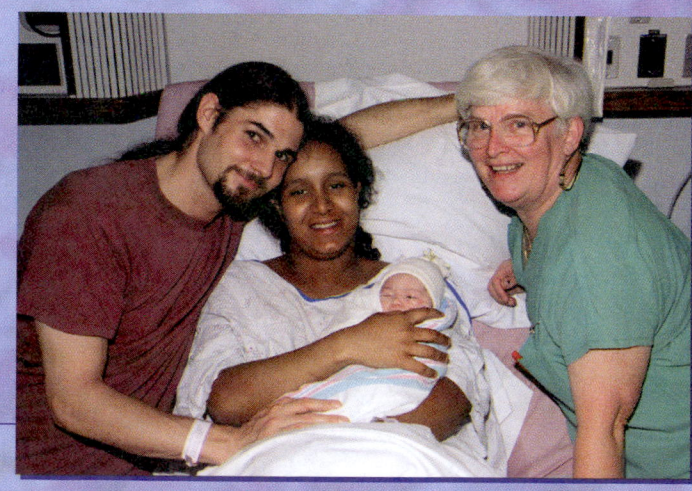

The happy family begins its life together.

Fetal Descent Assessment

Full dilation of the cervix is a function of descent; therefore, if there is continually a cervical lip, then the baby is not descending. Fetal descent is evaluated by performing a vaginal examination, or visually when the presenting part is at the perineum. When the cervix is fully dilated while the presenting part is still relatively high (0 to +1 station) the woman may wish to defer pushing efforts until after the fetal head has descended further. The second stage can be divided into a passive phase and an active phase. In the passive phase of the second stage, the woman does not yet have any urge to push. Descent does not require pushing. During this phase, the fetal head should be allowed to descend by means of involuntary uterine contractions (primary powers). This action is called *laboring down,* and it helps to prevent stress on the fetus and exhaustion of the mother from extended pushing time. In the active phase of the second stage, pressure on S2 to S4 creates the urge to push; therefore, the woman should begin her expulsive efforts (secondary powers). There are no benefits to pushing before the active phase of the second stage of labor. Visible signs of descent include bulging of the perineum and crowning (Figure 25-22).

Psychological Considerations

The start of the second stage often is a relief for the laboring woman because she can now take a more active part in delivering her baby by augmenting the involuntary primary powers (uterine contractions) with secondary powers (pushing). Instead of panting through each contraction and fighting the almost uncontrollable urge to push, she can concentrate all her energies on pushing out the infant. Being able to push gives the woman a feeling

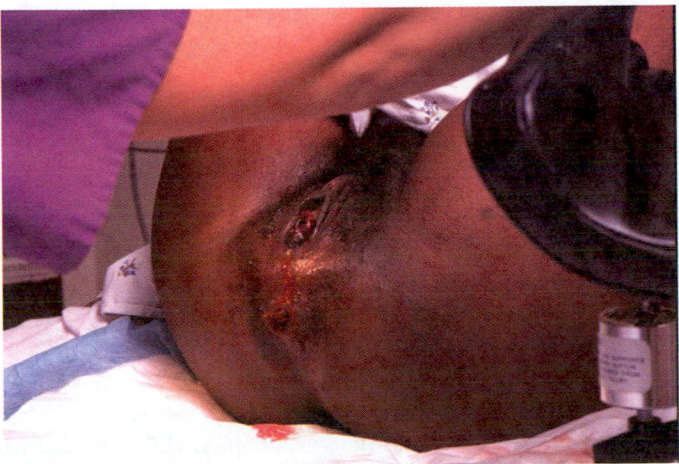

Figure 25-22 A bulging perineum is a visible sign of fetal descent.

of having some control over her labor (Box 25-12). The woman's perceptions are narrowed to the extent that she is all absorbed in the effort of pushing with contractions. Between contractions she should be encouraged to close her eyes take a deep cleansing breath and completely relax to conserve her strength for the next expulsive effort. The woman may experience nausea and may perspire with the effort of pushing.

The number of visitors permitted in a hospital room will vary and, as the time of delivery approaches, the nurse should ask the woman whom she would like to attend the delivery. This can best be done when visitors have temporarily stepped out of the room, so that the woman does not feel obliged to allow someone to see the delivery if she really does not want them there. The nurse can be an advocate for the woman by being the gatekeeper and ensuring that the woman's wishes in this regard are met.

Maternal Positioning

The nurse assists with maternal positioning to facilitate fetal descent and promote comfort. Several position options are available during pushing. The most commonly used position in the United States is the semi-Fowler's position in which the head of the bed is elevated about 45 degrees and the woman grasps her flexed knees or ankles. Epidural anesthesia has probably contributed to this semi-recumbent positioning. Women can benefit from pushing in a more upright position, which can be accomplished by leaning forward on a supported bedside table, a squat bar, or a birthing ball. Repeated studies have shown that upright positions, such as walking or standing, benefit both mother and fetus. These positions have a favorable effect on uterine contractility and reduce pain and perineal trauma (Mayberry, 2000). A lateral position also can be used for pushing and delivery. The pushing position used depends on the desires of the client and also requires flexibility on the part of the nurse and physician or nurse-midwife. Arbitrary limits on the second stage of labor should be abandoned if both the mother and fetus are doing well and progress is being made.

To assist with effective breathing and pushing, the nurse can ascertain which techniques the woman has learned in her prenatal classes and reinforce them. The woman is urged to listen to her body and bear down when she feels the urge to do so. The desire to bear down is an involuntary response to the pressure of the presenting part on the stretch receptors of the pelvic muscles. One drawback to this urge-to-push method is that the woman who has received epidural anesthesia may never feel the need to push. If the woman is not aware of contractions because of epidural analgesia, she needs to be coached to push during each contraction. Her partner may help by

Box 25-12 Pushing Technique

1. Encourage spontaneous bearing down. Allow the mother to rest until the fetal head has descended low enough in the pelvis to stimulate Ferguson's reflex (a reflex stimulated by stretch receptors in the pelvic floor, which usually occurs at a +1 station that stimulate in the mother an involuntary urge to push).

2. Consider fetal station and position in addition to dilation in determining a woman's readiness for pushing.

3. Discourage prolonged maternal breath-holding (more than 6 seconds) during pushing.

4. Encourage four or more pushes per contraction.

5. Support rather than direct the woman's involuntary pushing efforts, whether they include grunting, groaning, exhaling, or breath-holding for less than 6 seconds (Figure 25-23).

6. Validate the normalcy of sensations and maternal sounds.

7. The woman who has received epidural anesthesia may require more directed support for her expulsive efforts during the second stage.

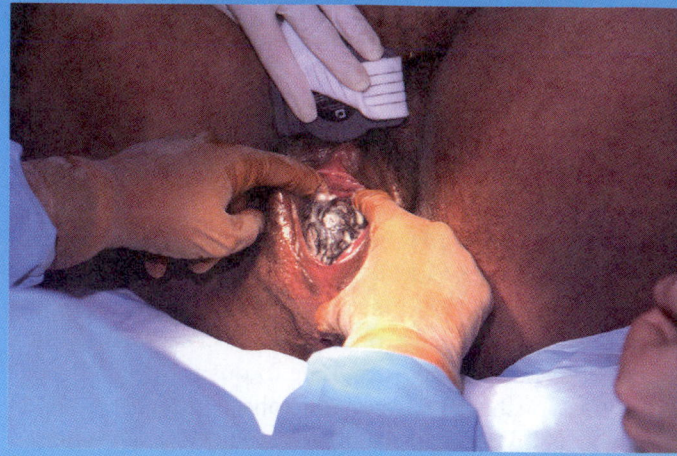

A.

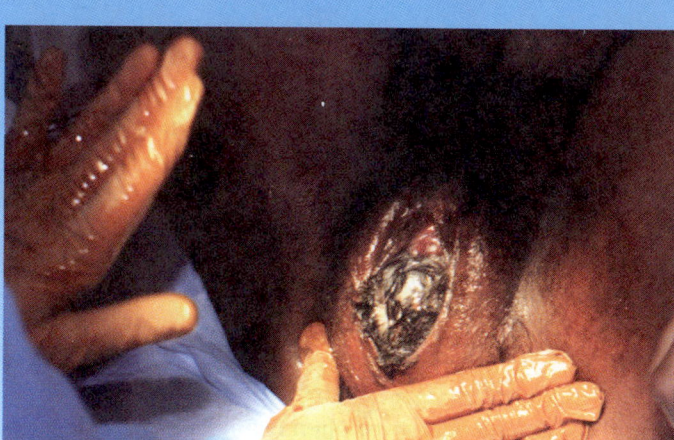

B.

Figure 25-23 A. The perineum is stretched as the infant's head crowns. B. The health care provider supports the woman's efforts by encouraging her to stop pushing between contractions.

supporting the woman's head or shoulders during pushing, wiping her brow with a cool damp cloth, and offering words of encouragement. The nurse and partner need to understand that because of the stress of labor, pain, and exhaustion, it is not uncommon for the woman to say things that she would not otherwise say. The primary provider is kept apprised of progress or lack of progress, as indicated. The woman, her partner, and family are kept informed of her progress, the expected sequence of events, and the delivery routine.

As the fetal head descends, bulging of the perineum occurs and rectal mucosa is exposed. Any stool in the rectum will be expelled. The fetal head passes under the pubic arch, and the vertex is visible as it pushes open the vaginal introitus, which is known as **crowning**.

Other Team Members

Other personnel required to be present during delivery will depend on the needs of the mother and infant as well as the protocol of the facility. If the woman is receiving epidural anesthesia, some facilities require a Certified Registered Nurse Anesthetist (CRNA) to be present during the delivery. The CRNA is there in case a bolus of analgesia is needed and to remove the epidural cannula immediately after the third stage is over and perineal repairs are completed.

If the amniotic fluid is meconium-stained, some facilities require that a neonatologist or a neonatal clinical nurse specialist be at the delivery to provide endotracheal suction to the newborn and ascertain whether meconium was aspirated by the baby. Other personnel that may be required, depending on the particular protocol are a surgical technician to assist with the instrument table and a nursery nurse to receive the baby. It is the primary nurse's responsibility to ensure that the primary caregiver and other health care team members as appropriate are notified of the impending delivery and are called in time.

Nursing Responsibilities in Preparing for Delivery

The client is never left alone during the second stage of labor; therefore, the nurse must anticipate the need for equipment and supplies. An instrument table is prepared and the individual requirements of the physician or nurse-midwife are considered (Figure 25-24). Other necessary items include a table containing sterile delivery instruments and an antiseptic such as Betadyne, adequate lighting, and oxygen and suction equipment for both mother and newborn. The radiant warmer or incubator should be prewarmed and spread with warmed baby blankets and a knit cap. Identification labels are prepared according to hospital protocol. Four identical identification bracelets usually are used for labeling the baby (two), mother, and partner. Two vials of oxytocin (Pitocin), 10 U, should be on hand for administration to the mother after the placenta has been delivered.

The nurse adjusts the birthing bed, delivery table, or operating table to accommodate the client and health care provider (who also may require a stool). In a physician-assisted delivery the client's legs often are supported in stirrups and the lower section of the delivery bed removed (Figure 25-25). A woman who has received epidural analgesia may have difficulty moving her legs; therefore, the nurse must ensure that the woman's legs are completely secure in the stirrups. It is not advisable for the client's legs to be placed in stirrups until the baby's head is almost crowning and the primary caregiver nurse is present in the

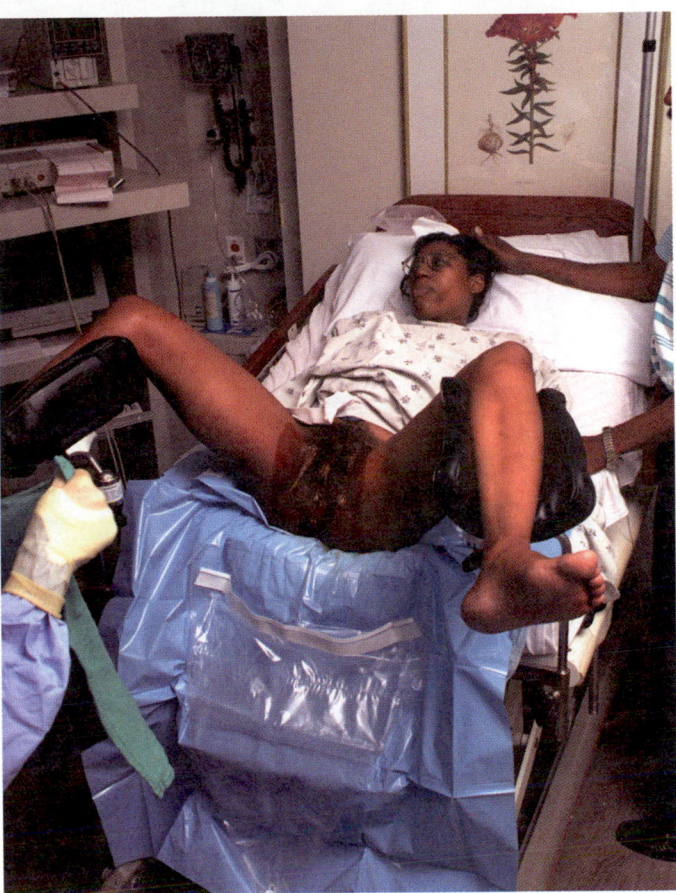

Figure 25-25 This woman is ready to deliver, with her legs supported in stirrups, the perineal area cleansed, and the foot of the bed removed.

delivery room, at which time the woman's legs are secured in the stirrups and the lower part of the delivery bed is removed. In a nurse-midwife-assisted birth, the bed is not broken down and stirrups are not commonly used.

For the birth, the nurse wears a waterproof gown and a mask with an eyeshield. Just before the birth, the nurse dons sterile gloves and cleanses the maternal perineum with prepackaged Betadyne-soaked sponges, using sterile technique as per the hospital policy and procedure (Figure 25-26).

The nurse and client's partner continue to support and encourage the woman in her expulsive efforts, instructing her to modify her breathing and pushing technique as indicated. Xylocaine 1% local anesthetic should be available in case the primary caregiver nurse decides that **episiotomy**, an incision into the perineum, is necessary to shorten the length of the second stage.

Episiotomy and Nuchal Cord

At the time of crowning, when the largest diameter of the fetal head first becomes visible, the perineum is stretched

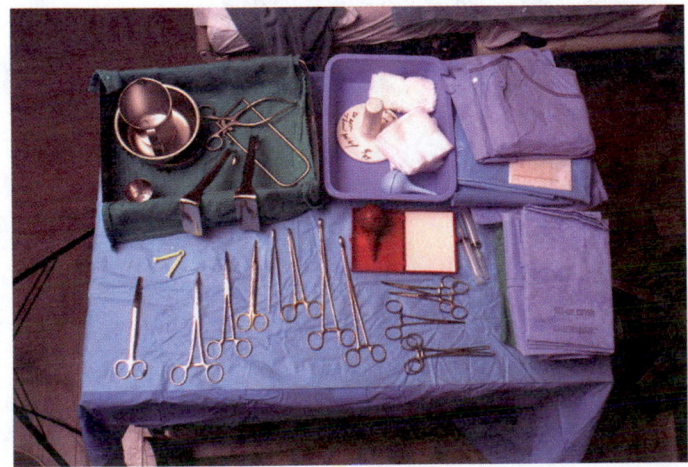

Figure 25-24 Delivery instrument table.

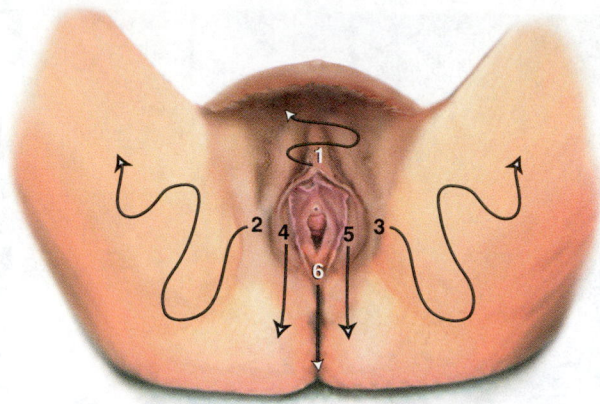

Figure 25-26 Perineal scrub; clean from the vagina outward, that is, from 1 to 6, moving bacteria away from and not toward the vagina.

extremely thin and may tear, particularly in the case of a nulliparous woman. Episiotomy is performed when a 3- to 4-cm diameter of fetal head is visible, before the perineal floor undergoes excessive stretching (Cunningham, 1997) (Figure 25-27). Local anesthesia can be injected before the episiotomy.

The episiotomy incision is made in the midline downward (median or midline episiotomy), or it begins in the midline and is directed laterally and downward away from the rectum (mediolateral episiotomy) (Figure 25-28). A straight, neat episiotomy incision is easier for the primary caregiver to repair than is a ragged laceration; however, research has shown that liberal use of episiotomy is not associated with a lower frequency of severe perineal tears (Anthony et al., 1994).

After episiotomy has been performed, the fetal head often is delivered with the next contraction. The infant's head is born by extension (see mechanism of labor in Chapter 23) and the primary caregiver feels around the infant's neck for **nuchal cord**, which is umbilical cord that has become wound once or more times around the infant's neck (Figure 25-29). If the cord can be felt around the neck, it often is loose enough to be pulled over the infant's head while the mother is instructed not to push. During the brief pause for restitution of the fetal head to take place, the primary caregiver may suction the mouth and nares of the infant before the infant's first breath. If the amniotic fluid has been stained by meconium, the infant's mouth and nares should be suctioned using a suction catheter to ensure that any meconium in the mouth or nose will not be aspirated (Figure 25-30). If the nuchal cord is tightly wound around the infant's neck the physician or nurse-midwife may need to double clamp and cut the cord to allow the infant to be delivered. Delivery time, date, and sex of the infant are noted on the mother's chart and on the infant labels (Figure 25-31).

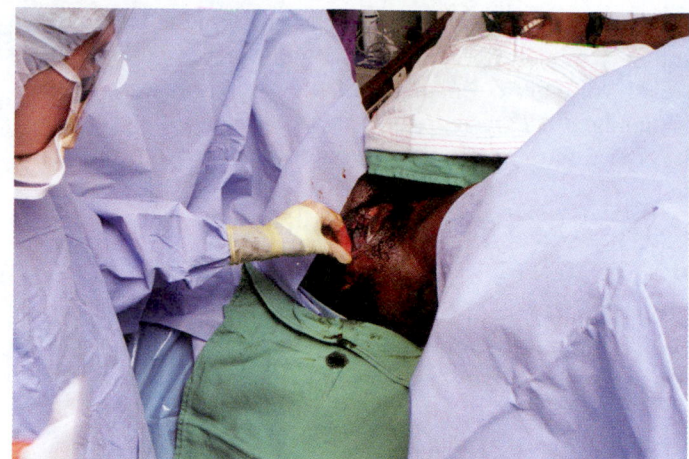

A.

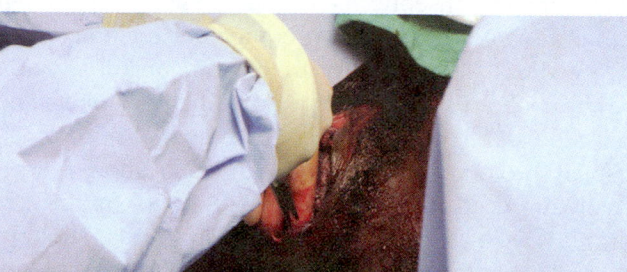

B.

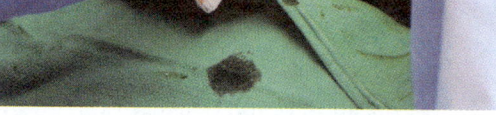

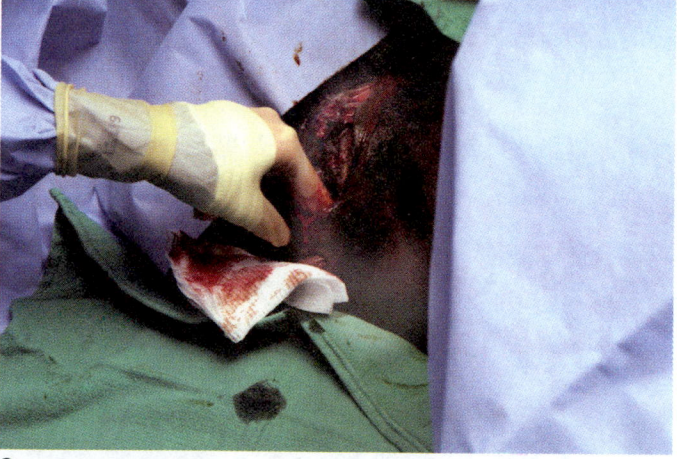

C.

Figure 25-27 Episiotomy procedure. A. Stretching of the perineum is assessed. B. Median incision is made. C. Some bleeding occurs.

Meconium Aspiration

In utero, the fetus has two normal "breathing" patterns by which it moves amniotic fluid into and out of the lungs:

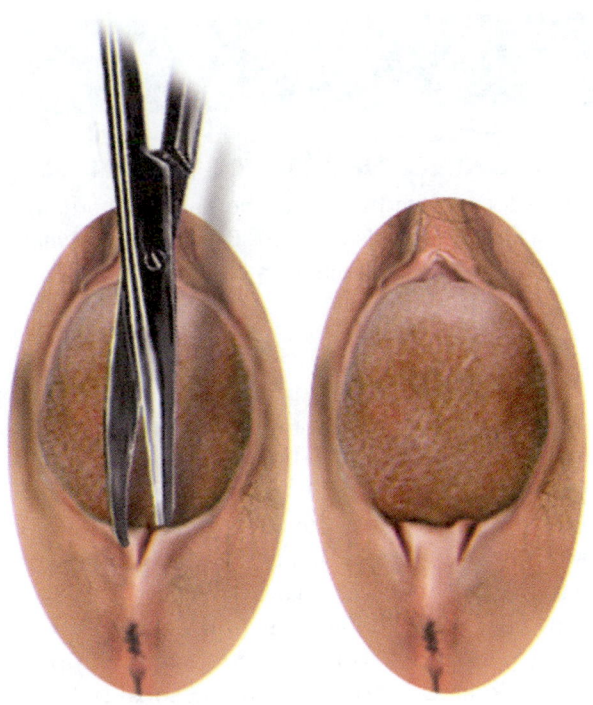

Figure 25-28 Episiotomy.

shallow regular breathing (90% of the time) and deep ir-regular breathing (10% of the time). In the presence of hy-poxia, the fetus may be stimulated to make compensatory gasping respirations. Hypoxia may result in passage of meconium, and the meconium-stained amniotic fluid can be aspirated into the fetal lungs if gasping respirations are stimulated by asphyxia.

When there is thick meconium in the amniotic fluid, the primary caregiver may order **amnioinfusion**, introduc-tion of warm normal saline or lactated Ringer's solution into the uterus by way of an IUPC, in an attempt to thin out the meconium and prevent meconium aspiration by the fetus.

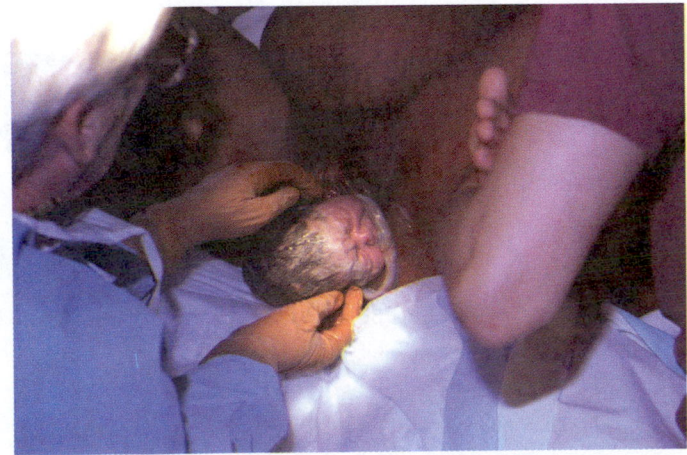

Figure 25-29 Birth of the fetal head with nuchal cord.

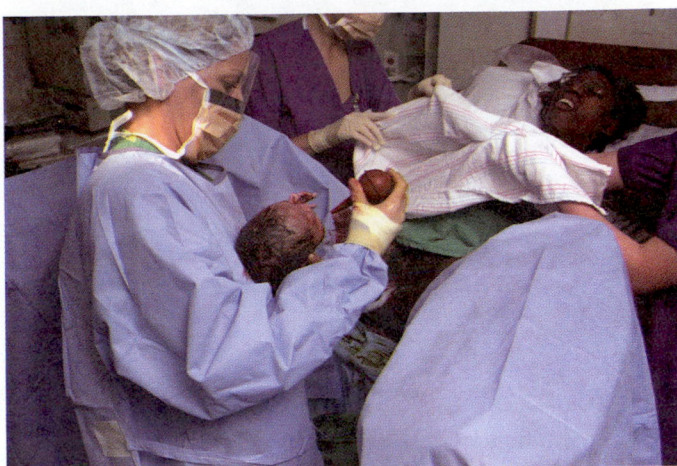

Figure 25-30 This infant was born so rapidly that there was no time to suction the mouth and nares until after the delivery was completed.

At delivery, the neonatology personnel should be present to provide prompt resuscitation and oxygenation as necessary. As the fetal head appears, the woman should be asked to refrain from pushing so that the primary care-giver can clear the airway, using a DeLee suction catheter, before the infant takes its first breath. The neonatology

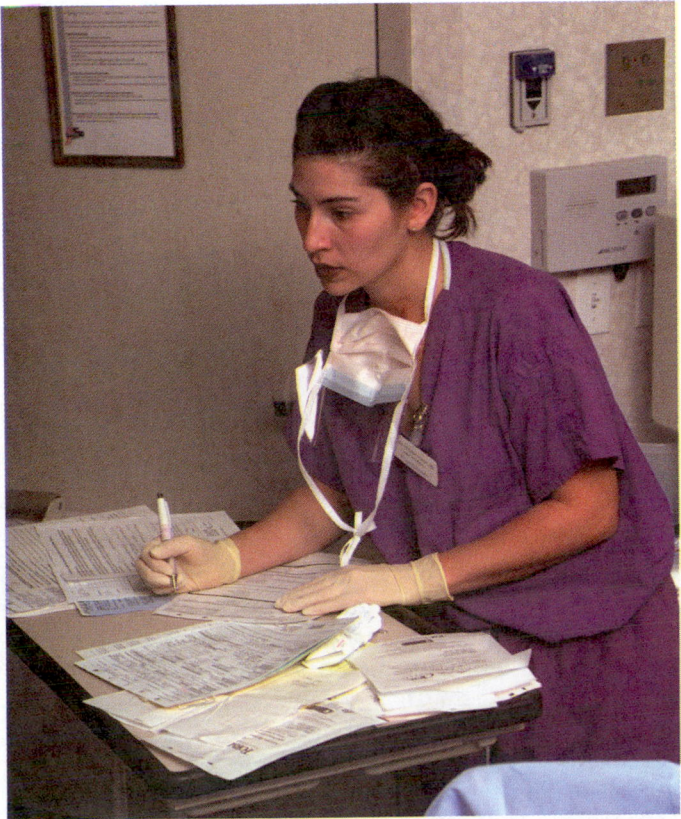

Figure 25-31 The nurse documents the delivery date, time, and the infant's gender on the mother's chart.

personnel may need to intubate the infant to clear the airway of meconium by way of an endotracheal tube.

Third Stage

The **third stage of labor** begins with delivery of the infant and ends with delivery of the placenta. This process may take up to 20 minutes. The nurse's attention at this time is directed toward newborn care.

Newborn Care

The time of birth is noted in the delivery record and the newborn's chart. When indicated, oral, pharyngeal, or endotracheal suctioning is performed according to the hospital policy, procedure, and protocol. Ideally, the infant is laid on the mother's abdomen and quickly covered with warm blankets to prevent heat loss by evaporation. The primary caregiver hands the infant directly to the nurse, who (wearing waterproof gown, mask, and sterile gloves), receives the infant into a sterile baby blanket. The nurse places the infant either into an incubator or beneath a radiant heater to prevent loss of body heat by evaporation while the infant is being dried. When necessary, the mouth and nares are again cleared by use of a suction bulb. In the neutral thermal environment of the incubator or infant warmer, the infant is dried thoroughly and a cap placed on the infant's head for extra warmth. As the nurse dries the infant, respiratory effort, color, and muscle tone can be observed. The action of drying the infant with warm baby blankets acts to stimulate the baby to breathe deeply and cry. Lightly flicking the soles of an infant's feet also will stimulate an infant to cry.

While drying the infant the nurse notices any rib, sternal retractions, "grunting" sounds or nasal flaring, which indicate respiratory compromise. Heart rate is checked by

Nursing Tip

CHECKING NEWBORN HEART RATE

Place a finger and thumb at the base of the umbilical cord. Count the pulsations for 6 seconds and multiply by 10 to calculate the infant's heart rate.

placing the thumb and two fingers over the base of the umbilical cord and counting the pulsations, which should be within the range of 110 to 160 bpm. Skin temperature should be 97.8°F (36.5°C). While assessing respirations and heart rate, the nurse conducts a gross physical examination (Table 25-6). The infant should be crying and becoming pink. The infant's hands and feet usually are still slightly blue. This condition is known as **acrocyanosis** and may persist for 7 to 10 days. Respiratory support is initiated, if required, according to the hospital policy, procedure, and protocol. Respiratory support includes administration of oxygen or ventilation by bag or mask. Obvious abnormalities, such as spina bifida, cleft palate, and extra digits, are documented. The number of vessels in the umbilical cord also are noted; the umbilical cord should have two arteries and one vein.

The **Apgar score**, a numerical expression of the newborn's well-being, is assigned at 1, 5, and 15 minutes after birth as the neonate's immediate adaptation to extrauterine life is monitored (Table 25-7). The newborn is given a score of 0 to 2 in each of the following five categories: respiratory effort, heart rate, muscle tone, reflex irritability, and skin color.

Newborn laboratory studies vary according to the hospital protocol but might include cord blood samples if the mother is Rh-negative or has type O blood group. Cord blood for neonatal blood type and Rh factor is obtained by

Nursing Alert

"FLOPPY" INFANT, NOT BREATHING

When receiving an infant from the delivering primary caregiver: if the infant is "floppy" (lacking muscle tone) and is making no respiratory effort, it is wise to assume that the infant is already experiencing secondary apnea and therefore will be unresponsive to stimulation. Artificial ventilation with positive-pressure oxygen must be initiated at once. The nurse should not waste time by trying to stimulate the infant to cry but should call immediately for the neonatologist and nursing assistance, while administering bag and mask ventilation with 100% oxygen.

Table 25-6 Newborn Evaluation at Delivery	
Assess	**Normal Findings**
Respirations	Rate 30–60 breaths per minute, irregular No retractions No grunting
Apical pulse	Rate 120–160 beats per minute
Temperature	97.5°F (36.5°C)
Skin color	Body pink, with bluish extremities
Umbilical cord	Two arteries and one vein
Gestational age	Should be >37 weeks to remain with the parents for an extended time

Table 25-7 Apgar Scoring System

Sign	Score		
	0	1	2
Respiratory effort	Absent	Slow, irregular	Good crying
Heart rate	Absent	Slow, below 100 beats per minute	Above 100 beats per minute
Muscle tone	Flaccid	Some flexion of extremities	Active motion
Reflex irritability	None	Grimace	Vigorous cry
Color	Pale blue	Body pink, blue extremities	Completely pink

the birth attendant while awaiting placental separation (Box 25-13). Cord blood gas analysis to evaluate biochemical status may be requested if the infant has a low Apgar score (Figure 25-32).

If the Apgar is less than 9 at 5 minutes, the infant should be stabilized rather than remaining with the mother in the LDR. Other situations that would require stabilization by the neonatal personnel include the following: "Grunting" respirations or rib retractions, nasal flaring, heart rate below 120 bpm or above 160 bpm, pallor, serious congenital anomalies such as spina bifida, a mother who is insulin-dependent, less than 38 weeks' gestational age, or small for gestational age appearance.

After the Apgar evaluation, identification procedures are completed according to the hospital policy, procedure, and protocol (Figure 25-33). Usual identification includes taking the footprints of the infant and a fingerprint or thumbprint of the mother, and labeling. A common

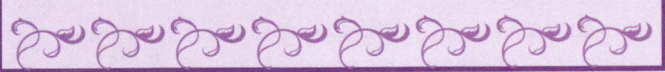

Critical Thinking

What is This Infant's Apgar Score?

The infant has just been delivered, and the physician hands the infant to you. You immediately lay the infant beneath the radiant heat lamp and begin your initial assessment as you dry the infant. The infant is breathing but not crying and the hands and feet are blue. The heart rate is 120 beats per minute, and the respirations are 30 breaths per minute and irregular. The infant's arms and legs are floppy. When you suction the mouth, the infant begins to cry more vigorously.

What is the 1-minute Apgar score that you will assign to this baby?

Answer: 6 (respiratory effort, 1; heart rate, 2; muscle tone, 0; reflex irritability, 2; skin color, 1).

Box 25-13 Procedure for Collection of Umbilical Cord Blood for Blood Gases

1. Before delivery, request that a 6- to 8-in segment of umbilical cord be clamped, cut, and passed off the surgical field as soon as possible after delivery.

2. One person is needed to attend the delivery and care for the neonate; another is needed to collect the blood samples.

3. Prepare a cup or Ziplock® bag of crushed ice, two 1-mL insulin syringes with 23-gauge needles and rubber stoppers, two laboratory slips, and two specimen labels.

4. Don gloves and goggles.

5. Using a bevel-down approach, aspirate 1 mL of blood from one of the umbilical arteries first.

6. Remove air bubbles: Air contamination has no effect on pH, partial pressure of carbon dioxide, or bicarbonate but may increase the partial pressure of oxygen (Gaskins & Goldkrand, 1994).

7. Remove the needle from the syringe with a hemostat, and cap the syringe with the rubber stopper.

8. Repeat the process with the umbilical vein (Figure 25-32). Compare the color of the blood in the syringes. The pinker blood is venous, and the darker blood is arterial.

9. Label each syringe with name, identification number, source, and time; place both syringes in the bag of ice.

10. Expedite delivery of the blood samples to the laboratory for blood gas analysis.

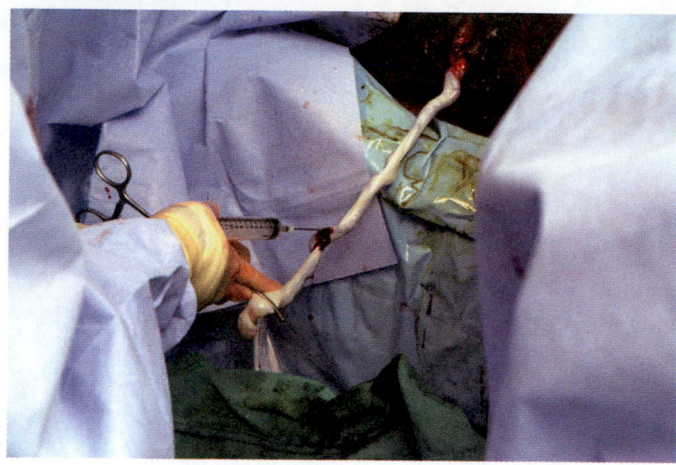

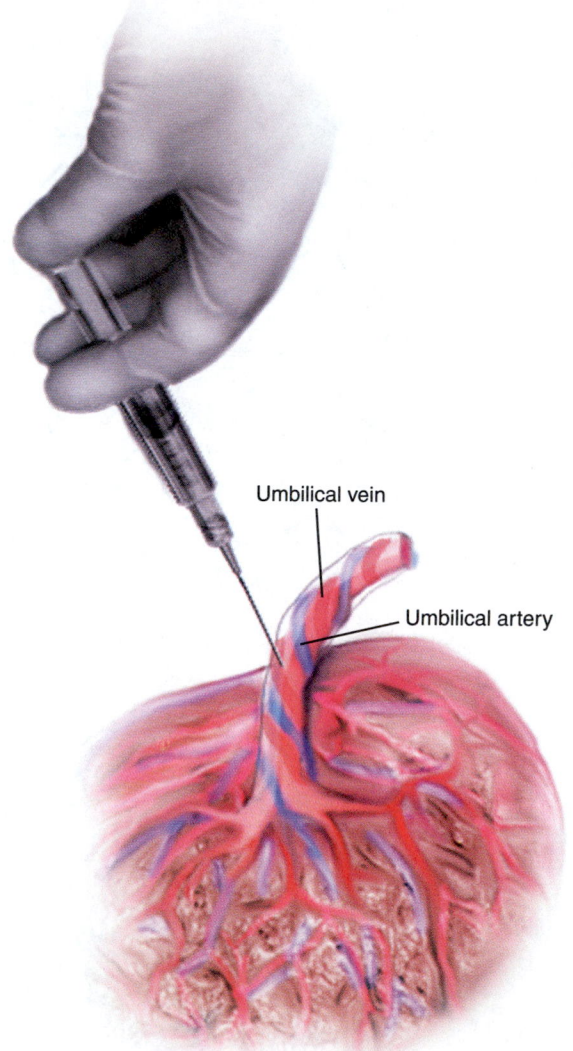

Umbilical vein

Umbilical artery

Figure 25-32 Aspiration of umbilical cord blood.

labeling protocol involves preparation of a set of four identically numbered waterproof bracelets with the mother's name, sex of the baby, physician or nurse-midwife of record, and the date and time of delivery. The baby wears two bands and the mother and her partner wear the others.

Delivery of the Placenta

The third stage of labor begins after the birth of the newborn and ends with delivery of the placenta. The priority at this time is the complete separation and expulsion of the placenta and prevention of hemorrhage from **uterine atony**, which is inability of the uterus to contract. After the baby is born, the height of the fundus is ascertained by palpating the abdomen. As long as the uterus remains contracted and there is no bleeding, the policy is one of watchful waiting for signs of placental separation. Separation of the placenta may take as long as 20 minutes but more often takes place within 1 to 10 minutes of the birth. During the waiting time the physician or nurse-midwife may examine the cervix and vagina and perform any necessary perineal repairs; however, repairs usually are undertaken after the third stage is complete. Contractions during the third stage of labor are of much less intensity than are those experienced during the second stage.

The placenta is attached to the endometrium by numerous fibrous villi, which break when uterine contractions cause the placental site to shrink. If the uterus remains flaccid, the placental site does not contract and thus the placenta cannot detach from the endometrium. Attempts to deliver the placenta, before it detaches from the uterus, by using cord traction or fundal pressure can result in tearing of the cord or membranes or inversion of the uterus. **Inversion of the uterus**, turning the uterus inside out, results in serious hemorrhage and shock. Indications that the placenta has separated from the uterine endometrium are the following (Cunningham, 1997):

- A firmly contracting fundus.
- Globular shape of the uterus as the separated placenta descends into the lower uterine segment.
- A small spurt of blood from the vagina.
- Apparent lengthening of the umbilical cord at the introitus as the placenta descends into the lower uterine segment.

When signs of placental separation are evident, the mother should be asked to bear down for the final time (Figure 25-34). Whether the shiny fetal surface of the placenta appears first (Schultze mechanism) or the dark roughened maternal surface shows first (Duncan mechanism) is of no consequence (Cunningham, 1997) (Figure 25-35). Perineal

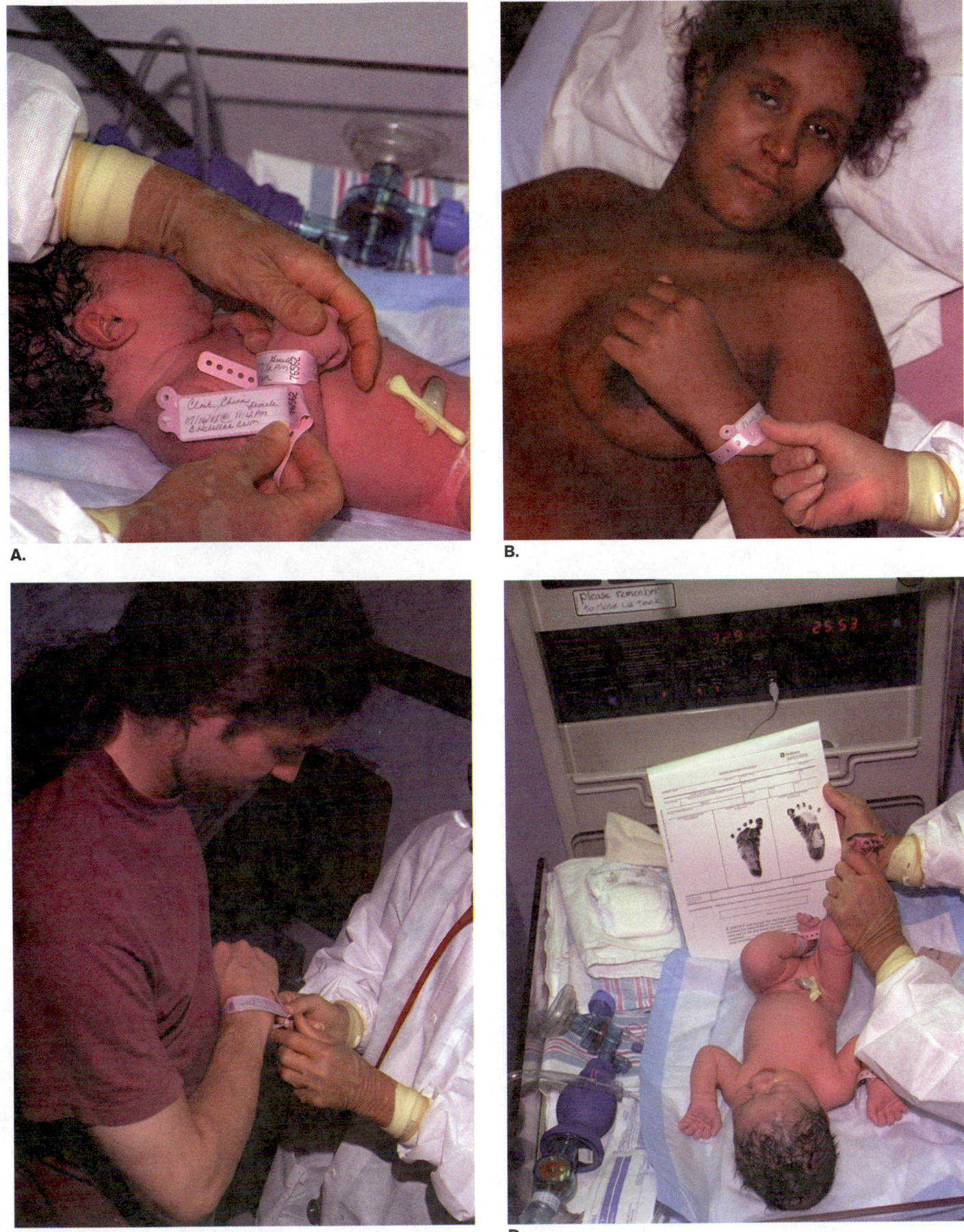

Figure 25-33 Matching idendification bands are placed on the (A) infant, (B) mother, and (C) father; (D) the infant's footprints are taken.

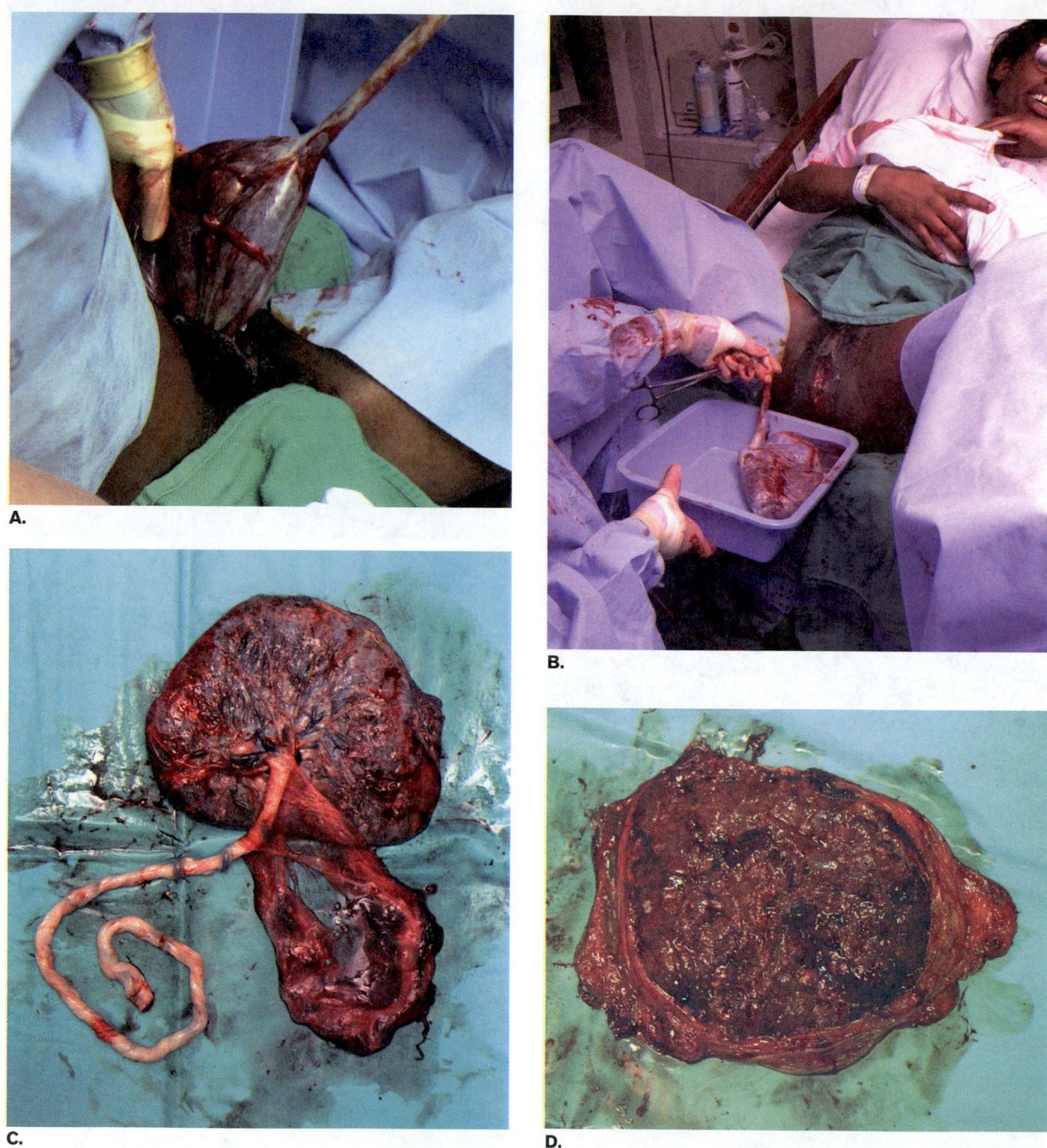

A.

B.

C.

D.

Figure 25-34 A. Delivery of the placenta. B. Inspection of the placenta. C. Fetal side (note empty amniotic sac). D. Maternal side.

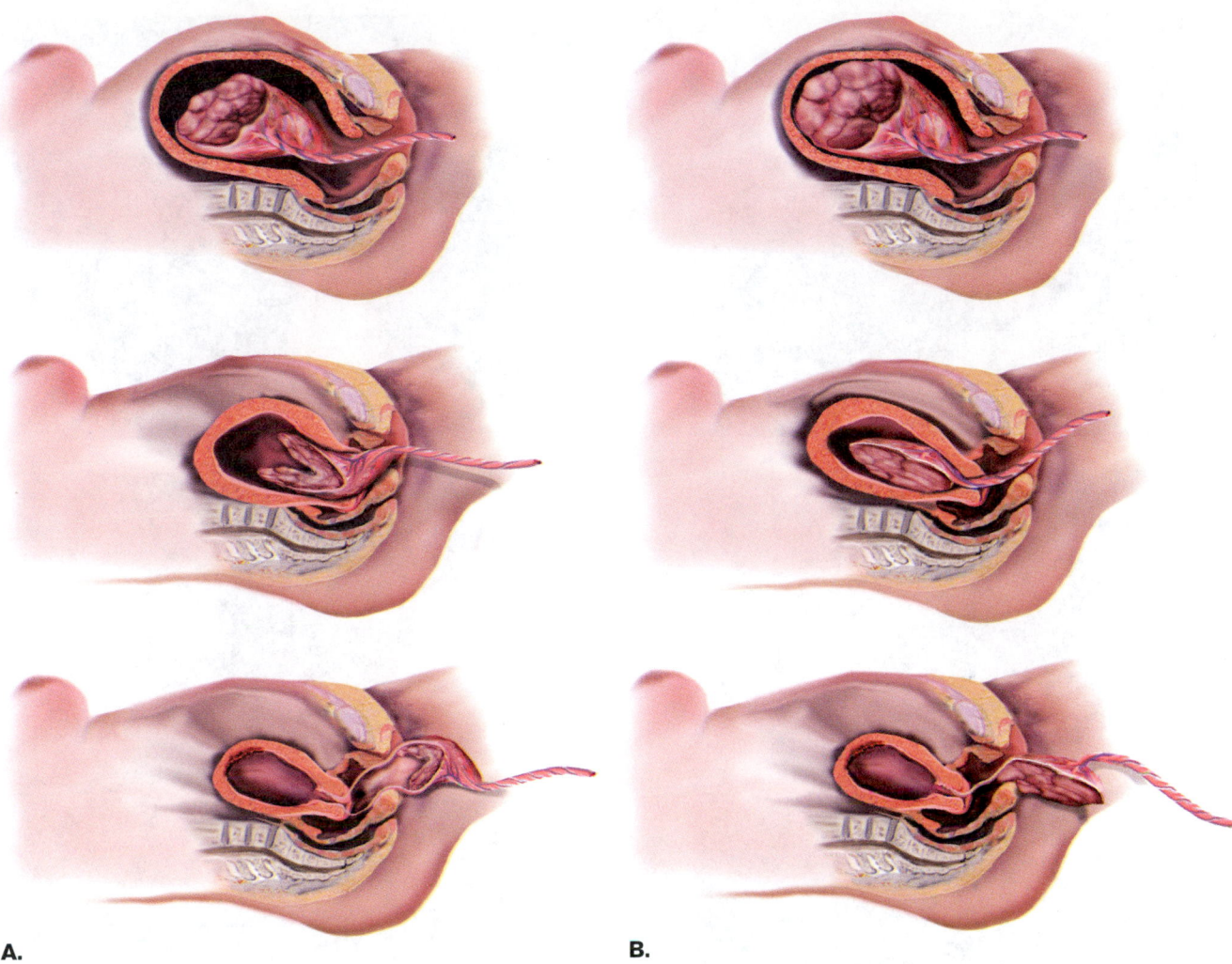

Figure 25-35 Placental separation. A. Schultze mechanism. B. Duncan mechanism.

repairs for laceration (tear in the perineum, vagina, or cervix caused by childbirth) and episiotomy are then performed (Figure 25-36).

Oxytocin Administration

Oxytocin is given at the end of the third stage of labor, according to the hospital policy and procedure. The purpose of oxytocin administration is to prevent postpartum hemorrhage by stimulating the uterus to contract (Table 25-8). If the woman has an IV line, a frequent protocol is to add of oxytocin (Pitocin), 20 U, to 1 L lactated Ringers solution and infuse over 40 to 60 minutes. A second liter of oxytocin (Pitocin), 20 U, in 1 L lactated Ringers solution or 5% dextrose lactated Ringers solution is sometimes given at a rate of 125 mL/h.

The placenta and membranes are examined by the primary caregiver for completeness, and the placenta may be sent for pathological examination. Cultures or tissue specimens are obtained as per the request of the primary caregiver and according to the hospital protocol.

The time of delivery of the placenta, its condition, and any abnormal characteristics are recorded in the Delivery Record. The amount of blood loss during delivery is estimated by the physician or nurse-midwife and noted in the Delivery Record by the nurse. The average blood loss at vaginal delivery is up to 500 mL (ACOG, 1998). The mother's perineum is cleansed gently and a sterile peripad applied. The degree and type of episiotomy or laceration is recorded in the Delivery Record (Table 25-9). An ice pack should be applied to the perineum to prevent swelling and pain, particularly if there are lacerations or an episiotomy. The lower portion of the delivery bed is replaced, and the woman's legs are carefully and slowly removed from the stirrups and placed back on the bed. If the woman has received epidural analgesia, it is discontinued and the cannula removed by the CRNSA. Warm blankets can be provided for comfort. All care is documented in the delivery record (Figure 25-37).

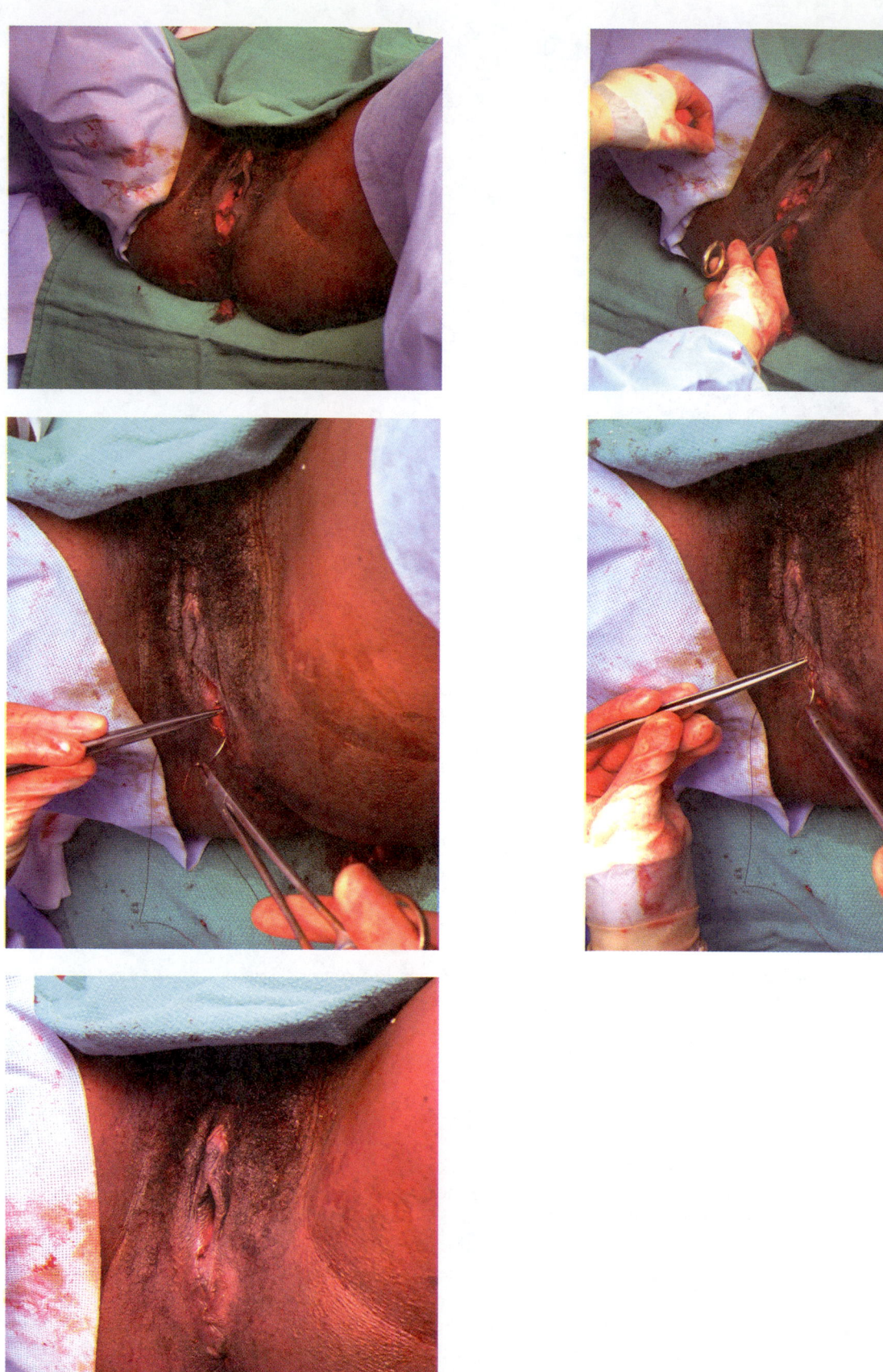

Figure 25-36 Perineal repair for laceration and episiotomy.

Table 25-8 Oxytocin Administration After Delivery of Placenta

Oxytocin (Pitocin)	Polypeptide hormone.
Action	Increases myometrial contraction by increasing the availability of intracellular calcium. Binds to oxytocin receptors in the decidua and myometrium.
Indication	Delivery of the placenta.
Dosage and route	Oxytocin, 20 U, in 1 L lactated Ringer's solution or dextrose 5% lactated Ringer's solution. Administer the first liter at a rapid rate. When a second liter of solution is ordered, administer at 125 mL/h. Oxytocin for control of postpartum bleeding may be diluted and administered by IV, or 10–20 U IM.
Adverse effects	With too rapid an infusion, tachycardia may occur; hypotension or hypertension also may occur. The antidiuretic effect may cause oliguria, fluid overload, arrhythmia, water intoxication, nausea, vomiting, or headache.
Nursing considerations	Assess the fundus for contraction. Assess the amount of lochia. Monitor vital signs, record intake and output, and assess the bladder.

Fourth Stage (Recovery)

The recovery phase immediately after delivery of the placenta often is referred to as the fourth stage of labor. This is a misnomer because labor and delivery are completed with the expulsion of the placenta. The fourth stage is the critical time that begins after delivery of the placenta and ends when the mother's systems have stabilized, usually 1 to 4 hours later.

Newborn-Family Attachment

The recovery period is a time of relative peace after the exertion and activity of labor and delivery. It also is a time of becoming acquainted with the newborn and for initial bonding to take place. Newborn-family attachment is promoted by encouraging touch and eye contact as soon as possible after delivery and by giving the family time to hold and admire the baby. Maternal bonding behaviors include smiling and talking softly to the baby, holding it up to her face and making eye contact, and breast-feeding. If the mother displays a negative behavior toward the baby, such as refusing to hold it or look at it, further exploration and supportive follow-up are warranted as are documentation and communication with the other nurses caring for the family.

Nursing Tip

NURSING DIAGNOSES, POSTPARTUM

Appropriate nursing diagnoses during this stage are the following:

- Deficient fluid volume related to hemorrhage as evidenced by blood loss secondary to uterine atony or perineal trauma.

- Impaired skin integrity secondary to median episiotomy.

- Interrupted family process related to addition of a new member.

- Grieving related to the birth experience not being as was expected, or the newborn not being the desired sex, as evidenced by the mother refusing to hold the newborn.

- Risk of uterine and perineal infection related to bacterial invasion secondary to trauma during labor and delivery, episiotomy, and extended time with ruptured membranes.

- Health-seeking behaviors related to newborn care, self-care, normal postpartum physiologic occurrences as evidenced by the client asking questions.

Table 25-9 Lacerations of the Birth Canal

Degree	Involvement
First	Fourchette, perineal skin, and vaginal mucous membrane
Second	Fourchette, perineal skin, vaginal mucous membrane, and fascia and muscles of the perineal body
Third	A second-degree tear involving the anal sphincter
Fourth	A third-degree tear extending through the rectal mucosa to expose the lumen of the rectum

✳ Hollister™

Labor and Delivery Summary
Hollister Maternal/Newborn Record System **Page 1 of 2**
To order call: 1.800.323.4060   Re-order No **5712**

Labor Summary

G	T	Pt	A	L	Type and Rh	EDD
III	II	o	o	II	o+	7/4/96

Prenatal Events ☐ None
- ☐ No Prenatal Care
- ☑ Preterm Labor (≤ 37 Weeks)
- ☐ Postterm Labor (≥ 42 Weeks)
- ☐ Previous Cesarean
- ☑ Prenatal Complications *Restricted activity*
- ☑ *Terbutaline 2.5mg. p.o. 32-36 wks*

Intrapartal Events
Maternal
- ☐ Febrile (≥ 100.4°F/38°C)
- ☐ Bleeding—Site Undetermined
- ☐ Preeclampsia (mild) (severe)
- ☐ Seizure Activity
- ☑ Medications   ☐ None

Date	Time	Medication	Dose	Route
6/23	1510	Oxytocin (titrated)		IV pump
6/23	1630	Bicitra	30cc	p.o
6/23	1325→	Marcaine	0.25%	CEA

- ☐ Transfusion _____ units
  Blood Component _____
- ☐

Amniotic Fluid
- ☑ SROM ☐ AROM Date 6/23 Time 0100
- ☐ Premature ROM ☐ Prolonged ROM
- ☑ Clear *initially*
- ☑ Meconium-Stained (describe) *light during 2nd stage*
- ☐ Bloody
- ☐ Foul Odor
  - ☐ Cultures Sent _____ Time ____
- ☐ Polyhydramnios
- ☐ Oligohydramnios
- ☐ _____

Placenta
- ☐ Placenta Previa
- ☐ Abruptio Placenta
- ☐ _____

Labor
- ☐ Precipitous Labor (< 3 hrs)
- ☐ Prolonged Labor (≤ 20 hrs)
- ☐ Prolonged Latent Phase
- ☐ Prolonged Active Phase
- ☑ Prolonged 2nd Stage (> 2.5 hrs)
- ☐ Secondary Arrest of Dilatation
- ☐ Induction   ☑ None
  - ☐ AROM   ☐ Oxytocin ☐ ____
- ☐ Augmentation   ☐ None
  - ☐ AROM   ☑ Oxytocin ☐ ____

Labor Summary (Cont'd.)
Fetus
Gestational Age (Wks) 38 3/7 By Dates
                      38 3/7 By Ultrasound

Presentation   **Position**
- ☑ Vertex | R | O | A |
- ☐ Face/Brow
- ☐ Breech ☐ Frank ☐ Complete
  - ☐ Single Footling
  - ☐ Double Footling
- ☐ Transverse Lie ☐ Back-up ☐ Back-Down
- ☐ Compound
- ☐ Unknown
- ☐ Cephalopelvic Disproportion (CPD)
- ☐ Cord Prolapse

Monitor ☐ None   FHR   UC
  External   ☑   ☑
  Internal   ☑   ☐
- ☑ STV ☑ Present ☐ Absent
- ☐ LTV _____
- ☐ Fetal Bradycardia
- ☐ Fetal Tachycardia
- ☐ Sinusoidal Pattern
- ☑ Accelerations ☑ Spont. ☐ Uniform
- ☑ Decelerations ☑ Early   ☐ Late
                   ☑ Variable ☑ Prolonged
- ☐ Scalp pH ≤7.2
- ☐

FM Discontinued 6/23 Time 1946
FHR Prior to Delivery 20/110 bpm Time 1945

Delivery Data
Support Person Present ☑ Yes ☐ No
Delivery Location
  ☐ LDR ☑ LDRP ☐ DR
  ☐ Birthing Room ☐ OR
  ☐ _____

Method of Delivery
- ☑ Vaginal ☐ VBAC
  Number Previous Cesareans ____
- ☑ Vertex
  - ☐ Spontaneous
  - ☑ Assisted | R | O | P | to | R | O | A |
    - ☐ Manual Rotation
  - ☑ Forceps (type *Simpson*)
    - ☑ Outlet ☐ Low ☐ Mid
  - ☐ Vacuum Extraction
- ☐ Breech (type _____)
  - ☐ Spontaneous
  - ☐ Partial Extraction (assisted)
  - ☐ Total Extraction
  - ☐ Forceps Assist
    - ☐ Piper ☐ _____
- ☐ Cesarean
  - ☐ Scheduled   ☐ Emergency
  - ☐ Primary   ☐ Repeat (x____)
  - ☐ Other
Operative Indication
  - ☐ Previous Uterine Surgery
  - ☐ Failure to Progress

Method of Delivery (Cont'd.)
Operative Indication (Cont'd.)
- ☐ Placenta Previa
- ☐ Abruptio Placenta
- ☐ Fetal Malpresentation _____
- ☐ Non reassuring FHR Pattern _____
- ☐ Other _____
Uterine Incision
- ☐ Low Cervical, Transverse
- ☐ Low Cervical, Vertical
- ☐ Classical
- ☐ Hysterectomy ☐ No ☐ Yes
- ☐ Tubal Ligation ☐ No ☐ Yes
Skin Incision
- ☐ Vertical
- ☐ Pfannenstiel

Episiotomy ☐ None
- ☑ Midline
- ☐ Mediolateral L R
- Laceration/Episiotomy Extension ☐ None
- ☐ Periurethral
- ☐ Vaginal
- ☐ Cervical
- ☐ Uterine
- ☑ Perineal ☐ 1° ☐ 2° ☐ 3° ☑ 4°
- Repair Agent Used *Ch ōō*

Placenta
- ☐ Spontaneous
- ☐ Expressed
- ☐ Manual Removal
- ☐ Adherent (type _____)
- ☐ Uterine Exploration
- ☐ Curettage
Configuration
- ☐ Normal
- ☑ Abnormal *short cord*
Weight 680 gms
Disposition *To lab*

Cord
- ☑ Nuchal Cord (x 1)
- ☐ True Knot Length _____ cms
- ☐ 2 Vessels
- ☑ 3 Vessels
Cord Blood ☑ To Lab ☐ Refrig ☐ Discard
Lab ☐ Type + Rh ☐ Cultures ☐ Coombs
    ☑ pH ☐ _____

Surgical Data
Sponge Counts Correct
☑ N/A ☐ Yes ☐ No _____
Needle Counts Correct
☑ N/A ☐ Yes ☐ No _____

J Hall RNC (Signature)   Date Completed 6/23/96

LABOR AND DELIVERY SUMMARY FORM #5712 (Page 1 of 2) 696

Figure 25-37 Labor and Delivery Summary. Courtesy of Hollister Incorporated.

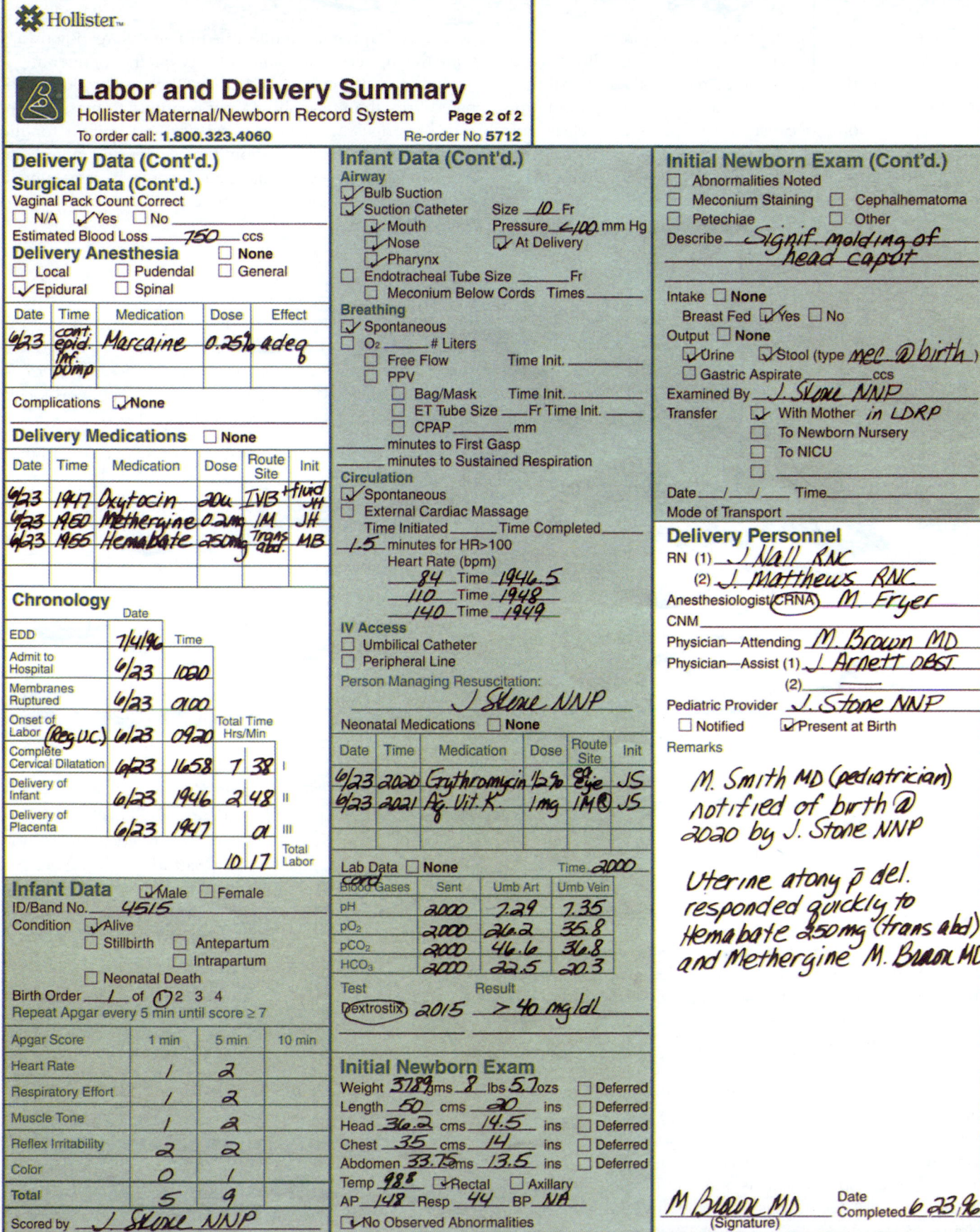

✳ Hollister™

Labor and Delivery Summary
Hollister Maternal/Newborn Record System   **Page 2 of 2**
To order call: **1.800.323.4060**   Re-order No **5712**

Delivery Data (Cont'd.)
Surgical Data (Cont'd.)
Vaginal Pack Count Correct
☐ N/A   ☑ Yes   ☐ No _____
Estimated Blood Loss ___750___ ccs
Delivery Anesthesia   ☐ **None**
☐ Local   ☐ Pudendal   ☐ General
☑ Epidural   ☐ Spinal

Date	Time	Medication	Dose	Effect
6/23	cont. epid. Inf. pump	Marcaine	0.25%	adeq

Complications ☑ None

Delivery Medications   ☐ **None**

Date	Time	Medication	Dose	Route Site	Init
6/23	1947	Oxytocin	20u	IVB +fluid	JH
6/23	1950	Methergine	0.2mg	IM	JH
6/23	1955	Hemabate	250mg	trans abd.	MB

Chronology

	Date	Time	
EDD	7/4/96		
Admit to Hospital	6/23	1020	
Membranes Ruptured	6/23	0100	
Onset of Labor (Reg UC)	6/23	0920	Total Time Hrs/Min
Complete Cervical Dilatation	6/23	1658	7 38	I
Delivery of Infant	6/23	1946	2 48	II
Delivery of Placenta	6/23	1947	01	III
			10 17	Total Labor

Infant Data   ☑ Male   ☐ Female
ID/Band No. _4515_
Condition ☑ Alive
   ☐ Stillbirth   ☐ Antepartum
              ☐ Intrapartum
   ☐ Neonatal Death
Birth Order _1_ of ①2 3 4
Repeat Apgar every 5 min until score ≥ 7

Apgar Score	1 min	5 min	10 min
Heart Rate	1	2	
Respiratory Effort	1	2	
Muscle Tone	1	2	
Reflex Irritability	2	2	
Color	0	1	
Total	5	9	

Scored by _J. Stone NNP_

Infant Data (Cont'd.)
Airway
☑ Bulb Suction
☑ Suction Catheter   Size _10_ Fr
   ☑ Mouth   Pressure <100 mm Hg
   ☑ Nose   ☑ At Delivery
   ☑ Pharynx
☐ Endotracheal Tube Size ____Fr
   ☐ Meconium Below Cords   Times ___
Breathing
☑ Spontaneous
☐ O₂ _____ # Liters
   ☐ Free Flow   Time Init. _____
   ☐ PPV
     ☐ Bag/Mask   Time Init. _____
     ☐ ET Tube Size ___Fr Time Init. ___
     ☐ CPAP _____ mm
_____ minutes to First Gasp
_____ minutes to Sustained Respiration
Circulation
☑ Spontaneous
☐ External Cardiac Massage
   Time Initiated _____ Time Completed _____
_1.5_ minutes for HR>100
   Heart Rate (bpm)
     _84_ Time _1946.5_
     _110_ Time _1948_
     _140_ Time _1949_
IV Access
☐ Umbilical Catheter
☐ Peripheral Line
Person Managing Resuscitation:
     J. Stone NNP
Neonatal Medications   ☐ **None**

Date	Time	Medication	Dose	Route Site	Init
6/23	2020	Erythromycin	1/2%	eye	JS
6/23	2021	Aq. Vit. K.	1mg	IM ®	JS

Lab Data ☐ None   Time _2000_

Cord Blood Gases	Sent	Umb Art	Umb Vein
pH	2000	7.29	7.35
pO₂	2000	26.2	35.8
pCO₂	2000	46.6	36.8
HCO₃	2000	22.5	20.3

Test	Result
Dextrostix 2015	> 40 mg/dl

Initial Newborn Exam
Weight _3789_ gms _8_ lbs _5.7_ ozs ☐ Deferred
Length _50_ cms _20_ ins ☐ Deferred
Head _36.2_ cms _14.5_ ins ☐ Deferred
Chest _35_ cms _14_ ins ☐ Deferred
Abdomen _33.75_ cms _13.5_ ins ☐ Deferred
Temp _98.8_ ☑ Rectal ☐ Axillary
AP _148_ Resp _44_ BP _NA_
☑ No Observed Abnormalities

Initial Newborn Exam (Cont'd.)
☐ Abnormalities Noted
☐ Meconium Staining   ☐ Cephalhematoma
☐ Petechiae   ☐ Other
Describe _Signif. molding of head caput_

Intake ☐ **None**
   Breast Fed ☑ Yes ☐ No
Output ☐ **None**
   ☑ Urine   ☑ Stool (type _mec @ birth_)
   ☐ Gastric Aspirate _____ ccs
Examined By _J. Stone NNP_
Transfer ☑ With Mother _in LDRP_
     ☐ To Newborn Nursery
     ☐ To NICU
     ☐ _____
Date __/__/__ Time _____
Mode of Transport _____

Delivery Personnel
RN (1) _J. Nall RNC_
   (2) _J. Matthews RNC_
Anesthesiologist/(CRNA) _M. Fryer_
CNM _____
Physician—Attending _M. Brown MD_
Physician—Assist (1) _J. Arnett OBST_
     (2) _____
Pediatric Provider _J. Stone NNP_
☐ Notified   ☑ Present at Birth
Remarks

M. Smith MD (pediatrician) notified of birth @ 2020 by J. Stone NNP

Uterine atony p̄ del. responded quickly to Hemabate 250mg (trans abd) and Methergine M. Brown MD

M. Brown MD
(Signature)   Date Completed _6/23/96_

Figure 25-37 *(continued)*

Some women wish to breast-feed immediately after the baby is born. At this time, the newborn usually is quite alert and amenable to breast-feeding. Suckling the baby as soon as possible after the birth is desirable from the mother's viewpoint because it stimulates the release of oxytocin, which helps the uterus to contract and thereby prevents hemorrhage. Refer to Chapter 30 for a complete discussion of breast-feeding.

After the excitement and stress of labor and delivery, the recovery time is an appropriate time to review events with the parents and give positive reinforcement. The nurse encourages verbalization of the birth experience and provides explanations so that the client and family can better incorporate these events into their life experience. During this time it is not unusual for the mother to apologize to the nurse for making "too much" noise or for being irritable during labor. The nurse can promote positive recall of the birth experience by commending the woman for her efforts and reassuring her that she fulfilled her part well. The objective is for the woman to remember her childbirth experience as an empowering and satisfying event.

Maternal Status

As the mother's organs begin the task of readjusting to the nonpregnant state, careful observations are recorded by the nurse. The priority of care during the recovery period is prevention of hemorrhage from the placental site.

In LDR settings, the woman remains in the labor and delivery area for 1 to 2 hours of intense observation. Findings during these first 2 hours are charted in the Obstetric Recovery Record according to the hospital protocol (Figure 25-38). Handwashing precedes assessment. Nonsterile latex gloves are worn when the perineum is inspected or when there is a possibility of contact with mucous membranes, skin that is not intact, blood, or other body fluids. Hands are washed again after removal of gloves.

Uterus

The uterus is assessed every 15 minutes for the first hour. The woman is positioned with knees flexed and head flat. The nurse uses one hand to stabilize the uterus just above the symphysis pubis and the outer edge of the other hand to locate the fundus. Position of the fundus is noted in relation to the umbilicus and recorded as centimeters above or below the umbilicus. During the fourth stage, the fundal height usually is at the level of the umbilicus. Placement of the uterus also is noted in relation to midline. Consistency is noted: If the uterus is not firm, it is referred to as *boggy,* and the fundus is massaged gently in a circular motion until the uterus contracts and becomes firm (Figure 25-39).

Clots are expelled at this time by the nurse placing both hands on the mother as if for measuring fundal height and applying gentle but firm pressure downward with the upper hand while observing the perineum for amount and size of expelled clots. Once the fundus is palpated firm, the nurse should not continue to massage because overmassaging is unnecessary and painful for the woman. A full bladder should be suspected when the uterus requires repeated massage to contract, remaining at the level of the umbilicus or above and being displaced to one side.

Lochia

Lochia is monitored every 15 minutes for the first hour, and the findings are recorded. The nurse notes the amount, color, and presence of clots. The red lochia encountered during this stage is known as lochia *rubra.* A standardized method for estimating the amount of lochia after delivery was devised by Jacobson (1985):

- Scant: Blood on tissue only when wiped or less than a 2-in stain.
- Light: Less than a 4-in stain on the peripad.
- Moderate: Less than a 6-in stain on the peripad.
- Heavy: A saturated peripad within 1 hour.

A perineal pad that is completely soaked with blood contains about 68 to 80 mL of blood (Lugenbiehl et al., 1990). When lochia is heavy, pads and linens should be saved for inspection by the physician or nurse-midwife. Continuous bleeding in the presence of a well-contracted uterus indicates soft tissue damage or retained products of conception such as placental tissue or membranes.

Prevention of Hemorrhage

Hemorrhage from the placental site is controlled by contraction of the uterus. Anything that impedes contraction of the uterus may result in postpartum hemorrhage. Assessments are designed to identify events that presage postpartum hemorrhage. The loss of at least 500 mL of blood is considered postpartum hemorrhage. The uterus is palpated at 15-minute intervals to ensure it is firm. A well-contracted uterus will not fill with blood. The peripad is

Nursing Alert

CHECKING FOR HEMORRHAGE

When assessing a newly delivered woman for bleeding, always look beneath her buttocks. Sometimes the perineal pad is barely soiled because blood is running down and pooling beneath the mother. The client may be completely unaware that she is hemorrhaging.

✳ Hollister™

Recovery Flow Record
Hollister Maternal/Newborn Record System
To order call: **1.800.323.4060**   Re-order No **5713**

Maternal Data
Admitted **6/23/96** Time **1020**

G.	T.	Pt.	A.	L.
III	III	0	0	III

Delivered **6/23/96** Time **1946** Age **35**

☑ Vaginal ☐ VBAC ☐ Cesarean (☐ Scheduled ☐ Emergency)
☐ Tubal Ligation ☐ _____
Episiotomy ☐ None ☑ Midline ☐ LML ☐ RML
Perineal Laceration/Extension ☐ None ☐ 1° ☐ 2° ☐ 3° ☑ 4°
Abdominal Incision ☑ No ☐ Yes _____
Anesthesia **continuous epidural infusion pump**
Complications **Prolonged 2nd stage ROP assisted → ROA**
Mother's Physician **M Brown MD** Planned LOS **1 day**

Infant Data
☑ Male ☐ Female
ID/Band No. **4515** Name _____
Condition ☑ Live/Normal ☐ Live/Abnormalities Noted
☐ Fetal/Neonatal Death
Feeding ☑ Breast ☐ Bottle
Location ☑ With Mother ☐ Nursery ☐ _____
Adoption ☑ No ☐ Yes
Problems Identified ☑ None

Visitors Present ☐ None ☑ **parents & siblings**

Maternal Assess

Medication Allergy/Sensitivity ☐ None (Identify) **Demerol**

Time	Temperature	Pulse	Respirations/O.Sat.	Blood Pressure	Level of Consciousness	Fundus	Bladder	Abdomen	Lochia	Perineum	Leg Movement	Pain	Intake (PO cc's)	Output (Urine cc's)	Response to Infant	Comments	Init
2015	99	88	16/97	120/70	2	F/u	F	NA	Mod	Ed/Ec	1	1	—	—	3	Reviewed infant ID band info c̄ mother	LM
2030		84	18	114/68	2	F/u	F	NA	Mod	Ice Ed.	1	1	—	—	4	Line of ecchymosis marked	LM
2045		81	18	118/76	2	F/u	F	NA	Mod	Ice Ed.	1	1	—	450	4	Bladder palp.↑ Foley cath. inserted-450cc	LM
2100		80	16	112/76	2	F/u	E	NA	Sc	Ice Ed.	1	1	chips	Foley 375	4	<3 v. pads mod. sat. since 2015	LM
2130		76	16	118/78	2	F/u	E	NA	Sc	Ice	2	1	240	Foley	4	No change in line of ecchymosis Enjoying dinner	LM
2200	99	76	16	120/78	2	F↓	E	NA	Sc	Ice	2	1	240	Foley 100	4	1 v-pad mod sat. in ½ hr.	LM
2215				120/78	2	F↓	E	NA	Sc	Ice	2	1	100		4	Breast feeding infant	LM
																Pericare given - Supplies rev'd.	LM

Intake (IV)

Start Date	Time	Solution	Amount cc's	Medication/Dose Added	Initials	Infused Date/Time	Amount
6/23/96	1947	F#3 LR	1000	Oxytocin 20u	LM	6/23/96/2340	1000
6/23/96	2340	F/A	(350)	Oxytocin 10u	JJ	6/24/96/0200	350

Medication

Time	Medication	Dose	Route/Site	Initials
2016	Cefotan	gms II	IV p.o.	LM
2015	Marcaine 0.25%	cont. epid. inf pump		LM

Released By **L MAX RNC** Date **6/23/96** Time **2215**
Transferred To **Mother/baby care team - LDRP** Time **2215**
Report To **J. Jones RNC** Time **2215**

L. Max RNC Signature

Infant Assess

Time	Temperature axillary	Pulse	Respirations	Skin Color	Muscle Tone	Behavior State	Feeding	Urine	Stool	Gastric	Comments	Init
2015	98⁸	144	40	P	2+	QA	@ Br	0	0	0	Skin: skin contact c̄ mother - breast feeding c̄ approp. suck & swallow	LM
2030		140	44	P	2+	QA	—	0	0	0	Swaddled and to dad	LM
2045		146	46	P	2+	S	—	0	0	0	Infant supplies reviewed c̄ parents	LM
2100		144	42	P	2+	S	—	0	0	0	Siblings here to visit	LM
2130	98	148	46	P	2+	S	—	0	0	0	J. Stone NNP in to assess infant	LM
2200		148	46	P	2+	S	—	0	0	0		LM
2215		148	48	P	2+	C	Br	0	0	0	Eagerly suckles @ breast	LM

Transferred To **Mother/baby care team** Time **2215**
Report To **J. Jones RNC** Time **2215**
L. Max RNC Signature

Initials	Signature	Initials	Signature
LM	L Max RNC		
JJ	J Jones RNC		

RECOVERY FLOW RECORD FORM #5713 696

Figure 25-38 Recovery Flow Record. Courtesy of Hollister Incorporated.

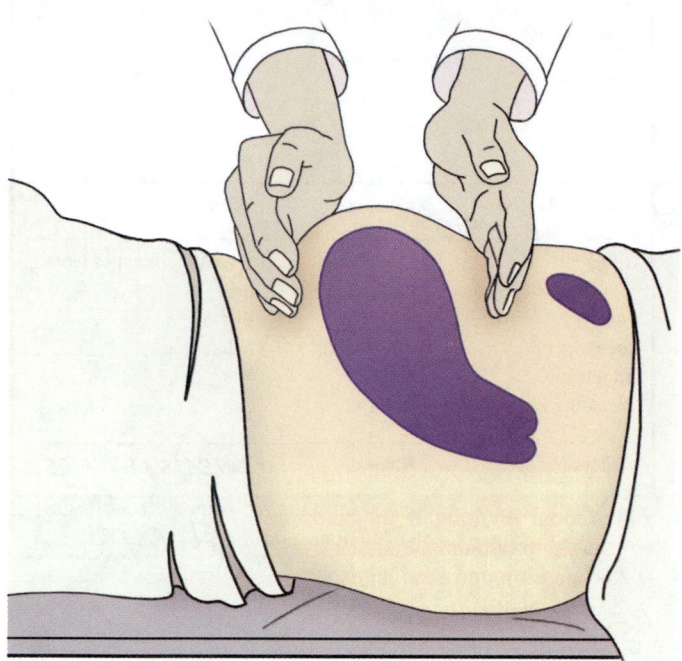

Figure 25-39 Recovery assessment of the fundus.

checked every 15 minutes to monitor lochia. The fundus normally is firm or can become firm after gentle massage and expulsion of any clots that have accumulated within the uterus. Certain factors are associated with postpartum uterine atony:

- Rapid labor.
- Prolonged first and second stages of labor.
- Forceps or vacuum extraction.
- Overdistention of the uterus (owing to hydramnios, multiple gestation, or large fetus).
- Previous postpartum hemorrhage.
- Advanced maternal age.
- Parity of four or more.
- Abruptio placentae or placenta previa.
- Induced labor.
- Preeclampsia and eclampsia.

Perineum

The perineum is observed every 15 minutes for the first hour to assess the episiotomy site or laceration repair to ensure it is intact and for edema, bleeding, and hematoma. Ice packs provide comfort and prevent swelling.

Bladder

The woman may have difficulty voiding spontaneously owing to bruising of the meatus or the effects of epidural anesthesia. The nurse should palpate the bladder for filling every 15 minutes during the first hour. When the mother's

Nursing Tip

MAKE SURE THE BLADDER IS EMPTY

When your client is to be transferred after the recovery hour from an LDR room to a busy postpartum unit (with a higher nurse-client ratio), it is prudent to have the woman empty her bladder before she is transferred. A client who has not voided after delivery is at risk for hemorrhage secondary to uterine displacement by a full bladder.

vital signs are stable and she is not suffering the effects of sedation or anesthesia, she may be assisted to the bathroom to void. Alternatively, a bedpan may be offered. Urine is measured and the time of voiding recorded. A full bladder usually causes the uterus to become boggy and be displaced to the right, and may lead to increased bleeding. When the woman is unable to void even though the bladder is palpable, or the uterus is displaced, catheterization is necessary.

Blood Pressure

Recording of blood pressure provides a database for possible diagnosis of complications such as hypertension. Under normal circumstances, few alterations in blood pressure are seen and pressure readings should return to prelabor levels within the first hour of vaginal delivery. Blood pressure is monitored every 15 minutes for the first hour, or more frequently if the client's condition warrants (AAP & ACOG, 1997).

Heart Rate

Pulse readings are recorded every 15 minutes for the first hour, and rhythm and regularity are assessed. The pulse usually returns to the prelabor rate within the first hour after vaginal delivery. If the nurse detects tachycardia, dehydration or infection should be ruled out.

Temperature

A temperature reading is taken during the first hour. It is not unusual for the woman's temperature to increase to at least 100.4°F (38°C) owing to the dehydrating effects of labor; however a higher temperature than this should be reported to the primary caregiver.

Psychosocial Status

The mother may be emotionally and physically exhausted but at the same time elated. She may be talkative and eager to phone friends and relatives with news of the newborn. Women often feel hungry immediately after delivery; however, food usually is withheld until after the recovery hour.

Pain

The mother may experience abdominal cramping commonly referred to as afterpains as the uterus contracts. Oxytocin administration after delivery of the placenta also will stimulate uterine contractions, and the nurse can explain to the woman the rationale for oxytocin administration and how this may cause some cramping. Analgesics should be administered according to the hospital policy, procedure, and protocol.

Maternal Teaching

The mother should be instructed in palpating her own uterus and how to massage it when necessary. The nurse can guide the woman's hand so that she can feel the firm contracted uterus (about the size of a grapefruit). It often is less uncomfortable for the mother to massage her own fundus than for this to be done by the nurse; however, teaching the mother in no way relieves the nurse of the responsibility of checking the fundus for firmness every 15 minutes during the recovery hour. It should be stressed that neither the woman nor the nurse should massage the fundus if it already is firm. Before she gets out of bed for the first time, the woman should be cautioned to call for a nurse to assist her.

Transfer to the Postpartum Unit

In some hospitals the mother remains in the same room for labor, delivery, recovery, and the postpartum period and the same nurse may care for the mother and infant. At other institutions the care may be handed over to a postpartum nurse. Many hospitals take the newborn to a nursery for 4-hours' transition time, during which the infant is observed closely. If the baby is to go to the nursery, the LDR nurse should encourage the partner to accompany it. When the father goes with the infant to the nursery, the mother may feel more at ease because she knows a family member is in attendance.

Recovery from Anesthesia

If the woman is to be transferred from the LDR to the postpartum unit, she should not be discharged from the LDR until her vital signs are stable. If she received epidural analgesia, she should be sufficiently recovered from its effects to be able to move both legs and raise her hips in order to move from the delivery bed to a gurney. Effects of an epidural may take several hours to completely dissipate; therefore, the mother should be instructed to call for

nursing assistance before getting out of bed the first time. A complete verbal report is given to the nurse coming on duty.

PRECIPITOUS DELIVERY

Occasionally, labor progresses so rapidly that the infant is delivered before the primary caregiver can attend, and therefore, the labor and delivery nurse assists the woman in giving birth. This is referred to as a **precipitous delivery**. The two most important concepts that the nurse must bear in mind when assisting a woman in the absence of the primary caregiver, is to support the fetal head as it descends, preventing it from popping out quickly, and to ensure that the newborn has a patent airway.

Nursing Alert

NURSING INTERVENTIONS DURING PRECIPITOUS DELIVERY

1. Instruct the woman to pant with contractions if the fetal head is crowning.

2. With a gloved hand, apply gentle pressure against the fetal head to maintain flexion and prevent it from popping out quickly. Support the perineum with the other hand.

3. When the fetal head is born, instruct the woman to pant and not to push. Suction the fetal nares and mouth with a bulb syringe.

4. Insert two fingers along the back of the fetal neck to check for a nuchal cord. If present, pull it over the infant's head. If the cord is too tight to pull over the infant's head, clamp it twice and cut between the clamps. Unwind the cord from around the neck.

5. While requesting the woman to push gently, exert gentle downward pressure on the head and neck to assist in the birth of the anterior shoulder. Then exert gentle upward pressure to assist with the posterior shoulder. Support the rest of the infant's body as it is born.

6. Place the newborn on the maternal abdomen, and dry the infant with warm blankets. Keep the newborn covered.

7. Check the firmness of the fundus and observe for bleeding.

8. Watch for signs of placental separation.

DELIVERY IN A NONHOSPITAL SETTING

Childbirth that occurs too rapidly for the mother to get to the hospital is referred to as **emergency childbirth**. Because there may be a certain amount of panic on the part of the mother and those with her, it is important that the person helping the mother remain calm and reassuring. Someone should call 911 as soon as possible so that help will be on the way. Most infants born under such nonconventional circumstances do very well, although they are at risk for cold stress. If there are other persons willing to give assistance, here are some main points to keep in mind.

1. Someone must be designated to take notes as the events unfold. The primary helper can dictate as the events unfold so that times will be accurate. Important information to record during emergency birth includes:
   a. Time the membranes ruptured, color of the amniotic fluid, and any unusual odor.
   b. Fetal position and presentation.
   c. Time of delivery.
   d. Presence or absence of the nuchal cord and the number of loops.
   e. Apgar scores at 1 and 5 minutes after birth.
   f. Resuscitation efforts, if needed.
   g. Condition of the infant.
   h. Sex of the newborn.
   i. Time of delivery of the placenta and its appearance.
   j. Amount of bleeding.
   k. Woman's condition: interventions to control bleeding and condition of the perineum.

2. Try to ensure some privacy.

3. If the mother is lying on the floor, put something beneath her such as towels, a blanket, or layers of newspaper.

4. Help her to remove her clothing as necessary.

5. If you have a few minutes and the head of the infant is presenting, it is best to have the mother push between contractions rather than at the height of the contraction. This will help to prevent tearing. Positioning the mother on her side also will lessen the intensity of the contractions and lessen the pressure, which, in turn, will help prevent the infant's head from popping our precipitously. A lateral position and pushing between contractions also will lessen the risk for perineal tearing.

6. Place your hand against the infant's head to provide support and to prevent it from popping out precipitously.

7. Check whether the amniotic sac is intact. If it is, then try to tear the sac so the newborn will not breathe in amniotic fluid with the first breath. Sometimes the fetal membranes are covering the infant's face and are too slippery to be grasped. It this is the case, break the membranes when the head is out by inserting a finger into the infant's mouth.

8. When the infant's head is out, have the mother relax and stop pushing while external restitution takes place. Watch as the infant's face turns toward the mother's inner thigh.

9. While restitution is taking place, feel around the infant's neck for a possible nuchal cord. If you feel the cord, and it is loose, slip it over the infant's head.

10. After restitution there is no need for manipulation of the shoulders unless more than 3 or 4 minutes has passed since the birth of the head. Placing your hands on each side of the infant's head, covering the ears, and pushing gently down on the head toward the floor may help free the anterior shoulder, and then lifting up the infant may facilitate birth of the lower shoulder.

11. The infant must be supported as it emerges. Hold the newborn at the level of the uterus to facilitate blood flow through the umbilical cord. Bring the infant up onto the mother's abdomen and cover it with whatever is available, preferably a clean cloth or towel. Wipe the infant's nose and mouth with a cloth or towel.

12. It is essential to keep the infant warm at all times. The best way to do this is to lay the infant skin to skin on the mother and cover them both. While the mother is holding the infant close to her body, stimulate the infant to cry by gently drying the skin with the cloth. Assign an Apgar score without exposing the infant to cold air. There is no need to tie or cut the umbilical cord. It will stop pulsating within a few minutes.

13. If the infant is showing no signs of spontaneous respiration, rescue breathing must begin (adult mouth over infant's nose and mouth).

14. To facilitate separation of the placenta and membranes, by contraction of the uterus, the mother should be encouraged to put the infant to her breast at this time. Suckling of the infant stimulates uterine contractions through release on oxytocin from the pituitary gland.

15. Watch for signs of placental separation. When the placenta has separated, have the woman give one slow steady push and catch the placenta in your hands. Gently twist the placenta so that the trailing membranes will twist to form a rope as they slowly separate from the uterus. Try not to let the membranes tear away from the placenta.

Case Study/Care Plan

THE CLIENT WITH PAIN DURING A VAGINAL DELIVERY

Maria Brown, a 26-year-old gravida 3, para 2, is admitted to the labor and delivery unit at 41 weeks' gestation. Maria says that she thinks her "bag of waters" has broken. The nurse orientates Ms. Brown and her boyfriend to the labor, delivery, and recovery room (LDR). After Ms. Brown has undressed and put on a hospital gown, external fetal heart rate (FHR) monitoring is begun. The FHR has a baseline of 140 beats per minute (bpm) and good variability.

The nurse has Maria sign a consent form and proceeds with the interview and assessment. No risk factors are identified from the prenatal record and the nursing assessment. A vaginal examination indicates Maria's cervix is 80% effaced and 3 cm dilated. The presenting part is vertex at −1 station. No amniotic sac is palpated, and there is clear fluid draining from the vagina and pooling in the bed. Nitrazine paper, when touched to the wet bed linen, turns deep blue, indicating the presence of amniotic fluid. When asked the time the membranes ruptured, Maria indicates that they have been ruptured for 2 hours. The nurse-midwife is notified and states that she is en route to the hospital.

Maria's labor continues uneventfully. Blood is drawn for routine laboratory tests. Maria's temperature is taken every 2 hours. Various measures are employed to ensure her comfort during the first few hours. She ambulates up and down the hall with her boyfriend, and he brings her back to the LDR every 30 minutes for intermittent fetal monitoring. After 3 hours of labor, Maria says that she would like to rest in bed. The nurse and Maria's boyfriend help her into a comfortable lateral position and support her with extra pillows.

At 5 cm dilation, Maria becomes increasingly uncomfortable and requests epidural anesthesia. The nurse starts IV lactated Ringer's solution, 1 L, to infuse over the next 30 minutes. The anesthesiologist briefly interviews Maria as the nurse positions her to receive the epidural anesthesia. The boyfriend helps to support Maria in the required position.

Thirty minutes after the epidural is placed and Maria is feeling comfortable once more, vaginal examination reveals the cervix to be 8 cm dilated, 100% effaced, and the vertex at 0 station. At this time, the FHR decelerates from the 140 bpm baseline to 90 bpm, and then to 60 bpm. Maria's blood pressure is 94/44 mm Hg. The nurse quickly turns Maria on her side and opens the IV to give a rapid bolus of fluid. Oxygen is started by way of a non-rebreather mask, at 10 L/min. After 2 minutes, Maria's blood pressure is 100/54 mm Hg, and the FHR has returned to baseline. After a 500-mL bolus of IV fluid has been infused, the nurse slows the rate to 125 mL/h. Vaginal examination reveals the cervix still 8 cm dilated, 100% effaced, but the vertex is at +1 station. A fetal scalp electrode is placed for internal FHR monitoring. The amniotic fluid remains clear, and Maria is afebrile. A Foley catheter is inserted and attached to bedside drainage. Intake and output are recorded carefully.

Labor continues uneventfully for the next 3 hours, when Maria is fully dilated and the presenting part is at +2. Because of the effects of the epidural, Maria does not have an urge to push. The nurse instructs Maria how to support her knees, and to push when there is a contraction. After 1 hour of pushing, a viable male is delivered and placed skin to skin on the mother's abdomen. Maria's boyfriend, the baby's father, is able to cut the umbilical cord. The Apgar scores are 8/9/9. The placenta and membranes are delivered complete 5 minutes later. Total blood loss is 250 mL; the perineum is intact although swollen. An ice pack is applied. Maria and her boyfriend are jubilant as she prepares to breast-feed their new son.

Assessment

MB is 26 years old and in labor with her third baby. External fetal monitoring is in progress and the FHR shows average variability, with a baseline of 140 bpm. Vaginal examination reveals MB's cervix is 3 cm dilated, 80% effaced, and vertex presentation at −1 station. Membranes are ruptured, and the amniotic fluid is clear. Contractions are moderate in intensity. MB is gasping with each contraction and sometimes verbalizing pain.

(continued)

Nursing Diagnosis

Pain related to uterine contractions and cervical dilation as evidenced by MB's facial contortion and gasping when uterine contractions occur and her statement: "I am really hurting now."

Expected Outcome Maria will verbalize decreased discomfort with uterine contractions and experience a degree of relaxation.

Planning The nurse must take into account the length of time Maria's labor is likely to endure (she is only 3 cm dilated), and structure care to help Maria cope with labor progress.

Nursing Interventions	Rationales
1. Assess the MB's preparation for labor.	1. Patients who have attended childbirth preparation classes often use psychoprophylactic methods to reduce pain.
2. Teach MB breathing techniques during early labor.	2. Controlled thought and focused breathing will increase relaxation. Patients are more receptive to teaching during early labor.
3. Encourage MB's boyfriend in methods that may help to reduce her discomfort: offering fluids, ice chips as ordered, back rubs, assist MB into comfortable position, give praise.	3. Measures are often more effective when effective when delivered by a familiar person. Studies have shown that a support person helps to reduce the length of labor.
4. Provide comfort measures.	4. Ambulation, back rubs, change of position, extra pillows, warm shower, and other comfort measures help to reduce the discomfort of labor.
5. Explain what analgesics and anesthesia are available for use during labor and mode of administration.	5. Explanation of pharmacological methods of pain control will provide knowledge to help MB make decisions about analgesia and anesthesia.
6. Assist in the placement of an epidural catheter, if ordered.	6. Regional anesthesia provides analgesia and anesthesia during labor and delivery.
7. Keep MB aware of her progress and review the process of labor.	7. Knowledge that she is making expected progress will allay anxiety and increase coping.
8. Encourage regular voiding to decrease the chance of distention.	8. Bladder distention can increase discomfort during contractions and impede the progress of labor.
9. Encourage conscious relaxation between contractions.	9. Fatigue contributes to increased pain perception and inability to cope with pain.

Evaluation MB verbalizes decreased discomfort with her contractions during early labor with the assistance of her boyfriend and the nurse, who supplied back rubs, extra pillows, encouragement, information, assistance in positioning, and ambulation. As labor progressed, and after receiving information about analgesia and anesthesia, MB made the decision to have epidural analgesia. After the epidural was placed, MB was able to rest peacefully and stated: "I can no longer feel any pain with my contractions."

16. Wrap the placenta and place it together with the infant; it will provide some warmth.

17. Check the firmness of the uterus. The fundus may be massaged to stimulate contractions and decrease bleeding.

18. Clean the area under the mother, and inspect the perineum for lacerations. Bleeding from lacerations may be controlled by pressing a clean peripad against the perineum and instructing the woman to keep her thighs together.

Web Activities

- What information can you find on the Doulas website?
- Outline client teaching tips drawn from the Lamaze internet offerings.

Key Concepts

- Nursing care of the laboring woman is very complex because the nurse must ensure the well-being of the mother and fetus throughout the labor process.
- Although labor and delivery are normal physiologic events, there is a great potential for negative outcomes.
- In many birthing units, the nurse is the sole health care provider with which the client interacts throughout labor.
- The nurse who provides intrapartum care must have a thorough understanding of the labor process as well as signs of fetal status to identify actual or potential labor complications.
- Initial and ongoing assessment for risks and changes in condition are of paramount importance.
- Every woman deserves to have the most positive birth experience possible considering her condition.
- Interventions that provide relaxation and comfort to the laboring woman facilitate the birth process.
- Every woman deserves to know her birth experience was special.

Review Questions and Activities

1. What should the nurse ask first about the amniotic sac?
a. Presence of bloody show
b. Time the membranes ruptured
c. Frequency of contractions
d. Appearance of the fluid

The correct answer is d.

2. Estelle is encouraged to change positions to promote comfort. Which position should not be used during labor?
a. Lateral position
b. Squatting position
c. Standing position
d. Supine position

The correct answer is d.

3. Which of the following structures are involved when an episiotomy is performed?
a. Glans clitoris
b. Labia minora
c. Levator ani muscle
d. Labia majora

The correct answer is c.

4. Which of the following is an expected characteristic of amniotic fluid?
a. Deep yellow color
b. Clear, with small white particles
c. Nitrazine test shows acidic result
d. absence of ferning

The correct answer is b.

5. When planning care for a woman whose membranes have ruptured, the nurse recognizes that the woman is at increased risk for:
a. hemorrhage
b. precipitous labor
c. supine hypotension
d. intrauterine infection

The correct answer is d.

6. When assessing a woman in the first stage of labor, the nurse recognizes that the most conclusive sign that uterine contractions are effective would be:
a. dilatation of the cervix
b. presence of capput succadeneum on the vertex
c. rupture of amniotic membranes
d. increase in bloody show

The correct answer is a.

7. The nurse who performs vaginal examinations to assess a woman's progress in labor should:
a. perform an examination at least once every hour during the active phase
b. perform the examination more frequently if vaginal bleeding is present
c. wear two clean gloves for each examination
d. discuss the findings with the woman and her labor partner

The correct answer is d.

8. The nurse knows that the second stage of labor has begun when the:
a. Amniotic membranes rupture
b. Cervix cannot be felt during a vaginal examination
c. Woman experiences a strong urge to bear down
d. Presenting part is below the ischial spines

The correct answer is c.

9. The most critical nursing action when caring for the newborn immediately after birth is:
a. Keeping the newborn's airway clear
b. Fostering parent-newborn attachment
c. Drying and wrapping the newborn in a blanket
d. Recording the time of birth and Apgar score

The correct answer is a.

10. The nurse prepares to administer oxytocin to a woman, after expulsion of the placenta, to:
a. Relieve pain
b. Stimulate uterine contraction
c. Prevent infection
d. Facilitate rest and relaxation

The correct answer is b.

References

American Academy of Pediatrics & American College of Obstetricians & Gynecologists. (1997). *Guidelines for perinatal care* (4th ed.). Elk Grove Village, IL:

American Collect of Obstetricians and Gynecologists (ACOG). (Dec. 1995). *Dystocia and the augmentation of labor* (ACOG Technical Bulletin No. 218). Washington, DC: American College of Obstetricians and Gynecologists.

American College of Obstetricians and Gynecologists (ACOG). (1995). *Fetal heart rate patterns: Monitoring, interpretation, and management* (ACOG Technical Bulletin No. 207). Washington, DC: American College of Obstetricians and Gynecologists.

American College of Obstetricians and Gynecologists (ACOG). (1996). *Hypertension in pregnancy* (ACOG Technical Bulletin No. 219). Washington, DC: American College of Obstetricians and Gynecologists.

American College of Obstetricians and Gynecologists (ACOG). (Sept. 1997). *Smoking and women's health* (ACOG Educational Bulletin No. 240). Washington, DC: American College of Obstetricians and Gynecologists.

American College of Obstetricians and Gynecologists (ACOG). (March 1997). *Thromboembolism in pregnancy* (ACOG Educational Bulletin No. 234). Washington, DC: American College of Obstetricians and Gynecologists.

American College of Obstetricians and Gynecologists (ACOG). (1998). *Postpartum hemorrhage* (ACOG Educational Bulletin No. 243). Washington, DC: American College of Obstetricians and Gynecologists.

Anthony, S., Buitendijk, S. E., Zondervan, K. T., van Rijssel, E. J., & Verkerk, P. H. (1994). Episiotomies and the occurrence of severe perineal lacerations. *British Journal of Obstetrics & Gynaecology, 101,* (12), 1064–1067.

Association of Women's Health, Obstetric and Neonatal Nurses (AWHONN). (1998). *Standards and guidelines* (5th ed.). Washington, DC: Association of Women's Health, Obstetric and Neonatal Nurses.

Berensen, A. B., Wiemann, C. M., Wilkinson, G. S., Jones, W. A., & Anderson, G. D. (1994). Perinatal morbidity associated with violence experienced by pregnant women. *American Journal of Obstetrics and Gynecology, 170,* (6), 1760–1766.

Cunningham, F. G. (Ed.). (1997). *Williams Obstetrics* (20th ed.). New York: NY: Graw-Hill.

Fraser, W. D., Turcot, L., Krauss, I., & Brisson-Carrol, G. (2000). Amniotomy for shortening spontaneous labour (Cochrane Review). In *The Cochrane Library, Issue 1.* Oxford: Updated Software.

Friedman, E. A. (1970). An objective method of evaluating labor. *Hospital Practice, 5,* (7), 83.

Gaskins, J. E., & Goldkrand, J. W. (1994). Air contamination in umbilical cord blood sampling. *American Journal of Obstetrics & Gynecology, 171,* (6), 1546–1549.

Gazmararian, J. A., Lazorick, S., Spitz, A. M., Ballard, T. J., Saltzman, L. E. & Marks, J. S. (1996). Prevalence of violence against pregnant women. *Journal of the American Medical Association, 275,* (24), 1915–1920.

Hilliard, P. J. (1985). Physical abuse in pregnancy. *Obstetrics & Gynecology, 66,* 185–190.

Hodnett, E. D. (2000). Caregiver support for women during childbirth (Cochrane Review). In *The Cochrane Library, Issue 1,* Oxford: Updated Software.

Kohl, S. (1997). Neonatal herpes virus infection. *Clinics in Perinatology, 24,* (1), 129–150.

Lowe, N. K. (1996). The pain and discomfort of labor and birth. *Journal of Obstetric, Gynecologic, and Neonatal Nursing, 25,* (1), 82–92.

Lugenbiehl, D. L., Brophy, G. H., Artigue, G. S., Phillips, K. E., & Flak, R. J. (1990). Standardized assessment of blood loss. *Maternal Child Nursing, 15,* 241.

Manogin, T. W., Bechtel, G. A., & Rami, J. S. (2000). Caring behaviors by nurses: Women's perceptions during childbirth. *Journal of Obstetric, Gynecologic, and Neonatal Nursing, 29,* (2), 137–168.

Mayberry, L. J., Wood, S. H., Strange, L. B., Lee, L., Heisler, D. R., & Nielson-Smith, K. (1999). Managing second-stage labor. *AWHONN Lifelines, 3,* (6), 28–34.

McFarlane, J., Parker, B., & Soekew, K. (1996). Physical abuse, smoking, and substance abuse during pregnancy: Prevalence, interrelationships, and effects on birth weight *Journal of Obstetric, Gynecologic & Neonatal Nursing, 25,* (4), 313–320.

Murray, M. (1997). *Autopartal and Intrapartal Fetal Monitoring* (2nd ed.). Albuquerque, NM: Learning Resources International, Inc.

Parker, B., McFarlane, J. & Soekew, K. (1994). Abuse during pregnancy: Effects on maternal complications and birth weight in adult and teenage women. *Obstetrics and Gynecology, 84,* (3), 323–328.

Queenan, J., & Hobbins, J. (Eds.). (1996). *Protocols for high-risk pregnancies* (3rd ed.). Cambridge, England: Blackwell Science.

Roberts, S. W., Cox, S. M., Dax, J., Wendel, G. D., & Leveno, K. J. (1995). Genital herpes during pregnancy: No lesions, no cesarean. *Obstetrics & Gynecology, 85,* (2), 261–264.

Salamalekis, E., Loghis, C., Panayotopoulos, N., Vitoratos, N., Giannake, G., & Christodoulacos, G. (1997). Non-stress test: A fifteen-year clinical appraisal. *Clinical & Experimental Obstetrics & Gynecology, 21,* (2), 79–81.

Scott, J., DiSaia, P., Hammond, C., & Spellocy, W. (Eds.). (1994). *Danforth's obstetrics and gynecology* (7th ed.). Philadelphia, PA: J. B. Lippincott.

Teixeira, M., Fisk, N. M., & Glover, V. (1999). Association between maternal anxiety in pregnancy and increased uterine artery resistance index: Cohort based study. *British Medical Journal, 318,* 153–157.

Vintzileos, A. M., Nochimson, D. J., Guzman, E. R., Knuppel, R. A., Lake, M., & Schifrin, B. S. (1995). Intrapartum electronic fetal heart rate monitoring versus intermittent auscultation: A meta-analysis. *Obstetrics & Gynecology, 85,* (1), 149–155.

Wadhwa, P. D., Porto, M., Garite, T. J., Chicz-DeMet, A., & Sandman, C. A. (1998). Maternal corticotropin-releasing hormone levels in the early trimester predict length of gestation in human pregnancy. *American Journal of Obstetrics and Gynecology, 179,* 1079–1085.

Suggested Readings

Apgar, V. (1966). The newborn (Apgar) scoring system: Reflections and advice. *Pediatric Clinics of North America, 13,* 645.

Carroli, G., & Belizan, J. (2000). Episiotomy for vaginal birth (Cochrane Review). In *The Cochrane Library Issue 1*. Oxford: Updated Software.

Hall, S. (1997). The nurse's role in the identification of risks and treatment of shoulder dystocia. *Journal of Obstetrics, Gynecology, and Neonatal Nursing, 26,* (1), 25–32.

Horger, E. (1995). Shoulder dystocia. *Female Patient, 20,* (12), 12–58.

Jacobson, H. (1985). A standard for assessing lochia volume. *Maternal-Child Nursing, 10,* (3), 174–175.

Parker, B., & McFarlane, J. (1991). Identifying and helping battered pregnant women. *American Journal of Maternal Child Nursing, 16,* (3), 161–164.

Tucker, S. M. (1996). *Pocket guide to fetal monitoring assessment* (3rd ed.). St. Louis, MO: Mosby.

Resources

American Academy of Husband-Coached Childbirth, P.O. Box 5224, Sherman Oaks, CA 91413, 800-442-4784

American College of Obstetricians and Gynecologists (ACOG), 409 12th Street, SW, Washington, DC 20024, 800-762-2264, www.acog.com

American Society for Reproductive Medicine, 1209 Montgomery Highway, Birmingham, AL 35316, 205-978-5000, www.asrm.com

March of Dimes Birth Defects Foundation, National Foundation/March of Dimes, 1275 Mamaroneck Avenue, White Plains, NY 10605, 914-428-7100, 888-663-4637 (MODIMES), www.modimes.org

Maternity Center Association, Inc., 281 Park Avenue South, 5th Floor, New York, NY 10010, 212-777-5000

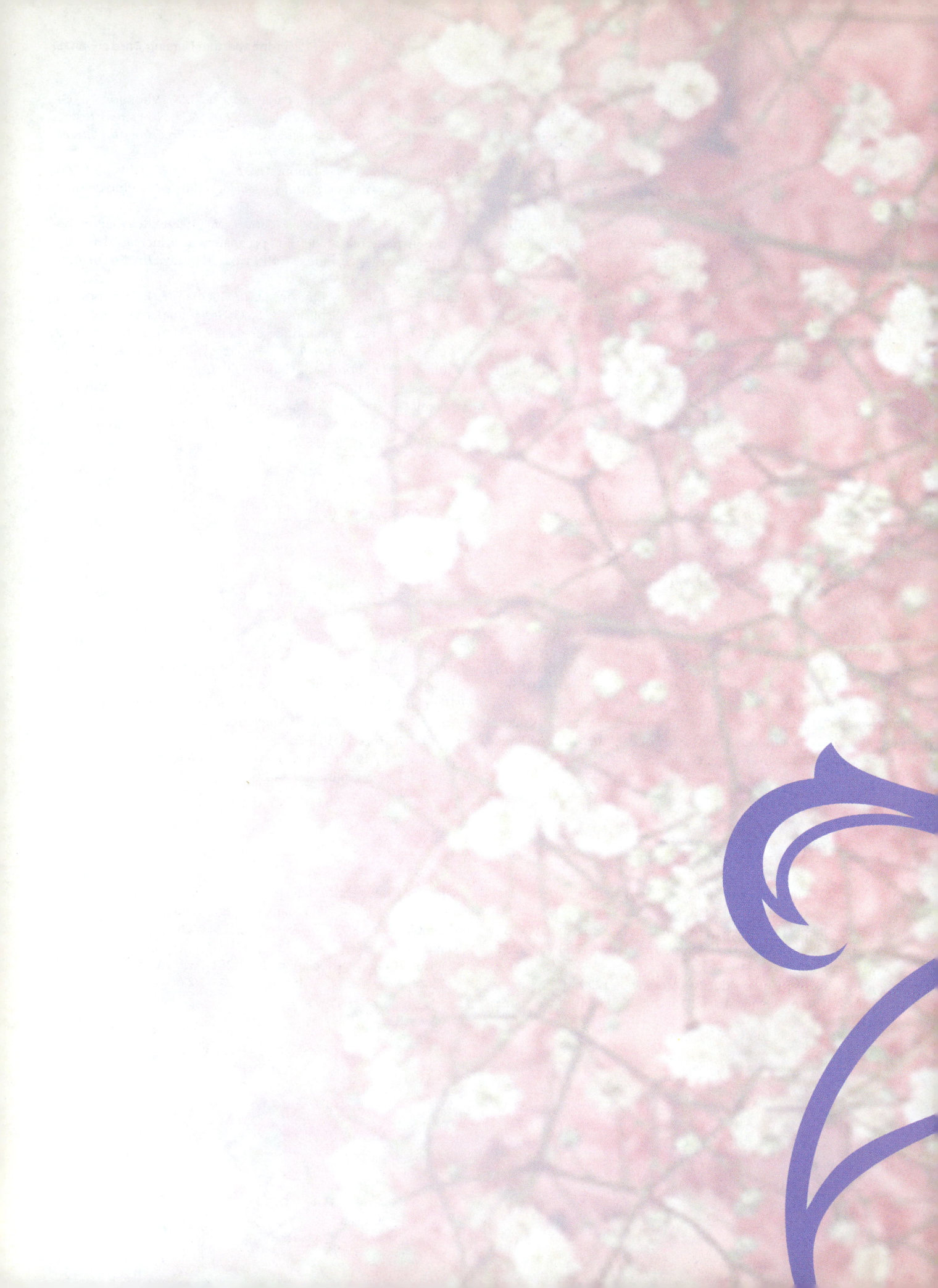

CHAPTER 26

High-Risk Births and Obstetric Emergencies

Complications arise suddenly and often quite dramatically in obstetrics. Complications can transform a routine antepartum or intrapartum experience into an emergent situation, with both maternal and fetal well-being at stake. Because of the ever-present potential for complications to arise, the obstetric nurse should possess strong critical thinking skills coupled with anticipatory preparations that allow immediate intervention. The nurse must incorporate these skills and preparations without compromising the birthing environment in which the client and her family are seeking to participate. Balancing the goals of positive birth experiences with acute and intensive support of maternal and fetal status can be quite a challenge for the professional nurse. As you review the following questions, reflect on your own personal views, experiences, and coping mechanisms:

- *How do I feel about being responsible for the fetus whose status may be difficult to assess because of limited available assessment data?*

- *How do I react in emergency situations?*

- *Have I ever been present during a cesarean section? How did I feel?*

- *Have I ever been present at a delivery where complications occurred? How did I respond?*

- *Have I or has anyone close to me experienced a perinatal loss, had a baby born with a birth defect, or had an infant injured at birth? How do I feel about that experience now?*

- *How do I feel about comforting a client who will have or has had a baby requiring intensive care, or who has had an infant who will not or did not survive?*

Key Terms

Abruptio placentae
Amniotic fluid embolism
Amniotomy
Anencephaly
Breech presentation
Brow presentation
Cephalopelvic
  disproportion (CPD)
Contracted maternal
  pelvis
External cephalic version

Face presentation
Fetal distress
Hydrocephalus
Hypertonic labor
Hypotonic labor
Intrauterine pressure
  catheter (IUPC)
Kleihauer-Betke test
Labor augmentation
Long-term variability
  (LTV)

Malposition
Malpresentation
Multiple gestation
Oligohydramnios
Placenta percreta
Placenta previa
Polyhydramnios
Precipitate labor
Short-term variability
  (STV)
Shoulder dystocia

Shoulder presentation
Transverse lie
Turtle sign
Umbilical cord
  compression
Umbilical cord prolapse
Undulating variability
Uterine rupture
Vasa previa
Velamentous insertion of
  the cord

Competencies

Upon completion of this chapter, the reader should be able to:

1. Identify selected dysfunctional labor patterns and the nursing interventions to enhance maternal and fetal well-being.

2. Identify and differentiate the common fetal malpositions and malpresentations. Discuss the assessment data relative to confirming the fetal position. Explain the delivery concerns for each of the malpositions and malpresentations.

3. When fetal distress occurs, integrate the nursing process by focusing on assessment, diagnoses, and implementation of appropriate interventions to achieve the desired outcomes. Describe the evaluation parameters that will verify successful implementation.

4. Discuss the assessment data found in clients who have experienced uterine rupture and the plan for implementing care and evaluation of outcomes.

5. Compare and contrast the assessment parameters found with placenta previa and abruptio placentae. Differentiate the plans of care and evaluations of outcomes.

6. Discuss the assessment findings that indicate a prolapsed umbilical cord and the emergent implementation of required interventions.

7. Identify the hemorrhagic conditions that predispose obstetric clients to coagulopathies, such as disseminated intravascular coagulation, or DIC.

8. Discuss the maternal and fetal implications when a diagnosis of oligohydramnios or polyhydramnios has been confirmed. Identify the contributing causes of both of these abnormal volumes of amniotic fluid.

9. Describe the assessment data indicative of amniotic fluid embolism and two critical factors impeding maternal survival.

Pregnant clients at risk for or who incur obstetric emergencies are dependent on the entire health care system to support their needs during pregnancy, labor, and delivery. Because of the constant interaction with the professional nurse during the labor and delivery process, clients and their support persons anticipate and trust that the nurse will be ready to identify problems that develop and intervene immediately. The goal is clear: a positive outcome for both mother and child. That goal, however, is not always easily achieved.

Integration of the nursing process into the high-risk obstetric setting can be challenging. Assessment of clients includes reviewing historical and prenatal data; completing a maternal physical assessment; assessing fetal status; and obtaining pertinent emotional, cultural, developmental, and educational data. The development of outcomes or goals must be done with regard to the current plan of medical management. Nursing plans and interventions may combine one-on-one interactions, such as massaging and positioning clients, with highly technical skills, such as maternal-fetal monitoring and management of multiple medications to augment labor. Evaluation of the process depends on the confirmation of assessment data, success of the nursing interventions, and comparison of the actual with the desired maternal-fetal outcomes.

The obstetric nurse working in labor and delivery often provides care in an atmosphere of a relaxed home environment. The nurse's initial interactions with the client and her significant others include acknowledging their hopes and dreams for their expected baby. The expectations of the client and her support persons for the pregnancy, labor, and delivery are affected by various factors: family structure; cultural aspects, including language barriers; educational levels; and religious beliefs. The relationship that develops between the nurse and client often is a personal one that may last throughout the labor and delivery experience. The nurse must take the time to establish rapport and trust with the client. Rapport may enable the nurse to accomplish necessary interventions quickly and efficiently, while minimizing the client's fear and anxiety (Manogin, Bechtel, & Rami, 2000). The nurse also must be able to recognize the many feelings that the woman may experience as an obstetric patient at high risk. These feelings vary with the person and the chronicity of the problem but may include a sense of entrapment or being held prisoner, boredom, loss of control, reversal of the role of caregiver to one of being cared for, and frustration with the limitations imposed by bed rest and hospitalization. The nurse is challenged to incorporate interventions that minimize negative feelings and support optimal coping (Gupton, Heaman, & Ashcroft, 1997). Establishing a strong relationship between the nurse and client, and the client's support persons, confirms the nurse's role as a client advocate during the course of care.

Assessment of maternal-fetal status is critical. The total clinical picture should incorporate data from both the mother and fetus that offer reassurances of maternal stability and fetal well-being. The assessment process is very dynamic in the intrapartum period because changes that compromise the maternal-fetal status may occur in minutes. Interventions also are completed quickly and often have results requiring immediate evaluation. Quick interventions, however, should not be the result of an incomplete assessment. Complete assessment of critical information best enables the nurse to formulate diagnoses, intervene appropriately, and achieve successful and timely outcomes.

REFLECTIONS FROM A NURSE

"The miracle of birth is an awesome experience. To participate and support a client throughout the course of her labor and delivery is rewarding. Encountering and overcoming the challenges of high-risk situations, complications, and obstetric emergencies to achieve a positive birth outcome truly result in a victory for the obstetric health care team! Regardless of the outcome, providing professional, supportive, and compassionate care is equally challenging."

The intensity and speed of the labor and delivery process may at times produce a feeling of being overwhelmed in clients, support persons, and even the nurse. These feelings become more intense as high-risk situations, complications, or emergent situations arise. It is important for the nurse to remain calm, use critical thinking skills, communicate clearly, and intervene appropriately. To help increase the efficiency of interventions during an emergent situation, the nurse should anticipate client needs; ready equipment and other personnel; and put in place well-established lines of communication with the physician or Certified Nurse Midwife (CNM), nursery, anesthesia services, and additional team members.

Several conditions make the intrapartum period one of high risk. Conditions that will be addressed in this chapter include dysfunctional labor patterns, fetal malpresentation, maternal and fetal structural anomalies, multiple gestation, fetal distress, uterine rupture, placental anomalies, umbilical cord anomalies, and amniotic fluid anomalies. Each condition requires astute nursing care to ensure positive maternal and fetal outcomes.

DYSFUNCTIONAL LABOR PATTERN

A **dysfunctional labor pattern** is a labor processes that does not proceed normally. Normal labor is characterized by uterine activity that causes cervical change in effacement and dilation and fetal descent, resulting in a vaginal delivery (Cunningham et al., 1997). Dysfunctional labor patterns often are medically classified as labor dystocias (Bashore, 1992). Labor dystocias are ranked as the leading cause of primary cesarean sections at approximately 43%

(Cunningham et al., 1997). Labor dystocias during the first stage of labor occur in 8% to 11% of vertex presentations. They occur at approximately the same rate during the second stage of labor (Wiznitzer, 1995). Hypertonic labor, hypotonic labor, and precipitate labor are three types of dysfunctional labor patterns, or dystocias, attributed to uterine dysfunction.

Hypertonic Labor

Hypertonic labor is classified as an "abnormality of the expulsive forces" of the uterus in *Williams Obstetrics* (1997). The pattern of uterine activity includes uterine irritability, poor resting tone, and contractions occurring at a frequency of closer than every two minutes. Whereas this pattern of uterine activity is painful to the pregnant client, it usually is not effective in causing the cervical changes necessary for labor to progress and the fetus to descend. Maternal and fetal factors that contribute to hypertonic labor include primiparous labor, fetal presentation other than cephalic, persistent occipitoposterior position (Joshi & Bharadwaj, 2000), flexion of the fetal head, and increased fetal size. Up to 50% of the time however no attributable cause for the dysfunction can be clearly identified (Cunningham et al., 1997).

The consequences of a hypertonic uterine pattern may include maternal exhaustion and inadequate pain relief from prolonged uterine activity, a prolonged latent or active phase of labor, increased risk for maternal or fetal infection when the membranes have ruptured, and increased risk for maternal or fetal injury.

Medical management of hypertonic labor patterns may be approached in more than one way. The physician or CNM may choose to allow the client to rest using hydration and sedation, which also will reduce uterine irritability and allow reevaluation of uterine activity (Cunningham et al., 1993). When the membranes have already ruptured, resting the client is not an option. The physician or CNM also may choose to use oxytocin to stimulate a more effective contraction pattern (Bashore, 1992). When oxytocin is used to enhance ineffective uterine activity, the procedure is called **labor augmentation** (Payton & Brucker, 1999).

The nursing process begins with thorough maternal and fetal assessments. Data that will assist in confirming a hypertonic uterine pattern focus first on assessment of uterine activity. Manual palpation of uterine activity and the uterine activity recording found on the external fetal monitor tracing provide valuable information to the nurse. Contraction activity may occur closer than every two minutes, with poor uterine relaxation between contractions. The contractions usually will not feel firm even at peak intensity, although the client may voice variable levels of discomfort. The pelvic examination should include assessment of cervical dilation and effacement and fetal station,

Critical Thinking

Oxytocin and Propanolol

A 1996 study reported the comparison of oxytocin augmentation alone with oxytocin augmentation accompanied by the additional administration of intravenous (IV) push doses of propanolol in the treatment of dysfunctional labor. The study results were favorable, with the group receiving both oxytocin and IV propanolol having fewer cesarean sections. In addition, no increase in poor maternal or fetal delivery outcomes were reported. The outcomes of this study will change the management of dysfunctional labor patterns. What is your opinion of the value of the oxytocin-propanolol combination?

Sanchez-Ramos, L., Quillen, M. J., & Kaunitz, A. (1996). Randomized trial of oxytocin alone and with propanolol in the management of dysfunctional labor. *Obstetrics and Gynecology,* 88, (4), 517–520.

presentation, and position. Failure to observe changes in the cervix or fetal descent in the presence of irritable uterine activity indicates an ineffective pattern of labor. Membrane status must be assessed. When the membranes have ruptured, the risk for infection becomes a consideration in the client's medical management. Augmentation is the primary medical management of a hypertonic pattern of labor when the membranes have ruptured.

Fetal tolerance to the contraction pattern also must be assessed (Box 26-1). Assessment is accomplished through ausculation or, better, intermittent or continuous external fetal monitoring. When fetal monitoring is employed, data used to make the assessment include fetal heart rate baseline, the presence of heart rate variability, the presence and type of periodic changes, and any nonperiodic changes (Feinstein & McCartney, 1997). Maternal vital signs, including temperature and input and output status, may offer information about her physical tolerance of the labor pattern. The assessment also should indicate the client's level of knowledge, particularly of the labor experience, and the cultural and religious considerations that may affect her response to the labor process.

Nursing diagnoses for a client experiencing a hypertonic labor pattern may include the following:

1. Risk for infection (maternal or fetal) related to prolonged latent labor process, as evidenced by maternal fever of 100.4°F, maternal tachycardia, fetal tachycardia, or a combination of these (Feinstein & McCartney, 1997).

Box 26-1 Fetal Monitoring Terms and Parameters

Baseline Data

Rate: Maintained for a minimum of 10 minutes.
 Normal: 120–160
 Tachycardia: >160
 Bradycardia: <110
Fetal Heart Rate Variability: The heart rate changes from beat to beat or over an extended period of time measured in one-minute intervals that indicate central nervous system status.
 Short-term variability (STV): Measured in beat-to-beat changes in the baseline as either present or absent. Only measurable with internal mode of fetal monitoring.
 Long-term variability (LTV): Measured in minute intervals from the baseline and rated as follows: decreased, 0–5 bpm; average, 6–25 bpm; or marked, >25 bpm (on a 3-point scale).
 Undulating variability: Waveform variation that is repetitive and almost uniform in appearance, including sinusoidal and pseudosinusoidal patterns.

Rhythm

 Regular
 Irregular
Periodic Changes: Heart rate changes in response and relation to the occurrence of uterine activity.
Accelerations*: Variations upward from baseline. Presence, frequency, peak, and duration of accelerations are assessed.
Decelerations*: Variations downward from baseline. Presence, frequency, shape, type classification, depth, and durations are assessed.
 Variable: Frequency and timing in relation to contractions, shape, and duration vary.
 Early: Shape and occurrence are more uniform before or with contractions; "mirroring."
 Late: Shape and occurrence also are uniform but begin during or after contractions.
 Prolonged: >2 minutes but <10 minutes in duration.

---

*Accelerations and decelerations also may occur without a defined relationship to the contraction and are then termed nonperiodic or spontaneous in occurrence.
Adapted From Feinstein, N., & McCartney, P. (1997). *AWHONN: Fetal heart monitoring principles and practices*, 2nd ed. Dubuque, IA: Kendall/Hunt.

2. Acute pain (maternal) related to uterine irritability and prolonged labor, as evidenced by frequent or persistent maternal requests for pain relief, frequent uterine contractions, poor uterine resting tone, and failure of the cervix to dilate 1- to 2-cm/h on cervical assessment.

3. Deficient knowledge of labor processes and variations related to inexperience and unfamiliarity with intervention options, as evidenced by client questions and an inability to cooperate with requested interventions.

4. Fatigue (maternal) related to a prolonged labor process, as evidenced by an inability to rest between contractions, inadequate pain relief, client statements of exhaustion, and client inability to cooperate with requested interventions.

5. Impaired gas exchange (fetoplacental) related to hyperstimulation of the uterus with oxytocin augmentation, as evidenced by nonreassuring fetal tracing inclusive of severe variable decelerations; late decelerations; bradycardia; or loss of long-term or short-term variability, or both. Inadequate fetoplacental oxygenation as a result of uterine hyperstimulation can adversely affect the fetus (Feinstein & McCartney, 1997).

6. Anxiety related to unfamiliar experiences, surroundings, and unexpected medical nursing interventions, as evidenced by client verbal and nonverbal behaviors.

Desired outcomes are based on the nursing diagnoses developed for the client. Prevention of risks for problems or resolution of actual problems are addressed in the following outcome statements:

1. Client and fetus will not experience infection related to a prolonged labor process.

2. Client will verbalize effective pain relief without demonstrating adverse maternal or fetal response to the selected interventions.

3. Client and support persons will verbalize an understanding of the uterine pattern; plan of care to address it; and expected outcomes, including the projected mode of delivery. The client also will be able to participate in and cooperate with requests from the nurse.

4. Client will not experience exhaustion related to prolonged fatigue during a hypertonic labor pattern.

5. Fetus will not exhibit **fetal distress**, a nonreassuring fetal heart rate response to the intrauterine environment as a result of the hypertonic labor pattern or oxytocin augmentation of labor.

6. Client will demonstrate effective coping behaviors in response to heightened anxiety.

Achieving the above outcomes requires ongoing assessment and support of the client by the professional nurse. The nurse must assess maternal-fetal status and relay the pertinent information to the attending physician or CNM. Critical elements include monitoring of uterine activity, results of the pelvic examination (changes in cervical dilation or fetal descent), maternal vital signs, and fetal heart rate data. Changes in maternal-fetal status may alter the current medical plan of management. For instance, if the initial medical plan was to rest the patient and on reassessment the fetal heart rate data are of concern, the physician or CNM may decide to augment the labor pattern and move toward delivery.

Assessment data should include ongoing monitoring for signs of infection. The fetal heart rate and the maternal temperature, heart rate, and respirations may increase with the onset of infection. Fetal tachycardia is most frequently the result of maternal fever or maternal or fetal infection (Feinstein & McCartney, 1997). Monitoring maternal input and output reduces the likelihood of dehydration being a cause of maternal fever and maternal or fetal tachycardia. Monitoring of the input and output also is critical when oxytocin is administered because of its antidiuretic effect and the potential for water intoxication (Payton & Brucker, 1999; Cunningham et al., 1997). Ongoing maternal-fetal assessments become even more imperative once the membranes rupture and this barrier of defense is no longer intact.

Anxiety can increase catecholamine secretion and thus lead to a dysfunctional labor process (Feinstein & McCartney, 1997). Aside from the physiologic effects, anxiety im-

pacts the client's perception of the birth experience and can further impact the resolution or successful integration of the events into her adaptation from pregnancy to parenthood. Lack of knowledge can increase the anxiety levels of both the client and her support persons. Thus, all interventions should be explained in a manner best understood by the client and questions should be encouraged and answered. Initially establishing rapport with the client and her support persons is fundamental in developing trust. In turn, trust can allay fears and reduce anxiety. A trusting relationship also makes it easier for the client to follow instructions and better participate in the labor process. When the client and her support persons feel the nurse is aware and respectful of their level of knowledge and any cultural or religious considerations, they are more likely to cooperate and actively participate in the plan of care. Finally, when they believe the nurse is knowledgeable and capable of managing the client's care, the labor experience is more likely to be perceived as being positive, regardless of the need for technical intervention (Manogin, Bechtel, & Rami, 2000).

The nurse can help provide pain relief by using physical comfort measures such as position changes, lower back rubs, counterpressure at the lower back during a contraction (pressing the fist firmly into the identified pressure point low on the back), and administration of analgesic medications. The physical presence of the nurse along with sincere encouragement may further alleviate anxiety that may enhance pain perception (Manogin, Bechtel, & Rami, 2000). An explanation about the medications and the likely responses after administration may further reassure the client regarding pain relief. Ensuring that the environment is conducive to rest by reducing external stimuli (e.g., lowering lighting levels, reducing the volume on noise-producing equipment, and turning off televisions) is another intervention the nurse can use. Although the nurse does not insert or administer epidural anesthesia, assisting with adequate hydration, assessing baseline vital signs, positioning the client, and evaluating maternal-fetal responses to the effects of the epidural anesthesia are all within the nursing role. Finally, the nurse can help the client achieve adequate pain relief and reduce fatigue by evaluating her responses to the medications, regional anesthesia, and physical comfort measures taken, and by promoting rest opportunities between contractions.

When the physician orders oxytocin to augment labor, the nurse should ensure that the orders and protocols for administration are observed. Adding the correct amount of oxytocin to the IV solution and administering it to the client by IV pump through a piggyback approach to the main IV line are all important steps in this process. Monitoring the maternal-fetal responses to the augmentation process is critical because the increase in dosage is titrated to these responses. Some protocols require dosage increases of a set amount of milliunits every 15 to 30 minutes until an effective labor pattern is achieved. The parameters may be established by the individual physician after a low-dosage regimen or may follow a high-dosage regimen. The administration rate of a low-dosage regimen is 0.5 to 2 mU/min and is increased by the nurse every 15 to 40 minutes, with a maximum dosage limit between 20 and 40 mU/min. When a high-dosage protocol is ordered, the starting rate may be 6 mU/minute, with increases every 20 to 40 minutes and a maximum dosage of 40 mU/min (Payton & Brucker, 1999). Regardless of the protocol, the nurse should try to ensure the occurrence of regular contractions of moderate to firm intensity that last 30 to 60 seconds every 2 to 5 minutes, without causing maternal or fetal compromise.

Once an effective labor pattern is established and cervical change occurs, the physician may choose to perform an **amniotomy**, which is artificial rupture of the membranes to further augment the labor process (Figure 26-1). When assisting with the amniotomy, the nurse should ensure that the fetal heart tracing remains stable and note the color, amount, particulate matter in, and odor of the fluid. At that time, fetal monitoring options may include internal monitoring modes to increase the accuracy of uterine activity assessment (intrauterine pressure catheter [IUPC]), fetal heart rate assessment (fetal spiral electrode [FSE]), or both. Having the amniotomy hook, internal monitoring devices, sterile gloves, appropriate monitor cables, towels, and fresh hip pads readily available will enhance the efficiency of the procedure. Although the modes of data attainment may have changed, the nurse is still responsible

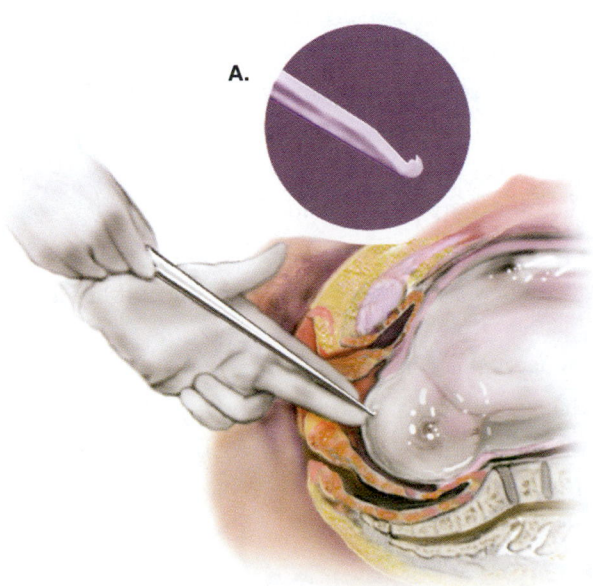

A.

B.

Figure 26-1 A. Disposable amnihook to rupture membranes. B. Technique for amniotomy.

for ongoing maternal-fetal assessments as the client progresses through labor.

Evaluation of maternal-fetal status ensures that the interventions employed have been effective. Medical management and nursing interventions may need to be altered or continued based on the findings of the evaluation.

1. Are signs of infection present? Are maternal and fetal vital signs stable? Is the fetal heart rate tracing reassuring, with long-term variability and accelerations present?

2. Is the client's pain relieved? Does she state there is less pain? Does she appear less distressed? Is there less uterine irritability, or is there better uterine relaxation between contractions? Are the contractions less frequent? If an epidural is in place, is it intact? Has the client stated she has adequate pain relief from the epidural without demonstrating hypotensive responses, fetal bradycardia, or prolonged decelerations?

3. Does the client understand what is happening? Does she ask appropriate questions? Is she cooperative? Does she verbalize understanding? Do her support persons verbalize an understanding of the process? Do they express confidence in the management of care?

4. Does the client rest between contractions? Does she verbalize resting between contractions? Does she participate in her care?

5. Does the client's labor pattern become effective? Is there cervical change? Is there fetal descent? Are the maternal-fetal responses to the augmentation of labor reassuring or stable?

6. Has the client and her support persons coped with the process of labor and the associated interventions effectively? Has she verbalized relief or reduction of anxiety?

A hypertonic uterine pattern of labor may evolve into a normal labor pattern, and the client eventually will deliver vaginally. In contrast, an ineffective pattern of labor may continue, necessitating a cesarean section either as a result of arrested labor or because the maternal or fetal status shows evidence of compromise. The professional nurse must continuously assess maternal-fetal status and communicate this information to all health care providers to optimize outcomes. Readiness to initiate alternative interventions in the event the desired outcomes are not achieved is essential. The physician or CNM, anesthesia services, nursery, and all health care personnel required at the delivery should be kept abreast of the client's changing status. Finally, the nurse is responsible for recording the following: assessment data, interventions employed, maternal-fetal responses, and evaluations of outcomes.

Hypotonic Labor

Hypotonic labor refers to uterine contractions that are inadequate in terms of frequency, intensity, or duration. Hypotonic labor tends to occur during the latent or active phase of labor. The client experiences contractions that are ineffective in causing cervical dilation or effacement, or fetal descent. Risk factors that contribute to the occurrence of a hypotonic labor pattern include large fetal size, fetal malpresentation, and early or repeated maternal sedation in labor. Recent concerns have been voiced regarding epidural administration as a contributing cause of hypotonic labor patterns. Current studies do not support the claim that epidural anesthesia negatively impacts labor, although it is frequently used for pain management in clients with ineffective labor patterns because of increased need for adequate pain relief (Thompson, et al., 1998). In another study, Clark, et al., (1998) further found that epidural anesthesia did not increase the rate of cesarean sections in women with dystocia managed actively with oxytocin. Similar findings were the result of a study by Bofill et al., (1997). The significance of these studies impacts the nurse in two ways. Epidural anesthesia is a viable pain relief intervention that is monitored throughout its duration of action by the nurse. In addition, each study acknowledges the need for strict active management of the labor method that employs the high-dosage oxytocin protocol. This method requires the nurse to intensively monitor maternal-fetal responses and oxytocin titration based on uterine activity. The results of a hypotonic labor include prolonged latent labor, prolonged active labor, or both; increased risk for maternal or fetal infection; increased risk for fetal compromise from insufficient reserve; maternal fatigue and exhaustion; and the need for additional medical, technical, and nursing interventions, including altering the client's desired birth plan.

Medical management of the hypotonic labor pattern is similar to that used for the hypertonic labor pattern. The physician or CNM may choose to allow the client to rest by administering hydration and sedation and then reevaluate her later for cervical changes, fetal descent, and improved uterine contraction activity. The other management option is to augment the labor with IV piggyback administration of oxytocin, amniotomy, or both.

Nursing considerations for the client with hypotonic labor include assessment information obtained from the monitoring of uterine activity and the pelvic examination. Maternal vital signs and fetal status must be assessed and monitored closely for changes that may indicate either complications or progression of labor. The nursing assessment should explore the client's level of formal or experiential knowledge, cultural and religious considerations, influence of support persons, and her perceived fear and anxiety level.

As with the hypertonic labor pattern, the nursing diagnoses for hypotonic labor address the risk for maternal and fetal infection. Prolonged labor processes related to hypotonic labor patterns also can impair fetoplacental gas exchange relative to the sheer duration of the labor process and the lack of further fetal reserve (Feinstein & McCartney, 1997). Maternal pain and fatigue and knowledge deficit of the client and her support persons also are risk factors in hypotonic labor. The client may incur heightened anxiety, particularly when it seems as if little to no progress is being made. The desired outcomes for these diagnoses also will be similar to those for hypertonic contraction patterns. The ultimate outcome is for the client to deliver vaginally, without evidence of maternal or fetal compromise.

The nursing plan and interventions employed also are similar to those used for hypertonic labor patterns. Continuous monitoring for signs of maternal or fetal infection and fetal intolerance to oxytocin augmentation is imperative. Implementation of client comfort measures, use of labor pain relief methods, emotional support of the client and her support persons, and ongoing client teaching are instrumental throughout the labor process. The nurse must always anticipate alternative outcomes that require rapid intervention. Communication and documentation of assessment data, interventions, and evaluations also are necessary. Communication and documentation cannot be overstressed in an area where dramatic changes may occur very rapidly.

In evaluating outcomes the nurse should ask pertinent questions of the situation.

- Have the outcomes been achieved or are further interventions required?
- Is the medical management of the client changing?
- Will the nursing interventions need to change to support the medical management?
- Is the maternal-fetal status stable?
- Is the client coping effectively?
- Are her support persons able to support her and participate in her care?
- What is the delivery outcome?
- Is the neonate stabilized easily at birth?
- Is the mother able to initiate bonding interactions with her newborn?

Precipitate Labor

Precipitate labor refers to a labor pattern that progresses rapidly and ends with delivery occurring less than three hours after the onset of uterine activity. Maternal and fetal contributory factors for precipitate labor include maternal

Research Highlight

Prediction of Difficult Birth

Purpose

A total of 1,692 clients were evaluated in early labor, and predictions were made for easy labor-vaginal birth, difficult labor-vaginal birth, or improbable vaginal birth-cesarean section.

Method

The prediction was based on clinical evaluation of pelvic dimensions, and fetal measurements by sonography at term.

Findings

The combined prediction that a client would have either a difficult labor-vaginal birth or cesarean section was very accurate (362 out of 370, or 97.8%). However, the separate prediction of difficult labor-vaginal birth and a cesarean section was less accurate, although still significant (73.4% and 90.2%, respectively).

Nursing Implications

Careful evaluation of a client in early labor could help to recognize the dystocic labor-delivery and early indication for cesarean sections. This would avoid unnecessary and prolonged labor without necessarily increasing the cesarean section rate.

Abitbol, M. M., Bowen-Ericksen, M., Castillo, I., & Pushchin, A. (1999). Prediction of difficult vaginal birth and of cesarean section cephalopelvic disproportion in early labor. *Journal of Maternal Fetal Medicine 8* (2): 51–6.

multiparous status, small fetus, relaxed pelvic and vaginal musculature, and a history of rapid labors with previous deliveries. Maternal and fetal risks include a delivery out of asepsis, maternal soft tissue injuries, and fetal injuries from rapid expulsion at delivery. Medical diagnosis and management include a readiness on the part of the entire health team for the delivery, particularly when the client has a history of rapid labor. The American College of Obstetricians and Gynecologists (ACOG) acknowledges that a history of rapid or precipitous labors is a reason for medical induction to ensure a hospital delivery and increase the likelihood for a controlled delivery that minimizes the potential for maternal and fetal injuries.

The nursing assessment of the client should include a thorough history of gravidity, length of previous labors, and delivery outcomes. Uterine activity should be assessed by palpation, fetal monitoring, or both. Precipitate delivery may occur as a result of pelvic relaxation; however, intense and frequent contractions may contribute to rapid progression of labor. When uterine relaxation is inadequate, fetoplacental gas exchange may be compromised. Assessment of fetal position using Leopold's maneuvers, review of ultrasonography information for position, and estimation of fetal weight may provide information regarding the likelihood of rapid delivery. The pelvic examination will reveal information on cervical status, fetal station, and adequacy of pelvic outlet. Subsequent examinations will denote changes, and a rapid or significant change may be a predictor of a short labor process. Assessment of patient responses, such as intensity of behavior, bearing down, and increased anxiety, may reveal a need for the nurse to reevaluate the progression of labor. Fetal tolerance to labor should be assessed continuously. Maternal vital signs are significant for baseline information because women who experience particularly intense, precipitous labor and deliveries are at a higher risk for amniotic fluid embolism and uterine atony after delivery than are women who do not (Cunningham et al., 1997).

Nursing diagnoses for the client experiencing precipitous labor and delivery include a recognition of risks for the following: maternal or fetal soft tissue injury related to rapid descent and expulsion, maternal or fetal infection if delivery occurs outside of aseptic surroundings, and maternal hemorrhage if atony results after delivery. The nurse also must consider maternal pain and anxiety. The goals of these client outcomes are to avoid the risks of soft tissue injury, infection, and hemorrhage, while reinforcing maternal comfort and attempting to reduce or limit anxiety.

Nursing care involves vigilant attendance, preparations for delivery in advance, client comfort measures, and education and emotional support for the client and her support persons. The onset of rapid labor can be frightening and overwhelming. When uterine relaxation is minimal, little reprieve between contractions is provided. Thus, the opportunity of resting, refocusing, and preparing for the next contraction is limited. Communication with the physician or CNM and all other team members anticipated at delivery must be clear, concise, and timely to avoid the lack of critical support personnel during delivery.

The nursing plan of care and interventions should include continuous reassessment of maternal-fetal status. Any change in status, maternal or fetal tolerance, or sign of impending problems must be communicated in a timely manner to the physician or CNM and all other required health care providers. The nurse should inform the client of any change in the plan of care. As changes are made, the nurse should explain all procedures and offer reassurance to the client of the readiness of the health care team for delivery. Visually seeing the nurse set up for the anticipated delivery may reassure the client and her support persons that the nurse trusts their concerns and is responding by preparing for the birth of their baby. Teaching or reinforcing relaxation techniques may assist the client in optimizing rest periods between contractions. Rapid labor may prevent the client from obtaining regional anesthesia; however, small IV dosages of pain medication may be ordered when cervical dilation has not progressed to the second stage of labor or immediately preceding this stage. When medication is administered, maternal responses and vital signs and fetal heart rate responses should be evaluated. The nurse also should anticipate successful relaxation and a resulting rapid delivery when providing pharmacologic interventions. When labor progresses too rapidly for even small amounts of pain medication, the nurse can support the client by staying with her and encouraging and assisting her into a comfortable position. After delivery, monitoring maternal vital signs, assessing the uterine fundus for uterine atony, and observation for signs of soft tissue hematoma or increased vaginal bleeding that may indicate a hidden laceration should be done at frequent intervals (every 15 minutes, if stable; more frequently, if there are concerns). The nurse should assess the neonate for soft tissue injuries and monitor vital signs to ensure stability after delivery.

Evaluation of client outcomes involves answering the questions that recognize the success of the established outcomes.

- Did the neonate have bruising, swelling, or signs of injury after delivery?
- Is the mother demonstrating signs of hematoma, lacerations, or increased bleeding?

- If lacerations were present, are the repairs intact with heavy bleeding evident?
- Are maternal vital signs stable?
- Is the mother or neonate demonstrating signs of infection?
- Did the delivery occur in an appropriate setting?
- Are temperatures and respiratory efforts within normal limits?
- Are there signs of maternal hemorrhage after delivery?
- Is the fundus firm and at the umbilicus?
- Is excessive fundal massage required to increase fundal tone?
- Did the client demonstrate reduced anxiety with the nursing support interventions?
- Did the client verbalize enhanced relaxation or reassurance with the nursing interventions?
- Did the client verbalize or demonstrate reduced pain?
- Were pharmacologic interventions helpful?
- Were the maternal-fetal responses reassuring, without evidence of vital sign or fetal heart rate compromise?
- Were nonpharmacologic comfort interventions helpful to the client?

FETAL MALPRESENTATION AND MALPOSITION

Fetal malpresentation and malposition may interfere with the progression of labor and fetal descent. **Malpresentation** refers to a fetal presenting part other than the vertex and includes breech, transverse, compound, shoulder, face, and brow presentations. Malpresentations may be identified late in pregnancy or may not be discovered until the initial assessment during labor. Fetal **malposition** refers to a position other than an occipitoanterior position. Malpositions include occipitotransverse, occipitoposterior, and oblique, or acynclytic, positions of the fetal head in relation to the maternal pelvis. Fetal malpositions are assessed during labor. Fetal malpresentation or malposition may pose risks to maternal-fetal well-being and may necessitate operative vaginal delivery, cesarean section, or other interventions to accomplish delivery.

Breech Presentation

Breech presentation occurs when the fetal buttocks, legs, feet, or a combinations of these parts present first into the maternal pelvis. Classifications of breech presenta-

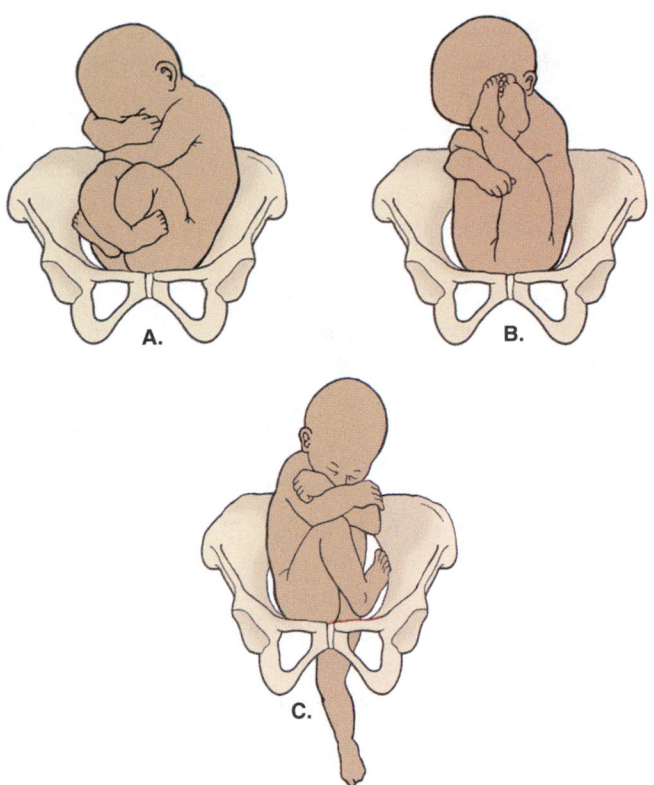

Figure 26-2 Breech presentations. A. Complete. B. Frank. C. Footling.

tion include complete, frank, and footling (double or single) (Figure 26-2). The complete breech presentation is best described as when the thighs are flexed on the abdomen and the legs are upon the thighs. In the frank breech presentation the fetus appears as if it is folded in half, with its feet in its face and the buttocks presenting. The fetal legs are extended in the frank breech presentation, unlike the crossed legs found in the complete breech presentation. The fetus in the footling breech presentation has one or both feet presenting first in the maternal pelvis followed by the buttocks. Breech presentation is frequently found in pregnancies of 28 weeks' gestation and less; however, it is documented in approximately 3% to 4% of term pregnancies (Toth & Jothivijayrani, 1999; Acien, 1995; Albrechtsen, Rasmussen, Dalaker, & Irgens, 1998). Of breech presentations, 65% are frank, 25% are footling, and the remaining 10% are complete breech presentations.

The most common contributing factors to malpresentation and malposition include prematurity; fetal anomalies, such as **hydrocephalus** (increased circulating cerebrospinal fluid, resulting in an increase in the size of the fetal head) and **anencephaly** (failure of the fetal brain, skull, and head to fully develop; this condition is incompatible with life); multiple gestation; placental placement abnormalities; maternal uterine or pelvic abnormalities; and **polyhydramnios**, a condition in which the amount of amniotic fluid in the uterus is increased to two or more liters within the third trimester (Toth & Jothivijayrani, 1999). Advanced maternal age also has been associated with an increased incidence of breech birth (Acien, 1995 Rayl, Gibson & Hickok, 1996).

Maternal risks from breech labor and delivery include prolonged difficult labor, potential for soft tissue injury, lacerations, and need for cesarean section. Fetal risks from breech delivery exceed maternal risks for injury. Even without fetal anomalies present that can be exacerbated by a vaginal delivery, risks to the fetus include umbilical cord prolapse, with compression and resultant hypoxia; brachial plexus injuries; and fetal head and neck injuries from entrapment.

Medical management of the client with a suspected breech presentation includes plans to confirm the fetal presentation. Sonography also is used to screen for apparent anomalies and obtain an estimate of the fetal weight. The physician or CNM will find these data to be instrumental in determining the best plan of care for the client. The physician or CNM will determine whether a vaginal trial of labor or cesarean section is in the best interests of both the mother and fetus. In some cases, there is an attempt to perform **external cephalic version**, which is a procedure by which the physician manipulates the fetus externally through the maternal abdomen to turn the fetus from the abnormal presentation to a cephalic presentation. Most breech presentations are delivered by cesarean section due to the dwindling number of skilled physicians able to safely deliver breech babies (Cunningham et. al, 1997). Cesarean delivery is commonly used in the following circumstances: (1) a large fetus; (2) any unfavorable shape of the maternal pelvis; (3) a hyperextended fetal head; (4) maternal indications for delivery including pregnancy-induced hypertension (PIH) or ruptured membranes for 12 hours or more without labor; (5) uterine dysfunction; (6) footling presentation; (7) a healthy, viable preterm fetus of 25 to 26 weeks or more with the mother in active labor or in need of delivery; (8) severe fetal growth restriction; (9) previous perinatal death or children suffering from birth trauma; and (10) a request for sterilization (Cunningham et al., 1997). Trial of labor may be attempted when estimated fetal weight is equal to or less than previous delivery weights (2,500 to 3,800 g), pelvic assessment reveals adequacy of the outlet, the position is frank breech, the fetal head is flexed, and the gestational age of the fetus is 36 weeks' or more (Toth & Jothivijayrani, 1999).

During the initial assessment the nurse should take into account the gestational age of the fetus, keeping in mind that breech presentations are more frequently found in premature gestations. The nurse should review the client's prenatal history and enquire if a breech presentation has already been suspected or diagnosed, if there is a multiple gestation, or if there has been a prenatal diagnosis of fetal or maternal anomalies. Initial assessment of the gravid abdomen with Leopold's maneuvers may reveal a suspicion of breech presentation. Auscultation of the fetal heart rate at or above the umbilicus may increase this suspicion of a noncephalic presentation. Finally, pelvic assessment may further increase or confirm a breech presentation by palpation of feet, buttocks, or genitalia. Confirmation of presentation with a limited sonographic scan may be permitted as an institutional protocol. Suspicion of breech presentation during the initial maternal assessment should be relayed to the physician or CNM. Care should be taken to avoid rupturing the membranes because there is an increased risk of prolapsed umbilical cord with a noncephalic presentation.

Nursing diagnoses in the management of breech presentation include the risk for fetal injury related to hypoxia from cord prolapse and injury to the fetal head, neck, soft tissue, and nerves related to traumatic delivery. Potential maternal problems include the risk for hemorrhage and infection related to soft tissue injury or lacerations from operative vaginal or cesarean delivery. Maternal pain, anxiety, and knowledge level are actual diagnoses routinely addressed in all laboring patients.

Maternal and fetal outcomes evolve from both medical and nursing management. The medical plan of care and nursing interventions strive to prevent fetal hypoxia, fetal injury, and maternal hemorrhage and infection. These critical interventions are provided concurrently while promoting physical comfort, ensuring adequate pain management, and offering both emotional and educational support for each obstetric client at high risk.

In order to achieve these outcomes, the professional nurse must continuously monitor and update the maternal-fetal assessment and relay the information to the physician. To prevent injury from cord compression related to prolapse and avoid artificially rupturing the membranes, pelvic examinations should be conducted with care. The nurse also should instruct the client to report suspicion of her membranes rupturing. When membranes rupture spontaneously, the nurse should assess for the presence of the umbilical cord in the vaginal vault. The fetal heart rate should also be assessed to ensure it is stable and within normal range. When the medical plan includes a cesarean section, all health team members required at the surgery should be notified. When a vaginal trial of labor is the plan, the nurse should have a double delivery setup available. A double setup consists of a vaginal delivery table setup and a cesarean section instrument table ready to be opened in the surgical suite. Special instruments such as Piper forceps should be in the room, if not open on the instrument table. The nursery personnel should be made aware of any complicating factors, such as prematurity or fetal anomalies.

Pain interventions should be implemented according to the client's assessed needs. Position changes, back massage, IV medication per physician orders, and regional anesthesia may be used to relieve maternal pain during labor. Labor support, reassurance, client education, and validation of client response to the comfort interventions are all interventions the nurse may employ for pain relief. For cesarean section, regional anesthesia is used when possible to minimize fetal anesthetic effects that could occur with a general anesthetic. The nurse's role may include assisting with client positioning for insertion of the regional anesthetic. Although the client is monitored by the anesthesiologist throughout the cesarean section, monitoring during recovery is within the scope of the nurse's role.

Client anxiety may be heightened by the discomfort of the labor and threat of the unknown. Assessment of baseline knowledge, feelings, and perceptions helps the nurse reassure and educate the client to reduce anxiety. Validating information with the client provides appropriate feedback to promote her emotional and physical support during breech labor or a cesarean section. Manogin, Bechtel, and Rami (2000) reported that providing the laboring client with information about her status and the plan of care for delivery enables her to incorporate the information into her experience and develop a healthier, positive perception of the delivery process.

The nurse caring for the client with breech presentation may be required to function in the role of a circulating nurse during the cesarean section. This role includes preparing the client for the operative procedure (shaving when ordered, insertion of a Foley catheter, and preanesthesia fluid loading) and transporting her, as necessary. The circulating nurse supports the needs of the anesthesiologist and obstetrician during the delivery, records sponge and instrument counts, documents occurrences during the procedure, and ensures both equipment and team readiness to receive the neonate. A cesarean section performed for breech presentation may require additional supplies. Obtaining verification of special requests for supplies from the obstetrician promotes readiness. These supplies may be present in the operative suite unopened, unless needed. After the case is completed, the nurse also may be required to monitor the client during the recovery period.

When a client undergoes a trial of labor for vaginal breech delivery, similar preparations should be anticipated. The physician may request additional personnel to assist with delivery or additional supplies. The labor process may be prolonged related to lack of a firm presenting part to enhance dilatory processes. Augmentation may be required to avoid dystocia, which can result in heightened discomfort and anxiety. The nurse's meticulous attention to client responses to labor discomfort will not only promote client support and better meet pain needs but also should reduce anxiety. At delivery, the physician may request administration of amyl nitrite or nitroglycerin to obtain rapid uterine relaxation should head entrapment become apparent. Having the requested medication readily available reduces delays at a critical time in the delivery.

After delivery, vaginal or operative, rapid feedback to the mother regarding the status of the neonate offers reassurance and reduces additional anxiety. Neonatal assessment for soft tissue injuries, swelling, lack of mobility, and lack of flexion of the extremities is critical once respiratory support and thermoregulation are established. Any deviation from normal neonatal assessment should be reported to the nursery or neonatal staff receiving the infant.

Evaluations of the maternal-fetal outcomes answer several questions.

- Did the fetal heart monitoring provide reassuring rates, accelerations, and variability?
- Did the client experience frank or occult prolapse and compression of the umbilical cord?
- Did the neonate demonstrate effective respirations or require minimal support at delivery?
- Did the neonate experience injury at delivery?
- Was assessment rapid, and were interventions initiated immediately?
- Did the client express adequate pain relief verbally or nonverbally?
- Did maternal-fetal status remain stable throughout pharmacologic interventions?
- Did the client express comfort with the plan of care?
- Were questions by the client asked and answered?
- Did the client verbalize reduced anxiety?
- Did maternal vital signs remain stable?
- Did fluid balance remain stable?
- Did the client experience hemorrhage?
- Did the client experience laceration or hematoma?
- Was aseptic technique observed?
- Did the client or fetus demonstrate signs of infection?

Shoulder Presentation

Transverse lie involves the fetus assuming a more horizontal position in the uterus. This type of lie results in a **shoulder presentation** in which the presenting part of the fetus is the shoulder or combination of shoulder, arm, and hand (Figure 26-3). When the fetal back faces the maternal abdomen, it is referred to an acromiodorsoanterior position. When the fetal back faces the maternal back, it is referred to as an acromiodorsoposterior position. Cunning-

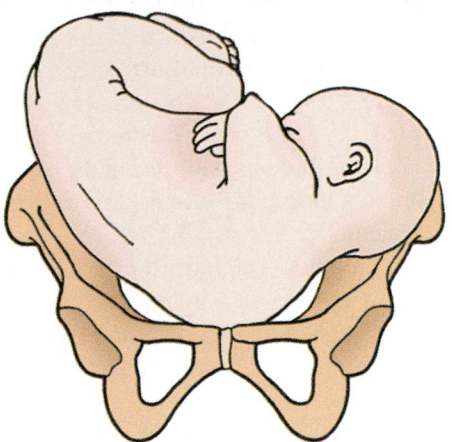

Figure 26-3 Shoulder presentation.

ham et al. (1997) has identified the incidence of transverse lie with shoulder presentation as 1 in 420 singleton deliveries. Common contributing factors for transverse lie and shoulder malpresentation include grand multiparity (as a result of relaxed abdominal musculature), prematurity, multiple gestation, placenta previa, polyhydramnios, and abnormalities of the maternal pelvic structure. When this presentation is identified antenatally, external cephalic version may be attempted to reposition the fetus into cephalic or even breech presentation. Risks to the client include uterine rupture, a high probability of cesarean section, and sepsis if the fetal arm prolapses after membrane rupture and returns through the uterus during cesarean section. Fetal risks include umbilical cord prolapse and fetal injury from attempted and failed version. Medical management is aimed at confirming the transverse lie and shoulder presentation. The usual plan of care is cesarean section once the malpresentation is confirmed.

The nursing assessment is instrumental as a first indicator of malpresentation. A review of maternal prenatal history may promote identification of risk factors. Initial abdominal assessment with Leopold's maneuvers often will identify the transverse or oblique lie. Pelvic assessment may reveal a very high presenting part or no presenting part at all. Care should be exercised to prevent accidental rupture of membranes because this malpresentation also carries a high risk of umbilical cord prolapse. Fetal heart rate assessment should be performed, and the nurse may locate the fetal heart rate at the umbilicus or laterally to it.

From the data obtained in the nursing assessment, the nursing diagnoses should address the risk for the following: fetal injury related to hypoxia from prolapsed umbilical cord or uterine rupture; maternal injury related to hemorrhage from uterine rupture; infection from prolonged labor, with eventual chorioamnionitis; and postoperative infection.

Once malpresentation has been confirmed the nursing plan of care is based on the medical plan of management. Preparation for cesarean section must be completed before the physician attempts external version because the potential for injury exists. Otherwise, the nurse will repeat the interventions for the breech malpresentation in preparing, accompanying, assisting, and monitoring the operative recovery of the client.

Outcome evaluation validates the following: neonatal physical stability at delivery, maternal physical stability during and after cesarean section, maternal coping with and understanding of procedure, and the absence of signs of infections postoperatively.

Face Presentation

Face presentation occurs when the fetal head is hyperextended and the fetal face descends into the pelvis, as opposed to the flexed position, resulting in fetal vertex presentation. **Brow presentation** occurs when the area between the anterior fontanelle and the fetal eyes descends first (Figure 26-4). *Williams Obstetrics* (1997) reports the incidence of face presentation as 1 in 600, or 0.17%. Brow presentation is described as occurring less frequently than does face presentation at a rate of 0.02%, or 1 in 4,470 births. Contributing causes are less clearly defined for face and brow presentations but do include maternal multiparity, fetal macrosomia, fetal anencephaly, and abnormalities of the maternal pelvis. Brow presentation is presumed rare because of its expected conversion

to face or occiput presentation to allow vaginal delivery. Unless the maternal pelvis is generously adequate or the fetus is small, persistent brow presentation is not a viable presentation for vaginal birth (Cunningham et al., 1997). This fact may increase the likelihood of prolonged or difficult labor, and failed vaginal delivery, and increases the potential for surgical delivery. Fetal risks for both of these presentations include significant facial edema and bruising and the potential for aggressive interventions at the time of vaginal delivery.

Medical management is expectant in nature, meaning that the client is allowed to labor and her progress is evaluated (Shields & Medearis, 1992a). As stated previously, the brow presentation usually will convert to face or vertex presentation so the fetus can pass through the pelvis. Oxytocin augmentation may be employed for dystocia. When arrested dilation or descent occurs, medical management may then be operative delivery. Aggressive interventions involving midpelvic manipulation are not currently recommended because they increase fetal morbidity and mortality (Shields & Medearis, 1992).

The nursing assessment should include client history, including perinatal diagnosis of any anomalies or multiple gestation. Estimated gestational age should be documented and verified. Auscultation or fetal monitoring indicates fetal well-being. The pelvic assessment is the one most likely to reveal a nonvertex presentation by palpation of the soft facial features or anterior fontanelle to brow. Sonography may be performed to confirm position, flexion, hyperextension, and fetal size.

The nursing diagnoses for the face or brow presentation are similar for all cephalic labors, plus the risk for fetal injury related to the difficult delivery and the potential for infection should operative vaginal or cesarean delivery become necessary. The outcome for the client based on the first additional diagnosis is that the fetus will not incur permanent injury. Realistically, little can be done to avoid the facial edema associated with a face delivery. The other specific diagnosis addresses maternal well-being and absence of postdelivery infection.

The nursing plan should address both vaginal and cesarean delivery potentials. The nurse must continuously monitor maternal labor progress, fetal well-being, and maternal pain and coping behaviors. Ongoing labor assessment allows early identification of abnormal labor processes so that the physician or CNM may intervene with orders for augmentation when deemed appropriate. When augmentation is ordered, nursing actions include careful IV medication administration and monitoring of uterine activity to prevent hyperstimulation, while promoting an effective labor pattern. The nurse also must continuously reassess the fetal response through fetal heart rate monitoring. Communication with the physician or CNM by the nurse is instrumental to being a client advocate. The

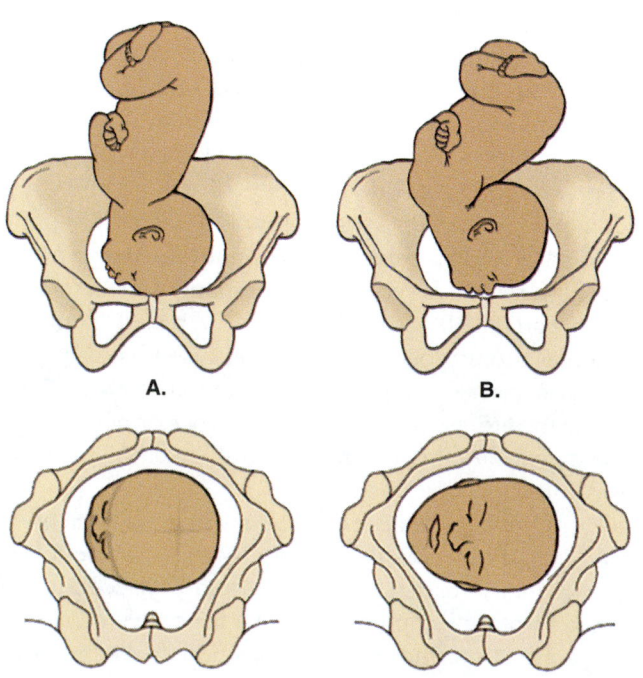

Figure 26-4 A. Brow presentation. B. Face presentation.

nurse must assess client pain responses, offer comfort interventions, administer pain medications as ordered, assist with regional anesthesia, and monitor the client after administration of anesthesia. In order to educate and reduce anxiety, the nurse may offer explanations to the client and support persons regarding the plan of care; reason for augmentation; and expectations regarding face or brow presentation, particularly fetal appearance. Offering reassurance and maintaining a vigilant presence also will help reduce anxiety in the client and her support persons. Preparation in advance for operative vaginal delivery with any additional instruments, such as forceps or vacumn suction devices, ensures readiness and reduces potential delays if complications were to arise. In addition, communication with the other health team members promotes ready availability of support for the neonate once delivered. When cesarean section is required the nurse must prepare quickly and efficiently, while monitoring maternal-fetal status. As before, the nurse probably will assume the role of circulating nurse during the cesarean section or operative vaginal delivery, and possibly will assume the role of recovery nurse after the procedure. The continuity of the nurse's attendance should reassure the client and limit anxiety throughout the delivery process.

Evaluation of the outcomes unique to face and brow presentations addresses the neonate's stability and presence or absence of injury. Evaluation of maternal pain management and anxiety requires obtaining feedback verbally and observing behavioral responses. Periodic evaluation throughout labor and delivery allows for revision or reinforcement of the nursing interventions to better meet the emotional and educational needs as well as the physical care of the client and her fetus.

Malpositions

Malpositions include persistent occipitoposterior and persistent occipitotransverse positions, which result from fetal rotation as the fetus descends through the pelvis. When the extension process is incomplete, the rotational process also may be incomplete. Fetal and maternal contributing factors include macrosomia and pelvic abnormalities, respectively. A malposition may result in increased discomfort during labor, particularly back pain; prolonged, abnormal labor; soft tissue injury; lacerations; or an extensive episiotomy incision. The fetus in a malposition may experience extensive caput and molding from the sustained occipitotransverse or occipitoposterior position. Catput succedaneum is swelling of a portion of the fetal head most commonly occurring when the head is in the lower portion of the birth canal after the resistance of a rigid vaginal outlet is encountered (Cunningham et al., 1997).

Molding refers to the movement of the bones in the skull of the neonate to fit through the maternal pelvis.

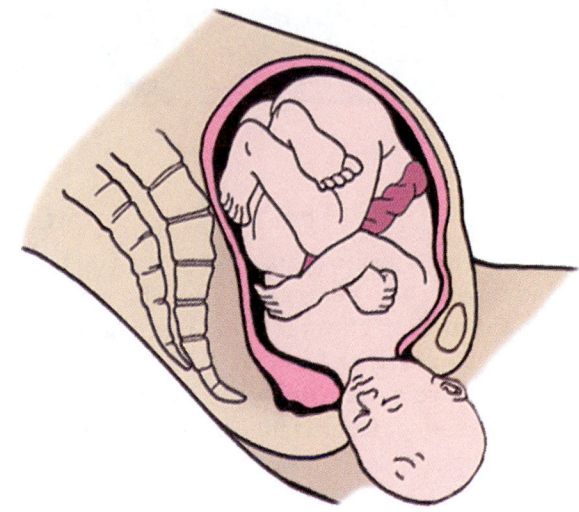

Figure 26-5 Shoulder dystocia.

The degree to which the neonate's head is capable of molding may make the difference between successful vaginal delivery and cesarean section (Cunningham et al., 1997). When the fetus has macrosomia, the potential exists for shoulder dystocia. Shoulder dystocia is a condition in which the fetal shoulders are large and cannot be delivered spontaneously by the maternal pelvis (Figure 26-5). Most cases of malposition resolve spontaneously, and less than 10% fail to resolve (Cunningham et al., 1997). Those cases that do not resolve may be managed with operative vaginal delivery, including outlet forceps to assist delivery in the occipitoposterior position, forceps rotation of the fetal head to an occipitoanterior position, and manual rotation of the fetal head for subsequent delivery (Thompson, 1995; Hankins & Rowe, 1996). When arrest of descent occurs and macrosomia or abnormal pelvic outlet is suspected, the physician may choose delivery by cesarean section.

The nursing assessment should include the historical, physical, emotional, and educational information necessary to plan for the holistic support of the client, her fetus, and her support persons. The history should include information that may indicate macrosomia, such as maternal diabetes, excessive weight gain, results from sonography showing large for gestational age status, and a history of an infant with macrosomia. A history that includes prolonged labor or operative vaginal delivery also may indicate the potential for a malposition to occur. The experienced obstetric nurse may be able to assess malposition during the pelvic examination by denoting fetal suture line and fontanelle position in relation to the maternal pelvis. However, assessment becomes much more difficult once significant caput is present. Fetal heart rate monitoring for well-being and labor tolerance should be performed. Uterine activity assessment is necessary to ensure adequacy of

Case Study/Care Plan

CLIENT WITH FETAL MALPRESENTATION

Linda is a 29-year-old gravida 2, para 1001 at 39 5/7 weeks' estimated gestational age. She arrives in labor and delivery with her partner, Tim. She states that she is having contractions every 5 minutes and denies that her membranes have ruptured. Her first baby weighed 6 pounds, 7 ounces and was born after 14 hours of labor. Her physician has voiced concern that this baby appears much bigger than that based on ultrasonography, Leopold's maneuvers, and fundal height measurements. After orientation to her room and the unit, Linda is assessed for labor status. External fetal monitoring is applied. Fetal heart tones are located at the maternal umbilicus and are in the 130s. Accelerations are present. Maternal vital signs are the following: temperature, 98°F, pulse, 88; respirations, 18; and blood pressure, 120/72. Pelvic examination reveals cervical dilation of 4 cm, 80% effaced, and −2 station with palpable intact membranes. The presenting part feels softer than a vertex (fetal skull), raising the suspicion of a breech presentation.

 The nurse finds that critical elements of the assessment are suspicions of a larger baby than the first, who weighed 6 pounds, 7 ounces. In addition, fetal heart tones are located around the maternal umbilicus. Finally, the presenting part seems more like a breech presentation, which is a malpresentation. The cervical dilation of 4 cm may play a role in the face of spontaneous rupture of membranes. In such a case, if the breech presentation is not well applied to the cervix, prolapse of the umbilical cord could occur.

Assessment

- 39⅚ weeks'
- P 88
- BP 120/72

- T 98°F
- R 18
- 4 cm dilated

Nursing Diagnosis

Risk for injury (fetal) related to possible umbilical cord prolapse with spontaneous rupture of membranes, soft tissue injury, or nerve compression from macrosomia or a complex delivery owing to malpresentation, as evidenced by signs of acute fetal cord compression or fetal trauma after operative or cesarean birth.

Expected Outcome   Fetus will not incur injury from cord prolapse or complex delivery maneuvers.

Planning   Alert care team to potential risks and prepare for emergency procedures.

Nursing Interventions	Rationales
1. Report to the physician or CNM suspicion of malpresentation. Supplemental confirmation of large baby is also important because a vaginal breech delivery is probably not the option of choice for this client due to large fetal size.	1. Medical management is necessary to carefully assess fetal presentation, fetal size, maternal pelvic size, and mode of delivery.
2. Order and report ultrasonography results to the physician or CNM.	2. Information about presentation and fetal weight is critical to determining course of action.
3. Monitor maternal vital signs and fetal tolerance to labor.	3. Constant monitoring of maternal and fetal well-being is most important in fetal malpresentation.
4. Instruct the client to report any sensation of ruptured membranes and to be alert for potential prolapse of the umbilical cord.	4. With a breech presentation, a significant fetal risk includes umbilical cord prolapse.

(continued)

Evaluation   Fetal vital signs are stable and cord did not prolapse before delivery. Fetal tracing showed no cord compression. No fetal injuries, bruising, brachial nerve compression, or hip problems were noted.

Nursing Diagnosis

Risk for infection (maternal) and injury related to operative procedure, as evidenced by postoperative infection, hemorrhage, or hematuria.

Expected Outcome   Client will not experience postoperative infection or injury from operative delivery.

Planning   Prepare client for post-delivery care procedures so that she may anticipate and accept nursing care measures.

Nursing Interventions	Rationales
1. Preoperative procedures to minimize the risk for infection and operative injury may include abdominal shaving and preparation and insertion of an in-dwelling Foley catheter.	1. These steps will reduce the risk of infection.
2. Give Tim appropriate scrubs and position for procedure to support Linda without contaminating surgical setup.	2. Partner participation in the birth process must be in line with the need to maintain a sterile environment.
3. After surgery, carefully monitor the client according to postanesthesia unit standards to minimize the risk of postoperative complications.	3. Febrile morbidity is rather frequent after cesarean deliveries because of postpartum infection.

Evaluation   Maternal vital signs are stable and there is no maternal fever or signs of infection, hemorrhage, or shock.

Nursing Diagnosis

Anxiety (maternal and family) related to altered plans for childbirth experience and unfamiliarity with the management of breech presentation, as evidenced by client verbalization and nonverbal behaviors.

Expected Outcome   Client and support persons will verbalize concerns regarding birth plans, alterations, and possible management, while demonstrating effective mechanisms for coping with the stress of the labor and delivery process.

Planning   Work with client and partner so they understand and accept the delivery options that are now likely.

Nursing Interventions	Rationales
1. Remain in the room with the client while the attending physician or CNM visits with the client and family, and listen to the plan of care and how it is presented.	1. This enables the nurse to reinforce the plan of care with the client and family.
2. Answer client questions regarding the attendance of her partner, Tim, at the scheduled cesarean section and access to infant after delivery.	2. Client education and support reduces anxiety and stress.

Evaluation   Client and family verbalized and demonstrated effective coping with the altered plan of a cesarean section.

(continued)

contractions and early identification of signs of abnormal labor. Client complaints of pain may be focused on her back when the fetal position is occipitoposterior. Assessing the location of pain allows better intervention and provides indications of fetal position. Client level of knowledge, fear, and anxiety also should be assessed.

The nursing diagnoses address fetal injury, maternal injury, maternal pain, anxiety, and knowledge deficits. The outcomes seek prevention and resolution of these potential or actual problems. Nursing interventions include ongoing assessment of maternal-fetal status and the progression of labor. Particularly useful in converting malpositions in labor are maternal position change laterally or onto her hands and knees in the form of a knee-chest position (Smith, Ou, Chen, & Su, 1997). In addition, nursing support for pain management, containment or reduction of anxiety, and client education are essential interventions. Because of the likelihood and intensity of back labor, nursing support should include a variety of comfort measures, including position changes; low back counterpressure during contractions; and the use of, if permitted and requested, epidural anesthesia. IV anesthesia also is helpful but should not be used late in labor to avoid fetal sedation and fetal respiratory depression at delivery. Additional

needs for vaginal delivery, such as forceps or vacumn suction devices, should be anticipated and equipment made available. Evaluations should obtain the objective and subjective feedback necessary to determine whether interventions have been successful or require revision. Interventions are successful when no fetal or maternal trauma occurs, pain is adequately managed, and the clients anxiety and educational needs are met.

MATERNAL AND FETAL STRUCTURAL ABNORMALITIES

Variations in maternal and fetal structural proportions that may result in high-risk deliveries include cephalopelvic disproportion and macrosomia.

Cephalopelvic Disproportion

Cephalopelvic disproportion (CPD) exists when the maternal pelvis cannot accommodate the fetal head as it descends. A contracted maternal pelvis and fetal macrosomia contribute to CPD (Bashore, 1992). A **contracted ma-**

ternal pelvis refers to abnormalities in measurements that fall short of those required for an average delivery. Congenital or acquired (from trauma) pelvic deviations may exist. Relative CPD is said to exist when the fetus is larger than the maternal pelvic inlet-outlet or when the fetal position places the head at an angle that is larger than the size the pelvis can facilitate. Relative CPD is particularly important when considering the mode of delivery for subsequent pregnancies. A 1998 study that reviewed cesarean deliveries for CPD showed that 68% of the women successfully delivered their subsequent neonate vaginally and 47% had larger babies (Impey & O'Herlihy, 1998). This data should encourage practitioners, including nurses, not to predetermine the mode of delivery for clients attempting trial of labor who have a history of cesarean section for CPD. Contracted maternal pelvic outlets are reported in less than 1% of the delivering population. The reported incidence of macrosomia using 4,000 g as the weight index is 5.1%. Using 4,500 g as the weight index, the incidence is 0.4% (Cunningham et al., 1997).

Contributing factors for CPD include congenital non-gynecoid pelvic (flattened, narrow, or irregular) shape or post-traumatic contractures as a result of a crushed or fractured pelvis. The risks to the laboring client are a prolonged and painful labor and failure of the cervix to dilate or the fetus to descend, with resultant need for operative delivery. The potential also exists for maternal uterine rupture from prolonged thinning of the lower uterine segment during a nonprogressive but active labor process. Fetal risks include extensive caput and molding from the prolonged labor; fetal intolerance, with resultant hypoxia from the prolonged labor; and the potential for birth injury related to a difficult and traumatic delivery.

Medical management will carefully assess pelvic and fetal sizes. Sonography may be beneficial, although estimates of fetal weight with very large fetuses are not very reliable. X-ray pelvimetry measures were more commonly used several years ago but offer true pelvic measures. The management of labor may be expectant when labor activity is adequate, or augmentation may be attempted when the contraction pattern is not regular or firm. At the point of delivery in CPD, the physician may attempt outlet forceps delivery or vacuum suction to assist in delivering the fetus vaginally. When measurements or these interventions are not satisfactory, or the fetal heart rate demonstrates intolerance of the delivery process, the physician may order preparations for cesarean delivery.

The nursing assessment history may help identify a pelvic adequacy problem. Risk factors are maternal diabetes, previous prolonged labor, previous fetal or maternal trauma at delivery, previous need for operative vaginal delivery (extensive episiotomy, use of forceps or vacuum extraction), and previous cesarean delivery. Leopold's maneuvers may reveal a fetus that is not well descended into the maternal pelvis. Pelvic examination that identifies caput or molding, particularly while the fetus remains at station 0 or higher, may indicate a problem. Pelvic examination by the nurse that fails to reveal cervical change hourly despite regular contractions that are moderate to firm in intensity also may be significant in identifying CPD. These assessment variables help to indicate potential CPD; however, they do not preclude the initial thorough and complete assessment of maternal-fetal status or the dynamic elements that are reassessed every 5, 15, 30, or 60 minutes, depending on the stage of labor, client risk status, and fetal tolerance (Feinstein & McCartney, 1997).

Nursing diagnoses address the risks for maternal and fetal injury and infection and the concerns for maternal pain, anxiety, and lack of knowledge during labor and delivery. Desired outcomes designate that no fetal or maternal injury or infection will occur, and adequate pain and anxiety management and appropriate education will be achieved.

While the nursing interventions to meet the above outcomes may seem routine, the dynamics of the potential problem require the nurse to be alert for changes that are either reassuring or nonreassuring in nature. The individualization of the emotional and educational support as well as the unique interaction between the nurse and each client prevent the experience from being routine or less than challenging. The client experiencing CPD or relative CPD may experience a prolonged labor process and require extensive medical intervention for an operative vaginal delivery, or she may need to undergo a cesarean section. The nurse does not control the medical management of labor and eventual delivery; however, assisting the client to achieve optimal delivery outcomes with a minimum of negative occurrences is a nursing role. Evaluation of successful or less than successful outcomes provides the nurse with feedback from which new interventions or further support can be applied.

Macrosomia

Macrosomia is a cause of relative cephalopelvic disproportion. The increased size of the fetus can make passage through an adequate-sized pelvis difficult or impossible. As stated previously, macrosomia is more common than are contracted maternal pelvic disorders, with a 5.1% incidence (Cunningham et al., 1997). When the fetus does descend, the passage may be further complicated by delivery of the fetal head but then halted abruptly because of shoulder dystocia. Shoulder dystocia occurs when the fetal shoulder width is so large that it is not deliverable beneath the maternal symphysis pubis without additional delivery intervention or fetal injury. Shoulder dystocia occurs when the anterior shoulder of the fetus is aligned with the anteroposterior line of the pelvis and becomes lodged behind

REFLECTIONS FROM A MOTHER

"I was feeling very alone as I neared my due date. I had friends, but the father of my baby was not involved. My parents tried to be supportive. However, they were not pleased with my status as a single pregnant woman. When I arrived in labor and delivery in active labor, I was scared and hurting terribly from my contractions. When the nurses saw the heart beat on the monitor everything began to happen very fast. I had three people working on me at the same time. I had an oxygen mask on my face, and the smell of plastic was awful. My parents' faces had looks of concern and fear. They stood away from me while everyone was busy working on me. I was so scared!

Then I saw Marta. She is a nurse who was called into my room when the other nurses saw my baby's heart beat recording. She calmed everyone down, and they worked fast without panic. She explained what was happening and why. She assured me my doctor was aware of what was happening and was coming immediately. She asked me if I had questions, and then she asked my parents. She brought my mother to one side and let her hold my hand. Up until then, my mother and I had said little to each other because of her disappointment in me. Now, however, we just held hands and prayed my baby would be okay.

Marta seemed to calm everyone. When my baby did not respond to the oxygen, IV fluids, and all the different positions they had me move to, she appeared concerned but did not panic. My doctor came in and confirmed her expectations for a cesarean section. Even though everything happened very fast, I trusted Marta. She stayed with me and encouraged me throughout my surgery. She showed me my baby as soon as he was ok. She explained to me the things that were around me. I wasn't scared with everyone working around me, because she told me they would help my baby adjust to being outside. I have a healthy son, Aaron, because the labor and delivery team worked so hard and fast. I have a good memory of my experience because of Marta."

---

the symphysis pubis, the alignment is appropriate but the size of the shoulders prevents anterior shoulder progression toward delivery, or the posterior shoulder becomes lodged behind the sacral promontory (Hall, 1997). The delivery of the shoulders can be extremely difficult for the mother to experience, and fetal injury may be impossible to prevent regardless of the skill and experience of the physician or CNM. Shoulder dystocia is considered an obstetric emergency (Hall, 1997; Wagner, Nielsen, & Gonik, 1999). The reported incidence of shoulder dystocia varies from 0.2% to 2% because of variable definitions of true shoulder dystocia. Within this range, the low percentages are attributable to those cases requiring classic delivery maneuvers and the high percentages are based on fetal weights with documentation of shoulder dystocia (Cunningham et al., 1997; Hall, 1997).

The literature shows that the most frequent risk factor leading to shoulder dystocia is macrosomia (Cunningham et al., 1997; Hall, 1997; Lewis et al., 1998; Wagner, Nielsen, & Gonik, 1999). Other risk factors include concurrent maternal diabetes, a history of a previous large infant, prolonged second stage of labor, and excessive weight gain during pregnancy (Toohey et al., 1995; Lewis et al., 1998). Less clear as risks but still frequently believed to be contributory are advanced maternal age, previous history of gestational diabetes, multiparity, short maternal stature, and maternal obesity (Hall, 1997; Lewis et al., 1998). Two acronyms summarize the risk factors that should be assessed routinely: Diabetes Obesity Postterm Excessive (DOPE) fetal or maternal weight gain, and Age + DOPE (ADOPE) (Cunningham et al., 1997; Hall, 1997).

Risks to the client that are related to shoulder dystocia include soft tissue injury; bladder injury; cervical, vaginal, or perineal lacerations; separation of the symphysis pubis; uterine rupture; postpartum hemorrhage; and cesarean section (Hall, 1997). Risks to the fetus include fractures of the clavicle and humerus and nerve damage, resulting in Erb's or Klumpke's palsy. Erb's palsy affects mobility of the upper arm; Klumpke's palsy affects mobility of the lower arm and hand and tone. The fetus also may experience increased intracranial pressure, hypoxia, acidosis, and asphyxia (Cunningham et al., 1997).

Medical management is determined by early identification of risk factors and consideration of delivery options. Both early elective induction and scheduled cesarean section have been evaluated for delivery of infants with macrosomia whose mothers have diabetes, with variable results (Gonen et al., 1998; Conway & Langer, 1998; Wagner, Nielsen, & Gonik, 1999). These measures are anticipatory in nature. Many times, however, shoulder dystocia must be dealt with at the time of occurrence.

Nursing considerations are significant in the recognition of and intervention for shoulder dystocia. The nurse's initial and ongoing assessments during labor may be the first data indicating shoulder dystocia. Labor delays, particularly with fetal descent, should be communicated to the physician or CNM. Pronounced caput or molding even at a relatively high station (above zero) may also be indicative of impending shoulder dystocia. Observation during maternal pushing may allow recognition of the turtle sign. The **turtle sign** occurs when the fetal head pulls back instead of completing the external rotation process and progressing forward into the maternal perineum. The appearance is as if the head is retracting back into the shell of the pelvis. Once the head is delivered, the inability to deliver the anterior shoulder beneath the symphysis pubis with gentle traction is diagnostic of shoulder dystocia (Hall, 1997; Cunningham et al., 1997).

The nurse should remain with the physician or CNM and call from the room for assistance. Once shoulder dystocia is recognized, constant monitoring of fetal status at one-minute intervals is essential. Fetal acidosis can begin after five minutes. The fetus may experience low Apgar scores or signs of asphyxia after only 7 to 10 minutes (Hall, 1997). Several maneuvers may be used by the physician or CNM to complete the delivery process. It is essential that the nurse remain calm to assist in delivery, reduce the client's anxiety, and facilitate client cooperation while these maneuvers are being attempted (Hall, 1997; Simpson, 1999).

The McRoberts maneuver requires maternal position changes in which the client's legs are bent at the knees and hyperflexed against her abdomen to straighten the sacrum and alter the angle, allowing for the anterior shoulder to be dislodged (Figure 26-6). Preferably two nurses assist the mother, with one nurse supporting each leg in the hyperflexed position while the physician or CNM attempts to complete the delivery. When reviewed as a first procedure used for reducing shoulder dystocia, the McRoberts maneuver was successful in 47% of cases. The

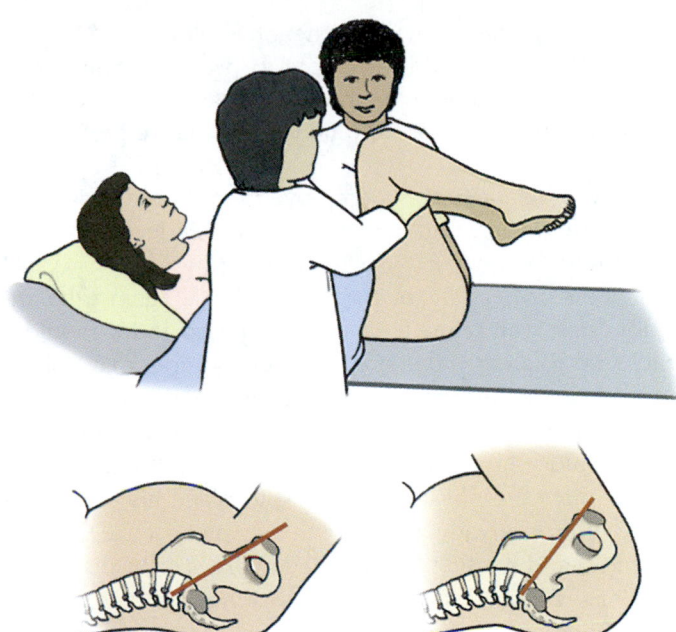

Figure 26-6 In the McRoberts maneuver, the client's legs are bent at the knees and hyperflexed against her abdomen. The result is straightening of the sacrum and altering of the angle, allowing the shoulder to dislodge.

remaining deliveries reviewed required additional interventions (Gherman et al., 1997).

Suprapubic pressure is another procedure used that the nurse may be requested to perform. By applying suprapubic pressure either in an oblique or lateral approach (Rubin technique) or posteriorly and laterally (Mazzanti technique), the anterior shoulder may be compressed and slip beneath the symphysis pubis (Figure 26-7). These techniques may be combined with maternal pushing, or the client may be requested not to push and

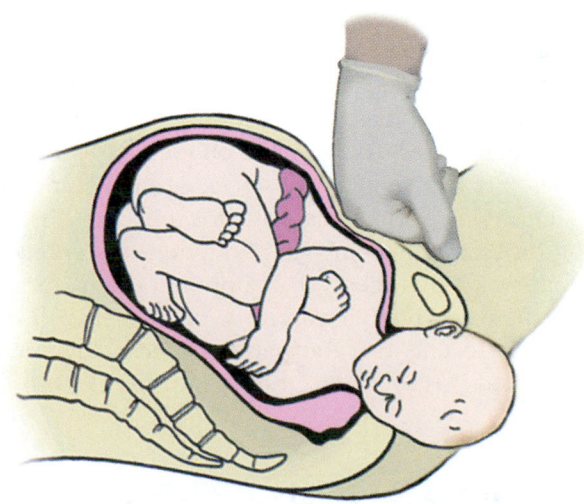

Figure 26-7 Suprapubic pressure may release shoulder dystocia.

rely only on the traction of the physician or CNM. The client's bladder should be empty to prevent trauma. The nurse may have already emptied the bladder before delivery, or the physician or CNM may do so before performing these maneuvers.

The other maneuvers employed for shoulder dystocia are more invasive in nature. They include the Woods corkscrew maneuver in which the physician or CNM places his or her fingers within the vagina against the anterior chest wall of the fetus to push the posterior shoulder back and rotate it 180 degrees. Either shoulder may deliver as a result of this maneuver. The physician may request that the nurse apply suprapubic pressure to keep the anterior shoulder in an adducted position. The Rubin maneuver requires the physician or CNM to place his or her fingers within the vagina against the scapula of the anterior shoulder and rotate it forward 180 degrees. This maneuver also may be used to rotate the posterior shoulder anteriorly. Once again, the nurse may be requested to provide suprapubic pressure. When the rotational maneuvers are unsuccessful in dislodging the shoulders and delivering the fetus, the physician may then attempt to deliver the posterior arm. In this procedure, a hand is inserted into the vagina to the posterior arm and traces the path to the elbow, allowing flexion, retrieval, and delivery of the arm. This procedure allows for room to dislodge the anterior shoulder. This maneuver may result in fracture of the fetal humerus. When these maneuvers fail, the fetal head may be rotated to direct occipitoanterior position and pressure applied to replace the head within the pelvis for retrieval through emergent cesarean section. The person supporting the head will remain in that position until the cesarean is complete and the fetus delivered. The morbidity is much higher with this procedure; however, the alternative may be stillbirth when the shoulders cannot be delivered vaginally (Hall, 1997; Cunningham et al., 1997).

Nursing diagnoses include risks of fetal injury and fetal hypoxia, risks of maternal injury and infection, as well as the usual nursing diagnoses. The outcomes seek to prevent negative outcomes from occurring. Interventions during the labor process focus on the ongoing assessment that indicates possible shoulder dystocia, communicating concerns effectively, remaining with the physician or CNM, calling for help, remaining calm, offering reassurance and information to the client and support persons, assisting with maneuvers, notifying nursery personnel, and documenting the events that transpired as accurately and systematically as possible (Hall, 1997; Simpson, 1999).

MULTIPLE GESTATION

Multiple gestation refers to the carrying of more than one fetus during the same pregnancy (Figure 26-8). With the in-

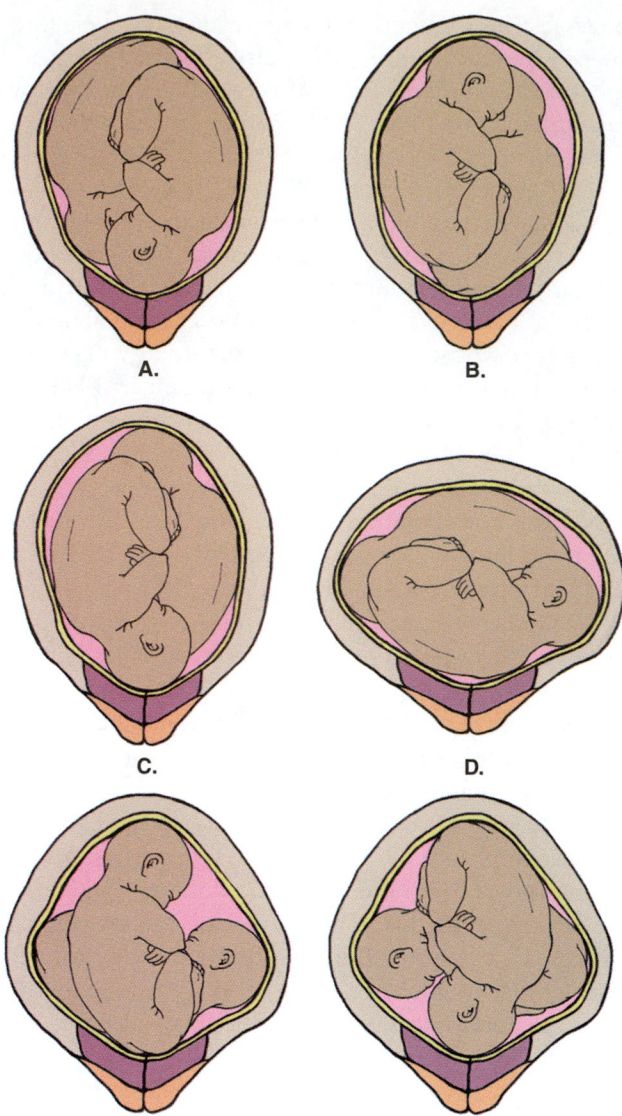

Figure 26-8 Twin fetuses can assume any number of presentations.

crease in infertility management and assisted reproductive technology, such as in vitro and gamete transfer technology, the incidence of twins, triplets, and higher-order gestations (quadruplets, quintuplets, and so on) has increased significantly. Bowers (1998) reviewed the 1995 U.S. statistics and found there were 96,736 neonates born alive as twins, 4,551 as triplets, 365 as quadruplets, and 57 as quintuplets or higher-order multiple births. In 1990, the reported incidence of twins was 1 in 43 live births and that of triplets was 1 in 1,341 live births. Ovulation induction and assisted reproductive technology are identified as the causes of 83% of triplet pregnancies and 95% of quadruplet pregnancies (Eganhouse & Petersen, 1998). Higher-order pregnancies, inclusive of triplets, have increased rapidly at approximately 11% a year since 1997 (Bowers, 1998).

Multiple fetus pregnancies are evaluated for separate amnions and chorions. Shared amnion and chorions allow for shared placental circulations and physical entanglement issues. Shared placentas, amnions, and chorions are the result of monozygotic splitting. *Williams Obstetrics* reports that *monozygotic twinning,* (when twins occur from a single ovum and may share a single placenta, amnion, and chorion) occurs in approximately 1 in 250 births (Cunningham et al., 1997). Most triplet pregnancies are reported as trizygotic (separate chorions and amnions); however, assisted reproductive interventions have increased the likelihood of monozygotic triplets (Eganhouse & Petersen, 1998).

The increase in the number of multifetus pregnancies is attributed to advanced maternal age as the result of delaying pregnancies and infertility requiring ovulatory stimulation medications and assisted reproductive technologies (Bowers, 1998). With additional fetuses come additional risks, which increase with each additional fetus in the pregnancy. The major risks in all multiple gestations are prematurity and low birth weight. Bowers (1998) reported that 47.9% of twin gestations and 87.8% of all higher-order gestations end before the 37th week, unlike singleton pregnancies. Other problems are also increased, with twin gestations experiencing an overall complication rate at least twice that of singleton pregnancies. Triplets and higher-order multiples experience much higher complication rates than do twins. Over 92% of higher-order multiples fall into the low-birth-weight category, and 35% are reported as having very low birth weights (Bowers, 1998). In addition, the infant death rate for higher-order multiples exceeds that of singleton gestations by 12 times.

Among the fetal risks are *conjoining abnormalities* (when twins have incomplete separation and demonstrate a common organ or portion of the body), placental abnormalities, twin-to-twin transfusions, and discordant fetal growth (when the growth of one twin exceeds that of the other(s) by at least 25%). Cerebral palsy and other neurologic impairments, stillbirth, glucose instability at birth, and birth injuries also occur more frequently (Cunningham et al., 1997). Fetal mortality ranges from 9.8% to 13.6% (Eganhouse & Petersen, 1998). Perinatal mortality is described as being five times higher for twin gestations than for singleton pregnancies (Ellings, Newman, & Bowers, 1998).

Maternal complications of multiple gestations also increase with the number of fetuses carried. All of the physiologic changes that occur to the client carrying a singleton gestation are increased to the extreme with multiple gestations. These include cardiac output, diastolic blood pressure, plasma volume, and venous distention. In contrast, maternal cardiac reserve, pulmonary residual volumes, and even gastrointestinal tone and motility are decreased (Bowers, 1998). Problems that can occur with pregnancy, such as anemia, pyelonephritis, cholelithiasis and cholesta-sis, peripartum cardiomyopathy, and fatty liver disease, are more likely to occur in women with multiple gestations; and preexisting chronic problems affecting any organ system are likely to be exacerbated (Bowers, 1998). Maternal challenges also include increased nutritional demands, increased discomforts and compromises from uterine distention, and the risk for preterm labor. The complications that result from treating these problems also are challenges for the client. Preeclampsia, uterine atony after delivery, and postpartum hemorrhage are also risks the client with multiple gestation faces (Shields & Medearis, 1992b; Ellings, Newman, & Bowers, 1998). Psychosocial risks for the client and support persons include the incorporation of the multiple fetuses into the client's and the family's pregnancy plan and adaptation; acceptance as a high-risk obstetric patient; altered activities, including prolonged hospitalizations; financial concerns related to the loss of income and hospital costs; and the overriding fear of potential fetal loss (Bowers, 1998; Sather & Zwelling, 1998). The potential for anxiety and depression related to all of the concerns listed is well documented in families of multiple gestations (Leonard, 1998).

Medical management of the multiple gestation surrounds early diagnosis, monitoring of maternal and fetal well-being, and interventions as indicated in the face of complications. Medical surveillance may rely on laboratory values (for anemia), sonogram data (to assess fetal growth, chorionicity, and complications such as entanglement of cords) (Aisenbrey, 1995), fetal viability and cervical assessment (for stable labor status). Intrapartum management of multiple gestations may consider vaginal delivery for twins; however, many twins and all higher-order gestations are delivered by cesarean section.

Nursing considerations for the client and her support persons experiencing a multiple gestation are numerous. Whether the client is receiving nursing care in a high-risk antepartum hospitalization, is trying to halt the threat of preterm labor, or is in labor and delivery for her high-risk delivery, the nurse will be an integral part of a multidisciplinary team. The focus of care is to minimize or prevent antepartal and intrapartum complications (Bowers, 1998). The need for emotional support also is tremendous (Sather & Zwelling, 1998). The thoroughness of the nursing assessment is critical to identify even subtle concerns or changes in maternal-fetal status. The assessment should focus on maternal stability, fetal well-being with serial nonstress testing, and the absence or presence of uterine activity recorded on the fetal monitor. Psychosocial assessment should address the client's adaptation to the multiple pregnancy, the current situation, anticipatory grief processes, basic knowledge, coping skills, the ability to cooperate with the plan of care, and her support system (Bowers, 1998; Sather & Zwelling, 1998). An awareness of the potential for peripartum depression is particularly important. The nurse may facilitate the client in seeking additional support that may reduce the likelihood of impaired maternal-infant attachment or even neglect or abuse (Leonard, 1998). The nurse may become the hub of the team by communicating needs, problems, plans, and readiness to other team members, such as the physician, the neonatal nursery team, social services, pastoral care, lactation support persons, and postpartum caregivers. An additional benefit to the client is provided through the nurse's consistent presence in an organized and calm environment (Bowers, 1998). Readiness for delivery and the necessary fetal and neonatal support are essential to prevent delay in resuscitative efforts or stabilization of all neonates. Perioperative procedures should be strictly observed to reduce the potential for infection. Provision of information and answering of questions should be done to meet the client's and support person's educational needs and reduce anxiety.

Evaluations of outcomes for the client and her neonates in a multiple gestation require review of the events.

- Was preterm labor halted long enough to achieve fetal viability, growth, and optimal survival?
- Did the delivery result in minimal problems for the fetuses and mother?
- Were the emotional needs of the client and her family met?
- Were resources consulted to assist with social and economic challenges?
- Were spiritual needs, inclusive of grief, addressed and supported?

The challenge of providing care for the client with multiple gestation is becoming more frequent and requires that the nurse provide highly technical care coupled with careful attention to the emotional well-being of the whole family.

FETAL DISTRESS

Nonreassuring fetal status, inclusive of the term **fetal distress**, refers to the response of the fetus to the antepartum or intrapartum uterine environment. Distress refers to the lack of fetal reserve or presence of fetal hypoxia, acidosis, or asphyxia. The fetal monitor tracing may demonstrate repetitive late decelerations; loss of variability; increasing baseline; or deep prolonged decelerations, with failure to return to baseline. A low scalp pH may indicate distress. A poor biophysical profile score also may indicate fetal compromise.

Any pregnant client may demonstrate a nonreassuring fetal status. It is safe to assume however that obstetric clients with high-risk conditions, such as prematurity, post-

maturity, infectious processes, hemorrhagic conditions, and preeclampsia, are more likely to experience problems. Fetal risk factors include permanent injury or death as a result of sustained hypoxia, with resultant acidosis and asphyxia. Maternal risks include the potential for operative vaginal or cesarean section, once the condition is diagnosed, and the resultant complications.

Concurrent medical management depends on whether the client is antepartal or intrapartal and the extent of the nonreassuring data. For example, when a client who is antepartal undergoes a fetal nonstress test that is nonreactive, despite adequate maternal hydration and various fetal stimulation interventions, the physician or CNM may

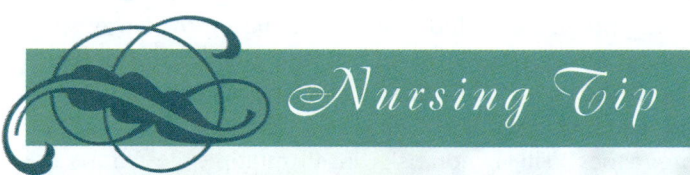

Nursing Tip

FETAL SURVEILLANCE KEY

Nonstress Test

A noninvasive test using an external fetal monitor to note fetal response, oxygenation, and autonomic functioning. A reactive nonstress test exists when two fetal heart rate accelerations of 15 bpm lasting for 15 seconds occur in a 20-minute period. Accelerations may occur spontaneously after fetal movement or other stimulation methods. A nonreactive test fails to demonstrate these accelerations and may indicate a need for further testing (Halle, 1993).

Contraction Stress Test

Use of the external fetal monitor to evaluate the fetal response to the stress of contractions. The challenge is to achieve three moderate-intensity contractions lasting 40 to 60 seconds in 10 minutes and note the fetal response. The contractions are achieved by client nipple stimulation or IV administration of an oxytocin piggyback drip. The desired response is referred to as a negative test. The occurrence of repetitive late decelerations is referred to as a positive test and indicates the need for intervention, usually delivery (Halle, 1993).

Biophysical Profile

Combines a nonstress test with ultrasound evaluation of fetal movement, breathing, tone, and amniotic fluid measures, with a scoring system from 0 to 2.

Halle, J. (1993) Diagnostic evaluation of high risk pregnancies. In S. Mattson & J. Smith (Eds.) (Chapt. 11). *NAACOG: Core curriculum for maternal newborn nursing.* Philadelphia, PA: W. B. Saunders.

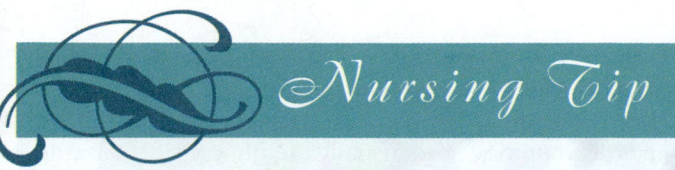

AMNIOINFUSION

Amnioinfusion may be ordered to be performed at a bolus rate (up to 800 mL at one instillation); continuous flow rate (3 mL/min); or combination of an initial bolus (600 to 800 mL at 10 to 15 mL/min followed by continuation at 3 mL/min), with a subsequent continuous flow rate. Amnioinfusion requires ruptured membranes and an intact intrauterine pressure catheter (IUPC), preferably a double-lumen one. You must:

1. Check the functioning of the IUPC.

2. Connect the primed tubing by way of the controller pump to the instillation port of the IUPC. Set the rate for bolus or continuous flow.

3. Use warmed solution, which is standard practice; some policies require a warmer to maintain temperature.

4. Monitor the maternal abdomen for tension, the perineum for outflow of fluid on the hip pad, and the fetal tracing for symptomatic relief of cord compression.

5. Discontinue as per orders or if complications arise (e.g., no fluid return and fetal intolerance).

6. Document preinfusion data, amount, maternal fetal response, and tolerance to amnioinfusion.

Adapted from a protocol in Schmidt, J. (1997). Fluid check: Making the case for intrapartum amnioinfusion. *AWHONN: Lifelines, 1,* (7); 47–51.

choose to obtain a biophysical profile or other evaluation of the fetus. In contrast, when a client who is antepartal demonstrates **oligohydramnios** (less than 5 cm total of four quadrant measurements) on a biophysical profile along with a nonreactive stress test, the physician or CNM may choose to deliver. A client who is intrapartal and demonstrates deep variables in labor may respond to interventions and continue without additional problems. In contrast, the client who is intrapartal and demonstrates deep variables, decreasing variability, lack of accelerations, and delayed return to the baseline may require immediate delivery.

Nursing assessment of fetal status is critical. Fetal heart rate baseline, variability, the presence of periodic or nonperiodic accelerations, the presence of periodic or nonperiodic decelerations, depth, and duration should all be assessed in detail. Maternal status that can affect fetal response, including position, maternal infection, hydra-

tion, uterine activity, blood pressure and medication, also must be assessed. Psychosocial elements, such as anxiety, pain, and lack of knowledge, also may affect maternal tolerance and thus fetal oxygenation.

The nursing plan is based on the initial and ongoing maternal-fetal assessment. Nursing interventions specifically used to increase fetal oxygenation may include use of maternal position changes to either side or even a modified knee-chest position to relieve pressure on the umbilical cord in utero. The nurse may apply supplemental oxygen by face mask at 8 to 10 L/min to enhance maternal-fetal oxygenation; increase IV fluid hydration to correct dehydration or dilute oxytocin stimulatory effects; and reduce or discontinue oxytocin uterine stimulation, particularly in the face of hyperstimulation. The nurse may be able to increase the accuracy of fetal monitoring by applying an internal fetal electrode for direct electrocardiogram monitoring or inserting an intrauterine pressure catheter (IUPC) to accurately assess intrauterine pressure during contractions and at rest. Application of these devices may be done by individual order, standing order, or critical pathway orders. Application should be done by the physician, CNM, or a nurse with additional expertise and experience. Each institution has policy parameters for performing these procedures based on the nursing practice act of the state and community norms. The nurse may be requested to start, maintain, and monitor an *amnioinfusion,* which is an invasive procedure that instills warm fluid into the uterine cavity by infusion pump to increase fluid volume and relieve pressure on the umbilical cord. This procedure also serves to dilute thick meconium and therefore may reduce the likelihood of meconium aspiration syndrome (Schmidt, 1997). Finally, in the face of nonreassuring responses, the nurse needs to make preparations for an emergent delivery.

Although not specific for fetal distress, the nurse also must incorporate general nursing monitoring and support interventions for client well-being. It is critical that the nurse maintain excellent channels of communication with the physician or CNM to discuss maternal-fetal status, interventions, and results. The intervention process should be calmly explained to reassure the client and support persons, convey concern and confidence in the interventions, and help reduce the overall level of anxiety. Finally, communication with the neonatal team is also important so that the members can prepare for any neonatal resuscitative efforts.

UTERINE RUPTURE

Uterine rupture involves a separation of the uterine wall that may allow protrusion of fetal parts into the maternal abdomen. A longitudinal rupture, sometimes referred to as a classic rupture, occurs over the body of the uterus and is an acute emergent situation. Maternal shock and fetal distress may quickly become apparent to the nurse providing care. Uterine rupture of a low transverse segment over a scar from a previous low transverse cesarean section may have less acute symptoms; however, all ruptures place the mother and fetus at risk. Ruptures are classified as complete and incomplete. A complete rupture extends into the peritoneal cavity; an incomplete rupture maintains peritoneal integrity. Dehiscence refers to the separation of the old scar line and does not result in protrusion of fetal parts into the peritoneal cavity (Cunningham et al., 1997).

The rate of uterine rupture varies by institution, with reported incidences ranging from 1 in 1,280 to 1 in 3,000 deliveries (Cunningham et al., 1997). One 10-year review from Singapore has revealed an incidence of 1 in 6,331 deliveries, with a ratio of three previous cesarean scarred uteri to one unscarred uterus (Chen, Tan, & Yeo, 1995). The incidence of rupture in an unscarred uterus is even less common, and has been reported in one study as 1 in 16,849 deliveries (Miller, Goodwin, Gherman, & Paul, 1997). Contributing factors to uterine rupture include a previous cesarean scar, major surgery involving the uterus, such as a myomectomy; congenital abnormality of the uterus; grand multiparity; and use of oxytocin or protaglandins (Al Sakka, Dauleh, & Al Hassani, 1999; Caughey et al., 1999; Kirkendall, Jauregui, Kim, & Phelan, 2000; Cunningham et al., 1997; Miller, Goodwin, Gherman, & Paul, 1997). Rupture also has been reported when forceps were used (Miller, Goodwin, Gherman, & Paul, 1997). Blunt trauma also has been associated with spontaneous uterine rupture (Cunningham et al., 1997). There have been reports, although rare, of spontaneous rupture of the unscarred primigravid uterus in the absence of uterine trauma or an infectious process. The second such case ever recorded was associate with an abnormally implanted placenta (**placenta percreta**; abnormal placental attachment that completely penetrates the uterine myometrium) in the second trimester and occurred as a spontaneous acute event (Imseis, Murtha, Alexander, & Barnett, 1998).

Maternal consequences of rupture include hypovolemic shock, bladder injury, anemia, emergent hysterectomy, anemia, transfusion, bowel injury, and death; fetal and neonatal outcomes include low Apgar scores, brain damage, intrapartal death, and neonatal or infant death (Kirkendall, Jauregui, Kim, & Phelan, 2000). Admissions to the neonatal intensive care unit and increased neonatal acidosis at delivery also have been associated with uterine rupture (Menihan, 1998).

Medical management of uterine rupture includes identification of risk factors, such as the client being a candidate for vaginal birth after cesarean section; careful management of all intrapartum patients; and surgical intervention and repair, as indicated. Clients who have had previous cesareans sections are evaluated carefully, including previous scar documentation, before undergoing a trial of labor after cesarean (TOLAC) section. Clients with longitudinal uterine scars usually are not considered candidates for TOLAC. Clients with low transverse uterine scars, an adequate pelvis, and an appropriate-sized fetus without indication of malposition or malpresentation may be considered candidates for TOLAC. Management of prostaglandins and oxytocin should follow accepted medical standards of care. Many institutions require the ready availability of the physician or CNM when oxytocin is being administered during labor. Medical awareness of signs and indications of possible uterine rupture and ready availability for surgical intervention are necessary to ensure optimal maternal-fetal outcomes. Finally, repair of any sustained injuries and possible hysterectomy coupled with appropriate volume and blood replacement are part of the medical management of the client experiencing uterine rupture.

Nursing considerations for providing care for the client with potential uterine rupture is to identify risk factors with a thorough nursing assessment. Maternal history should be reviewed for previous cesarean section and type of uterine scar (longitudinal or low transverse), previous uterine surgery (such as a myomectomy in which uterine fibroids were removed), and trauma. Nursing assessment should focus on maternal uterine activity, especially contraction frequency, intensity, duration, and resting phases. When oxytocin is being administered, care should be taken to avoid hyperstimulation of the uterus. The client's abdomen also should be assessed for signs of abdominal trauma, bruising, tenderness, pain, and rigidity. Maternal vital signs may indicate shock with an elevated pulse, shallow respirations, and decreasing blood pressure. Maternal complaints of acute pain without interruption or evidence of fetal distress may support suspicion of uterine rupture.

Nursing diagnoses specific for uterine rupture identify the risks for injury to both mother and fetus from hemorrhage, shock, sustained hypoxia, hypovolemia, and acidosis. Nursing diagnoses also should address the emotional and educational needs of the client and family. Grief challenges should be included among the nursing diagnoses.

Nursing interventions center around prevention of uterine rupture induced by aggressive use of oxytocin, immediate recognition and stabilization of the client experiencing this obstetric emergency, and notification of the physician or CNM (and team members) to perform an emergency cesarean and possibly a hysterectomy. During this urgent situation the nurse should remain calm, offering explanations and reassurances to the client and informing the family of the status of the mother and fetus. Specific interventions to stabilize the client include monitoring maternal vital signs, ensuring IV access with fluid volume replacement, discontinuation of oxytocin, placement of an oxygen face mask at 10 L/min, and monitoring fetal status. Immediate laboratory tests should include, at minimum, a complete blood count (CBC), platelet count, typing, and crossmatching. Operative preparations, including insertion of a Foley catheter, are managed urgently. The nurse also may need to assist in obtaining and administering blood products as ordered.

PLACENTAL ABNORMALITIES

Placental abnormalities also may contribute to a high-risk delivery or obstetric emergency. Placental abnormalities may be related to the implantation depth or site in the uterus; early separation from the uterine wall; or developmental problems, such as poor attachment of the cord, veins, or arteries to the body of the placenta. All of these placental abnormalities place the client and fetus at risk for hemorrhage, hypoxia, and even death. The incidence of hemorrhage related to placental abnormalities varies related to differing definitions but ranges somewhere between 3% and 7% (Cunningham et al., 1997).

Placenta Previa

Placenta previa is a condition in which the placenta implants low in the uterus (Figure 26-9). It is referred to as a *complete placenta previa* when the cervical os is completely covered by the placenta. When the cervical os is only partially covered, it is called a *partial previa*. When the placenta borders on the edge of the cervical os, it is referred to as a *marginal previa*. A placenta that implants

very close to the edge is called a *low-lying placenta* (Cunningham et al., 1997; Schmidt, 1993). The incidence of placenta previa is reported to be between 0.33% and 0.5% (Crane et al., 1999; Cunningham et al., 1997). The problem with such low implantation is that as the uterus contracts or the cervix dilates, the placenta is separated from the cervix and bleeding occurs. Acute or chronic bleeding may adversely affect the mother and fetus. Acute, dramatic bleeding places the mother and fetus at risk for hypovolemia, shock, and diminished perfusion. Chronic bleeding over the second and third trimester may result in impaired fetal perfusion and growth. Ultrasonography may identify placenta previa in the second trimester before the first episode of antepartum or intrapartum bleeding. As the gestation advances, however, as many as 90% of marginal and low-lying placentas resolve (Ricci, 1992). Placenta previa demonstrates a higher rate of abnormal implantation in the uterus. *Placenta acreta* refers to abnormal implantation to the myometrium. *Placenta increta* extends into the myometrium. *Placenta percreta* implants through the myometrium. These conditions further increase the risk for hemorrhage, uterine injury, and infection (Cunningham et al., 1997). With the exception of low-lying placentas and some marginal presentations, cesarean section is the mode of delivery for clients with placenta previa.

Contributing factors to placenta previa include previous placenta previa, advanced maternal age, multiple gestations, multiparity, uterine scars from previous cesarean sections, abortions, and endometriosis (Cunningham et al., 1997). Smoking also has been associated with increased risk for placenta previa (Cunningham et al., 1997; Andres, 1996). Consequences for the pregnant client include acute or chronic hemorrhage accompanied by resultant anemia

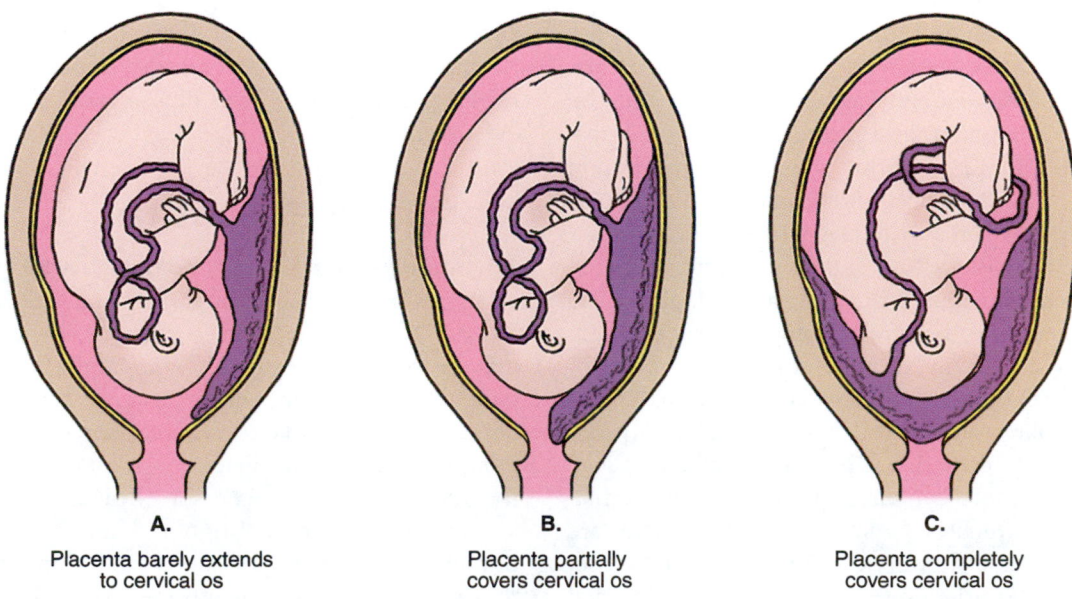

A.	B.	C.
Placenta barely extends to cervical os	Placenta partially covers cervical os	Placenta completely covers cervical os

Figure 26-9 Placenta previa. A. Low implantation (marginal). B. Partial placenta previa. C. Total placenta previa.

and coagulopathies, including disseminated intravascular coagulopathy (DIC). Additional maternal risks include the potential that the previa has abnormally implanted as a placenta acreta, increta, or percreta. These conditions not only necessitate emergent cesarean delivery but require hysterectomy (Cunningham et al., 1997; Lin, et al., 1998). Fetal risks include impaired placental perfusion that may inhibit growth and survival. Complications reported by Crane et al. (1999) include preterm delivery, respiratory compromise, anemia, and a higher rate of congenital defects.

Medical management strives to identify placenta previa before the onset of bleeding; however, this is not always successful. Even when placenta previa is identified, the onset of bleeding is not always predictable. Acute bleeding episodes may be managed initially in the hospital; after bleeding cessation, if maternal-fetal status is deemed stable, home management may be attempted (Love & Wallace, 1996). Close monitoring of maternal-fetal status with blood tests to evaluate hemodynamic stability is necessary for maternal and fetal well-being, regardless of whether the client is hospitalized or is managed on an outpatient basis. Outpatient management requires frequent office visits and concurrent home health care. When maternal-fetal status is nonreassuring or the client is approaching term, cesarean delivery is performed.

Nursing considerations when managing an obstetric client who is bleeding include identification of the source or cause of the hemorrhage and stabilization of the client and fetus until cesarean section can be performed. Assessment data should include review of prenatal history, predisposing risk factors to suggest previa, other antepartum bleeding events, maternal Rh-factor status, and whether $Rh_o(D)$ immune globulin (RhoGAM) was received if indicated. The current assessment should include when the bleeding began, the amount, the duration, whether or not the bleeding was associated with pain, and the presence or absence of fetal movement. Vaginal bleeding should be assessed for color, amount, and presence of clots. The assessing nurse should not perform a vaginal examination in the presence of bleeding. Fetal monitoring should be performed to assess for signs of fetal well-being or nonreassuring fetal status. Blood for initial laboratory testing should be drawn to evaluate hemodynamic stability. The nurse may anticipate orders for a complete blood count, typing, and crossmatching. Clotting studies, such as prothrombin time (PT), partial thromboplastin time (PTT), fibrinogen, fibrin split products and fibrin degradation products also may be performed. A **Kleihauer-Betke test** may be performed to denote evidence of fetal cells in the maternal circulation, which is significant for clients who are Rh negative. The nurse should be aware of the acute onset of abdominal or referred pain that may indicate a placental abruption co-existing with or instead of placenta previa.

Unit-based ultrasonography may allow confirmation of the placental abnormality and provide better information with which to plan care.

Nursing interventions include ongoing maternal-fetal assessment, establishment of IV access with a large-bore cannula in anticipation of transfusions, continuous monitoring of maternal vital signs, maternal pulse oximetry, oxygen supplied by face mask at 10 L/min, and insertion of an in-dwelling Foley catheter for strict intake and output measures. Assessment of bleeding can be obtained by weighing the hip pads before and after use and by counting the total number of saturated pads. As a rule, 1 g is equivalent to 1 mL. Positioning the client laterally to increase good circulatory return is useful. The nurse should perform these interventions while explaining the reasons for them and offering information about the procedures as they occur. The nurse may offer reassurance to the client and family by giving feedback about the fetus.

If the client stabilizes and stops bleeding, she may remain in the hospital or eventually return home on strict bed rest, with home health nursing support. Maintaining a client on bed rest for an extended period of time causes challenges for client mobility, strength, loss of control, coping mechanisms, and heightened anxiety. When the client with placenta previa is near term or continues to bleed, preparations for cesarean delivery and the associated communications, setup, and preparations are carried out while informing and involving the client and family as much as possible. The client with known placenta previa who has been bleeding chronically may actually be quite relieved with the aspect of impending delivery; the client with newly diagnosed placenta previa who has acute bleeding may be highly anxious and frightened. These differences should be assessed by the nurse to individualize client and family support. Finally, nursing considerations should include spiritual and grief support, as indicated, keeping in mind that uncontrolled acute hemorrhage may result in maternal or fetal illness, permanent injury, and even death.

Abruptio Placenta

Abruptio placenta is a condition in which the placenta separates prematurely from the uterine wall (Figure 26-10). Partial abruption involves a portion of the placenta and may be very small or nearly completely separate. In complete abruption, the entire placenta separates from the uterus. When complete placental separation occurs, fetal demise is certain and maternal morbidity is high. Hemorrhage is the chief characteristic of placental abruption. The bleeding may be frank, bright red, and associated with abdominal tenderness, as in a classic abruption. The abruption may be hidden beneath the placenta and concealed, without apparent vaginal bleeding. Pregnancies can con-

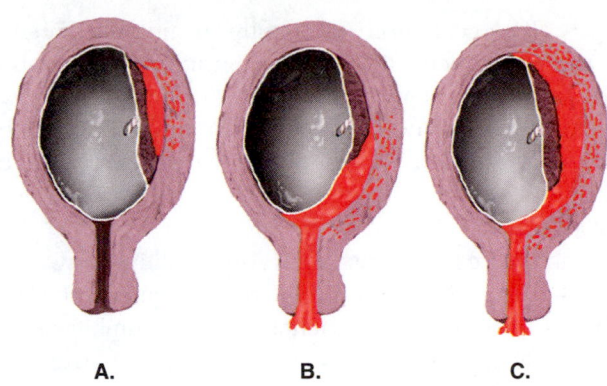

A.   **B.**   **C.**

Figure 26-10 Abruptio placenta A. Central abruption, concealed hemorrhage. B. Marginal abruption, external hemorrhage. C. Complete abruption, external hemorrhage (could also be concealed).

tinue with partial concealed abruptions that do not exceed 50% of the placental surface. When abruption of more than 50% of the placenta occurs, fetal perfusion usually is very severely compromised and the fetus will die in utero (Anath, Berkowitz, Savitz, & Lapinski, 1999). The incidence of abruption ranges from approximately 1 in 100 to 1 in 200 deliveries (Anath, Berkowitz, Savitz, & Lapinski, 1999; Cunningham et al., 1997). Abruption recurs in subsequent pregnancies up to 16% of the time (Schmidt, 1993). Misra and Ananth (1999) has reported that initial abruption rates average 1.7%, whereas rates in second pregnancies average 2.2%.

Factors that contribute to the development of abruption include advanced maternal age and advanced parity. Abruption also occurs more frequently in African American women than it does in Caucasion or Hispanic women. The most significant contributing factor, however, is maternal hypertension (Cunningham et al.,1997; Schmidt, 1993). There seems to be no difference in potential for abruption based on whether maternal hypertension is chronic and preexisting or acute, as in preeclampsia. Other risk factors for abruption include smoking, preterm premature rupture of membranes, external trauma from motor vehicle accidents, internal trauma from insertion of an IUPC, maternal cocaine use, uterine leiomyomas beneath placental implantation, and a short umbilical cord (Andres, 1996; Misra & Anath, 1999; Reis, Sander, & Pearlman, 2000; Handwerker & Selick, 1995; Cunningham et al., 1997; Schmidt, 1993). Maternal risks include shock, severe anemia related to hemorrhage, hypovolemia, risk for DIC, risk for embolism during the placental separation process, and death. Fetal risks include fetal growth impairment when the abruption is small and chronic; prematurity; severe hypoxic insults resulting in permanent neurologic damage; and intrauterine fetal demise (Anath, Berkowitz, Savitz, & Lapinski, 1999).

Medical management centers around the earliest possible identification of abruption, emergent cesarean delivery when the fetus is still alive, and maternal hemodynamic stabilization. When the abruption is minimal and maternal-fetal status is stable, an attempt at expectant management to allow fetal maturing may be considered cautiously, with emergent cesarean delivery an ever-present probability (Cunningham et al., 1997). Tocolysis may be provided to control uterine irritability and contractility that may increase the process of placental separation (Cunningham et al., 1997; Towers, Pircon, & Heppard, 1999). When the fetus is no longer alive in utero, vaginal delivery may be attempted with regard to maternal coagulopathy (DIC) that predisposes her to significant hemorrhage (Corbett & Fonteyn, 1995). Hypovolemia is treated with IV fluids and blood product replacement (cryoprecipitate, packed erythrocytes, and platelets), as indicated.

Nursing considerations in the care of the client experiencing an abruption depend on a thorough but efficient nursing assessment, keying in on risk factors that may signal this potential emergency. The nurse should also explore habits and events leading up to the point of maternal symptoms, such as abdominal trauma, cocaine use, or a history of heavy smoking. During the physical assessment the nurse should pay special attention to maternal vital signs, especially in the face of hypertension or shock indices (hypotension, tachycardia, and tachypnea); vaginal bleeding; and uterine tenderness, rigidity, or hypertonic response. Noting an increase in abdominal girth may alert the nurse that the client is bleeding into the uterine muscle, resulting in a Couvelaire uterine hematoma. Vaginal bleeding should be assessed with a hip pad count, with before and after weights of the pads being documented. Monitoring the fetal status is critical to establishing fetal well-being or identifying fetal distress as close as feasible to the onset of compromise. Particular attention should be paid to the presence of tachycardia, bradycardia, late decelerations, sinusoidal pattern, and loss of variability. IV access with a large-bore catheter is essential for delivery of lactated Ringer's solution and blood products. Necessary laboratory tests include a CBC, a platelet count, clotting studies, typing, crossmatching, baseline electrolyte and chemistry studies, and liver and renal functions studies. An in-dwelling Foley catheter should be inserted, with strict measurement of intake and output. Pulse oximetry monitoring should be used, if available, and supplemental oxygen delivered by face mask. When the maternal hemodynamic status is not stable or oliguria is not corrected with administered fluids and blood products, the client may require hemodynamic monitoring with a central venous line or pulmonary catheter. The mode of delivery depends on maternal-fetal status and maternal clotting status. If the fetus is alive, the nurse may anticipate an emergent cesarean. If the fetus is not alive, a vaginal delivery may be in order, with oxytocin stimulation required. When oxytocin is ordered, careful titration must be observed to prevent further uterine trauma (Cunningham et al., 1997). In the midst of rapid medical and nursing interventions employed to stabilize the client and her fetus, the nurse must also provide the vital information necessary to quickly educate and reassure the client and her family. In the event of fetal demise, grief and spiritual support also must be considered. This aspect of care is particularly challenging because the family may have numerous unanswered questions as they try to cope with overwhelming grief related to the loss of their baby and uncertainty regarding maternal survival.

Other Placental Anomalies

Other placental abnormalities may contribute to poor fetal outcome, because maternal hemorrhage may go undetected until it is discovered at or after delivery. These abnormalities may be developmental or the result of superimposed trauma, such as from hypertensive episodes. Hypertension, either chronic or pregnancy-induced, may cause placental injuries called *infarcts*. These areas of tissue injury are no longer able to facilitate placental circulation. When these areas of damaged placental tissue are large or numerous, perfusion to the fetus may be compromised. Fetal growth may be affected over an extended period of time. Fetal heart tracings on the monitor may be nonreassuring, particularly during the stress of labor. Such fetal intolerance may result in fetal distress and necessitate cesarean section.

UMBILICAL CORD ANOMALIES

Developmental errors may occur as the umbilical cord joins into the placenta. **Velamentous insertion of the cord** refers to the junction of the cord at the edge of the placenta. The vessels separate into the membranes before reaching the insertion site. This abnormality can result in chronic altered fetal perfusion. More significantly, this abnormality can undergo trauma and compression during labor and delivery, resulting in rupture and hemorrhage. **Vasa previa** involves the cord vessels crossing the cervical os and results in significant compression and possible rupture from the pressure of the fetal head during descent. Fetal compromise may include hypoxic injury, hemorrhage, hypovolemia, and death. Before the ability to diagnose vasa previa in the antepartum period, the mortality rate was 33% to 100% (Oyelese et al., 1998). Both velamentous insertion and vasa previa tend to accompany other placental abnormalities, such as placenta previa and bilobed or irregularly developed placentas. These abnormalities also occur more frequently in multiple pregnancies and pregnancies that result from in vitro fertilization. With the advent of more detailed ultrasonography, vasa previa and cord abnormalities may now be detected before labor, allowing for an alternative form of delivery in highly suspicious cases (Oyelese et al., 1998; Lee et al., 2000).

Umbilical cord events and abnormalities may occur that result in a high-risk pregnancy or emergent status. Problems may be developmental, as in an umbilical cord having only two vessels instead of three. The absence of one of the umbilical cord arteries occurs in 0.72% to 0.85% of delivered infants, and it occurs more frequently in Caucasian women and even more frequently in women who have diabetes (Cunningham et al., 1997). Labor and delivery may proceed without any indication of problems until the neonate's cord stump is assessed at delivery and found to have only two vessels. Antenatally, sonography currently can screen for the presence of a three-vessel cord at the anatomic scan performed during the second trimester. Although this abnormality is not a problem during labor and delivery, neonates with only two vessels in the cord have been found to have a higher incidence of multisystem abnormalities (spinal, gastrointestinal, renal, and cardiac). Other cord problems may become evident during labor, such as cord length. Whereas *Williams Obstetrics* (Cunningham et al., 1997) identifies the average cord length as 55 cm, the variances range from 0 to 300 cm. Higher risks of rupture, abruption, and inversion of the uterus are associated with a short umbilical cord. An exceptionally long umbilical cord may result in fetal entanglement, with an intrauterine fetal demise being the result. **Umbilical cord compression** involves pressure applied to the umbilical cord. Compression can occur as the presenting part presses against the cord on descent or from entanglement or looping around a body part, such as the neck or shoulder, or from the existence of a true knot. Fetal perfusion is interrupted as cord compression increases or persists. Cord compression has been associated with nonreassuring fetal tracings, low Apgar scores, meconium-stained fluid, emergent cesarean section or operative vaginal delivery, neonatal resuscitation, and admission to the neonatal intensive care unit (Jauniaux, Ramsay, Peellaerts, & Scholler, 1995; Larson, Rayburn, Crosby, & Thurnau, 1995). Longer cords also may incur a true knot (occurring in 1.1% of cords) or prolapse during labor once the membranes rupture. **Umbilical cord prolapse** occurs when the cord precedes the presenting part into the birth canal (Figure 26-11). Fetal position, multiple fetuses, artificial rupture of the membranes, and fetal activity may contribute to the likelihood of a prolapsed cord. Maternal risks include hemorrhage, uterine inversion accompanied by profound shock, and trauma from emergent interventions. Fetal risks include decreased or obliterated perfu-

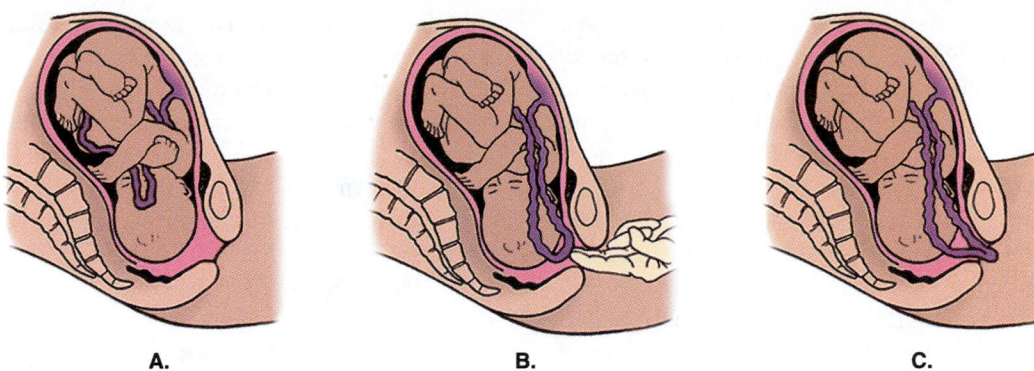

Figure 26-11 Prolapsed cord. A. Occult (hidden, cannot be seen or felt). B. Complete (cannot be seen but may be felt). C. Visible (can be seen protruding from vagina).

sion, hypoxic injury, and death. The incidence of umbilical cord prolapse has been reported to be as frequent as 1 in 426 births or 0.4% to 0.5% (Murphy & MacKenzie, 1995; Cunningham et al., 1997). The prolapse may be either frank, with obvious fetal response and the umbilical cord found in the vagina or protruding from the introitus vaginae, or the prolapse may be occult, compressed between the presenting part and the cervix and not discovered until the time of delivery. Time is essential once a prolapse is suspected or confirmed. Delays in intervention for a prolapsed cord can result in fetal injury or death. Prabulos and Philipson (1998) reported that in a review of 26,545 cases of cord prolapse, a significant percentage of negative fetal outcomes still occurred despite diagnosis-to-delivery times averaging 11 minutes, 9 minutes less than the average vaginal delivery time of 20 minutes from diagnosis of cord prolapse to delivery of the baby. This study emphasized the need to deliver emergently once a diagnosis of prolapse has been made and also raised questions about the possibility of other variables contributing to negative neonatal outcomes.

Medical management of cord compression and prolapse involves early recognition, intervention, and delivery to avoid fetal compromise or death. Medical management of prolapse is an obstetric emergency. Umbilical cord compression can be managed conservatively as long as the fetal tracing is reassuring. When fetal intolerance becomes evident, alternative medical management may become necessary, including emergent cesarean section.

Nursing considerations focus on assessment of risk factors and evidence to support concerns about fetal perfusion. Most significant will be the fetal response recorded on the monitor tracing. Cord compression may be accompanied by variable decelerations that become deeper, wider, or return slowly to the baseline. Loss of variability or increasing baseline may signify loss of fetal reserve and indicate fetal compromise. In a frank cord prolapse, an acute and sustained bradycardia, decreasing fetal baseline,

or prolonged deceleration may be observed on the tracing. The pelvic examination also may assist the nurse to identify risk factors. When the presenting part is not well applied to the cervix or when a malposition or malpresentation (e.g., in breech and transverse lie presentations) is present, the client is at high risk for prolapse of the umbilical cord. Cord compression may be more apparent in the client with oligohydramnios, a condition in which the amniotic fluid volume equals 5 cm or less of the estimated total volume at or near term. A client with ruptured membranes also may experience more frequent compression because limited fluid is available to prevent pressure on the cord in utero. When the nurse suspects a prolapse, a pelvic examination should be performed. When the umbilical cord is palpated, the nurse can attempt to gently lift the presenting part away from it, thus permitting cord perfusion to resume. Once this is done, the examiner should not remove the examining hand. Fetal monitoring should continue, and the client either may be positioned with her head slightly downward or assume a modified knee-chest position to further remove the presenting part off of the cord. The nurse should call for assistance while remaining with the client. It is important to explain to the client what is happening and why the interventions are being performed. Supplemental oxygen with a face mask should be added to enhance placental fetal perfusion. Frank cord prolapse is an emergent condition. An emergent cesarean section is needed to deliver the fetus before significant circulation is interrupted and fetal hypoxia and acidosis occur.

Vaginal deliveries sometimes occur when the prolapse is occult, or hidden. In these cases, deep, broad variables may be observed on the fetal tracing. Maternal position changes and supplemental oxygenation with a face mask may provide some relief of the cord compression and enhance circulating oxygen until delivery occurs. If the fetal tracing becomes nonreassuring or demonstrates loss of fetal well-being, the physician may choose to perform operative vaginal delivery with low outlet forceps or vacuum suction if delivery is imminent. A cesarean section may be necessary if labor is early. Having supplies available for these options is a part of the anticipatory preparations the nurse can make once the fetal monitor tracing becomes suspicious for problems.

The nurse providing care for the client experiencing cord compression may employ similar interventions, with maternal position changes from side to side or even a modified knee-chest position. The client may benefit from oxygen supplementation by face mask. The nurse may be asked to start and maintain an amnioinfusion to instill fluid within the uterus to replace the cushioning effect of amniotic fluid and relieve cord compression. The nurse should carefully monitor labor progression. When labor is progressing rapidly, the fetus may better tolerate the effects of cord compression. When cord compression is significant in early labor or during a sluggish labor, the fetal tracing may become nonreassuring before vaginal delivery is feasible. It is particularly important that the nurse complete preparations for delivery, including notifying the nursery personnel and having resuscitation supplies available in the event the fetus has respiratory depression from chronic cord compression. Emotional support and educational information are helpful to reduce or alleviate patient anxiety that accompanies high-risk situations.

AMNIOTIC FLUID ABNORMALITIES

Problems with amniotic fluid also can make a pregnancy and delivery high risk. Amniotic fluid amounts that deviate from normal can result in complications for the client and her developing fetus. Abnormal amounts of amniotic fluid are referred to as polyhydramnios (or hydramnios) and oligohydramnios. Amniotic fluid embolism is a critical event with an unclear cause. These three amniotic fluid aberrations can result in significant maternal and fetal complications.

Polyhydramnios

Polyhydramnios refers to an increased amount of amniotic fluid within the uterus. An amount of 2 L at term is considered to be polyhydramnios (Cunningham et al., 1997). This measurement is often based on clinical assessment of uterine size and perceived amount of fluid using Leopold's maneuvers. Another way of measuring polyhydramnios is to calculate the amniotic fluid index, which measures a pocket of amniotic fluid in each of the four quadrants using sonography. If the sum of the measures in the four quadrants exceeds 24 cm, the client is diagnosed

with polyhydramnios. The advent of routine sonography has offered a more objective way to evaluate amniotic fluid volume. The reported incidence of occurrence is approximately 0.9%, with most cases identified as mild hydramnios (Cunningham et al., 1997).

The occurrence of polyhydramnios has been associated with maternal diabetes; multiple gestations; and maternal isoimmunization, with resultant fetal hydrops (Kellogg, 1993). Polyhydramnios is also found in the fetus with neural tube malformations such as spina bifida or anencephaly, with increased fluid loss through meningeal membranes, gastrointestinal problems that interfere with the normal swallowing and absorption of amniotic fluid (Cunningham et al., 1997). Maternal effects of polydramnios include general discomfort from overexpansion of the uterus, respiratory compromise, uterine irritability from overdistention, premature labor, and uterine rupture. Fetal risks include premature delivery, cord prolapse, malpresentation, macrosomia, and cesarean delivery (Kellogg, 1993; Panting-Kemp et al., 1999). A 1998 study that evaluated the incidence of complications and hydramnios found a higher number of antepartum and postpartum deaths, abruptio placentea, fetal distress, meconium-stained fluid, low Apgar scores, and chorioamnionitis, as well as the problems listed previously (Maymon et al., 1998). An earlier study had concluded similar findings in hydramnios when the condition was persistent throughout the second and third trimesters. When hydramnios resolved in the third trimester, the incidence of negative outcomes decreased significantly (Golan et al., 1994b).

Medical management of the client with polydramnios is related both to an identified cause and symptomatic complaints. When hydramnios is severe, amniocentesis to remove fluid is performed. The procedure is carried out with ultrasound guidance, and the amount of fluid is measured and recorded. Otherwise, medical management addresses the client and fetus at the time of labor (i.e., prematurity, maternal diabetes, fetal anomalies, and so on).

Nursing considerations also depend on the contributing causes and maternal symptoms. For instance, when the client is admitted in preterm labor, the nursing care focuses on tocolysis, fetal and maternal monitoring, and prevention of therapy side effects. In addition to the cause of hydramnios, if known, client comfort is a particularly important nursing issue. Maternal comfort in late pregnancy is always challenging, and the addition of more amniotic fluid that causes further uterine distention and dyspnea is even more so. Elevation of the head of bed, pulse oximetry, and humidified oxygen supplementation by nasal cannula may be beneficial in late antepartal care. Oxygen by face mask is still preferred in labor. Fetal monitoring may be difficult related to the additional uterine expansion and bulk. Leopold's maneuvers also may be more difficult because of the taut abdominal skin and the large volume of fluid to try and "feel through." Once delivery is inevitable, the neonatal team should be notified of the premature labor and anticipated fetal anomalies. The client experiencing hydramnios has the additional challenges of coping with increased physical discomforts; causative factors, such as diabetes; and the overriding concern for the well-being of the infant. The chronicity of the condition may be extremely fatiguing and become comparable to the client on extended bed rest for multiple gestation or preterm labor. Diligent client education, emotional support, and encouragement are nursing interventions that may assist the client to better cope with her situation.

Oligohydramnios

Oligohydramnios refers to the amniotic fluid being significantly less than expected for pregnancy. The volume measurement is 500 mL or less between 32 and 36 weeks' gestation, or an amniotic fluid index of 5 cm or less (Kellogg, 1993; Cunningham et al., 1993). Sonography has allowed early identification of oligohydramnios along with follow-up surveillance of the client with persistent oligohydramnios. Oligohydramnios identified early in the pregnancy has a more negative prognosis relative to the cause and chronicity of the condition (Cunningham et al., 1997). The incidence varies with the associated cause; however, a 1994 study found a rate of 0.58% in a review of 25,000 obstetric clients (Golan, 1994b). A more recent study of 6,423 pregnancies found an occurrence rate of 2.3% (Casey et al., 2000).

Contributing causes toward the development of oligohydramnios include fetal anomalies, especially of the renal system. Fetal anomalies were attributed as being the cause in over 50% of cases of oligohydramnios in the second trimester of pregnancy and almost 25% of cases in the third trimester (Shipp et al., 1996). Fetal renal agenesis (known as Potter's syndrome), or the failure of the fetal kidneys to develop, is associated with severe chronic oligohydramnios. The renal agenesis is accompanied by pulmonary hypoplasia. The fetal renal and pulmonary systems are significant in maintaining and rebuilding amniotic fluid volumes (Cunningham et al., 1997). Without their existence or development, the fetus is compressed within the uterus. Renal agenesis is an anomalous condition that is incompatible with life outside the uterus. Other fetal problems that contribute to oligohydramnios include renal system obstruction and polycystic kidneys. Maternal factors that contribute to oligohydramnios are hypertension; leaking or premature rupture of membranes; and most frequently, gestations that continue beyond 41 weeks (Cunningham et al., 1997).

Perinatal outcomes reported in a study examining the various complications included increased rate and need for labor induction, increased stillbirths, nonreassuring fetal heart rate tracings, neonatal intensive care unit admissions, meconium aspiration, and neonatal death (Casey et al., 2000). Cesarean section and an Apgar score of less than 7 at 5 minutes were found more frequently in clients with oligohydramnios (Chauhan et al., 1999). Increased rates of maternal hypertension, second trimester bleeding, fetal intrauterine growth retardation, fetal skeletal and renal system anomalies, and perinatal mortality were reported in a 1994 study (Golan et al., 1994a). Even borderline amniotic fluid levels ranging between 5 and 10 cm on the amniotic fluid index have been associated with increased intrauterine growth problems and perinatal complications (Banks & Miller, 1999). *Idiopathic* (meaning unknown cause) oligohydramnios without associated fetal growth problems as followed on surveillance sonography did not demonstrate a higher incidence of fetal complications other than premature delivery in a 1997 study reported by Garmel et al. (1997).

Medical management of the client with oligohydramnios includes early diagnosis with anatomy surveillance for anomalies. When maternal conditions such as hypertension and postdate gestation are contributory, evaluation for delivery must be considered. Use of the biophysical profile may augment the practitioner's plan of care by providing feedback on fetal well-being. When oligohydramnios results from premature leaking or rupture of membranes, medical care may be expectant. That is, maternal-fetal status is monitored for stability and infection while the opportunity is provided for amniotic fluid to accumulate. When signs of infection are apparent, delivery plans replace expectant management to minimize the risk of sepsis. When oligohydramnios is severe or associated with fetal anomalies, the client and family must be informed and prepared for the likely outcomes.

Nursing considerations in the care of the client with oligohydramnios are determined by assessment data related to the cause of the oligohydramnios and the medical plan of care. When expectant management is the plan, nursing considerations include thorough maternal-fetal assessment, with the fetal tracing providing critical information on fetal status. Monitoring for signs of infection in the event the membranes are leaking or ruptured also is a nursing concern. The client with hypertension may be on strict bed rest and required to undergo repeated surveillance sonograms and nonstress tests. Anticipatory grief support may be the most important support offered to the client with a fetus that has significant anomalies. When delivery is planned, the nurse can anticipate orders for an amnioinfusion to relieve cord and fetal compression and thus reduce overall stress during labor. Ongoing fetal monitoring may reveal deep variables and prolonged decelerations related to severe umbilical cord compression. Maternal position changes may be futile relative to the uterine compression of the fetus in severe cases of oligohydramnios

Critical Thinking

Cardiopulmonary Resuscitation in Labor and Delivery

- Are you currently credentialed in cardiopulmonary resuscitation?
- Have you recently reviewed the unit policies?
- Do you know where your cart or supplies are?
- Remember the ABCs? They are the same.

Airway: How do you insert an oral airway? Can you obtain a seal and secure a chin lift position?
Breathing: How do you use a self-inflating resuscitation bag? How many ventilations should be done?
Circulation: What are the landmarks to be assessed to ensure proper hand placement on the patient's chest wall? What is the proper position for a pregnant patient receiving CPR? How many compressions should be done each minute for an adult?

but should be attempted to achieve optimal fetal response. Supplemental oxygenation may benefit fetal perfusion and can be administered by face mask. IV hydration should be maintained to avoid perfusion complications that increase fetal stress. As in all high-risk delivery settings, the neonatal team should be ready in the event neonatal resuscitation is required.

Promoting parental grief and acceptance of their loss in the event the fetus or neonate does not survive is a critical nursing concern. The nurse should assess the parental needs and readiness for grieving and provide adequate time for the parents to see, hold, and bond with their infant with privacy, respect, and any requested spiritual support. Many facilities have protocols for perinatal loss support that include photographs, time together, burial layettes, and memory books with a lock of hair and handprints and footprints of their baby. Recognizing that all persons grieve differently should provide insight into how to implement and observe such a protocol without offending or upsetting the mother and family if they are not ready or are unable to participate in such a personal farewell. In some cases, the memorabilia is collected and saved in a labeled envelope in case the parents desire it at a later time.

Amniotic Fluid Embolism

Amniotic fluid embolism is a very rare but life-threatening condition. Amniotic fluid embolism involves the presence of an embolus composed of amniotic fluid along with

particulate matter (such as vernix caseosa, lanugo, meconium, and other fetal cells) that enters the maternal circulation and causes acute respiratory distress, cardiovascular collapse, severe coagulopathy, shock, and death (Austin, 1993). The reported occurrence is 1 in 65,000 deliveries, and the maternal mortality rate is up to 80%. A 1995 review of national registry records reported a maternal mortality rate of 61% (Clark et al., 1995). A more recent study in 1999 reviewed approximately 1.1 million deliveries and identified an incidence of 1 per 20,646 deliveries and an associated maternal mortality rate of 26.4% (Gilbert & Danielsen, 1999). Half of all maternal survivors of amniotic fluid embolism have significant neurologic sequelae (Locksmith, 1999). The embolic event occurs during or immediately after delivery when the placenta separates from the uterine wall and maternal veins are open for transport of the embolus. Intrauterine pressures are favorable for transport of the embolus, especially when there is aggressive uterine stimulation; tumultuous, hypertonic labor; or placental abruption. Amniotic fluid embolism is more common when the labor has been precipitous or strong; when premature placental separation makes maternal access available sooner; and when more particulate matter, such as meconium, is available to compose the embolus (Cunningham et al., 1997). Studies repeatedly have reported classic responses of maternal respiratory distress, cardiovascular collapse, shock, and coagulopathy; however, the similarities between amniotic fluid embolism and anaphylaxis or septic shock are identified as possible potentiators that increase the mortality rate (Clark et al., 1995; Locksmith, 1999; Weiwen, Ningyu, Lanxiang, & Yu, 2000).

Clinical presentation of an amniotic fluid embolism is abrupt and spontaneous and includes complaints of respiratory difficulty and pain, cyanosis, and chest pain, with rapid onset of shock and cardiovascular collapse (Weiwen, Ningyu, Lanxiang, & Yu, 2000). In the previously cited study, the time of onset of symptoms to the time of death was reviewed. Thirty-nine percent of mothers died within one hour of onset of symptoms, and one-third died within the first 30 minutes. Women who survive are at significant risk of neurologic impairment from severe hypoxemia. If delivery has not been completed, the fetus is at the same risk of hypoxemia and subsequent damage or death.

Medical management depends on recognition of the clinical symptoms and is supportive in nature because there is no known curative protocol (Locksmith, 1999). Rapid intervention involves immediate and aggressive resuscitation to maintain oxygenation; volume replacement; monitoring of cardiac output and vital signs; and transfusions of cryoprecipitate, fresh frozen plasma, and packed erythrocytes and platelets to control the coagulopathy (Cunningham et al., 1997). When delivery has not occurred, it must be performed surgically and immediately if the fetus is to survive.

Nursing considerations include astute assessment of maternal-fetal status throughout the third and fourth stages of delivery. Attention should be focused on vital sign stability and any maternal complaints of shortness of breath, chest pain, heightened anxiety, and sensation of impending doom. Other assessment data include listening to breath sounds, observing for increased bleeding from the perineum or incision, and monitoring the level of maternal consciousness. The nurse should never leave an unstable or deteriorating patient. Calling for assistance and emergency supplies such as the crash cart should be done immediately on identification of maternal problems. The first interventions are based on the classic ABCs of resuscitation: **a**irway, **b**reathing, and **c**irculation. Maintaining or reestablishing an airway is first and foremost, and may be as simple as initially applying an oxygen face mask at a rate of 10 L/min. However, maintaining the client's airway may progress rapidly from oxygen supplementation to manual ventilation with a self-inflating resuscitation bag, and finally to assisting with intubation and support by ventilator. Circulation and perfusion are maintained with IV fluids, chest compressions if cardiac arrest occurs, and assisting with defibrillation as necessary. Multiple pressor drugs may be ordered to help maintain blood pressure and promote adequate perfusion. Continuous monitoring of maternal vital signs is critical. Pulse oximetry should be used until a pulmonary catheter and an adjunctive arterial line are put in place for accurate cardiac output assessment and monitoring of blood gases. The nurse can anticipate orders for various laboratory tests, including CBC, platelet count, typing, crossmatching, a clotting panel (PT, PTT, fibrinogen, fibrinogen split products, and fibrin degradation products), and chemistry panels to assess electrolyte stability and renal function. An indwelling Foley should be inserted, with strict intake and output monitored hourly. Receiving and following through with orders for the various blood products and strict compliance with administration procedures also are nursing responsibilities. Monitoring ongoing blood loss and recording of amounts are important factors is estimating replacement needs.

REFLECTIONS FROM A NURSE

"Labor and delivery was my passion! I had just attained a level of clinical comfort as an experienced labor and delivery nurse. I had participated in numerous high-risk deliveries, started IVs in almost nonexistent veins, protected seizing patients from self-injury, managed Pitocin and magnesium sulfate, transfused blood, and raced my patients to the OR like lightning in an emergent situation. I prided myself on bonding with the clients, their families, and even their newborns.

Then entered our newest admission. Kate was 31 and in labor with her first child. She and her husband, Scott, were so excited about their baby. They worked together in labor, and her labor was tough. Strong contractions were exhausting but she coped well with minimal pharmacologic intervention. She pushed hard to deliver a strong, loud, healthy boy weighing in at 9 pounds. They were oblivious to the repair as it was in progress. Within 10 minutes of the placental delivery, she began complaining of chest pain and acting so anxious. Her color paled and she became diaphoretic. We had to initiate resuscitation in another few minutes. Minutes felt like hours. The ABCs of CPR rang in my ears. The response of everyone was admirable and quick, but futile. Later as I would clean and prepare Kate for her return to her horrified husband, I reviewed the process and wondered what else could have been done. I hugged him, cried with him, and told him how sorry I was.

Still later as I reviewed my chart and followed the process for closing a chart that would undergo immediate risk review, I tried to retrace the events to explore one more time what could have been done. Nothing. How humbling that thought. We are but human. We did all that could be done. Alone, on my way home, I cried for us all; Kate, Scott, their newborn son, my colleagues, and myself."

The resuscitative process can be overwhelming to the health care team. The process certainly will be a terrifying experience for the family and support persons who witness a cardiovascular arrest, significant hemorrhage, and the incredibly aggressive response. Because such events are unexpected, the scene can appear chaotic as supplies and team members are rapidly assembled and participate in the resuscitative efforts. Quick explanations about the situation to the family and support persons should be provided. They may be asked to move to an area in the room where they can remain close or to wait outside the room. Available space in the room or hospital policies may determine where the family and support persons will be asked to stay. Whenever possible, a social worker or spiritual counselor should remain with the family to provide support while resuscitative efforts continue. If the client is stabilized and placed on ventilatory support, the family should be allowed to see her before she is transferred to the intensive care unit. If the client does not survive, the family should receive grief support and be allowed to spend time saying farewell. If the fetus does not survive, the family's grief will be further increased. If the neonate survives, support will be needed to enable a healthy adaptation with the surviving family.

Most of the time, obstetrics is a happy nursing specialty area. In the event of maternal or fetal death, the health care team must deal with their own personal feelings of loss and possibly failure. It may be helpful for a grief or spiritual counselor to meet with the team that was involved to assist them with coping, both personally and professionally. Review of all resuscitations can be expected as a part of risk management and quality improvement requirements. Careful review of the chart documentation, including entering of any late entries, should also be done after a resuscitation.

Web Activities

- Visit ACOG's and AWHONN's websites. Do they include information specific to some of the dysfunctional labor patterns discussed in this chapter? Compare information regarding the nurse's role v. the physician's role.

- Search the internet for information for parents of multiples. Are there chat rooms? Support groups? Toll-free numbers? Resource materials, such as books and videos?

Key Concepts

- Dysfunctional labor patterns include hypertonic, hypotonic, and precipitate labor patterns. Oxytocin may be used to regulate and normalize a dysfunctional labor pattern.

- Malpositions include occipitotransverse and occipitoposterior. Malpresentations include breech, acromion, face, brow, and transverse presentations. Persistent malpositions and malpresentations place mother and fetus at risk for cesarean section or operative vaginal delivery.

- Fetal distress indicates fetal intolerance to the intrauterine environment, labor, or both. When left untreated, the fetus can experience hypoxic injury, acidosis, and death. Nursing interventions focus on increasing fetal oxygenation and perfusion.

- Uterine rupture is more likely to occur in a scarred uterus and may result in fetal death and maternal shock and hemorrhage. Uterine hyperstimulation may contribute to rupture.

- Placenta previa and abruptio placentae are hemorrhagic conditions of pregnancy. Placenta previa frequently presents as silent, nonpainful bleeding that may initially occur in the second and third trimesters. Abruptio placentae is more frequently acute and associated with abdominal pain. Complete placenta previa necessitates cesarean section, as does acute abruption. Abruption of over 50% is incompatible with fetal survival. Two consequences of abruption include DIC and a higher risk of amniotic fluid embolism.

- Prolapsed umbilical cord is an obstetric emergency. When unrelieved, the cord compression may result in fetal death.

- Abruption, uterine rupture, and amniotic fluid embolism predispose the obstetric client to DIC.

- Oligohydramnios refers to less than normal amniotic fluid volume in the second and third trimesters. Fetal cord compression, intolerance to labor, and negative fetal outcomes are increased in clients with oligohydramnios. This abnormality is frequently found in pregnancies with fetal anomalies. Maternal factors include hypertension and postdatism.

- Polyhydramnios refers to a greater than normal amniotic fluid volume and can result in maternal respiratory compromise, fetal malpresentation, and cord prolapse. Polyhydramnios is frequently found in pregnancies with maternal diabetes, multiple gestation, and isoimmunization.

❦ Amniotic fluid embolism is a rare event with a high maternal mortality rate as a result of obstetric shock from cardiopulmonary collapse and hemorrhagic coagulopathy. The physiologic response is comparable to anaphylactic and septic shock.

Review Questions and Activities

1. Ms. J. is an obstetric patient who is in observation status in labor and delivery. Her contractions are occurring irregularly every 2 to 10 minutes. She states that she has had contractions like these for 9 hours. She is afebrile, and her vital signs are stable: pulse, 90; respirations, 18, and blood pressure, 114/72. The fetal heart rate is in the 140s, the baseline tracing demonstrates several accelerations, and no decelerations are noted. What other assessment information should you gather to assist in formulating diagnoses and a plan of care for Ms. J?

2. Ms. P. is a 32-year-old gravida, para 2002. She arrives in labor and delivery breathing, panting, and holding her abdomen near the suprapubic region. She tells you her membranes ruptured 10 minutes ago and that she now feels the urge to push. As you take her to a bed, you continue to gather additional information and discover she had her last baby en route to the hospital after a 30-minute labor. Without a pelvic examination performed, what action might you take?

3. Ms. R. is a gravida 2, para 1001. She has been completely dilated and at +1 station for 2 hours. She had an epidural and was unable to push well with contractions. She has begun to feel the pressure sensation and believes she can push better now. The fetal heart rate is in the 130s with long-term variability present, no decelerations noted, and an occasional acceleration observed. Ms. R.'s vital signs are stable. What interventions might you try to enhance her pushing efforts? What signs might you observe that may indicate a problem with fetal descent?

4. Ms. B. is a gravida 3, para 1011. She is 36 5/7 estimated gestational age with a twin gestation and presents with contractions that are 3 minutes apart, lasting 45 seconds, and moderate to firm in intensity. The twins' heart rates are identified at the right lower quadrant and left upper quadrant and range in the 130s and 150s, respectively. Discuss the assessment information you require for a safe labor and delivery process for this client. What factors may affect her mode of delivery and outcomes?

5. Ms. K. is a gravida 2, para 1001, and is attempting a trial of labor after having a cesarean section. Her

original cesarean was 4 years ago for arrested descent. She complains of intense burning pain over the parapubic region. What other assessment parameters must you evaluate to identify a uterine rupture? What preparations have you already completed knowing this client has had a previous cesarean section and is undergoing trial of labor?

6. Ms. T. arrives in the labor and delivery unit by stretcher from an ambulance. Her vital signs follow: pulse, 120; respirations, 24 and shallow; blood pressure, 84/50 and faint. She complains of acute abdominal pain that began abruptly 1.5 hours ago. She has a very scant amount of bright red bleeding. Fetal heart tones are auscultated in the 90s. What do you suspect has occurred? Formulate a priority-based plan to ensure the best outcome for Ms. T. and her fetus.

7. As you begin your shift you receive a report on Ms. A. She is a gravida 4, para 0030, at 37 2/7 estimated gestational age, with a history of late pregnancy losses for unknown reasons. She is currently in a low Fowler's position, on continuous fetal monitoring, and having contractions of moderate intensity that are 4 minutes apart and last for 45 seconds. While you review her fetal monitor tracing, you note that the baseline is in the 120s. You do not note any accelerations and, in fact, notice late decelerations occurring after each contraction for the last 15 minutes. Identify interventions to attempt to alleviate this nonreassuring pattern. Are there other tests to reinforce your concerns or establish a sense of well-being in the client?

8. Ms. F. presents to labor and delivery in active labor. Examination finds that she is 4 cm dilated, has 80% effacement with bulging membranes, and the presenting part is at −3 station. Fetal heart tones are reactive in the 130s to 140s, with accelerations present. As you enter laboratory requisitions at the desk, you note on the central monitor that the fetal heart rate is now in the 90s. You return to find Ms. F. saying she just was going to call you because her membranes have ruptured. What are your next actions in a prioritized order?

9. Ms. Y. is a 26-year-old gravida 3, para 3003, who just delivered 15 minutes ago. You are assessing her vital signs and talking with her about her baby while the physician repairs her perineal laceration when she suddenly looks worried and tells you she cannot breathe well. You note that she has become pale and clammy in this few moments. Her vital signs are reflecting changes with a pulse that is increasing and at 106, a blood pressure that is decreasing and at 88/56, and respirations that are shallow and rapid at 28. She is gasping and looks panicky. What do you suspect is occurring? Discuss the prioritized interventions and complications that may arise secondary to her immediate diagnosis.

References

Abitbol, M., Bowen-Ericksen, M., Castillo, I., & Pushchin, A. (1999). Prediction of difficult vaginal birth and of cesarean section for cephalopelvic disproportion in early labor. *Journal of Maternal Fetal Medicine, 8,* (2), 51–56.

Acien, P. (1995) Beech presentation in Spain, 1992: A collaborative study. *European Journal of Obstetrics, Gynecology and Reproductive Biology, 62,* (1), 19–24.

Aisenbrey, G., Catanzarite, V., Hurley, T. Spiegel, J., Schrimmer, D., & Mendoza, A. (1995). Monoamniotic and pseudomonoamniotic twins: Sonographic diagnosis, detection of cord entanglement, and obstetric management. *Obstetrics and Gynecology, 86,* (2), 218–222.

Albrechtsen, S., Rasmussen, S., Dalaker, K., & Irgens, L. (1998). The occurrence of breech presentation in Norway 1967–1994. *Acta Obstetrics and Gynecology Scandinavia, 77,* (4), 410–415.

Al Sakka, M., Dauleh, W., & Al Hassani, S. (1999). Case series of uterine rupture and subsequent pregnancy outcome. *International Journal of Fertility and Women's Medicine, 44,* (6), 297–300.

Anath, C., Berkowitz, G., Savitz, D., & Lapinski, R. (1999). Placental abruption and adverse perinatal outcomes. *Journal of the American Medical Association, 282,* (17), 1646–1651.

Andres, R. (1996). The association of cigarette smoking with placenta previa and abruptio placenta. *Seminars in Perinatology, 20,* (2), 154–159.

Austin, D. (1993). Labor and delivery at risk. In S. Mattson & J. Smith (Eds.), (Chapt. 34). *NAACOG: Core curriculum for maternal newborn nursing.* Philadelphia, PA: W.B. Saunders.

Banks, E., & Miller, D. (1999). Perinatal risks associated with borderline amniotic fluid index. *American Journal of Obstetrics and Gynecology, 180,* (6), Part 1, 1461–1463.

Bashore, R. (1992). Dystocia. In N. Hacker & J. Moore, (Eds.), (Chapt. 23). *Essentials of obstetrics and gynecology,* 2nd ed. Philadelphia, PA: W.B. Saunders.

Bofill, J., Vincent, R., Ross, E., Martin, R., Norman, P., Werhan, C., & Morrison, J. (1997). Nulliparous active labor, epidural analgesia and cesarean delivery for dystocia. *American Journal of Obstetrics and Gynecology, 177,* (6), 1465–1470.

Bowers, N. (1998). The multiple birth explosion: Implications for nursing practice. *Journal of Obstetric, Gynecologic and Neonatal Nursing, 27,* (3), 302–310.

Casey, B., McIntire, D., Bloom, S., Lucas, M., Santos, R., Twickler, D., Ramus, R., & Leveno, K. (2000). Pregnancy outcomes after antepartum diagnosis of oligohydramnios at or beyond 34 weeks' gestation. *American Journal of Obstetrics and Gynecology, 182,* (4), 909–912.

Caughey, A., Shipp, T., Repke, J., Zelop, C., Cohen, A., & Lieberman, E. (1999). Rate of uterine rupture during a trial of labor in women with one or two prior cesarean deliveries. *American Journal of Obstetrics and Gynecology, 181,* (4), 872–876.

Chauhan, S., Sanderson, M., Hendrix, N., Magann, E., & Devoe, L. (1999). Perinatal outcome and amniotic fluid index in the antepartum and intrapartum periods: A meta-analysis. *American Journal of Obstetrics and Gynecology, 181,* (6), 1473–1478.

Chen, L., Tan, K., & Yeo, G. (1995). A ten year review of uterine rupture in modern obstetric practice. *Annals Academy of Medicine in Singapore, 24,* (6), 830–835.

Clark, A., Carr, D., Loyd, G., Cook, V., & Spinnato, J. (1998). The influence of epidural analgesia on cesarean delivery rates: A randomized, prospective clinical trial. *American Journal of Obstetrics and Gynecology, 179,* (6), Part 1, 1527–1533.

Clark, S., Hankins, G., Dudley, D., Dildy, G., & Porter, T. (1995). Amniotic fluid embolism: Analysis of the national registry. *American Journal of Obstetrics and Gynecology, 172,* (4), Part 1, 1158–1167.

Conway, D., & Langer, O. (1998). Elective delivery of infants with macrosomia in diabetic women: Reduced shoulder dystocia versus increased cesarean deliveries. *American Journal of Obstetrics and Gynecology, 178,* (5), 922–925.

Corbett, J., & Fonteyn, M. (1995). Treating disseminated intravascular coagulation. *American Journal of Maternal Child Nursing, 20,* (5), 290.

Crane, J., van de Hof, M., Dodds, L., Armson, B., & Liston, R. (1999). Neonatal outcomes with placenta previa. *Obstetrics and Gynecology, 93,* (4), 541–544.

Cunningham, F., MacDonald, P., Gant, N., Leveno, K., Gilstrap III, L., Hankins, G., & Clark, S. (1997). *Williams Obstetrics,* 20th ed. Stamford, CT: Appleton & Lange.

Eganhouse, D., & Petersen, L. (1998). Fetal surveillance in multifetal pregnancy. *Journal of Obstetric, Gynecologic and Neonatal Nursing, 27,* (3), 312–321.

Ellings, J., Newman, R., & Bowers, N., (1998). Prenatal care and multiple pregnancy. *Journal of Obstetric, Gynecologic and Neonatal Nursing, 27,* (4), 457–465.

Feinstein, N., & McCartney, P. (1997). *AWHONN: Fetal heart monitoring principles and practices,* 2nd ed. Dubuque, IA: Kendall/Hunt.

Garmel, S., Chelmow, D., Sha, S., Roan, J., & D'Alton, M. (1997). Oligohydramnios and the appropriately grown fetus. *American Journal Perinatology, 14,* (6), 359–363.

Gherman, R., Goodwin, T., Souter, I., Neumann, K., Ouzounian, J., & Paul, R. (1997). The McRobert's maneuver for the alleviation of shoulder dystocia: How successful is it? *American Journal of Obstetrics and Gynecology, 176,* (3), 656–661.

Gilbert, W., & Danielsen, B. (1999). Amniotic fluid embolism: Decreased mortality in a population-based study. *Obstetrics and Gynecology, 93,* (6), 973–977.

Golan, A., Lin, G., Evron, S., Arieli, S., Niv, D., & David, M. (1994a). Oligohydramnios: Maternal complications and fetal outcome in 145 cases. *Gynecologic and Obstetric Investigation, 37,* (2), 91–95.

Golan, A., Wolman, I., Sagi, J., Yovel, I., & David, M. (1994b). Persistence of polyhydramnios during pregnancy: Its significance and correlation with maternal and fetal complications. *Gynecology and Obstetric Investigation, 37,* (1), 18–20.

Gonen, O., Rosen, D., Dolfin, Z., Tepper, R., Markov, S., & Fejgin, M. (1998). Induction of labor versus expectant management in macrosomia: A randomized study. *Obstetrics and Gynecology, 89,* (6), 913–917.

Gupton, A., Heaman, M., & Ashcroft, T. (1997). Bed rest from the perspective of the high-risk pregnant woman. *Journal of Obstetric, Gynecologic and Neonatal Nursing, 26,* (4), 423–430.

Hall, S. (1997). The nurse's role in the identification of risks and treatment of shoulder dystocia. *Journal of Obstetric, Gynecologic and Neonatal Nursing, 26,* (1), 25–32.

Halle, J. (1993). Diagnostic evaluation of high-risk pregnancies. In S. Mattson & J. Smith (Eds.), (Chapt. 11). NAACOG: *Core curriculum for maternal newborn nursing.* Philadelphia, PA: W.B. Saunders.

Handwerker, S., & Selick, A. (1995). Placental abruption after insertion of catheter tip intrauterine pressure transducers: A report of four cases. *Journal of Reproductive Medicine, 40,* (12), 845–849.

Impey, L., & O'Herlihy, C. (1998). First delivery after cesarean delivery for strictly defined cephalopelvic disproportion. *Obstetrics and Gynecology, 92,* (5), 799–803.

Imseis, H., Murtha, A., Alexander, K., & Barnett, B. (1998). Spontaneous rupture of a primigravid uterus secondary to placenta percreta. *Journal of Reproductive Medicine, 43,* (3), 233–236.

Joshi, R., & Bharadwaj, A. (2000). Occiputposterior vertex in labor, an under recognized cause of dystocia. *Obstetrics and Gynecology, 95,* (4), suppl. 1, S 40.

Jauniaux, E., Ramsay, B., Peellaerts, C., & Scholler, Y. (1995). Perinatal features of pregnancies complicated by nuchal cord. *American Journal of Perinatology, 12,* (4), 255–258.

Kellogg, B. (1993). Placental development and functioning. In S. Mattson & J. Smith, (Eds.) (Chapt. 5). *NAACOG: Core curriculum for maternal newborn nursing.* Philadelphia, PA: W.B. Saunders.

Kirkendall, C., Jauregui, I., Kim, J., & Phelan, J. (2000). Catastrophic uterine rupture: Maternal and fetal characteristics. *Obstetrics and Gynecology, 95,* (4), suppl. 1, 74.

Larson, J., Rayburn, W., Crosby, S., & Thurnau, G. (1995). Multiple nuchal cord entanglements and intrapartum complications. *American Journal of Obstetrics and Gynecology, 173,* (4), 1228–1231.

Lee, W., Lee, V., Kirk, J., Sloan, C., Smith, R., & Comstock, C. (2000). Vasa previa: Prenatal diagnosis, natural evolution and clinical outcome. *Obstetrics and Gynecology, 95,* (4), 572–577.

Leonard, L. (1998). Depression and anxiety disorders during multiple pregnancy and parenthood. *Journal of Obstetric, Gynecologic and Neonatal Nursing, 27,* (3), 329–337.

Lewis, D., Edwards, M., Asrat, T., Adair, C., Brooks, G., & London, S., (1998). Can shoulder dystocia be predicted? Preconceptive and prenatal factors. *Journal of Reproductive Medicine, 43,* (8), 654–658.

Lin, C., Adamczyk, C., Montag, A., Zelop, C., & Snow, J. (1998). Placenta previa percreta involving the left broad ligament and cervix. A case report. *Journal of Reproductive Medicine, 43,* (9), 839–843.

Locksmith, G. (1999). Amniotic fluid embolism. *Obstetric and Gynecologic Clinics of North America, 26,* (3), 435–444.

Love, C., & Wallace, E. (1996). Pregnancies complicated by placenta previa: What is appropriate management? *British Journal of Obstetrics and Gynecology, 103,* (9), 864–867.

Manogin, T., Bechtel, G., & Rami, J. (2000). Caring behaviors by nurses: Women's perceptions during childbirth. *Journal of Obstetric, Gynecologic and Neonatal Nursing, 29,* (2), 153–157.

Maymon, E., Ghezzi, F., Shoham-Vardi, I., Silberstein, T., Wiznitzer, A., & Mazor, M. (1998). Isolated hydramnios at term gestation and the occurrence of peripartum complications. *European Journal of Obstetrics, Gynecology and Reproductive Biology, 77,* (2), 157–161.

Menihan, C. (1998). Uterine rupture in women attempting a vaginal birth following prior cesarean birth. *Journal of Perinatology, 18,* (6), Part 1, 440–443.

Miller, D., Goodwin, T., Gherman, R., & Paul, R. (1997). Intrapartum rupture of the unscarred uterus. *Obstetrics and Gynecology, 89,* (5), Part 1, 671–673.

Misra, D., & Ananth, C. (1999). Risk factor profiles of placental abruption in first and second pregnancies: Heterogenous etiologies. *Journal of Clinical Epidemiology, 52,* (5), 453–461.

Murphy, D., & MacKenzie, I. (1995). The mortality and morbidity associated with umbilical cord prolapse. *British Journal of Obstetrics and Gynaecology, 102,* (10), 826–830.

Ou, X., Chen, X., & Su, J. (1997). Correction of occipito-posterior position by maternal posture during the process of labor. *Chung Hua Fu Chan Ko Tsa Chih, 32,* (6), 329–332.

Oyelese, K., Schwarzler, P., Coates, S., Sanusi, F., Hamid, R., & Campbell, S. (1998). A strategy for reducing the mortality rate from vasa previa using transvaginal sonography with color Doppler. *Ultrasound Obstetrics and Gynecology, 12,* (6), 434–438.

Panting-Kemp, A., Nguyen, T., Chang E., Quillen, E., & Castro, L. (1999). Idiopathic polyhydramnios and perinatal outcome. *American Journal of Obstetrics and Gynecology, 181,* (5), Part 1, 1079–1082.

Payton, R., & Brucker, M. (1999). Drugs and uterine motility. *Journal of Obstetric, Gynecologic and Neonatal Nursing, 28,* (6), 628–638.

Prabulos, A., & Philipson, E. (1998). Umbilical cord prolapse: is the time from diagnosis to delivery critical? *Journal of Reproductive Medicine, 43,* (2), 129–132.

Rayl, J., Gibson, P., & Hickok, D. (1996). A population-based case-control study of risk factors for breech presentation. *American Journal of Obstetrics and Gynecology, 174,* (1), Part 1, 28–32.

Reis, P., Sander, C., & Pearlman, M. (2000). Abruptio placentae after auto accidents. A case control study. *Journal of Reproductive Medicine, 45,* (1), 6–10.

Ricci, J. (1992). Antepartum hemorrhage. In N. Hacker & J. Moore, (Eds.) (Chapt. 14). *Essentials of obstetrics and gynecology,* 2nd ed. Philadelphia, PA: W.B. Saunders.

Sanchez-Ramos, L., Quillen, M., & Kaunitz, A. (1996). Randomized trial of oxytocin alone and with propanolol in the management of dysfunctional labor. *Obstetrics and Gynecology, 88,* (4), 517–520.

Sather, S., & Zwelling, E. (1998). A view from the other side of the bed. *Journal of Obstetric, Gynecologic and Neonatal Nursing, 27,* (3), 322–328.

Schmidt, J. (1997). Fluid check: Making the case for intrapartum amnioinfusion. *AWHONN: Lifelines, 1,* (7), 47–51.

Schmidt, J. (1993). Hemorrhagic disorders. In S. Mattson & J. Smith (Eds.) (Chapt. 28). *NAACOG: Core curriculum for maternal newborn nursing.* Philadelphia, PA: W.B. Saunders.

Shields, J., & Medearis, A., (1992a). Fetal malpresentations. In N. Hacker & J. Moore (Eds.) (Chapt. 20). *Essentials of obstetrics and gynecology,* 2nd ed. Philadelphia, PA: W.B. Saunders.

Shields, J., & Medearis, A., (1992b). Multiple gestation. In N. Hacker & J. Moore (Eds.) (Chapt. 21). *Essentials of obstetrics and gynecology,* 2nd ed. Philadelphia, PA: W.B. Saunders.

Shipp, T., Bromley, B., Pauker, S., Frigoletto, F., & Benacerraf, B. (1996). Outcome of singleton pregnancies with severe oligohydramnios in the second and third trimesters. *Ultrasound Obstetrics and Gynecology, 7,* (2), 108–113.

Simpson, K. (1999). Shoulder dystocia. Nursing interventions and risk management strategies. *MCN American Journal of Maternal Child Nursing, 24,* (6), 305–310.

Thompson, J. (1995). Forcep deliveries. *Clinical Perinatology, 22,* (4), 953–972.

Thompson, T., Thorp, J., Mayer, D., Kuller, J., & Bowes, W. (1998). Does epidural analgesia cause dystocia? *Journal of Clinical Anesthesia, 10,* (1), 58–65.

Toohey, J., Keegan, K., Morgan, M., Francis, J., Task, S., & deVeciana, M. (1995). The "dangerous multipara": Fact or fiction? *American Journal of Obstetrics and Gynecology, 172,* (2), Part 1, 683–686.

Toth, P., & Jothivijayrani, A. (1999). Obstetrics: Breech Delivery. (Chapt. 8). In University of Iowa Family Practice Handbook, 3rd ed. P25-8 html.Virtual Hospital.

Towers, C., Pircon., R., & Heppard, M. (1999). Is tocolysis safe in the management of third trimester bleeding? *American Journal of Obstetrics and Gynecology, 180,* (6), Part 1, 1572–1578.

Wagner, R., Nielsen, P., & Gonik, B. (1999). Shoulder dystocia. *Obstetric and Gynecologic Clinics of North America, 26,* (2), 371–383.

Weiwen, Y., Ningyu, Z., Lanxiang, Z., & Yu, L. (2000). Study of the diagnosis and management of amniotic fluid embolism: 38 cases of analysis. *Obstetrics and Gynecology, 95,* (4), suppl. 1, S38.

Wiznitzer, A. (1995). Obstructed labor and shoulder dystocia. *Current Opinions in Obstetrics and Gynecology, 7,* (6), 486–491.

Suggested Readings

Hankins, G., & Rowe, T. (1996). Operative vaginal delivery: Year 2000. *American Journal of Obstetrics and Gynecology, 175,* (2), 275–282.

McDougall, R., & Duke, G. (1995). Amniotic fluid embolism syndrome: A case report and review. *Anaesthesia Intensive Care, 23,* (6), 735–740.

Richey, M., Gilstrap, L., III, & Ramin, S. (1995). Management of disseminated intravascular coagulation. *Clinics in Obstetrics and Gynecology, 38,* (3), 514–520.

Turley, G. (1993). Essential forces and factors in labor. In S. Mattson & J. Smith (Eds.) (Chapt. 14). *NAACOG: Core curriculum for maternal newborn nursing.* Philadelphia, PA: W.B. Saunders.

Resources

American College of Obstetricians and Gynecologists (ACOG), 409 12th Street, P.O. Box 96920, Washington, DC 20090-6920, www.acog.com

Association of Women's Health, Obstetric and Neonatal Nurses (AWHONN), Suite 740, 2000 L Street, NW, Washington, DC 20036, U.S.: 800-673-8499, Fax: 202-728-0575, Canada: 800-245-0231, www.awhonn.org

National Association of Neonatal Nurses (NANN), Suite 450, 701 Lee Street, Des Plaines, IL 60016, 847-299-NANN (6266), Toll-free: 800-451-3795, Fax: 847-297-6768, E-mail: info@nann.org

National Organization of Mothers of Twins Clubs, Inc. (NOMOTC), P.O. Box 23188, Albuquerque, NM 87192, 505-434-MOST, E-mail: NOMOTC@aol.com, www.nomotc.org

Resolve Through Sharing, 765-456-5429

Sidelines National Support Network, P.O. Box 1808, Laguna Beach, CA 92652, 714-497-2265, E-mail: Sidelines@sidelines.org, www.sidelines.org

Twins Magazine, Suite 400, 5350 South Roslyn, Englewood, CO 80111-2125, 888-55-TWINS, www.twinsmagazine.com

CHAPTER 27

Birth and the Family

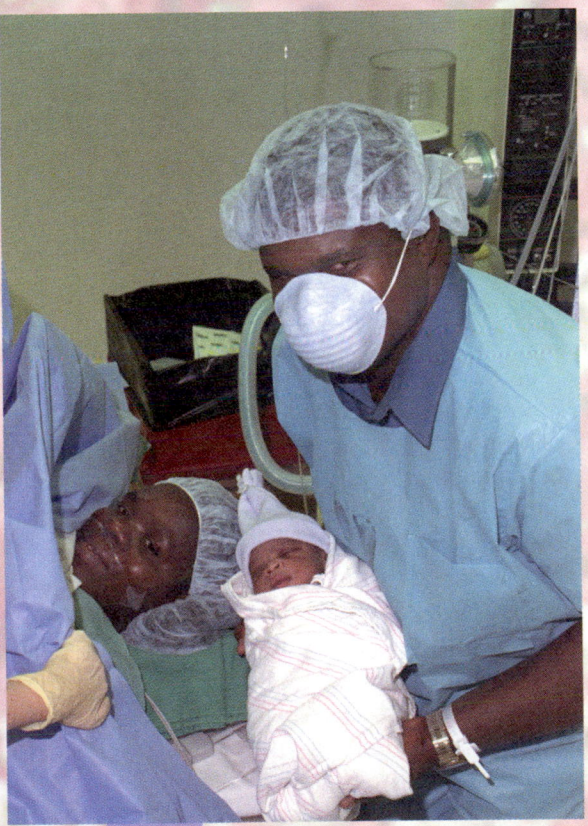

Working with childbearing families is one of the most rewarding challenges in nursing practice. During this time, the nurse has an opportunity to assist clients and families in developing coping strategies that will help them reach their full potential as individuals and a family unit (Maushart, 1999; von Klitzing, Amsler, Schleske, Simoni, & Bergin, 1996). Families are more open, receptive to education, and willing to make changes in their lives during the childbearing years than during any other time in their lives (Maushart, 1999; von Klitzing et al., 1996; Hawkins & Gorvine, 1985). This is also a time when the nurse discusses important issues about reproductive health. While assisting a family during labor, birth, and the immediate postpartum period, the nurse has an opportunity to examine the client's personal views, choices, and experiences. The most effective maternal-newborn nurses integrate a sensitivity to their own response to birth with the skills they need to assist families in moving through their particular experience.

Consider the following questions as you examine your personal feelings regarding birth.

- *What are my personal experiences with birth?*

- *If I have given birth, or if I have been present at the birth of a child, were there professionals who were helpful to me in having the birth experience I desired?*

- *What were the qualities of these professionals?*

Key Terms

Couvade	Cultural competence	Developmental crisis	Situational crisis
Crisis	continuum	Ecologic environment	

Competencies

Upon completion of this chapter, the reader should be able to:

1. Discuss the effect of an uncomplicated birth experience on mothers and fathers.
2. Compare the effect of an uncomplicated birth experience for primiparous and multiparous families.
3. Describe the potential effect of a new birth on siblings.
4. Discuss the effect of birth within a multigenerational family.
5. Explain how to identify the needs of a family that is experiencing a complication of birth.
6. Discuss the relevance of assessing the family's response to birth when identifying infants at risk for child abuse and neglect.
7. Apply the nursing process in the assessment of the family's response to birth, the identification of adaptive and maladaptive processes, the development of a plan of care that supports positive responses or assists the family in developing appropriate responses, and the evaluation of the care provided.
8. List community resources available to postpartal families that can assist in coming to terms with the birth experience.

The moment of birth is a transition point, a line of demarcation between life before the baby and life with the baby. No matter how well prepared a woman or her family believes they are for this transition, the reality of the experience of birth is impossible to predict. Each birth is unique, each infant unlike any other. The congruence of the quality of the labor and the specific qualities of the birth and the infant with the expectations of the participants determines the response of family members to the birth (Maushart, 1999). One important family experience during the birth process is fear for the life or health of the mother and the infant.

The location of birth can affect the family's response. The family that is invested in a noninterventional style or unconventional place of birth, such as the home setting, may experience anxiety and stress if the birth occurs in a hospital. A sudden change in birth venue, whether from home to hospital, birth center to hospital, or hospital birthing room to operating room generates disequilibrium in the family as it struggles to come to terms with expectations that are not mirrored by reality.

The responsiveness of the birth site to the needs of the family influences their experience. "Ownership" of the birth experience is perceived differently in different settings. The home environment is under the control of the family and parents; the birth center environment is usually constructed to allow the family to control events to a certain extent; and hospital sites are governed by administrative rules that tend to remove the locus of control from clients and families. Depending on the philosophy of the institution, families can be limited not only in choices about how to birth but about who may be present. Table 27-1 offers insight into some of these philosophies. Some institutions and some professionals are more restrictive than others. Reasons for these variations may be based in theory or on the personal experience and perspective of the professionals involved (DeVries, Wrede, Teijlingen, & Benoit, 2001).

Assessment of the family member's immediate response to the birth experience sets the stage for nursing interventions during the postpartum period. By using the nursing process and thoroughly understanding the diverse aspects of nursing, obstetric, psychological, sociologic, educational, and political theory that intersect during the time of birthing, the nurse can choose culturally competent interventions that assist the family in moving through their birth experience (Cross, Bazron, Dennis, & Isaacs, 1989).

Table 27-1 Potential Effects of Birth Site Philosophy on Family Birth Experience

Birth Site	Philosophy	Effect on Family Birth Experience
Home	This is the family's personal space. The family owns and operates the space.	The family controls who is present in the space where the birth occurs. The family assumes responsibility and contracts with the birth attendant. The family controls issues such as clothing worn during labor, fluid, nutrition, and ambient music. Supportive people are present at the family's request.
Birth Center	The center owns and operates the space. When beginning prenatal care the family contracts with the center for services. Self-care and participation in decision making are expectations of the relationship.	The family has control over the experience in collaboration with the center staff and policies. Responsibility is shared. The family controls issues such as clothing worn during labor, fluid, nutrition, and ambient music. Supportive people are present at the family's request.
Hospital	Corporately owned with strict visitation policies dictated by nursing and administration. Governed by infection-control policies.	Institutional policy governs where the birth occurs, who and how many people may be present; who those persons may be; how long they may stay; available food and fluids; clothing worn, and how the family can use music or other support strategies. Obstetrical medical policy dictates whether oral nutrition is available and if technology is used routinely. The family has as much control as they are willing to exercise within the boundaries of the institutional policies.

HISTORICAL ASPECTS OF BIRTH AND THE FAMILY

The history of birthing is an interesting one. Cultural and family practices and beliefs around childbearing have been passed from generation to generation. In the United States, the 20th century, the location for birth moved from the home to medical institutions. There were many contributing factors, including the development of medicine as a science, the trend away from using midwives to using doctors to care for women during pregnancy and birth, the development of medications and anesthetics, the redefinition of hospitals as places of healing where services were available that could not be provided in the home, the growth of hospital beds, the advent of hospitalization insurance, and the redefinition of birth as an illness requiring specialized care. By the 1950s, most women gave birth in the hospital with the latest technologies, including twilight sleep (a combination of sedation and anesthesia for the birth itself). Rural and non–Caucasian women continued to birth at home during this time, probably because of lack of proximity to hospitals and the segregation of many facilities (DeVries et al., 2001).

In the 1960s, the natural childbirth movement grew, partially from the women's movement and partially as a result of some women's desire to reclaim control over their childbearing experiences. During the next 20 years, changes were made in who could accompany a woman in labor (fathers and the infant's siblings), where the birth could take place (in a labor or birth room as opposed to a traditional delivery room), and how long the hospital stay

would be. In the 1970s, the Birth Center Movement began as families asked for a place of birth that was home-like but had some medical technology available. And during that time, the number of practicing nurse-midwives began to grow (DeVries et al., 2001; Simkin, 1996).

Family centered maternity care developed in the 1970s and 1980s as hospitals and obstetric professionals responded to the growing demands of families to participate in birth and to the growing amount of research that supported the positive outcomes for families when their personal and cultural needs were met (Simkin, 1996).

The history of birth in the United States has substantial implications for maternity nursing practice. In each of the following sections of this chapter, consideration is given to the historical changes that have affected family participation in the birth process.

CULTURAL CONSIDERATIONS IN A FAMILY'S RESPONSE TO BIRTH

Worldwide, pregnancy and birth are perceived from either a wellness or an illness viewpoint. Racial, religious, ethnic, political, economic, and technologic advancement all influence perspectives of childbirth. Over time, culturally specific practices have developed that enable family members to deal with this time of vulnerability for the mother and her child and of change for the family and community. The way a family experiences birth is influenced by the values of the culture than they are born in to and the congruence of that orientation with the culture in which they birth (Esposito, 1999).

Birth sites and those individuals who staff them have their own orientation to childbearing, which is influenced by the same factors. Given the mobility available to individuals and families today, it is quite likely that a family from one culture gives birth in a place unlike their homeland and is cared for by attendants who come from still other environments. Based on the interactions of the individuals in these multicultural situations, the potential exists for powerful, positive, growth-enhancing outcomes for the family and the practitioners and also for negative, personally destructive outcomes.

A **cultural competence continuum** is a progressive description of the ability of an individual or institution to respond to the individual, culturally specific needs of people. Table 27-2 illustrates the layers of a cultural competence continuum from cultural incapacity through cultural competence (Cross et al., 1989). Individuals or agencies can fall anywhere on this continuum and therefore have a positive or destructive interaction with a family during the birth experience. Nursing professionals have a responsibility to assess where they fall on the cultural competence

continuum and seek opportunities to move forward toward cultural competence.

THEORETICAL APPROACHES TO THE STUDY OF THE FAMILY

A family's adaptation and response to a birth can be viewed through different frameworks. Systems theory, developmental theory, and crisis theory each provide a context for understanding a family's growth and change.

Systems Theory

Systems theory describes the relationship of the individual and the multiple forces with which the individual interacts throughout life. Each person is a part of multiple larger groups and contributes to the totality of those groups. The family is the primary group. As a system the family is influenced by its individual members and responds to the feedback from other systems and the social network in which it is maintained. As both the individual member and

Table 27-2 A Cultural Competence Continuum

Cultural destructiveness	Attitudes, policies, and practices, including person interactions that are destructive to cultures and consequently, to the individuals within the culture. For instance, belittling ritual practices and denying access to culturally acceptable healers.
Cultural incapacity	Attitudes, policies, and practices, including personal interactions that are not intentionally destructive but which reflect a lack of ability or capacity to help clients of other cultures. For instance, restricting a laboring woman to only one "helper" or stereotyping women based on their behavioral response to labor pains.
Cultural blindness	Functioning with the belief that skin color and culture make no difference at all and that all people are the same. Usually characterized by the belief that the helping approaches used by the dominant culture are universally applicable. This approach ignores the cultural strengths of a family, encourages assimilation, and blames the family for not "fitting in."
Cultural pre-competence	Individuals and agencies recognize their weaknesses in providing services to families of other cultures and seek to develop approaches to meet some of the needs of some of the families. Characterized by the ability to ask, "How can I help?" This level is indicative of beginning the process of becoming culturally competent but shows a lack of information and clear knowledge of how to proceed.
Cultural competence	Individuals and agencies that accept and respect the differences of the varied families they serve. They see the differences between cultures and within cultural subgroups, each distinct from each other and having important strengths. Such individuals are able to engage in self-assessment regarding culture, pay careful attention to the dynamics of difference between their cultural orientation and that of their clients, and are continually expanding their cultural knowledge and resources.
Cultural proficiency	Advanced cultural competence. Every culture is held in high esteem. Individuals and agencies conduct research and develop new therapeutic approaches based on culture. They advocate for cultural competence and improve relations in their own agencies and communities. For instance, the development of a culturally specific doula program would address the individual needs of families giving birth.

Adapted from Cross, T., Bazron, B., Dennis, K., & Isaacs, M. (1989). Towards a culturally competent system of care: Vol. 1. National Technical Assistance Center for Children's Mental Health, Georgetown University, Washington, DC.

the group interact with other organizations and individuals in the environment, adaptive changes occur. In this way, the family system responds and contributes to its environment. By balancing the needs of the individual and the collective group, the family dynamically progresses through life (Cox & Paley, 1997).

Individual systems have boundaries that define their identity and maintain their integrity. Those boundaries change as members are added or removed (Figure 27-1). As the number of persons in this system changes the relationships among the remaining members change. For instance, when a couple has a child, they move from a dyadic system to a triadic one. This alters lines of communication, the number of members for which the system is responsible, and the amount of input the system receives from its members.

The family is the first social context to which an individual belongs. However, the interactions of the family do not occur in isolation from other social interactions that present opportunities and risks for the development and well-being of the family and its members (Patterson, 1999). By envisioning the family as a microsystem within the context of the larger environment of community, culture, religion, socioeconomic class, and geographic group, a family can be seen as central to its **ecologic environment** (the total of the macrosystems within which a family resides) (Cox & Paley, 1997; Patterson, 1999).

Family systems have four central functions, which affect their members and the society of which the family is part. These functions are: (1) family formation, which provides a sense of belonging, direction for life, and identity for its members; (2) economic provision for the basic needs of food, clothing, shelter, and other resources for its members; (3) nurturance, education, and socialization, which provide physical, psychological, social, and spiritual

development and instills social values and norms; and (4) protection, which provides care for young and vulnerable members (Patterson, 1999). The ability of the family to fulfill these responsibilities for its members and for society depends to a large extent on its relationship with the macrosystem.

Birth represents a change in the family system—in its constellation and its internal communications—and challenges the family's ability to provide the basic necessities and protection for its members. This is a time when the family system interacts with the medical care system and other institutional systems and a time when the relationships with employment systems may change. At the time of birth, the nurse is in a unique position to facilitate the dynamic changes the family is going through by being sensitive to the cultural, economic, and physiologic issues confronting the family members; by assisting them in navigating the medical system; and by supporting them in making choices that improve their level of functioning.

Developmental Theory

Families, like individuals, go through developmental stages. Family structure changes with the addition of members during the childbearing cycle or through adoption, and when family members leave, such as a young adult leaving home or the death of a family member. Family functions change and family roles are negotiated as members move from dependency to contribution and then become more independent (Patterson, 1999). At birth, the family is in the process of moving from one developmental stage to another. For instance, at this time a two-person family must move from the stage of independence to a stage of nurturance, with the addition of a totally dependent new member. This transition to parenthood disrupts the balance the family has achieved and requires learning new roles and strategies for coping. While working with families during labor and birth, the nurse has the opportunity to provide anticipatory guidance that will assist the family during this transition (Patterson, 1999; Belsky & Kelly, 1994).

Crisis Theory

A **crisis** can be defined as a situation in which a family or individual's balance is disrupted, requiring development of new coping strategies. Erikson first used the term **developmental crisis** in describing the adjustment of the individual to new stages of development (Erickson, 1963). In his work, Erikson describes the work involved in of each developmental crisis, or turning point, as the individual moves from birth to death. The key to successfully resolving the crisis is reduction in the anxiety level generated by the person's move from homeostasis to disequilibrium and back to equilibrium, once the turning point is

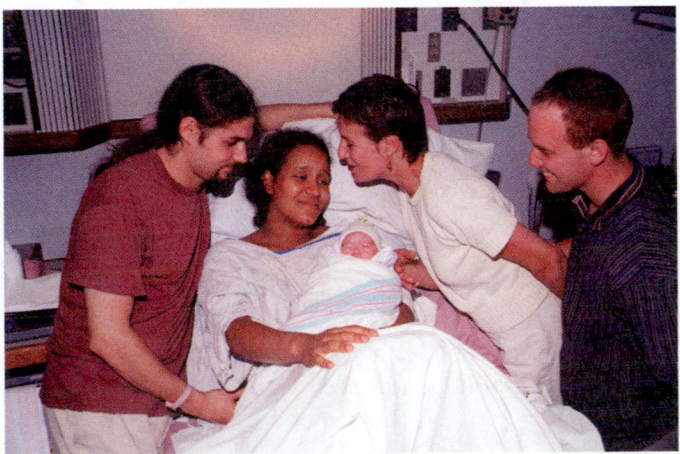

Figure 27-1 The birth of a child presents the extended family with new opportunities for growth and bonding.

successfully negotiated (Maushart, 1999; Erickson, 1963; Elkind, 1994).

In moving chronologically from one stage to the next, the individual either completes the work of the developmental stage, which provides the foundation from which to do the work of the next stage, or the individual remains stagnant at that stage, interfering with progress to the next stage. The result of not negotiating the crisis point in the life cycle is that the state of disequilibrium continues. This state of disequilibrium, or constant anxiety, is what prevents the person from functioning optimally and moving on developmentally to the next stage (Maushart, 1999; Hawkins & Gorvine, 1985). Pregnancy, birth, and parenting, viewed from this theoretical framework, are developmental crises, or turning points, in human growth and development (Mercer, 1995).

These same events can be viewed as situational crises in the life cycle. A **situational crisis** is an event or situation that occurs in a person or a family's life, which requires the adaptation or acquisition of new coping mechanisms. Using Erickson's theoretical framework, the adaptations that a 16-year-old needs to make in life to accommodate pregnancy and parenting are added to the adaptations necessary to work through the developmental stage of adolescence (Erickson, 1963).

Families, whatever their configurations, can be viewed as systems that move through the same kinds of crisis as individuals (Maushart, 1999). As individuals come together to form family groups, they move through developmental stages in much the same way that individuals do. At each turning point, the family seeks to develop strategies with which to cope with its life in a way that maintains the homeostasis or equilibrium of the family. The family group experiences the same movement from equilibrium to anxiety and back to equilibrium as the individual does. The family's success or failure in developing higher levels of coping is dependent on the success of its members in achieving equilibrium and is influenced by culture, environment, and family history (Maushart, 1999; Belsky & Kelly, 1994).

Birth represents a crisis or turning point for the family. The family brings to the birth room all its baggage, hopes, expectations for the experience of birth, expectations for the baby, and projections for the future. As the birth unfolds, there is congruence or lack of congruence with family member's expectations (Cross, et al., 1989; Esposito, 1999; Mercer, 1995). Perhaps the labor is longer than expected and the time commitment of the family is an issue, or perhaps there is more pain or noise than family members expected or can tolerate.

NURSING IMPLICATIONS

The nursing process is a valuable framework for working with families. Using the nursing process, the nurse gathers data and assesses the response of the family unit to birth and of individual family members. Based on these observations, decisions can be made about the level of positive or negative response and a specific plan can be developed in collaboration with the family to identify the goals of the individual members and of the family as a system. With an understanding of the needs and goals of the family, the nurse can choose appropriate interventions, which may include referrals to other health care professionals, and design a strategy for evaluating the progress of the family as they journey toward meeting their goals.

At the time of birth, the nurse must assess each family member's response to the experience. This is a time of heightened awareness, when potential risks to mother, infant, and family system can be identified, and a time when positive responses can be reinforced.

In promoting a positive response to the birth, the nurse must validate the family's experience. Listening is the first step. Secondly, the nurse must understand that, because most families have limited experience with the birth process and medical procedures, their own perceptions of the events are reality for them. Reinforcing positive responses to the birth, the infant, and the support of the family is an important strategy in helping a woman integrate the events that have occurred. Assisting the woman and her family in identifying those events that were consistent with their expectations and helping them to find honest adaptations to those events that were inconsistent with their expectations helps to promote a positive response to the birth.

Because the current trend in postpartum stays for women who give birth in a hospital or birth center facility have significantly shortened, with the range from 24–48 hours in an uncomplicated vaginal birth to 72 hours for an uncomplicated cesarean birth, the evaluation of the outcome of interventions may require follow-up with outpatient services or home visiting (Wallace, Green, Jacos, Paine, & Story, 1999). This is an important collaborative piece of the plan. Use of the nursing process is highlighted in each of the following sections that describe the family response to birth.

EFFECT OF BIRTH ON THE FAMILY

Each member of the birthing family experiences a period of adaptation after the birth of a new member. An individual's response is shaped by personal experience, history, cultural background, and developmental stage.

Maternal Adaptation

Labor and birth encompass a proportionately short period in a woman's life. However, no other experience has the intensity of physical and emotional feelings or represents such a profound life change (Simkin, 1996; Rubin, 1984). A woman's self-concept is affected by the congruence of her birth experience and her expectations. Ego strength is enhanced by a birth, which leaves the woman with a sense of accomplishment, some sense of control, and positive reinforcement from family. In contrast, an experience that does not meet expectations or that leaves the woman with a sense of loss of control may foster feelings of frustration, disappointment, or shame (Mercer, 1995; Katz-Rothman, 1996).

The maternal response to an uncomplicated birth experience is colored by her previous birth experiences and her expectations for this birth. During a comparatively short period, the woman has an intense physical experience that is totally outside of her control. Her body acts on its own in ways she might not have anticipated. Choices in dress, food, and activity may be dictated by the stage of labor, institutional policy, and provider preference. The amount of control that a woman perceives that she has during the birth process and the degree of pain she feels both have direct relationships to her feelings about that experience and to her self-concept (Mercer, 1995). Data obtained from focus groups with postpartum women indicate that when labor and birth go well, the mother and baby had no problems and the woman felt supported and involved in care. They felt emotions ranging from happy to delighted and indicated that the commonly used term "satisfied" was in no way descriptive enough regarding how they perceived the care they received. On the other hand, when things did not go well, the woman felt unsupported and uninvolved and when the outcomes were less than expected, feelings ranged from disappointed to devastated (Proctor, 1998).

The timing of the birth, whether at term or postterm, affects the mother's response to birth. A woman who has given birth to an infant at term may be happy, tired, and interactive with her baby and family. In contrast, a woman experiencing the birth of an infant during the 2 weeks past her due date may be fearful, unwilling to touch or interact with her baby, and disappointed with herself and her body's inability to perform correctly and on time (Mercer, 1995). The fact that delivery within 42 weeks' gestation is within the realm of normal may not be reassuring enough for a woman who has been looking to the estimated date of delivery (EDD) as the marking point of the end of pregnancy.

The duration of labor has an effect on the woman's response to the experience. It may be obvious that a long labor can leave a woman exhausted and depleted of resources at the birth. However, a precipitous birth experience is physically tumultuous and may be frightening in its intensity.

The difficulty of the delivery is another variable that influences the mother's response (Figure 27-2). A normal

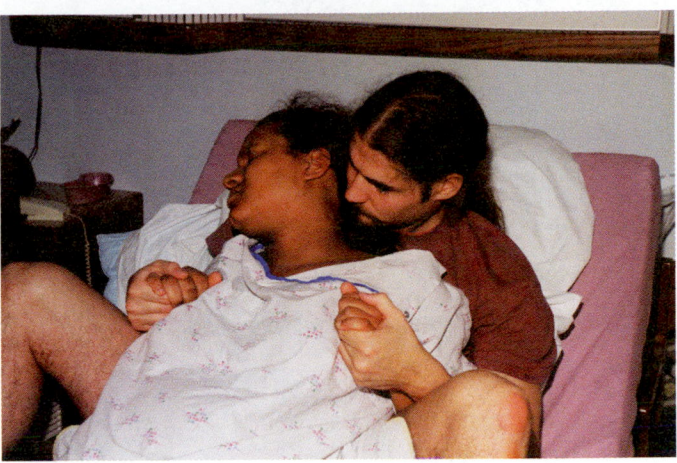

Figure 27-2 The difficulty of the delivery may influence a couple's response to the birth process.

vaginal birth can be perceived to be difficult. Women who are unprepared for the feeling of extreme perineal pressure as the head crowns may be frightened. Women, who have received regional anesthesia for labor and whose practitioner has allowed the anesthesia to wear off to allow the natural pushing reflex to return, may perceive the birth as difficult. A situation that requires manipulation by the birth attendant, for example, shoulder dystocia, may cause the mother to experience fear for herself, her baby, and her birth. Immediately after such an experience, the woman may feel relief that all is well, disappointment that this was not the birth experience she expected, or anger that she or her infant could have been hurt.

Theories of Maternal Adaptation

Rubin, Lederman, Mercer, and others have described the developmental tasks of pregnancy and have discussed how the completion or noncompletion of these tasks affects a woman's labor, birth, and parenting experience. While many of these tasks are nonsequential, there appear to be three that must be accomplished in a certain order. Building one upon the other, the woman first accepts the reality of her pregnancy during the first trimester; second, develops a relationship with the unborn child during the second trimester; and third, prepares for the unknown experience of giving up the fetus and meeting her newborn. Women who do not complete these tasks before delivery may not be fully psychologically equipped to move into their role as mother (Mercer, 1995; Rubin, 1984; Lederman, 1984).

Rubin (1984) discusses the immediate response of the mother to her infant. After months of fantasizing, the woman meets her newborn at the moment of birth (Rubin, 1984). The congruence of that real infant with her fantasy affects her response and her incorporation of the child into her reality. From observation and client inter-

REFLECTIONS FROM A MOTHER

"Becoming a mother is the most life-altering and wonderful experience a woman can have. It becomes who you are, and everything you do in life becomes secondary to that, requiring extraordinary ability to balance it all. While pregnant or awaiting the arrival of a child through adoption, you can read and read about how your relationship with your spouse will change and how you need to maintain that relationship with your spouse. What I'd never read about and wish I'd known more about is that your spouse changes, too, from becoming a parent. And that in a sense, you will fall in love again with this new person, who is now a father and showing tenderness toward the child you carried for 9 months.

A pleasant surprise is how all of your relationships change as you evolve into a mother. Suddenly, to everyone in your life, you are someone's mother, with the expectations of that role in their eyes (and that's different for so many people). And then you are the other things around that—daughter, daughter-in-law, professional, friend, sister, brother. All of the continuous emotional growth in my life that stems from being a mother has, in most cases, helped me be a more empathetic daughter, daughter-in-law, professional, friend, and sister, and to realize the powerful effect a mother's nurturing has on the entire world—in a way only a mother can do it."

views, Rubin describes the stages of attachment between mother and child that the mother experiences. These stages are: "taking-in" describing the early postpartum period; "taking-hold" during the later postpartum period around a week after birth; and "letting go" the final incorporation of the maternal role. Moving from touching the infant with her fingertips to using finger pads and then palmar surfaces to encircle the infant, the woman brings the baby close to her body again. The "en face" position, where the mother places the infant on the bed at her eye level and turns face to face with the baby, was found to occur in women who had a positive self-image (Mercer, 1995).

A woman may also feel a sensation of loss, once the infant is delivered and outside of her body. Rubin observed women positioning infants on their abdomen immediately after birth and continuing to hold the baby in this manner when lying down for some weeks thereafter. She hypothesized that holding the baby this way might be a compensation for a sense of loss of the internal feeling of the fetus in the uterus, which these women continued to describe feeling for several months (Rubin, 1984).

Rubin describes labor as a period when time and space lose congruence with reality. Contractions, their length and frequency, measure time. Perception of space narrows almost to the woman's body boundaries. How she incorporates those around her into her experience is influenced by her cultural background and style of coping with life. Some women want to be surrounded and touched, others want to be left alone. Her perception of safety and the intensity of the experience influence who and what else she can attend to and allow into her "space" (Rubin, 1984).

In her research describing women's birth experience, Simkin (1996) found that women remember their labor and birth with unusual clarity for up to 20 years after the event. The benefits of continuous labor support have been documented by several authors (Scott, Klaus, & Klaus, 1999; Fowles, 1998). Women who feel they were surrounded by supportive people in labor have been shown to have more positive feelings about their experience, use less pain medication, and be more likely to choose to breastfeed their baby and to breastfeed for a longer period of time. During the later postpartum period, these women are less likely to experience depression and more likely to exhibit higher levels of self-esteem and demonstrate increased sensitivity to the needs of their infants (Scott et al., 1999; Scott, Berkowitz, & Klaus, 1999; Hodnett, 1994).

Nursing Process

Hawkins and Gorvine (1985) used the "crisis model" to develop a useful framework for maternal-newborn nurses to use in assessing family responses to birth and in planning appropriate interventions for postpartum women and their families. They discuss the risks to the postpartum woman in negotiating this time of crisis and how to develop the coping strategies required to enter the role of parent. Those women who meet this challenge experience a reduction in anxiety as they achieve equilibrium in the resolution of the pregnancy and birth. Those women unable to achieve equi-

Client Education

Self Care for Postpartum Families

Recent work by Jeanne Watson-Driscoll and Deborah Sichel (1999) describes the effects of birth on brain chemistry and the ability of the woman to adapt to the new family relationships postpartum. To enable women to address the emotional challenges of this period, these researchers have developed a self-care program that can maximize the woman's ability to develop effective coping strategies during the postpartum period. The program is called NURSE and provides the following guidelines to use in developing a plan with the woman:

- N—Nourishment: Maintain basic nutrition, using the food pyramid as a guide, to provide the brain with appropriate vitamins and basic nutrients. Discuss a multivitamin supplement with your midwife or physician. Be sure to include adequate amounts of alpha–3 omega fatty acids, such as those found in fish proteins, because they are important for nerve cell functioning and, through modulating chemical nerve transmission, may have mood-stabilizing effects.

- U—Understanding: Work with the new mother and family to develop strategies that provide support in the form of listening, validating feelings and nurturing each other. Identify family resources for backup, such as the phone numbers of counseling services and community support groups.

- R—Rest and relaxation: Adequate rest and sleep are essential for the brain to restore itself biochemically. New parents may become sleep-deprived if they do not actively plan rest periods and sleep when the infant sleeps. Planning for rest periods and for taking turns at getting up with the infant may be important strategies to protect against sleep deprivation.

- S—Spirituality: Each woman and family has experiences and activities that nourish their souls. Planning to include such activities, which can be as simple as buying fresh cut flowers to place in a living space or listening to soulful music, addresses this need.

- E—Exercise: It is well-documented that physical exercise causes the release of endorphins, which cause a feeling of well-being. A daily exercise regimen can be as simple as taking the newborn out together for a walk.

librium experience a continuing level of anxiety, which interferes with achieving the role of mother and the development of successful parenting skills (Hawkins & Gorvine).

Nursing interventions in this model are designed to enable postpartum women and their families to develop successful coping strategies for this new dimension of their lives by using what they bring to the experience with them as well as resources available through their extended family and community. Examples of resources that a woman brings to the childbirth experience may include: previous coping mechanisms, nutritional status (which influences her physiologic ability to adapt to birth), and belief system. Examples of external resources include family and friends, community support groups, social services, and religious organizations (Hawkins & Gorvine, 1985).

Assessment

Relevant clinical, demographic, and social data can be gathered from the medical record or the client herself, including:

- Cultural background
- Gravidity and parity
- Prenatal course (complications or lack thereof)
- Social situation, including housing, income, presence of partner, gender of partner, and extended family
- Work situation, type, and job title
- Recorded plans for infant feeding and postpartum care

While interacting with the woman during labor and birth, the nurse should gather data, such as the following:

- Conduct and length of labor
- Type of birth, vaginal or operative
- If the mother holds the infant immediately after birth
- What the mother says to the infant, e.g., "I am so glad to see you" or "you nearly killed me"
- If the mother looks at the infant

Research Highlight

Labor Concerns of Mothers 2 Months After Delivery

Purpose

The majority of the research about family adjustment to birth is found in the social, behavioral, and family therapy disciplines. Reva Rubin's descriptive studies of women's immediate response to birth remain the hallmark of qualitative observations in the research of maternal role attainment (Rubin, 1984). Subsequent studies have built on Rubin's observations and have shown how changes in society, medicine, and the family affect adaptation to motherhood.

Methods

As part of a larger study that examined the development of maternal role identity, Eileen Fowles (1998) described the contribution of the experience of labor and birth to a woman's self-esteem in maturing into the maternal role. In this qualitative study, the researcher asked women at 9-weeks postpartum to respond to the following open-ended question: "Is there anything about your labor and delivery that is still bothering you?"

From September 1992 through June 1993, a convenience sample of women was obtained from the prenatal classes held in three hospitals in the Midwest for the larger study. The institutions were distributed throughout the area. Women included in the sample were ages 18 to 35, primiparous, in the last 3 months of pregnancy without any complications, living with the father of the baby, and English-speaking. One hundred fifty-seven women (93% of the women who were given a prenatal questionnaire), remitted a completed postnatal questionnaire, and 77 of these women completed the open-ended question. The analysis of the 77 completed open-ended responses is the data for the study.

Analysis of the Data

Qualitative research methods provide insight into the areas of emotional, social, and experiential phenomena in health care. Qualitative research questions explore what happened and how and why, and in so doing, often generate theories and hypotheses and show relationships and patterns that may result in conceptual frameworks for looking at observed phenomena.

Through qualitative analysis, themes and concepts were identified from the questionnaire responses and divided into major or minor categories. Relationships between categories and subcategories and among subcategories were examined.

(continued)

- How the mother touches the infant (e.g., does she progress from fingertips to encircling the infant, or turn away or hold the infant away from her body?)
- How the mother interacts with her support network

Nursing Diagnosis

Nursing diagnoses represent the nurse's decision about the data gathered. Diagnoses commonly seen include impaired parenting related to inability to bond with newborn, and anxiety about feelings of loss.

Outcome Identification

Outcomes can be described in terms of short- and long-term goals. For example:

- The mother demonstrates positive interaction with her newborn.
- The client discusses the difference between postpartum "baby blues" and the symptoms of depression.
- The client and her partner identify childcare options within their extended family and community for babysitting.

Research Highlight (continued)

Findings

Two major themes, positive experiences and frustrations, were identified from the women's responses, and within each major theme, several subcategories were identified, which helped to explain and support the major theme.

The theme of "positive experiences" was expressed by 12 of the women and related to who helped the women in labor and to specific actions by birth attendants that were supportive and professional.

A theme of "frustrations" was expressed by 42 of the women and was related to pain, lack of control, lack of knowledge (feeling uninformed), and negative perceptions of caregivers.

Nursing Implications

The results of this study are consistent with those of Simkin (1996), who found that women remember and are influenced by their birth experiences long after the event. Actions by health care professionals identified in this study that contributed to a positive feeling and were most helpful were those that promoted self-confidence and that made the women feel cared for and respected. Women who reported feelings of frustration felt that health care professionals did not help them feel in control of events, did not provide adequate information, and were not helpful in decreasing pain.

Generalization of the results of this study is limited for two important reasons. First, the sample was a convenience sample, not randomized, and limited to one area of the country, and second, the phrasing of the question focusing on things "still bothering you" may have elicited excess negative responses, as reflected in the distribution of 12 responses focused on positive aspects and 42 focused on negative aspects.

However, the message for nurses remains clear. Women remember the behaviors of their primary caregivers, and these behaviors greatly influence women's ultimate perception of their birth experience. Nursing actions that promote self-confidence, communicate sensitivity and caring, and provide information about what is happening and why are pivotal in helping women perceive the birth experience positively, regardless of the method of delivery. The concept of family-centered maternity care was developed to help professionals and institutions meet the individualized needs of families. Birth is an experience that either fosters growth and coping or has negatively effects on the mother and other family members. This study highlights the effects that the birth experience has on women and the important role that the nurse's choice of behavior plays in influencing women's memories.

Planning

With the client, the nurse identifies those strategies that will assist the client in meeting short- and long-term goals. Strategies range from bedside education and reading materials to referral to a visiting nurse service or social services.

Interventions

Nursing interventions can assist the mother in developing a realistic interpretation of her birth experience and may include:

- Encouraging the mother to talk about what she experienced
- Describing the birth of the baby, if she was not able to see it in a mirror
- Helping the mother distinguish between what she thought happened and what actually occurred
- Assisting the woman to inspect the infant
- Encouraging the mother to hold her baby

Evaluation

The ability of the nurse to evaluate the success of the interventions varies, depending on the length of interaction with the family. Observations of behaviors that meet stated goals may be possible. Additionally, referral to collaborative agencies or providers may be necessary to evaluate the progress toward long-term goals.

Paternal Adaptation

The history of the participation of men in birth experiences has been affected by sex role definitions, cultural mores, economic status, politics, and social expectations. Some cultures have prescribed activities for fathers during pregnancy and childbirth. However, to a great extent throughout most of history, men have been excluded from participation in the childbearing process (Jordan, 1990; Heggenhougen, 1980).

In earliest history, men waited outside the tent or the cabin or the bedroom, while the women labored and were delivered by female attendants. In the 19th and 20th centuries, men waited outside the house or in hospital waiting rooms to be told "what their wife had had." Before the 1970s, little, if any, exploration was done of expectant or new fatherhood as a developmental process. All attention was focused on the maternal experience (Jordan, 1990a).

As the attendants at birth moved from the female midwife at home to the physician in a hospital, the presence of men in the birth room became more acceptable, at least for those male physicians performing their duties. Heggenhougen (1980) looked at the role of fathers in childbirth from an anthropologic perspective. He described the research of leading anthropologists about the cultural role of men in childbirth. **Couvade** is a term used to describe the physiologic responses a man has to his partner's pregnancy and those ritual actions that men perform during pregnancy and childbirth (Heggenhougen, 1980). In some traditional cultures, male behaviors range from weight gain, particularly in the abdomen, to nausea and vomiting and specific acts during labor and birth, such as acting out of contractions or holding the birthing woman as she pushes. The behavior enacted during labor may be an effort to divert the pain of childbirth from the woman to help her deliver with less effort (Nichols & Humenick, 2000; Pryia, 1992).

In industrialized societies, there is a common notion that, because conception is a shared experience, birth should be no less so. This perspective was influenced by the growth of the women's movement and the changing view of men's role in the family. Fathers were provided with specific tasks for labor by the prepared-childbirth movement. This ability to take an active part in birth is viewed by families and health professionals as an important step in consolidating the family unit (Nichols & Humenick, 2000; Pryia, 1992).

To better understand the father's response to pregnancy and parenting, Jordan (1990a) reviewed related literature from other helping disciplines and found that pregnancy is a developmental experience for men that parallels that of women during the reproductive and parenting cycles. Essential tasks for the father in each trimester include integrating the physical and emotional changes in his mate, reworking his own relationship with parent figures, and the reality of fatherhood at the time of introduction to his baby. Specific issues for men develop from their perspective of the outsider or the one who is not physically involved with the growing pregnancy. Fathers may be anxious about loss of income when the woman stops working in a two-income family and his ability to provide for a new family constellation. He may have feelings of inadequacy in childcare activities because of lack of exposure and concern about the change in status he may experience in the relationship as he anticipates sharing his partner with the new family member (Jordan, 1990b). The level of anxiety for a father and his feelings of helplessness may be increased when the pregnancy is unplanned and he feels as though he was unable to plan for these significant events (Clinton & Keiber, 1993; Hall, 1995).

The decision to share the birth experience is one that fathers do not take lightly. This is one subject about which men have traditionally been deprived of information. Fear of the unknown, discomfort with "female" bodily processes, and inability to cope with his partner's pain all influence the man's decision to attend the birth. In some areas of Western society today, this trend is to almost demand the father's participation in labor and birth whether he is comfortable with it or not. Palkovitz (1987) explored the motives for fathers attending birth in 37 primiparous couples. She identified a variety of motives that developed from the father's beliefs about their roles as partners, their social reference points, and their expectations for the experience (Palkovitz, 1987).

Paternal Role Attainment

While the fetus becomes real to the mother as she feels it move, the father does not perceive the reality of the child until after the birth, when his perception moves from secondhand, or vicarious, to face-to-face, seeing and holding the baby after birth. According to Jordan, "Seeing the infant emerge from his mate's body through vaginal or cesarean birth was a powerful experience for each father. Birth proved that this infant had been the growth within the mother's abdomen. Fathers then sought physical similarities to validate [that] the child was theirs" (Jordan, 1990b). The father's progressive touching behaviors, be-

REFLECTIONS FROM A FATHER

"Becoming a father is the greatest thing that ever happened to me. Children are an absolute blessing. It struck me, however, on the birth of my second daughter, how different the experience was from the birth of my first daughter. When Madeline was born (after 20 hours of labor, my wife would want pointed out), I couldn't stop crying. I was incredibly happy and relieved that everything went well, but I was simply overwhelmed with raw emotion. By contrast, when my second daughter was born (9 hours of labor), my wife and I couldn't stop laughing. We were both thrilled, relieved, and emotional, but this time we expressed it through laughter. It was so bad that, when my wife went into hard labor, she got the giggles. That has always struck me as an odd contrast."

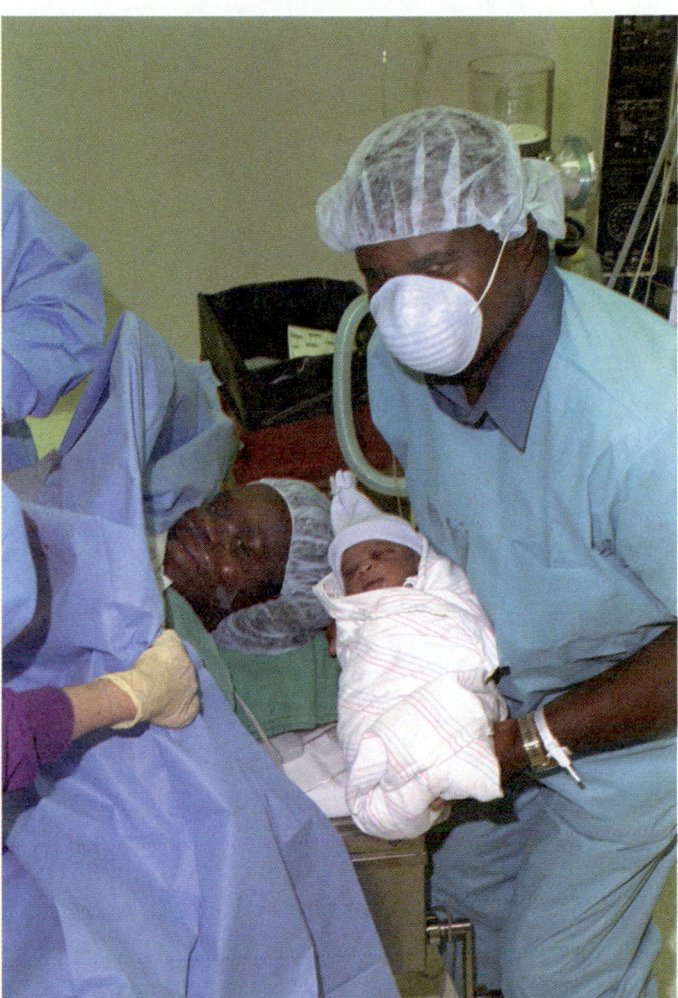

Figure 27-3 Immediately after his wife's cesarean delivery, this father begins to bond with his newborn son.

ginning with the fingertips, progressing to full palmar touch and enfolding in the arms, which mimics the behavior of the mother, were identified by Tomlinson, Rothenberg, and Carver (1991). These behaviors demonstrate the incorporation of the child, from first touch, into the body space of the father as he validates the reality of the child (Figure 27-3).

There is agreement in the literature that pregnancy and birth represent a turning point or crisis for the father in ways that are both similar and dissimilar to the mother (Elkind, 1994; Jordan, 1990a, 1990b; Teichman & Lahan, 1987; Hall, 1995; Deimer, 1997; Duncan, 1995). Like his partner, the father's coping mechanisms are challenged. He loses his equilibrium as the life he has come to know is altered by the experience of this pregnancy and birth, and he struggles individually and in concert with his partner to develop new strategies of coping that bring equilibrium back to his world (Hawkins & Gorvine, 1985). The length of the labor, the level of pain endured by his partner, the mechanism of birth, and the location of birth all affect the reaction a father has to the birth experience.

The experience of the father at birth may be a different one from that of the mother (Nolan, 1996). He must be a participant and an observer of the changes experienced by his partner. The early relationship of the father and his child and the father as parent with his partner in this new family constellation is significantly influenced by the emotional experience of birth (von Klitzing et al., 1996).

The experience of fathers is also influenced by attitudes of the health care providers who interact with him during the birth experience. Jordan (1990b) found that fathers predominantly felt treated as peripheral to the mother by health care professionals. Their needs were addressed only as they related to the woman. In this way, the man felt excluded from active participation in the birth. Inclusion of the father as an active participant in the support system and provision of care to the laboring woman significantly increased the father's investment in the labor and birth. Nurses working closely with the laboring couple have an unparalleled opportunity to assist the father in having a positive birth experience, which can bolster his self-concept and help him lay the foundation for effective coping as a parent.

Nursing Implications

When working with families, it is important for the nurse to understand the father/partner's role, which may be evidenced by his participation in the prenatal course and previous birth experiences. While interacting with the father, the nurse should observe his physical relationship to his partner (does he physically soothe her, massage her back, or sit by the bed without touching her?) and listen to his interaction with the laboring woman (does he coach her, encourage her, and share her experience?). His coping strategies and desire to hold or touch his newborn may also be indicative of his view of his new parental role. Positive adaptations may be seen in the father's identifying ways in addition to feeding that he can participate in the care of his newborn, and the father's participation in identifying childcare options.

Nursing interventions that can assist the father in developing a realistic interpretation of his birth experience might include: including the father in discussions about the decisions being made with the laboring woman, providing the father with explanations about what is happening, encouraging the father to cut the umbilical cord, and encouraging the father to hold the baby with the mother, to enfold both of them in his arms (Figure 27-4)

Sibling Adaptation

The participation of siblings in birth has a history similar to that of fathers. The acceptance of children in the birth setting has been influenced by social attitudes regarding children, economics, cultural beliefs, and the politics of birthing institutions.

In cultures in which extended families live in close proximity and pregnancy is an accepted developmental rite of passage, children are more likely to be a part of the group experience of birth. The presence of alternative caretakers, such as older children or other family members, and geography has dictated whether children were sent away from the home when birth occurred.

Developmental Issues

Children's perceptions of birth are limited by their developmental stage. Erickson's work describes the cognitive ability of children, which progresses from self-enteredness to other-centeredness and from fantasy to concrete thought and expression. At each of these stages of development, the child is increasingly able to focus on the events going on around him or her and to understand what is happening (Erickson, 1963).

Preschool children may not be attentive to the activities of the adults around them. In the birth setting, they may be focused on their dolls or toys, ignoring the adults

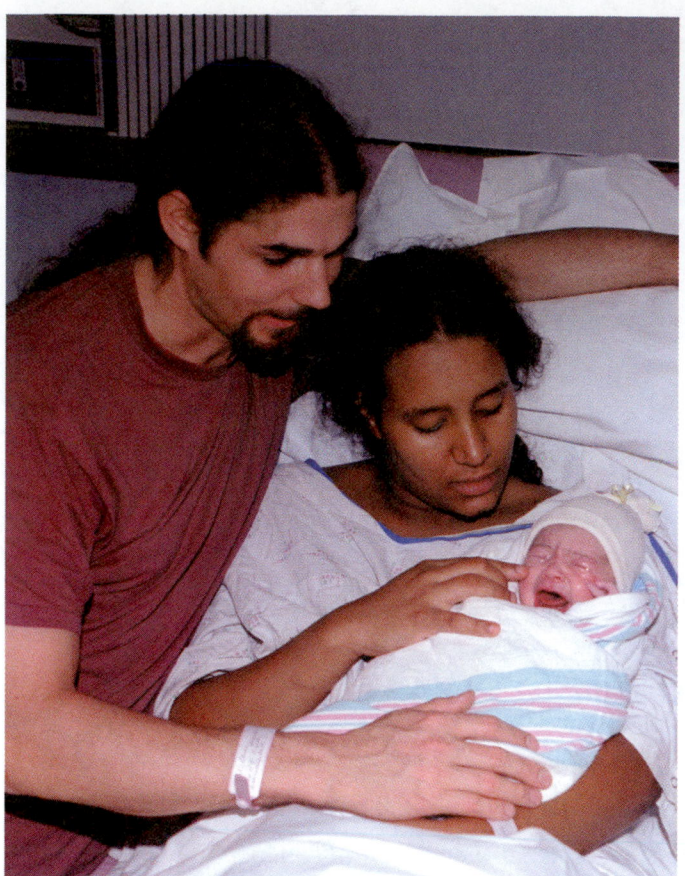

Figure 27-4 This father welcomes his daughter to the world by enfolding the mother and baby in his arms.

around them. School-aged children may be bothered by the noise of a birth setting. They may perceive their mothers' pain and, in some way, take responsibility for not being able to assuage it. Adolescents may be able to be supportive or may identify with the bodily functions inherent in the birth process and personalize the events (Erickson, 1963).

A mother's relationship with each child is different, changing with the addition of another child. The older children must alter their current relationship with mother and with each other to accommodate the new baby (Mercer, 1995). Therefore, children may perceive the birth as threatening and as invading their space and interfering with their relationships within the family. Alternatively, the new baby may be perceived as a welcome playmate. The child may not immediately understand the dependence of a newborn and may be excited to have a new friend.

The participation or attendance at birth of older children is determined on the basis of the dynamics of the individual family and institutional and provider policy. In families where the cultural norm is that children are peripheral to the adults until they become old enough to be

Nursing Alert

CHILDREN ATTENDING A BIRTH

If children are present during labor and delivery, one adult (other than professional staff) must be present for each child to provide safe and adequate supervision.

Nursing Tip

NURSING INTERVENTIONS THAT CAN ASSIST SIBLINGS AT BIRTH

- Providing simple factual explanations of events at the level of the child's understanding
- Answering questions posed by the children as simply and honestly as possible
- Orienting the children to the birth environment as early as possible before the intensity of the experience clouds their vision
- Allowing the children to move in and out of the birth environment at will
- Assuring that there is a competent adult present, other than the staff, whose only responsibility is to meet the needs of the children
- Encouraging the parents to interact with the children as much as possible so that the children see that the parents are safe
- Interacting with the child or children as much as possible
- Providing simple explanations to the children about procedures that they see their mother undergoing
- Creating a space for the child or children (perhaps at the head of the bed rather than at the foot of the bed) that allows them to interact with their mother but preserves her modesty
- Providing positive reinforcement for the decisions the child makes relative to his or her participation in the labor and birth and his or her response to the newborn

treated as adults, there may not be an issue: the children will not have the option to attend the birth. In families where the cultural norm is to include children in the dynamics of change, they may have been incorporated into the family experience of pregnancy and may be present for all or part of the birth. In some families, the adults want the children to be active participants; however, the children may be uninterested (Nolan, 1996).

The birth site has a major effect on the presence of siblings at birth and the level of their participation. At home in a familiar environment, children may move in and out of the birth room, interspersing normal activities with looking in on what is happening. Depending on the length of labor and the time of delivery, children may even sleep through the birth. In a birth center environment, children are usually accommodated as space allows and should be accompanied by an adult who is not involved with supporting the birthing woman. It is not possible to predict children's reactions to labor and birth, so it is essential that a responsible adult be available to meet their needs or even to remove them from the setting, if necessary.

In more traditional hospital birth settings, the children's presence is dictated by institutional and infection control policy. Most hospitals require some preparation for children who will attend a birth. This may take the form of a puppet show, a hospital tour, viewing a video, or attending a series of classes with parents. Parents are told of the need to be alert to health concerns, such as viral illnesses, that would prevent the older children's participation, and some institutions may require proof of health screening and up-to-date vaccination status of children who wish to attend.

Sometimes the opinion of the birth attendants or other professional staff dictates whether children can be present. Individual professionals may have personal feelings about children viewing birth. These feelings or opinions may or may not be theoretically supported. To address the effect that self-interest has in the politics of birth, health care providers must distinguish their own needs and opinions from those of the birthing family. This enables them to implement a plan of care that safely meets the needs of families and their children (Kuhn & Kopcinski, 1984; Brown, 1996).

Grandparent and Extended Family Adaptation

Adults view pregnancy, birth, and childrearing from the perspective of their own experience. "Birth baggage" refers to the feelings one has about one's own child birth experience. Included in this "baggage" are all the feelings about needs that were met or unmet. The expectations of birth held by grandparents are colored by the experiences they had during childbirth experiences. Many women were not afforded the opportunity to process their feelings about what happened during their own labor and delivery, for example, the pain they had or how helpless they may have felt (Figure 27-5). These unresolved feelings affect

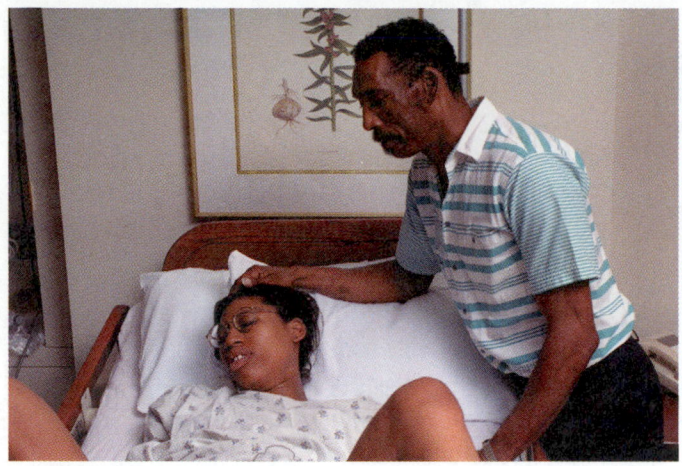

Figure 27-5 To help his daughter through her labor and delivery, this father, soon to be a grandfather, needed to be open-minded to the changes in practice that have occurred since his children were born.

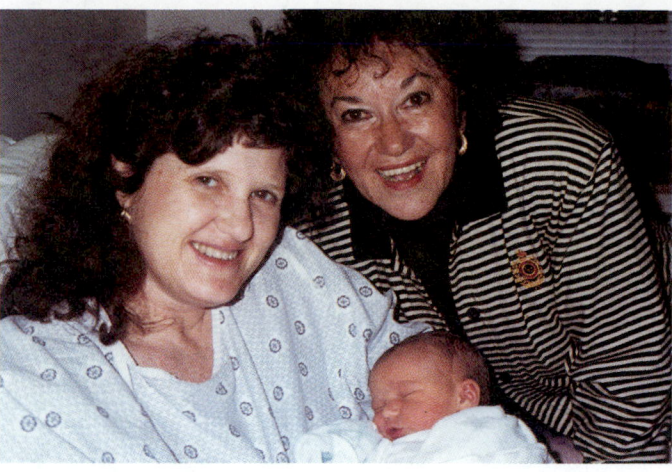

Figure 27-6 Birth: three generations.

the amount of energy available and the kind of support grandparents, siblings, aunts, and uncles can give to the birthing woman and her family (Simkin, 1996). A woman who was not given a choice about the use of medication may not understand her daughter's desire for an unmedicated delivery. A man who waited in the waiting room during the birth of his children may not understand the desire of his son to be present at delivery. Alternatively, extended family members who were not able to birth as they would have liked or who may, for example, have had emergency operative deliveries may be strongly supportive of the choices made by the birthing family.

Grandparents who have successfully negotiated the life stages preceding having children will be ready to view the birth as an addition to their own lives. Grandparents who have not completed the appropriate developmental tasks may not be ready to see themselves as "old enough to be grandparents." By the same token, aunts and uncles who are comfortable with their developmental stage in life will have a different response to the birth of a new generation than those who have not completed their own developmental work. "I'll be a great aunt but I am not a Great Aunt!" may be the response of a woman, present at the birth of her niece's child, who is not ready to view herself as a member of an older generation (Erickson, 1963).

Family members may be so overwhelmed by the experience of birth that they may have strong emotional reactions. The family's response to birth and their ability to provide positive reinforcement to the birthing woman is dependent on their usual coping styles (Figure 27-6). Birth provides an opportunity for families to develop more effective coping mechanisms (Hawkins & Gorvine, 1985).

The birthing woman, her partner, and the baby are the first responsibility of the nurse. The response of the family

to birth is a complex, multifaceted issue. "Birth baggage" or other experiences of individual family members may prevent them from bringing positive energy to the birth environment. While it is the mother who defines the family and dictates who is present at the birth, family members who are unable to be supportive or who are interfering with the mother's ability to cope with labor should be politely escorted to a waiting area.

Prolonged Labor and Assisted Delivery

Birth, by its very nature, is an unpredictable experience. Any deviation from expectations can leave the woman and her family feeling unfulfilled or detract from their feelings of confidence and wholeness. For the birthing woman, a prolonged labor may indicate to her that her body won't work correctly. A delivery assisted by forceps, vacuum, or episiotomy may place her in a position of loss of confidence in her body, loss of integrity of her body boundaries, or a sense of unfulfillment or of ineptitude (Hawkins & Gorvine, 1985).

For a partner, a prolonged labor and difficult delivery may challenge his or her self-concept as a protector. The persistent feeling of helplessness in the face of the events of birth can influence the partner's response to the newborn. A partner who feels guilty about not protecting the woman from the difficulties of the birth may experience anger or frustration. The nurse is in a pivotal position to help partners come to terms with their feelings of disappointment and frustration and to avoid displacing these feelings on each other. By using communication skills to engage partners in a discussion about the experience and validating their frustrations and fears, the nurse can guide

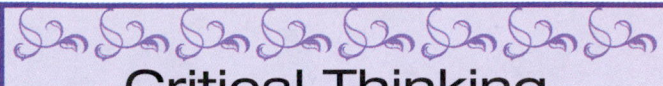

Critical Thinking

A New Mother

J.L. is a 21-year-old primapara single woman who has just given birth to an 8-lb baby boy. Her pregnancy was obstetrically uncomplicated. However, her social situation was not stable during the last trimester. Her partner, the baby's father, moved to another state and refused to communicate with her; she moved in with her parents, who have been supportive of the pregnancy and her decision to continue as a single parent. Her parents accompanied her in labor; her mother was her primary support person. Because she had an uncomplicated labor and birth, J.L. will be discharged from the hospital after 48 hours.

Discuss appropriate nursing assessments that will indicate the level of risk that J.L. has for difficulty in adjusting to her role as a mother.

What are the strengths of this situation that will ultimately assist J.L. in adjusting to her role as a new mother?

How can you assess the response of the grandparents to the birth of their grandson?

What are two immediate and two long-term interventions that you can implement to assist this family?

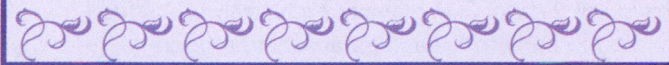

the partners to an understanding of their response and channel that energy in to positive activities to assist the new mother, such as breastfeeding support.

Cesarean Delivery

Cesarean delivery may be perceived as the ultimate inability of the woman's body to perform the normal function of giving birth. Not only did her body fail to deliver normally, but she also loses the integrity of other body systems for varying lengths of time. A cesarean birth means that the woman's motor system is temporarily impaired; her mobility is affected by anesthesia, pain, and the presence of intravenous lines or drains; her systems of elimination are altered as she recovers from Foley catheterization and decreased bowel motility; and the pain of the childbirth experience continues for a longer period of time than anticipated, as incisional pain and the discomforts of postoperative exercises (Hawkins & Gorvine, 1985).

DiMatteo, Morton, Lepper, Damush, Carney, Person, & Kahn (1996) reviewed research describing early and long-term sequelae of the cesarean birth experience for women. Women delivered by cesarean section held their

babies later after delivery than those who delivered vaginally; however, they held them for a longer period of time. Women delivering by cesarean felt less satisfied with their birth experience than those delivered vaginally, and initially, cesarean-birth mothers viewed their babies in a less positive light.

Response of the At-Risk Family

DeMeir, Hynan, Harris, and Manniello (1996) evaluated the incidence of posttraumatic stress disorder (PTSD) in mothers who experienced a high-risk birth. Using six measures of perinatal stressors, which included (1) gestational age of the baby, (2) birth weight, (3) length of hospital stay for the baby, (4) a postnatal complication rating for the infant, and (5) and (6) Apgar scores at 1 and 5 minutes, they predicted the occurrence of PTSD. The authors found that mothers of premature and term infants who required neonatal intensive care reported significantly more symptoms of PTSD than mothers of term infants who were born without stress factors present. The researchers found that the difficult birth experience left scars within the woman's psyche, which affected them and their coping abilities for many years (DiMatteo et al., 1996). This profound affect on the mother's life is consistent with long-term memory of birth experiences that Simkin perceived in her interviews with women (Simkin, 1996).

Older children in a family that has experienced a difficult birth may blame themselves for interfering or causing the problem. How a child perceives the events surrounding a difficult birth depends on age and developmental stage (Erickson, 1963). Feelings may range from exclusion if they planned to participate and could not, to fear for the life of their mother as they observed her in pain and the reactions of other adults around her.

The extended family fears for the safety of both the mother and the baby. Maternal grandparents fear for their daughter and her infant. They may feel guilt for nonsupport or the level of support they gave their child. The experience may seem to confirm their fears that their child isn't normal and that there is some undiagnosed reason that she is not able to birth normally, for which they are responsible. They may feel they did not do enough. Alternatively, they may be angry with the partner or obstetric professionals for not protecting their daughter from harm or illness.

The family reaction to a difficult birth experience also has implications for the relationship each member has with the new infant. In a family where the infant is blamed for the pain or the type of delivery, the infant is potentially at risk for neglect or abuse, such an infant is termed a "vulnerable infant." DeMier and colleagues (1996) found parental hypervigilance to be sequelae, both in the immediate postnatal

Case Study/Care Plan

A GROWING FAMILY

G.P. is gravida 3, para 3 (G3, P3), a Native American woman who has delivered at the New Market Birth Center and is now 2 hours postpartum.

After a 15-hour labor and without the use of medications, Dahlia Louise was born over an intact perineum, weighing 8 pounds, with an Apgar score of 9 at 1 and 5 minutes. The baby breathed spontaneously and was delivered onto the mother's abdomen. M.P., the father, was present, providing labor support throughout, and cut the umbilical cord. During the labor and birth, specially recorded taped music was played; the family explained to the nurse that the pieces were special spiritual songs that promoted peacefulness and inner strength.

Also present during labor and for the birth were both sets of grandparents; Marc, the couple's 8-year-old son; and Jean, the couple's 4-year-old daughter.

During the labor and birth, Jean slept, colored, and roamed around the center, appearing unconcerned with the events in the birth room. Marc was actively involved, giving his mother ice chips and timing contractions, while his father provided physical support. The grandparents alternated sitting in the family room, visiting and observing activities in the birth room, and going out for provisions. Much of their conversation was about the changes in birth practices and worries about the safety of out-of-hospital birth. After the birth, they gathered in the birth room, cooing over the baby and praising G.P. and M.P. for their accomplishment.

Postpartum assessments have been within normal limits. The midwife has done a newborn examination that yielded results that were within normal limits. The mother has been to the bathroom and eaten. The baby has had a stool and passed urine.

The family plans to leave the birth center at 12 hours postpartum to return home. They live in a single-family dwelling with two flights of stairs. M.P. has to return to work in 2 days. G.P. plans to exclusively breastfeed her baby, as she did her first two children, and has already put the baby to breast, establishing a good latch-on. G.P. plans to return to work in 6 weeks and to place the infant in daycare with her 4-year-old daughter.

Assessment

- No contributory medical or surgical history
- Pregnancy at term without complications
- Postpartum recovery without complication
- Newborn examination (within normal limits), baby has passed urine and meconium
- Multiparous family, apparently prepared for the birth experience and comfortable with participation from all members, each member having a proscribed role
- Family does not have a plan for support after discharge

Nursing Diagnosis

Interrupted family processes related to the birth experience

(continued)

period and on a continuing basis as a parenting style on the part of women who experienced a high-risk birth. Some families may become overprotective of the infant in an attempt to shield them from further trauma.

Identification of negative responses to the mother or child in the birth setting may be the first sign of risk to the infant for neglect or abuse. In families in which the mother is not be the primary caretaker, for example, if the mother is a single adolescent, the nurse must include the grandmother, or other identified primary caretaker, in the birth experience. This provides an opportunity for the person to bond with the infant and for the nurse to observe the response and interaction of the birth mother, infant, and primary caretaker. If inappropriate behavior is identified, early referral and intervention can be accomplished, reducing the risk to the infant.

Expected Outcomes	1. The client and family will validate their experiences during labor and birth. 2. The family will develop support strategies, using community and family support systems. 3. Before leaving the birth center, G.P. will discuss specific strategies that she can employ to help her organize life at home to reduce stress. 4. The client and family will discuss the warning signs of postpartum depression. 5. At 3 days and 1 week postpartum, the family will not exhibit signs of dysfunction related to the birth experience.
Planning	The nurse can include the family and siblings in planning care that will reflect the needs of the family as a whole.

Nursing Interventions	Rationales
1. The nurse will encourage the individual members of the family to talk about how they felt during the labor and birth.	1. At this time, the nurse will validate feelings and provide accurate information about events.
2. The nurse will provide referrals to home visiting nursing services for intervals at 24 hours postdischarge and 3 days postpartum to assess the mother, newborn, and family adjustment. The nurse will also provide a pediatric referral to the pediatrician of the mother's choice of 48 hours postpartum for newborn assessment and relevant testing.	2. This assists the family in identifying community resources, such as church, to enlist in providing postpartum support services.
3. The nurse will discuss specific options, such as the NURSE program, to help the client manage stress.	3. These strategies offer resources to the client to learn how to manage stress.
4. The nurse will discuss the specifics of the signs of postpartum depression.	4. This helps the client become independent and assists the family in recognizing symptoms that should be addressed.
5. The nurse will make follow-up phone calls to the client at 3 days and 1 week postpartum and document the success of the care plan for this family or identify problems needing resolution.	5. To assess family adjustment and offer assistance if needed.

Evaluation	Family adjustment is facilitated by actions of the nurse that foster maternal self-confidence and family support. By beginning with validation of the birth experience, the nurse can identify feelings of satisfaction or dissatisfaction and congruence or dissonance with actual events. Helping the family put the experience in perspective before they leave the birth site is a preventive measure. Assisting the family to identify and develop support systems after discharge is preventive and supportive. Evaluating the family at proscribed intervals allows the nurse to address developing issues before they lead to dysfunction.

RESPONSE TO LOSS AT BIRTH

Loss of an infant at birth can be viewed from several perspectives. One is the incongruity of the experience with the expectations of the parents: the loss, so to speak, of the perfect baby. The stillbirth of a fetus is another type of loss, which is discussed in detail in chapter 37. Finally, the birth of an infant that is to be relinquished, either to adoption or because the woman cannot keep the child (for example, an incarcerated mother) is a different type of loss.

Any type of loss engenders a process of grieving in the parents and family. The value placed on the pregnancy and the newborn influences the depth and intensity of the emotions. The intensity of loss felt in the family who has labored through the process of infertility treatment may be stronger and more prolonged because they are forced to deal with the emotional rollercoaster of assisted fertility (Woods & Esposito-Woods, 1997).

Kübler-Ross (1969) identified stages of grieving, through which individuals move, as they try to come to terms with death and loss. These include denial that the event has occurred; anger directed at anyone deemed responsible, including self, God, the midwife or doctor; the hospital, other family members; bargaining by trying to find alternatives to accepting the reality of the event; resolution to the facts; and, finally, acceptance. In the birth setting, the most likely stages that the nurse sees and assists the family with are anger, denial, and bargaining. The entire process can take days, months, years, or, for some families, remain forever unresolved.

Birth mothers and fathers fantasize about what their baby will look like and how it will act. This is a way of rehearsing for parenthood (Rubin, 1984; Lederman, 1984). The newborn they meet at birth, while not an imperfect baby, will not look like the baby of their fantasies. It is necessary for the parents to give up and grieve for the imagined perfect baby and move into acceptance of the real baby, wrinkled and covered with vernix. This happens quite quickly. So quickly, in fact, that the nurse may miss the cues that may be present during transition of labor or the second stage, such as the mother saying that she cannot push or holding her legs tightly together. Once she is able to hold the infant, validating the number of fingers and toes and the resemblance to her partner or to other family members are ways of coming to accept the newborn.

Even after an uncomplicated birth experience, a woman may grieve the loss of the fetus as a part of her body. For 9 months, the fetus was a part of her body space. She may grieve the loss of that sensation similarly to the loss of an appendage, even as she is joyful in embracing her newborn (Rubin, 1984).

Loss Through Adoption

In some instances of open adoption, adoptive parents develop a relationship with the birth mother or parents. In these cases, the birth experience may be shared with the adoptive parents. Even in a normal, uncomplicated birth, the nurse is working with two families in flux, one experiencing the joy of expansion, the other perhaps a combination of relief and grief. Assessment of each family and their coping mechanisms is a challenge for the nurse. Immediate strategies to incorporate both sets of parents in the birth room may include bringing the adoptive mother to the bedside of the birth mother and encouraging them to initially hold the baby together and gradually encouraging the birth mother to move the infant into the arms of the adoptive mother. Allowing the birth mother to express her feelings, perhaps by crying, with acceptance and support may occur simultaneously with the adoptive mother's joyful tears.

One area that has not been written about in great detail is the loss felt by parents who relinquish their birth child. Fathers in particular are left out of the literature. Deykin, Patti, and Ryan (1988) interviewed 125 birth fathers about their feelings about relinquishing the child to adoptive parents. Loss of the child continued to be an unresolved issue of grieving for the fathers many years later. Menard (1997) looked at the role of the birth father who is relinquishing his child in a perinatal setting from the perspective of the social services. There is a delicate balance that must be kept to address the needs of the father in this situation, along with the needs and rights of the mother, the child, and the adoptive family. Nurses as care providers in the birth setting are in a pivotal position to help birth fathers and mothers own the decisions they have made and develop coping strategies. Additional investigation should be done in this area to enable nurses in the birth setting to develop appropriate interventions for families that are relinquishing their newborns.

Loss Through Special Circumstances

An unusual situation for the nurse to encounter is one in which the birth mother is relinquishing her child to another family or foster care because she is incarcerated. A woman who is pregnant when arrested for committing a crime or who is pregnant when sentenced will not, in most instances, be able to stay with her newborn after birth. In a few prisons, such as Bedford Hills Correctional Facility in Bedford Hills, New York, programs have been developed for pregnant and parenting prisoners (Felter-Wernsdorfer, Nass, & Weingrad-Smith, 2000). However, for the majority of incarcerated women, within days or hours after birth, they will have to relinquish their baby to someone else's care and be separated from their newborn for extended periods of time. Whatever their crime, a woman relinquishing her child right after birth will grieve and exhibit behaviors related to sadness and loss (Wismont, 2000).

Response of Health Care Professionals

The professional and institutional response to loss at birth has changed dramatically over the years. Historically, in an effort to "spare" the mother and parents, women were anesthetized for delivery and stillborn babies were whisked out of sight. Infants slated for adoption were removed from the delivery room quickly to protect the mother from seeing or hearing the child and feeling the sadness of her decision. Today most institutions have perinatal grief teams, which are specially developed teams of nurses, social workers, and others who are available to assist families and staff with the issues of grieving. Rather than trying to brush the experience away, we know today that it is necessary for families to come to closure with the loss of the baby to develop effective coping strategies for continuing their lives.

Web Activities

- Visit the websites listed in the Resources. What information is offered on assisting new families through the adaptation process when a new member is born?

- Locate Internet sources designed for families who are losing a child to adoption or because of incarceration of the parent.

Key Concepts

- Nursing care of the birthing woman and her family is based on an understanding of the theoretical framework of the family's response to birth.

- Appreciating the history and development of family participation in birth helps the nurse assess and plan for individual needs of families.

- A family's response to birth reflects their culture, belief system, and style of coping with changing life circumstances.

- Birth is a crisis, or turning point, in life that challenges the family to adapt their lifestyle coping mechanisms. This is an unprecedented time, during which the nurse has the opportunity to assist the family in moving into a new stage.

- Appropriate nursing interventions may be developed only after careful assessment of the individual family member's developmental stage and coping ability.

- An understanding and acceptance of the nurse's personal experience and response to both the birth experience, and the loss of an infant at birth help assure that these issues do not interfere with the nurse's ability to meet the needs of the client and family.

Review Questions and Activities

1. Describe Reva Rubin's theory of maternal response to birth.

2. Define birth as a "crisis," or turning point, for families.

3. Discuss the impact of birth on the father, siblings, and grandparents.

4. Go to a hospital that has a "grief team." Describe the organization of the team and the roles of the different members. What role do nurses play? What are the specific activities the team engages in that assist the woman and her family? What follow-up is provided by the team to the families?

5. Discuss how personal unresolved feelings that a nurse may have about birth can interfere with his or her ability to assist the family in reaching their goals for birth.

6. List three specific areas for nursing research regarding a family's immediate response to birth.

7. What are the potential implications for a female infant if the parents were invested in the sex of their child being male?

8. In what specific ways can a normal, uncomplicated birth be an empowering experience for the woman, her partner, and her family?

9. Discuss the implications of the birth experience for older children. List nursing interventions that can assist children in appreciating the experience.

10. Define "couvade" and discuss modern rituals that fathers may go through during the birth experience.

References

Belsky, J., & Kelly, J. (1994). *The transition to parenthood.* NY, NY: Bantam Doubleday Dell.

Brown, C. (1996). Freedom of choice: An expression of emerging power relationships between a childbearing woman and her caregiver. *International Journal of Childbirth Education, 11,* (3), 12–16.

Clinton, J. F., & Kelber, S. T. (1993). Stress and coping in fathers of newborns: Comparisons of planned versus unplanned pregnancy. *International Journal of Nursing Studies, 30,* (5), 437–43.

Cox, M. J., & Paley, B. (1997). Families as systems. *Annual Review of Psychology, 48,* 243–267.

Cross, T., Bazron, B., Dennis, K., & Isaacs, M. (1989). Towards a culturally competent system of care: Vol I. Washington, DC: *National Technical Assistance Center for Children's Mental Health.* Georgetown University Child Development Center.

Deimer, G. A. (1997). Expectant fathers: influence of perinatal education on stress, coping, and spousal relations. *Research in Nursing & Health, 20,* (4), 281–293.

DeMier, R., Hynan, M., Harris, H., & Manniello, R. (1996). Perinatal stressors as predictors of symptoms of posttraumatic stress in mothers of infants at high risk." *Journal of Perinatology, 16,* (4), 276–280.

DeVries, R., Wrede, S., van Teijlingen, E., & Benoit, C. (Eds.) (2001). *Birth by design.* New York: Routledge.

Deykin, E. Y., Patti, P., & Ryan, J. (1988). Fathers of adopted children: A study of the impact of child surrender on birthfathers. *American Journal of Orthopsychiatry, 58,* (2): 240–248.

DiMatteo, M. R., Morton, S., Lepper, H., Damush, T., Carney, M., Person, M., & Kahn, K. (1996). Cesarean childbirth and psychosocial outcomes: A meta-analysis. *Health Psychology, 15,* (4), 303–314.

Duncan, D. (1995). Fathers have feelings, too. *Modern Midwife, 5,* (1), 30.

Elkind, D. (1994). *Ties that stress: The new family imbalance.* Cambridge, MA: Harvard University Press.

Erickson, E. (1963). *Childhood and society,* 2nd ed. NY, NY: W.W. Norton & Co.

Esposito, N. (1999) Marginalized women's comparisons of their hospital and freestanding birth center experiences: A contrast of inner-city birthing systems. *Health Care for Women International, 20,* 111–126.

Felter-Wernsdorfer, R., Nass, J., & Weingrad-Smith, J. (2000) Educational experience in a correctional facility. *Journal of Midwifery and Women's Health, 45,* (4), 314–317.

Fowles, E. (1998). Labor concerns of women two months after delivery. *Birth, 25,* (4), 235–240.

Hall, E. O. (1995). From fun and excitement to joy and trouble— An explorative study of three Danish fathers' experiences around birth. *Scandinavian Journal of Caring Sciences, 9,* (3), 171–179.

Hawkins, J., & Gorvine, B. (1985), *Post partum nursing: Health care of women.* NY, NY: Springer.

Heggenhougen, H. K. (1980). Father and childbirth: an anthropological perspective. *Journal of Nurse Midwifery, 25,* (6), 21–26.

Hodnett, E. D. Support from caregivers during childbirth. In: Neilson, J. P., Crowther, C. A., Hodnett, E. D., Hofmeyr, G. J.,

Keirse, M. J. N. C. (Eds.). *Pregnancy and childbirth module of the Cochrane database of systematic reviews.* Issue 2.

Jordan, P. (1990a). Laboring for relevance: Expectant and new fatherhood. *Nursing Research, 39,* (1), 11–16.

Jordan, P. (1990b), First-time expectant fatherhood: nursing care considerations. *NAACOGS Clinical Issues in Perinatal & Womens Health Nursing, 1,* (3), 311–316.

Katz-Rothman, B. (1996). Women, providers, and control. *JOGNN, 25,* 253–256.

Kübler-Ross, E. (1969). On death and dying. NY, NY: Macmillan.

Kuhn, J., & Kopcinski, E. (1984). Siblings at birth: Professional philosophy and preparations. *Health Care for Women International, 5,* (4), 223–232.

Lederman, R. P. (1984). Psychosocial adaptaton in pregnancy: Assessment of seven dimensions of maternal development. NJ: Prentice-Hall.

Maushart, S. (1999). *The mask of motherhood: How becoming a mother changes everything and why we pretend it doesn't.* NY, NY: W.W. Norton & Company.

Menard, B. J. (1997). A birth father and adoption in the perinatal setting. *Social Work in Health Care, 24,* (3/4), 153–163.

Mercer, R. T. (1995). *Becoming a mother: research on maternal role identity from Rubin to the present.* Springer Series: Focus on Women. NY: Springer.

Nichols, F. Humenick, S. (2000). *Childbirth education: Practice, research, and theory.* NY, NY: Harcourt Health Sciences.

Nolan, M. (1996). The birth of Natasha—one labour: Two very different experiences. *Modern Midwife, 6,* (2), 6–9.

Palkovitz, R. (1987). Fathers' motives for birth attendance. *Maternal-Child Nursing Journal, 16,* (2), 123–129.

Patterson, J. M. (1999). Healthy american families in a postmodern society: An ecological perspective. In Wallace, H., Green, G., Jaeos, K., Paine, L., & Story, M. (1999). *Health and welfare for families in the 21st century.* Sudbury, MA: Jones & Bartlett.

Proctor, S. (1998). What determines quality in maternity care? Comparing the perceptions of childbearing women and midwives. *Birth, 25,* (2), 85–93.

Pryia, J. V. (2000). Birth traditions and modern pregnancy. In Nichols F., & Humenick S. (2000). *Childbirth education: Practice, research and theory.* NY, NY: Harcourt Health Sciences.

Rubin, R., (1984). Maternal identity and the maternal experience. NY, NY: Springer.

Scott, K., Berkowitz, G., & Klaus, M. (1999). A comparison of intermittent and continuous support during labor: A meta-analysis. *American Journal of Obstetrics and Gynecology, 180:* 1054.

Scott, K., Klaus, P., & Klaus, M. (1999). Obstetrical and postpartum benefits of continuous support during childbirth. *Journal of Women's Health and Gender-Based Medicine, 8,* (10), 1257–1264.

Sichel, D., & Watson-Driscoll, J. (1999). Women's moods. NY, NY: William Morrow.

Simkin, P. (1996). The experience of maternity in a woman's life. *JOGNN, 25,* 247–252.

Teichman, Y., & Lahav, Y. (1987). Expectant fathers: Emotional reactions, physical symptoms and coping styles. *British Journal of Medical Psychology, 60,* (Pt 3): 225–232.

Tomlinson, P. S., Rothenberg, M. A., & Carver, L. D. (1991). Behavioral interaction of fathers with infants and mothers in the immediate post partum period. *Journal of Nurse Midwifery, 36,* (4), 232–239.

Von Klitzing, K., Amsler, F., Schleske, G., Simoni, H., & Burgin, D. (1996). Effect of psychological factors in pregnancy on the development of parent-child relations. 2. Transition from prenatal to postnatal phase. *Gynakologisch-Geburtshilfliche Rundschau, 36,* (3), 149–155.

Wallace, H., Green, G., Jaros, K., Paine, L., & Story, M. (1999). *Health and welfare for families in the 21st century.* Jones and Bartlett Sudbury, MA.

Wismont, J. (2000). The lived pregnancy experience of women in prison. *Journal of Midwifery and Women's Health, 45,* (4), 292–300.

Woods, J., & Esposito-Woods, J. (1997). *Loss during pregnancy or in the newborn period: Principles of care with clinical cases and analyses.* Pitman, NJ: Jannetti.

Resources

American College of Nurse-Midwives, 818 Connecticut Avenue NW, Suite 900, Washington, DC 20006, Phone: (202) 728-9860, Fax: (202) 728-9897, info@acnm.org, www.midwife.org

Association of Women's Health, Obstetric, and Neonatal Nurses, (AWHONN), 2000 I, St. NW Suite 740, Washington, DC 20036, Phone: (800) 637-8499, www.awhonn.org

March of Dimes, Education Services, 1275 Mamaroneck Avenue, White Plains, NY 10605, Phone: (888) MODIMES, www.modimes.org

National Center for Education in Maternal and Child Health, 2000 15th St North, Suite 701, Arlington, VA 22201-2617, Phone: (703) 524-7802, www.ncemch.org

National Maternal and Child Health Clearinghouse, Sponsored by DHHS Health Resources Administration, Phone: (888) 434-4MCH, www.nmchc.org

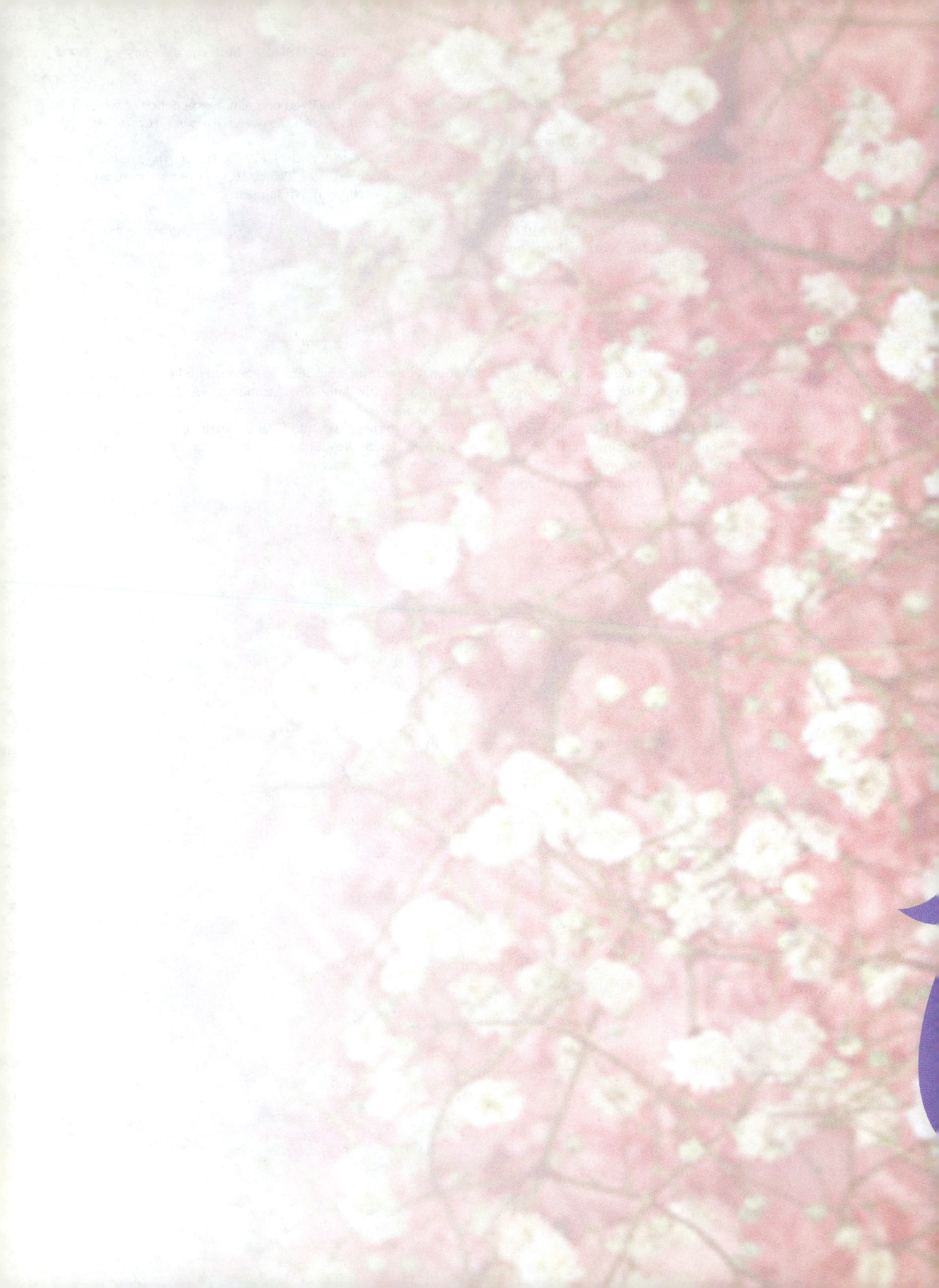

UNIT VII

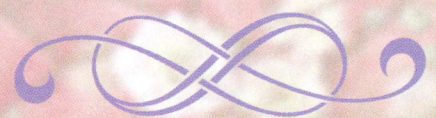

Postpartum Health and Nursing Care

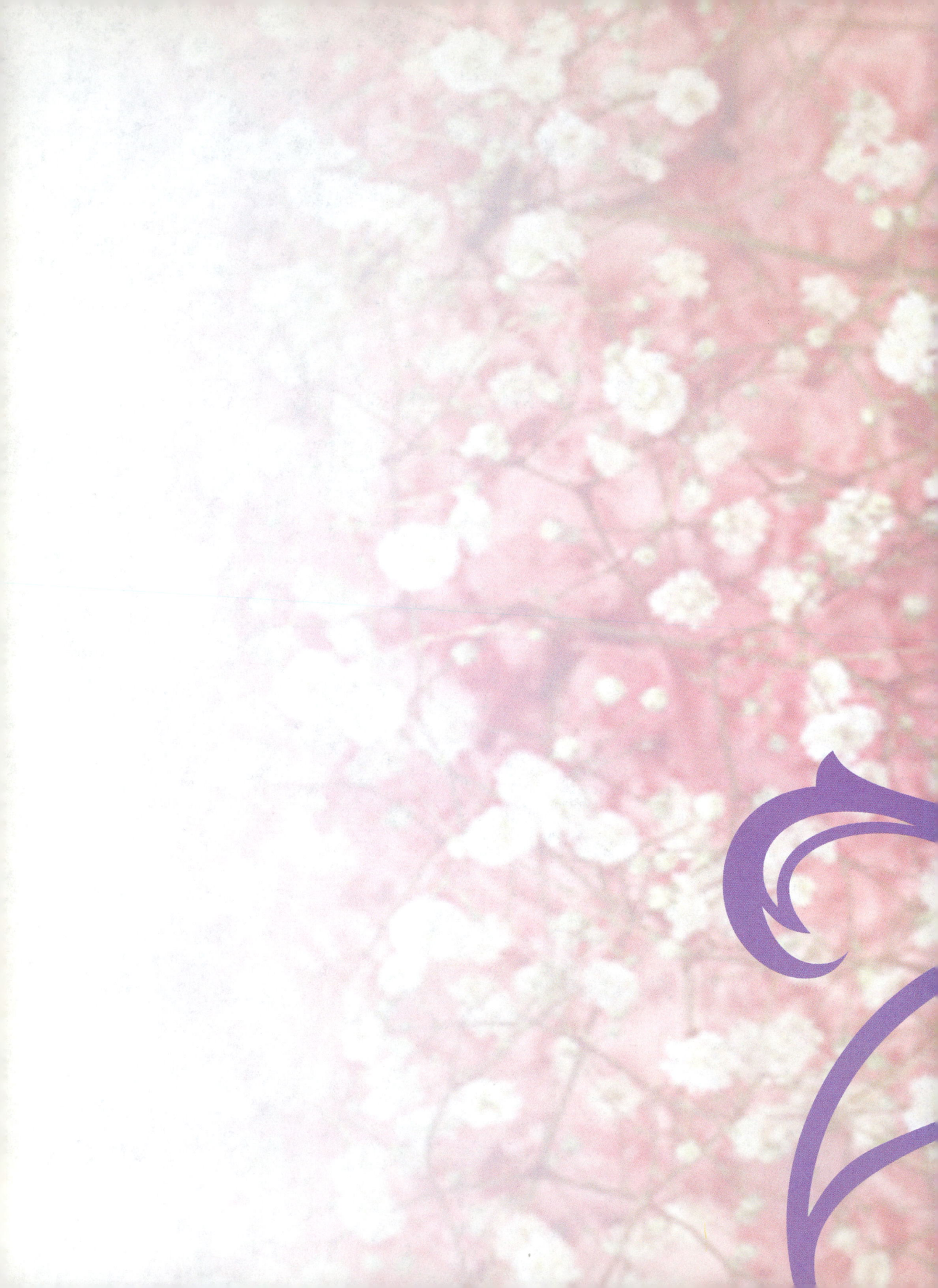

CHAPTER 28

Normal Postpartum Nursing Care

*I*n today's society, many women place great importance on body image and thinness. Immediately after delivery, the postpartum woman may be shocked and discouraged when she discovers her body appears "as if she were still pregnant." Use the following questions to assist the new mother in sorting through her personal feelings:

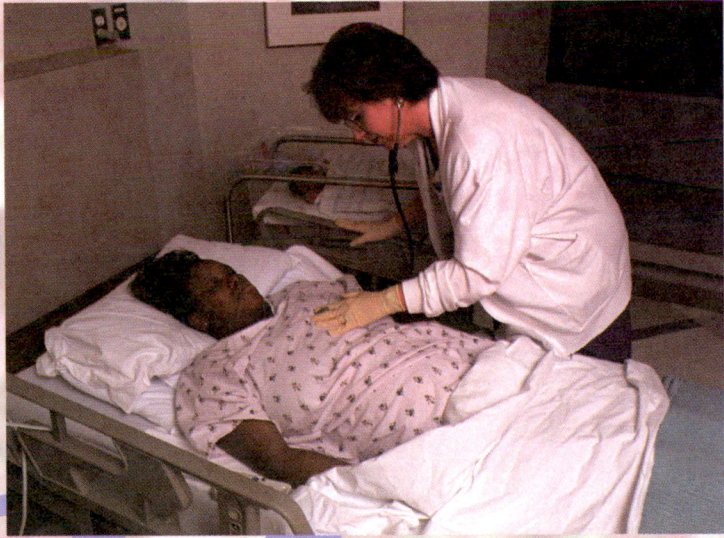

- *How do you feel about your delivery?*
- *How does your body feel?*
- *How do you feel about the shape of your abdomen?*
- *What do you think about still fitting into the clothing you wore during pregnancy?*
- *Are you interested in learning about postpartum exercises?*
- *What are your plans to get back to your prepregnancy figure?*

Key Terms

Afterpains	Engorgement	Lochia	Puerperium
Atony	Episiotomy	Mastitis	Residual urine
Boggy	Fundus	Puerpera	Striae
Diastasis recti	Involution	Puerperal sepsis	Subinvolution
Endometritis			

Competencies

Upon completion of this chapter, the reader should be able to:

1. Define the key terms.
2. Determine a systematic, logical approach to postpartum assessment.
3. Identify the expected values and clinical assessments to be evaluated in the care of the woman postpartally.
4. Summarize the systemic physiologic changes women experience after childbirth.
5. Identify and describe appropriate nursing interventions for the woman postpartally.

The puerperium, or the postpartum period (fourth trimester), lasts from delivery of the placenta to approximately 6 weeks afterward. During the postpartum period, the woman is referred to as the **puerpera**. The immediate postpartum period consists of the first 24 hours after delivery. The early postpartum period lasts from the second day after birth to the end of the first week. The postpartum period continues until 6 weeks postpartum.

The obstetric nurse will see the pregnant client experience various physiologic and psychosocial changes when she makes the transition from a pregnant woman to a mother on delivery. Postpartum nursing care often is considered routine; however, it encompasses a wide range of nursing care that includes psychological and physiologic assessment and intervention and provision of infant care.

The needs of the client and her family in the postpartum period can best be met through coordinated multidisciplinary care. Physicians, midwives, nurses, social workers, lactation consultants, and others must ensure that clients receive the services they need. The responsibilities of the obstetric nurse in caring for the client postpartally include being able to make relevant assessments, plan and implement a family-centered plan of care, and evaluate the effectiveness of her care. The nurse also has the potential to significantly affect the client's postpartum health by presenting self-care and infant care education, preparing for hospital discharge, and providing follow-up for the mother and infant.

POSTPARTUM CARE

The birth of a child most often is a joyous occasion for the family. Unless complications occur the father or significant other and other supportive family members and friends should be encouraged to remain with the mother and infant after birth. Interaction between the family and infant should be facilitated by encouraging members to hold the infant and point out special physical characteristics. If the mother is not breast-feeding, the father or other siblings may provide infant feedings. The bonding or family-infant interaction provides an initial introduction to each other.

Mother-Baby Nursing

The postpartum nurse may need to be prepared to care for both the mother and her infant. Some hospitals continue to offer a traditional postpartum unit and separate nursery. In this type of setting the postpartum nurse is responsible for caring for the mother, whereas another nurse cares for the infant. Many facilities (i.e., birth centers) have now transitioned to family-centered maternity care (FCMC) in which the nursing philosophy is based on the concept of mother-baby nursing or couplet care (Phillips, 1997). The approach to care in this nursing strategy is based on the family being the primary caregivers. The mother's well-being is interdependent with that of her newborn as they adjust to multiple physical, cognitive, and psychosocial changes during the postpartum period (Box 28-1). One team of health care providers (e.g., a nurse and technician

Box 28-1 Practicing Mother-Baby Nursing

The benefits of mother-baby nursing for the family and newborn include the following:

- Facilitating earlier establishment of biologic rhythms with flexible feeding and sleeping cycles.
- Fostering breast-feeding.
- Decreasing the incidence of cross-infection.
- Providing individualized, one-on-one care.
- Promoting the mother's role and attachment.
- Increasing educational opportunities.
- Fostering continuity of care and reduction of confusion of messages between caregivers.
- Promoting the mother's learning about her newborn and self-care capabilities.
- Increasing maternal self-confidence in caring for her newborn.
- Eliminating anxiety about whether the newborn is properly cared for.

The benefits of mother-baby nursing for the nursing staff include the following:

- Streamlining responsibilities of care and teaching.
- Increasing nursing involvement and responsibility for patient care and learning.
- Increasing accountability.
- Improving communication between the family and caregivers.
- Replacing fragmented care with continuity of care.
- Eliminating duplication of services.
- Facilitating discharge planning.
- Increasing efficiency and productivity.
- Improving teamwork and interdisciplinary communication.
- Increasing job satisfaction through the provision of individualized care, a more stimulating work environment, and positive feedback from families.

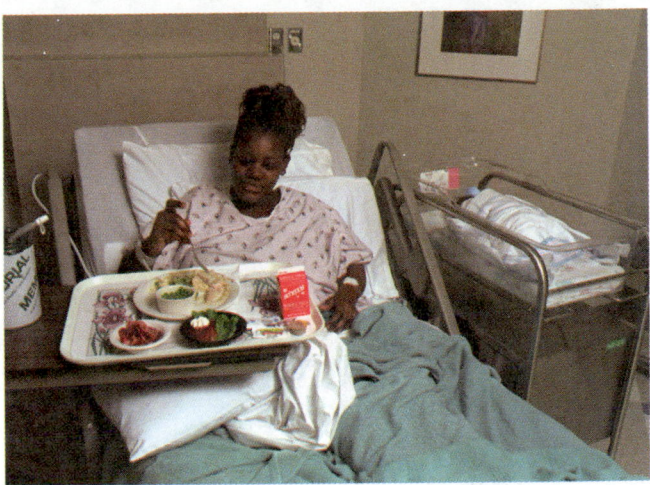

Figure 28-1 The practice of rooming-in allows mother and baby to be together throughout the day.

role of the "mother-baby nurse" involves early parent-infant interaction, demand feeding, flexible care schedules, personalized parenting education, and family visitation.

In addition to mother-baby nursing, there is a separate concept of rooming-in, whereby the infant remaining in the mother's room at her bedside is permitted and encouraged (Figure 28-1). The infant rooms in with the mother unless medically contraindicated or the mother is unable to care for her infant owing to medical problems or emotional difficulties.

Infant Security

An important aspect of postpartum care is infant security. Cases of infant abduction have directed hospitals to institute infant safety and security systems. The nursing staff must be alert and educate mothers and families about proper security and identification processes (Figure 28-2). The nurse should always check the identification bands on both the mother and infant when providing care.

Hospital Length of Stay

The usual hospital length of stay for mothers having normal vaginal delivery is 24 to 48 hours. Some hospitals, along with third-party insurance companies, previously dictated early discharge without consideration of the mother's needs. Today, the mother and newborn are protected in regard to the length of hospital stay after childbirth based on the Newborns' and Mothers' Health Protection Act of 1996. Under this federal law, third-party insurance companies cannot restrict benefits for hospital stays in connection with childbirth to less than 48 hours after a vaginal delivery and 96 hours after a cesarean delivery. The attending provider is permitted to discharge the

or aide) cares for both the mother and her newborn as a unit, viewing them as an interdependent couplet.

A gradual shift has occurred from the nurse providing all the newborn care while the mother watches, to the mother independently caring for her newborn. Education about self-care and newborn care is integrated during the nurse's daily physical care for the couplet. The expanded

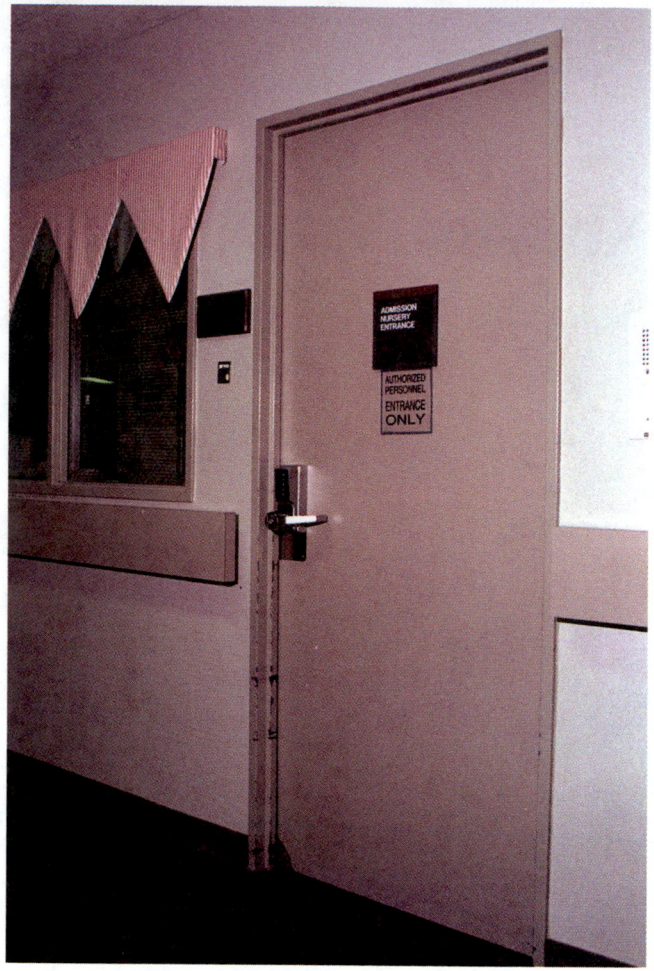

Figure 28-2 Security measures in the postpartum unit and nursery always are in force.

client earlier if the client agrees. The 48-hour period begins at the time of delivery. If the mother delivers outside the hospital and is later admitted, the period begins at the time of admission. The newborn's 48-hour length of stay is independent of the mother's hospital stay.

Thus, the Health Protection Act impacts the way health care is delivered. Compared with years ago, mothers now have less time to recover from the birth process while under professional supervision. Nurses, in turn, have less time to ensure that new mothers are physiologically stable, able to safely provide care for themselves and their new infants, and able to assume the responsibilities of motherhood. Because the purposes of hospitalization after birth are to (1) identify maternal and neonatal complications and (2) provide professional assistance at a time when the mother is likely to need supportive care (American Academy of Pediatrics [AAP] & American College of Obstetricians and Gynecologists [ACOG], 1997), it is essential that the postpartum nurse effectively completes the nursing process to successfully attain an optimal outcome.

Critical Thinking

Practicing Family-Centered Maternity Care

Progressive new hospitals have transitioned obstetric services to offering family-centered maternity care (FCMC) (Phillips, 1997). This style of care philosophizes that health includes not only physical dimensions but social, spiritual, psychological, and economic dimensions as well (in comparison with the more traditional model in which the health care professional has a paternalistic attitude about what families need and want).

The elements of FCMC are based on principles designed to promote greater family self-determination, decision-making capabilities, and control. The families are empowered to be responsible for their own care. The family is recognized as a whole unit and care is not necessarily limited to the nuclear family.

- How can you collaborate with families while providing appropriate care and education in respect to their structure, cultural background, and racial and ethnic group?
- How can you be flexible, accessible, and responsive to the needs of families while also respecting their privacy?

CLINICAL ASSESSMENT

Before providing care for the postpartum client, the nurse should review the medical record for the antepartum and intrapartum histories. A nursing report from the labor and delivery nurse should communicate pertinent information regarding the intrapartum course. Information such as length of labor, estimated blood loss, and the presence of episiotomy will alert the postpartum nurse to potential complications.

The nurse should be prepared to provide physical and psychosocial nursing care. The new mother may want to discuss the events of her child's birth in the immediate postpartum period. Retelling what happened during birth validates the events for her and gives the nurse an idea of the mother's state of mind. Active listening by the nurse may elicit potential problems that may occur later in the postpartum period, (e.g., "I pushed for 3 hours. I am so tired, and now my bottom really hurts.")

During the entire hospital stay, the nurse must incorporate client teaching in all aspects of nursing care. Although the new mother may be emotionally and physically overwhelmed after birth, she must be provided information and educated. The sensitive nurse will instruct the mother with each step and will explain the reasoning for doing it. (For example, the nurse might say, "I am checking your lochia. It should normally be bright red for the first 3 days.") Client education after birth is important and should be provided at the same time the nursing care is being performed. Ensuring privacy before examining the client will convey respect and may help ease the new mother's fears.

Nursing Approach to Cultural Sensitivity

The nurse also should remember to approach the client with sensitivity, taking cultural and religious practices into consideration. For example, some clients may have deep beliefs regarding personal hygiene and modesty or foods to eat (i.e., hot versus cold). The nurse should consult a reference guide, such as *Cultural Assessment* by Geissler (1998), that addresses cultural considerations for the type of patient population she serves in her community. This guide annotates health care beliefs, predominant sick care practices, health team relationships, food practices and intolerances, birth and death rites, infant feeding practices, and child rearing practices for many nationalities.

In addition to cultural differences, the nurse may find herself unable to communicate to her client if the woman speaks a different language. A family member or professional interpreter may assist in relaying important information to the client.

Vital Signs

The recovery period normally lasts for the first few hours after delivery and until the client is stable. Depending on the protocol of the particular unit, the nurse should measure vital signs every 15 minutes for the first hour, every 30 minutes for the second hour, at the third and fourth hour, and then every 8 hours thereafter (Association of Women's Health, Obstetric and Neonatal Nurses [AWHONN], 1996). Close monitoring assists in identifying potential complications, such as hemorrhage and infection. Clients who received some type of conductive anesthesia (e.g., an epidural or spinal) should be monitored during recovery by trained staff in an area with appropriate resuscitative equipment.

Blood Pressure

The client's blood pressure may demonstrate negligible if any changes in the postpartum period. Within the first 6 hours the blood pressure should stabilize to or remain consistent with the client's baseline before delivery. Blood pressure may be lowered owing to the effects of analgesia or anesthesia. Hypotension may result from administration of epidural anesthesia or hemorrhage. Signs of orthostatic hypotension may include dizziness or faintness immedi-

Critical Thinking

Cultural Differences in Postpartum Care

Soon after childbirth, American women are encouraged to get out of bed, ambulate, and care for themselves. Other cultures treat new mothers differently.

A new mother on the Japanese island of Goto Archipelago will stay in bed for 1 month after delivering her baby (Epstein, 2000). It is normal in this culture to have an extended postpartum recovery period. Female relatives, such as grandmothers, aunts, and others, take turns "mothering" the mother and her infant until she feels ready to care for her baby herself.

Based on anthropologic research, historical tribes also mothered new mothers for the first year postpartum (Griffin, 2000). They treated the mothers with massage to help them relax and to restore normal circulation. Massage also was thought to facilitate musculoskeletal healing. Some mothers were treated to a daily full-body massage for the first 3 months after birth.

The balance of hot and cold is part of a belief system in many cultural groups, such as Chinese, Filipinos, and Hispanics. They believe there are natural external factors that must be kept in balance to maintain health. To restore a disrupted balance, for example, the treatment is to apply the use of opposites. To treat a so-called hot condition, such as a fever, the person should eat cold foods, such as fresh vegetables, dairy products, and meats. To treat a so-called cold condition, such as a headache, the person should eat hot foods, such as eggs, cheese, chocolate, and aromatic beverages.

How would you incorporate these beliefs and practices into your nursing care to ensure that your practice embodied cultural sensitivity?

ately after sitting or standing. Hemorrhage in the postpartum client may be difficult to identify because the blood pressure may be within normal limits. Blood volume increases 30% during pregnancy, and therefore, time is needed for it to return to prepregnancy volumes. The postpartal client may be in moderate shock before blood pressure changes occur; thus, a decrease in blood pressure may be a late sign of hemorrhage.

Blood pressure elevation may be related to oxytocin administration or excessive use of medications (AWHONN, 1996). Hypertension may be the result of pregnancy-induced hypertension (PIH), anxiety, or essential hypertension. When a client has PIH, her blood pressure values may remain elevated 5% above the norm until 4 days postpar-

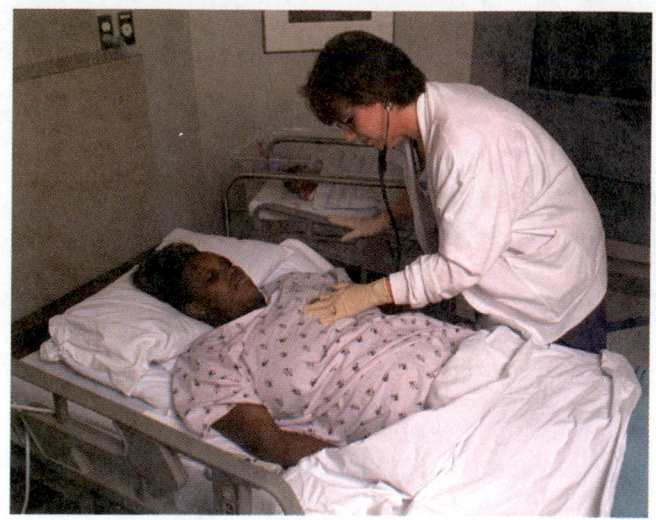

Figure 28-3 The nurse assesses the apical pulse of the postpartum mother.

tum (AWHONN, 1996). Clients with PIH should be monitored more frequently, measuring blood pressure every 4 hours for the next 48 hours because the risk for seizures may continue into the postpartum period.

Pulse

Owing to increased blood volume during pregnancy, normal findings for pulse rate may be slightly bradycardic (50 to 60 beats per minute [bpm]) immediately after birth owing to increased blood volume (AWHONN, 1996). A heart rate greater than 100 bpm may indicate pain, fever, anxiety, dehydration, infection, or hypovolemia (Figure 28-3).

Respiratory Rate

Without the presence of respiratory disease or medications, such as an epidural narcotic, the normal respiratory rate should be 16 to 24 breaths per minute. Epidural narcotics include fentanyl and morphine, both of which depress the respiratory rate to less than 12 breaths per minute. The nurse

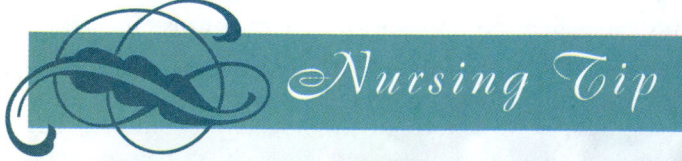

VITAL SIGNS

Despite a stable blood pressure, the presence of both tachycardia and tachypnea may suggest hypovolemia secondary to early hemorrhage. In a client with hypertension, it may be difficult to determine hemorrhage because blood pressure may appear normal when she actually may have hypovolemia.

POSTPARTUM SHIVERS

Shivering immediately after delivery may be caused by chills or an infection. Many women experience tremors or shaking, sometimes uncontrollably. Changes in hormones, adrenaline, and the physiology of the body cause shivering. You should assess the client's vital signs and risk factors for infection. Once infection has been ruled out, reassure the client that the tremors are normal and soon will pass. Placing a warm blanket over her can reduce the shivering.

should carefully monitor the respiratory rate and have a narcotic antagonist (e.g., naloxone [Narcan]) readily available.

Temperature

The client's oral temperature should range from 36.2°C to 38°C (98°F to 100°F). A temperature greater than 100.4°F in the first 24 hours after delivery may indicate dehydration (Figure 28-4). A temperature greater than 38°C (100.4°F) 6 hours apart after the first 24 hours after delivery for 2 consecutive days may indicate a postpartum infection (AWHONN, 1996). Unless proved otherwise, fever in the postpartum period suggests the presence of an in-

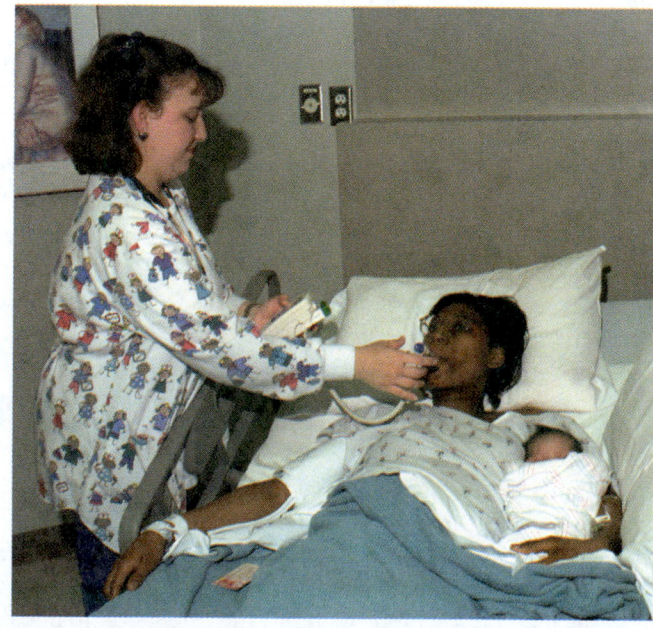

Figure 28-4 The nurse should assess the new mother's temperature regularly in the early postpartum period because fever may suggest an infectious process.

fectious process, usually somewhere in the genitourinary tract (Williams & Cooper, 1993).

Physical Assessment

The nurse should follow an organized method when examining the postpartum client. This manner provides a consistent, quality approach to nursing care. The acronym BUBBLE-HE can serve as a helpful reminder of the elements in a postpartum assessment. BUBBLE-HE stands for:

- Breasts
- Uterus
- Bladder
- Bowel
- Lochia
- Episiotomy
- Homan's sign
- Emotional status

The nurse should assess these elements every 8 hours, along with vital signs (AWHONN, 1996).

Breasts

After delivery, on palpation breasts usually are enlarged, soft, and warm and contain only a small amount of colostrum, the precursor of milk. The nipples should be intact without redness, tenderness, cracks, or blisters. Colostrum may be expressed. If the mother is not breast-feeding, the breast changes as a result of pregnancy regress after 1 to 2 weeks postpartum.

The mother may experience breast **engorgement** (enlargement and filling of the breasts with milk), which may begin as a tingling sensation in her breasts, 2 to 4 days after delivery. In the presence of prolactin hormone, the breasts begin to fill with milk or become engorged. Engorged breasts are secondary to increased vascularity and lymph and venous stasis. The breasts feel very full, tender, and uncomfortable until the milk is either released through infant sucking, manual expression, or pumping. The discomfort from engorged breasts normally subsides once stimulation to produce milk is decreased. The nursing mother's breasts should be inspected and palpated for the presence of inverted nipples, cracks, blisters, fissures, and tenderness (Figure 28-5).

When a client chooses to bottle-feed her infant, the nurse should teach the client about lactation suppression. Suppression can be achieved through a variety of methods: decreasing stimulation to the breasts (e.g., securely binding the breasts with a snug support bra and with a an ace bandage if more support is needed), avoiding warmth (e.g., hot shower water) on the breasts, and applying ice packs to the breasts. The mother can take acetaminophen

Client Education

Breast Care in Nonlactating Women

For the nonlactating client to successfully care for her breasts, you should teach her the following:

- Do not manually express milk from the breasts.
- Do not stimulate the nipples.
- Wear a tight-fitting bra.
- Use ice packs to constrict the superficial blood vessels.
- Take analgesics to minimize discomfort.
- Do not take medications (e.g., bromocriptine [Parlodel]) to suppress lactation because they may cause adverse side effects.

(Tylenol) for breast discomfort. These methods can be used until milk production stops.

Uterus

Immediately after delivery the uterus begins the process of **involution** or reduction in size. It generally takes 6 weeks for complete physiologic involution and for the reproductive system to be restored to its nonpregnant state, except for the nursing mother's breasts. **Subinvolution**, or the failure of the uterus to return to a nonpregnant state, occurs when the process of involution is prolonged or stopped as a result of hemorrhage, infection, or retained placental parts.

Uterine involution involves the return of the uterus to a nonpregnant condition—diminishing in size and weight—and anatomic location back into the pelvis (Figure 28-6). The endometrial decidua is shed, as noted by the lochial vaginal bleeding. By the end of the 3 weeks postpartum, the endometrial lining and site of the placental attachment should have returned to a nonpregnant state. The placental site usually is completely healed without scarring by the 6 weeks postpartum.

Immediately after delivery, the uterus weighs about 1,000 g (2 lb, 4 oz), measuring 14 by 12 by 8–10 cm, which is two to three times the nonpregnant size (Table 28-1). At the end of 6 weeks postpartum, the uterus weighs 50 to 100 g (AWHONN, 1996). Breast-feeding or breast stimulation assists in hastening the speed of uterine involution. There generally is no difference between primiparas and multiparas regarding healing time. Multiparas may have less abdominal muscle tone, however, and the cervix does not completely return to its closed nonpregnant appearance. The parous cervix is easily distensible and appears as a slit.

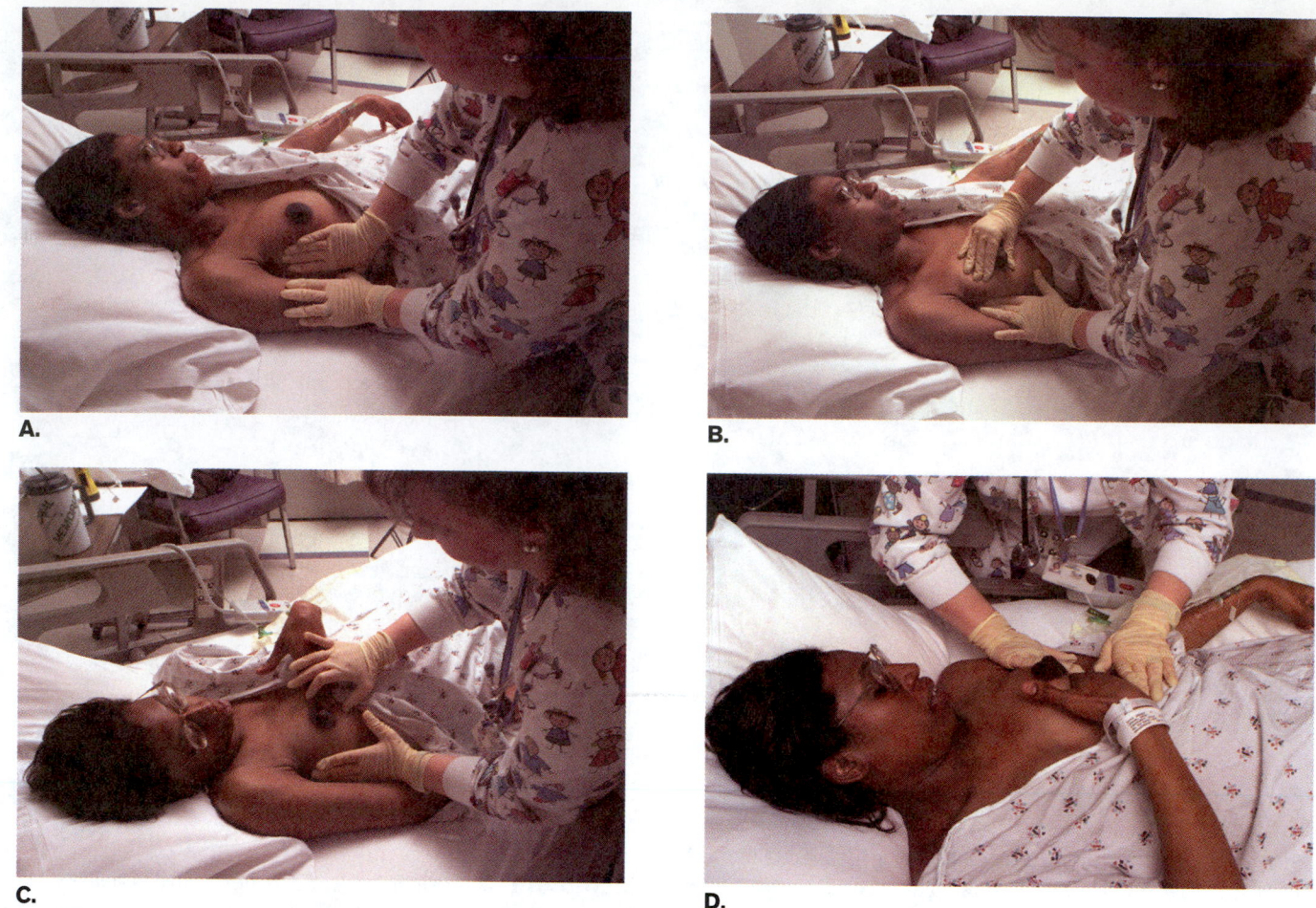

Figure 28-5 Postpartum breast assessment. A. The nurse palpates the breast for tenderness and lumps, which may indicate a plugged milk duct. B. The nipples are assessed for inversion, cracks, blisters, and tenderness; colostrum may be expressed during compression of the areola. C. Showing the new mother how to assess her breasts is an important element of postpartum teaching. D. After assessing the first breast, the nurse examines the second breast.

Assessment of the Fundus

When assessing the location and firmness of the uterine **fundus**, the top portion of the uterus, the nurse should place the client in a supine position with the bed flat. Using a two-handed approach, the nurse places one hand beneath the uterus to support it, while using the other hand to cup the fundus (Figure 28-7).

Immediately after delivery, the fundus usually can be located midline at the level of or one to two fingerbreadths below the umbilicus. Immediately after birth, the fundus should be at or below the level of the umbilicus. The fundus is approximately 1 cm below the umbilicus at 12 hours after delivery. After the first postpartum day the fundus descends or involutes 1 to 2 cm (0.4 to 0.8 in) each day. Finally, the fundus is nonpalpable as it gradually descends into the true pelvis on or about 9 days postpartum.

Assessments may be documented using the abbreviations ML (midline) at "U + 2, U + 1, @U, U-1, U-2" from the umbilicus. There may be individual variations in the as-

sessment of the fundal location from one examiner to the next owing to differences in fingerwidths (Figure 28-8).

The fundus should be massaged for firmness (Box 28-2). Fundal massage provides the opportunity to maintain contraction of the uterine blood vessels where the placenta was once attached, preventing potential hemorrhage and expelling placental fragments and blood clots (Figure 28-9). If it is not firm or palpable, the fundus may feel soft or **boggy**. A boggy uterus may be related to an overdistended uterus or structural anomalies (e.g., fibroids). A fundus that remains boggy is a warning sign of uterine atony and potential postpartal hemorrhage.

The position of the fundus also should be noted if it is midline or displaced to the left or right of the umbilicus. If the bladder is full, the fundus may be displaced higher and to the right of the umbilicus. Because the broad and round ligaments were greatly stretched during pregnancy and become very lax after the loss of the enlarged uterus after delivery, the uterus is easily displaced by an overfilled blad-

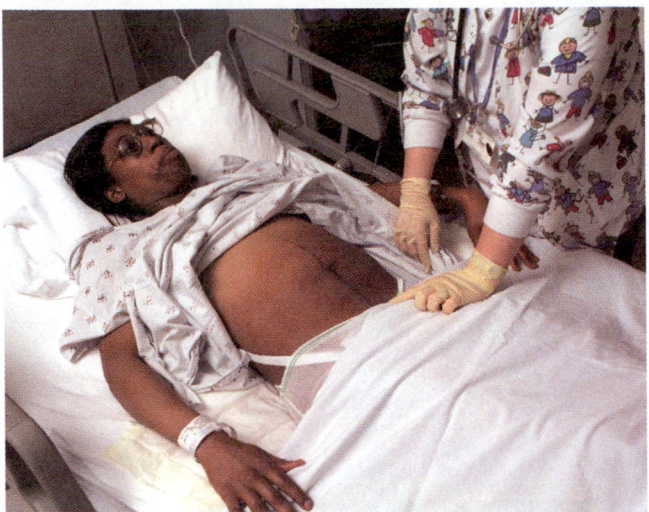

A. Primipara

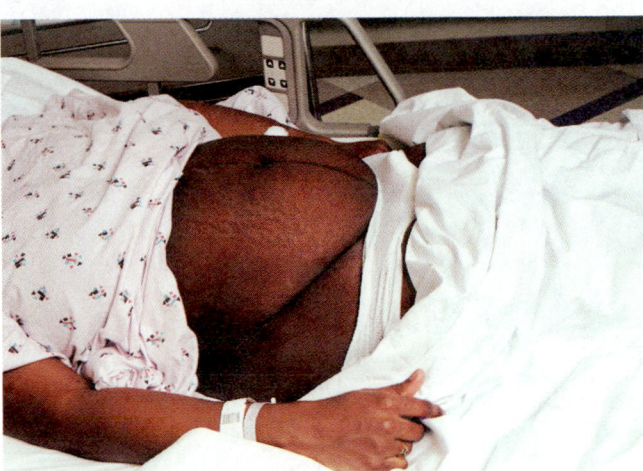

B. Multipara

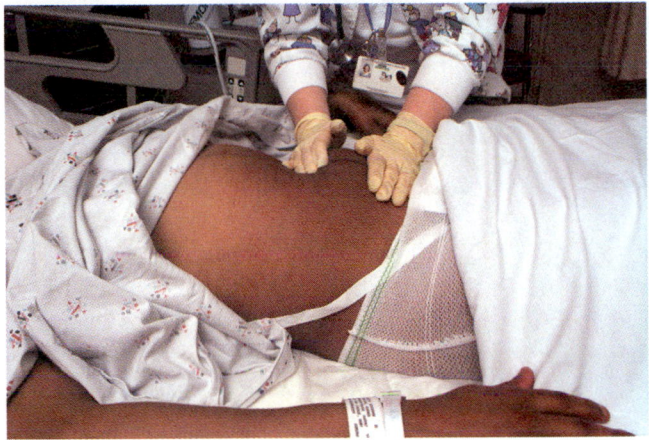

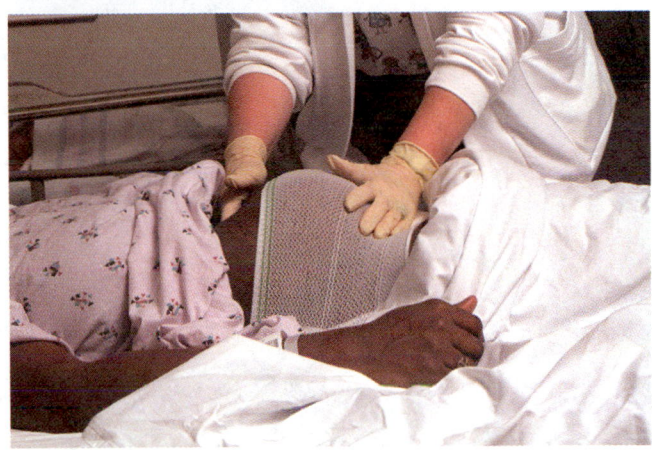

Figure 28-6 Uterine involution 4 hours after delivery in the primipara (A) and the multipara (B). Note the size and shape of the abdomen (top), and the size of the palpated uterus (bottom).

der. Women who have had several pregnancies or large babies may have a large uterus that is palpated higher than is normally expected.

Management of Bleeding

After delivery of the placenta, 20 to 40 U of oxytocin (Pitocin) often are added to the mainline intravenous (IV) solution if an IV is in place. Oxytocin is prescribed to hasten uterine contractility and control bleeding (Spratto

and Woods, 2001). When IV access is not present, other options include administering oxytocin (10 U) intramuscularly (IM), initiating early breast-feeding, or performing nipple stimulation (Table 28-2).

When the uterus remains boggy despite fundal massage and oxytocin administration, other reasons for bleeding

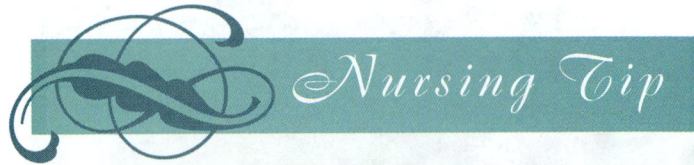

Nursing Tip

ASSESSING BLEEDING

Postpartum hemorrhage should be considered if a pad is saturated with blood within 15 minutes or two pads within 30 minutes (AWHONN, 1996). A slow, steady seepage of blood also may lead to postpartum hemorrhage.

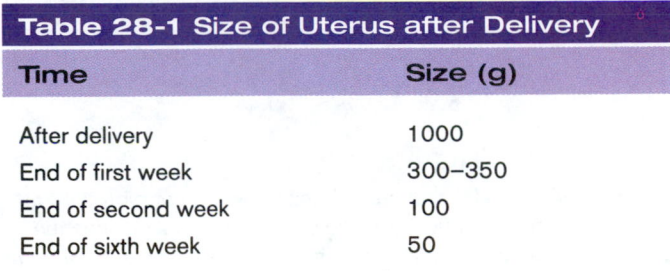

Table 28-1 Size of Uterus after Delivery	
Time	**Size (g)**
After delivery	1000
End of first week	300–350
End of second week	100
End of sixth week	50

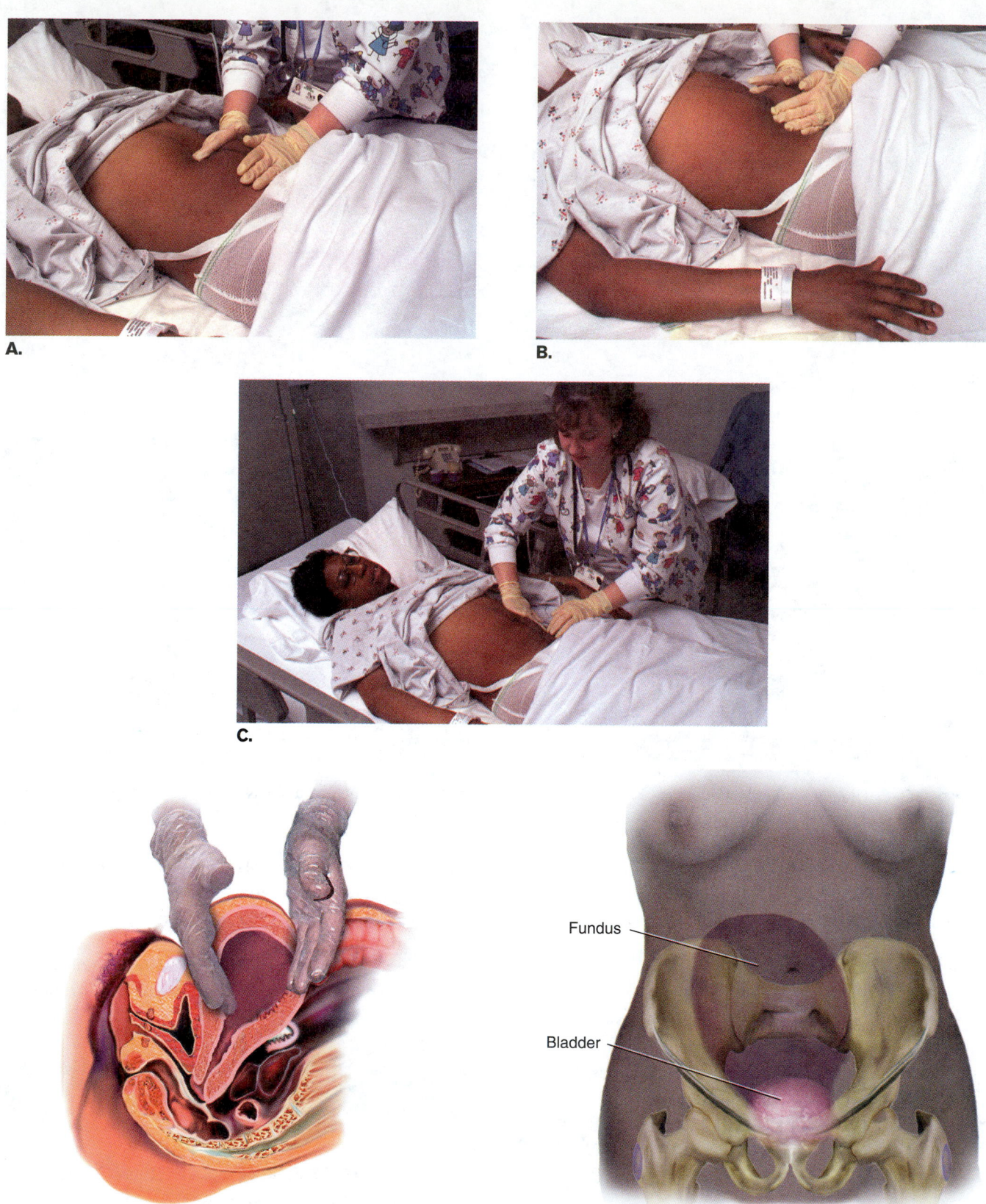

Figure 28-7 Assessment of the fundus. A. The nurse supports the uterus with her left hand held beneath it while cupping the fundus (top of the uterus) in her right hand. B. The nurse palpates the uterus to determine if it is firm or boggy. C. The nurse assesses the position (midline or displaced to the left or right) of the uterus, which must be done at each fundal assessment. D. View of the uterus during fundal assessment. E. A full bladder displaces the uterus and prevents its contraction.

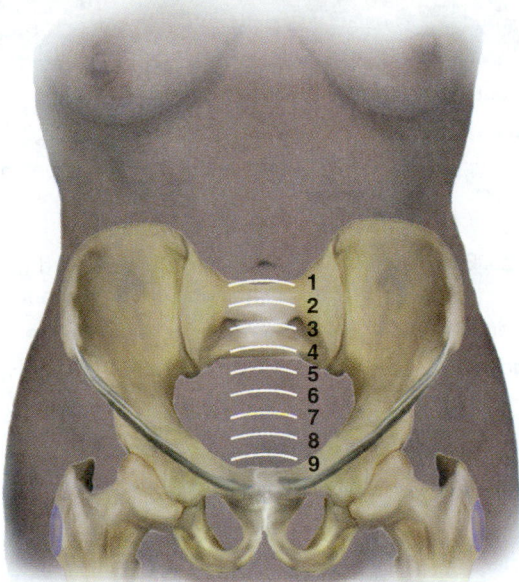

Figure 28-8 Height of the fundus after delivery; numbers indicate postpartum day and level of fundus, in fingerwidths, in relation to the umbilicus.

must be determined. When bleeding continues, a second pharmacologic agent, such as an ergot preparation, should be considered. Methylergonovine (Methergine), 0.2 mg, may be given IM to clients who do not have a current history of high blood pressure (Table 28-3).

Another medication useful in controlling bleeding is a prostaglandin called carboprost tromethamine (Hemabate) (Table 28-4). Hemabate often is used when fundal massage and second-line medications such as methylergonovine do not stop the hemorrhage.

Assessment of Uterine Pain

Abdominal cramping or **afterpains** are caused by uterine tonic contractions, which are the efforts of the uterus to expel blood clots and placental fragments. The contractions are enhanced with oxytocin. A history of multiple gesta-

Nursing Alert

PRECAUTIONS FOR METHYLERGONOVINE

Methylergonovine should only be given to clients who *do not* have high blood pressure. Take a blood pressure reading before administering the medication. If the patient with hypertension or risk of hypertension has a blood pressure greater than normal parameters, do not give the medication.

Box 28-2 General Approach to Fundal Massage

- Ensure that your hands are warm and clean.
- Inform the client what you are going to do.
- Determine if the client needs to empty her bladder. A full bladder impedes uterine involution.
- Put the client in a supine position with her legs slightly flexed.
- Gently touch the client's abdomen to decrease tension on it.
- Tell the client you are going to place (cup) one hand on top of the symphysis pubis to support and hold the lower part of the uterus.
- Place (cup) the other free hand on the fundus.
- Gently palpate the fundus and massage with a downward, steady pressure. If you cannot locate the fundus, move your hand higher or lower as needed. The fingers should lay flat on top of the abdomen while massaging. Do not massage for more than a few minutes because overstimulation of the fundus may cause muscle fatigue and continued agony.
- Note the consistency of the fundus that is, whether it is soft and boggy or firm. The firm fundus will feel hard like a softball.
- If the fundus is soft, massage it until it contracts and becomes firm.
- Teach the client how to massage the fundus.
- Note the location of the fundus. When the fundus is greater than the level of the umbilicus, the nurse should assess for the possibility of uterine filling with blood or blood clots and uterine displacement by a distended bladder.
- It is best to observe the perineum at the same time you palpate the fundus to note the amount and color of lochia or clots that may be discharged during massage. The bleeding may increase during massage.
- Replace the old peripad, as needed.
- Cover the client and reposition her in the bed, as needed.
- Document findings in the client's medical record.

tion, multiparity, or uterine overdistention usually is associated with afterpains.

The uterus of the primipara woman tends to remain in a better or more prolonged state of contraction compared

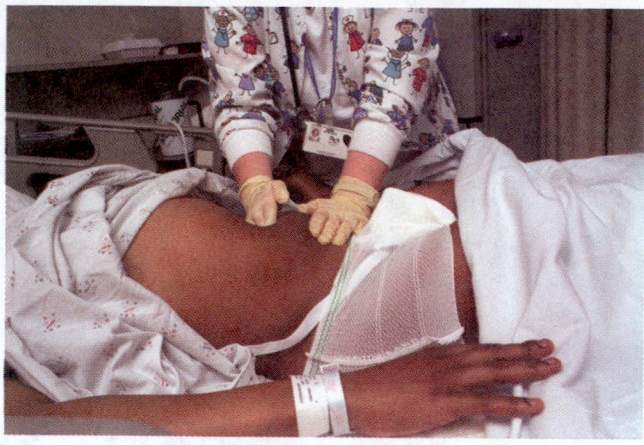

Figure 28-9 Fundal massage helps the uterus return more quickly to its prepregnancy state; massage also helps prevent hemorrhage and expel placental fragments and blood clots.

Table 28-2 Pharmacology in the Postpartum Period: Oxytocin (Pitocin)	
Therapeutic Class	Oxytocic agent
How Supplied	10 µ/mL ampule or vial
Indications for Use	Induces or stimulates labor, controls postpartum bleeding, induces completion of an incomplete or inevitable abortion
Chemical Effect	Causes selective potent stimulation of the smooth muscles of the uterus and mammary glands
Therapeutic Effect	Induces labor; reduces postpartum bleeding
Dosage	When used postpartum: IV, 10 to 40 µ, are added to 1,000 mL of D₅W, D₅LR, lactated Ringer's solution, or 0.9% normal saline at a rate of 20–40 mµ/min or a rate necessary to control bleeding; IM, 10 µ
Side Effects	Anaphylaxis, fatal a fibrinogenemia, hypertension, increased heart rate, arrhythmias hypersensitivity, nausea and vomiting, water intoxication from prolonged IV infusion
Nursing Considerations	Monitor for fluid overload, coma, or seizures; monitor intake and output; note amount and color of lochia; do not give as an IV bolus; no effects on breast-feeding infant

Data from Spratto, G. R., & Woods, A. L. (2001). *PDR nurse's drug handbook.* Albany, NY: Delmar Thomson Learning.

Table 28-3 Pharmacology in the Postpartum Period: Methylergonovine (Methergine)	
Therapeutic Class	Oxytocic agent
How Supplied	IM or IV, 0.2 mg/mL; PO, 0.2 mg
Indications for Use	Manages and prevents postpartum hemorrhage by producing firm uterine contractions
Chemical Effect	Stimulates rate, tone, and amplitude of uterine contractions
Therapeutic Effect	Stops postpartum hemorrhage
Dosage	IM, 0.2 mg, every 2 to 4 h; IV, 0.2 mg, slow IV push over 1 min; PO, 0.2 mg three to four times a day 2 to 7 d
Side Effects	Dizziness, headache, seizures, hypertension, palpitations, thrombophlebitis, dyspnea, diaphoresis, nausea and vomiting, uterine tetany
Nursing Considerations	Monitor blood pressure and other vital signs for evidence of shock or hypertension while administering IV; abdominal cramps may continue for 3 h after administration; may dilute IV dose up to 5 mL of normal saline; not recommended for use in lactating women

Data from Spratto, G. R., & Woods, A. L. (2001). *PDR nurse's drug handbook.* Albany, NY: Delmar Thomson Learning.

with that of a multipara woman. Thus, the multipara woman's afterpains will seem more intense, contracting vigorously at regular intervals. Afterpains usually become milder after 3 days. When abdominal pain becomes significantly more intense or the uterus is tender to palpation, the nurse should assess for further indications of problems, such as **endometritis**, an infection of the uterine lining. Severe pain that is not relieved by medications should be reported to the health care provider.

If the third stage of labor is mismanaged by pulling on the cord before readiness of the placenta to detach from the uterine wall, uterine inversion or prolapse may occur. Although rare, this is a life-threatening occurrence that requires emergency measures and immediate notification of the physician. The client may go into shock. The uterus must be reinserted immediately by returning it to a normal position in the pelvis, a procedure that must be performed by a physician.

Bladder

In the immediate postpartum period, the bladder is congested, edematous, and hypotonic from the effects of

Table 28-4 Pharmacology in the Postpartum Period: Carboprost Tromethamine (Hemabate)	
Therapeutic Class	Oxytocic; uterine stimulant
How Supplied	IM, 250 μg/mL
Indications for Use	Prevents and treats postpartum hemorrhage not managed by conventional methods
Chemical Effect	Produces immediate strong uterine contractions
Therapeutic Effect	Stops postpartum hemorrhage
Dosage	IM, 250 μg/mL, deep IM every 1.5 to 3.5 h, may increase to 500 μg if bleeding is not controlled; total dosage should not exceed 12 mg
Side Effects	Nausea, vomiting, diarrhea, fever, chills
Nursing Considerations	Monitor drug's effectiveness by evaluating uterine contractions and cessation of bleeding; may prophylactically administer an antidirrheal drug, such as diphenoxylate and atropine (Lomotil)

The newly delivered mother requires ample fluids. Nursing responsibilities include teaching her to empty the bladder often after birth to assist in controlling pain and bleeding. Immediately after delivery, the client should be assisted to the bathroom the first two or three time to protect against falls; the nurse must monitor her for dizziness and faintness (Figure 28-10). Early ambulation and comfort facilitate urination. After delivery the client should be able to urinate within 4 hours, at least 150 mL, with complete emptying of the bladder (AWHONN, 1996). The nurse should note complaints of urinary frequency, dysuria, and retention. The primary provider should be notified if the woman has not voided 6 to 8 hours after delivery.

The nurse should closely observe for bladder distention and adequate emptying after urinary efforts. After urination, the fundus should be repalpated for location to ensure appropriate emptying of the bladder. The bladder normally should be nonpalpable. If the bladder remains distended, the client may be retaining residual urine. **Residual urine** is defined as urine remaining in the bladder after elimination. Residual urine can result in urinary tract infection.

The nurse may need to perform a straight catheterization when the client cannot urinate, the bladder remains distended, and the client is uncomfortable. The judgment to perform a straight catheterization depends on the client's

labor. Unless a urinary tract infection is present, these effects should resolve within 24 hours of delivery. Considerable diuresis—up to 3,000 mL—may follow for several days after delivery, decreasing by 3 days postpartum (AWHONN, 1996). The diuresis results from the decreasing production of aldosterone hormone (sodium retention decreases and urine production increases) and the body's method of removing excess fluid. The renal pelvis and ureters, stretched and dilated during pregnancy, return to normal by the end of 4 weeks postpartum.

In the immediate postpartum period, urinary distention, incomplete emptying, and residual urine are complications that result in a full bladder. These complications are related to an edematous perineum, pain, reflex spasms, and bladder desensitization. A full bladder interferes with uterine contractions and increases the risk for hemorrhage.

Risk factors for these problems include: episiotomy (surgical incision to enlarge the vaginal opening for delivery of the infant's head), perineal edema or tenderness, long labor, assisted vaginal delivery (forceps or trauma may cause neural blockage), lacerations, previous catheterization (secondary to pain and swelling associated with an episiotomy), and anesthesia (bladder tone may be temporarily lost, resulting in urinary retention and diminished perception of bladder fullness).

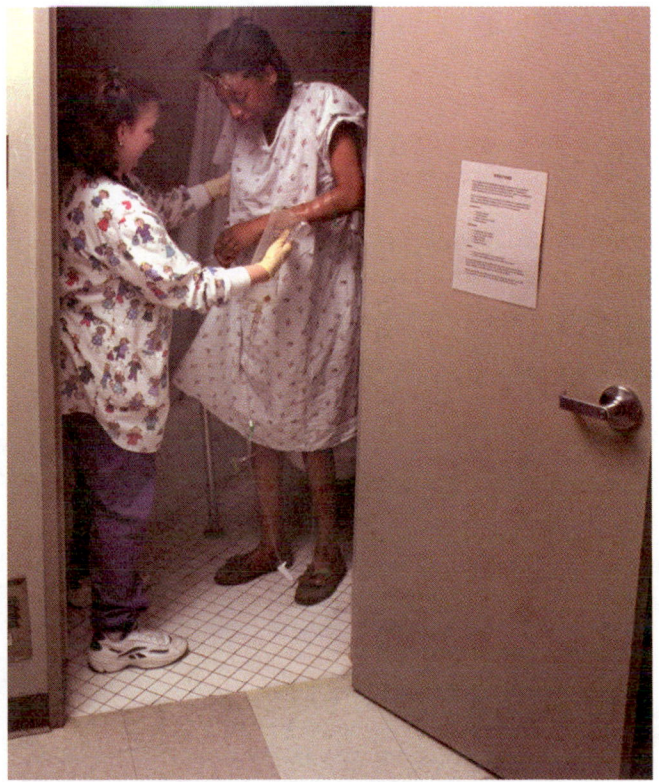

Figure 28-10 The nurse should assist the new mother the first few times she attempts to ambulate after delivery.

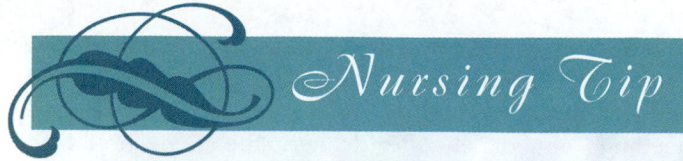

URINATION AFTER DELIVERY

The newly delivered client may need assistance in urinating. Actions, such as mental relaxation, taking an analgesic before voiding, drinking fluids, running the tap water, blowing bubbles through a straw in a glass, pouring water over the perineum, concentrating on relaxing part of the perineum using pelvic tightening exercises (Kegel's), or standing in the shower, may aid in stimulating urination. A few drops of peppermint oil in the toilet water also is helpful in stimulating the urge to urinate.

Critical Thinking

Voiding after Delivery

Marissa, your newly delivered 30-year-old grava 2, para 2, mother, is unable to void 5 hours after delivery. She received an epidural when she was 5 cm dilated, and a Foley catheter was inserted after the epidural when she was unable to void. She quickly progressed though labor, delivering a 9 lb, 7 oz baby boy.

- Which methods would you use in assisting your client to urinate?
- Which nursing intervention must be performed if the client is unable to void spontaneously?
- Which other assessments should you monitor if the client has a distended bladder?

circumstances: the degree of bladder distention, location of the displaced uterus, amount of bleeding, amount of fluid or IV intake since the last voiding, and the techniques used to encourage voiding. When all of these parameters are not extreme or have not been met, catheterization should be delayed an hour or so until further assessment.

An indwelling catheter should be inserted when the client cannot empty her bladder completely. An increased incidence of bacteriuria exists with an indwelling catheter. An indwelling catheter inserted before cesarean delivery generally is kept in place for 24 hours.

Bowels

The client's appetite typically will return to normal immediately after delivery, with the new mother usually becoming hungry 1 to 2 hours after delivery. If there are no complications from anesthesia, diet habits with regular food may be resumed. The client who had vomited during labor

may not have an appetite. The nurse should encourage her to increase her fluid intake and choose foods high in potassium and protein. Especially after a long and difficult labor, the new mother needs nourishment with food and fluids to regain her strength.

A woman's nutrition continues to be important throughout the postpartum period, regardless of choice of infant feeding methods. The physical stresses of labor and delivery and the psychological demands of being a new mother take a toll on her body. The client may need a diet high in protein and iron if she has experienced postpartum hemorrhage. Adequate dietary protein and iron facilitates tissue healing and restore iron levels from the normal hemoglobin hemodilution of pregnancy.

The client's bowel pattern should remain unchanged after a vaginal delivery, with a bowel movement normally occurring by 2 or 3 days postpartum. Often, a woman may defecate while pushing during the second stage of labor. When gastric motility does not return by 2 or 3 days after delivery, constipation may occur. The nurse should assess the client's abdomen for nondistention, softness, and bowel sounds.

Constipation in the early postpartum period may occur owing to decreased bowel motility during labor, postpartum fluid loss, prelabor diarrhea, the side effects of medication and anesthesia, and the self-restraint or hesitancy to defecate owing to perineal or rectal discomfort. For women who have had an episiotomy, fear of tearing the stitches may lead to or exacerbate the occurrence of constipation.

The client's possible inhibition must be assessed because it may lead to fecal impaction. The nurse should ex-

Nursing Alert

DETECTING A DISTENDED BLADDER

When the bladder is full and distended, on palpation it will feel like a ballottable cystic mass or rounded bulge. The mound may fluctuate as does a water-filled balloon. Dull percussion may be heard over the symphysis pubis. A full bladder tends to displace the uterus up and to the right. Lochia may be more than normal because the uterus is unable to contract effectively. A distended bladder takes longer to regain its original tone because muscle tone may have been lost as a result of stretching.

USE OF ENEMAS AND SUPPOSITORIES AFTER DELIVERY

Do not administer enemas or suppositories to women who have experienced a fourth-degree laceration.

plain that the stitches are inserted in layers and assure the client that the normal effort of bearing down with rectal pressure will not affect the episiotomy. The client should be encouraged to drink six to eight 8-oz glasses of fluids daily and eat a high-fiber diet (e.g., whole grains, legumes, vegetables, and fruits). Warm sitz baths, topical anesthetics (e.g., chloroprocaine [nesacaine]), and stopping medications that cause constipation (e.g., Tylenol with Codeine) are helpful interventions to lower the chances of constipation.

When constipation is severe, administering an analgesic and a stool softener (e.g., docusate [Colace]) before ambulation may assist in facilitating a bowel movement. Many health care providers order a mild prophylactic laxative, such as magnesium hydroxide (Milk of Magnesia), 30 mL/day, for women who have had a fourth-degree laceration. If the client has not yet had a bowel movement by 2 to 3 days postpartum, mineral oil, bisacodyl suppository (Dulcolax), or Fleet enema may be prescribed to stimulate intestinal activity.

Hemorrhoids

Examination of the bowels includes assessment for the presence of hemorrhoids. Hemorrhoids present during pregnancy may enlarge during labor. If the hemorrhoids are too large, they may cause pain if they become thrombosed and may subsequently cause constipation. Treatments with witch hazel or a topical anesthetic spray may relieve discomfort.

Lochia

The usual uterine discharge of blood, mucus, and tissue after childbirth is called **lochia.** Lochia contains the sloughing of decidual tissues, including erythrocytes, epithelial cells, and bacteria. Lochia is assessed according to its amount, color, and change with activity and time. The duration of lochia is not affected by breast-feeding or the use of oral contraceptives (Bowes, 1996).

The descriptive name of lochia changes concomitantly with the changes in color. *Lochia rubra* is the term given for the discharge in the first 3 days after delivery. Lochia rubra is small to moderate in amount and having a bright-

red color, secondary mainly to decidual tissue and bloody content. The color becomes progressively paler. Small clots may be present.

Lochia serosa, which occurs 4 to 10 days after delivery, is a watery, pink, or brown-tinged color, which is lighter in amount than is lochia rubra. Lochia serosa primarily contains serous fluid, leukocytes, erythrocytes, and decidual tissue.

The lochia transitions into *lochia alba,* a whitish-yellow creamy discharge on days 10 to 17. Many women may have minimal discharge by day 14; however, it is not uncommon for lochia alba to last until 6 weeks postpartum (Bowes, 1996). Lochia alba consists of a mixture of leukocytes, decidual tissue, and decreasing fluid content. The nurse should inform the client that there likely will be an episode of heavy vaginal bleeding between days 7 to 14 when the placental eschar sloughs off (Bowes, 1996).

The flow of lochia rubra is evaluated by examining the blood saturation on a peripad that occurs in 1 hour or less. The nurse should document her assessment of lochia using the descriptive term and the amount of blood saturation. Descriptions of lochia can be scant (less than 2.5 cm, or 1 in), light/small (less than 10 cm, or 4 in), moderate (less than 15 cm, or 6 in), or heavy/large (one pad saturated within 15 to 30 min) (Figure 28-11).

Determining the exact amount of blood on a peripad can be a challenge. Health care providers often mistakenly underestimate blood loss. Quantifying blood loss is a learned skill that should be practiced to accurately assess blood loss. Factors influencing objectivity and consistency in reporting include education of personnel and type of pad used.

Saturation of a pad within 15 to 30 minutes may indicate hemorrhage. When the client is bleeding heavily, the nurse needs to ensure that the blood is not coming from another source, such as a cervical or vaginal laceration. Lacerations are more highly suspected when heavy bleeding continues despite a firm uterus. The nurse also should check under the woman's buttocks for bleeding on the underpad and bed sheets.

The peripad, along with the Chux or pads used, may be weighed (1 g = 1 mL fluid). Blood tests can be used as an indicator of blood loss. A complete blood count (CBC) may indicate a 1.0 to 1.5 g/dL decrease in hemoglobin and a 3% to 4% decrease in hematocrit, which is consistent with a loss of 500 mL of blood (AWHONN, 1996).

The amount of lochia varies with position changes but should continually decrease throughout the first 4 to 6 weeks postpartum. The blood pools in the vaginal vault when the client is recumbent and drains when standing up. Clot formation occurs as a result of the pooling in the uterus or vagina. An increase in bright-red bleeding and the passage of clots also may occur during physical activity or breast-feeding. Lochia with a reddish color that

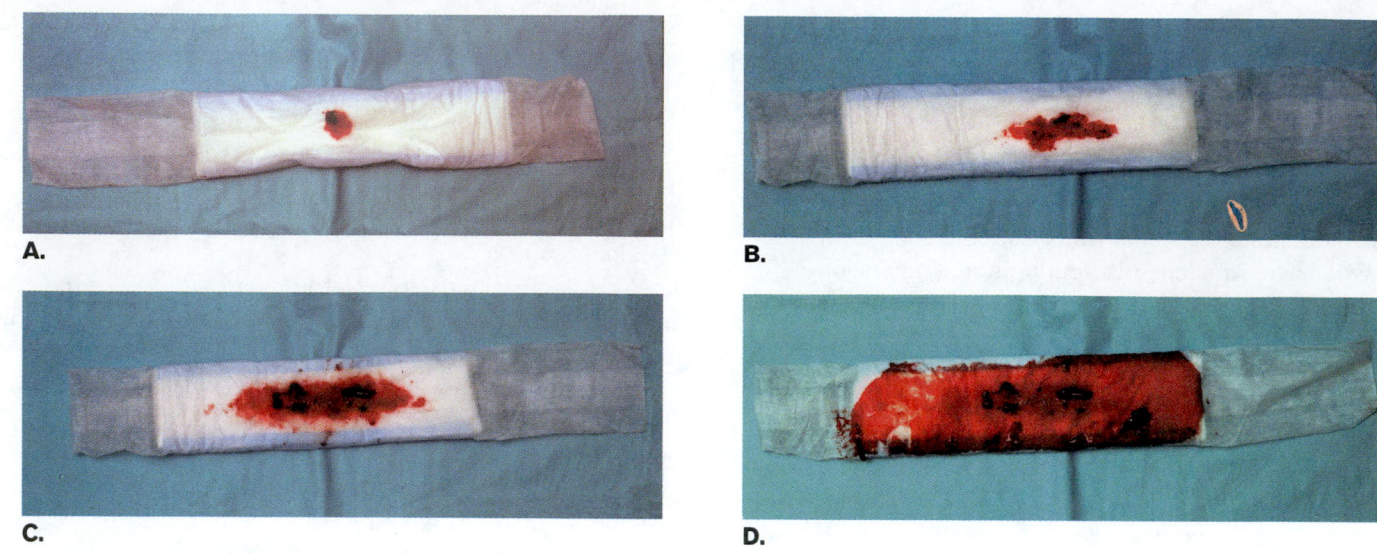

Figure 28-11 Assessment of lochia is based on the amount of blood saturation on a peripad. A. Scant. B. Light/small. C. Moderate. D. Heavy/large.

persists after 2 weeks of delivery may indicate subinvolution of the placental site or retained placental parts; this finding must be reported to the physician (Bowes, 1996).

The client should be instructed to notify the nurse if blood clots larger than 1 cm or roughly the size of a silver dollar are passed. Nursing actions include assessing the fundus for firmness and amount of lochia (Figure 28-12). When clots persist the nurse should notify the health care provider because an examination may be required to evaluate for other sources of continued bleeding.

Lochia has a characteristic menstrual-like musky or fleshy smell. A foul-smelling discharge, along with other indicators, such as fever and uterine tenderness, may suggest an infection, such as endometritis. Lochia serosa emits

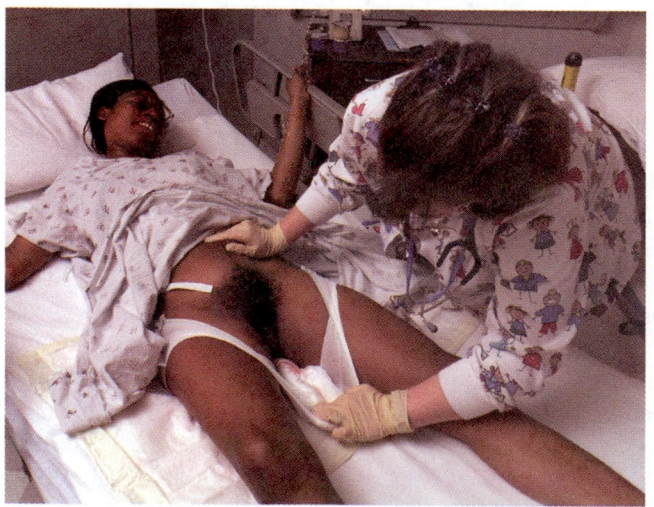

Figure 28-12 The nurse places a hand on the fundus while assessing the amount of lochia.

the strongest odor, which increases if mixed with perspiration. Because lochia is an excellent medium for bacterial growth, clients should be taught to change the peripad at every urination.

The first menstrual period usually begins within an average of 8 weeks after delivery for most nonlactating women. The timing may be delayed from 2 to 18 months in breast-feeding mothers; however, ovulation may occur without the onset of the first menstrual period (AWHONN, 1996). Thus, it is possible for a woman to become pregnant before the return of menses. Consistent, continuous breast-feeding increases prolactin levels, thus postponing the resumption of ovulation. Once breast stimulation decreases, prolactin levels decrease and FSH and LH hormone levels increase, inducing ovulation.

Client education includes teaching the client to report signs and symptoms of problems, such as foul-smelling lochia, heavy flow or change in normal flow, presence of large clots, and lochia rubra that continues past 4 days postpartum or that returns after initial cessation.

Episiotomy

An **episiotomy** is the surgical incision made to enlarge the vaginal opening for delivery of the baby's head. Depending on client preference, situation, and provider preference and judgment, some women experience delivery with an episiotomy. The episiotomy is incised midline down the center of the perineum, rather than mediolaterally, which extends in a diagonal angle to either the left or right side. With or without an episiotomy, the perineum also may suffer from lacerations during childbirth. Lacerations are classified as first, second, third, or fourth degrees (Table 28-5).

Table 28-5 Classification of Perineal Lacerations

Classification	Description
First degree	Involves only the skin and superficial structures above the muscle
Second degree	Extends into the perineal muscles
Third degree	Reaches into the anal sphincter muscles
Fourth degree	Continues into the anterior rectal wall

To assess an episiotomy and the condition of the perineum, it is best to have the client lie on her side, flexing her upper leg toward her hip. The nurse can then lift the buttocks to expose the perineum. Using a good light source, such as a gooseneck lamp or flashlight, facilitates visualization of the incision and repair (Figure 28-13). The REEDA (redness, edema, ecchymosis, discharge, and approximation) scoring scale can be used when assessing the episiotomy. At the client's request, the nurse can provide a mirror to show her the episiotomy to help dispel fears and misconceptions about healing of the perineum. (See Postpartum Complication for assessment and care of a perineal hematoma.)

Care of the vulva includes applying ice packs to the perineum for the first 24 hours to help decrease edema and pain. Ice packs also assist in constricting blood vessels, minimize the risk of hematoma formation, and decrease muscle irritability and spasm (Bowes, 1996). Ice packs should not be applied directly to the skin; they should be wrapped with an absorbent disposable type of covering.

After the first 24 hours after delivery, a sitz bath with warm water or moist heat may be used to reduce the local discomfort caused by perineal trauma and an episiotomy.

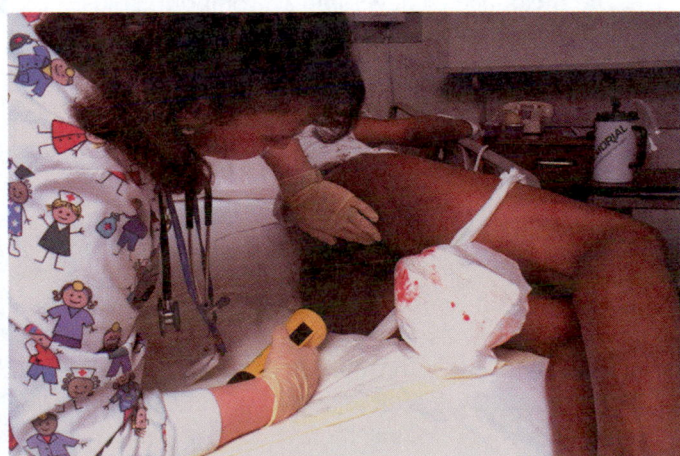

Figure 28-13 The nurse inspects the episiotomy site with the client lying on her side.

Nursing Tip

REEDA SCALE

Use the REEDA acronym as a nursing tool when evaluating an episiotomy (Davidson, 1974). REEDA stands for redness, edema, ecchymosis (purplish patch of blood flow), discharge, and approximation (closeness of the skin edges).

This tool used to assess healing is based on a 3-point scale; a score of 3 signifies an assessment of very poor wound healing. On the first postpartum day, the score may range from 0 to 3; by the second week postpartum, the score should be 0 to 1.

The change from cold to warm therapy enhances vascular circulation and healing. The sitz bath may be used until the episiotomy heals. Use of a heat lamp two or three times a day also will assist in the healing process (Box 28-3).

The client should be taught perineal hygiene, including daily washing with warm water and mild soap. The perineum should be cleansed after each voiding and bowel movement. A squeeze-bottle filled with warm tap water may be used to clean the perineum. The water should be comfortably warm on the wrist (approximately 38°C, or 100°F). The nozzle should be directed toward the perineum. The perineum should be wiped from the anterior to the posterior, or in a front-to-back motion, to avoid contamination from the anal region. Practices such as changing the peripad frequently (after each voiding and bowel movement or at least four times a day, removing the pad from front to back, and hand washing will help decrease the risk for infection and promote wound healing for episiotomy and repaired lacerations. Soiled pads should be placed in an appropriate disposal container.

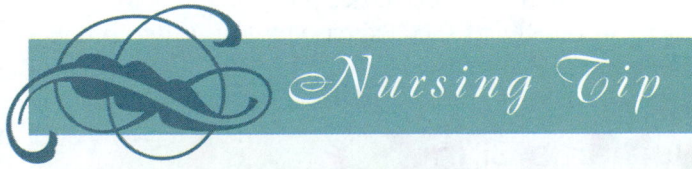

Nursing Tip

USING ICE PACKS

Many commercially prepared ice packs are available; however, an inexpensive way to make an ice pack is right on your unit. A condom or latex glove filled with crushed ice and wrapped with a disposable paper towel can be used as an ice pack. Fresh ice will easily mold on the woman's body; however, frozen packs will last longer before they begin to melt.

Box 28-3 Nursing Care of the Episiotomy: Sitz Bath and Heat Lamp

Sitz Bath

- Inform the client about the rationale and process of using a sitz bath.
- Remove the contents from the package.
- Clamp the tubing.
- Fill the enclosed bag with warm water.
- Hang the bag on a hook by the toilet.
- Fill the container half-way with warm water.
- Lift the toilet seat.
- Place the container on the toilet with the overflow opening facing toward the back.
- Attach the tube into the opening in the container.
- Instruct the client to sit atop the container for 15 to 20 min.
- Adjust the water level and temperature of the water by opening the clamp and releasing more water into the container.
- Instruct the client to dry the perineum and apply a clean peripad when finished.
- Empty the container.
- Clean the container and allow to dry.
- Assess the perineum.
- Document the use of a sitz bath and assessment of the episiotomy site.

Heat Lamp

- Obtain a lamp with a 40-W bulb.
- Inform the client about the rationale and process of using a heat lamp.
- Instruct the client to empty the bladder, cleanse the perineum with a squeeze-bottle, and apply a clean peripad.
- Prepare the client on the bed in a lithotomy or side-lying position, with appropriate drapes as needed.
- Cover the lamp with a towel.
- Position the lamp 50 cm (20 in) away from the perineum.
- Tell the client to use the lamp for a 20-min period three times a day.
- Instruct the client to apply a clean peripad when finished.
- Assess the episiotomy site when treatment is completed.
- Document use of the heat lamp and assessment of the episiotomy site.

Immediately after delivery, the vagina appears edematous, bruised, stretchable, and may gape at the introitus. By weeks 4, the vaginal ruggae return. Always remaining slightly larger than in the prepregnant state, the vagina returns to its prepregnant state by 6 to 8 weeks postpartum. The nurse should teach the client how to perform perineal exercises, such as Kegel's exercises, to assist in restoring vaginal and perineal tone and elasticity and to help reduce urinary incontinence. (See Exercise for instructions on performing Kegel's exercises.)

Homan's Sign

Assessment of the extremities should include examination of varicosities, deep tendon reflexes (DTRs), tenderness, and presence of edema or nodular areas on the legs. DTRs should be no greater than +1 to +2. Brisk DTRs (+3 to +4) may present hyperactive reflexes suggestive of PIH. Pretibial or pedal edema may be present, especially in the client with PIH.

Preconditions of blood hypercoagulability, severe anemia, traumatic delivery, and obesity are risk factors for developing superficial or deep vein thrombosis. Pain, erythema, or local swelling on the legs, especially the calves, may signify thrombophlebitis. The nurse should assess for Homan's sign as a positive indicator of thrombophlebitis (Figure 28-14). Early ambulation in current practice reduces the incidence of developing thrombophlebitis.

In addition, the client's legs should be assessed for sensation and mobility when epidural or spinal anesthesia has been administered. After delivery, the epidural infusion should be discontinued and the epidural catheter removed by the anesthesiologist or certified nurse anesthetist. (The catheter may be left in if the client will be undergoing a postpartum tubal ligation after delivery.) The nurse should assess for continuing abatement in the effects of the epidural or spinal anesthetic by determining the level at which the client feels sensation. The nurse may place a needle or sharp object on the client's torso to determine the level of tactile sensation, which should begin to approach T-11 or T-12 within the first hour of delivery. With appropriate return of mobility, the client should be able to move her toes and lift her buttocks off the bed within 2 to 4 hours after the discontinuation of the anesthesia.

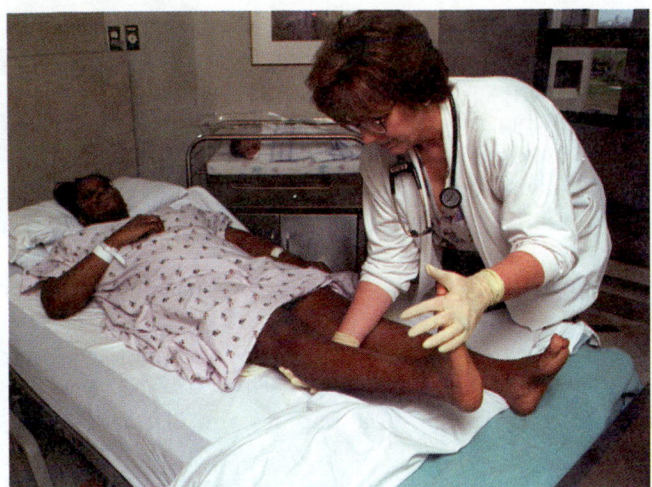

Figure 28-14 The nurse assesses for Homan's sign by checking for calf pain when the foot is flexed.

Emotional Status

Many times the client experiences a sense of elation immediately after the birth of her baby. She is excited and relieved that labor is finally over. The mother may want to relive the experience by talking about the labor. If she went through a particularly long and painful labor and delivery, however, she also may be exhausted and need sleep and rest to restore her body to health. In this "taking-in phase," the mother wishes to meet her own rest and nutritional needs before focusing her energy on her newborn. Chapter 29 provides a more in-depth description of the psychosocial phases the woman usually experiences after childbirth.

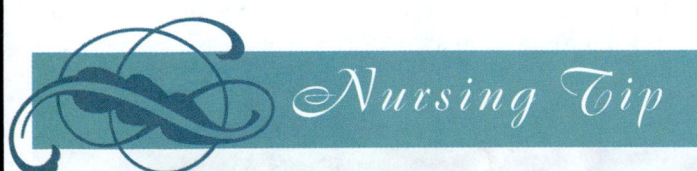

ASSESSING HOMAN'S SIGN

Homan's sign is assessed by straightening the client's leg flat on the bed. Place one hand on the knee, applying gentle pressure to keep the leg straight. Place the other hand on her foot, gently flexing the foot toward the body. The leg may be more easily examined when the woman slightly bends her knees and places the foot flat on the bed. The feeling of calf pain on flexion in either foot is a positive sign of thrombophlebitis. Use both hands on either side of the leg to palpate the calf for warmth and tenderness. Examine the calves for redness, hardness, or nodules along a vein. In addition, check the ankle and pretibial areas for edema.

PREVENTION OF THROMBOPHLEBITIS

Clients who remain in bed up to 8 hours should perform leg exercises to prevent formation of clots (thrombus) in the legs, which can develop into thrombophlebitis or thromboembolism. Deep vein thrombosis (DVT) is a severe condition in that a clot formed in the deep pelvis leg veins may fragment from the original clotted site and lodge into the lungs as pulmonary embolus. Superficial thrombophlebitis is noted as a hard, painful, warm, and red vein. Unlike DVT, there is little potential for pulmonary embolism with superficial thrombophlebitis.

Teach clients to flex and extend both feet and legs alternately while in bed. In a rhythmic motion, press then relax the backs of the knees into the mattress. Clients should also be taught other ways to prevent thrombus formation, such as keeping the legs uncrossed while seated, not flexing the legs at the groin, resting the legs without putting pressure on the back of the knees, wearing support hose or antiembolism stockings when varicosities are present, and padding pressure points during lithotomy positions.

Assess the client for signs of pulmonary embolism: dyspnea, coughing, and chest pain.

OTHER ASSESSMENTS

In addition to the basic postpartum assessments addressed in the approach using the acronym BUBBLE-HE, other important body systems need to be examined.

REFLECTIONS FROM A FAMILY

"The recovery period was difficult for me. I waited 9 months to be able to hold my baby for the first time, but I didn't get the chance to do it. I was bleeding a lot after the delivery so the doctor was rubbing real hard on my belly. I just couldn't deal with holding my baby when I was bleeding."

Hemodynamic Status

A CBC may show marked leukocytosis, predominantly neutrophils, both during and after labor. The leukocyte count may increase during labor up to 25,000/mm³, increase to as high as 30,000/mm³ during a prolonged labor, and remain elevated for the first 2 days postpartum (AWHONN, 1996). The average leukocyte count is 14,000 to 16,000/mm³. A possible infectious process should be ruled out in the presence of such increased counts or an increase of more than 30% from baseline during the first 6 hours after delivery.

Hemoglobin, hematocrit, and erythrocyte levels may fluctuate during the first postpartum days. When considerable blood loss occurs, the levels may decrease below those measured before labor. Immediately after delivery the hematocrit begins to rise increase owing to hemodilution, increase in plasma volume, and dehydration. By 4 to 5 weeks, the hematocrit returns to normal values of 37% to 47% (AWHONN, 1996).

Blood coagulation normalizes a few days after delivery; profiles secondary to PIH remain elevated. Findings may include uterine clot formation at the placental attachment site or pooled blood in the uterine cavity. It takes 3 to 4 weeks for the blood volume to return to prepregnant levels, depending on the amount of blood lost during delivery. Cardiac output remains increased for at least 48 hours after delivery.

Integumentary System

The newly delivered client may wonder if the stretch marks or **striae** on her breasts, thighs, and abdomen will ever go away. The striae eventually fade to a pale color but may never completely disappear, especially in dark-skinned women (Figure 28-15). Massaging lotion, such as aloe vera, may assist in lightening the color. Skin discolorations that appeared during pregnancy (e.g., chloasma) usually disappear toward the end of pregnancy. However, hyperpigmentation of the areolae and linea nigra may be permanent (Cashion, 1997).

After giving birth, the mother may complain of perfuse perspiration, especially at night, which is normal during the first week as the body rids itself of excess fluid from pregnancy. The nurse should try to keep the mother warm and dry.

Some women may note an eruption of mild acne from hormonal changes (AWHONN, 1996). Women who suffered from pruritic urticarial papules and plaques of pregnancy, or PUPPP, will note a rapid regression of this uncommon pregnancy rash within 1 to 2 weeks after delivery (Gordon & Landon, 1996). Topical steroids is the standard treatment for controlling the intense pruritus.

Other changes include hair loss for the first 2 months after delivery. The mother may become concerned with the large amount of hair found at the bottom of the tub or shower; the nurse should reassure her that this is normal owing to hormonal changes. The increase in fine hair usually disappears; however, coarse or bristly hair may remain (Cashion, 1997). The rapid decrease in estrogen also induces the regression of vascular abnormalities, such as palmar erythema and spider angiomas.

Musculoskeletal System

Because the abdomen stretches during pregnancy, the mother's abdominal walls relax or become flaccid after delivery. When visually assessing and palpating the abdomen and fundus, the nurse may notice some degree of muscle separation, called **diastasis recti**, along the center of the abdomen. This separation is due to pressure from an enlarging uterus and may increase with each subsequent

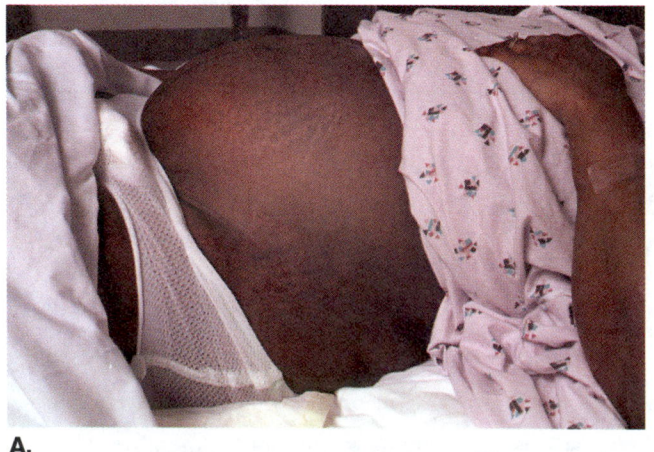
A.

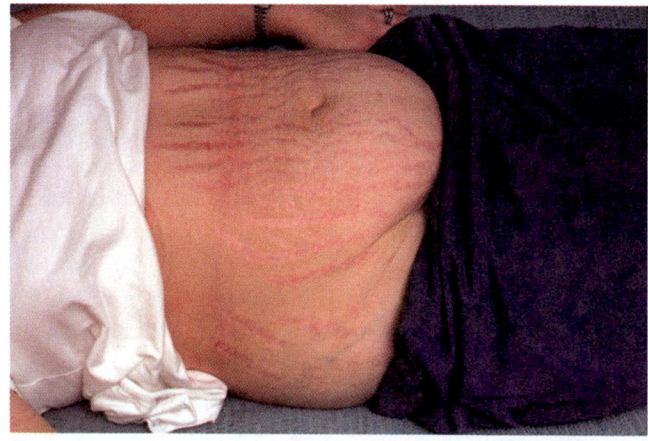
B.

Figure 28-15 Postpartum striae, or stretch marks, in (A) dark-skinned and (B) light-skinned clients.

Research Highlight

Differences between Primigravida and Multigravida Mothers in Sleep Disturbances, Fatigue, and Functional Status

Purpose

To determine whether differences occur in levels of functioning in primigravida compared with multigravida mothers.

Methods

A secondary analysis of a descriptive longitudinal study was done using an available sample of 31 pregnant women (primigravida, 12; multigravida 19). The mothers were tested during the third trimester and the first month postpartum for their level of functioning in the household, sleep efficiency, and fatigue and vitality.

The level of functioning was determined by the Inventory of Functional Status tool, an 11-item, Likert-type instrument by which the subjects rate their ability to perform certain activities of daily living. On a four-point scale, subjects described their ability to perform activities, such as cooking and shopping, from "not at all" to "fully."

Measurements of sleep disturbance were conducted using a sleep efficiency index taken from an electroencephalogram (EEG) machine during two consecutive nights during the two time periods in the study.

Fatigue and vitality were measured by a self-reporting tool called the VAS Fatigue scale, consisting of 18 items along a 100-mm visual analogue line. Subjects rated 13 items relating to fatigue and 5 items related to vitality.

Findings

Primiparas experienced increased fatigue, less vitality, and decreased sleep efficiency over time compared with multiparas. Multigravidas, indeed, experienced increased levels of household functioning compared with primigravidas.

Nursing Implications

It is important for nurses to provide anticipatory teaching to first-time mothers to help them transition into motherhood. Integrating the new role as mother may be more difficult for the primipara than expanding the already acquired role of mother may be for the multipara woman.

Water, M. A., & Lee, K. A. (1996). Differences between primigravidae and multigravidae mothers in sleep disturbances, fatigue, and functional status. *Journal of Nurse-Midwifery, 41,* (5), 364–367.

pregnancy. The severity depends on the client's general physical condition, muscle tone, timing between pregnancies, parity, and other circumstances that distend the uterus and abdomen. Multiple gestation, macrosomia, and hydramnios also distend the uterus to a larger than average size, making it difficult for the client to regain her prepregnant muscle tone.

Many mothers complain of fatigue after childbirth. They require time to recuperate and recover from the effects of labor and delivery. Primiparas and multiparas often have different physical and emotional needs. (See the accompanying Research Highlights.)

Activity

Once the puerpera is stable, the nurse should encourage her to ambulate often. The advantages of early ambulation are well established (Box 28-4). Women who deliver vaginally often are able to ambulate to the restroom within a few hours of delivery.

Although the nurse must be ready to assist a patient out of bed, the client should be offered the use of a wheelchair, when necessary. Before rising from the bed, the client should be assessed for dizziness and motor weakness from weak knees or legs. Ask the client how she feels

Box 28-4 Advantages of Early Ambulation

In general, the client will feel better and stronger if she begins to ambulate early after delivery. The following are the specific medical advantages of early ambulation:

- Fewer bladder infections.
- Less frequent constipation.
- Decreased incidence of deep vein thrombosis.
- Decreased incidence of pulmonary embolism.

Nursing Tip

PAMPERING YOURSELF POSTPARTUM

Suggest to the new mother to prepare a "Personal Postpartum Pampering Plan Checklist" to follow once she returns home after childbirth. A sample plan follows:

- Ask friends and family to cook meals (double menus, and freeze half). Ask friends to bring food if they are coming to visit, or let them cook for you when they arrive.
- Wear a gorgeous bathrobe, or wear comfortable clothing.
- Take a warm, soothing bath. Have someone else watch your baby during this break.
- For routine household chores, hire cleaning help ask friends or family, or hire a neighborhood teenager.
- Get out of the house. Go shopping. Take a walk in the park. Go to the local fitness club. Call other new mothers to accompany you, and take the babies together.
- Take frequent naps.
- Enjoy your baby.

when she rises from a recumbent position and if she is able to stand straight without assistance. When the mother is very tired or has received an epidural or analgesics that may cause drowsiness, she may not have the ability to stand and walk independently. When assisting the client in getting up from bed for the first time, the nurse should accompany her because she may experience orthostatic hypotension and be at risk of falling.

The client should be encouraged to return to normal activities of daily living as soon as possible. She should be able to provide independent self-care before going home. Once home, depending on the physician's instructions, she may perform light household chores. Family members or friends should take on the primary responsibility for major household chores, however, such as meal preparation. The client should be cautioned against driving for 10 to 14 days, especially if she received anesthesia or is taking analgesics that cause drowsiness. When episiotomy has been performed, the client should shower instead of using a tub until the incision has healed and the flow of lochia has diminished.

Exercise

Although vigorous exercise should be delayed until the client feels well-recovered, a woman who has had an uncomplicated vaginal delivery can begin moderate exercise soon afterward. The client may perform mild stretching and flexing of muscles, especially abdominal muscles, which may relieve tension and muscle strain (Figure 28-16). Care should be emphasized because joints do not stabilize until 6 to 8 weeks postpartum. Other safe exercises include Kegel's exercises, deep breathing, and pelvic tilts. Exercising too much and too soon may result in an increase in bright-red vaginal blood flow. The client must not lift anything heavier than her baby for the first 2 weeks after childbirth. She should avoid climbing stairs for about 2 to 3 weeks.

A safe healthy exercise program should include 30 to 60 minutes of aerobic exercises that increase the heart rate at least four times a week. Even exercising 1 hour a day, such as taking a brisk walk while pushing the baby in a stroller or carrying the infant in a sling will burn off 400 calories. The exercises should include abdominal and back strengthening exercises to support the organs, protect the back, improve posture, and improve appearance. Abdominal exercises can include those that isolate different abdominal muscles, such as stomach crunches. The addition of weight-lifting training for all major muscle groups at least three times a week will assist in building muscle. Muscles operate at a much higher metabolic rate than does fat therefore more calories are burned (Gilbert, 2000).

New mothers may report that they do not have the time or ability to exercise. The nurse can suggest that she find another mother to trade babysitting favors or a neighborhood teen to help watch the baby. New baby strollers allow the mother to jog or run with her baby. The mother may not fit into the clothing she wore at very early in her pregnancy. Although she may not relish the idea of wearing maternity clothes again, she can wear pants with an elastic waist and a loose top.

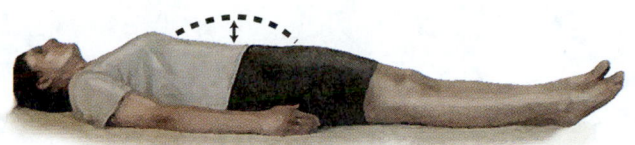

A. Deep breathing

Breathe deeply, expanding your abdominal muscles; then slowly exhale, tightening your abdominal muscles.

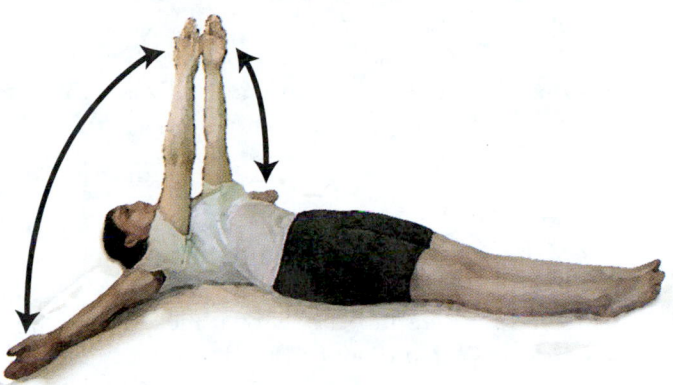

B. Arm raises

Place your arms at right angles to your body: slowly raise them, touch your hands together, then slowly lower your arms.

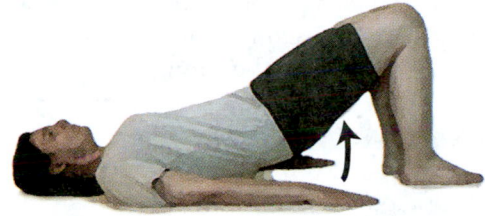

C. Pelvic tilt

Place your arms at your sides and your feet flat on the floor. Tighten abdominal and buttock muscles, press back into floor, then tilt pelvis toward ceiling.

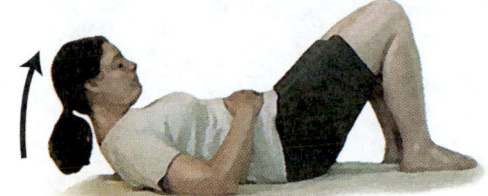

D. Head raises

Lie with your knees flexed, feet flat on the floor. Contract your buttocks, lift your head.

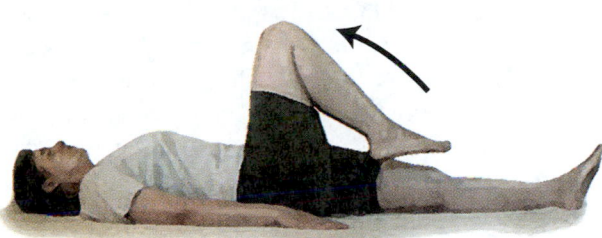

E. Knee flexes

Flex one knee towards your abdomen; lower your foot towards the floor, then straighten your leg.

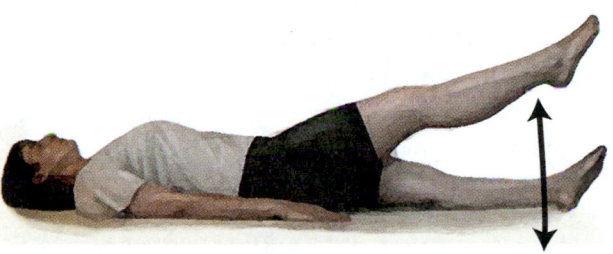

F. Leg raises

Straighten legs and point toes. Slowly raise then lower one leg and then the other using your abdominal muscles.

Figure 28-16 Postpartum exercises

Weight Loss

Although the client's figure does not automatically return to prepregnancy form, there is immediate loss of weight after delivery, representing the combined weights of the infant, placenta, and amniotic fluid. Average weight loss is 12 to 15 lb after delivery. An additional 5 lb is lost during the first week postpartum owing to extracellular fluid diuresis. Another 10 lb may be lost in the next 6 weeks.

Most women return to their prepregnancy weight 6 months after delivery; however, postpregnancy weight loss is difficult to achieve for some women. The client's ability to lose weight is related to the amount of weight gained during pregnancy, number of pregnancies, smoking, and the opportunity to return to work outside the home.

Exercises that flatten the stomach muscles and eating a healthy diet will help the client return to her prepregnant size and weight. The client should keep in mind that because the skin has been stretched greatly during pregnancy, the abdomen may not return to a totally flat appearance. The stretched muscles also may not return completely. First, the client should set goals and tailor her exercise and nutrition programs to her needs. She should include foods from the four basic food groups, increase her fluid intake, and avoid eating junk food.

The main approach to losing weight should be to change her metabolism gradually with a healthy diet. She should avoid fad and starvation diets that include in their regimens the practice of skipping meals. She should calculate her basic daily caloric needs, which is the number of calories of balanced nutrition she can consume to maintain a feeling of well-being without gaining weight. The diet should contain 1,500 calories or more, while the client

Client Education

Performing Kegel's Exercises

Pregnancy, childbirth, and being overweight can weaken the pelvic floor muscles and cause leaking of urine and stool. The muscles are weak if the client notes symptoms such as leaking urine when she sneezes, coughs, or lifts heavy objects. As with other muscles, exercises can make the pelvic floor muscles stronger. The pelvic floor muscles between the legs attach to the front, back, and sides of the pelvic bone. Two pelvic muscles do most of the work. The largest muscle stretches as does a hammock; the other is shaped like a triangle.

You should teach the client to perform Kegel's exercises properly. The client should be instructed to find the muscles that are stretched using two methods:

1. She should try to stop and start the flow of urine when sitting on the toilet.

2. She should imagine she is trying to stop passing gas or complete a bowel movement. She should squeeze the rectal muscles she would use. She will feel a pulling sensation when she is using the correct muscles.

There are two types of Kegel's exercises: quick and slow. In doing the quick ones, the client should tighten and relax the muscles rapidly. In doing the slow ones, she should tighten the muscles for 5 to 10 seconds and then relax.

The client should work up to doing 10 to 15 repetitions each time, three times a day. It is important to instruct the client about the following:

- She should not overdo exercising the muscles.
- She should not hold her breath.
- She should take care not to tighten other muscle groups, such as the stomach, buttocks, and legs. Squeezing the wrong muscles can put more pressure on the bladder control muscles.

Kegel's exercises can be done anywhere: sitting in a chair while watching television, standing in the kitchen cooking, or sitting in a car while stopped at a red light. The client should do the exercises in three different positions: sitting, lying, and standing. Doing so makes the muscles the strongest.

The client should be advised to have patience in seeking results. Improvement in bladder control may not occur for 3 to 6 weeks but may occur earlier. The client should try to tighten her muscles before sneezing, lifting, or jumping to protect them from more damage.

---

simultaneously increases the intensity and duration of exercise (Sears & Sears, 2000). Breast-feeding mothers need at least 500 extra calories for lactation. Abstaining from only one nonnutritious snack a day (e.g., one chocolate chip cookie contains about 100 calories) will reduce the daily caloric intake by 500 calories, or 3,500 calories a week, which is enough to lose 1 lb of weight. The mother can keep track of her success by monitoring her eating habits and weekly weight loss.

The client must approach losing weight in positive way and try to do it slowly (about 1 lb a week). The slower the weight loss, the better she will feel and the more likely the weight will stay off. The exercise program will invigorate her physically and mentally. Although the changes will be gradual, she will feel satisfied with herself once she reaches her weight and fitness goals.

Sexuality

There is no prescribed time when to resume sexual intercourse after childbirth. Mothers are warned to avoid sexual activity until their episiotomy has healed, which can take 6 weeks or more, or until they are comfortable and desire to have sex. Some women feel like resuming sexual activity as early as 2 weeks after birth; others may wait for 5 or 6 months until they are ready physically and emotionally. Bleeding and infection are less likely to occur once 14 postpartum days have passed. Because of perineal discomfort or swelling, some mothers often wait to resume sexual intercourse until after the 6-week checkup.

Several factors affect a woman's desire for sexual activity after the birth of her child. The birth experience places incredible stress on the body. Episiotomy stitches (if present) will have tightened the vagina, making it less elastic at first so that intercourse may hurt the first time after delivery. Breast-feeding mothers may have decreased estrogen production, leading to vaginal atrophy and dryness, making sexual intercourse difficult and painful.

The physical demands of taking care of a newborn infant with frequent feedings often leave both parents deprived of sleep. The new father may feel some cautiousness because he may be afraid of hurting his partner

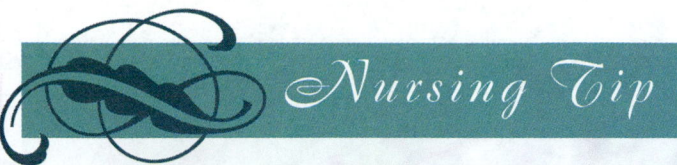

TIPS FOR MAKING SEXUAL INTERCOURSE AFTER BIRTH EASIER

You can give the client the following tips to educate her on how to make sexual intercourse easier after delivery:

- Try positions that may be more comfortable for the newly delivered mother. The woman-on-top position gives her greater control over the depth of penetration and allows her to move in a way that is most pleasurable for her.

- Use a water-based lubricant to ease vaginal dryness.

- Try having sex at different times of the day if you are too tired when you go to bed at night.

- Move your baby into another room to preserve the privacy and intimacy of your bedroom.

- If sex is too painful, engage in noncoital sex as a safe and satisfying alternative.

- Keep the lines of communication open by talking about and exploring new ways to satisfy each other physically.

Critical Thinking

Too Tired for Sex

New parents often feel overwhelmed by the birth of a child, which brings major changes into their lives. Suddenly, there are numerous diaper changes and 2 a.m. feedings. New parents may complain of their baby crying during the night, every night. They stagger into bed, knowing that the next feeding is right around the corner. Because of sleep deprivation, the last thing they may be thinking about is having sex.

You can teach the client that after a few months, the new baby will settle into a routine. Inform her that the baby's new schedule eventually will allow her and her partner to again have a satisfying sexual life. Provide the client with solutions for the problems that new parents face in resuming their sexual relationship. One solution is not to confine sex only to nighttime hours. The partners should try to make time for each other during the day, for example, when the baby is napping. They can try waking up earlier in the morning to provide themselves with some quiet, private time to enjoy before facing the responsibilities of the day.

How would you counsel new parents who confide their frustration in resuming regular sexual relations?

---

during sexual activity. Both partners must communicate openly about their feelings and discuss what is compatible and what is painful. It is important to convey to each other that a lack of interest or hesitancy is not indicative of a lack of interest or love in their marriage. The first attempts at sexual closeness can include massaging, cuddling, and touching without requiring penetration. Both partners will need to be sensitive and approach sex slowly according to their own timetable (Mayo, 2000).

The nurse should teach the new mother that, as a rule, it is acceptable to wait to have sexual intercourse after childbirth until both partners feel comfortable and secure. Sex after childbirth may not be exactly the same as it was before but can be satisfying. The client should use a water-based lubricant, such as K-Y jelly, for vaginal dryness to assist in making sexual intercourse easier and more pleasurable. The new mother may experience feelings of unattractiveness and loss of sexual appeal. She may be inhibited and hesitant to resume sexual openness with her partner. The nurse should inform the mother that these feelings are natural and that she should take it slowly and be patient with herself. The mother who is nursing may feel a decreased sex drive because breast-feeding produces lower levels of estrogen, the hormone that stimulates the sex drive. The breasts also are more sensitive to

stimulation and might be tender to touch. The milk might leak or let-down might occur during breast stimulation and orgasm; wearing a nursing bra or nightgown or having a towel nearby may help with this problem.

Contraception

Many women may not think about contraception immediately after birth, or they may be waiting for their 6 week check-up, or for the return of mensus. However, many women resume sexual activity prior to the 6 week check-up and may get pregnant before return of mensus. Therefore, it is important for the nurse to discuss contraception before discharge from the hospital.

The decision about contraception depends on many things: the client's and her partner's motivation, the number of children desired, the state of the client's health, whether she is breast-feeding, and the couple's religious beliefs.

The use of oral contraceptives while lactating is controversial (Bowes, 1996). It is thought that oral contraceptives can suppress milk production. When prescribed, providers often suggest starting contraceptives after breast-feeding has been firmly established. The mother who is not breast-feeding can begin to take oral contraceptives as early as 2 to 3 weeks after delivery.

Other choices in steroid contraception include depot medroxyprogesterone acetate (DMPA), which is given IM every 3 months. The major advantages of this method are patient convenience and easy administration. Another form is the insertion of levonorgestrel subdermal implants (Norplant). The normal time of insertion is 4 to 6 weeks postpartum; insertion also can be done immediately after delivery. In one study, implants placed 4 weeks after delivery showed no effects on lactation (Bowes, 1996).

If the client chooses to use a barrier method, such as a diaphragm, she will need to be fitted for the proper size at her 6-week postpartum checkup even if this method was used previously. The cervix will require time to return to the more normal prepregnancy size. The breast-feeding woman will experience vaginal dryness and tightness secondary to involution, which will make fitting more difficult. Use of the diaphragm also requires a spermicidal lubricant.

If an intrauterine device (IUD) is the method of choice, it usually is inserted after the 6-week postpartum checkup. Some providers may decide to insert it in the immediate postpartum period because fewer perforations occur when it is inserted between weeks 1 and 8; however, the risk of expulsion is higher, with rates from 10% to 21% (Bowes, 1996).

If the couple is undecided on the method of family planning or is postponing oral contraceptive therapy until 6 weeks, the use of condoms or in combination with spermicides may be a good choice. If the couple is sure about permanent sterilization, this can often be accomplished during a cesarean delivery or 24 to 48 hours after delivery. The timing must be carefully planned. Immediate postpartum sterilization often is associated with guilt and regret (Bowes, 1996). If the couple decides to postpone the procedure until 6 to 8 weeks after delivery, it will provide them time to ensure their infant is healthy and to be sure they are making the correct decision.

Pain Management

After delivery, the mother is at risk for various types of discomfort. She may complain of perineal discomfort, uterine cramping, sore nipples, or a headache if she received incorrectly administered spinal anesthesia. A great source of discomfort is from the afterpains related to uterine contractions.

Postpartum medications commonly given for episiotomy or uterine pain may be oral nonsteroidal anti-inflammatory drugs (NSAIDS), such as ibuprofen (Motrin), 400 to 800 mg orally every 4 to 6 hours as needed. Acetaminophen with codeine (Tylenol with Codeine) may be

Nursing Tip

RELIEVING AFTERPAINS

Suggest to the client an exercise called mini head lifts that can assist in managing afterpains. The client should be instructed to lie down with her knees bent. She should take a deep breath and as she exhales, lift her chin so it rests on her chest. She should perform the head lifts 5 to 10 times each time afterpains are felt, several times a day, to encourage uterine contraction.

given for more severe cramping. Emptying the bladder every hour or so is an effective measure to reduce afterpains. Another useful method is for the client to lie on her abdomen with a pillow against her lower abdomen because this creates pressure that keeps the uterus contracted (Jordan, 1998).

Topical anesthetics (e.g., Chloroprocaine [Nesacaine]) may provide temporary relief from episiotomy pain. The anesthetic spray should be used sparingly 3 to 4 times a day after voiding. As previously mentioned, ice packs and sitz baths also may provide relief for the mother. (See the accompanying Client Education box for herbal remedies.)

Immune System

Before discharge, the nurse should check the client's record for proper immunization status, particularly against rubella. If the mother is rubella nonimmune with a titre below 1:8, she should be vaccinated before leaving the hospital. The client must sign a consent form to receive the vaccine. Because the effects of congenital rubella syndrome (CRS) have devastating teratogenic effects on a fetus, it is important that the nurse counsel the client

Nursing Alert

ASSESSING UNRELIEVED PERINEAL PAIN

When medications do not relieve complaints of perineal pain, you should assess the site more carefully. Pain unrelieved by other means may indicate a possible perineal hematoma. Episiotomy pain normally is reduced and asymptomatic by 3 weeks after delivery. The postpartum client with a perineal hematoma will be in severe pain, often unable to sit comfortably.

Client Education

Perineal Comfort Measures

A midwife suggests alternative nonpharmacoligic methods of relieving perineal discomfort:

- Use of herbal mixtures for postpartum perineal discomfort: shepherd's purse, uva-ursi (bearberry), comfrey leaves and roots, sea salt, *Calendula* flowers, rosemary, lavender flowers, fresh garlic, myrrh, and ginger.

- A tea bag concoction with powdered comfrey and plantain on the perineum can relieve perineal tearing and soreness. The mixture can be placed in unbleached paper coffee filters and sealed or infused together (sewed by hand or glued). Pour boiling water over the coffee filter and tea bag in a small bowl and let steep for about 10 minutes. Check the temperature and when comfortable, press out some of the excess water and apply directly onto the perineum. Leave on until it becomes cold. Dip it into the warm water again, and use the other side. Can be repeated with the same tea bag three times on each side.

- A homemade-type recipe called "people paste" or "goose poops" is placed directly on the area causing the most discomfort. The base is made of three equal parts of powdered slippery elm, goldenseal, and myrrh. Comfrey and plantain can be added for vaginal tears. Clover powder can be added for stronger pain relief. Honey, molasses, aloe vera, and water can be added to the base. Combine the mixture, keeping it a little on the dry side so it can be shaped into a teardrop shape. Place the mixture on the perineum when relief is needed.

- Soothing sitz bath herbs that can be used include a mixture of 2 oz of comfrey, 1 oz of uva-ursi (helps prevent infection), one eighth to one fourth cup of sea salt, 1 oz of shepherd's purse, and 1 clove of garlic.

- Place lukewarm comfrey tea in a squirt-bottle to cleanse the perineum in the bathroom to help reduce healing time.

- Use frozen pads soaked with comfrey tea to reduce pain and swelling. Make a strong pot of comfrey tea. Bring about 2 quarts of water to a boil; remove from heat; and add 8 to 10 large, fresh, clean comfrey leaves, or 0.5 to 1 oz dried leaves. Let steep overnight or at least 4 to 5 hours. Fold 4 to 6 sanitary pads in half and hold the top and bottom ends together, with the adhesive on the inside, or cut up oversized pads to make two smaller ones. Dip the pads into tea, soaking the middle. Lay dipped pads side by side in a container (a shallow baking pan or plastic container). Place waxed paper or saran wrap on top of the pad layer and then make another dipped pad layer on top of that (like making a lasagna). The wax paper will keep the pads separated and prevent them from sticking together. Place the entire container of pads in the freezer. To use, wrap one frozen pad in a soft, white paper towel, washcloth, or layers of sterile gauze to prevent freezer burn. Place in a waterproof pair of underwear (e.g., Kotex Personals) or disposable underwear. Wear the underwear with the frozen pad. Use a new pad each time you void or for about 45 to 60 minutes until it becomes soggy.

- Use tea tree oil to promote tissue healing, relieve itching, and reduce the risk for infection. Mix three drops of tea tree oil (essential oil only) and 1 cup of distilled water. Place in a spray-bottle and mist onto the perineum.

Source: http://gentlebirth.org/archives/pppericr.html

against becoming pregnant again before receiving the vaccine—if she has declined to receive it in the hospital—and for the next 2 to 3 months after receiving the vaccine (ACOG, 1992). The client should know that she may experience a brief period of rubella-like symptoms such as a rash, lymphadenopathy, joint symptoms, and a low-grade fever 5 to 21 days after the vaccination. The vaccine is safe to give to breast-feeding mothers.

Unsensitized mothers who are $RH_o(D)$-negative and have given birth to an infant who is Rh-positive also should receive 300 μg of $RH_o(D)$ immune globulin (RhoGAM) within 72 hours of delivery (Table 28-6) (ACOG, 1990b).

Table 28-6 Pharmacology in the Postpartum Period: Rh$_o$(D) Immune Globulin Vaccination

Pharmacologic Class	Immune serum
Therapeutic Class	Anti-Rh$_o$(D)-positive prophylaxis agent
How Supplied	IM, 300 μcg vial (standard dose); 50 μg vial (microdose)
Indications for Use	Anti-Rh$_o$(D)-positive prophylaxis agent during situations such as abortion, miscarriage, ectopic pregnancy, postpartum
Chemical Effect	Suppresses active antibody response and formation of antibodies to antigens from Rh-positive fetal blood, which results in erythroblastosis fetalis
Therapeutic Effect	Blocks the adverse effects of Rh-positive exposure; prevents sensitization and subsequent development of antibodies to antigens from Rh-positive fetal blood, which results in erythroblastosis fetalis
Dosage	300 μg vial (standard dose) IM if fetal erythrocyte count <15 mL; provide more than one vial if fetomaternal hemorrhage is >15 mL
Side Effects	Low fever, anaphylaxis, discomfort at injection site
Nursing Considerations	Must administer medication within 72 hours of delivery; obtain confirmation of fetal blood type from sample of cord blood and maternal blood type before administration
Client Teaching	Ensure client knows the reason for receiving RhoGAM
Laboratory Finding	Rh$_o$D is negative and direct Coombs is negative test, give RhoGAM

RhoGAM is administered even if the mother received RhoGAM in the antepartum period. Depending on the extent of the hemorrhage and exchange of maternofetal blood, a larger dose of RhoGAM may be necessary.

Although standard precautions should be practiced with all clients, particular care must be taken with the postpartum client who has the human immunodeficiency virus (HIV) or acquired immunodeficiency syndrome (AIDS). Personal protective gear (e.g., latex gloves and safety glasses) should be worn to prevent the transmission of blood and other bodily fluids. The nurse should advise the mother to avoid contact of her bodily fluids with her

Client Education
Congenital Rubella

Although the incidence of congenital rubella has decreased over the years, about 10% to 20% of women are susceptible. Congenital rubella is a serious disease, with the fetus experiencing severe physical abnormalities.

You have the opportunity to teach the client that if she is not immunized, the rubella virus can cross the placental barrier. The frequency and intensity of infection depends on the timing of the infection. The more severe infections occur in the first 4 weeks of pregnancy, that is, at a time when she will not know she is pregnant. During this time, half of infants exposed to the virus will become infected. The rate decreases to less than 1% when the infection occurs after the first trimester.

Inform the client that a wide variety of severe abnormalities result from congenital rubella syndrome. The four most common problems are deafness, eye defects, central nervous system (brain) defects, and cardiac malformations (patent ductus arteriosus). Other abnormalities include a small head (microcephaly), mental retardation, susceptability to pneumonia, small size (intrauterine growth restriction), enlarged liver, and blood dyscrasias (hemolytic anemia and thrombocytopenia).

You can instruct the client about prevention. Prevention of congenital rubella can be obtained by receiving the rubella vaccine. About 95% of women who receive it become immunized. Inform the client that there are only a few rare side effects from the vaccine, for example, a low-grade fever, fatigue, and arthralgia. When the vaccine is given immediately after delivery the effects may be delayed for up to 21 days (Bowes, 1996). The vaccine is not contraindicated in women who are breast-feeding.

infant's mucous membranes and open skin areas. The client also should be cautioned not to breast-feed and thus take the risk of transmitting HIV to her infant (Duff, 1996). Clients with HIV or AIDS may receive medications postpartally, such as zidovudine.

Family Considerations

When a subsequent child is born into the family, the other children must adjust to the new family member. Mothers

Client Education

Receiving RhoGAM During Pregnancy

You should educate the client by telling her that if she has Rh-negative blood, she may need to receive RhoGAM after delivery. If the father's blood is Rh-positive, the blood of the baby also may be Rh-positive. If the baby has Rh-positive blood, small amounts of the baby's blood may have escaped into the mother's bloodstream during delivery. Natural antibodies are then released into the bloodstream as the body tries to destroy the foreign Rh-positive cells from the baby. When this happens, the client will become permanently sensitized to Rh-positive blood cells. If she has an Rh-positive baby in a future pregnancy, her body will have sensitized antibodies that will attack her baby's blood cells during pregnancy. Her baby may then develop a disease called erythroblastosis fetalis.

Instruct the client that to avoid this potentially fatal disease in an unborn baby the immune globulin RhoGAM should be given after the first pregnancy. Once her body becomes sensitized, it can never be reversed, even if given RhoGAM. Once she receives RhoGAM, future pregnancies with Rh-positive babies will not be affected because her blood will be free from anti-Rh-positive antibodies.

who have other children should be encouraged to include them in the bonding process. Other children, depending on their ages, will be curious about their new brother or sister.

Older siblings may be jealous of a new baby in the family and thus may demonstrate sibling rivalry. Signs of such behavior may include squabbling or jealousy among brothers and sisters, rejection of the new baby, anger, and introversion. An only child and children under 5 years of age may resent the new baby and may exhibit regressive behavior such as bed-wetting and biting. For instance, the toddler who is potty-trained, may revert back to dirtying the diaper, or the school-aged child may begin sucking on a pacifier again or begin biting others. This is the child's way of coping with a situation that he or she may not be able to handle in any other way. The other children may be jealous and afraid that the new baby will take away their mother's and father's love and attention.

Sibling rivalry is normal. When children live together, they often feel a need to compete and thus display emo-

tions of jealousy and anger. In some instances, sibling rivalry can be positive because small doses of competition can be healthy by teaching children how to negotiate. Children can learn to love someone and still be able to disagree with their point of view.

To minimize sibling rivalry, caregivers should begin to discuss the new baby's arrival before the actual birth. The other children should be encouraged to take part in preparation for the baby's arrival. Another suggestion is on birth of the infant, the older brother or sister can receive a present from the new baby as a way to show them they are important and loved. Care activities such as diaper changes and feedings can include an older sibling (Figure 28-17). Even toddlers can help by bringing a clean diaper to mommy, and so on.

At times when she is not caring for her newborn, the mother should plan on reserving personal time for herself and older children. The new mother needs time to rest and possibly reflect on the changes in her life and family. Although a newborn infant demands a great amount of attention, the new mother needs to ensure that she spends time with her other children. Her children need to know that their mother still loves them and has time for them.

Family pets (i.e., a dog or cat) also can begin to act strangely when a new baby is brought into the home. They also can be prepared to adjust to the change. Before bringing the baby home from the hospital, allow the pet to sniff the baby's scent on a piece of the baby's clothing or receiving blanket. This way, the animal can become familiar with the smell.

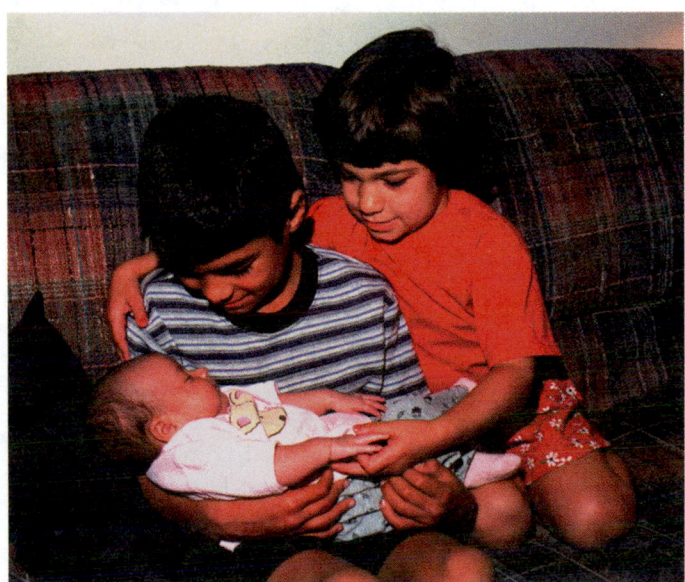

Figure 28-17 Encouraging older siblings to be involved in the new baby's care through simple tasks such as holding, comforting, and playing with the new baby may help them feel less threatened by this new family member.

Research Highlight

Sibling Behavior with a Newborn: Parents' Expectations and Observations

Purpose

To investigate parents' expectations and perceptions of their firstborn child's behavior before and after the birth of their second child.

Methods

As part of a larger longitudinal study, a sample of 70 couples with one child aged 6 years or younger completed two questionnaires plus a demographics form at home during two time periods (late in pregnancy and about 4 weeks after the birth of the second child). Both developed by Gullicks, the first questionnaire was the Older Child Expectation (27 items)/Older Child Observations inventories (23 items) and the second one was the Sibling Behavior Inventory (50 items). The questions were the same at both times, although those dealing with pregnancy were asked only the first time. For each question on the Older Child Expectation/Older Child Observation inventory, the parents rated behaviors at the two different times, responding on a 5-point scale ranging from 1, "Will almost never behave that way," to 5, "Will almost always behave that way."

Findings

The authors determined that "Parents expected their firstborn child's behavior to be more negative than they actually observed it to be." There were similar levels of appropriate behaviors particular to the developmental level in their firstborn before and after the second child's birth.

Nursing Implications

Findings indicated that parents expected less positive behavior from their first child, with behaviors changing little over time. Working closely with parents, nurses may help guide parents toward realistic expectations of their firstborn child, helping to encourage positive behaviors and coping with the arrival of the baby as a new member of the family.

Gullicks, J. N., & Crase, S. J. (1992). Sibling behavior with a newborn: Parents' expectations and observations. *Journal of Obstetric, Gynecologic, and Neonatal Nurses, 22,* (5), 438–443.

Documentation

Daily care of the woman after delivery encompasses assessments of the same parameters, such as episiotomy, lochia, and so on. If written in narrative format, the nurse may use the acronym BUBBLE-HE to assist her in ensuring all pertinent assessments are charted completely at least every shift or more frequently, depending on the client's acuity and the facility's policy on nursing documentation (Figure 28-18). In general, nursing documentation should follow the nursing process.

Flowcharts facilitate the documentation process (Figure 28-19). The use of flowcharts and graphs provide the ability to quickly note trends and changes from one shift to another. Columns at the top of the flowchart provide ease

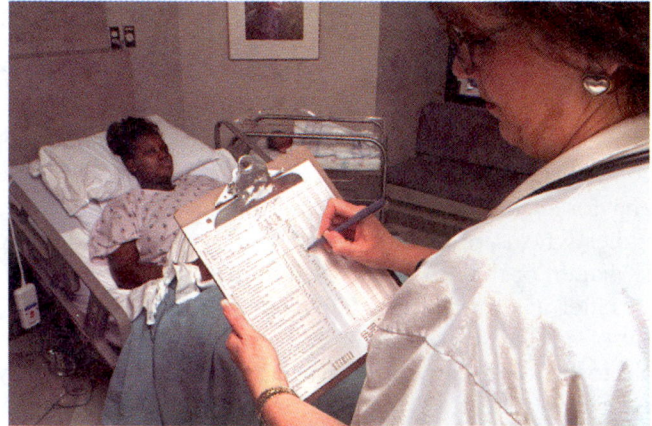

Figure 28-18 Careful documentation is the closing step of each assessment encounter.

Date														
Date														
Time														
Initials														
Breasts														
Fundus														
Lochia														
Perineum														
Diet														
Activity														
Bowels														
Bladder														
Homan's Sign														
Emotions														
IV														
Meds														

Legend:

Breasts
S=Soft
F=Filling
E=Engorged
NT=Nontender
T=Tender

Fundus
F=Firm
B=Boggy
@ U +/−
ML=Midline

Lochia
Sc=Scant
Sm=Small
M=Moderate
L=Large
R=Rubra
S=Serosa
A=Alba

Perineum
N=Normal
E=Edematous
B=bruised
H=Hemorrhoids
  present
IP=Icepack in
  use
S=Sitz bath in use

Diet
NPO
Reg=Regular
CL=Clear
Liquid
ADA=Diabetic

Activity
AL=Up AdLib
BR=Bed rest

Bowels
BM=Bowel
  Movement
F=Flatus

Bladder
QS=Voiding
  quantity
Sufficient
F=Foley
  Catheter

Homan's Sign
−=Negative
+=Positive
BL=Bilaterally

Emotions
N=Normal
S=Sad
H=Happy
N=Neutral
O=Other

Figure 28-19 Sample Postpartum Assessment Flowchart.

in checking off a box or placing the nurse's initials, as appropriate.

POSTPARTUM COMPLICATIONS

In caring for the low-risk healthy woman after delivery, the nurse must monitor and prevent the development of complications that may occur during the puerperium. The most common complications discussed in this section include hemorrhage, perineal hematoma, and infection.

Postpartum Hemorrhage

Obstetric hemorrhage is the most common complication in the postpartum period and is one of the three leading causes of maternal morbidity and mortality in the United States (ACOG, 1990a). Hemorrhage may be classified as early or late. Acute or early hemorrhage may occur within the first 24 hours after delivery, with the first 2 hours being the most crucial. Late hemorrhage occurs after 24 hours after delivery and before 6 weeks postpartum. Late postpartum hemorrhage is most likely to present on days 6 to 14 after delivery (ACOG, 1990a). Normal blood loss during an uncomplicated vaginal delivery is 500 mL or less (Benedetti, 1996). Hemorrhage is defined as blood loss greater than 500 mL for a vaginal delivery; however, providers tend to underestimate the measured blood loss. Hemorrhage is greater than the normal blood loss. The diagnosis of postpartum hemorrhage is based on the clinician's judgment of estimated blood loss.

Causes for early hemorrhage include retention of placental fragments, uterine atony or hypotonia, trauma or lacerations of the birth canal or lower genital tract, systemic coagulopathies, uterine inversion, and uterine rupture. Other risk factors are cesarean delivery, unusually large episiotomy, use of operative devices (e.g., forceps and vacuum extraction), precipitous labor, atypically attached placenta, and fetal demise. Risk factors for bleeding caused by uterine rupture include previous uterine surgery and internal podalic inversion (ACOG, 1990a).

The most common reason for early postpartum hemorrhage, accounting for 80% to 90% of the cases, is uterine **atony**, or lack of uterine muscle tone. Uterine atony occurs when the uterus fails to contract and becomes boggy. The failure to contract leads to continued bleeding from the site of placental insertion. Risk factors for uterine atony include the following:

- Uterine overdistention (e.g., from hydramnios, multiple gestation, or macrosomia)
- Uterine anomaly
- Poor uterine contractility (often present in women with high parity, rapid or prolonged labors, Pitocin-

induced or augmented labors, use of uterine-relaxing medications [e.g., halogenated agents, magnesium sulfate, or general anesthetics], chorioamnionitis, and a history of uterine atony)

- Placentas that do not separate wholly at the site usually leave behind fragments that prevent adequate uterine contraction and subsequently lead to bleeding. Risk factors for retained placental fragments include the following:
- Mismanagement of the third stage of labor
- Second trimester delivery related to an immature placenta
- Abnormal uterine anatomy
- Abnormal placental implantation (e.g., placenta accreta or placenta percreta)
- Abnormal placental implantation site (e.g., succenturiate lobe)
- Placental malformation

Another cause for bleeding are tears or lacerations of the birth canal from the following (ACOG, 1990a):

- Operative or instrumental deliveries (e.g., vacuum extraction and forceps delivery)
- Precipitous delivery
- Abnormal tissue or scarring (e.g., conization secondary to abnormal cervical cells)
- Extensions of perineal lacerations
- Varices
- Hematomas of the vulva or vagina
- Abnormalities of the soft tissue

Bleeding also may be related to systemic coagulopathies, such as disseminated intravascular coagulation (DIC). The risk of DIC is higher in women having PIH, abruptio placenta, clotting abnormalities, thrombocytopenia, fetal demise or retention of a dead fetus, amniotic fluid embolism, and infectious processes, and in whom anticoagulants have been used.

SIGNS OF DISSEMINATED INTRAVASCULAR COAGULATION

Bleeding from other nongenital sites in the body, such as venous puncture sites, may suggest the development of disseminated intravascular coagulation (DIC).

Table 28-7 Signs and Symptoms of Shock

Signs and Symptoms	Causes
Hypotension	• Stroke volume and cardiac output
Tachycardia, weak thready pulse	• Symptomatic vasoconstriction; chemoreceptor stimulation, progressing to medullary respiratory stimulation secondary to metabolic acidosis
Decreased pulse pressure	• Stroke volume
Cool, pale, clammy skin	• Peripheral vasoconstriction
Cyanosis	• Excessive vasoconstriction of reduced hemoglobin in blood
Oliguria or anuria	• Renal perfusion
Extreme thirst	• Extracellular fluid
Hypothermia	• Metabolism
Apathy, lethargy, confusion, coma	• Cerebral blood flow, acidosis
Irritability and anxiety	• Epinephrine secretion; hypoxia

ASSESSING FOR DECREASED PERFUSION

To subtly test for decreased perfusion in the extremities, squeeze the hypothenar area of the hand for 1 to 2 seconds and then release the pressure. If the client has a normal volume, the skin will initially blanch and then return to a normal color after 1 to 2 seconds. Circulatory refill in the blanched hand will be delayed in the client with a 15% to 25% volume deficit.

Postpartum hemorrhage can be very rapid, and often is very dramatic. Health care providers must be able to recognize the signs and symptoms early and respond immediately. During the immediate postpartum period the nurse bears great responsibility in assessing for potential hemorrhage. Knowledge of predisposing factors and careful examination of the client alert the nurse to the potential for hemorrhage and help anticipate it, preventing further complications. Many cases of postpartum shock are not recognized until the client is in moderate to severe shock, which requires more aggressive treatment to reverse. Table 28-7 lists the signs and symptoms seen in shock and the reasons for these conditions. Table 28-8 differentiates among mild, moderate, and severe shock.

Management of acute hemorrhage includes determining the cause of the bleeding, estimating blood loss, and trying to control the bleeding. Hemorrhage often occurs immediately before or after delivery of the placenta (Beneditti, 1996). Treatment of hemorrhage is based on identification of the classification and percentage of blood loss (Table 28-9).

Clients with Class 2 hemorrhage will begin to demonstrate clinical signs, such as tachycardia or tachypnea (Beneditti, 1996). Tachypnea is considered a nonspecific and early sign of mild volume deficit. Minute ventilation often is double its normal rate and should be interpreted as a sign of impending problems. Blood pressure changes include orthostatic hypotension and decreased perfusion to the extremities. The pulse pressure begins to narrow; when it decreases to 30 mm Hg or less, the client may be experiencing further volume loss (Beneditti, 1996).

The pregnant client with a Class 3 hemorrhage will begin to exhibit marked tachycardia (120 to 160 bpm) and tachypnea (30 to 50 bpm). Overt hypotension is present, and the nurse may note cool clammy skin. The client with a greater than 40% blood loss has a Class 4 hemorrhage. The nurse may not be able to detect a blood pressure in a

Table 28-8 Classifications of Hemorrhagic Shock

Signs and Symptoms	Blood Pressure	Pulse	Respiration	Skin	Urinary Output	Level of Consciousness
Mild	Normal or hypertensive	Increased, tone becoming weaker	Increased, deep	Cool and pale	Normal (average 30 mL/h)	Alert, oriented, mildly anxious
Moderate	Systolic, 60–90 mm Hg	Tachycardic, tone becoming irregular	Tachypneic, becoming shallow	Cool, pale, and moist	Decreased (10–22 mL/h)	Oriented, increasing anxiety and restlessness
Severe	Systolic, <60 mm Hg	Tachycardic, thready and irregular	Tachypneic, irregular	Cool, clammy, central cyanosis	Oliguric (<10 mL/h)	Lethargic

Table 28-9 Classifications of Hemorrhage

Class	Percent of Blood Loss	Estimated Blood Loss (mL)
1	15	<900
2	20–25	1200–1500
3	30–35	1800–2100
4	40	>2400

Nursing Alert

HEMABATE PRECAUTIONS

You should not administer carboprost tromethamine (Hemabate) when a client has a history of bronchospasms. Carboprost tromethamine is a prostaglandin that stimulates smooth muscles, such as the lungs, to contract. When given, clients usually develop diarrhea. You should use medications such as diphenhylate and atropine prophylactically to prevent diarrhea.

patient with profound shock. Pulses often are absent and urine output is minimal (oliguria) to none (anuria). Examination of the hematocrit may assist in estimating a large blood loss if it significantly changed from the previous baseline. Significant hematocrit changes will not occur until after 4 hours of the time of hemorrhage (Beneditti,

1996). The client also may exhibit signs of air hunger, anxiety, visual disturbances, and unusual thirst.

The overall goal in postpartum hemorrhage management is to prevent cardiovascular collapse—the bleeding must be controlled immediately. If the cardiac output decreases, renal blood flow will be compromised. The physi-

Critical Thinking

Beliefs about Blood Transfusions

You must be attuned to the client's cultural or religious values regarding health care. Members of some groups, such as the Jehovah's Witness faith, have deep religious convictions against receiving blood transfusions because doing so directly violates their beliefs. Blood transfusion is forbidden for them by Biblical passages noted in the following citation: "Only flesh with its soul—its blood—you must not eat" (Genesis 9:3-4); "[You must] pour its blood out and cover it with dust" (Leviticus 17:13-14); and "Abstain from . . . fornication and from what is strangled and from blood" (Acts 15:19-21). These beliefs include not accepting homologous or autologous whole blood, packed red blood cells, white blood cells, or platelets. The religious understanding of the Jehovah's Witness does not absolutely prohibit the use of other components such as albumin and immune globulins. Nonblood replacement fluids, such as colloid or crystalloid fluids, are allowed.

Health care professionals face this challenge as a major health issue. There are over half a million (and the numbers are increasing) Jehovah's Witnesses in the United States who do not accept blood transfusions. A liability concern for health care personnel exists; however, Jehovah's Witnesses will take adequate

legal steps to relieve liability as to their informed refusal of blood. Many physicians and hospital officials previously viewed refusal of a transfusion as a legal problem and sought court sanctions to proceed as they saw fit medically. Current medical literature indicates changes in attitudes of medical professionals. Nonetheless, the medical community has been trying to adapt other methods of treatment and practice the doctrine of treating the "whole person."

Caring for minors presents the greatest concern, often resulting in legal action against parents under child-neglect statutes. However, many people believe that Jehovah's Witnesses seek good medical care for their children. These parents urge that the legal and medical community give consideration to the family's religious beliefs.

How would you feel if your client is bleeding heavily and urgently needs a blood transfusion to replace her volume deficit?

Source: Jehovah's Witnesses Official Web Site. (2000). *Jehovah's Witnesses: The surgical/ethical challenge.* [On-line], Available: www.watchtower.org/library/hb/jw_surgical_ethical.htm. Reprinted with permission from *Journal of American Medical Association* (1981). *246*, (21), 2471–2472.

cian will play a major role in evaluating the reason for hemorrhage. A careful exploration of the uterus for retained placental parts and the cervix and vagina may show the source of bleeding.

Intravenous access should be available to administer fluids, medications, and replacement blood products, as needed. Pharmacologic agents to control bleeding include ergovine and synthetic prostaglandins. Packed erythrocytes most commonly are ordered to expand blood volume; other blood products, such as whole blood, platelets, fresh frozen plasma, and cryoprecipitate, also may be used. A CBC and typing and crossmatching for erythrocytes may be ordered as well as a coagulation profile (prothrombin time, partial thromboplastin time, platelets, fibrinogen, fibrin split products, and a clot retraction test). Blood products normally are given when the hemoglobin is 7 g/dL or less. If all else fails, surgical intervention with laparatomy may be indicated (Beneditti, 1996).

The nurse, along with the provider, should continually try to keep the client informed of her current medical status, especially as interventions are performed in an urgent manner. The nurse should explain what the actions being taken are and why they are being performed. The nurse should assist the client into a supine position, with legs slightly elevated to facilitate blood return to the heart. Other interventions include avoiding administering sedatives, analgesics, or other central nervous system depressants because they depress the vasomotor center. Overheating also should be avoided because it causes vasodilation.

Late hemorrhage occurs 24 hours or more after delivery and is defined as a sudden increase in bleeding 8 to 14 days postpartum (Bowes, 1996). At a time when the lochia transitions to lochia serosa, the client may experience a return to lochia rubra. The bleeding usually lasts for a short period of time and is self-limiting. Subinvolution at the placental site, vulvar hematomas, and infection (endometritis) are some of the reasons for the delayed or late bleeding. Of all cases, 40% are caused by retained placental parts (Bowes, 1996). Ultrasonography assists in identifying retained placental fragments, and suction evacuation is performed to remove the fragments.

Pelvic Hematoma

Pain that does not go away despite treatment with analgesics should be examined more closely. A common cause of severe perineal pain is the presence of a hematoma. This condition is potentially dangerous because blood loss may not be visible. Hematomas may be categorized into three types: vulvar, vaginal, and retroperitoneal.

The most common hematoma is located on the vulva, which forms when ruptured arteries and veins in the superficial fascia seep into the nearby vulvar tissue (Bene-

detti, 1996). Signs of a vulvar hematoma are local pressure; discoloration, such as ecchymosis (bluish-purplish); and a visible outline of a hematoma (Figure 28-20). Blood loss is subacute and the client may complain of perineal pain. Management involves surgical incision and evacuation of the blood and clots. Once sutured, the space is compressed with a large sterile dressing. An indwelling urinary catheter inserted at the start of the procedure should remain in place for 24 to 36 hours.

Trauma to maternal soft tissues during delivery (e.g., by the use of forceps) may result in formation of a vaginal hematoma. Large amounts of blood usually do not form. The client frequently complains of severe, unrelenting rectal pain. On examination, a large bulging mass may be protruding into the vagina. A large enough vaginal hematoma can make urination difficult. A vaginal hematoma is treated with incision and evacuation. The incision need not be closed; a vaginal pack is used to put pressure on the incision edges and is removed after 12 to 18 hours (Benedetti, 1996).

Least common but most dangerous to the mother are retroperitoneal hematomas. They occur when one of the vessels from the hypogastric artery is lacerated. A large amount of bleeding may ensue until the signs and symptoms of hypotension or shock are noted. Treating this life-threatening hematoma requires surgical exploration and ligation of the lacerated vessels (Benedetti, 1996).

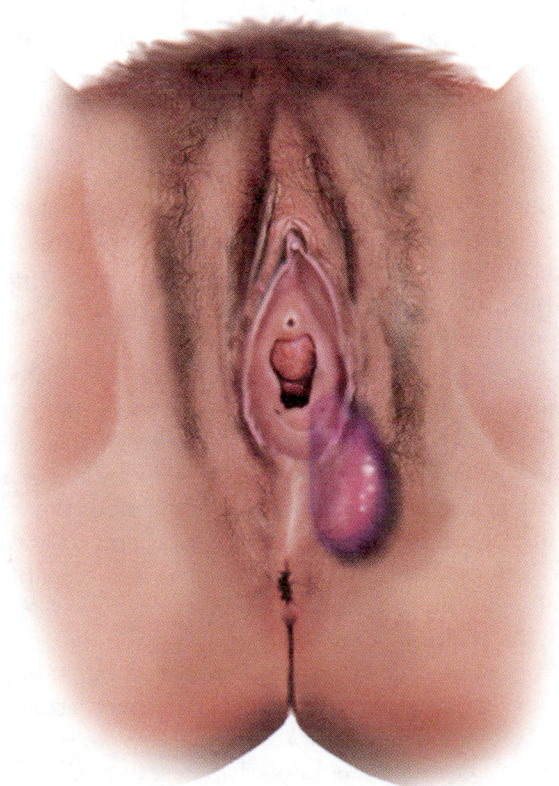

Figure 28-20 Hematoma of the vulva.

It is important for the nurse to examine the perineal area with the client in a supine as well as side-lying positioning to adequately detect a hematoma, especially when a new mother presents with severe perineal pain. Opened hematoma sites should be kept clean, with frequent pad changes. Smaller hematomas usually are allowed to resolve spontaneously, with ice packs used for comfort.

Many health care providers may order a postpartum CBC to evaluate hemoglobin and hematocrit values, especially if blood loss is significant. Otherwise, no other laboratory tests are required until clinical indications dictate.

Postpartum Infections

Postpartum infections, commonly known as **puerperal sepsis**, involve infections of the genital organs that occur during the first 6 weeks after childbirth. Postpartum infections are the leading cause of nosocomial infections and maternal morbidity and mortality (Clark, 1995). Postpartum infection is significant in that it delays mother-infant bonding and breast-feeding, the hospital stay is prolonged, or re-admission occurs. Nurses have the opportunity to identify women at risk for infection and recognize the subtle and early signs and symptoms. Because of early discharge, the nurse also must provide preventive care and anticipatory teaching to minimize the risks.

The classic definition of postpartum infection is an oral temperature greater than 38°C (100.4°F) taken twice 6 hours apart on any two of the first 10 days postpartum, excluding the first 24 hours after delivery (Bowes, 1996). Postpartum infections may occur within or outside of the pelvis. Pelvic infections include endometritis (the most common), pelvic cellulitis, pelvic abscesses, hematomas, and septic pelvic thrombophlebitis. Extrapelvic infections are those that occur in the urinary tract, at the episiotomy site, in the breasts (mastitis), or in the legs (thrombophlebitis). Refer to Table 28-10 for a description of the most common postpartum infections.

The causes of postpartum infections are related to anatomic and microbiologic factors. Microorganisms may enter the body at the site of the placental implantation. The infection then becomes systemic. With prolonged rupture of membranes, endogenous or exogenous flora may enter and ascend the vagina, causing infection. Dilation of the cervical canal after delivery makes it susceptible to bacterial invasion from normal flora.

The duration of labor (>18 hours), route of delivery, and colonization of amniotic fluid are the strongest predictors of developing a puerperal infection. Other factors that predispose clients to infections are obesity, anemia, malnourishment, cigarette smoking, diabetes, drug abuse, and immunosuppression. Other risk factors for developing infection include the following (Bowes, 1996):

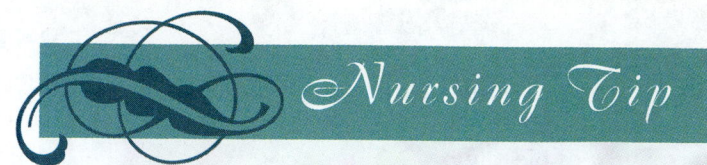

POSTPARTUM URINE CULTURES

Postpartum women often have midstream urine contaminated with lochia. When obtaining a clean-catch urine specimen to evaluate the client for a urinary tract infection, you should instruct the client in the proper technique. Because catheterization increases the risk of infection, it should be avoided.

To obtain a clean-catch urine specimen, instruct the client to separate the labia with two fingers of one hand. Using the other free hand, she should clean the labia with sterile wipes moving from front to back. The client should try to wipe three times: once on each side of the urethra along the labia and the third in the middle, cleansing the urethra. The specimen can then be collected.

- Cesarean section (changes in hemostasis; the incision site becomes a focal point for infection)
- Frequent vaginal examinations intrapartum (greater chance of introducing microorganisms)
- Prolonged delivery after rupture of membranes (>24 hours)
- Internal fetal monitoring (fetal scalp electrodes, intrauterine pressure catheter)
- Positive amniotic fluid culture (*Escherichia coli* and *Klebsiella* are commonly obtained from cultures of amniotic fluid)

Physical examination of the client with a suspected infection includes assessment of a change in the color, amount, odor, and consistency of the lochia. The episiotomy, if present, should be examined for redness, warmth, edema, tenderness, or disruption in the wound incision. The nurse should assess for fundal tenderness or pain when massaged. Costovertebral tenderness that may suggest pyelonephritis should be ruled out. Vital signs may indicate elevated temperature and tachycardia. Laboratory findings from blood, cultures, urinalysis, and culture and sensitivity tests may indicate the presence of infection. Culture reports will help determine the diagnosis and type of antibiotic therapy needed.

General Approach to Management of Infection

Infection with a single organism is rare. Broad spectrum antibiotics directed at multiple organisms often are administered prophylactically for cesarean sections and

Table 28-10 Common Postpartum Infections

Infection	Definition	Causative Organism	Comments	Clinical Findings	Management
Endometritis	• Infection of endometrium, lining of uterus	• *Escherichia coli* • *Chlamydia trachomatis* • *Gardnerella vaginalis* • *Mycoplasma hominis*	• Major risk factor: cesarean section (C/s) (especially after laboring or rupture of membrane [ROM]) • Incidence increases with presence of bacterial vaginosis • Degree of fever can indicate extent of infection	• Uterine distention or tenderness • Abdominal pain • Malaise, lethargy • Nausea and vomiting • Anorexia • Foul-smelling lochia • Fever, chills • Tachycardia • Anemia • Increased leukocytes with shift to the left • Increased erythrocyte pedimentation rate	• Broad spectrum antibiotics (double or triple) • If single antibiotics: high-dose Clindamycin or cephalosporins for 24–72 h • Supportive treatments • Rest • Hydration • Analgesia
Wound site	• Infections include various sites • Episiotomy • C/S, at abdominal incision site	• *E. coli* • *Mixed group A streptococcus* • *Clostridium perfringens*	• Encompasses infections of C/S, episiotomy, lacerations, and so on • Usually develops after hospital discharge • Risk factors: -Obesity -Diabetes -Prolonged labor -Prolonged ROM -Frequent vaginal examinations -Chorioamnionitis -Immunodeficiency -Hematoma formation	• White line along the episiotomy • Edema • Skin discoloration • Erythema • Warmth • Tenderness • Seropurulent drainage • Wound edge separation • Fever • Pain • Lochia odor • Lochia color change	• Re-admission • Debride wound; excise all necrootic tissue • Open and drain abdominal wound; pack as required • Antibiotics (if late onset, then no antibiotics) • Cephalosporins • Penicillin-resistant drugs • Vancomycin • Comfort measures • Frequent perineal care • Sitz baths • Warm compresses • Client teaching • Frequent pad changes • Good handwashing technique • Wipe "front to back" (avoid cross-contamination) • Modify activities • No isolation precautions from infant • Self-care • Adequate diet and fluids
Urinary tract infection (UTI)	• Infection of bladder or ureters	• *E. coli* • *Other gramnegative aerobic bacilli* • *Other enterococci*	• Most common extrapelvic infection • Risk factors: -Bladder hypotonia -Urinary stasis -Intermittent catheterization -Epidural anesthesia	• Manifestations of lower UTI: -Dysuria -Frequency -Urgency -Low-grade fever -Bladder overdistention	• Monitor for client complaints of infrequent or insufficient urination, discomfort, burning, foul-smelling urine • 10-d antibiotic therapy

(continued)

Table 28-10 Continued

Infection	Definition	Causative Organism	Comments	Clinical Findings	Management
Urinary tract infection (UTI) *(continued)*			• High number of pelvic examinations • Genital tract injury • History of UTI • Bacteriuria • Operative delivery • Anatomic disorders • Impaired bladder function; bacteria ascends from perineal or vaginal site into urethra	• Suprapubic pain • Urinary retention • Hematuria • Pyruia • Manifestations upper UTI: -Flank pain -Costovertebral tenderness -Urinalysis -Leukocytes -Nitrites -Bacteria >100,000/mL in a CCUA	• Ampicillin • Cephalosporin • Analgesia • Hydration • Outpatient treatment (except for pyelonephritis) • Client teaching • Monitor temperature, pulse, bladder function, urine appearance • Self-care measures • Report complications • Preventive measures • Avoid carbonated drinks (increased alkalinity) • Drink acidic fluids (cranberry, plum, apricot, prune juices) • Wipe from "from to back" • Increase fluid intake • Urinate frequently
Thrombophlebitis (so-called milk legs): • Septic pelvic thromobophlebitis (SPT) • Deep vein thrombosis (DIC)	• Inflammation of lining of blood vessel owning to blood clot formation, usually in deep veins in legs, thighs, or pelvis		• SPT is the least common infection • SPT frequently occurs with wound infection, especially when no client response to antibiotics • DVT incidence: -1:1,000 in vaginal deliveries -3–4:1,000 in assisted deliveries -25:1,000 in cesarean sections • Risk factors for SPT and DVT: -Venous stasis from remaining in bed for prolonged period -Increased coagulapathy -Blood vessel damage	• SPT • Pain 2–4 postpartum in groin, upper or lower abdomen, flank area • Moderate fever • Guarding • Tachycardia • Ropelike, tender mass near uterus • Gastrointestinal distress • Decreased bowel sounds • DVT • Rapid onset • Severe pain and swelling • Redness, warmth, tenderness in calves or legs • Hardness or nodules along a vein • Varicosities • Positive Homan's sign	• SPT • Laboratory tests: complete blood count, chemistry, coagulation profile, cultures • Chest X-ray film, computerized tomography scan • Re-admission • Anticoagulation therapy with heparin • Antibiotics • Supportive care • Rest • Hydration • Analgesia • Evaluation respiratory status every 2–4 h • Breath sounds • Rales (from pulmonary edema) • Monitoring of coagulation profile • Prothrombin time, partial thromboplastin time

Table 28-10 Continued

Infection	Definition	Causative Organism	Comments	Clinical Findings	Management

Mastitis (continued)	• Infection of lactating breast	• *Staphylococcus aureus*	• Preventable infection
			• Found most often in Caucasian multiparous women
			• Found in 7%–11% of lactating women
			• Symptoms usually occur 2–4 weeks postpartum
			• Presentation might be mild and almost chronic or severe and acute
			• Risk factors:
			  -Damaged nipples
			  -Failure to empty breasts adequately
			  -Primiparity
			  -Stress
			  -Breast abnormalities
			  -Skin infections
			  -Increased maternal age
				• Sudden onset of flulike symptoms
				• Chills, fever
				• Tachycardia
				• Achiness
				• Headache
				• Malaise
				• Nausea and vomiting
				• Unilateral local breast pain
				• Warmth, swelling, redness
				• Axillary adenopathy
				• Clogged milk ducts
				• Endemic mastitis
				• Red, inflamed
				• V-shaped area
				• Leukocytosis
					• Antibiotics
					• Dicloxacillin
					• Complete emptying of breasts
					• Use of breast pumps
					• If not breast-feeding, bind breasts
					• Supportive measures
					• Moist heat or ice to the local area
					• Hydration
					• Analgesics
					• Assess breast-feeding technique
					• Client teaching on preventive measures
					• Proper infant position for correct latch-on and sucking
					• Breast-feed every 2–3 h
					• Avoid nipple shields
					• Try to avoid supplemental feedings and pacifier use
					• Change wet nursing pads
					• Avoid tight clothing, underwire bras, infant carriers that may block milk ducts or prevent breasts from emptying adequately
					• Avoid practices that put pressure on breasts:
					  -Sleeping on stomach
					  -Gripping breasts tightly when nursing
					  -Resting infant on the breast while supine
					  -Infant's hand on breast while feeding
					  -Pressing breast tissue away from infant's nose during feeding
					  -Stopping milk flow by pressing on areola

(continued)

Infection	Definition	Causative Organism	Comments	Clinical Findings	Management
Mastitis *(continued)*					• Empty breasts completely; avoid milk stasis • Manually express milk if milk duct is blocked • Avoid cracked nipples • Use larger or different cut of bra for comfort

prolonged rupture of membranes. The issues of treatment and timing of the treatment, however, vary among health care providers. With the high incidence of antibiotic-resistant organisms, antibiotic medications should be used as a last resort. Health care providers should identify measures to prevent infection and encourage herbal and holistic means of increasing the immune response. General nursing practice in preventing infection is targeted at maintaining health with diet, exercise, and diligent hygiene practices, such as good hand-washing technique.

The nurse can provide anticipatory teaching to help clients prevent infection. The client should be instructed on how to use a squeeze-bottle with warm water after using the toilet to better cleanse the area and on how to wipe anteriorly to posteriorly. Perineal pads should be changed in the same manner, that is, removed from anterior to posterior, and should be replaced each time she goes to the bathroom. Client education includes the side effects of therapy, prevention of spread of infection, maintenance of adequate fluid intake, adherence to the prescribed treatment regimen, the signs and symptoms of worsening infection, and when to contact her provider.

Caregivers also should be cognizant of preventing the transmission of infection among staff and clients. Standard precautions and careful conscientious hand-washing should be practiced. Shared equipment (e.g., heat lamps and tubs) should be thoroughly cleaned and disinfected. Staff members with signs of infection (i.e., respiratory infection) should refrain from providing direct client care.

Endometritis

Endometritis is an infection of the uterine lining occurring from pathogens that ascend from the lower genital tract (Bowes, 1996). Endometritis occurs in 2% of vaginal deliveries and 10% to 15% of cesarean deliveries. When endometritis presents after 1 to 2 days after delivery, the

causative agent usually is group A streptococcus. Infections that occur after 3 or 4 days usually are caused by anaerobic organisms, such as *Escherichia coli* (Bowes, 1996).

The client with endometritis may complain of symptoms of lower abdominal pain, chills, anorexia, malaise, and a malodorous vaginal discharge. The nurse should assess for fever, abdominal tenderness, and mucopurulent vaginal discharge. Laboratory studies will include a CBC, urine culture, and blood cultures.

Prompt IV antibiotic therapy is used to treat suspected endometritis. Treatment is continued until all symptoms have been resolved for 48 hours, including fever. A combination of clindamycin and gentamycin usually is ordered, which will provide coverage for aerobic and anaerobic organisms (Bowes, 1996). Single antibiotic therapy may be prescribed with either a cepholasporin or extended spectrum penicillin (Bowes, 1996).

Mastitis

An infection of the breast, **mastitis**, usually involves the ducts and lactiferous glands of the breast. Mastitis usually is endemic in nature, resulting from *Staphylococcus aureas*, which comes from the infant's mouth (Clark, 1995). It is not harmful to the infant. Other causes of mastitis include cracked nipples, missed or shortened feedings, and consistent pressure placed on the breast (Kimm, 1997). Incomplete emptying of the breast will result in the breasts being overly full and, subsequently, development of plugged milk ducts. The nurse should teach the client steps to prevent mastitis.

The client most often will present with complaints of swollen tender breasts around 5 or 6 weeks postpartum but as early as 2 weeks (Bowes, 1996). The breast (normally unilateral) will feel very warm, with areas that may appear reddened with hardened nodules. The client may report a sudden onset of flulike symptoms, including

Preventing Mastitis

You should instruct the breast-feeding mother to avoid missing or shortening feeding times. She should be mindful of the times her baby begins to suddenly sleep longer at night, begins an irregular nursing pattern (nursing a lot one day and less the next), she begins to supplement feedings with formula, or she begins to give the baby a pacifier frequently.

The client should be instructed to avoid putting pressure on the breasts. She should try not to sleep on her stomach or hold her baby too tight against her chest while feeding. She should be told that shoulder straps from purses and diaper bags may place pressure on her breast. The client should make sure her bra fits correctly. Underwire bras may cause a problem. Thick breast pads or breast shells also may make her bra too tight.

Instruct the client to pay attention to proper positioning and how her baby is latching on. She can massage the hardened area to try to open plugged milk ducts. Finally, she should be sure to take care of herself by getting enough rest. Mastitis often is the first sign a new mother is doing too much and not taking care of herself. She should try cutting back on activities and start relying on family members and friends to help.

aching joints, malaise, nausea, vomiting, severe headache, chills, and fever (Overfield & Tully, 1997). Mastitis resulting from an endemic nature may be characterized by a demarcated V-shaped area of redness and inflammation (Clark, 1995).

The nurse should instruct the client with mastitis to continue breast-feeding. If she prefers, the client may continue to express milk either though pumping or manual expression to ensure complete emptying of the affected breast. The client will require increased fluids and ample time to rest. The nurse should instruct the client to place warm compresses on the affected area and take NSAIDs to relieve pain and fever. The mother should avoid supplementing with infant formula, nipple shields, and pacifiers (Clark, 1995). Nursing pads should be changed when they become wet. Antibiotic therapy using penicillin, ampicillin, or dicloxacillin (Bowes, 1996) often is prescribed to complete the treatment. When mastitis recurs, the infant's throat may be cultured to determine if the baby is reinfect-

ing the mother. Reassure the mother that although the course of mastitis may be very painful and frustrating for her and her baby, the infection will eventually resolve within a few days of antibiotic treatment.

CLIENT EDUCATION

Client education comprises much of the nurse's responsibilities and postpartum nursing practice. With shortened hospital stays, the nurse must streamline her teaching methods, assessing the new mother's and family's personal teaching needs. Client interactions should become more efficient, focusing on communicating knowledge to clients. The focused interactions should be directed toward desired client outcomes, empowering the woman and her family. Ideally, the nurse should assess the mother's current knowledge regarding self-care and infant care because the mother's prior experiences with pregnancy and infant care may change the direction of the nurse's teaching plans.

Depending on the facility, client teaching may incorporate a wide range of methodologies. Group classes scheduled for specific times of the day enable educating many clients at one time. One-on-one teaching may be more effective for those mothers requiring individual attention but is not realistic in terms of cost. Closed-circuit television programs also provide a medium of individualized education in the privacy of the client's room. Various printed materials and videotapes are widely available commercially. Specific information developed by the hospital also may be available.

Before being discharged the new mother must learn how to care for herself and her infant (Figure 28-21). Self-care topics include those activities that help her to manage, anticipate, and recognize health problems or danger

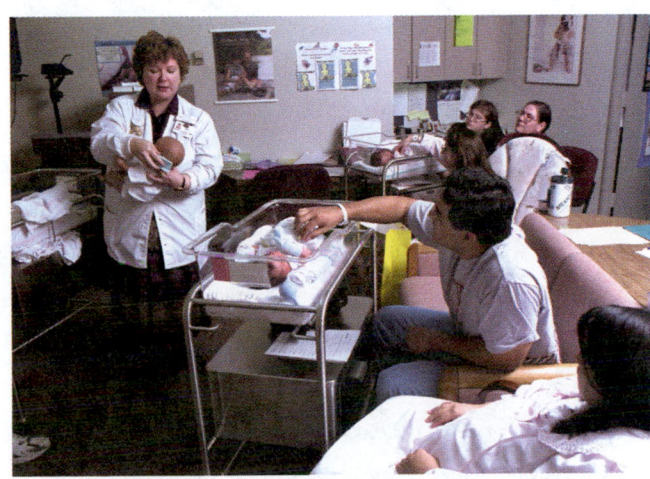

Figure 28-21 Infant care, self-care, and family adaptation are topics typically covered in postpartum education classes.

Box 28-4 List of Community Resources
- Hospital advice lines.
- Newborn clinics for follow-up.
- Visiting nurse and public health nurse home visits.
- Private free services.
- Library-loan books and videos.
- Client educational materials and resources.

signs. Infant care encompasses activities such as feeding, dressing, and recognition of health problems.

General instructions, in addition to other client education discussed throughout this chapter, should be given to the client. The nurse should also instruct the client on warning signs of complications after delivery. Suggestions for community resources for support and education also should be offered (Box 28-4).

Client Education

General Discharge Instructions

You should provide these general discharge instructions to the new mother:

- Take it easy when you go home.
- Do not lift anything heavier than your baby. Do not move furniture or vacuum for the first few weeks. No driving for the first 2 weeks or until approved by your physician. Limit stair climbing to only when necessary for the first 2 weeks.
- Get lots of rest. Sleep when the baby sleeps.
- Take advantage of offers of help from others.
- Ignore housework for the first few weeks. Enjoy your baby.
- If you have an episiotomy, avoid having sexual intercourse until it heals or until your bottom feels better. You may need to use a lubricant to help with dryness.
- Try to take older siblings' feelings into consideration.
- Take your medications as prescribed.
- Keep your postpartum follow-up appointment.
- Call your health care provider if you have any of the warning signs of sickness.

Client Education

Warning Signs of Illness after Delivery

You should inform the client to call her provider if she experiences any of the warning signs of sickness after she is discharged from the hospital:

- Fever greater than 100.4°F.
- Severe pain, redness, or swelling in the episiotomy or cesarean section incision.
- Foul-smelling vaginal discharge.
- Increased bleeding; soaking of a peripad more than once an hour or a large amount of bright-red lochia after your discharge has turned dark red or pink.
- Passing of several large clots greater than the size of a half dollar coin.
- Backache or severe abdominal pain or cramping (unrelieved by medication), or pain in the episiotomy or perineal area.
- Reddened, tender, swollen breasts that may have hardened lumps (may be related to flulike symptoms).
- Pain, redness, and swelling of your legs.
- Burning when you urinate, or frequent urination.
- The blues or crying that lasts for days.
- Depression that is severe or does not go away.
- Thoughts of harming your baby.
- Suicidal thoughts.

As part of the discharge process, the nurse may use a facility-specific checklist to ensure all care has been provided (e.g., birth certificate completed, laboratory testing obtained, and teaching handouts and pertinent information received). The nurse should ensure the client is instructed on any discharge medications ordered and where to obtain them. Some women may continue to take their prenatal vitamins and iron until the postpartum checkup, especially if the hematocrit is low. If the woman experienced a third- or fourth-degree laceration, she may be prescribed a stool softener. The provider may order over-the-counter or prescription pain medication for home use.

Before discharge the new mother should leave the hospital with a follow-up clinic appointment already in hand or with clear instructions on how to obtain one. A postpartum follow-up examination usually is scheduled for 6 weeks after delivery. The examination may be sched-

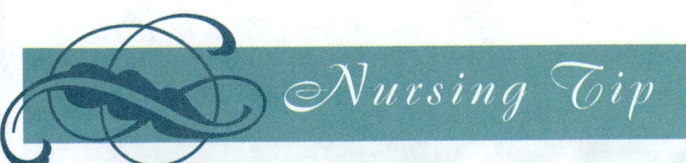

ASSESSMENT OF LIGHT BLEEDING WEEKS AFTER DELIVERY

At the 6-week postpartum checkup the provider will perform a Pap smear, which may cause light bleeding.

Some women may experience light bleeding for up to 3 months postpartum, which is considered normal when the following criteria are present:

- The uterus has returned to its normal size.
- No fever is present.
- Clots or tissue is not being passed.
- The client is not feeling exceptionally fatigued.
- No foul odor is associated with the bleeding.

Postpartum bleeding also can be caused by exercise, sexual intercourse, and breast-feeding. Certain oral contraceptives and depot provera cause postpartum spotting. The bleeding also can be the start of the first menstrual period.

uled for as early as 2 or 4 weeks if the client has experienced complications.

The provider will perform a complete well-woman examination, checking the client's physical and emotional health. The follow-up includes an examination of the epi-

REFLECTIONS FROM FAMILIES

"I fell in love with my baby after she was born. I couldn't wait to be the best mother I could be to her. However, I happen to be the main breadwinner in the family. It would cost us financially if I were to stop working or even only work part-time.

After the normal 6 weeks of maternity leave, I have to return to work. I am torn between having to return to work so soon and being able to stay at home with my baby. I want to be able to see her crawl or sit for the first time. It won't be fair if the day-care provider experiences my child's milestones before I do."

siotomy (if one was performed), Pap smear, bimanual examination, and breast examination. The client will have an opportunity to ask questions and discuss concerns. If not already done, the client should discuss her contraceptive options at this time.

EARLY DISCHARGE

Hospital stays for new mothers have decreased to an average of 48 hours or less (based on client preferences). To qualify for early discharge, it must be determined that the mother is at low risk and has had an uncomplicated antepartum and intrapartum course and a normal vaginal delivery. Guidelines for discharge vary with each hospital. Each facility should have policies in place that identify the circumstances and processes that must occur for the new mother and infant to be discharged early from the hospital. The Guidelines for Perinatal Care (AAP & ACOG, 1992) state specific criteria that must be met before a mother and her infant may qualify for early discharge from the hospital (Box 28-5). Refer to the Chapter 32 Newborn for more guidelines regarding infant-care client teaching.

Before the new mother's discharge, the postpartum nurse should include an assessment for adequate support at home (Figure 28-22). Does she a designated support person available to help with the household duties, such as cleaning and preparing meals? The new mother may become overwhelmed with the responsibility of caring for herself and her new infant without adequate support.

The nurse should be cognizant of other referrals for services the client may require. For example, consultations with a nutritionist, physical therapist, nursery nurses, social services, home care services, maternal-child clinical nurse specialist, or lactation expert may be of benefit to the client. Referrals for high-risk care and follow-up and community resources for breast-feeding assistance (e.g., La Leche League) also are available. Many of these services are not covered by insurance, except for those for high-risk mothers. The local community may have programs (e.g., "First Steps") designed to assist high-risk clients, such as adolescents and women in low-income families. Canada has several programs ("Healthiest Babies Possible" and "Brighter Futures") that begin prenatally and continue postnatally for these clients.

Social services may help coordinate the discharge process by obtaining needed psychosocial support, monetary assistance, and referrals to community resources. Mothers who meet the criteria (i.e., financial and physical needs) for such services may qualify for food supplied by federal programs, such the Special Supplemental Nutrition Program for Women, Infants, and Children (WIC). First-time mothers may benefit from a family-advocacy nurse specialist who may provide counseling on parenting. Family-advocacy nurses focus on the high-risk client who may require further follow-up, including home visits and

Box 28-5 Criteria for Early Discharge

Mother

- Uncomplicated pregnancy, labor, birth, and postpartum course.
- No evidence of premature rupture of membranes.
- Stable blood pressure and no fever.
- Ability to ambulate.
- Ability to void without difficulty.
- Intact perineum without third- or fourth-degree perineal laceration.
- Hemoglobin level greater than 10 g.
- No significant vaginal bleeding (mild to moderate).

Infant

- Term infant (37–41 weeks) with birth weight of 2,500–4,500 g
- Normal findings on physical assessment.
- Normal laboratory data, including negative results for Coombs test and hematocrit.
- Stable vital signs.
- Stable temperature.
- Successful feeding (normal suckling and swallowing).
- Apgar score greater than 7 at 1 and 5 minutes.
- Normal voiding and stooling.
- Newborn screening test completed.

ensuring the new parents obtain the necessary cognitive and performance skills to care for their infant.

HOME VISIT GUIDELINES

With high health care costs impacting postpartum hospital stays, the new mother may benefit from home visits from a community health nurse or family-advocacy nurse specialist after hospital discharge. Often, a hospital postpartum teaching program with limited nurse-client interactions cannot address all the client's learning needs in 48 hours or less. The client also may not be ready to learn after delivery. A postpartum home visit program may provide a safe and economical alternative to extended hospital stays.

Referrals for a home visit should be assessed during the discharge planning process and discussed with the client. Clients at risk for complications should be identified early and plans made accordingly. The home visit also can provide support and address concerns the mother may have after leaving the hospital. The visiting nurse may provide a positive impact on the new mother. The new parents, especially a primipara mother, may require extra encouragement and instructions on infant care. Self-esteem and self-confidence are valuable elements in the mother's adaptation to the maternal role. The nurse can help build these characteristics though education and demonstration.

The visiting nurse should assess the mother's physical well-being and self-care activities. Assessments should include the following: normal changes in lochia pattern, uterine involution, appropriate bowel and bladder functioning, rest and activity patterns, pain management, nutrition, infection, and coping. The nurse may be able to identify problems with episiotomy healing or development of mastitis.

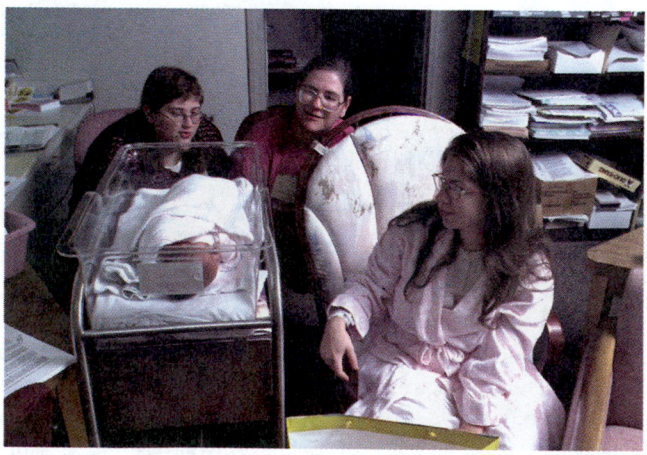

A.

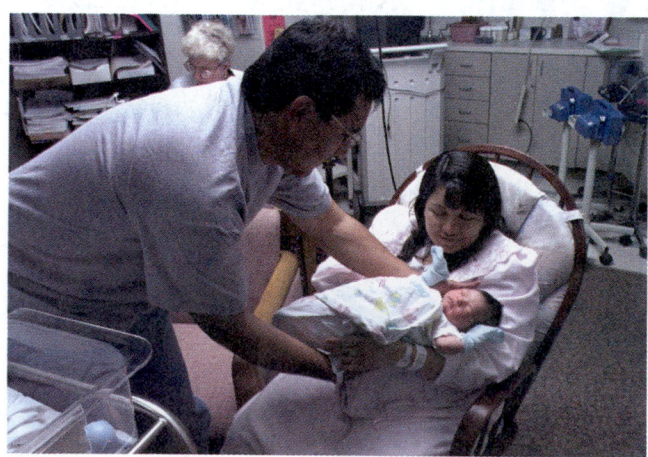

B.

Figure 28-22 Discharge planning includes assessment of the new mother's support systems. A. This single mother may benefit tremendously from the support and experience of her mother and sister. B. This new father is eager to assume an active role in his newborn son's life.

Case Study/Care Plan

THE CLIENT WITH POSTPARTUM BLEEDING AND PAIN

Cristina, grava 4, para 4, is a married, 32-year-old, Hispanic woman who gave birth to a healthy, term baby boy at 8:48 a.m. by forceps delivery. Her membranes ruptured 6 hours before the start of active labor. She had an episiotomy with a second-degree laceration. The estimated blood loss was 450 mL. Apgar scores were 8 and 9 at 1 and 5 minutes after birth. No resuscitation was required. The infant weighed 9 lbs, 10 oz., and was 21 in long. During the intrapartum course, Cristina received only IV analgesia for pain relief. She was catheterized once when she was unable to urinate. She quickly progressed through labor, totaling only 5 hours and 22 minutes for the entire labor. Her perineum was moderately swollen.

During fundal massage the first hour after childbirth, the nurse noted the peripad was saturated with a large amount of lochia rubra. The fundus was boggy, firmed up on massage, but became soft again once massage was discontinued. The location of the fundus was U+2 deviated to the right side. Christina had not voided for the past 4 hours. The client was awake, alert, and mildly tired after labor. Vital signs were as follows: blood pressure 105/72 mm Hg, pulse 94 bpm, respirations 20 breaths per minute, and temperature 99.2°F. An IV of lactated Ringer's solution with 20 U of oxytocin is infusing at 125 mL/h. Bowel sounds are present and active. She complains of moderate cramping. She plans to breast-feed. Her husband is at her bedside holding their new baby.

Assessment

Cristina presents with two major nursing problems related to bleeding and pain. First, she delivered a large infant by forceps delivery, making her at risk for bleeding. The bleeding may be caused by atony secondary to uterine distention and lacerations from the use of forceps. Having a full bladder and delivering rapidly also are risk factors for bleeding. Second, the client is a multipara who previously has experienced very uncomfortable afterpains. Her discomfort is increased with her episiotomy and, most likely, the full bladder.

Nursing Diagnosis

Deficient fluid volume related to postpartum hemorrhage secondary to uterine atony.

Expected Outcome	• Maintain a firm fundus within normal assessment parameters.
	• Saturate no more than one pad an hour during the recovery period.
	• Maintain normal fluid balance as evidenced by vital signs and hematocrit within normal limits.
Planning	Closely observe normal fluid volume balance within the first 24 to 28 hours following delivery.

Nursing Interventions	Rationales
1. Monitor fundal height, position, and tone as per the protocol. Massage as appropriate.	1. Ensures the uterus remains firmly contracted.
2. Monitor amount, color, and type of lochia as per the protocol. Note the amount of blood saturated on the peripad and on the pad under the buttocks and bed sheets. Weigh peripads as necessary.	2. Obtains an accurate estimate of blood loss.
3. Observe for vital sign changes and report acute or critical values to the primary care provider.	3. Ensures prompt identification and treatment of complicating.
4. Ensure adequate IV access. Administer IV fluids with oxytocin as ordered.	4. Maintains uterine tone and involution after delivery.

(continued)

5. Interventions beyond nursing may be necessary.

5. Administer other medications as needed if bleeding continues. If bleeding continues despite above actions, notify provider for further evaluation.

6. Moniter levels.

6. Obtain hemoglobin and hematocrit levels as ordered.

7. To prepare for transfusion if needed.

7. Ensure or prepare for administration of blood or blood products. Obtain blood for typing and cross-matching.

Evaluation Cristina's bleeding may decrease to a small amount of lochia rubra 12 hours after delivery; however, the nurse must continue to assess for bleeding until discharge. Ongoing evaluation may demonstrate that although the fundus remains firm, the continuation of moderate vaginal bleeding and changing vital signs may indicate bleeding coming from an overt site, such as an overlooked vaginal or cervical laceration.

Nursing Diagnosis

Urinary retention related to trauma to tissues secondary to childbirth and perineal discomfort.

Urinary Retention

Expected Outcome • Resume normal bladder function as evidenced by minimal urinary output of greater than 150 mL per voiding and absence of urinary distention.

Planning Work with client to set time-bound goals for voiding.

Nursing Interventions	Rationales
1. Assess the time and amount of last voiding.	1. Provides baseline data.
2. Palpate symphysis pubis and evaluate location of fundus in relation to the umbilicus the first 8 hours after delivery.	2. Notes bladder distention.
3. Asisst client to ambulate to bathroom if able, providing privacy as needed. Palpate bladder after voiding.	3. To assure adequate emptying.
4. Offer various methods to encourage urination. Use ice packs to decrease perineal discomfort.	4. Instructing in various bladder management techniques increases likelihood of client finding successful method.
5. If unable to void, perform straight catheterization as ordered.	5. To avoid urinary stasis and retention.
6. Encourage minimum fluid intake of 2,000 mL/d.	6. Maintains hydration.

Evaluation If Cristina continues to experience urinary retention, she may be discharged with an indwelling catheter or be taught how self-catheterization. Christina's input and output are within targeted parameters within 6 hours.

Nursing Diagnosis

Accute pain related to uterine cramping (normal uterine involution), perineal pain, and breast tenderness.

Expected Outcome • Experience pain relief or moderate control of pain.

• Verbalize methods of satisfactory pain relief.

• Obtain restful pain-free-periods and the ability to return to normal activities of daily living and self-care.

(continued)

| Planning | Plan care procedures to minimize disruptions in client rest; ask client about her preferred methods of pain management (therapy, guided imagery, medications, and so forth). |

Nursing Interventions	Rationales
1. Assess location, intensity, and duration of pain. Determine pain. Determine pain intensity by asking the client to describe her pain on a scale from 1 to 10, with 10 being the strongest intensity of pain.	1. Clarifies client's interpretation of the pain experience.
2. Administer the appropriate prescribed analgesia to the client. A combination or altering different prescribed medication also may be effective in controlling pain if the client is very uncomfortable (e.g., nursing frequently).	2. Regularly administered medications may control the pain more effectively.
3. Support client's use of nonpharmaceutical pain control, such as patterned breathing, touch therapies, and visualization.	3. These may provide effective pain relief avoiding rests associated with medications.
4. Provide ice packs to the perineum for the first 24 hours after delivery, then warm therapy with sitz baths afterward.	4. Reduces inflammation and promotes healing.
5. Provide ordered anesthetic sprays or creams as desired.	5. Reduces discomfort.
6. Instruct the client to position herself differently while sitting or lying in bed.	6. Position changes may alter pain levels.
7. Ensure proper positioning and latch-on when breast-feeding. Instruct client to massage colostrum into nipples to sooth them.	7. Proper positioning and breast care will alleviate discomfort.
8. Encourage rest and relaxation strategies.	8. These will help reduce pain and tension and facilitate let-down response.

| Evaluation | Christina continued to experience uterine cramping 6 hours after delivery; it intensified significantly when she breast-fed her son. Lying on her side to nurse seemed to dull the intensify of the afterpains. |

Infant care issues include the method and success of feeding, be it breast-feeding or bottle-feeding; sleep patterns; safety; cord care; circumcision care, if applicable; bowel and bladder elimination; bathing, dressing and diapering; infection; and skin integrity. Problems such as jaundice and infection of the umbilical cord site may be identified and treated early. Other topics to discuss include postpartum exercise, fertility and sexuality, and infant anticipatory guidance regarding behavior and development.

Because emotional changes (i.e., postpartum blues) may not be manifested until after discharge, assessing how the mother is coping at home is very important (Box 28-6).

Box 28-6 Assessing Emotional Changes at Home

- What is the mother's demeanor? Is she happy? Is she able to cope with the demands of motherhood?
- Is she getting enough rest? Does she look and behave as if she is tired?
- How does she act toward her baby and other children in the house?
- Does she have support and help available?
- How does the home environment appear?

NURSING IMPLICATIONS

Health care facilities may choose to use a critical pathway in providing direction in client care. Other facilities may choose to use the traditional nursing care plan. The nursing care plan should clearly delineate the process of assessing client information, developing a nursing diagnosis, performing the interventions, and evaluating the outcomes of that intervention. Depending on the documentation policies of the institution, the nursing care plan may be a preprinted care plan with common obstetric nursing problems. The nurse caring for the postpartum client should be able to individualize the care plan to meet her client's needs.

Web Activities

- Which online site provides information on recovering from labor and delivery?

- Which resources on the Internet can you find regarding general postpartum care?

- Where can you find information on how to perform Kegel's exercises?

- Where can you find a sample postpartum exercise routine?

- Where can you find a website that offers recipes for cooking large quantities of food that you can place in the freezer?

- Where can you find information regarding obtaining maternity leave from your employer?

Key Concepts

- Although pregnancy is considered to be wellness-oriented, the postpartum nurse must use clinical decision-making and critical thinking skills to provide safe, high-quality nursing care.

- Vital signs indicative of problems, such as hemorrhage and infection, are important elements in the assessment of the client postpartally.

- A systemic evaluation of postpartum women consists of examining the breasts, uterus, bladder, bowels, lochia, episiotomy, Homan's sign, and emotional status.

- Uterine involution to nonprepregnant size and return of other pregnancy changes to normal functioning occur 4 to 6 weeks after delivery.

- Postpartum hemorrhage, often attributable to uterine atony, is most often prevented with astute fundal and lochia monitoring.

- Although eager to lose her pregnancy weight, the new mother must approach weight loss and exercise slowly and in a healthy manner.

- Various approaches to pain relief can include traditional pharmacologic interventions as well as holistic alternative treatments.

- Before discharge the nurse must ascertain the client's immune status; the Rh-negative mother who delivered an infant who is Rh-positive should receive RhoGAM, and the mother who is rubella nonimmune should be immunized with rubella vaccine before her next pregnancy.

- Because of short hospitalizations, the postpartum nurse should try to identify key self-care and infant-care information that the new mother needs and wants to learn; the nurse should guide her teaching plan toward meeting these needs.

- The nurse incorporates consideration of client and family needs into planning her nursing care, including being aware of cultural diversity.

- Throughout the hospital stay, the nurse should educate and counsel the client (and family) as she encourages the client to progress toward confident, independent care of herself and her new baby.

Review Questions and Activities

The following review questions relate to the previous case study. Melanie Jones is the day shift registered nurse caring for Cristina for the first 12 hours after delivery.

1. Cristina was unable to urinate 4 hours after delivery. Which risk factors did she have that would predispose her to having problems?

a. Delivery of a male infant
b. Forceps delivery
c. Blood loss of 450 mL
d. Rapid labor

The correct answer is b.

2. Which of the concepts regarding assessment of vaginal bleeding are incorrect?
   a. Lochia rubra is a normal characteristic the first few days after delivery.
   b. The passage of a large amount of bright-red blood with multiple clots is a normal finding the first 24 hours after delivery.
   c. Blood may accumulate in the vaginal vault and gush out when the client moves from a horizontal to a vertical position.
   d. Bleeding usually is controlled with up to 40 U of oxytocin added to an IV bag of fluids.

The correct answer is b.

3. Which intrapartum factor put Cristina at risk for increased bleeding?
   a. Ruptured membranes more than 4 hours before the start of active labor

b. Catheterization
c. Overdistended uterus
d. Administration of a narcotic analgesic

The correct answer is c.

4. Nursing actions that can help relieve Cristina's complaints of pain may include:
   a. Applying ice packs to the perineum for the first 24 hours after delivery
   b. Administering an analgesic, such as ibuprofen, for relief of uterine cramping
   c. Ensuring the client is able to completely empty her bladder after delivery
   d. All of the above

The correct answer is d.

5. Lochia undergoes changes over the course of a few weeks. What does lochia consist of during the first 24 hours?
   a. A large amount of bright-red blood
   b. A small amount of light-pink blood
   c. A large amount of brownish-white blood
   d. A small amount of brownish-white blood

The correct answer is a.

References

American College of Obstetrics and Gynecology (ACOG) Technical Bulletin. (1990a). *Diagnosis and management of postpartum hemorrhage.* pp. 1–5.

American College of Obstetrics and Gynecology (ACOG) Technical Bulletin. (1990b). *Prevention of D isoimmunization.* pp. 1–4.

American College of Obstetrics and Gynecology (ACOG) Technical Bulletin. (1992). *Rubella and pregnancy.* pp. 1–8.

American Academy of Pediatrics (AAP) and American College of Obstetricians and Gynecologists (ACOG). (1992). *Guidelines for perinatal care* (4th ed.). Washington, D.C. and Elk Grove, IL: American Academy of Pediatrics and American College of Obstetrics and Gynecology.

Association of Women's Health, Obstetrics, and Neonatal Nurses (AWHONN). (1996). *Compendium of postpartum care.* Washington, D.C.: Association of Women's Health, Obstetrics and Neonatal Nurses.

Beneditti, T. J. (1996). Obstetric Hemorrhage. In S. G. Gabbe, J. R. Niebyl, & J. L. Simpson (Eds.). *Obstetrics: Normal and problem pregnancies.* (pp. 692–713). New York, NY: Churchill Livingston.

Bowes, W. A. (1996). Postpartum care. In S. G. Gabbe, J. R. Niebyl, & J. L. Simpson (Eds.). *Obstetrics: Normal and problem pregnancies.* (pp. 692–713). New York, NY: Churchill Livingston.

Cashion, K. (1997). Normal postpartum. In D. L. Lowdermilk, S. E. Perry, & I. M. Bobak. (Eds.). *Maternity and women's health care* (6th ed.). St. Louis, MO: Mosby.

Clark, R. A. (1995). Infections during the postpartum period. *Journal of Obstetric, Gynecologic, and Neonatal Nurses, 24,* (6), 542–548.

Davidson, N. R. S. (1974). REEDA: Evaluating postpartum healing. *Journal of Nurse Midwifery, 19,* (2), 6–8.

Duff, P. (1996). Maternal and perinatal infection. In S. G. Gabbe, J. R. Niebyl, & J. L. Simpson (Eds.). *Obstetrics: Normal and problem pregnancies.* (pp. 692–713). New York, NY: Churchill Livingston.

Epstein, B. A. (June 6, 2000). New baby, new stress. *The Doctor's Office.* [On-line], Available: www.allkids.org/Epstein/Articles/New Baby Stress.html.

Geissler, E. M. (1998). *Cultural assessment.* St. Louis, MO: Mosby.

Gilbert, S. (2000). *How do I lose the excess weight?* [On-line], Available: http://health.yahoo.com/healthc/pregfaq/how do I lose the excess weight .html.

Gordon, M. C., & Landon, M. B. (1996). Dermatologic disorders. In S. G. Gabbe, J. R. Niebyl, & J. L. Simpson (Eds.). *Obstetrics: Normal and problem pregnancies.* (pp. 1184–1187). New York, NY: Churchill Livingston.

Griffin, N. (June 25, 2000). *After-the-birth mother care.* [On-line], Available: http://wospace.cnation.com/Health/Hlth MotherCare.html.

Health Care Financing Administration. (June 21, 2000). *The newborns' and mothers' health protection act of 1996.* [On-line], Available: http://my.webmd.com/content/dmk/dmk article 5462944.

Higgins, P. (2000). Postpartum complications. In S. Mattson, & J. E. Smith (Eds.). *Core Curriculum for Maternal-Newborn Nursing* 2nd Ed. Philadelphia, PA: W. B. Saunders.

Jordan, P. (1998). Losing belly after childbirth. [On-line], Available: www.allhealth.com/health/followup/print/0,4197,6936 968,00.html.

Kimm. (1997). *Mastitis.* [On-line], Available: www.parentsoup.com/experts/leche/110797B.html.

Mayo, M. (June 6, 2000). Sex after baby. Nashville Parent Magazine.

Overfield, M. L., & Tully M. R. (1997). Newborn nutrition and feeding. In D. L. Lowdermilk, S. E. Perry, & I. M. Bobak. *Maternity and women's health care* (6th ed.). St. Louis, MO: Mosby.

Phillips, C. (1997). *Mother-baby nursing.* Washington, DC: Association of Women's Health, Obstetrics, and Neonatal Nurses.

Sears, W., & Sears, M. (2000). *Postpartum basics: Getting your body back.* [On-line], Available: www.2.parentsoup.com/firstyear/articles/postpartum/body/0,5302,,00.html.

Simpson, K. R., & Creehan, P. A. (1996). *Perinatal nursing.* Philadelphia, PA: Lippincott.

Thomas, L., Ptak, H., Giddings, L. S., Moore, L., & Opperman, C. (1990). The effects of rocking, diet, modifications, and antiflatulent medication on postcesarean section gas pain. *Journal of Perinatal Neonatal Nursing, 4,* (3), 12–24.

Water, M. A., & Lee, K. A. (1996). Difference between primigravidae and multigravidae mothers in sleep disturbance, fatigue, and functional status. *Journal of Nurse Midwifery, 41,* (5), 364–367.

Williams, L. R., & Cooper, M. K. (1993). Nurse-managed postpartum home care. *Journal of Obstetrics, Gynecologic, and Neonatal Nurses, 22,* (1), 25–31.

Suggested Readings

Alspach, J. G., & Williams, S. M. (1995). *Core curriculum for critical care nursing.* Philadelphia, PA: W. B. Saunders.

Association of Women's Health, Obstetrics, and Neonatal Nurses (AWHONN). (1991). Postpartum nursing care: Vaginal delivery. *OGN nursing practice resource.* Washington, D.C.: Association of Women's Health, Obstetrics, and Neonatal Nurses.

Bailey, P. H., Maciejewski, J., & Koren, I. (1993). Combined mother and baby care: Does it meet the needs of families? *Canadian Journal of Nursing Research, 25,* (3), 29–39.

Beger, D., & Loveland Cook, C. A. (1998). Postpartum teaching priorities: The viewpoints of nurses and mothers. *Journal of Obstetric, Gynecologic, and Neonatal Nurses, 27,* (2), 161–168.

Bick, D. E., & MacArthur, C. (1995). Attendance, content, and relevance of the six week postnatal examination. *Midwifery, 11,* 69–73.

Bond, L. (1993). Physiological changes. In S. Mattson, & J. E. Smith (Eds.). *Core curriculum for maternal-newborn nursing.* Philadelphia, PA: W. B. Saunders.

Brasner, S. (1998). *Advice from a pregnant obstetrician: An insider's guide.* New York Hyperion Books.

Braveman, P., Egerter, S., Pearl, M., Marchi, K., & Miller, C. (1995). Problems associated with early discharge of newborn infants. Early discharge of newborns and mothers: A critical review of the literature. *Pediatrics, 96,* (4 Pt 1), 716–726.

Brooten, D. (1995). Perinatal care across the continuum: Early discharge and nursing home follow-up. *Journal of Perinatal and Neonatal Nursing, 9,* (1), 38–44.

Brooten, D., Knapp, H., Borucki, L., Jacobsen, B., Finkler, S., Arnold, L., & Mennuti, M. (1996). Early discharge and home care after unplanned cesarean birth: Nursing care time. *Journal of Obstetrics, Gynecologic, and Neonatal Nursing, 25,* (7), 595–600.

Brown, L. P., Towne, S. A., & York, R. (1996). Controversial issues surrounding early postpartum discharge. *Nursing Clinics of North America, 31,* (2), 333–339.

Brown, S. G., & Johnson, B. T. (1998). Enhancing early discharge with home follow-up: A pilot project. *Journal of Obstetrics, Gynecologic, and Neonatal Nursing, 27,* (1), 33–38.

Bucher, L., Williams, S., Hayes, E., Morin, K., & Sylvia, B. (1997). First-time mothers' perceptions of prenatal care services. *Applied Nursing Research, 10,* (2), 64–71.

Conversations with Colleagues. (1997). *Lifelines.* p. 27.

Cunningham, F. G., MacDonald, P. C., Gant, N. J., Leveno, K. J., & Gilstrap III, L. C. (1993). The puerperium. In K. Licht (Ed.). *William's obstetrics.* (pp. 459–473). Norwalk, CT: Appleton & Lange.

Dalby, D. M., Williams, J. I., Hodnett, E., & Rush, J. (1996). Postpartum safety and satisfaction following early discharge. *Canadian Journal of Public Health, 87,* (2), 90–94.

De Sevo, M. R. (1997). Keeping the faith: Jewish traditions in pregnancy and childbirth. *Lifelines, 1,* (4), 46–49.

Doenges, M. E., & Moorhouse, M. F. (1996). *Nurses pocket guide: Nursing diagnoses with interventions* (5th ed.). Philadelphia, PA: F. A. Davis.

Dowswell, T., Piercy, J., Hirst, J., Hewison, J., & Lilford, R. (1997). Short postnatal hospital stay: Implications for women and service providers. *Journal of Public Health Medicine, 19,* (2), 132–136.

Druelinger, L. (1994). Postpartum emergencies. *Emergency Medicine Clinics of North America, 12,* (1), 219–237.

Edwards, N. C., & Sims-Jones, N. (1997). A randomized controlled trial of alternative approaches to community follow-up for postpartum women. *Canadian Journal of Public Health, 88,* (2), 123–128.

Evans, C. J. (1991). Description of a home follow-up program for childbearing families. *Journal of Obstetrics, Gynecologic, and Neonatal Nurses, 20,* (2), 113–118.

Evans, C. J. (1995). Postpartum home care in the United States. *Journal of Obstetric, Gynecologic, and Neonatal Nurses, 24,* (2), 180–186.

Freedman, L. H. (1999). *Birth as a healing experience: The emotional journey of pregnancy through postpartum.* Old Saybrook, CT: Harrington Park Press.

Gagnon, A. J., Edgar, L., Kramer, M. S., Papageorgiou, A., Waghorn, K., & Klein, M. C. (1997). A randomized trial of a program of early postpartum discharge with nurse visitation. *American Journal of Obstetrics and Gynecology, 176,* (1 Pt 1), 205–211.

Gazmararian, J. A., Koplan, J. P., Cogswell, M. E., Bailey, C. M., Davis, N. A., Cutler, C. M., & Heath, A. (1997). Maternity experiences in a managed care organization. *Health Affairs, 16,* (3), 198–208.

Gillerman, H., & Beckham, M. H. (1991). The postpartum early discharge dilemmas: An innovative solution. *Journal of Perinatal and Neonatal Nursing, 5,* (1), 9–17.

Gjerdingen, D. K., Froberg, D. G., & Kochevar, L. (1997). Changes in women's mental and physical health from pregnancy through six months postpartum. *Medical Care, 35,* (5), 507–521.

Grullon, K. E., & Grimes, D. A. (1997). The safety of early postpartum discharge: A review and critique. *Obstetrics and Gynecology, 90,* (5), 860–865.

Gulanick, M., Gradishar, D., & Puzas, M. K. (1994). *Plans of care for specialty practice: Obstetric and gynecologic nursing* Albany, New York: Delmar.

Gulanick, M., Gradishar, D., Puzas, M. K., & Gettrust, K. V. (1994). *Obstetric and gynecologic nursing: Plans of care for specialty practice.* Albany, NY: Delmar Publishers.

Handfield, B., & Bell, R. (1995). Do childbirth classes influence decision making about labor and postpartum issues? *Birth, 22,* (3), 153–160.

Health Care Financing Administration. (June 21, 2000). *The newborns' and mothers' health protection act of 1996.* [On-line], Available: http://my.webmd.com/content/dmk/dmk article 5462944.

Higgins, P. (1993). Postpartum complications. In S. Mattson, & J. E. Smith (Eds.). *Core Curriculum for Maternal-Newborn Nursing.* Philadelphia, PA: W. B. Saunders.

Howard, J. Y., & Berbiglia, V. A. (1997). Caring for childbearing Korean women. *Journal of Obstetrics, Gynecologic, and Neonatal Nursing, 26,* (6), 665–671.

Idarius, B. (1999). *The homeopathic childbirth manual: A practical guide for labor, birth, and the immediate postpartum period.* Talmaze, CA. Idarius Press.

Iovine, V. (1997). *The girlfriend's guide to surviving the first year of motherhood.* New York Perigree.

Lewis-Copeland, C. (1997). *Mother's first year: A realistic guide to the changes and challenges of motherhood.* Berkeley, CA. Berkeley Publishing Group.

Mandl, K. D., Brennan, T. A., Wise, P. H., Tronick, E. Z., & Homer, C. J. (1997). Maternal and infant health: Effects of moderate reductions in postpartum length of stay. *Archives Pediatric Adolescent Medicine, 151,* (9), 915–921.

Margolis, L. H., Kotelchuck, M., & Chang, H. Y. (1997). Factors associated with early maternal postpartum discharge from the hospital. *Archives Pediatric Adolescent Medicine, 151,* (5), 466–472.

McGovern, P., Dowd, B., Gjerdingen, D., Moscovice, I., Kochevar, L., & Lohman, W. (1995). Time off work and the postpartum health of employed women. *Family Medicine, 27,* (9), 592–598.

Moran, C. F., Holt, V. L., & Martin, D. P. (1997). What do women want to know after childbirth? *Birth, 24,* (1), 27–34.

Noble, E. (1995). *Essential exercises for the childbearing year: A guide to health and comfort before and after your baby is born* (4th ed.). Harwich, MA. New Life Images.

Persily, C., Brown, L. P., & York, R. (1996). A model of home care for high-risk childbearing families. Women with diabetes in pregnancy. *Nursing Clinics of North America, 31,* (2), 327–332.

Placksin, S. (2000). *Mothering the new mother: Women's feelings and needs after childbirth a support and resource guide.* New York, NY. Newmark Press.

Prodromidis, M., Field, T., Arendt, R., Singer, L., Yando, R., & Bendell, D. (1995). Mothers touching newborns: A comparison of rooming—in versus minimal support. *Birth, 22,* (4), 196–200.

Ruchala, P. L., & Halstead, L. (1994). The postpartum experience of low-risk women: A time of adjustment and change. *Maternal Child Nursing Journal, 22,* (3), 83–89.

Samselle, C. M., Seng, J., Yeo, S., Killeon, C., & Oakley, D. (1999). Physical activity and postpartum well-being. *Journal of Obstetric, Gynecologic, and Neonatal Nurses, 28,* (1), 41–49.

Simpson, K. R., & Creehan, P. A. (1996). *Perinatal nursing.* Philadelphia, PA: Lippincott.

Smith-Hanrahan, C., & Deblois, D. (1995). Postpartum early discharge: Impact on maternal fatigue and functional ability. *Clinical Nursing Research, 4,* (1), 50–66.

Spratto, G. R., & Woods, A. L. (2001). *PDR nurse's drug handbook.* Albany, NY: Delmar.

Stover, A. M., & Marnejon, J. G. (1995). Postpartum care. *American Family Physician, 52,* (5), 1465–1472.

Thomas, L., Ptak, H., Giddings, L. S., Moore, L., & Opperman, C. (1990). The effects of rocking, diet, modifications, and antiflatulent medication on postcesarean section gas pain. *Journal of Perinatal Neonatal Nursing, 4,* (3), 12–24.

Troy, N. W., & Dalgas-Pelish, P. (1997). The natural evolution of postpartum fatigue among a group of primiparous women. *Clinical Nursing Research, 6,* (2), 126–139.

Water, M. A., & Lee, K. A. (1996). Difference between primigravidae and multigravidae mothers in sleep disturbance, fatigue, and functional status. *Journal of Nurse Midwifery, 41,* (5), 364–367.

Welt, S. I., Cole, J. S., Myers, M. S., Sholes, D. M., Jr., & Jelovsek, F. R. (1993). Feasibility of postpartum rapid hospital discharge: A study from a community hospital population. *American Journal of Perinatology, 10,* (5), 384–387.

Wheeler, L. (1997). *Nurse-midwifery handbook: A practical guide to prenatal and postpartum care.* Philadelphia, PA: Lippincott Williams & Wilkins.

Williams, L. R., & Cooper, M. K. (1996). A new paradigm for postpartum care. *Journal of Obstetrics, Gynecologic and Neonatal Nurses, 25,* (9), 745–749.

Placksin, S. (2000). *Mothering the new mother: Women's feelings and needs after childbirth a support and resource guide.* New York, NY. Newmark Press.

Resources

www.avsc.org/pregnancy/pppcreco.html
www.unmc.edu/Community/noo/bowelbladder.htm
www.ctw.org/babywprkshop/checkli.../0,3158,cG9zdHBhcnR1b Sw0NTE4MA==,00.htm
www.alexian.org/progserv/babies/mothercare/momcare3.html
www.bayfront.org/explore/wwallabout/wwpreg27.html
www.unmc.edu/Community/npp/uterus.htm

www.depend.com/incont edu center/living with incont/ kegel exercises.asp
http://pregnancy.miningco.com/health/pregnancy/library/blpostexer.htm
http://busycooks.about.com/food/busycooks/library/features/blfrzmyrec.htm
www.parentsplace.com/pregnancy/maternityleave/qa/0,3105,59 004,00.html

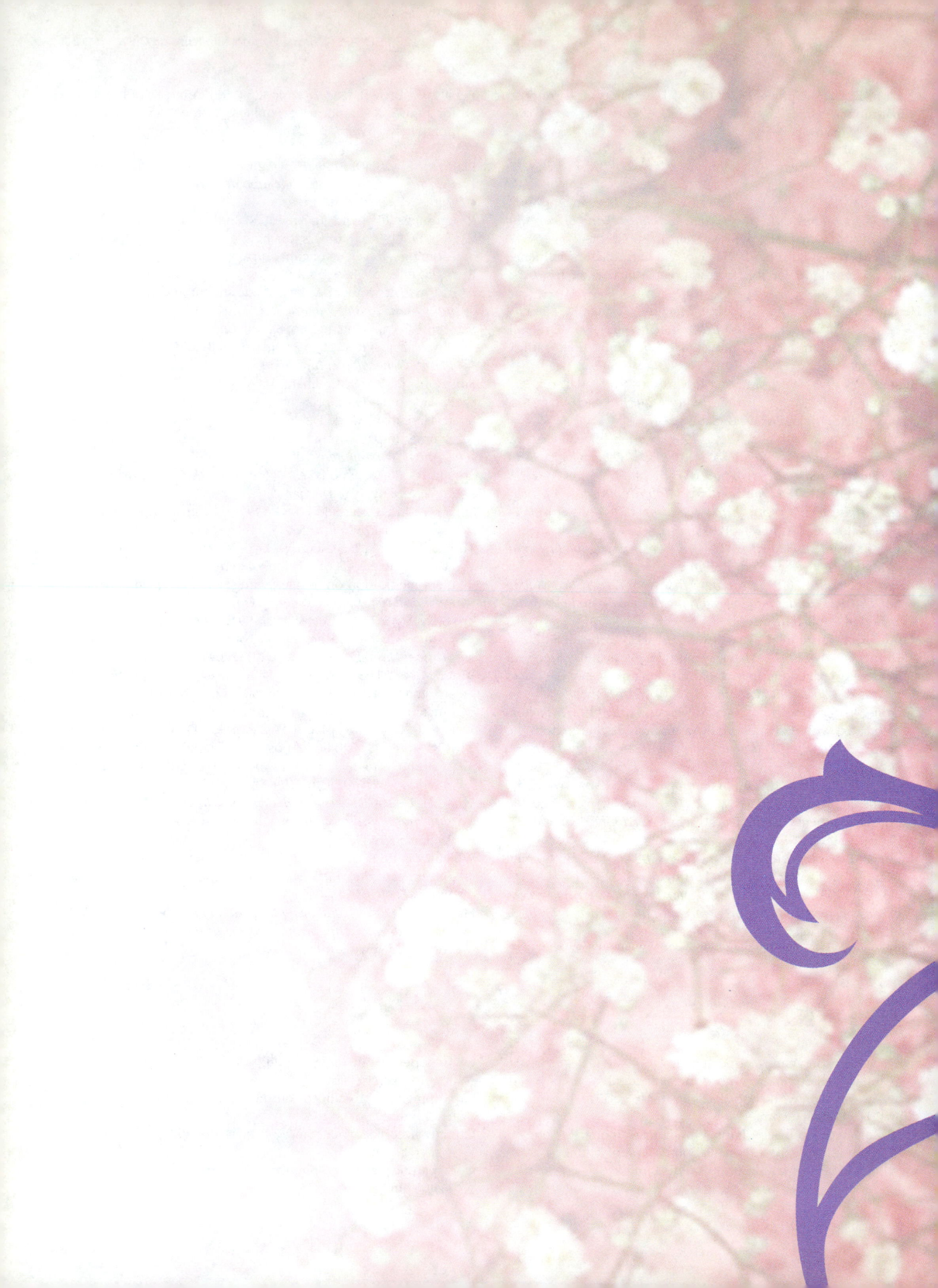

CHAPTER 29

Postpartum Family Adjustment

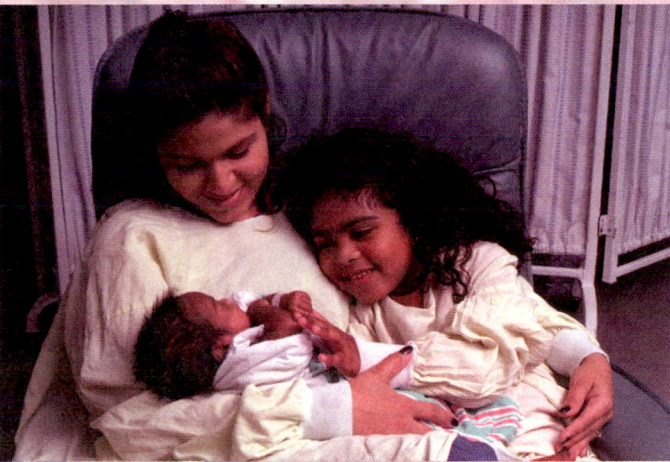

Working with families as they adjust to a new baby is challenging and requires perception and excellent assessment skills to identify needs before they become problems. Answer the following questions to increase your awareness of the needs of families during the postpartum period.

- *How has my new role as a student nurse affected my perception of others?*
- *How do I feel as I adjust to my role as a student nurse?*
- *How comfortable am I with my new role?*
- *What factors helped to make my role transition easier?*
- *What factors slowed the process of my role transition?*
- *Who helped support me with my role transition?*
- *How can I apply what I learned to help others with their role change?*

Key Terms

Attachment	Kangaroo care	Role attainment	Sleep-wake cycle
En face	Letting-go phase	Role transition	Taking-hold phase
Engrossment	Maternal-infant bonding	Role mastery	Taking-in phase

Competencies

Upon completion of this chapter, the reader should be able to:

1. Describe the attachment process.
2. Identify theories related to maternal and paternal attachment behaviors.
3. Identify infant behaviors that enhance the attachment process.
4. Outline three phases of maternal role adjustment.
5. Assess maternal and paternal role adjustment.
6. Describe sibling adjustment.
7. Describe the grandparent's role.
8. Examine cultural variations related to parental role transition.
9. Assess the impact of adolescent pregnancy on developmental tasks.

The birth of a baby is one of life's most exciting and challenging events. Brazelton (1981) pointed out that parenthood is an opportunity for personal growth and maturity, because a baby presents parents with the task of becoming a family with all the feelings and responsibility that entails. Adapting to the role of parent can be challenging, because developmental tasks must be successfully accomplished to integrate the new role. **Role transition**, or the process of adopting new behaviors related to change and developmental tasks, involves not only the birth of a firstborn child for the new parents but also the expanding of the family. Since family adjustment and attainment of developmental milestones are complex, health care providers can be helpful in helping families make these transitions.

Adaptation to parenthood is not an easy process. There has been a great deal of research about the developmental course of early attachment relationships (Waters, Posada, Crowell, & Lay 1994). **Attachment** is the process of connecting with another human being. Ideally, a mother's attachment to her offspring is a strong bond that lasts a lifetime. Attachment usually begins during pregnancy and intensifies as the pregnancy progresses and a fantasy child is perceived.

In the period after birth, or the postpartum period, the mother-infant acquaintance begins as the infant is compared to the child who was perceived in the womb. This "getting-to-know-you" period is characterized by behaviors that initiate the attachment process. Researchers speak of this period as a time when parents begin to identify with their newborn. It is a time when parents begin to integrate the newborn into their lives as they reconcile the fantasy child with the real child and begin to view their role as parents.

Adams & Cotgrove (1995) reported that the mother-child attachment pattern is generally established by age 1 and the effect of early attachment exerts a powerful influence on the child's future development. They also point out that the established attachment pattern directly affects the child's future psychological health, marital relationships, and the relationship the child will have with his or her children. Early intervention by health care professionals can assist in preventing impaired attachment.

MATERNAL-INFANT ATTACHMENT

Major theoretical ideas stem from early studies examining infant attachment to mother figures. In 1958, John Bowlby introduced a biologic model that identified secure attachment to a parental figure as being necessary for normal child development (Biringen, 1994). Bowlby's definition of attachment is based on the formation of an affectionate

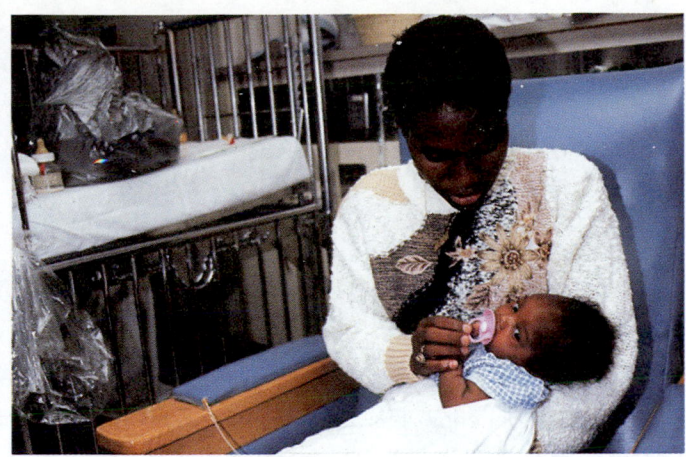

Figure 29-1 Meeting the newborn's physical needs is an important step in the maternal-infant attachment process.

link between a child and its mother figure that occurred during the child's first year of life. The identified attachment behaviors were crying, sucking, smiling, and clinging. These behaviors initiated attachment interactions between an infant and its mother. Thus, by meeting the child's physical needs, mutual satisfaction resulted and the foundation for maternal-infant attachment was laid (Figure 29-1).

Mary Salter Ainsworth, a colleague of John Bowlby, also studied infant attachment to a primary caregiver. She reported that an infant must have sufficient interaction with a mother figure to become attached. Ainsworth is best known for her "strange situation" experiment that tested the strength and style of an infant's attachments to its primary caregiver. As the infant grows, a strong attachment to a specific mother figure is seen around 8 months of age, when the child exhibits "stranger fear" (Ainsworth, 1997).

The attachment process does not occur overnight. Brazelton (1981) reported that parents often believe in the romanticized version of parenthood characterized by instinctive, instantaneous attachment, which is not necessarily immediate, but often a continuing process. Early research conducted by Klaus and Kennel (1982) examined maternal attachment and found that the period when a mother falls in love with her baby was not easily identified. They reported it was common for mothers to experience distress and disappointment if they did not experience feelings of love for their infants in the first minutes or hours after birth. Many of the mothers studied developed an affection for their infant within the first week; however, the onset of maternal feelings of affection toward their infant was delayed if labor was painful, amniotic membranes were ruptured artificially, or the mother had received narcotic drugs for pain relief.

Klaus and Kennel (1982) referred to the first hour following birth of an infant as a period when maternal-infant attachment begins and labeled this attachment as **maternal-infant bonding**. In the past, much emphasis was placed on early mother-infant bonding as being instantaneous and crucial. Troy (1993) found that a relationship between mother and infant occurred when the infant was first held, regardless of how long after delivery the holding occurred. The mothers in the study were found to develop feelings of maternal attachment towards their infant anywhere from 10 minutes to 2.5 days after the delivery. Crouch and Manderson (1995) reported that the ideal birth experience does not always occur and the expectations of women regarding instant bonding with their newborn may be incongruent with the actual experience, causing feelings of guilt and anxiety. They also pointed out that maternal attachment develops over an extended period and the term "bonding" has a wide range of meanings related to process and outcome. Because a mother's physical and emotional state can be adversely affected by exhaustion, pain, anesthesia, the absence of support persons, or an unwanted outcome, a delay or block in the attachment process can occur.

While most of the early research focused on observed infant behavior, models and assessment tools were developed to examine mother-infant interactions. Researcher Kathryn Barnard (Tomey & Alligood, 1998) developed a model that identified caregiver-parent characteristics that promoted attachment. These were: a sensitivity to cues, the alleviation of distress, and provision of growth-fostering situations. These characteristics were compared to infant characteristics, which were identified as: clarity of cues and responsiveness to caregiver. Barnhard also developed a satellite-training project in which 4,000 nurses, throughout the nation and in foreign countries, were taught how to use a series of standard child assessment instruments. Her child health assessment interaction theory has been widely used to assess parent-child interactions. This theory is based on 10 theoretical assertions:

1. The goal of assessment is to identify problems in which intervention would be most effective.
2. Environmental factors are important for determining the child's health outcomes.
3. The caregiver-infant interaction reflects the nature of the child's environment.
4. The caregiver brings to the caregiver-infant relationship a basic style and level of skills that is readily influenced by the infant's responses as well as environmental support.
5. The process of mutual modification is one in which the parent's behavior influences the child and, in turn, the child influences the parent, so that both are changed.

6. The adaptive process is more modifiable than the mother's or infant's basic characteristics, and nursing intervention should lend support to the mother's sensitivity in response to her infant's cues, rather than try to change her characteristics or style.

7. It is important to promote the child's learning by permitting child-initiated behaviors and reinforcing the child's attempt at a task.

8. A major goal for the nursing profession is to support the child's caregiver during the first year of life.

9. Assessment of interactions is important.

10. Assessment of the child's environment is important.

By encouraging early maternal-infant contact, nurses can provide an environment that fosters attachment behaviors (Figure 29-2). Klaus (1998) examined early mother-infant emotional ties and found that maternal-infant attachment may be biochemically modulated through oxytocin stimulated in the mother by the infant sucking. Newborn infants have the ability to crawl toward the breast to initiate suckling. The close contact aids in thermoregulation of the infant. In addition, by encouraging attachment behaviors, such as early contact, suckling, and *rooming-in,* infant abandonment was reduced. Rooming-in involves the infant remaining in the mother's room throughout hospitalization. Mothers who had early and extended infant contact through rooming-in arrangements were found to interact with their infant more and exhibited more touching behavior (Prodromidis, Field, Singer, Yando, & Bendell, 1995). In contrast, maternal reluctance to engage in attachment behaviors may occur if the mother has min-

Critical Thinking

Mother-Infant Attachment and Early Infant Contact

The concept of early contact immediately after birth has been discussed as a necessary experience for mother-infant attachment. However, some mothers are too exhausted during the first hour after a difficult labor and delivery or deliver a high-risk infant, who is immediately taken to the nursery. Do you think these mothers experience less attachment toward their infant? Do you think they feel a sense of loss, depression, and anxiety because they missed an experience that has been promoted as important to the mother-child relationship? Is the first hour a critical period or can maternal-infant attachment behaviors be postponed? If so, how long can the postponement be? Is there a long-term negative effect on mother-child attachment if early contact does not occur, as in the case of an ill newborn? Do you think the presence of a support person enhances the attachment process? How can nurses facilitate early maternal-infant contact? What nursing behaviors may interfere with early maternal-infant contact?

imal contact with the infant or if the infant is unwanted, has a disorder, or was born after a difficult labor and delivery. Diamond (1995) reported that the presence of a father in the role of protective watchfulness has been observed to facilitate a nurturing environment for the mother and infant that promotes the development of maternal-infant attachment.

Maternal Adjustment and Role Attainment

The postpartum period is a time for mothers to adjust to the new role of motherhood as the attachment process continues. During this time, the mother experiences many psychological and physiologic changes. It is a critical transition period for initiating maternal role attainment. Nurses can assist the mother and family with role transition by understanding maternal **role attainment**, which is the process of accomplishing the developmental tasks of a new social role. Classic research by Reva Rubin (1984) explored the process of maternal role attainment. Her published work describes the relationship between maternal identity and role attainment. According to Rubin, after the

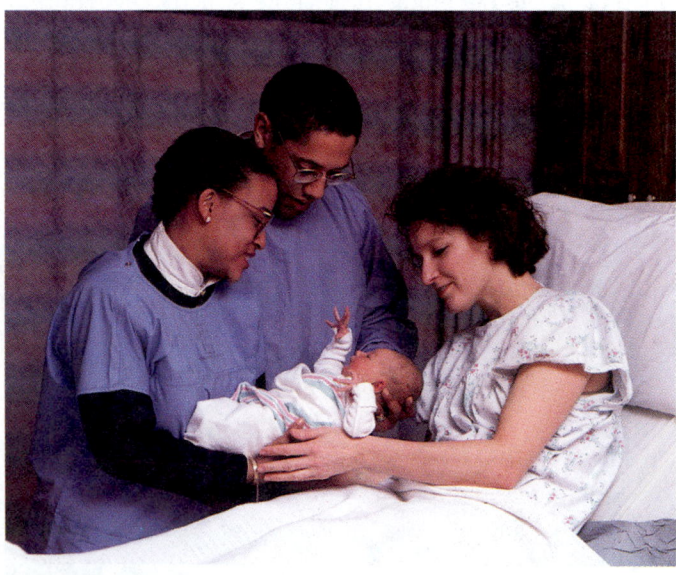

Figure 29-2 The nurse can help create an environment conducive to parental attachment behaviors by encouraging early parent-infant contact.

Table 29-1 Rubin's Phases of Maternal Adjustment	
Phase	**Maternal Characteristics**
Initial: *Taking-in*	Passivity and dependence Preoccupation with self Reviews the reality of giving birth Compares infant to her "fantasy child" Concerned with rest, food, and comfort
Second: *Taking-hold*	Resumes control over her life Concerned about self-care Interested in caring for her newborn Begins to gain self-confidence
Third: *Letting-go*	Maternal role attainment Relationship adjustments

delivery, the mother shifts her attention from an inward focus that is characteristic of labor and delivery to focusing outward on her relationship with her infant. This relationship is personal and unique between a mother and her infant. Rubin identified three adjustment phases involved in the process of assuming the maternal role (Table 29-1).

Taking-In Phase

The **taking-in phase** of maternal adjustment is characterized by basic maternal needs for food, care, and comfort. The mother's initial goal is to recover physically from the birth; depending on cultural variances, this period may be characterized by a dependency on others to meet needs related to rest, comfort, and nutrition. These needs must be met before the mother can begin to care for her infant. Psychologically, the mother is "taking-in" the reality of having given birth. It is not uncommon for the mother to be talkative as she relives the birth of her child with a sense of euphoria. Some mothers may express a sense of unreality as they view their infant and wonder, "Is this really *my* baby"? Some mothers may feel disappointment as they compare the infant with the perceived "fantasy child." Fatigue and physical exhaustion commonly follow the initial euphoric feelings. It is not uncommon for mothers in this stage to exhibit little interest in providing care for their infant. They frequently are content to be a passive observer of their infant's care. The nursing focus at this stage is to provide a quiet, restful environment to facilitate the mother's recovery and promote mother-child interaction.

Taking-Hold Phase

Following the initial phase of dependency, mothers move on to the **taking-hold phase**, which occurs after they

have had a chance to rest and have received relief from discomfort. This phase may begin 24 to 48 hours after delivery. Characteristically, mothers in this phase begin to show an increased interest in participating in their infant's care. However, it is not uncommon for some mothers, especially first-time mothers, to continue to exhibit dependency behaviors. Cultural beliefs also influence the transition to this stage. The primary goal of a mother at this stage is achieving self-confidence in caring for her infant. Mothers usually exhibit a keen interest in assessing their infant's cues and begin to participate in the infant's care as their confidence increases. First-time mothers may take longer to achieve the level of confidence needed.

Today, with early hospital discharge, this phase often occurs earlier or may occur after discharge. The nursing focus in this phase is to foster self-confidence by helping mothers learn infant care. It is not unusual for many new mothers to feel anxious and fearful as they begin to assume care of their infant. Nurses can facilitate learning by collaborating with the mother to establish goals that can help her learn to care for herself and her newborn. It is important to begin by assessing learner readiness and level of understanding. Also, it may be helpful to incorporate a support person in the teaching process (Figure 29-3) and to reinforce learning by providing resources, such as printed materials, videos, lactation consultant referrals, and a written summary of what was taught. Berger and Loveland Cook (1998) suggested that learning can be facilitated by addressing topics in the hospital that were initially presented in prenatal classes and by reinforcing these topics through outpatient classes or group sessions. Nurses have a key role in assisting the mother to feel confident in her ability to care for herself and her newborn. It is important to assess learning needs and provide positive reinforcement during the teaching-learning process. By praising the mother's accomplishments, the nurse can foster maternal

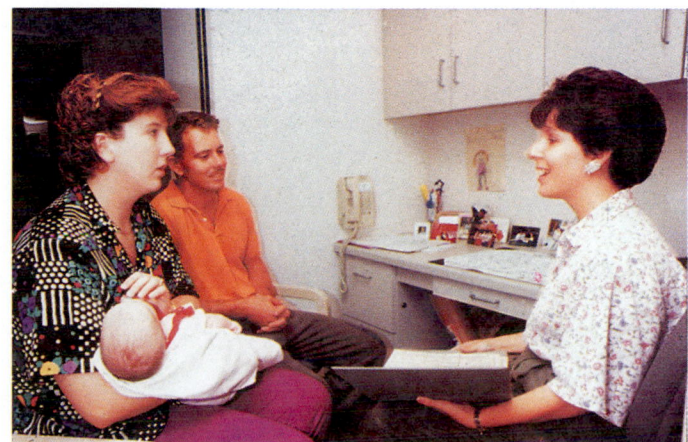

Figure 29-3 Including support persons in postpartum teaching encourages parental self-confidence.

confidence in the mother's ability to care for herself and her infant.

Letting-Go Phase

Mothers move last to the **letting-go phase**. This phase is characterized by role attainment and relationship adjustments. It may take several weeks to reach and is influenced by cultural beliefs. Maternal role attainment often occurs slowly, as maternal self-confidence increases and maternal-child attachment strengthens. However, not all mothers go home with their infants. Their infant may be ill and hospitalized or given up for adoption, which can lead to a situational crisis. Nurses must be aware that maternal role attainment is affected by such factors as maternal age, cultural beliefs, a difficult delivery, postpartum complications, a sick or impaired infant, or a lack of adequate support systems. Prenatal expectations that conflict with actual experiences may directly impede maternal role adjustment. The goal of the "letting-go" stage is to achieve relationship and role stability.

Role Attainment

Researcher Ramona Mercer was influenced by the work of Reva Rubin. Mercer's research looked at maternal role attainment in diverse populations: adolescents, older mothers, ill mothers, mothers of children with anomalies, families experiencing antepartal stress, parents at high risk, and mothers who have had a cesarean section. Her research focused on factors that affect maternal role attainment from delivery to 12 months postpartum. Tomey and Alligood (1998) presented Mercer's theoretical framework as a useful guide for assessing maternal role attainment:

1. Increased maternal age appears to be an asset in child care behavior.

2. The older the woman, the more experience she has had in acquiring new roles.

3. Greater knowledge and early experiences enhances competency in moving to new roles.

4. The maternal role is socially accepted as an adult role but is inappropriate for the psychologically immature teenager.

5. The events of labor and delivery have the potential to affect the mother's self-esteem in either a positive or negative way along with the experience of early interaction with her infant.

6. Social stress has been correlated to complications of pregnancy and parenting.

7. A relationship exists between the woman's support system and her mothering capability.

8. The woman's ego strength, self-confidence, and nurturant qualities have been observed to be basic determinants of her capacity as a mother.

9. Maternal illness during pregnancy or birth affects the woman's self-esteem and drains energy that would otherwise be available for mothering.

10. Child-rearing attitudes, how parents handle irritating child behaviors, and parent-child interaction and communication all sharply differentiate abusive from nonabusive parents.

11. Mothers who rate high in adaptive maternal behavior have been observed to have infants with easy temperaments.

12. Culture and socioeconomic levels affect the maternal role.

13. Attainment of the maternal role may be accomplished in 12 months.

During maternal-infant interaction, the mother often displays a heightened awareness and interest in exploring her infant. Maternal attachment behaviors, such as holding the baby close, cuddling, stroking, making eye contact, and talking softly to the infant can serve to facilitate maternal role attainment. Nurses can promote maternal-infant attachment by encouraging the mother to hold her infant closely, with skin-to-skin contact, and giving the mother time to see and hold her newborn. Skin-to-skin contact, often referred to as **kangaroo care** (Figure 29-4), has many beneficial effects, especially with the premature infant, in whom it was found to facilitate neurobehavioral development, promote parenting interventions, decrease maternal stress, and enhance maternal confidence (Ludington-Hoe & Swinth, 1996). Nurses can also facilitate maternal role attainment by carrying out a complete assessment of family interactions and available support systems. Mothers should be encouraged to verbalize concerns and identify stressors that may impede maternal role attainment. By using therapeutic communication skills and active listening, nurses can develop a collaborative plan of

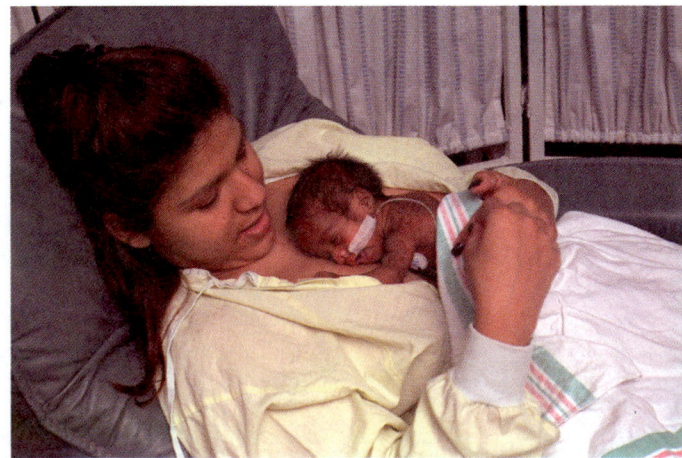

Figure 29-4 Kangaroo care (skin-to-skin contact) promotes bonding and attachment, which is especially important for the premature infant.

PROMOTING ATTACHMENT BEHAVIORS

Nurses have a special role in promoting maternal-infant attachment behaviors:

1. Always refer to the infant by name.
2. Unwrap the infant and initiate exploration of the infant's body.
3. Answer concerns that the parents may have (such as those regarding cord care or circumcision).
4. Encourage the mother to pick up and hold her infant.
5. Encourage the mother to hold her infant in a *enface* (face-to-face) position.
6. Talk directly to the infant in a calm, soothing voice.
7. Use the infant's grasp reflex to hold onto the mother's finger.
8. Demonstrate comforting techniques, such as gentle patting and rocking (Figure 29-5).
9. Assess the mother's readiness to learn infant care.
10. Point out the infant's response to maternal stimulation.

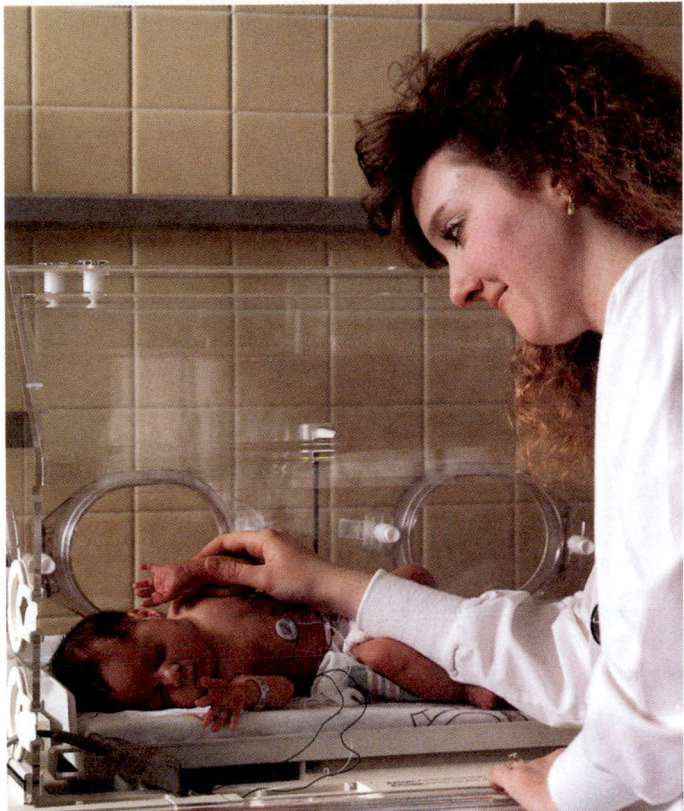

Figure 29-5 Nurses should help parents of high-risk infants to find ways to bond with and comfort their newborns.

care and initiate referrals to support services when indicated.

The importance of understanding maternal attachment behaviors and role attainment cannot be underestimated. Carter-Jessop and Yoos (1994) reported that understanding the beliefs parents hold about parenting may yield more important information than observing parenting behaviors. The researchers also emphasized that early intervention to encourage communication between the parents can promote positive role adjustment. A randomized, controlled trial by Midmer, Wilson, and Cummings (1995) studied the effects of middle-trimester parenting communication classes on postpartum anxiety, marital satisfaction, and adjustment. Classes contained didactic sessions, role-playing sessions, and value-clarification exercises. The researchers found that prenatal parenting communication classes had a significant positive effect on postpartum anxiety, marital satisfaction, and adjustment. Since many hospitals offer prenatal classes for breastfeeding, childbirth, and sibling adjustment, perhaps the findings of this study could pave the way for nurses to develop prenatal parenting communication classes.

Maternal adjustment to role change is dependent on many factors. Gjerdingen and Chaloner (1994) examined factors affecting maternal role adjustment at 1 month postpartum and found correlations among maternal fatigue, lack of sleep, concerns about appearance, infant illnesses, and poor mental health. They reported that adverse effects on postpartum adjustment were related to previous mental problems, physical problems, poor general health, poor social support, fewer recreational activities, young age, and low income. A maternal mental health study by Beck (1996) examined the interactions of postpartum depressed mothers with their infant. The findings showed that depressed mothers went through the motions of mothering, were emotionally detached from their children, and failed to respond to their infants' cues. Parental responsibilities, guilt, irrational thinking, and anger overwhelmed these mothers.

Postpartum adjustment difficulty may be related to the depletion of energy stores, lack of sufficient sleep, hormonal shifts, and an overwhelming sense of responsibility. A study conducted by Smith-Hanrahan and Deblois (1995) focused on maternal fatigue and found that severe fatigue affected 25% of the mothers at 1 and 6 weeks postpartum. Merchant, Affonso, and Mayberry (1995) reported two psychosocial factors, i.e., marital adjustment and childcare stress, significantly influenced maternal depression at 9 months and pointed to the need to follow mothers beyond

REFLECTIONS FROM A MOTHER

"When I delivered my first baby at age 21, my husband was not able to attend the birth because of a military assignment. After the delivery of our son, the nurse gave him to me to hold and encouraged me to put the baby to breast. However, I really did not want to nurse at that time, because I was in too much pain from a difficult delivery and was upset about not having my husband with me. I felt so guilty about not having an immediate attachment to my baby; it felt like I was looking at someone else's baby. These feelings made me feel like crying; I thought I was being a bad mother. With extreme feelings of guilt, I asked the nurse to take the baby and give me some pain medication. She seemed to disapprove of my unwillingness to nurse my baby. It made me feel so sad and confused."

---

the traditional 6-week postpartum checkup. Thus, nurses must adequately assess maternal physical and mental health and social support structures to establish early interventions and referrals that assist mothers with maternal role adjustment. During postpartum visits, the nurse must observe the mother for signs of fatigue, feelings of sadness, or inability to cope with infant demands. Nurses were found to be more aware than physicians of the emotional effect of postpartum depression, and nurses who demonstrated empathic understanding were more aware of the postpartum depressive phenomenon (Lepper, DiMatteo, & Tinsley, 1994).

Seven characteristics that enhance nurses' caring for depressed mothers were identified (Beck, 1995):

1. Having sufficient knowledge about postpartum depression.
2. Using observation and intuition to recognize depression.
3. Providing hope to mothers.
4. Taking time to listen to the mother's concerns.
5. Initiating referrals.

Client Education

Helping Parents Adjust to Parenthood

Adjusting to the birth of a baby involves many changes, both physiological and psychological. It is important that parents:

- Recognize that adjusting to parenthood takes time.
- Discuss feelings with support persons.
- Obtain adequate rest and nutrition.
- Use community resources.
- Seek out support from family and friends.
- Understand postpartum and newborn care.
- Refer to written plans of care for postpartum and newborn care.
- Keep postpartum and newborn followup appointments.

6. Providing continuity of care.
7. Having empathic understanding.

Because of shorter hospital stays, nurses should be aware of the availability of outpatient maternity support services to assist mothers with postpartum transition (Figure 29-6). Fishbein and Burggraf (1998) studied the concerns of early postpartum discharge and reported that

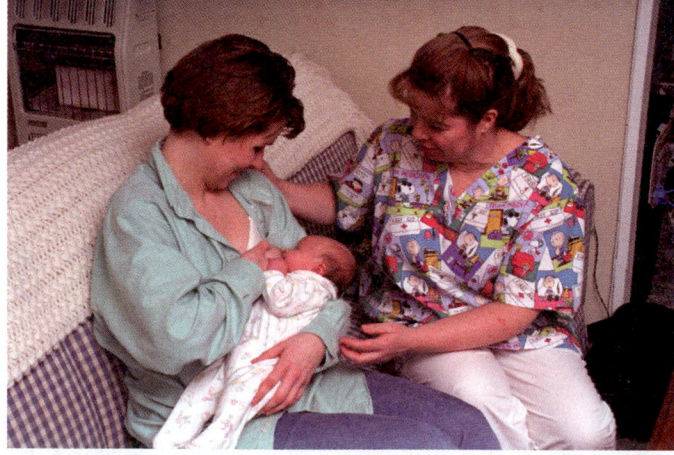

Figure 29-6 Outreach programs that include home visits are especially helpful to new parents who are adjusting to their new family.

Research Highlight

Prenatal and Postnatal Attachment: A Modest Correlation

Purpose

To determine whether a correlation exists between prenatal and postnatal attachment.

Methods

Participants (228 women) were recruited from childbirth education classes. Most of the women were young, Caucasian, well-educated, married, and employed. The Prenatal Attachment Inventory (PAI) was administered to measure attachment before birth. The Maternal Attachment Inventory (MAI), the How I Feel About my Baby Now Scale, and the Maternal Separation Anxiety Scale were used to measure maternal attachment after birth.

Findings

One hundred ninety-six women completed the inventories and scales. A correlation was found between the Prenatal Attachment Inventory and the Maternal Attachment Inventory ($r = 0.41$, $p < 0.0001$). The modest size of the correlation suggests other factors influenced postnatal scores. One factor of marital status was found to significantly influence both the PAI and MAI scores. Single women had higher prenatal attachment scores than married women. Mean maternal attachment scores were higher for single women that for women who were living with a partner.

Nursing Implications

Because the findings indicate that a modest correlation exists between prenatal attachment and postnatal attachment, nurses should support the natural progression of attachment but not attempt to intervene to reach high levels of prenatal attachment, which may interrupt a natural process causing disappointment and self-blame. Instead, nurses should promote the mother's self-esteem, reassure her that maternal-child attachment is a lifelong process, and provide interventions that promote confidence related to being a good mother.

Muller, M. A. (1996). Prenatal and postnatal attachment: A modest correlation. *JOGNN, 25,*(2), 161–166.

early postpartum concerns were related to fatigue and physiologic concerns such as perineal sutures, breast care, etc. They found that over half of the respondents would use outpatient postpartum resources if they were offered. Thus, nurses should be aware of the availability of outpatient services for postpartum mothers. In some communities, nurses have answered the need by establishing postpartum outreach programs. These programs include home visits, telephone contact, information lines, lactation information, mother-infant outpatient care, and parent support groups (Evans, 1995). Additionally, nurses have been instrumental in creating online resources to assist parents. These Internet websites provide parents with information related to pregnancy, delivery, the postpartum period, and newborn care.

PATERNAL ADJUSTMENT

Marks and Lovestone (1995) found that the common experience during the months immediately following childbirth is contrary to the idealized images of parenthood, and the process of attaining the role of father is influenced by the man's internal and external experiences as well as his relationship with the infant's mother, who acts as mediator in the father-infant relationship. Grant, Duggan, Andrews, and Serwing (1997) gave support to the effects of maternal influence on paternal role attainment when they reported that maternal expectations of the father's role during infancy were dependent on the strength of the parents' relationship and the mother's desire for the father's participation. Initial research by Jordon (1990) examined paternal role attainment and found that a father's quest towards role identification and relevance involved three steps:

1. Initial acceptance of the reality of the pregnancy.
2. Being recognized by his mate in the role of father.
3. Becoming more involved as a father.

Ferketich and Mercer (1995) reported that inexperienced, first-time fathers, at 4 and 8 months following birth of their child, had greater anxiety and depression than experienced fathers and that a sense of mastery and family functioning were predictors for paternal role competence. Nurses can facilitate paternal adjustment by encouraging fathers to participate in childbirth preparation classes, during which they are given an active supportive role. In years past, fathers assumed a passive role, sitting in a waiting area anxiously awaiting the birth. Today, their role as coaching partners allows them the opportunity to experience the birth process with the mother and be actively involved in attachment behaviors immediately after birth.

Similar to maternal attachment, paternal attachment is a gradual process that occurs over weeks or months. Paternal attachment is usually manifested by **engrossment** behaviors, in which the father exhibits an intense interest in his newborn. Most fathers display a feeling of pride and satisfaction as they begin to develop a strong attraction toward their child. One study of paternal parenting attitudes revealed a decrease in happiness at 3 months postpartum, which may be related to the effects of fatigue and stress that result from added responsibilities (Tiller, 1995). Fathers need assistance in adjusting to role change. Nurses can guide fathers by including them in maternal and infant care. After delivery, the father should be encouraged to hold his newborn and private time should be provided for the couple to absorb the reality of the birth experience as they become acquainted with their newborn. By including the father as a support person, many fathers continue to assist the mother and are usually very interested in learning how to care for their infant (Figure 29-7). Some fathers take leave from work to help their partner at home. By providing opportunities to learn infant care and addressing concerns, nurses can assist in guiding fathers to reach paternal role attainment. Nurses have also been successful in developing prenatal and postnatal classes for fathers, and some hospitals have adopted policies whereby fathers can room-in with their partner and newborn.

Anderson (1996) explored fathers' experiences of becoming connected to their infant. They identified three major categories as important in the initial attachment between the father and newborn. These categories were identified as: making a commitment, becoming connected, and making room for baby. Paternal-infant attachment begins with the acceptance of the pregnancy as a reality. Participation in childbirth preparation classes facilitates pa-

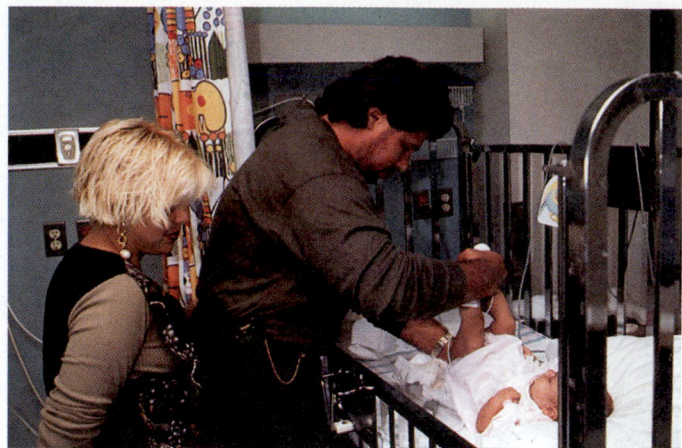

Figure 29-7 Most fathers are eager to learn how to care for their newborn.

ternal antenatal attachment behaviors and prepares the father for the birth process and the needs of the expanding family.

Minton & Pasley (1996) examined the relationship between paternal role identity and involvement in child-related activities. They found that nonresidential fathers felt less competent and satisfied in their paternal role but had higher scores on role identity that correlated with more frequent involvement with their children. It is interesting to note that fathers of high-risk newborns perform significantly more infant care ($p < 0.005$) and were found to have a better adjustment to parenthood ($p < 0.0381$) at 1 month after discharge than fathers of healthy newborns. There were no differences found at 3 months after discharge (Brown, Rustia, & Schappert, 1991).

While it may not be easy for a father to adjust to his new role when the infant is healthy, the adjustment is more difficult when the infant is ill or disabled. Western cultural expectations promote male toughness during hard

REFLECTIONS FROM A FATHER

"When my daughter was born I was elated and very proud. In the early weeks, there was little chance for me to play with her because all she did was sleep and eat. Then one day, when I was changing her diaper, she looked directly at me and smiled. I felt extreme love and attachment. I was hooked for life."

Critical Thinking

Transition to Fatherhood

Male emotions are not well accepted in Western culture. Men are taught to be strong, and crying is thought to be a sign of weakness. Do you think that fathers experience strong emotional feelings at the birth of their child? How do you feel when you see a man cry? Are men conditioned to hold in their emotions? What is the result of emotional restraint? What do you think is the impact of the added responsibilities on the new father? How can the nurse help the father adjust? How does culture influence the father's response?

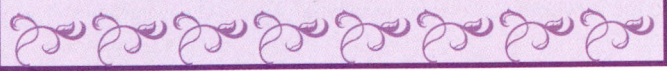

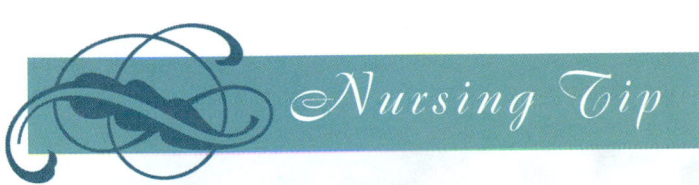

ASSISTING PARENTAL ROLE ADJUSTMENT

1. Establish rapport early to promote effective communication and verbalization of positive and negative feelings.
2. Assess the goals of the parents and include them in the planning process.
3. Give parents a feeling of empowerment by giving them choices regarding participation in maternal and infant care.
4. Encourage alone time with the infant to explore and get acquainted.
5. Promote rooming-in for the infant and the mother's partner to foster knowledge of their infant's normal patterns and encourage touching and holding behaviors.
6. Assess readiness to learn and participate in providing care.
7. Identify support figures and encourage involvement.
8. Encourage sibling visitation where possible.
9. Refer to community classes for parenting, nutrition, new fathers, infant massage, or similar activities.

times. Little boys are often scolded for crying and peers may call them sissies. Finding support for conflicting difficult emotions when dealing with ill or disabled newborns may be difficult. Many men grieve inwardly, and depression is often hidden. May (1996) found that fathers of children with chronic illness or disability often felt isolated as they came to terms with loss and were required to strengthen caretaking capabilities. Thus, it is important for nurses to help fathers adjust to their role by taking time to listen to their concerns, letting them know it is acceptable to express their emotions, and showing them how they can become involved in the care of the child with special needs. By slowly introducing fathers to the care needs of their child and assessing their readiness to participate, nurses can reduce role strain and enhance family adjustment. It is also important to refer the grieving father to resources, such as support groups for fathers or counseling services. Today's technology provides online support resources that may be acceptable to the grieving father.

INFANT BEHAVIORS INFLUENCING ATTACHMENT

As a new mother begins to get acquainted with her newborn, infant behavioral cues can assist in facilitating maternal-child attachment. Nurses should be aware of infant behaviors to assist parents to understand their infant's cues and to recognize when their infant is most receptive to stimulation. Brazelton (1981) identified six stages in the infant's **sleep-wake cycle** that affect alertness and responsiveness: deep sleep, light sleep, drowsiness, quiet alertness, active alertness, and crying (Table 29-2). A mother must be able to identify an infant's state of quiet alertness when they are most responsive to stimulation. During this state, the infant responds to stimulation with a widening of the eyes and increased alertness; this is an optimum time for maternal-infant interaction. When placed in a face-to-face (*en face*) position, the infant is able to briefly focus on the mother's face and attend to her vocal sounds. Infants often are seen to move their body in synchrony with the mother's voice. Brazelton (1981) identified this behavior as mutual regulation. When stimulated, the infant responds with coordinated, synchronous body movement and may imitate vocal sounds and facial gestures. Also, the face-to-face position is an important position for optimal interaction. Failure to assume the *en-face* position may be an early symptom of maternal maladjustment.

Mothers should recognize infant behavior when overstimulation occurs: infants take a break from the interaction and intermittently look away to reduce the intensity of the interaction when overstimulated. Nurses can assist parents to recognize infant behaviors to optimize parent-newborn interactions and facilitate the attachment process.

Table 29-2 Newborn Sleep-Wake States

State	Observed Activity
Deep sleep	Very little movement Occasional startle motion Regular breathing
Light sleep	Some body movements Eye fluttering Smiles occasionally Irregular breathing
Drowsiness	Mild startle movements Intermittent eyelid opening Glazed eyes
Quiet alertness (most attentive state)	Some increase in activity Widening of the eyes More alert face
Active alertness	Increased motor activity Fussiness Decreased attention to stimulation Increased reaction to discomfort
Crying	Increased motor movement Extreme response to discomfort

Data from Brazelton, T. B. (1984) *Neonatal behavioral assessment scale*, 2nd ed. London: Heineman.

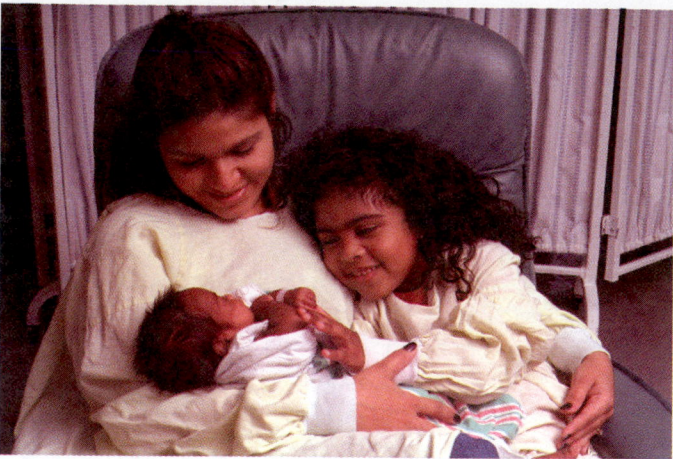

Figure 29-8 Encourage parents to introduce older siblings to the newborn as soon as feasible.

SIBLING ADJUSTMENT

Another challenging aspect of adjustment for the growing family involves the adjustment of siblings. Brazelton (1981) pointed out that small children can recognize changes in their mother as she becomes more internalized during the pregnancy, and it is not unusual for these children to turn elsewhere for nurturing. When a newborn is introduced into the family structure, siblings must adjust and assume the role of the older brother or sister. Anxiety and feelings of jealousy may occur as the sibling reorganizes his or her place in the family. It is not unusual to see regression to earlier behaviors, such as bed wetting and thumb sucking. Jealousy may also be used to gain parental attention. Sibling adjustment can be made easier if the parents involve the older child in a sibling preparation class. Nurses have developed these classes to assist the child in adjusting when they visit the hospital nursery and are addressed as the "big brother" or "big sister." In many areas, older children are permitted to attend the birth. The sooner the older child is involved in the preparation for a new family member, the more positively involved they are likely to be (Brazelton, 1981). By allowing visitation time for older children to greet their new sibling, nurses can foster behaviors that initiate a positive attachment (Figure 29-8). This attachment is further strengthened by finding ways in which the older child can carry out the role of "big brother" or "big sister" through participation in the infant's care. Older children can feel important when they help by retrieving supplies or carrying the diaper bag. Many parents find it helpful to set aside special time alone with the older child in a play activity. During this time, the older child should be encouraged to express their feelings.

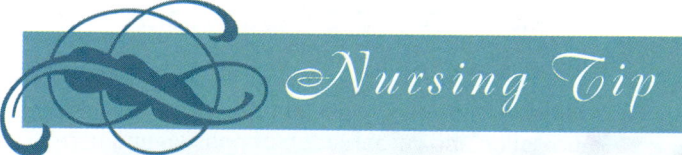

Nursing Tip

SIBLING VISITATION POSTPARTUM

Early inclusion of older siblings helps to facilitate adaptation of older children to their new role and promotes a sense of being a family.

1. Promote early contact with the newborn to facilitate integration into the family unit.

2. Enhance the older sibling's feeling of importance within the family as a "helper."

3. Include the sibling in a celebration party to promote a feeling of belonging.

4. Take precautions against cross-infection by questioning parents to see if their older child has been exposed to a communicable disease in recent weeks or presently has symptoms of a infection, such as vomiting, coughing, runny nose, fever, diarrhea, or rash.

5. Educate parents regarding sibling handwashing to promote safe sibling contact with the newborn and facilitate appropriate sibling attachment behavior.

Client Education

Strategies for Managing Sibling Rivalry

Observed Behavior: Regression

Strategy

Regression is a coping mechanism whereby the child returns to a coping behavior of an earlier stage of development. This is a normal behavior for young children to exhibit in times of stress. Behaviors such a thumb sucking, temper tantrums, and increased dependency help the child cope with stress. Be patient, don't scold, and use a calm, caring approach. With time, the behavior will pass.

Observed Behavior: Jealousy

Strategy

This is a normal behavior when young children see a new baby taking most of the parents' time. Set aside special times for outings with the older child. Don't address negative coping behaviors. Focus on encouraging the older child to express feelings through verbalization, drawings, or play. Listen attentively and help older children sort out their feelings. Most of all, older children need to feel important and loved.

Observed Behavior: Anger or Tantrums

Strategy

Recognize this as attention-getting behavior. Ignore the tantrum by avoiding eye contact and moving out of view, but nearby. Do not make statements such as, "Stop acting like a baby," or threaten to spank the child. If anger is directed toward harming the baby, set rules in a calm manner; "time out" may be enforced. Encourage positive interactions with supervision and give praise for positive behavior. Involve the older child by asking them to get supplies and to help by carrying the diaper bag, and praise the child for being a big helper (Figure 29-9). Never leave an angry child unattended near the newborn. With time, love, positive involvement, and rule setting, the problem behaviors will pass. Older children need praise, hugs, and a parent's undivided attention to help them adjust to the change.

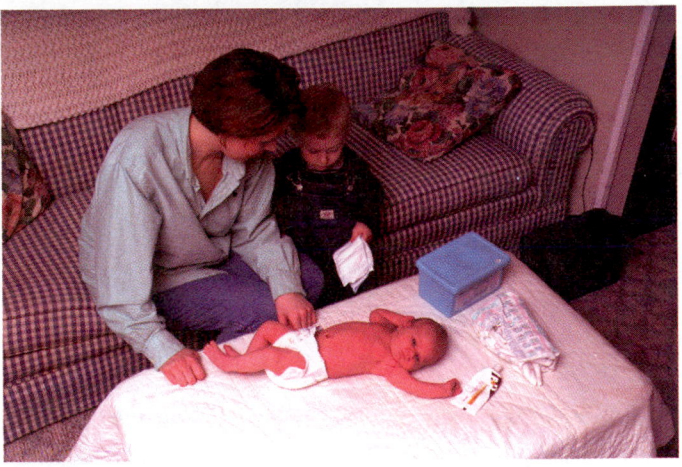

Figure 29-9 Older siblings feel important if they can help care for the new baby through simple tasks, such as retrieving a clean diaper.

GRANDPARENT ADJUSTMENT

Grandparents can be a source of support for new parents. Grandparents are unique in that they have the experience to assist new parents as they adjust to the role of parent (Figure 29-10). A grandmother's expertise can be helpful to a new mother as she learns to care for her infant. Having someone who has raised children is a valuable source of information and support that can lessen the anxiety of new parents and give the mother a chance to rest and focus on her role.

However, the role change can be a stressful time for both the parents and grandparents. It is not unusual for grandparents to be unsure of how much involvement they should have. Many grandparents are still employed and

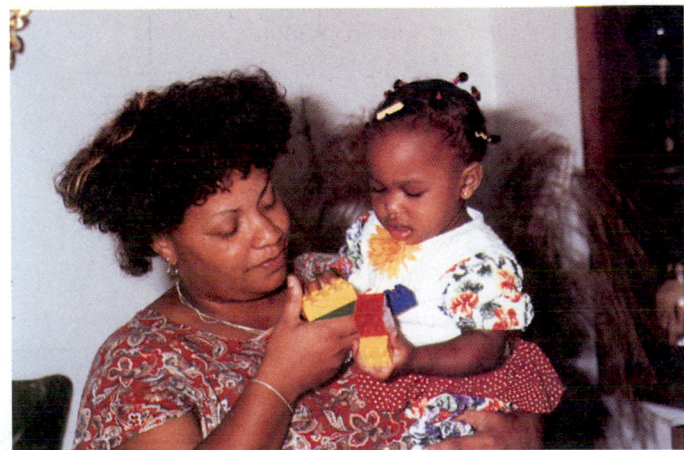

Figure 29-10 Grandparents can be a source of help and wisdom for new parents and sometimes may even take over the parenting role, if the new parents are unable to manage the responsibilities.

REFLECTIONS FROM
AN OLDER SIBLING

"I was about age 4½ when my younger brother Joey was born, but I still remember that day. (Boy, do I remember that day!) Let's just say it involves a grandma, bathroom cleanser, and one really upset (spoiled) little girl. . . .

Picture it: the Bronx, 1982. A cute little girl storms into the bathroom at her grandparents' home, a bathroom complete with a claw-footed bathtub and difficult-to-manage locks. She was feeling particularly high-spirited (ok, evil) on that day, the first day my mother had ever left me for such a long time. I didn't care that she had been in labor for hours with her first 'normal' delivery, (being of the difficult type, I was delivered by cesarean section.) I was determined to wreak havoc and take all of my emotion out on my poor, gentle grandma. So I did what any protesting individual does: I staged a 'sit in,' right in my grandparents' bathroom. And I did the unspeakable: I locked myself in. Needless to say, my grandma was a little nervous for a while. But that stopped when she became extremely worried after the third hour. I heard my mild-mannered grandma become a fire-breathing dragon right on the other side of that thick oak door. She began screaming for me to open the door and to stay away from everything in the bathroom. But like the protestors of the 60s, I held tight. I even chanted a little. But after the sixth hour, I became hungry and eventually figured out how to open the difficult lock. My grandma, so relieved that I wasn't dead from drinking the bathroom cleanser, was ecstatic.

And I've been a 'protestor' ever since."

---

unable to provide assistance, or they may give unsolicited advice and spoil the child with gifts. This can be a source of disagreement between the parents and grandparents. Today, many grandparents are active with their own lives and may not demonstrate the expected interest and involvement with their grandchild. In addition, today's mobile society has made it difficult for many grandparents to have close contact with their children because they live too far away. Thus, the parent-grandparent relationship can be a challenging one.

The inclusion of grandparents is a personal decision the couple makes and is based on relationship factors, distance, economics, and cultural expectations. Many cultures rely heavily on the grandmother to be actively involved in a child's life. Likewise, many grandparents are excited about their new role as it adds a positive dimension to their life. Today, there is a growing trend in society for grandparents to assume the parenting role because of their child's single parenthood, divorce, illness, or substance abuse. A study by Kelley and Damato (1995) reported that the experience of parenting grandchildren was emotionally rewarding but psychologically and physically stressful. However, some of the respondents reported an improvement in their emotional health as they provided care for their grandchildren. Those who found the experience to be psychologically stressful found that they were restricted in their social life. Some felt isolated from friends and resented being tied down. Repressed anger and depression often occurred. Physically, many reported being too old to be able to keep up with the demands of childrearing. However, some reported that the rewards of doing the right thing gave them joy but that they felt heartache when their grandchild questioned why they did not live with their mommy and daddy. Many of the respondents reported their other adult children as their greatest support, but 54% reported difficulty in relationships with their other children, who often expressed feelings of envy and resentment about the time spent with the grandchild. In addition, 15% reported that nurses or teachers were a source of support. In another study, Patterson (1997) examined the involvement of the maternal grandmother with the children of an adolescent child. Interestingly, 72% of the children were found to be securely attached to their grandmothers, and 44% of the children were securely attached to their mother. Thus, a grandparents' role change to parenting grandchildren is an important support but causes stress for many grandparents, who, at this stage in life, feel they should be free from the burdens of raising children.

FACTORS AFFECTING ROLE MASTERY

Role mastery involves successful attainment of developmental goals. Duvall (1971) outlined task-oriented goals that are to be mastered at each stage in the life cycle. In the stage of *family with infants,* the developmental tasks to be completed are to provide a safe, nurturing home and adapt to new roles and relationships. Transition to parenthood is a crucial time when parents must assess their perception of themselves while striving to successfully complete developmental tasks. Parents need to realistically appraise and successfully integrate their new role to prevent a crisis. Thus, the nurse should assess the parent's emotional and physical needs. By encouraging parents to verbalize their feelings, the nurse can help them clarify their perception of their role as parent and assist them to set realistic goals towards role mastery.

Role mastery is dependent on developing competence in infant care, successfully assessing and meeting the infant's needs, integrating the infant into the family structure, and redefining relationships with a spouse, children, and extended family members. These tasks can be overwhelming and difficult for new parents to achieve. A study conducted by Sullivan (1997) focused on maternal problem solving and found that mothers were often not certain of their infant's problem even after comforting them and that nurses must use planned and unplanned encounters to effectively teach mothers about their infants. Also, including fathers in the teaching process increased their comfort level with infant care and assisted them in supporting their partner. Leathers, Kelley, and Richman (1997) reported that high levels of maternal depressive symptoms were related to the mother's perception of low levels of emotional support from her partner along with low control and gratification in the parenting role. Stamp (1994) analyzed three dimensions salient to the appropriation of the parental role: (1) the accuracy of role expectations, (2) the facilitation of role enactment, and (3) the openness in role negotiation with one's spouse. Self-esteem was found to be a major predictor for maternal role competence for both primiparas and multiparas (Mercer & Ferketich, 1995).

Critical Thinking

The Impact of Adolescent Pregnancy

Adolescence is a time of change when many teens are trying to develop a sense of identity and begin to move toward independence. Do you think adolescent pregnancy impedes the developmental process? Do you think pregnant adolescents suffer from low self-esteem? Do you think adolescents can successfully attain the maternal role? Do you think single adolescent mothers are able to parent effectively? Do you think adolescent mothers can successfully adapt to the role of mother if they actively participate in planning interventions? Do you think adolescent mothers need close follow-up during the postpartum period? Do you think the unwed father should play an active supporting role throughout the pregnancy and after birth?

the teen mother's concerns, include her in health care decisions, collaborate with her when planning interventions, and include support persons to assist the teen mother throughout the pregnancy, delivery, and postpartum period to facilitate positive adjustment. The adolescent's ability to adapt to the pregnancy and respond with realistic expectations depends on effective sources of support to assist her to clarify feelings and set realistic goals.

Burke and Liston (1994) reported that the experience of parenting could give the adolescent a sense of responsibility and an opportunity for growth (Figure 29-11). The researchers also found that adolescents identified the baby's father as their key support person. Diehl (1997) reported that paternal involvement was a significant factor in fostering a positive interaction between adolescent moth-

THE POSTPARTUM ADOLESCENT MOTHER

Adolescence is a time of great change as teens address developmental milestones of independence and strive to achieve self-identity. When developmental progress is interrupted, a situational crisis occurs that affects the entire family. An unplanned pregnancy during the teen years generally results in a major personal and family crisis. The pregnancy can block the adolescent's successful completion of developmental tasks and can put a teenage mother in a state of crisis as her sense of identity becomes blurred. The pregnant adolescent has an increased dependence on others at a time when she is striving for independence. Nurses can assist the pregnant adolescent by fostering independence and a sense of self. It is important to listen to

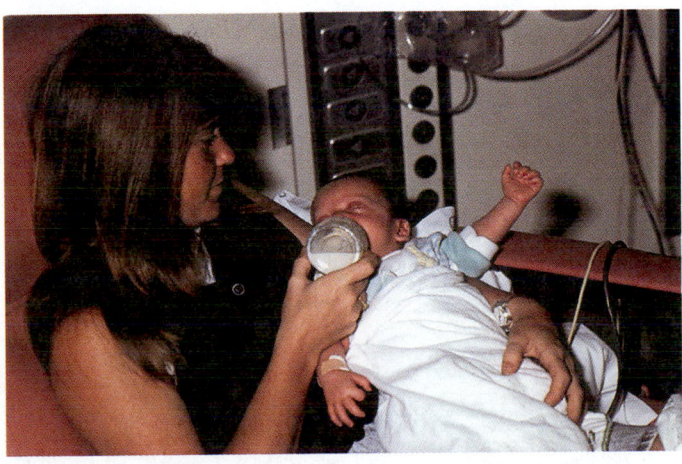

Figure 29-11 This teenage mother is accepting the responsibility of caring for her newborn.

Research Highlight

Depressive Symptoms, Stress, and Social Support in Pregnant and Postpartum Adolescents

Purpose

To prospectively assess the incidence and course of depressive symptoms among pregnant and postpartum adolescents and explore the roles of stress and social support.

Methods

Participants (n=125) were pregnant teenagers who were enrolled in a pregnancy and parenting program during the third trimester of pregnancy and followed through for 4 months postpartum. Depressive symptoms were measured with self-administered instruments during the third trimester, and at 2 and 4 months postpartum. The teens were predominantly African American (93%) and were from 12 to 18 years of age. Assessments were received from 114 teens at 2 months and 108 at 4 months postpartum.

Findings

During the third trimester, 42% reported significant depressive symptoms, and stress levels increased significantly from the third trimester to the postpartum period ($p < 01$). There was a positive association between stress and depression. Lower rates of stress and depression occurred when the teen mother received social support from her mother or the infant's father. Conflict with the infant's father was seen in conjunction with increased depressive symptoms.

Nursing Implications

Social support is important in decreasing stress and depressive symptoms among teenage mothers. Early identification of depressive symptoms, increased stress levels, and a lack of support is important in helping teen mothers to receive early intervention through support services and referrals.

Barnet, B., Joffe, A., Duggan, A. K., Wilson, M. D., & Repke, J. T. (1996). Depressive symptoms, stress, and social support in pregnant and postpartum adolescents. *Archives of Pediatric & Adolescent Medicine, 150* (1), 64–69.

---

ers and their children. Bloom (1998) examined the role of the father in adolescent pregnancy. The findings supported Rubin's theory of maternal identity formation in that a close and satisfying relationship with the father of the baby had a positive influence on adolescent maternal-infant attachment behaviors. When possible, it is important to involve the father as a support person for the adolescent mother to facilitate positive role transition.

CULTURAL CONSIDERATIONS

Culture is the value or belief system of a group of individuals and directly affects maternal role transition. Western culture, in past years, encouraged a long hospitalization for the mother to recover from delivery. This time, known as the "lying-in period," was several weeks, during which the mother was expected to maintain bedrest and rely on nurses and family for assistance. It was not unusual for the mother to maintain bedrest for 7 days and to stay in the hospital for 10 to 14 days. Problems with thrombophlebitis were commonplace.

Today's fast-paced society places emphasis on preparing for the birth, but little time is given to recovery. Mothers now experience short hospital stays that are referred to as "drive-through" delivery. However, many Eastern cultural traditions continue to support the "lying-in" concept, and these families are stressed by Western cultural expectations. Nurses should take time to ask women about their

Research Highlight

An Early Intervention Program for Adolescent Mothers

Purpose

To improve health outcomes in a vulnerable population of adolescent mothers and their infants.

Method

The effects of an early intervention program (EIP) were compared with the interventions of traditional public health nursing care. Participants (n=63) were provided intensive early interventions by means of four prenatal classes and approximately 17 home visits by specially trained public health nurses. Interventions addressed health issues, sexuality and family planning, life skills, the maternal role, and social support systems. Participants (n=58) in traditional public health nursing care received three home visits regarding intake, prenatal care, and postpartum and well-baby care information.

Findings

Early program interventions indicated a reduction in premature birth rates for both groups compared with national data for adolescent mothers. In addition, there were fewer days of infant hospitalization during the first 6 weeks postpartum for the EIP participants. Thus, both traditional and intensive early intervention in adolescent pregnancy significantly improved perinatal outcomes.

Nursing Implications

Both the traditional and intensive EIPs improved perinatal outcome in terms of infant birth weight and gestational age. The teaching of self-care and the initiation of referrals for prenatal care were common aspects of both programs. The more intense and frequent nursing contacts maintained through prenatal classes, home visits, and telephone interactions seemed to have a positive influence on infant outcome. The adolescents who received the intensive intervention program had an opportunity to discuss their concerns about their infants and other issues. The environment created was one that allowed the adolescent to develop rapport with and a sense of trust in their health care provider. The planned activities served to facilitate maternal role adaptation and heighten awareness of infant behavior and development. The program was shown to be cost-effective by decreasing infant morbidity and hospitalization because of prematurity.

Koniak-Griffin, D., Mathenge, C., Anderson, L. R., & Verzemnieks, I. (1999). An early intervention program for adolescent mothers: A nursing demonstration project. *JOGNN, 28* (1), 51–59.

cultural practices to individualize the teaching plan and help them recover from the birth.

New examples of cultural traditions (Schott & Henley, 1996) that affect the postpartum period include:

- Traditional African-Caribbean mothers are expected to rest for 2 weeks after giving birth and to avoid chilling. Thus, they may not want to shower. Breastfeeding is seen as best for the baby, and it is not uncommon to squirt a little breast milk into the infant's irritated eyes. Support is obtained from older women in the family. Food preferences for the new mother include the main dietary staple of starchy vegetables, such as potatoes, yams, rice, and plantains. Fish is the main protein source, and spices are always included. Western hospital food is considered bland.

- Traditional Chinese mothers are viewed as being in a period of *yin* (cold) and require hot foods for at least a month to recover from the birth. A special broth of sweet black vinegar, ginger, and stewed pigs' trotters is served with a freshly boiled egg. The postpartum period is seen as a rest period of 1 month, with emphasis on serenity and harmony and avoidance of any stress. Traditionally, men are not present during labor and birth and the woman receives support from her mother or other married women in the family. Modesty is an important consideration, because some families believe the husband should stay away on grounds of modesty. In many cases, bottle feeding is preferred because it is seen as an indication of high financial status compared with breastfeeding, which is mostly seen in poor families. A study by Chong-Yeu Liu-Chuang (1995) explored the practice of the Chinese ritual, *Tso-Yueh-Tzu* (doing-the-month), which is a 30-day postpartum seclusion observed by Taiwanese women. During this time, physical care was provided by an older family member and focused on promoting emotional stability. However, today's modern career women have been experiencing difficulty with this ritual and rely heavily on their husband.

❧ Traditional South Asian women from India, Pakistan, Bangladesh, and Sri Lanka regard childbearing and raising of children as a woman's greatest fulfillment and the act that permits the bride to be accepted into the groom's family. Older women of the family are important for support and guidance and have firm expectations that the new mother will follow their advice. It is traditional for newly delivered mothers to go to their parents' home for postnatal seclusion. During this time, mothers are expected to rest and be cared for by other women in the family for 6 weeks. The emphasis is on sleep, warmth, and good food. The mothers are also encouraged to stay in bed and request help. Their baby may be in bed with them or may be with them only for feeding. Breastfeeding is highly regarded and expected to continue for at least 1 year, but many do not believe in giving colostrum to the baby. It is believed that if mothers do not follow the expected routine, the mother's long-term health and emotional well-being will suffer. The husband is expected to stay with his parents during this time. The Western practice of initiating bonding by placing the baby on the mother's abdomen is particularly distressing to some women because they believe that the baby is covered with impurity from the birth canal and should be washed before handling.

❧ In traditional Hispanic culture, mothers rely heavily on their partner for assistance. A study by Khazoyan and Anderson (1994) studied Hispanic women and found that they expected their partner to have an active role in the birth by being nearby and offering words of love, encouragement, and support, which they believed enhanced the mother's inner strength and promoted calmness. During the postpartum period, Hispanic women observe a lying-in period, during which they receive help from their mother and grandmother. Health restoration focuses on correcting imbalances by ingestion of proper foods, medications, or herbal remedies. Certain foods, such as pork, are considered to be "hot" and to upset balance within the body. Foods that are defined as "hot" or "cold" are an individual preference. Thus, the nurse should assess individual preferences and needs and respect them accordingly. Also, nurses should recognize that the grandmother has a great deal of influence in the decisions made regarding postpartum care.

Cultural Assessment

Nurses need to be aware of how to conduct a sensitive cultural assessment, which is critical in providing care for today's ethnically diverse population (Campinha-Bacote, 1995). To provide care for people of different cultures, nurses must be knowledgeable and culturally competent (Leininger, 1996). Seideman, Jacobson, Primeaux, Burns, & Weatherby (1996) outlined important cultural aspects to consider, using a Native American family as an example:

❧ Native American families differ from each other in their traditional beliefs and family structure.

❧ Generally, grandparents have an important role in parenting grandchildren.

❧ Extended family networks remain constant.

❧ Problems with parents and tradition occur when there is marriage with other tribes or ethnic groups.

❧ Distrust of Caucasian caregivers can interfere with interactions.

❧ Time is expected to be spent in establishing rapport before beginning an assessment.

❧ Learning by observation is preferred because asking questions is considered rude and intrusive.

❧ Unhurried observation is the best assessment approach.

❧ Positive reinforcement regarding observed strengths is important.

❧ Addressing areas that need improvement is best done in a neutral, indirect manner.

❧ A genuine interest in understanding the Native American culture is desirable.

❧ Referrals are more successful if a Native American professional or a person who is appreciative and sensitive to the culture is recommended.

NURSING PROCESS

For the postpartum family, the nursing process is an ongoing process that is used to develop an individualized plan of care. It involves careful collection of a database that supports a problem-solving approach to client care. The nursing process identifies areas in which the postpartum family requires nursing intervention.

Assessment

Family assessment begins with the initial nurse-family interaction, and focuses primarily on maternal and father-partner assessment. When taking a history and observing family dynamics, nurses begin to identify problem areas for collaborative intervention.

Maternal Assessment

Assessment of maternal behaviors that reflect a positive adjustment to the maternal role must take into consideration the expected behaviors of the "taking in" and the "taking hold" phases. Early indicators of a positive maternal adjustment include that the mother:

- Appears concerned when the infant cries and seeks to hold the infant.
- Uses eye contact in a face-to-face position when holding the infant.
- Is interested in getting to know the infant by gently exploring.
- Handles the infant lovingly and talks affectionately.
- Wants to review the birth and comments positively about the birth experience.
- Demonstrates a positive relationship with her partner or support person.

If the mother displays a negative attitude, does not have eye contact with the infant, does not want to hold the infant, or expresses anxiety and a lack of interest in the infant, maladaption may be occurring. Nurses should assess maladaptive behaviors, therapeutic communication skills, help the mother to clarify her feelings, and assess cultural beliefs that may be affecting postpartum behaviors. What may seem to be rejection behaviors may well be an accepted cultural norm. Other factors that must be considered are the mother's perception of the maternal role, her physical and emotional status, stressors that may be affecting role attainment, lack of support systems, young age, and poor coping mechanisms.

Father or Partner Assessment

The family-centered approach to postpartum care allows the nurse to view family dynamics. Paternal adaptation depends on a feeling of being included. Assessment of the father's perception of the birth and his behavior as a support person can give insight into the status of family adjustment. Many fathers want to discuss their feelings but are denied the opportunity when attention is focused primarily on the mother and infant. Fathers should be given the opportunity to express their feelings and to participate in the attachment process. By assessing the father's readiness to participate, nurses can assist in fostering the protective, watchful environment many fathers display.

Nursing Diagnosis

Identification of actual or potential problems early in the postpartum period is necessary for effective planning and intervention. On the basis of assessment data, cultural influences, spiritual needs, medical considerations, and family interactions, problem areas are analyzed and nursing diagnoses are developed. Examples of common nursing diagnoses that affect maternal role attainment are anxiety, fear, deficient knowledge, ineffective breast-feeding, ineffective role performance, and impaired parenting.

Outcome Identification

Outcomes for nursing interventions lay the pathway for nursing care. Goals are set through mutual determination of priorities between the nurse and the mother. The expected outcome or goal is specifically to reduce or eliminate the identified problem within a specified time frame. For example, if a mother is afraid to interact with her newborn, the nurse and mother need to explore the cause, identify the relationship of the cause to the problem, and assign priority to attainable goals. Identified outcome criteria act as a pathway for nursing interventions. An example would be: the nursing diagnosis of knowledge deficit related to inexperience with infants could have as one possible goal that the mother is able to demonstrate proper infant positioning during feeding.

Planning

Mutual planning involves assessing problem areas, considering expected outcomes, and setting realistic goals within a specified time period. Individualized nursing plans of care are established to include nursing actions, available resources, and client willingness to participate. For example, when developing a plan for a mother who is unsure about breastfeeding, the plan of care could include a referral to a resource, such as a lactation consultant.

Nursing Intervention

An individualized plan is based on identification of reasonable actions that can achieve desired outcomes. These actions may be independent nursing actions or collaborative actions involving other members. Actions are developed to resolve or lessen an identified problem and provide direction for nurses and other health care

Box 29-1 Nursing Care of the Postpartum Family

Nursing Diagnosis

Ineffective coping (potential) related to maturational crisis as evidenced by inability to meet role expectations.

Goal

The mother will begin to demonstrate positive coping behaviors by discharge.

Outcome

The mother is able to express feelings and set realistic goals and role expectations.

Intervention

Take time to explore the mother's role expectations.

Nursing Diagnosis

Risk for impaired parent, infant, or child attachment related to anxiety associated with the parent role as evidenced by lack of desire to interact with the infant.

Goal

The family will begin the attachment process by discharge.

Outcome

Parents are able to demonstrate attachment interactions with their infant.

Intervention

Slowly involve parents in infant care, guiding them from passive observers to active participants.

Nursing Diagnosis

Deficient knowledge related to lack of experience with infant care as evidenced by anxiety and hesitancy to provide infant care.

Goal

The parents will begin to provide infant care.

Outcome

Parents are able to initiate infant care before hospital discharge.

Intervention

Mother will demonstrate correct cord care.

professionals. Examples of interventions directed towards assisting the mother with role performance may include:

1. Using therapeutic communication to encourage verbalization of feelings and clarification of areas of concern.
2. Assessing cultural beliefs and incorporating them in maternal and infant care.
3. Involving the mother, her partner, and support persons in discharge planning.
4. Incorporating alternative therapies to reduce stress, such as music, massage, or guided imagery.
5. Referring parents to community resources, such as parenting classes, breastfeeding classes, or father's support classes.
6. Referring to counseling services as indicated.

Evaluation

Evaluation involves appraisal of identified outcomes and goals to decide if the goals have been reached (Box 29-1). Evaluation of goal achievement starts by assessing the client and gathering data to determine if outcomes have been reached or need adjusting. Questions to consider are whether or not the identified problems have been resolved or to what extent they still exist. Are there new problems to consider? Were the outcomes, goals, and interventions appropriate for this client? Were the nursing interventions consistently followed? What changes need to be made in the plan of care? Factors that hindered or helped goal attainment can be identified by interviewing the client and the family. Does the family need to be more involved in assisting with goal attainment? Is a planned conference with members of the health care team needed? If the client has achieved the established goals, and no new problems are present, the plan of care is considered successful and the client is in a stabilized health pattern.

Web Activities

- What sites could you recommend to new families who are looking for self-help information, chat rooms, or other electronic information sources?

- Is there a listing on the Internet of books, videos, or other media on postpartum adjustment? Are these resources available in your local library or through purchase from a website?

Case Study/Care Plan

POSTPARTUM TEEN MOTHER

Megan is a 16-year-old primigravida who delivered an 8-lb. girl by cesarean section. She is unwed and has no contact with the baby's father. She was in her junior year in high school, until her parents sent her to another state to live with an aunt for the last trimester and delivery. The parents are busy with their professional careers and have no interest in raising a grandchild. Because they are attorneys, they were able to arrange for adoption.

On the day following delivery, Megan was found crying. She told the nurse that she wanted to see her baby but was afraid to hold her. She expressed a desire to stay with her aunt and keep the baby. She also wanted to finish high school and get a job. Her aunt has been very loving and supportive, but she is raising three children alone as a divorced parent and cannot take on the added responsibility. Megan asked the nurse for pain medication while looking sadly at and holding her swollen abdomen. She tearfully said she would never get her figure back.

Assessment

Subjective data obtained through the interview process:

- Client was sent away to have her baby and give it up for adoption.
- Client is an unwed adolescent.
- Client desires to finish high school.
- Client has expressed a desire to keep her baby.
- Client desires to see her infant and is afraid to hold her.
- Client has no contact with the baby's father.
- Client has busy parents who give her monetary support and arranged the adoption.
- Client has an aunt who is supportive but unable to care for her niece and newborn.
- Client requested pain medication.
- Client states she will not get her figure back.

Objective data obtained through observation:

- Client is tearful and crying.
- Client looks anxious when talking about the baby.
- Client is holding her hands over incisional area.
- Client looks at the physical changes in her body.

Nursing Diagnosis

Pain related to cesarean incision as evidenced by supporting the incisional area and requesting medication.

Expected Outcome Client will have significant pain reduction within 1 hour after medication administration.

Planning Collaborating with client, determine how pain medication is to be administered and how often.

Nursing Interventions	Rationales
1. Assess need for pain medication using a scale from 1 to 10. Use guided imagery to refocus and enhance medication effectiveness.	1. Relief of pain is achieved with pharmacologic and nonpharmacologic means.

(continued)

Evaluation Pain medication schedule is effective in reducing client's pain within 1 hour after administration.

Nursing Diagnosis

Ineffective coping related to personal vulnerability in a situational crisis as evidenced by ineffective coping skills, and lack of support.

Expected Outcome Client will be able to clarify feelings and improve coping skills by discharge.

Planning By collaborating with client and support services, determine interventions to increase coping with situational crisis.

Nursing Interventions	Rationales
1. Take time to listen and assist to clarify feelings and improve coping skills. Address situational crisis via referral to a social worker.	1. Showing respect to client by listening and offering referrals will encourage confidence and realistic view of situation.

Evaluation Client is able to collaborate with social worker through family counseling to clarify feelings, improve coping skills, and set realistic goals regarding situational crisis by discharge.

Nursing Diagnosis

Anxiety related to situational crisis as evidenced by conflict with adoption issue.

Expected Outcome Client will demonstrate use of alternative relaxation techniques to reduce anxiety by discharge.

Planning Collaborating with client, determine methods to reduce level of anxiety.

Nursing Interventions	Rationales
1. Encourage ventilation of feelings; take time to listen. Incorporate alternative relaxation techniques, such as music, therapeutic touch, or focal breathing.	1. Encouraging verbalization of feelings and relaxation exercises will help to lessen anxiety.

Evaluation Client is able to effectively carry out alternative relaxation techniques to reduce anxiety by discharge.

Nursing Diagnosis

Disturbed body image related to physical changes as evidenced by concern about appearance.

Expected Outcome Client will demonstrate an understanding of postpartum body changes and exercise and nutritional program by discharge.

Planning Collaborating with the client, determine actions to increase realistic perception of self through physical and nutritional interventions.

Nursing Interventions	Rationales
1. Address concerns related to physical changes. Review postpartum exercise program, which may include yoga or walking. Refer to dietitian if calorie reduction is indicated.	1. Realistic understanding of physical changes promotes acceptance of body image. Knowledge of available resources assists in maternal adjustment.

Evaluation Client is able to understand physical changes during postpartum and incorporate a progressive exercise program by discharge.

Key Concepts

- The parent-child attachment process occurs over a period of time.
- Role adjustment to parenthood involves developmental task attainment.
- Maternal adjustment passes through three phases.
- Newborn sleep-wake behaviors influence the attachment process.
- Paternal adjustment occurs over time and is related to maternal influences.
- Siblings are affected by role change and seek nurturing by significant others.
- Grandparent's role adjustment may be positive or negative depending on the situation.
- Nurses need to be aware of cultural influences that affect parental role adjustment.
- Postpartum adolescents require assistance in achieving role adjustment and meeting the developmental tasks of adolescence.
- The nursing process provides a mechanism for assessing individual and family role transition.
- Alternative therapies can assist in maternal adjustment.

Review Questions and Activities

1. What does it mean to be a parent?
2. What nursing actions facilitate parent-child attachment?
3. How can nursing theory be applied to maternal role attainment?
4. How can culture affect maternal role attainment?
5. List infant behaviors that can facilitate the parent-child attachment process.
6. Compare and contrast paternal and maternal role attainment.
7. What community resources are available in your community to assist teen mothers?
8. What role do new grandparents have?
9. How can sibling adjustment be facilitated?
10. List 10 indicators of positive maternal adjustment.
11. Identify three salient dimensions related to paternal role attainment.

References

Adams, L., & Cotgrove, A. (1995). Promoting secure attachment patterns in infancy and beyond. *Professional Care of Mother & Child, 5,* (6), 158–160.

Ainsworth, M. S. (1997). The personal origins of attachment theory: an interview with Mary Sister Ainsworth. *Psychoanalytic Study of Children,* (52), 386–405.

Anderson, A. M. (1996). The father-infant relationship: becoming connected. *Journal of the Society of Pediatric Nursing,* (2), 82–92.

Barnet, B., Joffe, A., Duggan, A. K., Wilson, M. D., & Repke, J. T. (1996). Depressive symptoms, stress, and social support in pregnant and postpartum adolescents. *Archives of Pediatric & Adolescent Medicine, 150,* (1), 64–69.

Beck, C. T. (1996). Postpartum depressed mothers' experiences interacting with their children. *Nursing Research, 45,* (2), 98–100.

Beck, C. T. (1995). Perception of nurses' caring by mothers experiencing postpartum depression. *Journal of Obstetric, Gynecologic, & Neonatal Nursing, 24,* (9), 819–825.

Berger, D., & Loveland Cook, C. A. (1998). Postpartum teaching priorities: the viewpoints of nurses and mothers. *Journal of Obstetric, Gynecologic, and Neonatal Nursing, 27,* (2), 161–168.

Biringen, Z. (1994). Attachment theory and research: Application to clinical practice. *American Journal of Orthopsychiatry, 64,* (3), 404–420.

Bloom, K. C. (1998). Perceived relationship with the father of the baby and maternal attachment in adolescents. *Journal of Obstetric, Gynecologic, & Neonatal Nursing, 27,* (4), 420–429.

Brazelton, T. B. (1984). *Neonatal behavioral assessment scale,* 2nd ed. London: Heineman.

Brazelton, T. B. (1981). *On becoming a family: The growth of attachment.* New York: Dell.

Brown, P., Rustia, J., & Schapper, P. (1991). A comparison of fathers of high-risk newborns and fathers of healthy newborns. *Journal of Pediatric Nursing,* (4), 269–273.

Burke, P. J., & Liston, W. J. (1994). Adolescent mothers' perception of social support and the impact of parenting on their lives. *Pediatric Nursing, 20,* (6), 593–599.

Campinha-Bacote, J. (1995). The quest for cultural competence in nursing care. *Nursing Forum, 30,* 19–25.

Carter-Jessop, L., & Yoos, L. (1994). Parental thinking: Assessment and applications in nursing. *Maternal Child Nursing, 22,* (2), 49–55.

Chong-Yeu, L. C. (1995). Postpartum worries: An exploration of Taiwanese primipara who participate in the Chinese ritual of Tso-Yueh-Tzu. *Maternal-Child Nursing, 23,* (4), 110–122.

Crouch, M., & Manderson, L. (1995). The social life of bonding theory. *Social Science Medicine, 41,* (6), 873–844.

Diamond, M. J. (1995). Someone to watch over me: The father as the original protector of the mother-infant dyad. *Psychoanalysis and Psychotherapy, 12,* (1), 89–192.

Diehl, K. (1997). Adolescent mothers: What produces positive mother-infant interaction? *Maternal-Child Nursing, 22,* 88–95.

Duvall, E. (1971). *Family development,* (4th ed). Philadelphia: J.B. Lippincott.

Evans, C. J. (1995). Postpartum home care in the United States. *Journal of Obstetric, Gynecologic, & Neonatal Nursing, 24,* (2), 180–186.

Ferketich, S. L., & Mercer, R. T. (1995). Predictors of role competence for experienced and inexperienced fathers. *Nursing Research, 44,* (2), 88–95.

Fishbein, E. G., & Burggraf, E. (1998). Early postpartum discharge: How are mothers managing? *Journal of Obstetric, Gynecologic, & Neonatal Nursing, 27,* (2), 142–148.

Grant, C. G., Duggan, A. K., Andrews, J. S., & Serwing, J. R. (1997). The fathers role during infancy: Factors that influence maternal expectations. *Archives of Pediatric & Adolescent Medicine 151,* (7), 705–711.

Gjerdingen, D. K., & Chaloner, K. M. (1994). The relationship of women's postpartum mental health to employment, childbirth, and social support. *Journal of Family Practice, 38,* (5), 456–472.

Jordon, P. L. (1990). Laboring for relevance: Expectant and new fatherhood. *Nursing Research, 39,* 11–16.

Kelley, S. J., & Damato, E. G. (1995). Grandparents as primary caregivers. *Maternal-Child Nursing, 20,* 326–331.

Khazoyan, C. M., & Anderson, N. L. (1994). Latinas' expectations for their partners during childbirth. *Maternal-Child Nursing, 19,* 226–229.

Klaus, M. (1998). Mother and infant: Early emotional ties. *Pediatrics, 102,* (5), 1244–1246.

Klaus, M. H., & Kennel, J. H. (1982). *Parent-infant bonding,* (2nd ed.) St. Louis: C. V. Mosby.

Knoiak-Griffin, D., Mathenge, C., Anderson, L. R., & Verzemnieks, I. (1999). An early intervention program for adolescent mothers: A nursing demonstration project. *Journal of Obstetric, Gynecologic, & Neonatal Nursing, 28,* 51–59.

Leathers, S. J., Kelley, M. A., & Richman, J. A. (1997). Postpartum depressive symptomology in new mothers and fathers: Parenting, work, and support. *Journal of Nervous & Mental Disorders, 185,* (3), 129-139.

Lamp, J. M., & Howard, P. A. (1999). Guiding parents' use of the Internet for newborn education. *Maternal Child Nursing, 24,* (1), 33–36.

Leininger, M. (1996). Culture care theory, research, and practice. *Nursing Science Quarterly, 9,* (2), 71–78.

Lepper, H. S., DiMatteo, M. R., & Tinsley, B. J. (1994). Postpartum depression: How much do obstetric nurses and obstetricians know? *Birth, 21,* (3), 149–154.

Ludington-Hoe, S. M., & Swinth, J. Y. (1996). Developmental aspects of kangaroo care. *Journal of Obstetric, Gyneclogic, & Neonatal Nursing 25,* (8), 691–700.

Marks, M., & Lovestone, S. (1995). The role of the father in parental postnatal mental health. *British Journal of Medical Psychology, 68,* 157–168.

May, J. (1996). Fathers: The forgotten parent. *Pediatric Nursing, 22,* (3), 243–246, 271.

Mercer, R. T., & Ferketich, S. L. (1995). Experienced and inexperienced mothers' maternal competence during infancy. *Research in Nursing, 18,* (4), 333–343.

Merchant, D. C., Affonso, D. D., & Mayberry, L. J. (1995). Influence of marital relationship and child-care stress on maternal depression symptoms in the postpartum. *Journal of Psychosomatic Obstetrics, & Gynaecology, 16,* (4), 193–200.

Midmer, D., Wilson, L., & Cummings, S. (1995). A randomized, controlled trial of the influence of prenatal parenting education on postpartum anxiety and marital adjustment. *Family Medicine, 27,* (3), 200–205.

Minton, C., & Pasley, K. (1996). Fathers' parenting role identity and father involvement: A comparison of nondivorced and divorced nonresident fathers. *Journal of Family Issues, 17,* (1), 26–45.

Muller, M. A. (1996). Prenatal and postnatal attachment: A modest correlation. *Journal of Obstetric, Gynecologic, & Neonatal Nursing, 25,* (2), 161–166.

Patterson, D. L. (1997). Adolescent mothering: Child-grandmother attachment. *Journal of Pediatric Nursing, 12,* (4), 228–237.

Prodromidis, M., Field, T., Arendt, R., Singer, L., Yando, R., & Bendell, D. (1995). Mothers touching newborns: A comparison of rooming-in versus minimal contact. *Birth 22,* (4), 196–200.

Rubin, R. (1984). *Maternal identity and the maternal experience.* New York: Springer.

Seideman, R. J., Jacobson, S., Primeaux, M., Burns, P., & Weatherby, F. (1996). Assessing American Indian families. *Maternal-Child Nursing, 21,* 274–279.

Shott, J., & Henley, A. (1996). *Culture, religion, and childbearing in a multiracial society.* Boston: Reed Educational and Professional.

Smith-Hanrahan, C., & Deblois, D. (1995). Postpartum early discharge: Impact on maternal fatigue and functional ability. *Clinical Nursing Research, 4,* (1), 50–66.

Stamp, G. H. (1994). The appropriation of the parental role through communication during the transition to parenthood. *Communication Monographs, 61,* (2), 89–112.

Sullivan, J. M. (1997). Learning the baby: A maternal thinking and problem-solving process. *Journal of the Society for Pediatric Nursing, 2,* (1), 21–28.

Tiller, C. M. (1995). Fathers' parenting attitudes during a child's first year. *Journal of Obstetric, Gynecologic, & Neonatal Nursing, 24,* (6), 508–514.

Tomey, A. M., & Alligood, M. R., (Eds). (1998). *Nursing theorists and their work,* 4th ed. St. Louis: Mosby.

Troy, N. W. (1993). Early contact and maternal attachment among women using public health care facilities. *Applied Nursing Research, 6* (4), 161–166.

Waters, E., Posada, G., Crowell, J. A., & Lay, K. L. (1994). The development of attachment: From control system to working models. *Psychiatry, 57,* (1), 32–42.

Suggested Readings

Barclay, L., Everett, L., Rogan, F., Schmied, V., & Wyllie, A. (1997). Becoming a mother—an analysis of women's experience of early motherhood. *Journal of Advanced Nursing, 25,* (4), 719–728.

Beck, C. T. (1998). A review of research instruments for use during the postpartum period. *Maternal Child Nursing, 23,* (5), 254–261.

Beck, C. T. (1999). Available instruments for research on prenatal attachment and adaptation to pregnancy. *Maternal Child Nursing, 24,* (1), 25–32.

Collins, C. (1998). Yoga: Intuition, preventive medicine, and treatment. *Journal of Obstetric, Gynecologic, & Neonatal Nursing, 27,* (5), 563–567.

Logsdon, M. C., & Davis, D. W. (1998). Guiding mothers of high-risk infants in obtaining social support. *Maternal Child Nursing, 23,* (4), 195–199.

Miles, M. S., Holditch-Davis, D., & Shepherd, H. (1998). Maternal concerns about parenting prematurely born children. *Maternal Child Nursing, 23,* (2), 70–75.

Olson, S. L. (1998). Bedside musical care: Applications in pregnancy, childbirth, and neonatal care. *Journal of Obstetric, Gynecologic, & Neonatal Nursing, 27,* (5), 569–574.

Rees, B. L. (1995). Effect of relaxation with guided imagery on anxiety, depression, and self-esteem in primiparas. *Journal of Holistic Nursing, 13,* (3), 255–267.

Roye, C. F., & Balk, S. J. (1997). Caring for pregnant teens and their mothers, too. *Maternal Child Nursing, 22,* 153–157.

Rogan, F., Schmeid, V., Barclay, L., Everitt, L., & Wyllie, A. (1997) Becoming a mother—developing a new theory of early motherhood. *Journal of Advanced Nursing, 25,* (5), 877–885.

Starn, J. R. (1998). Energy healing with women and children. *Journal of Obstetric, Gynecologic, & Neonatal Nursing, 27,* (5), 576–583.

Stern, D. (1998). Mothers' emotional needs. *Pediatrics, 102,* (5), 1250–1252.

Tiedje, L. B. (1998). Alternative health care: An overview. *Journal of Obstetric, Gynecologic, & Neonatal Nursing, 27,* (5), 557–562.

Resources

Baby Business: http://www.sdx-tech.com/baby

Baby Center: http://www.babycenter.com

Baby Engine (search engine): http://www.novasight.com/babyeng/index.htm

Carnation Baby: http://www.carnationbaby.com

Childcare Experts National Network: http://www.childcare-experts.org

Family.com: http://www.family.disney.com

Family Education Network: http://www.familyeducation.com

HealthSeek: http://www.healthseek.com

Infoseek Kids and Family Channel: http://www.infoseek.com/kidsandfamily

Johnson & Johnson: http://www.jnj.com

National Center for Fathering: http://www.fathers.com

The National Parenting Center: http://www.tnpc.com

Newwellness: http://www.netwellness.org

Pampers Parenting Institute: Total Baby Care: http://www.pampers.com

Parenthood Web: http://www.parenthoodweb.com

Parenting Q&A: http://www.parenting-qa.com

Parentsoup: http://www.parentsoup.com

Parentsplace: http://www.parentsplace.com

Welcome Addition Online: http://www.welcomeaddition.com

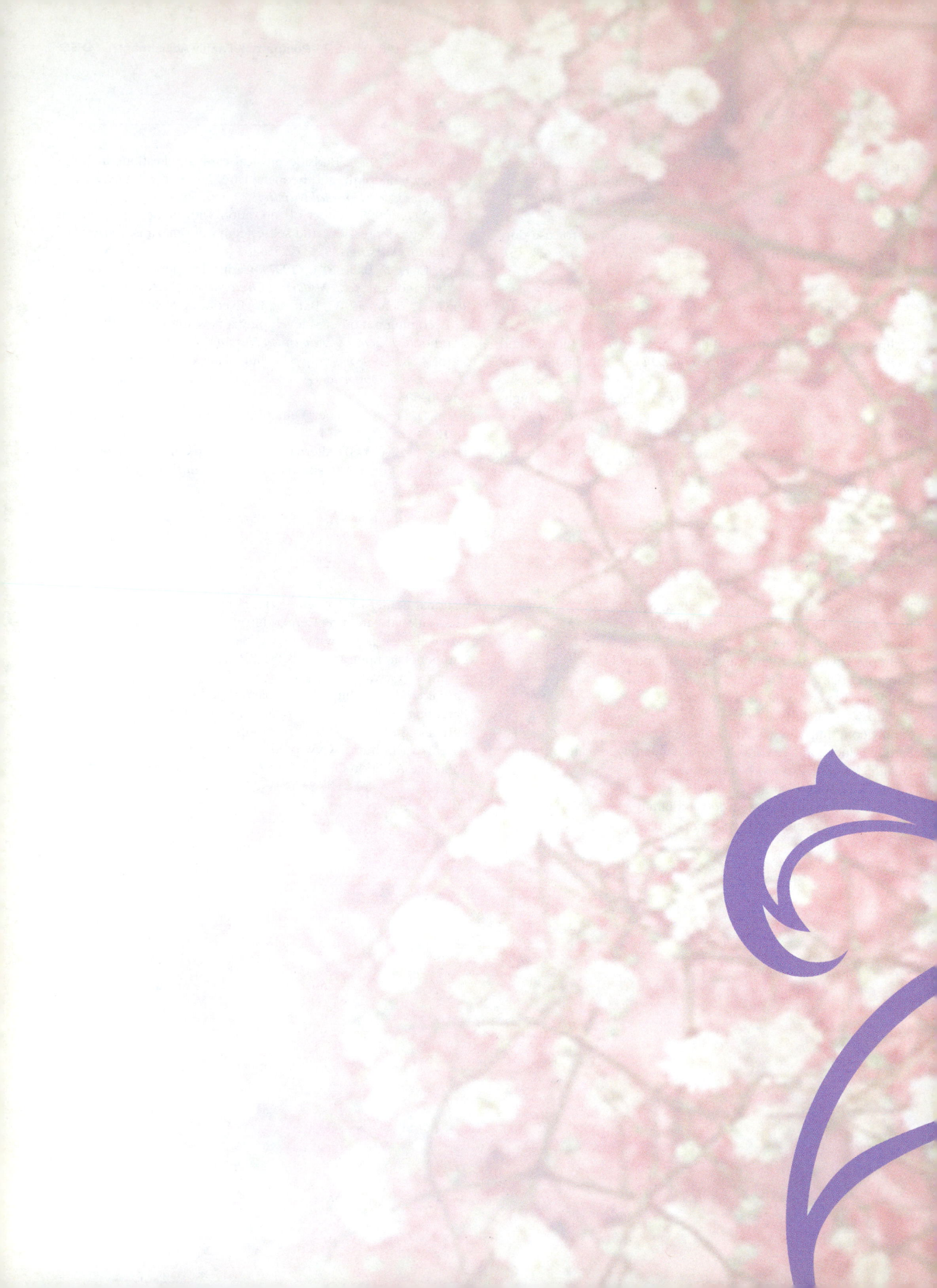

CHAPTER 30

Lactation and Nursing Support

H elping new mothers and mothers-to-be with breast-feeding decisions requires the nurse to examine her own biases regarding feeding methods. Working with mothers and families to support the decision that is best for them and their infants can have an empowering effect on these new mothers.

- *Do I really believe that "breast is best"?*

- *Which feeding method would I choose for my own infant?*

- *Do I feel embarrassed to see a woman breast-feed in public?*

- *How do I feel when trying to help a woman breast-feed for the first time?*

- *Do I feel angry when a client doesn't do what I think is best for her or her infant?*

- *Can I allow a client to tell me how she really feels without judging her?*

- *Do I respect cultural beliefs about breast-feeding that may not be scientifically sound?*

Key Terms

Alveoli	Hindmilk	Let-down reflex	Relactation
Areola	Lactation consultant	Mastitis	Rooting reflex
Colostrum	Lactogenesis	Mature milk	Transitional milk
Engorgement	Latching-on	Oxytocin	Weaning
Foremilk	La Leche League	Prolactin	Wet nurse
Galactopoiesis			

Competencies

Upon completion of this chapter, the reader should be able to:

1. Identify the health and financial benefits related to breast-feeding.
2. Explore the motivations and perceived barriers related to breast-feeding.
3. Describe effective strategies to promote breast-feeding in a culturally sensitive manner.
4. Develop interventions that lead to successful breast-feeding outcomes.
5. Delineate nursing responsibilities for patient education and informed consent related to breast-feeding decisions.
6. Assess the nutritional status of the breast-fed infant.
7. Describe the physiology of lactation.
8. Apply the nursing process to the woman who is breast-feeding.

The health, nutritional, and psychologic benefits of breast-feeding are widely recognized in the medical, lay, and scientific communities. Breast-feeding is the infant feeding method recommended by the American Academy of Pediatrics, American Public Health Association, and American Dietetic Association for the first 12 months after birth (American Academy of Pediatrics, 1997). The practice guidelines of the American Academy of Pediatrics are straightforward and supported by solid research. These recommendations include the following:

- Newborns should be nursed when they show signs of hunger (crying is identified as a late sign of hunger). Newborns should be nursed approximately 8 to 12 times every 24 hours until satiety.

- No supplements should be given to newborns unless a medical indication exists. Supplements and pacifiers should be avoided if used at all, and only used after breast-feeding is well established.

- Exclusive breast-feeding is ideal and sufficient to support optimal growth and development for approximately 6 months.

- Gradual introduction of iron-enriched solid foods in the second half of the first year should complement breast milk.

- Breast-feeding should continue for at least 12 months, and thereafter for as long as mutually desired.

Breast-feeding provides the optimal nutrition for infants during the first year of life when there is rapid physical and developmental growth. In addition to providing essential nutrients, breast-feeding provides unique opportunities for positive interactions and bonding between infants and mothers. A woman's decision to breast-feed is determined by many factors. Feeding her new infant can be an exciting, satisfying, and personally empowering experience for many women. The nurse can provide vital support to women who choose to breast-feed and do not have role models in their families who have successfully breast-fed. This area of health care is one in which the nurse and other health care professionals really can make a difference that has long-lasting effects. Breast-feeding will result in immediate positive health outcomes for infants and mothers. The financial savings of increasing the number of infants who are breast-fed will be realized immediately by the families and the entire health care system.

Promotion of breast-feeding has become a worldwide health goal for all nations because of the many unique components found only in human milk (WHO/UNICEF, 1994). The priority health goal for the United States, as published in the "Healthy People 2010" document, is to increase breast-feeding for infants among all women, especially those who have low incomes and are African American, Hispanic, Native American, and Alaskan Native (U. S. Department of Health and Human Services, 2000). Specifically, the goal is to increase the number of women who initiate breast-feeding in the early postpartal period to at least 75%, with a 50% continuation rate at 5 to 6 months (U. S. Department of Health and Human Services, 2000).

In the 1970s the deleterious effects of manufactured formula on infant health and survival became better appreciated throughout the world, and the role of advertising became increasingly suspect. For decades the World Health Organization (WHO) has included as a part of their Code for Infant Feeding, a statement designed to protect developing countries from being inundated with formula advertising, which discourages breast-feeding. In many Third World countries that have poor sanitation and contaminated water supplies, infant survival depends on being nourished at the breast (WHO/UNICEF, 1994). In 1998, in a controversial step, the United Nations (U.N.) revised its breast-feeding recommendations because of the soaring rates of human immunodeficiency virus (HIV) infection in much of the world. In 1997, HIV transmission through breast-feeding accounted for up to one third of the 600,000 children infected, according to UNAIDS, the U.N. agency that developed the policy (Weinberg, 2000). The U.N. has issued recommendations intended to discourage women who are HIV-positive from breast-feeding by informing them about the risk of transmission to their babies through breast milk and about the alternative use of formula. Some experts have voiced concern that the increased use of formula will result in other deadly infections because of the use of contaminated water that may occur in formula preparation (Altman, 1998).

HISTORY OF BREAST-FEEDING

Historically, writings on breast-feeding can be found in the Bible and in many ancient texts of Greece, Rome, Egypt, and the European world. A wet nurse (a woman employed to breast-feed an infant not her own) was used when the mother died or when a child was abandoned. Hammurabi's code from about 1800 B.C. contained regulations on the practice of wet nursing, that is, nursing another woman's infant for pay. In 1472, Paul Bagellardus, a Renaissance medical writer in Padua, described the characteristics of a good wet nurse. In the 1700s, French orphanages were staffed by carefully selected wet nurses. From 1500s to 1700s, however, many wealthy English women did not nurse their infants but used wet nurses and fed in-

fants cereal or bread gruel from a spoon. The death rate in foundling homes from feeding infants cereal or bread gruel approached 100% (Lawrence, 1999).

The benefits of breast milk from the biologic mother have long been well known. Over two thousand years ago, Hippocrates wrote, "One's own milk is beneficial, other's harmful" (Lawrence, 1999). Breast milk was commonly accepted as the best milk for infants until 1884, when physicians and chemists entered the field of infant feeding. The competition among infant formula manufacturers was launched by the end of the 19th Century. In the United States, during the 1920s, women were encouraged to raise their infants scientifically, which led to the conclusion that prepared foods, such as formula, were superior because they could be measured and calculated to meet specific dietary requirements (Lawrence, 1999).

The benefits of breast-feeding have been scientifically supported beginning in the 1970s. Since then, more women have been nursing their infants. Statistically, however, the numbers of women who breast-feed are far from those proposed by the health goals stated in the "Healthy People 2010" document (U.S. Department of Health and Human Services, 2000).

Epidemiology

Breast-feeding rates are higher among women who are Caucasian, of higher socioeconomic status, older, married, and have a high educational level. Women who are African American, single, younger, unmarried, enrolled in the federal Special Supplemental Nutrition Program for Women, Infants, and Children [WIC], working outside the home, and of low educational level are less likely to initiate breast-feeding (McClurg-Hitt & Olsen, 1994). These mothers and infants of low-income status have a high risk of morbidity and mortality and would benefit most from breast-feeding because of the health, financial, and psychologic advantages.

In the United States the breast-feeding rate among highly educated women in families of high socioeconomic status is encouraging (54%); however, among women who are less educated, of low-income status, and members of a minority the rate is lower (30%). Ironically, infants born into poverty are exactly those who would benefit most from the protection that breast-feeding affords (Ryan, 1997). Figure 30-1 illustrates the breast-feeding rates of three cultural groups in the United States.

Incidence

The Ross Products Division of Abbott Laboratories has been a significant resource for breast-feeding statistics since 1955. The Ross Mothers' Survey is an ongoing mail survey that is sent to new mothers at the time their new

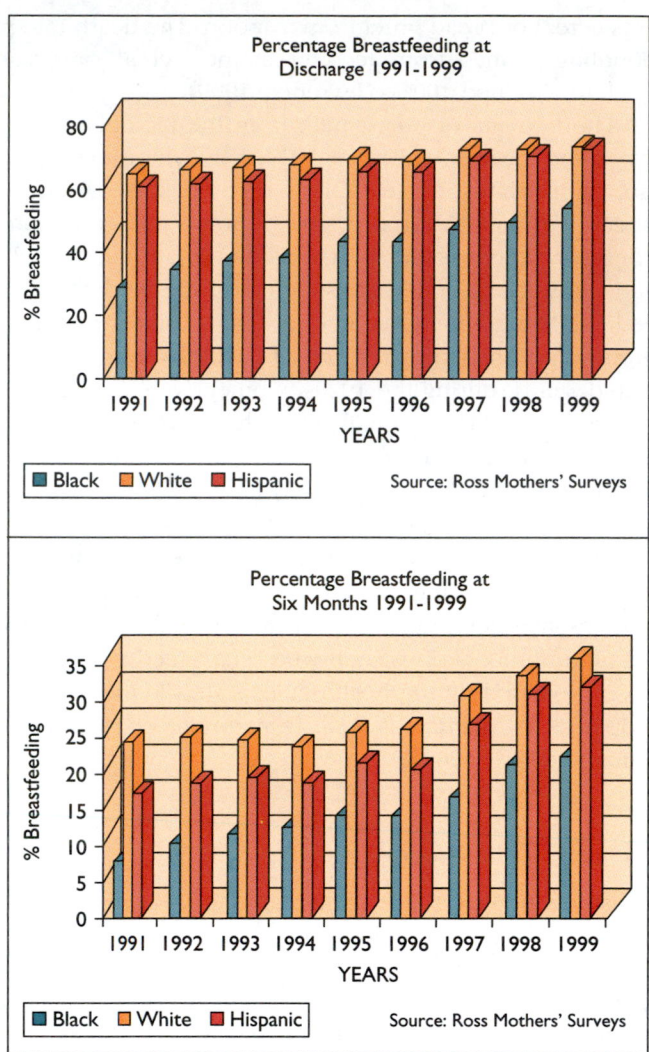

Figure 30-1 Breast-feeding rates in the United States. (Source: Ross Mothers' Survey).

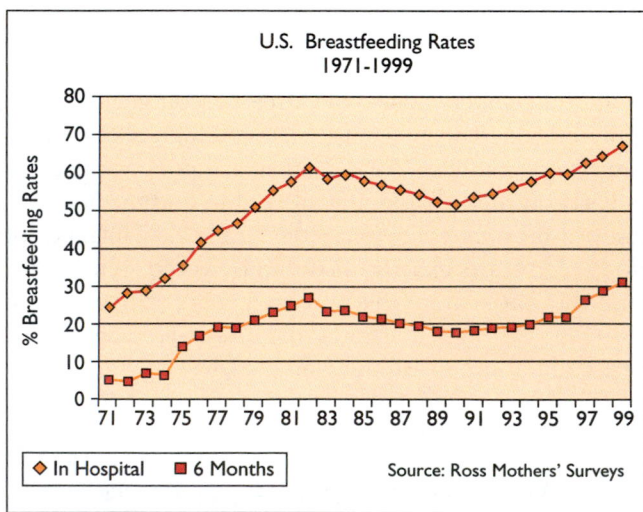

Figure 30-2 Breast-feeding rates in the United States: 1971–1999. (Source: Ross Mothers' Survey).

infant is 6 months of age. Results of the survey are weighted based on selected demographic variables associated with adoption of breast-feeding behaviors. Since 1992, more than 725,000 new mothers have received this questionnaire annually (Ryan, 1997). Figure 30-2 shows the change in breast-feeding rates over the past 30 years, as reported in the Ross survey.

Prevalence

Breast-feeding rates differ greatly by region of the United States in which the mother resides, with higher rates in the West and lower rates in the East and Southeast. Western states, such as Washington and California, have breast-feeding initiation rates as high as 98% on discharge from the hospital. In contrast, some Southern states, such as Mississippi, have much lower rates than the national average (Mothers Survey, 2000).

Socioeconomic Status and Ethnic Patterns

According to the Ross Mothers' Survey, breast-feeding rates are lowest among African American infants, infants born into homes with annual incomes of less than $10,000 per year, and mothers with only a grade-school education. All demographic categories experienced increases in breast-feeding initiation rates from 1990 to 1999. The groups with the historically lowest breast-feeding initiation rates experienced the largest increases during the same time period. (Ryan, 1997). This increase in breast-feeding rates can be attributed to the promotion efforts of many nurses and other health care workers.

Cultural Values, Beliefs, and Traditions

In human beings, breast-feeding behavior is highly variable from one culture to another. Different cultures have different "rules" about lactation. Cultural tradition dictates the initiation, frequency, and cessation of breast-feeding.

Within the United States there are many regional and ethnic cultures. Dealing effectively with these various groups requires that the nurse be knowledgeable about and sensitive to the cultural influences contributing to the values and beliefs of each client. Persons who have immigrated to the United States may have come from a culture in which traditionally all infants are breast-fed. After coming to the United States, however, some of these women may feel that bottle-feeding is more modern and therefore better for their infants. Other women may adopt formula-feeding because they want to be more like Americans, and perceive that bottle-feeding is the custom in the United States. Some women may choose breast-feeding because it seems more natural to them and is healthier for infants and because the women enjoy the closeness that breast-feeding provides.

It is clear that culture and economics greatly influence decisions regarding infant feeding. Breast-feeding behavior is highly variable from one culture to another. Variables such as the degree of body contact, how often an infant is held, and how the infant is carried vary greatly from culture to culture. Studies of world societies reveal that North American and European women are concerned about the beliefs that it is indecent to expose the breast, children are spoiled by holding them too much, and early weaning is a sign of maturity in a child (Lawrence, 1999). Many women rely on knowledge obtained from their immediate families and the experiences of women in the community when making decisions about infant care and feeding. It is generally believed that a mother's decision regarding infant feeding is based on beliefs about growth and development. Considering the variability among ethnic groups, however, many researchers are recognizing the roles culture and ethnicity play in those decisions (Underwood et al., 1997).

Many factors are related to a woman's personal choice of infant feeding method. Her attitude, personality, cultural belief, biologic adaptation, genetic endowment, response of her infant, past interpersonal relationships, family support, and previous pregnancies all contribute to the decision-making process regarding infant feeding. Conflicts regarding the function of the breast as a sexual organ versus an organ for infant nourishment may play an important role in the choice of feeding method.

In Stuart-Macadam and Dettwyler's (1995) book on the biocultural perspectives of breast-feeding, cultural forces that conflict with breast-feeding are presented as perspectives influencing human behavior. These authors propose that infant feeding practices are influenced by geography and culture. In many countries of the world (such as Finland) breast-feeding is the norm, and no infant formula is manufactured. In some developing countries, safe formula feeding is almost impossible because of contaminated water supplies.

Women from other cultures, such as Filipino, Mexican American, and Vietnamese, do not give **colostrum** (thin fluid in the breast from pregnancy into the early postpartal period, which is rich in antibodies and high in protein) to newborns. Women in these societies prefer to wait until their milk is established to initiate breast-feeding. In some cultures, colostrum is believed to be "old" milk that has been in the breast too long or milk that is contaminated and must be removed and disposed of before the infant is put to the breast (Lawrence, 1999). In some Asian cultures the infant is only given boiled water until the mother's milk supply is established.

Modesty is important for the Mexican-American mother, and some women will avoid breast-feeding in

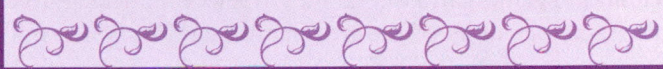

Critical Thinking

Cultural Views on Colostrum

Clients from some cultures, such as Hispanic, Navajo, Filipino, and Vietnamese, will not give their infants colostrum. These women begin breast-feeding only after the transitional milk comes in and therefore will reject attempts to begin breast-feeding behavior in the immediate postpartum period.

How can nurses ensure good breast-feeding outcomes and still respect cultural differences, values, and beliefs?

public because they find it embarrassing. In Western cultures, breasts are regarded as sexual objects and the biologic role of the breasts for infant nutrition is downplayed. African American women breast-feed at much lower rates than do Caucasian and Hispanic women. Most Muslim women breast-feed because the Qur'an encourages it until the child is 2 years old (Hutchinson & Baqi-Aziz, 1994). Many research studies have collected data on attitudes toward breast-feeding in an attempt to understand the cultural and ethnic differences that influence breast-feeding decisions. The nurse needs to be aware of and understand the impact of culture on infant feeding methods to evaluate the effect of the belief or value on breast-feeding decisions.

Research studies on breast-feeding have examined the factors that influence adoption of breast-feeding (initiation), factors that seem to predict the length of time a woman will continue breast-feeding (duration), and how much supplementation of formula will be used along with breast-feeding (exclusivity). The purpose of these studies is to be able to predict the women who will breast-feed successfully compared with women who will not do so. This information can then be used to design interventions that will increase breast-feeding in the groups of women who are less likely to choose breast-feeding.

BIOLOGY OF LACTATION

Lactation is the biologic completion of the reproductive cycle. Starting at about 16 weeks' gestation the breast develops and prepares for full lactation. In the first few postpartal hours and days the breast responds to hormones and the stimulation of the infant's sucking to produce and release milk.

Anatomy of the Breast

Nurses caring for new mothers need to have accurate knowledge about the anatomy and physiology of the lactating breast to facilitate the client's understanding. Prepared with adequate knowledge, the client will be able to achieve a successful breast-feeding experience.

The breasts or mammary glands are specialized sebaceous glands located in the superficial fascia between the second rib and sixth intercostal cartilage. The pectoral and anterior serratus muscles lie beneath each breast. Cooper's ligaments support the breast, extending from the deep fascia to the skin covering each breast. The breasts are composed of adipose, fibrous, and glandular tissues. Deep within the glandular tissue are the treelike branching **alveoli** (secretory units of the mammary gland in which milk production takes place), or acini, arranged in a series of 15 to 42 lobes. Lobes are separated by adipose and fibrous tissues and are arranged like spokes converging on the central nipple. Each lobe is made up of many lobules. The lobules are made of many grapelike clusters of alveoli (acini) around small ducts. The ducts combine to form larger lactiferous ducts that open on the surface of the nipple (Figure 30-3).

At the center of each breast is the nipple, a conic elevation composed of erectile tissue that becomes more rigid during sexual excitement, pregnancy, and lactation. Each nipple contains 15 to 25 lactiferous ducts that end as small orifices near the tip of the nipple (Figure 30-4). The tissue surrounding the nipple is heavily pigmented and called the **areola**. Montgomery's tubercles, small papillae, are located in the areola. These tubercles secrete a substance that lubricates the nipples and areola during pregnancy and lactation.

The blood supply to the breast is mainly from the internal mammary artery (60%). The lateral thoracic artery, intercostal arteries, and branches of the axillary and subclavian artery supply the remaining 40% of blood supply (Figure 30-5). Innervation of the breasts is from the branches of the fourth, fifth, and sixth intercostal nerves. Sensory fibers innervate the smooth muscles in the nipple, areola, and skin.

Lymphatic drainage of the breasts is mainly due to the axillary and parasternal nodes along the internal thoracic artery (Figure 30-6). The lymphatics originate in the lymph capillaries of the mammary connective tissue and drain through the breast tissue. Some drainage goes to the opposite breast, liver, intraabdominal nodes, and subclavicular nodes deep to the clavicle (Lawrence, 1999).

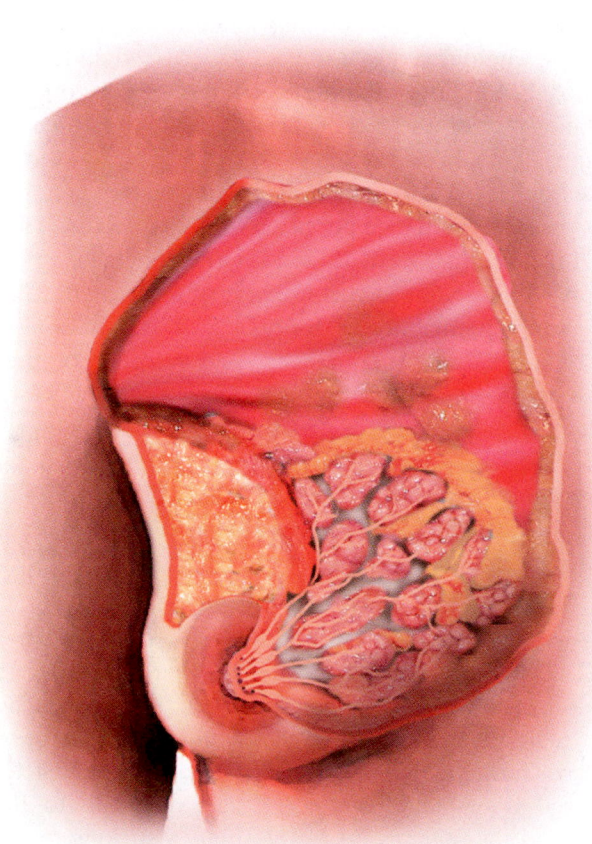

Figure 30-3 Anatomy of the breast.

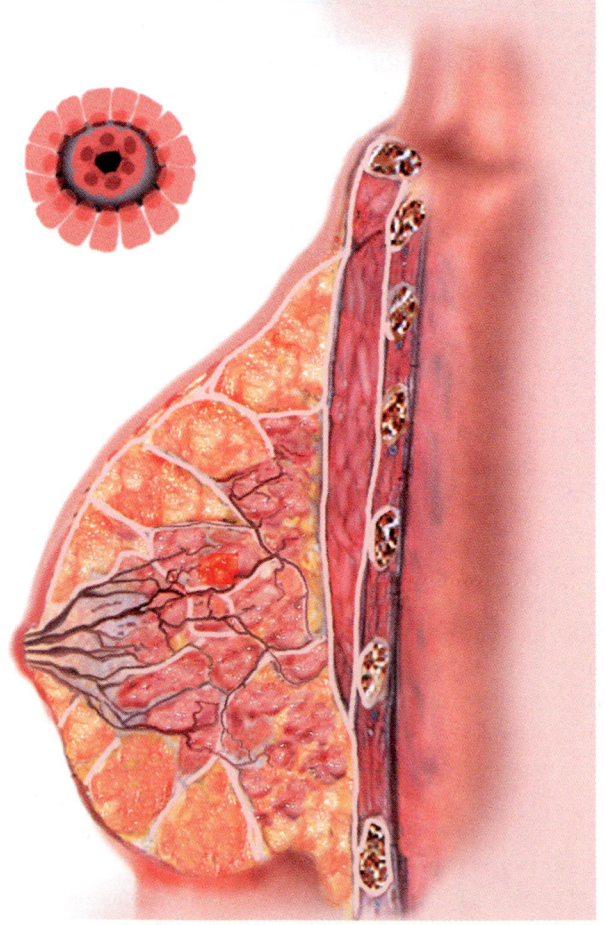

Figure 30-4 Duct system of the breast.

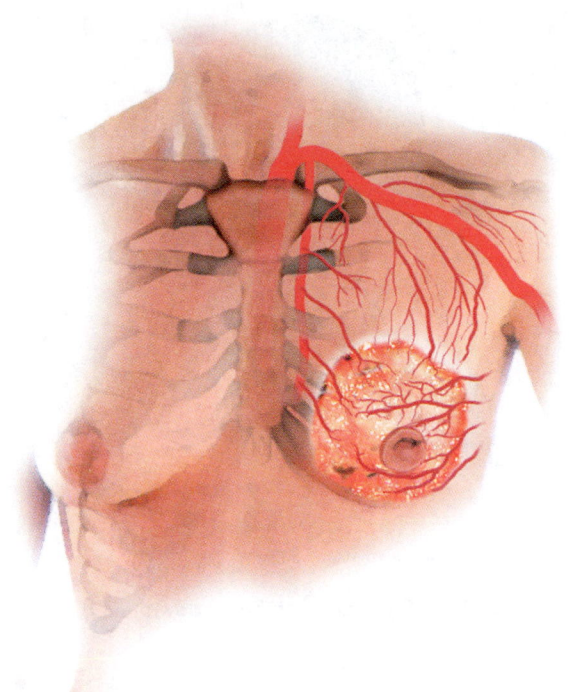

Figure 30-5 Blood supply to the breast.

Physiology of Lactation: Hormones and Processes

One of the biologic functions of the breasts is to supply nourishment and protective antibodies to infants during the lactation process. Cyclic hormonal stimulation of the breast occurs during each menstrual cycle, puberty, and

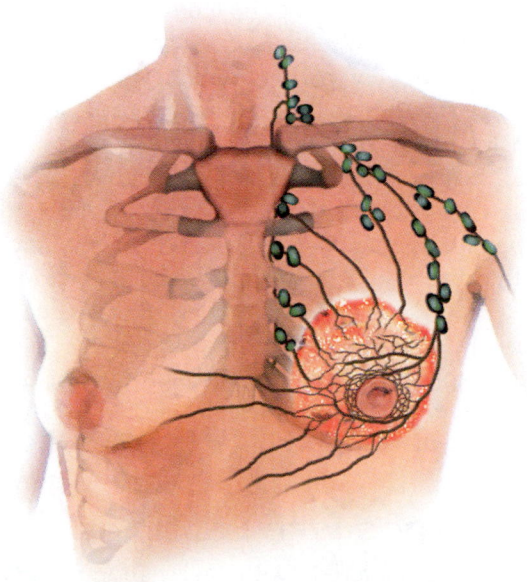

Figure 30-6 Lymphatic drainage of the breast.

especially pregnancy and lactation. The nonpregnant breast does not ordinarily secrete any milklike substance but may enlarge slightly during the menstrual cycle. During pregnancy, changing levels of circulating hormones profoundly change the growth of the ducts, alveoli, and lobes in the breasts. During lactation, the breast tissue is characterized by large numbers of alveoli. After lactation, when milk is no longer removed from the breast by the infant, the alveoli gradually collapse and adipose tissue increases. The hormonal control of lactation can be described under three main headings: **mammogenesis**, or mammary growth; **lactogenesis**, or initiation of milk secretion; and **galactopoiesis**, or the maintenance of established milk secretion.

Lactogenesis

Complex nervous and endocrine factors are involved in the establishment of milk production in the first 2 to 5 days postpartum (lactogenesis) and in maintenance of lactation (galactopoiesis). Childbirth results in a rapid decrease in estrogen and progesterone and an increase in prolactin secretion. **Prolactin** is a hormone produced by the pituitary gland that triggers milk production by stimulating the alveolar cells of the breast. Prolactin levels increase in response to tactile stimulation of the breast, such as in response to sucking by the infant.

The synthesis of human milk involves a cellular site at which the epithelial cells of the acini are active in milk production (Figure 30-7). Most milk is synthesized during the process of suckling. The cellular components of human milk are enzymes, proteins, fats, ions, water, and glucose.

Let-down Reflex and Milk Ejection

The infant's sucking also stimulates the release of oxytocin. **Oxytocin** is a hormone produced by the posterior pituitary that stimulates uterine contractions and release of milk from the mammary glands. Oxytocin increases the contractility of the myoepthelial cells that line the walls of the mammary ducts, resulting in the let-down reflex (Figure 30-8). The **let-down reflex** is the ejection of milk from the breast and milk flow toward the nipple triggered by nipple stimulation or emotional response to the infant. Once lactation is well established, prolactin decreases while oxytocin and suckling continue to be important in maintaining milk supply.

Three main hormones are involved in the lactation process: human placental lactogen (HPL), human growth hormone (HGH), and prolactin. The progressive increase in prolactin during pregnancy parallels the increase in HPL. HGH is thought to have a synergistic effect with prolactin and glucocorticoids in the maintenance of lactation. Both prolactin and oxytocin release is accomplished by nipple stimulation. Milk ejection involves both neural and

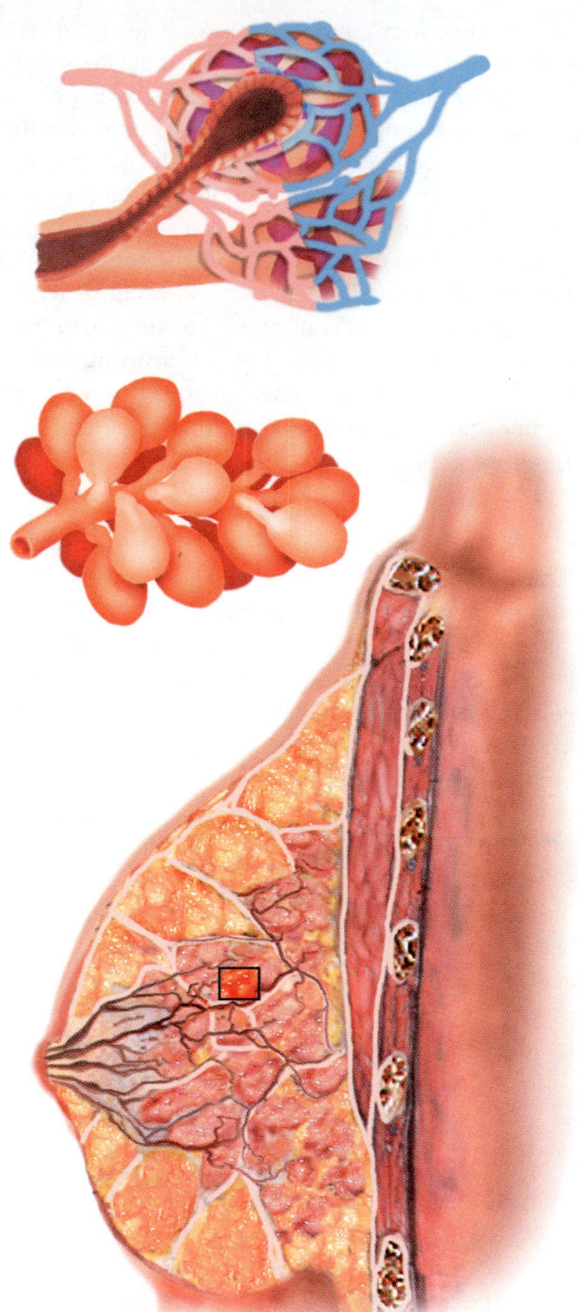

Figure 30-7 Physiology of lactation.

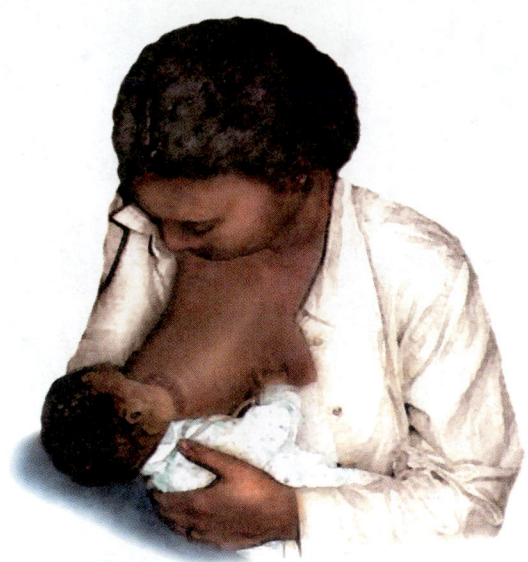

Figure 30-8 Physiology of the let-down reflex.

endocrinologic stimulation and response. A neural afferent pathway and an endocrinologic efferent pathway are required. Interference with the ejection reflex usually is due to psychologic inhibition caused by stress of some kind, such as disapproval of breast-feeding by a family member.

Galactopoiesis

The nurse also needs to teach the new mother that because breast milk is based on supply and demand, the best way to increase breast milk supply is for the infant to demand more by nursing often. It therefore follows that the more supplementation with formula or glucose water is used, the less the demand. Thus, the supply diminishes. The nurse should advise the new mother to avoid giving supplemental bottles because doing so will interfere with establishing her milk supply and may cause *nipple confusion* (the inability of the infant to go from bottle to breast and vice versa). Encouraging night feedings and preparing the client for infant growth spurts (that usually occur 10 to 14 days, 6 weeks, 3 to 4 months, and 6 months) will reduce concern about the lack of an adequate milk supply.

The client also needs to be taught that breast-feeding usually requires the infant to be fed every 2 to 3 hours during the first 3 to 4 weeks. Frequent demand for feedings may concern the new parents, and they may wonder if the infant is getting adequate nutrition. Signs of adequate intake include 8 to 10 wet diapers in 24 hours, frequent stooling, steady weight gain, and contentment after breast-feeding. The stools of breast-fed infants differ from those of formula-fed infants in color and consistency. Stools from the breast-fed infant are golden yellow, sweet smelling, and loose or liquid in consistency. Breast-fed infants usually regain their birth weight by 14 days of age, then gain approximately 15 g/d (0.5 oz/d) in the first 6 months of life. Birth weight usually is doubled by approximately 5 months of age (Riordan & Auerbach, 1999).

Interference with Lactation

Many factors can interfere with the lactation process. Physical factors, medical conditions, poor diet, and maternal anxiety all can contribute to unsuccessful breast-feeding.

Anxiety

Mothers who are breast-feeding may experience some problems coping with their new maternal role and may develop fears or anxieties. For example, mothers may worry about not producing enough milk, particularly during the first few days of breast-feeding and during infant growth spurts. The nurse can help prepare the new mother to handle these fears by reminding her that these emotions are common and can be expected as the infant's demand may occasionally exceed the supply for a few days. Milk production for these growth spurts will correct itself quickly when the breast is offered more often and for longer periods of time.

New mothers need to be reassured that all infants cry as a way of communicating and that crying is not a sign that the breast milk is inadequate. Frequently, it may be necessary to remind new mothers that retreating to a private area to breast-feed may help them relax and be able to reduce the stresses surrounding new motherhood. If someone in their environment is causing stress or anxiety, such as a relative, it may be best to deal with that person in an open and direct manner to correct the uncomfortable situation.

Medical Problems

The breast-feeding mother who has a serious medical condition or who suddenly develops a condition that requires hospitalization or management with surgery presents an unusual situation. It is obvious that the medical condition must be addressed promptly; however, it is also important to treat the mother as a lactating woman. Questions must be answered such as whether or not the condition is life-threatening or contagious and will the drugs necessary for treatment pass into the breast milk and adversely affect the infant? The other questions that must be taken into consideration are what is the prognosis for recovery and how long will recovery take. When the prognosis is poor and drugs prescribed for the mother are contraindicated in the infant, the decision must be made to discontinue breast-feeding. However, abrupt cessation of breast-feeding can cause a an influenza-like syndrome in the mother that may confuse the medical picture (Lawrence, 1999).

Nutrition and Fluid Intake

Breast-feeding mothers will need approximately an additional 500 cal/d compared with mothers feeding their infants artificial formula (Figure 30-9). Approximately 2,500 cal/d are needed while lactating. This calorie intake can be met through a properly balanced diet. A daily increase in some food groups, such as meat and dairy products, is of great importance. A daily increase in fluids, calcium, protein, and folic acid also is essential. A proper diet promotes a good supply of milk and good maternal health.

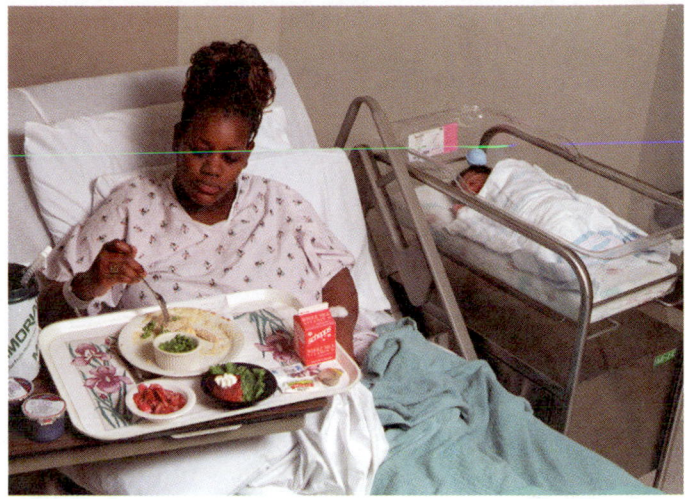

Figure 30-9 Breast-feeding mothers need an additional 500 cal/d.

Prenatal vitamins also may be continued. Fluid requirements can be met by drinking at least six 8-oz glasses of water or caffeine-free drinks every day (Figure 30-10). Increasing fluid intake above normal levels, however, will not increase the milk supply (Reifsnider & Gill, 2000).

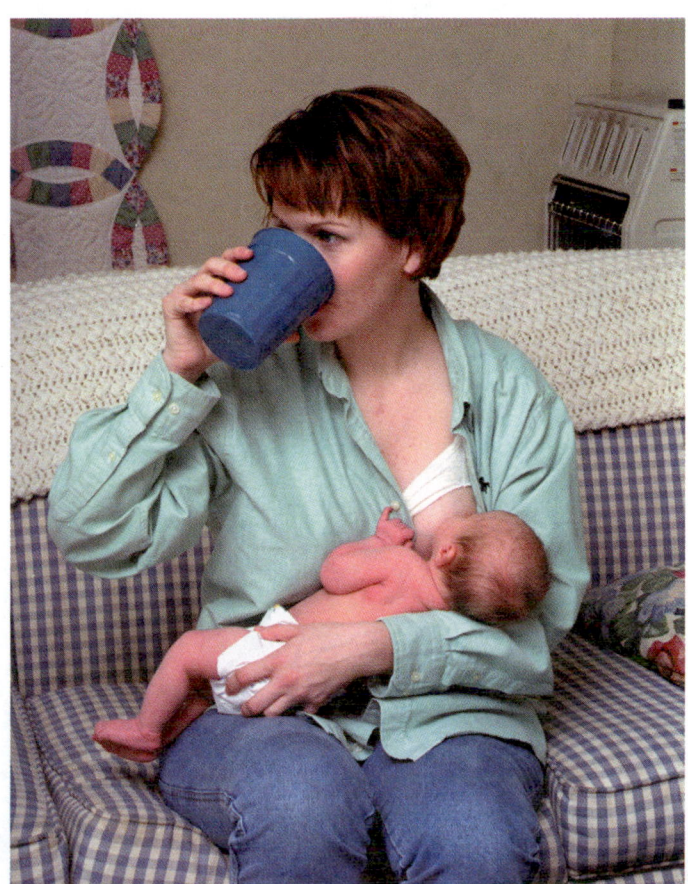

Figure 30-10 Increased fluid intake is especially important for the breast-feeding woman.

REFLECTIONS FROM A FATHER

"My wife breast-fed all three of our children. I enjoyed watching her develop a close bond with each child as they nursed. I admit that sometimes, as a new dad, I felt left out. So we decided that my role was to burp the baby during and after each feeding. I loved this! Feedings became a family event, each of us with our own important role to play."

Mechanics of Lactation

The nurse working with the breast-feeding mother must be knowledgeable about the basic anatomy and physiology of breast-feeding, know how to assist the new mother with early feedings, and help with interventions for common problems. Although breast-feeding is a natural process, breast-feeding skills must be learned and practiced. It may help to tell the new mother that she and her infant are both learning new skills. The nurse can promote successful breast-feeding through timely interventions to correct any problems before they undermine the mother's confidence in her ability to feed her baby.

Maternal

The nurse should help a new mother initiate breast-feeding without making her feel like a failure for not knowing these skills. The mother needs to find a comfortable position before beginning so that she can relax. She will enjoy breast-feeding much more and experience the let-down reflex more easily when comfortable. Next, she must position her infant so that she and her infant are comfortable and the breast is supported. She needs to cup her breast in one hand with all four fingers underneath and the thumb on top, making sure that the fingers and thumb are not touching the areola, while supporting the baby's head with the other hand (Figure 30-11).

When the mother touches the baby's lips with her nipple she will activate the rooting reflex in her baby, and the infant will open the mouth wide (Figure 30-12a). The mother can pull the baby's head to her breast, and the infant will latch on to the nipple (Figure 30-12b). Correct latching-on will occur when the nipple and most of the areola are in the baby's mouth, and the baby's lips are pursed out as opposed to tucked under, forming solid suction. The sucking may cause discomfort for the first few

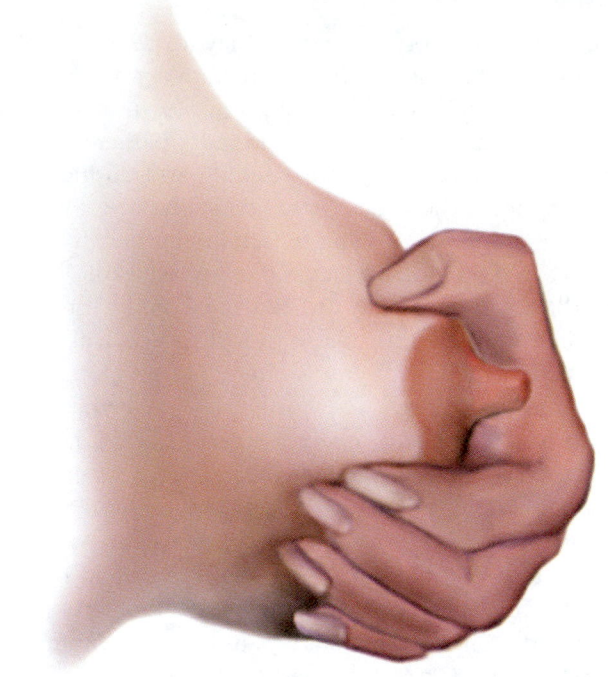

A.

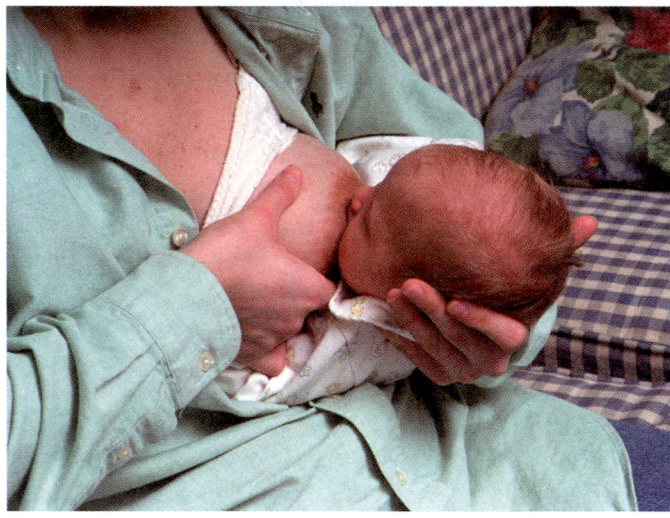

B.

Figure 30-11 C-hold technique. A. Hand placement. B. Position of infant.

seconds; however, the discomfort will stop when the baby settles into a rhythmic sucking pattern (Methodist Hospital, 1999).

Research suggests that nipple soreness is not related to the length of time the infant is at the breast but to improper positioning or improper removal of the infant from the breast (Mohrbacher & Stock, 1997). Inserting a finger into the corner of the sucking infant's mouth to break the suction will facilitate removing the infant without damage to the nipple (Figure 30-13).

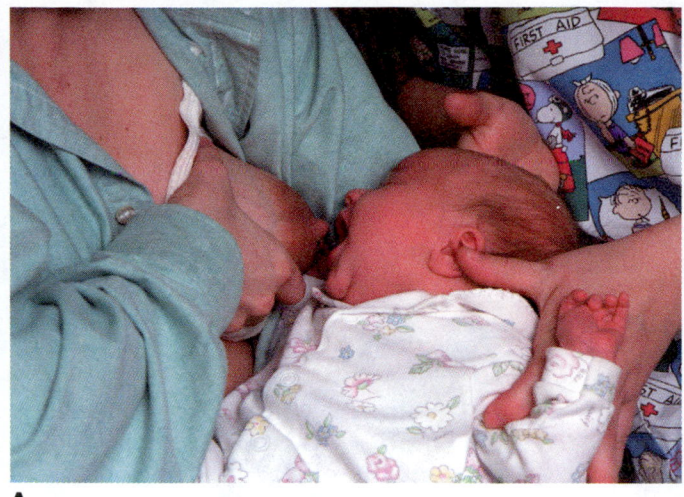

A.

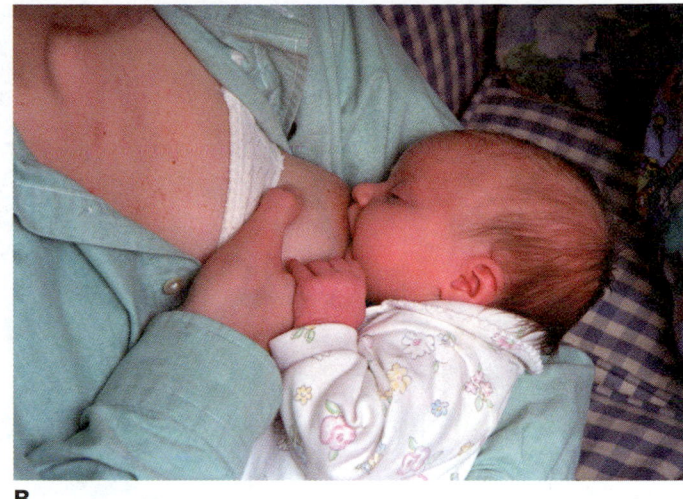

B.

Figure 30-12 Initiating latch-on. A. Touching the baby's lips with the nipple stimulates the rooting reflex. B. Once the baby opens the mouth wide, the mother can pull the baby's head to her breast.

After removing the infant from the breast, the mother needs to be taught how the infant may be burped in any one of three positions (Figure 30-14). Burping will allow any swallowed air to be released from the infant's stomach. The mother should position the infant upright, with the head resting on the mother's shoulder. The mother can then rub or pat the infant's back with her hand, while supporting the infant's buttocks with her other hand. A mother may prefer to burp the infant by placing the infant face down across the mother's lap. While holding the infant's head with one hand, the mother can rub or pat the infant's back with the other. An infant also may be burped by holding the infant upright on the mother's lap, supporting the head from the front with one hand and patting or rubbing the back with the other.

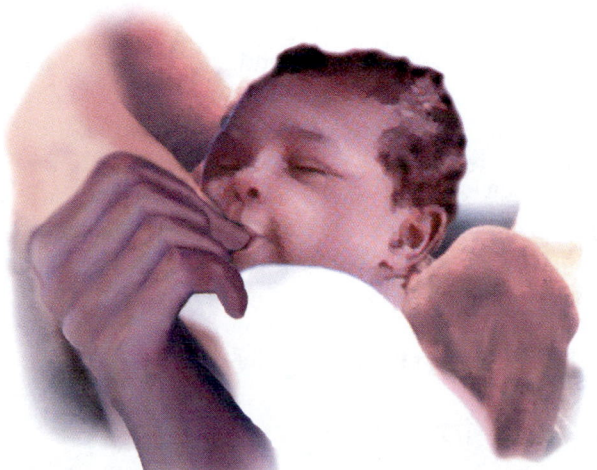

Figure 30-13 Removing the infant from the breast.

Infant

In order to determine if the neonate is ready to be breast-fed, the nurse or mother can test the rooting and sucking reflexes (Figure 30-15). Stimulation of the rooting reflex can be accomplished by stroking the infant's cheek toward the lips. The infant should turn toward the side that is being stroked. The mother can insert her finger into the infant's mouth and gently stroke the soft palate to trigger the sucking reflex. Sucking should be strong, and the tongue should curve around the finger. When the infant sucks strongly on the mother's finger, breast-feeding can begin. Researchers such as Smith et al. (1988) have used ultrasound studies to observe the dynamics of breast sucking. These studies have confirmed that sucking patterns differ in bottle-fed versus breast-fed infants. The tongue presses the nipple against the hard palate, forcing milk from the ducts and sinuses (Figure 30-16).

Latching-on

The nurse can help the new mother by teaching her to position her infant's nose at the level of her own nipple and then to brush the nipple across the baby's lower lip. Doing so will cause the infant to open the mouth wide (**rooting reflex**), allowing the mother to bring her nipple in toward the upper part of the infant's mouth. The rooting reflex is the normal response of the newborn to move toward whatever touches the area around the mouth. The rooting reflex facilitates proper **latching-on** (proper attachment of the infant to the breast for feeding) to the entire areola, not just the end of the nipple. Riordan and Auerbach (1993) state that for early feedings both breasts should be offered at each feeding to stimulate milk production quickly. Each

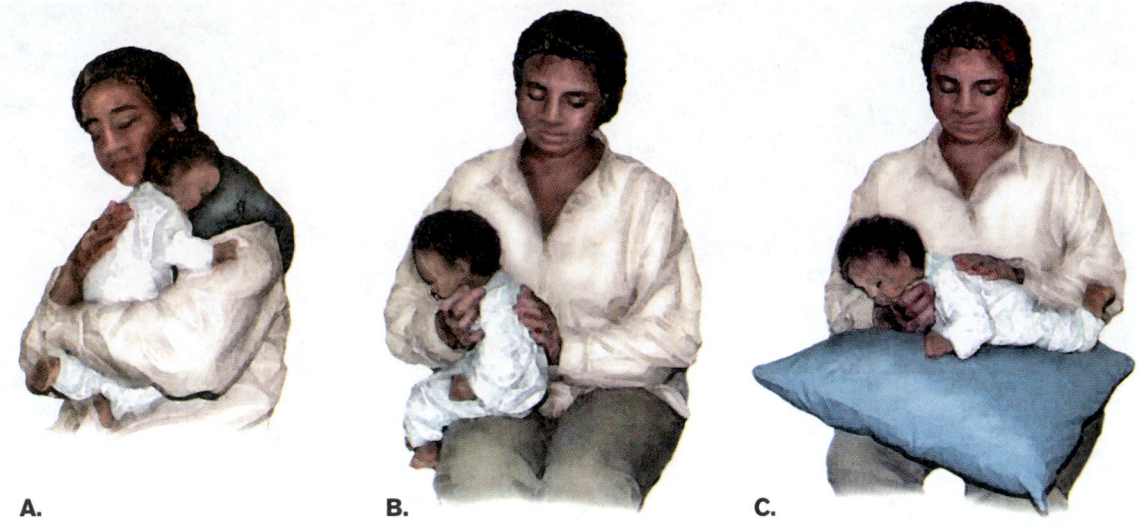

Figure 30-14 Burping positions. A. Supported on the shoulder. B. Upright on the lap. C. Face down across the lap.

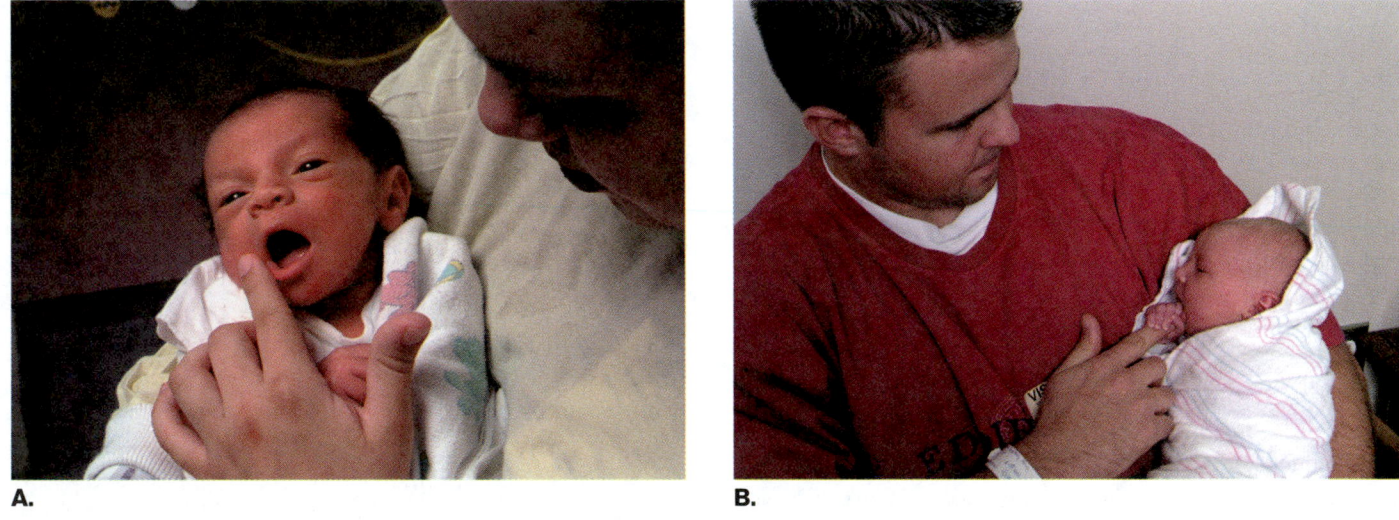

A.

B.

Figure 30-15 Judging readiness to nurse. A. Stroking the cheek next to the baby's mouth elicits the rooting reflex. B. This newborn is attempting to suck on her father's finger.

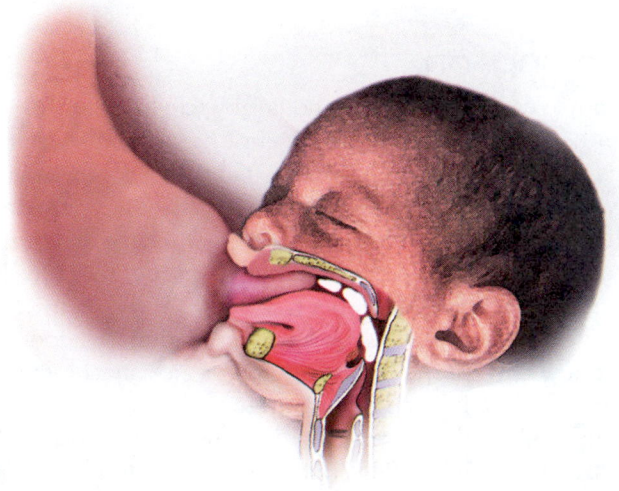

Figure 30-16 Proper positioning for successful latch-on.

breast should be offered frequently for at least 15 minutes every 2 hours or on demand, whichever occurs first. After breast-feeding is established the client should let the infant complete a feeding on one breast before offering the other. As milk volume adjusts to the infant's needs this pattern may change, depending on the infant's requirements during growth spurts. Frequently, mothers will report feeling very relaxed, almost sleepy, during breast-feeding. This relaxed state is a side benefit of the hormone oxytocin, which also stimulates the let-down reflex.

Nursing Implications

Most mothers who are breast-feeding for the first time have a possible nursing diagnosis of ineffective breast-feeding related to deficient knowledge about breast-feeding. The

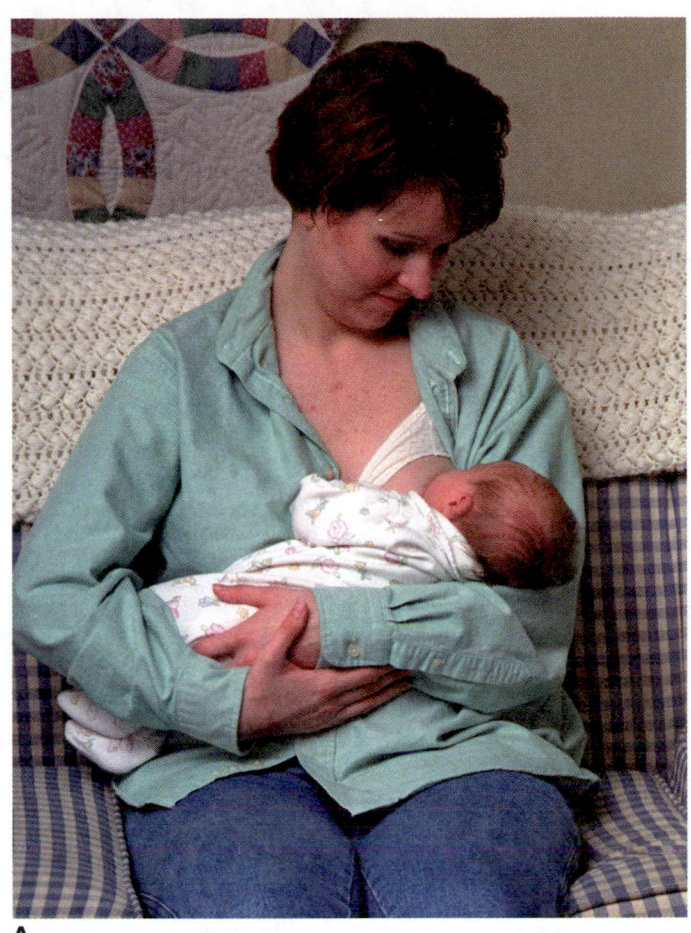

A.

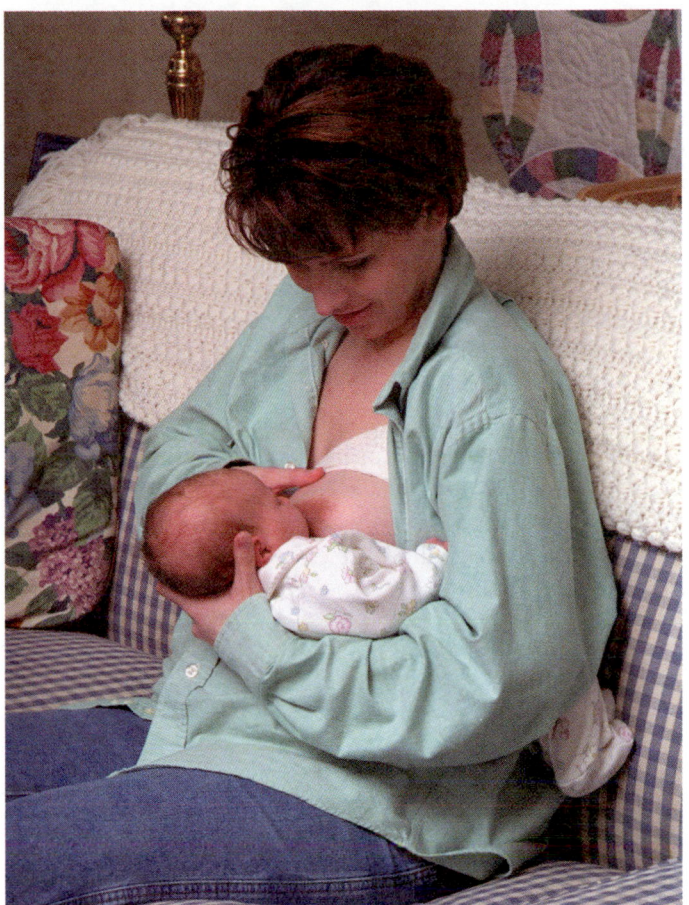

B.

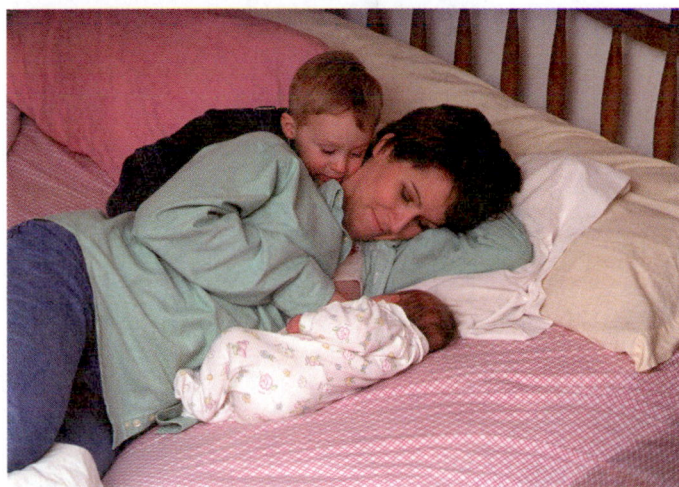

C.

Figure 30-17 Breast-feeding holds. A. Cradle hold.
B. Football hold. C. Side-lying hold.

nurse can take advantage of the opportunities to teach the new mother during the postpartal stay. For the healthy full-term newborn, no contraindications exist to feeding immediately after delivery. Most infants are highly responsive and eager to suck during the first 30 minutes after delivery. The nurse can use this time to teach and help initiate successful breast-feeding behaviors.

When working with a new mother, the nurse should always stay at her eye level to decrease the anxiety that any new activity causes the learner. Proper positioning at the breast can decrease the problem of ineffective breast-feeding by teaching the mother different comfortable positions that enhance feeding behaviors. The mother should be made as comfortable as possible either in her bed or chair and given as much privacy as needed. Mothers who have delivered by cesarean section usually need more help to find a comfortable position because of the abdominal incision and the pain related to movement. The woman may need to void before beginning to breast-feed, and she should be instructed to wash her hands each time she nurses her infant.

There are three common breast-feeding positions that can be used by most mothers. These positions are the cradle hold, the football hold, and the side-lying position (Figure 30-17).

ISSUES RELATED TO BREAST-FEEDING

According to the American Academy of Pediatrics policy statement (1997, pp. 1035–1039), "Extensive research, especially in recent years, documents diverse and compelling advantages to infants, mothers, families, and society from breastfeeding and the use of human milk for infant feeding. These include health, nutritional, immunologic, developmental, psychological, social, economic, and environmental benefits."

Benefits

The benefits of breast-feeding include but are not limited to superior species-specific feeding that provides optimum infant growth, health, and development. Breast milk also has been shown to decrease the incidence and severity of many childhood illnesses, provide a protective effect against several diseases, and enhance cognitive development. A number of research studies indicate there are health benefits for mothers who breast-feed. In addition to these individual benefits, breast-feeding provides significant social and economic benefits to the nation. These include reduced health care costs and reduced employee absenteeism (American Academy of Pediatrics, 1997).

Maternal Benefits

Maternal benefits include lactational amenorrhea, which promotes a longer period of decreased fertility after the birth of an infant, and less blood loss from menstruation. New research demonstrates that lactating women have an earlier return to prepregnant weight, improved bone remineralization, reduction in hip fractures in the postmenopausal period, and reduced rates of ovarian cancer and premenopausal breast cancer (American Academy of Pediatrics, 1997).

Promotion of Involution

Breast-feeding has many benefits for the mother. The release of oxytocin during breast-feeding causes the uterus to contract, hastening the involution of the uterus to its prepregnant state (Figure 30-18). This same action also reduces the chances of postpartal hemorrhage by keeping the uterus contracted.

Assistance in Weight Control

Breast-feeding promotes weight loss after delivery because of the great expenditure of energy and calories needed during lactation. The nursing mother should increase her caloric intake by 200 cal over the pregnancy requirements. This increase in calories results in a 500-cal increase from her prepregnancy requirements. An intake of 2,500 to 2,700 cal/d is required for most women during lactation (Dewey, 1993).

Psychologic Benefits

Breast-feeding also provides new mothers with many psychosocial advantages. The increased levels of oxytocin in

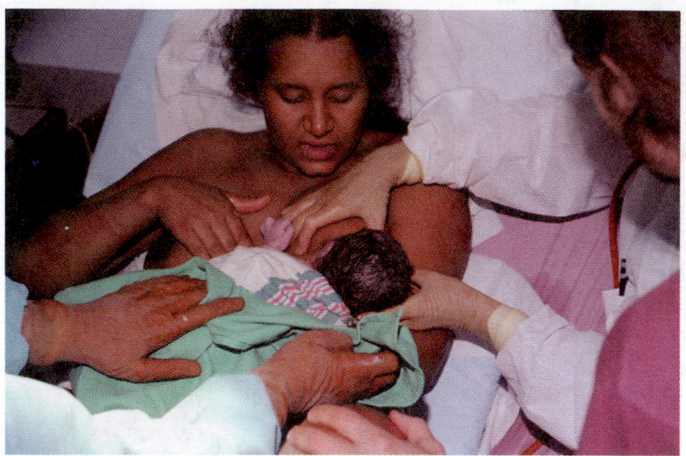

Figure 30-18 Breast-feeding immediately after delivery stimulates involution of the uterus.

the nursing mother's bloodstream are believed to coincide with more even mood responses and increased feelings of maternal well-being (Lawrence, 1999). Many researchers believe that increased levels of oxytocin promote maternal-infant bonding and protective behavior. Many animal and human studies have provided documentation for this belief. One study in female rats demonstrated increased maternal behaviors after oxytocin administration (Pedersen, 1992). Breast-feeding enhances attachment by providing many opportunities for direct skin contact, eye contact, and closeness between mother and baby. This increased time of closeness helps mothers learn their infant's cues and needs and also helps the new mother to slow down and relax during feedings. Many lactation consultants will attest to the fact that as the mother's milk "lets down," many times the mother will close her eyes and almost fall asleep. Successfully breast-feeding also will increase the new mother's sense of accomplishment and self-esteem as she sees her infant being nourished and comforted by breast-feeding (Lawrence, 1999). Many women have reported that this contact has long-lasting, positive results on her feelings as a competent and powerful woman.

Many researchers have looked at the relationship between postpartum depression and the infant feeding method. Mothers with depression had more problems breast-feeding and tended to think that the infant did not want their milk or did not like it (Riordan & Auerbach, 1999).

Several authors, including Klaus et al. (1995) have cited a calming effect on mothers during breast-feeding as a positive outcome of breast-feeding behavior. These authors hypothesize that a cascade of interactions between the mother and baby occurs with early skin-to-skin contact, suckling, rooming-in, and increased maternal oxytocin levels. Manipulation of estrogen, progesterone, and prolactin has been studied to detect maternal behavior enhancement or inhibition by each. Klaus et al. (1995) have stated that early and continuous mother-infant contact appears to decrease infant abandonment and increase the length and success of breast-feeding. The long-term psychophysiologic response of unrestricted nursing is a more even mood cycle compared with the mood swings associated with the menstrual cycle. The long-term benefit of amenorrhea for as long as the woman continues breast-feeding is one of the more desirable effects of breast-feeding.

Contraceptive Benefits

Exclusive breast-feeding has been found to delay ovulation and thus acts as a natural birth control method. Breast-feeding makes a women less likely to conceive; however, the degree of protection depends on many variables, such as hormonal levels, nipple stimulation, and frequency of feedings. After delivery, levels of progesterone and estrogen decrease, allowing the gradual return of secretion of luteinizing hormone and follicle-stimulating hormone. Ovulation and a return to fertility typically will occur within 4 to 6 weeks in the nonnursing mother. Breast-feeding extends the normal period of anovulation by sending impulses to the hypothalamus that decrease the release of gonadotropins. Decreasing gonadotropin levels suppress ovulation by preventing follicle development. Prolactin also plays a direct role in preventing ovulation by making the ovaries less responsive to luteinizing hormone and by suppressing the effects of estrogen (Lawrence, 1999). Lactational amenorrhea is regarded as a period of natural infertility after childbirth and during lactation.

The Lactional Amenorrhea Method (LAM) of family planning is based on the principle that a "woman who continues to fully or nearly fully breastfeed her infant and who remains amenorrheic during the first 6 months postpartum is protected from pregnancy during that time" (Perrez, Labbok, & Keenan, 1992, p. 968). LAM allows clients to take advantage of the natural decrease in fertility provided by breast-feeding. The woman who desires the use of this method of contraception needs to continue to fully or nearly fully breast-feed her infant, must remain amenorrheic, and must be feeding frequently (including during the night) for the method to work (Lawrence, 1999).

Long-term Benefits

Research studies also have found a link between breast-feeding and a decrease in the development of breast cancer in women who have breast-fed. Newcombe et al. (1994) state that there clearly is a protective effect of lactation on the development of breast cancer among premenopausal women. In another study of 521 Asian women, breast-feeding was found to play a protective role

against breast cancer, regardless of confounding effects of age at first pregnancy, parity, and closely related factors (Yoo, Tajima, & Kuroishi, 1992).

According to a report recently issued by the Society of Gynecologic Oncologists, National Cancer Institute, and Office on Women's Health of the U.S. Department of Health and Human Services, ovarian cancer rates have remained the same for almost 50 years. However, the good news is that women who have breast-fed have a 50% decreased risk for developing ovarian cancer (O'Brien, 1998).

Cost Savings

Breast-feeding saves money for families, taxpayers, and the health care system. Infant formula is expensive. The cost of formula is about twice that of the extra food needed by the lactating mother (Jarosz, 1993.) Providing formula to women who are not breast-feeding costs the WIC program, and thus the U.S. taxpayers, a large amount of money every year. WIC is the largest purchaser of infant formula, buying 40% of all formula sold in the United States. In 1991, the cost of formula given to WIC participants for free was $404 million (Riordan, 1997) (Table 30-1). There are some costs to the family associated with breast-feeding. A breast pump is needed, as are plastic bags and bottles for milk storage.

Riordan (1997) suggests that if breast-feeding were universal, 5,000 lives would be saved in the United States annually. The financial implications are staggering. The costs of increased morbidity and mortality include medical costs, physician visits, medicine, and hospitalizations. The hidden costs associated with these problems are lost wages to parents of sick children and increased premiums for health care insurance. The savings associated with reducing the number of otitis media infections in children is estimated at $660 million in the United States alone. Table 30-2 examines additional health care costs for four medical conditions frequently seen in infants.

Table 30-1 Hidden Costs of not Breast-feeding

Decreased intellectual development	Incalculable
Infant formula distributed by the Women, Infants, and Children (WIC) program annually	$2,665,715
Increased parental absenteeism	Incalculable
Increased potential for additional pregnancies	Incalculable
Prenatal and postnatal care for increased pregnancies	Incalculable

Adapted from Riordan, J. (1997). The cost of not breastfeeding: A commentary. *Journal of Human Lactation, 13*, (2), 93–97.

Table 30-2 Additional U.S. Health Care Costs for Four Medical Conditions Owing to not Breast-feeding

Condition	Annual Health Care Costs
Infant diarrhea	$291.3 million
Respiratory syncytial virus	$225 million
Insulin-dependent diabetes mellitus	$9.6–124.8 million
Otitis media	$660 million
Total costs	>$1 billion

Adapted from Riordan, J. (1997). The cost of not breastfeeding: A commentary. *Journal of Human Lactation, 13,* (2), 93–97.

Maternal-Infant Attachment

Breast-feeding provides ideal opportunities for mother-infant interactions, which include closeness, touching, holding, talking, mutual gazing, and reciprocal socialization. Attachment is the development of an enduring relationship between the infant and the caregiver (Klaus, Kennell, & Klaus, 1995). Breast-feeding increases the quantity and quality of early contact between the mother and her infant, thus enhancing the strength of the relationship. Studies on the psychologic benefits to the infant suggest that breast-feeding may increase the emotional union between mother and infant. Widstrom et al. (1990) measured the psychophysiologic responses of mothers who were breast-feeding or bottle-feeding to their infants' signals. Mothers who were breast-feeding were physiologically more relaxed, were more likely to interact with their infants, and expressed greater satisfaction with the feeding experience.

Benefits to the Infant

Breast milk has been called the perfect food for infants because it contains all necessary nutrients in readily bioavailable forms, while providing many immunologic components at the same time. Human milk is considered a living tissue, such as blood, and is capable of affecting biochemical systems, increasing immunity, and even destroying pathogens (Newman, 1995). The main selling point for manufacturers of infant formula continues to be the comparison of how closely the product conforms to the gold standard of breast milk.

Nutritional Benefits

Breast-feeding provides infants many nutritional benefits. Breast milk supplies all the nutrients, vitamins, and minerals needed by the infant until 6 months of age. Breast milk is nonallergenic, and its composition varies according to the age and needs of each infant. Mothers of infants born preterm make milk that is higher in fat because the pre-

Critical Thinking

Comparison of Breast Milk with Formula

- Breast milk is nutritionally superior to formula.
- Breast milk contains immunoglobulins, enzymes, and leukocytes to protect against infection.
- Breast milk is less expensive than formula.
- Breast milk is easily available at a perfect temperature and with no preparation.
- Breast milk may reduce allergies.
- Breast-feeding may enhance mother-infant attachment.
- Breast-feeding promotes the development of jaw and facial muscles.
- Breast milk reduces the risk of bacterial contamination.

How can a nurse help promote breast-feeding as a superior feeding method among all women of childbearing age?

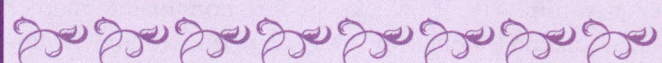

term infant needs more fat content for myelination of the neurons of the undeveloped neurologic system.

Components of Breast Milk. Breast milk is composed of lactose, lipids, polyunsaturated fatty acids, and amino acids, such as taurine, and has a whey-to-casein ratio that facilitates digestion, absorption, and full use when compared with formulas (Worthington-Roberts & Williams, 1993). Research also suggests that the high levels of cholesterol may trigger the production of specific enzymes that may reduce the harmful effects of cholesterol on the cardiovascular system (Worthington-Roberts & Williams, 1993). Breast milk provides infants with minerals in more appropriate amounts than do formulas. The iron in breast milk, although much lower in concentration, is more readily digestible and more fully absorbed than that found in formulas. The iron in breast milk is sufficient to supply the infant's needs for the first 4 to 6 months of life. Giving an infant iron supplements during this period can actually decrease the ability of lactoferrin to enhance iron absorption and protect against infection. According to the American Academy of Pediatrics Committee on Nutrition (1992), the only supplements a breast-fed baby will need are vitamin D and fluoride beginning at 6 months of age.

The caloric needs of the newborn range from 105 to 110 cal/d per kilogram of body weight, or 50 to 55 cal/d per pound, and are divided among protein, carbohydrates, and fat. Water requirements are high (140 to 160 mL/d per

Research Highlight

Does Breast-feeding Protect Against Diabetes Mellitus?

Purpose

To note a link between infant feeding method and insulin-dependent diabetes mellitus.

Methods

While many advocates of breast-feeding can and do correctly cite studies indicating that breast-feeding reduces children's risk of developing insulin-dependent diabetes mellitus (IDDM), many are not aware of the ongoing debate among researchers on this issue. The first report associating breast-feeding with a reduction in risk for juvenile onset IDDM was published in 1984 by Borch-Johnson et al. This study observed that Norwegian children born during the years when breast-feeding rates were high were less likely to develop IDDM than were children born in years of low breast-feeding rates. Since that time, more than 90 articles have been published in this area, some supporting and some refuting this association.

Findings

Most of the studies were case-controlled studies, in which characteristics of children with IDDM were compared with those of healthy children. Many of these studies indicated that children with IDDM were breast-fed for a shorter duration or were exposed to cow's milk proteins earlier than were healthy children. These relationships remained statistically significant after controlling for confounding factors such as maternal age and education. However, other studies found no association (Meloni et al., 1997).

Nursing Implications

Findings indicate that scientific truths are not validated overnight but are a result of an evolutionary process. You must be prepared to critically evaluate all studies, even when they do not support your point of view. Staying current with the latest research increases your credibility, promotes communication with professional colleagues, and increases your knowledge of breast-feeding.

Heinig, M. J. (1997). Staying abreast of the latest scientific controversies: Infant feeding and insulin-dependent diabetes mellitus. *Journal of Human Lactation, 13,* (2), 91–92.

---

kilogram of body weight, or 64 to 73 mL/d per pound). Fluid needs also increase during illness and hot weather (Worthington-Roberts & Williams, 1993). The protein requirement per unit of body weight is greater in the newborn than at any other time of life. The recommended daily allowance (RDA) for protein during the first 6 months is 2.2 g per kilogram of body weight. Carbohydrates should provide at least 40% of the total calories in the newborn's diet. At least 15% of the newborn's calories should be provided by fat (triglycerides). The fat in human milk is easier to digest and absorb than is that in cow's milk (Behrman, Kliegman, & Arvin, 1996).

Natural Variation in Composition of Human Milk. Over 200 constituents have been identified in breast milk, and researchers are just beginning to understand the

impact that these changing constituents have on the infant. Moreover, milk composition changes as the infant nurses at each feeding.

Formula-fed infants gain weight faster than do breast-fed infants because larger quantities of food are needed to obtain the same nutrients. The nutrients in breast milk are more easily obtained because breast milk is completely digested. Bottle-fed infants usually regain their birth weights within 10 days. Breast-fed infants may not regain their birth weights until 14 days after birth. Formula-fed infants generally double their birth weight by 4 months, and breast-fed babies double their weight at about 5 months (Lawrence, 1999).

Transitional milk is produced at the end of colostrum production and immediately before mature milk comes into the breast. **Foremilk** is the thin, watery breast milk secreted at the beginning of a feeding. Foremilk is low in calories but high in water-soluble vitamins. **Hindmilk** is the thick, high-fat breast milk secreted at the end of a feeding. Hindmilk is ejected approximately 10 to 15 minutes after the initial "let down" and has the highest concentratation of calories. Hindmilk is thicker and richer in appearance than is foremilk owing to its higher fat content essential for the infant's proper growth and development. **Mature milk** is breast milk that contains 10% solids for energy and growth.

The nutritional needs of the infant vary with the unique differences of each stage of the new baby's development. Breast milk supplies all of the nutrients to meet the ever-changing demands of the baby from newborn to toddler stage. The infant's diet must provide adequate calories and must include sufficient protein, carbohydrates, fat, water, vitamins, and minerals to meet the rapid rate of both physical and mental growth and development (Lawrence, 1999).

Long-Term Benefits

Epidemiologic research shows that human milk may provide a possible protective effect against sudden infant death syndrome (SIDS), insulin-dependent diabetes mellitus, lymphoma, Crohn's disease, ulcerative colitis, allergic diseases, and other chronic digestive diseases. Breast-feeding also has been related to enhancement of intelligence and visual acuity (American Academy of Pediatrics, 1997).

Immunologic Benefits

The immunologic benefits of breast-feeding for infants include varying degrees of protection against many types of infections. Breast-feeding has a positive effect on the overall health of the infant because it provides increased protection from meningitis, sepsis, otitis media, and respiratory and gastrointestinal (GI) diseases. For years, physicians have believed that infants who are breast-fed contract fewer infections than do those who receive formula because breast milk contains no bacteria. Research has now demonstrated that human milk actively helps newborns avoid disease in a variety of ways. These benefits are due to the many components of colostrum and breast milk present in varying amounts, depending on the specific environment of the mother-baby dyad. Colostrum is the thin fluid present in the breast from pregnancy into the early pospartal period. Colostrum is rich in antibodies, which provide protection from many diseases; high in protein, which binds bilirubin; and acts as a laxative, speeding the elimination of meconium and helping loosen mucus.

Breast-feeding helps protect the infant by maximizing the baby's defenses against the contaminated environment outside of the uterus. Newborns do not have adequate levels of immunity to protect themselves against infection by pathogens of all types.

Newborns have a deficiency of neutrophils, which are necessary in the early phagocytic response to injury. Deficiencies of specific immunoglobulins also predispose newborns to infection, particularly in the first 4 to 6 weeks of life. The infant receives passive immunity to bacterial toxins from the placenta through immunoglobulin E (IgE). Immunity against common viral infections, such as measles, may last 4 to 8 months; whereas immunity to certain bacteria may last only 4 to 8 weeks. The newborn is normally deficient in immunoglobulins M (IgM) and A (IgA). These immunoglobulins are thought to protect against gram-negative entero-organisms and some viruses and to supply protection on the secretory surfaces of the respiratory, urinary, and GI tracts (Newman, 1995). These immunoglobulins are found in human milk and are transferred to the newborn during breast-feeding. Cells contained in human milk include macrophages, polymorphonuclear leukocytes, lymphocytes (T- and B-), neutrophils, and epithelial cells.

The intestinal flora of the breast-fed newborn is strikingly different from that of the formula-fed infant. Researchers have shown that colostrum and human milk contain a specific factor called bifidus factor that supports the growth of *Lactobacillus bifidum*. The presence of this type of bacillus offers protection against many intestinal disorders, such as diarrhea and necrotizing enterocolitis (NEC). NEC is generally associated with gram-negative organisms, especially *Klebsiella*. According to Lawrence (1999), colonization of breast-fed infants with *Klebsiella* does not occur. Breast-feeding protects against infection through the provision of host resistance factors in human milk, including immunoglobulins, lactoferrin, bifidus factor, and lymphocytes. Exclusive breast-feeding also reduces the likelihood of exposure to infection that arises when contaminated food is introduced (Kovar, Serdula, Marks, & Fraser, 1984) (Table 30-3).

Breast milk has been shown to combat many types of infections, such as cholera and salmonella, staphylococcal, and viral infections. Lipase found in human milk has been found to inactivate protozoans that also may cause many disease processes. Human milk also protects against intestinal and respiratory pathogens without causing inflammation. The antiallergic properties of human milk have been studied in an attempt to discover how antibodies are formed by the infant's immune system (Lawrence, 1999).

Immediate Protection against Environmental Infectious Agents. The collection of antibodies transmitted to the infant is highly targeted against pathogens in the child's immediate surroundings. The mother synthesizes specific antibodies when she inhales or ingests an environmental disease-causing agent. The antibody she produces is specific to that agent and binds to a single protein or antigen present in the infant's immediate environment,

Table 30-3 Immune Benefits of Breast Milk

Leukocytes	Benefits
Neutrophils	May act as phagocytes by ingesting bacteria
Macrophages	Kill microbes in infant's intestinal tract
B lymphocytes	Produce antibodies against specific microbes
T lymphocytes	Kill infected cells directly and strengthen immune response

Molecules	Benefits
Bifidus factor	Promotes growth of harmless bacteria to stop growth of harmful bacteria
Antibodies secretory immunoglobulin A	Bind microbes in gut to prevent passage into other tissues
Firbronectin	Assists macrophages and repairs damaged tissues in gut
B_{12} binding protein	Reduces bacteria by decreasing vitamin B_{12}
Fatty acids	Destroy virus membranes
Interferon gamma	Promotes antimicrobial activity of immune cells
Hormones and growth factors	Enhance maturity of infant's digestive tract
Lysozyme	Kills bacteria by attacking cell wall
Lactoferrin	Reduces available iron, thus reducing growth of bacteria
Oligosaccharides	Bind to microorganisms before they can attach to mucosa surfaces
Mucins	Interfere with attachment of bacteria and viruses to mucosal surfaces

Source: Adapted from: Newman, J. (1995). How breast milk protects newborns. *Scientific American*, 76–79.

thus protecting the infant against those specific infectious agents most likely to cause illness (Newman, 1995). Therefore, if an older sibling develops an upper respiratory infection, the mother will make antibodies to protect her new infant against the specific bacteria or virus causing the infection. Secretory IgA has antiviral, antibacterial, and antigenic-inhibiting factors. Secretory IgA decreases the permeability of the intestines to macromolecules that cause disease. Many other components of breast milk inhibit the growth of both bacteria and viruses. Lactoferrin, *L. bifudum*, lysozymes, and many other immunoglobulins, such as one that acts against poliomyelitis, are present and offer immunity to various disease-producing substances.

Passive Immunity with Childhood Implications. Human milk is a biochemically unique substance perfectly adapted to each individual infant's needs. The

Nursing Alert

ASSISTING WITH BREAST-FEEDING
When teaching clients about breast-feeding, you should wear disposable gloves while:

- Assisting new mothers to breast-feed immediately after delivery.
- Handling the mother's breasts during expression of milk.
- Handling breast pads.
- Handling breast milk for storage or milk banking.

You must wash your hands before and after gloving!

breast milk that is made by each mother is individually suited to meet the needs of her infant. Mortality rates of breast-fed infants clearly are lower in all studies and countries than are the rates of formula-fed infants. Mortality rates are lower at all ages for breast-fed infants. The incidence of illness (morbidity) in artificially fed infants, particularly in Third World countries, is equally impressive. Formula-fed infants have a 50% greater chance of becoming sick enough to require hospitalization than do breast-fed infants. Breast milk provides immunologic protection against death from infectious diseases, such as diarrhea, respiratory infections, otitis media, and pneumonia. Breast milk also offers some protection against allergies and SIDS.

Sudden infant death syndrome is the leading cause of death in infants after 1 month of age. A 3-year multicenter study of SIDS in New Zealand reported on in 1993 found four modifiable risk factors: sleeping prone, maternal smoking, lack of breast-feeding, and the infant sharing a bed. New Zealand launched a major prevention program to educate the public about these risk factors (Scragg, Mitchell, & Tonkin, 1993).

Psychologic Benefits

The psychosocial benefits of breast-feeding have been studied by many researchers. Maternal-infant attachment appears to be enhanced owing to the close skin-to-skin contact that occurs during breast-feeding behavior. The newborn's sense of touch is highly developed at birth, and the tactile stimulation of breast-feeding contributes to the infant's sense of closeness and comfort.

BARRIERS TO LACTATION

Barriers or deterrents to breast-feeding may be biologic, psychologic, or social in nature. The risk-to-benefit ratio of breast-feeding compared with bottle-feeding must be

Research Highlight

Breast Milk and Subsequent Intelligence Quotient in Children Born Preterm

Purpose

To determine whether nutrition in early life has a long-term influence on neurodevelopment.

Methods

Babies under 1,850 g at birth admitted to the special-care baby units at five hospitals in England were entered into four parallel trials of preterm infant feeding. Mothers chose whether or not to provide breast milk for their infant within 72 hours of delivery. The researchers collected information about family structure, social class, mother's education, pregnancy, labor, delivery, and the neonatal period. Intelligent quotient (IQ) was assessed with the Wechsler Intelligence Scale for Children. Testing was done at 18 months and at 7.5 to 8 years of age.

Findings

Children who had consumed mother's breast milk in the early weeks of life had as significantly higher IQ at 7.5 to 8 years than did those who received no maternal milk. An 8.3 point advantage (over half a standard deviation) in IQ remained even after adjustment for differences between groups in mothers' education and social class ($P < 0.0001$).

Nursing Implications

Findings indicate that the differences in IQ may be attributed to docosahexaenoic acid (DHA). DHA is the primary structural fatty acid of the gray matter of the brain and retina of the eye. It is a critical building block essential for normal brain and eye development. DHA is found naturally in breast milk but is not present in formula available in the United States, providing another excellent reason to promote breast-feeding among all women. This study also has implications for manufacturers to add DHA to their infant formula. Research studies comparing cognitive and physical development of breast-fed with bottle-fed children have revealed many interesting differences. More body activity, a more alert state, and a stronger arousal reaction in breast-fed newborns have been reported by researchers both in England and the United States. The longer the infant was nursed, the more profound the differences. In several studies using achievement tests to test IQ, children who were breast-fed for 4 to 6 months scored significantly higher than did children who were bottle-fed. It appears that there are specific proteins, amino acids, and fatty acids that contribute to enhanced brain development in the breast-fed infant (Lucas et al., 1992).

Lucas, A., Morley, R., Cole, T., Lister, G., & Leeson-Payne, C. (1992). Breast milk and subsequent intelligence quotient in children born preterm. *The Lancet, 339,* 261–264.

assessed by the woman and her health care provider to arrive at the best decision for both the mother and her infant.

Biologic Barriers

Although most women are physically capable of breast-feeding, a biologic problem may occasionally interfere with lactation. The problem can be due to abnormal anatomy such as unilateral or bilateral hypoplasia. Acquired abnormalities of the breasts from trauma, burns, or radiation also may interfere with lactation. Patients with biologic barriers must be carefully evaluated on a case-by-case basis to determine if lactation is possible.

Maternal Barriers

Maternal barriers to breast-feeding can be due to physical problems, medical or disease conditions, hormonal factors, or psychiatric disorders. Insufficient milk supply may be attributed to many factors, including insufficient glandular tissue, diet, illness, fatigue, psychologic factors, drugs, and smoking. When these factors have been ruled out, the cause may involve imbalances in hormone production or secretion. Low prolactin levels cause poor milk production, and low or inhibited oxytocin release causes a poor milk-ejection reflex (Bodley & Powers, 1999).

Psychiatric problems can interfere with lactation and rarely may require hospital admission. The incidence of psychiatric disorders increases dramatically in the postpartum period. Studies in postpartum women who were clinically depressed have revealed that two of three have major depression. Although breast-feeding mothers have been found to be more relaxed and have less mood swings, a mother experiencing depression may find breast-feeding difficult (Lawrence, 1999).

Maternal Breast Surgery

Augmentation mammoplasty has become an acceptable surgical procedure that can have implications for the breast-feeding mother. Breast-feeding can be successful when there is no destruction of breast tissue or interruption of ducts, nerve supply, or blood supply to the breast tissue or nipple. After extensive research the Food and Drug Administration (FDA) has concluded that it is not necessary to remove intact implants when a woman wishes to breast-feed.

Reduction mammoplasty is a surgical procedure to reduce the size of very large breasts. This type of surgery is more destructive to breast tissue than is augmentation because of the necessity of replacing the nipples symmetrically, which requires interruption of the milk ducts.

Breast surgery for nonmalignant tumors usually does not preclude breast-feeding unless the ductal structure has been interrupted. Women with a periareolar incision have a fivefold risk of lactation insufficiency (Lawrence, 1999).

Nipple Inversion

Flat or inverted nipples do not preclude breast-feeding and may respond to breast shells. Breast shells are vented plastic disks with holes in the center and a dome cover that allows the nipples to evert (Figure 30-19). The shell is slipped into the cup of a brassiere. The shells can be worn during the last trimester by women who choose to do so. However, research has shown no significant difference between groups of women who have used breast shells and groups who have used exercises that pull and stretch the nipple (Hoffman exercises) before delivery. Physicians caution women to avoid nipple stimulation because of the possibility of causing uterine contractions or preterm labor (Lawrence, 1999).

Nipple shields made of silicone are now frequently used to help women gradually pull out the inverted nip-

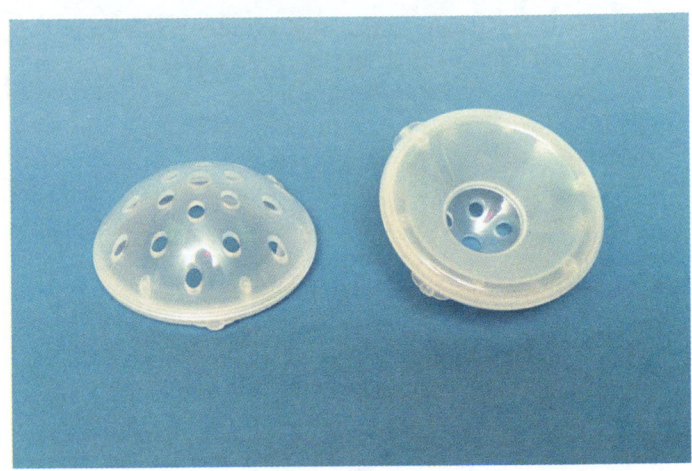

Figure 30-19 Breast shells.

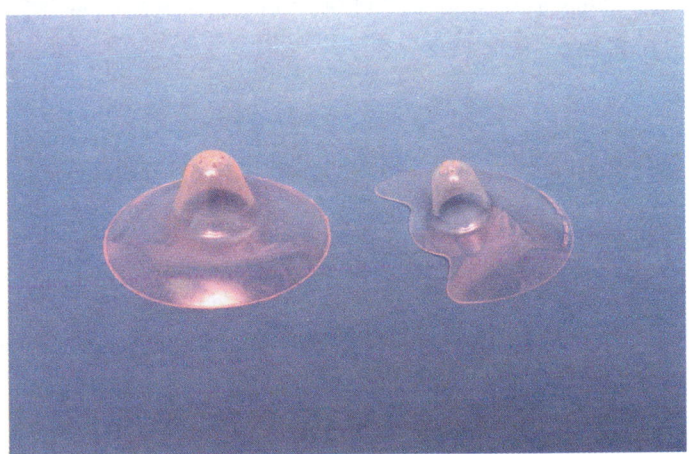

Figure 30-20 Nipple shields.

ples to allow the infant to latch on to a nipple that is more difficult to grasp (Figure 30-20). The mother is taught to pump her breasts after each nursing session to build up her milk supply while using the nipple shields. After the nipples are everted and the milk supply is built up the mother is encouraged to gradually wean the infant to the bare nipple (Martin, 2000).

Nipple Sensitivity

Most women will quickly adapt to the nursing experience naturally; however, often there may be nipple discomfort or pain during the initial breast-feeding sessions. Nipple sensitivity during breast-feeding is created by the negative pressure on the ductules within the breast, which are not yet filled with milk. The most common cause of nipple discomfort in the first few days is improper positioning. The nurse can help the mother to prevent discomfort by stressing proper positioning and making sure that the areola is grasped by the infant and not just the nipple. Occasionally the maternal tissues are unusually tender and delicate. Applying breast milk to the nipple at the end of the feeding and allowing it to dry is helpful to most mothers. Nipple shields, a device worn over the nipple and areola while the infant is sucking, do offer some protection to sensitive nipples. However, nipple shields should be used with caution because it is sometimes difficult to wean the infant back to the bare breast and the shields may decrease milk production (Riordan & Auerbach, 1999).

Hormonal Barriers

Confusion about the compatibility of contraceptives with breast-feeding may pose a barrier that influences the feeding decision for some women. Use of a contraceptive method in a breast-feeding mother is a particularly important decision, because ovulation may occur before the onset of menses and some methods may interfere with milk production. Nonhormonal methods, such as condoms, cervical caps, and diaphragms, can be effective in preventing pregnancy when used correctly and consistently. Spermicides may be used in the postpartum period; however, the medication may be transferred to the maternal blood, and minute amounts can be passed on in breast milk. No adverse effects have been observed in infants. It is also helpful to discuss the hormonal effect of lactation on the vagina. Vaginal dryness from hormonal influences during breast-feeding may cause dyspareunia for some nursing mothers. Vaginal lubricants, such K-Y jelly, can sometimes help alleviate this problem. A sudden change in vaginal lubrication can sometimes indicate ovulation.

Intrauterine devices (IUDs) are a very effective method of contraception available to nursing mothers. According to FDA regulations, however, IUDs can be inserted only after uterine involution is complete. Periodic abstinence using symptomatic and temperature methods to detect ovulation also may be used during breast-feeding. Tubal ligation after delivery also can be compatible with breast-feeding but usually requires anesthesia for the procedure. According to Hale (1999), because many anesthetic medications have brief half-lives, rapid redistribution from the plasma to other remote sites (adipose tissue, muscle, and so on), or both, the overall amount of exposure of the breast-feeding infant is quite small. When pain medication is given postoperatively it can be given immediately after the infant is fed to permit the level to peak before the next feeding. Medications used should be limited to short-acting drugs that are excreted within 4 hours and that the newborn is able to excrete (Martin, 2000).

Hormonal contraceptive methods must be used in the breast-feeding mother with caution because some hormonal methods will interfere with milk production. Oral contraceptives containing only progestin are very effective when used in combination with breast-feeding. A small amount of hormone passes to the infant; however, no known adverse effects have been reported (Adams, 2000).

In 1981, the American Academy of Pediatrics approved the use of combination oral contraceptives in women electing to breast-feed once lactation is well established. Estrogen has been reported to reduce milk supply in several studies (Lawrence, 1999; Riordan & Auerbach, 1999). Therefore, alternative contraceptive methods should be considered as a first choice in lactating women, particularly during the first 6 weeks postpartum. The WHO has suggested that the combination oral contraceptive should not be the first choice for women who are lactating (World Health Organization, 1988, 1994).

Depot medroxyprogesterone acetate (Depo-Provera) does not suppress milk production and is an effective contraceptive method for breast-feeding women. Subdermal implants that contain the progestin levonorgestrel do not affect the breast-fed infant and may be inserted at 6 weeks postpartum after lactation is established (Lawrence, 1999).

Decreased Lactogenesis

"**Relactation** is the process by which a woman who has given birth but did not initially breastfeed is stimulated to lactate" (Lawrence, 1999, p. 555). Historically, relactation has been used to provide nutrition to an infant whose mother has died. A relative or friend would take on the care of the infant at the breast. Many women who have adopted infants have the desire to breast-feed. Mothers of premature infants also have expressed the desire to breast-feed their infants after the time in the neonatal intensive care unit is over. Pharmacologic manipulation of lactation has been used to induce breast-feeding. Some medications seem to work only if the breast has been stimulated by pregnancy, whereas other drugs have been used to increase prolactin levels in the absence of pregnancy. Drugs such as thyrotrophin-releasing hormone, and drugs that block hypothalamic catecholamines, such as phenothiazines, reserpine, meprobamate, and amphetamines, have been used to manipulate lactation (Lawrence, 1999). The use of an electric breast pump and frequent nursing of the infant with various lactation devices also will help establish lactation. Milk production by mothers of premature infants has been evaluated by many researchers who have concluded that frequent expression is significantly associated with greater milk production (Brown, 1996).

Infant Barriers

Most normal full-term infants can breast-feed with only minor adjustments. The infant with a medical or surgical problem presents a need for special interventions that ensure adequate newborn nutrition.

Prematurity

Low-birth-weight and premature infants present unique nutritional problems. Optimal growth for premature infants is considered to be the growth curve they would have normally followed if they had remained inside the uterus. Although human milk provides the ideal nutrients, it would require an inordinate, physiologically infeasible volume to achieve adequate amounts of some nutrients. These needs can be met by artificial formula or supplementation.

Preterm milk has been found to contain special properties that are uniquely suited to meet the needs of the premature infant (Figure 30-21). Preterm milk contains higher levels of fat, protein, and other necessary nutrients than term milk. Many mothers of preterm infants need to be given instructions on how to build up their milk supply with electric breast pumps. The milk may be used to feed very low-birth-weight infants by feeding tube until the infant is strong enough to nurse on his own.

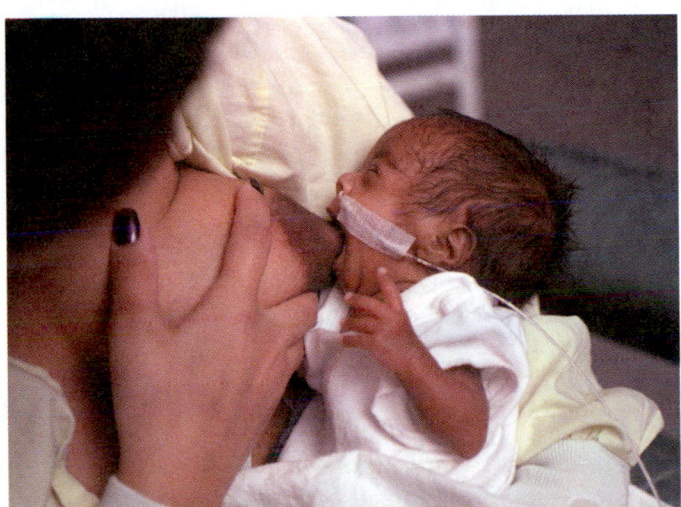

A.

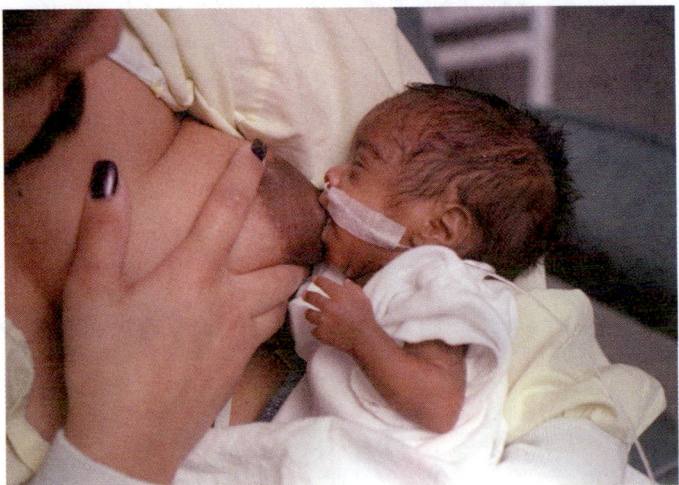

B.

Figure 30-21 This preterm infant, who has been gavage feeding, is trying breast-feeding for the first time. A. The mother elicits the rooting reflex, and the baby responds by opening the mouth wide. B. The baby gets the nipple into the mouth but not much of the areola.

The protective properties of human milk against infection are considered a very important reason to provide human milk to preterm infants. NEC is an acute inflammatory disease of the GI mucosa commonly seen in the premature infant. Human milk has been associated with a decreased incidence of this very serious condition (Lawrence, 1999). When the infant nurses at the breast, there is a large outpouring of 19 different GI hormones in both the mother and infant, including cholecystokinin and gastrin. These hormones stimulate the growth of the baby's and mother's intestinal villi and increase the surface area for the absorption of calories with each feeding. The increased gut motility with each breast-feeding episode also removes a large amount of meconium from the infant's colon, with its large load of bilirubin (Ulvnas-Moberg, 1989).

Recent research has demonstrated that the use of small, thin, silicone nipple shields in preterm infants significantly increases milk transfer (Meier et al., 2000). Immature feeding behaviors, such as short, ineffective sucking bursts and falling asleep easily, predispose premature infants to underconsumption of breast milk. The nipple shield makes it easier for the preterm infant to stay latched on to the breast and extract milk. This research demonstrated that not only did milk intake increase significantly but the use of nipple shields also resulted in most mothers breast-feeding for a longer duration than did mothers who had not used shields.

Illness and Disability

Infants who have been compromised in utero or during delivery will need special treatment. Infants who will have the best outcomes when breast-feeding can be maintained are those experiencing postmaturity, fetal distress, and hypoxia; acute illnesses, such as fever; or contagious diseases. Some problems such as galactosemia or inborn errors of metabolism may require that breast-feeding be terminated.

Down syndrome or other congenital anomalies may make breast-feeding more difficult. Breast-feeding in these infants will require patience and support of the mother and infant by all members of the health care staff. Feeding of any sort may be greatly hindered by abnormalities of the jaw, nose, or mouth, such as cleft lip or cleft palate. These infants may need to have surgical correction during the first few weeks of life. The mother may have to express or pump her breast milk and offer it by dropper when sucking is ineffective (Lawrence, 1999).

Hypoglycemia

Hypoglycemia during the early neonatal period of a term infant is defined as a blood glucose concentration of less than 35 mg/dL, or a plasma concentration of less than 40 mg/dL. Hypoglycemia occurs because the infant's glucose supply is stopped when the cord is cut. Signs of hypoglycemia include jitteriness; irregular respiratory effort; and cyanosis, apnea, feeding difficulty, and lethargy. Many nurseries routinely obtain a blood glucose test soon after birth because hypoglycemia can sometimes by asymptomatic. Infants at high risk require more frequent testing (Lawrence, 1999).

According to the International Lactation Consultants Association's guidelines for breast-feeding management during the first 14 days (1999), hypogycemia during the first 3 hours after delivery usually has a physiologic cause. These guidelines further state that early, frequent breast-feeding helps prevent lowered blood glucose levels. Because colostrum contains 18 cal/oz compared with 6 cal/oz for 5% glucose water, newborns are less likely to experience hypoglycemia when feeding is not supplemented with glucose water after delivery. Colostrum also has higher levels of protein than does glucose water and therefore has a stabilizing effect on blood glucose levels.

Jaundice

Physiologic jaundice is a normal occurrence in 50% of term and 80% of preterm newborns. Neonatal jaundice occurs because the newborn has a high rate of bilirubin production. The number of fetal erythrocytes per kilogram of body weight is greater than in an adult, and there is considerable reabsorption of bilirubin from the neonate's intestine. Meconium is extremely high in bilirubin and is a source of reabsorbed bilirubin. Jaundice appears 24 hours after delivery in an otherwise healthy infant. Although many causes for physiologic jaundice have been investigated, research has documented that the number of breast-feedings during the first 3 days of life relates to bilirubin levels. The greater the number of breast-feedings, the lower the bilirubin levels (Lawrence, 1999). The newborn should be fed at least 8 or more times a day. Colostrum is a natural laxative and promotes the excretion of meconium, thus decreasing bilirubin levels.

Psychologic Barriers

Bryant (1992) conducted extensive qualitative research using focus groups throughout the United States in an effort to determine which perceived barriers are keeping women with low incomes from breast-feeding. Bryant analyzed data and found several consistent responses among these women:

- Lack of confidence in their ability to breast-feed. Many women lacked confidence in their ability to produce adequate quality or quantity of breast milk.
- Embarrassment. The embarrassment that many women feel when nursing in front of others is a major deterrent to breast-feeding.
- Loss of freedom. Many women feel that breast-feeding will prevent them from going to work, school, or social events.
- Concerns about dietary and health practices. Many women feel that they will have to change many of the things that they like to do in order to breast-feed.
- Influence of family and friends. Many women do not feel that they have the courage or strength to go against the negative influence of family members or friends.
- Women expressed many other concerns, such as pain, fear of disfigurement, sexual feelings about breasts, invalid medical concerns, and a lack of social support.

Modesty

According to Bryant (1992) many women view their breasts as sexual objects and associate them with their ability to attract and please men. Because of these feelings many women are apprehensive about breast-feeding in front of other people, particularly men. Women may worry that nursing their infant in public will arouse men, make

---

Nursing Alert

MANAGEMENT OF EARLY PHYSIOLOGIC JAUNDICE WHILE BREAST-FEEDING

You should:

- Monitor all infants for initial stooling.
- Initiate breast-feeding early and frequently.
- Discourage water, dextrose water, and formula supplementation.
- Monitor weight, voidings, and stooling associated with breast-feeding.
- When the bilirubin level approaches 15 mg/dL, stimulate stooling by feeding the infant more often and stimulate breast milk production with pumping. When the bilirubin level exceeds 20 mg/dL, use phototherapy.

No evidence exists that early jaundice is associated with an abnormality of the breast milk; therefore, withdrawing breast milk is indicated only when jaundice persists for more than 6 days, the bilirubin level increases to above 20 mg/dL, or the mother has a history of having had an affected infant (Lawrence, 1999).

Client Education

Sexuality and the Breast-feeding Woman

Sexual stimulus can trigger the milk ejection reflex in breast-feeding women, particularly during orgasm. This "let-down" of milk during sexual relations may have either a negative or positive effect on the sexual partner. Psychologic conflicts in the partner may be a result of misunderstanding of the "let-down" reflex. Practical solutions to unwanted spraying of milk - "let-down" during sexual relations include the following:

- Breast-feeding the infant immediately before sexual relations.

- Expressing milk before beginning sexual relations.

- Explaining the biologic phenomenon to couples, thus avoiding negative reactions.

- Teaching couples that oral and manual manipulation and fondling of the breasts during love-making need not be restricted (Lawrence, 1999).

Lack of Confidence

Some women lack confidence in their abilities to produce an adequate supply of nutritious breast milk. Few women understand the mechanics of breast milk production and are easily influenced by stories from other women whose milk "dried up" or couldn't satisfy their child's nutritional needs because it was too weak, blue in color, or too thin. If these stories come from an important social influence, such as a grandmother, they may take on special significance because of the possibility that the problem may have been passed on genetically to the new mother.

When women lack confidence in their own ability to make adequate and nutritious breast milk, they frequently will begin supplementing with formula. Doing so creates a downward spiral in breast milk production that becomes a self-fulfilling prophecy. Because infant formulas have labels that list the ingredients, many women will trust these products more than their own bodies. Not being able to accurately measure the amount of breast milk the infant is taking during nursing also seems less scientific than being able to measure formula taken in ounces, leading women to worry about the amount of milk being produced.

Educational materials on breast-feeding usually depict women as being confident, secure, and completely in control of their lives. Use of promotional materials that picture average and minority women may help overcome these worrisome perceptions. Helping the woman analyze and resolve her fears and concerns about breast-feeding can build her confidence and self-esteem.

their husbands or boyfriends jealous, or look disgusting to others. Women say they will feel uncomfortable breast-feeding in front of anyone unless they are sure their breasts are not exposed. Finding a private place to breast-feed while out in public is a very real concern for many women. Women may resent being forced to hide in restrooms or cars to keep from feeling embarrassed by breast-feeding.

The nurse can help allay these fears by teaching the woman how to breast-feed discreetly by demonstrating how to cover her breasts while she is nursing and assuring her that most women are apprehensive about breast-feeding in front of others but usually adjust quickly once they begin to nurse. If she is one of the women who does not adjust, she can pump her breast milk and give the baby a bottle when she is in public.

A small proportion of women feel they cannot even consider breast-feeding because they associate the breast with sexual arousal. These women may consider the idea of putting their baby's mouth on the breast as disgusting. Survivors of sexual abuse also may have unresolved issues about the breasts and may not be able to breast-feed their infants.

Social Barriers

Social support has been recognized as a very important component of successful breast-feeding. Social support has been defined as input directly provided by another person (or group) that moves the receiving person toward goals that the receiver desires (Baranowski et al., 1983). In order for breast-feeding support to succeed, it is necessary to have a person desiring to learn how to breast-feed and a support person who can teach the skills that must be achieved. Social support can be provided by a nurse, a lactation consultant, a family member, friends, peers, or a significant other. Factors influencing attitudes and social support include personal networks, attitude of the baby's father, health care provider's attitudes and help, and maternity ward policies and practices (Figure 30-22). The nurse plays an important role in facilitating the new skills necessary to promote successful breast-feeding because the nurse frequently has the most direct and personal contact with new mothers. However, some mothers complain that nurses frequently give conflicting information or may be ill-prepared to offer advice (Hill, 2000).

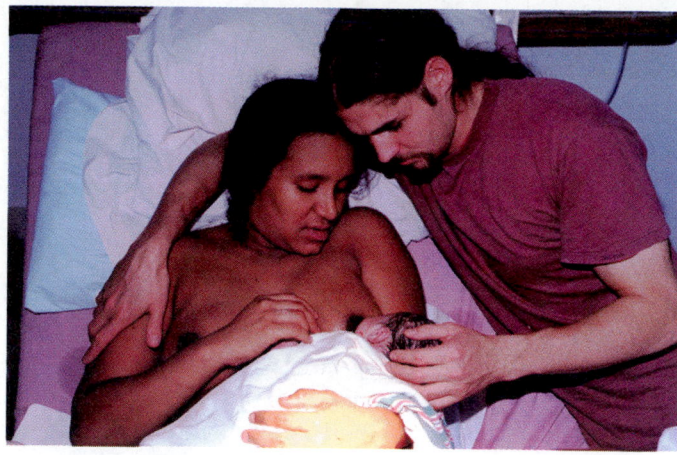

Figure 30-22 Involvement of the baby's father or other support persons in the breast-feeding process is more likely to result in successful breast-feeding.

Lack of Social Support

The negative influence of family and friends or lack of social support is associated with a decrease in breast-feeding initiation and duration (Raj & Plichta, 1998). Studies of socioeconomic factors associated with lower breast-feeding rates include women who are unmarried, single, widowed, or divorced. For many women, especially teens, who may not have a strong support network, peer support groups and lactation consultants have been shown to increase both initiation and duration of breast-feeding.

Misperceptions and Misconceptions

Many women have misinformation about breast-feeding and may decide it is not an option for them. Stories from other women that suggest breast-feeding is painful or may even permanently disfigure the breasts can be real barriers. Some women have heard that contraceptives cannot be used while breast-feeding and may bottle-feed because of this misconception. Nurses need to elicit the client's misconceptions and misperceptions to deal with them effectively. Simply saying, "Tell me what you have been told about breast-feeding" will help the client state her concerns in a nonthreatening environment (Bryant, 1992).

Other Barriers

In addition to personal and social barriers to breast-feeding, subliminal messages linked to specific hospital policies and institutional procedures also can play an important role in feeding decisions.

Hospital Policies

Many studies have looked at the effect of formula supplementation on breast-feeding outcomes. Most of these stud-

Critical Thinking

Breast-feeding Myths

Can you answer clients' questions about breast-feeding myths? What information would you offer to counter each myth? Research and continue to dispel myths about breast-feeding.

- Women do not need to drink large amounts of fluids to produce large amounts of breast milk.
  Advice is simple: Drink fluids when thirsty.
- Women do not need to restrict the food they eat while breast-feeding.
  Advice is simple: There is no need to eliminate foods from the diet unless consumption of a certain food, such as onions, is followed by symptoms in the breast-fed baby, such as excessive crying or gas.
- A mother can drink alcohol in moderation and continue breast-feeding.
  Advice is simple: There is no need to completely eliminate drinking alcohol while breast-feeding.
- It is safe and recommended that mothers and babies sleep together if the infant is kept supine and soft materials are not allowed in the bed.
  Advice is simple: Co-sleeping is safe and facilitates breast-feeding for mother and baby unless the parents use medications that impair arousal (Heinig, 2000).
- Breast-feeding does not make breasts sag or become disfigured.
  Advice is simple: Wear a good supportive bra.
- A mother's anger will ruin or curdle her milk.
  Advice is simple: Angry feelings may cause mothers to feel tense and the infant may sense this tension; however, the quality of the breast milk will not be affected (Lamaze International, 1998).

ies have reported a decrease in milk supply that seems to be directly related to the amount of supplementation of formula. A study by Bliss et al., (1997) clearly showed that mothers who requested formula in the hospital and requested a discharge pack of formula were more likely to discontinue breast-feeding than were mothers who exclusively breast-feed. Other studies have looked at the effect of giving formula samples on discharge from the hospital. Simpson (1999) found that mothers who were given for-

Client Education

Working and Breast-feeding

You should teach the client to consider the following information for successfully combining working with breast-feeding:

- Take full advantage of maternity leave to establish a supply of milk.
- Keep in mind that breast-feeding can reduce the amount of sick days taken because breast-fed infants usually are sick less often then are formula-led infants.
- Try to introduce a bottle once you have a milk supply established (in 4 to 6 weeks) to prepare the baby for bottle-feeding during the day by someone else.
- Purchase or rent a high-quality, automatic, electric breast pump.
- Purchase a double-pumping kit with the electric pump so that both breasts can be expressed simultaneously in only 10 to 15 minutes (Figure 30-23).
- Gradually become familiar with the process by simulating the pumping schedule to be used at work for 2 weeks before returning to work.
- Breast-feed once in the morning; pump every 2 to 3 hours at work; and then breast-feed as soon as possible on returning home, during the evening, and at bedtime.
- Try to find a private area if a pumping room is not available at your place of employment.
- Store the breast milk pumped at work in a refrigerator or cooler. Milk can be kept refrigerated for 72 hours; it also can be labeled, dated, and frozen for 6 months when kept in the deep-freeze section of the freezer.

You can teach the mother to keep the following in mind:

- Pumping the breasts at work can be easy, fast, and painless.
- Many working mothers combine breast-feeding and bottle-feeding with few problems.
- Your child-care provider can feed the baby breast milk from a bottle while you are at work.
- Breast-feeding creates a special bond between you and the baby that no one else can have.
- Plan and commit yourself to breast-feeding because it is a worthwhile endeavor for your baby.

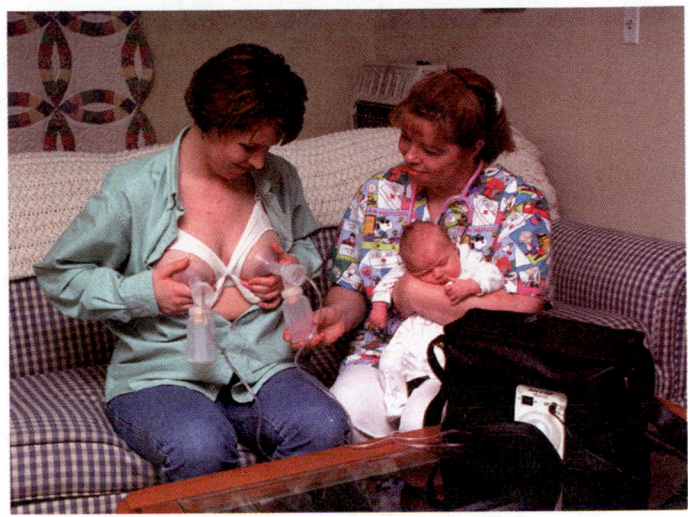

Figure 30-23 Expressing milk from both breasts simultaneously is a time saver for the busy mother.

mula discharge packs were significantly less likely to be breast-feeding at 1 month and were more likely to have introduced solid foods by 2 months.

One of the possible explanations for the breast-feeding problems associated with formula supplementation is a phenomenon called *nipple confusion*. This problem seems to be related to the fact that infants must use a completely different method of sucking to extract milk from the breast compared with the bottle and therefore have problems changing from one to the other. While sucking at the breast, the infant's tongue moves in a peristaltic motion from front to back, causing milk to be squeezed out of the nipple. When an infant sucks on an artificial nipple, the tongue pushes forward against the nipple to control the milk flow. Some breastfed babies make the necessary adjustments without problems; however, others do not and push the mother's nipple out of the mouth.

Many lactation consultants recommend the use of special nipples to help infants switch between breast-feeding and bottle-feeding. A specially designed nipple made of silicone that is broad, soft, and naturally shaped allows infants to suckle using their tongues and lips, similar to the way they use their muscles when breast-feeding.

Other hospital policies that can negatively affect breast-feeding include taking the newborn to a transitional nursery immediately after delivery, no rooming-in policy, routine supplementation of breast-feeding infants in the nursery, inconsistent or contradictory advice from hospital staff, and infants being allowed to nurse only on a strict hospital schedule. The woman who wants to breast-feed her infant may need to find out about the breast-feeding policies of the hospital before she chooses where to deliver.

Return to Work

The largest number of women choosing to breast-feed today are women who intend to return to work (Bar-Yam, 1998). Some women may feel that returning to work is a barrier to breast-feeding because of the added commitment and effort needed to combine work and breast-feeding the baby. Most companies have a written policy that establishes how long the maternity leave will be extended, and many companies find it beneficial to support breast-feeding to keep a high-quality workforce (Bar-Yam, 1998). The new mother must make decisions about child care and whether to continue breast-feeding after returning to work. Although breast-feeding will require some extra commitment and effort, many women find that the rewards far outweigh the difficulties.

The most important thing a new mother can do to get ready to return to work is to learn how to stimulate the production of milk. Frequent feedings and emptying the breasts completely increase milk production because these actions signal the breasts that there is a need for more milk. About 2 weeks before returning to work, the new mother should start pumping after and between feedings, and begin to store the breast milk in the freezer so that an adequate supply will be available to the baby's caregiver. Returning to work gradually or leaving the baby with a sitter for practice sessions will help to make an easier transition for both baby and mother.

Choosing a person to care for the baby who supports the mother's commitment to breast-feeding is an important first step in preparing to return to work. The client who plans to breast-feed after returning to work will need anticipatory guidance and support. The client can breast-feed when she is home and pump her milk while at work. She can leave breast milk for the infant to be given by a babysitter while she is away. The client's work wardrobe should include clothing that will allow her easy and private access to her breasts so that pumping while at work will be as easy as possible. Breasts may also leak during the first few weeks after returning to work. To help minimize leakage, instruct the client to press against the nipples when she feels the tingling feeling associated with the let-down reflex. The client also may want to place breast pads in her bra so that the milk will not stain her clothing. Wearing patterned clothing or bringing along a sweater to wear over other clothes also will prevent embarrassment if leaking occurs.

Nursing More Than One Child

Many women may wonder if pregnancy, multiple births, or being unable to establish lactation immediately after delivery are barriers to successful breast-feeding. Pregnancy can and does occur while lactating. It is possible to lactate throughout pregnancy and then to nurse both infants at

REFLECTIONS OF A NEW MOTHER OF TWINS

"During an interview with a new mother of twins, she was asked how in the world she could possibly breast-feed twins. The mother replied with absolute sincerity: 'I breast-feed because it is the easiest way to feed two babies. How would I ever keep up with bottles and formula for both of them? This way I can nurse both of them at once. It just makes good sense'!"

the breast postpartum. This is presently happening often enough to be called *tandem nursing.* The amount of nourishment provided to the first child depends on age and the other supplements being given. It has been shown that both infants can be nourished at the breast without any apparent adverse effect on either infant (Lawrence, 1999). The mother should be advised to get adequate rest, nourishment, and psychologic support to help her cope with the added demand on her both physically and mentally.

It is also possible for a mother to nurse twins and triplets (Figure 30-24). Research reports the fact that a single mother can provide adequate nutrition for more than one infant (Mohrbacher, & Stock, 1997). If the mother can nurse both twins at once the time needed to feed twins can be minimized. The mother will need adequate nutrition, rest, help, and support from relatives and friends to care for twins during the first busy year of life. The breast is capable of responding to nutritional demands placed on it by more than one infant, and many mothers of twins report that breast-feeding is much easier than trying to keep up with bottles for more than one infant.

CONTRAINDICATIONS TO BREAST-FEEDING

When discussing the contraindications to breast-feeding, it is necessary to examine the specific conditions that put the mother or infant at risk. The risk-to-benefit ratios must be weighed by the clinician and mother to arrive at the best decision for both mother and child. Life-threatening or severely debilitating illnesses in the mother may necessitate avoiding lactation.

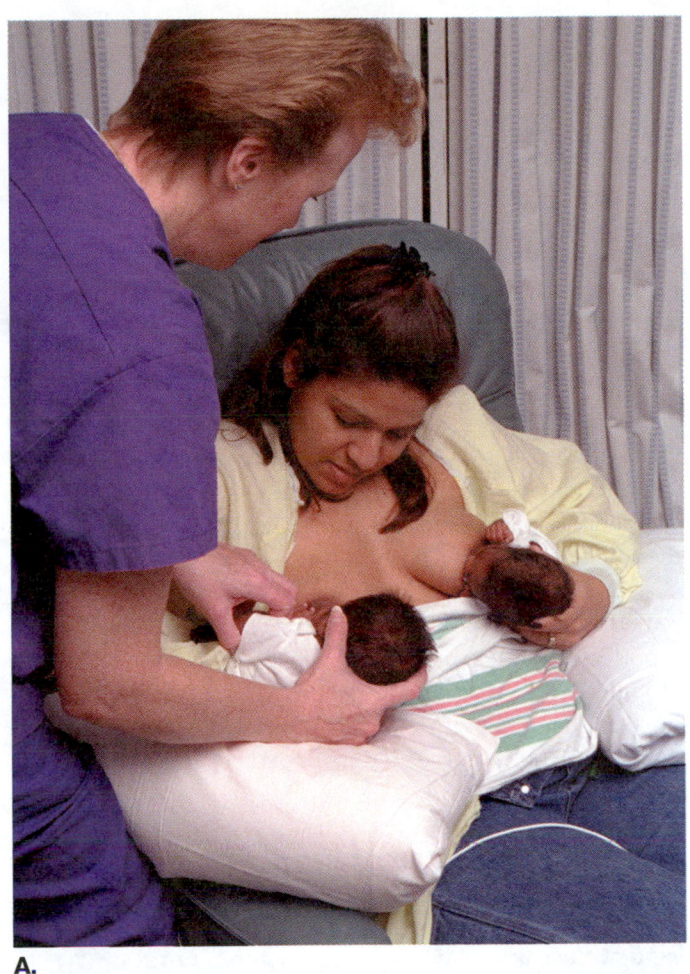
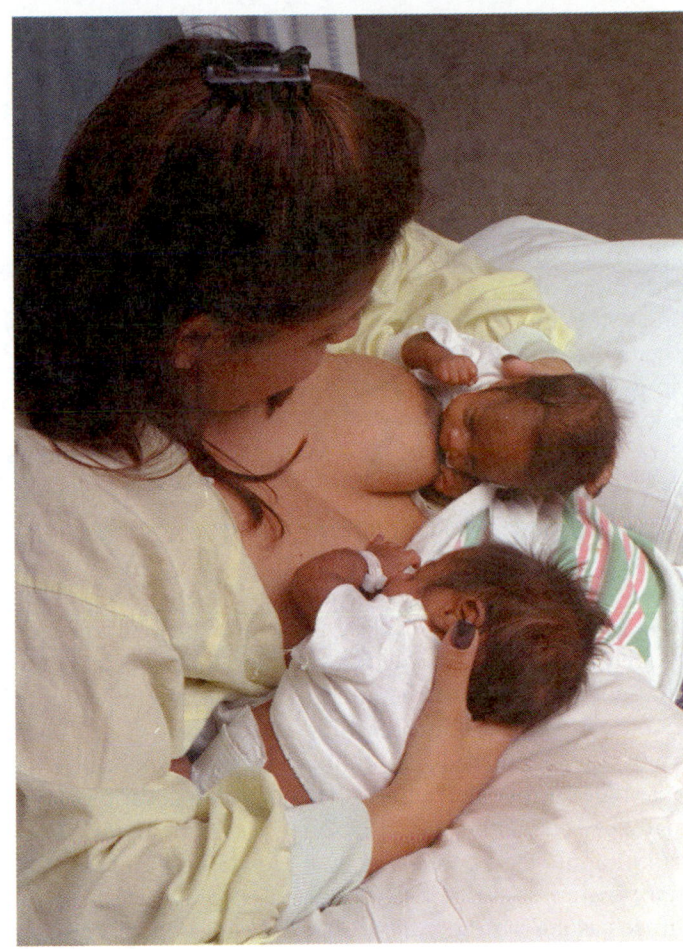

A.

B.

Figure 30-24 Breast-feeding multiples. A. The nurse is helping this mother of triplets with her efforts at breast-feeding two babies at once. B. This mother and her babies will learn how to breast-feed together.

Maternal Disease

A new mother with a diagnosis of breast cancer should not nurse her infant so that the mother can begin definitive treatment for the disease. Breast-feeding is incompatible with chemotherapeutic agents. The question has been asked whether tumor cells can be transmitted to the infant by breast milk? At the present time no documented evidence exists of women with breast cancer having RNA of tumor virus in their milk (Lawrence, 1999).

Hepatitis B virus transmission from mother to infant has been described in several studies worldwide (Centers for Disease Control and Prevention, 1998). All infants born to mothers who have active disease or are carriers now receive both hepatitis B immune globulin (HBIG) immediately after birth plus a dose of human hepatitis B vaccine, followed by a second dose at a week of age or later. The Committee on Infectious Disease of the American Academy of Pediatrics states that newborns of mothers who test positive for hepatitis B and who have received the HBIG vaccine may be breast-fed (Lawrence, 1999).

Hepatitis C virus is the major agent causing blood-transmitted forms of non-A, non-B hepatitis. Because of the probable transmission of the hepatitis C virus into breast milk, the chance of chronic liver disease, and the lack of effective treatment, breast-feeding is not recommended when a mother is infected with the virus (Lawrence, 1999).

Cytomegalovirus (CMV) has been identified in human milk of women with the CMV antibody. However, the risk of CMV infection or other serious complications to the infant of a lactating women with CMV in her milk is negligible because the milk also contains appropriate antibodies that protect the infant.

Studies on acquired immunodeficiency syndrome (AIDS) have found that breast milk has been implicated in person-to-person transmission of the HIV virus. The Center for Disease Control and Prevention (CDC) and the U.S. Public Health Service recommend that women in the United States who test positive for the HIV antibody should not breast-feed to avoid postnatal transmission to a child who may not have been infected in utero or during delivery. In Third World countries where infant mortality from diarrhea and other diseases is 50%, breast-feeding is still the feeding method of choice (Lawrence, 1999; Popkin et al., 1990).

In the United States, human T-cell leukemia virus type I (HTLV-I) is a disease endemic in intravenous drug users and their sexual partners. Transplacental transmission of HTLV-I is virtually nonexistent; however, evidence exists of horizontal transmission through breast milk. Therefore, breast-feeding is not recommended for women who test positive for HTLV-I and for any mother who is abusing drugs because of the possibility of the infant receiving substantial amounts of the drug through breast milk (Lawrence, 1999).

Infant Disease

Most breast-fed infants are healthy, and many illnesses are less severe than those described previously; however, an infant may be born with a disease or may develop an illness after birth. Diarrhea and intestinal tract disease are much less common in breast-fed infants; however, if they occur, the infant should continue on breast milk if at all possible. Human milk is a physiologic solution that normally causes neither dehydration nor hypernatremia. Colitis in infants may be caused by a metabolic disorder; a dietary insult; some types of bacteria; and several types of viruses, such as the rotavirus. Respiratory tract illnesses and otitis media are less likely in the breast-fed infant. However, infants who develop respiratory tract illnesses can be maintained on the breast. The advantages of breast milk are the presence of antibodies and many neutralizing agents that protect the infant from many common childhood illnesses (Lawrence, 1999).

Drugs and Medications

Riordan and Auerbach (1999) emphasize the three "knows" about drugs and human milk:

1. Most drugs pass into breast milk.
2. Most medications appear only in small amounts in breast milk.
3. Few drugs are contraindicated for breast-feeding mothers.

Many variables affect the passage of drugs into breast milk: amount of drug taken, frequency and route of administration, timing of the dose in relationship to feeding the infant, and characteristics of the drug involved.

The effects of the drug on the infant are influenced by the infant's age, amount of milk ingested, frequency of feedings, and degree of absorption that occurs in the infant's GI tract. Lawrence (1999) suggests that long-acting

forms of drugs be avoided and that drugs be administered immediately after the women has nursed her baby so that peak levels of the drugs will occur long before the next feeding time. Lawrence also suggests that infants be carefully assessed for drug reactions and that when alternative drugs are available that are less likely to pass into breast milk, they be used.

The mother who is breast-feeding should always inform her physician that she is doing so to avoid harming the infant. Information on potential effects of drugs given during lactation can be obtained from the American Academy of Pediatrics Committee on Drugs, 1994. Some drugs also may affect breast milk volume and therefore must be used cautiously. When dispensing medications to a nursing mother, the health care provider should always weigh the benefits of the medication against the possible risks to the infant (Table 30-4).

Herbs and herbal teas currently are very popular remedies for a variety of problems. Many herbs have been reported to enhance milk production (Lawrence, 1999). Mothers should be aware of the effects of herbal compounds that are ingested and the possible reaction in the breast-feeding infant. The nurse needs to inquire about all

Table 30-4 Drug Recommendations During Lactation

Contraindicated Drugs	Drugs to Use Cautiously
Bromides	Atropine
Chloramphenicol	Barbiturates
Cocaine	Chloral hydrate
Coumadin	Dihydrotachysterol
Crack cocaine	Ergonovine
Cyclophosphamide	Ethinyl estradiol
Diazepam	Medroxyprogesterone acetate
Dicumarol	Methadone
Diethylstilbestrol	Metronidazole
Ergot alkaloids	Nalidixic acid
Gold salts	Nitrofurantoin
Heroin	Norethisterone
Indomethacin	Phenothiazines
Iodides	Quinine
Lithium carbonate	Senna
Methotrexate	Sulfonamides
Methylergonovine	Thiazide diuretics
Phenylbutazone	
Radioactive Iodine	

Source: Hale, T. (1999) *Medications and mothers' milk*, Amarillo, TX: Pharmasoft.

foods and beverages when taking a medical history. When excessive amounts of any herbal substance are being consumed, its contents need to be checked. Education of the lactating client on avoidance of plants and herbs that may adversely affect her newborn is an essential nursing intervention.

According to the National Institute on Drug Abuse (1998) persons with the highest rate of illicit drug use are those between the ages of 18 and 25 years. Of women between 18 and 34 years of age, 30% reported using an illicit drug during the past year. Most breast-feeding women do not use drugs. Because some do, however, it is important that the nurse have accurate information to inform these women about the possible adverse effects of specific drugs on breast-feeding and newborns (Riordan & Auerbach, 1999).

Marijuana is probably the most common illegal drug used today by breast-feeding women. It is estimated that 5% to 15% of pregnant women use or have used marijuana. Although impairments in DNA and RNA have been reported in laboratory animals, there are no reports of infant health problems solely from marijuana use during lactation. Thus, the question is raised of whether a woman should be advised not to breast-feed if she refuses to give up smoking marijuana. Although not an ideal situation, there is little evidence that marijuana causes serious harm; therefore, it may be better for these mothers to continue to breast-feed rather than wean their babies (Riordan & Auerbach, 1999).

Cocaine use in the United States has dramatically increased because it has become less expensive, and the more popular form known as crack cocaine has emerged. This drug is entirely different from marijuana. Cocaine harms the fetus and the nursing infant. Cocaine is highly lipid-soluble and readily crosses into human milk. For at least 36 hours after the mother's last use of cocaine, the results of tests on milk samples will be positive for cocaine and its metabolites. Infants exposed to cocaine can exhibit irritability, vomiting, tachycardia, and seizures. Therefore, the recommendation is very clear: cocaine should never be used by a mother who is breast-feeding. A mother who uses cocaine is putting her infant at risk for great harm and also may have the baby removed from her custody if legal action is pursued (Hale, 1999–2000).

Amphetamines are readily transferred to breast milk, and levels in the infant may be three times higher than maternal blood levels. Despite these high levels in a large study of 100 mothers taking amphetamines, no adverse changes occurred in the infants' behavior (Riordan & Auerbach, 1999).

The effects of alcohol on the infant of a mother who is breast-feeding seem to be directly related to the amount of alcohol ingested by the mother. When the mother who is breast-feeding drinks a small amount of alcohol, the alcohol may not affect the infant or may cause a little sedation.

One study in mothers who were breast-feeding and who drank alcohol found the motor development of their infants to be slower; however, no effect on the infants' mental development was noted (Little, 1989).

PROBLEMS ENCOUNTERED WITH BREAST-FEEDING

There are many problems that can result in a nursing diagnosis of ineffective breast-feeding. Many of the so-called breast-feeding problems are merely normal phenomena that simply need to be addressed and worked through. The fact that breast-feeding problems have received so much attention probably accounts for the reluctance of many women to even give breast-feeding a chance. By focusing on the problems and not the rewards, health care professionals are doing a great disservice to clients and their infants. Nurses can offer anticipatory guidance to new mothers and support them with referral services after discharge, if necessary.

Client Education

Milk Supply

You must teach clients to cope with fears about adequate milk supply:

- Remember that the more milk the baby removes from the breasts, the more will be produced.
- Expect to breast-feed every 2 to 3 hours until the milk supply is established.
- Do not skip feedings or supplement feedings. Night feedings are necessary to establish adequate milk supply for the first few weeks after delivery.
- Breast-feed for at least 15 to 20 minutes so that the baby will receive the rich hindmilk.
- Try to rest and relax as often as possible, and accept offers from friends and family for help.
- Offer both breasts to the infant at every feeding.
- Eat an adequate healthy diet, and drink plenty of liquids.
- Remember that infant growth spurts are to be expected and are only temporary.

REFLECTIONS FROM A CLIENT

When talking to a new mother who had been breast-feeding for 3 months, she shared this story of how difficult it was to learn to trust her body to make good-quality and an adequate quantity of breast milk.

"During the first 4 weeks I would breast-feed my baby every 1 to 2 hours all day long. By night-time my breasts felt completely empty. I was afraid to put my baby to sleep for the night when she might be hungry or starving to death, so each night I would breast-feed first and then offer a bottle of formula. She would sometimes take one ounce and then go off to sleep. When I took her back for her well-baby check-up at 6 weeks, her weight was off the top of the chart. I decided to confess to the pediatrician that I had been supplementing. When I told him how much formula she was taking each day, he laughed and said, 'If you think your baby is gaining this much weight from one ounce of formula a day, you must be kidding me.' Then he said, 'Your breast milk is what is making this child gain weight so well.' From that day on, I never supplemented again because I finally trusted and believed in my own body. It was just a matter of gaining confidence in myself."

Many of the problems can be avoided if the nurse provides anticipatory guidance in assessing and planning the care of the new mother who wishes to breast-feed. The nurse's role in working with the woman who is breast-feeding includes developing a plan of care that includes teaching of proper feeding techniques and interventions to correct any related problems.

Maternal Problems

Mothers may experience some difficulties when beginning to breast-feed. Most complications can be avoided if the mother receives appropriate guidance, education, and support during initiation of breast-feeding after delivery. Early recognition and resolution of problems are essential to prevent disruption of breast-feeding. Because the nurse usually is the first person to interact with the new mother, the nurse is in a unique position to offer timely assessment, help, and effective interventions.

Cracked or Sore Nipples

Sore nipples are another common concern for breast-feeding mothers. Sore nipples usually are due to improper infant attachment, although some soreness is normal during the first few days or weeks of breast-feeding. Letting the nipples air dry after feeding, applying a few drops of breast milk to the nipples after feeding, and avoiding soaps and other drying agents usually will relieve soreness. Probably the most important intervention for this concern is observing the placement of the infant on the breast and helping the mother to ensure the infant is on the areola and not just the nipple.

Nipple soreness may be decreased by encouraging the mother to rotate positions when feeding the infant. Changing position alters the focus of greatest stress and promotes more complete breast emptying. Nipple soreness also can develop because of faulty infant sucking habits. Nipples can develop bruises, scabs, or blisters during improper sucking episodes when the nipple is rubbing against the roof of the infant's mouth. Nipples can be chewed because of improper positioning when the baby is just getting on the nipple and not the areola, resulting in cracked and tender areas near the base. Mothers need to be taught how to get the baby's mouth wide open and on the areola and how to remove the infant without causing more damage to the nipple. Nipple soreness also can result in cracked nipples. Cracked nipples need to be assessed for fissures, and the breast-feeding position must be observed. The mother may want to begin the feeding session with the nipple that is less sore or may need to temporarily use a nipple shield made of silicone to allow time for the nipple to heal.

The mother needs to be made aware that nipple soreness is most uncomfortable during the first few minutes of breast-feeding. Because the let-down reflex takes a few minutes to occur, she needs to try to keep nursing long enough for the milk to begin flowing. When the infant is overeager because of extreme hunger, nipple pain can be compounded. Feeding more often and applying ice to the nipples before beginning may help.

The best way to care for the nipples is simply to apply some breast milk to them at the end of the feeding and allow them to air dry. The use of creams or ointments is discouraged. Washing the nipples with plain water (no soap) prevents drying and helps healing. If the mother's nipples are irritated by clothing, breast shields or pads may be worn under the bra.

When a mother has persistent sore nipples, candidiasis is a possibility. It is caused by a fungus, *Candida albicans,* also called *Monilia* or thrush when it occurs orally. This condition should be suspected when the mother has been breast-feeding without discomfort and then suddenly complains of very sore nipples, itching, burning, or pain deep in the breast. When the mother has signs of deep pink inflammation on her nipples, the infant's mouth also needs assessment for signs of white patches. Treatment of all infected areas in both mother and baby are necessary to eliminate the infection and prevent reinfection (Heinig & Francis, 1999). Antifungal medication is given by mouth to the infant, and the mother must apply antifungal cream to her nipples before each breast-feeding (Riordan & Auerbach, 1999).

Inverted Nipples

Assessment of the mother's nipples for protractility when stimulation occurs can be done by asking the mother to gently pinch her nipple and observing each as it everts (Figure 30-25). Inverted nipples can be successfully treated during the prenatal period by using breast shells that exert a gentle suction on adhesions anchoring the nipple. This will usually allow the inverted nipple to protrude when the baby latches on (Riordan & Auerbach, 1999). If a mother has flat or inverted nipples, a breast shield made of thin latex may help to draw the nipple out but may reduce milk transfer to the infant by 22% (Lawrence, 1999). The use of an electric breast pump also may help pull the nipple out before the infant tries to latch on. The mother should also be encouraged to help shape the nipple by using her hands or apply ice before feedings.

Breast Engorgement

Breast **engorgement,** which results in swelling and fullness, occurs in all women who are lactating from three to seven days after delivery. Engorgement usually involves

the vascular system as blood flow is increased to the breasts to prepare for milk production after delivery (Figure 30-26). The breasts are described as full, red, warm, and uncomfortable. This type of engorgement will subside on its own within 3 to 5 days and is a natural response.

Another type of engorgement involves overdistention of breast milk in the alveola. This overdistention may be

Client Education

Prevention and Treatment of Engorgement

You should teach the client how to prevent engorgement:

- Breast-feed the infant frequently, 8 to 12 times in 24 hours to prevent discomfort and mastitis.
- Avoiding supplements of water or formula for the first 3 to 4 weeks.
- Express milk when feedings are missed.
- Gradually wean the baby.

You should teach the client how to treat engorgement:

- Apply hot, moist towels to the breasts for 2 to 5 minutes, or take a hot shower before nursing.
- Hand express some milk to soften the areola after using moist heat, making it easier for the baby to attach to the breast.
- Use gentle breast massage before and during breast-feeding.
- Avoid bottles, pacifiers, and nipple shields during this period, which can cause nipple confusion for the infant.
- Apply cold compresses to the breasts after feeding to relieve discomfort.
- Use relaxation techniques before and during feeding.
- When the baby will only take one breast at a time, use a breast pump or hand express milk from the other breast during engorgement periods.
- Use a breast pump or hand express milk to soften the areola when the baby cannot latch on to the nipples because the breasts are too full.

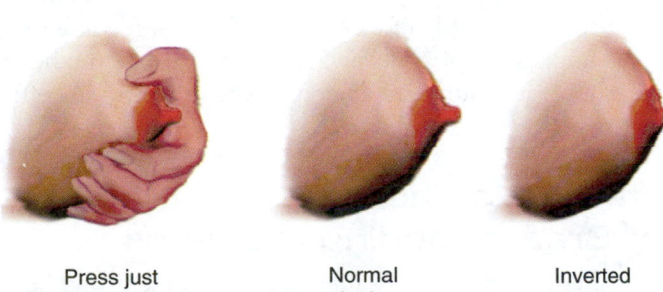

Press just behind areola

Normal nipple protraction

Inverted nipple

Figure 30-25 Assessing for nipple inversion.

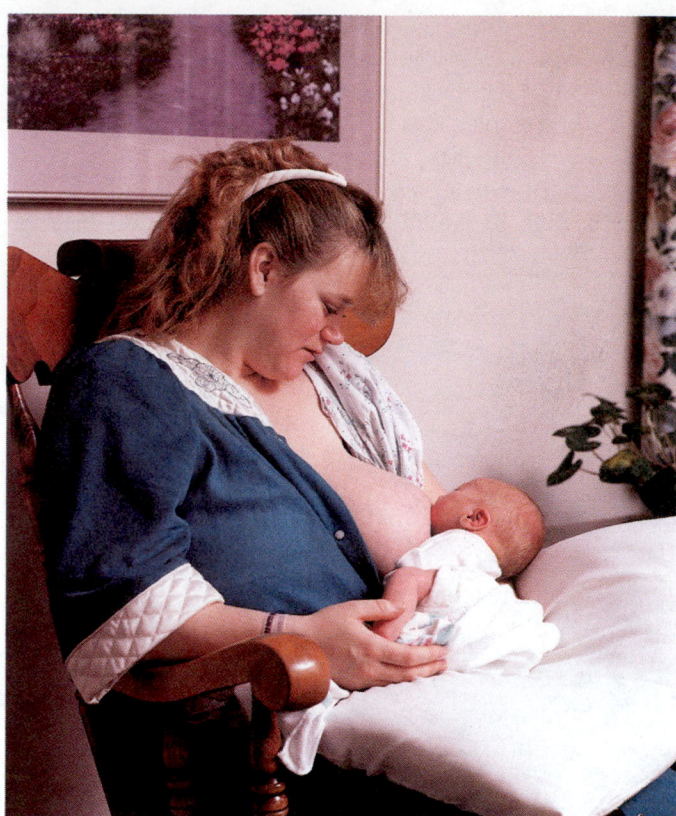

Figure 30-26 Breast-feeding is the best relief for breast engorgement.

due to restricted sucking time, large volumes of milk, or incorrect infant attachment. Some mothers experience plugging of one or more milk ducts, especially during or after engorgement. This problem is manifested by a lumpy area of tenderness in the breast and also is referred to a "caked breasts." Treatment consists of the use of heat, breast massage, and frequent breast-feeding to ensure complete emptying of the breast (Lawrence, 1999).

Mastitis

Mastitis is an infection of the breast generally caused by *Staphylococcus aureus* and seen primarily in women who are breast-feeding. The most common source of the bacteria is the infant's mouth. This infection usually occurs after discharge from the hospital; therefore, the client needs to be taught symptoms and preventive measures before discharge. The symptoms of mastitis are erythema, swelling, and pain, usually occurring in the upper outer quadrant of the breast. Enlarged and painful axillary lymph nodes also may be present. The woman with infectious mastitis also may present with influenza-like symptoms, such as fever, and a headache, along with a reddened and painful area in the breast.

Many factors may contribute to the development of mastitis and most can be prevented: poor drainage of milk;

cracked or damaged nipples; a tight bra or improper breast support; poor hygiene; engorgement; or a change in the infant's feeding habits, such as sleeping through the night or being ill. The nurse can help prevent mastitis by teaching proper breast-feeding techniques, encouraging mothers who are breast-feeding to wear a good supportive bra, and teaching methods of preventing milk stasis.

New mothers should contact their physician, nurse practitioner, or Certified Nurse Midwife immediately if they experience signs of mastitis. A diagnosis of mastitis usually is based on symptoms and physical examination. Treatment consists of feeding the baby frequently or pumping the breasts, bed rest, increased fluid intake, a supportive bra, local application of heat, medications for pain, and with a 10-day course of antibiotics (Lawrence, 1999). Most antibiotics are safe for the breast-feeding mother. If the antibiotic can be given to an infant, it is then safe to give the breast-feeding mother. However, because most antibiotics transfer into breast milk, the antibiotic may cause loose stools or candidiasis in both the mother and infant (Riordan & Auerbach, 1999).

Mastitis occasionally may develop into an abcess that needs to be incised and cultured. If breast-feeding becomes impossible, it is necessary to maintain the mother's milk supply and prevent engorgement by using an efficient pump to remove the milk.

Alternative Therapy for Breast-feeding Problems

There are many alternative therapies for problems mothers have with their breasts when breast-feeding. Rapid healing has been achieved by applying breast milk to the mother's nipples and allowing it to dry. Applying tea bags mois-

Research Highlight

Effects of Cabbage Leaf Extract on Breast Engorgement

Purpose

To compare the effectiveness of cabbage leaf extract and a placebo in the treatment of breast engorgement in lactating women.

Methods

In a double-blind experiment with a pretest-posttest design, 21 participants received a cream containing cabbage leaf extract and 18 received a placebo cream.

Findings

The placebo and treated groups reported receiving equal relief, with the two groups showing no difference on all outcome measures. However, mothers perceived both creams to be effective in relieving discomfort. Feeding had a greater effect than the application of cream on relieving discomfort and decreasing tissue hardness.

Nursing Implications

It is recommended that lactation consultants encourage mothers to breast-feed if possible to relieve the discomfort of breast engorgement.

Roberts, K., Reiter, M., & Schuster, D. (1998). Effects of cabbage leaf extract on breast engorgement. *Journal of Human Lactation, 14,* (3), 231–236.

---

tened in warm water is receiving new acceptance. The tannic acid in the tea helps toughen the nipples, and the warmth promotes healing.

Lawrence (1999) reports that application of cabbage leaves is a favorite treatment for breast engorgement that has been handed down for generations. Two reports in the literature are cited. Treatment consists of application of refrigerated cabbage leaves to the breast, leaving the nipple exposed. The leaves are left on for 20 minutes or until wilted. Whether it is the coolness of the leaves or some innate property of the leaves that helps the engorgement is yet to be proved.

Many herbs and foods have been used to encourage and promote the flow of milk and to treat some of the problems of breast-feeding. Simple teas such as raspberry leaf, alfalfa, and comfrey are used to stimulate a plentiful supply of breast milk and a relaxed mother and infant. All leafy greens such as parsley, watercress, and green beans are considered helpful in maintaining lactation. Other herbs and leaves, including hops, are thought to increase milk production.

Nursing mothers may rely on herbal products to help produce more or a better quality of milk. However, the scientific efficacy of these remedies is limited. Few data exist on the excretion of herbal products into breast milk. Some common herbal remedies, such as chamomile, have been used for thousands of years and are considered safe for use during lactation by the FDA. However, many other common herbs are considered dangerous and should be avoided while breast-feeding: aloe vera, basil, black cohosh, bladderwrack, comfrey, ginseng, licorice, and golden seal (Kopec, 1999).

Many poultices, compresses, and soaks also are recommended as being beneficial to stimulate circulation and ease pain in sore breasts. The use of warm compresses soaked in a variety of herbs and leaves is suggested as a remedy for sore nipples, clogged milk ducts, engorgement, and mastitis (Hoffman, 1992).

The use of relaxation techniques, such as deep breathing, imagery, and body massage, also can be used to promote relaxation and thus the "let-down" reflex. Accupressure massage techniques also can be used to help create relaxation and decrease stress and anxiety. Many women find that they need a quiet, private place to breast-feed their infant to allow the flow of milk to occur. A warm, relaxing bath or shower also will stimulate the flow of milk.

After the first few weeks, the let-down reflex occurs more easily and just the thought, sight, or sound of the infant frequently will trigger milk flow.

Return to Work: Pumping, Storing, and Supplementation

When a mother wishes to breast-feed and is unable to nurse her baby because the infant is premature or she must return to work, she can express the milk either manually or with a breast pump. During the postpartum period, if a baby is unable to nurse at the breast, the mother needs frequent breast stimulation to help establish her milk supply. She should use an electric breast pump with a double setup (pumps both breasts at once) at least 8 times in a 24-hour period (Riordan & Auerbach, 1999). The milk obtained can be refrigerated and given by gavage or fed from a tiny plastic cup made especially for premies, until the infant is able to nurse on its own.

There are many kinds of breast pumps on the market (Figure 30-27). Breast pumps generate a suck-release action by way of a flange that is placed over the areola. The milk obtained is passed into a reservoir. The new mother should be taught to use a breast pump before leaving the hospital postpartum unit. The new mother should be taught to first wash her hands and gather all equipment, which should be clean. The let-down reflex can be triggered before beginning to pump by rolling the nipple between the thumb and forefinger for a minute or two. Pumping, using an electric pump on each breast for at least 10 minutes every 3 to 4 hours around the clock, will stimulate milk production. Milk can then be transferred to sterile containers and frozen until needed. Breast pumps can be hand pumps, which are inexpensive but inefficient. Battery-operated pumps are more efficient than hand pumps but also are more expensive. Electric pumps are the most efficient but are very expensive. Most agencies now offer clients the option of renting an electric breast pump that is easy to use and very efficient in collecting and stimulating milk production. Most hospitals offer new mothers a list of suppliers of these types of pumps.

Milk also can be expressed manually by squeezing toward the nipple using the thumb and fingers around and above the areola and rotating 360 degrees around the breast (Figure 30-28). Massaging the breasts and nipples to stimulate the let-down reflex will help make the milk flow more readily.

Breast milk should be stored in clean plastic containers because leukocytes in the milk adhere to glass containers and thus their protective effect may be lost. When breast milk is frozen, leukocytes are destroyed. To safely use frozen breast milk, it must be thawed by running warm water over the container and then shaking it well to return the milk to suspension. It should not be warmed in

Client Education
Breast Milk Storage

For the client to successfully store breast milk, the nurse must teach the following about storage and preparation of the breast milk:

1. Refrigerated breast milk must be stored at 40°F or below and used within 72 hours.
2. Frozen breast milk must be stored at 0°F or below and used within 6 months.
3. To thaw frozen breast milk, run warm water over the container and shake it to return the milk to suspension.
4. Frozen breast milk that is thawed must be refrigerated at 40° or below and used within 24 hours.

a microwave oven because doing so causes uneven heating and may burn the infant.

Many businesses are now starting to provide comfortable, private places that allow new mothers to nurse their infants or to pump breast milk to be given to their infant at a later time. These pumping rooms, with breast pumps and refrigerators for breast milk storage, are being offered to employees by companies that realize the health benefits and resulting cost savings that can result from encouraging their female employees to breast-feed their infants. Because many new mothers must return to work before they are ready to wean their infants, it is imperative that these mothers be allowed the time and opportunity to remove the breast milk to prevent the breast engorgement. The newest electric pumps are extremely effective in removing the milk, and most mothers can finish pumping in 20 to 30 minutes. This type of support from employers can enable new mothers to continue their commitment to breast-feeding while maintaining their commitment to their jobs.

Weaning

The decision to stop breast-feeding and either place the infant on a bottle or a cup (**weaning**) may be considered a potential problem by the mother. In fact, some women have heard horror stories about the difficulties of weaning and are afraid to even try breast-feeding because of these fears. Women who are comfortable with breast-feeding and understand the weaning process will know when the time comes to wean because of sensitivity to the child's cues. In our society weaning frequently occurs very early

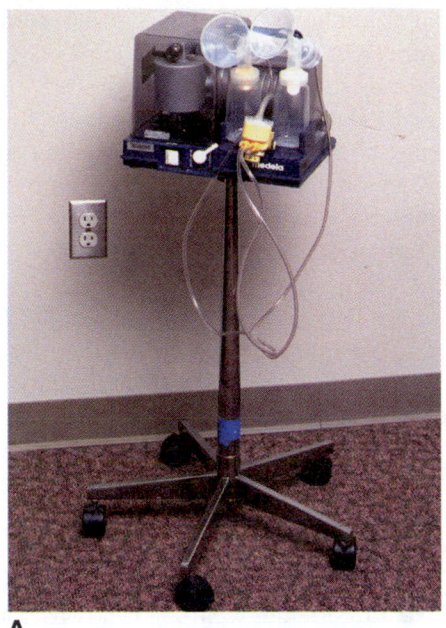
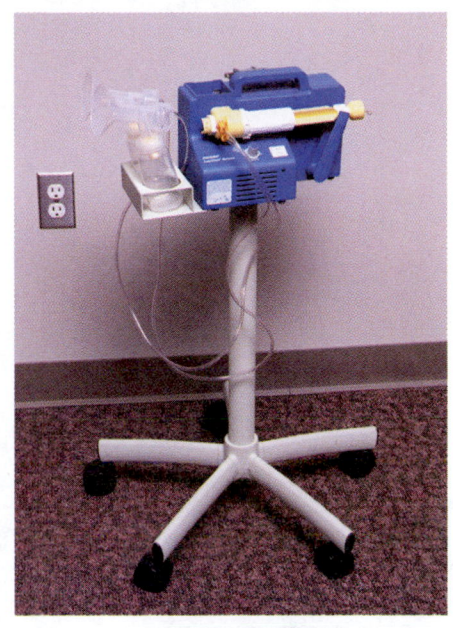

A.

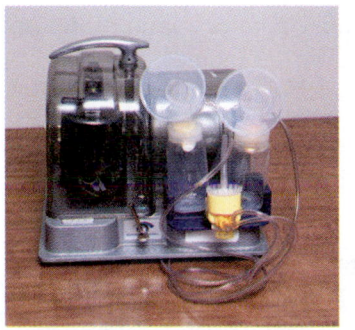
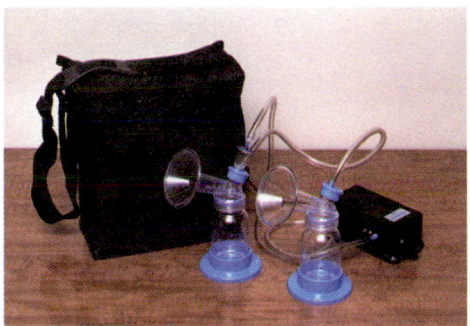
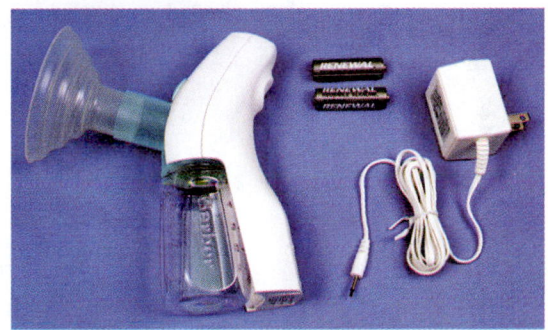

B.

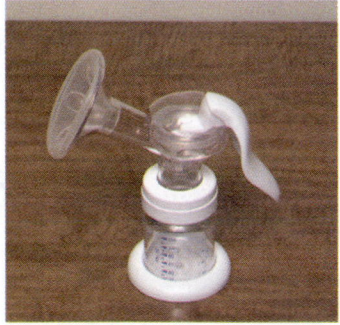
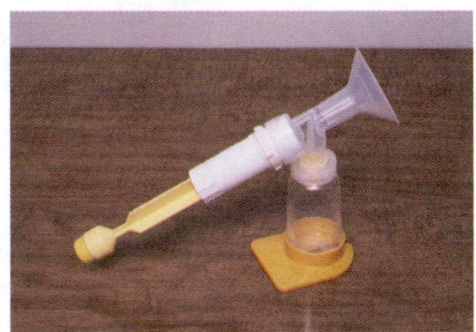
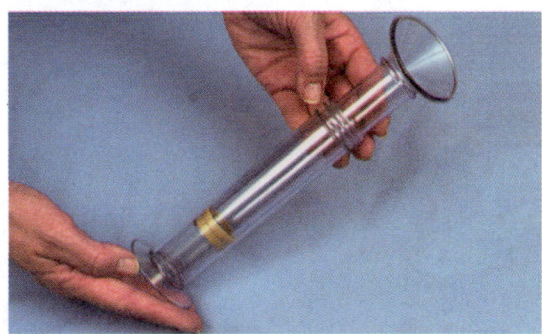

C.

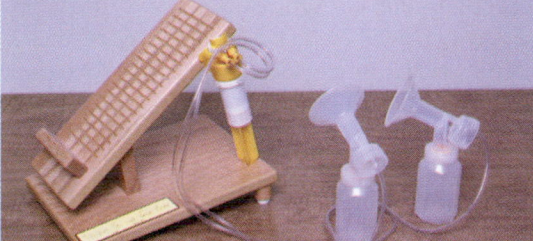

D.

Figure 30-27 Breast pumps. A. Hospital pumps.
B. Electric and battery-operated pumps. C. Manual pumps.
D. Foot-operated pump.

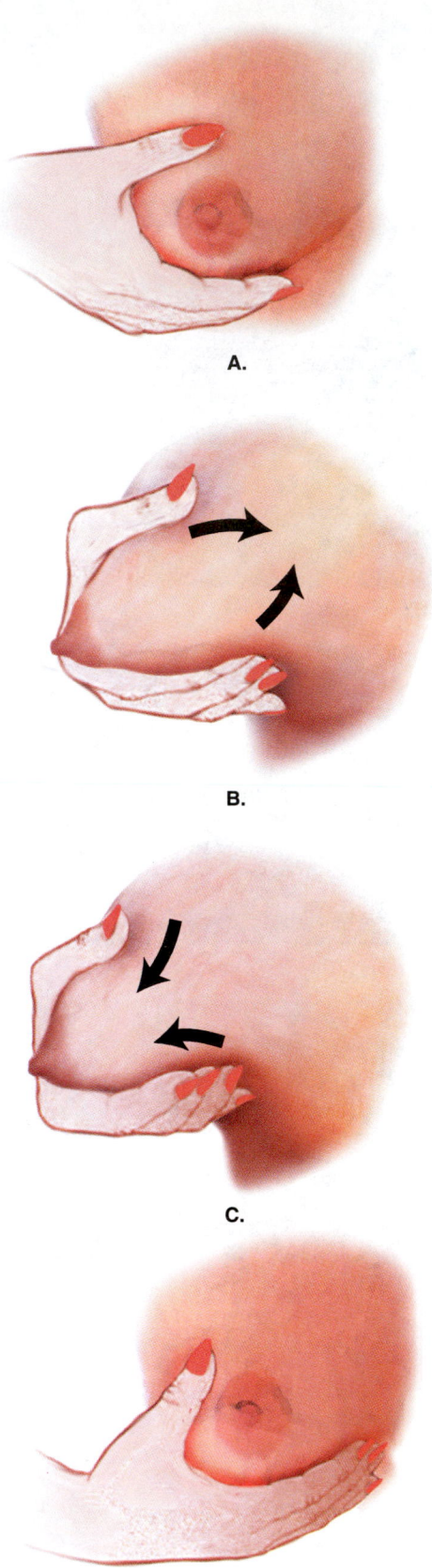

Figure 30-28 Manual expression of breast milk. A. Grasp your breast in a C-hold. B. Squeeze your thumb and fingers together, while pushing fingers toward the chest wall. C. Maintain hand position, and push your fingers toward the nipple. D. Shift thumb and fingers an inch away from their first location and repeat the process, working your way around the entire breast.

in the infant's life. The latest recommendation from the American Academy of Pediatrics is to breast-feed for one year (American Academy of Pediatrics, 1997). The slow method of weaning by gradually substituting one cup or one bottle for one breast-feeding session over days or weeks helps prevent breast engorgement and allows the infant to slowly adapt to the new feeding method (Lawrence, 1999).

Early introduction of solid and semisolid infant foods varies depending on the culture. Worldwide there is a high rate of breast-feeding initiation and too early supplementation with other foods. At some time, every breast-fed infant reaches a point when breast milk alone can no longer meet his or her nutritional needs, and solid foods are necessary. Three types of weaning have been described:

1. Gradual weaning takes place slowly over several weeks or months.
2. Deliberate weaning is a conscious effort instituted by the mother to end breast-feeding at a certain time.
3. Abrupt weaning is an immediate cessation of breast-feeding, usually initiated by the mother.

The timing and type of weaning can affect the infant's health and may even be associated with a feeling of being rejected in either the infant or the mother.

RESOURCES FOR BREAST-FEEDING MOTHERS

An important breast-feeding promotion strategy that has developed to help provide support for women's breast-feeding efforts is the lactation consultant. **Lactation consultants** are specially trained health care providers whose primary focus is assisting new mothers in establishing breast-feeding. These consultants provide a variety of services, including individual consultations, collaboration with other health care providers to develop a plan of care for new mothers, teaching classes, and instruction on the use of products such as breast pumps. These consultants also serve as informational sources, researchers, and data collectors and may help in developing special breast-feeding programs.

The U.S. Department of Agriculture, Food and Consumer Service (USDA/FCS), which promotes good nutrition for women and children, sponsors the WIC program. For a woman to be eligible for WIC, she must be at nutritional risk as designated by her individual state of residence and meet federal poverty level income qualifications. This program has provided formula free of charge and food stamps that can be redeemed for nutritious fruits, dairy products, and vegetables. Many people felt that giving free formula promoted the choice of bottle-feeding among women with low incomes. Since 1989, each state has been required by the USDA to spend a specified amount on breast-feeding promotion and support. Since that time, many new programs have been set up to encourage mothers on the WIC program to breast-feed their infants. The WIC program strongly supports breast-feeding and encourages mothers to nurse their infants through its nutrition education, breast-feeding promotion, and special food packages for nursing women and their other children (McClurg-Hitt & Olsen, 1994).

Recently, due to extra funding, the Secretary of Agriculture announced a new program, "Loving Support Makes Breastfeeding Work." This program will encourage mothers on the WIC program to begin and continue breast-feeding by providing more breast-feeding materials, referrals, and professional support. These programs are designed to increase public awareness and support of breast-feeding and provide technical assistance to WIC professionals in helping mothers breast-feed. WIC has tried many innovative projects to help promote and support breast-feeding. Programs of peer counselors who have been trained to assist new mothers have met with great success (Kistin, Abramson, & Dublin, 1994).

Many national and international organizations also are available that use the media to promote breast-feeding worldwide. The World Alliance for Breastfeeding Action was formed in 1991 as a group that coordinates international breast-feeding advocacy efforts by its members, which include organizations such as the International Lactation Consultants Association (ILCA) and International Breastfeeding Association (IBFAN). Two of the most notable activities are coordinating World Breast-feeding Week during the first week of August each year and lobbying for breast-feeding at international conferences (Bailey, 1997). *The Journal of Human Lactation* is a scientific journal devoted entirely to the publication of research and information on breast-feeding. Many books also are available to

LALECHE LEAGUE

LaLeche League is a self-help group for breast-feeding mothers with members around the world. LaLeche sponsors workshops and has an extensive publication list. The organization consists of small neighborhood groups in all major cities and rural areas. LaLeche group leaders also are available for additional information and support. The groups usually have a lending library and newsletter.

ILCA

The International Lactation Consultant Association (ILCA) promotes breast-feeding awareness among health care providers and the public. The ILCA also helps define the scope of practice of lactation consultants. The ILCA publishes the *Journal of Human Lactation.*

help not only the health care professional but also new mothers. Dr. Ruth Lawrence is considered a leading authority on breast-feeding and has written a book entitled *"Breastfeeding: A guide for the medical profession"* (Lawrence, 1999).

Clients may be referred to resource groups, which provide education, support, and public awareness of breast-feeding. The ILCA promotes breast-feeding awareness and helps define the scope of practice of lactation consultants. **LaLeche League** is a self-help group for breast-feeding mothers and is available worldwide. Members also are available for individual consultation and support.

NURSING IMPLICATIONS

Currently, nurses are faced with the challenge of providing care that is based on the most current evidence available. Evidence-based practice in nursing is a fairly new concept and allows nursing to move away from basing interventions on rituals, unverified rules, anecdotes, opinions, traditions, customs, intuition, or unit culture. Organizations such as the Association of Women's Health, Obstetrics and Neonatal Nurses (AWHONN) and the ILCA are introducing evidence-based guidelines to help nurses change practices so that the care they offer women and infants is the most effective and safest they can provide.

Internet technology can now be used for clinical decision-making, creating policies and protocols, patient and staff education, and researching information. With over a million web sites available, however, accessing electronic sources can be an overwhelming task. The Cochrane Pregnancy and Childbirth database is an ongoing meta-analysis of evidence documenting effective health care practices for childbearing women and their infants (Callister & Hobbins-Garbett, 2000). One example of the importance of using evidence-based practice is a breast-feeding publication produced by ILCA in 1999, "Evidence-based guidelines for breastfeeding management during the first fourteen days." This publication can be used to change hospital policies such as routine supplementation of breast-feeding with water, dextrose water, or infant formula by providing the research evidence that contradicts such a policy (Heinig, 1999).

Although most women in the United States know that breast milk is best for infants, the breast-feeding rates still remain low. Traditional education programs that promote breast-feeding have not adequately influenced the adoption of breast-feeding in a large segment of the population. Social marketing is a communications strategy that has been used in the commercial market for many years to convince the public to purchase items such as cars and clothing. Recently, the social marketing strategy has been used to promote several socially beneficial products, such as exercise and smoking cessation.

The use of social marketing techniques to encourage breast-feeding among women with low incomes was conceptualized by Carol Bryant, an anthropologist and researcher, who created a company called Best Start. Best Start was organized to research, develop, and provide a multifaceted campaign aimed at new mothers, family members, health professionals, and the community at large. The materials that were designed can be obtained and used by a variety of breast-feeding promotion programs at a low cost (Bryant, Bailey, and D'Angelo 1989). This company, in cooperation with the USDA/FCS, has recently announced a pilot project in 10 states to include:

- Formative research.
- Development of a national breast-feeding resource guide and community organizer's kit.
- Training of WIC staff in coalition building, use of media, breast-feeding counseling strategies, and other aspects of breast-feeding promotion.
- Implementation of a state-wide media campaign (ILCA Globe Newsletter, 1997).

Overcoming Barriers

Prenatal education should begin as early as possible so that breast-feeding information can be presented to each client as often as possible to clear up misinformation and resolve doubts. Most women make their infant feeding decisions before becoming pregnant or during the first trimester (Grossman et al., 1990). Although most women know breast-feeding is best for infants many women have specific barriers that keep them from trying to breast-feed.

Education

Most women decide on an infant feeding method either before getting pregnant or during the first trimester. Therefore breast-feeding education programs need to be designed to provide information either preconceptually or during the early prenatal period. Breast-feeding education can be accomplished by formal classes, informal discussions, printed materials, video tapes, and even by way of the Internet (Riordan, 2000). Educational programs should emphasize the benefits of breast-feeding and the potential hazards of formula-feeding. A complete promotion program has two essential components. First, counseling on how to overcome barriers to breast-feeding must be provided. Second, educational sessions must be held covering the mechanics of breast-feeding, how to deal with common breast-feeding problems, and how to assess adequate nutrition in the infant.

Another attempt to increase breast-feeding initiation in hospitals is shown in Box 30-1.

Cultural Negotiations

The nurse and other health care providers need to provide culturally appropriate care and guidance when helping

---

Box 30-1 The WHO/UNICEF "Ten Steps to Successful Breastfeeding"

Hospitals that are willing to adopt 10 specific steps and complete an accreditation process are then named "Baby-Friendly" hospitals. These 10 steps follow:

1. Have a written breast-feeding policy that is routinely communicated to all health care staff.
2. Train all health care staff in the skills necessary to implement this policy.
3. Inform all pregnant women about the benefits and management of breast-feeding.
4. Help mothers initiate breast-feeding within a half hour of birth.
5. Show mothers how to breast-feed and maintain lactation, even when separated from their infants.
6. Give newborn infants no food or drink other than breast milk, unless medically indicated.
7. Practice rooming-in (keeping the infant in the mother's room), and allow mothers and infants to remain together 24 hours a day.
8. Encourage breast-feeding on demand (whenever the infant is hungry).
9. Give no pacifiers.
10. Foster the establishment of breast-feeding support and refer mothers on discharge from the hospital or clinic.

WHO/UNICEF. (1994). Protecting, promoting and supporting breastfeeding: The special role of maternity services. *A joint statement by WHO/UNICEF,* Geneva, 1989, World Health Organization.

DECISION TO BREAST-FEED

When working with pregnant women who may be interested in learning about breast-feeding, you can:

- Begin with open-ended questions to elicit the client's specific concerns. For example, "What do you know about breast-feeding?"

- Acknowledge her concerns and reassure her that her feelings are normal. For example, "Many women worry about that same thing."

- Educate each woman using carefully targeted messages that address specific concerns.

new mothers breast-feed. The nurse needs to consider breast-feeding beliefs about health, support or resource persons, parenting responsibilities, and infant care. Because breast-feeding is a sensitive and personal matter for all women, it is important to assess attitudes toward modesty and cultural norms for each woman. Breast-feeding in a public place or in the presence of other people is an extremely sensitive issue for most women. Teaching women that breast-feeding can be accomplished in a modest manner and acknowledging variations in comfort are essential to successful feeding experiences.

In many cultures, colostrum is viewed as "old" milk that is not healthy for infants. In other cultures, this first milk is viewed as "poison" or "pus" that must not be given to babies. Nurses need to assess beliefs about colostrum in each client and attempt to educate the client while being careful not to insult her cultural beliefs. Well-meaning efforts to acculturate women to the nurse's beliefs may actually disrupt breast-feeding efforts. It is important to demonstrate understanding and value of the client's beliefs while helping her establish successful breast-feeding behaviors (Riordan & Auerbach, 1999).

Facilitating the Process

A renewed interest in the first minutes, hours, and days of life has been stimulated by several behavioral and physiologic observations in both mothers and infants. A special area of study on bonding has focused on increasing mother-infant time together by keeping newborns on the mother's chest in skin-to-skin contact during the first hour after birth.

Research has demonstrated that when infants are immediately dried (except the hands) with warm towels and it is clear they have good color and are active and normal,

they can go safely to their mothers. At this time the warm and dry infant is placed between the mother's breasts or on her abdomen. The mother's chest is able to maintain the infant's body temperature quite nicely. One of the most significant findings in this early period is related to breast-feeding. Six of nine studies have revealed that when a mother wants to breast-feed, is permitted to have early contact with her infant and an opportunity for suckling in the first hour of life, and is rooming-in with her infant, she is more successful at breast-feeding than mothers who do not have these experiences (Widstrom, Wahlberg, & Mathiesen, 1990).

One of the most exciting observations made is the discovery that newborns have the ability to find their

SUPPORTING BREAST-FEEDING

You should encourage breast-feeding by:

- Enthusiastically promoting and supporting breast-feeding.

- Simplifying breast-feeding. There is no need to eat or drink differently because only an additional 500 cal/d are needed along with a normal amount of fluid, six 8-oz glasses a day.

- Helping women understand the ability of their infant to communicate readiness to feed, latch on, and breast-feed well.

- Talking about parenting styles that promote and facilitate breast-feeding, such as holding and cosleeping.

- Communicating the rewards and benefits of breast-feeding after returning to work.

- Discussing ways women can influence their workplace to become breast-feeding-friendly.

- Working to change hospital practices that sabotage initiation of breast-feeding, e.g., providing formula discharge packs, separation from the baby, and lack of adequate help to initiate breast-feeding.

- Encouraging the media to present breast-feeding as positive and normal.

- Keeping informed regarding new breast-feeding knowledge.

Lamaze International. (1998). A special report on breastfeeding. *ASPO/Lamaze, 1,* (7), 3.

Critical Thinking

Informed Consent for Infant Feeding Decisions

In order for women to make an informed decision about infant feeding methods, mothers must be given facts about the nutritional and immunologic needs of the infant that can best be met by human milk, potential benefits to the mother, and potential risks associated with formula-feeding. The nurse is required to give the parents complete information, document that she has done so, and record the mother's choice in her medical record.

How can you make sure that your client makes informed decisions regarding health care for herself and her family?

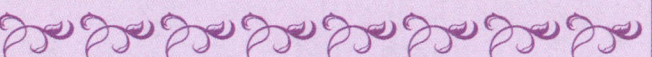

control postpartal bleeding, and hastens involution of the uterus. The infant will be most interested in breast-feeding within the first 20 to 30 minutes after birth, and the colostrum will begin to provide immunologic benefits immediately. The infant's digestive system will be stimulated by 19 different GI hormones, and passage of meconium will be enhanced by the ingestion of colostrum. The milk supply will be stimulated, and attachment between mother and baby will be increased (Ivnas-Mobert, 1989).

Research has examined many variables that have an effect on breast-feeding initiation and duration. Several studies have collected data on the length of time between delivery and the first breast-feeding session. Most of these studies have found that the sooner breast-feeding is initiated after delivery the better the outcomes. All studies found that both early initiation of breast-feeding and frequent feedings contribute to longer breast-feeding duration (Lawrence, 1999). There appears to be an "early window of opportunity" for the infant's sucking to stimulate prolactin receptors, which enhance milk production (Riordan & Auerbach, 1999).

mothers' breast on their own and decide for themselves when to take their first feeding (Klaus & Klaus, 1998). Infants use the taste and smell of the amniotic fluid on their hands to make a connection with a substance on the nipple. This scenario may take place in a matter of minutes, or within 30 to 60 minutes. Because the mother and infant are kept together both immediately after birth and during rooming-in, the new mother learns to recognize the infant's readiness for feeding and can feed the infant on demand. These signals of hunger from the infant include lip smacking, flow of saliva, finger sucking, and mouthing movements (Buransin, 1991).

Prenatal Decision-making

The most effective time to prepare for breast-feeding is early in the prenatal period or even preconceptually. An early conference with the pregnant woman's health care provider will allow time for discussion regarding the importance of breast-feeding and the benefits to mother and infant. An examination of the breasts is part of good prenatal care. If any anatomic abnormalities are observed, they can be discussed at that time. The health care provider can supply literature on breast-feeding and answer questions during the prenatal visits. There is no specific prenatal preparation of the breasts or nipples proved to be effective in relieving initial discomfort associated with breast-feeding. Breast shells have been found to be effective in treating women with flat or inverted nipples (Lawrence, 1999).

The First Feeding

Early feedings after birth are important for several reasons. The infant's suckling stimulates uterine contractions, helps

Critical Thinking

Early Interventions

Swedish researchers have shown that the normal infant, when dried and placed nude on the mother's chest and then covered with a blanket, will maintain body temperature, cry significantly less than an infant placed in a bassinet, and crawl to the breast and latch on within the first hour. It seems likely that each of these features—crawling ability, decreased crying, and warming capabilities of the mother's chest—are adaptive and have evolved genetically over more than 400,000 years to help preserve the infant's life (Christensson, Selis, & Moreno, 1992).

When the infant suckles from the breast, there is a large outpouring of 19 different GI hormones in both the mother and infant, including cholecystokinin and gastrin, which stimulates growth of the baby's and mother's intestinal villi and increases the surface area for the absorption of calories with each feeding. These responses were essential for survival thousands of years ago when periods of famine were common (Uvnas-Moberg, 1989).

- How can you change hospital policies that are not based on evidence?
- Where can you access current evidence-based practice research?

Early Postpartum Period

When working with a new mother immediately after delivery, the nurse can begin her assessment of the nursing mother and infant during the initiation of the first breast-feeding session. A systematic assessment of several breast-feeding episodes provides the nurse with the opportunity to teach the new mother, provide anticipatory guidance, and plan for the need of follow-up care both in the hospital and after discharge. During these initial sessions the nurse should evaluate maternal and infant cues, latch-on, positioning, and maternal and infant responses to the feeding episode. As the mother prepares to feed her infant, the infant's level of hunger and state of arousal must be evaluated.

This is a good time to teach new parents about the cues that infants may use to communicate their needs. Breast-feeding is designed to be led by the baby. Babies are born capable of communicating readiness to eat in many ways. Crying is actually a late sign of hunger. Early signs of hunger include rapid eye movements, hand to mouth movements, mouth and tongue movements, body movements, and small sounds. Responding to these feeding cues, rather than waiting for crying, results in a baby and mother who are relaxed and a baby who is not too frantic to latch on and feed properly (Lamaze International, 1998). For a sleepy baby it may be necessary to show the new mother some easy ways of increasing the infant's alertness. Activities such as rubbing gently, taking the infant out of the blanket, and moving and talking to the infant usually will stimulate infants to come to a more awake state. For an overly hungry or upset infant, rocking or talking quietly may provide an opportunity for the infant to calm down so that breast-feeding can begin.

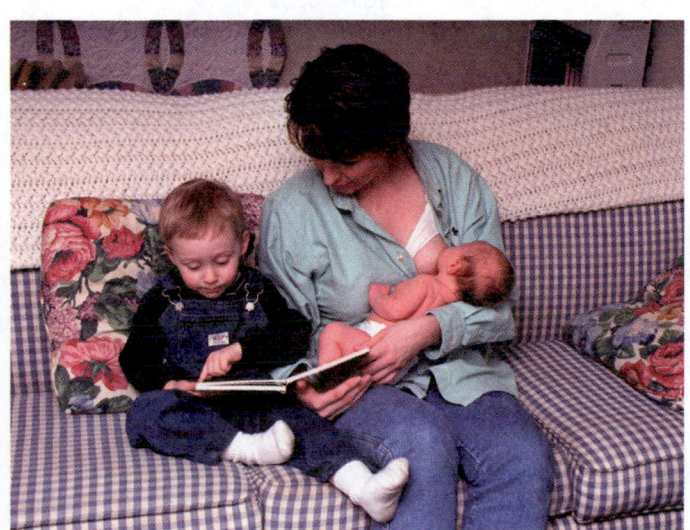

Figure 30-29 Nurses can help new mothers learn to balance the many demands on their time.

Discharge Planning

Early discharge from the hospital markedly reduces the time to teach beginning breast-feeding skills and assess how well the baby is nursing. Many hospitals are now beginning to provide support and follow-up by using telephone calls and home visits. In endeavoring to prevent premature weaning and help new mothers deal with common problems (Figure 30-29), hospitals are now providing written instructions on breast-feeding and telephone numbers of community referrals and resources (Riordan & Auerbach, 1999).

NURSING PROCESS

The nurse can use the nursing process to provide a framework to help guide the assessment, nursing diagnosis, planning, implementation, and evaluation of the nursing pair. The nursing process is a systematic method that uses information in a meaningful way to plan care for the patient in an optimal manner.

Breast-feeding is an interdependent, constantly evolving, and reciprocal relationship between mother and infant. Nurturing mothers and babies during the initiation of breast-feeding can help new mothers learn the skills necessary for successful and satisfactory infant feeding. Although most women have made a decision about whether to breast-feed or bottle-feed by the time they have delivered, some women may just need information and encouragement to decide to breast-feed their infants.

Assessment of the Nursing Pair

Some factors that attract women to breast-feeding are consistent with their aspirations to be good mothers. Mothers want to protect their children from disease and have heard about the benefits that breast-feeding offers in protecting their children. Most mothers also want to be close to their infants and establish a special bond with them that no one else can. Mothers also enjoy the special moments that breast-feeding and motherhood allow them to experience.

Assessment of the Mother

Although the process of breast-feeding is natural, many of the skills and techniques must be learned by both the mother and infant. Nurturing mothers so that they can nourish their newborn should be done through education. Nurses need to dispel myths and misconceptions about breast-feeding and help the new mother embrace her natural inclination to provide her infant with the best nutrition possible.

ASSESSMENT CHECKLIST FOR THE BREAST-FEEDING MOTHER

You should document the following in the breast-feeding client:

1. Maternal vital signs.
2. Maternal and infant intake and output.
3. Maternal position and comfort level during breast-feeding.
4. Condition of nipples and breasts.
5. Maternal sensations during breast-feeding (tingling).
6. Maternal understanding of breast care and nutrition.
7. Maternal understanding of assessment of adequate infant intake.
8. Maternal understanding of proper infant positioning.
9. Maternal understanding of pumping methods.
10. Maternal and paternal attitudes toward breast-feeding.

You should teach the mother the signs that the infant needs to be seen by a health care provider:

1. The infant is putting out scant or no urine.
2. The infant has infrequent stools, less than four a day by end of first week.
3. The infant is very fretful and never appears satisfied after feedings.
4. The infant is lethargic, i.e., hard to awaken.

5. The infant does not make swallowing sounds during feedings.
6. The infant is not gaining weight.

Initially the neonate's intestines contain meconium, which is a dark, thick, greenish-black tarry stool. Normally, the infant will pass the first meconium stool within the first 24 hours. Early and frequent breast-feeding stimulates the passage of stool much earlier and helps decrease bilirubin reabsorption from the meconium in the infant's intestinal tract. The type of infant feeding determines the characteristics of subsequent stools. Formula-fed infants pass pasty, pale-yellow stools with a strong odor. Formula-fed infants may have problems with constipation owing to a more solid stool formation than breast-fed infants. Breast-fed infants pass stools that are golden yellow, sweet smelling, and more liquid in consistency. Breast-fed infants have more frequent bowel movements than do formula-fed infants because breast milk is more easily digested than formula.

You should assess the following factors in the infant:

- Excessive drooling, coughing, gagging, or respiratory distress.
- Time spent at the breast.
- Sucking reflex.
- Signs of lactose intolerance, e.g., cramping, distention, and diarrhea.
- Response after a feeding session.

Nursing Diagnoses

Nursing diagnoses provide the basis for the selection and implementation of nursing interventions to help the client achieve satisfactory outcomes. The following are potential nursing diagnoses for the client who is breast-feeding. The following nursing diagnoses related to breast-feeding are diagnostic labels approved by the North American Nursing Diagnosis Association (NANDA):

- Effective breast-feeding: the state in which a mother-infant dyad/family exhibits adequate proficiency and satisfaction with the breast-feeding process.
- Ineffective breast-feeding: the state in which a mother or child experiences difficulty with the breast-feeding process.

- Interrupted breast-feeding: a break in the continuity of the breast-feeding process as a result of the inability or inadvisability to put the baby to breast for feeding.

Outcome Identification

A client outcome is a statement of the progression toward goal achievement. Collaborative planning with the new mother helps promote goal attainment. The breast-feeding mother would expect to progress toward the outcome of providing her infant with optimal nutrition supplied by breast milk in a specific time period.

Planning

After assessing the client and formulating the nursing diagnoses, the nurse must develop and implement a plan of care. Interventions are planned strategies, based on scientific rationale, devised by the nurse to assist the client in meeting the client's desired outcomes. Planning for breast-feeding clients would include discussion of proper feeding methods and infant positioning, and client demonstration of breast-feeding to assess the client's abilities.

Planning statements for breast-feeding mothers would include statements such as:

- The nursing plan for teaching breast-feeding information will include a discussion of proper feeding techniques and positioning, written materials, and a client demonstration of breast-feeding.

- The nurse's role includes teaching of proper feeding techniques and help in correcting any related problems.

Nursing Intervention

Implementation is the execution of the interventions that were devised during the planning stage. The nurse should use respect, empathy, and understanding when working with clients to encourage collaboration in this planning process. Many new mothers need help in ensuring proper positioning of the infant, correct attachment, and assistance in establishing a breast-feeding pattern.

Evaluation

Evaluation is the last phase of the nursing process. During the evaluation, the client's progress in reaching outcomes is determined. The nurse, in collaboration with the client, evaluates the effectiveness of the plan of care. The nurse evaluates both subjective and objective data on an ongoing basis. When the client's outcome goals have been met, then the plan of care has been effective. When the client's outcome goals have not been met, then the nurse and client must revise the nursing plan to include different interventions.

Evaluation of the breast-feeding plan of care would include statements such as the following:

- The client was able to demonstrate proper breast-feeding techniques.

- The client was able to explain proper self-care methods.

- The client was able to list signs and symptoms that would require medical care.

- The client was able to demonstrate proper pumping techniques.

- The client was able to list the signs that her infant was obtaining adequate breast milk.

- The client showed no signs of breast problems.

- The client was able to state support systems available to her after discharge.

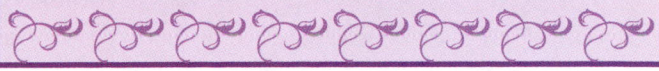

Case Study/Care Plan

THE CLIENT WITH INTERRUPTED BREAST-FEEDING

Judy Martin, aged 31, delivered her first child, a boy weighing 7 lb, 4 oz, 15 hours ago. Ms. Martin had a traumatic delivery and ran an elevated temperature of 102°F during the birth. Her infant was taken to the neonatal intensive care unit (NICU) for a sepsis workup to rule out infection. During Ms. Martin's first attempt at breast-feeding in the NICU, the infant had a difficult time latching on and both became agitated and anxious. Ms. Martin's nipples are slightly inverted, and her infant is having trouble latching on. Ms. Martin calls the nurse and is crying and very upset. She says that every time she attempts to nurse her infant, "He acts like I am killing him." She says either she has to have help today or she is going to quit breast-feeding.

Assessment

Subjective Data

- Client denies prenatal problems.
- Client states that because she had an elevated temperature (102°F) during a prolonged (more than 20 hours) labor and vaginal delivery, her infant was taken to NICU to rule out sepsis.
- Client states that the nurses have told her that her infant cannot be brought to her room for 48 hours.
- Client states that she had a very traumatic delivery, has a fourth-degree episiotomy, and is in pain.
- Client states she is a registered nurse and "really wants to breast-feed as soon as possible because she knows it is best for the baby."

Objective Data

- Client is a para 0, gravida 1, delivered at 39 weeks' gestation.
- Client vital signs: temperature, 98.8°F; pulse, 90; respirations, 20; blood pressure 110/80 mm Hg.
- Client has an intravenous infusion of 1000 mL lactated Ringer's with ampicillin, 500 mg, dripping at 100 mL/h.
- Client appears to be in pain when moving or sitting and needs help with ambulation.
- Breasts are soft; nipples have no cracks and are slightly inverted.
- Client is 15 hours post delivery.
- Infant is male, appropriate for gestational age.
- Infant's Apgar scores were 8 and 9.
- Gestational age assessment was 39 weeks.
- Infant weight is 7 lb, 14 oz, and length is 21 inches.
- Infant temperature is 98.2°F rectally.

Nursing Diagnosis

Interrupted breast-feeding related to possible illness in infant.

Expected Outcome	Client wants to breast-feed her infant successfully as soon as possible and plans on breast-feeding for 6 months.
Planning	Before leaving the hospital, the client will do the following:

1. Initiate breast-feeding behaviors as soon as the infant's condition allows.
2. Demonstrate proper breast-feeding techniques.
3. List three positions for breast-feeding.
4. Demonstrate appropriate techniques for attaching the infant to the breast.

(continued)

5. Maintain close contact with her infant.
6. Explain criteria to assess infant's hydration and weight gain status.
7. List proper pumping and storage techniques.
8. Discuss support resources she can use after hospital discharge.

Nursing Interventions	Rationales
1. Assist client to the NICU in a wheelchair to hold and breast-feed her infant as soon as permitted.	1. Client's physical condition requires assistance for ambulation.
2. Teach the client breast-feeding techniques, including positions and proper latching-on.	2. Many new mothers need help with the skills and techniques that must be learned for successful breast-feeding.
3. Provide the client with privacy and help in the NICU, as needed.	3. Privacy helps to allay some embarrassment and anxiety associated with breast-feeding for the first time.
4. Teach the client with information on infant nutritional assessment in short sessions using appropriate terms and language.	4. Teaching clients in short sessions helps prevent information overload and allows the client to process and remember the material presented.
5. Instruct the client on the use of breast pumps and milk storage.	5. The client may need to establish a milk supply with a pump and store her milk until the infant is discharged from the NICU.
6. Provide lists of breast-feeding resources and support available after discharge.	6. Written material allows the client to review information after discharge. Support for breast-feeding has been found to be an essential element in successful lactation.

Evaluation

- Client was taken to the NICU 15 hours after delivery to hold her infant and initiate breast-feeding.
- Client demonstrated proper breast-feeding techniques behind a movable screen, which provided privacy from the rest of the nursery.
- Client became anxious because her infant was unable to latch-on because of inverted nipples.
- Client was able to explain information provided to her, including proper pumping and storage of breast milk.
- Client stored the written materials in her suitcase for use after discharge.

Nursing Diagnosis

Ineffective breast-feeding related to poor latching-on.

Expected Outcome Client will effectively breast-feed her infant.

Planning
1. Client will call a lactation consultant today to obtain a visit to assess the breast-feeding pair.
2. Client will pump breast milk and use a specially designed nipple to feed the infant until the infant is able to latch on (a nipple specially designed to mimic the breast in both form and function).
3. Client will use a breast shield made of silicone to help the infant latch on and to stimulate the nipples to evert.
4. Client will use an electric breast pump to help maintain an adequate milk supply and to help pull out the nipples.
5. Client will have someone in her family take care of her and her infant when she is discharged to home to encourage rest and relaxation in new mother.

(continued)

Nursing Interventions	Rationales
1. Use a silicone breast shield to facilitate infant latching-on.	1. A silicone breast shield can protect sore nipples from further damage and make the nipples easier for the infant to grasp.
2. Apply ice compresses to the nipples just before feeding to stimulate them.	2. Ice numbs the nipples and makes them firmer and easier for the infant to grasp.
3. Lubricate the nipples with a few drops of expressed milk before feeding.	3. Expressed breast milk put on the nipples helps prevent tenderness.
4. Let the nipples dry thoroughly after feeding.	4. Air drying helps promote healing and comfort.
5. Apply warm tea bags to the nipples if soreness occurs.	5. Tannic acid in warm tea bags toughens the nipples, and the warmth promotes healing.
6. Avoid applying soaps to the nipples.	6. Soaps directly applied to the nipples can cause drying and cracking.
7. Encourage frequent feeding.	7. Frequent feedings help stimulate milk production, prevent stasis of breast milk, and reduce the risk of mastitis.
8. Use prophylactic breast massage after each feeding.	8. Breast massage helps prevent breast engorgement and stasis and promotes the let-down reflex and milk flow.
9. Express milk by using an electric breast pump, if necessary.	9. Expression of milk using an electric pump relieves overdistention and promotes milk drainage while maintaining the milk supply.
10. Take a warm shower.	10. Warm water promotes the let-down reflex and milk flow and enhances relaxation in the mother.

Evaluation   Ms. Martin met with the lactation consultant that day and felt very encouraged and more positive about continuing breast-feeding. Ms. Martin's infant nursed well with the breast shields in place and latched on well. Ms. Martin was aware that using breast shields can decrease milk supply and was instructed to gradually wean her infant off of the shields. She was also instructed that she should continue to pump after nursing to maintain milk supply. Ms. Martin continued to successfully breast-feed her infant and gradually weaned her infant to her own nipples.

Web Activities

- Which resources can you locate on the Internet for new mothers experiencing difficulties initiating breast-feeding?
- Where can a new mother locate a lactation consultant?
- Where can a new mother locate an electric breast pump?
- Where can a pregnant woman find a hospital that is "breast friendly"?

Key Concepts

- Breast-feeding provides unparalleled health benefits for infants and cost savings for mothers, families, the health care system, and taxpayers.

- Understanding the motivations and perceived barriers felt by many women can help health care professionals develop effective breast-feeding promotion strategies.

- When caring for a client whose culture is different from the nurse's culture, it is necessary to evaluate the impact of the client's values and beliefs on infant feeding practices.

- Interventions that lead to successful breast-feeding need to be individualized to fit the needs of each client.

- Promotion of successful breast-feeding requires that the nurse be sensitive to the needs of the mother so that a trusting relationship will permit the sharing of knowledge about techniques to facilitate lactation.

- Informed consent can only be obtained by providing women with both the advantages and disadvantages of breast- and formula-feeding.

- Although breast-feeding is a natural process, the necessary skills must be taught and learned by both mother and baby.

Review Questions and Activities

1. Compared with most prepared formulas, which does mature breast milk have?
   a. A thicker consistency
   b. More calories per ounce
   c. Greater immunologic value
   d. More nitrogenous wastes

   The correct answer is c.

2. How long after birth is colostrum replaced by transitional milk?
   a. 8 hours
   b. 12 to 24 hours
   c. 2 to 4 days
   d. 1 week

   The correct answer is c.

3. When should the nurse provide information about breast-feeding?
   a. First trimester
   b. Second trimester
   c. Third trimester
   d. First attempt at breast-feeding

   The correct answer is b.

4. What will a newborn do to indicate hunger to the mother who is breast-feeding?
   a. Wave the arms in the air
   b. Make sucking motions
   c. Have the hiccups
   d. Stretch the legs out straight

   The correct answer is b.

5. Which of the following hospital policies can interfere with breast-feeding duration?
   a. Distribution of formula samples
   b. Single-room maternity care
   c. Beginning breast-feeding during the first hour after delivery
   d. Encouraging mothers to feed on demand based on feeding readiness cues

   The correct answer is a.

6. A breast-feeding mother develops engorged breasts at 3 days postpartum. Which of the following actions would help reduce engorgement?
   a. Reducing fluid intake for 24 hours
   b. Breast-feeding her infant every 1 to 2 hours
   c. Avoiding use of a breast pump
   d. Skipping feedings to let her breasts rest

   The correct answer is b.

7. A new breast-feeding mother asks, "Is it true that breast milk will prevent my baby from catching colds and other infections?" Which reply can the nurse give that will reflect the results of current research?
   a. Breast-fed infants will have increased resistance to illness but may still get sick.
   b. Mothers of breast-fed infants do not have to worry about exposure to contagious diseases until breast-feeding stops.
   c. Breast milk offers no greater protection to breast-fed infants than does formula.
   d. Breast milk will give infants protection from all illnesses to which the mother is immune.

   The correct answer is d.

8. A new breast-feeding mother calls the nurse while breast-feeding her infant. The mother tells the nurse, "Something must be wrong. Every time I breastfeed my baby I feel like I am having labor pains again." Which of the following responses should the nurse give?
   a. "Your breasts are secreting a hormone that causes your abdominal muscles to contract."
   b. "Prolactin hormone is causing more blood to go to your uterus, resulting in pain."
   c. "The same hormone that is released in response to your baby's sucking and that causes the milk to flow also causes your uterus to contract."
   d. "You may have a small blood clot in your uterus, and you are trying to expel it."

   The correct answer is c.

9. When should a breast-fed infant be nursed?
   a. Every 4 hours
   b. Four to six times in 24 hours
   c. Eight to 12 times in 24 hours
   d. Every 3 hours, unless sleeping

   The correct answer is d.

10. Which of the following observations will allow a new mother to feel confident that her breast-fed infant is receiving enough milk?
    a. Six wet diapers in 24 hours, and four stools a day
    b. Three to four wet diapers in 24 hours and two stools a day
    c. One to two wet diapers in 24 hours, and six to eight stools a day
    d. No problem sleeping after nursing

    The correct answer is a.

References

Adams, D. (2000). Breastfeeding and oral contraceptives: Exploring opinions and the options. *AWHONN Lifelines, 4,* (3), 45–47.

Altman, L. (1998. July 26). AIDS brings a shift on breastfeeding: U.N. discouraging practice in women infected with H.I.V. *The New York Times,* pp. 1, 8.

American Academy of Pediatrics (1994). Committee on Drugs: The transfer of drugs and other chemicals into human milk (RE 9403). *Pediatrics, 93,* (1), 137–150.

American Academy of Pediatrics. (1992). Committee on nutrition: Follow-up of weaning formulas. *Pediatrics, 89,* 137.

American Academy of Pediatrics Work Group on Breastfeeding. (1997). Breastfeeding and the use of human milk. *Pediatrics, 100,* 1035–1039.

Baranowski, T, Bee, D., Rassin, D, Ricardson, C., Brown, J., Guenther, N., & Nader, P. (1983). Social support, social influence, ethnicity and the breastfeeding decision. *Society of Social Medicine, 17,* 1599–1611.

Bailey, D. (1997). World Breastfeeding Week 1997: "Breastfeeding: The Natural Way!" *International Lactation Consultant Association Globe,* Spring, 5, (2).

Bar-Yam, N. B. (1998). Workplace Lactation support, Part I: A return-to-work breastfeeding assessment tool. *Journal of Human Lactation, 14,* (3): 249–254.

Behrman, R., Kliegman, R., & Arvin, A. (Eds.). (1996). *Nelson's handbook of pediatrics* (15th ed.) Philadelphia, PA: W.B. Saunders.

Bliss, M., Wilkie, J., Adreolo, C., Berman, S., & Tebb, K. (1997). The effect of discharge pack formula and breast pumps on breast-feeding duration and choice of infant feeding method. *Birth: Issues in Perinatal Care and Education, 24,* 90–97.

Bodley, V., & Powers, D. (1999). Patient with insufficient glandular tissue experiences milk supply increase attributed to progesterone treatment for luteal phase defect. *Journal of Human Lactation, 15,* (4), 339–343.

Borch-Johnson, K., Joner, G., Mandrup-Poulsen, T., Christy, M., Zachau-Christiansen, B., Kastrup, K., & Newup, J. (1984). Relation between breastfeeding and incidence rates of insulin-dependent diabetes mellitus. A hypothesis. *Lancet 2,* 1083–1086.

Bromber Bar-Yam, N. (1998). Workplace lactation support, Part 1: A return-to-work breastfeeding assessment tool. *Journal of Human Lactation, 14,* (3), 249–254.

Brown, N. (1996). Use of human milk for low-birth-weight infants. Online *Journal of Knowledge Synthesis in Nursing, 3,* (27), 1–9.

Bryant, C., Bailey, D., & D'Angelo, S. (1989). *Best Start: A program brief.* Lexington, KY: Lexington-Fayette County Health Department.

Bryant, C. (1992). A strategy for promoting breastfeeding among economically disadvantaged women and adolescents. *NAACOG'S Clinical Issues in Perinatal & Women's Health Nursing, 3,* 723–730.

Buransin, B. (1991). The effect of rooming-in on the success of breastfeeding and the decline in abandonment of children. *Asia-Pacific Journal of Public Health, 5,* 217–220.

Callister, L., & Hobbins-Garbett, D. (2000). Cochrane pregnancy and childbirth database: Resource for evidence-based practice. *Journal of Obstetric, Gynecologic, and Neonatal Nursing, 29,* (2), 123–128.

Centers for Disease Control and Prevention. (1998). Guidelines for treatment of sexually transmitted diseases. *MMWR, 47,* 1–117.

Christensson, K., Selis, C., & Moreno, L. (1992). Temperature, metabolic adaptation and crying in healthy newborns' care for skin-to-skin. *Acta Paediatric, 81,* 488–493.

Crossette, B. (2000). Researchers raise fresh issues in breastfeeding debate. *New York Times on the Web,* www://nytimes.com.

Dewey, K. (1993). Maternal weight-loss patterns during prolonged lactation. *American Journal of Clinical Nutrition, 58,* 162.

Dewey, K., Heinig, M., Normmsen-Rivers, L. (1995). Differences in morbidity between breast-fed and formula-fed infants. *Journal of Pediatrics,* (5), 126, 696–702.

Hale, T. (1999–2000). *Medications and mother's milk.* Amarillo, TX: Pharmasoft Medical Publishing.

Hale, T. (1999). Anesthetic medications in breastfeeding mothers. *Journal of Human Lactation, 15,* (3), 185–194.

Hartley, B., & O'Connor, M. (1996). Evaluation of the "Best Start" breastfeeding education program. *Archives of Pediatric and Adolescent Medicine, 150,* 868–871.

Heinig, M. J. (2000). Bed sharing and infant mortality: Guilt by association? *Journal of Human Lactation, 16,* (3), 189–191.

Heinig, M. J. (1999). Evidence-based practice: Art versus science? *Journal of Human Lactation, 15,* (3), 183–184.

Heinig, M. J., & Francis, J. (1999). Mammary candidosis in lactating women. *Journal of Human Lactation, 15,* (4), 281–288.

Heinig, M. J. (1997). Staying abreast of the latest scientific controversies: Infant feeding and insulin-dependent diabetes mellitus. *Journal of Human Lactation, 13,* (2), 91–92.

Hill, P. (2000). Update on breastfeeding: Healthy people 2010 objectives. *MCN, American Journal of Maternal/Child Nursing, 25,* (5), 248–251.

Hoffmann, D. (1992). *The new holistic herbal.* Rockport, MA: Element.

Hutchinson, M., & Baqi-Aziz, M. (1994). Nursing care of the childbearing Muslim family. *Journal of Obstetric, Gynecologic and Neonatal Nurses, 17,* (2), 767–769.

International Lactation Consultants Association. (1999). Evidence-based guidelines for breastfeeding management during the first fourteen days. Raleigh, NC: International Lactation Consultant Association.

ILCA Globe Newsletter. (1997). Best Start and WIC cooperate to promote breastfeeding. *ILCA Globe, 5,* 2.

Ivnas-Mobert, K. (1989). The effects of breastfeeding on gastrointestinal absorption. *Scientific American, 7,* 78–83.

Jarosz, L. (1993). Breast-feeding versus formula: Cost comparison. *Hawaii Medical Journal, 52,* (1), 14–18.

Kistin, N., Abramson, R., & Dublin, P. (1994). Effect of peer counselors on breastfeeding initiation, exclusivity, and duration among low-income women. *Journal of Human Lactation, 10,* 11–15.

Klaus, M., Kennell, J., & Klaus, P. (1995). *Bonding: Building the foundation of a secure attachment and independence.* Reading, MA: Perseus Books.

Klaus, M., & Klaus, P. (1998). *Your amazing newborn.* Reading, MA: Perseus Books.

Kopec, K. (1999). Herbal medications and breastfeeding. *Journal of Human Lactation, 15,* (2), 157–161.

Kovar, M., Serdula, M., Marks, J., & Fraser, D. (1984). Review of the epidemiologic evidence for an association between infant feeding and infant health. *Pediatrics* (Task Force on Infant Feeding Practices), 615–638.

Lamaze International. (1998). A special report on breastfeeding. *ASPO/Lamaze, 1* (7), 3.

Lawrence, R. (1999). *Breastfeeding: A guide for the medical profession* (5th ed.). St. Louis, MO: Mosby.

Little, R. E. (1989). Maternal alcohol use during breast-feeding and infant mental and mother development at one year. *New England Journal of Medicine, 321,* 425–430.

Lucas, A., Morley, R., Cole, T., Lister, G., & Leeson-Payne, C. (1992). Breast milk and subsequent intelligence quotient in children born preterm. *The Lancet, 339,* 261–264.

Martin, C. (2000). *The nursing mother's problem solver.* New York: Fireside.

McClurg-Hitt, D., & Olsen, J. (1994). Infant feeding decisions in the Missouri WIC program. *Journal of Human Lactation, 10,* (4), 253–256.

Meier, P., Brown, L., Hurst, N., Spatz, D., Engstrom, J, Borucki, L., & Krouse, A. (2000). Nipple shields for preterm infants: Effect on milk transfer and duration of breastfeeding. *Journal of Human Lactation, 16,* (2), 106–114.

Meloni, T., La Vecchia, C., Marinaro, A., Negri, E., Mannazzu, M., Colombo, C, & Ogana, A. (1997). IDDM and early infant feeding: Sardinian case-control study. *Diabetic Care, 20,* 340–342.

Methodist Hospital. (1999). *Guidelines for breastfeeding your baby.* Houston, TX: Methodist Press.

Mohrbacher, N., & Stock, J. (1997). *The breastfeeding answer book.* Schaumburg, IL: La Leche League International.

Mothers Survey, Ross Products Division, Abbott Laboratories. (2000). *Breastfeeding Trends Through 1999.*

National Institute on Drug Abuse. (1998). *Drug abuse statistics: 1998 population estimates,* Washington, DC: Alcohol, Drug Abuse, and Mental Health, U.S. Public Health Service.

Newcombe, P., Storer, B., & Longnecker, M. (1994). Lactation and a reduced risk of premenopausal breast cancer. *New England Journal of Medicine, 330,* 81.

Newman, J. (1995). How breast milk protects newborns. *Scientific American,* 76–79.

O'Brien, C. (1998). Cooperative Study Focuses on Ovarian Cancer. *The Texas Medical Center News,* p. 11. August 15

Pedersen, C. (1992). Oxytocin activation of maternal behavior in the rat. *Annual New York Academy of Science,* 652–658.

Perez, A., Labbok, M., & Keenan, J. (1992). Clinical studies of the lactational amenorrhea method for family planning. *The Lancet, 339,* 968–970.

Popkin, B., Adair, L., Akin, J., Black, R., Briscoe, J., & Flieger, W. (1990). Breastfeeding and diarrheal morbidity. *Pediatrics, 88,* (6), 874–882.

Public Health Service. (1990). *Healthy People 2000 (National Health Promotion and Disease Prevention Objectives).* Washington, DC: U.S. Department of Health and Human Services, p. 123.

Raj, V., & Plichta, S. (1998). The role of social support in breastfeeding promotion: A literature review. *Journal of Human Lactation, 14,* (1), 41–45.

Reifsnider, E., & Gill, S. (2000). Nutrition for the Childbearing Years. *Journal of Obstetric, Gynecologic, and Neonatal Nursing, 29,* (1), 43–55.

Riordan, J. (2000). Teaching breastfeeding on the Web. *Journal of Human Lactation, 16,* (3), 231–234.

Riordan, J. (1997). The cost of not breastfeeding: A commentary. *Journal of Human Lactation, 13,* (2), 93–97.

Riordan, J., & Auerbach, K. (1999). *Breastfeeding and human lactation.* Sudbury, MA: Jones & Barlett Publishers.

Roberts, K., Reiter, M., & Schuster, D. (1998). Effects of cabbage leaf extract on breast engorgement. *Journal of Human Lactation, 14,* (3), 231–236.

Ryan, A. (1997). Electronic article: The resurgence of breastfeeding in the United States. *Pediatrics, 99,* (4), p. e12.

Scragg, L., Mitchell, E., & Tonkin, S. (1993). Evaluation of the cot death prevention programme in South Auckland. *New Zealand Medical Journal, 8,* 106.

Simpson, K. (1999). Should nurses offer discharge formula samples to women who plan to breastfeed? *MCN, The American Journal of Maternal Child Nursing, 24,* (4), 166–167.

Smith, W. E., Evenberg, A., Nowak, A. & Franken, E. A., (1988). Imaging evaluation of the human nipple during breastfeeding. *American Journal of Disabilities in Children 142,* (1), 76–78.

Underwood, S., Pridham, K., Brown, L., Clark, T., Frazier, W., Limbo, R., Schroeder, M., & Thoyre, S. (1997). Infant feeding practices of low-income African-American women in a central city community. *Journal of Community Health Nursing, 14,* (3), 189–205.

United States Department of Health and Human Services (2000). *Healthy People 2010.* Washington, D.C.: U.S. Government Printing Office.

Ulvnas-Moberg, K. (1989). The gastrointestinal tract in growth and reproduction. *Scientific American,* July, 78–83.

Weinberg, G. (2000). The dilemma of postnatal mother-to-child transmission of HIV: To breastfeed or not? *Birth, 27,* (3), 199–205.

WHO/UNICEF. (1994). Protecting, promoting, and supporting breastfeeding: The special role of maternity hospitals. *A Joint Statement by WHO/UNICEF.* Geneva, 1989, World Health Organization.

Widstrom, A., Wahlberg, W., & Mathiesen, A. (1990). Short term effects of early suckling and touch of the nipple on maternal behavior. *Journal of Early Human Development, 21,* 153–163.

World Health Organization. (1994). Progestin only contraceptives during lactation: Infant growth. *Contraception, 50,* 55–58.

World Health Organization. (1988). Special task force on oral contraceptives: Effects of hormonal contraceptives on breast milk composition and infant growth. *Study of Family Planning, 19,* 361–369.

Worthington-Roberts, B., & Williams, S. (1993). *Nutrition in pregnancy and lactation* (5th ed.). St. Louis: C.V. Mosby.

Yoo, K.-Y., Tajima, K., & Kuroishi, T. (1992). Independent protective effect of lactation against breast cancer: A case-control study in Japan. *American Journal of Epidemiology, 135,* 726.

Suggested Readings

Auerbach, G., & Riordan, J. (2000). *Clinical lactation: A visual guide.* Sudbury, MA: Jones & Barlett Publishers.

Biancuzzo, M. (1998). *Breastfeeding the newborn: Clinical strategies for nurses.* St. Louis: Mosby.

Grossman, L., Fitzsimmons, S., Larsen-Alexander, J., Sachs, L., & Harter, C. (1990). The infant feeding decision in low and upper income women. *Clinical Pediatrics, 29,* (1), 30–37.

Healthy People 2010. (1999). Healthy people 2010 objectives: http://web.health.gov./healthypeople/2010/object.htm.

Janke, J. (1993). The incidence, benefits and variables associated with breastfeeding: Implications for practice. *Journal of Obstetric, Gynecologic and Neonatal Nurses, 18,* (6), 22–29.

Libbus, K., & Kolostov, L. (1994). Perceptions of breastfeeding and infant feeding choice in a group of low-income mid-Missouri women. *Journal of Human Lactation, 10,* (1), 17–23.

Pryor, G. (1999). *Nursing mother, working mother: The essential guide for breastfeeding and staying close to your baby when you return to work.* New York: Harvard Common Press.

Snell, B., Krantz, M., Keeton, R., Delgado, K., & Peckman, C. (1992). The association of formula samples given at hospital discharge with the early duration of breastfeeding. *Journal of Human Lactation, 8,* (2), 67–72.

Stuart-Macadam, P., & Dettwyler, K. (Eds). (1995). *Breastfeeding biocultural perspectives.* New York: Aldine De Gruyer.

UNICEF. (1994). Barriers and solutions to the global 10 steps to successful breastfeeding: A summary of in depth interviews with hospitals participating in the WHO/UNICEF baby friendly hospital initiative interim program in the United States. *U.S. Committee for UNICEF,* April 1994.

Wiesenfeld, A., Malatesta, C., & Whitman, P. (1985). Psychophysiological response of breast and bottle-feeding mothers to their infant's signals. *Psychophysiology, 22,* 79.

Resources

American Academy of Pediatrics
www.aap.org/visit/breastww.htm
www.aap.org/advocacy/washing/brfeed.htm
www.pediatrics.org/cgi/content/full/99/4/e12
Website for Health People 2010 Document
www.health.gov/healthypeople
United States Government
www.house.gov
The Cochrane Pregnancy and Childbirth database is an ongoing meta-analysis of evidence documenting effective health care practices for childbearing women and their neonates.
www.hcn.net.au/cochrane
Association of Woman's Health, Obstetric, and Neonatal Nursing
www.awhonn.org

Organization of Certified Nurse Midwives
www.midwives.org
HealthWeb: Evidence-Based Health Care
www.uic.edu/depts/lib/health/hw/ebhc
National Guideline Clearinghouse
www.guidelines.gov
Cumulative Index to Nursing and Allied Health Literature (CINAHL)
www.cinalhl.com
Medline National Library of Medicine
www.nlm.nih.gov
Health STAR
www.nlm.nih.gov
www.parentsplace.com/expert/lactation

Resources for breastfeeding, La Leche League, 1400 N. Meacham Road, Schaumburg, IL 60173, 800-525-3242 (42-hour line), www.lalecheleague.org

International Lactation Consultant Association, 201 Brown Avenue, Evanston, IL 60202-3601, 708-260-8874

American Academy of Pediatrics, 141 Northwest Point Boulevard, Elk Grove, IL 60007-1098, 847-228-5005, www.aap.org

Academy of Breastfeeding Medicine

Special Supplemental Nutrition Program for Women, Infants, and Children (WIC), Food and Consumer Service, 3101 Park Center Drive, Room 819, Alexandria, VA 22302, 703-305-2286, www.usda.gov/fns/wic/html

Association of Women's Health, Obstetrics and Neonatal Nursing (AWHONN), 2000 L Street NW, Suite 740, Washington, DC 20036, 800-673-8499, www.awhonn.org

Human Milk Banking Association of North America (HMBANA), HMBANA Executive Office, P.O. Box 370464, West Hartford, CT 06137-0464, 800-232-8809

Baby Friendly Hospital Initiative, Baby Friendly USA, 8 Jan Sebastian Way, Unit 13, Sandwich, MA 02565, www.aboutus.com/a100/bfusa

National Alliance for Breastfeeding Advocacy (NABA), Breastfeeding as the Foundation for Health, http://members.aol.com/marshalact/Naba

World Breastfeeding Week, World Alliance for Breastfeeding Action (WABA), P.O. Box 1200, 10850 Penang, Malaysia

International Lactation Consultants Association (ILCA): Evidence-based guidelines for breastfeeding management during the first 14 days. Raleigh, NC

U.S. Representative Carolyn Maloney, Breastfeeding legislation in the 106th Congress, www.house.gov.maloney

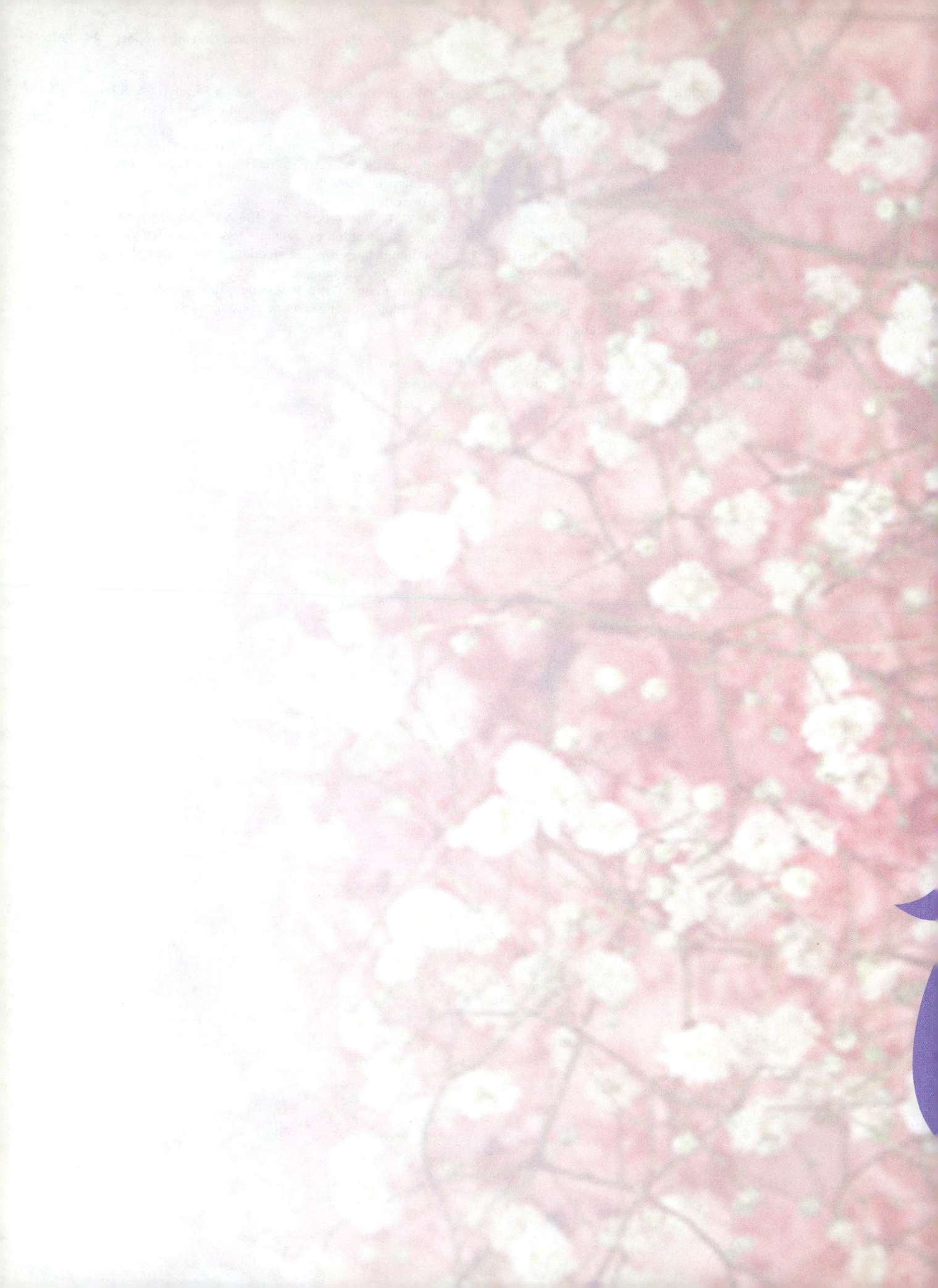

UNIT VIII

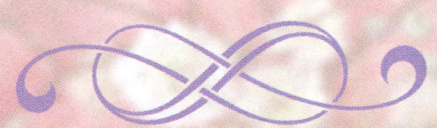

Newborn Development and Nursing Care

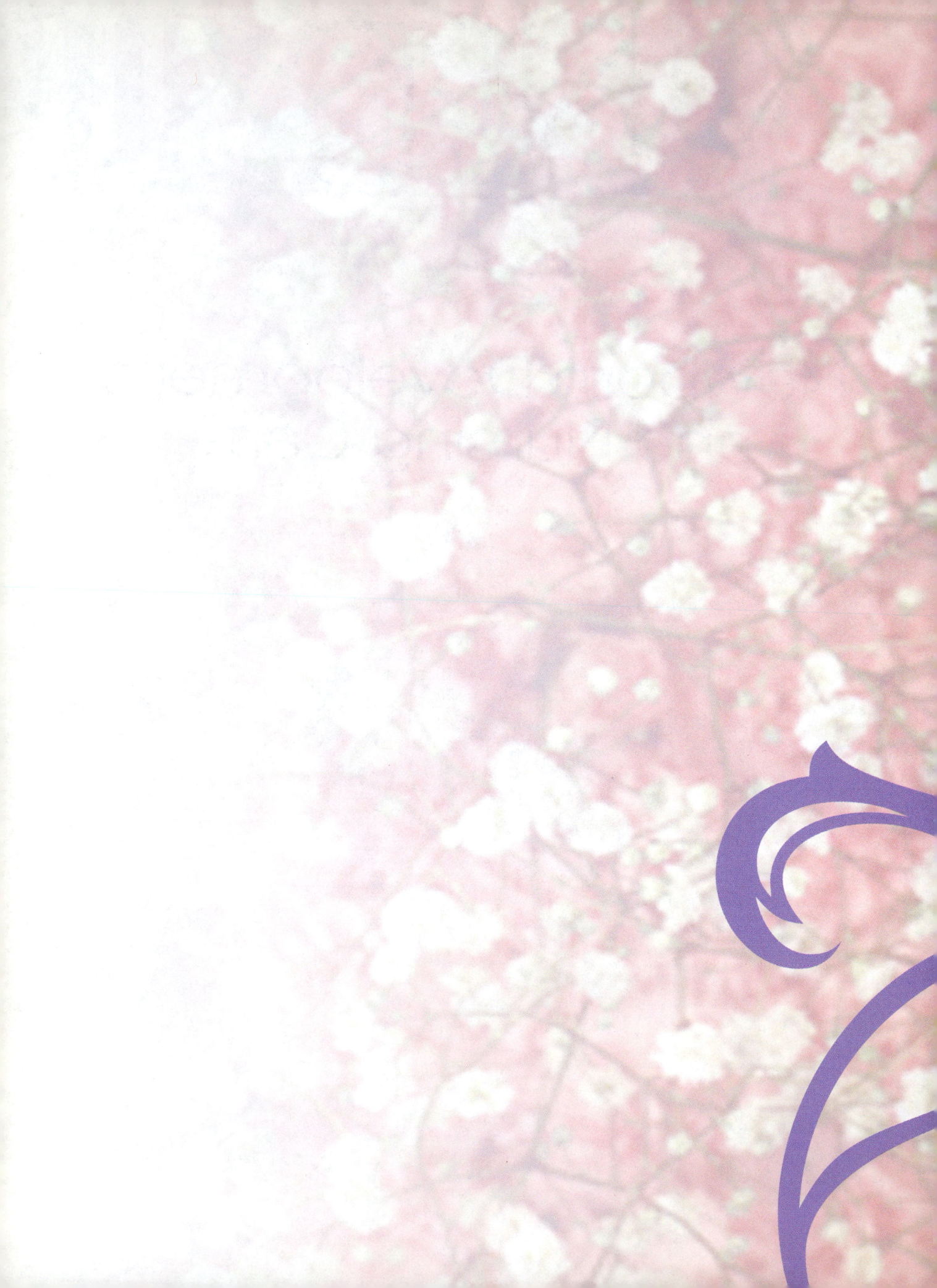

Physiologic and Behavioral Transition to Extrauterine Life

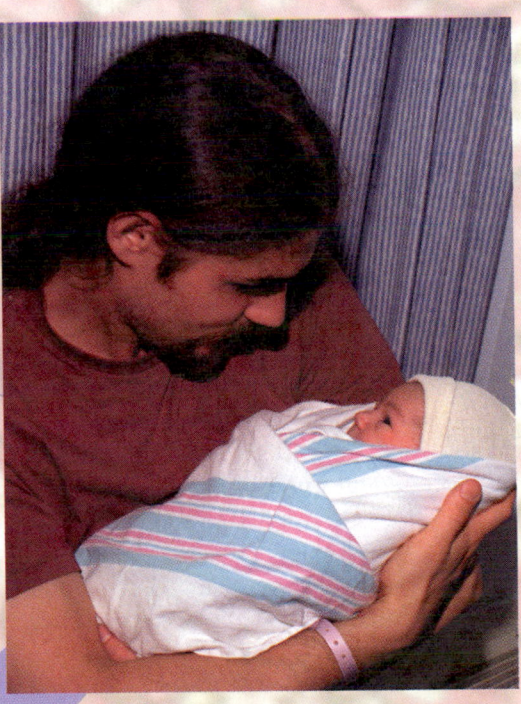

The journey to birth is nothing more than an incredible miracle of life. This journey requires a number of successful transitions if the newborn is to survive. In utero, the fetus is entirely dependent on the placenta to sustain physiologic functions and to provide nutrition necessary for optimal growth and development. Following birth, a number of major physiologic changes must occur if the infant is to make a successful transition to extrauterine life, including pulmonary, cardiovascular, and gastrointestinal changes.

The first few hours after birth of a baby are also a time of transition for the parents. Perinatal nurses play an important role in helping parents to make a successful transition to parenthood by facilitating positive parent-infant interactions and providing education on routine baby care. Anticipatory guidance and crisis intervention are also important aspects of the perinatal nurses' role in caring for parents who experience delivery complications or the birth of a sick newborn.

Key Terms

Asphyxia
Behavioral state
Congenital heart defects
Diaphragmatic hernia
Ductus arteriosus
Ductus venosus
Extrauterine life
Fetal circulation

Foramen ovale
Habituation
Hypoglycemia
Hypothermia
Hypovolemia
Meconium staining
Neutral thermal
   environment

Persistent pulmonary
   hypertension
Postnatal circulation
Preterm
Primary apnea
Pulmonary vascular
   resistance
Resuscitation

Secondary apnea
Sepsis
Surfactant
Systemic vascular
   resistance
Thermoregulation
Transient tachypnea of
   the newborn

Competencies

Upon completion of this chapter, the reader should be able to:

1. Describe the primary features of the fetal pulmonary and cardiac systems.

2. Identify the physiologic changes that occur at birth as the newborn makes the transition to extrauterine life.

3. Describe the neurobehavioral changes that occur during the first 12 hours after birth as the newborn makes the transition to extrauterine life.

4. Discuss the parenting and family issues that occur during the period of newborn transition to extrauterine life.

5. Understand the major complications that can occur during the transition process.

6. Discuss the effects of prematurity on the transition to extrauterine life.

7. Understand the role and responsibilities of the nurse during the transition process.

8. Discuss appropriate resuscitation of the asphyxiated infant, using the American Academy of Pediatrics and American Heart Association Neonatal Resuscitation Program guidelines.

Transitions by nature are challenging, but this is never more true than it is for transition from intrauterine to **extrauterine life**. In fact, the essence of life depends on this successful transition. Successful transition requires the initiation of spontaneous breathing; significant cardiopulmonary changes, including the shift from fetal to postnatal circulation; and a variety of other important adaptations, including but not limited to, thermoregulatory and metabolic adjustments. Failure of the infant to make a successful transition may result in varying degrees of morbidity or mortality.

Two major factors have contributed to today's awareness of the importance of the process of the infant's transition to extrauterine life in the first critical hours after birth. First, the technology and assessment techniques available to monitor the well-being of the fetus and the neonate have increased in sophistication, availability, and routine use. Strategies, such as fetal monitoring, sonography, and development of training and certification in the assessment

of fetal heart rate monitoring and resuscitation, have all heightened the awareness of the complexity of the physiologic changes the neonate undergoes in the hours before, during, and after birth. Second, the changes in health care policy that have led to shorter and shorter hospital stays for mothers and babies have created an increased need for careful assessment of the infant's transition process during the hours before discharge from the hospital (Behram, Moschler, Sayegh, Garguillo, & Mann, 1998).

This chapter, therefore, explores the physiologic changes that occur during the newborn's adaptation to extrauterine life and discusses common newborn complications that may impede the newborn's ability to adapt successfully. First, this chapter explores physiologic and neurobehavioral transitions of the newborn, at and immediately following birth. Common neonatal conditions and diseases that may interfere with the newborn's smooth transition to extrauterine life and require resuscitation and stabilization in the delivery room are discussed, as well as the effect of prematurity on pulmonary and cardiac transition. Finally, standards for resuscitation of newborns in the delivery room established by the American Academy of Pediatrics and the American Heart Association are discussed.

PHYSIOLOGIC TRANSITIONS OF MAJOR SYSTEMS

Physiologic transition from intrauterine to extrauterine life involves a number of major changes that are necessary for newborn survival. These include pulmonary, cardiac, thermoregulation, metabolic, and gastrointestinal changes.

Pulmonary System Transition

During uterine development, the placenta is the organ of respiration, with the lungs receiving little of the cardiac output (Guyton & Hall, 1996). The blood bypasses the lungs through shunt pathways, such as the ductus venosus, the ductus arteriosus, and the foramen ovale. This occurs primarily because of pressure gradient differences between pulmonary and systemic vascular systems. In the fetus, the lungs are a high-resistance, low-flow organ (Guyton & Hall, 1996).

Pulmonary vascular resistance (PVR) is the resistance in the pulmonary vascular bed against which the right ventricle must eject blood. High levels of fetal PVR are caused by a number of interrelated factors that promote constriction of the pulmonary capillaries. These factors include the thick muscular medial layer of the small pulmonary arteries (Sansoucie & Cavaliere, 1997), the low P_{O_2} levels normally present during fetal life (Pridjian, 1994), and possibly, the compression of the pulmonary capillaries by fetal lung fluid. The high level of PVR is also thought to be influenced by the absence of air-fluid interface in the alveoli, the lack of rhythmic distention of the lung, and the large amount of active vasoconstricting substances present within the pulmonary bed (Sansoucie & Cavaliere, 1997).

Because of this high-pressure gradient in the pulmonary system, the oxygenation of the fetus occurs in the placenta (Guyton & Hall, 1996; Nelson, 1994; Sansoucie & Cavaliere, 1997). The exchange of oxygen (O_2) and carbon dioxide (CO_2) within the placenta occurs by simple diffusion at the intervillous space (Sansoucie & Cavaliere, 1997). Differences in diffusion pressures of O_2 and CO_2 between the fetal and maternal sides of the placenta facilitate and regulate the exchange of gases between mother and fetus (Guyton & Hall, 1996; Pridjian, 1994). Because blood on the fetal side of the placenta has a lower (30 mm Hg) partial pressure of dissolved oxygen (P_{O_2}) than blood on the maternal side (50 mm Hg), oxygen readily diffuses from the maternal side of the placenta to the fetal side (Guyton & Hall, 1996). Blood on the fetal side of the pla-

centa, with a higher partial pressure of dissolved carbon dioxide (P_{CO_2}), is readily diffused to the lower pressure maternal side of the placenta (Guyton & Hall, 1996). In addition, with the exchange of gases, the relative changes in serum pH between the maternal and fetal sides of the placenta also contribute to fetal oxygenation (Guyton & Hall, 1996). For example, as CO_2 from the fetal circulation diffuses into the maternal circulation, the maternal P_{CO_2} increases and, correspondingly, maternal plasma pH falls. This increase in acidity interferes with the ability of maternal hemoglobin (Hgb) to bind oxygen and thereby promotes the transfer of the oxygen to blood on the fetal side of the placenta. Simultaneously, as the fetal blood loses CO_2 and the fetal pH increases, the fetal Hgb binds the oxygen released by the maternal Hgb more readily.

In addition to the simple diffusion processes just described, differences in O_2 content (i.e. dissolved and hemoglobin-bound O_2) and higher concentrations of fetal Hgb also serve to facilitate oxygenation in the fetus (Box 31-1). The O_2 content of the blood on each side of the placental membrane is determined in large part by the different affinities of maternal and fetal Hgb for O_2 (Pridjian, 1994). Oxygen-carrying capacity is enhanced by the increased presence of fetal Hgb. At any given P_{O_2}, fetal Hgb has a higher affinity for oxygen than does maternal adult Hgb (Guyton & Hall, 1996; Sansoucie & Cavaliere, 1997). Furthermore, the shift of the fetal oxyhemoglobin dissociation curve to the left of the maternal curve allows enhanced oxygen delivery to the peripheral tissues when capillary P_{O_2} is low (Guyton & Hall, 1996; Pridjian, 1994).

Pulmonary adaptation at birth is accomplished via a complex series of events that switches the function of respiration from the placenta to the lungs. Various metabolic and environmental factors are responsible for the onset of breathing in the neonate. Mild hypercapnia, hypoxia, and acidosis act as powerful stimuli for the onset of breathing in the newly born infant and result from the intermittent cessation of uteroplacental perfusion during contractions, which occurs during normal labor (Guyton & Hall, 1996; Nelson, 1994). While the decreased pH stimulates the respiratory center directly, the low level of pO_2

> **Box 31-1 Factors Enhancing Oxygen Delivery to Fetus**
>
> - Lower P_{O_2} on fetal side of placenta
> - Fall in level of maternal plasma pH from transfer of fetal CO_2
> - Increased fetal pH
> - Higher concentrations of fetal hemoglobin
> - Left shift of fetal oxyhemoglobin dissociation curve

and high level of pCO_2 stimulate the respiratory center via central and peripheral chemoreceptors. Other external stimuli that also enhance rhythmic breathing at delivery include the environmental factors of cold, light, noise, and touch (Nelson, 1994).

During pulmonary transition, fluid within the lung must also be cleared. During labor, fetal lung fluid is beginning to be reabsorbed. During vaginal delivery, the chest wall is compressed and approximately one-third of the fetal lung fluid is expelled via the trachea. Following delivery of the chest, the chest wall recoils causing inspiration of air and expansion of the lungs (Nelson, 1994). The transpulmonary pressure generated by the first breath drives the remaining fetal lung fluid into the interstitium, where it is absorbed through the lymphatic and pulmonary circulation (Donn & Faix, 1996; Guyton & Hall, 1996; Nelson, 1994).

The work of inspiration is mainly devoted to overcoming the surface tension of the walls of the terminal lung units at the air-liquid interface (Guyton & Hall, 1996; Nelson, 1994). On expiration, the ability to retain air depends on surfactant. **Surfactant** is a complete lipoprotein produced by type II alveolar pneumocytes and plays a role in lowering surface tension at an air-liquid interface (Guyton & Hall, 1996). As surfactant lowers surface tension in the alveolus at end-expiration, it stabilizes the alveoli and prevents collapse (Nelson, 1994). There is an increased functional residual capacity with each breath; thus, less inspiratory pressure is required for subsequent breaths (Guyton & Hall, 1996; Nelson, 1994).

The establishment of normal resting lung volume or functional residual capacity is important because of its role in allowing the PVR level to fall postnatally. With initial lung expansion, the pulmonary arterioles dilate in response to the increase in Po_2, and the PVR level falls (Guyton & Hall, 1996). With the abrupt lowering of resistance comes an equally abrupt increase in pulmonary blood flow (Guyton & Hall, 1996). Pulmonary vascular tone and blood flow are also modulated by vasoactive substances produced by the pulmonary endothelial cell. Prostaglandins and endothelium-derived relaxing factor are vasoactive substances that act directly to promote pulmonary vasodilation within the transitional pulmonary vasculature bed (Sansoucie & Cavaliere, 1997). As a result of the structural and physiologic adaptation of the pulmonary bed to lung inflation at birth, the lungs convert to a low-resistance, high-flow organ (Sansoucie & Cavaliere, 1997). Lung compliance continues to improve in the hours after delivery, secondary to the effects of circulating catecholamines. The increased levels of catecholamines (especially epinephrine) play important roles in increasing the release of surfactant at birth and in clearing the lungs by decreasing secretion of lung fluids and increasing their absorption through the lymphatic system. PVR progressively decreases until adult levels are reached at 2 to 3 weeks of age.

Cardiac System Transition

Cardiac transition from intrauterine to extrauterine life involves closure of fetal circulatory pathways and other cardiovascular adaptations that promote increased blood flow to the lungs for oxygenation and switch the fetal circulation to a postnatal (adult) circulatory pathway.

Fetal circulatory Pathways

Fetal circulation is anatomically and physiologically different than that of the infant in the extrauterine environment. This difference allows the oxygenation of the fetus to occur in the placenta rather than in the pulmonary system. Among the important differences are the existence of three anatomic shunts that, in utero, allow the most highly oxygenated blood to be preferentially delivered from the placenta to the brain and heart, while being diverted from the lungs (Donn & Faix, 1996; Guyton & Hall, 1996; Nelson, 1994; Sansoucie & Cavaliere, 1997). The three fetal circulatory shunts include the ductus venosus, the foramen ovale, and the ductus arteriosus. The **ductus venosus**, which connects the umbilical vein to the inferior vena cava, allows blood to bypass the liver. The **foramen ovale** allows blood entering the right atrium of the heart to go directly through the left atrium, left ventricle, and out the ascending aorta to immediately supply the brain, heart, and upper extremities. The **ductus arteriosus** shunts blood from the pulmonary artery to the descending aorta, bypassing the lung, to perfuse the lower body and return to the placenta for oxygenation. Figure 31-1 illustrates fetal circulation.

Blood oxygenated in the placenta travels to the fetus via a single umbilical vein. Fifty percent to 60% of the umbilical venous blood bypasses the liver through the ductus venosus to connect with the inferior vena cava (Sansoucie & Cavaliere, 1997). The other half passes through the liver and enters the inferior vena cava via the hepatic veins. To preserve the most highly oxygenated blood for the brain and heart, umbilical venous blood that bypassed the liver tends to stream separately from blood returning from lower portions of the body within the inferior vena cava (Sansoucie & Cavaliere, 1997). From the inferior vena cava, blood enters the right atrium. As a consequence of right atrium anatomy, the more highly oxygenated blood from the inferior vena cava tends to stream directly across the atrial septum via the foramen ovale to the left atrium (Donn & Faix, 1996; Guyton & Hall, 1996; Sansoucie & Cavaliere, 1997). Once in the left atrium, the blood from the right atrium mixes with a small amount of pulmonary venous return that arrives via the pulmonary veins. Blood from the left atrium passes through the mitral valve and enters the left ventricle, where it is pumped out through the aortic valve to the ascending aorta to perfuse the brain, heart, and upper extremities (Sansoucie & Cavaliere, 1997; Donn & Faix, 1996).

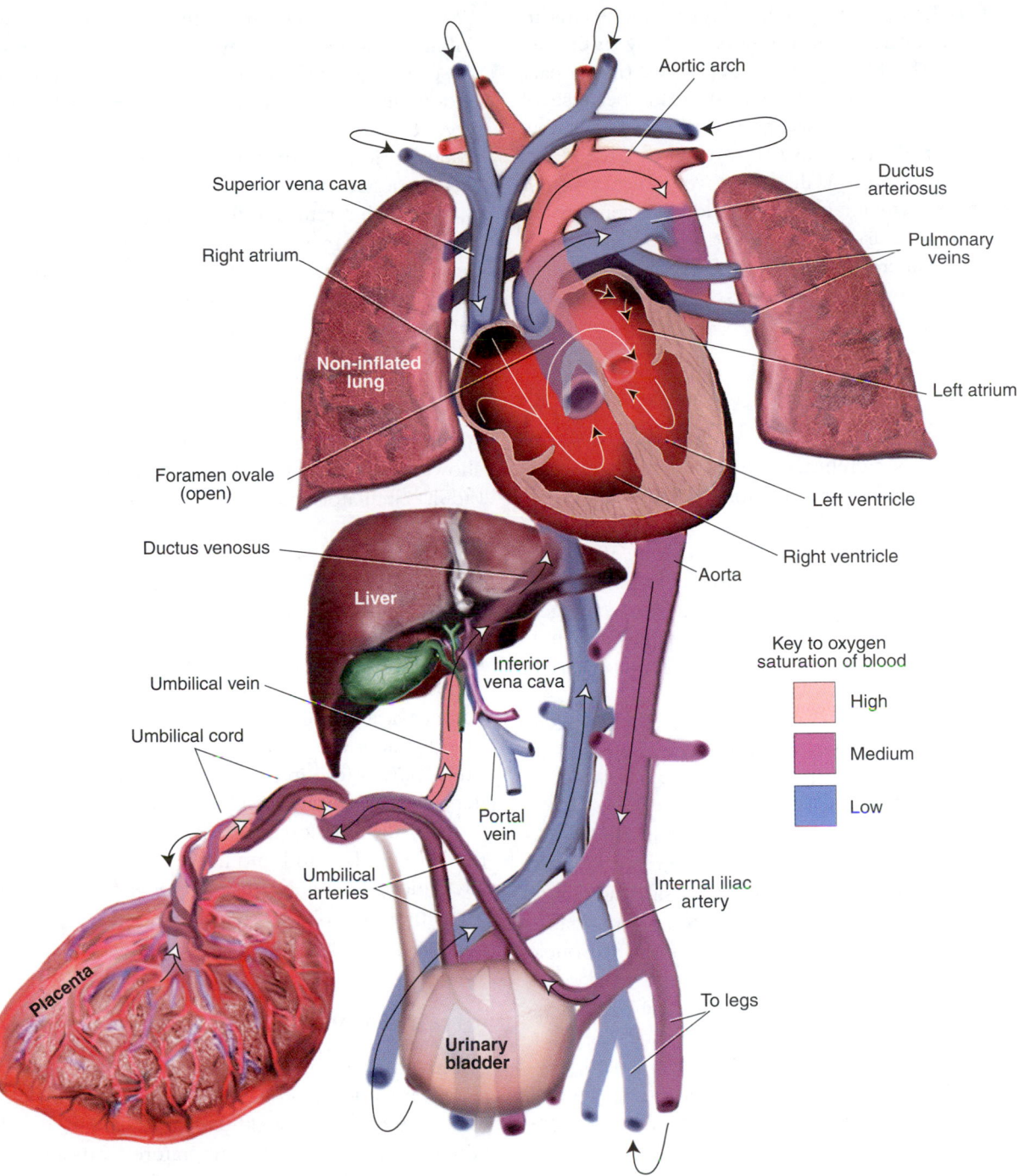

Figure 31-1 Fetal circulation. *Red* shows arterial blood, *dark purple* shows venous blood, and *light purple* shows mixed arterial venous blood.

Unoxygenated blood returning from the brain and upper extremities returns to the heart by way of the superior vena cava. In the right atrium, some mixing occurs between the unoxygenated blood from the superior vena cava and coronary sinus and the inferior vena caval blood not shunted directly into the left atrium via the foramen ovale (Donn & Faix, 1996). The majority of the blood enters the right atrium and flows to the right ventricle. The

right ventricle is the dominant ventricle in fetal life, ultimately ejecting about two-thirds of the total cardiac output to perfuse the lower body and placenta (Sansoucie & Cavaliere, 1997). From the right ventricle, blood crosses the pulmonary valve, but because of high pulmonary vascular pressures, most of the blood is directed away from the lungs. Approximately 12% of the blood flows into pulmonary veins to nourish the lung (Guyton & Hall, 1996).

The majority of blood bypasses the lungs via the ductus arteriosus, which connects the pulmonary artery to the descending aorta. The blood flows right to left (pulmonary artery to aorta) across the ductus arteriosus because of high pulmonary vascular resistance (PVR) levels and low systemic vascular resistance (SVR) (a result of low placental resistance) (Guyton & Hall, 1996). The patency of the ductus arteriosus is maintained by the low oxygen tension in utero and by the vasodilating effect of prostaglandin E_2 (Sansoucie & Cavaliere, 1997). Blood from the descending aorta supplies kidneys and intestines, divides into two arteries, and returns blood to the low-resistance placenta for oxygenation.

Cardiovascular Adaptation

The first breath has significant effects on cardiovascular function. With the onset of ventilation, there is a concomitant decrease in PVR and an increase in pulmonary vascular flow (Nelson, 1994; Sansoucie & Cavaliere, 1997). Increased alveolar oxygenation is accompanied by a further decrease in PVR. As a result of these pulmonary changes, the pressure in the right side of the heart falls and pulmonary venous return increases to the left atrium (Nelson, 1994).

With cord clamping and the loss of placenta circulation, **systemic (peripheral) vascular resistance** (SVR) increases and exceeds PVR (Donn & Faix, 1996; Nelson, 1994; Sansoucie & Cavaliere, 1997). As a result, pressures within the aorta and left heart increase significantly. The reversal of relative pressures leads to diminished right-to-left shunting across the foramen ovale, causing the flap to shut between the two atria within minutes or hours after birth (Donn & Faix, 1996; Guyton & Hall, 1996; Sansoucie & Cavaliere, 1997). Anatomic closure caused by the deposit of fibrin and cell products is usually completed during the first month of life; the structure becomes the fossa ovalis. Until the foramen ovale is anatomically sealed, anything that produces a significant increase in right atrial pressure can re-open the foramen ovale and allow a right-to-left shunt.

The ductus arteriosus also undergoes rapid change after birth. In contrast to the pulmonary arterioles, the muscular ductus arteriosus constricts in response to the postnatal increase in P_{O_2}; the decreased levels of or sensitivity to the dilating influences of prostaglandins (PGE_2, PGI_2); and the influence of certain vasoactive substances, such as endothelin 1 (Sansoucie & Cavaliere, 1997). Pressure changes within the cardiac chambers also lead to diminished flow across the ductus arteriosus. PVR rises and pulmonary vascular pressure falls within the first several hours after delivery, blood flow through the ductus arteriosus reverses and blood flows from left to right (from the descending aorta to pulmonary artery) (Guyton & Hall,

1996). Functional closure of the ductus is usually achieved within 96 hours in healthy, term newborns, and anatomic closure is generally completed within 4 months through endothelial and fibrous tissue proliferation (Guyton & Hall, 1996; Sansoucie & Cavaliere, 1997). As with the foramen ovale, during the functional closure stage, the ductus may be reopened under certain cardiopulmonary circumstances with a return to fetal circulation.

The third anatomic shunt, the ductus venosus, also undergoes change during the transition to extrauterine life. When the placenta is removed after birth, the ductus venosus constricts, as blood stops flowing through the umbilical vein (Guyton & Hall, 1996). Functional closure occurs within 2 to 3 days. Anatomic closure is achieved by fibrosis and is generally completed within 7 days, with the structure becoming the ligamentum venosum. Figure 31-2 shows the changes that shift fetal circulation to a postnatal (adult) circulatory pathway.

Postnatal Circulation

Once the placenta is removed, the neonate must change from a fetal circulatory pathway to a **postnatal (or adult) circulation** to survive in the extrauterine world. Systemic venous blood enters the right atrium from the superior vena cava and the inferior vena cava. Poorly oxygenated blood enters the right ventricle and passes through the pulmonary artery into the pulmonary circulation for oxygenation. The oxygenated blood returns to the left atrium through the pulmonary veins. This blood passes through the left ventricle and into the aorta to supply the systemic circulation. Following the oxygenation and perfusion of tissue beds, the blood returns to the right heart and the circulatory pathway is repeated.

Thermoregulation

Effective thermal management at the time of birth plays a significant role in promoting an optimal transition to extrauterine life. Most healthy term infants are capable of attaining a stable body temperature without difficulty if proper methods are employed in the delivery room to prevent heat loss postnatally. Newborns, however, are at a distinct disadvantage when it comes to their ability to maintain normal **thermoregulation** as compared with the older infant or child. First, the neonate has a much greater potential for losing body heat, primarily because of a large body surface area in relation to weight, as well as poor thermal insulation resulting from limited neonatal fat stores (Amlung, 1998; Guyton & Hall, 1996). Another disadvantage is that the neonate has a limited capacity for thermogenesis. Although the older child may use shivering to generate heat in the presence of thermal stress, the neonate has almost no ability to produce heat in this man-

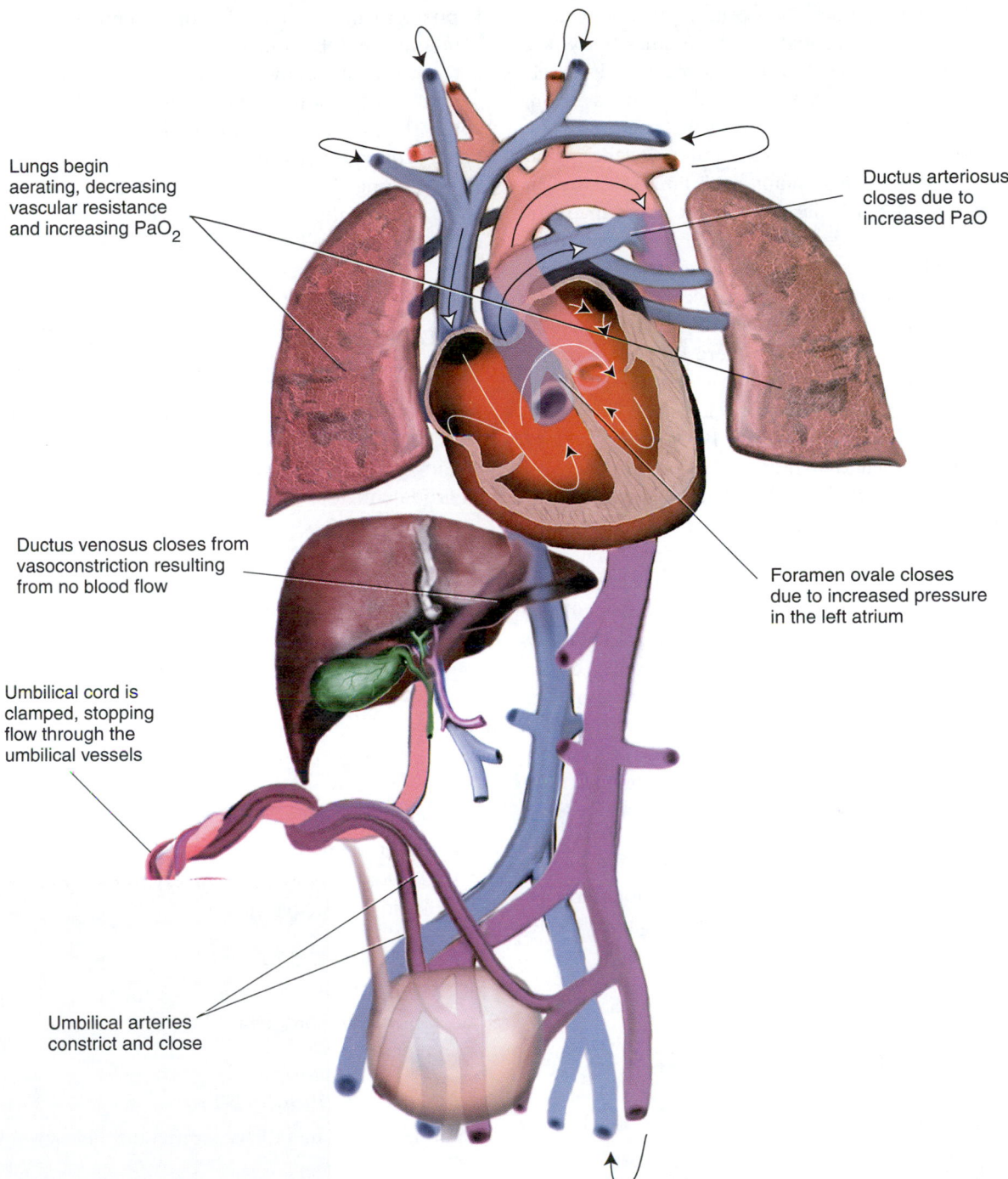

Lungs begin
aerating, decreasing
vascular resistance
and increasing PaO$_2$

Ductus arteriosus
closes due to
increased PaO

Ductus venosus closes from
vasoconstriction resulting
from no blood flow

Foramen ovale closes
due to increased pressure
in the left atrium

Umbilical cord is
clamped, stopping
flow through the
umbilical vessels

Umbilical arteries
constrict and close

Figure 31-2 The modifications that change fetal circulation to postnatal (adult) circulation.

ner (Amlung, 1998; Baumgart, 1996). The healthy, full-term neonate may use, to a limited extent, voluntary muscle activity to assume flexed postures, thereby minimizing heat loss through a reduction of exposed body surface area. The preterm infant, however, has almost no ability to generate heat through increased muscular activity, because motor immaturity often results in flaccid, extended postures (Amlung, 1998).

The primary source of heat production in infancy is chemical thermogenesis (Amlung, 1998; Baumgart, 1996; Hey, 1994). Heat production is activated in the presence of a cold stimulus (Baumgart, 1996). The hypothalamus responds by generating heat through the oxidation of glucose and free fatty acids (Amlung, 1998). In the healthy newborn, brown-fat metabolism is a primary mechanism of heat energy production in the first days of life (Amlung,

1998; Baumgart, 1996; Hey, 1994). Although brown fat is stored in small amounts throughout the infant's body, the majority of brown fat is located around the blood vessels and muscles in the neck, clavicles, axillae, and sternum (Figure 31-3). Brown fat also surrounds the major thoracic vessels and envelops the kidneys and adrenal glands (Amlung; 1998; Baumgart; 1996). Infants with limited brown-fat stores at birth are at particular risk for problems in maintaining a normal body temperature. Because brown fat stores are generally not complete until the last few weeks of gestation, preterm infants may be at risk for hypothermia (Amlung, 1998; Baumgart, 1996). In addition, brown-fat stores may have been consumed in utero for energy needs before birth in infants who are small for gestational age or who experience intrauterine growth retardation, thus also placing them at thermal risk (Amlung, 1998).

It has been estimated that heat loss in the delivery room may be as high as 0.2°C to 1.0°C per minute, depending on the infant's maturity and environmental conditions (Baumgart, 1996). This far exceeds maximal heat production in neonates and rapidly gives rise to the deleterious effects of hypothermia and cold stress. **Hypothermia** is defined as a rectal or axillary temperature below 97°F. In a cold environment, there is first a rise in oxygen consumption and endogenous heat production (Baumgart, 1996). If appropriate thermal interventions are not implemented promptly, heat loss exceeds heat production and the infant's skin and core temperature fall below the normal range (Baumgart, 1996). A body temperature outside the infant's neutral thermal range may result in development of hypothermia that has serious metabolic consequences for the infant, including the development of anaerobic metabolism, pulmonary vasoconstriction, tissue

hypoxia, metabolic acidosis, and eventually, hypoglycemia (Amlung, 1998; Baumgart, 1996).

Throughout delivery and the neonatal period, every newborn's thermoregulation needs must be carefully managed. The goal is to keep the infant in a **neutral thermal environment**, while maintaining a normal body temperature (Amlung, 1998; Baumgart, 1996). In a neutral thermal environment, the infant's axillary temperature is usually maintained in the range of 97°F to 99.5°F.

Nursing Process: Preventing Hypothermia and Maintaining a Neutral Thermal Environment

Full-term and preterm neonates are at risk for altered thermoregulation during the immediate postnatal period. This nursing process focuses on maintaining a neutral thermal environment for these infants.

Assessment

1. Assess factors related to the infant's risk of temperature fluctuation, including prematurity, sepsis, asphyxia, caregiving procedures, and high or low environmental temperatures. Assessment offers an opportunity to prevent cold stress.

2. Assess for potential or actual hypothermia by monitoring the infant's axillary temperature every 30 to 60 minutes after delivery until stable and then every 4 hours per nursery routine.

3. Monitor environmental room temperatures within the delivery room and nursery areas and readjust to avoid convective heat loss.

Nursing Diagnoses

Risk for imbalanced body temperature related to prematurity, abnormal disorders at birth, and exposure to cool environments.

Outcome Identification

Infant maintains an axillary temperature between 97°F and 99.5°F.

Planning

1. Identify the infant at risk for potential or actual temperature instability.

2. Prevent conditions that precipitate cold stress.

3. Provide a neutral thermal environment.

4. Teach parents how to maintain the infant's temperature.

Nursing Interventions

1. Minimize evaporative heat loss at delivery by immediately drying the infant and removing wet blankets.

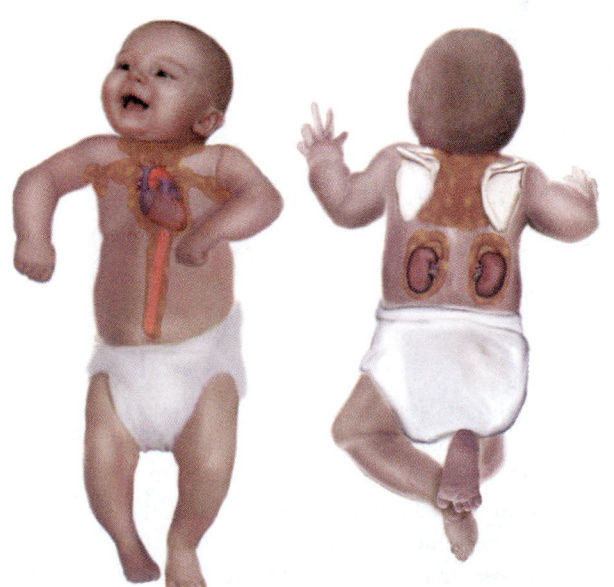

Figure 31-3 Distribution of brown fat in the newborn.

Research Highlight

Effect of Timing of Initial Bath on Newborn Temperature Regulation

The practice of ensuring that babies have a normal body temperature has been a principal component to successful transition to extrauterine life and to the reduction in infant morbidity and mortality within the last several decades. Think about caregiving events that might predispose an infant to thermal stress during the immediate newborn period. For example, bathing is a thermal stressor for newborns that may have implications for their health and well-being. Because of increasing concerns about the transmission of communicable diseases through blood or body fluid contact, research is being done to determine how early newborns can be bathed after birth without comprising their thermal stability.

Purpose

To determine the effect of early bathing on axillary temperature stability after the bath.

Method

Eighty healthy full-term newborns were randomly assigned to one of two bathing groups: 40 neonates were bathed at 1 hour after birth and 40 were bathed at 2 hours after birth.

Findings

The axillary temperatures of newborns bathed at 1 hour did not vary significantly from those of newborns bathed at 2 hours when axillary temperatures were compared at 10, 20, and 60 minutes after the bath.

Nursing Implications

To reduce the exposure of health care providers and family members to bloodborne pathogens, healthy full-term newborns can be bathed after 1 hour when appropriate care measures (e.g. swaddling, avoiding drafts, using radiant warmers, and placing newborns on warm surfaces to minimize heat loss during bathing) are taken to support thermal stability.

Source: Varda, K., & Behnke, R. (2000). The effect of timing of initial bath on newborn's temperature. *JOGNN, 29*, 27–32.

2. Use hat and warm blankets to swaddle infant during parent bonding.

3. Avoid placing infant directly in contact with cold surfaces, such as radiant warmer table or infant scale. This prevents heat loss by conduction.

4. Avoid placing infant in drafts. This prevents heat loss by convection.

5. If body temperature is unstable, place infant under radiant warmer or in incubator.

6. Use heat source when bathing infant. Wash only small sections of the body at a time, being careful to immediately dry the area before proceeding to the next area.

7. When placing infant in an open bassinet in nursery, dress infant warmly and cover with two or more blankets, as needed, to maintain normal axillary temperature.

8. Teach parents how to take their infant's axillary temperature and have them demonstrate the procedure. Talk with parents about causes of temperature fluctuation in newborns and how to prevent heat loss by appropriate clothing, avoiding drafts, and bathing techniques.

Evaluation

1. Assess and record the infant's axillary temperature every 30 to 60 minutes after delivery until stable and then every 4 hours per nursery routine.

2. Assess infant caregiving techniques in the delivery room and nursery and modify as necessary to prevent cold stress.

3. Assess infant's immediate environment for adequacy of thermal support, such as clothing and number of blankets.

4. Encourage parents' questions and requests for clarifications, and give demonstrations to ensure their knowledge of the infant's thermoregulation needs.

Healthy term infants are typically quite capable of thermal self-regulation when clothed and provided with a few ancillary support measures, such as swaddling. Swaddling minimizes heat loss by increasing insulation at the skin surface (Baumgart, 1996). Stocking caps may also assist the term infant in maintaining a normal body temperature, because they decrease heat loss from the large surface area of the head (Amlung, 1998; Baumgart, 1996).

Other methods of thermal stabilization focus primarily on minimizing heat loss that occurs in the infant's environment. A major source of thermal stress in babies occurs through evaporative heat loss. Drying the infant thoroughly after delivery, when the skin is wet with amniotic fluid, can minimize heat loss from evaporation. Additionally, when bathing the infant in the nursery, the nurse can minimize heat loss from evaporation by bathing the infant under a heat source and keeping as much of the infant covered with the bath towel as possible. When bathing the infant, the nurse should wash only small sections at a time, being careful to immediately dry the area before proceeding to the next area. Two other strategies nurses can use to minimize heat loss in the newborn period include avoiding drafts in the environment and pre-warming beds and infant scales that come into direct contact with the infant.

Metabolic Transition

In utero, the fetus is supplied with the necessary nutrients for growth and metabolic processes by the placenta and begins to prepare for postnatal energy demands. Primarily in the third trimester, the fetus begins the process of storing glycogen in the liver for conversion back to glucose during the immediate postnatal period (Brooks, 1997; Ogata, 1994). Although the fetal insulin response to maternal glucose load remains somewhat immature throughout gestation, fetal insulin also plays a role in stimulating fetal growth and body-fat deposition that is later used to maintain postnatal glucose homeostasis (Brooks, 1997; Ogata, 1994).

At birth, the continuous supply of glucose that diffused across the placenta is abruptly terminated. Although immediate newborn glucose levels are roughly equal to those of the mother, levels fall rapidly and reach their lowest point (approximately 40 mg/dL) within 1 to 3 hours in the healthy term newborn. Glucose levels begin to stabilize by 4 to 6 hours and typically are maintained in the range of 45

to 80 mg/dL. This rapid glucose homeostasis occurs as a result of glucose production from hepatic glycogen stores, a process known as glycogenolysis (Brooks, 1997). As hepatic glucose stores become depleted within the first couple of days after birth, the process of gluconeogenesis becomes more important for glucose production. Gluconeogenesis involves the formation of glucose by the liver from noncarbohydrate sources (Brooks, 1997). This transition to free fatty acids as the alternate fuel source is normally accomplished without incident in healthy term infants. However, the normal achievement of postnatal glucose homeostasis can be disrupted in high-risk infants who have low glycogen or fat stores, an increased glucose need, or immature hormonal regulation of glucose. These complications are discussed later in this chapter.

Gastrointestinal System Transition

The gastrointestinal tract undergoes major changes immediately after birth as a function of the initiation of respiration and the introduction of the first nutrients into the infant's gastrointestinal system. At birth, the infant's abdomen is relatively flat and bowel sounds are absent. With the initiation of respiration, the intestinal tract begins to fill up with air, the abdomen becomes more rounded and soft, and bowel sounds become audible with the stethoscope. This usually occurs within the first 15 minutes of life. Peristalsis may not be continuously audible over the next few hours but should be clearly initiated during the first period of reactivity. Some infants may pass meconium during this time, and voiding is common.

NEUROBEHAVIORAL TRANSITION IN THE FIRST 12 HOURS

The transition to extrauterine life begins with the birth of the infant and extends through the first 12 to 24 hours of life. It is a process in which the infant moves from a homeostatic metabolic state in the uterine environment to a homeostatic state in the extrauterine environment. It is a defined progression of events that is probably triggered by stimuli from the external environment. Before the early 1960s, detailed descriptions of the range of "normal" infant behaviors during this transition period were not available. It was, therefore, difficult to define the range of neonatal distress, to identify early signs of morbidity, or to evaluate the impact of clinical management decisions (Desmond, Franklin, Vallbona, Hill, Plumb, Arnold, & Watts, 1963). This concern led clinicians to begin systematically studying infant behavior during the first hours of life and describing the range of those behaviors (Arnold, Putnam, Barnard,

Desmond, & Rudolph, 1965; Desmond et al., 1963; Desmond & Rudolph, 1965). Observations in these studies began with the 1-minute Apgar evaluation, followed by a 10 to 15 minute observation period, during which routine care was provided. The infant was taken to the study nursery, where observations were taken every 15 minutes, including heart rate, respiratory rate, temperature, color, crying, activity, voiding, and stooling. The infant was observed for 6 to 18 hours, with follow-up examinations performed at 24 hours. From these studies, three basic patterns of activity were identified.

First Period of Reactivity

During the first few minutes after birth, the infant undergoes an intense period of activity and alertness that probably represents a sympathetic nervous system response to the intense stimulation of the labor and delivery process. The infant often responds with bursts of rapid, jerky movements of the extremities, alternating with periods of relative immobility. The infant may show high muscular tone during this period and demonstrate behaviors, such as finger splaying, arching, and hyperextension. The period is characterized by myoclonic movements of the eyeball, spontaneous startles and Moro reflexes, sucking activity, chewing, smacking and rooting, and fine tremors of the extremities. All of these behaviors indicate the infant's stress in coping with the sudden increase in environmental stimuli. During this period, the infant enters a state of alertness, peering intently at the surrounding people and environment. This may allow the infant to achieve and maintain eye contact with the parents or caregivers for brief periods of time.

This period of reactivity is also characterized by tachycardia and tachypnea. The infant's heart rate peaks in the first 2 to 3 minutes after delivery and typically falls over the first 30 minutes to 120 to 140 beats per minute. The respiratory rate remains rapid over the first hour, typically peaking at 1 hour and decreasing during the quiet period that follows the first period of reactivity. Some transient nasal flaring, chest retractions, and grunting are not unusual but should be decreasing by the end of the first period of reactivity. Fine rales and rhonchi are often heard in the first period of reactivity, usually clearing spontaneously within the first 15 minutes after birth.

Implications for Parent, Family, and Newborn Interaction

The first period of reactivity provides a unique opportunity to promote early family and newborn interaction. Two elements of the infant's behavior during this period are particularly conducive to this process. First, the infant is alert and responding to the immediate environment. This is a time in the infant's normal transition process when it is possible for the mother and father to hold and interact with the baby. If both mother and baby are stable, the family should be allowed a quiet time and place to be with their baby. The infant may be placed in the parents' arms in an "en face" (face-to-face) position to promote eye contact between parent and infant (Figure 31-4). This time of physical closeness and quiet interaction has been found to be intensely emotionally gratifying for many parents. The mother may also enjoy having skin to skin contact with the infant. The infant, clad only in a diaper, may be placed on the mother's chest and then covered with a blanket to maintain body temperature. This physical contact may also enhance the infant's physiologic organization (Ludington-Hoe, Hadeed, & Anderson, 1991).

Additional infant characteristics that may contribute to family and newborn interaction in this period of reactivity are sucking, rooting, and chewing behaviors. If the infant is to be breastfed, this is an opportune time to initiate

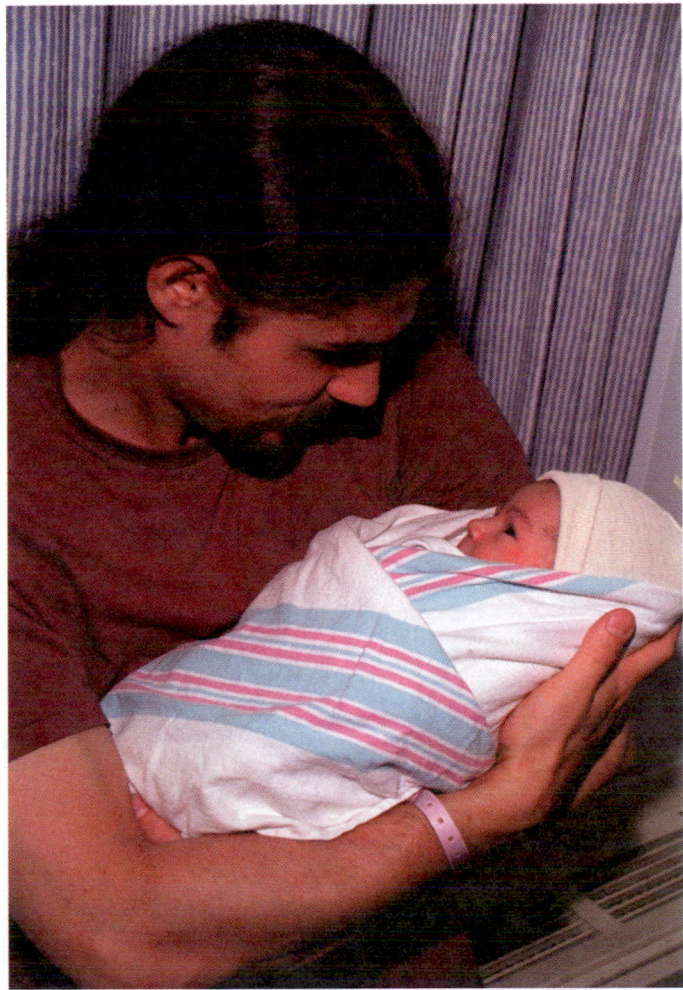

Figure 31-4 Father interacting with his alert newborn infant in the "en face" position.

suckling, using the infant's normal behaviors to promote a successful experience (Figure 31-5). Again, the determination of whether or not to initiate breastfeeding at this time must be made through the assessment of the physiologic stability of both the mother and the infant and the mother's emotional readiness and preferences.

Period of Decreased Activity

This period follows the first period of reactivity and probably represents a parasympathetic nervous system response as the environmental activity decreases and the infant's ability to cope with stimuli increases. During this period the infant's alertness gradually decreases and sleep may occur. Motor activity may reach a peak and then decline over this period. The infant continues to demonstrate some tics, twitches, and involuntary startles, although these should gradually diminish throughout this period. Muscle tone, which was high in the first period of reactivity, should begin to moderate. Movements should become

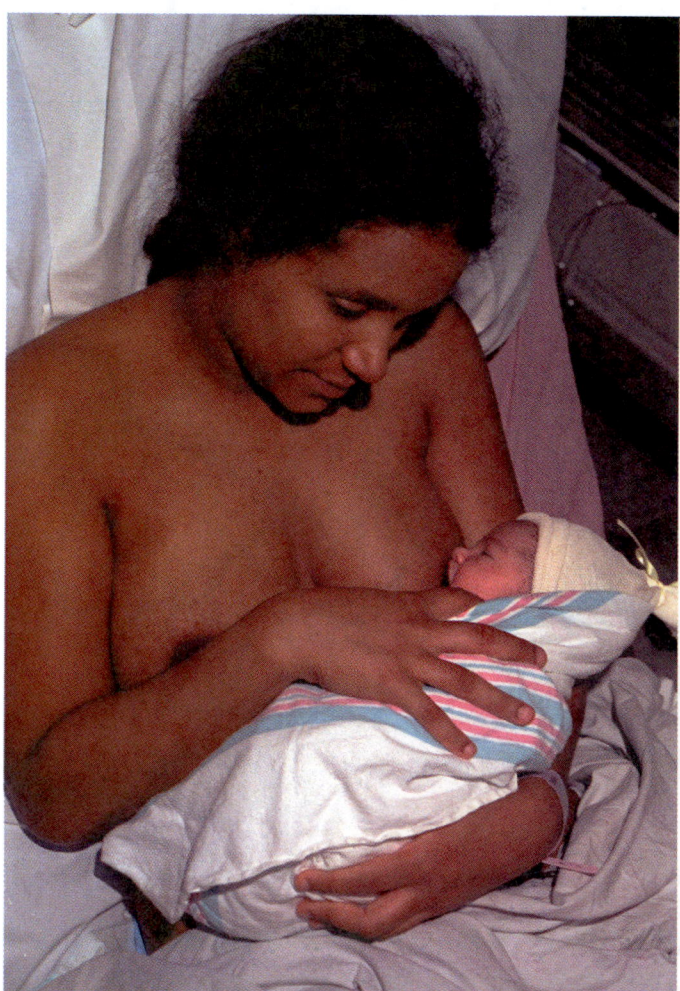

Figure 31-5 Full-term infant ready for breastfeeding at 30 minutes of age.

smoother, less jerky, and less frequent. The infant's heart and respiratory rates decline, and heart rate variability decreases. Respiratory symptoms, such as grunting, chest retractions, brief apneic periods, rales, and rhonchi, may still occur but should be diminishing during this period.

Implications for Parent, Family, and Newborn Interaction

Depending on hospital policy, mothers and infants may remain together during this period, or the infant may be taken to an observation nursery, where some of the initial assessment data is collected. This may be an opportunity for the parents to have some quiet time together and for the mother to rest. If the mother indicates a readiness to learn about her baby during this period, some teaching about the process of the baby's adjustment to extrauterine life, the initial assessment process, and the meaning of some of the infant's behaviors may be appropriate.

Second Period of Reactivity

The second period of reactivity begins as the baby awakens and shows an increased responsiveness to environmental stimuli. At this time the infant may show both heart and respiratory accelerations, particularly in response to environmental stimuli, such as loud noises, bright lights, voices, and touch. There may also be an increase in respiratory symptoms, such as transient grunting, retractions, rales, and rhonchi, although the frequency and severity should be less than that of the first period of reactivity and should gradually diminish throughout this second period. This period is also characterized by an increase in peristalsis and, frequently, the first passage of meconium, although this may have occurred earlier. At the same time, infants may show an increase in hiccoughs, gagging, and spitting up as they become more interactive with the environment and challenged by it. Motor activity increases during this stage but should not reach the level achieved in the first period of reactivity. Motor activity should also be smoother and more organized than in the first period. Muscle tone may increase in comparison to the period of decreased activity but should continue to moderate throughout this period.

Implications for Parent, Family, and Newborn Interaction

The pace and rhythm of parent, family, and newborn interaction during this transition period depends on the readiness and availability of all the involved parties for interaction. The onset of the second period of reactivity represents a time when the newborn is alert, active, and available. The mother's readiness or availability depends on her fatigue levels, her recovery from the delivery process, the amount and type of medication she has received, and her emotional status. It is common for the mother to desire to have her baby close and to want to participate in feeding and caring for the baby. It is equally normal for the mother to express a need for rest and recovery and to have minimal contact with the baby during this time. If the mother is ready for interaction with her baby, they should be provided with a quiet, comfortable environment in which to be together. The mother and father may have questions about behaviors they see in the baby at this time. If necessary, the parents should be helped to position the baby in a face-to-face position to promote interaction. Helping them to feed the baby or change a diaper are ways of strengthening their sense of competence in caring for their infant. Parents may also be encouraged to examine the baby and to ask any questions they may have.

Assessment Strategies and Newborn Competencies

The most widely used assessment strategies in this neonatal period are the Apgar score and the assessment of gestational age. Both of these assessment tools are discussed in detail elsewhere in this text and represent commonly used and valid one-time "snapshots" of the infant's status (Jepson, Talashek, & Tichy, 1991). However, adequate assessment of an infant's progress through the process of adjustment to extrauterine life requires that the nurse engage in serial observations of the infant. The determination that the infant is progressing normally through this transition period is based not on the observations of symptoms at one time point, but on the observation of an infant's pattern of moving toward more organized behaviors and an increase in the infant's ability to regulate his or her own physiologic responses. As an example, it is not uncommon for an infant to display symptoms such as grunting with respirations, chest retractions, or brief periods of apnea throughout the transition period. However, these symptoms should become less frequent and less severe over time. If these same symptoms appear to increase in frequency or severity over time, to continue beyond a normal transition period, or to be unresponsive to routine interventions, they may indicate a more serious medical complication and require a more extensive diagnostic workup and treatment.

Two infant neurobehavioral competencies, infant state and habituation, provide additional information regarding an infant's adjustment to extrauterine life. Infant state, or **behavioral state**, refers to the quality and level of alertness the infant demonstrates. Infant state is viewed as a range of alertness levels from sound quiet sleep through levels of drowsiness to levels of wakeful attentiveness and finally to hyperalert, agitated, or crying states. Infant state

stability provides a valuable window into the maturing nervous system and a useful assessment measure for evaluating neurobehavioral stabilization over the first 24 hours. Behavioral state is evaluated in terms of the range of states the infant is able to achieve and their duration and stability. In the first stage of reactivity, most infants are able to achieve an alert, wakeful state and are able to focus on a face or object for brief periods of time (Figure 31-6). These periods of alertness, however, may be interrupted by agitated movements, respiratory disturbances, and other signs of disorganization. The infant is likely to be distracted and reactive to environmental stimuli and to move rapidly from alert to drowsy to fussy states. During the period of decreased activity, the infant is likely to sleep but may continue to demonstrate involuntary movements and respiratory disturbances during the sleep state, rather than achieving a quiet, well-organized sleep state. Throughout the first 24 hours, the infant's ability to achieve and maintain an organized, quiet alert state and an organized quiet sleep state, as well as all of the intermediate states, should gradually increase. The nurse's observation of the change in the duration, stability, and range of the infant's state control is a valuable indicator of the infant's neurobehavioral intactness.

The concept of **habituation** refers to the ability of the infant to become adjusted or adapted to a specific environmental stimulus. When an infant is first confronted with an unexpected environmental stimulus, the infant responds with startles, twitches, tics, or respiratory instability. In a mature, well-organized baby, the reaction to the stimulus gradually decreases and the startles, twitches and other behaviors subside. This is called habituation. In the period immediately after birth, many infants are not able

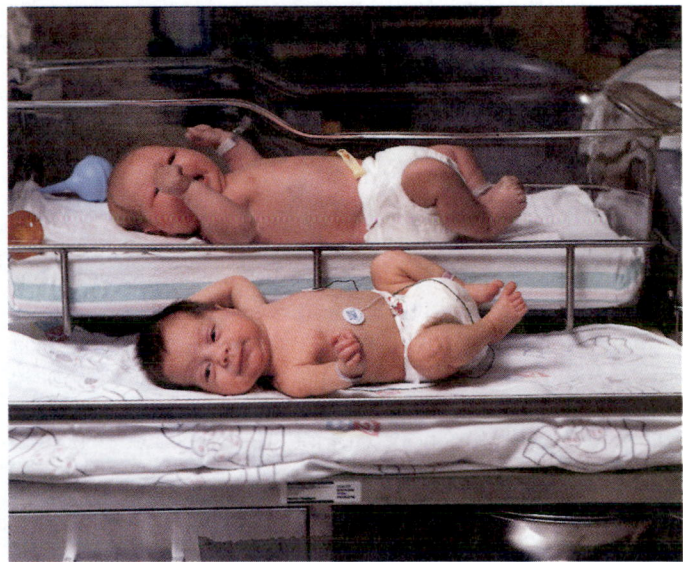

Figure 31-6 Newborn in organized, quiet, alert state during first 6 hours of life.

to habituate to an environmental stimulus. The startle reactions continue until the stimulus stops. Over the first 24 hours, the infant should increase the ability to habituate to environmental stimuli. This process, again, provides a useful indicator of the infant's neurobehavioral intactness.

COMPLICATIONS OF TRANSITION

Most healthy term newborns make the transition to extrauterine life without difficulty. However, this complex process does not always occur uneventfully. Complications occur that may be transient and require only minimal intervention or may represent a significant threat to the infant's well-being.

Common Complications

Conditions that may impede the newborn's smooth transition to extrauterine life include asphyxia, persistent pulmonary hypertension of the newborn, meconium staining, transient tachypnea of the newborn, hypoglycemia, and hypovolemia (shock). These are now discussed.

Asphyxia

One of the most serious of the complications of the transition process is asphyxia. **Asphyxia** is a metabolic process that arises from failure of the respiratory organ in the fetus or neonate. Failure of the organ of respiration leads to impairment of oxygen and carbon dioxide exchange. This results in hypoxemia, hypercarbia, and subsequently, acute respiratory acidosis. If such circumstances persist for a prolonged period, tissue hypoxia occurs, with superimposed metabolic acidosis. Without appropriate caregiver interventions to reverse and restore optimal gas exchange within the placenta or lung, permanent brain injury or death may result (Fisher & Paton, 1986; Kattwinkel, 2000).

Several prenatal and postnatal factors compromise the fetus and interfere with the physiologic transition to extrauterine life. Respiratory depression that leads to asphyxia may occur as a result of the reduction in placental perfusion or gas exchange or from umbilical cord accidents. Failure to establish spontaneous and effective respirations after birth may also result in postnatal asphyxia (Kattwinkel, 2000). In these circumstances fetal acid-base balance is normal at birth, but disturbances occur when adequate lung function cannot replace the detached placenta.

A classic series of events occurs when an infant becomes asphyxiated in utero or postnatally. The progressively severe clinical phases of asphyxia include primary apnea, gasping, and secondary, or terminal, apnea. By observing the infant's responses, the caregiver may be able to establish the duration and severity of the asphyxia episode, thereby determining the actions that are required to intervene in a timely and appropriate manner (Fisher & Paton, 1986; Kattwinkel, 2000).

During the initial period of deprivation of oxygen, the infant exhibits rapid breathing. If hypoxic conditions persist, the heart rate begins to fall, and the infant's respiratory efforts cease. This is referred to as **primary apnea**. During this period, blood pressure is normal or slightly elevated and pulses are palpable. Although the infant's tone gradually diminishes, the infant is still responsive to tactile stimulation and oxygen. If resuscitation is provided at this point, the infant responds quickly with gasping respirations, rapidly followed by the establishment of normal oxygenation (Fisher & Paton, 1986; Kattwinkel, 2000).

If the asphyxia progresses, the infant begins to demonstrate deep gasping respirations, indicative of serious acidemia and the need for immediate initiation of resuscitation with positive pressure ventilation. If, however, the asphyxia continues, the infant's heart rate progressively falls, the infant's blood pressure begins to drop, and the infant becomes almost flaccid. The infant's respiratory efforts become progressively weaker until respirations cease, and the infant enters into the period of **secondary apnea**. During this period, metabolic derangements are severe, with marked hypoxemia, hypbercarbia, and acidemia. Heart rate is extremely low, pulses are absent, and, without prompt intervention, death occurs. Tactile stimulation is ineffective for resuscitation of an infant in secondary apnea, thus requiring quick initiation of positive pressure ventilation with 100% oxygen. The infant usually becomes pink before the reestablishment of spontaneous respirations, because oxygenation is restored sooner than the brain can recover from the severely hypoxic event (Fisher & Paton, 1986; Kattwinkel, 2000).

Because primary and secondary apnea are often difficult to distinguish from one another, the health care provider should always assume the latter and initiate respirations using assisted ventilation. This approach facilitates rapid response to resuscitation efforts, ensures more rapid establishment of spontaneous respirations, and minimizes the potential for adverse neurologic outcomes (Fisher & Paton, 1986; Kattwinkel, 2000).

While the Apgar score has been widely used in the delivery room to evaluate the overall health status of the newly born infant, the Apgar score neither establishes nor rules out the presence of asphyxia. Apgar scoring frequently correlates poorly with the underlying acid-base status of the infant at birth. The need for resuscitation can be more accurately assessed by the evaluation of the infant's heart rate, respiratory activity, and color than by the Apgar score. Resuscitation, therefore, should not be delayed for the assessment of the 1-minute score but should be initiated immediately, based on criteria established by the American Academy of Pediatrics and the American Heart Association's Neonatal Resuscitation Program (Kattwinkel, 2000). **Resuscitation** of the newborn consists of emergency life-support measures, including airway management, positive pressure ventilation, chest compressions, medications, and thermal support. These criteria are discussed later in this chapter.

Persistent Pulmonary Hypertension of the Newborn

Persistent pulmonary hypertension of the newborn (PPHN), or persistent fetal circulation, is a condition characterized by a high level of PVR in the absence of recognizable cardiac, pulmonary, hematologic, or central nervous system disease (DeBoer & Stephens, 1997). It may be seen in conjunction with a patent ductus arteriosus and foramen ovale, resulting in a cycle of right-to-left shunting, hypoxemia of the arterial blood flow, and continuing or increasing pulmonary vasoconstriction. PPHN is seen most commonly in infants who are appropriate for gestational age and born at or near term. There is frequently a history of perinatal asphyxia or other pathologic event, such as meconium aspiration, pneumonia, or pneumothorax, that results in alveolar hypoxia with a subsequent increase in PVR. PPHN may also occur secondary to pulmonary hypoplasia when there is a decreased pulmonary vascular mass and a resultant increase in PVR. Maternal use of aspirin or other nonsteroidal anti-inflammatory medication during the third trimester of pregnancy has also been seen in conjunction with an increased incidence of PPHN.

Infants with PPHN demonstrate tachypnea, respiratory distress, and rapidly progressing cyanosis that may be aggravated by activity and stimulation of the infant. Infants with severe PPHN may develop systemic hypotension and cardiac failure. PPHN is treated primarily with administration of maximal amounts of oxygen and mechanical ventilation. PPHN may also be treated with inhalational pulmonary vasodilators (particularly nitric oxide) and extracorporeal membrane oxygenation (ECMO). Infants may need to be maintained in an environment of reduced stimulation or be sedated if stimulation and activity aggravate symptoms.

Meconium Staining

Meconium staining of amniotic fluid occurs in 10% to 15% of all deliveries (Whitsett, Pryhuber, Rice, Warner, & Wert, 1994). **Meconium staining** occurs when the fetus passes meconium during the labor or birth process, usually in response to some distress, such as an episode of asphyxia. It is most common in infants born postterm and occurs less commonly with decreasing gestational age. Meconium staining rarely occurs in infants born before 34 weeks' gestation.

The concern in the case of meconium-stained amniotic fluid is the possibility that the infant may aspirate the meconium. Aspiration of meconium can be a cause of serious pulmonary disease in neonates, either by causing an obstruction of the airways or by producing a chemical pneumonitis. These conditions may be severe and life-threatening, even in the healthy full-term infant. Complications resulting from meconium aspiration are increased if: 1) passage of meconium occurs before the second stage of labor, thus increasing the possibility that aspiration will occur; 2) the meconium-stained amniotic fluid is thick, increasing the severity of airway obstruction if aspiration occurs; and 3) on assessment of the newborn, meconium is noted below the vocal cords, indicating that some degree of aspiration has already occurred. Symptoms of clinical disease may be immediate and severe, requiring resuscitation in the delivery room, or may occur gradually over the first few hours after birth with the infant demonstrating respiratory distress and hypoxemia. PPHN may be observed in infants who develop severe meconium aspiration syndrome.

When meconium-stained amniotic fluid is noted, special measures should be taken to prepare for the delivery. An extra person may be necessary to help with the suctioning procedure, including assembling endotracheal tubes and suctioning equipment and monitoring the infant's physiologic status. If possible, the mouth, nose, and posterior pharynx should be suctioned immediately after the head is delivered and while the chest is still compressed in the birth canal. After birth, the need for tracheal suctioning of the infant's airway is determined by whether or not the infant is vigorous at birth (defined by strong respiratory effort, good muscle tone, and a heart rate of more

Critical Thinking

Newborn Resuscitation

Parents are often restricted from being present while their infant is being resuscitated in the newborn stabilization area adjacent to the delivery room. Ask yourself if this practice is done for the benefit of the newborn infant or for the comfort level of the health care team? Also ask yourself: If this was your baby, how would you feel if you were excluded from the newborn stabilization area while the health care team attempted to resuscitate or stabilize your infant? Would you be more frightened by the procedures being performed or by not knowing how your infant was responding to the intervention measures?

than 100 beats per minute) (Kattwinkel, 2000). If tracheal suctioning is required, the infant should not be stimulated to cry or inhale until the infant is intubated and suctioning has been performed. Prompt intubation and suctioning of the infant at delivery has reduced but not eliminated the occurrence of meconium aspiration syndrome.

Parents are often unprepared for complications at delivery. In the accompanying box, a father shares the experiences of one family whose baby had thick meconium staining and respiratory depression at birth. Nurses must partner with parents to ensure that hospital policies and practices facilitate the parents' right to be with their baby and to participate in their infant's care, as the clinical situation allows.

Transient Tachypnea of the Newborn

Transient tachypnea of the newborn (TTN) is a condition in which the infant presents with grunting, retractions, and an elevated respiratory rate at birth or shortly after. The condition is self-limiting, usually resolving

REFLECTIONS FROM A FATHER

"We were so excited that the time had finally come for my wife to deliver our firstborn son. Everyone was there, even my parents who lived 2 hours away by car. When my wife went into labor, the doctor said everything was fine. What we had not prepared for was meconium staining which the health care team members noted when my wife's bag of water broke. When he was delivered, the neonatal team 'wisked' our baby away to a separate room. The neonatal doctor said that I could come be with my baby as soon as they were certain that everything was okay. I didn't understand why I couldn't go with them. What were they doing to my baby that I shouldn't see? I think my wife and I were more frightened by not knowing what was going on and how our son was doing, than we would have been if I would have been allowed to go with them and observe and be with my son."

within 5 days. It is characterized radiographically by increased central vascular markings, hyperaeration, evidence of interstitial and pleural fluid, prominent interlobar fissures, and cardiomegaly. Because the condition is self-limiting, infants with TTN usually require only supportive care, mainly oxygen therapy and intravenous fluid supplementation. Rarely is short-term ventilation necessary. In addition, if maternal risk factors for sepsis or other causes for respiratory distress cannot be ruled out, infants are usually treated prophylactically with broad-spectrum antibiotics.

Although the symptoms of TTN are similar to behaviors in the normal process of transition to extrauterine life, the clinical progression is quite different. Shortly after delivery, infants with TTN demonstrate tachypnea, grunting, nasal flaring, rib retraction, and varying degrees of cyanosis. Many healthy infants also demonstrate some respiratory grunting and chest retractions initially, but these symptoms are usually resolved and the respiratory rate should be stabilizing by the end of the second period of reactivity, during which grunting, retraction, and increased respiratory rate should occur primarily in response to environmental stimuli, not when the infant is at rest. The increased respiratory efforts normally noted in the first and second periods of reactivity are related to the clearance of fetal fluid from the infant's lungs after birth and are not usually accompanied by cyanosis. In TTN, these symptoms may persist for several days and occur even when the baby is at rest. Nursing observations of the infant, then, should focus on whether these respiratory symptoms appear to be resolving through the first and second periods of reactivity or persisting at the same level or increasing in severity and whether the distress results in the need for oxygen therapy.

Hypoglycemia

Hypoglycemia is a relatively common complication in the early newborn period and one for which the nurse should be continually alert. Plasma glucose levels of less than 40 mg/dL should be considered hypoglycemic, although this level is somewhat arbitrary and has not been correlated with the glucose use rate of the infant or with severity of symptoms. Symptoms of hypoglycemia include jitteriness, tremors, apnea, cyanosis, limpness or lethargy, and in severe cases, convulsions.

Several groups of neonates are at particular risk for hypoglycemia. Infants who are born small for gestational age (SGA) have inadequate hepatic glycogen stores at birth. During intrauterine life, the nutrients available to these infants were necessarily channeled toward growth rather than being set aside for glycogen storage. At birth, then, little glycogen reserve is available to meet the infant's metabolic needs. Hypoglycemia is usually short-lived in these infants as nutrient intake is increased. Infants born prematurely are, similar to SGA infants, born with inadequate glycogen stores and are also vulnerable to hypoglycemic episodes. These infants have missed all or part of the third trimester of intrauterine development, during which much of the hepatic glycogen is stored. The younger the gestational age at birth, the less glycogen is present and the greater the risk for hypoglycemia. Furthermore, infants who are born both SGA and premature are at extremely high risk for hypoglycemia.

A third group of infants who have low glycogen stores at birth are those who have experienced perinatal stress. Stressful events, such as hypoxia, acidosis, and fluctuations in fetal blood pressure and flow, can increase catecholamine secretion in utero and subsequently increase mobilization of hepatic glycogen stores. At birth, these infants may have significantly depleted glycogen stores and are at increased risk for hypoglycemia.

Infants who experience a hyperinsulin state during intrauterine development, most commonly infants of diabetic mothers (IDM), carry over this hyperinsulin response to the extrauterine state. IDMs develop hyperinsulinism in utero in response to the mother's hyperglycemic state. In the neonatal period, the infants often have elevated plasma insulin concentrations and are hyperresponsive to increases in glucose levels. Infants with other conditions, including disorders of the pancreas and certain syndromes, may also have experienced a hyperinsulin state in utero and subsequently are at an increased risk for hypoglycemia postnatally.

Another group of infants at risk for hypoglycemia are those experiencing sepsis. Although the underlying mechanisms of this are not well understood, hypoglycemia or hyperglycemia are often the first indicators of sepsis in a neonate. An evaluation for sepsis should always be considered for infants with unexplained hypoglycemia.

The clinical management of infants susceptible to hypoglycemia begins with prevention and early identification. Although many neonates are asymptomatic, the symptoms most often described consist of respiratory distress, lethargy, apnea, or marked jitteriness (Brooks, 1997). Once the newborn is stabilized in the delivery room, feedings can be initiated as soon as possible after birth in healthy term infants. Such infants may be offered early breastfeeding or oral feedings with formula or glucose. Whenever hypoglycemic symptoms are observed or risk factors are present, glucose screening should be performed using a glucose oxidase strip or an approved blood glucose reflectance meter. If the screening test value is below 40 mg/dL, results should be confirmed with a laboratory venous blood glucose determination (Brooks, 1997; Ogata, 1994). Because asymptomatic or symptomatic hypoglycemia can result in serious neurologic sequelae to the neonate if untreated, it is recommended that therapy be initiated before obtaining the blood glucose test results. Asymptomatic infants may be offered a feeding and a glucose determination repeated 20 minutes after the feeding. Management of symptomatic infants is usually best accomplished by treatment with an intravenous bolus of glucose, followed by a continuous glucose infusion (Brooks, 1997; Levitt-Katz & Stanley, 1996). Blood glucose levels should be checked 20 minutes after intravenous therapy is begun and should be monitored until stable.

Hypovolemia

Hypovolemia (shock), or low blood volume, is a relatively uncommon but critical complication for the newborn. Acute hypovolemia may occur as a result of blood loss from the fetal side of the placenta secondary to placenta previa or abruptio placenta. These two maternal emergencies are discussed elsewhere in this text, but can lead to a severely compromised infant at delivery. The delivery room management of these infants is a critical part of their survival. Resuscitation equipment and personnel trained in neonatal resuscitation must be present in the delivery room as soon as one of these maternal emergencies is identified. Other possible causes of fetal or neonatal hemorrhage include umbilical cord rupture (secondary to precipitous delivery) or superficially implanted umbilical vessels. Hypovolemia may also be seen with intrauterine asphyxia without evidence of frank hemorrhage. While the healthy newborn can compensate for some blood loss, asphyxia disrupts the infant's ability to do so. In spite of this, most infants experiencing asphyxia do not progress to hypovolemia. However, almost all infants who develop hypovolemia have a history of intrauterine asphyxia.

Babies with hypovolemia appear pale and have weak pulses. They may have a persistently high or low heart rate. Their extremities may feel cold and they may have delayed filling of the capillaries after blanching under normal pressure (provided that core temperature is normal). Infants with hypovolemia may have persistent metabolic acidosis and their circulatory status often does not improve in response to effective ventilation, chest compressions, and epinephrine during resuscitation. The treatment for hypovolemia is blood volume expansion through repeated small infusions of normal saline, Ringer's lactate, or O-negative blood that has been cross-matched with mother's blood (if time permits before delivery).

Major Pathologies that Affect Transition

Three major diseases that may impede the newborn's smooth transition to extrauterine life include congenital heart defects, sepsis, and diaphragmatic hernia.

Congenital Heart Defects

Congenital heart defects, or structural malformations of the heart in the developing fetus, may limit or prevent the neonate from making a successful transition to extrauterine life. Difficulties in transition may not become apparent until the organ of respiration changes from the placenta to the lungs and fetal circulatory shunts close, particularly the ductus arteriosus (Sansoucie & Cavaliere, 1997). In neonates with congenital heart malformations, the ductus arteriosus often maintains blood flow between the pulmonary and systemic circulations after birth, allowing the cardiac defect to go unrecognized. With spontaneous closure of the ductus arteriosus during transition to extrauterine life, the status of a previously asymptomatic neonate may suddenly deteriorate as blood flow between the pulmonary and systemic circulations is abruptly terminated (Sansoucie & Cavaliere, 1997).

Characteristics of cardiac blood flow in utero have an important influence on the structure of the developing heart (Sansoucie & Cavaliere, 1997). Aberrant flow patterns in utero significantly affect the size and shape of the heart postnatally (Serwer, 1992). For example, if blood flow from the right to left atrium is decreased in fetal circulation, diminished growth of the left atrium and ventricle may result and the infant may demonstrate signs of hypoplastic left heart in the early newborn period, such as poor perfusion and a mottled appearance of the skin.

Development of the pulmonary vascular bed may also be affected by structural malformations of the heart. A fetus with pulmonary atresia in utero may have an underdeveloped pulmonary vascular bed that leads to a delayed decline in PVR postnatally and the devastating and often fatal development of PPHN in the immediate postnatal period (Sansoucie & Cavaliere, 1997).

Sepsis

Successful transition to extrauterine life may also be affected by the presence of viral or bacterial endotoxins that are acquired in utero, at birth, or during the early newborn period. **Sepsis** is defined as a clinical syndrome of systemic illness accompanied by bacteremia. Infants at risk for complications related to sepsis include the preterm infant and the infant born to a mother who experiences a prolonged period between rupture of membranes and delivery, fever, chorioamnionitis, or other characteristics suggesting infection (Lott & Kenner, 1998).

Circulating bacterial endotoxins, particularly group B streptococcal endotoxin, can exert effects on both systemic and pulmonary circulations, rendering the neonate vulnerable to the effects of septic shock and possibly even compromising the infant's survival, if aggressive medical interventions are not rapidly instituted. The progressive effects of endotoxin on the capillary beds may lead to failure to establish normal SVR as a result of decreased venous return to the heart and reduced cardiac output. This loss of effective blood volume within the circulatory system may further exacerbate tissue hypoperfusion and contribute to further cellular anoxia. Endotoxins also contribute to a rise in PVR and pulmonary congestion from increased capillary permeability. The effect of circulating bacterial toxins on the lung causes progressive compromise of pulmonary function with resultant hypoxemia. The infant who has sepsis at birth may exhibit apnea, poor respiratory effort, cyanosis, or frank signs of respiratory distress (Freij & McCracken, 1994). These infants may require initiation of oxygen and respiratory support, and all require the prompt initiation of antibiotics.

Diaphragmatic Hernia

Conditions requiring surgery may compromise the infant's ability to make a successful transition to extrauterine life. One of the most critical conditions requiring intense surgical intervention after delivery in the infant born with a diaphragmatic hernia. **Diaphragmatic hernia** is a condition in which the contents of the abdominal cavity are herniated into the thoracic cavity through a defect in the diaphragm. The herniation of the intestines into the chest cavity results in hypoplasia of the developing lung. The timing of the entry and the amount of abdominal contents that are herniated into the chest both determine the degree of pulmonary hypoplasia and degree of respiratory embarrassment experienced by the infant at birth. Most infants present with respiratory distress at birth or shortly after birth. Symptoms include cyanosis, increased work of breathing, and decreased breath sounds on the affected side. Heart tones may also be shifted from their normal point of maximal impulse. The abdomen is scaphoid as a result of the absence of intestines, and bowel sounds may be heard within the thoracic cavity. Cardiorespiratory symptoms exhibited by the infant are usually the result of decreased air exchange as a result of the pulmonary hypoplasia and thoracic compression of the lung. This leads to hypoxemia and increased PVR within the pulmonary capillary bed. With progressive increases in pulmonary vascular pressures and hypoxemia, right-to-left shunting through the fetal circulatory shunts is common. If the defect goes unrecognized, the infant is at serious risk for persistence of fetal circulation and pulmonary hypertension. The establishment of adequate oxygenation and systemic circulation are key components to infant survival and most infants require some measure of respiratory support, including oxygen, intubation, and positive pressure ventilation (Guzzetta, Anderson, Eichelberger, Newman, Rouse, Schnitzer, Boyajian, & Tomaski, 1994). If the infant with suspected diaphragmatic hernia requires prolonged positive pressure ventilation, ventilation should be delivered

Case Study/Care Plan

BIRTH OF INFANT WITH CONGENITAL DIAPHRAGMATIC HERNIA

A 3940-gram male infant was born to a 24-year-old woman at 40 weeks' gestation by spontaneous vaginal delivery. Apgar scores were 8 at 1 minute and 8 at 5 minutes. The infant did well initially; however, shortly after birth he developed cyanosis and respiratory distress and, 15 minutes later, required intubation and ventilatory support. On physical assessment, the abdomen was unusually flat (scaphoid). Breath sounds were diminished on the left, and heart sounds were shifted to the right side of the thorax. A chest x-ray film was done and revealed air-filled loops of intestine within the left side of the chest, confirming the presence of a left-side congenital diaphragmatic hernia. The priority nursing diagnosis is discussed below, though several other diagnoses would also apply.

Assessment

Term infant with respiratory distress, as evidenced by presence of cyanosis, ineffective breathing pattern requiring ventilatory support, and diminished breath sounds.

Nursing Diagnosis

Impaired gas exchange related to presence of congenital diaphragmatic hernia.

Expected Outcomes   Infant will maintain adequate gas exchange (until surgery can be performed) as evidence by lack of cyanosis, maintenance of arterial P_{O_2} of more than 60 mm Hg and P_{CO_2} of less than 45 mm Hg, clear breath sounds on unaffected side of chest, respiratory rate within normal limits (40 to 60 breaths per minute).

Planning
1. Frequent assessments to determine adequacy of gas exchange.
2. Provision of interventions (based on assessments and medical orders) to optimize effectiveness of breathing pattern and gas exchange.

Nursing Interventions	Rationales
1. Assess and record respiratory rate, breath sounds, and signs and symptoms of respiratory distress every 1 to 2 hours.	1. Monitors respiratory status.
2. Take samples and record results of arterial blood gas tests when indicated.	2. Determines adequacy of gas exchange.
3. Check and record oxygen and ventilator settings every 1 to 2 hours.	3. Provides baseline and measure of changing oxygen needs.
4. Assess patency of endotracheal tube by listening to breath sounds every 1 to 2 hours. Suction endotracheal tube, using sterile technique, as clinically indicated. Record characteristics of secretions and tolerance of procedure.	4. Ensures patency of ET tube.
5. Position infant on left side with head of bed elevated.	5. Optimizes gas exchange of unaffected lung and helps to encourage downward displacement of the abdominal contents.
6. Prevent infant from crying whenever possible by using comfort measures and sedation if ordered.	6. Crying allows the infant to swallow air, which will result in gastric and intestinal distention and increased respiratory distress.

(continued)

Nursing Interventions	Rationales
7. Ensure nasogastric tube is placed correctly and connected to suction.	7. Decompresses the stomach and minimizes respiratory distress.
8. Administer antibiotics as ordered.	8. Minimizes potential for infection related to planned surgery and invasive procedures.
9. Check and record results of chest x-ray film, if available.	9. Identifies existence of congenital diaphragmatic hernia.

Evaluation Describe breath sounds and any signs or symptoms of impaired gas exchange, and any successful measures used to decrease crying. Record nasogastric suction pressures and characteristics of drainage. Record medications administered as ordered, including antibiotic and sedative agents.

with an endotracheal tube rather than a bag and mask to prevent further respiratory embarrassment, which may result from distention of the gastrointestinal tract (Kattwinkel, 2000).

TRANSITION OF THE PREMATURE INFANT

A **preterm** neonate is defined as an infant born at less than 38 weeks' gestation. Successful transition to extrauterine life is much more complicated in infants born prematurely. In this section, the effects of developmental immaturity of the pulmonary and cardiac systems on adaptation of the preterm neonate to extrauterine life are discussed. The general approach to education of prospective parents of preterm neonates in the delivery room is also discussed.

Complications of Pulmonary System Transition

Developmental characteristics of premature newborns predispose them to respiratory complications in the transition to extrauterine life. One such characteristic is the developmental stage of the alveolar structures in the lungs. At the beginning of the third trimester of fetal development, the respiratory system of the fetus has reached the end of the canalicular period. At this point, alveolar ducts, a primitive form of the future alveoli, have formed and the lungs are becoming increasingly vascular. When these alveolar ducts are first formed, the walls of the ducts are thick. At the end of this period, the alveolar walls are beginning to thin, allowing the newly formed capillaries to push into the ducts as capillary loops. It is at this intersection of the capillary and the alveolar wall that the exchange of oxygen and carbon dioxide occurs. This period, at about 24 to 26 weeks

of gestation, is the first point at which respiration is possible, because some but not all of the infant's alveolar ducts have developed into thin-walled, vascularized terminal sacs. This developmental period determines the lower limits of viability for the premature infant. By the 28th week of gestation, most preterm infants have sufficient terminal air sac development to permit survival. However, the process of terminal sac development continues through the next period of lung development, called the terminal sac or saccular period (24 to 36 weeks gestational age). This period is characterized by rapid development of thin-walled terminal sacs and by a rapid proliferation of the capillary system, with increasing numbers of capillaries bulging into the air sacs. Throughout this period, the surface available for the exchange of oxygen and carbon dioxide is increasing correspondingly with the infant's capacity to sustain independent respiratory function. In the period from 36 weeks' gestation through early childhood, the pulmonary system is considered to be within the alveolar period of development, during which the walls of the terminal air sacs become extremely thin and take on the form of the mature pulmonary alveoli (Moore & Persaud, 1993).

Another major factor influencing the respiratory transition of the premature infant is the presence or absence of surfactant in the lungs. Surfactant is a substance secreted by the epithelial cells in the terminal air sacs, beginning at about the 28th week of gestation. This substance provides a surface tension–reducing action in the alveoli, which allows the alveoli to expand more easily on inspiration and prevents their collapse on expiration. The lack of adequate surfactant in the infant's alveoli is a primary reason for the development of respiratory distress in the premature infant and the need for mechanical ventilation. Synthetic forms of surfactant have now been developed. They are administered shortly after birth and have greatly reduced the need for mechanical ventilation (Lott, 1998).

An infant born early in the third trimester of gestation experiences compromised respiration not because of any existing disease but because of the normal immaturity of the developing respiratory system. It is the combination of inadequate terminal sac development, incomplete vascular development, and inadequate surfactant secretion that leads to the development of the life-threatening condition of respiratory distress syndrome (RDS), formerly called hyaline membrane disease. RDS is a primary cause of mortality and morbidity in the premature infant. The lower the gestational age of the infant at birth, the higher the incidence of RDS and, generally, the greater the severity of the condition. Infants with RDS present, at birth or within a few hours of birth, with signs of respiratory distress, including grunting, chest retractions, cyanosis, rales, nasal flaring, use of the accessory muscles of breathing, and an increasing oxygen requirement. Chest radiographic findings are characterized by atelectasis, air bronchograms, and diffuse reticular-granular infiltrates (Whitsett et al., 1994).

Complications of Cardiac System Transition

One of the common complications of cardiac transition to extrauterine life in the premature infant is the occurrence of a persistent patent ductus arteriosus (PDA). In the fetus, the ductus arteriosus forms a bridge between the pulmonary artery and the dorsal aorta, inserting at the aortic isthmus. At birth, the ductus is a muscular contractile structure. The closure of the ductus at birth depends on multiple factors, including the increase in oxygen tension, the level of circulating prostaglandins, and the available ductal muscle mass. Each of these factors is compromised by premature birth. The hypoxia characteristic of extreme prematurity and the immaturity of the alveolar development may contribute to high PVR, which acts to maintain the right-to-left shunting activity, causing the unoxygenated blood to bypass the pulmonary system and to return to systemic circulation. Conversely, as the PVR decreases after delivery, left-to-right shunting may occur, causing pulmonary venous congestion and, eventually, symptoms of congestive heart failure and an inability to wean from the ventilator or to reduce oxygen requirements. Prostaglandin E$_2$ (PGE$_2$) appears to be responsible for maintaining the patency of the ductus arteriosus during fetal life. Before term birth, there is a reduction in the levels of circulating PGE$_2$ that allows the constriction of the ductus. Infants born prematurely have high levels of circulating PGE$_2$, which tend to maintain the patency of the ductus after delivery (Lott, 1998).

Clinical manifestations of PDA depend in part on the size of the ductus (mild PDA may be asymptomatic) and the PVR level. Clinical presentation may include the classic continuous murmur (most commonly heard in the small premature infant) or a crescendo systolic murmur. Infants with severe PDA may demonstrate bounding peripheral pulses and widened pulse pressures and a hyperactive precordium. If the PDA persists, the infant may show signs of increasing congestive heart failure.

Indomethacin, administered intravenously, is used in the treatment of PDA in premature infants. If given early, indomethacin has been found effective in closing nearly 85% of PDAs (Flanagan & Fyler, 1994). Indomethacin acts to inhibit the production of PGE$_2$ and thereby promotes the closure of the ductus. Indomethacin is toxic to the kidneys and is contraindicated in infants with renal compromise, bleeding disorders, hyperbilirubinemia, and necrotizing enterocolitis. Surgical ligation of the PDA is indicated when treatment with indomethacin has not been successful or when such treatment is contraindicated.

Anticipatory Guidance for Prospective Parents of Preterm Neonates

Parents are often unprepared for emergency situations that occur during the birth of their infant. Because of the unanticipated nature of preterm births, parent counseling before delivery is often performed under less than ideal circumstances. However, every effort should be made to communicate effectively with the prospective parents. Medical terms, abbreviations, and percentages should be avoided as much as possible. Discuss with parents what to expect at delivery, possible complications, and the range of possible outcomes. The infant's chances for survival should also be discussed, and the uncertainties regarding the infant's outcome should be acknowledged. Most importantly, repetition may be necessary for parents to comprehend all this information, and an opportunity to review the information and ask questions should be provided. If neonatal intensive care unit (NICU) admission is anticipated, an opportunity to tour the NICU should be offered, if time permits (Gomella, Cunningham, Eyal, & Zenk, 1999).

RESUSCITATION AND STABILIZATION IN THE DELIVERY ROOM

The American Academy of Pediatrics and American Heart Association Neonatal Resuscitation Program sets the standard for the resuscitation and stabilization of babies who have cardiorespiratory depression at birth or who present with asphyxia (Kattwinkel, 2000). Key components of the program involve anticipating which infants may require resuscitation and having appropriately trained personnel

Client Education

Anticipatory Guidance for Expectant Parents of Premature Infants

Anticipatory guidance for prospective parents of preterm neonates should be geared toward brief explanations about the infant's probable condition, expected outcome, length of hospital stay, equipment, and policies and procedures of the NICU (Gomella, Cunningham, Eyal, and Zenk, 1999). Some points that may be discussed with parents of preterm infants include:

1. Most extremely preterm neonates have respiratory distress and require oxygen and ventilatory support to breathe effectively. Other problems commonly experienced by preterm neonates include metabolic problems, infection, necrotizing enterocolotis, patent ductus arteriosus, intraventricular hemorrhage, apnea, and bradycardia.

2. Chronic complications of prematurity include chronic lung disease, periventricular leukomalacia, intraparenchymal cysts, hydrocephalus, malnutrition, retinopathy of prematurity, and hearing impairment.

3. Although the risk of disability is higher in preterm infants than in the general population, the majority of preterm children do not develop a major disability. Learning disability, attention deficit disorder, minor neuromotor dysfunction, and behavior problems are more frequent in school-aged children who were preterm than in full-term controls.

4. The expected length of hospital stay for most preterm neonates is estimated to be 2 weeks before or after the baby's estimated due date.

and equipment available and ready to respond if the need arises. Generally, one trained caregiver should be available at every delivery in which a healthy newborn is expected, and two caregivers should be available if a problem is anticipated. A skilled resuscitation requires the combined efforts of two trained individuals who perform a coordinated series of steps based on an evaluation of the infant's condition and response.

After delivery of a healthy term infant, routine care should be provided, including warmth, clearing of the infant's airway, and drying to prevent heat loss. In addition,

Nursing Alert

UNIVERSAL PRECAUTIONS

When performing neonatal resuscitation in the delivery room, the infectious status of the mother and baby is often unknown and the risk of exposure to potentially harmful body fluids is relatively high. The Centers for Disease Control and Prevention recommends that all bodily fluids be treated as potentially infectious, including blood, urine, stool, saliva, vomitus, and, in the case at delivery, amniotic fluid. Masks and protective eyewear or face shields should be worn during procedures that are likely to generate droplets of blood or other bodily fluids, which are especially common during the birth process. Gloves and protective gowns should be worn during resuscitation and when handling the newborn immediately after delivery. Mechanical devices should be used when suctioning the baby's nose, mouth, and pharynx and when suctioning the infant for meconium. Bag-mask devices should be used instead of mouth-to-mouth resuscitation when positive pressure ventilation is required. Although relatively uncommon, endotracheal suctioning or umbilical catheter placement has at times produced potentially infectious splashes of sputum or blood, respectively, thus requiring caregivers to exercise extreme caution and proper precautions when performing these procedures on a newborn.

because of the concern about the transmission of communicable diseases through blood or body fluid contact, strict universal precautions should be followed for all infants.

Resuscitation of an infant should be provided if meconium is present, the infant is not breathing or crying, the infant lacks good muscle tone, the infant is cyanotic, or the infant is delivered prematurely. Initial steps in the resuscitation include thermal management, positioning, suctioning, and tactile stimulation. First, the infant should be placed under a preheated radiant warmer to prevent heat loss. The infant should be positioned on his or her back or side with the neck slightly extended to ensure an open airway. If meconium was present in the amniotic fluid and the baby is not vigorous at birth (defined by strong respiratory effort, good muscle tone, and a heart rate of more than 100 beats per minute), tracheal suctioning should be performed (Kattwinkel, 2000). The infant's mouth, and then the nose, should be gently suctioned, using either a bulb syringe or mechanical suction (Figure 31-7). The infant should then be dried and the wet linens removed.

Once the infant has been dried, suctioned, and positioned, resuscitative personnel should simultaneously evaluate the infant's respiratory effort, heart rate, and color

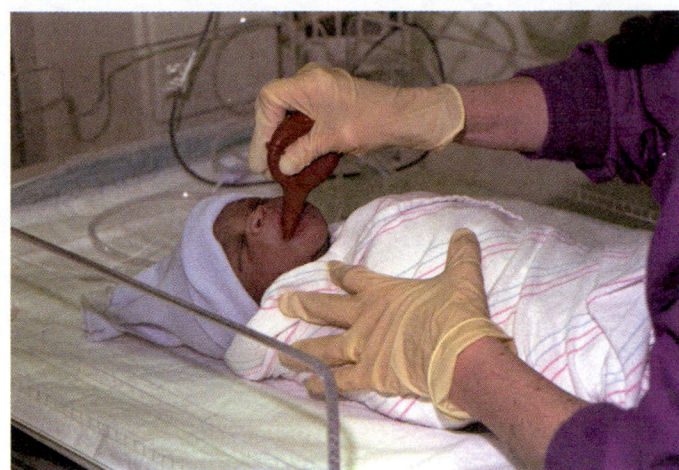

Figure 31-7 Bulb suction of post-term infant in delivery room.

(Kattwinkel, 2000). If central cyanosis is present but the infant is breathing spontaneously with a heart rate of more than 100 beats per minute, free-flow oxygen should be administered at 5 to 10 L/min, using either an oxygen mask or oxygen tubing held with a cupped hand over the infant's face (Kattwinkel, 2000) (Figure 31-8). If the infant remains cyanotic despite 100% free-flow oxygen, positive pressure ventilation should be initiated.

If the infant is not breathing or has inadequate respirations, tactile stimulation can be briefly provided by gently slapping the soles of the infant's feet or rubbing the infant's back. If the infant does not respond, mask-bag ventilation should be provided at a rate of 40 to 60 breaths per minute and continued until spontaneous respirations are established. The establishment of adequate alveolar ventilation is the cornerstone of the resuscitation process, because it promptly reverses many of the metabolic consequences of failure of the respiratory organ. Bag-mask

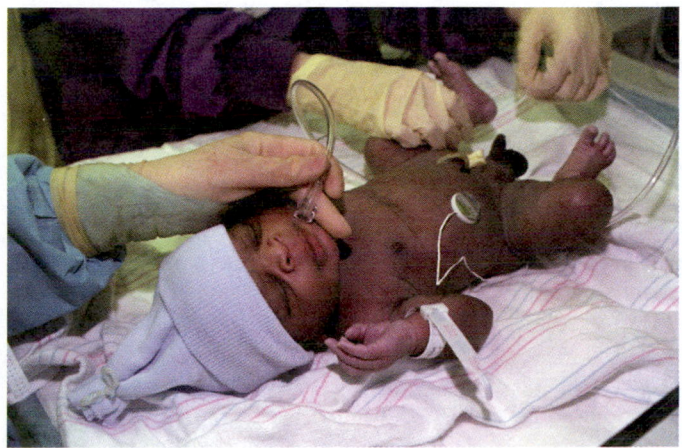

Figure 31-8 Newborn receiving free-flow oxygen in delivery room as therapy for central cyanosis.

Critical Thinking

Failure to Respond to Resuscitation Efforts

A 24-year-old primiparous woman is admitted to the obstetric unit in active labor at 41 weeks' gestation. No prenatal care was obtained during the pregnancy. Rupture of membranes occurred 2 hours ago, with thick, particulate meconium noted. Fetal monitoring discloses an abnormal fetal heart pattern that is unresponsive to maternal positioning and oxygen administration. A decision is made to perform an emergency cesarean section. At delivery, the baby is cyanotic, limp, and unresponsive, with a heart rate of 40 beats per minute.

1. What risk factors mean that this baby may require newborn resuscitation?

2. What personnel should be present at the delivery?

3. What equipment would you assemble in preparation for the delivery?

4. What are the steps you would take to resuscitate this infant?

5. If the infant's heart rate remains below 60 beats per minute despite ventilation, chest compressions, and medications, what assessment would you make to ensure that resuscitation efforts were being effectively delivered?

6. Complications of delivery and misdiagnosis or failure to diagnose in a timely fashion are indicative of a comparatively high rate of risk and litigation in perinatal health care. Given that you are certain that ventilation, chest compressions, and medications are being delivered appropriately, what other medical causes would you need to consider if the infant remains unresponsive to all resuscitative efforts?

ventilation should be given with enough pressure to provide an easy rise and fall of the chest and produce breath sounds. If bag-mask ventilation is performed for longer than a few minutes, an orogastric tube should be inserted and left in place, thereby preventing distention of the stomach and intestines and decreasing the risk of aspiration of gastric contents. If the infant is suspected of having a diaphragmatic hernia, prolonged positive pressure ventilation should be performed using a bag and endotracheal tube (Kattwinkel, 2000).

Positive pressure ventilation should also be performed any time that the heart rate is less than 100 beats per minute. If the heart rate is less than 60 beats per minute, despite 30 seconds of effective positive pressure ventilation with 100% oxygen, chest compressions should be initiated. The lower third of the infant's sternum, immediately above the xyphoid process, should be compressed to a depth of one-third the anterior-posterior diameter of the infant's chest and at a rate of 90/sec in conjunction with a ventilation rate of 30 breaths per minute (Kattwinkel, 2000). Chest compressions are the central tool in maintenance of circulatory function in the infant with persistent bradycardia during resuscitation. Maintenance of adequate circulatory function is a critical factor in determining survival and outcome. Because cardiac output and blood flow in the newborn are heart rate–related, resuscitation efforts should be made with great care to maintain the adequacy of circulatory function and minimize the devastating effects of tissue ischemia.

Positive response of the infant to resuscitative efforts is indicated by increasing heart rate, spontaneous respirations, and improving color. If the infant's condition continues to deteriorate or fails to improve despite assisted ventilation, the resuscitative team should check the adequacy of ventilation. If the chest movement is adequate and 100% oxygen is being administered, the infant may require endotracheal intubation to further stabilize his or her condition.

Although medications are rarely needed in newborn resuscitation, if the heart rate remains less than 60 beats per minute, despite 30 seconds of ventilation and another 30 seconds of coordinated chest compressions and ventilation, drugs may be indicated to improve the infant's circulatory status (Table 31-1). Although the umbilical vein is the preferred route of administration in the delivery room, epinephrine may also be administered by an endotracheal tube if an umbilical venous catheter or other intravenous catheter is not already in place.

Epinephrine (1:10,000) is currently used in resuscitation to increase heart rate, augment cardiac contractility, and increase PVR. Although sodium bicarbonate is not indicated during brief arrest, it may play a role if severe

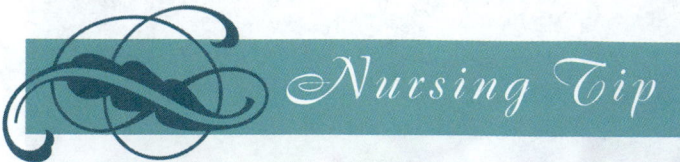

POSITIVE PRESSURE VENTILATION

Since establishing effective ventilation is the key to nearly all successful newborn resuscitations, the caregiver must be prepared to troubleshoot if the infant is not responding to positive pressure ventilation (Kattwinkel, 2000). Assessment must be done to ensure that chest movement is adequate. Common reasons why the chest may not be rising with each squeeze of the bag include:

- Inadequate face-mask seal
- Airway blocked because of improper head position or secretions
- Not enough pressure being used to ventilate the infant

If this happens when you are attempting to provide positive pressure ventilation, try using the following techniques:

- Reapply the mask to the infant's face
- Reposition the infant's head
- Suction secretions from the infant's nose, mouth, or oropharynx
- Increase ventilation pressure until there is an easy rise and fall of the chest

Table 31-1 Medications for Neonatal Resuscitation			
Medication	**Dose**	**Route**	**Rate**
Epinephrine (1:10,000)	0.1–0.3 mL/kg	Endotracheal tube Umbilical vein or other intravenous route	Rapid push
If hypovolemia, Normal saline or Ringer's lactate or O-negative blood	10 mL/kg	Umbilical vein or other intravenous route	Over 5–10 minutes
If severe metabolic acidosis, Sodium bicarbonate, 0.5 mEq/mL (4.2% solution)	2 mEq/kg	Umbilical vein or other intravenous route	Slowly; no faster than 1 mEq/kg/min

metabolic acidosis is suspected or proven by blood gas analysis. Sodium bicarbonate should not be used, however, until adequate ventilation has been established. If alveolar ventilation is inadequate, bicarbonate administration exacerbates acidosis and may be accompanied by a fall in cardiac output and increased lactic acid production by the gut.

Volume expanders are the third classification of drugs that are currently of proven value in newborn resuscitation, by means of increasing vascular volume and, subsequently, tissue perfusion. Volume expanders are indicated during resuscitation when there is evidence or suspicion of acute blood loss accompanied by signs of hypovolemia. A significant blood loss may be suspected if the infant has a pale color, weak pulse, persistently high or low heart rate, and if improvement in circulatory status is poor, despite resuscitation efforts (Kattwinkel, 2000). The recommended solution for acutely treating hypovolemia is normal saline, but other acceptable volume expanders include Ringer's lactate, O-negative blood that has been cross-matched with mother's blood, or emergency-release O-negative blood.

If the infant continues to deteriorate despite effective resuscitative efforts, other possible causes that should be explored include depressed respiratory drive, airway malformations, congenital heart disease, and lung problems, such as pneumothorax or diaphragmatic hernia.

Web Activities

- What online resources are available to support the American Academy of Pediatrics and American Heart Association's Neonatal Resuscitation Program? (see http://www.aap.org/profed/nrp/nrpmain.htm)

- What information can you locate on the Internet about transition to extrauterine life that both parents and nurses can use?

- What parent support groups can you locate on the Internet for families of full-term or preterm infants who require neonatal intensive care?

Key Concepts

- Fetal circulation differs from that in the newborn in three major respects: minimal blood flow through the lungs, presence of placental circulation, and presence of anatomic shunts.

- Gas exchange in the placenta occurs by simple diffusion at the intervillous space. Two factors favoring oxygen diffusion from the mother to the fetus include oxygen pressure gradients across the placenta and higher concentrations of fetal hemoglobin.

- Three anatomic shunts divert oxygenated blood to organs performing life-sustaining functions. The ductus venosus connects the umbilical vein to the inferior vena cava and allows blood to bypass the liver; the foramen ovale allows blood entering the right atrium of the heart to go directly to the left atrium, left ventricle, and out the ascending aorta to immediately supply the brain; and the ductus arteriosus shunts blood from the pulmonary artery to the descending aorta, thus bypassing the lungs.

- Several changes at birth occur that switch the organ of respiration from the placenta to the lung, including the onset of ventilation with a concomitant decrease in pulmonary vascular resistance and increase in pulmonary blood flow, rise in blood oxygen content, and loss of placental circulation, resulting in an increase in systemic (peripheral) vascular resistance.

- Effective thermal management at the time of birth plays a significant role in promoting an optimal transition by the neonate to extrauterine life.

- Physiologic and behavioral transition to extrauterine life in the immediate newborn period occurs in three phases: initial period of reactivity, period of relative inactivity, and second period of reactivity.

- Conditions that may impede the newborn's smooth transition to extrauterine life include asphyxia, persistent pulmonary hypertension of the newborn, meconium staining, transient tachypnea of the newborn, hypoglycemia, and hypovolemia (shock).

- Asphyxia is a metabolic process that arises from failure of the respiratory organ in the fetus or neonate. This impaired gas exchange results in a complex combination of hypoxemia, hypercapnia, acidosis, and ischemia.

- The Apgar score neither establishes nor rules out the presence of asphyxia. Resuscitation should be immediately initiated when indicated and not delayed for assessment of 1-minute Apgar score.

- Major pathologies that may impede the newborn's smooth transition to extrauterine life include congenital heart defects, sepsis, and diaphragmatic hernia.

- Developmental immaturity of the pulmonary and cardiac systems may impede the preterm neonate's adaptation to extrauterine life.

- Nurses must partner with parents to ensure that hospital policies and practices facilitate the parent's right to be with their baby during the crisis period and to participate in their infant's care, as guided by parent preference and the clinical situation.

- The American Academy of Pediatrics and American Heart Association's Neonatal Resuscitation Program provides recommendations for resuscitation of infants, including thermal support, airway management, establishment of breathing and circulation, and medications as clinically indicated.

Review Questions and Activities

1. During normal transition from fetal to postnatal circulation, all of the following cardiopulmonary changes must occur in the neonate *except:*
   a. The placenta is removed and SVR decreases
   b. Lung expansion occurs and PVR falls
   c. Ductal blood flow becomes left-to-right
   d. Increased left atrial pressure

   The correct answer is a.

2. An infant in primary apnea would exhibit which of the following signs?
   a. Gasping before becoming pink
   b. Heart rate around 50 beats per minute
   c. Pulses poor or absent
   d. No response to tactile stimuli

   The correct answer is a.

3. Which of the following statements is true concerning asphyxia?
   a. The Apgar score is a good indicator of the presence or absence of asphyxia
   b. Poor perfusion accompanied by asphyxia is caused by volume depletion
   c. The acidosis associated with asphyxia is primarily metabolic in origin
   d. Ischemia has a more profound effect on tissue oxygenation than hypoxemia does

   The correct answer is d.

4. In the delivery room, an infant presenting with no spontaneous respiratory effort and an Apgar score of 2 probably has:
   a. Primary apnea
   b. Secondary apnea
   c. Narcotic depression
   d. Retained fetal lung fluid

   The correct answer is b.

5. Which of the following statements is *false* regarding the transition from a fetal to a postnatal circulatory pathway?
   a. The major determinant of the direction of shunting through fetal circulatory pathways is the relationship between SVR and PVR

   b. Shunting of blood from right-to-left during transitional circulation may result in pulmonary congestion
   c. In fetal circulation, blood is ejected from both the right and left ventricle into systemic circulation
   d. A major determinant of the resistance to blood flow in the pulmonary circuit is alveolar hypoxia

   The correct answer is b.

6. High PVR in utero is maintained by the presence of all of the following factors *except:*
   a. Small pulmonary arteries, which contain little muscle mass
   b. Absence of air-fluid interface in the alveoli
   c. Absence of rhythmic distention of the lung
   d. Low resting oxygen tension in utero

   The correct answer is a.

7. A term infant develops severe respiratory distress within minutes after birth. On physical examination, the chest is hyperexpanded and the point of maximal impulse (PMI) is shifted to the right. Which of the following is the most likely cause for this infant's respiratory distress?
   a. Diaphragmatic hernia
   b. Congenital pneumonia
   c. Right-sided pneumothorax
   d. Meconium aspiration

   The correct answer is a.

8. Which of the following statements is *true* concerning thermoregulation in the newborn?
   a. The infant's core body temperature is an accurate assessment of neutral thermal environment
   b. Hypoxia blunts the infant's metabolic response to cold stress
   c. An infant in an incubator is in a neutral thermal environment when the randomly set air temperature maintains the infant's axillary temperature at 97.5°F to 99.5°F
   d. The zone of thermal neutrality is wider in the infant with a very low birth weight

   The correct answer is b.

9. The method of heat loss in which heat is lost to cool surfaces in direct contact with the infant is called:

a. Radiation
b. Convection
c. Conduction
d. Evaporation

The correct answer is c.

10. The neonate with an axillary temperature of 96.5°F is at increased risk of developing all of the following *except:*

a. Metabolic acidosis
b. Hypoglycemia
c. Hypotension
d. Hypoxemia

The correct answer is c.

References

Amlung, S. R. (1998). Neonatal thermoregulation. In C. Kenner, J. W. Lott, and A. A. Flandemeyer (Eds.) *Comprehensive neonatal nursing: A physiologic perspective, 2nd ed.,* (pp. 207–219). Philadelphia: W. B. Saunders.

Arnold, H. W., Putnam, N. J., Barnard, B. L., Desmond, M. M., & Rudolph, A. J. (1965). The newborn: Transition to extrauterine life. *American Journal of Nursing, 65,* (10), 77–80.

Baumgart, S. (1996). Thermal regulation in the fetus and newborn. In A. R. Spitzer (Ed.) *Intensive care of the fetus and neonate,* (pp. 401–416). St. Louis: Mosby.

Behram, S., Moschler, E. F., Sayegh, S. K., Garguillo, F. P., & Mann, W. J. (1998). Implementation of early discharges after uncomplicated vaginal deliveries: Maternal and infant complications. *Southern Medical Journal, 91,* (6), 541–545.

Brooks, C. (1997). Neonatal hypoglycemia. *Neonatal Network, 16,* (2), 15–21.

DeBoer, S. L., & Stephens, D. (1997). Persistent pulmonary hypertension of the newborn: Case study and pathophysiology review. *Neonatal Network, 16,* (1), 7–13.

Desmond, M. M., & Rudolph, A. J. (1965). Progressive evaluation of the newborn infant. *Postgraduate Medicine, 73,* 207–212.

Desmond, M. M., Franklin, R. R., Vallbona, C., Hill, R. M., Plumb, R., Arnold, H., & Watts, J. (1963). The clinical behavior of the newly born. *Journal of Pediatrics, 62,* (3), 307–325.

Donn, S. M., & Faix, R. G. (1996). Delivery room resuscitation. In A. R. Spitzer (Ed.) *Intensive care of the fetus and neonate,* (pp. 326–336). St. Louis: Mosby.

Fisher, D. E., & Paton, J. B. (1986). Resuscitation of the newborn infant. In M. H. Klaus & A. A. Fanaroff (Eds.). *Care of the high-risk neonate, 3rd ed.,* (pp. 31–50). Philadelphia: W. B. Saunders.

Flanagan, M. F., & Fyler, D. C. (1994). Cardiac disease. In G. B. Avery, M. A. Fletcher, & M. G. MacDonald (Eds.) *Neonatology: Pathophysiology and management of the newborn,* 4th ed., (pp. 516–559). Philadelphia: J. B. Lippincott.

Freij, B., & McCracken, G. (1994). Acute infections. In G. B. Avery, M. A. Fletcher, & M. G. MacDonald (Eds.) *Neonatology: Pathophysiology and management of the newborn,* 4th ed., (pp. 1082–1116). Philadelphia: J. B. Lippincott.

Gomella, T. L., Cunningham, M. D., Eyal, F. G., & Zenk, K. E. (Eds.) (1999). *Neonatology: Management, procedures, on-call problems, diseases, and drugs, 4th ed.,* (pp. 209–212). Stamford, CT: Appleton & Lange.

Guyton, A., & Hall, J. (1996). *Textbook of medical physiology,* 9th ed. Philadelphia: W. B. Saunders.

Guzzetta, P. C., Anderson, K. D., Eichelberger, M. R., Newman, K. D., Rouse, T. M., Schnitzer, J. J., Boyajian, M., & Tomaski, S. (1994). General surgery. In G. B. Avery, M. A. Fletcher, & M. G. MacDonald (Eds.) *Neonatology: Pathophysiology and management of the newborn, 4th ed.,* (pp. 914–951). Philadelphia: J. B. Lippincott.

Hey, E. (1994). Thermoregulation. In G. B. Avery, M. A. Fletcher, & M. G. MacDonald, (Eds.) *Neonatology: Pathophysiology and management of the newborn, 4th ed.,* (pp. 357–365). Philadelphia: J. B. Lippincott.

Jepson, H. A., Talashek, M. L., & Tichy, A. M. (1991). The Apgar score: Evolution, limitations, and scoring guidelines. *Birth 18,* (2), 83–91.

Kattwinkel, J. (Ed.) (2000). *Textbook of neonatal resuscitation,* 4th ed. Elk Grove Village, IL: American Academy of Pediatrics & American Heart Association.

Levitt-Katz, L. E., & Stanley, C. (1996). Disorders of glucose and other sugars. In A. R. Spitzer, (Ed.) *Intensive care of the fetus and neonate,* (pp. 982–992). St. Louis: Mosby.

Lott, J. W. (1998). Assessment and management of cardiovascular dysfunction. In C. Kenner, J. W. Lott, and A. A. Flandemeyer, (Eds.) *Comprehensive neonatal nursing: A physiologic perspective, 2nd ed.,* (pp. 306–335). Philadelphia: W. B. Saunders.

Lott, J. W., & Kenner, C. (1998). Assessment and management of immunologic dysfunction. In C. Kenner, J. W. Lott, and A. A. Flandemeyer, (Eds.) *Comprehensive neonatal nursing: A physiologic perspective,* 2nd ed., (pp. 496–519). Philadelphia: W. B. Saunders.

Ludington-Hoe, S. M., Hadeed, A. J., & Anderson, G. C. (1991). Physiological responses to skin-to-skin contact in hospitalized premature infants. *Journal of Perinatology, 11,* (1), 19–24.

Moore, K. L., & Persaud, T. V. N. (1993). *The developing human: Clinically oriented embryology, 5th ed.,* (pp. 226–236). Philadelphia: W. B. Saunders.

Nelson, N. (1994). Physiology of transition. In G. B. Avery, M. A. Fletcher, & M. G. MacDonald, (Eds.) *Neonatology: Pathophysiology and management of the newborn, 4th ed.,* (pp. 223–247). Philadelphia: J. B. Lippincott.

Ogata, E. (1994). Carbohydrate homeostasis. In G. B. Avery, M. A. Fletcher, & M. G. MacDonald, (Eds.) *Neonatology: Pathophysiology and management of the newborn, 4th ed.,* (pp. 568–584). Philadelphia: J. B. Lippincott.

Pridjian, G. (1994). Fetomaternal interactions: Placental physiology and its role as a go-between. In G. B. Avery, M. A. Fletcher, & M. G. MacDonald, (Eds.) *Neonatology: Pathophysiology and management of the newborn, 4th ed.,* (pp. 126–143). Philadelphia: J. B. Lippincott.

Sansoucie, D. A., & Cavaliere, T. A. (1997). Transition from fetal to extrauterine circulation. *Neonatal Network, 16,* (2), 5–12.

Serwer, G.A. (1992). Postnatal circulatory adjustments. In R. A. Polin and W. W. Fox, (Eds.) *Fetal and neonatal physiology,* (pp. 710–721). Philadelphia: W. B. Saunders.

Whitsett, J. A., Pryhuber, G. S., Rice, W. R., Warner, B. B., & Wert, S. E. (1994). Acute respiratory disorders. In G. B. Avery, M. A. Fletcher, & M. G. MacDonald, (Eds.) *Neonatology: Pathophysiology and management of the newborn, 4th ed.,* (pp. 429–452). Philadelphia: J. B. Lippincott.

Suggested Readings

McCollum, L. (1998). Resuscitation and stabilization of the neonate. In C. Kenner, J. W. Lott, and A. A. Flandemeyer, (Eds.) *Comprehensive neonatal nursing: A physiologic perspective, 2nd ed.,* (pp. 190–206). Philadelphia: W. B. Saunders.

Niermeyer, S. (Ed.). (2000). International guidelines for neonatal resuscitation: An excerpt from the guidelines 2000 for cardiopulmonary resuscitation and emergency cardiovascular care: International consensus on science. *Pediatrics, 106,* (3), 1–16.

O'Neill, (Eds.) *Core curriculum for neonatal intensive care nursing, 2nd ed.* (pp. 40–62)

Varda, K., & Behnke, R. (2000). The effect of timing of initial bath on newborn's temperature. *JOGNN, 29,* 27–32.

Zabloudil, C. (1999). Adaptation to extrauterine life. In J. Deacon and P. O'Neill, (Eds.) *Core curriculum for neonatal intensive care nursing, 2nd ed.,* (pp. 40–62).

Resources

American Academy of Pediatrics, Division of Life Support Programs, 141 Northwest Point Blvd., P.O. Box 927, Elk Grove Village, IL 60009-0927, (800)433-9016, extension 6798, http://www.aap.org/

National Association of Neonatal Nurses, 4700 W. Lake Avenue, Glenview, IL 60026-1485, (800)451-3795 or (847)375-3660, http://www.nann.org/

Assessment and Care of the Normal Newborn

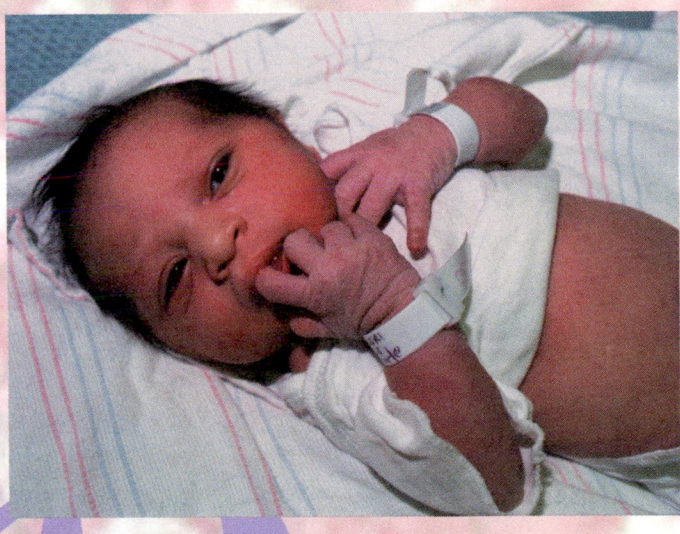

Nursing care of mothers and their newborn infants is often thought to be the most joyous and rewarding experience for the nurse because a brand new person is welcomed into the world. Although nursing care of the newborn after transition is focused on the health of the infant, the nurse has the opportunity to be involved with the parents of the infant and to interact with other family members to plan for the infant's future well-being within the family unit. Use the following questions to examine your personal feelings regarding nursing care of newborn infants:

- *How would I feel if I were the nurse caring for an infant who would not stop crying?*
- *How would I feel as a new mother if no one were to tell me whether my baby were doing well and when I might see him?*
- *How would I feel as a nurse if I were caring for an infant who was not feeding well?*
- *How would I feel if I were a new mother of a baby who was sick or had a physical abnormality?*
- *How would I feel if I were the nurse caring for a mother and her newborn and I overheard a family member say something to the mother that would affect the infant's health and safety at home?*

Key Terms

Acrocyanosis
Anal wink reflex
Anterior fontanel
Caput succedaneum
Cephalhematoma
Chorioamnionitis
Coarctation of the aorta
Cyanosis

Developmental dysplasia
  of the hip (DDH)
Epispadias
Erythema toxicum
Hypospadias
Imperforate anus
Lanugo
Macrocephaly

Meconium
Microcephaly
Milia
Mongolian spots
Mottling
Patent ductus arteriosis
  (PDA)
Polydactyly

Posterior fontanel
Postterm infant
Preterm infant
Pustular melanosis
Syndactyly
Tachycardia
Tachypnea
Term infant

Competencies

Upon completion of this chapter, the reader should be able to:

1. Perform a full physical examination and gestational age assessment on a newborn infant to provide an accurate account of the infant's status to its mother and father.

2. Describe the unique characteristics and behaviors of a newborn infant to its parents and other family members.

3. Demonstrate to all family members proper holding and positioning of infants for safety and to prevent injury.

4. Discuss factors with the parents and family that may place the infant at risk for illness, and suggest parental interventions for illness prevention.

5. Explain feeding and elimination schedules to parents to alleviate any concerns.

6. Anticipate parental anxieties related to caring for their new infant during the neonatal period and develop a teaching plan for parents to address these anxieties.

7. Incorporate family values and ethnic and religious perspectives in teaching plans for infant care and health maintenance visits.

Preparing for a healthy infant preoccupies a mother-to-be during the time that she is pregnant until the time of delivery, when the physiologic forces of contractions and the process of labor disrupt her fantasies and redirect her attentions. Her first glimpse of her infant reassures her that the journey from the womb to the world was accomplished safely (Rubin, 1984). As the mother holds her newborn for the first time, she celebrates this new life with the infant's father and other family members. The nurse in charge of the infant's care can safeguard this moment in family life by not intruding or interrupting the family's opportunity to be with their newest member.

After the parents and family members have the opportunity to touch, hold, and interact with their infant, the nurse can address any concerns related to the infant's condition or behavior. The interaction of the nurse with all family members at this time forms the basis for the nursing assessment of the family's ethnic or cultural perspectives

regarding the infant. This assessment is incorporated into the nurse's teaching plans for the parents and the family regarding caring for the infant at home.

Before the introduction of the infant to the parents and the family, the nurse uses assessment skills to determine the physical health of the infant and its physiologic stability after transition. This chapter describes the complete examination of the infant and the gestational age determination with size parameters that describes the physical condition of the infant. Findings that may place the infant at risk for injury or infection or that warrant further investigation alert the nurse to develop strategies for intervention. In addition, guidelines are presented for continued nursing assessments of the infant while the infant remains under the nurse's care. Finally, factors to consider in the determination of parental and family perspectives are delineated to provide a comprehensive assessment of the parental and family environment. The design of this chapter provides knowledge of the skills in newborn assessment so that the nurse can intervene when necessary and implement infant care strategies that address parental concerns and family considerations.

ASSESSMENT AFTER TRANSITION

Nursing assessment of the newborn infant after transition continues to be a critical factor in determining the infant's adjustment to the extrauterine environment. Transition of the newborn immediately after delivery in the nursery or in another special care environment is conducted according to the institutional protocol. Time frames for this transitional period are adjusted for the individual infant's condition and accurate assessment of the infant's physiologic stability. Transition of newborn infants usually encompasses the first 4 to 6 hours of life (Seidel, Rosenstein, & Pathak, 2001). Nursing concerns after the transitional period are directed toward balancing the need for observation and assessment of the newborn infant with the needs of the mother and family to have their infant with them.

REFLECTIONS FROM A NURSERY NURSE

"I had gone to the mother's room to pick up her infant for the end of shift report. The mother was adamant that her infant was not going anywhere. She informed me that this was her baby, and if I touched her baby, she would call hospital security and accuse me of kidnapping. I was speechless. I didn't know what to do, so I left her infant in her room and made my report to the next shift. I went home and thought about what the mother had said, her rights as the mother of this infant, and hospital policies interfering with parental rights to their infants. I decided that my role as a nurse was to facilitate the opportunities for infants, mothers, and families to be together and that I needed to adjust my thinking and approach to accomplish this."

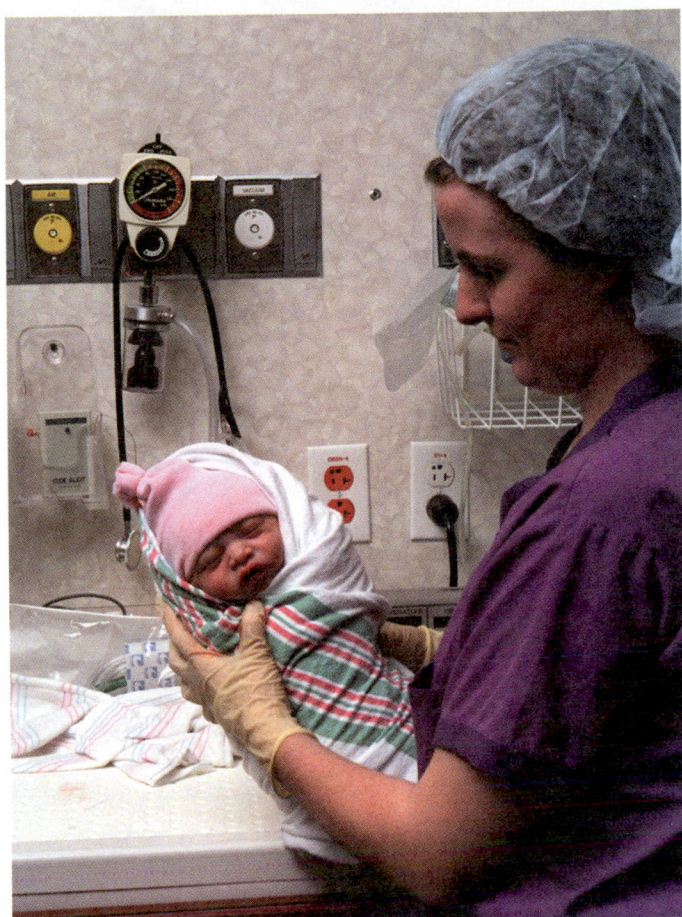

Figure 32-1 Knit caps and swaddling in a blanket help newborns maintain body heat.

Temperature

During the transitional period, the nurse determines that the infant is physiologically stable by skilled examination and assessment of the infant's thermoregulatory effort, cardiac system, and respiratory system. Infants received from the delivery room are usually swaddled in blankets with stocking caps to prevent chilling (Figure 32-1). To maintain body temperature, the infants are placed immediately in a temperature-controlled isolette or on a radiant warmer. Body temperature is assessed by recording axillary temperature or attaching the infant to a thermoprobe and recording monitor. Rectal temperatures are no longer routinely done on infants because the insertion of the rectal thermometer into the anus of an infant risks damage to the rectal lining and may break the thermometer. Anal patency is no longer confirmed by insertion of a thermometer. It is assessed by examination of the anus and visual confirmation of stool being excreted through the anal opening (Seidel et al., 2001). Axillary infant temperature should be maintained between 36.5°C to 37.6°C (97.7°F to 99.7° F) (Wong, Hockenberry-Eaton, Wilson, Winkelstein, Ahmann, & DiVito-Thomas, 1999).

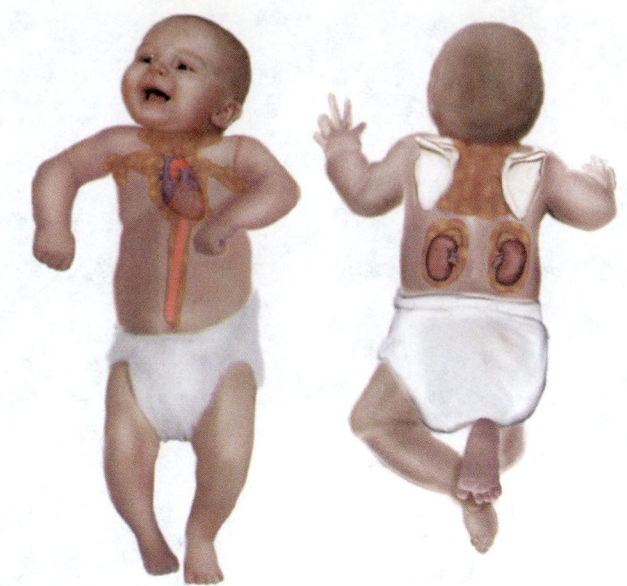

Figure 32-2 Brown-fat distribution in the newborn.

The infant's ability to maintain body heat is related to controlling the factors that produce heat loss in the newborn infant. The organ system that occupies the largest surface area on an infant is the skin, placing the infant at risk for heat loss by evaporation to the environment. Placing the infant in a warm environment minimizes this risk. In spite of the rise in newborn birth weight, leading to larger infants, the subcutaneous fat layer is thin, offering no insulation against heat loss and no adequate energy source to raise body temperature. Warm environments coupled with decreased infant stimulation and energy expenditures assist the infant in maintaining body temperature. Infants who are chilled are not able to produce body heat through shivering but can produce body heat through an alternative mechanism. This alternative mechanism involves stimulating the metabolism of brown fat (Figure 32-2), a special adipose tissue in newborns, located between the scapulae, around the neck, in the axillae, behind the sternum, around the kidneys, and surrounding some of the major arteries (Wong et al., 1999). The location of brown fat in the axillae may cause a transient rise

Nursing Tip

BROWN FAT

It is important to keep the neonate warm to avoid excess energy expenditure. Brown fat is the infant's last defense mechanism against hypothermia.

in axillary temperature that the nurse may misinterpret as a rise in infant core body temperature. Assessments of infant temperature after transition provide the nurse ample opportunities for a determination of the infant's ability to control its temperature within the environment.

Cardiovascular System

Assessment of the cardiovascular system after the transitional period is directed to the infant's ability to convert fetal circulation to postnatal circulation. Fetal circulation during pregnancy was dependent on shunting blood flow through the foramen ovale, the ductus arteriosus, and the ductus venosus. As the infant breathes on his or her own, the inspired oxygen enters the pulmonary vasculature and pulmonary vascular resistance decreases, leading to an increase in pulmonary blood flow to the chambers on the left side of the heart. This, coupled with the increased systemic blood circulation from the placenta during cord clamping, leads to reversal of fetal blood flow because the heart now undergoes postnatal ventricular contraction (Wong et al., 1999). Reversing blood flow through the fetal shunts ultimately results in their closure, and backflow through the shunts results in heart murmurs that are often called "flow murmurs." The nurse monitors these events by carefully auscultating heart sounds, determining heart rate, checking peripheral pulses, and observing skin color changes indicative of improving cardiac perfusion to the extremities.

During the course of transition, the nurse would expect the infant's heart rate to decrease from highs of 150 to 160 beats per minute to a regular pattern and rate between 130 and 140 beats per minute. The infant heart adjusts to the increased blood flow through the ventricles and becomes more efficient at pumping blood through them. Peripheral perfusion is evaluated by the presence of peripheral pulses, capillary refill, and skin color. The nurse identifies the characteristics of peripheral pulses related to strength, rhythm, and bounding qualities; compares pulses bilaterally; and times capillary refill (rapid refill is 3 seconds or less). Skin color should remain pink or healthy and may appear "rosy" as capillary circulation improves.

Respiratory System

Nursing assessment of the infant's respiratory system after transition begins with observing the infant's respiratory effort, listening to the sounds made while the infant is breathing, and auscultating all lung fields. Air entering the infants' lungs after delivery competes with fluid remaining in the alveolar spaces. The majority of this fluid in the lungs and aveoli is removed by pulmonary capillaries, the lymphatic system, and the labor and delivery process. Surfactant reduces the surface tension of the fluid and allows air to enter the aveoli for gas exchange (Wong et al., 1999).

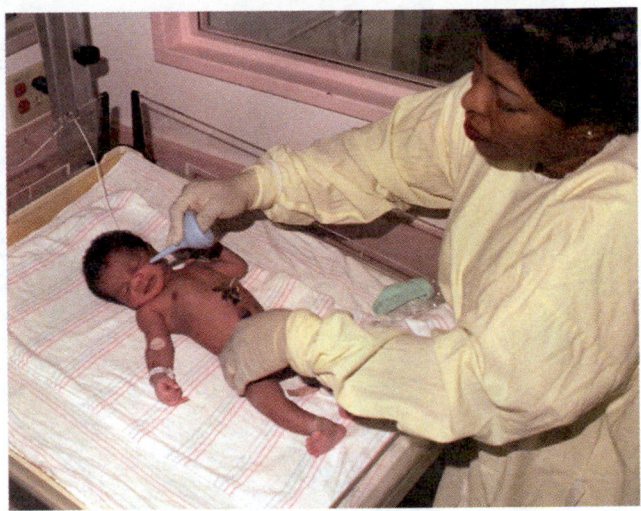

Figure 32-3 Infants who blow bubbles through their mouth or nose should be suctioned with a bulb syringe.

Fluid remaining in the lungs may cause a condition called transient tachypea of the newborn (TTN) characterized by a rapid respiratory rate (above 60 breaths per minute) with no other symptoms of respiratory distress, for example, intercostal or sternal retractions, nasal flaring, or grunting. Grunting is an audible sound made by the infant while undergoing inspiration and expiration. Normal breathing occurs quietly. TTN is characterized by fluid in the lung fissures and streaky parenchymal changes with hyperinflation of the lungs on a chest X-ray (Seidel et al., 2001). Normally, with no treatment other than careful observation, a repeat chest X-ray 24 hours later reveals a clearing of the fluid and a resolution of the hyperinflated lung state.

Observation of the infant in the supine position assists the nurse in the evaluation of the infant's respiratory effort. Symmetrical chest movements, use of accessory muscles, a labored or unlabored appearance, and intercostal or sternal retractions are noted. Infants breathe primarily through their nose, and visual inspection can confirm this. Those infants who have evidence of bubbles around the mouth or who appear to be blowing bubbles through their nares can be relieved by using a bulb syringe to clear the oropharynx or the nasal passages (Figure 32-3). Lung fields should be auscultated anteriorly and posteriorly while gently rolling the infant onto each side. Breath sounds are noisy, and the

sound radiates and echoes throughout the entire chest because of the thinness of the chest wall. Until respiratory and hemodynamic stability is achieved, at approximately 12 to 24 hours of life, it is difficult to determine the presence of rales or rhonchi in lung fields because of the echoing and radiation of the auscultated sounds.

Nasal patency can be confirmed by gently occluding one naris at a time with the infant's mouth closed and observing for a rise in the chest, indicative of the infant's ability to inhale air into the lungs through an intact nasal passageway. Infants who have difficulty with this maneuver may have choanal atresia, a malformation of the bucconasal membrane, leading to obstruction of the nasal passageway. Choanal atresia is confirmed by being unable to insert a small catheter (a No. 8 French feeding tube is preferred in newborns) into an infant's nares. Bilateral choanal atresia produces cyanosis when the infant's mouth is closed and disappears when the mouth is open or the infant is crying. Unilateral choanal atresia may not be identified until rhinorrhea (nasal discharge) occurs in early childhood, obstructing the naris that is patent (Seidel et al., 2001). Choanal atresia is a developmental anomaly occurring during gestation, and it may be accompanied by other defects. Positive findings of choanal atresia should be reported immediately, and the infant should be examined for other anomalies, the most common being CHARGE association (Box 32-1).

General Nursing Care

Once the nursing assessment of body temperature and the cardiac and respiratory systems is made and established as stable over time, the nurse notes whether the infant has received ophthalmic and vitamin K prophylaxis and a first bath.

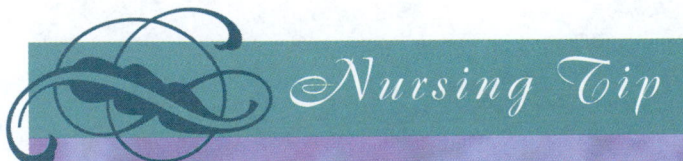

Box 32-1 Characteristics of CHARGE Association in the Newborn

C = Coloboma, a malformation of the iris and pupil, which affects the retina and the optic nerve

H = Heart defect

A = Choanal atresia

R = Retardation, physical and mental

G = Genital hypoplasia

E = Ear anomalies

Infants with CHARGE association may need an emergency tracheostomy or surgical repair of the atresia. They experience difficulty in feeding and responding to light (vision problems) or sound stimulation (hearing problems) and have episodes of peripheral and central cyanosis. Additionally, these infants may have decreased kidney function because embryonic development of ears and kidneys occurs at the same time. Nursing care focuses on reducing environmental stressors that irritate or excite the infant because these infants may have compromised breathing patterns and circulatory problems.

Nursing Alert

EYE DISCHARGE

Any eye irritation or discharge persisting for more than 24 hours should be reported immediately to rule out chemical conjunctivitis from eye prophylaxis.

1% silver nitrate solution, and 1% tetracycline, which are effective against infection. Silver nitrate solution stains the periorbital area black when the infant blinks and can be removed with a moist wipe. All three ointments or drops cause a chemical conjunctivitis of the eyes within the first 24 hours of life. The nurse observes a matting of the eyelashes and, possibly, a yellowish discharge that can be removed with a moist wipe. The discharge and irritation to the eyes ceases after 24 hours.

Vitamin K Prophylaxis

Prophylactic injection of vitamin K (0.5 to 1.0 mg phytonadione) is given by intramuscular injection into the infant's thigh during the first hour of life to stimulate production of vitamin K by the bacteria in the infant's intestine (Figure 32-5). At delivery, the intestine of the infant is considered to be sterile, or without normal bacteria. Once the **meconium** stool has passed, the intestinal lining and mucosal cells rapidly adjust to metabolize food and excrete food by-products. Bacterial formation stimulates production of vitamin K, a cofactor in the normal clotting process, from the infection given to the neonate. Infants may develop a

Ophthalmic Prophylaxis

Ophthalmic prophylaxis is given according to institutional protocol in ointment or drop form to prevent gonococcal and chlamydial infection in neonates (Figure 32-4). Choices for ointments or drops include 0.5% erythromycin,

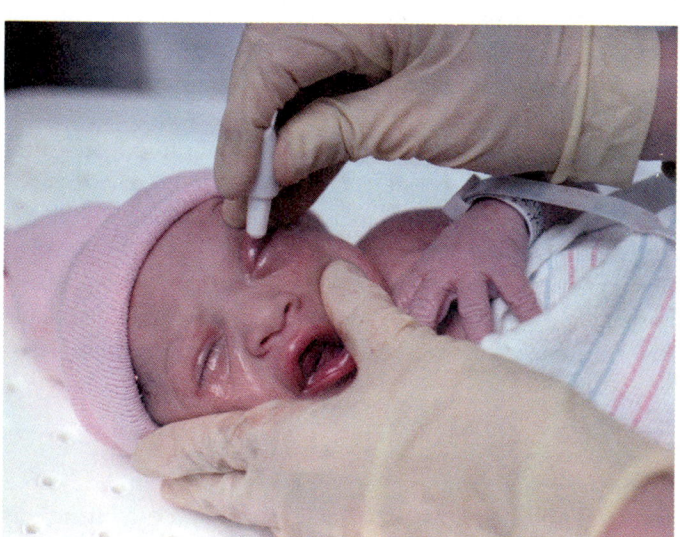

Figure 32-4 Ophthalmic prophylaxis prevents gonococcal and chlamydial infection in the newborn.

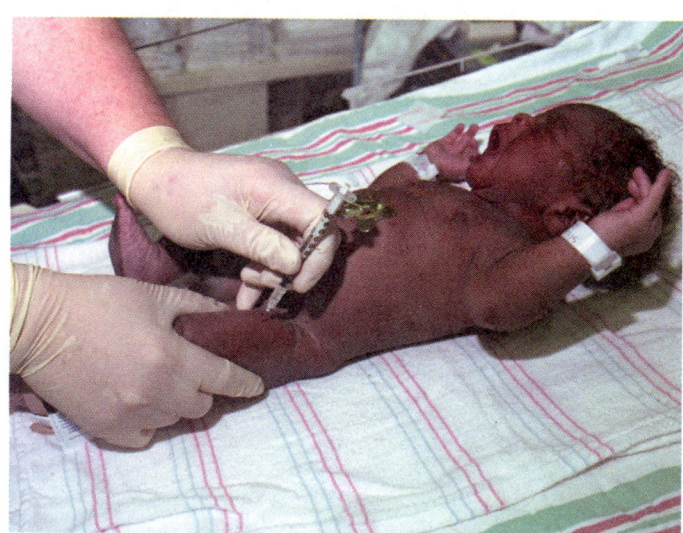

Figure 32-5 Administration of vitamin K.

REFLECTIONS FROM A NURSE

"I was the nurse caring for a mother and her new-born son in the rooming-in area of our postpartum unit. I remembered this mother because she was so upset that she delivered here instead of at home. All she wanted to do was go home. She didn't want anything done for the baby. I think she was worried about it costing more money. I brought her the consent form to sign for the vita-min K injection and the eye ointment and she re-fused. She said her baby didn't need it. I went back to the nurse practitioner in charge, who sub-sequently conferred with the physician. The nurse practitioner and I went back to see the mother and explain to her that she had the right not to sign the consent form but that she needed to be fully in-formed before she made that decision. The nurse practitioner told the mother that there was a 10% risk of intraventricular hemorrhage in her baby's head during the first year of life without prophylaxis vitamin K and also explained the importance of the eye ointment to protect her baby's corneas. Mom said she would think about it. Later that day, before she left with her infant, she asked for both the eye ointment and vitamin K for her baby. I thought to myself, 'I'm so glad she thought about what her baby needed, instead of her own frustration at being here.'"

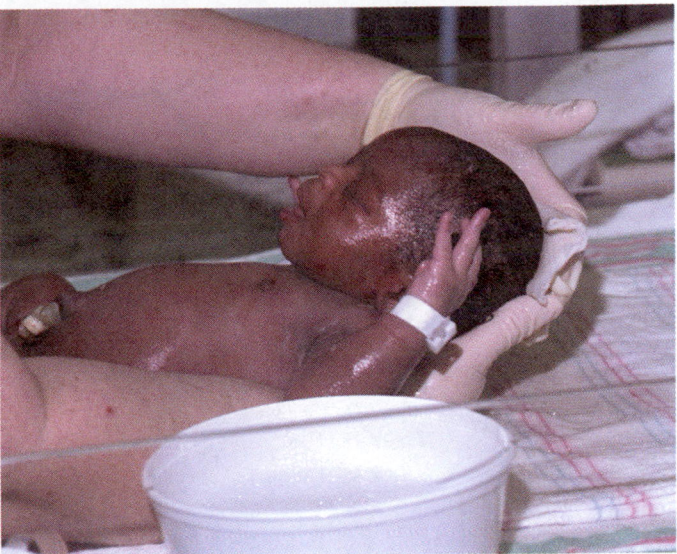

Figure 32-6 A newborn's first bath.

residues on the skin (Figure 32-6). The nurse should antic-ipate any chilling effect from the circulating air or the bath and take precautions to ensure that the infant is kept warm and dried quickly. Institutional protocol may recommend painting of the umbilical cord with a bacteriostatic dye. Some institutions have discontinued this procedure be-cause the dye does not hasten the drying process of the cord or prevent umbilical cord infections. If the painting is done, the nurse must inspect and record the number of cord vessels present before the painting. It is difficult to in-spect the cord for the presence of vessels when it has dye on it or when the cord has partially dried.

After being bathed and swaddled in blankets, the infant is ready to be examined in more detail. Nurses

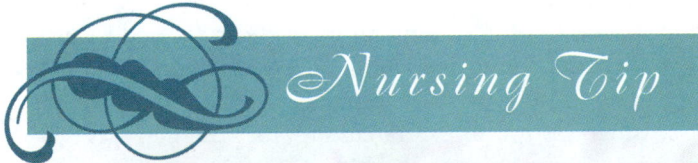

Nursing Tip

UMBILICAL CORD VESSELS

The infant should have an umbilical cord with three vessels, two arteries, and one vein. Two-vessel cords (one artery, one vein) must be reported immediately: they are associated with renal and cardiac anomalies. Ultrasound examinations and echocardiograms are recommended in these cases to confirm any abnor-mality that might be present. The most common renal abnormality characterized by a two-vessel cord is renal agenesis, which affects the infant's urinary out-put because a kidney, usually the left, fails to develop normally in utero.

vitamin K deficiency within 2 to 3 days following birth if the vitamin K prophylaxis is not given. Severe conse-quences may occur in infants not given vitamin K, because central nervous system hemorrhages commonly occur (Taeusch & Ballard, 1998).

First Bath

The first bath is given in warm water with a mild soap to remove amniotic fluid, blood, vaginal secretions, and other

Table 32-1 Critimal Pathway for Timing of Newborn Assessment

Assessment	Age (hrs)					
	0–4	4–8	8–12	12–24	24–36	36–48
Laboratory	Blood type Coombs' Test (Cord Blood) Glucose blood level	–	–	–	–	–
Assessment						
Gestational age	–	–	X	–	–	–
Physical	–	–	X	X	X	X
Vital signs	HR>130	HR-100–130	X	X	X	X
	RR<60	X	X	RR 40–60	X	X
	T>97°F	X	X	X	X	X
Skin color	White-pink	Pink	X	X	X	X
Interventions	Radiant warmer Blankets	Feeding	Position	X	X	X
Nutrition	None or breastfeeding	Water	Formula or breast	X	X	X
Medication	Vitamin K Eye prophylaxis	Cord Dye	–	–	Hepatitis B vaccine	X
Activity	Sleep	Awake	Active-Alert	X	X	X
Safety	Airway identification	Position	X	X	X	X
Teaching	–	Bulb syringe First bath	Feeding	Cord care	Skin Care	Diaper rash
Discharge planning	–	–	–	Breastfeeding	Illness	Follow-up
	–	–	–	Feeding	X	Car seat
	–	–	–	Car seat	X	Follow-up
	–	–	–	Neonatal screening	X	
	–	–	–	Follow-up	X	

Second neonatal screening done at 2-wk follow-up visit.
RR, respiratory rate; HR, heart rate; T, temperature.

perform several different assessments on newborns after delivery. The first assessment is accomplished during the transition, the first 4 to 6 hours of the infant's life. The infant is monitored for temperature and cardiac and respiratory stability during transition. After transition, the nurse performs a full physical examination, including a general assessment, physical examination, and gestational age assessment. Once this examination has been completed, the infant is monitored for any changes through periodic nursing assessments done at each nursing shift, brief examinations two or three times during the shift, and interactional assessments with the mother, father, and other family members. The purpose of all these assessments is to ensure the infant's physical and biologic stability and assist the nurse in planning for the family's adaptation to and care for the infant (Table 32-1).

GENERAL ASSESSMENT

Visual inspection of the infant in the crib forms the basis for a general nursing assessment. From inspection, the nurse can determine the infant's body position, skin color,

respiratory effort, relative size and length, and state of mind (asleep, awake, quiet-alert, or alert) and evaluate security measures in place to guarantee the identity of the infant and protect it from abduction. Infants in the nursery have nurses who are charged with the care of infants who are not at mother's bedside. Infants rooming-in with mother are cared for by the mother with the assistance of the nursing staff when needed.

Position

A newborn's position leaves clues as to its innate position of comfort. Many infants adopt their in utero position after delivery to enhance their feelings of security after separating from mother during the birth process. The normal body position of the newborn is flexion of both upper and lower extremities. The flexion of the upper extremities allows infants to touch their face with their hands, suck their fingers, and explore their new environment.

Lower extremities may be extended, fixed in one position from delivery position, or flexed. Usually, positioning in newborn infants is symmetrical. Asymmetrical posi-

POSITIONING OF INFANTS

The American Academy of Pediatrics (2000) recommends that all infants be placed to sleep in a non-prone position to prevent Sudden Infant Death Syndrome (SIDS). Placing infants in the supine position offers the best protection against SIDS. When using the side-lying position, caretakers are advised to bring the dependent arm forward to lessen the likelihood of the infant rolling to the prone position.

tioning may suggest an initial nursing assessment of injury related to birth trauma and may warrant further investigation. Failure to move an extremity or diminished extremity movement, unilaterally or bilaterally, would be a cause for concern.

Skin Color

Skin color becomes a vital part of the general nursing assessment because the newly born infant may show signs of jaundice or cardiovascular instability in the first several days of life. Jaundice in the newborn is characterized by a gradual yellowing of the skin that develops from head to toe. Visual jaundice in a newborn infant less than 24 hours old is considered to be "pathologic jaundice" or "hemolytic jaundice" and most likely results from serious blood incompatibility between the mother and the infant. "Physiologic jaundice" or "non-hemolytic" jaundice is the gradual yellowing of the skin in newborn infants that occurs after 24 hours of life, which may have a non-hemolytic cause. The three most common of these causes are: 1) the failure to adequately process bilirubin through inadequate intake or elimination, 2) traumatic birth injuries, and 3) minor blood incompatibilities. The neonatal jaundice that occurs with breastfeeding is usually not seen in the early postpartum period; this type of jaundice becomes visible in newborns that are approximately 1 week old and may persist during the entire course of breastfeeding.

N u r s i n g   A l e r t

JAUNDICE

Visible jaundice in a newborn infant under 24 hours of age must be reported immediately. A rate of rise in bilirubin levels of more than 0.5 mg/dL per hour should be investigated.

Additionally, congenital heart defects may be initially detected by skin pallor that does not improve with time. Skin color in all infants should be pink, indicating successful cardiac perfusion to the extremities. **Acrocyanosis** is common in newborns, localized to the hands and feet (Figure 32-7). Central cyanosis in the newborn has been described as a blue tint of the lips, gums, tongue, fingertips, and toes, with pallor noted underneath the eyes and on the cheeks. This is an indication that the newborn has a circulatory problem and needs immediate attention and investigation into the suspected cause of the cyanosis. Stimulating the infant to cry, changing the infant's position to increase movement, or gently patting the soles of the feet should result in a rapid pinking of the skin to a red color as the infant increases respiratory and heart rate. The length of time the infant takes to return to the previous skin color forms the basis for the visual nursing assessment of the infant's cardiovascular system.

While the development of jaundice and pallor are the most critical problems found during the nursing assessment of skin, neither jaundice nor pallor of the skin can be determined accurately without knowing the infant's normal skin color. Infants of color, particularly African American and Hispanic infants, may have skin colors that have yellow tones that may make it difficult for the nurse to determine normal skin color. Strategies to improve the accuracy of assessment of infant skin include using more than one light source, examining all skin surface areas of the infant, and palpating over bony prominences. Light sources in areas where infants are examined vary in intensity from overhead room lights and hallway lights to lights in radiant warmers and fluorescent lights. Nurses who examine infants using more than one light source can identify skin color more accurately. Examination of the entire skin surface of the infant, paying particular attention to the palms, soles of the feet, lips, and behind the ears, adds to the

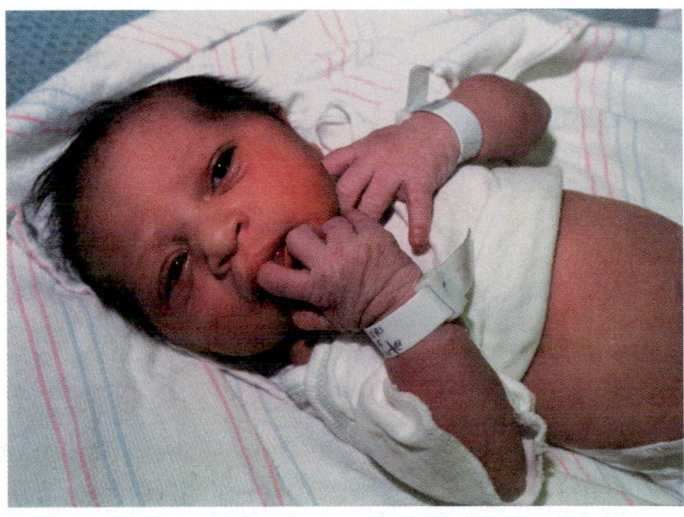

Figure 32-7 This newborn's hands show acrocyanosis.

REFLECTIONS FROM A NURSE

"It was two days before St. Patrick's Day and I had just finished the physical examination on a newborn girl with bright red hair and creamy white skin. I showed her off to everyone in the nursery, because you just don't see a lot of newborns with red hair. We (the nurses) joked that she came just in time for St. Patrick's Day. When I took her to her mother, I had to go in the room twice because I didn't see any Caucasian mothers in the room. I pulled her mother's chart and checked the ID bracelets just to make sure. I presented her to her mother, who was a very dark-skinned African American woman. She told me that all her babies had been born with red hair and this one looked like all of her other babies! I admitted my awkwardness and it gave me the opportunity to talk with this mother on a completely different level about her baby and her other children. I was so glad I had this experience. It totally changed my thinking about skin color in babies."

accuracy of the determination of normal skin color for the infant. Brief palpation of the infant's bony prominences, including the nose, sternum, sacrum, wrist, and ankle, by applying gentle pressure for 1 second yields the normal white color of blanching (first stage), followed by the "true skin color" (second stage), and ending with the skin color that reflects the ethnic heritage of the infant (third stage). Second-stage skin color (determined by using this method) that is not pink or pink-white and remains yellow or pale white is indicative of jaundice or pallor.

Body Size

Infant size is visually approximated for head-to-toe length and abdominal girth. The nurse's opinion as to whether the infant is small, medium, or large is later correlated with the graphed size classification. These physical parameters form the foundation for all future assessments of growth and development. The nurse also visually con-

firms that the head of the infant appears to be the largest body part.

Reactivity

The infant's reactions confirm the neuromuscular development of the infant. Is the infant asleep, awake, awake and quiet, or alert? Is the infant beginning to respond to the nurse by looking and moving extremities? Or is the infant actively alert, starting to fuss and cry? These are all discrete behavioral levels of awareness, or states (Brazelton, 1973), and require the infant to progress or regress from one to the other. The official behavioral state terms are deep sleep, light sleep, drowsy, quiet alert, considerable motor activity, and crying (Brazelton, 1973) (Figure 32-8). The implication of this assessment is that the term infant has developed a mature neuro-organizational system that eases the transition from one behavioral state to another (D'Apolito, 1991). Term infants exposed to cocaine in utero have lost the ability to change behavior levels in an orderly manner. Their behavior is erratic and disorganized, with excessive responses to stimuli and lengthy or absent transition periods between behaviors (Napiorkowski, Lester, Frier, Brunner, Dietz, Nadra, & Oh, 1996).

Observing the infant's response to the presence and voice of the nurse confirms the infant's responsiveness and behavioral organization levels. Infants who are irritable or who appear to be overreacting to voices, touch, or movement need comforting to assist them in calming their behavior. Swaddling in blankets, cuddling, rocking, and holding infants are interventions that the nurse can implement in the nursery. A complete physical examination should not be done on infants who are already irritated, because the examination leads to further disruption and disorganization of the infant's behavior.

Identification

All infants born in birthing centers, health care institutions, or hospitals are monitored to prevent misidentification, switching, or abduction. It is estimated that 12 to 18 infants are abducted by non–family members or strangers from health care facilities each year (Schuman, 1999). All nurses must become familiar with the infant security system used in their area of practice. Identification bracelets, "name-alert" cards for mothers with the identical last name, video cameras, door alarms, name badges to identify institutional personnel, and other sensing devices are often used to allay parental fears about the whereabouts and safety of their infant (Figure 32-9). Postpartum nursing units and nurseries traditionally receive many daily visitors because friends and family members want to welcome and see the new arrival. Increased traffic patterns between these two nursing units lead to crowding and increased opportunities for security violations. Nurses must also be alert to the

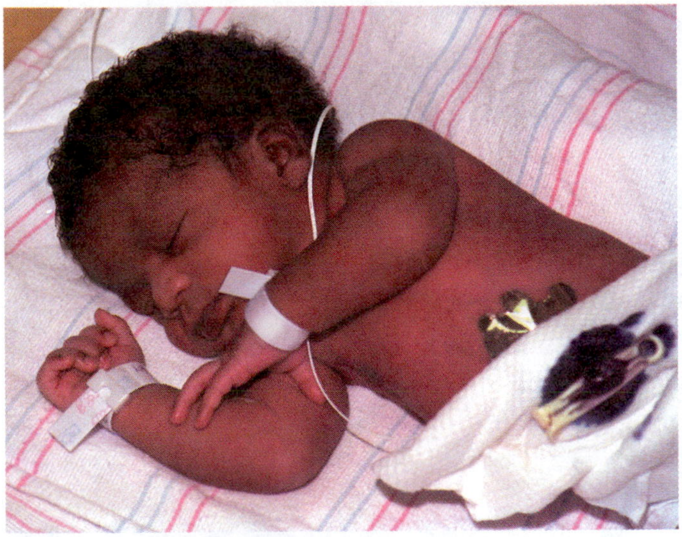

Figure 32-8 Behavioral states of the newborn. A. Light sleep; B. Drowsy (Courtesy of Mead Johnson Nutritionals); C. Quiet alert; D. Crying.

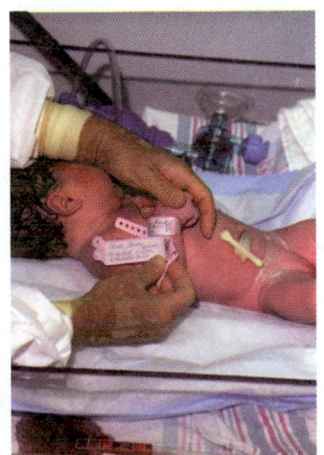
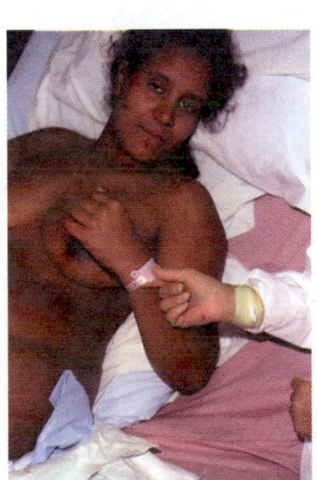
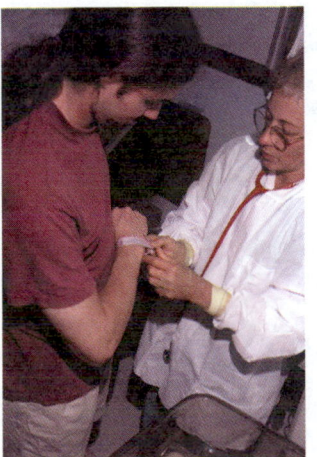
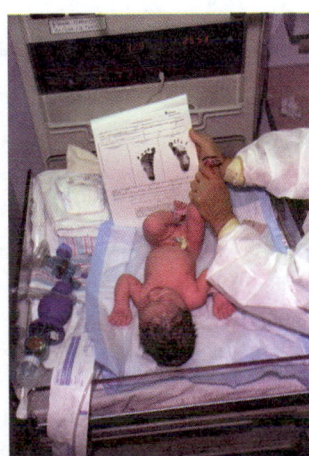

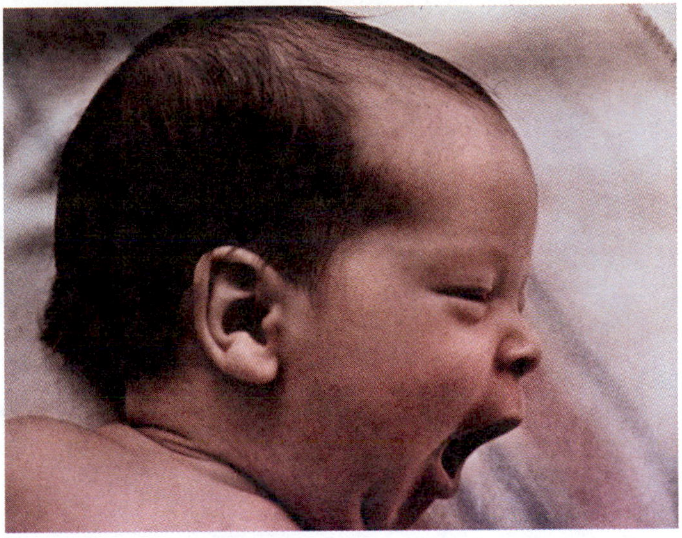

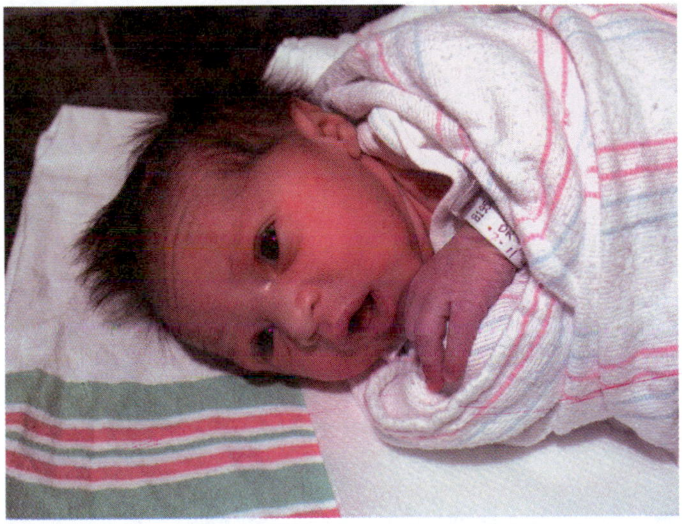

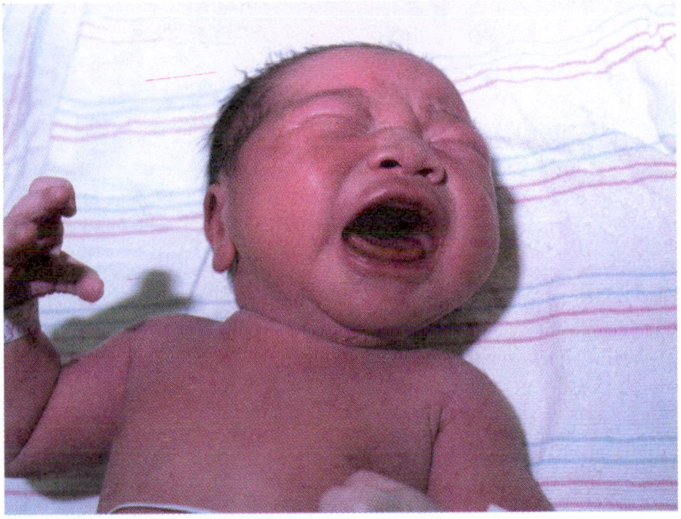

Figure 32-9 Matching identification bands are placed on infant, mother, and father; infant is footprinted.

Box 32-2 Preventing Infant Abductions

1. The identity of mothers of newborn infants is verified by their identification bracelet or other institutional device for identification.

2. Infants are identified by wearing two identification bracelets or one bracelet and another device (sensor or tag) (Figure 32-10). These security devices are placed on the infant in the delivery room. The nurse must verify that all identification devices, in addition to name cards, paperwork, charts, or anything else placed in proximity to an infant, belongs to that infant.

3. All identification devices of a mother and her infant are checked by the nursing staff before an infant is matched to its mother for visits or rooming-in. These devices are continuously re-checked by the nursing staff at the end and at the beginning of each nursing shift.

4. Transportation of infants from one unit to another or to another department for examination should be done only by authorized nursing staff, who should remain with the infant until the examination is complete and return the infant to its original location.

5. The infant should not be left by nursing staff with anyone but the birth mother, unless an official agency involved with parents and family has stipulated to the contrary. This includes persons claiming to be the mother's sister or spouse, father of the infant, grandmother, family relative, or adoptive mother.

6. When the birth mother is ill and is unable to take care of her infant, the father assumes responsibility for the infant and receives an identification bracelet to be matched with the infant's. In many hospitals, the father routinely receives an ID bracelet as well.

7. Family members or relatives may only see the infant while it is in the nursery. The mother's written permission is required for them to be able to hold or feed her infant in the nursery under nursing staff supervision.

8. The mother of the infant is instructed by the nursing staff never to give her permission to let someone that she does not know take or hold her infant.

9. All nursing staff are identified through their identification badges, not by the clothes that they wear. Nursing staff must continually reinforce their identity with mothers of newborns and be available to accompany them at all times for their security and safety.

10. All nursing staff should be aware of the institutional code for infant abduction and the procedures to follow should this event occur.

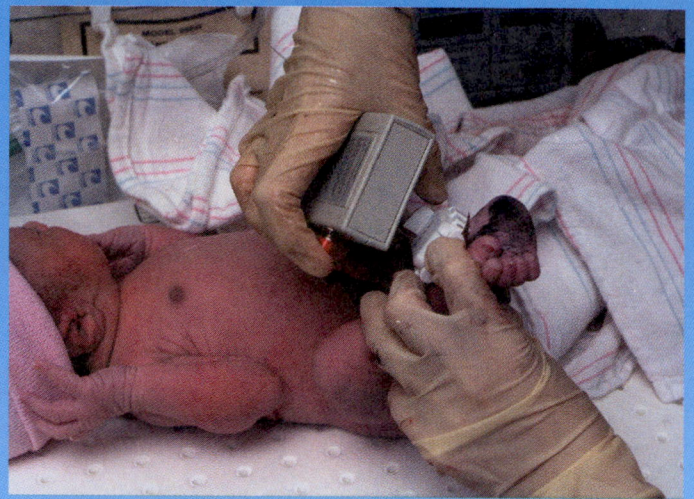

Figure 32-10 Application of a heel sensor.

location of the infant at all times and continually share this knowledge with the mother. Refer to Box 32-2.

PHYSICAL EXAMINATION

After the general nursing assessment is complete, the nurse begins the physical examination of the infant if the infant appears calm or resting. The manipulation and examination of the infant should not stress or irritate the infant.

Weight, Measurement, and Vital Signs

The infant's weight in grams and length in centimeters was determined in the delivery room and during the transitional period. Average weight for a term newborn infant is 3400 g (range, 2500 to 4300 g) and average length is 49.6 cm (range, 45 to 54 cm) (Fox, 1997). The frontal-occipital circumference (FOC) is measured in centimeters with a

Newborn Assessment

*O*nce the infant enters the nursery, the nurse conducts a complete head-to-toe physical assessment to determine the infant's health status. The pictures in this story are arranged in order of priority, from most to least important. Each of these photos can be compared to the Ballard scale.

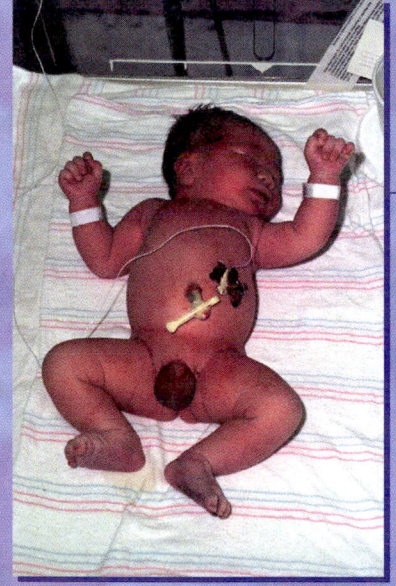

A general inspection is done first to identify abnormalities. A normal newborn assumes a flexed position.

Skin is inspected for color and texture. A full-term infant may display signs of skin dryness and cracking. Acrocyanosis may be present in the hands and feet but should diminish.

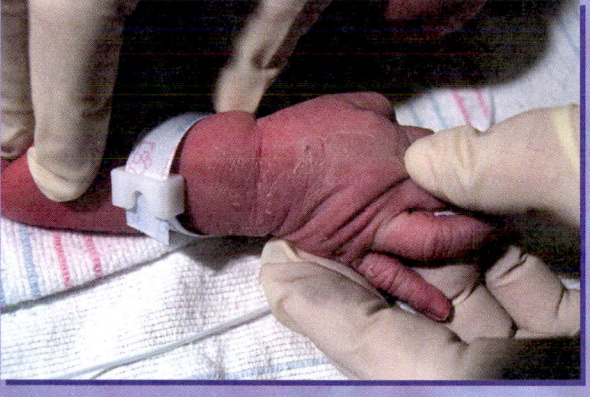

The newborn's heart is auscultated for rate and rhythm.

The lungs are auscultated to ensure expansion of both lungs and absence of rales or rhonchi.

Sometimes suctioning is required to remove residual fluid from the infant's mouth.

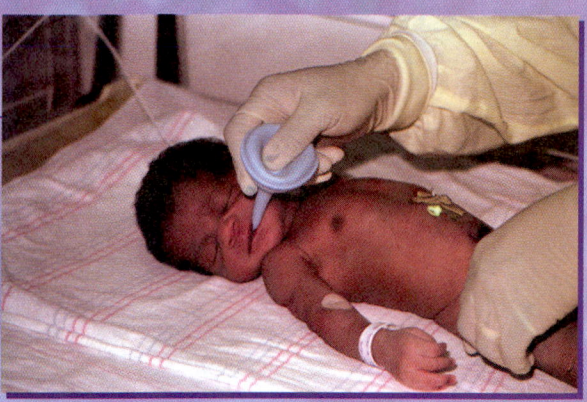

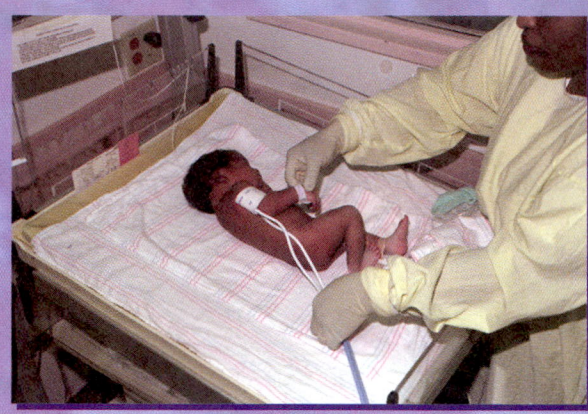

The newborn's first blood pressure measurement is taken.

The axillary body temperature is taken.

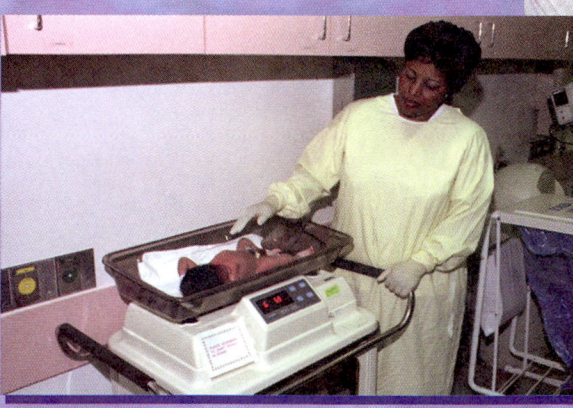

The newborn is weighed.

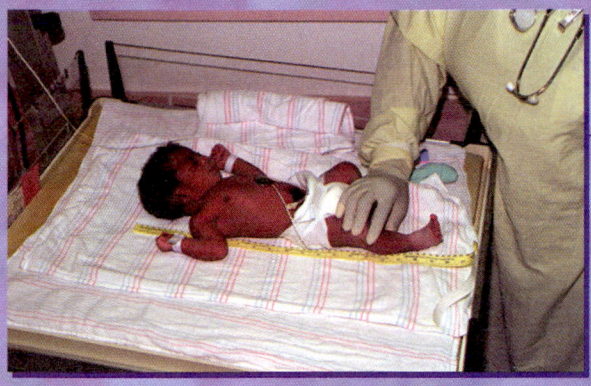

The infant's head-to-toe length is measured.

The infant's head circumference is measured.

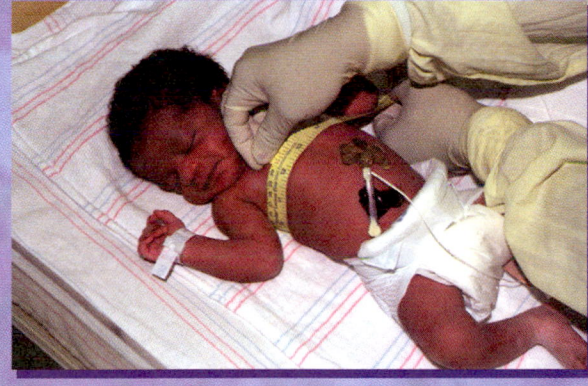

The infant's chest circumference is measured.

The infant's abdominal circumference is measured.

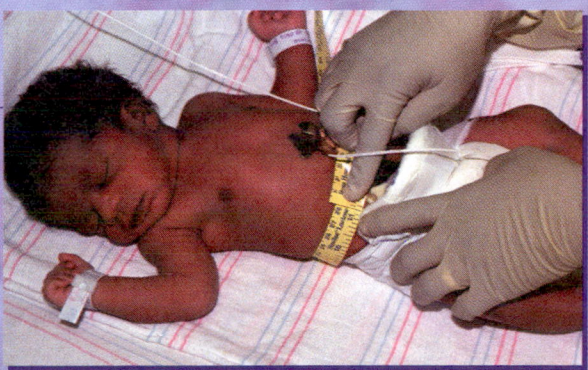

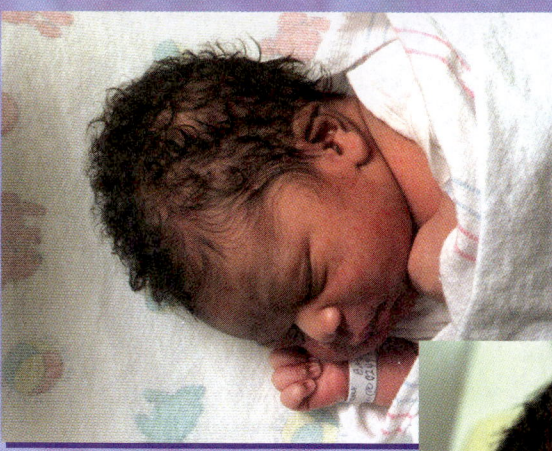

The infant's head is inspected for molding and suture lines are palpated.

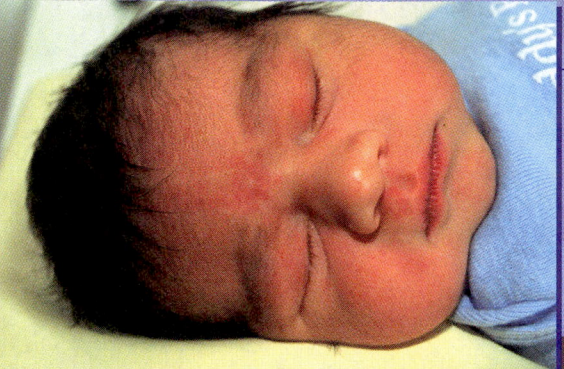

The face is inspected for symmetry, birth marks, milia, and nevi ("stork bites") over the forehead and eyelids.

The mouth is inspected for natal teeth and abnormalities of the hard and soft palate; the tongue should be at midline.

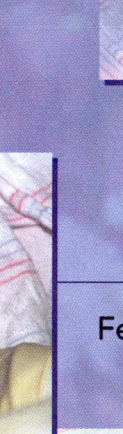

Femoral pulses are palpated.

Brachial pulses are palpated.

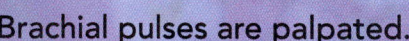

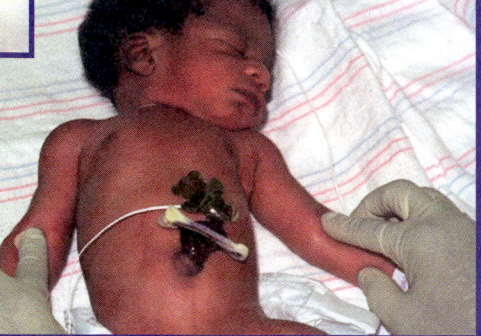

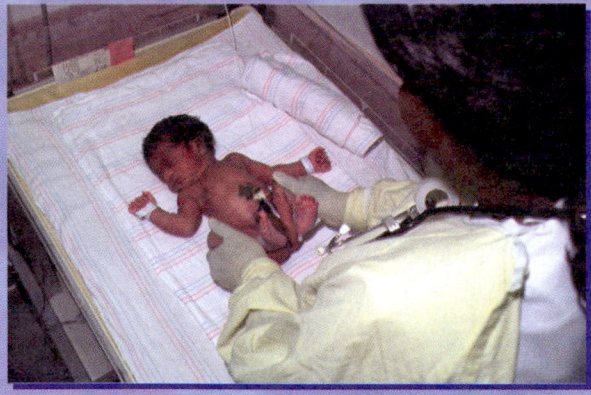

Ortolani's maneuver is done to check for hip dislocation.

Inspection of the genitalia. The nurse is palpating the scrotum to check for descent of the testes.

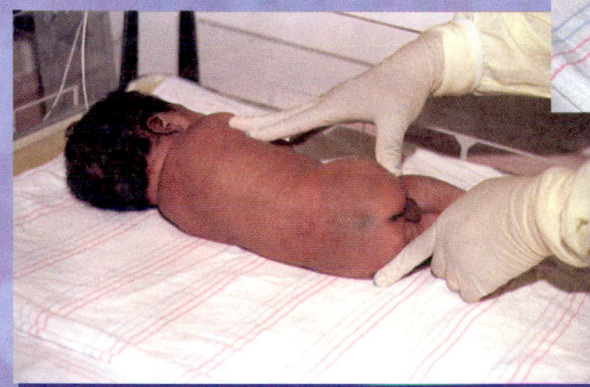

The spine and skin on the back are inspected for alignment, breaks in skin, moles, birth marks, or markers along the spinal column. This infant has a Mongolian spot near the base of the spine; this is a normal finding.

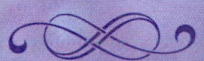

During the examination, the nurse will check certain reflexes. The presence of these reflexes suggests maturity of the neonatal neurological system.

This is the rooting reflex. The infant turns his head and opens his mouth when the perioral area is stimulated.

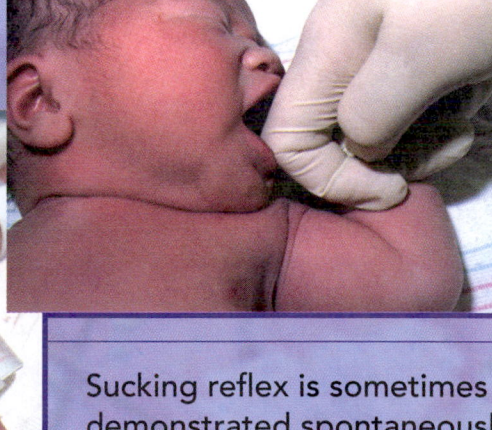

Sucking reflex is sometimes demonstrated spontaneously during the examination.

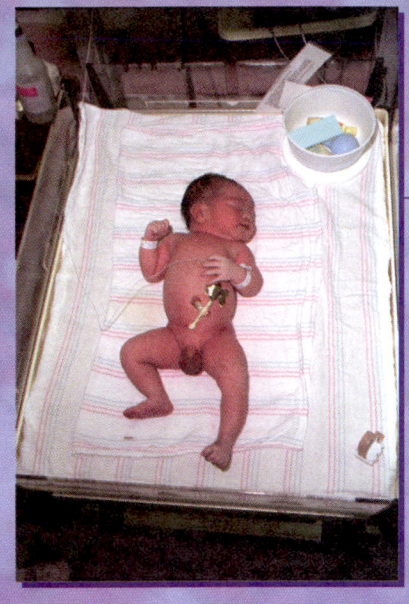

The tonic neck or fencing reflex—note the leg extension and the partial extension of the arm on the side the head is turned to, and the flexion of the arm and leg on the opposite side.

The grasp reflex is assessed.

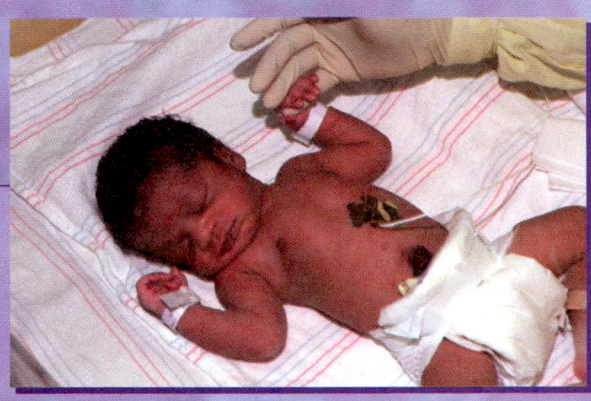

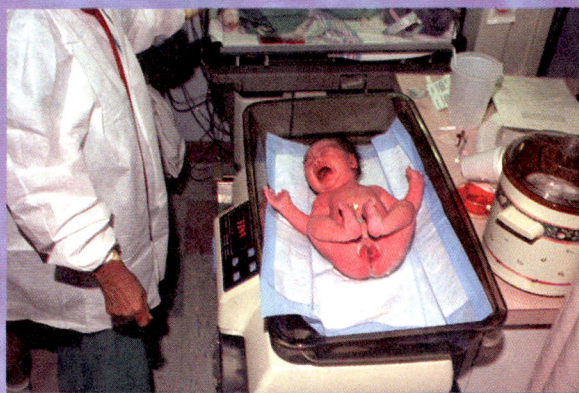

The Moro reflex is assessed.

The head lag or traction reflex is assessed.

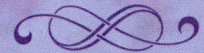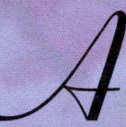

Assessment of Physical Maturity Using the Ballard Scale

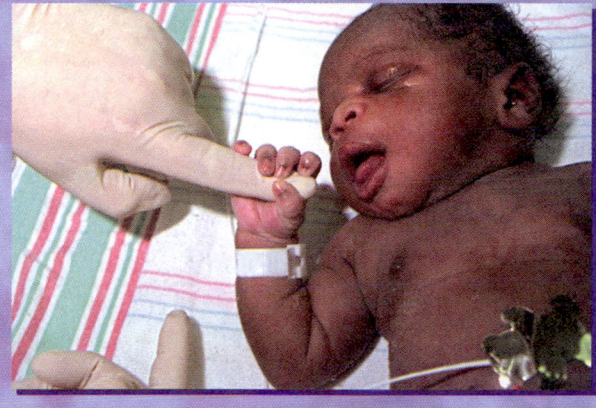

Skin is assessed using the six parameters of the Ballard Scale. This post-term newborn shows skin cracking and peeling.

The amount of lanugo is estimated using the six parameters of the Ballard Scale.

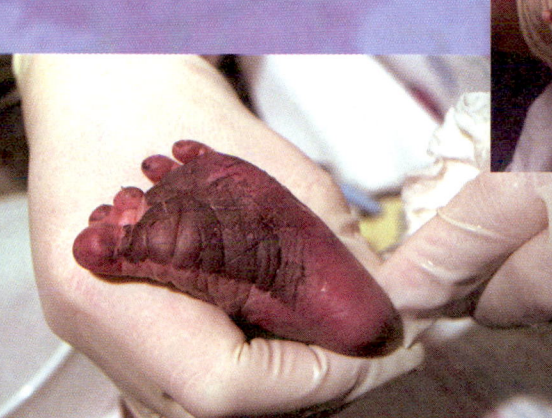

The plantar surface of the foot is assessed for creases.

Maturity of nipple buds is estimated.

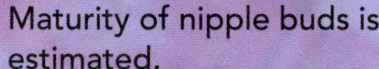
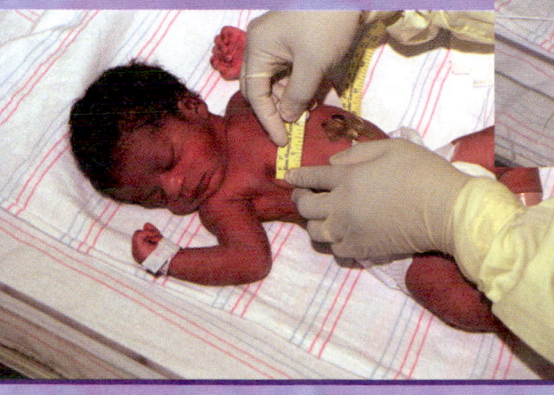

Nipples are measured.

The amount of cartilage in the ear is assessed.

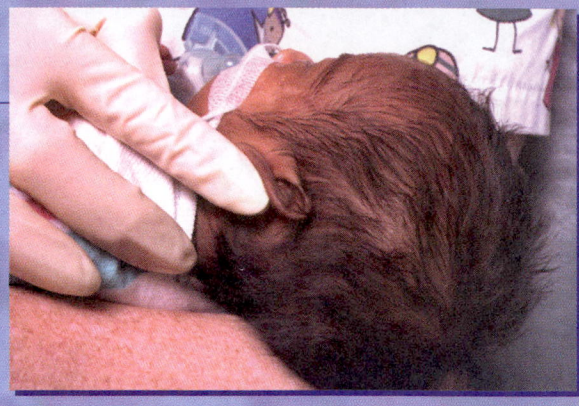

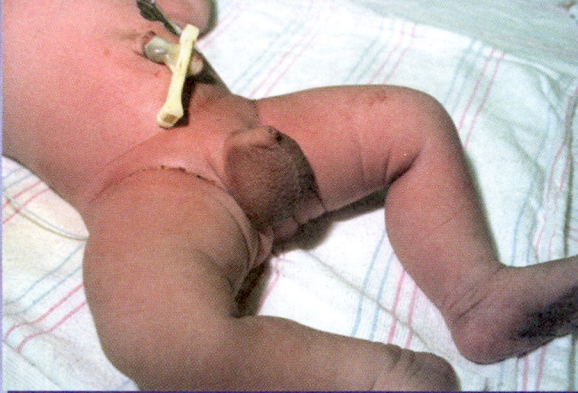

The male genitalia are assessed to determine if the testes have descended and if rugae are present.

The female genitalia are assessed to determine maturity of development of the labia and clitoris.

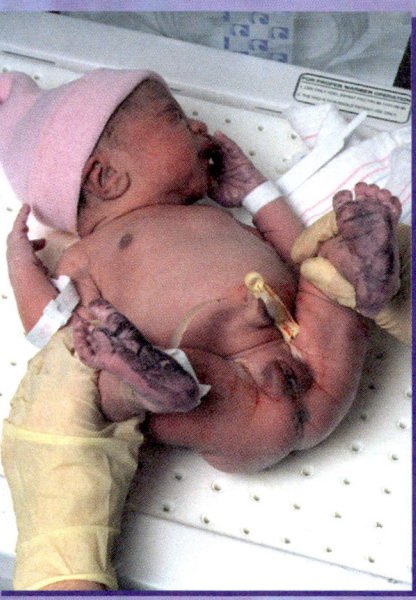

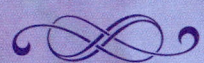

*A*ssessment of Neuromuscular Maturity

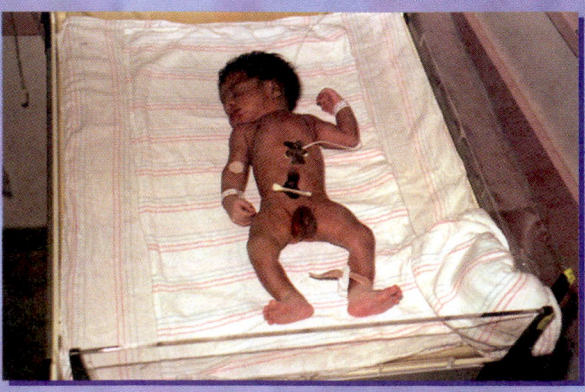

Degree of flexion is determined.

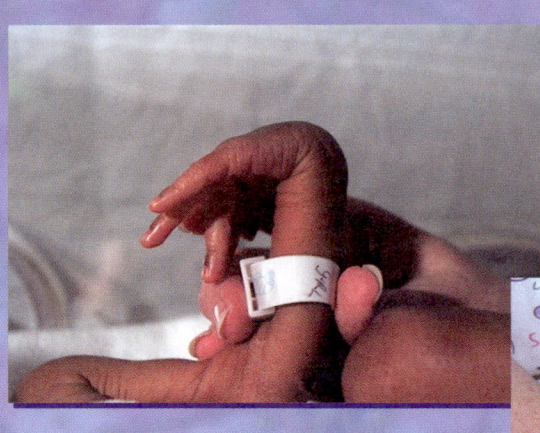

Square window determination.

Popliteal angle.

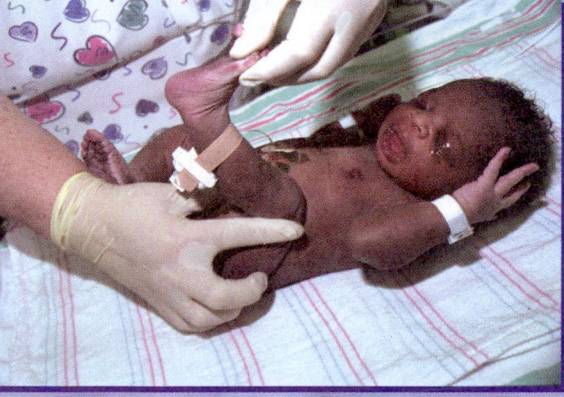

Scarf sign in term infant.

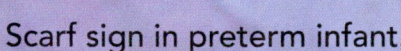

Scarf sign in preterm infant.

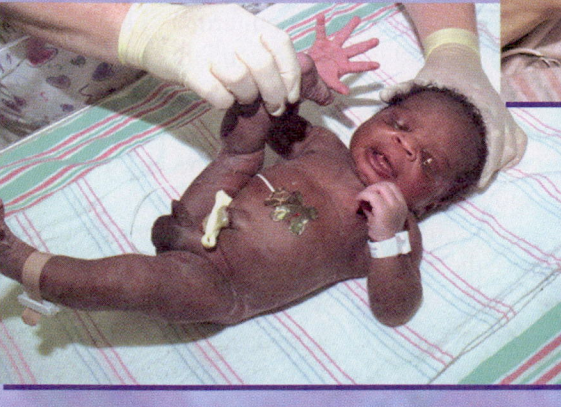

Heel to ear.

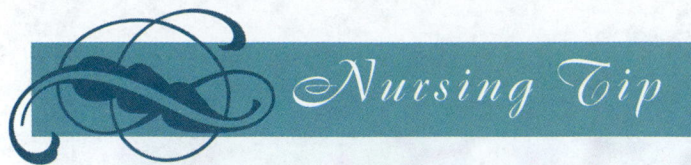

CALCULATING POUNDS FROM GRAMS AND INCHES FROM CENTIMETERS

Infant weight is usually a whole number indicating how many grams the infant weighs. Divide this number by 1000: 1000 g = 1 kg = 2.2 lbs. Multiplication of the number of kilograms by 2.2 yields the number of pounds of infant weight. Less than 1 pound can be converted to ounces by remembering that 16 ounces = 1 pound. One can multiply the grams by 0.0022 to convert to pounds. To convert grams to ounces, divide the grams by 28.35. For example a 7 pound 8 oz baby would be 3402 grams. The length of the infant in centimeters is divided by 2.5 to convert centimeters to inches: 1 in. = 2.5 cm.

measuring tape to determine head size. The measuring tape is gently placed around the infant's head at the largest part of the occipital area and gathered over the forehead, resting on top of the eyebrows. The largest of three attempts is recorded by the nurse. Normal head circumference for a term infant at birth ranges from 33 to 38 cm (Johnson & Oski, 1997). The weight, length, and head circumference measurements are plotted against the gestational age of the infant to determine the size category of the infant (Figure 32-11). Size categories are small for gestational age (SGA), appropriate for gestational age (AGA), and large for gestational age (LGA).

Vital signs are taken by the nurse and charted. Heart rate and respiratory rate are determined by auscultation. Temperature is recorded with an axillary thermometer or tympanic membrane thermometer. Blood pressure is checked on both the thigh and the arm of the infant. Systolic blood pressures range from 50 to 90 mm Hg and diastolic blood pressures range from 20 to 60 mm Hg (Fox, 1997). The systolic blood pressure of both the thigh and arm should be equal. A decrease of 10 mm Hg or more in the thigh in comparison to the arm may indicate **coarctation of the aorta**. This may also be indicated with a systolic blood pressure of more than 90 mm Hg (Fox, 1997).

Gestational Age Assessment

Since 1967, when the American Academy of Pediatrics recommended that all newborns be classified by birth weight and gestational age, the modification of the Dubowitz scoring system by Ballard, Khoury, Wedig, Wang, Eilers-Waisman, & Lipp (1991) remains the most popular method for determining gestational age. This examination provides a score of neuromuscular and physical maturity that can be mathematically extrapolated onto a corresponding age scale to reveal the gestational age in weeks. Other gestational age examinations include fundal height before delivery, ultrasonography, and eye lens vascularity. Approximation of gestational age at delivery can be obtained by date of the mother's last menstrual cycle. This information is not as accurate as physical examination for gestational age. Gestational age assessments are often done by nurses on normal newborns and reported in the infant's chart.

The Ballard Gestational Age by Maturity Rating (Ballard et al., 1991) consists of two scoring systems: neuromuscular maturity and physical maturity of six characteristics each. Scores from each system are added together and mathematically extrapolated on the maturity rating scale to determine the gestational age by examination (Figure 32-12). The systems scored reflect the decreasing flexibility of muscles and joints in prematurity and the return to original positioning after movement indicative of a mature term infant. This examination is usually performed by the nurse within the first 12 hours of life and is more accurate when done on term infants between 10 and 36 hours of life (Gagliardi, 1993). It is not necessary to perform this examination in any order of categories to be assessed.

Maturity may occur at different rates among these categories. A score of 4 in one category does not mean that all subsequent categories must be scored as a 4. The examiner may strongly feel that a half-score is needed in one particular category because the infant exhibits a characteristic that falls between two scoring options. This is a valid choice, and half-scores are seen quite often in these assessments. These assessments are illustrated in the accompanying photo story.

Posture: Posture is the natural position that the infant assumes on its back. Both arm and leg positions are assessed in this category, and this is matched to the best picture of upper and lower extremities for scoring.

Square window: Wearing gloves, the examiner uses his or her thumb to gently press the infant's wrist and palm toward its forearm. Either the angle that the wrist and the third and fourth fingers make against the forearm or the angle that the wrist and thumb make against the forearm is used for scoring purposes.

Arm recoil: This category is scored by the lateral or inferior extension of both arms after flexing them at chest level. After release from extension, the amount of return to original position is observed by the nurse and scored. This assessment is often used to confirm brachial plexus injuries or fractured clavicles in the newborn when movements of the arms are observed to be unequal.

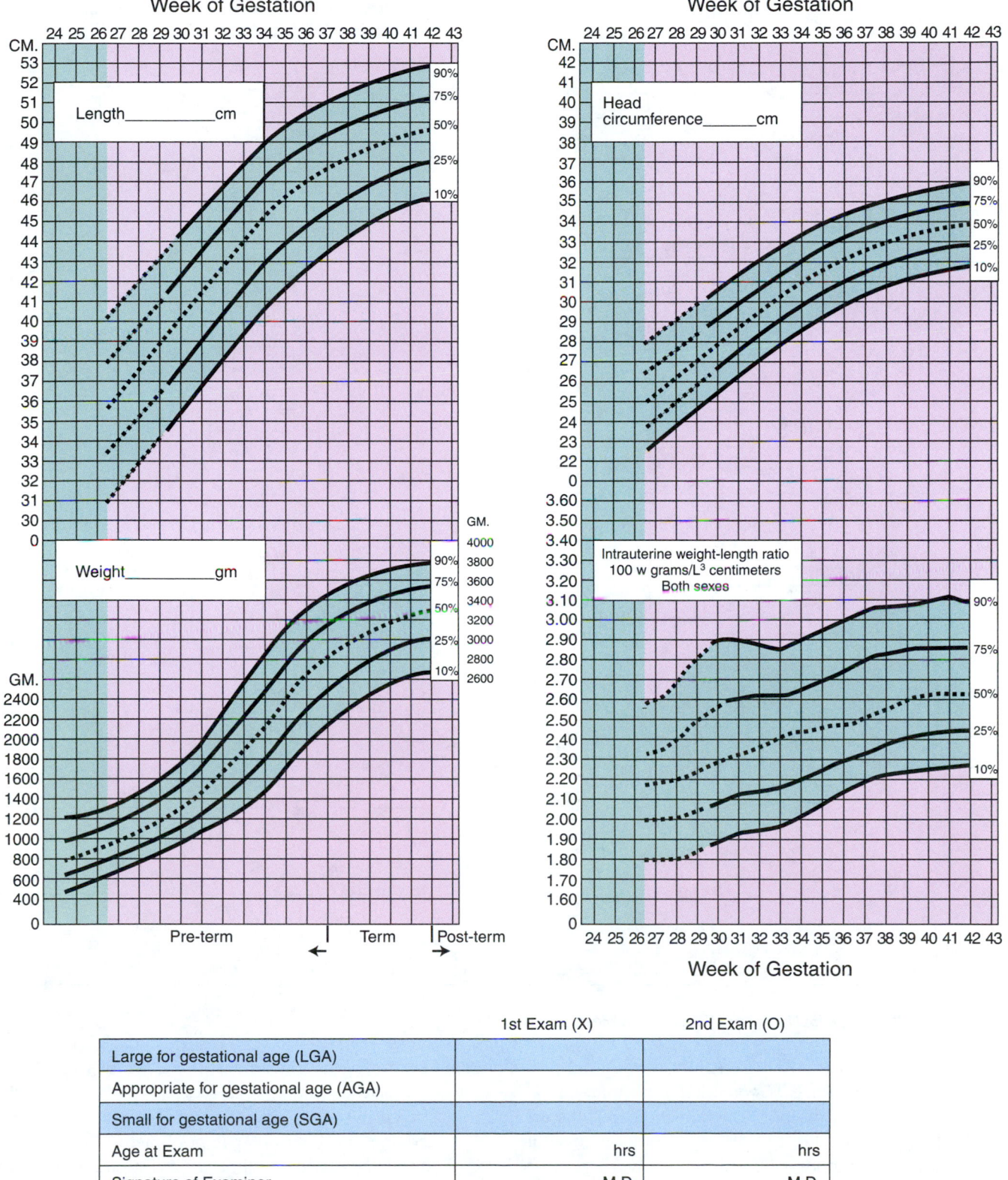

CLASSIFICATION OF NEWBORNS -
BASED ON MATURITY AND INTRAUTERINE GROWTH
Symbols: X - 1st Exam   O - 2nd Exam

	1st Exam (X)	2nd Exam (O)
Large for gestational age (LGA)		
Appropriate for gestational age (AGA)		
Small for gestational age (SGA)		
Age at Exam	hrs	hrs
Signature of Examiner	M.D.	M.D.

Figure 32-11 Gestational age assessment (Courtesy of Mead Johnson Nutritionals).

NEWBORN MATURITY RATING & CLASSIFICATION
ESTIMATION OF GESTATIONAL AGE BY MATURITY RATING
SYMBOLS: X - 1ST EXAM   O - 2ND EXAM

Gestation by Dates _____ wks

Birth Date _____ Hour _____ am/pm

APGAR _____ 1 min _____ 5 min

NEUROMUSCULAR MATURITY

	-1	0	1	2	3	4	5
Posture							
Square Window (wrist)	>90°	90°	60°	45°	30°	0°	
Arm Recoil		180°	140°-180°	110°-140°	90°-110°	<90°	
Popliteal Angle	180°	160°	140°	120°	100°	90°	<90°
Scarf Sign							
Heel to Ear							

PHYSICAL MATURITY

Skin	sticky friable transparent	gelatinous red, translucent	smooth pink, visible veins	superficial peeling and or rash few veins	cracking pale areas rare veins	parchment deep cracking no vessels	feathery cracked wrinkled
Lanugo	none	sparse	abundant	thinning	bald areas	mostly bald	
Planiar Surface	heel-toe 40 - 50min: -1 <40 min: -2	>50mm no crease	faint red marks	anterior transverse crease only	creases ant. 2/3	creases over entire sole	
Breast	imperceptible	barely perceptible	flat areola no bud	stippled areola 1-2mm bud	raised areola 3-4mm bud	full areola 5-10mm bud	
Eye/Ear	lids fused loosely: -1 tightly: -2	lids open pinna flat stays folded	sl. curved pinna; soft slow recoil	well curved pinna; soft but ready recoil	formed and firm instant recoil	thick cartilage ear stiff	
Genitals Male	scrotum flat, smooth	scrotum empty faint rugae	testes in upper canal rare rugae	testes descending few rugae	testes down good rugae	testes pendulous deep rugae	
Genitals Female	clitoris prominant labia flat	prominant clitoris small labia minora	prominant clitoris enlarging minora	majora & minora equally prominant	majora large minora small	majora cover clitoris and minors	

MATURITY RATING

score	weeks
-10	20
-5	22
0	24
5	26
10	28
15	30
20	32
25	34
30	36
35	38
40	40
45	42
50	44

SCORING SECTION

	1st Exam=X	2nd Exam=O
Estimating Gest Age by Maturity Rating	Weeks	Weeks
Time of Exam	Date ___ Hour ___ am/pm	Date ___ Hour ___ am/pm
Age at Exam	Hours	Hours
Signature of Examiner	M.D.	M.D.

Figure 32-12 New Ballard score (Courtesy of Mead Johnson Nutritionals).

Popliteal angle: This is the assessment of the angle created when the knee is extended. The infant is assessed in the supine position with the pelvis flat and the thigh of one leg resting on the abdomen while the knee is extended by exerting upward pressure on the heel of the leg with the examiner's finger until resistance is met.

Scarf sign: This is placement of the infant's hand to the opposite shoulder. It is scored by observing where the elbow of the arm that was moved falls. The dotted line in the scoring category picture represents the sternal border or midline. In the supine position, the infant's hand is grasped between the thumb and first finger of the nurse's hand and, in one sweeping movement, the nurse attempts to place the hand on the opposite shoulder. Using a finger, the nurse marks on the infant's chest where the elbow of the infant falls and scores this category accordingly.

Heel-to-ear: This category assesses hip flexibility in infants. With the infant in the supine position, with the pelvis on a flat surface, one leg is gently extended and moved toward the infant's head on the corresponding side. When resistance is met, the visual distance between the ear on the infant's head and the great toe of the foot, along with the leg position, is scored. Infants who experienced breech positioning or who are suspected of having **developmental dysplasia of the hip (DDH)** may show a great amount of flexibility in this category.

Skin: Scoring in this category is based on palpation and visual inspection. Skin texture, transparency, relative thickness, and flaking and peeling of the epidermis are noted. Transparency, defined as skin through which veins can be seen, is evident in premature (preterm) infants and disappears with increasing maturity. Flaking of skin and peeling with wrinkles occurs in post-term infants.

Lanugo: Lanugo is the fine hair seen mostly on the backs and arms of premature infants. It eventually thins out in the lumbar region and disappears, leaving small traces on the shoulders. Stroking the infant's back while in the prone position will assist the nurse in identifying the lanugo that still exists apart from the infant's natural body hair. Mexican-American infants normally have thin, dark body hair that may cover their entire back and shoulders. This needs to be distinguished from real lanugo, which is lighter in color and softer and curls at the ends.

Plantar surface: Creases on the soles of both feet are scored according to the extent to which the creases cover the soles. The best way to visualize the extent of plantar creases is to gently curl the infant's toes toward the heel, and determine the score.

Breast: The amount of breast tissue is approximated by gently measuring the tissue present on the infant using a measuring tape in millimeters or by grasping the tissue between the examiner's the thumb and forefinger. In addition, the bud and areola are inspected for size and stippling. Lastly, the area of breast tissue is palpated to determine its elevation from the chest wall.

Eye and ear: Eyelids should be open and should open easily in the mature infant. Ears are inspected for incurving of the pinna and palpated for a determination of the thickness of cartilage. The upper lobe recoil is performed bilaterally to validate the return to the posterior upright position when moved anteriorly and inferiorly. As pinnal incurving occurs from the top of the lobe down toward the bottom of the lobe, some mature infants may only have the upper portion of the pinna on the ear lobe curved in, with the remainder flat. The nurse may want to look at the ears of the infant's parents and other family members before scoring this category.

Genitalia: Both male and female genitalia are assessed with the infant in the supine position and the legs abducted. At approximately 35 weeks gestational age, the testes descend into the scrotum from the inguinal canal and rugae start to appear as creases on the surface of the scrotum. Deep creases gradually develop as crevices on the scrotum as the infant becomes more mature. Visualization of a pendulous scrotum occurs in the supine position with the lower extremities abducted. In this same position, female infants can be assessed for the covering of the clitoris and the size of the labia majora. The distance between the edges of the labia majora and how much of the female genitalia is covered can also be visualized and scored.

Once the scoring is complete on the Ballard Newborn Maturity Rating, the scores from both the neuromuscular and physical maturity categories are totaled. This score is compared mathematically to the gestational age (in weeks) through a simple proportionate formula that equates the score range with the gestational age in weeks and calculates the exact position of the score within that range. Nurses should note that maturity scoring does not directly translate to gestational age in weeks. Often examiners make this mistake and estimate an infant's age at birth to be much younger than it is. An infant determined to be

Nursing Tip

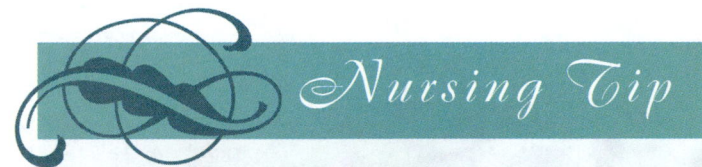

HOW TO CALCULATE GESTATIONAL AGE

Your newborn's gestational age examination score of 34 falls between the scores 30 and 35 and occupies $\frac{4}{5}$ of the score range from 30 to 35. Correspondingly, the exact age in weeks must also occupy $\frac{4}{5}$ of the age score range of 2 between 36 and 38. Solving this simple ratio equation, you note that $\frac{4}{5}$ of 2 equals $1\frac{3}{5}$, which, multiplied by 7 (days in a week) and added to 36, reveals a gestational age of $37\frac{4}{7}$ weeks for a maturity score of 34.

less than 37 weeks' gestational age is called **preterm**, or premature. An infant whose score falls between 37 weeks' and 42 weeks' gestational age is called **term**, and the infant that is scored beyond 42 weeks' gestation is called **post-term**.

Systems Assessment

The nursing assessment of the newborn infant's physical characteristics begins after completion of the general assessment and the gestational age assessment. The examination is initiated by placing the infant in the supine position and usually proceeds from the assessment of the skin first, followed by a head-to-toe examination. This assessment follows the inspection, light palpation, deep palpation, and auscultation sequence of nursing assessments except when the abdomen of the infant is examined. Inspection, then auscultation, followed by light and deep palpation is the proper sequence to follow when examining the abdomen. The examination may be performed on a radiant warmer to preserve infant temperature stability, in the infant's crib in the nursery, or at the mother's bedside. Performing this examination at the mother's bedside allows the nurse to introduce the mother to her infant and display the unique characteristics of this infant to the mother. It also allows the nurse to begin the interactional assessment of the mother and infant by observing the mother's attention to her infant, talking to her infant, tone of voice used, and holding position.

Integumentary System

The skin and all the other elements of the integumentary system, i.e., hair and nails, are examined for color, texture, distribution, disruptions, eruptions, and distinguishing characteristics or birth marks. When performing the skin

assessment, the nurse should make sure that the room is well-lit and be willing to use extra light sources for accuracy. The color of a newborn's skin should be pink, indicating good peripheral cardiac perfusion. After blanching over bony prominences, the underlying skin color should be pink-white before it returns to its natural pigmentation. Skin color can also be assessed by a visual inspection of the infant's mouth, tongue, and gums. These areas should always display a healthy pink-red color, darkening to bright red when the infant is crying.

Common Variations

Wearing gloves, the nurse inspects and lightly palpates the scalp and body hair for texture and distribution. Mexican-American, Asian, and African American infants are often born with a full head of scalp hair and have some body hair on their back, shoulders, and buttocks. Hair is described as fine, thick, curly, or straight and the color and location are noted (Figure 32-13). Mexican-American and Asian newborns have dark, straight hair at birth. The hair on African American newborns is usually tightly curled and softer in texture. Eyelashes and brows are also inspected. Nail beds are examined on both fingers and toes for shape, length, and color. Many infants are born with long fingernails that may cause facial scratches as the infant feels and explores using fingers (Figure 32-14). Scratching by a newborn infant is controlled by placing mittens on the hands because newborn nails are very soft and flexible and difficult to trim with accuracy.

Infant skin should feel soft and smooth in term infants, and leathery with cracking and peeling in post-term infants. Breaks in the skin are noted to be either disruptions or eruptions. Disruptions include any break in skin integrity, including lacerations, electrode marks, and peeling layers. Forceps deliveries or vacuum extractions may

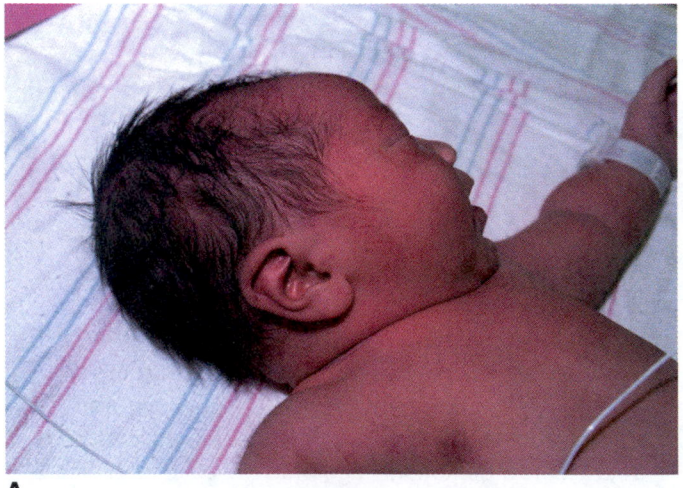
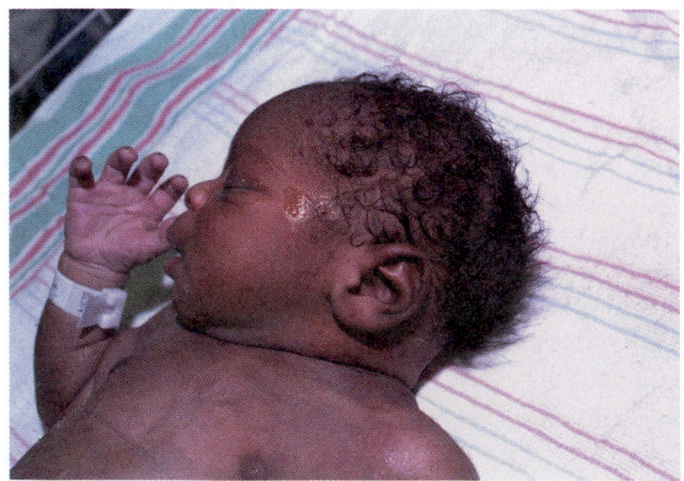

A.   B.

Figure 32-13 Newborn hair varies in texture, from straight (A) to curly (B).

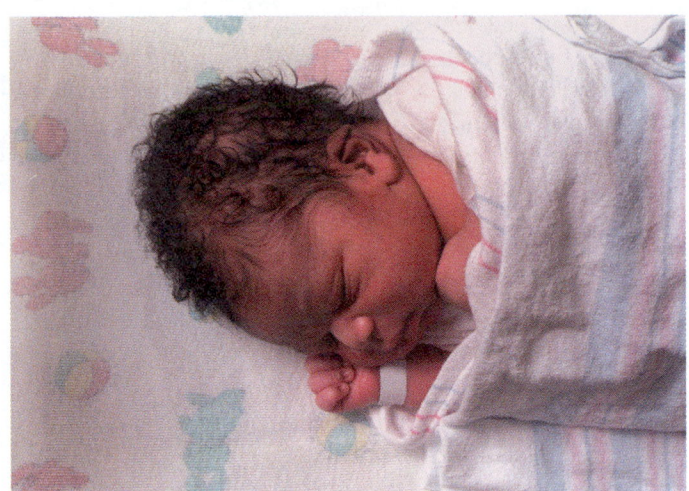

Figure 32-14 This newborn has facial scratches from long fingernails.

break the skin on the scalp or face, leaving marks or bruises. Scalp electrode monitors leave small puncture sites in the infant's scalp that may not have a scab covering them at the time of the nursing assessment. Skin peeling is common in those infants classified as post-term. Frequently, infants are born with a condition called **pustular melanosis**, in which small pustules are formed before delivery. The pustule disintegrates, leaving behind a small residue (scale) in the shape of the pustule, which later develops into a small flat spot called a macule, 1 to 2 millimeters in diameter. These small macules are numerous, look brown similar to freckles, are located on the chest and extremities, and appear to be a rash (but are not). Pustular melanosis is more commonly seen on African American infants than on Caucasian infants.

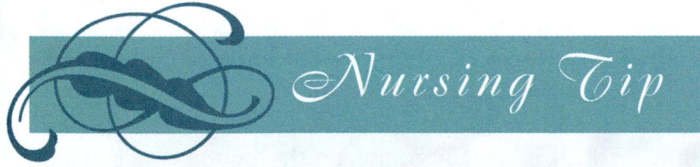

NAIL LENGTH IN NEWBORNS

Nurses who are experienced in examining newborns report: "the longer the nails, the more mature the baby." They are basing this observation on the time of development of fingernails and toe nails, which occurs late in the third trimester of pregnancy.

A greenish color around the nail bed of a finger or toe may indicate **meconium** staining from in utero exposure to meconium before or during delivery. Two other places where the nurse would see meconium staining on a newborn infant are the umbilical cord and the ear canals.

Some of the skin eruptions that occur in the early neonatal period are classified as normal variations. Small, singular, white papules that appear to be tiny pimples may be seen on a newborn's face, particularly on the chin. This skin condition is called **milia** and is one form of a sebaceous cyst. One or two white, pinhead-sized inclusion cysts may be seen on the penis or the scrotum of male infants or on the areola of female infants. Separate from milia and inclusion cysts, the infant may have acne, a skin eruption that usually occurs with puberty but, in infancy, is related to excessive amounts of maternal hormones. Neonatal acne eventually disappear from the infant's cheeks and chest. The most common normal skin eruption seen in newborns is **erythema toxicum**, a rash that generally occurs on the face and chest first and spreads to the rest of the body. The cause of this rash is unknown, and it may persist on the infant for a month after delivery. It begins with small, irregular, flat patches of redness on the cheeks and progresses to singular, small, yellow pimples on an erythematous base, as it moves to the chest, abdomen, and extremities. This skin condition appears particularly disturbing and frustrating to parents because there is no treatment to speed up its departure. It appears, remains, and disappears on its own schedule.

Another skin eruption is a blister formation on the fingers, wrist, or upper lip of the infant from sucking before and after delivery. These are not cause for alarm, and parents need to be reassured that these blisters or calluses will go away.

Distinguishing characteristics of the newborn's skin are either normal variations in skin color, birth marks, or evidence of birth trauma from the delivery. Normal variations in skin color include the dark blue, grey, or purple diffuse color seen on the buttocks of infants called **Mongolian spots**, which also appear on their shoulders, forearms, wrists, and ankles (Figure 32-15). These spots will

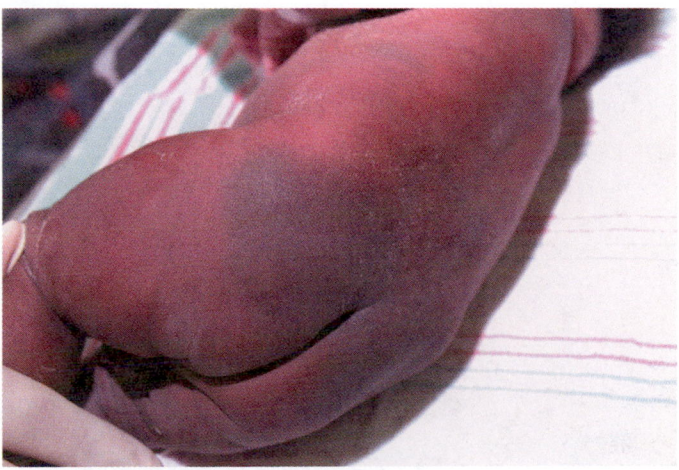

Figure 32-15 Mongolian spots.

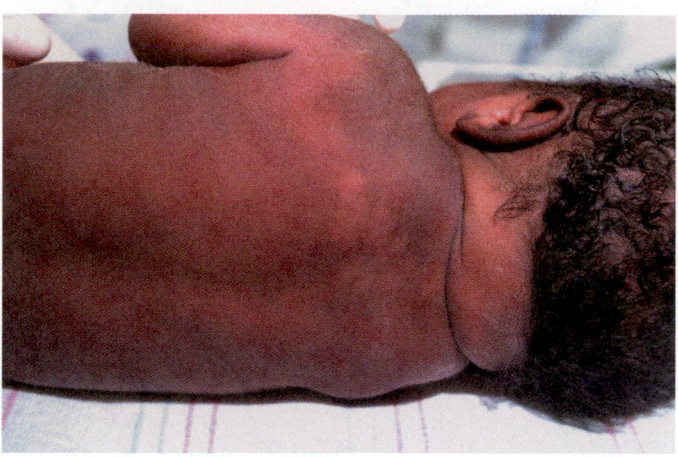

Figure 32-16 Mottling.

fade and disappear as the infant grows older. Some new-born skin shows a "cobblestone" appearance of pink-white areas outlined with a darker pink border (Figure 32-16). This **mottling** (called cutis marmorata) of the skin is common in newborns and results from the infant's vaso-motor response to a lowered environmental temperature outside the womb. As the newborn adjusts to extrauterine life, this mottling disappears. Additionally, maternal hor-mones during labor and delivery may cause a normal darkening of the skin in the genital areas of both male and female infants.

Birth marks on a newborn infant are different from other marks that are the result of trauma to the infant from the delivery process. Birth marks are usually small, flat areas of color that may be white, tan, brown, red, or blue. Borders may be irregular. The nurse documents the loca-tion and color of the birth mark (Figure 32-17). Any area of colored skin that contains hair or is located at the midline of the infant anteriorly or posteriorly should be investi-gated for underlying tissue involvement. A white or pale

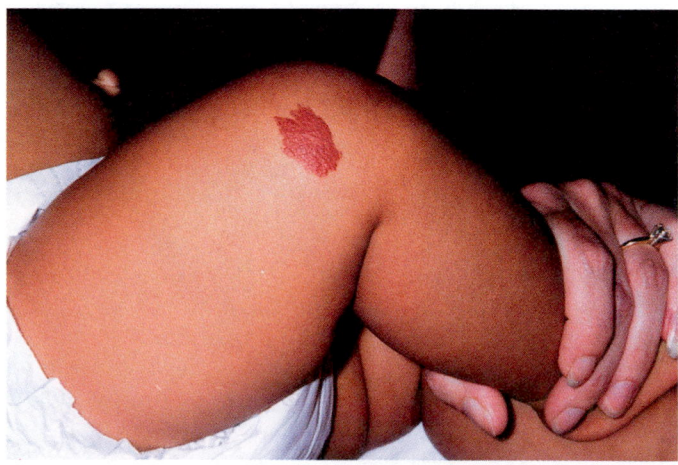

Figure 32-17 Birth mark.

patch of skin usually represents an area of hypopigmenta-tion and, by itself, is not an indicator for concern. How-ever, numerous areas of hypopigmentation, including patches that have a leaf pattern, must be reported immedi-ately. These patches may be found on the chest, back, ex-tremities, and in the axilla. A neurologic condition, tuber-ous sclerosis, may be suspected in infants who have a hypopigmented skin patch that resembles a patterned leaf. Tan spots on the skin are often called cafe-au-lait marks and are very difficult to see on an African American infant. Many infants are born with these, and it is only a signifi-cant finding when the nurse counts six or more that are larger than 1 centimeter in diameter. Infants with these large cafe-au-lait spots at birth may be at risk for develop-ing type I neurofibromatosis and need observation during infancy for any tumors that develop underneath the skin.

Brown skin marks or brown nevi (singular, nevus) are birth marks in which the color may vary from brown to in-tense black. Nevi have been thought to be an early form of a precancerous lesion (Seidel et al., 2001), and parents are taught by nurses to observe and report any change in color, shape, size, or elevation of these marks during the lifetime of their child.

A red birth mark, or nevus flammeus, is often seen at the nape of the neck ("stork bite") and on the face be-tween the eyebrows or on the eyelids, nose, or upper lip. Appearing pale red in color, the nevus flammeus often has an irregular border or "splash mark" appearance. Red birth marks often turn bright red when the infant is crying, and gradually fade as the infant gets older. Other red birth marks observed in infancy are capillary hemangiomas, which may appear as red, raised lesions anywhere on the infant's body. They also contain areas of purple, blue, or white skin within the lesion. The nurse can address the parents' concern about this lesion by explaining that it will grow larger, undergo a process of involution, and then gradually disappear during the first year of life. These le-sions are not surgically removed unless they interfere with a vital system or are located on the face.

A blue nevus is a small, discrete blue or blue-black birth mark. It is usually found on the buttocks and hands and feet. This nevus is often mistaken for a Mongolian spot when located on the buttocks. It is differentiated from a Mongolian spot by its distinct borders and brighter color, which is different from the darker diffuse purple-blue-gray coloring over a general area characteristic of Mongolian spots. They are usually no larger than one centimeter in diameter.

Common Problems

Marks on an infant that are the result of birth trauma are usually characterized by the initial red imprint of the trau-matizing instrument (e.g., forceps) and their color follows the normal progression of the skin color changes with a bruise. Common areas to inspect for birth injuries are the scalp, face, shoulders, arms, legs, and feet. Marks from birth trauma are commonly seen in large infants when it is difficult to deliver the head or rotate the shoulders. Infants whose delivery position is breech or whose presenting parts are either the legs or feet can often show extensive bruising or edema from attempts to deliver the infant. In some cases, birth trauma may not be evident by a difference in skin color or edema at the injury site. These infants become extremely irritable when their position is changed or during simple extremity movements. Observation of infant behavior when the nurse examines the skin of the infant in the prone and supine position may lead the nurse to further investigate additional areas.

The presence of petechiae on the infant's skin that cannot be attributed to birth injury or trauma must be investigated further. Petechiae may represent an underlying infection, a hemorrhagic process, or congenital condition (congenital rubella). Petechiae should be reported immediately because many of the causes may be life-threatening to the infant if left untreated.

Purple or dark red marks that are extensive and differ from nevus flammeus are called port wine stains. Port wine stains are usually found on the head over the eyelid along the trigeminal nerve tract. These birth marks usually do not cross the midline and may be seen on the trunk or extremities. Neurologic assessments should be performed on all infants with port wine stains. Parents can be reassured that pulse-dye laser surgery can achieve cosmetic correction of the lesion at a later age (Seidel et al., 2001).

Colored skin lesions that contain two distinct areas of color, are extensive, cover a large amount of body surface, or contain hairs or a tuft of hair should be evaluated by a dermatologist. These skin lesions may indicate a defect in the underlying structures, and often ultrasound is indicated to evaluate the tissue underneath the skin. Skin nevi that contain hairs or a tuft of hair are called hairy nevi and, when present on the posterior surface midline in conjunction with the spinal column, may indicate a vertebral defect. The nurse should inspect and palpate the spinal column and sacrum for dimpling or depressions in the skin that may also be an indication of a vertebral defect. Spinal ultrasound examination of the spinal vertebrae is necessary to confirm any defects that would indicate the presence of spina bifida or spina bifida occulta.

Small crops of blisters or a single blister found on full examination may require further evaluation. Blisters that are not located on the thumb or hand (sucking blisters) or on the extremities in conjunction with other lesions indicative of pustular melanosis are a cause for concern. Groups or crops of blisters on a presenting part of the infant's body are caused by exposure to herpes as the infant passed through the birth canal. The most common location for these blisters is on the infant's scalp, near the hair-line, or around the scalp electrode monitor site. Because this condition can be life-threatening to the infant, this finding must be reported immediately.

Newborn skin color that remains red or dark pink may be an indication of plethora. Plethora may be caused by polycythemia vera or hyperthermia. Polycythemia vera is a condition in which an increased number of red blood cells in the infant's bloodstream occurs as a result of backflow of maternal blood into the infant when the cord was cut. This diagnosis can be confirmed by a capillary hematocrit value of 65 or greater and a venous hematocrit of 60 or more (Seidel et al., 2001). Treatment of polycemia vera includes admission to the intensive care unit for monitoring and a partial exchange transfusion.

Hair patterns may present a problem in infancy. Hair distribution is described in the nursing assessment, and the nurse notes the texture, color, and distribution. Visually, the nurse determines any disruptions to the distribution of hair or any areas that contain hair that is not uniformly distributed over the scalp with distinct hairlines. Hair that extends over the forehead, blurring the forehead and shortening the distance between the hairline and the eyebrows, raises a concern because of its association with congenital syndromes. Particular attention should be directed toward those areas of hair that are lighter in color, sections of hair colored very differently in comparison to the rest of the scalp hair, and hair patterns that appear to have a circular design (whorls). White hair patches in the midst of darker colored scalp hair and circular hair patterns may indicate a defect in underlying structures or be initial findings in congenital syndromes. These findings should be documented by the nurse and reported immediately for further evaluation.

Nursing Implications

An accurate assessment of the infant's skin allows the nurse the opportunity to prepare for conditions that might adversely affect the infant and to show common skin variations on the infant to the parents and any other family members that are present. New parents are especially concerned about "marks" or "spots" on their babies, and the nurse can address these concerns as well as remove any fears that the parents or family members may have voiced.

Head, Ears, Eyes, Nose, and Throat

The head, ears, eyes, nose, and throat (HEENT) of the infant are examined next, after the skin has been assessed. Visual inspection guides the nursing assessment of this system. The nurse inspects the face for symmetry and placement of eyes, nose, lips, mouth, and ears. The shape of the eyes, nose and mouth are also examined, and any

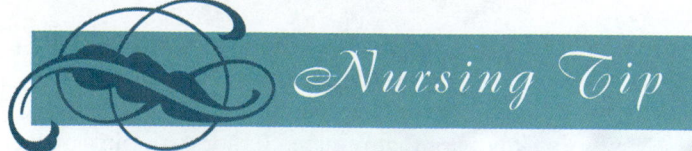

NEWBORN EXAMINATION

The nurse should wash her hands and don clean gloves before touching the newborn during the examination.

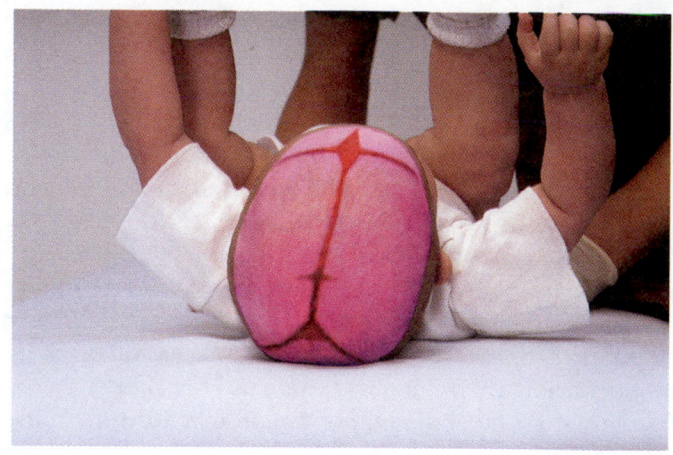

Figure 32-18 Sutures and fontanels.

movements of the lips and eyelids are observed. Damage to cranial nerve VII (facial nerve) from trauma during the delivery process can result in one side of the mouth or tongue drooping, unequal cheek muscle movement or lack of appropriate eyelid movement. Ear shape, size, and position on the head can be examined from profile head positioning as well as the en-face position. Low-set ears bilaterally may indicate the need to examine the infant for other physical characteristics of syndromes. It is common for infants to be born with one ear set a little lower than the other. Eyes are described in terms of color and spacing on the forehead, and whether lids are open or closed. Nares should be open bilaterally, and the nasal bridge should not have a lateral deviation resulting from the delivery process. Upper and lower lip formations should be approximately the same size with the same color as the tongue and buccal mucosa inside the mouth. A chin should be visible and more prominent when the infant's head is placed in the profile position. A small jaw (micrognathia) viewed from the profile position may cause concern about proper tooth development, sucking, swallowing, and later tongue movement inside the mouth for speech.

Common Variations

Palpation begins with the head to determine the spaces between suture lines, the width of the fontanels, and the location and extent of edema from the delivery process. The sutures are felt as bony ridges, with spacing between them to indicate the distance between the borders (Figure 32-18). The **anterior fontanel** is a diamond-shaped open space formed by the anterior-posterior sagittal and frontal sutures and the lateral coronal suture. The area of the fontanel can be determined by feeling its borders and using the nurse's finger for measurements; 2.5 cm, or 1 inch, is the distance from the tip of the finger to the first finger joint). Some infants may have fairly large anterior fontanels (from 5 to 7 cm), and conversely, others may have small anterior fontanels (from 1 to 2 cm). The **posterior fontanel** is a small, triangular-shaped space formed by the sagittal suture and the posterior lateral suture and called the lambdoidal suture. This fontanel is usually 1 cm at its widest point and, on palpation, may be closed, with only a slight indentation

at the initial examination. This is not an unusual finding. The anterior fontanel must be open to provide for the expansion of the bones of the skull for brain growth during the first year of life. Spaces between suture lines are reflective of the molding process necessary to deliver the head of the infant and may extend to all suture lines, including the frontal suture in the middle of the forehead. Fontanels should be palpated by the nurse for an assessment of intracranial pressure. Fullness without bulging, either palpated or visible, is a sign of normal intracranial pressure. Bulging fontanels in infants with large head circumferences are characteristic of increased intracranial pressures, most likely associated with hydrocephalus.

Soft-tissue edema or swelling from delivery may be palpated during the examination of the head (Figure 32-19). Edema that is fairly diffuse and crosses suture lines is called **caput succedaneum** and usually disappears during the first several days of life. Edema that appears to be localized, giving the infant's head the appearance of growing a horn on one side, is called a **cephalhematoma**. This represents a subperiosteal hemorrhage that does not cross suture lines. The skin in the area may or may not have a reddened color. As this material is slowly broken down and resorbed, the shape of the head may remain "lumpy" for a month after birth and the infant may show signs of jaundice from the metabolism of broken red blood cells from the hemorrhage.

The face, including eyes, nose, and ears, is palpated to confirm shape and size. Eyelids are opened manually to check color of the iris, sclera, and conjunctiva. Tiny pinpoint scleral hemorrhages may be noted in the inner or outer canthus of the eyes and are common after delivery. Small amounts of a yellowish discharge that appear to originate from the conjunctiva and stick to the eyelashes, along with swollen eyelids, indicate that the infant has received eye prophylaxis. Bilateral red reflexes are assessed with an ophthalmoscope and recorded.

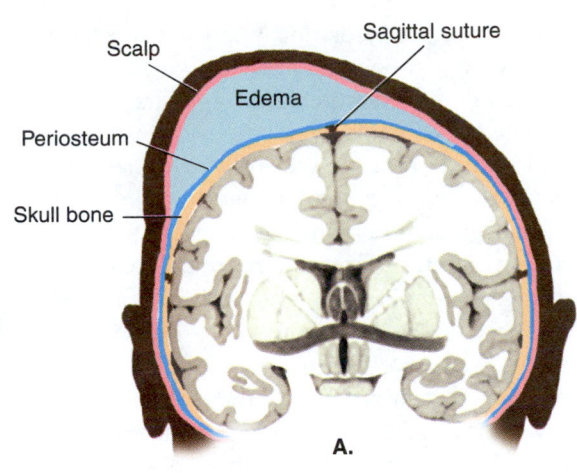

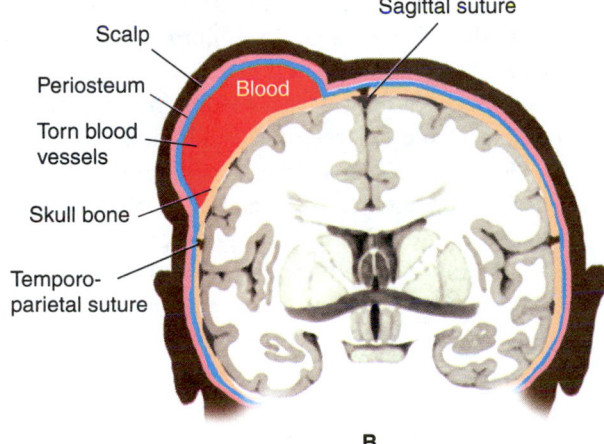

Figure 32-19 A. Caput succedaneum;
B. Cephalhematoma.

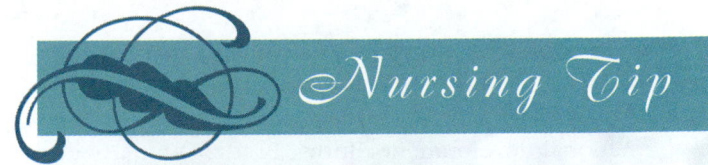

ABSENCE OF RED REFLEX

Absence of a red reflex on physical examination of a newborn infant on one or both eyes constitutes an ophthalmic emergency because of the interference with the transmission of light to the retina. Appropriate nursing and medical personnel are notified immediately: early suppression of optic nerve function from obstructed light pathways may cause blindness.

throat, tongue, and uvula visualized. The throat is palpated externally to check for the presence of an enlarged thyroid gland and to ensure the trachea is at midline. Neck rotation is assessed through inspection of head movement and with gentle passive rotation by the examiner. Limitations to neck rotation may be a torticollis, which manifests as the head held to one side with the chin pointing to the other side, or a congenital defect in the cervical vertebrae. Since any limitation in neck movement has serious consequences for the infant, this must be reported immediately.

The ears are palpated to determine the thickness of the ear lobe and pinna, and irregular or unsymmetrical shapes are noted. Two common preauricular ear malformations are ear pits and ear tags. Ear pits are tiny pinholes located near the upper curved border of the pinna. These

Gross vision in the infant may be evaluated by holding the examiner's face approximately 10 inches from the infant's face and determining the infant's ability to direct his or her gaze to the nurse's face and readjust the gaze when the nurse moves. The nasal bridge is palpated for symmetry and presence of any fracture that might have occurred during the delivery process. The mouth is opened and inspected and gums are palpated for the presence of neonatal teeth lying underneath the gum surface. Visible neonatal teeth should be assessed for looseness and may have to be removed to prevent aspiration (Figure 32-20). The uvula should be at midline. A bivalved or two-lobed uvula is an indication that there may be a cleft in the palate. During the mouth assessment, the infant's ability to suck can be tested by inserting a gloved finger into the mouth to feel the strength of the sucking motion. At the same time, the infant's hard and soft palate can be assessed for size, shape, and cleft formations. Cleft formations may be palpated as an actual opening or a notched ridge. High-arched palates may be an indication of difficulties in swallowing and may affect later speech development. The gag reflex should also be elicited and the back of the mouth,

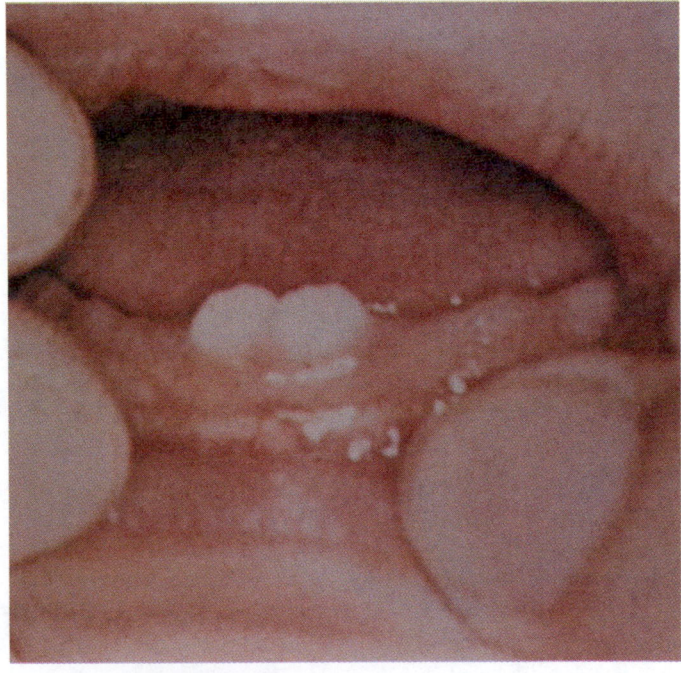

Figure 32-20 Neonatal teeth (Courtesy of Mead Johnson).

may represent a small sinus tract between the skin and underlying structures. They result from the imperfect fusion of the tubercles of the first and second brachial arches during gestational development (Burns, Brady, Dunn, & Starr, 2000). The nurse should examine ear pits carefully to determine if there is a layer of skin covering the opening or the pit is open at its bottom. Ear pits that are draining fluid or appear to be at risk for infection require surgical repair. Ear tags are tags of skin shaped like bulbs that project from the surface of the skin. Removal by a plastic surgeon for cosmetic purposes is recommended because these areas often contain microcapillaries that bleed when severed. Ear canals are inspected for patency and gross hearing assessed by ringing a bell near each ear.

Common Problems

HEENT findings that necessitate further investigation are asymmetrical, unusual, or may be indicative of defects in underlying structures or congenital syndromes. The examination findings that are the most problematic for the infant are those that are immediately visible to the nurse examiner. Down syndrome is often identified in the early newborn period during the HEENT exam by the positive physical findings of a flattened (not round) occiput; a broad nasal bridge; upward slanted eyes with epicanthal folds; low-set ears; a prominent, enlarged tongue; a high, arched palate; and a small chin. In addition, the infant may exhibit Brushfield's spots, which are whitish spots on the iris of the eye. Cleft lip and cleft palate appear as open separations of the lip, mouth, nose, and hard or soft palate and are associated with a bivalved uvula. These clefts involve facial disfigurement, and the parents and family members are sensitive to other persons observing their infant. Malformations of the ears that involve missing lobes or lack of an ear canal also increase parental sensitivity unless they are covered by the infant's hair.

A careful nursing assessment of the eyes reveals several conditions that have the potential to adversely affect the infant's condition. In the visual inspection of the eye, any deviation from the normal white color of the sclera should be noted. Sclera that appear to have a bluish color may be indicative of a congenital condition called osteogenesis imperfecta, which affects the integrity of the structure of the bones. Infants with this condition may already have fractures from the trauma of delivery and must be handled carefully. Yellowing of the sclera appears last in the progression of jaundice in the newborn infant. The yellow color should alert the nurse to increased bilirubin levels in the newborn and the possible need for immediate intervention, including intravenous fluids and phototherapy. Examination of the iris of the eye may show a disruption, called a coloboma, that looks like a keyhole in the distinct circle of the iris and pupil that will affect vision in that eye. A yellow or white shad-

owy covering of the iris and pupil that occludes the red reflex may be a congenital cataract, which requires immediate referral. A red reflex that appears to be white in color, called *leukocoria* or "white eye," instead of the normal red or red-orange color may be caused by a neuroblastoma, which requires immediate medical attention. Congenital glaucoma manifests as eyes that appear to be protruding slightly from the periorbital area and feel hard and firm on palpation. This is an ophthalmic emergency because eye drops are required to decrease intraocular pressure to preserve vision.

A detailed examination of the eyes, nose, and upper lip may also reveal facial features characteristic of alcohol-related birth defects (ARBD). Short palpebral fissures, a small upturned nose, a flattened nasal bridge, and a thin upper lip with a wide, smooth philtrum are the most prominent features of ARBD (Jones, 1997). These infants demonstrate poor growth, a small head (**microcephaly**), small chins, and mental retardation (Taeusch & Ballard, 1998). Previously, these characteristics were referred to as fetal alcohol syndrome (FAS) or fetal alcohol effects (FAE) indicating the range of physical and mental effects that maternal alcohol consumption has on the developing fetus. The incidence of ARBD is 1 to 2 infants per 1000 live births and it may occur with the consumption of as little as three ounces of alcohol per day (Taeusch & Ballard, 1998). The incidence is much higher (1 in 50 live births) in Native American populations (Abel & Sokol, 1987). After delivery, these infants may exhibit jitteriness, irritability, and poor feeding that are related to their alcohol exposure. Nursing care of these infants is directed toward comforting mechanisms and decreasing environmental stimuli that would surprise or startle an infant prone to irritability.

Nursing Implications

The examination of the head, face, eyes, ears, nose, and throat is one of the most important examinations for nursing. The infant's head and face are the only body parts that are visible to the outside world when the infant is wrapped in or covered with blankets. The parents, family visitors, and strangers form their impression of the infant by viewing the head and face. Unfortunately, many congenital defects and syndromes affect parts of the head and face. Normal variations (for example, large or protruding ears, hair color, and birth marks) that often are the result of familial inheritance are also compared to other infants. Accurate assessments of the head and face will guide the nurse to address parental concerns.

Respiratory System

The infant's respiratory efforts are first assessed visually by the nurse noting the symmetry of chest movements. At this time, the chest is also inspected for placement and size of

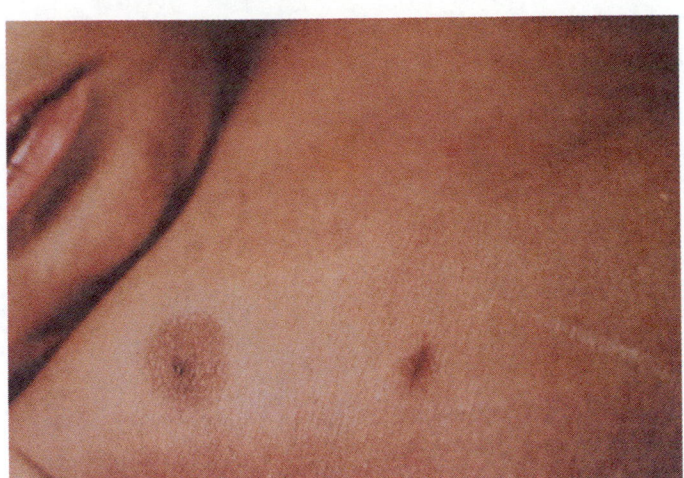

Figure 32-21 Accessory nipple (Courtesy of Mead Johnson).

breast tissue. Maternal hormones crossing the placenta during labor and delivery may cause an enlargement of breast tissue even in male infants. Breast tissue and nipples should be aligned with the mid-clavicular line, which is an imaginary line that is one-half the distance from midline (the sternum) to the lateral border of the chest wall formed by the rib cage. Breast tissue that is placed between the mid-clavicular line and the lateral chest wall is called "wide-spaced nipples." Wide-spaced nipples have been associated with several congenital syndromes, particularly Down syndrome. Additionally, the infant may have smaller extra nipples either above or below the primary nipples. The extra nipples, called accessory nipples, do not enlarge with puberty and may be removed at a later age for cosmetic reasons (Figure 32-21).

Common Variations

Relative ease of breathing can be determined by examining the infant lying in a supine position and observing the pattern of breathing, counting the respirations, and determining whether or not accessory muscles are needed for quiet breathing. The nurse may notice very slight sternal retractions during normal respirations in the infant. On palpation, the xiphoid process may be prominent or appear to protrude underneath the skin. Parents need reassurance that as the infant grows, this small piece of the sternum will not get bigger or pierce the skin. Infants are known to have irregular breathing rates with apneic spells that may last up to 15 seconds. Parents need to be warned by the nurse that infants do have apneic spells with normal breathing. Otherwise, they may become frightened that their infant is not breathing. Taking several respiratory rates during the physical examination may be required to get an accurate picture of the infant's respiratory effort. Respiratory rates under 60 breaths per minute in a term

newborn infant are considered normal. Rates between 60 and 70 breaths/min that are not caused by crying episodes and that persist need further examination.

Common Problems

Infants who appear to have marked sternal or intercostal retractions with breathing and look like they are expending energy ("working hard to breathe") need a prompt respiratory assessment. Palpation of the anterior lung fields may reveal a birth injury, a fractured clavicle or rib, which may be causing an increased respiratory rate resulting from pain at the injury site. Rib injuries may also be visualized as asymmetrical respiratory movements of the chest wall. The shape of the chest may be inspected for deformities that might interfere with normal lung expansion. Funnel chest (pectus excavatum) and pigeon chest (pectus carinatum) result from an abnormal development of the ribs and sternum. Auscultation of all lung fields anteriorly and posteriorly can confirm the respiratory rate (instead of counting abdominal movements) as well as detect adventitious breath sounds from congestion. Upper airway congestion from mucus and residual amniotic fluid can be differentiated from lower airway congestion by auscultation of the infant's nose. Noisy breath sounds heard from the nose are usually indicators that the congestion exists in the nasal passages, throat, and upper bronchus rather than in the middle or lower lobes of the lungs. The nurse can use a bulb syringe to clear nasal and throat passages of fluid and mucus to ease breathing efforts by the infant. Retractions decrease as breathing becomes easier.

Retractions that do not disappear may be an indicator of respiratory distress in the infant. Respiratory distress is a symptom of many conditions in the newborn infant that should be investigated immediately. The infant may have a congenital respiratory condition, which is usually a narrowing of an airway; a congenital heart condition that interferes with the capacity of the lungs to supply oxygen to the blood for circulation; or an infection acquired from the mother. All of these conditions are life-threatening to the infant, and they require nursing and medical interventions.

Nursing Implications

Respiratory rates in newborns between 60 and 70 breaths per minute require continual observation by the nurse. The infant breathes faster when moving, irritated, or crying. The respiratory rate should be taken when the infant is calm or quiet. As with transient tachypnea of the newborn, a rapid respiratory rate in a quiet infant may be a temporary adjustment to extrauterine life. However, the nurse must be alert to the development of additional symptoms, i.e., nasal flaring, grunting, or intercostal

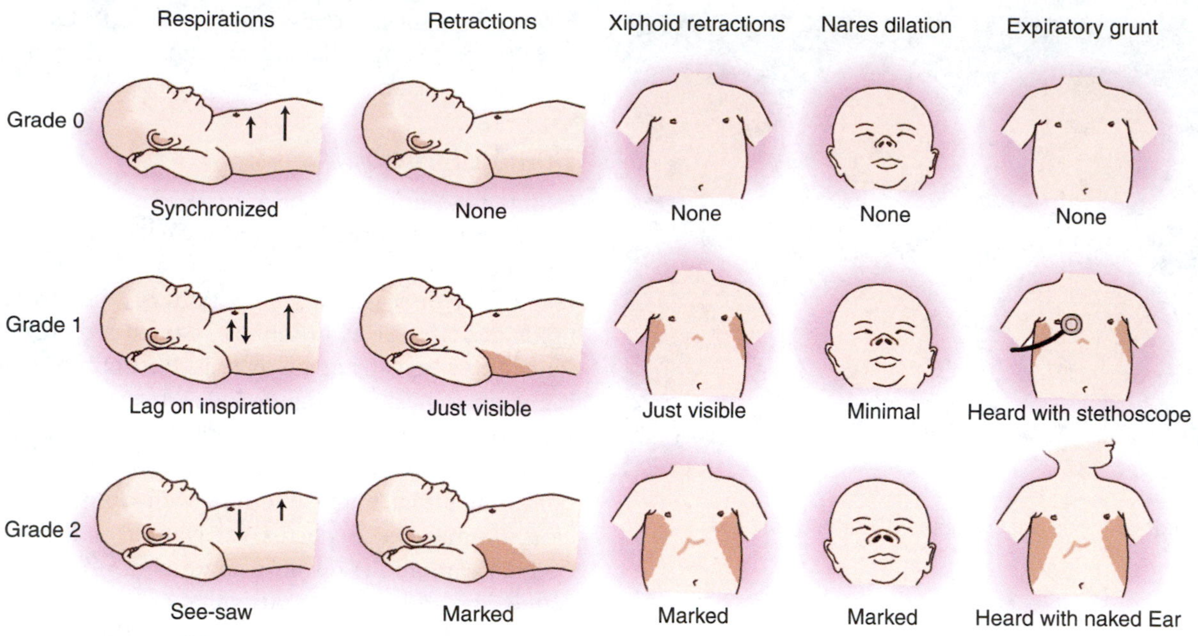

	Respirations	Retractions	Xiphoid retractions	Nares dilation	Expiratory grunt
Grade 0	Synchronized	None	None	None	None
Grade 1	Lag on inspiration	Just visible	Just visible	Minimal	Heard with stethoscope
Grade 2	See-saw	Marked	Marked	Marked	Heard with naked Ear

Figure 32-22 Silverman-Anderson index of respiratory distress.

retractions, that would indicate the development of a more serious condition (Figure 32-22). The nurse should monitor skin color and capillary refill of both upper and lower extremities to complete the nursing assessment of the efficiency of the respiratory system. The nurse must determine whether additional symptoms indicate a condition of respiratory distress in the infant or whether the absence of additional symptoms indicates that the infant is approaching respiratory stability.

Cardiovascular System

The cardiovascular system is best assessed by the nurse visually and by auscultation. Visual assessment includes skin color of the trunk of the infant and the skin color of the extremities. Color should be pink and increase to red when the infant cries or moves its extremities. Visual inspection of the lips, mouth, gums, and buccal mucosa is the best indicator of cardiac perfusion. The chest is palpated for any thrills, heaves, and the point of maximum impulse (PMI). In newborns, the PMI by auscultation occurs at the apex of the heart near the third or fourth left intercostal space. Heart rate is counted and heart rates above 160 beats/min are called **tachycardia**. The heart rate normally should fall in the range of between 120 and 150 beats/min. Capillary refill in fingers and toes is examined by pinching the end of the finger or toe and counting the seconds until the skin returns to its normal color. Normal refill times are less than 3 seconds. Refill times of more than 3 seconds may indicate a shunting of the circulation away from the periphery towards the trunk of the infant. All peripheral pulses are palpated for bilateral symmetry, strength, and rate. Pulses that continue to be strong and bounding as distance from the

heart increases may be an indication of a cardiovascular problem. Special attention is given to femoral pulses. These are checked one at a time and compared to the brachial pulses. Any decrease in the strength of the pulse between the brachial pulses and the femoral pulses may be an indication for a cardiac condition called coarctation of the aorta. Coarctation of the aorta is a narrowing of a portion of the aortic arch. The aorta is the main transport vessel for oxygenated blood to the upper and lower portions of the body. A narrowing of the aortic arch causes diminished blood flow patterns and may be suspected in infants with diminished or decreased femoral pulses.

Common Variations

All areas of the heart, i.e., the aortic, pulmonic, tricuspid, mitral, base, and apex, are examined by auscultation. Infant heart rates vary: they slow down with rest and speed up with activity or crying. Term infants usually maintain a heart rate of between 110 and 160 beats/min; rates lower than 100 beats/min are indicative of bradycardia and rates higher than 160 beats/min are considered to be tachycardia (Seidel et al., 2001). Either persistent bradycardia or tachycardia must be reported to the nursing staff responsible for the infant. Initially, infant heart rates are difficult to hear. The chest wall in infancy is thin and heart sound transmission has a tendency to be noisy and obscured by the infants' respirations. Patience and continued listening by the nurse are often necessary to determine the heart rate as well as any extra sounds or murmurs. Murmurs are often heard in newborns less than 24 hours old near the sternal border at the level of the left second or third intercostal space. A increasing amount of sound (crescendo)

Critical Thinking

The Newborn After Transition

You are performing a cardiac assessment on an infant who is 8 hours old. Auscultation of the heart reveals a soft heart murmur heard throughout systole and a heart rate of 170 beats/min. The infant appears large in size and has no visible congenital anomalies. Skin color is pale-pink with a capillary refill time of 3 seconds in both upper and lower extremities. Pulses are equal bilaterally, rhythm is regular, and you note that pedal pulses are especially strong, close to bounding.

- What do bounding pulses mean in a newborn infant?
- Are your physical exam findings normal or abnormal at this time?
- Which is the best nursing action to take next?

1. Continue observation of this infant and repeat your assessment in 30 minutes.
2. Ask a nursing colleague to verify your physical examination findings.
3. Report your findings to the medical staff immediately.
4. Repeat your assessment to confirm your findings.

The best response is number three. Bounding pedal pulses, a heart rate increased above normal, and a soft systolic murmur indicate increased cardiac contractility in the presence of blood backflow through fetal shunts. This "increased workload" for the heart may lead to cardiac failure if not evaluated immediately. While confirmation of findings may be an appropriate action, examination findings can always be confirmed by the medical staff on duty. The nurse must learn to trust her own assessment skills and judgment in patient care situations that require immediate decisions. Signs of cardiac failure in newborns infants may be very subtle at first, and the nurse must be alert to any cardiac findings that are questionable.

occurring through systole is the usual sound pattern heard. The sound from an infant with **patent ductus arteriosus** (PDA) will gradually disappear when the ductus closes, within 2 to 3 days. Murmurs that persist beyond the second day of life and whose sound has changed to a more definitive whoosh pattern are not characteristic of an open ductus and require a cardiac evaluation.

Common Problems

The most common heart murmur in infancy is the ventricular septal defect (VSD) in which there is a small hole in the wall of the ventricle between the right and left chambers of the heart. The sound of the murmur is created by the heart pumping blood and the blood leaking through this hole. Small defects produce louder murmurs because of the buildup in pressure in the chambers from the blood leaking through with each contraction. Large defects produce softer murmurs as blood flow through the hole is greater, reducing the pressure buildup. The majority of ventral septal defects close without surgical correction as a result of the normal cardiac growth during the first year of life. Mothers of newborns with heart murmurs need to be reassured that most heart murmurs noted in infancy are not fatal nor do they require surgery, which are their biggest fears.

Cardiac insufficiency, leading to heart failure, occurs when the infant is unable to properly oxygenate and circulate blood. Nurses may suspect this condition in irritable infants with persistent pallor, rapid breathing, and cyanosis around the lips. Pulse oximetry readings of less than 94% oxygen saturation are cause for concern. An infant whose oxygen saturation falls below 90% must be placed on a cardiac and respiratory monitor in an intensive care unit. Infants who exhibit these symptoms may have heart defects with normal heart functions as long as the ductus remained open. As the ductus starts to close on day 2 or 3 of life, their cardiac condition becomes unstable and compromised. In these infants, a murmur develops on day 2 of life, which is the first indication of a cardiac problem. Infants who develop cardiac instability within the first 2 days of life are those infants who have a genetic karyotype of trisomy 13, 18, or 21 or tetralogy of Fallot. Tetralogy of Fallot consists of four specific cardiac anomalies: transposition of the aorta and pulmonary artery, right ventricular hypertrophy, pulmonary stenosis, and ventricular septal defect (Taeusch and Ballard, 1998). Newborns with tetralogy of Fallot are stable after birth, have no murmurs on auscultation, and maintain cardiac perfusion as long as their ductus arteriosus remains open. Medical and nursing staff refer to these infants as "pink tets." When the ductus begins to close after 24 hours of life, severe cardiac instability occurs, with the development of central cyanosis. These infants are placed on a cardiac monitor in an intensive care unit, receive intravenous fluids with medication to preserve cardiac output, and undergo a full cardiac and surgical evaluation.

Nursing Implications

The accurate assessment of the heart and cardiovascular system in a newborn is necessary for the determination of present and future cardiac stability of the infant. Nurses who examine newborns develop the knowledge and

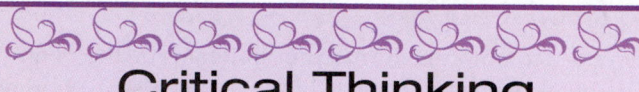

Critical Thinking

Newborn Heart Defect: What Do You Say?

You are reading an infant's chart and discover that the health care provider suspects a cardiac defect, has ordered an ECG, and has called a pediatric cardiologist to examine the infant. When you bring the infant to the mother, she tells you that she feels great, is ready to go home, and has called the father of the baby to come pick them up.

• What would you say to this mother?
• What might you say to the physician?

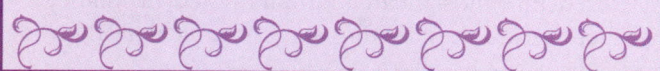

expertise to detect cardiac conditions often before the medical staff is aware of them. Nurses are also the key personnel that parents and family members contact who have concerns about the health of their infant. Cardiac problems in infancy cause severe anxiety in both parents. The major role of nurses beyond the cardiac assessment of newborns is to develop skills in communication to convey to parents and other family members the nature of the problem, the steps being taken, and the health and welfare of their infant.

Abdomen

The abdomen of a newborn infant in the supine position appears round, full, and bilaterally symmetrical. The umbilical cord should be clamped securely with no oozing of blood or it will need to be re-clamped. The cord should be examined for the presence of three vessels, two arteries, and one vein. Umbilical cords with fewer than three vessels should be reported to the charge nurse and medical staff. Large cords that have thickened areas of gelatinous material are referred to as having Wharton's jelly. Infants' abdomens may look distended from the presence of stool that has not yet been eliminated. After inspection of the relative size and shape of the abdomen, and watching abdominal breathing patterns, auscultation for bowel sounds in all four quadrants is begun. Several areas in each quadrant are assessed, because bowel obstruction in the newborn may present initially as a lack of bowel sounds in a small area of the bowel. Auscultation for the gastric bubble and the heart sounds of the abdominal aorta completes this part of the examination.

Common Variations

Light and deep palpation of the abdomen allows the nurse the opportunity to assess the integrity of the abdominal contents of the infant. Light palpation begins with the end of the sternum and the xiphoid process, proceeding midline to the seat of the umbilicus on the abdomen. As palpation proceeds along the midline, a diastasis rectus, or a thinning of the abdominal wall along the midline may be palpated. A diastasis rectus can also be visualized as a "furrow" formation, or elongated lump, at midline when the infant is crying. Last, the circumference of the umbilicus can be palpated for hernias. The umbilical cord should be firmly seated in the abdominal wall, but there may be a separation between the cord and the abdominal wall, called a hernia. Hernias are measured by finger-tips to determine if they are large or small. Umbilical hernias are common in newborn infants, and small ones often close on their own when infants grow larger. Palpation is continued along the midline below the umbilicus to the symphysis pubis. Some umbilical hernias extend inferiorly and the size of the hernia may be misjudged.

Light palpation of the abdomen continues from midline to the costal margins (rib cage) to determine the presence of masses or enlarged organs. The small size of the newborn abdomen facilitates this examination as a result of the lack of space for enlarged organs or extra material (tumors or masses). Deep palpation is used to outline specific organs and their borders. The liver border, felt just below the right costal margin should be smooth and firm and not extend more than 2 centimeters below this margin. The spleen, tucked underneath the left costal margin, is only palpable at the tip of the organ, 1 centimeter below the costal margin. Positive palpation findings on a newborn's spleen are a cause for concern because organ enlargement must be present for the spleen to be palpated beyond its tip. Kidneys may be palpated at a right angle to the umbilicus at midline, located 1 to 2 centimeters above the umbilicus. However, they may be missed because of their small size. The bladder wall should be smooth and can be palpated at midline, inferior to the umbilicus.

Common Problems

Assessment findings that indicate a serious abdominal condition in the newborn are abdominal distention, absent bowel sounds, discharge from the umbilical cord or site, and palpation of an abdominal mass. Abdominal distention may appear to involve the entire abdominal surface or small areas of bulging. The nurse may notice enlarged abdominal veins in a distended abdomen. Light and deep palpation may reveal stool in the colon, which is not cause for alarm. Areas of abdominal bulging that shift when the infant is moved in the supine position may indicate the presence of fluid in the abdomen. Light pressure on the abdomen below the costal margin may generate a fluid wave to the opposite costal margin. This requires immediate attention by the medical staff to determine the source of the fluid in the abdomen.

Auscultatory sounds that are diminished or absent in the abdomen are indicators of potential circulatory problems. Auscultation of the abdominal aorta at midline above the umbilicus gives the listener an impression of circula-

tion to the abdominal organs and lower extremities. Diminished sounds may indicate decreased circulatory efforts, as in coarctation of the aorta. Decreased blood flow would affect the kidney's ability to filter blood and form urine, and the bowel's ability to digest nutrients and undergo peristalsis. Absent bowel sounds in an area of the abdomen would indicate a portion of the bowel that is not functioning and requires immediate attention. Necrotizing entercolitis is a severe abdominal condition of newborns, resulting from inadequate circulation to the bowel, the destruction of the intestinal mucosa, and complete loss of bowel function. Loss of bowel function leads to intestinal obstruction and secretion of toxins from tissue that has been destroyed. This condition is life-threatening and requires immediate surgical intervention.

Inspection of the umbilicus and umbilical cord for discharge or leakage is done to detect signs of infection. Umbilical cords that have not been stained with the bacteriostatic dye are pale yellow. Green staining of umbilical cords occurs when the infant has passed meconium before delivery. The base of the umbilical cord should be clean and dry with no discharge or leakage of blood. The presence of a discharge must be reported immediately because it is an indicator of infection. Stool and urine from the diaper area should not leak out of the diaper and be in contact with the cord or the base of the cord. When this occurs, careful cleansing is required. An extra cord clamp can be applied if there is a blood leak. The abdominal wall surrounding the seat of the cord is inspected for redness. A circular area of redness around the base of the cord on the abdomen is a symptom of omphalitis, an infection of the base of the cord that requires antibiotic therapy.

Palpation of an abdominal mass or an enlarged abdominal organ in the newborn is facilitated by the infant's usually small abdominal girth. Masses or enlarged organs require immediate attention and investigation. The mass can be confirmed by an ultrasound examination, and medical management can be instituted at this time. In the newborn period, abdominal masses are usually a form of neuroblastoma, and the cause can be confirmed by biopsy. The most common enlarged abdominal organs are the liver, spleen, and kidneys. These findings can also be confirmed by ultrasound examination. The organs may be enlarged from an associated obstructive process or congenital malformation.

Nursing Implications

In addition to the cardiac and respiratory assessment, the assessment of the abdomen is vitally important in the newborn as the site of digestion and the beginning processes of elimination. The nurse develops auscultation and palpation skills to ensure the integrity of the abdominal organs and to detect any causes for concern. The nurse can anticipate the parental expectation that a round, full "tummy"

Nursing Alert

DISTENDED ABDOMEN

The essential tool for nursing assessment of the distended abdomen in a newborn is palpation. Abdomens that are distended can be palpated easily; they feel soft and pliable. A distended abdomen that the nurse is unable to palpate because of the rigidity of the abdominal wall is a medical emergency. This condition is often referred to as "acute abdomen," and the infant is often inconsolable.

on their baby indicates a healthy baby, and teach the parents the signs and symptoms of abnormal conditions of the abdomen.

Genitalia and Anus

Both male and female genitalia are visualized and assessed with the infant in the supine position with its hips abducted. The scrotum of male infants in this position can be determined to be pendulous with descended testes. Flattened or depressed areas of the scrotal sac may indicate that a testis that has not descended. Testes are palpated in the scrotal sac by placing the nurse's second finger at the posterior midline of the scrotum and the thumb on the anterior midline. The index finger and thumb can easily palpate the left side of the scrotum for the presence of a testis, and the third finger and the thumb can likewise palpate for a testis on the right scrotum. Palpation in this manner ensures that one testis is not mistaken for two by being passed from side to side. This technique also allows for gently stroking of the inguinal canal with the respective finger and thumb if a testis is not felt in the scrotal sac. The nurse can bathe the inguinal canal with warm soapy water when a testis can not be located. Warm water has tendency to make a testis "pop up" in the canal and become more visible. One or both undescended testes that cannot be located in the inguinal canal in an infant older than 35 weeks' gestational age is an indication for an urologic evaluation of the infant.

Female genitalia are inspected with the hips of the infant abducted while lying in a supine position. The labia majora are visualized first and the extent to which they cover the remaining tissues of the female genitalia indicates the maturity of the infant. In most female infants at term, the borders of the labia majora meet and the clitoris is covered completely. In some term infants, the development of the genitalia may lag behind other systems and the nurse may see the labia minora and the clitoris uncovered.

Inspection of the anus and palpation of the anal opening occurs at the same time as the genitalia are assessed. Hopefully, the infant will have a stool during the nurse's examination, so that the nurse can validate that the anus is patent and that the stool does, indeed, come out of one and only one anal opening. Stool appearing in a female infant from the vaginal opening results from a rectovaginal fistula, an opening between the rectum and the vagina. The anus is palpated by spreading the tissue around the anal opening and feeling the musculature around the opening. At this time, any rectal tears from the passage of stool in the anal ring may be noted and the **anal wink reflex** elicited. While the infant is in the prone position, the buttocks are stroked from side to side with the index finger of the nurse. The buttocks draw together and "wink" at the point of the anal opening, validating the anatomic position. This reflex is used to evaluate anal openings in females that are closer than 1 centimeter from the vaginal opening. Anal openings too close to vaginal openings do not develop the appropriate muscle strength needed to assist in evacuating the rectum as the infant grows older. The "wink" reflex indicates where the normal anal opening should be positioned for future surgical correction.

Common Variations

In male infants, the nurse may discover that palpation of the scrotum for testes is impossible because the scrotal sac is swollen and distended, preventing accurate palpation. Fluid accumulation in the scrotal sac causes this and can be verified by transillumination of the scrotum. However, the nurse must first verify that the enlarged scrotum does not contain trapped bowel. Careful auscultation of the scrotum for bowel sounds will confirm this condition. If bowl sounds are present, it must be reported and confirmed immediately because this a medical emergency for the infant. If bowl sounds are not present, the nurse can then proceed with transillumination of the scrotum. A penlight or an ophthalmoscope is used as the light source pressed against the scrotum to transilluminate it in a darkened room. Fluid appears as a yellow-orange reflection and, occasionally, a small, dark, round testis can be seen. The nurse must note that a scrotal or testicular mass does not transilluminate and report it immediately. Fluid in the scrotal sac is gradually be reabsorbed over the infant's first several weeks of life, and the mother can be reassured that the scrotum will eventually have a more normal size and appearance.

Palpation continues in male infants to include the shaft of the penis in order to estimate penile length. Normal male infants are born at term with a penis that measures about 2 centimeters. The foreskin (prepuce) is lightly retracted to inspect the urethral opening and the location of the opening on the glans. The nurse may notice a cheesy coating called *smegma,* of the glans underneath the foreskin. Vertical urethral openings (urethral meatus) may be seen instead of round openings and are a symptom of **hypospadias** when they are not centered on the glans and are located instead on the ventral surface (Figure 32-23). Hypospadias repair when indicated is accomplished by using the excess foreskin to re-fashion the meatus. All newborn males suspected of having hypospadias are not to be circumcised. **Epispadias** is the condition in which a vertical urethral opening is located on the dorsal surface of the penis instead of the glans.

Many female infants have a white, thick cheesy substance, called vernix caseosa, between the labia; this is not a cause for concern. A small, triangular-shaped piece of tissue may be visualized between the labia. This is a *hymenal tag* and decreases in size as the infant grows larger. Gentle palpation of the labia majora and labia minora allows for visualization of the hymenal area. It is not unusual at this time to see a white mucoid discharge in the vaginal area as well as a small amount of blood. Maternal

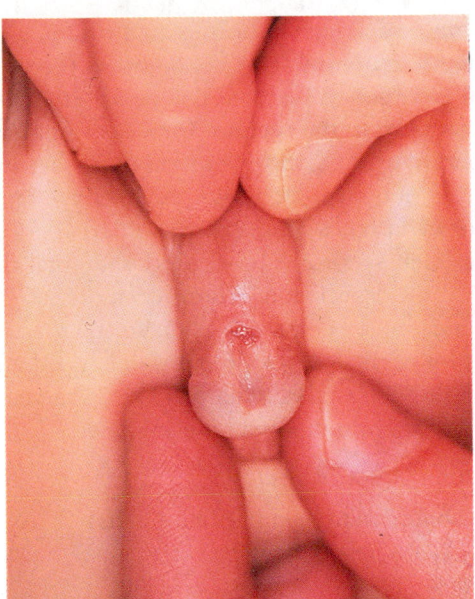

Figure 32-23 Hypospadias. (Courtesy of Dr. James Mardell, chief surgeon, urology, Albany Medical College, Albany, NY).

hormones crossing the placenta create this discharge and bleeding that mimics a period in female infants. This is normal, and parents need to know how to clean the genitalia of their infants and not to be frightened when they see small amounts of blood. It usually takes about a week for a female infant to eliminate the influence of maternal hormones. Females may also have a smegma discharge between the labia.

Common Problems

The nursing assessment of the male genitalia is focused on the determination of whether they are normal. Swelling or

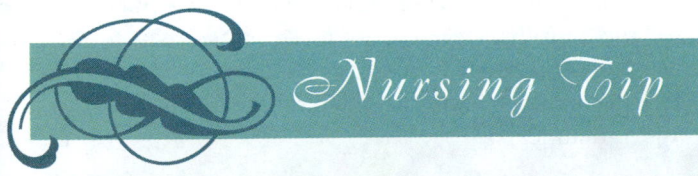

BLOOD IN THE DIAPER

Blood in the diaper of a newborn can be a concern for the nurse and frightening for the parents. The location of the blood can indicate the source of the bleeding. Blood that appears near the top of the diaper is most likely oozing from the umbilical cord. Blood that appears in the middle of the diaper in female infants is most likely bleeding that mimics a period from maternal hormones. Blood in the middle of a diaper on a male infant may be the result of a urine stream through a bruised penis from delivery or indicate a more serious problem to be investigated.

edema from the delivery process may impede this assessment. Bruising of the scrotum can occur with breech presentations, and palpation must be done carefully. Infants of color, particularly African American infants, have dark-skinned scrotums. Examination of the scrotal sac should reveal two testes. Undescended testes may be located in the inguinal canal and become problematic when they do not descend into the scrotal sac. Inguinal hernias are difficult to palpate in infancy. They are usually discovered when a loop of the infant's bowel becomes trapped in the scrotal sac. The scrotum enlarges, does not transilluminate, and exhibits characteristic bowel sounds when auscultated. This condition must be reported immediately, because surgical repair is necessary to save the bowel. A darkened area of the scrotum surrounding one testis with edema may be testicular torsion, in which the spermatic cord and tunica vaginalis twist before attachment of the tunica vaginalis to the scrotum (Juretschke, 2000). This condition in infancy is extremely rare, carries a high risk of testicular loss, and requires immediate surgical intervention (Juretschke, 2000).

Inspection and palpation of the penis determines penile length and completes the assessment of normal male genitalia. A penis less than 2 centimeters long indicates *micropenis* and may be associated with a pituitary tumor or insufficiency. Structures that resemble a penis in a female or ridges that mimic labia on a male require immediate investigation as ambiguous genitalia. In cases in which definite genitalia of either sex cannot be determined, genetic studies are performed in addition to testing for adrenal insufficiencies. Labeling of the infant as a "boy" or a "girl" prematurely leads the parents to treat the infant according to the label already given, which may be contrary to the genetic evidence.

The two most prominent concerns in the assessment of the female genitalia are an enlarged clitoral hood and imperforate hymen. Hormones crossing the placenta may cause the clitoris to be slightly enlarged. A large clitoris that appears hood-shaped and elongated, resembling a penis, may be the result of excess androgen stimulation. This is one symptom of congenital adrenal hyperplasia. Testing for precursors of adrenal corticosteroids and electrolytes for normal kidney function need to be initiated immediately. Edema from the birthing process may interfere with the examination of the labia majora and labia minora. Careful separation of the labia should reveal the urethral opening and an intact vaginal introitus. An imperforate hymen is a muscle wall that obstructs the vaginal opening. This condition will need surgical correction for future release of menses during normal menstrual cycles.

Inspection of the anal opening in both male and female newborns may reveal skin tags on the anal ring or an anal ring without an opening. The skin tags or other hemorrhoid-like tissues may cause discomfort or bleeding in the diaper when the infant is stooling. The lack of either

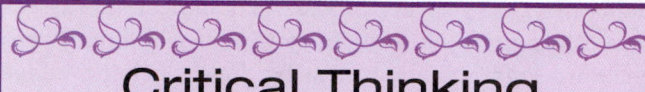

Critical Thinking

Ambiguous Genitalia

You are the nurse taking care of twins in the nursery. The twins are the fifth and sixth children of a young couple who desperately wanted to have a boy, since all their previous children were girls. The twins were born weighing 2200 g and 2250 g and appear to be normal boys. They have been in the nursery for the last 3 weeks, steadily gaining weight before discharge. As you read through the chart, you notice that one of the nurses palpated a high-arched palate on one twin and described a low-set ear. The medical team ordered chromosomal studies, which were reported last week. There was no evidence of trisomy, however, both of the twins had female karotypes. Abdominal ultrasound tests revealed the presence of ovaries and a uterus in both infants. Nursing staff conversations with the parents revealed their intentions to raise the infants as boys. What is the best approach for you to take when you talk with the parents today?

- Do you think that the parents are ignoring the test results?
- Do you think the parents will ever accept the test results?
- Which of the following do you think is the best response?

1. "Do you have any questions for me about the care of your babies?"
2. "I would like to talk with you about the test results and what they mean for your babies."
3. "I have made an appointment for you to see the genetics counselor this afternoon about your babies."
4. "I have asked the genetics counselor to meet with us and help me talk to you about your babies."

The best response is 4. The first response ignores the issue. The second response is repeating the same information the parents have heard before. They are not ready to listen to or hear what the test results mean. The third response takes control away from the parents and places them in a situation that they did not request. The fourth response offers the parents an opportunity to express their feelings and identifies any misunderstandings that they might have.

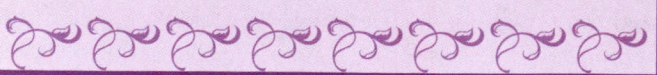

an anal ring or an opening in the anal ring is a condition called imperforate anus. This condition in the newborn is a surgical emergency because the newborn is unable to evacuate stool from the rectum. In 50% of newborns who have imperforate anus, this condition occurs as an isolated event and is not associated with other congenital malformations or syndromes (Taeusch & Ballard, 1998). A common congenital syndrome associated with anal malformations is VATER association. Three or more of the major abnormalities must be present to make the diagnosis, and prognosis for normal development is enhanced after surgical correction (Taeusch & Ballard, 1998). Characteristics of VATER association in the newborn include:

V = vertebral abnormalities

A = anal abnormalities (imperforate anus)

T = tracheal abnormalities

E = esophageal abnormalities (tracheal-esophageal fistulas)

R = renal and radial abnormalities

Nursing care of newborns with VATER association is directed toward proper newborn positioning for arm and spinal defects as well as promotion of breathing efforts through a partially compromised trachea. Additionally, nursing efforts to ensure nutritional intake and elimination are emphasized.

Nursing Implications

Nursing assessment of the genitalia of newborns forms the basis for parental interaction with the infant. The determination of sex is done briefly by inspection only in the delivery room and communicated to the parents. A detailed inspection and further examination is the responsibility of the nurse in charge of the newborn's care. Parents want to see that their infant is normal and looks normal. Any observed difference increases their anxiety. The nurse must have the sensitivity to address these issues with the parents and be prepared to correct misinformation that would affect the parents' ability to interact with their infant in a positive manner.

Circumcision of Male Infants

Circumcision of male infants is usually performed in the nursery and is the personal choice of parents based on their cultural, ethnic, and religious perspectives. Circumcisions for religious purposes may be performed at another site, and elective circumcisions during the first 2 weeks of life may be performed in a private office or clinic. In each case, the role of the nurse is to inform the parents of the risks and benefits of the procedure and address concerns to achieve a fully informed decision. Risks for the infant include infection, hemorrhage, skin dehiscence, adhesions, urethral fistula, and pain (Wong et al., 1999). Benefits to the infant are decreased incidence of urinary tract infections in the first 3 months of life (Schoen, Colby, & Ray, 2000) and possible prevention of penile cancer (Wong et al., 1999). In the circumcision procedure, part of the foreskin is removed by clamping and cutting with a scalpel (Gomco or Mogen clamp) or using a plastic ring with a string tied around it to trim off the excess foreskin (Plastibell). Small sutures or pressure from the plastic ring are used to prevent bleeding and promote wound closure.

Nursing care of the circumcised infant is directed toward providing pain relief before the procedure; comfort before, during, and after the procedure; and skilled observation for bleeding or voiding difficulties. It is the responsibility of the nurse to examine the equipment before the procedure for cleanliness and matching parts. Substitute parts that are not made by the same manufacturer may slip and cause the infant additional discomfort. For at least 2 hours before the procedure, the infant is given nothing by mouth to prevent vomiting or aspiration. Pain relief measures to be considered are: a local dorsal penile nerve block; application of EMLA cream (topical mixture of anesthetics), approximately 1 to 2 g, for 60 minutes before the procedure under an occlusive dressing; and a ring block. EMLA cream is used as a topical anesthetic without nerve blocks and also used with nerve blocks to anesthetize the site of injection. Proper pain relief requires that the cream be applied for at least 1 hour prior to the procedure and the application site varies with the nerve block used. The cream is applied to the foreskin and base of the penis for the dorsal penile nerve block and the foreskin and shaft of the penis for the ring block. The cream should be replaced if the infant urinates during the topical anesthetic period. The penis and scrotum are gently cleaned with a mild soap and warm water and dried. The cream is re-applied to the area required for anesthesia.

The infant is gently restrained during the circumcision procedure on a special board or apparatus with Velcro straps that limit extremity movement near the operative field. The nurse may consider shielding the infants' eyes from the lights, playing soothing music in the background, or stroking the infant's head, shoulders, or upper extremities during the procedure. Pacifiers soaked in a sugar-water solution dissolve 1 tablespoon sugar in 4 tablespoons of sterile water) have been shown to be effective in distracting infants from the procedure (Wong et al., 1999). Once the procedure is complete, the infant is released from the restraints and comforted by the nurse, if the parents are not present. The infant is brought to the parents as soon as possible after the procedure. The choice of dressings or treatments of the circumcision site depends on the method of circumcision. Petroleum jelly (Vasoline) or A & D ointment is applied with 4 × 4 gauze as a dressing to cover the site when a clamp has been used to cut the foreskin. No dressings are needed when the

Plastibell is used. The nurse applies the diaper loosely over this area to prevent any rubbing, pressure, or friction on the penis. When the infant is brought to the parents, the nurse explains the procedure, allows the parents to

Client Education
Circumcision Care

The nurse instructs the parents to carefully apply and remove the diaper over the circumcision site to prevent rubbing. During the first 24 hours, it is recommended that the site be checked by the parents or the nurse every 30 minutes for the first 2 hours and then every 2 hours afterward (Williamson, 1997). The site is checked for excess bleeding or swelling, and the diaper can be felt for dampness to indicate the infant has urinated. The infant must demonstrate an ability to void after the procedure, because edema at the operative site may occlude the urethra or the urethral meatus. Dressings, if present, are changed at least three times in the first 24 hours. The old dressing is removed; the area gently wiped clean with a warm, damp gauze and dried; and a fresh dressing with jelly or ointment applied. Infant acetaminophen (Tylenol) drops are continued every 4 to 6 hours for the first day after the procedure. They are discontinued when the parents feel that their infant is no longer displaying signs of discomfort, pain, or irritability. On the second day, a yellowish exudate appears, which is part of the healing process. The nurse instructs the parents not to remove this or disrupt it when cleansing during the dressing change. Dressing changes are continued for three days after the procedure. If the parents do not notice any swelling, discharge, bleeding, or reddening of the penis, they may discontinue dressing changes but need to watch the area very closely for the next week. The parents may want to change the infants' diapers more frequently to avoid the healing penis being exposed to stool in the diaper. The nurse emphasizes that discharge, swelling, or redness indicates signs of infection. Parents who report less than six diaper changes a day need to be concerned that their infant is having difficulty voiding after circumcision. Signs of infection, failure to void adequately, or excessive bleeding from the operative site must be reported immediately to their health care provider.

A Circumcision Story

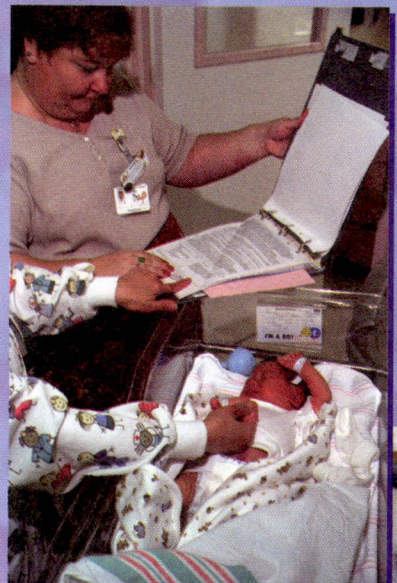

The nurse checks the infant's identification band against the signed consent form.

A circumcision restraint board safely immobilizes the infant during the procedure.

The uncircumcised penis and genital area are exposed.

The physician dons sterile gloves.

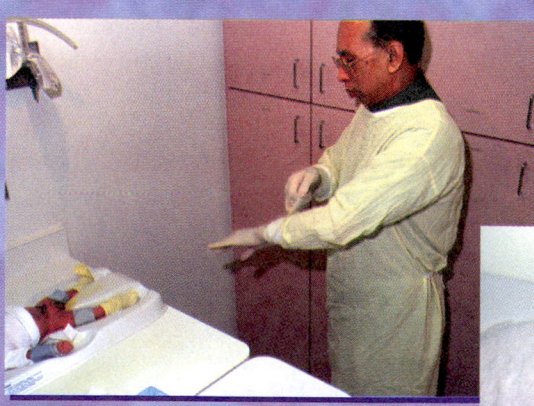

Antiseptic solution is applied to reduce the risk of infection.

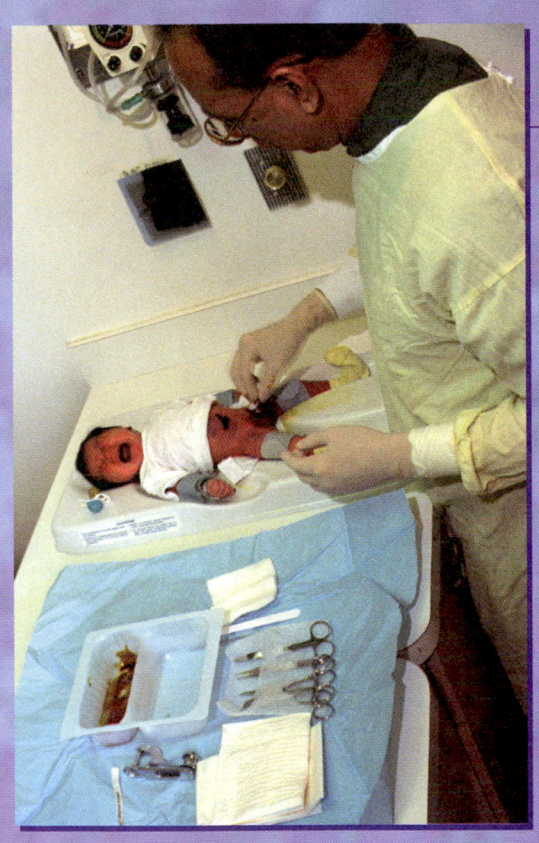

This baby is expressing his opinion of the procedure.

Infants are often offered a pacifier or other soothing measure to help calm them during the procedure.

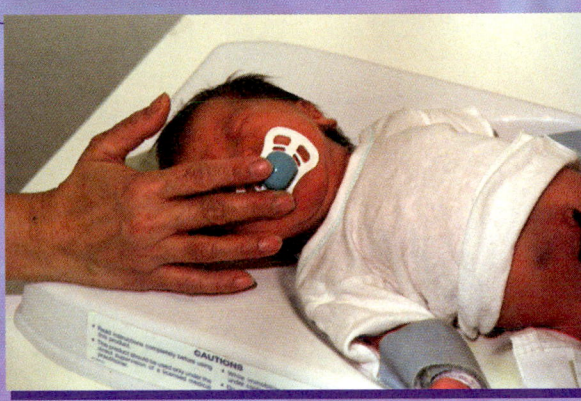

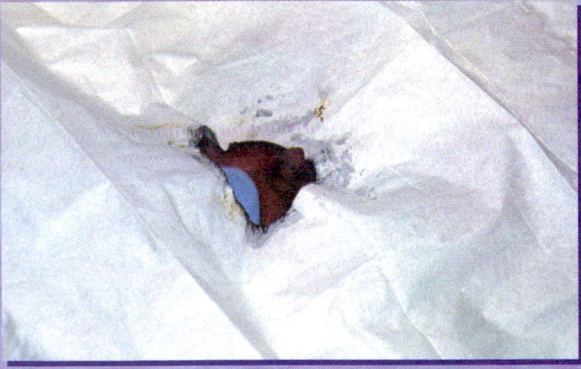

A sterile drape is applied to provide a sterile field.

Kelley clamps are used to extend the prepuce.

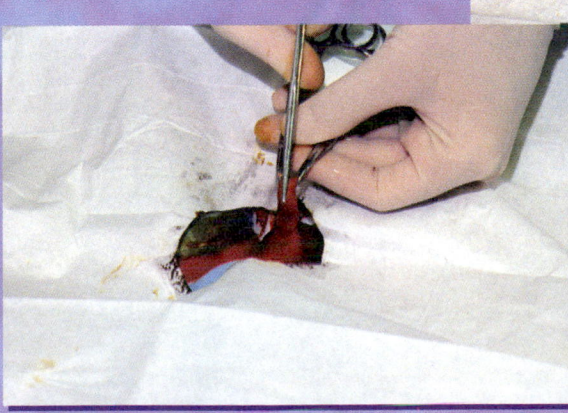

A small incision is made in the prepuce.

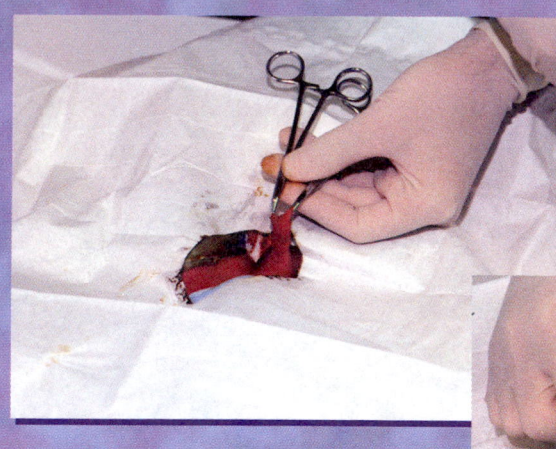

The incision will help accommodate use of the circumcision cone.

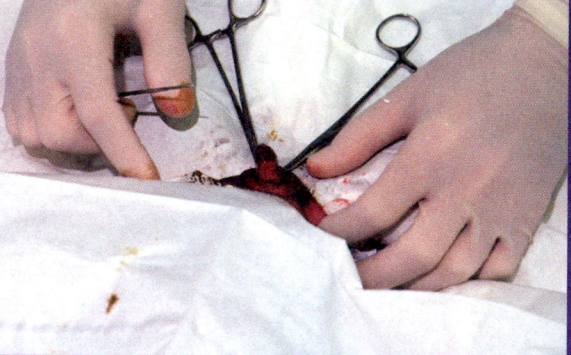

The clamps are left in place as the prepuce is retracted over the glans.

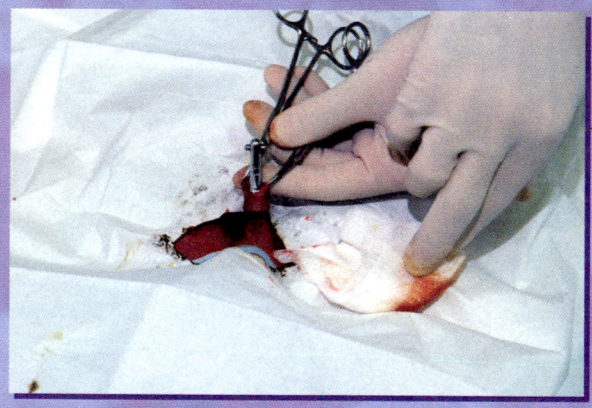

A circumcision cone is placed over the exposed glans penis and the prepuce is drawn up around it.

The clamp is applied and tightened for 3–5 minutes to reduce bleeding and circulation in the prepuce.

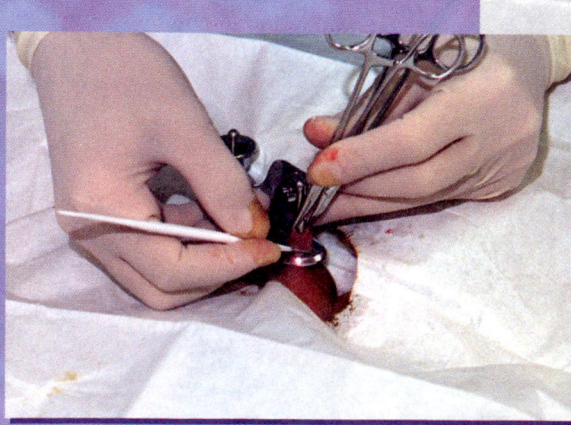

The prepuce is cut away at its base.

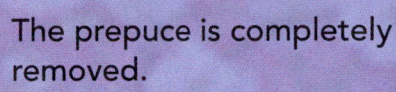

The prepuce is completely removed.

After removal of the cone, the newly exposed glans penis is gently swabbed with sterile gauze.

Sterile dressing is carefully applied to protect the circumcision area.

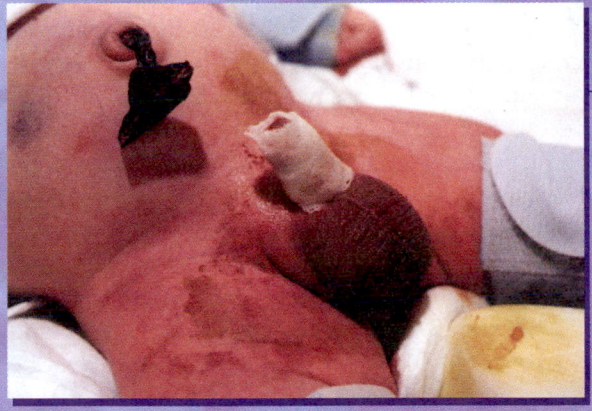

The newly circumcised penis will be completely healed within about a week.

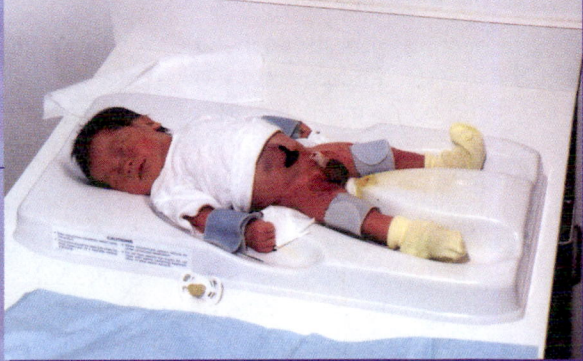

The infant rests following the procedure.

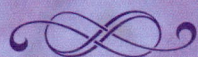

inspect the circumcision site, addresses their concerns, and instructs both parents on circumcision care.

Musculoskeletal System

The musculoskeletal system is on constant display when the infant is moving and exploring its environment. From extending legs and kicking to extending arms and sucking on fingers, the infant is discovering that it can move. Visual inspection of the infant reveals any movements that are compromised by injury or birth trauma. Stretching of the extremities often leads the infant to extend the toes and fingers: this confirms movement for the examiner. The nurse carefully observes the extremities for differences in size or length. Acondroplasia is a congenital condition that nurses observe first in newborns who have a small thoracic cage, lack the ability for elbow extension, and appear to have shortening of the humerus and femur (Jones, 1997). These infants are often referred to as dwarfs and have respiratory and neurologic problems in addition to their skeletal defects.

Watching the infant move in the supine position and then changing the infant to the prone position gives the nurse a good indication of muscle strength and tone. Failure to move the lower extremities may suggest a lesion or damage to the spinal cord. Asymmetrical movement may indicate nerve damage or a fracture from birth trauma. A newborn infant who does not move or feels "floppy" when turned over may have hypotonia, or decreased muscle tone, from a period of anoxia either in utero or during labor and delivery. Hypertonia, or increased muscle tone, in the presence of small, brief tremors, twitches, or myoclonic jerks, is a characteristic of neonatal abstinence syndrome (Wong et al., 1999). The newborn expresses withdrawal symptoms of drug exposure through these movements. The nurse, through careful inspection and observation, can identify elements of the musculoskeletal examination for further evaluation.

Common Variations

After inspection, palpation of the musculoskeletal system begins with the shoulders and moves inferiorly to the feet. Muscles and bones are palpated for symmetry and amount of tissue present. Joint rotations are checked by gently passive range of motion. Neck rotation is the first and most important motion to be examined. Infants must exhibit full neck rotation passively. Neck rotation may be hindered by torticollis, in which the head is held to one side with the chin pointing to the other side, or by congenitally missing portions of a cervical vertebra. As infants grow and develop, they turn their head to discover the location of sound and begin "tracking" the sound with their eyes. Proper neck rotation assists in the refinement of hearing and in the development of sight. Head lag is assessed by

gently pulling the infant up and watching its head gently fall back as it clears the surface of the crib. In this position, the nurse can also inspect the neck to make sure that there is no thyroid bulge. This maneuver also assists the nurse in evaluating upper body muscle tone and strength in the arms and shoulders.

The second most important joint to assess in newborns is the hip joint. Developmental dysplasia of the hip (DDH) can easily be missed in a newborn and, if not treated, can go on to interfere with the infant's future ability to retain balance and walk. Hips are evaluated by inspection of skin folds on the thighs in the supine and the prone positions. Asymmetrical skin folds may indicate a hip problem. Leg length and knee height are also inspected for unevenness. Palpation of the hips begins with the nurse gently moving the lower extremities in a kicking motion in order to ease the infant's distress during the hip evaluation. The nurse places her hands on the infant's thigh with the tips of her fingers encircling the head of the femur and her thumb and index finger securing the knee joint. From this position, the Barlow maneuver exerts a downward pressure on the head of the femur in an attempt to dislodge the head of the femur from the acetabulum. The Ortoloni maneuver is either a circular rotation of the femoral head or an inward-outward motion that attempts to "relocate" the head of the femur displaced by the Barlow maneuver in the acetabulum (Figure 32-24). Normal hip joints are moved easily and the nurse may feel crepitus or a slight grinding (a hip click) as the head of the femur is manipulated in the socket. Hip dysplasia is very common in infants who had in breech position in utero or breech deliveries. It is confirmed by the inability to move the leg easily in the hip joint and by feeling the head of the femur come out of the hip socket (a hip "clunk"). Many infants who had breech presentations have hyperextended knee joints that give the appearance of hip dysplasia but, on examination, the head of the femur remains firmly in the socket of the acetabulum. These leg positions gradually return to normal flexed positions. The nurse may examine the infant's hips and feel looseness in the hip joint even when the femoral head remains secure in the joint. Maternal hormones during pregnancy and delivery not only cause joint laxity in mothers but also can affect the joints of their infants.

The remaining joints are assessed by passive range of motion and by observing the infant moving or being moved. The last joint to be assessed is the ankle joint. Position of the infant during pregnancy may lead to bowed legs, ankle deformities, or unusual positions of the feet. Pronation (inward turning) of the feet in newborns is common and gently stroking the infant's insole will illustrate for the nurse the ease at which the infant's foot assumes a normal position. A severely pronated foot that the nurse is unable to place in normal alignment is inspected for the

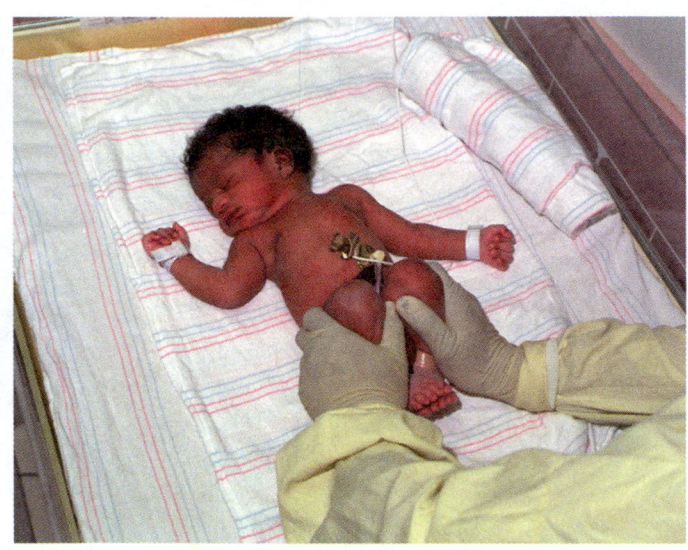
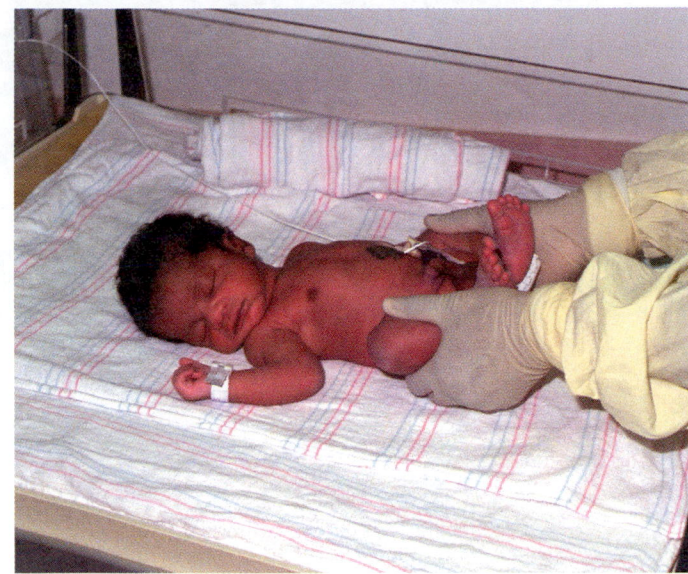

Figure 32-24 Ortoloni maneuver.

posterior alignment of the heel and the knee. Medial displacement of the heel from the posterior knee alignment may indicate the presence of a *club foot,* which can be confirmed on X-ray films. A club foot is usually placed in a cast during the early days of infancy, and mothers are instructed by the nurse in the care of the cast. Parents who express concern about their infant's feet "turning in" can be shown a simple exercise (stroking the outside of the infant's foot) that encourages the foot into a straight position.

Common Problems

Before any musculoskeletal assessment of the newborn infant, the nurse must inspect and palpate for broken bones. The infant should not be moved or positioned until this is done. The most common bone fracture is the clavicle, which occurs during delivery when the shoulders of the infant do not rotate easily. Palpation of both clavicles can confirm a separation between the ends of the bone at the fracture site or crepitus. Symptoms of fractures are swelling or edema at the fracture site, a bruise at the site, or infant irritability when moved. Experienced nurses who care for infants recognize the difference between an infant's fussiness at being disturbed and cries of pain. Other common fracture sites include the humerus, the ribs, and the skull. Definitive diagnosis is always made from X-ray films. Fractured clavicles heal by themselves over time, and the mother is taught to position the infant on the side opposite the injury. Special care is taken by the nurse to teach parents how to hold and support their infant's head and shoulders until the fracture heals. Humeral fractures are usually casted; rib fractures may be wrapped; and skull fractures are usually monitored in an intensive care unit.

Developmental dysplasia of the hip (DDH) results from a flattening of the acetabulum during pregnancy from its normal round, cup-like shape. This usually results from the infant in utero remaining in a breech position with legs extended upward during the period when bone growth occurs. The outer portion of the acetabulum becomes flat instead of curling around the head of the femur. The ability to secure the leg in the hip socket is lost. DDH can be diagnosed on physical examination by positive findings on the Barlow and Ortoloni maneuvers, unequal leg length, unequal knee height, and abnormal gluteal fold counts anteriorly or posteriorly. Diagnosis is confirmed by X-ray of the hip. Treatment for DDH involves placing the legs of the infant in abduction in a special harness, called a Pavlik harness. This harness remains on the infant for approximately 3 to 6 months, until new bone growth forms around the head of the femur and creates the normal cup-shaped hip socket.

Some infants may have extra digits and toes (**polydactyly**) or digits and toes that appear to be linked together by webbing of the skin (**syndactyly**). Extra digits on the hand are often located below the fourth finger attached to the palm by a thin cord of skin. They appear to have the same size as the fourth finger and may even have a fingernail. These digits need to be palpated by the nurse for the presence of bone. Bone indicates that surgical removal is necessary. The lack of bone is an indication that the extra digit may be tied off with suture silk. Tying off occludes the capillary, preventing circulation to the digit, and the digit undergoes necrosis and eventually falls off. Extra digits and toes tend to run in families, and parents will often describe relatives, other infants, or previous personal experiences with them. Webbing of toes does not interfere with balance or walking, and many parents do not choose to have the toes surgically freed from each other. Webbing of fingers is usually corrected for cosmetic and functional reasons.

Hands are inspected for palmar creases. These creases were noted earlier in the gestational age examination of the feet, but not of the hands. Three to four curved palmar creases are usually noted in normal newborns. A single, straight crease appearing in the middle of the palm is called a simean crease. These creases, unilaterally or bilaterally, by themselves are not an indicator of a special condition. However, with the presence of other symptoms, they may be associated with congenital syndromes, particularly Down syndrome.

Nursing Implications

The nursing assessment of the musculoskeletal system identifies the movement abilities of the newborn infant as well as movement limitations resulting from malformations or birth trauma. Through this assessment, the nurse determines the appropriate positioning for the newborn, exercises to enhance future abilities (if needed), and further follow-up or diagnostic evaluations. The nurse can raise parental awareness of their infant's movements, teach parents and family members proper holding and resting positions, and reinforce specific care needs of the newborn after discharge.

Neurologic System

The neurologic assessment concludes the physical assessment of the newborn infant. This assessment consists primarily of reflexes and other movements from which the nurse estimates the level of neurologic function. Reflexes can be divided into minor and major reflexes. Minor reflexes include: finger grasp, toe grasp, rooting, sucking, head righting, stepping, and tonic neck. Major reflexes indicate normal neurologic function; they are the gag reflex and the Babinski, Moro, and Galant reflexes.

Common Variations

Finger or palmar grasp is tested by watching infants curl their fingers around an object (usually the smallest finger of the nurse) placed across the palm. Plantar grasp by the toes is assessed in exactly the same manner, placing the object on the sole of the foot. Rooting and sucking are noted by stroking the infant's cheek and observing the infant turn toward the finger, open his or her mouth, and suck on an object placed in its mouth. Head righting is evaluated by lifting the infant in the prone position and gently stroking the back along the spinal cord. The normal infant attempts to hold the head up and arch the back at the same time. The stepping reflex is demonstrated by holding the infant upright with legs flexed and brushing

the soles of the feet on a flat surface. The infant picks up his or her feet and puts them down again in a stepwise fashion, imitating walking. The tonic neck reflex is often called the "fencing" reflex. The infant, in the supine position, extends the arm and leg on the side to which the head and jaw is turned and flexes the arm and leg on the opposite side.

The major reflexes need to be evaluated carefully by the nurse. A successful gag reflex is necessary for an infant to be able to expel material from the back the throat to avoid choking. Eliciting the Babinski reflex involves the upward stroking of the plantar surface of the foot from the heel to the toe, applying a slight pressure. Proper response to this stimulation is the incurving of the toes as in the plantar grasp with uncurling and fanning out (stretching out) of all the toes. The Moro reflex can be tested at the same time the head lag is assessed. As the infant head is elevated off the surface a release is mimicked and the bilateral arm extension and leg flexion movements that are indicative of the correct Moro response can be assessed. It is inappropriate to check this reflex in infants by making a loud clap sound to "startle" them. The responses of the infant may not be consistent with the Moro movements because the infant reacts to the movement of air across their body generated by bringing hands together in order to clap or to the sound of the clap itself.

The Galant reflex, or trunk incurvation reflex, is observed when the infant is held in a prone position and the lateral aspect of the leg is slowly stroked from below the knee superiorly to the buttocks. The infant reacts by moving its buttocks toward the side that is stroked in a curving movement. When this reflex is elicited correctly, the reaction is quite dramatic. The nurse can use this reflex to demonstrate to parents the capabilities of their infant.

Common Problems

The most common neurologic injury seen in newborns is at the brachial plexus from difficulties experienced rotat-

THE GALANT REFLEX

This reflex occurs when the infant is held securely in the prone position with its arms and legs dangling off the surface of the crib. The infant's legs are gently extended from a flexed position before the reflex motion is attempted. Leg extension is necessary to see the proper incurvation of the trunk and buttocks.

ing and delivering the infant's shoulders. This injury can be differentiated from shoulder dystocia, which is noted in newborns as temporary decreased movement and muscle tone in a shoulder and upper arm that improves rapidly after delivery. A form of brachial plexus injury, Erb's palsy, is easily detected from the position of the arm in the supine position. The infant's arms are normally flexed and moving. An infant with Erb's palsy has one or both arms extended in the supine position with hand extension. The arm does not spontaneously move into a flexed position. Palpation of the extremity reveals decreased muscle tone, decreased grasp reflex, and negative arm recoil on the affected side. This arm position has been called the "waiter's position" because it imitates a waiter with the arm at the side and the hand held out for a tip. The majority of brachial plexus injuries resolve within the first 2 weeks of life. The nurse assesses grasp and muscle tone frequently in these infants to monitor the resolution. Positioning of the infant requires placing the arm gently in flexed position at rest and supporting the arm while holding. Mothers can assist in the resolution of this injury by performing simple arm strengthening exercises that passively flex and extend their infant's arm at each diaper change.

Infants that have severe neurologic injuries from the birthing process or during embryonic development are assessed in neonatal intensive care units. Newborn infants who have difficulty breathing, moving extremities, or lack appropriate muscle tone are monitored closely on this unit. Brain damage or paralysis of extremities may result from periods of *anoxia* (oxygen deprivation) during development or during labor. Oxygen deprivation is one of the causes of cerebral palsy and may result in difficulties with swallowing, breathing, or movement in newborns. Manifestations of cerebral palsy in newborns occur in proportion to the amount of oxygen deprivation. The nurse may notice, at one extreme, an infant with a slight decrease in movement with diminished reflexes, and at the other extreme, no movement and no reflexes, with numerous differences between these extremes.

During the embryonic process, the brain and spinal cord are formed by the closure of the neural tube within the first 30 days of pregnancy. The failure of this tube to close at the posterior end results in a lesion that may contain a fluid or a section of the spinal cord. This condition is called spina bifida and is diagnosed during pregnancy. At birth, spina bifida presents as a skin-covered sac between the fifth lumbar and first sacral vertebrae posteriorly. The sac may contain an extension of the dura mater and fluid called a meningocele and usually does not result in any decrease in motor movement below the waist. A sac that contains dura mater, fluid, and part of the spinal cord is much more serious. This sac is called a myelomeningocele and does result in loss of bladder and lower bowel control and motor function below the waist.

Treatment of spina bifida varies according to the nature of the lesion. Usually, surgical closure of the lesion is required to prevent infection. A variation of spina bifida is called spina bifida occulta, which is a defect in the spinal vertebrae with no protrusion of the dura mater, fluid, or spinal cord that would interfere with motor function.

Incomplete closure of the anterior end of the embryonic neural tube causes a condition called anencephaly, which results in sections of the brain, forehead, skull, and occiput missing. Newborns with this condition are placed on respiratory and cardiac monitors to assess viability and shielded from visitors and curious onlookers.

Nursing Implications

Assessment of the neurologic system in newborns, particularly reflexes, is an important indicator of the newborn's development during pregnancy and the labor and delivery process. The developing fetus and the process of birth are vulnerable periods for the newborn, placing the newborn at risk for neurologic conditions that may be devastating to parents who are expecting a normal child. The nurse can be alerted to subtle changes in infant reactivity or the obvious signs of a neurologic deficit. Changes that warrant further investigation must be carefully communicated to the parents and preparations for care after discharge discussed with the parents and family members.

Body Size Classification

At the end of the physical assessment, the nurse measures the length of the infant from head to heel, with the infant's leg gently extended. This measurement, along with the head circumference and weight obtained in the delivery room, form the basis for the size classification for the infant. These measurements are plotted using the gestational age by examination, as determined earlier. Ideally, all three measurements, when plotted, fall on the same portion of the scale. Commonly, two out of the three measurements are similar. The infant's size is determined by which area two out of the three measurements fall, with the weight percentile range given preference. Infants whose scores fall on the graph under the tenth percentile are classified as small for gestational age (SGA). Infants whose scores fall between the tenth and ninetieth percentile are classified as appropriate for gestational age (AGA), and infants whose scores fall above the ninetieth percentile are classified as large for gestational age (LGA). Depending on where the graphed points fall, an infant may be additionally described as "borderline" LGA or AGA to illustrate extremes of the classification ranges.

After size classification is determined, the nurse must determine the accuracy of the graphing in comparison to

Critical Thinking

Newborn Size

Ask yourself the following questions:

1. What does the graph reveal as the largest part of the infant?

2. What does the physical examination reveal as the largest part of the infant? Is this the same result as the graph?

3. Are the length and head measurements falling at approximately the same percentile range on the graph?

4. Which two out of the three measurements graphed are the closest together in terms of the percentile range and why?

The head of the newborn infant should be the largest part by graph and visual examination. Length and head measurements should fall within the same range on the graph. Embryonic development proceeds from head to toe in utero. Head and length measurements that are close together on the graph suggest that the development of this newborn infant has proceeded normally during this pregnancy.

Any measurement that the nurse suspects is inaccurate should be measured again and plotted on the graph with a notation that the measurement was retaken for the official infant record. Once the physical assessment and size classification are complete, the nurse can report to the parents on the condition and characteristics of their infant. The nurse can bring the completed size graph to the parents to show them exactly where their infant's measurements fall on the graph.

the physical presentation of the infant recently examined. Because these measurements begin all future determinations of infant growth and development from growth curves, the nurse must develop an intuitive feeling that they are accurate.

ADDITIONAL ASSESSMENTS

After the initial physical examination, measurement, and size classification has been completed, the responsibility of the nurse changes to promoting opportunities for the parents and infant to interact and be with each other.

Periodic Shift Assessment

Periodic shift assessments are done at regular times, usually every 4 hours, to ensure infant physiologic stability and to alert the nurse to any changes in the newborn's condition. Parents can provide information, which along nursing expertise, and judgment of the newborn's condition all part of ongoing assessment. The medical staff should be informed immediately of any changes in the condition of the newborn.

Periodic assessments include vital signs; body weight; feeding and elimination details; hydration status; respiratory and cardiac function, and hip movements for DDH. Vital signs during the first 24 hours of life include: a heart rate that averages between 100 and 130 beats/min, a respiratory rate below 60 breaths/min, and a body temperature above 97°F. Blood pressure is usually not included in the periodic assessment, unless specifically ordered. Weight after the first 24 hours of life should show a loss, as the newborn is expending energy to breathe, maintain cardiac circulation, eat, and eliminate urine and stool. Diapers are checked for urine and the presence and color of stools. Stools should reflect a gradual change in color and consistency, from the dark-colored, thick meconium stools to brown-yellow, pasty transitional stools, and finally to yellow, loosely formed stools (Figure 32-25). Hydration status can be assessed through noting skin turgor and changing diapers. Newborns should have six to ten diaper changes a day for urine, but the stool content in these diapers may vary. The newborn respiratory and cardiac systems are assessed by the nurse at every periodic assessment. The nurse is particularly alert for signs and symptoms of respiratory distress, including intercostal retractions, noisy breathing, sternal retractions, nasal flaring, central cyanosis, tachypnea, and irritability. During the cardiac assessment, the nurse should listen carefully for any arrhythmias and heart murmurs. Murmurs that persist beyond the first 24 hours of life need further evaluation. Lastly, the nurse performs the Barlow and Ortoloni maneuvers to screen for DDH. Positive findings should be reported immediately if the nurse notes new findings at this time. The nurse records in her notes the results of her periodic assessment and tells the parents that the newborn infant is stable and normal.

Quick Examination

Quick examinations are performed when the nurse relieves another nurse and assumes the care of a newborn, either for a short period or for the remainder of the shift. The nurse assesses physiologic stability by examining the lungs and heart of the infant and taking its temperature. The nurse compares these findings with the documentation in the newborn's chart and the nursing report re-

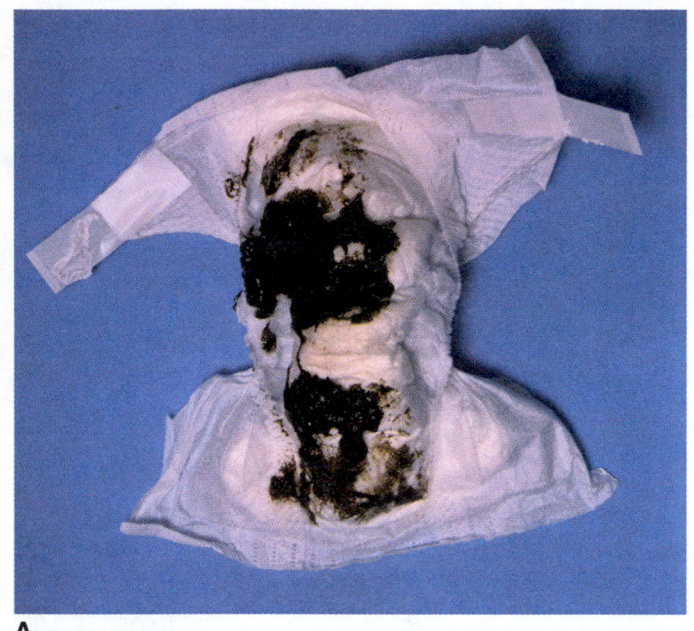

A.

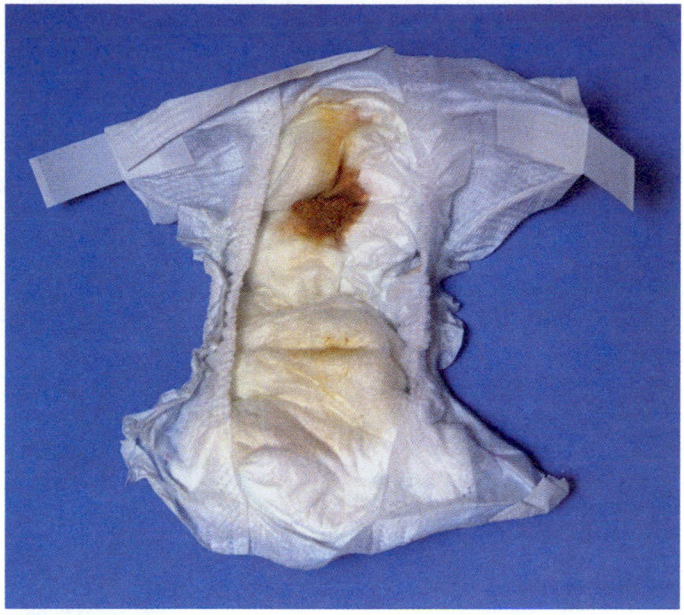

B.

Figure 32-25 A. Meconium stool; B. Breast-milk stool.

ceived on the status of this newborn. The nurse also should notice the reactivity of the newborn and record the state of the infant as asleep, awake, quiet, active, or irritable. Quick examinations are also performed on newborns when a nurse notices a odd behavior or something in passing that the nurse feels is unusual and should be assessed. This is a skill developed by nurses with experience in caring for newborns. These nurses have the ability to form an opinion about a newborn's condition from a quick look at a newborn at a mother's bedside or in the nursery.

Interactional Assessment

The interactional assessment of the newborn involves an assessment of the infant's reactivity to the environment and parental interaction with the infant. The newborn's reaction to the extrauterine environment fluctuates widely over the first 10 days of life, as the physiologic systems adjust to regular patterns of breathing, circulation, feeding, elimination, and sleeping (Pressler & Hepworth, 1997). There are six behavioral states: 1, deep sleep; 2, light sleep; 3, drowsy; 4, quiet alert; 5, considerable motor activity; and 6, crying (Brazelton, 1973). The nurse is aware of these newborn behavioral states and does the handling and examinations of the newborn during state 3 or state 4. Newborns who are at state 5 or state 6 are too irritable to be easily examined, because the examination intensifies and prolongs the motor activity and crying. The nurse can intervene by cuddling the infant, talking to the infant in a soothing voice, and waiting until the infant calms down. During the interactional assessment, the nurse notes the

state of the infant, any changes, and the length of time the infant takes to go from one state to another. This timeframe assists the nurse in forming an assessment of the infant's neurologic organization in the early days of life. Substance abuse during pregnancy interferes with and prolongs the newborn's ability to move from one state to another. These newborns are often described as "irritable" or difficult" by parents who spend a great amount of time and effort attempting to calm them.

The nurse observes the interaction between the parents, family members, and the newborn. The nurse initiates attachment of the newborn to the parents and the family and the attachment of the parents and the family to the newborn with the first bedside visit. The newborn is placed in the arms of the parents, and the nurse describes the infant's unique qualities and features. Common parental reactions to newborn infants include touching their infant, exploring and examining all of the body parts, massaging the infant's abdomen, stroking the face, and cuddling (Wong et al., 1999). This process assists the parents in identifying "their baby" and begins the attachment of the mother to the newborn. At this time, the nurse can instruct and demonstrate holding positions for the infant (Figure 32-26).

The involvement of the father and siblings is actively promoted by the nurse as part of the interactional assessment. Paternal engrossment has been defined in the research literature as the father's ability to be preoccupied and interested in the newborn infant (Wong et al., 1999). Fathers want to be able to touch, explore, and hold their infant. The nursing role in promoting the early stages of paternal attachment is to allow private time between both

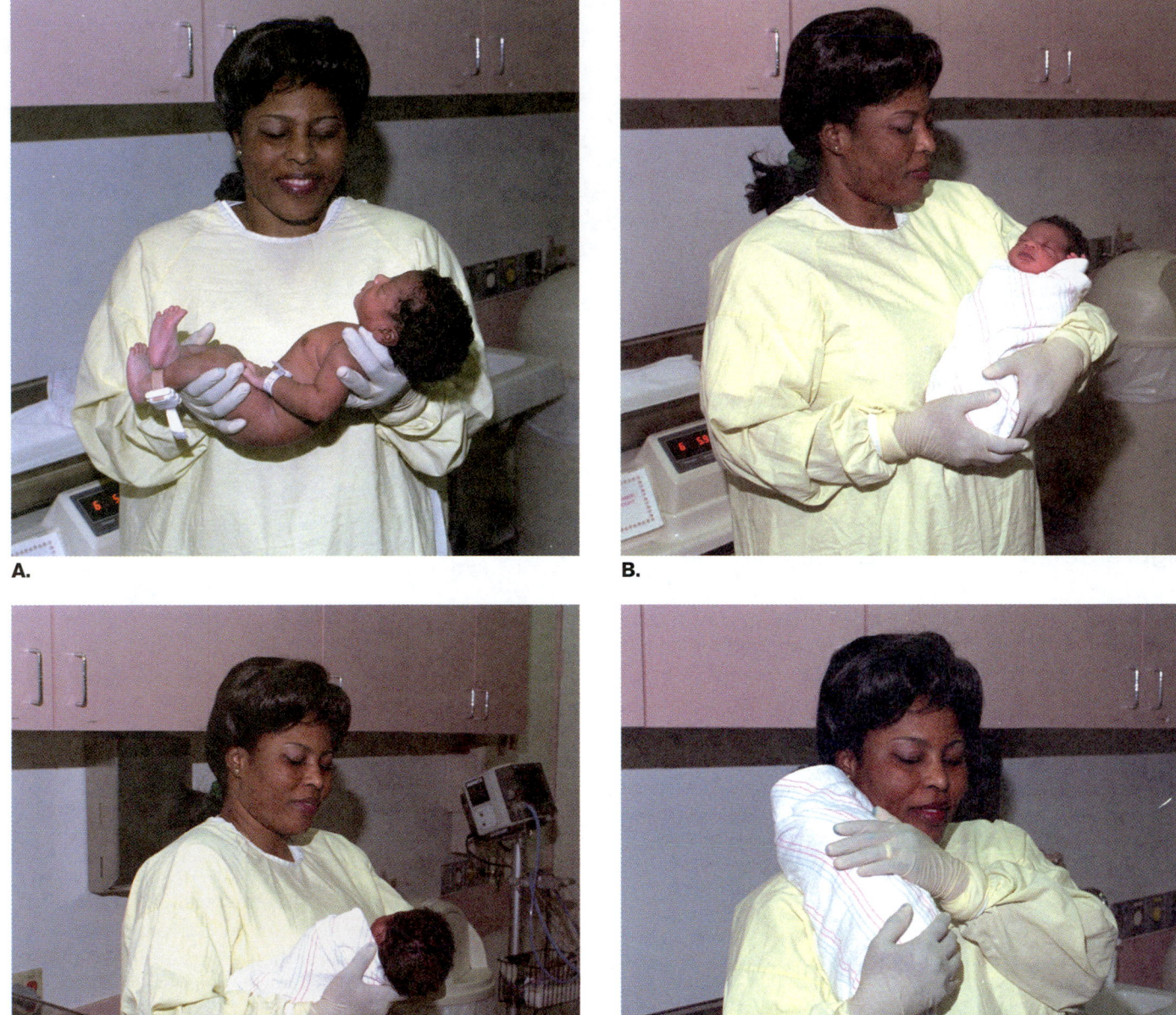

Figure 32-26 Proper holding of a newborn. A. Head and knee supported; B. Cradle hold; C. Football hold; D. Shoulder hold.

parents and their newborn. The nurse may accomplish this objective by bringing the newborn and leaving it at the mother's bedside, closing the door to the mother's room, and taking siblings on a tour of the hospital or down to the cafeteria or gift shop. Children react differently to newborns, depending on their age. School-aged and younger children focus on the newborn's face and touching the infant instead of holding the infant. The nurse can teach sib-

lings proper holding of the infant and infant transfer with the parent's permission.

The interactional assessment of the newborn and the family is accomplished by the nurse at least once a shift. The nurse notes the state of the newborn, the family members present, who is holding the newborn, and the reactions to the newborn by the holder or other family members. The nurse can use this time to address any concerns

Newborns after delivery are able to see best at a distance of 8 to 10 centimeters from an object. The holding position for newborns that maintains this distance and that has parent and infant facing each other is called the *en face* position. The advantage of this position is that the newborn can gaze on the holder and attend to something that can be seen. Placement of arms and hands for holding a newborn depends on which side the newborn is to be held. For the left side, the left arm encircles the head and shoulders of the newborn with the left hand holding the left thigh of the infant. The right arm encircles the legs and the right hand supports the newborn's back. The nurse emphasizes that the head of the infant must be supported at all times, because of the inability of the infant's neck muscles to support the head at this time. The nurse can demonstrate head support to the parents by wrapping a hand around the infant's neck and placing the thumb and third or fourth finger underneath the newborn's jaw on both sides if its head. For feeding, the newborn can be held in the mothers lap at a 45° angle to promote swallowing and decrease air going into the newborn's stomach. For transferring the infant from one person to another, the nurse can actively illustrate the transfer. The nurse holds and supports the infant and walks to the parent for transfer. The infant is placed in the parents outstretched arms and not released until the parent informs the nurse that he or she has control of the infant. Release before that time may cause the infant to be dropped, because the parent does not have a secure enough hold on the infant. The nurse emphasizes that one of the most important aspect of holding positions is the opportunity for parents to interact with and talk to their infant.

the parents or family have regarding their infant. The nurse should assess how well the family has understood the instructions on infant holding and positioning and, if necessary, reinforce and support efforts to follow the nursing instructions. Parental or familial interactions that the nurse observes with the infant that are not positive or are neglectful should be reported and confirmed by other nursing staff.

FACTORS THAT PLACE THE INFANT AT RISK

Besides the physical assessment of the infant, the nurse also evaluates other influences and conditions that impact on the health and well-being of the infant. These influences and conditions are evaluated for every infant, even those infants that are rooming-in with their mothers. It is during this evaluation that the nurse develops a plan of care for the infant and parents.

Physical

Physical factors that are assessed in the newborn period relate to birth injuries, congenital conditions, and temperature control. Bruising, edema, lacerations, and bone fractures are conditions that are detected on the initial physical assessment. The nurse plans care for the infant based on minimizing further injury to the site by proper positioning or protecting the injury site with antibiotic ointment or a gauze bandage. Teaching projects for the parents are designed to alleviate concern and anxieties, continue appropriate care regimens, and emphasize follow-up visits. Congenital physical conditions, such as malformations of the extremities or a cleft lip and palate combination, require special nursing sensitivity to the requirements of the infant. The infant requires special care and protection from curious onlookers who are not family members.

The last physical influence on an infant's health is the infant's ability to maintain its body temperature. Infant body temperature should range between 97°F and 100°F axillary temperature. Body temperatures of less than this value may indicate that an infant is too cold and needs to be re-wrapped. An infant with a body temperature outside this range should be evaluated for possible sepsis. Temperatures are taken about 30 to 45 minutes after nursing interventions. Repetitive low or high temperatures in a newborn infant may indicate an infectious process. Parents can be taught how to read a thermometer and to take their baby's temperature properly. The nurse can give the parents guidance for assessing temperature at home and appropriate actions to take in the event that temperature is outside the normal range.

Psychological

During the period of recovery from labor and delivery, the mother may be unable to care for the newborn infant and need assistance from the nurse, the father, or other family members. The mother may require intravenous fluids or medication that interfere with her ability to hold, cuddle, or breastfeed her newborn. Pain, uterine cramping, and discomfort from an incision site may contribute to positioning difficulties for the mother. Mothers admitted to intensive care units for observation and monitoring of symptoms experienced during labor and delivery are not able to care for their newborns. Visits to these units for the family members and the newborn are limited by the policies of the unit.

Psychological conditions that place an infant at risk are those conditions that inhibit interactions between the infant and the parents or primary caretaker, such as separation, rejection, or sensory or neural disorders. Mothers and fathers who are eager to see, hold, stroke, and explore their newborn are learning to accept this new tiny person into their life. Other parents may be disinterested, disappointed in the physical appearance or gender of the infant, or unable to adjust to having an infant with a physical problem. A normal, healthy infant is the dream of all parents. Anything that disrupts this image of the baby, whether it is the physical condition of the infant, medical or nursing statements concerning the infant, or the infant's behavior, may cause the parents to change their responses to the infant (Stern & Hildebrandt, 1986). This places the infant at risk for inappropriate caregiver interaction and possible neglect.

Family

The family constellation and organization are important in planning for care of the newborn. The nurse is able to gather information from parents and other family members concerning their plans after discharge, household arrangements, services needed, and follow-up care. Families with little financial support can be referred to community agencies and services for assistance. This assistance may include formula or food for breastfeeding mothers (Women, Infants, & Children [WIC] programs), diapers, housing or shelter, transportation, and health care for the mother and infant. Young mothers, especially teenagers, may be eligible for teen clinics that provide resources and follow-up services for them.

The nurse can assess the reactions of the siblings to the newborn and initiate interventions to help the parents introduce the infant to siblings. The nurse plans for the care of the infant and designs teaching projects to facilitate the understanding and participation of all family members within the unique family situation that is presented.

Environment

In addition to observing the parental and family dynamics, the nurse plans for newborn care by eliciting information about the home environment. Environmental conditions that place the newborn at risk are smoking in the home, inadequate heating or cooling, lack of kitchen facilities, water from a well, and pets. Infant exposure to second-hand smoke is believed to cause respiratory infections in infancy. Smokers are encouraged not to smoke around the infant and, preferably, to smoke outside rather than in the

home. Temperature regulation is important for the newborn. Newborns can become chilled or overheated if placed near ceiling fans, window air conditioners, or space heaters or when left in cars. The best position for the newborn is at the opposite end of a room from the fan, air conditioner, or heater. Space heaters are not recommended, owing to the danger of fire. However, many older, unheated homes use them for heat, and parents must be made aware of the danger and the necessity of flame-retardant clothing for infants. Infants should not be left unattended in cars because cars may overheat in the summer. Parents should be asked whether or not they have kitchen facilities, i.e., a refrigerator, stove, and running water. Formula and breast milk should be refrigerated and reheated on a stove or under running hot water. Water from a well should be tested every year to make sure that it is safe for consumption. Pets, especially long-haired dogs and cats, carry dander and hairs that might cause future allergies and sensitivities in newborns.

Illness and Infection

Infants of mothers whose delivery took longer than 18 hours after the rupture of membranes are at risk for a septic infection. Infants of mothers who had infections before delivery or who had a body temperature during labor above 100.4°F are at risk for infection (Mitchell, Steffenson, Hogan, & Brooks, 1997a).

The most common maternal illness at delivery is **chorioamnionitis**, which is an infection of the amniotic fluid surrounding the infant in utero before delivery. It is detected by the appearance of foul-smelling amniotic fluid at delivery, uterine tenderness, maternal fever and tachycardia, and infant tachycardia (Mitchell et al., 1997a). Newborn infants of mothers with these symptoms should be evaluated thoroughly for developing signs and symptoms of infection, which, in newborn infants, include lethargy, decreased appetite, jaundice or pallor, fever or chilling, increased respiratory or heart rate, or a general appearance of not "looking well" (Mitchell, Steffenson, Hogan, & Brooks, 1997b). Newborn infants with suspected infection are examined, tested, and often started on antibiotics. Infants with confirmed infections are placed on a prescribed intravenous antibiotic regimen for 7 to 10 days.

One of the causes of chorioamnionitis is group B streptococcal (GBS) infection which is the leading cause of bacterial meningitis and sepsis in newborns. GBS and *Escherichia coli* infections account for 70% of all cases; *Listeria monocytogenes* is the causative agent in 5% of cases (Taeusch & Ballard, 1998). Early onset of meningitis in the newborn infant is usually caused by exposure to infection in utero or during passage through the birth canal. Women usually are tested for GBS colonization during their prenatal care, usually after 35 weeks of pregnancy. Many women exhibit no symptoms of infection but can transmit the infec-

CULTURALLY APPROPRIATE CARE

Optimal care practices for infants should be attuned to the family's cultural and ethnic environment without sacrificing the infant's health and well-being. Achieving this delicate combination results in the provision of culturally sensitive care (Andrews, 1992) and creates a maternal and familial impression that the nurse understands and appreciates the relationship of this newborn infant to the family and their environment.

tion to their fetus during labor and delivery if membranes have ruptured (Mitchell et al., 1997a). Mothers known to be colonized with GBS before delivery are treated with intravenous penicillin G every 4 hours during labor (Mitchell et al., 1997a). Newborn infants of these mothers are monitored closely for the first 48 hours after delivery for early presentation of the infection. Treatments for suspected early-onset infection include immediate intravenous antibiotic therapy, obtaining cerebrospinal fluid and blood samples for culture, complete blood cell counts with differential, and a chest X-ray film. Rapid nursing assessment and medical intervention are needed to prevent some of the devastating sequelae from this neonatal infection.

NURSING IMPLICATIONS

Nursing care of the newborn infant after delivery is based on an accurate assessment of the infant's physical condition and any other factors affecting its health and well-being. The infant's physical condition is determined from the physical examination and additional frequent assessments of behavior, feeding, and elimination patterns. Familial and maternal conditions necessitating special procedures or treatment regimens are incorporated into the nursing plan of care.

Promotion of Physiologic Stability

The primary nursing goal in the care of the newborn infant is the maintenance and promotion of physiologic stability. Body temperature control, positioning, creation of a non-stressful environment, and establishing regular routines for newborn infants are the major concerns of nurses during the first several days of life. Creating a non-stressful environment is important for the development of infant behavior and reactivity patterns. Elimination of noise from beepers, monitors, telephones, televisions, and radios help to soothe a distressed infant. Carpeting reduces noise from

traffic and dimming the lights reduces glare and assists infants in opening their eyes more easily. Infants who are fussy and irritable require a response from a caregiver that may consist of touching, talking to the infant, or holding or rocking them. The earliest beginnings of Erikson's trust versus mistrust developmental stage begins shortly after birth, when the infant senses that someone responds to his or her needs. To assist nurses in providing this response, nurseries often encourage foster grandmothers and other volunteers to feed and hold newborn infants when their mothers are unable to do so.

Newborn Care

The care of the healthy newborn focuses on the feeding and elimination pattern of the infant and the parent's adjustment process to the care demands of a new infant. Nurses are able to prepare new parents for their future life at home with a new baby by using anticipatory guidance and by teaching skills in baby care. Nurses are often the first health care provider to answer parents' concerns about their infant. During the period after delivery, the nurse must not only assess the health and well-being of the infant but also to determine how well the parents are coping with the new and frequent demands for their attention and time.

Sleep and Activity

Newborn infants spend the majority of their time sleeping and brief periods awake and actively exploring their environment. It is not unusual for newborns to sleep 16 hours a day. Proper sleeping conditions for infants are placement in the supine position on a flat surface without a pillow and covered with a blanket in a crib or bassinet separate from the parents' bed. Sleeping infants should be protected from air currents generated from ceiling fans and air conditioners that may lower their body temperature. Infant sleep-wake periods do not always coincide with a parent's need for rest. Often, parents are awakened several times during the night by an infant needing feeding or attention. The first several months of an infant's life are spent trying to establish a sleep-wake schedule that allows both parents and infant to rest. The most common complaint of parents during the neonatal period is lack of adequate sleep. Encourage parents to rest while their infant is sleeping, instead of catching up on housework, chores, or the demands of other children or the partner (Ruchala & Halstead, 1994). Nurses can play a role in acknowledging parental frustrations during this time by being receptive to inquiries and providing guidance toward positive interactions between infant and family during this time. Infants who are awake and alert can respond to voices and noises and need sound and touch stimulation to begin to explore their environment. The more an infant is able to interact with family members and explore the surrounding environment, the easier it becomes for the infant to achieve developmental milestones and develop a unique personality.

Cord and Skin Care

Umbilical cord and skin care are additional concerns of new parents. The umbilical cord may or may not be stained with a bacteriostatic dye, but it is left clamped when the parents take the infant home. The clamp prevents blood from oozing from the cut cord and remains in place until the cord has dried and shriveled. Nurses can teach parents to look for cord discharge, redness, or oozing, which may be signs of infection. At each diaper change, the cord is swabbed with alcohol on a cotton ball at its base, where it attaches to the umbilicus, and the diaper is folded around the base, leaving the cord exposed to air. Somewhere between 7 and 14 days after delivery, the cord will fall off, leaving behind a moist stump inside the umbilicus, usually yellow in color. This stump requires application of alcohol or warm water and drying to continue the drying process of the stump for another 3 to 5 days after the cord has fallen off.

Many new parents may have cultural practices regarding the umbilical cord. Some families may attach belly bands, coins, cotton balls, or other objects to the umbilical cord to prevent umbilical hernias. Families should be encouraged to keep the area clean, dry, and open to the air as much as possible in keeping with their cultural beliefs.

The nurse can demonstrate proper cleansing of the diaper area with a warm, moist cloth, followed by drying with another cloth, and then replacing the diaper. Infant skin may feel dry to parents; the nurse can recommend a lotion that is hypoallergenic to be applied in a thin coat two or three times a day. Vasoline petroleum jelly and baby oil are not recommended as skin lubricants because they retain moisture and prevent air from contacting the skin. Parents are taught by the nurse to sponge-bathe their infant until the time when the cord falls off. Warm water and a mild soap is used to sponge-bathe the infant from the neck down. The infant's face is cleansed with warm water because the skin on the face has less natural oil and is subject to drying if soap is used. The parents are taught to bathe their infant in sections, drying each section before they proceed to another. This preserves the infant's body heat. Baby shampoo is used for washing the infant's hair. After shampooing and drying, the infant's head is covered. Hooded bath towels are available at stores that specialize in infant clothing and are ideal for keeping the infant's head warm after the bath. Lotion may be applied after the bath. After the cord falls off, the infant can be held securely in a shallow basin for bathing. Bath time can be a special time for parents to interact and play with their infant.

Diaper dermatitis results from mechanical irritation of the skin, the pH of urine, and decreased air circulation inside the diaper. Improper cleaning of the genital area and infrequent changes are all predisposing factors for the development of a diaper rash (Singleton, 1997). Once a reddening of the skin in the irritated area occurs, the best treatment includes washing the area with warm water, drying thoroughly between diaper changes, eliminating cornstarch or other baby powders, leaving the diaper open the area exposed to air several times a day, and the use of A & D Ointment or petroleum jelly, which is washed off at each diaper changes (Singleton, 1997). Diaper rash that does not improve with these remedies within 2 to 3 days should be evaluated by a health care provider.

Criteria for Discharge

Newborn infants are often discharged with 24 to 48 hours of delivery, depending on the policies of the institution. Federal law requires insurance coverage for newborns for 48 hours after a normal vaginal delivery and 72 hours after a caesarean section delivery. The responsibility of the nurse caring for a newborn is to determine if the infant and the family meet the criteria for discharge. First, the infant must be physiologically stable. The infant should be a term infant; appropriate or large for gestational age; maintain an axillary temperature above 97°F, a heart rate between 100 and 150 beats/min, and a respiratory rate of less than 60/min; successfully pass urine and stool; feed consistently; and have normal findings on physical examination and periodic assessments (Burns et al., 2000). Second, the parents and family members should be knowledgeable in the care and feeding of the infant, signs and symptoms of illness, community resources for assistance, and locations with appointments for follow-up care. The nurse ensures that the prenatal screening has been done and recommends smoke detectors in the home, a safe sleeping position, and an infant car seat for the trip home (Burns et al., 2000). Infants, parents, and families that meet these criteria can be safely discharged at 48 hours after delivery or less (Banks & Thorne, 1997). Infants who do not meet the criteria should have parents referred to the medical staff for advice and guidance.

Web Activities

- Visit the American Academy of Pediatrics website for guidelines on newborn care.
- Search the Internet for the website of a hospital in your geographic area. What resources do they include for expectant parents and new parents?

Research Highlight

Effect of Early Newborn Discharge

Purpose

To examine the effects of "Great Starts" early discharge follow-up on the future use of the urgent care clinic by newborn's parents before the 2-week newborn examination.

Methods

The rule of use of urgent care services was examined through record review. Included were record's of 315 infants whose parents had participated in the "Great Starts" program. These records were compared with 324 newborn records who were born prior to the initiation of the program. These records were examined for use of urgent care services prior to their 2-3 week newborn checkup. The "Great Starts" program consisted of one appointment to the clinic within 2-3 days of discharge, at which time groups of 8-10 mothers, with their newborns, discussed infant concerns.

Findings

In the control group, 188 (58%) of 324 infants had urgent care clinic visits during the first 2 weeks of life. 90/315 (28%) In the period after the "Great Starts" program, 90 (28%) of 315 infants had urgent care clinic visits in the first 2 weeks of life.

Nursing Implications

The parents indicated that the normal 2-week visit after discharge was "too long to go" to address their concerns about their infant. This study presented an alternative for parents and assisted them in increasing their knowledge and ability to care for their infant. Because newborns are often discharged early from hospitals, in spite of the mandated 48-hour stay, parents have limited opportunities to have their concerns addressed within this timeframe. Once the newborn is discharged, there is no source for parental information except the check-up at 2 weeks of age or an urgent care facility. Nurses have the opportunity to be involved in collaborative efforts to provide cost-effective alternative sources and resources for these parents.

Nursing examinations of the newborn infant, including the physical and interactional assessments, form the foundation for the beginning of an infant's life. The nurse applies knowledge and expertise to alleviate parental concerns about the health of their newborn infant, shares with them the unique characteristics of the infant, instructs parents on the care of their newborn, and supports the sociocultural traditions of the family in regard to caring for newborn infants.

Nelson, V. R. (1999). The effect of newborn early discharge follow-up program on pediatric urgent care utilization. *Journal of Pediatric Health Care, 13*(2), 58–61.

Key Concepts

🐾 The newborn's large surface area of skin, thin layer of subcutaneous fat, predisposes the infant to heat loss. Subsequently, nursing efforts are focused on assessing infant body temperature and maintaining normal temperatures by using blankets or radiant warmers.

🐾 Newborn cardiovascular and respiratory stability in the extrauterine environment is achieved after transition, usually around 12 hours of life.

🐾 The hemodynamic changes in the newborn cardiac system after delivery may lead to "flow murmurs" heard on auscultation, which normally disappear after 24 hours.

🐾 Nurses perform four assessments on newborns when they are physiologically stable. These assessments are the full physical examination, periodic or shift assessment, the quick examination, and the interactional assessment.

🐾 The full physical assessment of the newborn includes a general assessment, measurement of vital signs, body weight and measurements, and a full physical examination.

🐾 The periodic shift assessment is done at regularly scheduled intervals. The nurse evaluates vital signs and weight, feeding and elimination, hydration status, cardiac and respiratory function, and checks for hip DDH.

🐾 The quick examination is performed by the nurse who takes over the care of a newborn from another nurse. This examination is done when a nurse notices a particular behavior or cry from a newborn that needs further investigation. Body temperature, cardiac and respiratory status, and activity and irritability of the infant are assessed.

🐾 The interactional assessment involves an estimate of the newborn's reactivity to being handled and to the environment as well as evaluation of familial interactions.

🐾 The assessment of the newborn's body temperature, skin, and cardiac and respiratory status are the best indicators of newborn physiologic stability.

🐾 The assessment of the musculoskeletal and neurologic systems provides the nurse with indications of disruptions in embryonic development or problems related to trauma experienced during labor and delivery.

🐾 The accurate examination of the newborn genitalia provides parents with an indication of their newborn's gender and the opportunity for the nurse to reinforce what is "normal" with parents.

🐾 Factors that may dispose the newborn to injury or infection are evidence of birth trauma, maternal infection during pregnancy or delivery, and unsafe handling of the infant by family members.

🐾 Family or psychological factors that place the infant at risk are maternal inability to provide care, paternal noninvolvement, language barriers, and sibling rivalry.

🐾 Environmental barriers that affect the well-being of newborns include a lack of kitchen and water resources, smokers in the home, pets, and inadequate or dangerous heating or cooling systems.

🐾 Nursing care of newborns after delivery focuses on the promotion of physiologic stability, providing opportunities for optimal nutrition, protection from injury and infection, and enhancing appropriate interactions between the parents and the infant.

Review Questions and Activities

1. All of the following are assessed by the nurse after transition except:
   a. Temperature
   b. Body weight
   c. Heart rate
   d. Respiratory rate

   The correct answer is b.

2. The best response to a parent's question regarding the skin or hair color of their infant is:
   a. "The color of the skin or hair reflects what the infant inherited from the parents."
   b. "Skin or hair color always darkens during infancy."

   c. "The color of skin or hair in a newborn is not an accurate picture of inherited characteristics."
   d. "Newborn skin and hair color may change so that is difficult for you to picture the changes before they occur."

   The correct answer is d.

3. Which is the true statement regarding heart murmurs in the newborn period?
   a. Heart murmurs that sound the loudest on auscultation indicate large heart defects.
   b. Heart murmurs that are soft and barely audible on auscultation indicate small heart defects.

c. Heart murmurs that appear on day 2 or 3 of life need further evaluation.

d. Heart murmurs that are noted on the initial physical examination always disappear by day 2 or 3 of life.

The correct answer is c.

4. All of the following are signs of respiratory distress in the newborn *except:*
   a. Hyperglycemia
   b. Nasal flaring
   c. Grunting
   d. Intercostal retractions

The correct answer is a.

5. Which of the following findings on the physical examination of a newborn is the clearest abnormal finding?
   a. Heart murmur
   b. Tachypnea
   c. Pronated feet
   d. Hypotonia

The correct answer is d.

6. Which of the following findings on the physical examination of the newborn may be normal findings?
   a. Heart murmur
   b. Erb's palsy
   c. Leukocoria
   d. Bivalved uvula

The correct answer is a.

7. All of the following are assessed during the musculoskeletal examination *except:*
   a. Muscle tone
   b. Torticollis

c. Stepping
   d. Range of motion

The correct answer is c.

8. All of the following may be causes of infant irritability *except:*
   a. Substance abuse
   b. Hunger
   c. Injury
   d. Heart defects

The correct answer is d.

9. Which of the following positively influence the care of a newborn by family members?
   a. Feeding the newborn in the supine position in the crib.
   b. Leaving the newborn in the nursery to be cared for by nursing staff.
   c. Allowing the parents numerous opportunities to be with and care for their infant.
   d. Removing all objects and jewelry placed on the infant by family members.

The correct answer is c.

10. The nurse assesses the interaction between the parents and their newborn by observing all of the following *except:*
   a. Feeding position
   b. Display of affection between the couple
   c. Holding position
   d. Touching and stroking

The correct answer is b.

References

Abel, E. L., & Sokol, R. J. (1987). Incidence of fetal alcohol syndrome and economic impact of FAS: related anomalies. *Drug and Alcohol Dependence, 19,* (1), 51–70.

American Academy of Pediatrics. (2000). Changing concepts of Sudden Infant Death Syndrome: Implications for Infant Sleeping Environment and Sleep Position (RE 9946) *Pediatrics, 105,* (3), 650–656.

Andrews, M. M. (1992). Cultural perspectives on nursing in the 21st century. *Journal of Professional Nursing, 8,* 7–15.

Ballard, J. L., Khoury, J. C., Wedig, K., Wang, L., Eilers-Waisman, B. L., & Lipp, R. (1991). New Ballard score, expanded to include extremely premature infants. *Journal of Pediatrics, 119,* 417–423.

Banks, J. M., & Thorne, M. (1997, June). *Early follow-up clinic: An NP clinic for the best start.* Paper presented at the meeting of the American Academy of Nurse Practitioners, New Orleans, LA.

Brazelton, T. B. (1973). *Neonatal behavioral assessment scale.* Philadelphia: Lippincott.

Burns, C. E., Brady, M. A., Dunn, A. M., & Starr, N. B. (2000). *Pediatric primary care* (2nd ed.). Philadelphia: W. B. Saunders.

D'Apolito, K. (1991). What is an organized infant? *Neonatal Network, 10,* (1), 23–29.

Fox, J. A. (1997). *Primary health care of children.* St. Louis: Mosby.

Gagliardi, L. (1993). Biased assessment of gestational age at birth when obstetric gestation is known. *Archives of Disease in Childhood, 68,* 32–34.

Johnson, K. B., & Oski, F. A. (1997). *Oski's essential pediatrics.* Philadelphia: Lippincott-Raven.

Jones, K. L. (1997). *Smith's recognizable patterns of human malformation* (5th ed.). Philadelphia: W. B. Saunders.

Juretschke, L. J. (2000). Unilateral testicular torsion. *JOGNN, 29,* 451–456.

Mitchell, A., Steffenson, N., Hogan, H., & Brooks, S. (1997a). Group B streptococcus and pregnancy: Update and recommendations. *MCN, 22,* 242–248.

Mitchell, A., Steffenson, N., Hogan, H., & Brooks, S. (1997b). Neonatal group B streptococcal disease. *MCN, 22,* 249–253.

Napiorkowski, B., Lester, B. M., Frier, C., Brunner, S., Dietz, L., Nadra, A., & Oh, W. (1996). Effects of in utero substance exposure on infant neurobehavior. *Pediatrics, 98,* 71–75.

Pressler, J. L., & Hepworth, J. T. (1997). Newborn neurological screening using NBAS reflexes. *Neonatal Network, 16,* (6), 33–46.

Rubin, R. (1984). *Maternal identity and the maternal experience.* New York: Springer.

Ruchala, P. L., & Halstead, L. (1994). The postpartum experience of low-risk women: A time of adjustment and change. *Maternal-Child Nursing Journal, 22,* (3), 83–89.

Schoen, E. J., Colby, C. J., & Ray, G. T. (2000). Newborn circumcison decreases incidence and costs of urinary tract infections during the first year of life. *Pediatrics, 105,* 789–793.

Schuman, A. J. (1999). Infant abductions: Preventing the unthinkable. *Contemporary Pediatrics, 16,* (10), 93–110.

Seidel, H. M., Rosenstein, B. J., & Pathak, A. (2001). *Primary care of the newborn* (3rd ed.). St. Louis: Mosby.

Singleton, J. K. (1997). Pediatric dermatoses: Three common skin disruptions in infancy. *Nurse Practitioner, 22,* (6), 32–50.

Taeusch, H. W., & Ballard, R. A. (1998). *Avery's diseases of the newborn* (7th ed.). Philadelphia: W. B. Saunders.

Williamson, M L. (1997). Circumcision anesthesia: A study of nursing implications for dorsal penile nerve block. *Pediatric Nursing, 23,* 59–63.

Wong, D. L., Hockenberry-Eaton, M., Wilson, D., Winklestein, M. L., Ahmann, E., & DiVito-Thomas, P. (1999). *Whaley & Wong's nursing care of infants and children* (6th ed.). St. Louis: Mosby.

Suggested Readings

Aronson, D. D., Goldberg, M. J., Kling, Jr., T. F., & Roy, D. R. (l994). Developmental dysplasia of the hip. *Pediatrics, 94,* 201–207.

Association of Women's Health, Obstetric, and Neonatal Nurses. (1998). *Standards and guidelines for professional nursing practice in the care of women and newborns* (5th ed.). Washington, DC: Association of Women's Health, Obstetric, and Neonatal Nurses.

Cottrell, B. H., & Grubbs, L. M. (1994). Women's satisfaction with couplet care nursing compared to traditional postpartum care with rooming-in. *Research in Nursing & Health, 17,* 401–409.

Curry, L. C., & Gibson, L. Y. (1992). Congenital hip dislocation: The importance of early detection and comprehensive treatment. *Nurse Practitioner, 17,* (5), 49–55.

deBecker, C. (1999). *Protecting the gift.* NY: NY Dial Press.

Dodd, V. (1996). Gestational age assessment. *Neonatal Network, 15,* (1), 27–36.

Eregie, C. O. (1991). Assessment of gestational age: Modification of a simplified method. *Developmental Medicine and Child Neurology, 33,* 596–600.

Freeman, C. K., & Lowe, N. K. (1993). Breastfeeding care in Ohio hospitals: A gap between research and practice. *Journal of Obstetric, Gynecology and Neonatal Nursing, 22,* 447–454.

Josten, L. (1990). Looking toward the year 2000: Implications for maternal and child health nursing. *Maternal-Child Nursing Journal, 19,* 83–92.

Mercer, R. T. (1995). *Becoming a mother: Research on maternal identity from Rubin to the present.* New York: Springer.

O'Kane, M. (1995). Evaluating cord care. *Nursing Times, 91,* (29), 57–58.

Pasquale, J. A., Brittain, L., Lenfestey, C. C., & Jarrett-Pulliam, C. (1996). Breastfeeding, dehydration, and shorter maternity stays. *Neonatal Network, 15,* (7), 37–43.

Stern, M., & Hildebrandt, K. A. (1986). Prematurity stereotyping: Effects on mother-infant interaction. *Child Development, 57,* 308–315.

Resources

American Academy of Pediatrics: www.aap.org
American Nurses Association: www.ana.org
Association of Women's Health, Obstetric, and Neonatal Nurses: www.awhonn.org

Information for parents including a chat room: www.babycenter.com
National Association of Neonatal Nurses: www.nann.org
For parents from Procter and Gamble: www.pampers.com
Society of Pediatric Nurses: www.pednurse.org

CHAPTER 33

Newborn Nutrition

Guidelines from the American Academy of Pediatrics recommend breast-feeding and human milk as the standard for optimal infant nutrition in the first year of life. These guidelines are emphasized and current alternatives are presented for infants when breast-feeding and human milk feeding are not possible. Use the following questions to examine your knowledge and attitudes about infant nutrition:

- *What is my understanding of the differences in breast-feeding compared with formula-feeding related to infant growth and development?*

- *What are my own personal feelings and attitudes regarding infant feeding decisions?*

- *How do my past experiences related to infant feeding influence my ability to offer unbiased counseling and instruction to mothers?*

- *Do I believe that most lactation and breast-feeding problems are preventable and, with proper knowledge and technical skills, can be overcome?*

Accretion
Antioxidant
Bioavailability

Calorimetry
Macronutrients

Micronutrients
Reducing agent

Renal solute load
Vegan

Upon completion of this chapter, the reader should be able to:

1. Understand the composition and function of basic nutrients in human milk compared with artificial infant formula.

2. Describe the expected growth rates for normal full-term infants based on type of milk (human or artificial formula) received in the early months of life.

3. Describe the physiologic signs of adequate milk transfer in the infant who is exclusively breast-fed.

4. Identify strategies to improve infant growth rates in the infant who is exclusively breast-fed when growth faltering is diagnosed.

The newborn infant requires dietary energy for adequate growth and development. Determining the optimal nutrition for the healthy newborn infant has required extensive scientific investigation for decades. Infant nutrition research repeatedly concludes that human milk and breast-feeding are the gold standard to which all other forms of infant feeding alternatives should be compared. Reflecting on recent advances and knowledge on the benefits of breast-feeding, the American Academy of Pediatrics (AAP) revised its policy statement regarding infant nutrition. The AAP identifies breast-feeding as the ideal method of feeding and nurturing infants and recognizes breast-feeding as primary in achieving optimal infant and child health, growth, and development (American Academy of Pediatrics [AAP], 1997).

GROWTH AND DEVELOPMENT

Growth is the standard by which infant nutrition is judged. Birth weight triples and length increases by 50% during the first year. Infant growth is especially rapid during the first few months of life when weekly weight and length gains approximate 200 g and 1 cm, respectively. Brain growth is profound, tripling in size during infancy to reach 90% of adult size at 2 years of age (Dobbing & Sands, 1973; Widdowson, 1991). Scientific evidence is emerging that different diets in early infancy can have long-term consequences (Barker, 1992; Sultan & Barker, 1994). This so-called nutritional imprinting or programming affects metabolism, development, and disease processes later in life (Lucas et al., 1990; Mott et al., 1995).

Human milk has the distinct capability of providing not only energy to fuel growth but unique properties ben-

REFLECTIONS FROM A NURSE

"For years, I routinely promoted bottle-feeding because it was easy to see how much formula the babies consumed. It also was easy to teach mothers how to prepare the formula. Then I began to learn more about how formula was developed and how the formula companies were researching the composition of breast milk. I became convinced that, whenever possible, the best food for infants is their mother's milk. After more reading, I now feel that the babies whose mothers are not breast-feeding, for whatever reason, also are getting good nutrition as the infant formulas are getting more and more sophisticated."

efiting the infant's immune system and health status. Immune properties, most specifically secretory immunoglobulin A (sIgA), present in human milk, protect the infant from infection (Wold & Hanson, 1994). Studies comparing morbidity rates among feeding types found a lower incidence of otitis media, respiratory, and gastrointestinal (GI) infections in breast-fed compared with formula-fed infants (Scariati, Grummer-Strawn, & Fein, 1997; Dewey, Heinig, & Nommsen-Rivers, 1995; Kakai et al., 1995; Beaudry, Dufour, & Marcoux, 1995). Furthermore, breast milk has a direct effect on the infant's immune system (Hahn-Zoric et al., 1990; Pabst & Spady, 1990). These observations may explain why some evidence exists that breast-feeding protects against insulin-dependent diabetes mellitus, Crohn's disease, rheumatoid arthritis, malignant lymphoma, and allergic conditions (Virtanen et al., 1991; Mayer et al., 1988; Gerstein, 1994; Koletzko et al., 1989; Mason et al., 1995; Davis, Savitz, & Graubard, 1988; Shu et al., 1995; Wright, Holbert, Taussig, & Martinez, 1995; van den Bogaard, van den Hoogen, Huygen, & van Weel, 1993; Porro et al, 1993; Saarinen & Kajosaari, 1995). Recently, the content of long-chain polyunsaturated fatty acids, such as docosahexaenoic acid (DHA), present in human milk but not in formula, have received a significant amount of investigation. It has been determined that the presence of these fatty acids affects the composition of cell membranes in the brain and retina and also might affect development of visual acuity in the infant (Makrides, et al., 1994; Farquharson et al., 1992; Makrides et al., 1995; Jorgensen et al., 1996; Carlson, Werkman, & Tolley, 1996).

In terms of infant growth, optimal patterns for infants have been proposed. Growth charts are used to monitor individual infant growth patterns. Charts currently used throughout the world are based on the U.S. National Center for Health Statistics (NCHS) reference data (U.S. Department of Health, Education and Welfare, 1977). For the first 2 years of life, these data are based on the Fels Longitudinal Study, conducted in Yellow Springs, Ohio, from 1929 to 1975 (Roche, 1992). These data have come under scrutiny for several reasons: 1) the low incidence of breast-fed infants in the cohort, 2) too infrequent measurements to capture adequate patterns of growth, and 3) the reference group used not being a representative sample.

It has been demonstrated in several studies that the growth patterns of breast-fed infants differ from the NCHS reference data (Binns et al., 1996; Dewey et al., 1995; Dewey, et al., 1992; Hitchcock, Gracey, & Gilmour, 1985). An explanation commonly given for this difference is that most infants in the NCHS cohort were formula-fed. In longitudinal studies continuing throughout the first year, breast-fed infants showed as rapid or more rapid weight gains compared with formula-fed infants during the first 2 to 3 months. In contrast, evidence from these data show formula-fed infants weigh more than do breast-fed infants during the later months of the first year. As a result of these findings, the World Health Organization (WHO) completed a comprehensive review in 1995 of the uses and interpretation of the growth standards currently in use. WHO concluded that the current NCHS growth reference is inadequate and recommended that a new international

Nursing Tip

INFANT ASSESSMENT FOR INSUFFICIENT LACTATION

Possible signs of insufficient lactation in the exclusively breast-feeding infant-mother dyad in the first month after delivery follow:

- Low urination pattern (at least six wet diapers a day is the norm).

- Low stooling frequency (at least three yellow-greenish, seedy, soft stools a day is the norm).

- Minimal breast changes after delivery (such as fullness and leaking of milk).

- Very irritable or sleepy infant, nursing less than seven times a day.

- Weight loss of more than 10% of the birth weight, or continued weight loss after day 10 of life.

For the bottle-fed infant intake of 4 oz or more of formula taken every 2-3 hours, 6-10 feedings per day is the norm.

Client Education

Feeding Readiness Cues

Confirm that parents know to respond to early feeding readiness cues:

- Sucking movements
- Sucking sounds
- Hand-to-mouth movements
- Rapid eye movements
- Soft cooing or sighing sounds
- Fussiness

growth reference for infants was needed to more accurately reflect the population and current health recommendations. Given the differences in growth patterns based on feeding mode, however, concern exists that a growth reference constructed to be representative of a whole population may not be useful for judging the growth of either breast-fed or formula-fed infants (Garza, Frongillo, & Dewey, 1994). WHO has concluded that a multicountry growth study specifically designed to develop a growth reference of lasting value is necessary. The new reference sample should be based on breast-fed infants living in healthy environments that do not limit their genetic growth potential (de Onis, Garza, & Habicht, 1997).

Until such time that new growth references are available, health care providers need to take into account differences in growth rates based on feeding mode (Figure 33-1). Clinicians need to make appropriate recommendations to parents when observing negative deviations from the NCHS reference. Misinterpreting the growth patterns of healthy breast-fed infants by advising mothers to supplement unnecessarily or to stop breast-feeding altogether has profound public health significance. A general guideline is

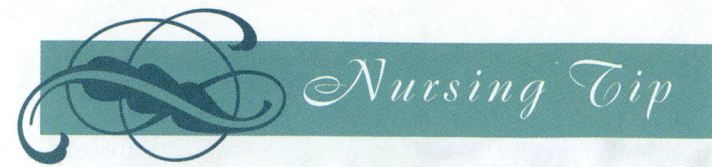

INFANT ASSESSMENT

A general approach to infant nutritional assessment follows:

1. Use an accurate electronic scale to measure weight.
2. Use a length board.

to note weight gain of 20 to 30 g/d (⅓ to ½ lb/wk) for the first 5 months, with a length gain of 0.80 to 1.07 mm/d (0.28 in/wk) and a head circumference increment of 0.3 cm/wk (Guo et al., 1991; Hamill et al., 1979).

Energy

Carbohydrates and fat meet the primary energy requirements for growth, metabolism, and activity. Protein also may provide energy. The most important function of protein in growth, however, is to provide the amino acids necessary for synthesis of body proteins and the hormones and enzymes that regulate metabolism (Carlson & Barness, 1996). Most of the data available with regard to total energy expenditure and balance have been defined from measurements of intake rather than determinations of energy need. Indirect **calorimetry** has been the most common technique used. This procedure measures energy production through the assessment of oxygen consumption and carbon dioxide production. Direct calorimetry, which directly measures heat loss from the infant, also has been used to assess expenditure but with far less frequency. A newer approach for assessing total energy expenditure is the doubly labeled water stable isotope technique. Validation studies have shown good correlation between the doubly labeled water technique compared with more conventional approaches to total energy expenditure (Jones et al., 1988; Roberts et al., 1986).

Because the composition and quantity of human milk consumed by infants vary, absolute requirements cannot be determined; however, normal ranges can be estimated. The current recommendations for energy requirements for a term infant are 108 kcal and 100 kcal per kilogram of body weight from birth through 6 months and 6 months through 12 months, respectively (National Research Council [NRC], 1989). These revised estimates reflect more accurately the infant populations receiving human milk (Prentice et al., 1988; Waterlow, 1988). The general compositions of human, bovine, and several infant formulas are compared in Table 33-1.

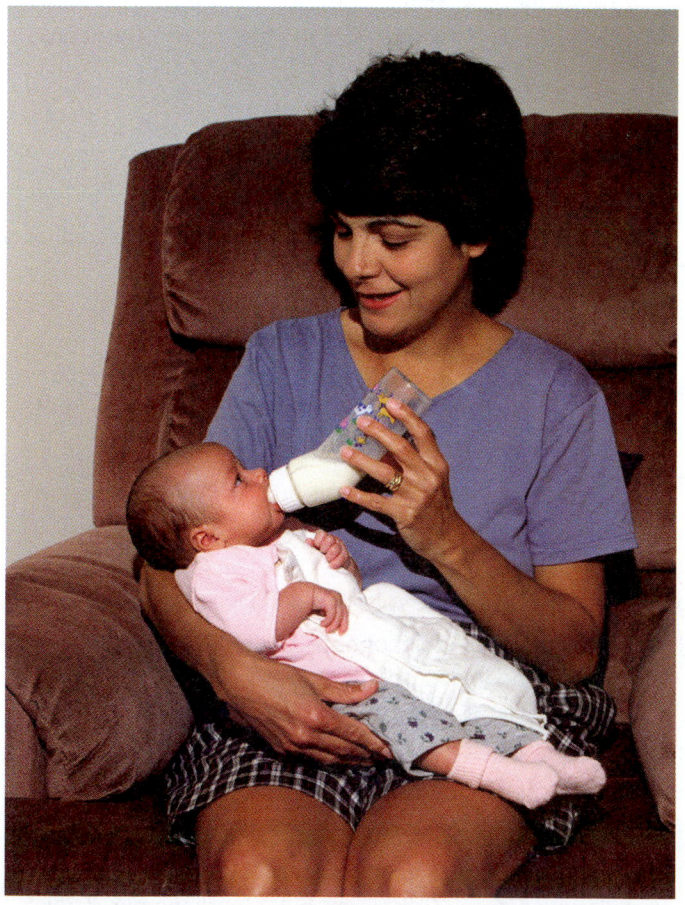

Figure 33-1 Adequate nutritional intake is noted by an infant's overall healthy appearance and steady growth rate.

Table 33-1 Composition of Human Milk and Formulas*

Selected Nutrients (100 mL)	Human Milk	Standard Cow's Milk–Based	Soy	Elemental	Preterm
		Formulas**			
Kcal	68	68	68	68	81
Carbohydrates (g)	7.2	7.0–7.3	7.0	7–9.1	9.0
Protein (g)	1.0	1.5	1.7–2.0	1.6–1.9	2.2–2.4
Fat (g)	3.9	3.6–3.8	3.6–3.7	2.7–3.9	4.1–4.4
Sodium (mEq)	0.78	0.8–0.96	0.9–1.4	0.7–1.4	1.4–1.5
Potassium (mEq)	1.34	1.43–1.87	1.9–2.1	1.7–2.0	2.1–2.7
Calcium (mEq)	28	42–51.9	60–71	43–71	134–146
Iron (mg)	0.03	1.2–1.3	1.2–1.3	1.2–1.3	1.5

*Commercial formulas average content: read individual labels for up-to-date quantity (Ross, Mead Johnson, and Stoe Brand formulas).
**Formulas with iron.

Protein

The amount of total energy intake utilized for growth is higher during the first 2 months of life than at any other time. During this most rapid period of postnatal growth, infants may use 60% of the protein they consume in producing new tissue. It has been calculated that about 45% of the dietary protein intake of human milk-fed infants comes from essential amino acids (NRC, 1989). In contrast, adults need only about 13% to 20% of their recommended protein intake in the form of essential amino acids.

There are significant differences in the digestibility and quality of human milk proteins compared with those of bovine milk-based formulas. The proportion of whey (supernatant) and casein (curd) in human milk is of interest. Human milk is more whey-dominant, with a whey-to-casein ratio of approximately 70:30 compared with 18:82 in bovine milk. In general, the whey fraction of soluble proteins is more easily digested and promotes more rapid gastric emptying (Billeaud, Guillet, & Sandler, 1990).

The type of proteins contained in the whey fraction differs in humans compared with bovine-derived formulas (Hambraeus, 1977). The major human whey protein is α-lactalbumin, a nutritional protein for the infant and a component of mammary gland lactose synthesis. Lactoferrin, lysozyme, and sIgA are specific human whey proteins involved in host defense and are present only in trace amounts in bovine-derived formulas. The major whey protein in bovine milk is beta-lactoglobulin, the protein implicated in bovine milk protein allergy and colic (Savilahti and Kuitunen, 1992; Jakobsson, Lindberg, Benediktsson, & Hansson, 1985).

In terms of protein requirements, doubts have been raised about whether the amount consumed by breast-fed infants is truly optimal (Foman, 1993). The theory has been put forth that the composition of human milk represents an evolutionary compromise between the need of the infant and the needs of the mother, and that the lower milk protein concentrations may protect the lactating mother from becoming nutritionally depleted. This theory was tested in an intervention study in Honduras in which infants were randomly assigned to be exclusively breast-fed for the first 6 months, or to receive preprepared solid foods (including egg yolk) in addition to breast milk beginning at 4 months (Dewey et al., 1996). Neither weight nor length gain from 4 to 6 months differed between groups, despite a 20% higher protein intake in the supplemented group. In another study, 20 healthy full-term infants, 10 of whom were breast-fed and 10 formula-fed, were followed longitudinally from birth to 24 weeks postnatal age (Motil, Sheng, Montandon, & Wong, 1996). Lean body mass and body fat were determined at 6-week intervals. The gross efficiency of nutrient utilization was calculated for each infant from the cumulative dietary intake and the change in body composition over time. Data revealed similar length and weight gains and lean body mass and body fat **accretion** (growth in size, especially by addition or accumulation) between breast- and formula-fed infants, despite significantly higher nitrogen and energy intakes of the formula-fed group. The gross efficiency of protein utilization for lean body mass deposition was almost twofold lower in formula-fed compared with breast-fed infants. Results from these studies indicate that human milk protein is not likely to be a limiting factor with regard to the growth of breast-fed infants from birth to 6 months.

Fat

The fats in human milk provide approximately 50% of the calories in the milk. The lipid profile consists of 98%

triglycerides, 1% phospholipids, and 0.5% cholesterol and cholesterol esters (Jensen & Jensen, 1992). In addition, fats are an integral part of all cell membranes, provide fatty acids necessary for brain development, and are the sole vehicle for fat-soluble vitamins and hormones in milk (Hamosh, 1988). The total fat content of human milk is approximately 3.5% to 4.5%; however, it is the most variable component of milk, varying in content throughout lactation, and within and between feedings. The fat content of human milk increases markedly during a single feeding from a breast, with the concentration of *hindmilk* (that milk produced toward the end of a nursing interval) typically being twice that of *foremilk* (lower-fat milk secreted from the breast prior to milk ejection). In addition, fat content increases during the day, with early morning milk having the lowest fat content. Total fat content increases gradually from colostrum (2.0%) through transitional milk (2.5% to 3.0%) to mature milk (3.5% to 4.5%) (Bitman et al., 1986).

Another major difference between the fat in human milk and that in infant formulas is the absence of long-chain (more than 18 carbons) fatty acids in infant formula. Additionally, only traces of cholesterol are present in infant formulas compared with an average amount of 10 to 15 mg/dL in human milk. Recently, two of these very long-chain fatty acids, arachidonic acid (AA) (20-carbon chain) and DHA (22-carbon chain), have received a significant amount of investigation, specifically their role in the developing retina and brain (Carlson, Werkman, & Tolley, 1996). These fatty acids are components of phospholipids found in brain and erythrocyte membranes. AA and DHA have been identified as affecting growth and development of cognition and vision (Uauy & Hoffman, 1991; Carlson, Werkman, Rhodes, & Tolley, 1993).

Human milk fat digestion and absorption are facilitated by the complex organization of the human milk fat globule, the pattern of fatty acids, their distribution on the triglyceride molecule, and the presence of bile salt–stimulated lipase (Hamosh, 1991; Innis, 1992; Jensen & Jensen, 1992). These features are especially important for the preterm infant. Because lipid deposition and accretion of specific lipids occur in the last trimester of intrauterine development, very low-birth-weight infants are deficient in both specific metabolites and the enzymes needed for fat digestion and metabolism.

Normal daily fat requirements for newborn infants are 3.3 to 6.0 g/100 kcal, which represents 30% to 54% of calories. Special attention should be given to providing sufficient essential fatty acids (linoleic and linolenic). Linoleic acid content should be a minimum of 1% to 3% of total kilocalories in current standard infant formulas. Linolenic is the precursor to DHA and should be 0.5% of the total kilocalories (European Society of Pediatric Gastroenterology and Nutrition [ESPGN], 1991). Owing to the special role of the long-chain fatty acids in neonatal brain development, and in normal nerve function at all ages, linolenic acid, AA, and DHA should be provided (Hamosh, 1991). It is interesting to note that several studies have shown that the fatty acid composition of the human milk lipid system is affected by maternal diet (Makrides, Neumann, & Gibson, 1996). For example, **vegan** mothers consuming no animal products and subsequently no DHA have low levels of DHA in their breast milk (Sanders & Reddy, 1992).

Carbohydrates

Carbohydrates provide fuel for fetal and neonatal metabolism, supplying both immediately usable and stored energy for macromolecular synthesis and tissue accretion (DiGiacomo, 1991). Approximately half of the glucose utilized is oxidized during normal metabolic processes whereas the remainder is used in nonoxidative pathways, such as in the synthesis of glycogen and fat (Denne & Kalhan, 1986). The neonatal brain is the major consumer of glucose, relying almost exclusively on glucose for its metabolism.

Lactose is the principal carbohydrate in human milk and provides approximately 50% of the energy content. Just as the two other major components of human milk have dual roles, so, too, does the carbohydrate component. Human milk carbohydrates have been shown to enhance infant immunity and brain development.

Dietary carbohydrates that resist intestinal enzymes are the main sources of carbon and energy for colonic bacteria. *Lactobacillus bifidum,* a strain of bifidobacteria, requires oligosaccharides from human milk for growth in the infant colon. This bifidobacteria represents 99% of total bacterial counts in the exclusively breast-fed infant by the end of the first week of life (Rasic & Kurmann, 1983). The lowering of pH in the gut aids in excluding enteropathic bacteria such as *Escherichia coli*. In contrast, the fecal flora of the bottle-fed infant resembles that of older children and adults, with less than 70% bifodobacteria and a higher intestinal pH.

Sialic acid (a monosaccharide residue) appears to play an important role in brain development. Approximately half of the 130 or so oligosaccharides present in human milk are sialylated (Sabharwal, Sjoblad, & Lundblad, 1991). Animal studies have revealed a significant proportion of this monosaccharide in the developing brain, with decreased concentrations of sialic acid during this early period being associated with irreversible impaired learning behavior (Morgan, Oppenheimer, & Winick, 1981). Investigators have shown that a high concentration of sialic acid exists in human milk in the first week of lactation, coinciding with a time of rapid synthesis of brain sialylated glycoproteins (Miller, Bull, Miller, & McVeagh, 1994). Additionally, lactose is a readily available source of galactose, which is essential to the production of the galactolipids, including cerebroside. These galactolipids are essential to the development of the central nervous system.

Water and Electrolytes

Water represents the constituent in the largest quantity in human milk, providing approximately 89 mL of preformed water in each 100 mL of milk consumed. Water is required by the infant to replace evaporative losses of water from skin and lungs and excretory losses from feces and urine. The first priority for water expenditures is for evaporative loss, and the second for urinary water necessary for the excretion of solutes. Estimated nonetenal water expenditures by full-term infants in a thermoneutral environment are presented in Table 33-2.

In the case of healthy full-term infants receiving adequate fluids, water intake is greatly in excess of requirements and diluted urine is excreted. At the same time, the amount of water excreted in the urine is determined by the renal solute load and renal concentrating ability. The sum of solutes that must be excreted by the kidney is termed the **renal solute load**. The renal solute load is of considerable importance in circumstances such as low fluid intake; abnormally high losses of water, for example, as those occurring with fever; hyperventilation; and diarrhea (Foman, 1993).

Sodium and chloride are major solutes of extracellular water, and potassium is a major solute of cellular water. The movement of water across cellular membranes and compartments occurs only as a result of the movement of these solutes. Absorption of amino acids and monosaccharides depends on absorption of sodium, and the intestinal secretions necessary for digestion of food are dependent on the secretion of chloride. Potassium is required for the transmission of nerve impulses and control of skeletal muscle contractility.

Estimates of requirements for sodium, chloride, and potassium (Table 33-3) are based on estimates of what is

Table 33-3 Recommended Daily Dietary Intake of Electrolytes for Healthy Infants

Age (mo)	Weight (kg)	Sodium (mg)	Chloride (mg)	Potassium (mg)
0–5	4.5	120	180	500
6–11	8.9	200	300	700
12	11.0	225	350	1,000
24	16.0	300	500	1,400

National Academy of Science. Food and Nutrition Board (1989) *Recommended Dietary Allowances*. Washington, D.C.: National Academy Press.

needed for growth and replacement of obligatory losses. These amounts depend on the rate at which extracellular fluid volume expands, a rate that varies with age.

The electrolyte compositions of human and bovine milks are given in Table 33-4. Human milk contains 7 mEq/L of sodium (range, 3 to 19 mEq/L) (Foman, 1993). Consumed at a rate of 750 mL/d, this provides the infant with an average of 120 mg/d (1.16 mEq/d per kilogram of body weight) from birth to 2 months of age and 0.8 mEq/d per kilogram of body weight from 3 to 5 months, which is considered more than sufficient. The potassium requirement for growth averages 65 mg/d for infants. An increase in lean body mass is a major determinant of potassium needs. Between 60 and 80 mEq are required for each kilogram of weight gained. The recommended dietary intake of chloride throughout the first year of life is 120 mg/d. The chloride intake of an infant consuming 750 mL/d of milk, providing 330 mg/L of chloride, is 248 g/d (Allen, Keller, Archer, & Neville, 1991).

Minerals

Calcium (Ca), phosphorus (P), and magnesium (Mg) homeostasis in the newborn involves hormonal influences that regulate the concentrations of these minerals in the infant. Most of the mineral content of the body is in tissues, with less than 1% of Ca, P, and Mg in the circulation.

Table 33-2 Nonrenal Water Expenditures of Full-Term Infants Under Thermoneutral Conditions at Different Ages

Route of Loss	Water expenditures (mL/d) 1 Mo	4 Mo	12 Mo
Evaporative loss	210	350	500
Fecal loss	42	70	105
Growth	18	9	6
Total	270	429	611

Adapted from Foman, S. (1993). *Nutrition of normal infants* (p. 92). St. Louis, MO: Mosby.

Table 33-4 Electrolyte Composition of Human and Bovine Milks

Component (mg/dL)	Human	Bovine
Sodium	15	58
Chloride	43	103
Potassium	55	138

Table 33-5 Serum Concentrations of Minerals in Neonates

Mineral	Normal Range (mg/dL)
Calcium	8–11
Magnesium	2.1 ± 0.3
Phosphorus	4–7.1

Data adapted from Itani, O., & Tsang, R. C. (1991). Calcium, phosphorus, and magnesium in the newborn: Pathophysiology and management. In W. W. Hay (Ed.). *Neonatal nutrition and metabolism.* St. Louis, MO: Mosby.

However, serum concentrations are useful because fluctuations from normal ranges often are associated with clinical symptoms. Normal serum concentrations of these minerals are presented in Table 33-5.

Blood calcium concentration is maintained within very narrow limits by the interplay of several hormones (1,25-dihydroxycholecalciferol, parathyroid hormone, calcitonin, estrogen, and testosterone), which control calcium absorption and excretion as well as bone metabolism. The 1% of calcium not found in the bone is essential in nerve conduction, muscle contraction, blood clotting, and membrane permeability. These extra skeletal levels of calcium are maintained at the expense of bone in the face of inadequate calcium intake or absorption. In the event of such circumstances, resultant demineralization of bone and reduction in strength occur.

Calcium homeostasis is closely linked with that of P and Mg. Longitudinal studies measuring Ca and P in human milk and maternal and infant sera show progressive increases in infant serum Ca in association with decreasing P content in breast milk and infant serum (Greer et al., 1982). In addition, progressive increases in serum Mg levels were seen in breast-fed infants in association with decreasing P content of the milk. Ca and P decrease over time during lactation (Anderson, 1992). Human milk provides optimal Ca, P, and Mg content for bone mineralization in term newborns. Cow's milk–based formulas generally have higher Ca content than does human milk to compensate for the poorer absorption rates of the formulas. Infants receive an average of 240 mg of Ca from 750 mL of human milk, approximately two thirds of which they retain. The retention of Ca from infant formulas based on cow's milk is less than one half. These differences in retention are reflected in the recommendations for Ca, P, and Mg for breast-fed and formula-fed infants outlined in Table 33-6.

Trace Elements

Whereas the macronutrients (protein, fat, carbohydrates, and major minerals) are essential components of body structure, energy sources and micronutrients provide protection against oxidative damage during cellular metabolism and have major roles in immune function. **Macronutrients** are any of the chemical elements, such as carbon, required in relatively large quantities for growth. **Micronutrients** are any of the chemical elements, such as iron, required in minute quantities for growth.

Iron, zinc, copper, manganese, selenium, molybdenum, chromium, and iodine are generally considered to be the essential trace minerals. Table 33-7 outlines the recommended daily intake of trace elements for infants.

Iron is a powerful oxidant and a constituent of hemoglobin, myoglobin, and a number of enzymes and, therefore, an essential nutrient for the infant. With stored iron, the term infant can maintain satisfactory hemoglobin levels from human milk without other iron sources during the first 4 months of life. After 6 months of age, infants should consume iron-fortified foods or iron-fortified formula to ensure adequate iron stores (Haschke et al., 1993). The recommended daily allowance (RDA) from 6 months to 3 years of age is set at 10 mg/d per kilogram of body weight for healthy infants and should not exceed a maximum of 15 mg/d. Iron deficiency anemia has been associated with impaired mental and motor development and should be prevented (Scheard, 1994).

Table 33-6 Recommended Dietary Intake of Calcium, Phosphorus, and Magnesium for Breast-Fed and Formula-Fed Infants

Age	1–6 mo		6–12 mo	
Mineral	Breast-Fed (mg)	Formula-Fed (mg)	Breast-Fed (mg)	Formula-Fed (mg)
Calcium	300	400	500	600
Phosphorus	300	300	500	500
Magnesium	40	60	40	60

Adapted from National Academy of Science. Food and Nutrition Board (1989). *Recommended Dietary Allowances.* Washington, D.C.: National Academy Press.

Table 33-7 Estimated Trace Element Requirements for Healthy Infants

Trace Element	1–6 Mo	6–12 Mo
Iron	6 mg	10 mg
Zinc	5 mg	5 mg
Copper	0.4–0.6 mg	0.6–0.7 mg
Manganese	0.3–0.6 mg	0.6–1.0 mg
Selenium	10 mEq	15 mEq
Molybdenum	15–30 mEq	20–40 mEq
Chromium	10–40 mEq	20–60 mEq
Iodine	40 mEq	50 mEq

Adapted from National Academy of Science. Food and Nutrition Board (1989). *Recommended Dietary Allowances*. Washington, D.C.: National Academy Press.

Table 33-8 Recommended Daily Dietary Allowances for Water-Soluble Vitamins for Infants

Vitamin	0–6 Mo	6–12 Mo
Vitamin C	30 mg	35 mg
Thiamin	0.3 mg	0.4 mg
Riboflavin	0.4 mg	0.5 mg
Niacin	5 mg NE	6 mg NE
Vitamin B_6	0.3 mg	0.6 mg
Folic acid	25 µg	35 µg
Vitamin B_{12}	0.3 µg	0.5 µg

National Academy of Science. Food and Nutrition Board (1989). *Recommended Dietary Allowances*. Washington, D.C.: National Academy Press.

Zinc is an essential component of many enzymes and plays a role in cellular immune function (Prasad, 1991). Because full-term infants exclusively breast-fed rarely show signs of zinc depletion, requirements must be satisfied by maternal milk levels. During the first month of life, breast-fed infants consume an average of 2 mg/d of zinc (Casey, Neville, & Hambidge, 1989). The dietary zinc requirement of infants consuming formula is higher than that of breast-fed infants because of lower bioavailability of the formula (Lonnerdal, Cederblad, Davidsson, & Sandstrom, 1984). Assuming an intake of 750 mL/d of formula, the recommended intake for formula-fed infants is 5 mg/d of zinc.

The remaining trace elements have received less investigation but are no less important in the enzymatic activity of the body. One consistent finding from studies of levels of trace elements in human milk is their variability between individuals and stages of lactation.

Water-Soluble Vitamins

The water-soluble vitamins (B and C vitamins) are, for the most part, present in the serum and, as the name implies, the fluid compartments of the body. With the exception of vitamin B_{12}, these vitamins are typically excreted in urine when blood concentrations are too high. The RDAs for water-soluble vitamins for infants are presented in Table 33-8.

Vitamin C (ascorbic acid) functions primarily as an **antioxidant** and a **reducing agent**. An **antioxidant** is a substance that slows down the oxidation of hydrocarbons, oils, fats, and so on, thus helping to check deterioration. A **reducing agent** is a substance that reduces another one, or brings about reduction, and is itself oxidized in the process. As a reducing agent, vitamin C serves as a cofactor for a number of essential enzymatic reactions (Hornig, Moser, & Glatthaar, 1988). In addition, vitamin C enhances iron absorption from the GI tract. Human milk is a rich source of vitamin C, containing approximately 43 mg/100 mL. Concentrations of ascorbic acid in human milk are generally considered to average approximately seven times those in plasma (Cummings, 1981). It is recommended that infant formulas contain at least 8 mg/100 kcal of vitamin C, providing approximately 30 mg/d.

Thiamin primarily serves as a cofactor for three enzyme complexes involved in carbohydrate metabolism (Moran & Greene, 1987). RDAs for thiamin are based on the mean thiamin concentration in human milk plus 2 standard deviations, which is 0.3 mg/L, or 0.4 mg/1,000 kcal.

Riboflavin serves as an essential component of flavoproteins. Flavoproteins function as hydrogen carriers in a number of critical oxidation-reduction reactions, such as energy metabolism, glycogen synthesis, erythrocyte production, and the conversion of folate to its active coenzyme (Moran & Greene, 1987). Requirements for riboflavin are related to nitrogen intake. The dietary allowance from birth to 6 months of age is set at 0.4 mg/1,000 kcal.

Niacin is converted in the liver to the active cofactors that play central roles in body metabolism in a wide range of oxidation-reduction reactions, including glycolysis, electron transport, and fat synthesis (Moran & Greene, 1987). Human milk contains approximately 1.5 mg of niacin and appears to be adequate to meet the niacin needs of the infant. The niacin RDA for formula-fed infants up to 6 months of age is 8 NE (niacin equivalent) per 1,000 kcal.

Vitamin B_6 serves as a cofactor for a large number of reactions involved in the synthesis, interconversion, and catabolism of amino acids and neurotransmission (McCormick, 1989). Most of the vitamin B_6 in human milk is in the form of pyridoxal (Hamaker, Kirksey, & Borschel, 1990). There is 12 to 15 µg/100 mL of vitamin B_6 in human

Table 33-9 Recommended Daily Dietary Allowances for Fat-Soluble Vitamins for Infants

Age (mo)	Vitamin A (μg RE)*	Vitamin D (μg)**	Vitamin E (mg)	Vitamin K (μg)
0–6	395	7.5	3	5
6–12	375	10	4	10

*1 retinol equivalent (RE) of vitamin A equals 3, 33 IU.

**10 g of vitamin D equals 400 IU.

Adapted from National Academy of Science. Food and Nutrition Board (1989). *Recommended Dietary Allowances.* Washington, D.C.: National Academy Press.

milk and 64 μg/100 mL in cow's milk. The RDA for infants under 6 months of age is 0.30 mg.

Folates function metabolically as coenzymes that transport single carbon fragments from one compound to another in amino acid metabolism and nucleic acid synthesis. Human and cow's milk both contain about 50 μg/L of folate. The needs of infants are adequately met by milk from humans and cow's milk.

Vitamin B_{12} functions as an enzyme in amino acid metabolism. The minimum RDA for infants is 0.3 μg/d the first year of life, when growth is rapid.

Fat-Soluble Vitamins

Vitamins A, D, E, and K are the fat-soluble vitamins, differing from the water-soluble vitamins in several ways. Fat-soluble vitamins are found in the fat component of milk and other foods and tend to move into the liver and adipose tissue and remain there, rather than being excreted as are water-soluble vitamins. Table 33-9 outlines the RDAs for the fat-soluble vitamins.

Vitamin A is essential for vision, growth, cellular differentiation, reproduction, and the integrity of the immune system (Goodman, 1984; West, Rombout, Van der Zijpp, & Sijtsma, 1991). In vitamin A deficiency, a keratinizing metaplasia of the mucus-secreting epithelial surface occurs and can result in overgrowth of bacteria and secondary infections (Sommer, 1994). The RDAs made by various groups are 350 to 400 μg/d (Joint Food and Agriculture Organization/World Health Organization Expert Committee, 1988, Food and Nutrition Board, 1989, Scientific Review Committee, 1990).

Vitamin D is essential for proper formation of bone and mineralization. The metabolite of vitamin D, 1,25-dihydroxyvitamin D, in concert with parathyroid hormone, is responsible for the mobilization and absorption of calcium, thereby promoting mineralization of the skeleton. Vitamin D is unique among nutrients because the body can synthesize it with exposure to sunlight. The level of 40 IU/100 mL, or 1.00 μg/100 mL, may provide adequate amounts in the fully breast-fed infant to meet the requirements of 40 IU, or 10 μg/d. The exception would be in-

fants whose mothers are not exposed to sunlight. It is recommended that these infants receive a daily supplement of 5 to 7.5 μg.

Vitamin E is an antioxidant similar in function to vitamin C but is fat-soluble. Its primary function is as a scavenger of free radicals, thereby protecting cellular membranes against oxidative destruction (Kelleher, 1991). Because the requirement for vitamin E is closely related to the intake of polyunsaturated fatty acids, the RDA of 3 mg for infants from birth to 6 months of age is based on the tocopherol concentration of human milk (Jansson, Akesson, & Holmberg, 1981).

Client Education

Bottle-Feeding the Neonate

- The bottle should be prepared (see Client Education: Preparation of Infant Formula) and allowed to come to room temperature, either by sitting out for half an hour or running warm water over the bottle.

- The neonate should be held in a comfortable position with the head elevated.

- The bottle should be held so the formula fills the nipple and no air is in the neck of the bottle (Figure 33-2).

- The infant should be burped at least twice during the feeding:

  —The infant may be upright on the shoulder.

  —The infant may be placed in a sitting position, with one hand supporting the chin and the other gently rubbing the back. This is the preferred position as it allows one to watch for regurgitation.

  —After a few minutes, resume feeding.

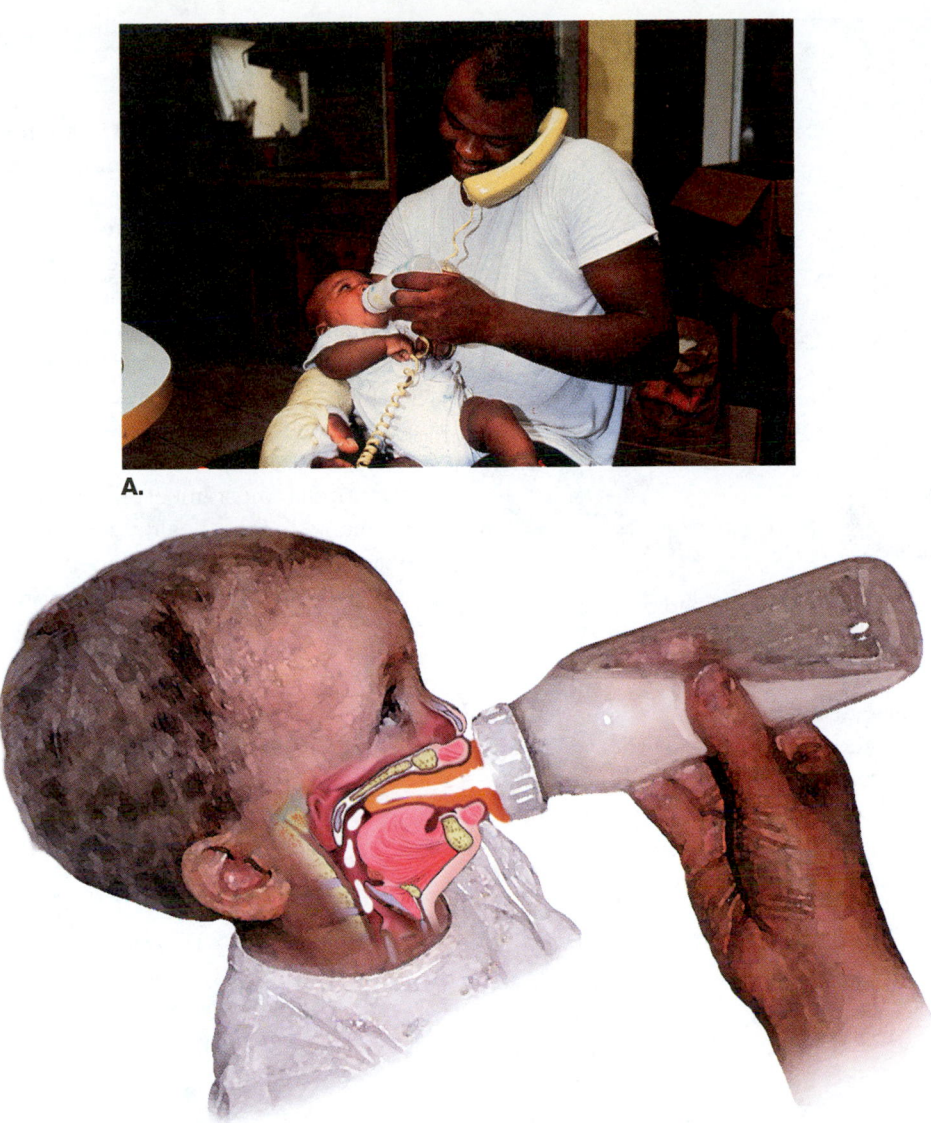

A.

B.

Figure 33-2 Proper bottle position for feeding. A. The baby should be held in a comfortable position with the head elevated. B. The bottle should be angled so that the nipple is completely covered with milk, preventing the baby from sucking air.

Vitamin K is a group of compounds essential for the formation of prothrombin and other proteins involved in the regulation of blood clotting. Owing to the low concentrations of vitamin K reported in human milk (2 μg/L), it is recommended that exclusively breast-fed infants receive a supplement at birth. Additionally, infant formulas should contain 4 μg/100 kcal of vitamin K (AAP, 1985).

BREAST-FEEDING

As previously stated, breast-feeding is the optimal choice of infant feeding by all major societies and agencies, including the AAP, American Dietetics Association, and WHO (Figure 33-3). These groups base their recommendations on the strong scientific evidence of decreased infant mortality in developing countries and decreased morbidity in developed countries seen in exclusively breast-fed infants compared with those fed human milk substitutes.

Lactation is a complex physiologic process under neuroendocrine control, whereas breast-feeding is the process by which milk is transferred from the maternal breast to the infant. Understanding the difference in these two interrelated processes is important when counseling the mother. Most lactation and breast-feeding problems are preventable and can be overcome with proper knowledge and technical skills (see Chapter 30). Prenatal visits should include discussion about infant feeding issues to provide an opportunity for parents to make an informed choice by gaining information. Allowing for open discussion of the facts helps diffuse the guilt that lack of knowledge or lack of support

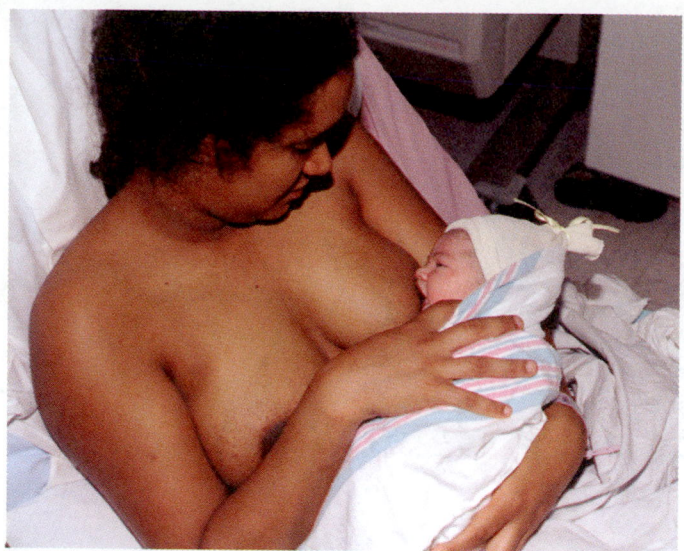

Figure 33-3 Breast-feeding is the method of choice for many new mothers.

from a physician or nurse about breast-feeding may cause. Studies have demonstrated that prenatal education and breast-feeding support from family, friends, and especially the infant's father, are associated with the mother's choice of breast-feeding, regardless of maternal age, ethnic group, educational level, or marital status. Prenatally, mothers are intensely focused on readiness for the birth experience, therefore breast-feeding instruction and information will need to be reviewed after delivery. The office and clinic environment can send a strong message to parents about the priorities of the clinician and staff. A clinic or hospital environment replete with formula advertisements in the form of posters, pads, and pencils gives a message that may undermine any verbal "lip service" paid to breast-feeding.

Critical Thinking

Bottle Propping

Feeding the infant by propping the bottle as the infant lies in the crib is not recommended. What are some of the reasons that this is not a good idea?

- The infant may regurgitate and aspirate the formula.
- Infants who nurse from propped bottles may develop bottle mouth syndrome.

Which other negative effects can you think of that are related to this manner of feeding?

COMMERCIAL INFANT FORMULA

No commercially processed infant formula has been developed that reproduces the immunologic properties, nutrient **bioavailability** (rate at which a nutrient enters the blood stream and is circulated to specific organs or tissues), digestibility, and nutritional effects of human milk. The composition of infant formula, however, has improved tremendously in the past 50 years as a result of a greater understanding of infant nutrient requirements, absorption, and metabolic activities. Continual research is under way to qualitatively enhance infant formulas (Lo & Kleinman, 1996).

When used as the sole source of infant nutrition, infant formula must meet all the energy and nutrient requirements for the healthy term infant. The AAP Committee on Nutrition has developed infant formula standards. The Food and Drug Administration regulations for infant formula are based on these standards. Additionally, the In-

Client Education

Preparation of Infant Formula

- The equipment should be gathered:
  - Bottles may be made of plastic or glass, or have plastic liners.
  - Nipples should allow a steady flow of formula but should not be so large as to cause the infant to swallow too fast.
  - Formula may be in ready-to-feed, concentrate, or powder form.
- The label should be checked to make sure the formula is in ready-to-feed or concentrate form.
- When powder or concentrate forms are used, they must be mixed according to the directions on the bottle.
- Either the ready-to-feed formula is poured directly into the bottles, or the concentrated or powdered formula is mixed in a clean container and then poured into the bottles.
- Once prepared, the formula may be stored in the refrigerator for up to 48 hours; if not used in 48 hours, it should be discarded.
- Formula may be left at room temperature for up to an hour and then should be discarded.

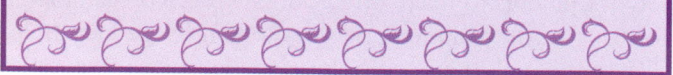

Research Highlight

Mothers' Ideas About the Infant Feeding Process

Purpose

To describe how mothers of preterm infants who were learning to nipple feed viewed their own as well as their infant's role in the feeding process.

Method

A descriptive, comparative study was undertaken in two neonatal intensive care units in the Midwest. A convenience sample of 22 mothers of very low-birth-weight infants was obtained. Interviews were undertaken in which mothers were rated on a 6-point scale concerning their thinking about their co-regulatory role in their infant's feeding. Videotapes also were obtained of the feeding procedure.

The instrument used for data collection was the Working Model of Feeding developed by Pridham, Schroeder, Van Riper, Thoyre, Limbo, & Mylnarczyk in 1999. It is a scale describing infant behaviors and maternal expectations concerning infant participation in feeding. The variables range from 1 in which infant participation in feeding is not regarded as a necessary or valued condition of feeding (the mother does not take the infant's perspective), through 6, in which the mother views the infant's participation as essential for the feeding to progress. Mothers with a score of 6 believed in being proactive during feeding to prevent distress and fatigue.

Findings

Scores ranged from 1 to 6, with a mean of 3.3 (SD = 1.4). Mothers with higher scores were more likely to be significantly older and their infants were at a younger gestational age at birth.

Understanding feeding from the maternal perspective may assist clinicians in developing strategies for teaching feeding skills. Rather than beginning teaching with how to feed, it may be more prudent to begin with examination of maternal ideas about learning to feed the infant at high risk.

Nursing Implications

Many times it is the nurse who has the initial contact with the mother who needs to begin feeding her infant who is at high risk after many days or weeks of alternative feeding methods. To discuss maternal attitudes before the onset of this process may eliminate significant barriers to the process.

Thoyre, S. M. (2000). Mothers' ideas about their role in feeding their high-risk infants. *Journal of Obstetric, Gynecologic, and Neonatal Nursing, 29,* (6), 613–624.

---

fant Formula Act mandates adherence to standards and quality control and requires that quantitative label declaration be made for 38 nutrients. The amount of each nutrient is added in formulas at higher concentrations than human milk to compensate for the lower bioavailability of nutrients from infant formula.

Commercially available infant formulas fall into several categories: 1) Standard cow's milk–based formulas; 2) soy-based and lactose-free formulas; 3) elemental, hydrolyzed protein, and free amino acid formulas; 4) premature infant formulas; and 5) specialty infant formulas, including those for metabolic disorders (Table 33-10). These formulas

come in powder, concentrate, or ready-to-feed forms. Health care providers should make sure that parents understand how to mix these formulas correctly to avoid hyperosmolar or overly dilute preparations, which can be dangerous (Wilcox, Florello, & Glick, 1993). When using a ready-to-feed formula after the infant is 6 months of age or living in an area with nonfluorinated water, a fluoride supplement may be required (AAP, 1985).

Standard cow's milk–based formula is the formula of choice for routine feeding when human milk or breast-feeding is not available (Klish, 1990) (Figure 33-4). These formulations modify whole cow's milk to reduce protein

Table 33-10 Commercial Infant Formula Selection

Formula	Criteria
Standard, cow's milk–based	Human milk not available
Soy, lactose-free	Galactose deficiency
	Vegan
Elemental, protein hydrolysate	Cow's milk allergy
	Intestinal malabsorption
Premature	Premature, low-birth-weight infants
Specialty	Metabolic disorders

and renal solute load. There are two categories, namely, casein predominant and whey predominant. Cow's milk is 80% casein and 20% whey, and the formulas derived from this are called casein predominant. Whey predominant formulas have been developed to provide a protein composition like that of human milk, 40% casein and 60% whey.

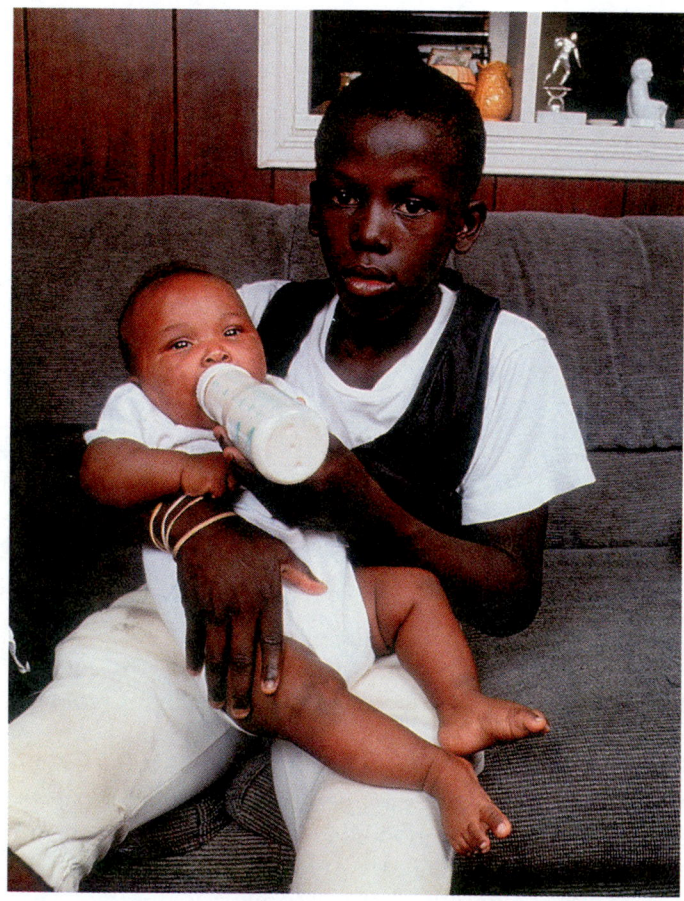

Figure 33-4 One of the benefits of bottle-feeding is that other family members, including siblings, can share in the responsibility of feeding the baby.

These "humanized" formulas are prepared by combining nonfat cow's milk with demineralized whey, a by product of cheese. In both types of standard formulas, lactose is added to provide a more appropriate energy ratio. Vegetable oils, as long-chain triglycerides, are added next as a fat source. To ensure adequate essential fatty acid intake, formulas should provide a minimum of 1% to 3% linoleic acid per kcal (ESPGN, 1991). Formulas have yet to include cholesterol or long-chain polyunsaturated fatty acids. At one quart of intake, 100% of the RDA can be met for vitamin and minerals. Iron-fortified standard formulas generally are well tolerated (Nelson et al., 1988) and should be used to provide adequate iron. With a caloric density of 67 to 70 kcal/dL (20 kcal/oz) these formulas should be offered as needed. The usual intake of 150 to 200 mL/d per kilogram of body weight provides 100 to 130 kcal/d per kilogram of body weight, resulting in a goal target weight gain of 20 to 30 g/d.

Soy-based, lactose-free formulas (ProSobee, Mead-Johnson; Bristol-Myers Isomil, Ross) originally were made from soy flour. Currently, manufacturers use a water-soluble soy protein isolate, which is purified to over 90% protein. Methionine is added to complete this protein. Corn syrup or sucrose is used as the carbohydrate source. These formulas are recommended to be used for their lactose-free status in infants with galactosemia lactose intolerance or vegetarian practices (AAP, 1983). However, these formulas are not designed for infants with cow's milk allergy because 30% of these infants also will be allergic to the soy protein. These formulas also are not recommended for preterm infants because the phytate fiber in the soy com-

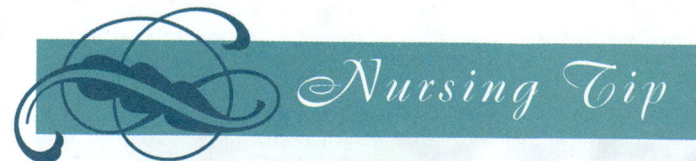

minerals that has been found to provide a safe, hypoallergenic source for infants who are allergic to the hydrolysates (Sampson, James, & Bernhisel-Broadbert, 1992).

The casein protein hydrolysates (Pregestimil and Alimentum) contain the carbohydrate source as glucose polymers and the fat source as a blend of long- and medium-chain triglycerides. The medium-chain triglycerides are added to enhance absorption because they do not require pancreatic lipase or bile salts for digestion. The formulas Nutramigen and Good Start do not contain medium-chain triglycerides. Vitamins and minerals are added to provide

---

Nursing Alert

WATER FOR FORMULA

If the water supply is not purified or there is any question about cleanliness, then:

1. Bottled or boiled water should be used to prepare the formula.
2. The equipment should be sterilized.

---

promises nitrogen and mineral balance for babies at high risk (Shenai et al., 1981). Calorie, protein, vitamin, and mineral needs can be met for infants consuming 1 qt/d. Also available is Lactofree (Mead-Johnson; Bristol-Myers) which is a lactose-free, protein formula from cow's milk.

Elemental, protein hydrolysates (Nutramigen and Pregestimil, Mead-Johnson Bristol-Myers; Alimentum, Ross) are designed to meet the needs of infants with documented cow's or soy protein allergy (Kleinman, Bahna, Powell, & Sampson, 1991; AAP, 1989; Lee & Heiner, 1986).

These formulas also have been used for infants with malabsorptive problems (Schwartz & Maedak, 1985). Manufacturers enzymatically hydrolyze the casein protein to remove large proteins that will be allergenic. The goal is to contain proteins of less than 1,200 molecular weight to be truly hypoallergenic. Free amino acids (L-cysteine, L-tyrosine, and L-tryptophan) are added to compensate for those removed in processing. A whey hydrolysate, i.e., Good Start (Carnation), is available but may contain proteins with molecular weights higher than 2,000 and may not be truly hypoallergenic. Infants that continue to exhibit bloody stools or cow's milk intolerance on the hydrolysate may benefit from free amino acid infant formulas (Vanderhoof et al., 1997). Neocate is a powdered infant formula composed of free amino acids, maltodextrins, long-chain triglycerides, medium-chain triglycerides, vitamins, and

---

Client Education

Methods for Infant Formula and Equipment Sterilization

Bottles must be sterilized if there is any question about the cleanliness of the water. There are two methods of bottle sterilization

Terminal Method

- The equipment is washed with soap and water.
- The formula is prepared according to directions.
- Bottles are filled; nipples are inverted, with caps loosely applied.
- Bottles are placed in a large pan, with 2 to 3 inches of water or in a bottle sterilizer.
- The pan is covered, and the water is boiled for 25 minutes.
- The bottles are allowed to cool, the lids screwed on, and the bottles stored in the refrigerator.

Aseptic Method

- The equipment is washed in soap and water and placed in a large pan or sterilizer.
- The equipment is boiled for 5 minutes.
- The water for mixing the formula is boiled separately for 5 minutes.
- The equipment is removed with tongs, and the formula is mixed in the sterilized pitcher.
- The prepared formula is poured into the bottles, lids applied, and stored in the refrigerator.

Nursing Alert

FOOD ALLERGY SYMPTOMS

1. Skin symptoms, such as swelling, hives, and skin rashes.
2. Colicky behavior, diarrhea, and blood in the stool.
3. Stuffy nose, and breathing difficulties.
4. Swelling of the mucous membranes of the mouth.
5. Anaphylactic shock.

100% of the RDAs for infants when intake is approximately 32 oz/d. Refer back to Table 33-1 for nutrient components.

Specialty formulas are made for infants with severe nutrient sensitivities (e.g., 3232A), or specific inborn errors of metabolism (e.g., phenol-free for infants with phenylketonuria. These products should only be used in consultation with a metabolic dietician and are beyond the scope of this review.

Premature formulas (Enfamil Premature Formula, Mead-Johnson; Similac Special Care, Ross) are designed specifically for the immature infant at high risk (Figure 33-5). Low-birth-weight infants are born without the benefit of the last trimester's supply of fat, minerals, and trace elements; therefore, requirements for intake are specialized to meet their needs (Neu, Valentine, & Meetze, 1990). Protein is more concentrated (2.2 to 2.4 g/dL) and contains 60% whey and 40% casein to provide enhanced digestibility and a better amino acid pattern. The carbohydrate source is a blend of 40% to 50% glucose polymers, with the remainder as lactose. Replacing half the lactose as glu-

cose polymers allows the formula to have an isosmolar formulation. Oil made up of long- and medium-chain triglycerides enhances digestibility. These 24 kcal/oz formulas with iron are recommended at an intake of 150 mL/d per kilogram of body weight to provide 100% of the RDAs of vitamins and minerals for preterm infants weighing less than 2,000 g and less than 35 weeks' gestation.

INTRODUCTION OF SOLID FOODS AND WEANING

Weaning is generally the term used to describe the introduction of semisolid or solid foods to the breast-fed or formula-fed infant. Several factors influence the introduction of solid foods and the weaning process, including the nutritional requirements of the infant, development and maturation of the infant, and foods available to supply the nutrients (Stordy, Redfern, & Morgan, 1996).

The introduction of semisolid foods should not take place too early for several reasons. Developmentally, the infant has an extrusion tongue reflex until 4 to 6 months of age, making solid feeding inappropriate. This protective reflex results in the infant pushing out with the tongue any semisolid or solid bolus of food. The practice of solid additions to the bottle, or so-called infant feeders, should also be avoided. In addition, solid foods add to the renal solute load and may contribute to higher plasma concentrations of sodium and urea (Wharton, 1996). As a result the infant will either reduce milk intake, which will compromise normal growth and development, or consume more calories than are needed, increasing the risk of childhood obesity. Some parents have started solids early believing that this practice will help the infant sleep through the night. However, feeding infants solids at bedtime is not related to nighttime sleeping patterns. Several well-controlled studies found that infants who receive solids before bedtime have the same sleep patterns as those who do not receive solids (Keane, Charney, Straus, & Roberts, 1988; Macknin, Medendorp, & Maier, 1989).

Conversely, the introduction of solids should not be delayed much beyond 6 months of age (AAP, 1980). For the breast-fed infant, mother's milk alone may be insufficient to meet the recommended energy and nutrient

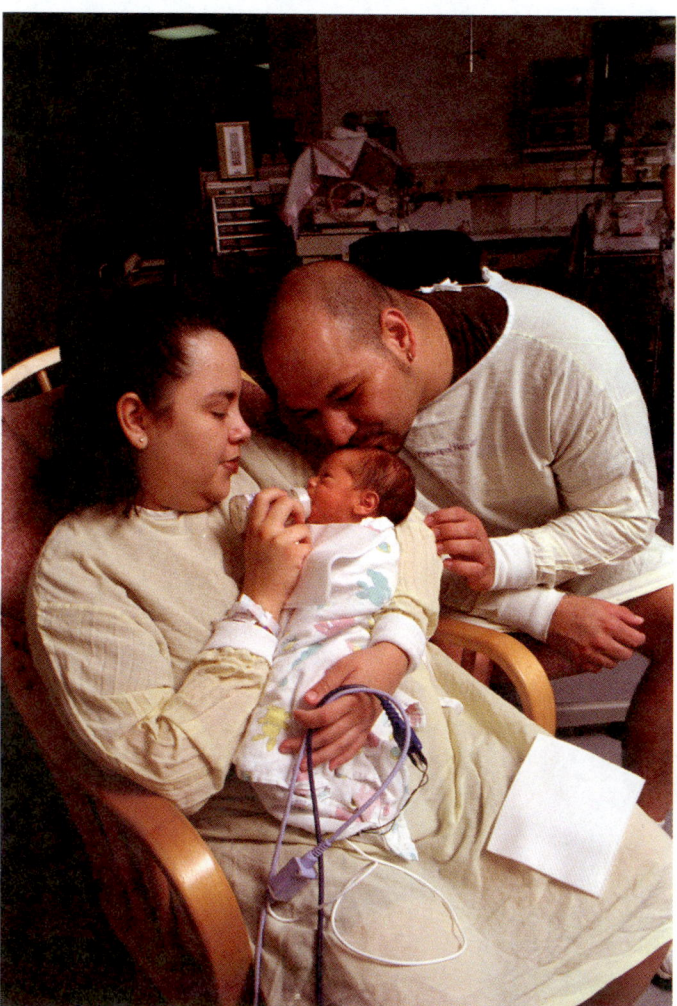

Figure 33-5 Special formulas are available for premature and high-risk infants.

> ### Nursing Alert
>
> #### CHOKING PREVENTION
> Avoid small items that can easily lodge in infant's airway, such as grapes, nuts, popcorn, watermelon, and seeds. Hotdogs also should be avoided.

Generally, routine vitamin supplements are not necessary for the fully breast-fed or formula-fed infant drinking 32 oz/d. Breast-fed infants receiving a limited amount of sunshine may require 44 IU/d of vitamin D. After 4 to 6 months, both breast-fed and formula-fed infants need iron; however, this need can be met by an iron-enriched diet or iron-fortified formula. Fluoride supplementation at 0.25 mg/d should be started once the teeth erupt (Foman and Ekshard, 1993) if the infants does not receive an adequate source of fluorinated water (AAP, 1986). Parents and caregivers should call their local water service to check how much fluoride is in the water.

needs, particularly in terms of vitamin D, iron, zinc, and copper. In addition, some infants who have not started to take food from a spoon by 6 months of age subsequently show considerable delay in adapting to the chewing and tongue-rolling action of the weaning from the milking action of the suckling.

Most mothers initially use manufactured weaning foods because of their convenience and their physical and nutritional properties. Because of the infant's need for iron at 6 months, iron-fortified rice cereal should be introduced first in quantities of 1 to 2 tablespoons/d mixed with breast

Critical Thinking

Infant Nutrition

You are asked to attend medical rounds in the neonatal unit. Infant nutrition is discussed. Several of the nurses, doctors, and residents have questions about the comparison of human milk and prepared formulas. How will you prepare for a continued discussion of this topic the next week?

- When comparing the constituents of human milk and formula, what are the benefits of human milk?
- What are some of the specialty formula preparations, and how do they differ from standard infant formula?
- What are some of the reasons that prepared formula would be used or recommended?

milk or formula (Poskitt, 1983; AAP, 1980). One food at a time should be introduced, waiting at least 3 days between each new food to watch for allergic reactions (e.g., hives, wheezing, gas, and blood in the stool). Oatmeal and barley cereal can then be introduced into the diet, again with portion sizes of 1 to 2 tablespoon per day. Orange, yellow, and green vegetables should be used next to provide increased vitamin A and C. Fruits can then be initiated, avoiding citris fruits (e.g., oranges and orange juice) until after 9 months of age. At 8 months of age, egg yolks and meats can be added to the diet. Avoid egg whites and fish until after 1 year of age because these foods can be highly allergenic. See Table 33-11 for a suggested schedule for introducing solid foods.

Foods based on the parents' meals usually are introduced next. Care should be taken to ensure food is small or mashed into pieces suitable for the baby. Cultural differences can play a role in the diet. Thus, caution should be observed when using home-prepared dishes that often are high in fat, carbohydrates, and sodium and low in iron and vitamin D (Stordy, Redfern, & Morgan, 1995; Mills & Tyler, 1992).

Careful attention to food preparation is essential when using commercially prepared foods to avoid exposure to botulism or lead from cans. Honey should be avoided because botulism spores tend to contaminate this product and can make the infant very ill. Other foods to avoid include nuts, grapes, popcorn, hard chopped carrots, celery, white bread (which can be very sticky), hard candy, and seeds. Cow's milk is recommended to begin after 1 year of age (AAP, 1992). Infants that begin too early are found to be iron deficient. Cow's milk also is inadequate source of folate, copper, linoleic acid, and vitamin C.

Infants on vegan diets should be assessed by a nutritionist because energy, protein, vitamins D, vitamin B_{12}, calcium, and zinc can be limited in their meals (Nutrition

Table 33-11 Recommended Timetable for Introducing Solid Foods	
Age (mo)	**Goal Intake**
6	1–2 tablespoons/d of iron-fortified rice cereal, increase to 4–5 tbsp/d, rice, oatmeal, or barley
7	Add 1–2 tbsp/d of yellow, green, or orange vegetables
8	Add 1–2 tbsp/d of strained meats or egg yolk
12	Add whole cow's milk Egg whites Seafood Orange juice

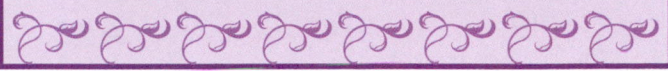

Box 33-1 Sample Menu for a 7-Month-Old Infant

A.M.	6 oz of milk
10 A.M.	2 oz of apple juice
Noon	1–2 tbsp of rice cereal
	1–2 tbsp of apple juice mixed in cereal
	6 oz of milk
3 P.M.	1–2 tbsp of banana
Dinner	1–2 tbsp of rice cereal
	1–2 tbsp of strained squash or pumpkin
Evening	6 oz of milk

Standing Committee of the British Pediatric Association, 1988). Menus and supplements should be provided to the caregivers to help them plan adequate nutrition. A sample menu for a 7-month-old infant is presented in Box 33-1.

NURSING IMPLICATIONS

The nurse needs to assess the particular nutritional needs of the infant. Prematurity, metabolic disorders, or sensitivities may require a specialized formula. The nurse also needs to assess the parent's choice of feeding. It is important to discuss this decision because the mother may have made the decision without adequate knowledge. Once these data have been gathered, the nurse may formulate nursing diagnoses regarding the infant's intake and the mother's knowledge and ability to feed the infant. Interventions may involve using a variety of techniques to deliver formula and trying different types of formula preparations. One of the most important interventions is to teach the mother to safely feed the infant, whether breast-feeding (covered in Chapter 30) or formula feeding. The nurse must monitor the infant feeding to ensure the infant is receiving adequate nutrition. The nurse can determine if the mother is able to prepare and properly feed her infant.

Web Activities

- Visit the websites of some of the formula manufacturers mentioned in this chapter. Compare the nutrient values they advertise for the different types of formula they offer, such as soy, nonfortified, and the like.

- Find a LaLeche League contact or support group in your geographic area by first visiting their web site.

- Go to www.tdh.state.tx.us/lactate/ position. Discuss your findings.

- What sources are available on the web that provide information about W.I.C.?

Key Concepts

- There are significant differences related to growth and development when comparing breast-fed and formula-fed infants.

- The nurse is expected to be able to assess adequate milk intake in the exclusively breast-fed infant during the first few weeks of life.

- Parents need to know how to assess early hunger cues in their newborn infant.

- Infant formulas are designed to meet the energy and nutrient requirements based on human milk as the gold standard or attend to particular needs such as prematurity and allergies.

Review Questions and Activities

1. Scientific evidence is emerging that relates the early diet of infants with long-term consequences. Which of the following are found in human milk but not in formula?
   a. Glucose
   b. DHA (docosahexaenoic acid)
   c. Sodium
   d. Magnesium

   The correct answer is b.

2. The milk protein whey is much easier to digest than is casein. In comparing human milk with bovine milk (the base for many formula preparations), the whey-to-casein ratio is different. Which ratio of whey to casein is best representative of human milk?
   a. 70:30
   b. 50:50
   c. 18:82
   d. 40:60

   The correct answer is a.

3. Which of the following statements about fat content in human milk is true?
 a. The fatty acid DHA is not dependent on maternal diet.
 b. Cholesterol levels are low in human milk.
 c. The fat content in human milk is consistent across feedings and individual mothers.
 d. Long-chain fatty acids in human milk have been related to cognitive function and vision.

The correct answer is d.

4. Infants need adequate carbohydrate intake for the following reasons with the exception of which?
 a. Energy for metabolism
 b. Energy for colonic bacteria
 c. Brain development
 d. Protein catabolism

The correct answer is d.

5. What are the fluid and electrolyte consequences of feeding an infant concentrated formula?

References

Allen, J. C., Keller, R. P., Archer, P., & Neville, M. C. (1991). Studies in human lactation: Milk composition and daily secretion rates of macronutrients in the first year of lactation. *American Journal of Clinical Nutrition, 54,* (1), 69–80.

American Academy of Pediatrics. (1985). *Pediatric nutrition handbook* (2nd ed.). Elk Grove Village, IL: American Academy of Pediatrics.

American Academy of Pediatrics. Committee on Nutrition. (1986). Fluoride supplementation. *Pediatrics, 77,* (5), 758.

American Academy of Pediatrics. Committee on Nutrition. (1989). Hypoallergenic infant formulas. *Pediatrics, 83,* 1068.

American Academy of Pediatrics. Committee on Nutrition. (1980). On the feeding of supplemental foods to infants. *Pediatrics, 65,* 1178.

American Academy of Pediatrics. Committee on Nutrition. (1983). Soy-protein formulas: Recommendations for use in infant feeding. *Pediatrics, 72,* (3), 359–363.

American Academy of Pediatrics. Committee on Nutrition. (1992). The use of whole cow's milk in infancy. *Pediatrics, 89,* 1105.

American Academy of Pediatrics. Committee on Nutrition. (1980). Vitamin and mineral supplemental needs in normal children in the United States. *Pediatrics, 66,* 1015.

American Academy of Pediatrics. Work Group on Breastfeeding. (1997). Breastfeeding and the use of human milk. *Pediatrics, 100,* (6), 1035–1039.

Anderson, R. R. (1992). Variations in major minerals of human milk during the first 6 months of lactation. *Nutrition Research, 12,* 701.

Barker, D. J. (1992). *Fetal and infant origins of adult disease.* London: British Medical Journal Publishing Groups.

Beaudry, M., Dufour, R., & Marcoux, S. (1995). Relation between infant feeding and infections during the first six months of life. *Journal of Pediatrics, 126,* 191–197.

Billeaud, C., Guillet, J., & Sandler, B. (1990). Gastric emptying in infants with or without gastro-oesophageal reflux according to the type of milk. *European Journal of Clinical Nutrition, 44,* 577–583.

Binns, H. J., Senturia, Y. D., LeBailly, S., Donovan, M., & Kaufer, C. K. (1996). Growth of Chicago area infants, 1985 through 1987. *Archives of Pediatric Adolescent Medicine, 150,* 842–849.

Bitman, J., Freed, L. M., Neville, M. C., Wood, D. L., Hamosh, P., & Hamosh, M. (1986). Lipid composition of prepartum human mammary secretion and postpartum milk. *Journal of Pediatric Gastroenterology & Nutrition, 5,* (4), 608–615.

Carlson, S. E., & Barness, L. A. (1996). Macronutrient requirements for growth. In W. A. Walker & J. B. Watkins (Eds.), (pp. 81–90). *Nutrition in Pediatrics* (2nd ed.). Boston, Massachusetts: Blackwell Science.

Carlson, S. E., Werkman, S. H., Rhodes, P. G., & Tolley, E. A. (1993). Visual-acuity development in healthy preterm infants: Effect of marine-oil supplementation. *American Journal of Clinical Nutrition, 58,* (1), 35–42.

Carlson, S. E., Werkman, S. H., & Tolley, E. A. (1996). Effect of long-chain n-3 fatty acid supplementation of visual acuity and growth of preterm infants with and without bronchopulmonary dysplasia. *American Journal of Clinical Nutrition, 63,* (5), 687–697.

Casey, C. E., Neville, M. C., & Hambidge, M. K. (1989). Studies in human lactation: Secretion of zinc, copper and manganese in human milk. *American Journal of Clinical Nutrition, 49,* 773–785.

Cumming, F. J. (1981). Effect of oral contraceptive use on ascorbic acid and vitamin A in lactation. *Journal of Human Nutrition, 35,* 249–256.

Davis, M. D., Savitz, D. A., & Graubard, B. I. (1988). Infant feeding and childhood cancer. *Lancet, 2,* (8607), 365–368.

de Onis, M., Garza, C., & Habicht, J. P. (1997). Time for a new growth reference. *Pediatrics, 100,* (5), e8.

Denne, S. C., & Kalhan, S. C. (1986). Glucose carbon recycling and oxidation in human newborns. *American Journal of Physiology, 251,* E71–E77.

Dewey, K. G., Cohen, R. J., Rivera, L., Canaguati, J., & Brown, K. H. (1996). Do exclusively breast-fed infants require extra protein? *Pediatric Research, 39,* 303–307.

Dewey, K. G., Heinig, M. J., & Nommsen-Rivers, L. A. (1995). Differences in morbidity between breast-fed and formula-fed infants. *Journal of Pediatrics, 126,* 696–702.

Dewey, K. G., Heinig, M. J., & Nommsen-Rivers, L. A., Peerson, J. M., & Lonnerdal, B. (1992). Growth of breast-fed and formula-fed infants from 0 to 18 months: The DARLING study. *Pediatrics, 89,* 1035–1041.

DiGiacomo, J. E. (1991). Carbohydrates: Metabolism and disorders. In W. W. Hay, Jr. (Ed.) (p. 93). *Neonatal nutrition and metabolism.* St. Louis, MO: Mosby-Year Book.

Dobbing, J., & Sands, J. (1973). The quantitative growth and development of the human brain. *Archives of Diseases of Children, 48,* 757–767.

European Society of Pediatric Gastroenterology and Nutrition [ESPGN], Committee on Nutrition. (1991). Comment on the content and composition of lipids in infant formulas. *Acta Paediatrica Scandinavia, 80,* 887.

Farquharson, J., Cockburn, F., Patrick, W. A., Jamieson, E. C., & Logan, R. W. (1992). Infant cerebral cortex phospholipid fatty-acid composition and diet. *Lancet, 340,* 810–813.

Foman, S. J. (1993). *Nutrition of normal infants.* St. Louis, MO: Mosby-Year Book.

Foman, S. J., & Ekshard, J. (1993). Fluoride. In S. J. Foman (Ed.) (pp. 299–310). *Nutrition of normal infants.* St. Louis, MO: Mosby-Year Book.

Food and Nutrition Board. (1989). *Recommended Dietary Allowances.* National Research Council. Commission on Life Sciences. Washington, DC: National Academy Press.

Garza, C., Frongillo, E. A., & Dewey, K. G. (1994). Implications of growth patterns of breast-fed infants for growth references. *Acta Paediatrica Supplement, 402,* 4–10.

Goodman, D. S. (1984). Vitamin A and retinoids in health and disease. *New England Journal of Medicine, 310,* 1023–1031.

Greer, F. R., Tsang, R. C., Levin, R. S., Searcy, J. E., Wu, R., & Steichen, J. J. (1982). Increasing serum calcium and magnesium concentrations in breastfed infants: Longitudinal studies of minerals in human milk and in sera of nursing mothers and their infants, *Journal of Pediatrics, 100,* (1), 59–64.

Guo, S., Roche, A. F., Foman, S. J., Nelsen, S. E., Chumlea, W. C., Rogers, R. R., Bamgartner, R. N., & Ziegler, E. E. (1991). Reference data on gains in weight and length during the first two years of life. *Journal of Pediatrics, 119,* 355–362.

Hahn-Zoric, M., Fulconis, F., Minoli, I., Moro, G., Carlsson, B., Bottiger, M., Raiha N., & Hansen, L. A. (1990). Antibody responses to parenteral and oral vaccines are impaired by conventional and low protein formulas as compared to breast-feeding. *Acta Paediatrica Scandinavia, 79,* 1137–1142.

Hamaker, B. R., Kirksey, A., & Borschel, M. W. (1990). Distribution of B-6 vitamins in human milk during a 24-h period after oral supplementation with different amounts of pyridoxine. *American Journal of Clinical Nutrition, 51,* 1062–1066.

Hambraeus, L. (1977). Proprietary milk versus human breast milk in infant feeding, a critical appraisal from the nutritional point of view. *Pediatric Clinics of North America, 24,* 7–35.

Hamill, P. B., Drizd, T. A., Johnson, C. L., Reed, R. B., Roche, A. F., & Moore, W. M. (1979). Physical growth: National Center for Health Statistics percentiles. *American Journal of Clinical Nutrition, 32,* 607–629.

Hamosh, M. (1988). Fat needs for term and preterm infants. In R. C. Tsang & B. L. Nichols (Eds.) (pp. 133–159). *Nutrition during infancy.* Philadelphia, PA: Hanley & Belfus.

Hamosh, M. (1991). Lipid metabolism. In W. W. Hay Jr. (Ed.) (p. 134). *Neonatal Nutrition and Metabolism.* St. Louis, MO: Mosby-Year Book.

Haschke, F., Vanura, H., Male, C., Owen, G., Pietschnig, B., Schuster, I., Krobath, E., & Huemer, C. (1993). Iron nutrition and growth of breast and formula-fed infants during the first 9 months of life. *Journal of Pediatric Gastroenterology and Nutrition, 16,* (2), 151–156.

Hitchcock, N. E., Gracey, M., & Gilmour, A. I. (1985). The growth of breastfed and artificially fed infants from birth to twelve months. *Acta Paediatrica Scandinavia, 74,* (2), 240–245.

Hornig, D. G., Moser, U., & Glatthaar, B. E. (1988). Ascorbic acid. In M. E. Shils & V. R. Young (Eds.) (pp. 417–435). *Modern nutrition in health and disease,* (7th ed.). Philadelphia, PA: Lea and Febiger.

Innis, S. M. (1992). Human milk and formula fatty acids. *Journal of Pediatrics, 120,* S56–S61.

Itani, O., & Tsang, R. C. (1991). Calcium, phosphorus, and magnesium in the newborn: Pathophysiology and management. In W.W. Hay (Ed.) (pp. 171–202). *Neonatal nutrition and metabolism.* St. Louis, MO: Mosby.

Jakobsson, I., Lindberg, T., Benediktsson, B., & Hansson, B. G. (1985). Dietary bovine beta-lactoglobulin is transferred to human milk. *Acta Paediatrica Scandinavia, 74,* (3), 342–345.

Jansson, L., Akesson, B., & Holmberg, L. (1981). Vitamin E and fatty acid composition of human milk. *American Journal of Clinical Nutrition, 34,* 8–13.

Jensen, R. G., & Jensen, G. L. (1992). Specialty lipids for infant nutrition. I. Milks and formulas. *Journal of Pediatric Gastroenterology and Nutrition, 1,* 232–245.

Joint Food and Agriculture Organization/World Health Organization Expert Committee. (1988). *Requirements of vitamin A, iron, folate, and vitamin B_{12}.* Geneva, Switzerland: Joint Food and Agriculture Organization/World Health Organization.

Jones, P. J., Winthrop, A. L., Schoeller, D. A., Filler, R. M., Swyer, P. R., Smith, J., & Heim, T. (1988). Evaluation of doubly labeled water for measuring energy expenditure during changing nutrition. *American Journal of Clinical Nutrition, 47,* (5), 799–804.

Jorgensen, M. H., Hernell, O., Lund, P., Holmer, G., & Michaelsen, K. F. (1996). Visual acuity and erythrocyte docosahexaenioc acid status in breast-fed and formula-fed term infants during the first four months of life. *Lipids, 31,* 99–105.

Kakai, R., Bwayo, I. A., Wamola, J. O., Ndinya-Achola, N. J. D., Anzala, A. O., & Plummer, F. A. (1995). Breastfeeding and immunity to intestinal infections. *East African Medical Journal, 72,* (3), 150–154.

Keane, V., Charney, J., Straus, J., & Roberts, K. (1988). Do solids help baby sleep through the night? *American Journal of Diseases of Children, 142,* 404–405.

Kelleher, J. (1991). Vitamin E and the immune response. *Proceedings of Nutrition Society, 50,* 245–249.

Kleinman, R. E., Bahna, S., Powell, G. F., & Sampson, H. A. (1991). Use of infant formulas in infants with cow milk allergy: A review and recommendations. *Pediatric Allergy Immunology, 2,* 146–155.

Klish, W. J. (1990). Special infant formulas. *Pediatrics in Review, 12,* (2), 55–62.

Koletzko, S., Sherman, P., Corey, M., Griffiths, A., & Smith, C. (1989). Role of infant feeding practices in development of Crohn's disease in childhood. *British Medical Journal, 298,* 1617–1618.

Lee, E. J., & Heiner, D. C. (1986). Allergy to cow milk: 1985. *Pediatrics in Review, 7,* (7), 195–203.

Lo, C. W., & Kleinman, R. E. (1996). Infant formula, past and future: Opportunities for improvement. *American Journal of Clinical Nutrition, 63,* 6465–6505.

Lonnerdal, B., Cederblad, A., Davidsson, L., & Sandstrom, B. (1984). The effect of individual components of soy formula and cows' milk formula on zinc bioavailability. *American Journal of Clinical Nutrition, 40,* 1064–1070.

Lucas, A., Morley, R., Cole, T. J., Gore, S. M., Lucas, P. J., Crowle, P., Pearse, R., Boon, A. J., & Powell, R. (1990). Early diet in preterm babies and developmental status at 18 months. *Lancet, 335,* 1477–1481.

Macknin, M. L., Medendorp, S. V., & Maier, M. C. (1989). Infant sleep and bedtime cereal. *American Journal of Diseases of Children, 143,* 1066–1068.

Makrides, M., Neumann, M. A., Byard, R. W., Simmer, K., & Gibson, R. A. (1994). Fatty acid composition of brain, retina, and erythrocytes in breast- and formula-fed infants. *American Journal of Clinical Nutrition, 60,* 189–194.

Makrides, M., Neumann, M. A., & Gibson, R. A. (1996). Effect of maternal docosahexaenoic acid (DHA) supplementation on breast milk composition. *European Journal of Clinical Nutrition, 50,* 352–357.

Makrides, M., Neumann, M. A., Simmer, K., Pater, J., & Gibson, R. A. (1995). Are long-chain polyunsaturated fatty acids essential nutrients in infancy? *Lancet, 345,* 1463–1468.

Mason, T., Rabinovich, C. E., Fredrickson, D. D., Amoroso, K., Reed, A. M., Stein, L. D., & Kredich, D. W. (1995). Breast feeding and the development of juvenile rheumatoid arthritis. *Journal of Rheumatology, 22,* (6), 1166–1170.

Mayer, E. J., Hamman, R. F., Gay, E. C., Lezotte, D. C., Savitz, D. A., & Klingensmith, G. J. (1988). Reduced risk of IDDM among breast-fed children: The Colorado IDDM Registry. *Diabetes, 37,* 1625–1632.

McCormick, D. B. (1989). Vitamin B_6. In M. E. Shils & V. Young (Eds.) (pp. 376–382). *Modern nutrition in health and disease.* (7th ed.). Philadelphia, PA: Lea and Febiger.

Miller, J. B., Bull, S., Miller, J., & McVeagh, P. (1994). The oligosaccharide composition of human milk: Temporal and individual variations in monosaccharide components. *Journal of Pediatric Gastroenterology and Nutrition, 19,* 371–376.

Mills, A., & Tyler, H. (1992). *Food and nutrient intakes of British infants aged 6–12 months.* London: HMSO.

Moran, J. R., & Greene, H. L. (1987). Nutritional biochemistry of water-soluble vitamins, In R. J. Grand, J. L. Sutphen, & W. H. Dietz, Jr. (Eds.) (pp. 51–67). *Pediatric nutrition: Theory and practice.* Boston, MA: Butterworths.

Morgan, B., Oppenheimer, J., & Winick, M. (1981). Effects of essential fatty acid deficiency during late gestation on brain N-acetyl-neuraminic acid metabolism and behaviour in the progeny. *British Journal of Nutrition, 46,* 223–230.

Motil, K. J., Sheng, H. P., Montandon, C. M., & Wong, W. W. (1996). Human milk protein does not limit growth of breast-fed infants. *Journal of Pediatric Gastroenterology and Nutrition, 24,* 10–17.

Mott, G. E., Jackson, E. M., DeLallo, L., Lewis, D. S., & McMahan, C. L. (1995). Differences in cholesterol metabolism in juvenile baboons are programmed by breast- versus formula-feeding. *Journal of Lipid Research, 36,* 299–307.

Nelson, S. E., Ziegler, E. E., Copeland, A. M., Edwards, B. B., & Foman, S. J. (1988). Lack of adverse reactions to iron-fortified formula. *Pediatrics, 81,* (3), 360–364.

Neu, J., Valentine, C. J., & Meetze, W. (1990). Scientific-based strategies for nutrition of the high risk low birth weight infant. *European Journal of Pediatrics, 150,* 2–13.

Nutrition Standing Committee of the British Pediatric Association. (1988). Vegetarian weaning. *Archives of Diseases of Children, 63,* 1286–1292.

Pabst, H. F., Spady, D. W. (1990). Effect of breast-feeding on antibody response to conjugate vaccine. *Lancet, 336,* 269–270.

Porro, E., Indinnimeo, L., Antognoni, G., Midulla, F., & Criscione, S. (1993). Early wheezing and breastfeeding. *Journal of Asthma, 30,* (1), 23–28.

Poskitt, E. M. (1983). Infant feeding. A review. *Human Nutrition Applied Nutrition, 37,* (4), 271–286.

Prasad, A. S. (1991). Discovery of human zinc deficiency and studies in an experimental human model. *American Journal of Clinical Nutrition, 53,* 403–412.

Prentice, A. M., Lucas, A., Vasquez-Velasquez, L., Davies, P. S., & Whitehead, R. G. (1988). Are current dietary guidelines for young children a prescription for overfeeding? *Lancet, 2,* (8619), 1066–1069.

Rasic, J. & Kurmann, J. (1983). Bifidobacteria and their role. *Experientia, 39,* (suppl), 22–50.

Roberts, S. B., Coward, W. A., Schlingenseipen, K-H., Nohria, V., & Lucas, A. (1986). Comparison of the doubly labeled water ($_2H_2{}^{18}O$) method with indirect calorimetry and a nutrient-balance study for simultaneous determination of energy expenditure, water intake, and metabolizable energy intake in preterm infants. *American Journal of Clinical Nutrition, 44,* (3), 315–322.

Saarinen, U. M., & Kajosaari, M. (1995). Breastfeeding as prophylaxis against atopic disease: Prospective follow-up study until 17 years old. *Lancet, 346,* (8982), 1065–1069.

Sabharwal H., Sjoblad S., & Lundblad A. (1991). Sialylated oligosaccharides in human milk and feces of preterm, full-term, and weaning infants. *Journal of Pediatric and Gastroenterology and Nutrition, 12,* 280–284.

Sampson, H. A., James, J. M., & Bernhisel-Broadbent, J. B. (1992). Safety of an amino-acid derived infant formula in children allergic to cow milk. *Pediatrics, 90,* (3), 463–465.

Sanders, T. A. B., & Reddy, S. (1992). The influence of a vegetarian diet on the fatty acid composition of human milk and the essential fatty acid status of the infant. *Journal of Pediatrics, 120,* S71–S77.

Savilahti, E., & Kuitunen, M. (1992). Allergenicity of cow milk proteins. *Journal of Pediatrics, 121,* S12–S20.

Scariati, P. D., Grummer-Strawn, L. M., & Fein, S. B. (1997). A longitudinal analysis of infant morbidity and the extent of breast-feeding in the United States. *Pediatrics, 99,* (6), e5.

Scheard, N. F. (1994). Iron deficiency and infant development. *Nutrition Reviews, 52,* (4), 137–146.

Schwartz, M. Z., & Maedak, K. (1985). Short bowel syndrome in infants and children. *Pediatric Clinics of North America, 32,* (5), 1265–1279.

Scientific Review Committee. (1990). *Nutrition recommendations. The report of the Scientific Review Committee,* Ottawa, Canadian Government Publishing Centre: Scientific Review Committee.

Shenai, J. R., Jhaveri, B. M., Reynolds, J. W., Huston, R. K., & Babson, S. G. (1981). Nutritional balance studies in very low birth weight infants: Role of soy formula. *Pediatrics, 67,* (5), 631–637.

Shu, X., Clemens, J., Zheng, W., Ying, D. M., Je, B. T., & Jin, F. (1995). Infant breastfeeding and the risk of childhood lymphoma and leukemia. *International Journal of Epidemiology, 24,* 27–32.

Sommer, A. (1994). Vitamin A: Its effect on childhood sight and life. *Nutrition Reviews, 52,* (2), 560–566.

Stordy, B. J., Redfern, A. M., & Morgan, J. B. (1995). Healthy eating for infants: Mothers' actions. *Acta Pediatrica, 84,* 733–741.

Stordy, B. J., Redfern, A. M., & Morgan, J. B. (1996). Weaning and weaning foods. In T. J. David (Ed.) (pp. 37–43). *Major controversies in infant nutrition*. International Congress and Symposium Series, 215, Royal Society of Medicine Press Limited.

Sultan,, H. Y., & Barker, D. J. P. (1994). Programming the baby. In Barker D. J. P., (Ed.) (pp. 14–36). *Mothers, babies and disease in later life*. London: British Medical Journal Publishing Group.

Uauy, R., & Hoffman, D. R. (1991). Essential fatty acid requirements for normal eye and brain development. *Seminars in Perinatology, 15,* 449–455.

U.S. Department of Health, Education and Welfare. (1977). *NCHS growth curves for children, birth–18 years.* (PHS 78-1650). Washington, DC: U.S. Government Printing Office.

van den Bogaard, C., van den Hoogen, H. J. M., Huygen, F. J. A., & van Weel C. (1993). Is the breast best for children with a family history of atopy? The relation between way of feeding and early childhood morbidity. *Family Medicine, 25,* 471–475.

Vanderhoof, J. A., Murray, N. D., Kaufman, S. S., Mack, D. R., Antonson, D. L., Corkins, M. R., Perry, D., & Kruger, R. (1997). Intolerance to protein hydrolysate infant formulas: an unrecognized cause of gastrointestinal symptoms in infants. *Journal of Pediatrics, 131,* 741–744.

Virtanen, S. M., Rasanen, L., Aro, A., Lindstrom, J., Sipploa, H., Lounamaa, R., Toivanen, L., Tuomilehto, J., & Akerblom, H. K. (1991). Infant feeding in Finnish children less than 7 years of age with newly diagnosed IDDM. Childhood Diabetes in Finland Study Group. *Diabetes Care, 14,* 415–417.

Waterlow, J. C. (1988). Basic concepts in the determination of nutritional requirements of normal infants. In R. C. Tsang & B. L. Nichols (Eds.) (pp. 1–19). *Nutrition during infancy*. Philadelphia, PA: Hanley & Belfus.

West, C. E., Rombout, J. H. W. M., Van der Zijpp, A. J., & Sijtsma, S. R. (1991). Vitamin A and immune function. *Proceedings of the Nutrition Society, 50,* (2), 251–262.

Wharton, B. A. & Scott, P. H. (1996). Distinctive aspects of metabolism and nutrition in infancy. *Clinical Biochemistry, 29,* (5), 419–428.

Widdowson, E. M. (1991). Growth and body composition in childhood. In E. Brunser, R. F. Carrazza, M. Gracey, B. L. Nichols, & J. Senterre (Eds.). *Clinical nutrition of the young child*. New York: Raven Press.

Wilcox, P. T., Florello, A. B., & Glick, P. L. (1993). Hypovolemic shock and intestinal ischemia: A preventable complication of incomplete formula labeling. *Journal of Pediatrics, 122,* (1), 103–104.

Wold, A. E., & Hanson, L. A. (1994). Defense factors in human milk. *Current Opinions in Gastroenterology, 10,* 652–658.

Wright, A. L., Holberg, C. J., Taussig, L. M., & Martinez, F. D. (1995). Relationship of infant feeding to recurrent wheezing at age 6 year. *Archives of Pediatric Adolescent Medicine, 149,* 758–763.

Suggested Readings

Dewey, K. G., Peerson, J. M., Brown, K. H., Krebs, N. F., Michaelsen, K. F., Persson, L. A., Salmenpera, L., Whitehead, R. G., Yeung, D. L., & the World Health Organization Working Group on Infant Growth. (1995). Growth of breast-fed infants deviates from current reference data: A pooled analysis of US, Canadian, and European data sets. *Pediatrics, 96,* (3), 495–503.

Gerstein, H. C. (1994). Cow's milk exposure and type I diabetes mellitus. *Diabetes Care, 17,* 13–19.

Kunz, C., & Lönnerdal, B. (1992). Re-evaluation of whey protein/casein ratio of human milk. *Acta Paediatrica Scandinavia, 81,* (2), 107–112.

Lawrence, R. A. (1999). *Breastfeeding: A guide for the medical profession*. (5th ed.). St. Louis, MO: C.V. Mosby.

Mohrbacher, N., & Stock, J. (1997). *La Leche League international's breastfeeding answer book*. LLLI, Schaumburg, IL: La Leche League International.

Riordan, J., & Auerbach, K. G. (1999). *Breastfeeding and human lactation*. (2nd ed.). Boston, MA: Jones & Bartlett Publishers.

Williams, C. P. (Ed.). (1998). *Pediatric manual of clinical dietetics*. Chicago, IL: American Dietetic Association.

Working Group on Cow's Milk and Diabetes Mellitus. (1994). American Academy of Pediatrics. Infant feeding practices and their possible relationship to the etiology of diabetes mellitus. *Pediatrics, 94,* 752–754.

World Health Organization Working Group on Infant Growth. (1995). An evaluation of infant growth. *Bulletin WHO, 73,* 165–174.

Resources

The Academy of Breastfeeding Medicine, P.O. Box 15945-284, Lenexa, KS 66285-5945, 913-541-9077, www.bfmed.org

American Dietetic Association, 216 W. Jackson Boulevard, Chicago, IL 60606-6995, 312-899-0040, www.eatright.org

Doulas of North America, 1100 23rd Avenue East, Seattle, WA 98112, 206-324-5440, www.dona.com

International Lactation Consultant Association, 4101 Lake Boone Trail, Suite 201, Raleigh, NC 27607, 919-787-5181, www.ilca.org

La Leche League International, 1400 N. Meacham Road, Schaumburg, IL 60173, 847-519-7730, www.lalecheleague.org

National Guideline Clearinghouse, 5200 Butler Pike, Plymouth Meeting, PA 19462, www.guideline.gov

CHAPTER 34

Newborns at Risk Related to Birth Weight and Premature Delivery

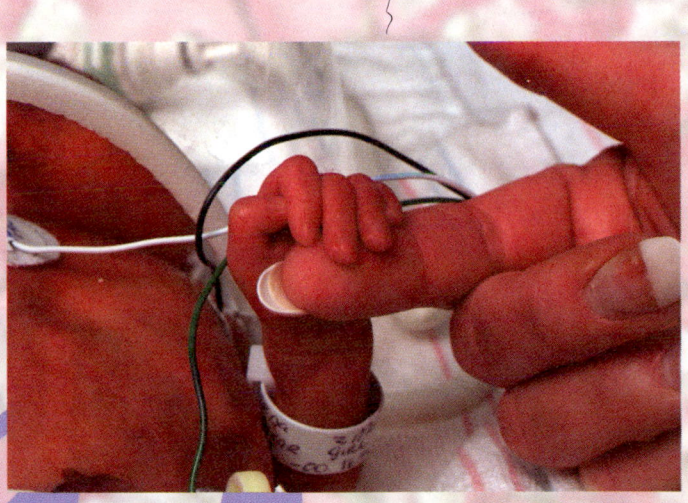

Nursing care of infants who are at risk for health problems related to low or high birth weight or to prematurity present unique nursing challenges. Although advances in care have improved survival, these infants are medically fragile. To work with these fragile infants, the nurse must be an advocate for neonates who cannot speak for themselves. Caring for these infants means being sensitive to the family unit as a whole. Use the following questions to examine your personal feelings about issues that may affect your response to the infant and family.

- *How do I feel about caring for an infant with potential long-term morbidity related to complications of prematurity?*

- *How can I facilitate the development of parent-infant bonding when an infant is severely ill?*

- *How do I feel about caring for an infant who has extremely low birth weight?*

- *Which ethical considerations should be considered in caring for a premature infant?*

- *How small is too small?*

Key Terms

Air-block syndrome
Apnea
Asymmetric intrauterine growth restriction
Auditory brain evoked response
Bilirubin
Bronchopulmonary dysplasia (BPD)
Containment
Disseminated intravascular coagulation (DIC)
Dysmotility
Extremely low birthweight (ELBW)
Gastroesophageal reflux (GER)

Gavage feeding
Hyaline membrane disease (HMD)
Hyperglycemia
Hyperkalemia
Hypernatremia
Hypoglycemia
Hypokalemia
Hyponatremia
Insensible water loss (IWL)
Intrauterine growth restriction (IUGR)
Intraventricular hemorrhage (IVH)
Jaundice
Large for gestational age (LGA)

Low birth weight (LBW)
Necrotizing enterocolitis (NEC)
Nephrocalcinosis
Neutropenia
Opsonization
Osteopenia
Patent ductus arteriosus (PDA)
Perinatal asphyxia profound
Periventricular leukomalacia (PVL)
Persistent pulmonary hypertension in the newborn (PPHN)
Plethora
Pneumatosis intestinalis

Prematurity
Preterm birth
Postconception age
Respiratory distress syndrome (RDS)
Retinopathy of prematurity (ROP)
Short bowel syndrome
Small for gestational age (SGA)
Symmetric intrauterine growth restriction
Total parenteral nutrition (TPN)
Ventricular peritoneal shunt (VPS)
Very low birth weight (VLBW)

Competencies

Upon completion of this chapter, the reader should be able to:

1. Compare the clinical characteristics of the infant who is small for gestational age with those of the premature infant.

2. List the problems that frequently affect the preterm infant.

3. Develop a plan of care for the infant who is small for gestational age.

4. Develop a plan of care for the infant who is large for gestational age.

5. Discuss parental challenges related to caring for their premature infant.

6. Illustrate the techniques and strategies that can be used to facilitate parent-infant bonding.

7. Discuss alternative care modalities for the premature infant.

8. Understand the ethical issues that may arise when providing care for the premature infant.

9. Review the long-term medical needs of infants who are small for gestational age or premature.

10. Discuss the rationale for thorough discharge planning to meet the needs of these infants.

This chapter highlights infants who are at risk as a result of low birth weight (LBW), birth weight higher than expected for a given gestational age, and prematurity. Infants who are born at birth weights below or above normal for their **postconceptional age** (age from conception described in weeks) are referred to as having intrauterine growth restriction (IUGR), being small for gestational age (SGA), or being large for gestational age (LGA). These conditions place the infant at risk for health problems, particularly when the infant also is premature. Although alterations in birth weight and prematurity may affect the same infant, the concepts are discussed separately for clarity.

THE SMALL FOR GESTATIONAL AGE INFANT

Infants termed **small for gestational age (SGA)** are those whose birth weight is lower than expected for the infant's gestational age. These infants are at high risk for multiple problems, including growth delays, feeding problems, thermoregulatory problems, respiratory problems, developmental delays, vision disturbances, and hearing impairment. The potential also exists for disruption of parent-infant bonding (Bernstein, Heimler, & Sasidharan, 1998). Nurses caring for mothers and their newborns should understand the unique challenges these infants and their families face.

Low birth weight often is linked to prematurity (post-conceptual age of less than 37 weeks). Infants who are premature have a number of risk factors related to gestational age (Figure 34-1). They also may have risks associated with birth weight that have long-term effects on the infant's health and the family unit. A group of infants at risk for problems separate from and often in conjunction with prematurity are those who are SGA. The infant who is SGA has not met the expected growth parameters for the gestational age at birth. The term implies that some intrinsic or extrinsic factor has affected the ability of the fetus to meet usual growth parameters.

It is important to recognize that the infant who is SGA is at risk for stillbirth, perinatal morbidity, and adverse effects in adulthood (Gardosi, 1997). These infants often require early delivery secondary to a hostile uterine environment. The fetus is compromised by deprivation of adequate nutrients and oxygen and is at risk for intrauterine death (Schaap et al., 1997).

The term **low birth weight (LBW)** can be defined as a birth weight less than 2,500 g. Each year, 20 million term infants are born with birth weights under 2,500 g (de Onis, Blossner, & Villar, 1998). The infant who is SGA has not achieved his genetic growth potential (Goldenberg & Cliver, 1997). Other terms used interchangeably with SGA are dysmaturity, fetal growth restriction (FGR), and intrauterine growth restriction (IUGR).

Intrauterine Growth Restriction

The term **intrauterine growth restriction (IUGR)** generally is reserved for infants who are at less than the 10th percentile at birth on standardized graphs in weight, length, and head circumference. Each year 30 million newborns are born who have growth restriction (de Onis, Blossner, & Villar, 1998). IUGR is classified as symmetric and asymmetric.

Symmetric Intrauterine Growth Restriction

The term **symmetric IUGR** is used when the measurements of the head, weight, and length are less than the 10th percentile. Symmetric IUGR implies that the cause of the growth restriction occurred early in pregnancy and was genetic or intrinsic in nature. Symmetric IUGR is more likely to result from an intrinsic cause, that is, something that affects the fetus from within and starts early in gestation. A poor prognosis is associated with major chromosomal disorders and congenital infection.

Asymmetric Intrauterine Growth Restriction

The term **asymmetric IUGR** is used when the measurements of the head circumference and length are in a higher percentile than is the measurement for weight. This growth pattern occurs later in pregnancy than does symmetric IUGR and may be caused by placental insufficiency, maternal malnutrition, or other extrinsic factors. Extrinsic factors are those that affect the fetus from the outside, such as maternal hypertension and low caloric intake. Outcomes are better in infants who have asymmetric IUGR compared with those who have symmetric IUGR. Asymmetric IUGR is more likely to be caused by extrinsic factors than is symmetric IUGR.

Factors Associated with Fetal Growth Restriction

A number of factors may affect fetal growth, including fetal, maternal, and placental factors. Some of these factors

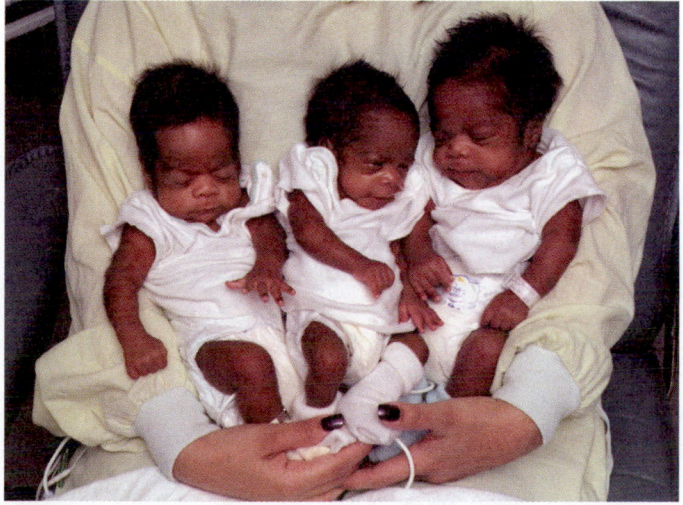

Figure 34-1 These male triplets were delivered before 37 weeks' gestation; now, at 6 weeks of age, they are each showing different rates of growth and weight gain.

are listed in the Nursing Alert. FGR may affect perinatal mortality and the infant's short and long-term morbidity.

Fetal Factors

Fetal factors are those that affect the genetic growth potential of the fetus. This potential may be affected by normal variations, such as race and gender. Multiple gestation also is associated with FGR (Goldenberg & Cliver, 1997; Sherear & Devon, 1997).

Infants with chromosomal anomalies such as trisomy 13 (Patau syndrome), trisomy 18 (Edward syndrome), trisomy 21 (Down syndrome) may be SGA. Congenital malformations such as anencephaly, gastrointestinal (GI) atresia, renal agenesis, and some cardiovascular defects may be implicated in LBW. Congenital infection may be implicated in infants who are SGA. Rubella may cause damage during organogenesis and may cause a decrease in cell number. Cytomegalovirus is associated with cytolysis and localized necrosis (Naeye, 1967). Inborn errors of metabolism, such as transient neonatal diabetes, galactosemia, and phenylketonuria, are associated with small fetal size.

Maternal Factors

Maternal factors include maternal hypoxemia, such as sickle cell disease, respiratory disease, cardiovascular disease, and living in a high-altitude environment. Other maternal factors include short stature, young maternal age, low socioeconomic status, primiparity, grand multiparity, and low pregnancy weight. Maternal exposure to teratogenic agents, such as alcohol, cigarette smoke, and anticonvulsant medications also may be implicated.

Placental Factors

Placental insufficiency is the leading cause of infants who are SGA because of the delivery of inadequate nutrients for appropriate fetal growth. Other physical attributes of the placenta and placental circulation also may affect fetal growth. Multiple infarcts, aberrant cord insertions, and small placental size may affect fetal growth.

Complications Associated with the SGA Infant

Infants who are SGA are at risk for many problems that range from perinatal asphyxia to hypoglycemia. Knowing that an infant is SGA can help anticipate, prevent, or provide early intervention for problems the infant may face. To determine whether an infant is at risk for the complications of the SGA infant the gestational age must be determined.

Assessment

Information from ultrasonography can be useful in establishing the predelivery diagnosis of IUGR. The fetal biparietal diameter, abdominal circumference, and femur length provide the obstetrician with information to determine appropriate fetal growth. Information from ultrasonography regarding placental morphology and amniotic fluid assessment and Doppler evaluation of blood flow through the umbilical vessels may contribute to determining the cause of the FGR and assessing the well-being of the fetus before delivery. Fetal lung maturity studies may identify potential respiratory problems at birth.

At birth the infant must be weighed and measured carefully. These measurements are then used to plot the infants' growth against standardized charts. The Colorado Growth Chart frequently is used in the United States (Battaglia & Lubchenco, 1967). Calculating the ponderal index is another way of determining appropriate growth (weight in grams divided by length to the third power). When the gestational age is in question the Ballard or New Ballard Score (Figure 34-2), which has been expanded to include extremely premature infants, may be used to help determine gestational age.

Care

Once the infant has been determined to be SGA, steps may be taken to anticipate problems and provide early intervention. Complications may include prematurity, birth asphyxia or birth depression, thermal instability, metabolic imbalances, and hematologic concerns. Birth depression encompasses infants who have low HR at birth. These infants may require intervention from caregivers to establish adequate HR an respirations.

At birth the infant is at risk for hypoxia from perinatal asphyxia profound, persistent pulmonary hypertension, and meconium aspiration syndrome. **Perinatal asphyxia profound** is metabolic acidosis at birth associated with

---

Nursing Alert

POTENTIAL COMPLICATIONS ASSOCIATED WITH FETAL GROWTH RESTRICTION

- Hypoxia
- Persistent pulmonary hypertension
- Meconium aspiration syndrome
- Hypothermia
- Hypoglycemia
- Hypocalcemia
- Polycythemia
- Hyperviscosity

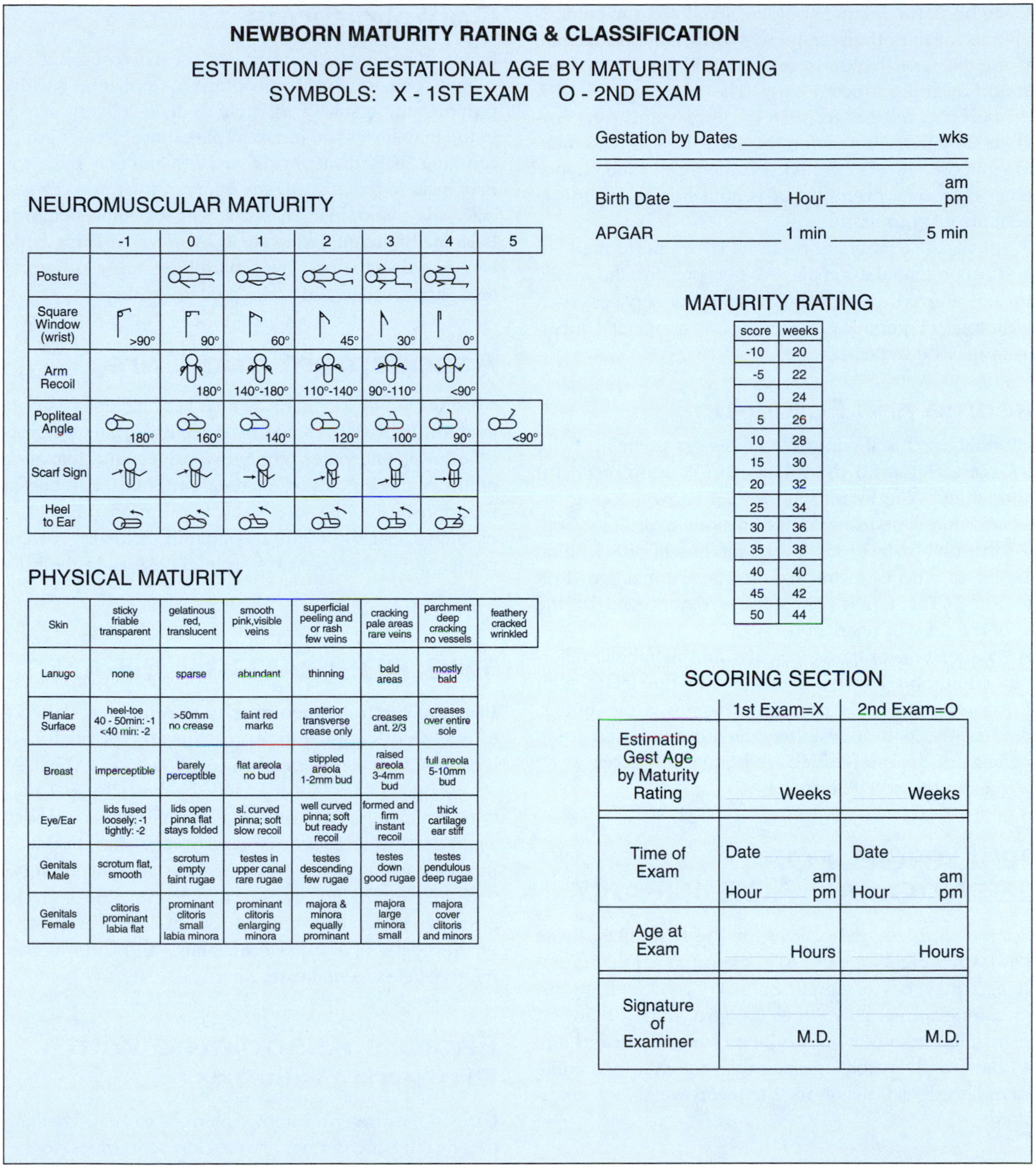

NEWBORN MATURITY RATING & CLASSIFICATION

ESTIMATION OF GESTATIONAL AGE BY MATURITY RATING
SYMBOLS: X - 1ST EXAM   O - 2ND EXAM

Gestation by Dates _____ wks

Birth Date _____ Hour _____ am / pm

APGAR _____ 1 min _____ 5 min

NEUROMUSCULAR MATURITY

	-1	0	1	2	3	4	5
Posture							
Square Window (wrist)	>90°	90°	60°	45°	30°	0°	
Arm Recoil		180°	140°-180°	110°-140°	90°-110°	<90°	
Popliteal Angle	180°	160°	140°	120°	100°	90°	<90°
Scarf Sign							
Heel to Ear							

PHYSICAL MATURITY

Skin	sticky friable transparent	gelatinous red, translucent	smooth pink, visible veins	superficial peeling and or rash few veins	cracking pale areas rare veins	parchment deep cracking no vessels	feathery cracked wrinkled
Lanugo	none	sparse	abundant	thinning	bald areas	mostly bald	
Planiar Surface	heel-toe 40 - 50min: -1 <40 min: -2	>50mm no crease	faint red marks	anterior transverse crease only	creases ant. 2/3	creases over entire sole	
Breast	imperceptible	barely perceptible	flat areola no bud	stippled areola 1-2mm bud	raised areola 3-4mm bud	full areola 5-10mm bud	
Eye/Ear	lids fused loosely: -1 tightly: -2	lids open pinna flat stays folded	sl. curved pinna; soft slow recoil	well curved pinna; soft but ready recoil	formed and firm instant recoil	thick cartilage ear stiff	
Genitals Male	scrotum flat, smooth	scrotum empty faint rugae	testes in upper canal rare rugae	testes descending few rugae	testes down good rugae	testes pendulous deep rugae	
Genitals Female	clitoris prominant labia flat	prominant clitoris small labia minora	prominant clitoris enlarging minora	majora & minora equally prominant	majora large minora small	majora cover clitoris and minors	

MATURITY RATING

score	weeks
-10	20
-5	22
0	24
5	26
10	28
15	30
20	32
25	34
30	36
35	38
40	40
45	42
50	44

SCORING SECTION

	1st Exam=X	2nd Exam=O
Estimating Gest Age by Maturity Rating	Weeks	Weeks
Time of Exam	Date _____ Hour _____ am/pm	Date _____ Hour _____ am/pm
Age at Exam	Hours	Hours
Signature of Examiner	M.D.	M.D.

Figure 34-2 New Ballard Score. Courtesy of Mead Johnson Nutritionals.

Apgar scores of 3 or less that persist after 5 minutes, multi-system organ dysfunction, and neurologic manifestations. **Persistent pulmonary hypertension in the newborn (PPHN)** is a condition in which abnormally elevated vascular pressures result in continuation of flow through fetal blood pathways such as the ductus arteriosus and foramen ovale. These infants should be delivered in a location where immediate access to resuscitation equipment and personnel who are expert in the resuscitation of high-risk newborns are available.

Once born, the infant should be stabilized and complications such as hypothermia, hypoglycemia, hypocalcemia, polycythemia, and hyperviscosity should be anticipated, screened for, and corrected early. The infant who is SGA should be observed for respiratory distress and care rendered as needed. Prevention of heat loss is essential. Blood glucose levels should be checked and hypoglycemia corrected promptly. A central hematocrit measurement also is important.

A physical examination should be performed to screen for congenital anomalies. When present, the family should be referred to appropriate specialty services, such as cardiology or genetics. Screening for congenital infection also may be indicated.

Outcome and Follow-up

The mortality risk is significantly higher for the infant who is SGA compared with the infant who is appropriate for gestational age. The infant who is SGA shows more gross motor and minor neurologic dysfunctions over time. Cognitive function also is lower for the infant who is SGA than for the infant who is appropriate for gestational age (Kok et al., 1998). The infant's outcome is determined by the cause of the growth restriction.

An association of cardiovascular and metabolic disorders in adulthood has been made with the infant with IUGR. More research is needed to improve the understanding of the pathophysiology, background, and long-term effects of the intrauterine environment (Barker, 1997; Westgren, Lingman, & Persson, 1997).

THE LARGE FOR GESTATIONAL AGE INFANT

In addition to infants who have low birth weights, those born at birth weights greater than expected for that gestational age may be at significant risk for complications. These complications may occur in utero, during delivery, or postnatally. Infants who are **large for gestational age (LGA)** have birth weights greater than the 90th percentile or 2 standard deviations above the mean weight for gestational age.

Associated Factors

Infants who are LGA are associated with diabetic mothers, are born to parents who are large, congenital syndromes such as Beckwith-Wiedemann syndrome or fetal complications such as hydrops fetalis. Mothers who have diabetes or Beckwith-Wiedemann syndrome produce hyperinsulinemic states in utero, thereby causing increased glucose levels in the fetal environment and resulting in increased weight gain by the fetus.

Complications

Infants who are LGA are at risk for macrosomatia and resultant cephalopelvic disproportion. Cephalopelvic disproportion may result in difficult vaginal delivery secondary to the inability of the infant to pass through the birth canal, resulting in birth asphyxia or birth trauma. Birth trauma may include brachial plexus injury, a fractured clavicle, facial palsy, shoulder dystocia, or subdural hemorrhage. Postnatally, infants who are LGA are at risk for hypoglycemia, polycythemia, hyperbilirubinemia, respiratory distress, and cardiac and congenital anomalies.

Assessment and Care

Nursing care of the infant who is LGA includes assessment for birth injury or respiratory difficulty, monitoring of glucose levels and other laboratory values, and management of any of these potential medical problems. Parents should be apprised of the potential complications and informed of changes in the infant's condition. Allowing parents to participate in the care of their infant assists in the bonding process.

THE PREMATURE INFANT

Preterm birth or **prematurity** is defined as delivery before 37 weeks' gestation. Approximately 8% of all births in the United States are preterm (AAP, ACOG, 1997).

Neonatal care has changed dramatically over the past two decades. In the 1980s, viability in infants was defined as those born at 28 weeks' gestation or later. In the 1990s, infants born at 24 to 25 weeks' gestation were surviving with less morbidity. These changes are due to technical advances in ventilatory management, better understanding of the needs of the preterm infant, and improvement in neurodevelopmental care.

Factors Associated with Preterm Delivery

Care of the preterm infant continues to be a challenge in the health care arena. Prematurity continues to be the leading cause of perinatal mortality in the United States (AAP, 1999). Many risk factors are associated with preterm labor and delivery. Some of these risk factors can be attributed to previous maternal history of a preterm birth, a spontaneous abortion, an incompetent cervix, or other uterine anomalies. Factors that occur during the pregnancy that put a woman at risk for preterm labor and delivery include multiple gestation (Figure 34-3), infection, premature rupture of membranes, adolescent pregnancy, polyhydramnios, and oligohydramnios (AAP, 2000).

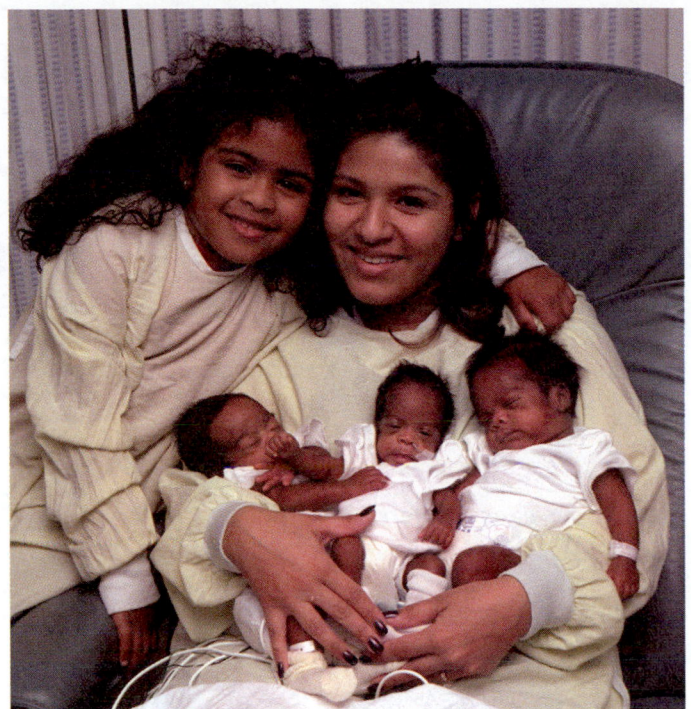

Figure 34-3 Multiple gestation is one risk factor for preterm delivery.

The lack of prenatal care also plays a role in preterm labor and delivery. Maternal habits, such as cigarette smoking, substance abuse, and poor diet, and social status also are areas in which we can change and improve outcomes.

Assessment of the Preterm Infant

Assessment of the high-risk infant is an important role of the bedside nurse. A systematic approach to the physical assessment of high-risk infants allows the neonatal nurse to determine the infant's condition and approximate gestational age quickly and efficiently. Continued evaluation reveals subtle changes that allow the caregiver to anticipate and manage problems early. It is important to determine the gestational age of the infant because doing so will provide valuable information in interpreting the physical examination and planning age-appropriate care. The physical examination also is important in the assessment of a premature infant. A careful head-to-toe assessment is important to determine the infant's condition. Ongoing observation allows the nurse to quickly recognize problems before they compromise the infant's well-being.

Gestational Age Assessment

Knowing the infant's gestational age assists the caregiver in anticipating problems that may occur after delivery. Gestational age must be considered in evaluating posture

muscle tone. Many details go into the assessment of an infant's gestational age. The results of the infant's examination may be compared with charts developed by Dubowitz and Ballard, who use a scoring sheet to evaluate neurologic characteristics, such as posture, and physical characteristics, such as skin thickness, to estimate the infant's gestational age (Ballard et al., 1991).

Neurologic Assessment

Neurologic assessment of the newborn includes evaluation of tone, activity, and reflexes. Tone develops by way of a caudalcephalic route. Knowing how reflexes mature with progressing gestational age can aid the nurse in developing a plan of care. For example, an infant's sucking reflex is evident at about 32 weeks postconception; however, a coordinated suck-swallow-breath pattern may not develop until about 34 weeks postconception. Encouraging nonnutritive sucking at 32 weeks postconception and introducing oral feedings at about 34 weeks postconception would be included in the care plan of an infant born at less than 32 weeks' gestation.

Physical Characteristics

The skin of a premature infant can be a clue to gestational age. Thin gelatinous skin is associated with infants who are less than 26 weeks' gestation. The skin becomes thicker and less translucent with increased gestational age. The presence or absence of lanugo, plantar creases, breast tissue, and ear cartilage provides other clues to the infant's gestational age (Figure 34-4). Eyes are fused before 24 weeks' gestation. Eyelashes and eyebrows appear at 20 to 23 weeks' gestation. Hair is fine and wooly and sticks together at 28 to 34 weeks' gestation. Before 28 weeks' gestation, the preterm female infant may have a prominent

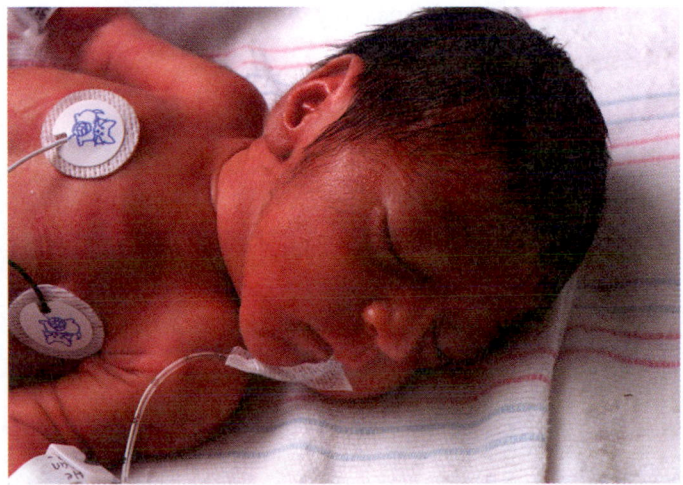

Figure 34-4 This preterm infant still has excess hair on the face, back, and arms.

REFLECTIONS FROM A NURSE

"As I wheeled the neonatal transport incubator into the recovery room I mentally prepared myself. I knew it would be a difficult first meeting for this baby and her mother. The mother had been in the hospital for 3 weeks now because of premature labor. It had seemed that the contractions were controlled, at least until tonight. The delivery was very fast; Dad didn't even have time to get to the hospital before the baby was born.

The baby was born at just 26 weeks' gestation, but smaller than expected. So many problems can affect a baby this size. We had to take her to the stabilization area right away; there was no time to show her to her mother. She needed to be warmed, to get oxygen, to be placed on a ventilator, to have IV access—these things are critical in the first minutes of a premature infant's life.

As I looked down at the baby I sighed. Even to me she looked tiny and helpless. A tube in her mouth was secured with tape, almost obscuring her face. Wires attached to electrodes were attached to her chest; a temperature probe was taped to her abdomen. An umbilical artery line for monitoring blood pressure and drawing blood for

laboratory tests and an umbilical venous line for administering intravenous fluids and medications were inserted into her umbilical cord and secured with tape. She was curled into the fetal position in a nest of blankets. The constant whoosh of the ventilator and beep of the cardiac monitor accompanied us.

I rolled the incubator to the mother's bedside and positioned it next to the mother's bed. Tears rolled down her face.

'She's so tiny,' she said.

'What's her name?' I asked.

'Sara,' she answered.

'Would you like to touch Sara?' I offered.

'I'm afraid I will hurt her,' she cried.

After assuring the mother that she would not hurt the infant and that in fact, Sara needed her touch, the mother agreed to touch her. I helped the mother to place her hand though the incubator porthole and touch Sara's hand. Sara's tiny fingers curled around her mother's finger. I saw a tiny smile shine through the tears, the first step of a long journey."

---

clitoris with small separated labia and the preterm male infant will have nondescended testes. Preterm males are prone to develop hydrocele and inguinal hernias and should be evaluated for these regularly.

Physical Assessment

The physical examination provides an opportunity for early recognition of problems. The nurse must be skilled in assessing the newborn for nonverbal cues. An experienced nurse can process multiple observations while examining individual systems. The nurse should develop a consistent approach to examination of the neonate that

covers all major systems. The sequence of the examination should be from least invasive to most invasive, for instance, observation would precede palpation.

A basic physical examination of a preterm infant should include the infant's color and skin condition. The baby's posture, activity, and state of arousal indicate his neurologic status. The respiratory rate and effort, heart rate, and presence or absence of murmurs, pulses, and perfusion are important information in assessing the infant's respiratory and cardiovascular status. The presence or absence of abdominal distension and bowel sounds are indicative of feeding tolerance. Prompt attention should be given to abnormalities observed during assessment.

Examination techniques used with the premature infant include inspection, auscultation, palpation, and transillumination. Observation requires patience and is an important skill to cultivate. Auscultation includes listening to sounds produced by the body that can be heard with the naked ear or a stethoscope. Palpation is examining by touch. Transillumination requires use of an instrument with an intense but cool light source. The light is placed against the infant's skin. Illuminated skin indicates the presence of air or fluid rather than solid matter.

When examining an infant, timing is important. The caregiver must know the infant's baseline values to evaluate changes in condition. The infant must be warm and positioned comfortably. The examination should be clustered with other caregiving activities to provide adequate rest intervals between care and before feedings.

Continuity of care is important in recognizing subtle changes in the infant's physical examination. Parents who visit frequently may be the first to note that something is different about their baby, and their observations should be viewed as important contributions to the evaluation database.

Because all systems are immature, premature infants are at risk for a number of complications. A head-to-toe physical examination includes a number of observations that may attest to the fact that the infant is immature. These observation in and of themselves may not be concerning. Putting a number of observations together, however, may indicate the need to assess an infant more closely for a specific condition common to premature infants. Complications commonly associated with premature infants are discussed in the systems review that follows.

Review of Systems

Potential alterations associated with prematurity are discussed by body system.

Cardiovascular System

The premature infant is at risk for a number of problems associated with the cardiovascular system. Two common problems encountered in the preterm infant are patent ductus arteriosus (PDA) and systemic hypotension.

Patent Ductus Arteriosus

A **patent ductus arteriosus (PDA)** results from the failure of the ductus arteriosus to close or from its reopening after closure. The ductus arteriosus is an artery that extends from the pulmonary artery to the aorta. It is part of the fetal circulation, allowing blood to bypass the lungs in utero. The ductus normally closes after birth. When the ductus arteriosus remains open after birth, a left to right shunt through the ductus may occur, which may lead to pulmonary edema. PDA with left to right shunt is associated with necrotizing enterocolitis (NEC), bronchopulmonary dysplasia, and intraventricular hemorrhage (IVC) (Davis et al., 1995).

A PDA is common in premature infants. The more premature an infant is, the more likely it is the infant will have a PDA. If left untreated the infant may require extended oxygen and ventilator therapy and may have difficulty gaining weight.

The nurse caring for a premature infant should be aware of the risk of a PDA and monitor the infant for symptoms. These symptoms include a murmur best heard in the second or third intercostal space at the left sternal border, a hyperactive pericardium, bounding peripheral pulses, and a widened pulse pressure.

A PDA is diagnosed by echocardiography. Treatment may be surgical ligation, or closure may be attempted using a prostaglandin inhibitor. The prostaglandin inhibitor commonly used is indomethacin (Davis et al., 1995).

Hypotension

Hypotension is a complication often seen in premature infants. It usually is associated with vasodilation after rapid rewarming or a response to an illness, such as sepsis. Morphine used for sedation may produce hypotension in the preterm infant. Hypotension is seen with hypovolemia after abruptio placenta, cord accidents, and internal bleeding. Hypotension is seen secondary to fluid shifts from intravascular to extravascular spaces in infants who have sepsis or who have had surgery. Cord accidents can occur due to rupture of cord, cord strippers, cutting without clamping, or knot in the end. Symptoms include tachycardia, pallor, poor capillary refill, poor peripheral pulses, and poor urine output. Treatment may be with volume expansion using 5% normal saline, albumin, or blood products. Vasopressor may be used to maintain the blood pressure at levels that will maintain renal perfusion and circulation.

Central Nervous System

The premature infant is at risk for a number of problems associated with the neurologic system. Common problems associated with prematurity are intraventricular hemorrhage, posthemorrhagic hydrocephalus, Periventricular leukomalacia (PVL), developmental delays, and hearing impairment.

Intraventricular Hemorrhage

An **intraventricular hemorrhage (IVH)** is an intracranial hemorrhage frequently associated with prematurity. The more premature the infant, the more likely it is the infant will have an IVH. The bleeding usually occurs within the first 3 days of life.

Box 34-1 Classification of IVH

Grade I: Subependymal germinal matrix hemorrhage

Grade II: Intraventricular extension without ventricular dilation

Grade III: Intraventricular extension with ventricular dilation

Grade IV: Intraventricular and intraparenchymal hemorrhage

The site of origin frequently is the subependymal germinal matrix (Bernstein, Heimler, & Sasidharan, 1998). This area of the brain is rich in capillary blood vessels. As the infant grows, the number of blood vessels decreases in size until about 36 weeks' gestation. The premature infant's body is unable to regulate blood flow in this area. Thus, changes in blood flow related to asphyxia, trauma, hypercarbia, or rapid fluid infusion may place a strain on the delicate vessels, causing them to rupture and bleed. Clinical factors associated with IVH are listed in the Nursing Alert.

Hypertension has been implicated as a factor in IVH. Sudden increases in blood pressure are associated with caregiving, such as suctioning, performing abdominal examinations, lumbar puncture, and starting an intravenous (IV) infusion. Rapid increases in blood pressure also may occur after correction of hypotension. The increased blood pressure may stress the vessel walls in the germinal matrix areas of the ventricles of premature infants.

Prevention of preterm delivery and use of antenatal steroids may reduce the incidence of IVH. Prompt resuscitation in the delivery room is an important factor in the prevention of IVH. Premature infants should be delivered in a location that has equipment and personnel available for expert resuscitation. The nurse caring for an infant who is at risk for IVH should take care to avoid activities that are likely to provoke rapid or excessive changes in the infant's blood pressure. Dim lighting, low noise levels, minimal handling, and care in the administration of fluids and medications are important. The head of the bed should be slightly elevated; the legs of the infant should not be raised higher than the head.

Infants who are at risk for IVH should be monitored for symptoms. These symptoms include a sudden deterioration in condition, oxygen desaturation, hypotension, bulging anterior fontanel, and hyperglycemia.

Diagnosis of IVH generally is made with portable ultrasonography using the anterior fontanel as a viewing window. The degree and extent of the IVH are classified from Grades I to IV. The grade describes the location and size of the bleed (Box 34-1). No increase in morbidity or mortality is associated with a Grade I or II IVH. Grade III may be associated with severe developmental delay. Infants with Grade IV are at high risk for death or severe developmental delay.

Intraventricular hemorrhage occurs in 15% to 40% of infants born at less than 32 weeks' gestation and who weigh less than 1,500 g at birth. Approximately 35% of infants with IVH develop posthemorrhagic hydrocephalus. In 65% of these infants the progression of ventricular enlargement will arrest spontaneously (Hansen & Snyder, 1998). The long-term outlook for these infants depends more on injury to the parenchyma than on the IVH and hydrocephalus.

Posthemorrhagic Hydrocephalus

After IVH, posthemorrhagic hydrocephalus may develop as a result of obstruction at the level of the ventricles or at the aqueduct of Sylvius. IVH also can impair absorption by way of the arachnoid villi owing to an inflammatory obliteration process in the posterior fossa (Hanson & Snyder, 1998). The obstruction results in overaccumulation of cerebrospinal fluid (CSF).

The daily care of a premature infant who has had an IVH should include keeping the head of the bed slightly elevated and assessing the fontanels and sutures (Roland & Hill, 1997). Head circumference measurements should be done weekly. Ventricular enlargement is monitored by serial ultrasonography.

Posthemorrhagic hydrocephalus may be associated with increased intracranial pressure. Signs of increased intracranial pressure include bulging fontanels and separated cranial sutures. Vomiting may be seen and may be forceful. An increase in the frequency and severity of apnea and bradycardia may be noted. Eyes may deviate downward.

Management of posthemorrhagic hydrocephalus depends on the rapidity of progression. A diuretic, such as acetazolamide, may reduce CSF production and is usually used in conjunction with furosemide. Infants treated with either diuretics or routine removal of CSF should be monitored closely for electrolyte imbalance and metabolic acidosis. Preliminary studies evaluating the use of fibrinolytic therapy have shown promise in the prevention of posthemorrhagic hydrocephalus (Roland & Hill, 1997). Surgical placement of a temporary draining device may be needed until the infant is ready for a **ventricular peritoneal shunt (VPS)** (a tunneled internal drain that empties into the peritoneal cavity). A ventricular to subgaleal shunt also may be used as a temporary device or until a VPS can be placed for long-term management (Roland & Hill, 1997; Hansen & Snyder, 1998).

Before discharge, parents of infants with VPSs should be taught to watch the infant for signs of increased intracranial pressure that could indicate shunt failure. Parents of infants with arrested posthemorrhagic hydrocephalus should also be taught the signs of increased intracranial pressure because late progression of hydrocephalus can occur (Hanson & Snyder, 1998).

Periventricular Leukomalacia

Periventricular leukomalacia (PVL) is a symmetric nonhemorrhagic lesion within the periventricular white matter of the brain. The pathogenesis of PVL is complex and not entirely understood. One possibility is that blood vessels in the periventricular white matter of the brain have limited capacity to expand during episodes of hypotension, allowing poorly perfused areas to of the brain to develop areas of infarction. Secondary hemorrhage into areas of infarction may occur with reperfusion. Another theory is that chemically mediated injury may occur with subclinical infection owing to an association between chorioamnionitis and positive blood cultures in the infant who subsequently develops PVL (Perlman, Risser, & Broyles, 1996).

Although PVL affects only 3% of preterm infants, it is associated with long-term neurologic morbidity, including seizures and spastic motor dysfunction (Perlman, Risser, & Broyles, 1996; Bernstein, Heimler, & Sasidharan, 1998; Volpe, 1997). Parents should be connected with resources for follow-up and treatment of associated neurologic sequelae and support groups.

Diagnostic techniques such as near-infrared spectroscopy may provide insights into the cause of PVL (Volpe, 1997). Once the pathophysiology is known, strategies to prevent PVL can be devised.

Hearing Loss

Cognitive development and social development are important aspects of developmental care. Because premature infants are at risk for otic nerve damage, resulting in hearing loss, it is important to assess the infant's ability to hear.

Nursing Alert

RISK FACTORS ASSOCIATED WITH HEARING IMPAIRMENT

- Asphyxia
- Congenital infection
- Hyperbilirubinemia
- Ototoxic drug administration
- Prolonged mechanical ventilation
- Persistent pulmonary hypertension
- Hydrocephalus
- Acidosis
- Sepsis
- High noise levels
- Bacterial meningitis
- Craniofacial anomalies

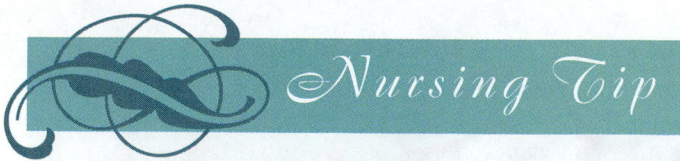

NOISE IN THE NICU

You can be instrumental in minimizing noise in the neonatal intensive care unit. Modifications such as using plastic trash cans, padding the top of the incubator, and keeping voices low help limit noise in the nursery (Figure 34-5).

Infants who are born prematurely are physiologically immature and at risk for a number of complications of prematurity, some of which are associated with the risk of hearing impairment. Some of the therapies used in the care of preterm infants are associated with the risk of hearing loss. Risk factors for hearing impairment include asphyxia, congenital infection, hyperbilirubinemia, administration of ototoxic drugs, prolonged mechanical ventilation, hydrocephalus, acidosis, sepsis, and noise levels in the neonatal intensive care unit (NICU).

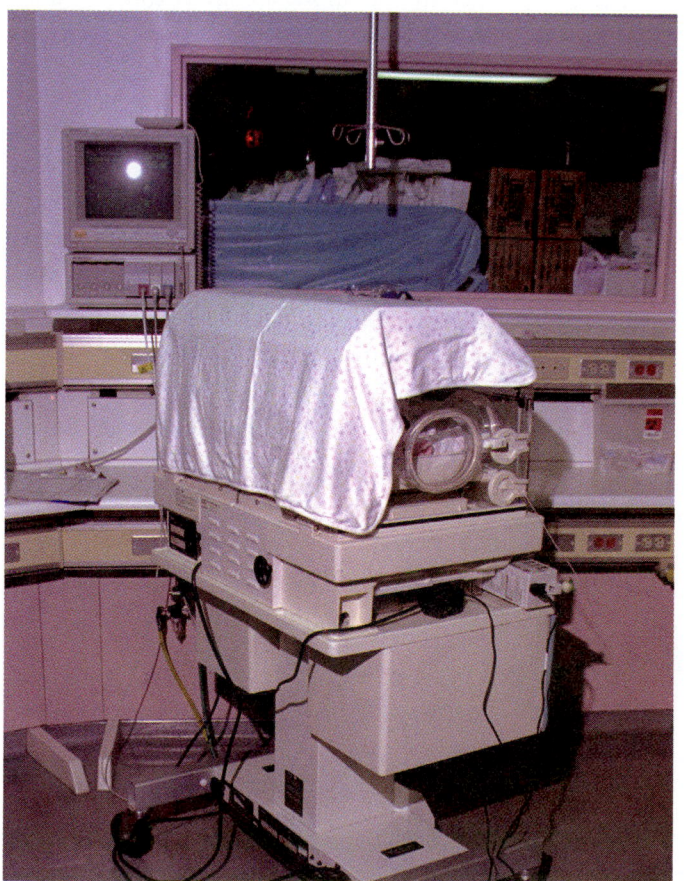

Figure 34-5 A pad wrapped around an incubator can help block light, cold, and noise to minimize environmental stimulation for the newborn.

The nurse should be alert to the infant's responses to sounds. If the infant does not respond to auditory stimuli, a hearing screening test should be performed. Automated oto-acoustic devices are used to screen infants for hearing impairment. An **Auditory Brain Evoked Response** test can be performed as well. It is a hearing test designed to screen newborns that records electrical potentials arising from the auditory nervous system. If the infant does not pass the test, follow-up with an audiologist is warranted.

To facilitate cognitive, social, and language development, an infant with hearing deficits may be fitted with hearing devices. The family should be taught communication skills, which will enhance the interactive process (Kenner, Amlung, & Flandermeyer, 1998).

Hematologic System

Nurses caring for preterm infants must have an understanding of the normal and abnormal conditions associated with the hematologic system. Acute and physiologic anemia, polycythemia, and coagulopathy often are found in the premature infant.

Anemia

Anemia can be defined as hemoglobin less than 13 g/dL in the first 28 days of life. Anemia may be present at birth or develop postnatally. It can be associated with blood loss, hemolysis, or decreased erythrocyte production.

Acute Anemia. Acute anemia is common and also may be associated with hypovolemia. Acute anemia may be caused by intrapartum events or frequent blood sampling for laboratory tests. Conditions related to blood loss in the fetus are fetomaternal transfusion or obstetrical bleeding from abruptio placenta, placenta previa, and abnormal insertion of the umbilical cord. After birth, blood loss may occur from a torn umbilical cord or internal hemorrhage in the newborn. Internal hemorrhage may include IVH or rupture of the liver or spleen during a traumatic delivery. Anemia also may result from hemolysis owing to chronic infection, isoimmune hemolytic disease, or inherited defects in the red cell membranes.

Acute anemia should be treated immediately. Symptoms include pallor, tachycardia, hypotension, and shock. The cause should be identified and treated, if possible. Laboratory evaluation may be helpful in identifying the cause when the maternal history does not include intrapartum bleeding.

Laboratory evaluation includes measuring hemoglobin and hematocrit levels. The hematocrit may be normal if blood is drawn immediately after an acute episode of bleeding; the true level of hemoglobin is masked because the blood loss is so rapid. As blood volume is restored (3 to 6 hours), the erythrocytes may be less dense and the hematocrit may be decreased. When large doses of volume are given to correct suspected hypovolemia, the hematocrit may be diluted.

Other laboratory evaluation includes a reticulocyte count. The reticulocyte count indicates if the anemia is chronic, such as in erythroblastosis fetalis, which is a hemolytic disease related to Rh incompatibility between mother and infant. In a chronic anemia the fetus rapidly replaces erythrocytes, which results in an increased reticulocyte count.

Erythrocyte morphology may give a clue to the cause of the anemia. For instance, an increased number of spherocytes may indicate an ABO incompatibility, or an increased number of erythroblasts may suggest hemolytic disease.

Direct and indirect Coombs tests on the infant is important to evaluate for maternal antigens to the infant's blood. These antigens may be seen in Rh disease, ABO incompatibilities, and minor blood group incompatibilities. The mother's blood may be tested to see whether fetal cells are present as seen in fetomaternal transfusions.

Physiologic Anemia. A physiologic anemia may develop from physiologic changes associated with the change from the production of fetal hemoglobin in utero to that of adult hemoglobin after birth. Physiologic anemia often is seen in the stable premature infant. The hematocrit reaches a natural low point as the infant's body transitions from the production of fetal hemoglobin to that of adult hemoglobin. The decrease in fetal hemoglobin prompts the postnatal increase in erythropoietin (Kenner, Amlung, & Flandermeyer, 1998). Erythropoietin then stimulates the production of erythrocytes.

The hematocrit reaches a low point at about 6 to 8 weeks in a premature infant. The infant may be pale but usually maintains a heart rate within normal range. Physiologic anemia does not require treatment unless the infant is dependent on oxygen, is having frequent blood drawn for monitoring, or is symptomatic of anemia. If decreased activity, poor feeding, tachycardia, dyspnea, tachypnea, or poor weight gain are present, the anemia is considered to be symptomatic (Chen, Wu, & Chanlai, 1995). Treatment generally consists of transfusion of packed erythrocytes. Human erythropoietin also may be used for treatment of anemia (Chen, Wu, & Chanlai, 1995; Kenner, Amlung, & Flandermeyer, 1998).

Polycythemia

Infants with polycythemia will have a peripheral hematocrit value of more than 75% or a central hematocrit value of more than 65%. Infants at risk are those with trisomy 13 (Patau syndrome), trisomy 18 (Edward syndrome), trisomy 21 (Down syndrome), twin-to-twin transfusion syndrome, and those who receive placental transfusion at birth. Infants whose mothers have diabetes also are at risk. Symptoms of polycythemia include lethargy, hypotonia, irritability, tremors, poor feeding, and **plethora** (deep rosy-red skin color). Cyanosis with crying, tachypnea congestive heart failure, heptomegaly, cardiomegaly, and jaundice is indicative of polycythemia. Polycythemia may be associated with hypocalcemia, hypoglycemia, and jaundice. When the hematocrit value is less than 70% and no symptoms are observed, the infant should be monitored. Complications of hyperviscosity are associated with infarcts in major organs. When the infant is symptomatic the hematocrit may be reduced by a partial exchange transfusion.

Coagulopathy

Clot formation requires an interaction between clotting proteins, platelets, and damaged blood vessels. Many conditions in the premature infant are associated with prolonged clotting times. Thrompocytopenia is one such condition that may occur with infection, isoimmune disorders, thrombotic disorders, necrotizing enterocolitis, and birth asphyxia. Maternal or infant medications may prevent clot formation by interfering with platelet function. Infection and asphyxia may be associated with **disseminated intravascular coagulation (DIC)**. This condition involves coagulation in the microvasculature that results in prolonged bleeding owing to the consumption of available clotting factors during the coagulation process.

Symptoms of coagulopathy include petechiae, ecchymosis, prolonged bleeding at puncture sites, pulmonary hemorrhage, and intracranial bleeding. Complications include anemia and hyperbilirubinemia related to breakdown of erythrocytes in entrapped hemorrhage. Management of coagulopathy includes identifying and treating the cause. Supportive measures include maintaining a normal blood pressure and provision of blood products if needed. Fresh frozen plasma, packed erythrocytes, and platelets may be transfused as needed.

Hepatic System

The liver of the preterm infant also is immature. Common hepatic problems associated with prematurity include hyperbilirubinemia and alterations in the metabolism of medications.

Hyperbilirubinemia

Hyperbilirubinemia implies excessive serum **bilirubin** (product of erythrocyte destruction that may be a result of a natural or a hemolytic process) and therefore is associated with a pathologic cause or outcome (Schwoebel & Sakraida, 1997). The physiology and etiology of bilirubin are discussed in Chapter 32.

Premature infants are prone to potentially high levels of bilirubin and may have **jaundice** (yellow tint to the skin related to increased bilirubin levels). Bilirubin levels increase earlier, reach peaks later (5 to 7 days) and remain elevated longer than in the term neonate as a result of several factors. These factors are low levels of the enzymes that bind to bilirubin, more rapid erythrocyte breakdown, and decreased albumin levels. The preterm infant also is at increased risk for reabsorption of bilirubin from the GI tract owing to poor GI motility, inability to feed, feeding intolerance, and delayed stooling.

Phototherapy is the treatment of choice for the management of hyperbilirubinemia in the preterm infant (Figure 34-6). Early intervention is recommended. Phototherapy may be started early on infants who have multiple bruises from delivery because serum bilirubin will increase as the blood in the bruise is broken down.

Issues of importance to the nurse caring for a preterm infant under phototherapy include maintenance of normal body temperature, ensuring eye patches are in place, monitoring of strict intake and output, managing IV fluid, monitoring bilirubin levels, assessing for signs of neurodevelopmental consequences, and educating the parents. Premature infants requiring phototherapy need increased maintenance fluids secondary to an increase in insensible water losses (IWLs).

The premature infant is at increased risk for neurologic injury because of immaturity of the blood-brain barrier and propensity for delayed clearance owing to delayed maturation of the normal physiologic mechanisms (Schwoebel & Sakraida, 1997). In addition, the potential for central nervous system (CNS) hemorrhage, hypoxia, and hypoglycemia increase the potential for bilirubin-related kernicterus. There is not a consensus on what bilirubin levels are dangerous to the preterm infant, but cautious management is necessary.

Gastrointestinal System

In utero, the GI tract processes large volumes of amniotic fluid, which aid in maturation. By 20 weeks' gestation the anatomic development of the GI tract is complete; functional capabilities develop later in gestation. Although some GI function is present at birth, regardless of gestational age, premature infants may have limitations in overall GI function. Common problems related to the immature GI tract include dysmotility, NEC, and gastroesophageal reflux (GER).

Dysmotility

The onset of peristalsis is at 28 to 30 weeks' gestation. Once feedings are initiated the infant must be monitored closely for **dysmotility**, or a slow rate of GI peristalsis. Environmental factors affect the development of the GI tract: colonization of bacteria and introduction of enteral feedings help to stimulate maturation.

Digestion and absorption of nutrients vary according to gestational age. Protein is remarkably well handled by the preterm infant, whereas carbohydrate absorption is

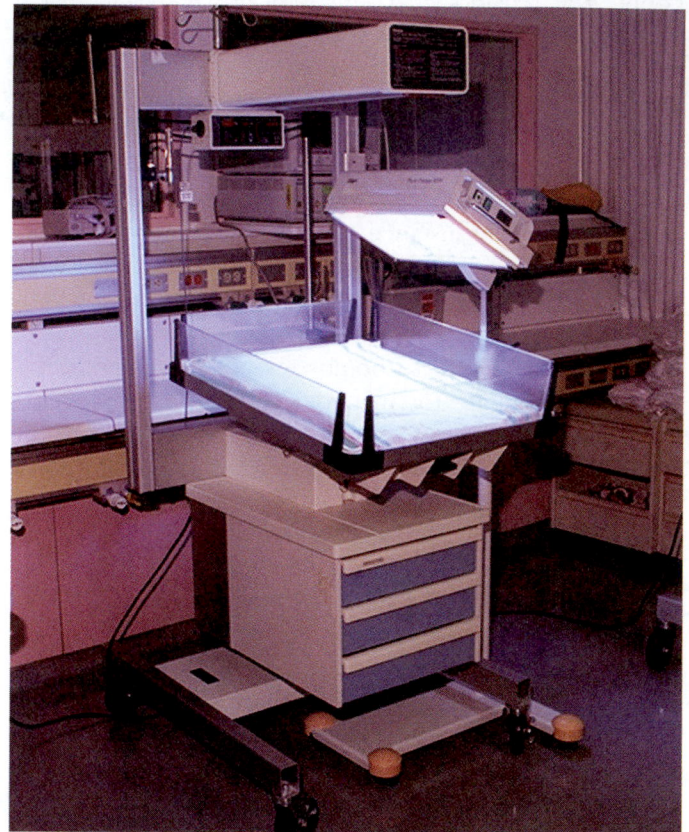

A.

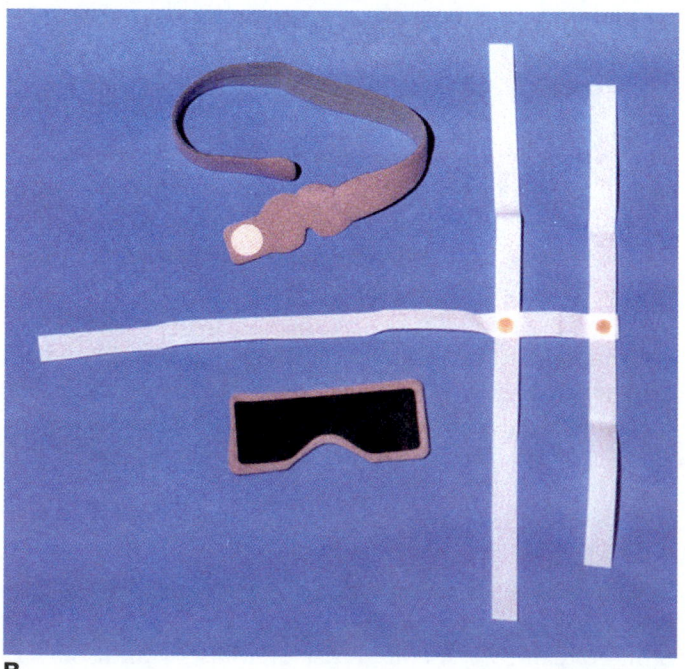

B.

Figure 34-6 A. Infant warmer with phototherapy light. B. Eye patches and phototherapy equipment.

limited because of lactase deficiency. Malabsorption of dietary fat is common secondary to a lack of small bile pools and pancreatic lipase. Early low-volume feedings have been shown to increase gut hormones thought to be important in intestinal maturation.

Motility of the GI tract changes during gestation and after birth. The gastroesophageal sphincter pressure increases from 28 weeks' gestation through the first week of life, and peristalsis of the small intestine improves during the third trimester (Merenstein & Gardner, 1998). Gastric emptying is decreased in preterm infants. The more premature the infant the greater the delay in passage of stool. Enteral feedings promote gastric emptying and the release of hormones that may improve peristalsis (Merenstein & Gardner, 1998).

Necrotizing Enterocolitis

Necrotizing enterocolitis (NEC) is a devastating disease process most commonly seen in premature infants but occasionally seen in compromised term infants. NEC is characterized by necrosis of the mucosal and submucosal layers of the GI tract. The exact pathogenesis remains unclear. Mucosal injury is thought to be the initial stage of this disease. The risk of mucosal injury in the neonate is associated with perinatal hypoxia; asphyxia; hypovolemia and rapid reperfusion; viscous blood with decreased flow to the GI tract, such as in polycythemia; and hypotension, with resultant decrease in blood flow.

Although prevention of NEC is of primary importance to the practitioner, the lack of a clear cause limits attempts to avoid the disease altogether. Prevention is aimed at preventing factors associated with NEC. Certain factors predispose infants to NEC; they are listed in the Nursing Alert. Changes in blood flow patterns to the GI tract are the most common cause of mucosal injury. Once mucosal injury has occurred the bowel lining becomes edematous. Hemorrhage and ulceration then occur followed by formation of a false membrane. Introduction of enteral feedings and overgrowth of normal GI flora (bacteria) cause an invasion in this already damaged bowel wall. Gas production occurs, which further weakens the mucosa, and gas becomes trapped in the interspace of the bowel wall. This trapped air is called **pneumatosis intestinalis** and is a hallmark of the disease process.

The infant may have subtle signs and symptoms or may deteriorate rapidly. The signs and symptoms can be divided into early onset, second stage, and late onset. Early symptoms include abdominal distention, gastric residuals, vomiting, and bloody stools. Lethargy, temperature instability, apnea, and bradycardia also may be present. When these conditions occur, delay in feedings is necessary and the infant should be monitored closely.

As the disease process worsens, fluid shifts from damaged intestinal mucosa into the abdominal cavity. Hypo-

Nursing Alert

RISK FACTORS FOR NECROTIZING ENTEROCOLITIS

- Prematurity
- Asphyxia
- Hyperosmolar feedings
- Polycythemia, hyperviscosity
- Rapid increase in the volume of feedings
- Enteric pathogenic microorganisms

volemia results, with a decrease in blood pressure and urine output. Late signs include erythema, edema, and abdominal tenderness. Thrombocytopenia occurs as platelets are consumed to help repair damaged bowel mucosa. The infant should be monitored for prolonged bleeding.

Management of this disease process should be begun at the earliest signs of difficulty. Management includes stopping feedings and starting IV fluids, gastric decompression with an orogastric tube, antibiotic therapy, strict measurement of intake and output, and replacement intravascular volume with blood or plasma. Resuscitation may be necessary. The infant should be monitored frequently for changes in clinical status. Radiographic views of the abdomen should be reviewed every 6 to 8 hours to assess for pneumatosis intestinalis. Laboratory evaluation includes complete blood count (CBC) with differential and platelet count, blood culture, serum electrolytes, blood urea nitrogen (BUN), creatinine and glucose, and a lumbar puncture for culture if the infant's condition permits.

If the infant's condition does not worsen in the first 3 days, feedings may be initiated slowly. If symptoms worsen, the infant should not be fed to rest the bowel. Total parenteral nutrition (TPN) with intralipids for nutrition and to promote healing will be initiated and IV antibiotics will continue for 7 to 14 days when indicated.

The infant is monitored closely for signs of perforation, leading to air in the peritoneal cavity. Surgical intervention is indicated when perforation occurs. Necrotic bowel is resected, and primary anastomosis or stoma is established. All efforts are made to preserve the length of the bowel. When perforation occurs, the mortality rate is 20% to 40%.

Complications of NEC include lactose intolerance, malabsorption, fungal infection, metabolic bone disease, cholestasis, and liver dysfunction. Late complications of NEC include strictures, fistulas, and abscesses. Recurrent signs and symptoms include chronic electrolyte imbalances and failure to thrive. **Short bowel syndrome** also may occur in NEC as a result of extensive resection of the GI tract, resulting in loss of absorptive surface that, in turn, results in diarrhea, dehydration, and poor growth.

Gastroesophageal reflux

Gastroesophageal reflux (GER) is defined as the return of gastric contents into the esophagus. The premature infant is at great risk for GER secondary to immature muscle tone, poor sphincter control, delay in gastric emptying, and increased intraabdominal pressure. Common signs of GER are vomiting, small wet burps, poor weight gain, apnea and bradycardia, esophagitis, and recurrent aspiration. Collaborative management is essential in GER. Nursing may include positioning the infant with the head elevated (Figure 34-7), frequent small-volume feedings, frequent burping during feedings, monitoring for apnea, and thickening formula. Medical management includes the use of agents to increase gastric emptying time and improve GI motility.

Immune System

Many factors put the preterm infant at high risk for infection. Two mechanisms are responsible for the infant's un-

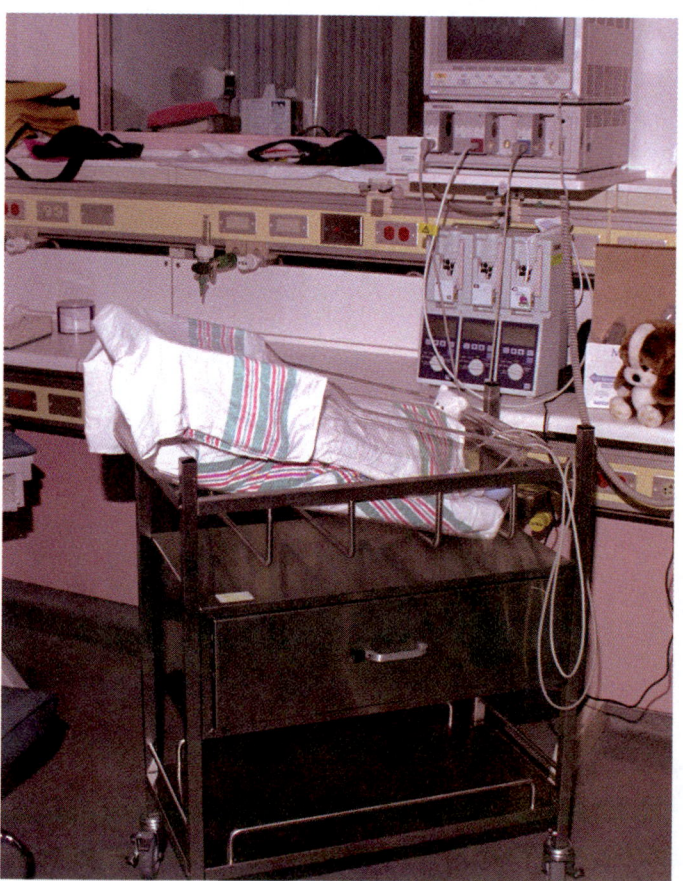

Figure 34-7 Elevating the head is one way of managing care for the infant with gastroesophageal reflux.

derdeveloped immune system: qualitative and quantitative neutrophil deficiency and impaired opsonization (Lott, 1994).

Neutropenia (decreased number of neutrophils) commonly is seen in infection from decreased neutrophil marrow progenitor cells and a decreased marrow neutrophil storage pool (Lott, 1994). Neutrophils also are less effective than they normally are during times of stress in the newborn.

Opsonization (the action of opsonins facilitating phagocytosis) is impaired secondary to lower immune complement and antibody levels. Maternal antibodies are the only source available and do not cross the placenta in large quantities before 32 weeks' gestation.

Infection

The most common risk factor for infection in the preterm infant is exposure to infections in utero. These infections are sometimes linked to the onset of preterm labor and delivery. Maternal risk factors for infection include health practices related to substance abuse, maternal illness, colonization with infection, active bacterial or viral infection, and fever during labor and delivery. Neonatal risk factors include prematurity, male gender, multiple gestation, and congenital abnormalities.

Infection is suspected in all infants born prematurely without a clear cause for the early delivery. Evaluation for infection may include a CBC with differential, blood culture, evaluation of tracheal aspirate (if intubated), gram stain culture, and a lumbar puncture for culture. Broad spectrum antibiotic therapy is initiated until the organism is identified. Length of treatment may vary from institution to institution.

The premature infant also is at risk for late-onset infection, which is one that occurs after the first 5 to 7 days of life. These are commonly nosocomial infections. Underlying illness, poor skin barrier, and immature immune status make the premature infant more susceptible to infection.

Prevention of late-onset infection is an important aspect of neonatal care. Nurses caring for premature infants must be diligent in good hand-washing technique and in instructing parents and other health care personnel to wash their hands thoroughly. Equipment should be cleaned before and after use to prevent spread of infection. Each infant should have his or her supplies to prevent cross-contamination. Overcrowding in a nursery also increases the risk for infection. Once an infant is admitted to the nursery, the infant's bed space should not be changed without careful deliberation. The nurse caring for a premature infant also should try to ensure that caregivers and family members avoid contact with the infant when they are ill. Screening siblings for illness when they visit the nursery with their parents is especially important (Figure 34-8).

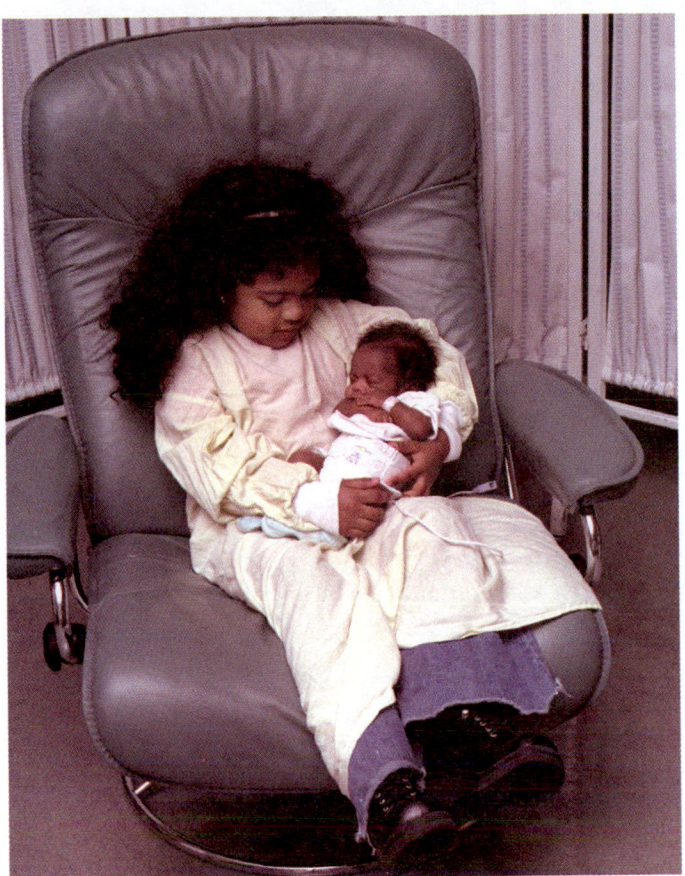

Figure 34-8 The triplet's big sister is allowed to hold only the infant who is showing the best growth rate and adaptation to extrauterine life.

Critical Thinking

Protecting Infants from Illness

Calling in sick is discouraged in hospitals. It is especially difficult in a neonatal intensive care unit because the unit may be left short-handed or substitute staff will be provided that cannot provide the level of care a staff nurse is trained to deliver. Even an expert neonatal nurse cannot complete the variety of tasks expected of full time personnel. Thus, calling in sick places an extra burden on co-workers.

You have read that infants who have low birth weights are susceptible to infection. In balancing personal pressure with the infants and co-workers' needs, what should you do if you wake up one morning with a fever? What should you do if you have had two previous absences and the third means a verbal counseling? What should you do if you know the unit is short-staffed?

The evaluation for late-onset infection is the same as for an early infection; suprapubic needle aspiration of urine for culture, a bladder tap also may be indicated. Increased incidences of meningitis and urinary tract infection also are seen in infants who have late-onset infections.

The infant may have varying signs and symptoms. Generalized symptoms are common, such as poor feeding, irritability, lethargy, and temperature instability. Signs of infection often include the following: respiratory symptoms, such as grunting, nasal flaring, retractions, increased respirations, and apnea; cardiovascular symptoms, such as bradycardia or tachycardia, decreased blood pressure, cyanosis, and mottling; and GI disturbances, such as diarrhea, abdominal distention, emesis, and increased residuals.

As in all pregnancies, mothers delivering premature infants must be screened for sexually transmitted diseases. If the mother has not been tested or if the prenatal chart is not available, the mother must be screened once hospitalized. Follow-up by nursery personnel is essential. Sexually transmitted diseases are treated the same way in preterm infants as they are in term infants.

The preterm infant also is at increased risk for fungal infections for several reasons. Prolonged treatment of the mother with antibiotics may increase yeast colonization in the mother's vaginal canal, thereby increasing the infant's exposure at delivery. These infants have multiple intravascular catheters in place for long periods of time, multiple courses of antibiotic therapy, and an immature immune response. Treatment with antifungal agents is common. These agents have effects on the renal and hematologic systems. Careful monitoring of potassium, BUN, creatinine, hematocrit, and platelet count is essential for early intervention should side effects occur.

Integumentary System

Skin care is an important aspect of care (Gordon & Montgomery, 1996). Skin functions as a barrier to infection and controls temperature and insensible water loss (Dollison &

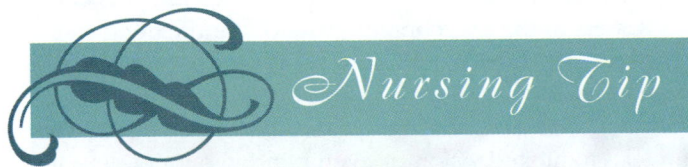

SOAP FOR BATHING

The natural acid mantle of the skin helps keep bacterial growth at a minimum. Nonalkaline soaps should be used for bathing the preterm infant to protect the acid mantle.

Beckstrand, 1995). At less than 34 weeks' gestation a preterm infant's skin is immature. Once the infant is born the skin matures over the first couple of weeks and begins to resemble that of a term infant. Because a premature infant's skin is fragile, it is subject to injury. Epidermal stripping, absorption of chemicals applied to the skin, and IV fluid infiltrates are common.

Epidermal Stripping

The skin of a preterm infant is more permeable because of its thin stratum corneum. The epidermis remains thin until 32 weeks' gestation. Collagen, which provides support to dermal structures and allows the skin to stretch, is unstable. Decreased cohesion between the dermis and epidermis exists. Epidermal stripping occurs easily because the adhesive of bonding agents may be greater than the bond between the epidermis and dermis. When the dermis is stripped, increased chemical absorption and increased fluid loss occur along with the potential for bacterial exposure. The use of pectin-based barriers helps prevent epidermal stripping. Placing the barrier under tape decreases the amount of epidermal stripping (Dollison & Beckstrand, 1995). Pectin-based barriers come in thin sheets that can be cut to the desired size and shape. The sheets stick to skin when warmed. Tape will pull on the barrier rather than the infant's skin.

Absorption of Chemical Agents

The thin skin of a premature infant allows chemicals to be readily absorbed through the skin. Nursing care includes avoidance or limitation of the use of adhesives and adhesive removers. Table 34-1 lists some chemicals that can be absorbed through the skin. Absorbable chemical agents should be removed from the skin with water.

Intravenous Fluid Infiltrates

Intravenous infiltrates are of particular concern in preterm infants because many solutions and medications can cause sloughing of the skin. Infection and scarring also can occur. Many premature infants require IV therapy because

Table 34-1 Effects of Absorbable Chemical Agents

Absorbable Chemical	Potential Effect
Isopropyl alcohol	Sloughing
Betadine	Transient hypothyroidism
Hexachlorophene	Central nervous system damage
Adhesive remover	Increased blood alcohol levels

of medical conditions that prevent full enteric nutrition or the need for pharmacologic therapy. Properly cleaning the site and protecting the IV to prevent infiltration necessitating multiple IV starts are important considerations. It is important for the nurse to remember that each needle puncture is a break in the integrity of the infant's skin and a potential source of infection.

The IV site should be checked at least every hour. When an IV infiltrate is detected, the IV should be discontinued immediately and the area of infiltrate elevated, if possible. Hyaluronidase may be used to limit sloughing in some cases. Phentolamine may help prevent tissue necrosis in dopamine solution infiltrates.

When the skin breaks down over a joint, scaring and development of a contracture may limit joint mobility in the future. A consultation with plastic surgery often is required for evaluation of the area and for recommendations on steps to take to minimize long-term sequelae.

Ophthalmologic System

As with other body systems, the eyes of a premature infant are still developing. The premature infant therefore is at risk for the development of vision problems.

Historically, premature infants developed retrolental fibroplasia (RLF), which resulted in blindness, as a result of exposure to high levels of oxygen. Changes in treatment modalities and development of sensitive monitoring equipment have essentially eradicated this illness; however, it is important for nurses caring for premature infants to be aware of the potential harm of indiscriminate use of oxygen.

With improved methods of treatment and equipment, smaller premature infants are surviving. These infants are at risk for retinopathy of prematurity. We now know the infant also is at risk for other eye problems.

Retinopathy of Prematurity

One of the most prevalent problems seen in premature infants is **retinopathy of prematurity (ROP)**. Before 32 weeks' gestation, vascularization of the retina is incomplete (Shapiro & Askin, 1999). The younger the infant the less vascularization has occurred. Once an infant is born, the vessels in the eye continue to grow and extend to the periphery of the retina. As these vessels grow there is risk for abnormal development of the eye vessels. This proliferation of blood vessels in the eye is known as ROP, which can lead to limited vision or even blindness if not detected and treated early. In severe ROP, treatment includes cryotherapy or laser photocoagulation to limit the development of the abnormal blood vessels. When these treatments fail the infant may require eye surgery to preserve some sight.

Infants who have birth weights less than 1,500 g or who are born at less than 28 weeks' gestation should be screened by a pediatric ophthalmologist for ROP at 4 to 6 weeks of life and then regularly until vascularization is complete. ROP occurs in 25% to 35% of surviving premature infants having up to 35 weeks' gestation. Blindness occurs in 3% to 5% (Bossi & Koerner, 1995; Bernstein, Heimler, & Sasidharan, 1998).

Other Eye Problems

Infants who have developed ROP at any stage are at risk for late retinal detachment and should be followed closely. Premature infants also are at risk for myopia, amblyopia, glaucoma, and strabismus (Bernstein, Heimler, & Sasidharan, 1998). Parents should be encouraged to keep postdischarge eye appointments so that vision problems can be identified early to preserve sight. The long-term implications on the quality of life of the infant and family are clear.

Renal System

The kidneys are responsible for elimination of toxins and regulation of fluid, electrolytes, and arterial blood pressure (Seaman, 1995). In utero the placenta acts as the organ of excretion, removing excess fluid and waste products from the fetus. The fetal kidney has a low glomerular filtration rate (GFR) that increases with gestational age. The GFR remains low until nephrogenesis is complete, at about 36 weeks' gestation. Infants born at less than 36 weeks' gestation have underdeveloped structures and decreased renal function. Renal function increases during the first week of life because of decreased renal vascular resistance and an increase in systemic blood flow. Increased renal function results in diuresis at about 5 days of life as the GFR increases and the infant excretes excess extracellular fluid. Although the GFR increases in the first week of life, it is lower in the preterm infant than in the term infant owing to a decreased number of nephrons (Seaman, 1995).

Careful monitoring of the renal status of premature infants is important so that problems are identified early and thus early intervention can be provided. Renal problems common to premature infants include oliguria, glucosuria, and nephrocalcinosis.

Oliguria

Urine flow depends on fluid intake. Normal urine output is 1 to 2 mL/h per kilogram of body weight (mL/kg/h). Oliguria can be defined as less than 1 mL/kg/h. Oliguria may be a symptom of inadequate fluid intake or acute renal failure. Acute renal failure in premature infants may be associated with perinatal asphyxia and multisystem organ failure. Urine output may be affected by hypoxemia, hypovolemia, acidosis, and mediations that impair renal blood flow. Sepsis sometimes is associated with renal failure.

An accurate urine output measurement is extremely important in monitoring renal well-being in infants; however, accurate measurements may be difficult to obtain. Nurses who care for premature infants have developed creative methods of checking output. One method involves weighing a dry and a wet diaper on a balance scale (Figure 34-9). The difference between the two weights is roughly the urine output.

In severe cases of oliguria a bladder catheter may be required for accurate measurement. In addition to urine output, renal function is evaluated by monitoring serum creatinine and hydration by monitoring BUN.

Glucosuria

Term infants may have a trace of glucose in the urine. Glucosuria is seen more frequently in premature infants in whom minor elevations in serum glucose allow spillage into the urine. Glucose in the urine sometimes is seen in premature infants who have an infection IVH, and in those receiving steroids.

An increased frequency of yeast dermatitis has been observed in infants with glucosuria. Keeping the skin area that comes into contact with wet diapers clean and dry is important in preventing cutaneous yeast infections. The nurse caring for the prematue infant should consider each diaper change an opportunity to observe the area for rash and skin breakdown. Yeast infections in the diaper area generally appear as redness in the creases with a papular rash, frequently with satellite lesions, that is, lesions extending beyond the reddened area. The treatment for yeast dermatitis is antifungal cream.

Nephrocalcinosis

Nephrocalcinosis is the formation of renal calculi, usually calcium oxalate (McCormick, Brady, & Keen, 1996). A hospitalized premature infant with a complicated medical history is at risk for nephrocalcinosis. Risk factors include prematurity and hypercalciuria, resulting from furosemide administration and calcium supplementation.

Diuretics often are used in the premature infant to treat congestive heart failure associated with PDA and to improve lung function in infants with certain lung diseases. A commonly used diuretic is furosemide. Premature infants need increased doses because of their low GFRs. Furosemide is associated with increased excretion of calcium and therefore may be associated with renal calcifications. When an infant is on long-term furosemide therapy, it is important to monitor renal function regularly. Ultrasonography of the kidneys may be done periodically to evaluate for the presence of renal calculi.

Fluid restriction, alkaline urine, and metabolic acidosis may contribute to the formation of nephrocalcinosis (McCormick, Brady, & Keen, 1996). Many preterm infants who are receiving diuretic therapy also will receive formula for premature infants that contains higher levels of calcium

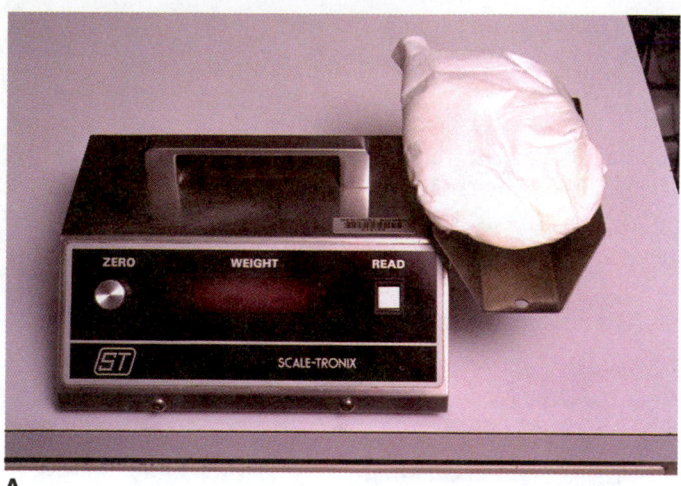

A.

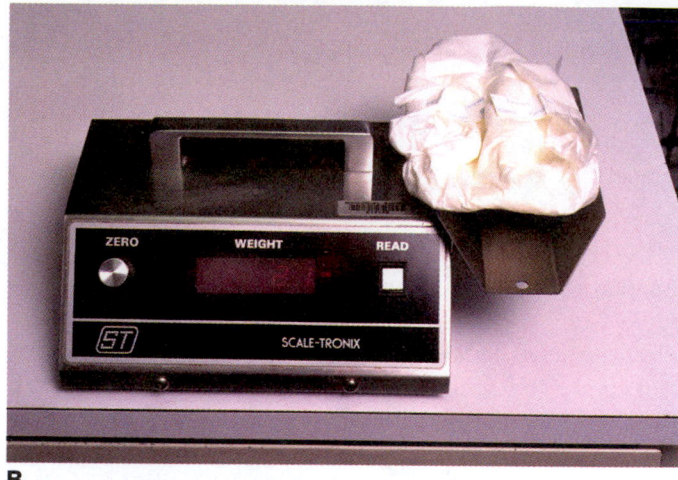

B.

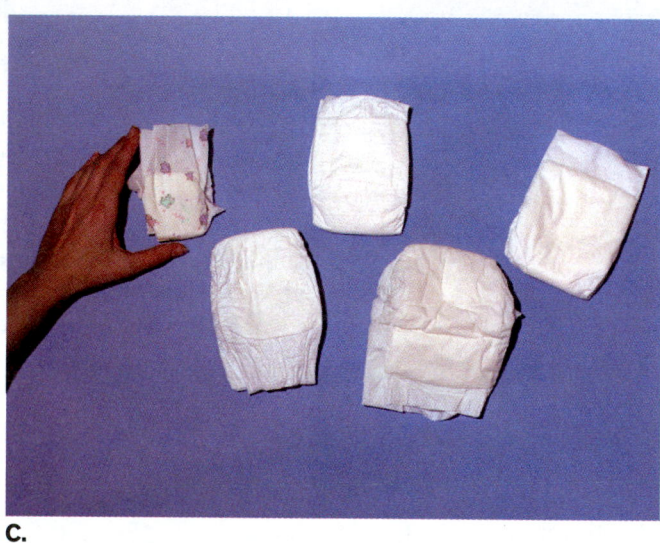

C.

Figure 34-9 Urine output can be measured by first weighing a clean diaper (A) and then a wet diaper (B); the difference is the infant's urine output. (C) The diaper of a premature infant is so small that this method of measuring urine output may prove a challenge.

and other minerals than does formula for term infants. Infants who are receiving diuretics because of a chronic lung condition may have fluid restrictions, placing them at an even higher risk for developing nephrocalcinosis.

When nephrocalcinosis is present, other diuretics also may be used, such as chlorothiazide and spironolactone. Chlorothiazide has a lesser effect on the infant's electrolyte values than does furosemide, and spironolactone is a potassium-sparing diuretic; however, electrolyte levels should be monitored, and replacement salts provided as required.

Respiratory System

Before birth the infant's lungs are filled with fluid and underperfused. The placenta acts as the organ of respiration for the fetus, providing for gas exchange. Most right ventricular output is shunted from the pulmonary artery across the ductus arteriosus into the aorta, bypassing the pulmonary circulation. (Kenner, Amlung, & Flandemeyer, 1998). Approximately 10% of blood flow goes to the fetal lung in utero.

Fetal lung fluid begins to be absorbed before birth, and the alveolar fluid secretion decreases near term. During labor this process accelerates. When the cord is clamped and with the first breaths, the alveoli are able to fill with air. Thus, lung volume is established. The lung fluid then moves to the interstitial space and is removed by the lymphatic and pulmonary blood vessels. Interruption of this process may result in a respiratory disease process in the newborn infant. Delivery of a preterm infant interrupts this process and may result in a respiratory disease state.

The most common problem in premature infants is respiratory distress. Premature infants may have respiratory distress syndrome (RDS), transient tachypnea of the newborn (TTN), retained fetal lung fluid, bronchopulmonary dysplasia (BPD), apnea of prematurity, air-block syndrome, pneumonia, or meconium aspiration syndrome. Respiratory problems may occur alone or in combination, or the premature infant may have one respiratory problem early in the course of treatment and another or others later.

Respiratory Distress Syndrome

Also called **hyaline membrane disease (HMD)**, **respiratory distress syndrome (RDS)** is the most common cause of respiratory disease in the preterm neonate. In rare cases, this disease also may be seen in infants of mothers with diabetes or term neonates with asphyxia. The disease manifests as surfactant deficiency characterized by collapsed alveoli and low lung volume.

Each year RDS is seen in over 40,000 infants and approximately 65% are infants of 30 weeks' gestation or less (Farrell & Wood, 1976). The disease process worsens with decreasing gestational age.

The premature lung is deficient in surfactant. Surfactant is essential in maintaining surface tension and preventing alveolar collapse. As surfactant is used up the premature lung becomes progressively atelectatic and underperfused, resulting in intrapulmonary shunting and hypoxia. Efforts to reduce the incidence and severity of RDS include the use of antenatal steroids and surfactant replacement therapy. Administering steroids to the mother prenatally seems to accelerate lung growth and maturity. The use of surfactant replacement helps to diminish the severity of RDS once the infant is delivered (Moise & Hanson, 1998; Casey, 1999).

Typical radiographs of the preterm infant with RDS reveal low volume lungs, with a granular appearance to the lung fields and air bronchography. Common forms of treatment include continuous positive airway pressure, positive end expiratory pressure to prevent lung volume loss during expiration, mechanical ventilation, high-frequency oscillatory ventilation, and surfactant replacement therapy (Kenner, Amlung, & Flandemeyer, 1998).

Transient Tachypnea of the Newborn

Transient tachypnea of the newborn (TTN) is not a common disease in the preterm infant. TTN lasts approximately 5 to 7 days, and the main symptom is tachypnea. Often, no underlying cause is identified.

Retained Fetal Lung Fluid

Retained fetal lung fluid is a disease process seen in term, near term, and preterm neonates resulting from the inability or failure to completely clear the lungs of fluid at birth. Retained fetal lung fluid often is mistaken for TTN. The lungs usually are mature.

The medical history often reveals a rapid vaginal delivery or delivery by cesarean section. The most common symptom is tachypnea; however, grunting, nasal flaring, and retractions also may be noted. The clinical course may be as short as 4 hours or up to 24 hours of age. Breath sounds generally are coarse on auscultation. Treatment includes oxygen therapy and fluid restriction. Occasionally, continuous positive airway pressure is needed (Figure 34-10).

Bronchopulmonary Dysplasia

One of the most common complications of respiratory disease in the preterm infant is **bronchopulmonary dysplasia (BPD)**. Infants who are born prematurely and require mechanical ventilation and oxygen therapy for a prolonged period of time are at risk for damage to the alveoli and lung tissue. Whereas the pathogenesis of BPD is multifactorial, the primary cause is immature pulmonary development with surfactant deficiency. Treatment of this pulmonary disease requires the use of mechanical ventilation, resulting in barotrauma to the small and large airways, interstitial damage, inflammation, fibrosis, and cystic changes.

Northway et al. (1967) described the pathology of BPD in four stages of progressive chronic changes in the lung, starting as early as the second to third day of life with patchy loss of cilia and advancing to necrosis of alveolar epithelium and severe bronchiolar metaplasia by 1 month of age. Toce et al. (1984) described a clinical and radiographic scoring system for preterm infants at 28 days of life or 36 weeks' postconceptual age. The scores range from normal to severe disease. Respiratory rate, retractions, oxygen requirement, carbon dioxide retention, and growth rate are evaluated. Radiographic changes range from cardiovascular abnormalities to lung hyperexpansion and fibrosis.

In the 1990s, an increase in the occurrence of BPD was seen. This increase is primarily a result of surfactant

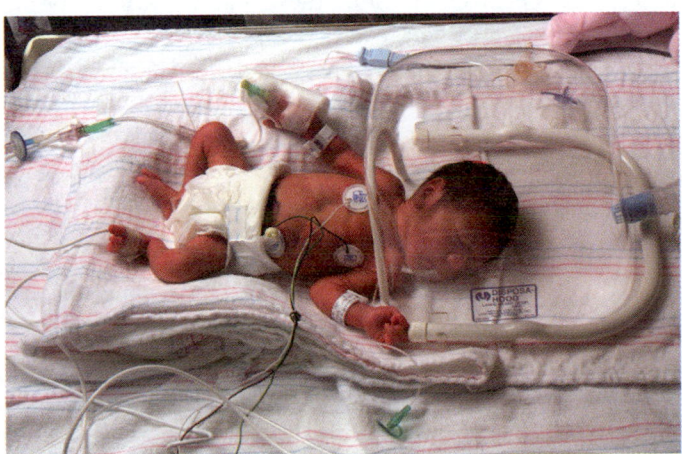

Figure 34-10 Premature infant receiving oxygen therapy through an oxygen hood.

replacement therapy and the ability to manage smaller preterm infants than in the past. These infants weight as little as 500 g and are delivered from 23 to 24 weeks' gestation.

Prevention of BPD is directed toward prevention of RDS by using prenatal steroids, managing preterm labor, and using ventilation strategies designed to reduce the effects of barotrauma. Other management strategies include closure of patent ductus arteriosus, fluid management, early diuretic therapy, and good nutrition. More recent strategies, including vitamin A supplementation, antioxidant therapy, and high-frequency oscillation, have reduced the severity of BPD.

Treatment strategies include a combination of modalities and require a multidisciplinary team approach. Fluid restriction in combination with diuretic therapy while providing adequate nutrition are tremendous challenges for all caregivers. Use of bronchodilators, steroids, and vasodilators is essential in controlling disease progression and managing symptoms.

Nursing care is aimed at providing a stable, developmentally sound environment to ensure optimal outcomes. Prevention of hypoxic episodes and close monitoring of the infant's tolerance to procedures and handling are essential. Clustering of care, use of containment during procedures, and sedation often are used to conserve energy expenditure. Energy conservation is extremely important to ensure adequate weight gain and optimal use of calories. Consistent caregivers are important both to the infant's social development and in order to be attuned to subtle changes in the infant's condition that can become serious if early intervention is not provided.

It is essential to have family involvement in the care of these infants who are developing socially and cognitively. Having family members provide routine care promotes attachment and allows the infant social contacts that are not medically oriented. Families must learn to provide the infant's care because many of these infants will go home with monitoring equipment and therapy that may be stressful for the family. A successful transition to home care is dependent on supporting the family structure while the infant is in the hospital.

The management and care of these fragile infants with chronic conditions present an ongoing challenge to neonatal caregivers. Research is needed to continue to improve outcomes in this population.

Apnea of Prematurity

Apnea is defined as the cessation of respirations for more than 20 seconds. Color changes and bradycardia may accompany apnea. Periodic breathing frequently is seen in the premature infant and is described as three or more pauses in respirations, with less than 20 seconds of respirations between pauses.

MAINTAINING AN APPROPRIATE THERMAL ENVIRONMENT

Maintenance of a neutral thermal environment is extremely important in the management of all aspects of caring for a premature infant.

Apnea may be classified as central or obstructive. Central apnea results secondary to the immature myelination of the neurons in the CNS. The chest wall in the premature infant is highly compliant, resulting in inadequate tidal volume. Obstructive apnea occurs when chest wall movement is evident but no airflow occurs in the nares.

Nursing management is directed toward control of the physical environment through temperature regulation and positioning. When positioning the preterm infant, it is extremely important to avoid neck flexion and thus airway obstruction. A good way to position an infant is prone, with neck and shoulder support to decrease flexion.

Exact documentation of the frequency of episodes, duration, severity, resolution, and intervention required is extremely important to determine a pattern, a cause, and adequacy of therapy. Many episodes of apnea may resolve on their own; however, others will require intervention. Intervention may include gentle tactile stimulation, such as stroking the foot. More vigorous stimulation may be needed and can be provided by rubbing the infant's back or soles of the feet. Use care not to rub vigorously enough to bruise the infant. Other interventions include oxygen therapy or positive pressure ventilation with bag and mask.

Medical management of apnea of prematurity includes treatment of the underlying disease process, supportive oxygen therapy, continuous positive airway pressure to increase end expiratory volume. Pharmacologic support is used to stimulate the chemoreceptors in the respiratory center of the CNS, relax bronchial smooth muscle, increase respiratory drive, and increase respiratory muscle activity. The most commonly used methylxanthines are aminophylline, theophylline, and caffeine.

Air-Block Syndrome or Pneumothorax

A complication of ventilation in the preterm infant is pneumothorax or **air-block syndrome**. Caused by alveolar overinflation and rupture, air enters the perivascular sheath and dissects along the blood vessels or along the trachea and bronchial tree. Maldistribution of air leads to overdistention in some alveoli and atelectasis in others. There are five types of air leakage: pneumomediastinum, pneumopericardium, pneumothorax, pneumoperitoneum, and subcutaneous emphysema. Air that enters the pulmonary interstitial tissue may lead to pulmonary interstitial emphysema (PIE).

Air leaks are caused by rapid changes in alveolar pressure and ventilation. In pulmonary disease the lung is stiff and noncompliant. The premature infant requires mechanical ventilation because of this disease process, thereby, increasing the risk of pneumothorax. The incidence of pneumothorax is decreased by minimizing inspiratory and mean airway pressures. Treatment of respiratory disease with surfactant and high-frequency ventilation has decreased the occurrence of air leakage in the preterm population (Carroll, 1991).

Signs and symptoms of pneumothorax in the preterm infant include decreased breath sounds on the affected side, changes in blood pressure, tachypnea, grunting, cyanosis, bradycardia, distant heart sounds, and irritability. It is more difficult to appreciate signs and symptoms of pneumothorax in the preterm infant because of resonance, chest wall compliance, and other disease processes.

Treatment requires evacuation of the extra pulmonary air and usually is an urgent surgical procedure. Nursing care requires continuous monitoring of blood pressure, heart rate, and oxygenation.

Pneumonia

The incidence of pneumonia in the preterm infant is greater than 10% (Lott, 1994) owing to immature immune response, extended hospitalizations, and prolonged ventilatory support. The mortality rate for perinatally acquired pneumonia is approximately 20%; for postnatal infections the rate increases to almost 50% (Lott, 1994).

The causes of neonatal pneumonia can be divided into three categories: transplacental infections that are mostly viral, such as cytomegalovirus, syphilis, tuberculosis, and listeria; perinatal infections that include group B *Streptococcus, Haemophilus influenzae, Escherichia coli, Klebsiella,* and *Chlamydia;* and postnatal infections, such as *Pseudomonas, Serratia, Staphylococcus aureus,* CMV, and respiratory syncytial virus (RSV).

Medical treatment requires broad spectrum antibiotics until the organism is identified. At that time antibiotic therapy is adjusted to suitable drugs for that organism.

Respiratory syncytial virus is the major cause of bronchiolitis and pneumonia in infants during the first 3 years of life (Lott, 1994) and is the most common cause of rehospitalization for the preterm infant. RSV is most prevalent during the months from winter to spring. Treatment in the infant who is mildly infected is aimed at supportive and symptomatic therapies. Ribavirin occasionally is used in infants with severe disease. Prophylactic immunization is available with palivizumab (Synagis) for infants most at risk for developing severe illness. Synagis is an intramuscular (IM) injection given once a month for 6 months and may be given in conjunction with other immunizations (AAP, 1998).

Meconium Aspiration Syndrome

Meconium aspiration is similar to RDS in presentation and radiographic findings and is caused by aspiration of meconium-stained amniotic fluid in utero or at delivery. Meconium aspiration syndrome rarely is found in premature infants of less than 36 weeks' gestation (Casey, 1999). Meconium aspiration results in a chemical pneumonitis, airway obstruction, and hyperinflation. Pneumonia, pulmonary hypertension, and pneumothorax are common complications.

SPECIAL CONSIDERATIONS IN CARING FOR THE INFANT AT HIGH RISK

Nurses in the NICU are in a position to provide physical care to infants and psychosocial care to families. This care involves facilitating parent-infant bonding, providing parent education, and serving as advocates for their patients—infants who cannot speak for themselves. Controlling the physical environment, meeting infants' physical and medical needs, and maintaining client records used in medical decision-making are important aspects of the nursing role (Figure 34-11).

Of particular importance in the NICU is alleviating parental anxiety and providing insights into the family's values and cultural preferences for the health care team. The nurse serves as the infant's protector when the parents are not at the bedside and as an interpreter for medical terminology. The following section addresses considerations that affect ill infants whether they are premature, have IUGR, or have other medical conditions.

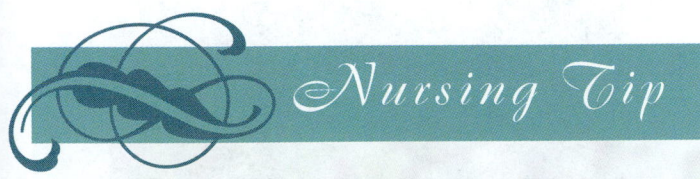

Nursing Tip

CHEST TUBE ASSESSMENT

1. Assess the chest tube insertion site: an occlusive dressing is used as a barrier to infection.
2. Assess chest tube patency: fluctuation of the water column may indicate patency.
3. Assess output: drainage should be minimal; drainage should not be bloody.
4. Evaluate the water seal: excessive bubbling indicates an air leak in the system.

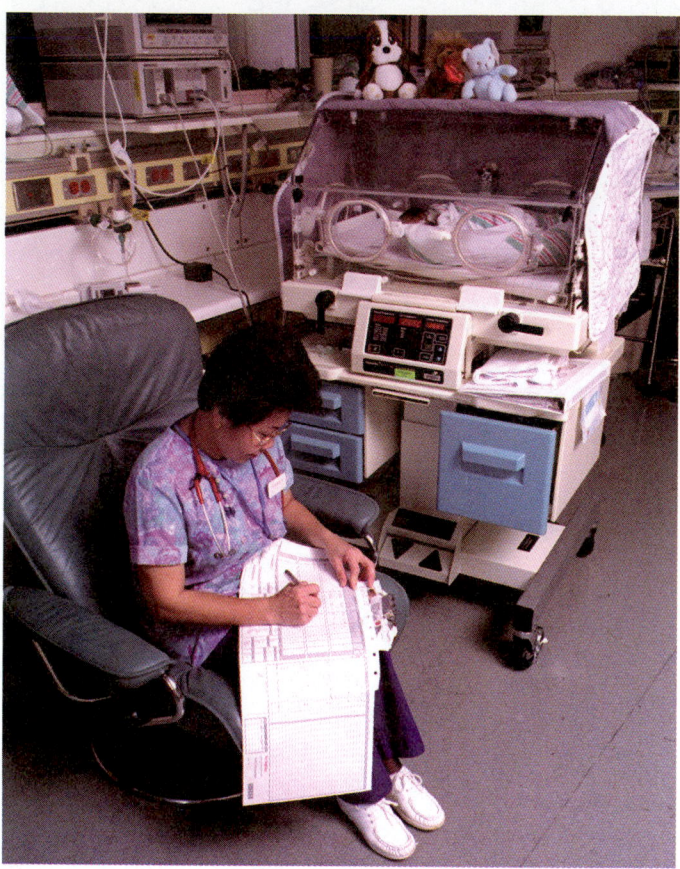

Figure 34-11 Documenting all care given to the high-risk infant is an important nursing responsibility.

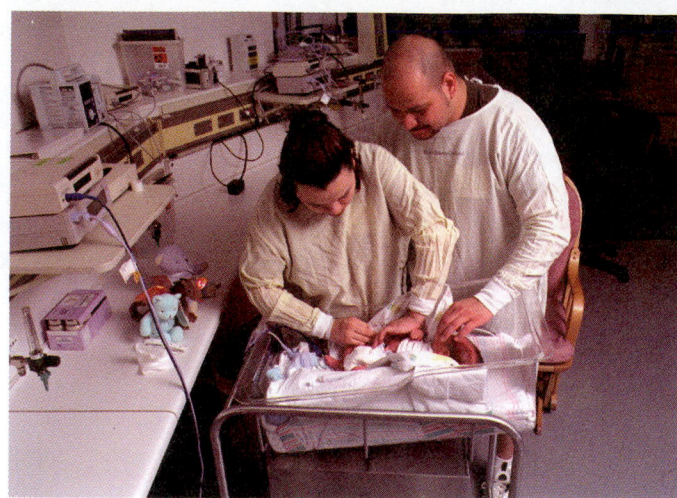

Figure 34-12 The nurse must remember the critical role that parents play in the at-risk infant's high-tech world.

Parental Anxiety

The birth of a premature infant is a challenge to parents who anticipated having an uneventful pregnancy, a normal delivery, and a healthy infant. Instead, the infant is ill, very small, and in a place filled with strange sounds and highly technical equipment (Figure 34-12). Hospital personnel are brisk, professional, and efficient; they speak rapidly, using medical jargon. It is easy for parents to feel as if they are unable to care for their infant and to experience a sense of isolation from the staff.

The technical component of care for the preterm infant is intimidating and often overwhelms parents. They may feel helpless because of the fragility of the infant. With support and education, parents become familiar with the equipment, staff, and routines. Once this occurs, parents are able to begin participating in the infant's care.

It is important for nurses who care for premature infants to promote family-centered care. The parent is the constant in the baby's life. The nurse should support the individuality and coping mechanisms of each family and should make each visit to the baby as pleasant as possible.

Information given to parents should be complete and clear. Specialized medical terms should be avoided, and any written materials should be provided in lay terms.

The developmental needs of the infant should be discussed. Teaching parents to recognize the unique personality of their infant and the infant's distress signals will foster parent-infant interaction and help provide confidence in parenting skills. Involving parents in the infant's care is very important (Figure 34-13).

Personalization of the infant's bedside, use of the infant's name, and a permissive visitation policy foster family involvement. Comfortable chairs, subdued lighting, and a quiet atmosphere may calm and sooth the baby and the parents.

Ethical Considerations

The goals of neonatal care are to preserve life, decrease morbidity, and relieve pain and suffering. Technologic advances have been a benefit to many and have allowed for

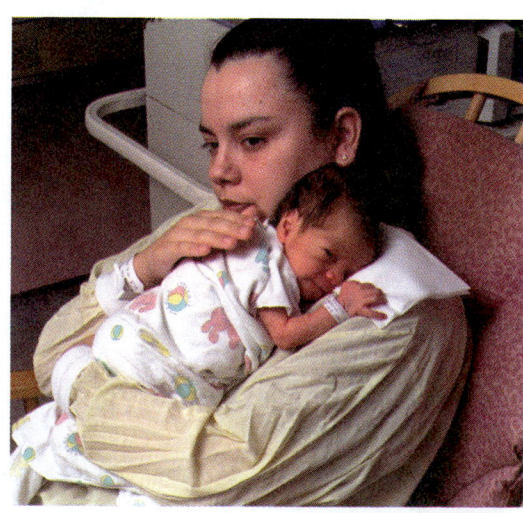

Figure 34-13 Parents will learn the cues to their infant's needs at each visit to the NICU.

the mortality and morbidity of premature infants to improve. These advances also have resulted in ethical dilemmas for all parties involved. How small is too small? Whose decision is it to resuscitate an infant born at 23 weeks' gestation? Should infants with lethal anomalies be resuscitated? These are just a few of the questions that face neonatal caregivers.

Nurses are the primary caregivers in the NICU. They need to maintain expertise and objectivity, while providing the family with a supportive and caring environment. These competing obligations make caring for the client more difficult. The role of the nurse should first be as client advocate, to ensure that the care the client is receiving is what is best for that client and the family.

In general, all infants at 24 weeks' gestation and above are considered viable. State and federal laws exist that mandate viability. In all instances, the parents should be given the information that is needed to make informed decisions about therapy and procedures. Most tertiary care centers have ethics committees that can be called on to assist in decision-making processes. The parents or anyone involved in the infant's care can request a committee meeting in which client information is presented, discussion of options occurs, and a collective decision can be made. The caregivers, social services, and support persons of their choice support parents through this process. Of utmost importance is to ensure that the decision is one the parents are comfortable with.

Thermoregulation

Maintenance of a normal body temperature is an extremely important aspect of nursing care of the preterm neonate. A healthy term infant is able to initiate temperature regulation by heat production within a few hours after birth. Term and preterm infants who are ill do not have this ability. The newborn can produce heat through four mechanisms: metabolic processes, voluntary muscle activity, peripheral vasoconstriction, and nonshivering thermogenesis (Kenner, Amlung, & Flandemeyer, 1998). The preterm infant is limited in the ability to produce heat as a result of decreased glycogen stores in the liver, decreased brown fat availability, small muscle mass, and increased body surface area.

The infant can lose heat by four modes of heat transfer: evaporation, conduction, convection, and radiation. It is important for nurses caring for premature infants to understand these concepts to prevent cold stress in infants (Box 34-2).

Evaporation is the loss of heat as water is lost from the skin to the environment. It is important to dry an infant rapidly after birth to prevent evaporative heat loss and cold stress. *Conduction* is the transfer of heat from one object to another when in direct contact. For example, placement on a cold scale to weigh the infant will result in heat from the infant's body being transferred to the scale. Placing a warm blanket on the scale first, and returning the dial to zero, before weighing the infant helps prevent conductive heat loss. Electronically warmed scales are available to help maintain the infant's temperature.

Convection is the loss of heat from an object to the environment. The use of servo-controlled incubators and neutral thermal temperature charts determines the best incubator temperature to prevent heat loss and minimize oxygen and calorie consumption so important in the care of the premature infant. When caring for an infant, use of portholes instead of opening the incubator door prevents rapid heat loss from the incubator. Open only the portholes of the incubator on one side at a time to prevent cross-ventilation and heat loss from the incubator. When nursed in a bassinet or on a warmer, the infant should be protected from drafts.

Radiation is the loss of heat between objects that are not in direct contact. A cold window near the infant's incubator would allow the wall of the incubator to cool. The infant would then lose heat to the cool incubator wall. The use of double-walled incubators and incubator covers helps prevent heat loss by radiation.

Once these conditions are controlled in the environment of a preterm infant, maintenance of body temperature is easier. Signs and symptoms of hypothermia and hyperthermia are outlined in Box 34-3. The consequences of hypothermia include hypoglycemia, pulmonary vasoconstriction, altered surfactant production, metabolic acidosis,

---

Box 34-2 Preventing Cold Stress in the Premature Infant

Evaporation	Conduction	Convection	Radiation
• Dry at delivery.	• Prewarm the bedding.	• Warm the environment.	• Avoid windows.
• Dry after bathing	• Use a warmed scale.	• Avoid drafts.	• Use incubator covers.
• Keep linens dry.	• Cover X-ray plates.	• Cover up the infant.	• Use a double-walled incubator.
• Use plastic-wrap blankets.	• Warm the diapers.	• Use head caps.	
• Use heat shields.	• Warm the water and cleansers.		
• Use humidified air.			

90%, whereas the term infant's is 80%. The extracellular fluid of the preterm infant is 50% to 55% compared with 45% in the term infant. The major routes of water losses are evaporative from the skin and lungs and excretory

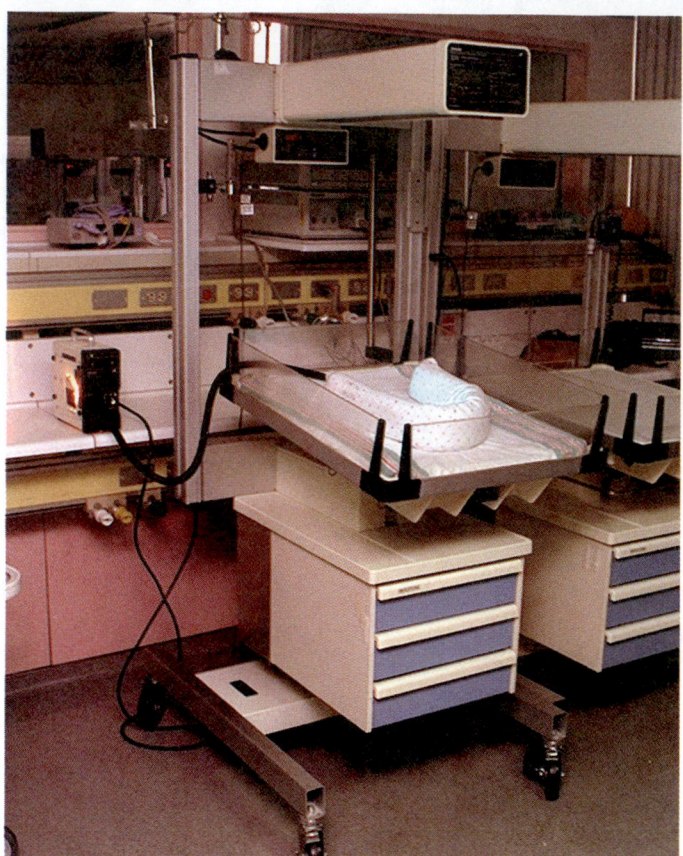

A.

hypoxia, and weight loss or poor weight gain (Blackburn & Loper, 1992).

When rewarming an infant who has been stressed by cold, it is important to increase the temperature gradually. Increase the ambient air temperature by 1 to 1.5 degrees until the infant's temperature is stable. Rapid rewarming may result in hypotension from peripheral vasodilation and apnea.

Consequences of hyperthermia include an increased metabolic rate, leading to increase oxygen consumption and dehydration from increased insensible water loss. Peripheral vasodilation may result in hypotension (Kenner, Amlung, & Flandemeyer, 1998). Seizures and apnea also may occur (Merenstein & Gardner, 1998).

All types of warming devices used in the care of preterm infants have benefits and risks. Shown in Figure 34-14 are a radiant warmer and one type of incubator. Heat shields, plastic-wrap blankets, hats, warming pads, and skin protectors are useful tools in temperature regulation. Skin-to-skin holding also is of benefit in heat conservation for infants and is discussed subsequently.

Nutrition and Fluid Management

Fluid and nutrition are essential to life. In the newborn who is ill, fluid and nutrition take on added importance because of the infant's large surface area, limited storage, and increased metabolic needs to maintain thermal homeostasis and for growth and development.

Fluid Management

The management of fluids in the preterm infant may become very complicated. Owing to their small size, large surface area, and immature skin barrier the premature infant may have large evaporative losses (insensible water losses). The preterm infant's total body water is 85% to

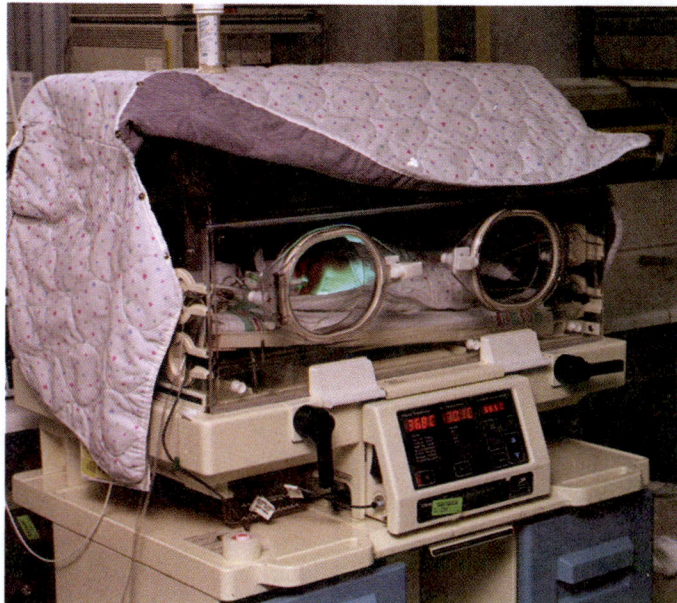

B.

Figure 34-14 A. Radiant warmer. B. Covered incubator with portholes.

from the urinary tract. Mechanisms that increase **insensible water loss (IWL)** include use of radiant warmers and phototherapy.

Fluid losses are inversely proportional to weight and gestational age. The smaller the infant the greater the fluid losses (Table 34-2). Measures to aid in decreasing IWLs include humidified air, which decreases IWL by 30%, and use of plastic blankets or shields, which decreases IWL by 50% (Costriano & Baumgart, 1986).

The overall goal of fluid management is threefold: to maintain normal body fluid composition and volume, to prevent overhydration and dehydration, and to replace ongoing water losses. Fluid needs in the first few days of life usually are higher in infants who have LBW than in larger premature infants or term infants. For example, an infant weighing less than 1,000 g initially may have a fluid requirement of 100 mL/kg/d, whereas an infant weighing 1,500 g would need only 80 mL/kg/d.

Strictly monitoring fluid intake and output is essential. Monitoring the infant's urine output by weighing diapers is necessary to assess fluid status. Evaluating laboratory values also is helpful. The following laboratory tests can assist in maintaining the delicate balance of fluids: serum electrolytes, BUN, and creatinine. Elevated sodium and BUN levels generally indicate a need for fluid. Elevated creatinine indicates renal dysfunction often owing to prematurity.

Weight loss is necessary and expected in the first few days of life (Figure 34-15). Generally, term infants may lose from 10% to 15% of their birth weights, whereas preterm infants may lose from 15% to 20% of their birth weights. This weight loss is caused by natural diuresis. It is essential to provide adequate nutrition during this time to prevent excess weight loss in an already compromised infant.

Because fluid balance is so important in premature infants and because very small amounts of fluid may add up to a significant volume, strictly measuring fluid intake and urine output is essential. All fluids are recorded and considered, including fluids that medications are mixed with and fluids used to flush IV lines and catheters. When

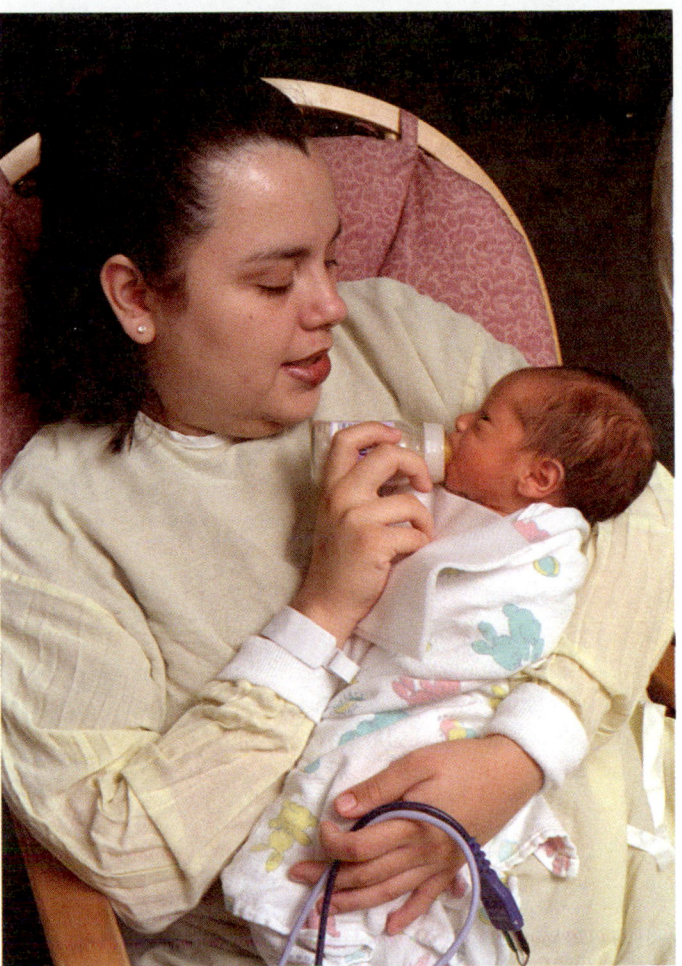

Figure 34-15 At 2 weeks of age, this preterm infant is starting to gain weight.

blood, blood products, and other volume-expanding fluids are used, the measurements also must be included in the infant's daily intake. Electronic pumps designed to administer fluid to a tenth of a milliliter are used to avoid overhydrating an infant. Failing to include medications and blood products in the intake, miscalculating fluid needs, entering an erroneous IV rate, or failing to adjust to decreased urine output in a timely manner can lead to fluid overload. Complications of fluid overload in the premature infant include pulmonary edema, PDA, congestive heart failure, IVH, and BPD.

Fluid management may be divided into short-term and long-term management. Those infants requiring IV fluids for the first few days of life generally are managed on a glucose solution, with the addition of electrolytes and calcium supplements. Very premature and acutely ill infants may require IV fluids for a prolonged period of time. These infants will need a **total parenteral nutrition (TPN)** solution that meets the requirements of carbohydrates, protein, electrolytes, vitamins, and minerals generally received through feedings. These needs generally are

Table 34-2 Fluid Losses in Incubator			
Weight (g)	Insensible Water Loss (mL/kg)	Urine (mL/kg)	Total (mL/kg)
<1,000	65	45	110
1,001–1,200	55	45	100
1,251–1,500	38	45	83
>1,500	17	45	62

met through TPN with intralipids for essential fatty acid requirements.

Various routes are available for parenteral fluid administration in the preterm infant. For short-term access, peripheral lines may be adequate. The nurse generally inserts a small-gauge Teflon catheter into a scalp or peripheral vein. Long-term access is necessary for **very low birth weight (VLBW)** infants, that is, infants weighing 1,500 g or less at birth; **extremely low birth weight (ELBW)** infants, that is, infants weighing 1,000 g or less at birth; and infants who are acutely ill. Long-term access may be achieved with umbilical venous catheters, percutaneous central venous catheters, or central venous catheters. Use of indwelling catheters increases the infant's risk for infection, bleeding, clot formation, and microemboli. Careful monitoring and aseptic technique are necessary.

Electrolyte Management

Electrolyte supplementation usually is not required in the first 24 hours of life and should not be given until urine output is established. The fluid losses from skin, lungs, and urine contain small amounts of electrolytes. By the second day of life maintenance electrolytes are required. At this time, 2 to 4 mEq/kg/d of sodium, potassium, and chloride may be added.

The infant who has VLBW lacks the ability to conserve sodium and potassium. Therefore, sodium requirements may be as high as 9 mEq/kg/d, and potassium requirements 8 to 10 mEq/kg/d. **Hyponatremia** (serum sodium less than 125 mg/dL) occurs secondary to sodium wasting with diuretic therapy, GI and renal tubular losses, fluid overload, syndrome of inappropriate antidiuretic hormone, sepsis, and congenital adrenal hyperplasia. **Hypernatremia** (serum sodium greater than 155 mg/dL) is most likely from dehydration or excessive sodium intake (Zenk, Sills, & Koeppel, 2000).

Hyperkalemia (serum potassium greater than 7 mg/dL) occurs as a result of low urine output and immature renal function, specifically distal tubular dysfunction. This condition is life-threatening. Preterm infants may present with electrocardiographic changes. Acidosis with a shift of potassium from the intracellular to the extracellular compartment is noted. Treatment includes discontinuation of potassium administration, increase in serum glucose levels, and insulin administration to shift the potassium into the intracellular compartment.

Glucose Homeostasis

Glucose is the main substrate necessary for energy, brain metabolism, and CNS integrity. During fetal life, glucose crosses the placenta and is the main source of energy for the growing fetus. After birth, neonates must maintain glucose homeostasis on their own.

Hypoglycemia

Owing to immaturity, the preterm infant's metabolism may not be capable of producing and regulating glucose. The preterm infant is at high risk for hypoglycemia secondary to rapid depletion of already low glucose stores and inability to produce and regulate glucose. **Hypoglycemia** is defined as serum glucose less than 40 mg/dL. Signs and symptoms of hypoglycemia include jitteriness, irritability, cyanosis, seizures, and apnea.

In term infants who are asymptomatic and nonstressed early feedings can be attempted. This option is less likely for a premature infant because of the inability to suck and lack of substrate for food absorption. At times, it may be appropriate to provide the early feeding by gavage, retesting 30 minutes after feeding. Infants who are symptomatic and most premature infants will require IV glucose followed by maintenance fluids. Glucose requirements for term and preterm infants weighing more than 1250 g initially begin at 6 to 8 mg/kg/min. is provided by 10% dextrose at 80 mL/kg/d. Preterm infants have a greater demand for glucose because of their large brain to body-weight ratio compared with term infants and older children (Haymond, 1989). Glucose levels are monitored until stable. Treatment of the underlying pathology is essential.

Hyperglycemia

Hyperglycemia is defined as a blood glucose greater than 125 mg/dL in the term infant and greater than 150 mg/dL in the preterm infant. Hyperglycemia is commonly seen in the premature infant. These infants are not able to tolerate a glucose infusion at the same rate as would a more mature infant. This intolerance is due a decrease in insulin release in response to glucose.

Sepsis, specifically gram-negative sepsis, also increases the risk for hyperglycemia. Certain drugs may cause an increase in glucose levels, including high levels of methylxanthines, which are used in the treatment of apnea of prematurity. Hyperglycemia may be a stress response as seen

---

Nursing Alert

RISK FACTORS FOR HYPOGLYCEMIA

- Decreased substrate availability
- Endocrine disorders
- Increased utilization
- Sepsis
- Central nervous system abnormalities

in neonates postoperatively. Steroid therapy also produces a hyperglycemic state in preterm infants.

In the infant who has LBW glucose infusions are initiated and increased gradually. Initial fluids are started at 2 to 4 mg/kg/min and gradually increased to 8 to 12 mg/kg/min, depending on the infant's tolerance and needs. The basal metabolic rate in preterm infants is higher than that in term infants and may require higher concentrations of glucose to meet these needs. If the preterm infant is unable to tolerate high glucose concentrations, insulin may be added to the fluids or given as a separate IV drip until levels are under control. In the first few days of life frequent monitoring of glucose levels is extremely important.

Feeding

Nutritional needs for premature infants often are complex. Accelerated needs for calories and minerals cannot always be met through the use of human milk or standard formulas. Approximately 50 to 60 kcal/kg/d are necessary for infants to maintain weight. The term infant may require 100 to 110 kcal/kg/d and the preterm infant from 110 to 140 kcal/kg/d for weight gain.

Formula Feeding

Formulas are available specifically designed for the preterm infant to provide high calorie intake per ounce and extra protein, vitamins, and minerals needed for growth and development (Figure 34-16). Human milk remains the feeding of choice for premature infants. Because of the infant's size and limitations related to the medical conditions, enteral intake may be restricted. Standard formula and human milk at the volumes tolerated by the infant may provide inadequate calories to sustain rapid growth and high metabolic needs. At limited volumes these feedings do not provide adequate minerals for bone mineralization, and **osteopenia** (bone mass below normal levels) may occur.

There are commercial formulas designed for premature infants and commercially prepared fortifiers available to add to expressed human milk that increase the calorie and mineral content of the milk. As the infant grows and is able to tolerate larger volumes of feedings, the formula may be changed to formula designed for term infants or to nonfortified human milk.

Breast Milk Feeding

Mothers who decide to provide breast milk for their infants need encouragement and support. Mothers must be educated on the correct expression and handling of breast milk. Many hospitals have nurses who specialize in lactation support available to assist these mothers. These lactation consultants are available to provide support to the

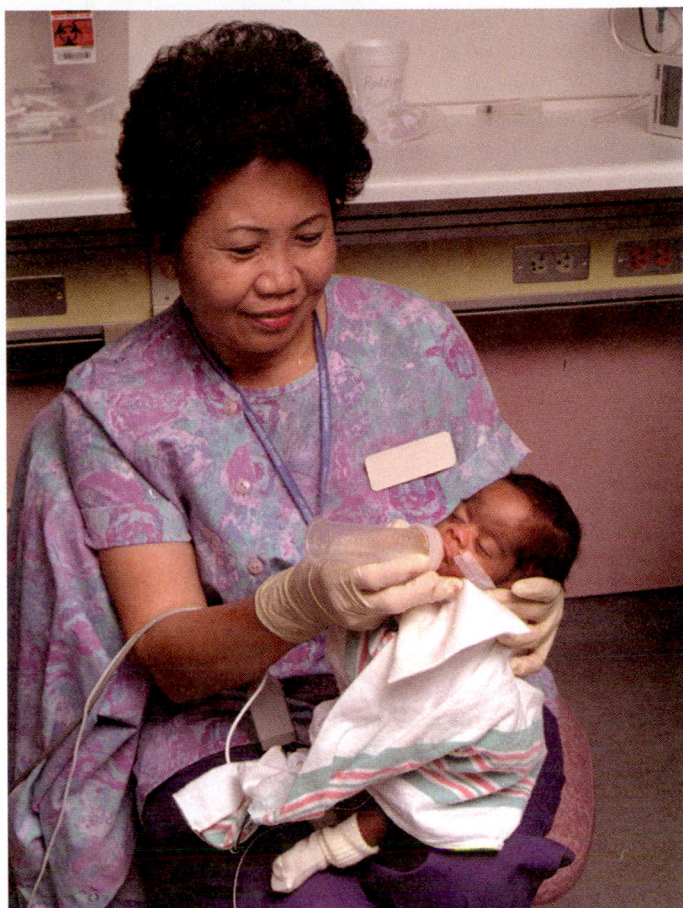

Figure 34-16 This preterm infant receives a specially designed formula to meet his nutritional needs; note placement of a nasogastric tube.

mothers during the transition from gavage feedings to breast-feeding when needed.

Initiating Feedings

Determining when to initiate feedings is dependent on several factors: the infant's clinical status, assessment of GI

PARENT EDUCATION

When teaching parents how to check orogastric feeding tube placement, teach them to place the end of the tube in a glass of water after checking placement. The water will bubble with each breath if the tube is in the trachea rather than the stomach. Being able to double-check placement may give parents more confidence in their ability to perform this skill.

motility, and nutritional needs. Once the infant's condition is stable and stooling has begun, enteral feedings usually may be introduced.

The feeding regimen may vary but generally depends on gestational age and weight. Preterm infants less than 31 week's gestation are unable to coordinate sucking and swallowing with respirations. Therefore, orogastric tube feedings are necessary (Figure 34-17). They may be given as a continuous hourly drip or by intermittent **gavage feedings**, usually every 2 to 3 hours, depending on the infant's tolerance (Box 34-4).

Very premature infants may be started on sterile water, human milk, or half-strength premature formula for the first feedings. These feedings are minute and are used to stimulated GI motility. Larger infants and premature infants who are more mature may be started on human milk or full-strength formula. Once the feedings have been initiated and tolerated, the caloric density and volume of feedings are gradually increased to full-strength 24-cal/oz formula, or fortifiers are added to human milk to increase caloric density to 24 cal/oz. Volume is gradually increased by 15 to 25 mL/kg/d until full feedings are established. A full enteral feeding for a premature infant is 150 to 160 mL/kg/d of premature formula or fortified human milk. Once the infant transitions to 20 cal/oz or nonfortified human milk, the infant must receive at least 180 mL/kg/d.

It is essential for the nurse to be aware of the infant's tolerance to feedings and changes in tolerance resulting from an increase in calories or volume. Signs and symptoms of feeding intolerance include increasing gastric residuals, bile in gastric aspirate, blood in gastric contents or stools, abdominal distention, change in bowel pattern or diarrhea, visibly dilated loops of bowel emesis, temperature instability, apnea and bradycardia, and hypoxia.

Infants between 32 and 35 weeks' gestation are generally assessed for readiness to feed by mouth. These include infants born at a younger gestational age and who

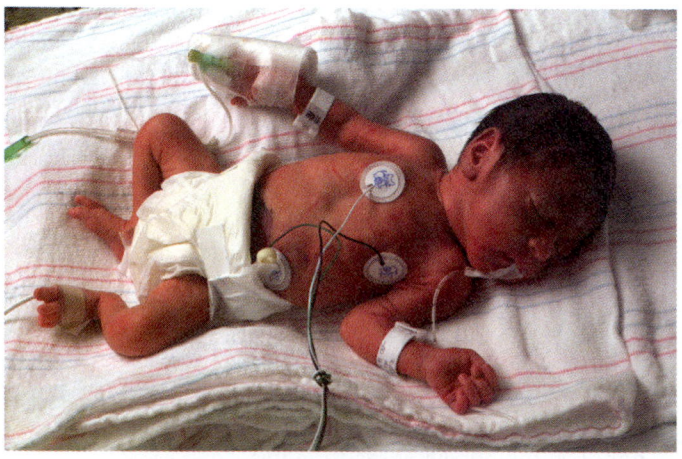

Figure 34-17 Premature infant with orogastric feeding tube.

are now 32 to 35 weeks by postconceptual age and infants who have just been born at this gestational age. If the infant does not demonstrate the ability to coordinate oral feedings (an adequate suck-swallow reflex and breathing) or does not have the stamina to feed orally, gavage feedings are indicated. As discussed in previously, volume is increased as tolerated by the infant.

During gavage feedings the infant will require oral stimulation to improve coordination and facial muscle tone. Offering a pacifier during gavage feeds may aid in the development of oral feeding skills (Figure 34-19). Non-nutritive sucking also may be achieved by suckling at the breast once the mother has manually expressed milk.

Occasionally, alternative formulas may be necessary. Because infants who have experienced bowel injury may not tolerate standard or premature formulas, use of elemental or basic formulas may be required. While an important adjunct for feeding high-risk infants, these formulas are not as high in calories and protein as are the premature formulas. When alternative formulas are used, supplementation with carbohydrates and protein is necessary to ensure optimal nutrition.

Pain Management in the Neonate

In 1979, the International Association for the Study of Pain defined pain as an unpleasant sensory and emotional experience associated with actual or potential tissue damage, or described in terms of such damage (Merskey et al., 1979). Pain is a very subjective experience. It is extremely difficult to identify the degree of pain of infants because of their inability to express pain. This inability of the infant to tell caregivers of their pain has led to failure of caregivers to recognize and treat pain in the neonatal population. According to Anand (1998), preterm and term infants demonstrate similar or even exaggerated physiologic and hormonal responses to pain compared with those observed in older children and adults.

The American Academy of Pediatrics (AAP) and the Canadian Pediatric Society (CPS) (AAP & CPS, 2000) jointly promoted a document to address the issue of pain management and prevention in neonates. In the past, the focus has been centered on treatment of pain rather than a systemic approach to reduce or prevent pain.

We now know that neonates have the neurologic capability to experience pain. The peripheral and spinal structures necessary for pain information transmission are present and functional between the first and the second trimesters. Therefore, infants born as early as 24 weeks' gestation are capable of feeling pain.

It has been proposed that untreated pain has adverse physiologic consequences and probable short-lived and long-term consequences (Shapiro, 1993). Adverse physio-

Box 34-4 Oral Gastric Tube Placement

A. Indications: Provision of enteric feedings when oral feedings are not possible.

  1. Immature suck-swallow reflex

  2. Abnormal gag reflex secondary to neurologic disease

  3. Inability to take full enteric feeding orally

  4. Abnormal respiratory pattern

  5. For gastric decompression

B. Contraindications

  1. Recent repair of esophageal fistula or perforation

C. Equipment

  1. Cardiac monitor

  2. Suction equipment and catheter

  3. 5- or 8-F feeding tube

  4. 3- or 5-mL syringe

  5. Stethoscope

  6. Gloves

  7. 1/2-in tape, Elastoplast, skin barrier

D. Procedure

  1. Wash hands.

  2. Put on gloves.

  3. Position infant on back.

  4. Monitor heart rate, oxygen saturations, and respiratory rate.

  5. Gently suction nares and oropharynx.

  6. Measure length for insertion by placing catheter tip from nose to stomach and estimating distance (Figure 34-18). Mark length on tube with tape.

  7. Moisten end of tube with sterile water.

  8. Place finger on anterior portion of tongue. Stabilize head.

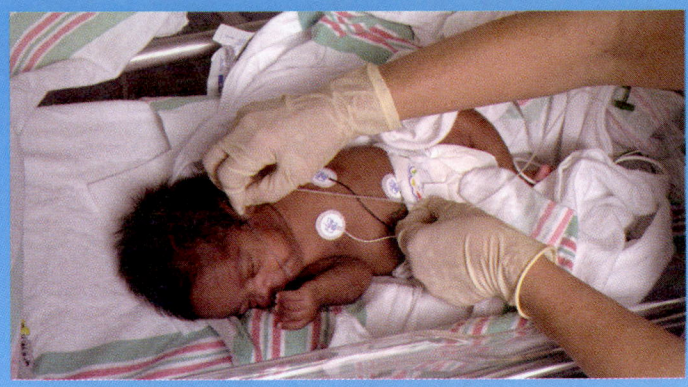

Figure 34-18 Measurement for a nasogastric feeding tube.

  9. Insert tube along finger into oropharynx.

  10. Gently advance tube to predetermined length.

  11. Use pacifier to stimulate suck-swallow if able.

    a. Do not advance if resistance is met.

    b. Stop procedure if signs of respiratory distress occur.

  12. Determine correct placement

    a. Inject 1 mL of air into catheter while auscultating over stomach.

    b. Aspirate contents; note amount and type.

  13. Secure catheter to infant's face using pectin-based skin barrier under tape.

E. Complications

  1. Apnea or bradycardia

  2. Hypoxia

  3. Perforation of posterior oropharynx, esophagus, stomach, or duodenum

  4. Aspiration or esophagitis

  5. Interference with suck reflex

logic consequences such as alterations in blood pressure and glucose may affect the development of IVH. More immediate effects may be feeding intolerance, inability of infants to interact with parents, and interruption of sleep-wake cycles. Potential long-term consequences include impairments of neurodevelopment, learning, and memory (Shapiro, 1993).

As caregivers, bedside nurses are the best advocates for neonates. Nurses must be aware of behavioral and physical signs neonates use to indicate pain. Behavioral changes include crying, facial changes, and gross motor movement (see the Nursing Tip). Physiologic and autonomic changes also occur that can indicate when infants are in pain. These changes may be subtle, or they may also indicate early signs of illness. These changes include increased heart and respiratory rates that when left untreated may advance to apnea and bradycardia, increased blood pressure, and palmer sweat. The very immature neonate may not show a response to pain and later have changes in heart rate, blood pressure, and oxygen saturation.

Several tools are available to aid the nurse in assessing neonatal pain. These tools use behavioral and physiologic

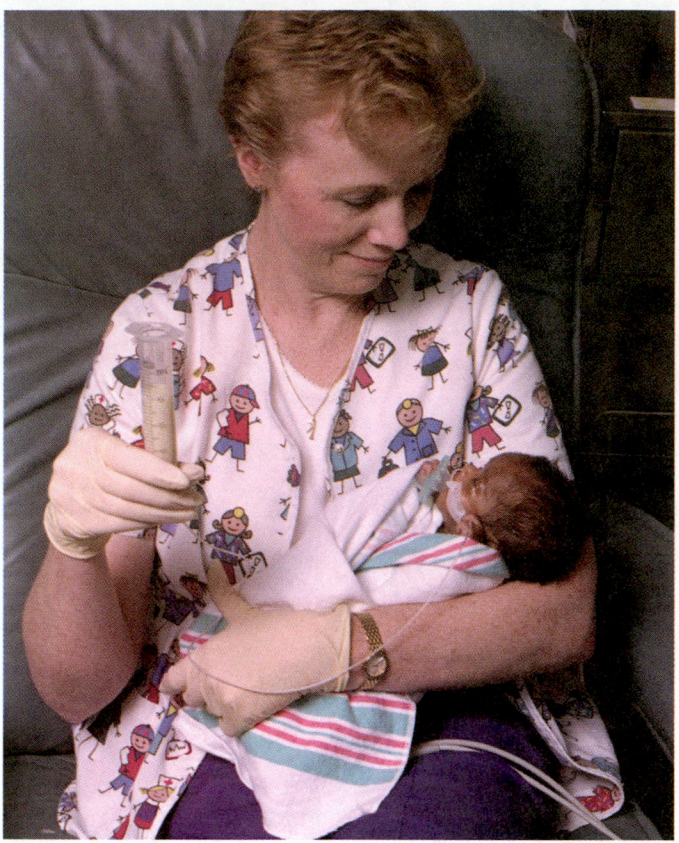

Figure 34-19 This premature infant sucks on a pacifier during his gavage feeding.

responses to pain or noxious stimuli. They are CRIES (Crying Requires Increases Expression Sleepless (Krechel & Bildner, 1995), the Premature Infant Pain Profile (PIPP) (Stevens, 1996), and the Neonatal Infant Pain Scale (NIPS) (Lawrence et al., 1993).

Pain management is an area of research on which neonatal caregivers have focused. Prevention or avoidance of noxious stimuli, use of nonpharmacologic measures,

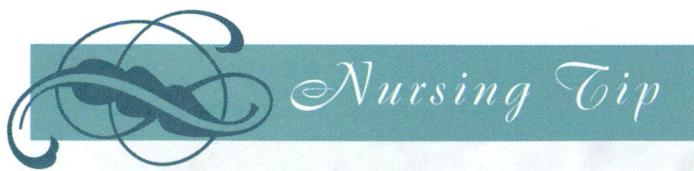

BEHAVIORAL SIGNS OF PAIN IN NEONATES

- Cry: change in frequency or pitch
- Facial changes: brow bulging, vertical furrows, eye squeezing, nasolabial furrow, and open lips
- Gross motor: attempt to withdraw from painful stimuli (near term infants),
- Limpness or flaccidity (preterm infants)

NONPHARMACOLOGIC MANAGEMENT OF PAIN

- Group blood draws
- Central venous access
- Noninvasive monitoring
- Expert staff for inserting IV lines and drawing blood

and pharmacologic treatment are integral parts of caring for our clients.

Changes in environment such as dim lighting and decreasing noise levels help decrease noxious stimuli and stress. Simple comfort measures aid in the neonate's ability to cope with painful interventions. These measures include containment, swaddling, nonnutritive sucking on a pacifier, and positioning to midline. These interventions may aid in the control of pain for minor procedures; they are not enough for moderately to severely painful procedures.

With the advances in neonatal care have come advances in anesthesia and training of personnel that have increased the safety and efficacy of anesthesia for neonatal procedures. The use of opioids has become more common in the NICU. Thus, caregivers must be aware of the potential for adverse effects on the respiratory, cardiovascular, and renal systems in neonates.

The goals of pain management are to minimize the intensity, duration, and physiologic cost to the neonate.

Drug Metabolism and Excretion

The liver and the kidneys are the major organs responsible for removal of drugs from the body. Whereas the metabolism and excretion of therapeutic drugs is well studied in healthy adults, the use of drugs in neonates is not well understood. Drug therapy must be carefully monitored for its tolerance and effect. In discussing drug metabolism absorption, distribution, clearance, and elimination must be considered.

Many factors affect drug absorption in the neonate. The route by which the drug given plays an important part. For example, for oral administration, the surface area of the intestinal tract is relatively small and the gastric emptying time is prolonged. The bile salt pool size is decreased, and bacterial colonization is not conducive to absorption. IM injection is not feasible long term owing to small muscle mass, poor peripheral perfusion, and decreased muscle activity. IV drug therapy is best tolerated by the neonate but in most cases requires prolonged IV placement with increased risk for infection.

Factors affecting drug distribution include increased body and extracellular water, decreased amount of plasma protein available for binding, decreased serum pH, and altered cardiac output.

In the preterm infant the liver and all other systems are immature. Hepatic function is decreased in neonates. There are varied hepatic pathways that mature at different points in gestation. Drug metabolism and elimination in the liver therefore depend on gestational age.

Renal elimination is directly correlated with the GFR. Extreme caution must be used in administering and monitoring drugs in premature infants. Drug therapy is tailored to the infant and may change daily.

Drug metabolism and elimination must be carefully monitored. Monitoring for therapeutic levels is essential to ensure that treatment is adequate and toxic levels are not reached. Standardized dosing regimens are common in neonates and calculated daily based on the infant's weight.

COMPLEMENTARY THERAPY

Neonatal nurses must be prepared to provide holistic family-centered care to the infants in their charge. Nurses can nurture clients and families by their caring and insight. There are nonpharmacologic therapies to enhance the experience of the infant and the family. Some are described in this section. The emphasis is on the premature infant and the infant's family because these infants are the ones hospitalized for long periods of time.

Developmental Care

Developmental care is a philosophic approach to the care of the premature infant. Premature infants may be hospitalized for a prolonged period of time and are subjected to many tests, procedures, and therapies during hospitalization. Developmental care is an approach designed to support the infant's efforts toward self-regulation.

Interventions include positioning, modification of the environment, and promotion of self-regulatory behaviors such as nonnutritive sucking (Engebretson & Wardell, 1997).

The reflexes and responses of a premature infant are consistent with postconceptual age. The infant continues to grow and develop postnatally. A need exists for early awareness and intervention to ensure normal musculoskeletal and developmental growth. Premature infants are prone to developing contractures and malposition of the extremities. Many infants require periods of sedation or paralysis owing their medical condition or require prolonged immobilization of a limb or extremity for medical interventions, such as percutaneous central lines. By being

aware of the potential for contractures to develop, the nurse can take measures to minimize risks.

Premature infants have undeveloped muscle tone. The more premature the infant the more hypotonic the infant will be. Tone will develop in the same sequence as in the term infant; however, flexor tone will not develop to the same degree. When premature infants are allowed to lie in a frog-legged position for long periods of time, with elbows flexed and shoulders abducted, the forward rotation of the shoulder may be limited (Figure 34-20). This limitation may interfere with the development of hand-to-mouth orientation. Prolonged positioning with the hips flexed, abducted, and externally rotated may cause hip dislocation or interfere with weight bearing later in life.

The infant's position should be changed regularly and frequently, about every 2 to 3 hours. Position changes should be documented to ensure a full range of positions. Gentle passive range-of-motion exercises may be provided as tolerated. Proper body alignment is essential. When turning, arms and legs should be held close to the infant's body.

Modifications of the infant's environment include indirect, soft, or dimmed lighting. A quiet environment is important. Padded incubator covers can help block out excess light and muffle noise. The inside of the cover should be dark and patterns limited to avoid overstimulation. Containment boundaries can give the infant a feeling of security, and soft bedding can aid in comfort.

Promoting self-regulatory behaviors includes clustering care to prevent fatigue and nonnutritive sucking. Nonnutritive sucking can provide infants who have LBW an opportunity to organize their behavior (Engebretson & Wardell, 1997). Nonnutritive sucking can be provided when the infant is irritable or receiving gavage feeds and after procedures to calm the infant (Figure 34-21). Once the infant is stable, nonnutritive breast-feeding can be introduced.

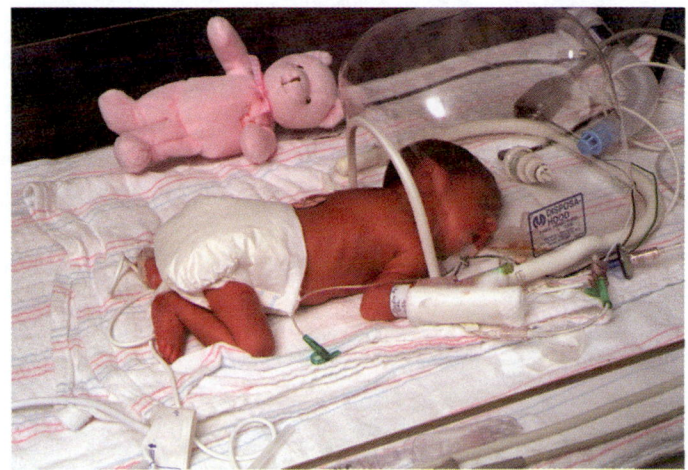

Figure 34-20 Frequent position changes for the premature infant will aid in development of good muscle tone.

Research Highlight

Development of a Pacifier for Low-Birth-Weight Infant's Nonnutritive Sucking

Purpose

As advances in neonatal care have improved the survival of smaller and smaller infants, nurses have had to modify care practices and equipment to accommodate the infant's size and level of development. The authors of this study developed and tested a pacifier specifically designed for infants who have very low birth weight.

Methods

Two aspects of pacifier design were addressed: size and shape. A natural approach was used to develop a pacifier similar to the infant's thumb. It was thought this shape would promote stimulation of the oral cavity and perioral region. Plaster molds of a preterm infant's palate and thumb were made and found to match. The model of the thumb was chosen as the pacifier design.

To determine the appropriate size for the pacifier, the sizes of thumbs, the infants' weights, head circumferences, and facial dimensions of 49 infants were obtained; thumb size was found to be proportional to weight. The mean values of these measurements were used to determine nipple length and circumference of the pacifier prototype. The addition of an angle upward was included to simulate the angle of the thumb.

Clinical trials were conducted in two phases to test the pacifier design. The first phase was to test a prototype nipple, which was attached to a commercial guard. The second phase was to test the completed nipple. The completed nipple was attached to a soft guard.

Infants who were average for gestational age, less than 2,500 g at birth, and free of anomalies that would interfere with sucking were included in the study; 36 infants were randomly assigned to either a prototype or a commercial pacifier. They were offered a pacifier while awake. Nurses in the neonatal intensive care unit served as clinical experts for the study. A nurse offered the pacifier and remained with the infant throughout the 30-minute observation time. Observation was of behavioral states using the 12-category Anderson Behavioral State Scale. Sucking patterns were noted, and the heart rate was measured and charted every 2 minutes. The pacifier was removed from the infant's mouth when signs of distress were observed.

Findings

In phase I, infants who received the prototype pacifier were found to be in a state of alert inactivity (a state suitable for feeding) significantly more often than were those in the group receiving the commercial pacifier. In the phase II clinical test, convenience samples of 20 infants were tested. The findings were positive for the acceptance of the pacifier: 100% of the infants sucked on the pacifier, 65% sucked vigorously, and 85% were in a sleep state after 20 minutes.

Nursing Implications

The infants in the clinical trials spent significantly more time in alert behavioral states associated with better feeding than did infants using the control pacifier. This increased alertness is an indication of behavioral organization. The pacifier is cost-effective and can be used successfully by parents to provide comfort to their infants. Use of this pacifier may contribute to earlier and better feeding patterns and improved growth.

Engebretson J. C., & Wardell D. W. (1997). Development of a pacifier for low-birth-weight infant's nonnutritive sucking. *Journal of Obstetric, Gynecologic, and Neonatal Nursing, 26,* (6), 660–664.

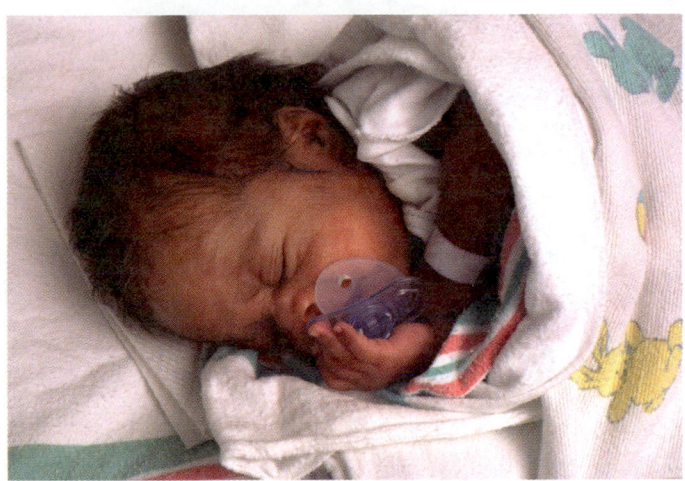

Figure 34-21 Nonnutritive sucking on a Wee-Thumbie pacifier helps this infant who has low birth weight remain calm and conserve energy.

All developmental interventions should consider the infant's gestational age. Older infants who are chronically ill should be provided with developmentally appropriate toys and activities. Parents should be involved as much as possible. A multidiciplinary team that includes physicians, primary nurses, infant occupational therapist, developmental specialists, and a speech pathologist may be needed to ensure the infant's developmental needs are being met. At discharge, preparing the infant for entry into society should be addressed in addition to the medical needs.

Early childhood intervention programs are federally funded programs designed to aid parents and infants in the transition from being hospitalized to going home. Team members include occupational therapists, physical therapists, and social workers. Infants are assessed for progression of developmental milestones, and parents are taught approaches to care to aid in the infant's development.

Therapeutic Touch

The newborn infant's sense of touch, temperature, and pressure are well developed. The major methods of communication are through touch and cry. The NICU environment and therapies consist of noxious stimuli, and the neonate may develop an aversion to touch. Noncaregiving touch is necessary and should be provided by parents and professionals. Parents should be taught to observe their infant's signals. Thus, they gain confidence in parenting skills and come to know and understand their infant's signals regarding what is and what is not tolerated.

Infant Massage

As the preterm infant matures, head-to-toe massage may be initiated. Infant massage consists of stroking at a rate of 12

to 16 strokes per minute and is thought to sooth the infant and stimulate respirations, circulation, and GI function. Varying the touch pattern maintains the infant's interest.

Containment

Containment is use of the hands to support the infant in a midline position during painful or noxious procedures. Also referred to as facilitated touch or gentle human touch, containment consists of a caregiver placing one hand on the infant's head and the other on either the infant's bottom or legs in a tucked position, and providing firm but gentle pressure (Figure 34-22). Containment has been shown to increase the infant's tolerance of procedures; provide faster return to baseline levels of vital signs on completion; cause less hypoxia, tachypnea, and tachycardia; and result in less energy expenditure.

Any of these forms of gentle touch help the preterm infant adapt to the environment and tolerate uncomfortable procedures. Therapeutic touch is needed during procedures to comfort the infant. Therapeutic touch is used at other times to provide the infant with pleasurable sensations and is especially effective when parents are involved. The infant may associate pleasurable sensations with the parents, facilitating attachment.

Kangaroo Care

Kangaroo care originated in Bogota, Columbia, as a necessity for providing preterm infants with warmth and

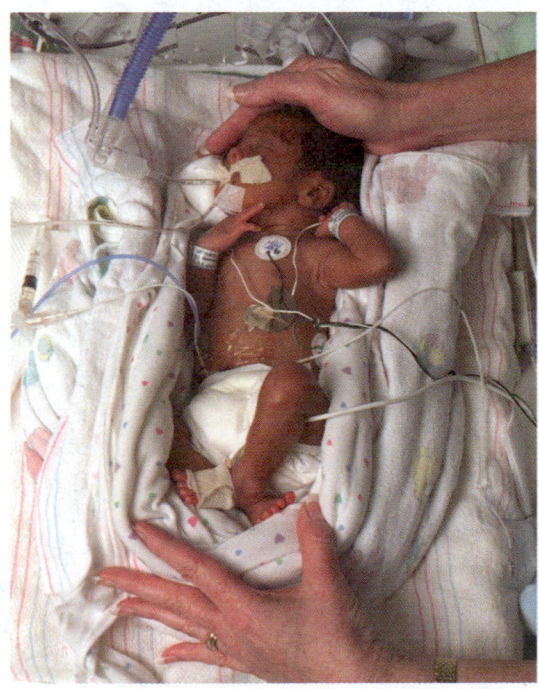

Figure 34-22 Containing the preterm infant in a midline position.

nutrition. Kangaroo care consists of a parent holding an infant, unclothed except for a diaper, upright on the mother's or father's chest. The parents are instructed to wear a shirt that opens in the front. This technique also is called skin-to-skin holding (Figure 34-23).

The benefits for the parents include feelings of well-being, feeling a part of their infant's care, enhanced parent-infant attachment, and self-confidence and self-esteem. The benefits for the infant include better weight gain, temperature regulation, decreased apnea, improved oxygenation, earlier discharge, increase in breast-feeding and increased supply, and earlier time to oral feeding. Kangaroo care, once viewed as an alternative therapy, is now common in most NICUs (Victor & Person, 1994).

Co-Bedding of Twins

Placing newborn twins together may provide support for the infants during transition to extrauterine life. Twins may be born with unique expectation of what constitutes a normal habitat, and their transition to extrauterine life may be facilitated by maintaining contact each other. This contact is thought to be supportive in nature (coregulating) (Nyquist & Lutes, 1998). Co-bedding is based on the premise that extrauterine adaptation of twin neonates is enhanced by

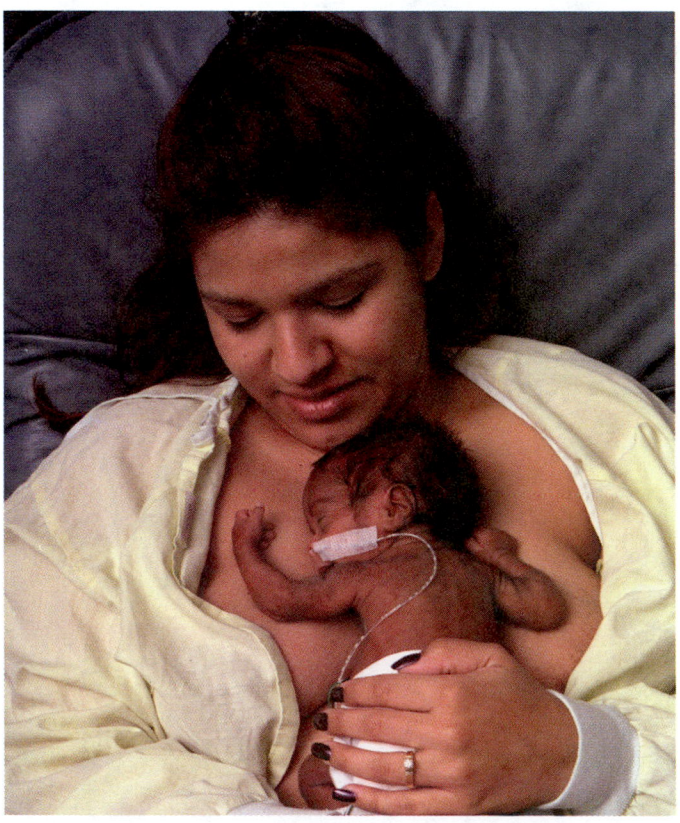

Figure 34-23 Kangaroo care, or skin-to-skin holding, has many benefits for the parent and infant.

continued physical contact with the other twin rather than the sudden deprivation of such stimuli (Nyquist, 1998).

An improvement in temperature regulation and behavioral states has been observed in co-bedding. Co-bedding may facilitate the development of similar circadian rhythm patterns and sleep-wake cycles. The effects of co-bedding and the value of supporting synchronized behavior in twins require additional evaluation (Nyquist, 1998).

NEONATAL TRANSPORT

Because care of small and premature infants requires specialized equipment and highly trained personnel, many infants require transport to regional centers where the needs of the infants can be met. Moving these infants requires an well-integrated system of assessment and perinatal transport.

Perinatal centers are designated according to their ability to handle complicated maternal and neonatal conditions. A level I center generally is a community hospital that is designed to care for the normal pregnant woman and delivery of a well newborn. A level II center is designed to handle more complex pregnancies and deliveries, and the nursery is prepared to care for infants with mild and intermediate conditions. A level III center is one that cares for the most complex obstetric and neonatal complications and conditions. A level III center also has the latest diagnostic techniques and the subspecialists necessary to care for infants with uncommon illnesses.

Maternal Transport versus Neonatal Transport

When a pregnancy is determined to be at high risk, plans can be made early to deliver the infant in a tertiary center. Mothers who go into premature labor may have no problems before the onset of labor. Transport of the pregnant mother to a center equipped to care for both her and the infant is the preferred method of transport.

When an infant is transported inside the womb there is no risk of exposure to cold stress or hypoglycemia, which are serious potential risks of neonatal transport. Transferring the pregnant woman who is in preterm labor allows the possibility of stopping labor on arrival at the tertiary care center.

Because high-risk deliveries may follow uneventful pregnancies, all hospitals must be set up to resuscitate and stabilize newborn infants. The American Heart Association and the American Academy of Pediatrics have developed a program called the Neonatal Resuscitation Program that addresses the needs of neonatal patients in the delivery room (AHA, AAP, 2000).

When a premature or infant at high risk is born at a level I or II perinatal center, a transport team with specialized equipment and training is required to move the infant to a regional center. Problems that develop during neonatal transport may be serious. Thermal stress, equipment failure, and other unexpected events may occur.

Neonatal Transport Team

Neonatal transport teams were developed to provide access to limited health care resources. They are composed of highly trained personnel experienced in the care of premature and infants at high risk. These teams extend the care of the level III perinatal center to the community with their expertise and specially designed equipment (Figure 34-24).

Members of the neonatal transport team assist the referring unit with stabilization of infants before transport. Infants must have the following before being transported: normal temperature, normal blood sugar level, and blood pressure within the normal range; stable airway, either breathing easily on their own or with an endotracheal tube in place; normal blood gas values, normal electrolyte values, and acid-base balance. When infection is suspected, treatment must begin before transport.

Parents should have the opportunity to see and touch their infant before transport. Small momentos of the infant are important. A lock of hair, the infant's footprints, or a picture may be given to the mother. Mothers should be encouraged to continue with plans for breast-feeding if that was their intent before delivery. Mothers should be encouraged to begin expressing breast milk as soon as possible after delivery and be referred to a lactation consultant or support group if the infant will not be able to breast-feed shortly after birth.

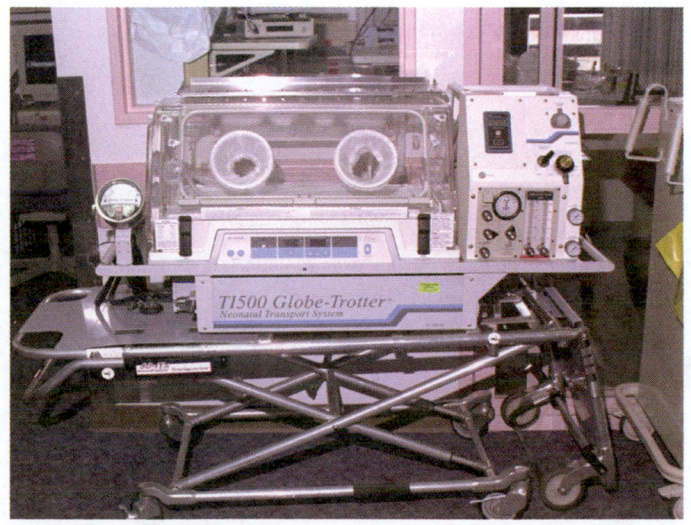

Figure 34-24 Transport incubator.

Back Transport

Level III nurseries often are located far from the parent's home. The location may make access difficult for some parents. Distance, traffic, weather, and parking costs are barriers to the nursery. When the infant no longer needs the expertise and support services offered by the level III nursery return transport should be considered as the infant's condition improves.

Return transport, or back transport, refers to transporting the infant back to the referral hospital for care until the infant is ready to go home. Return transport provides a number of advantages. The costs incurred at a community hospital are frequently lower than those at a tertiary center. If the infant is nearer the parents' home, they may have the opportunity to visit more frequently. Close proximity facilitates parent teaching and increases parents' familiarity with the care of their infant. The infant's pediatrician can assume primary care and facilitate discharge planning.

DISCHARGE PLANNING

Preparations for discharge of a high-risk preterm infant should begin on admission to the ICU. Many factors must be considered, and the discharge process often can be traumatic for the family. Providing a smooth transition for the infant and the parents is essential (Figure 34-25).

Criteria to be met before discharge include the infant's ability to maintain temperature in an open crib, steady weight gain, ability to breast-feed or bottle-feed, and absence of apnea or appropriate monitoring devices available at home. In some instances the infant may be discharged before being able to take all feedings orally. In these cases, the parents must be able to demonstrate the ability to provide alternate feeding strategies.

The parents must be educated in the proper care of their infant. To ensure proper caloric density the nurse caring for the infant should review feeding schedules, volumes, and preparation of formula. The nurse should teach the parents how to give medications needed by the infant after discharge, including dosing, accuracy, and administration. Parents who are taking their infant home on a cardiac, apnea, or saturation monitor need equipment training and training in cardiopulmonary resuscitation. Parents should be educated in infant safety. Parents also need to be taught to recognize signs of illness, when to call the pediatrician, and what to do in an emergency. Parents need a written record of the infant's diagnosis, any surgeries, and all discharge instructions, including treatments and medications.

The discharge process is a multidisciplinary team effort. Involvement of the primary nurse or advanced practice nurse, neonatologist, social services, respiratory services, occupational therapists, physical therapists, and appropriate consultants is essential for a smooth transition.

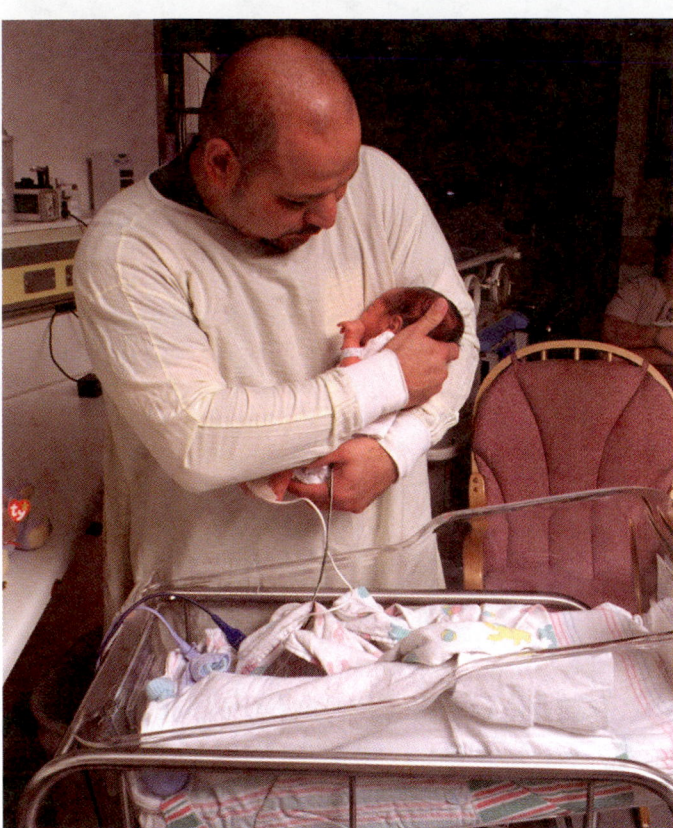

Figure 34-25 Parents need to develop comfort and confidence with their newborn before discharge.

Follow-up needs should be reviewed and their importance emphasized.

Resources are available in the community for parents of infants at high risk. Early childhood intervention programs provide for many of the follow-up services needed and are generally available nationwide. These programs also provide for transition from one stage of development to another. Support programs are common in urban areas, often through tertiary care centers and religious organizations. Financial planning must be addressed with the family early in the clinical course. Owing to advances in technology, smaller and sicker infants are surviving. Insurance provision often are used up while the infant is hospitalized. Assisting the family with the process of obtaining financial aide is critical, and social services play an integral part in this process. See Chapter 38 for further community services available to families of critical infants.

The most common causes of re-admission to the hospital include infection, specifically RSV; failure to thrive; profound apnea; and aspiration pneumonia.

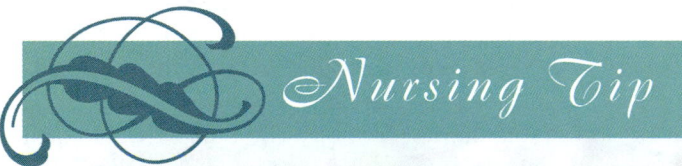

Nursing Tip

POTENTIAL DISCHARGE NEEDS FOR A PREMATURE INFANT

- Pediatrician capable of complex care
- Developmental follow-up
- Ophthalmologist
- Pulmonary specialists
- Speech and language
- Occupational therapists

Web Activities

The following websites have information concerning assessment of fetal status. Visit these sites for additional information.

- www.fetal.com
- www.medphys.ucl.ac.uk/mgi/fetal
- www.amnionet.com
- www.med.upenn.edu/meded
- www.public/berp/overview
- www.cpdx.com/cpdx
- www.virtualbirth.com
- www.sgvp.com
- www.docboard.org
- Search the Internet for websites offering information or some of the disorders discussed in this chapter, such as NEC, GER, BPD, and ROP.
- Visit the Internet to find support groups for parents of infants who are SGA, LGA, and premature. Do these sites have chat rooms? Information exchanges? Literature for sale?

Case Study/Care Plan

INFANT WITH IUGR

Daniel is a premature second twin born to a 34-year-old, gravida 3, para 2. Maternal prenatal laboratory results are A-positive blood type; nonreactive rapid plasma reagin testing; and negative results on testing for human immunodeficiency virus, hepatitis B surface antigen, and group B *Streptococcus.* The pregnancy was complicated by pregnancy-induced hypertension and twin gestation. His mother was treated during the pregnancy with apresoline and magnesium sulfate for control of her hypertension and with betamethasone (Celestone), a steroid that aids in the development of the fetal lung.

Daniel was delivered by cesarean section for severe IUGR at 33 weeks' gestation. He was assigned an Apgar score of 7 at 1 minute and 8 at 5 minutes. Daniel weighed 1,180 g at birth, his head circumference was 27 cm, his length was 38 cm. All parameters were less than the 10th percentile. He was vigorous at birth, cried at delivery, and then developed mild respiratory distress during the first few minutes of life.

Daniel was given whiffs of oxygen for cyanosis after delivery. He was placed in an oxygen hood for 2 days for treatment of TTN. For the first 2 weeks of life, Daniel had one to two episodes of apnea daily. He has had no apnea for the past 3 weeks.

Daniel's initial glucose level was 28 mg/dL. A glucose test was repeated after Daniel received an IV bolus of $D_{10}W$ and then was started on a continuous drip of $D_{10}W$. The repeated level was 57 mg/dL. Daniel was started on feedings of expressed breast milk on the second day of life. Human milk fortifier was later added to increase the caloric density of Daniel's feedings because of slow weight gain. Oral feedings were started at 1 week of life, corrected gestational age 34 weeks.

Daniel's parents live in a small town about 50 miles from the hospital where the NICU is located. His mother was transported to the obstetrical unit 3 weeks before his delivery. Daniel's parents were involved in his care as much as possible during his hospital stay. Daniel went home at 6 weeks of age.

Assessment

Daniel is at risk for a number of problems related to prematurity and fetal growth restriction. Not all complications affect all infants who are born early and smaller than expected for gestational age. All infants in this category, however, should be screened and monitored to be sure these complications are diagnosed early and appropriate steps taken to prevent or manage the problem. In addition, Daniel's family is at risk for problems related to separation anxiety, feelings of inadequacy to care for an ill infant, fear that he will not survive, and concerns for the financial strain this illness and hospitalization will place on the family.

Nursing Diagnosis

Impaired gas exchange related to retained fetal lung fluid or to surfactant deficiency as evidenced by increased oxygen requirement and work of breathing.

Expected Outcomes	Daniel will exhibit adequate gas exchange as evidenced by respiratory rate 40–60 breaths per minute; oxygen saturation greater than or equal to 92%; clear and equal breath sounds; mild to no retractions; and lack of nasal flaring and expiratory grunt.
Planning	Assure that trained medical healthcare team is available to care for infant, and that proper equipment and supplies are available and in working order. Anticipate potential for worsening of infant's condition requiring escalation of care.

(continued)

Nursing Interventions	Rationales
1. Place on radiant warmer with ISC control.	1. To minimize metabolic demands and oxygen consumption which are increased in temperature regulation.
2. Place on cardio-respiratory monitor and pulse oximeter.	2. To monitor vital signs and oxygen saturation.
3. Obtain arterial blood gas and chest x-ray if ordered. Report abnormal results.	3. Monitors levels of O_2 and CO_2 in the blood; monitors for potential respiratory complications due to fluid build-up in the lungs.

Evaluation   Monitor and record response to oxygen if used.

Nursing Diagnosis

Ineffective thermoregulation related to inadequate fat stores, large surface areas, and inability to shiver as evidenced by the need for assistance with temperature control.

Expected Outcome   Infant will maintain temperature within accepted range of 36.5 to 37.2. Infant will be free of apnea and bradycardia, and maintain adequate oxygenation.

Planning   Assure availability of equipment to provide a proper thermal environment for the infant. Assure availability of health care providers who are trained in the recognition of thermal stress and the use of equipment to provide thermal support for premature and ill infants.

Nursing Interventions	Rationales
1. Place infant on a radiant warmer with ISC control or into a preheated incubator set at a temperature appropriate for gestational age and weight.	1. Prevents hypothermia.
2. Monitor temperature on admission then hourly until stable. Continue to monitor temperature at regular intervals.	2. Provides baseline and monitors changes.
3. Observe for apnea, bradycardia, and color changes associated with temperature instability.	3. Respiratory and cardiac alterations require immediate attention; color change may be indication of significant temperature fluctuation.
4. Use caps and swaddling once temperature is stable.	4. Helps infant maintain normal temperature.
5. Avoid placing infant on cold surface such as scales without insulation.	5. Prevents hypothermia.
6. Avoid drafts during care giving activities.	6. Reduces heat loss.
7. Dry infant promptly following bathing.	7. Reduces chance of heat loss through evaporation.

Evaluation   Document temperature on nursing flow chart. Document interventions used to maintain temperature, and infant's response. Notify primary care provider of any abnormal temperatures.

Nursing Diagnosis

Risk for impaired parent-infant attachment related to separation as a result of illness.

Expected Outcomes   Parents will visit on a regular basis and demonstrate an interest in caring for their infant. They will ask appropriate questions about their infant's condition and express understanding, while participating in decisions about their infant's care.

(continued)

Planning	Assure health care providers are available who are trained in facilitation of parent-infant attachment and in crisis intervention. Provide a family-friendly environment to support attachment and family function.

Nursing Intervention	**Rationales**
1. Introduce parents to health care providers and to the nursery environment.	1. Will foster increased comfort level.
2. Avoid use of medical jargon when giving information.	2. Understanding is enhanced when information is presented at a level consistent with the current knowledge base.
3. Update parents on a regular basis regarding the condition of their infant.	3. Helps alleviate parental anxiety.
4. Encourage parents to name their infant and call the infant by name.	4. Emphasize the infant's individuality.
5. Encourage parents to bring in toys and pictures.	5. Personalizes the infant's bedside.
6. Offer the opportunity for parents to provide skin to skin holding of their infant.	6. Promotes bonding and attachment; gives infant feeling of security.
7. Encourage parents to participate in the care of their infant.	7. Helps parents assume ownership of their new roles.
8. Assure that appropriate referrals are made to Social Services, Psychological Services, etc.	8. Ensures that parents are aware of available resources.

Evaluation	Document family visits and phone calls, parent education and discharge planning, and any referrals made. Chart observations of family interactions with infant.

Key Concepts

- The smallest of changes in the care and management of infants who are preterm and have low birth weights may have profound effects on health.

- The American College of Obstetricians and Gynecologists (ACOG) and the World Health Organization report improvements in the management and prevention of preterm labor throughout the 1980s.

- The percentage of preterm births in the United States rose from 8.9% in 1980 to 10.2% in 1990.

- Prematurity is the cause of approximately 75% of neonatal deaths, and the costs of hospitalization and care have soared over the past decade.

- In addition to the technical care responsibilities of the nurse caring for infants at high risk is the responsibility of educating the parents and family and helping them to bond with their infant.

- In addition to the technical care of the preterm infant, it is the responsibility of the bedside nurse to educate

the parents and family. It is also the nurse's responsibility to aid the parents in bonding with their infant.

- The preterm infant's status may change very rapidly, therefore it is the nurse's assessment skills and ability to recognize changes in the infant's behavior that are crucial in identifying the disease process early in the course.

- Over the past decade we have seen remarkable changes in the management of preterm infants. Improvement in mortality and morbidity has been seen in infants as early as 24 weeks gestation.

- Neonatology encompasses the care of the very fragile preterm infant, and also caring for the ill term infant. The bedside nurse may care for an infant as small as 500 grams or an infant as large as 4000 grams.

- The nurse must be able to recognize the cues of a preterm infant that is stressed in order to prevent long term complications for that infant. These cues include but are not limited to crying, frowning, finger splay, decreased tone, and irritability. The cues may also be autonomic: variability in heart rate, respiratory rate and blood pressure are common.

🦢 It is extremely important for the bedside nurse to differentiate between the complications that may occur in the asymmetrical and symmetrical growth retarded infant, and in the large for gestational age infant.

🦢 The survival of smaller and younger gestation infants brings with it many ethical dilemmas that the caregivers and family must face. It is important for the nurse to identify and come to terms with these issues in order to assist the family in adjusting to the reality of their preterm infant.

Review Questions and Activities

1. Identify non-reassuring fetal heart rate patterns using electronic fetal monitoring and discuss the physiology and nursing interventions for each pattern.

2. What are the characteristics of a reassuring fetal heart pattern?

3. What is the difference between a screening test and a diagnostic test? Provide examples of each type of test used in care of the pregnant woman.

4. What are the indications for a non-stress test and how are the results interpreted?

5. Compare and contrast the non-stress test with the biophysical profile.

6. What is the purpose of a contraction stress test?

7. What are the goals of short-term fluid therapy?
   a. Prevention of hypoglycemia, limitation of negative fluid balance, and provision of protein sparing carbohydrates
   b. Prevention of hypoglycemia, provision of enough fluids to give a positive fluid balance, and to provide carbohydrates
   c. Provision of adequate glucose and fluids to prevent dehydration
   d. Replacement of insensible water losses

   The correct answer is a.

8. The major routes of water losses include:
   a. urine and stool
   b. Gastrointestinal losses
   c. evaporative from skin and lungs
   d. answers a and c

   The correct answer is d.

9. To be classified symmetric IUGR, what must the infant must be?
   a. less than the 10th percentile in birth weight
   b. less than the 10th percentile in birth weight and length
   c. diagnosed in utero by doppler ultrasonography

   d. less than the 10th percentile in birth weight, length and head circumference

   The correct answer is d.

10. What is the purpose of serial x-rays in-clients with necrotizing enterocolitis?
    a. Assessment of lung volume
    b. Assessment for pneumotosis or free air in the bowel
    c. To irradiate the infant
    d. To check for pneumonia

    The correct answer is b.

11. How is late onset infection defined?
    a. As onset of symptoms after day of life 14
    b. As onset of symptoms after day of life 5 to 7
    c. As onset of symptoms in the first few days of life
    d. As any infection occurring in the neonatal period

    The correct answer is b.

12. What are three common organisms of early onset infection?
    a. pseudomonas, staphylococcus epidermidus, and Escherichia Coli
    b. staphylococcus aureus, Klebsiella, and pseudomonas
    c. streptococcus pneumoniae, Escherichia Coli, and group B Streptococcus
    d. Haemophilus influenzae, staphylococcus epidermidus and candida albicans

    The correct answer is c.

13. What are the consequences of overhydration in the ELBW infant?
    a. Increased blood pressure, poor perfusion, and alkalosis
    b. Patent ductus arteriosus, hyperglycemia, bronchopulmonary dysplasia, and necrotizing enterocolitis
    c. Hypernatremia and acute renal failure
    d. Hypoglycemia and elevated heart rate

    The correct answer is b.

14. What causes compromise of the respiratory system of an infant born at 26 weeks gestation?
  a. The infant's chest wall is stiff and very compliant
  b. The infant's ribs have flexible cartilage
  c. The infant's intercostal muscles are underdeveloped

The correct answer is b.

15. Which are the common signs and symptoms of a patent ductus arteriosus in preterm infants?
  a. Murmur, widened pulse pressures, and increased heart size
  b. Weak pulses, normal blood pressure, and deterioration in ventilatory status
  c. Murmur, narrowed pulse pressure, and pulmonary edema
  d. clammy skin and thready pulse

The correct answer is a.

16. Which is the most common form of lung disease in the newborn?
  a. Meconium aspiration
  b. Retained fetal lung fluid
  c. Hyaline membrane disease
  d. Asthma

The correct answer is b.

17. Which intervention is utilized to keep oxygen consumption to a minimum during the re-warming process? Adjust the incubator:

  a. 1 to 1.5 degrees higher than the infant's temperature
  b. at 37 degrees
  c. at least 2 degrees higher than the infant's desired temperature
  d. at least 2 degrees lower than the infant's desired temperature

The correct answer is a.

18. What is true about post-hemorrhagic hydrocephalus?
  a. It is common with subarachnoid hemorrhage
  b. It always progresses rapidly
  c. It results when clot formation obstructs flow, and inflammation & debris impairs absorption

The correct answer is c.

19. What is included in the management of post-hemorrhagic hydrocephalus?
  a. serial lumbar puncture if non-communicating
  b. lasix alone
  c. acetazolamide

The correct answer is c.

20. Which risk factors decrease the incidence of respiratory distress syndrome?
  a. Prematurity and male gender
  b. Pregnancy induced hypertension and prenatal corticol steroids
  c. Diabetes and multiple gestation

The correct answer is b.

References

American Academy of Pediatrics Committee on Infections Diseases and Committee on Fetus and Newborn. (1998). Prevention of respiratory syncytial virus infections; update on the use of RSV-IGIV. *Pediatrics, 102,* (5), 1211–1216.

American Heart Association and American Academy of Pediatrics. (2000). Neonatal Revisitation Textbook. AHA; Dallas, TX.

American Academy of Pediatrics (AAP) & Canadian Paediatric Society (CPS). (2000). Prevention and management of pain and stress in the neonate. *Pediatrics, 105,* (2), 454–461.

Anand, K. J. (1998). Clinical importance of pain and stress in preterm neonates. *Biol Neonate, 73,* 1–9.

Ballard, J. L., Khoury, J. C., Wedig, K., Wang, L., Ellers-Walsman, B. L., & Lipp, R. (1991). New Ballard Score expanded to include extremely premature infant. *The Journal of Pediatrics, 119,* 417–423.

Battaglia, F. C., & Lubchenco, L. O. (1967). A practical classification of newborn infants by weight and gestational age. *J. Pediatrics, 71,* 159.

Bernstein, P. S., & Divon, M. K. (1997). Etiologies of fetal growth restriction. *Clinical Obstetrics and Gynecology, 40,* (4), 723–729.

Bernstein, S., Heimler, R., & Sasidharan, P. (1998). Approaching the management of the neonatal intensive care unit graduate through history and physical assessment. *Pediatric Clinics of North America, 45,* (1), 79–105.

Blackburn, S. T., & Loper, D. L. (1992). *Maternal, fetal and neonatal physiology: A clinical perspective.* Philadelphia, PA: W. B. Saunders.

Bossi, E., & Koerner, F. (1995). Retinopathy of prematurity. *Intensive Care Medicine, 21,* (3), 241–246.

Carroll, P. (1991). Pneumothorax in the newborn. *Neonatal Network, 10,* (2), 27–34.

Casey, P. M. (1999). Respiratory distress. In J. D. Deacon & P. O'Neill (Eds.), *Core curriculum for neonatal intensive care nursing* (2nd ed.). (pp. 118–150). Philadelphia, PA: W. B. Saunders.

Chen, J. V., Wu, T. S., & Chanlai, S. P. (1995). Recombinant human erythropoietin in the treatment of anemia of prematurity. *American Journal of Perinatology, 12,* (5), 314–318.

Costriano, A., & Baumgart, S. (1986). Modern fluid and electrolyte management of the critically ill preterm infant. *Pediatric Clinics of North America, 33,* 153.

Davis, P., Turner-Gomes, S., Cunningham, K., Way, C., Roberts, R. & Schmidt, B. (1995). Precision and accuracy of clinical and radiological signs in premature infants at risk for patent ductus arteriosus. *Archives of Pediatrics and Adolescent Medicine, 149,* (10), 1136–1141.

De Onis, M., Blossner, M., & Villar, J. (1998). Levels and patterns of intrauterine growth retardation in developing countries. *European Journal of Clinical Nutrition, 52,* (suppl) (1), S5–15.

Dollison, E. J., & Beckstrand, J. (1995). Adhesive tape versus pectin-based barrier use in preterm infants. *Neonatal Network, 14,* (4), 35–39.

Engebretson, J. C., & Wardell, D. W. (1997). Development of a pacifier for low-birth-weight infant's non-nutritive sucking. *Journal of Obstetric, Gynecologic, and Neonatal Nursing, 26,* (6), 660–664.

Farrell, P. M., & Wood, R. E. (1976). Epidemiology of hyaline membrane disease in the United States: Analysis of national mortality statistics. *Pediatrics, 58,* 167.

Gardosi, J. (1997). Customized growth curves. *Clinical Obstetrics and Gynecology, 40,* (4), 715–722.

Goldenberg, R. L., & Cliver, S. P. (1997). Small for gestational age and intrauterine growth restriction: Definitions and standards. *Clinical Obstetrics and Gynecology, 40,* (4), 704–714.

Gordon, M., & Montgomery, L. A. (1996). Minimizing epidermal stripping in the very low birth weight infant: Integrating research and practice to affect infant outcome. *Neonatal Network, 14,* (1), 37–44.

Hansen, A. R., & Snyder, E. Y. (1998). Medical management of neonatal post hemorrhagic hydrocephalus. *Neurosurgery Clinics of North America, 9,* (1), 95–104.

Haymond, H. W. (1989). Hypoglycemia in infants and children. *Endocrinology Clinics of North America, 18,* (1), 211–252.

Kenner, C., Amlung, S. R., & Flandermeyer, A. A. (1998). *Protocols in Neonatal Nursing.* Philadelphia, PA: W. B. Saunders.

Kok, J. H., den Ouden, A. L., Verloove-Vanhorick, S. P., & Brand, R. (1998). Outcome of very preterm small for gestational age infants: the first nine years of life. *British Journal of Obstetrics and Gynaecology, 105,* (2), 162–168.

Krechel, S. W., & Bildner, J. (1995). CRIES: A new neonatal postoperative pain measurement score. Initial testing of validity and reliability. *Pediatric Anesthesia, 5,* 53–61.

Lawrence, J., Alcock, D., McGrath, P., Kay, J., MacMurray, S. B., & Dulberg, C. (1993). The development of a tool to assess neonatal pain. *Neonatal Network, 12,* 59–66.

Lott, J. W. (1994). *Neonatal infection: Assessment, diagnosis, and management.* Santa Rosa, CA: NICU Ink.

Merskey, H. (1979). Pain terms: A list with definitions and notes on usage. Recommended by the IASP Subcommittee on Taxonomy. *Pain, 6,* (3), 249–252.

McCormick, F. S. C., Brady, K., & Keen, C. E. (1996). Oxalate nephrocalcinosis: A study in autopsied infants and neonates. *Pediatric Pathology & Laboratory Medicine, 16,* (3), 479–488.

Merenstein, G. B., & Gardner, S. L. (1998). *Handbook of neonatal intensive care* (4th ed.). St. Louis, MO: Mosby.

Moise, A. A.., & Hansen, T. N. (1998). In T. N. Hansen, T. R. Cooper, & L. E. Weisman, (Editors), *Contemporary diagnosis and management of neonatal respiratory diseases,* (2nd ed.). (pp. 79–95). Newton, PA: Handbooks in Health Care.

Naeye, R. L. (1967). Cytomegalic inclusion disease: the fetal disorder. *American Journal of Clinical Pathology, 47,* 738–744.

Northway, W. H., Jr, Rosan, R. C., & Porter, D. Y. (1967). Pulmonary disease following respiratory therapy of hyaline membrane disease: BPD. *New England Journal of Medicine, 276,* 357.

Perlman, J. M., Risser, R., & Broyles, R. S. (1996). Bilateral cystic periventricular leukomalacia in the preterm infant: Associated risk factors. *Pediatrics, 97,* (6 pt 1), 822–827.

Roland, E. H., & Hill, A. (1997). IVH and post hemorrhagic hydrocephalus. *Clinics in Perinatology, 24,* (3), 589–605.

Schaap, A. H., Wolf, H., Bruinse, H. W., den Ouden, A. L., Smolders-de Hass, H., van Ertbruggen, I., & Treffus, P. E. (1997). Influence of obstetric management on outcome of extremely preterm growth retarded infants. *Archives of Disease in Childhood, Fetal and Neonatal Education, 77,* (2), F95–99.

Schwoebel, A., & Sakraida, S. (1997). Hyperbilirubinemia: New approaches to an old Problem. *The Journal of Perinatal & Neonatal Nursing, 11,* (3), 78–97.

Seaman, S. L. (1995). Renal physiology part II: Fluid and electrolyte regulation. *Neonatal Network, 14,* (5), 5–11.

Shapiro, C. R. (1993). Nurses' judgment of pain in term and preterm newborns. *Journal of Obstetric, Gynecologic, and Neonatal Nursing, 22,* 41–47.

Shapiro, C., & Askin, D. F. (1999). Ophthalmologic disorders. In J. D. Deacon & P. O'Neill (Editors), *Core curriculum for neonatal intensive care nursing,* (2nd ed.). (pp. 597–615). Philadelphia, PA: W. B. Saunders.

Sherear, D. M., & Devon, M. Y. (1997). Fetal growth in multifetal gestation. *Clinical Obstetrics and Gynecology, 40,* (4), 764–770.

Stevens, B., Johnston, C., Petryshen, P., & Taddio, A. (1996). Premature infant pain profile: Development and initial validation. *Clinical J of Pain, 12,* 13–22.

Toce, S. S., Farrell, P. M., Leavitt, L. A., Samuels, D. P., & Edwards, D. K. (1984). Clinical and radiographic scoring systems for assessing bronchopulmonary dysplasia. *American Journal of Diseases in Children, 138,* 581.

Victor, L., & Persoon, J. (1994). Implementation of kangaroo care: Apparent-health care team approach to practice change. *Critical Care Nursing Clinics of North America, 6,* (4), 891–895.

Volpe, J. J. (1997). Brain injury in the premature infant: From pathogenesis to prevention. *Brain & Development, 19,* (8), 519–534.

Westgren, M., Lingman, G., & Persson, B. (1997). Cordocentesis in IUGR fetuses. *Clinical Obstetrics and Gynecology, 40,* (4), 755–763.

Zenk, K. E., Sills, J. H., & Koeppel, R. M. (2000). *Neonatal medication and nutrition: A comprehensive guide.* Santa Rosa, CA: NICU Ink.

Suggested Readings

American Academy of Pediatrics (AAP) and American College of Obstetricians and Gynecologists (ACOG). (1997). *Guidelines for perinatal care* (4th ed.). American Academy of Pediatrics and American College of Obstetricians and Gynecologists.

Bakewell-Sachs, S., & Porth, S. (1995). Discharge planning and home care of the technology dependent infant. *Journal of Obstetric, Gynecologic, and Neonatal Nursing, 24,* (1), 77–83.

Barker, D. J. P. (1997). The long-term outcome of retarded fetal growth. *Clinical Obstetrics and Gynecology, 40,* (4), 853–861.

Bersth, C. L. (1995). Minimal enteral feedings. *Clinics in Perinatology, 22,* 61.

Blackburn, S. (1995). Problems of preterm infants after discharge. *Journal of Obstetric, Gynecologic, and Neonatal Nursing, 24,* (1), 43–49.

Bissinger, R. (1995). Renal physiology: Structure and function. *Neonatal Network, 14,* (4), 9–19.

Bozzette, M. (1996). Respiratory syncytial virus infection in infants: A significant challenge for optimal care. *The Journal of Perinatal & Neonatal Nursing, 10,* (2), 72–87.

Brooks, C. (1997). Neonatal hypoglycemia. *Neonatal Network, 16,* (2), 15–21.

Chase, M. C. (1997). Neonatal hypoglycemia. *Mother Baby Journal, 2,* (5), 13–18.

Craigo, S. D., Beach, M. L., Harvey-Wilkes, K. B., & D'Alton, M. E. (1996). Ultrasound predictions of neonatal outcome in intrauterine growth restriction. *American Journal of Perinatology, 13,* (8), 465–471.

DellaPorta, K., Aforismo, D., & Butler-O'Hara, M. (1998). Co-Bedding of twins in the neonatal intensive care unit. *Pediatric Nursing, 24,* (6), 529–531.

Fletcher, M. A., & MacDonald, M. G. (1993). *Atlas of procedures in neonatology,* (2nd ed.) Philadelphia, PA: Lippincott.

Gibbins, S. A., & Chapman, J. S. (1996). Holding on: Parents' perceptions of premature infant's transfers. *Journal of Obstetric, Gynecologic, and Neonatal Nursing, 25,* (2), 147–153.

Gross, S. J. (1997). Intrauterine growth restriction: A genetic perspective. *Clinical Obstetrics and Gynecology, 40,* (4), 730–739.

Harrison, L., Olivet, L., Cunningham, K., Bodin, M. B., & Hicks, C. (1996). Effects of gentle human touch on preterm infants: Pilot study results. *Neonatal Network, 15,* (2), 35–41.

Hittner, H. M., Hirsch, N. J., & Rudolph, A. J. (1977). Assessment of gestational age by exam of anterior vascular capsule of the lens. *Journal of Pediatrics, 91,* (3), 456.

Kenner, C., Altimier, L., & Hess, D. J. (1998). Career opportunities for neonatal nurses. *Journal of Pediatric Nursing, 13,* (5), 317–325.

Kenner, C., Lott, J. W., & Flandermeyer, A. A. (1998). *Comprehensive neonatal nursing: A physiologic perspective.* (2nd ed.). Philadelphia, PA: W. B. Saunders.

Klaus, M., Fanaroff, A., & Martin, R. (1986). *Care of the high risk neonate* (3rd ed.). (pp. 96–112). Philadelphia, PA: W. B. Saunders.

Lott, J. W., & Kilb, J. R. (1992). The selection of antibacterial agents for treatment of neonatal sepsis, or which drugs kill which bug? *Neonatal Pharmacology Quarterly, 1,* (1), 31–41.

McCulloch, M. (1993). Neurological Disorders. In P. Beachy & J. Deacon (Eds.), *Core Curriculum for Neonatal Intensive Care Nursing.* (p. 412). Philadelphia, PA: W. B. Saunders.

Nyquist, K. H., & Lutes, L. M. (1998). Co-bedding twins: A developmentally supportive care strategy. *Journal of Obstetric, Gynecologic, and Neonatal Nursing, 27,* (4), 450–456.

Parker, L. A. (1995). Necrotizing enterocolitis. *Neonatal Network, 14,* (6), 17–25.

Pierce, S. F. (1998). Neonatal intensive care: Decision making in the face of prognostic uncertainty. *Nursing Clinics of North America,* (33), 2.

Premji, S. S. (1998). Ontogeny of the gastrointestinal system and its impact on feeding the preterm infant. *Neonatal Network, 17,* (2), 17–24.

Salfia, C. (1997). Placental pathology of fetal growth restriction. *Clinical Obstetrics and Gynecology, 40,* (4), 740–749.

Sokol, M. (1995). Creating a community of caring for families with special needs. *Journal of Obstetric, Gynecologic, and Neonatal Nursing, 24,* (1), 64–69.

Spinners, S., Gibson, E., Wrobel, H., & Sptitzer, A. R. (1995). Recent advances in home infant apnea monitoring. *Neonatal Network, 14,* (8), 39–46.

Thomas, K. (1994). Thermoregulation in neonates. *Neonatal Network, 13,* (2), 15–22.

Vandenberg, K. A. (1997). Basic principles of developmental caregiving. *Neonatal Network, 16,* (7), 69–71.

Whitaker, S. (1995). The art and science of home apnea monitoring in the 1990's. *Journal of Obstetric, Gynecologic, and Neonatal Nursing, 24,* (1), 84–89.

Wootton, J. C. (1999). World Wide Web resources for perinatal nursing. *Journal of Perinatal Neonatal Nursing, 12,* (4), 15–25.

Zelle, R. (1995). Follow-up of at-risk infants in the home setting: Consultation model. *Journal of Obstetric, Gynecologic, and Neonatal Nursing, 24,* (1), 51–55.

Resources

A.W.H.O.N.N. (1999). *Clinical competencies and education guide: Limited ultrasound examinations in obstetrics and gynecology/infertility settings.* Chicago: Association of Women's Health, Obstetrics, and Neonatal Nursing.

Murray, Michelle (1997). *Antepartal and intrapartal fetal monitoring.* Albuquerque: Learning Resources International Inc.

Sanders, R. (1996). *Structural fetal anomalies: The total picture.* St. Louis: Mosby.

Simpson, K. R. & Creehan, P. A. (1996). *Perinatal nursing.* Philadelphia: Lippincott.

www.neonatology-net.com

www.nichd.nih.gov/cochran

www.nichd.nih.gov/cochrane.neonatal

www.neonatology.org

www.pedsinreview.org

www.hawaii.edu/medicine/pediatrics/neoxray/neoxray.html

www.awhonn.org/about/index.html

www.nann.org

www.neonatology.org/career/default.html

www.inconnect.com/~bfam/neospan

www.parenttoparentnys.org/national%20directory.htm

www.preemieparenting.com/publications.htm

www.comeunity.com/premature/preemiepgs.html

www.parenttoparentnys.org/national%20directory.htm

www.preemieparenting.com/publications.htm

www.comeunity.com/premature/preemiepgs.html

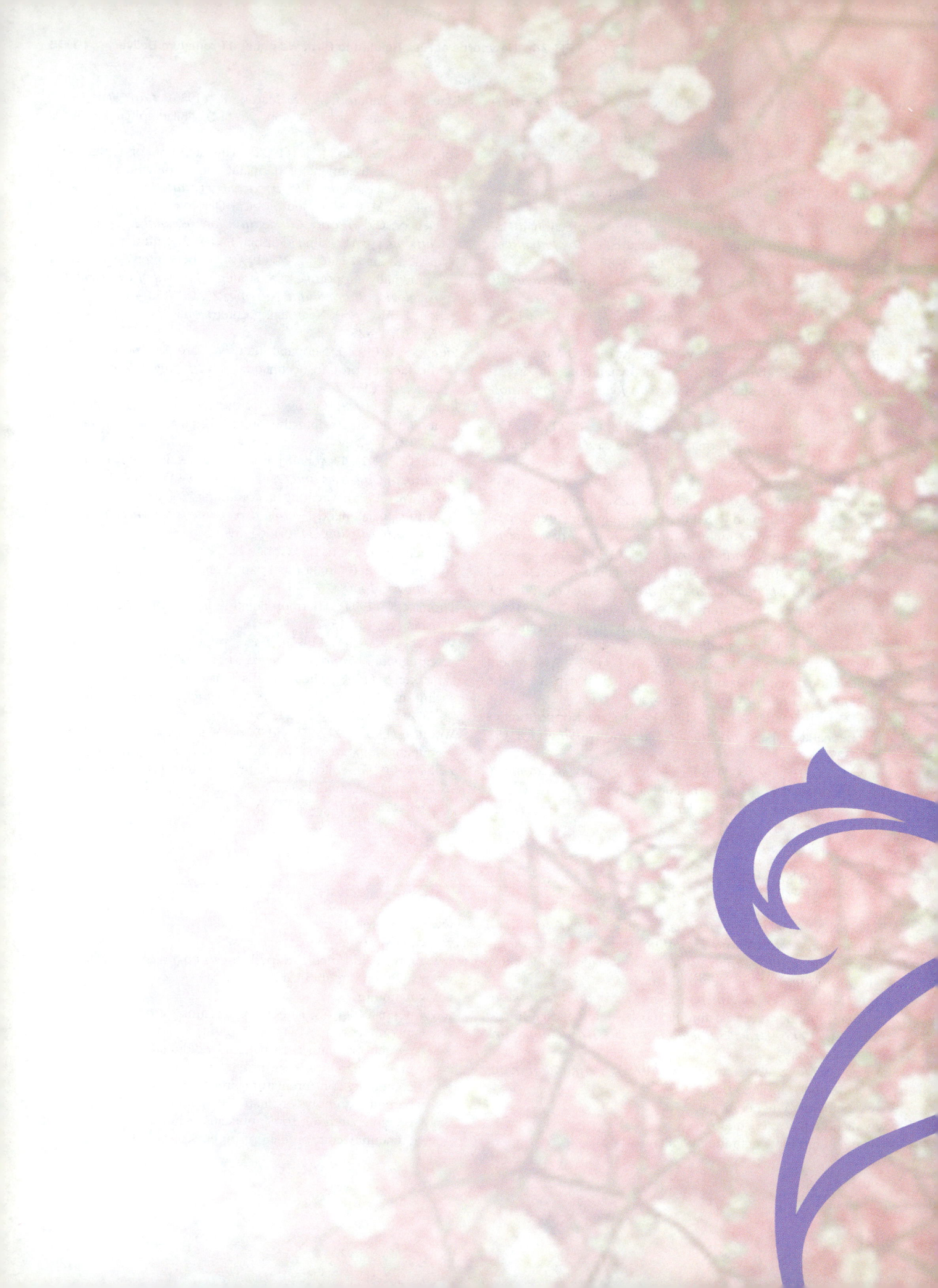

CHAPTER 35

Newborns at Risk Related to Congenital and Acquired Conditions

*D*uring a pregnancy, a family dreams of giving birth to the perfect child (or what they consider to be a normal child) both physically and mentally. The birth of a child with a congenital or acquired anomaly challenges those dreams and forces families to deal with a crisis for which they may be completely unprepared. As a nurse, you must tend to not only the physical needs of the infant and the family's need for knowledge, but also the psychological needs of the family as they strive to control the emotional upheaval that may result from this birth. You must also closely examine your own feelings and attitudes toward birth anomalies, so that you can effectively and sensitively guide families through the adaptation process.

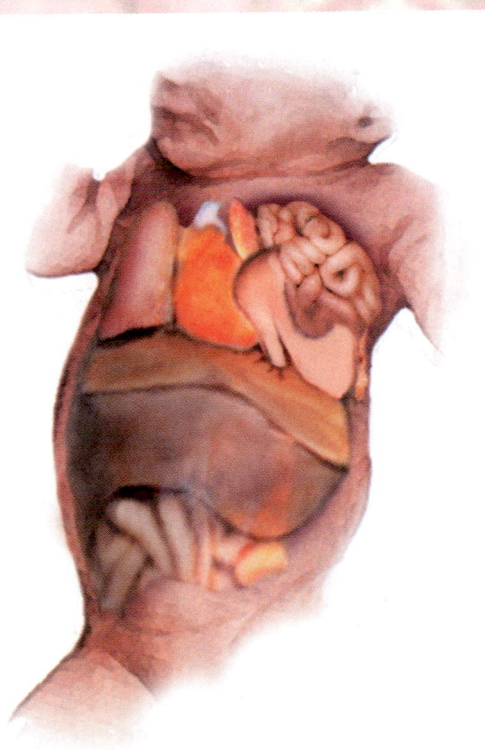

Key Terms

ABO incompatibility
Acquired disorder
Anencephalus
Brachial palsy
Choanal atresia
Cleft lip
Cleft palate
Clubfoot (talipes
    equinovarus)
Congenital disorder
Congenital heart defect
Developmental dysplasia
    of the hip (DDH)
Diaphragmatic hernia

Extracorporeal
    membrane
    oxygenation (ECMO)
Encephalocele
Epispadias
Erythroblastosis fetalis
Esophageal atresia
Exstrophy of the bladder
Facial palsy
Gastroschisis
Genetic disorder
Hydrocephaly
Hydrops fetalis
Hyperbilirubinemia

Hypocalcemia
Hypoglycemia
Hypospadias
Imperforate anus
Infant of a diabetic
    mother (IDM)
Intracranial hemorrhage
Jaundice
Kernicterus
Macrosomia
Maternal sensitization
Meningocele
Microcephaly
Myelomeningocele

Omphalocele
Pathologic jaundice
Phototherapy
Physiologic jaundice
Polycythemia
Rh incompatibility
Sepsis
Spina bifida
STORCH titer
Subarachnoid
    hemorrhage
Subdural hemorrhage
Tracheoesophageal
    fistula

Competencies

Upon completion of this chapter, the reader should be able to:

1. Identify the incidence, risk, anatomic anomalies, pathophysiologic markers, clinical manifestations, and potential complications of congenital or acquired defects in the neonate.

2. Develop a plan of care with specific nursing diagnoses and appropriate interventions for the neonate who is born with a congenital or acquired anomaly.

3. Design an educational plan to meet the needs of the parents and family of a neonate with a congenital or acquired anomaly.

4. Develop a therapeutic relationship to better meet the needs of the family of a neonate who is born with a congenital or acquired anomaly during this crisis.

5. Identify the incidence, risk, clinical manifestations, and potential complications of acquired disorders in the neonate.

6. Develop a plan of care with specific nursing diagnoses and appropriate interventions for the neonate with an acquired disorder.

The hope and expectation of every pregnant woman is to deliver a healthy, normal infant who will grow and develop into a mature adult who will someday make a contribution to society. Numerous factors, including heredity and the environment, can affect the outcome of a pregnancy. Some abnormalities or disorders can occur in a single or a few genes from either parent, from factors influencing the intrauterine environment, or from a combination of these.

A **congenital disorder** is an anomaly that results from genetic, prenatal, or environmental factors, or a combination of these, and is present at birth. A **genetic disorder** is an inherited defect that is transmitted from genera-

tion to generation. An **acquired disorder** is a condition that results from environmental factors rather than genetic circumstances.

This chapter describes the most common congenital and acquired disorders in the neonate and the immediate nursing care that is required, using the nursing process. In addition, the psychosocial impact of the disorders on the parents and family are presented. Both the perinatal and the neonatal team must anticipate and be ever cognizant of the needs, not only of the compromised neonate, but also of the infant's family. Parents should always be kept informed of their infant's condition and involved in care as soon and as often as possible.

CONGENITAL ANOMALIES

Congenital anomalies are abnormalities present at birth as a result of either genetic or prenatal environmental factors or both. Genetic anomalies are the result of hereditary factors and are transmitted from generation to generation. (See Chapter 13 for a detailed discussion of genetic disorders.)

Congenital defects occur in 3% to 4% of all live births (Wardinsky, 1994) but this number increases if one includes congenital defects that may not be diagnosed until later in childhood, such as developmental dysplasia of the hip (DDH). Major congenital defects are the leading cause of death in infants less than 1 year of age in the United States and account for 20% of all neonatal deaths.

Central Nervous System Anomalies

As one of the most complex systems of the body, the central nervous system (CNS) is subject to a multitude of congenital anomalies. The stages in the development of the nervous system must proceed in a predetermined order or a defect occurs. These stages can be affected by both genetic and environmental factors, or a combination of both.

The most common anomalies of the CNS occur during the primary neurulation period, which is during the first 3 to 4 weeks of gestation. These anomalies, termed "neural tube defects," occur as a result of failure of the neural tube to close. There has been steady decline in the number of children with all forms of neural tube defects as the result of prenatal diagnosis and termination of affected pregnancies (Golden, 1998). Recent evidence suggests that the nutrient folic acid promotes neural tube closure. Therefore, women considering conception are encouraged to begin taking folic acid supplements before conception and to continue with them until 12 weeks' gestation (Rayburn, Stanley, and Garrett, 1996). In 1993, the American Academy of Pediatrics recommended that folic acid be administered to all women of childbearing age (Rowe, 1995).

Encephalocele

Encephalocele is a herniation of the brain and meninges through an opening in the skull (Figure 35-1). This neural tube defect is readily visible at birth. Skin generally covers the encephalocele, but it may break open, increasing the risk for infection. Treatment consists of surgical intervention to replace brain contents and repair the defect. If hydrocephalus or enlargement of the head without enlargement of the facial structures is present, a ventricular shunting procedure is generally performed 7 to 10 days after the encephalocele has been repaired. The shunt is formed by placing a flexible tube into the ventricular sys-

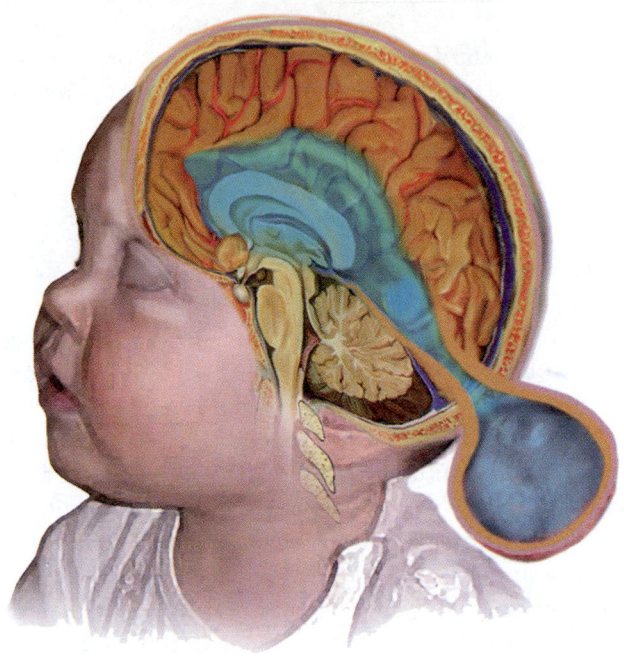

Figure 35-1 Infant with encephalocele.

tem of the brain, which diverts the abnormal accumulation of cerebrospinal fluid (CSF) into another area of the body, most often the abdominal cavity, where it can be absorbed. (Refer to the section on hydrocephaly in this chapter for nursing care of the infant with a shunt.)

Anencephaly

In **anencephaly**, there is a complete or partial absence of the cerebral hemispheres and skull. The exact cause of anencephaly is unknown; it occurs in 1 of 1000 live births (Paidas & Cohen, 1994). These infants are frequently stillborn or die within the first few days of life because they do not have any cerebral function. Nursing interventions are directed toward providing comfort measures until the infant dies from respiratory or cardiac failure. The families require a great deal of emotional and spiritual support in grieving the impending death of their newborn.

Microcephaly

Microcephaly is the condition in which there is a normal-sized head that contains a small brain. This condition can be either congenital or acquired. Congenital microcephaly may be seen in conjunction with a chromosomal abnormality; an intrauterine infection, such as rubella, cytomegalovirus, or toxoplasmosis; and maternal exposure to x-rays. The acquired form of microcephaly may result from maternal herpes, ischemic insults, or hypothyroidism. Diagnostic evaluation includes a **STORCH** titer, for syphilis, toxoplasmosis, other infections, rubella, cytomegalovirus, and herpes, and skull x-rays films. There is no treatment for this disorder, which generally results in mental retardation. Nursing care is predominantly supportive. The parents must be supported while they learn to cope with and accept this disorder in their newborn.

Hydrocephaly

Hydrocephaly is a condition that results from an excess accumulation of CSF in the ventricles of the brain and the subarachnoid space as a result of an imbalance between CSF production and absorption (Figure 35-2). Normal growth and development of the brain is altered because of the increased intracranial pressure (ICP) from the CSF fluid. This condition occurs in 3 to 4 of 1000 newborns (Shiminski-Maher & Disabato, 1994). Cesarean section may be necessary because of the enlarged head. This disorder is readily apparent at birth. The infant is born with an enlarged head, bulging fontanelles, separated skull sutures, and a prominent forehead with depressed eyes that are rotated downward, causing the "setting sun" sign.

Nursing care includes continuous observation and assessment of neurologic status of the infant. Ongoing observations must be carefully documented. The head should be supported while holding, turning, or positioning the infant. A flotation mattress or sheepskin is used under the infant to prevent skin breakdown and infection. Signs of increased ICP should be continuously assessed, and serial head circumference measurements should be plotted.

Surgical intervention includes the placement of a shunt from the ventricle in the brain to the peritoneum to allow for drainage of excess CSF. Postoperatively, the infant is positioned on the side opposite the shunt to prevent pressure and kinking of the shunt. The infant's bed is left in a flat position to prevent rapid loss of CSF and decompression. The long-term prognosis depends on the cause of hydrocephalus, the extent of tissue damage, and the success of the shunt procedure. Parents should be taught the care of the infant and shunt, including positioning and skin care, before discharge. They need to be edu-

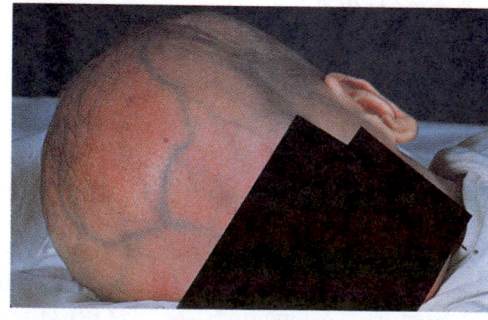

Figure 35-2 Hydrocephalus. (Courtesy of Armed Forces Institute of Pathology).

cated on the signs of increased intracranial pressure, shunt malfunction, skin breakdown, and infection.

Spina Bifida

Spina bifida is a common CNS defect that results from failure of the spinal cord to close. There are two categories: spina bifida occulta and spina bifida cystica. Spina bifida occulta is the failure of the spinal column to close when neither the cord nor the meninges herniate through the defect (Figure 35-3). This condition occurs in 10% to 30% of all live births (Kenner, Amlung, 1998).

Spina bifida cystica, which includes meningocele and myelomeningocele, has an incidence of 1 in 1000 live births (Kenner, Amlung, 1998). In a **meningocele**, there is an external sac that protrudes through the defect that contains meninges and CSF. However, the spinal cord and nerve roots are in their normal position. **Myelomeningocele** is the most common form of spina bifida cystica and occurs in 1 of 500 live births (Milhorat & Miller, 1994). In a myelomeningocele, the sac contains both meninges and

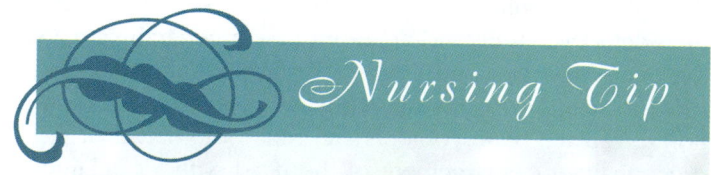

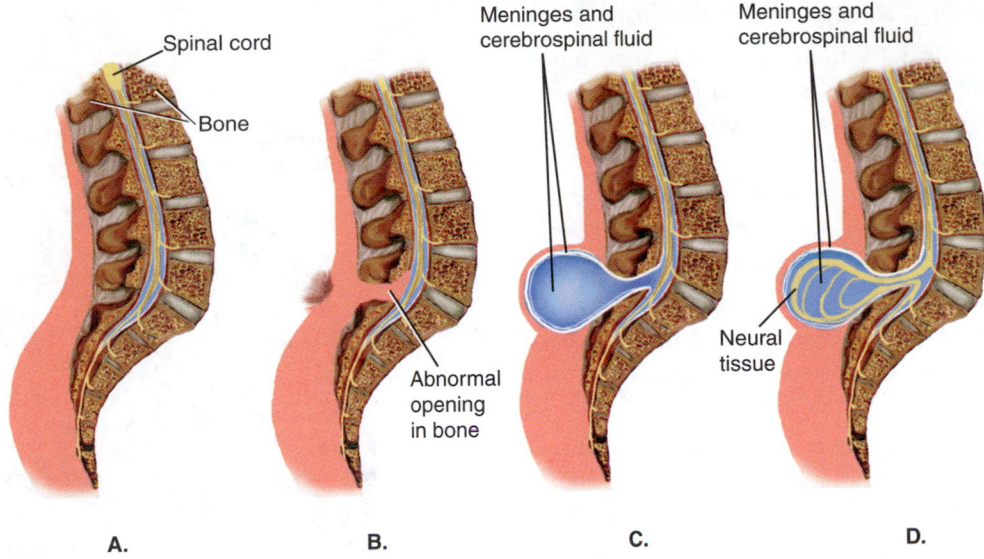

Figure 35-3 Spina bifida. A. Normal spine; B. spina bifida occulta; C. spina bifida with meningocele; D. spina bifida with myelomeningocele.

CSF, as in meningocele, but it also contains neural tissue. Myelomemingocele may arise at any point in the vertebral column from C1 to the coccyx but is most common in the lumbar, lumbosacral, and sacral segments.

Spina bifida may be diagnosed in utero through the testing of amniotic fluid. Elevated levels of alpha-fetoprotein (AFP) found in the amniotic fluid confirm the diagnosis of an open neural tube defect, such as spina bifida. The open defect allows leakage of CSF into the amniotic fluid, causing the elevated AFP levels. An ultrasound examination may also be performed to visualize the defect. If the diagnosis of spina bifida is not made in utero, it is usually apparent at birth. The head should be carefully examined for signs of hydrocephalus, and serial head-circumference measurements done. A computerized tomographic (CT) scan or magnetic resonance imaging (MRI) study may be performed to define the type and severity of hydrocephalus. Electromyography may assist in assessing the motor function of the lower extremities. In addition, an abdominal sonogram or intravenous pyelogram may be performed to rule out hydronephrosis (Milhorat & Miller, 1994).

Whenever possible, the spinal lesion should be closed within the first few hours of life. Prompt surgery is performed to prevent infection and halt any further loss of existing neurologic function. Since a high percentage of infants with neural tube defects develop hydrocephalus, a ventriculoperitoneal shunt is placed after the neural tube defect has been repaired.

Immediate nursing care includes placing the infant in a prone or side-lying position with rolled towels to prevent pressure on the sac and to protect the sac from tearing. Change the infant's position every hour to prevent

pressure on a specific area. The sac should be covered with a moist, sterile gauze dressing, and the skin around the defect should be cleansed and dried to prevent skin breakdown. The nurse should administer prescribed prophylactic antibiotic agents. The infant's bladder should be emptied, using Credé's method, at regular intervals to prevent stasis of urine in the bladder resulting from the loss of normal nerve innervation.

Postoperatively, nursing care involves assessing the infant for signs and symptoms of infection, increased ICP, and bowel and bladder assessment. The infant is placed in a prone or lateral position to keep pressure off the incisional area. Manual emptying of the bladder to stimulate urination is continued. Passive range of motion (ROM) exercises should be performed with the lower extremities; a physical therapist should be consulted for appropriate exercises. A number of orthopedic problems, such as foot deformities, dislocated hips, and kyphoscoliosis, can occur. Therefore, orthopedic status must be continually monitored and vigorous physical therapy must be initiated.

Assessing Newborn Urinary Elimination

1. Newborns usually void during delivery or immediately following delivery.

2. Urinary function may be suppressed for several hours after birth.

3. Newborns usually void 10–15 times each day by 2–3 days of life.

Warning signs

- failure to void within 24 hours

- concentrated, red, or rusty reddish brown urine

Assessing Newborn Intestinal Elimination

1. Newborns usually pass their first stool (meconium) by 8–24 hours. Meconium is passed for the first few days and is typically black or green in color, sticky, and tarlike.

2. By the second and third day the newborn passes transitional stools which are of thinner consistency than meconium, greenish-brown to yellowish-brown in color, and less sticky.

3. By the 5th day of life, the newborn typically passes 4–6 stools per day (frequency may vary from one stool per 2 days to 10 stools per day).

4. Breastfed newborns have yellowish (sometimes greenish) stools which are more liquid in consistency and frequent, while bottlefed infants tend to have more formed, pale stools.

Warning signs

- If no stool in 24 hours, consider impeforate anus

- Watery, green, excessive mucous, foul odor, and flatus may be evidence of intestinal problems or infection.

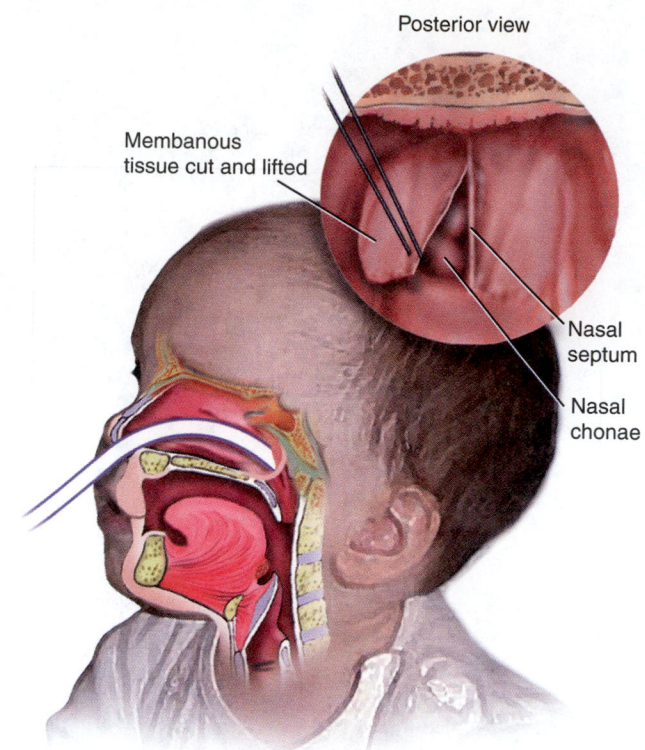

Figure 35-4 Choanal atresia, separation between the nose and pharynx.

Respiratory System Anomalies

The upper respiratory system begins forming early in the fourth week of gestation; formation of the lower respiratory system begins in the middle of that week. Malformations in the respiratory system can be life-threatening; therefore, recognition of these anomalies in the delivery room is imperative for proper treatment. The first few minutes of life are the most crucial, so ensuring adequate oxygenation during this period is necessary to the long-term positive outcome for the newborn.

Choanal Atresia

Choanal atresia is a condition in which there is a bony or membranous separation between the nose and the pharynx (Figure 35-4). Ninety percent of atresias are bony, and 10% are membranous. The incidence of choanal atresia is 1 in 5,000 to 7,000 births (Guzzetta, Anderson, Eichelberger, Newman, Rouse, Schmitzer, Boyajian, & Tomaski, 1994). Unilateral atresia is much more common than bilateral atresia, and the female-to-male ratio for affected infants is 2:1. Twenty to fifty percent of clients with choanal atresia have other anomalies; therefore, genetic consultation for these clients is recommended, along with a thorough search for additional anomalies (Miller, Fanaroff, & Martin, 1997). The most common anomalies are colobomata of the eyes, heart defects, renal anomalies, growth and mental retardation, ear deficits and gastroesophageal reflux (referred to by the acronym "CHARGE") (Coniglio, Manzione,& Hengerer, 1988).

Infants are nose breathers for the first 3 months of life. Choanal atresia may be immediately recognizable at birth by signs of respiratory distress, especially if the atresia is bilateral. One method that may be used in the delivery room to assess the infant for choanal atresia is passing a catheter through each nostril to check for patency. If the catheter does not pass bilaterally, the diagnosis of choanal atresia is made. Infants with choanal atresia may be cyanotic at rest, but their color improves when they open their mouth to cry. Nasal discharge is present.

If it is determined that the infant has bilateral choanal atresia, surgical intervention is an immediate necessity. Prognosis is excellent if there are no other concomitant related medical conditions. Unilateral choanal atresia is often not detected until the infant's nostril becomes occluded with secretions, such as during a cold.

Diaphragmatic Hernia

Congenital **diaphragmatic hernias** occur during gestational life when the diaphragm fails to close during the seventh or eighth week. The defect allows the abdominal organs to be displaced into the left side of the chest through an opening in the diaphragm (Figure 35-5). It occurs in 1 in 3,000 live births (Guzzetta, Anderson,

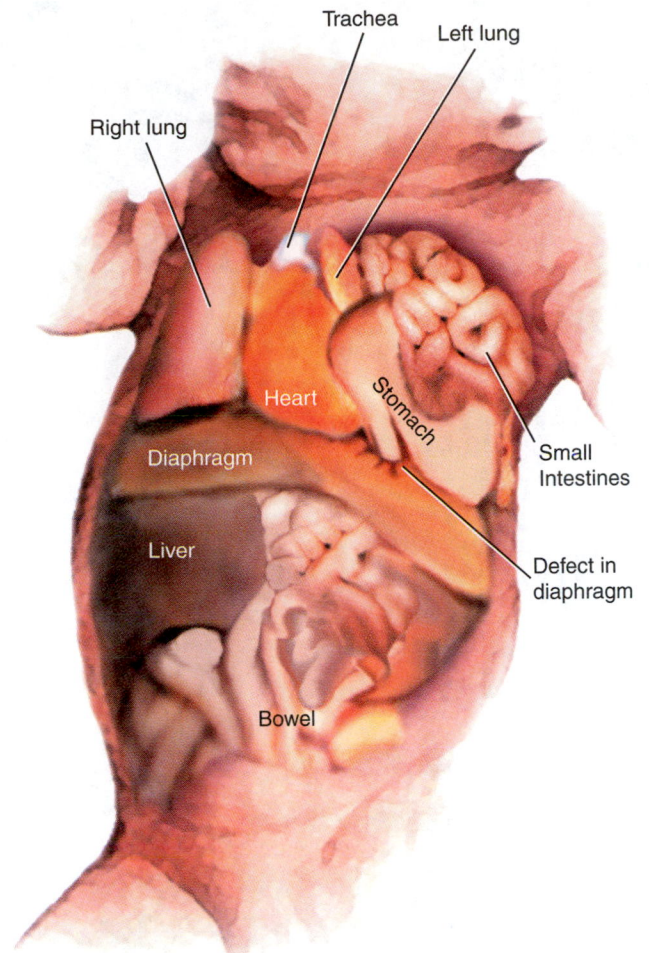

Right lung

Trachea

Left lung

Heart

Stomach

Diaphragm

Small Intestines

Liver

Defect in diaphragm

Bowel

Figure 35-5 Diaphragmatic hernia.

Eichelberger, Newman, Rouse, Schmitzer, Boyajian, & Tomaski, 1994) with equal frequency in male and female infants.

Prenatal diagnosis of congenital diaphragmatic hernia (CDH) may be made using an antenatal ultrasound technique as early as 26 weeks' gestation (Miller, Fanaroff & Martin, 1997). Surgical repair in utero has been completed at some perinatal centers, but this has not markedly changed the outcome (Holland et al., 1998). The presence of abdominal contents in the thoracic cavity during the embryonic period may prevent the normal development of lung tissue on the affected side. At birth, most affected newborns present with severe respiratory distress, because at least one of the lungs is unable to expand, or may not have fully developed (i.e., hypoplastic lungs). The respiratory distress progressively worsens as the stomach and bowels fill with air. Breath sounds are usually diminished or absent on the affected side and, instead, bowel sounds are audible in the chest. In 85% to 90% of cases, the hernia is on the left side because the liver fills the defects on the

right side (Holland, 1998). Physical examination of the newborn reveals a large or asymmetric chest and a flat relatively small abdomen.

Before surgery to repair the hernia is attempted, the infant's medical condition must be stabilized. Medical measures are taken to reverse hypoxia, hypercarbia, and metabolic acidosis. A nasogastric tube is inserted for gastric decompression. Mechanical ventilation with 100% oxygen is used to maintain functional respiratory status. If the infant's respiratory status does not improve, extracorporeal membrane oxygenation (ECMO) therapy may be required before the hernia repair (Guzzetta, Anderson, Eichelberger, Newman, Rouse, Schmitzer, Boyajian, & Tomaski, 1994). **ECMO** is a cardiopulmonary bypass therapy that allows the infant's lungs to rest and heal by exchanging blood gasses through a membrane oxygenator outside the body.

Preoperative nursing interventions include: positioning the newborn on the affected side with the head and chest elevated to allow for better expansion of the normal lung; placement of a gastric tube and connection to continuous low suction to keep the stomach and intestines decompressed; maintenance of oxygen and ventilatory support; and medication administration. Close and careful monitoring is essential at all times.

Once the infant is medically stable, surgical repair is performed. Postoperatively, maintenance of respiratory function is a high priority. Ventilatory support continues with careful monitoring for possible complications, such as pneumothorax and acid-base imbalances. Prognosis depends on the degree of pulmonary development and success of the closure. If the infant required mechanical ventilation during the first 18 to 24 hours of life, the survival rate is approximately 50%. If the infant with a diaphragmatic hernia did not experience any respiratory distress within the first 24 hours of life, survival rates reach 100% (Holland et al., 1998).

Cardiovascular System Anomalies

By the end of the third week of gestation, a functional cardiovascular system is in place to support further development of the embryo. Partitioning of the heart, a complex process, is completed by the end of the seventh week of gestation. Many women are not even aware that they are pregnant during this period. Formation of the cardiovascular system can be altered as a result of the presence of many factors, including genetic and environmental factors and some maternal medical conditions. A thorough maternal history and careful physical examination are important in the diagnosis of congenital heart disease (Figure 35-6).

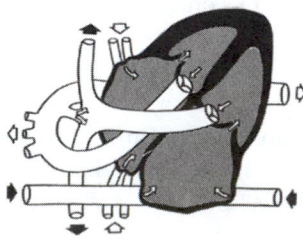
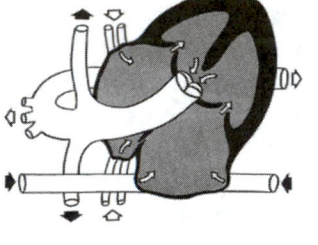
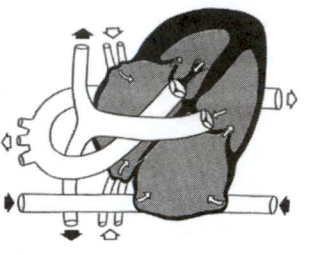
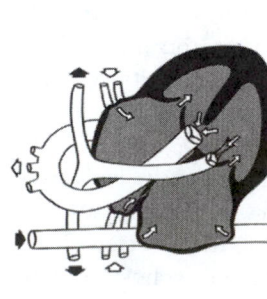
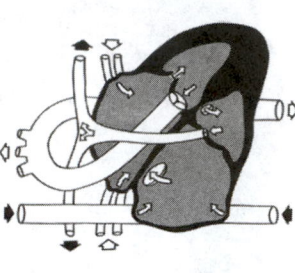
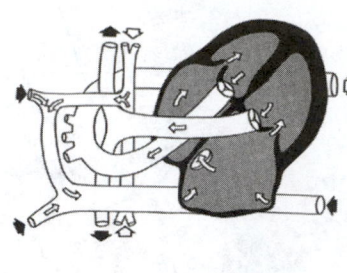

Patent Ductus Arteriosus

The patent ductus arteriosus is a vascular connection that, during fetal life, short-circuits the pulmonary vascular bed and directs blood from the pulmonary artery to the aorta. Functional closure of the ductus normally occurs soon after birth. If the ductus remains patent after birth, the direction of blood flow in the ductus is reversed by the higher pressure in the aorta.

Ventricular Septal Defects

A ventricular septal defect is an abnormal opening between the right and left ventricle. Ventricular septal defects vary in size and may occur in either the membranous or muscular portion of the ventricular septum. Due to higher pressure in the left ventricle, a shunting of blood from the left to right ventricle occurs during systole. If pulmonary vascular resistance produces pulmonary hypertension, the shunt of blood is then reversed from the right to the left ventricle, with cyanosis resulting.

Truncus Arteriosus

Truncus arteriosus is a retention of the embryologic bulbar trunk. It results from the failure of normal septation and division of this trunk into an aorta and pulmonary artery. This single arterial trunk overrides the ventricles and receives blood from them through a ventricular septal defect. The entire pulmonary and systemic circulation is supplied from this common arterial trunk.

Subaortic Stenosis

In many instances, the stenosis is valvular with thickening and fusion of the cusps. Subaortic stenosis is caused by a fibrous ring below the aortic valve in the outflow tract of the left ventricle. At times, both valvular and subaortic stenosis exist in combination. The obstruction presents an increased work load for the normal output of the left ventricular blood and results in left ventricular enlargement.

Coarctation of the Aorta

Coarctation of the aorta is characterized by a narrowed aortic lumen. It exists as a preductal or postductal obstruction, depending on the position of the obstruction in relation to the ductus arteriosus. Coarctations exist with great variation in anatomical features. The lesion produces an obstruction to the flow of blood through the aorta, causing an increased left ventricular pressure and work load.

Tetralogy of Fallot

Tetralogy of Fallot is characterized by the combination of four defects: 1) pulmonary stenosis, 2) ventricular septal defect, 3) overriding aorta, and 4) hypertrophy of right ventricle. It is the most common defect causing cyanosis in patients surviving beyond two years of age. The severity of symptoms depends on the degree of pulmonary stenosis, the size of the ventricular septal defect, and the degree to which the aorta overrides the septal defect.

Complete Transposition of Great Vessels

This anomaly is an embryologic defect caused by a straight division of the bulbar trunk without normal spiraling. As a result, the aorta originates from the right ventricle and the pulmonary artery from the left ventricle. An abnormal communication between the two circulations must be present to sustain life.

Atrial Septal Defects

An atrial septal defect is an abnormal opening between the right and left atria. Basically, three types of abnormalities result from incorrect development of the atrial septum. An incompetent foramen ovale is the most common defect. Blood from the right atrium passes through an atrial septal defect into the left atrium, mixes with oxygenated blood returning from the lungs, flows into the left ventricle, and is propelled into the systemic circulation. Improper development of the septum primum produces a basal opening known as an ostium primum defect, frequently involving the atrioventricular valves. In general, left to right shunting of blood occurs in all atrial septal defects.

Tricuspid Atresia

Tricuspid valvular atresia is characterized by a small right ventricle, large left ventricle, and usually a diminished pulmonary circulation. Blood from the right atrium returning from the body mixes with oxygenated blood returning from the lungs in the left atrium, flows into the left ventricle, and is propelled into the systemic circulation. The lungs may receive blood through one of three routes: 1) a small ventricular septal defect, 2) patent ductus arteriosus, and 3) bronchial vessels.

Anomalous Venous Return

Oxygenated blood returning from the lungs is carried abnormally to the right side of the heart by one or more pulmonary veins emptying directly, or indirectly through venous channels, into the right atrium. Partial anomalous return of the pulmonary veins to the right atrium functions the same as an atrial septal defect. In complete anomalous return of the pulmonary veins, an interatrial communication is necessary for survival.

Figure 35-6 Congenital heart abnormalities. (Used with permission of Ross Products, Division of Abbott Laboratories, Columbus Ohio.)

Congenital Heart Defects

Congenital heart defects (CHD) are anatomic abnormalities in the heart that are present at birth. The incidence of CHD is approximately 1% of births (Hoffman, 1995). There are more than 100 different types of cardiac anomalies; ventricular septal defects are the most common and constitute more than 20% of all CHDs. Transposition of the great arteries and coarctation of the aorta are the most common life-threatening anomalies. CHDs are the second major cause of death in the first year of life (premature birth, is the first).

The causes of CHDs are unknown, but both genetic and environmental factors are thought to influence their development. Infants with Down, Marfan, or Turner's syndromes frequently have related cardiac anomalies. Other factors linked to CHDs include maternal alcoholism; maternal rubella infection; maternal diabetes mellitus; maternal use of certain medications, including anticonvulsants, estrogen, progesterone, lithium, warfarin (Coumadin), or isotretinoin (Accutane); and exposure to x-rays. Prematurity, low birth weight, and congenital infections can also increase the risk for CHDs.

Major types of congenital cardiac defects are illustrated in Figure 35-6. CHDs are now categorized physiologically rather than as cyanotic or acyanotic (Wong & Perry, 1998). The four physiologic signs and the associated defects are listed in Table 35-1.

Assessment begins with a thorough review of the maternal history for risk factors that could predispose the infant to a congenital heart defect. The admitting nurse must carefully assess the infant's cardiovascular and respiratory functions and promptly report any abnormal findings. The infant is assessed for signs and symptoms of respiratory distress, including cyanosis, and congestive heart failure (CHF). In addition, a thorough assessment of the cardiac

Client Education
Congenital Heart Defects

Teach parents about the heart condition:

- Provide pictures and diagrams of the heart and then demonstrate the defect
- Provide written material on the specific heart defect

Instruct parents on medication administration:

- Provide a written schedule of times when the medication(s) should be administered
- Instruct on the purpose, dose, correct administration, and side effects of the medication(s). Inform parents about when to notify the physician.
- Allow parents to demonstrate their knowledge of medication administration (after instructions have been provided) to validate their understanding.

Educate parents about detecting these signs and symptoms and reporting them to the physician:

- Increased respiratory rate
- Breathing difficulties (such as nasal flaring or retractions)
- Excessive sweating
- Poor sucking
- Weight loss
- Poor feeding
- Cyanosis

Table 35-1 Physiologic Signs of Cardiac Defects	
Physiologic Sign	**Cardiac Defect**
Increase in pulmonary blood flow	Atrial septal defects Ventricular septal defects Patent ductus arteriosus
Obstruction to pulmonary blood flow	Coarctation of aorta Subaortic stenosis
Decrease in pulmonary blood flow	Tetralogy of Fallot Tricuspid atresia
Mixed blood flow	Complete transposition of great vessels Anomalous venous return Truncus arteriosus

rate, rhythm, and sounds should be conducted. Signs of CHF to look for include: tachycardia, tachypnea, gallop rhythm, diminished peripheral pulses, diaphoresis, edema, and hepatomegaly. Newborns exhibiting these signs require prompt diagnosis and appropriate therapy in a neonatal intensive care unit. Diagnostic tests used to obtain specific information about the defect and the need for surgical intervention include arterial blood gas analysis, chest x-ray studies, electrocardiogram (ECG), echocardiogram, and cardiac catheterization.

Nursing interventions include continuous monitoring of the infant's cardiac and respiratory status, maintaining a thermoneutral environment, administering oxygen as ordered, administering medications as prescribed, offering comfort measures to minimize crying when it precipitates cyanosis, and gavage feeding of the infant if necessary to decrease the workload of the heart. In addition, the nurse should inform the parents of the newborn's condition and management.

Before discharge, parents need experience in providing care and detailed instruction. Parents should be taught about their infant's heart defect, medication administration, and how to observe for signs and symptoms. In addition, home-based care should be instituted.

Gastrointestinal System Anomalies

Proper formation of the gastrointestinal (GI) system is necessary for the infant to support adequate nutrition and growth after delivery. During the fourth week of gestation, a primitive gut is formed. Many intricate steps are involved in the development of the complete GI tract, during which it is exposed to the possibility of formation of various anomalies. These malformations can occur anywhere in the GI tract and may be simple or complex. Knowledge of the signs and symptoms of GI anomalies is crucial because the nurse is often the first person to detect a problem.

Cleft Lip and Palate

Cleft lip or **palate** are terms that signify a congenital opening in the lip or palate, or both, that results from failure of the maxillary and premaxillary processes to fuse during the seventh to twelfth week of intrauterine life. This facial malformation is frequently seen in conjunction with other syndromes that occur in relation to avitaminosis or viral infections during the first trimester. Clefts of the lip or palate occur in approximately 1 in 600 to 700 Caucasian newborns. The incidence is double that rate in Asians and half that rate in African Americans. Cleft lip occurs more often in males and is generally located on the left side (Guzzetta, Anderson, Eichelberger, Newman, Rouse, Schnitzer, Boyajian, and Tomaski. 1994). The cleft deformity ranges from minor notching to complete separation of the entire lip and nasal floor (Figure 35-7). The defect may involve the lip, both the lip and palate, or only the palate, and may be unilateral or bilateral. Rarely is the defect located in the midline. The defect tends to occur more often in families in which a close relative also has the anomaly. Environmental factors, such as exposure to radiation or toxic substances, also play a part in contributing to the multifactorial nature of the defect.

Diagnosis of cleft lip may be made from physical appearance of the infant at birth. To determine if a cleft palate is present, the examiner inserts a gloved finger inside the newborn's mouth to feel the soft and hard palate.

Initial care of the child with a cleft lip or palate focuses on feeding. Feeding problems arise because of the infant's inability to create adequate suction and difficulty in swallowing. The infant with a cleft lip, is unable to hold onto and form a seal around the nipple. When feeding the infant, the bottle should be held while the infant's cheeks are grasped together to close the cleft. The infant should

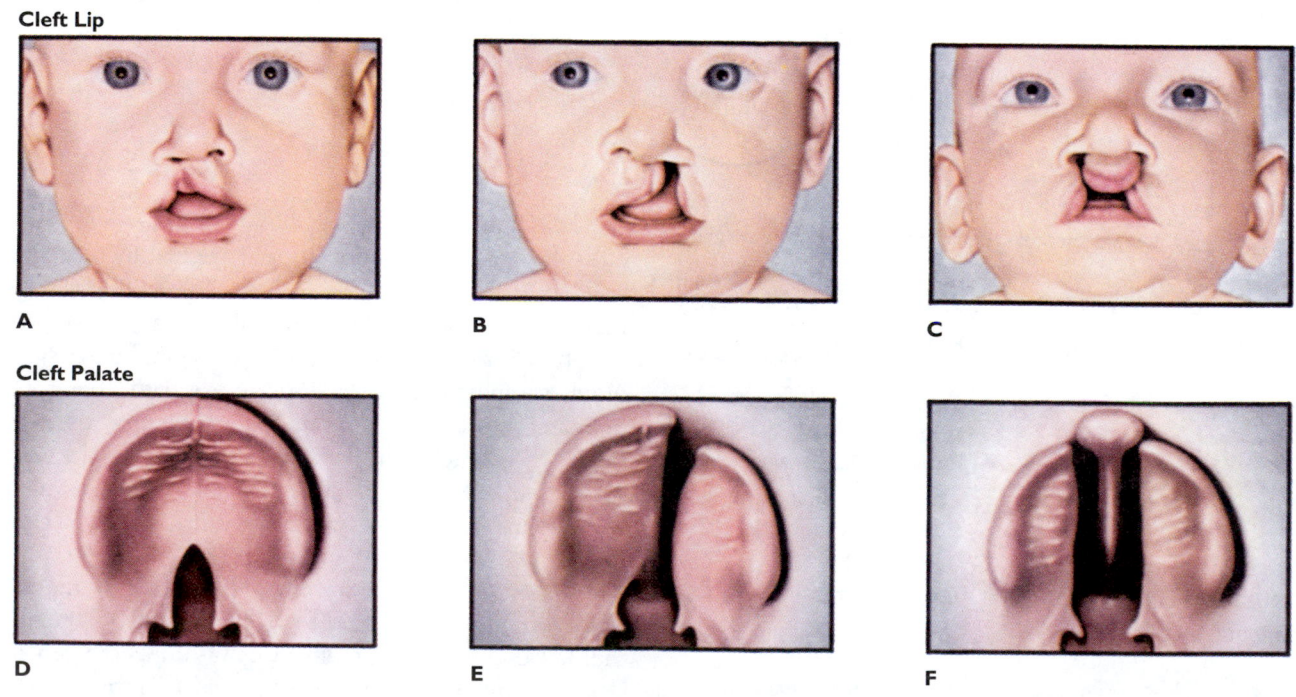

Figure 35-7 Cleft lip. A. Unilateral incomplete; B. unilateral complete; C. bilateral complete. Cleft Palate. D. Incomplete; E. unilateral complete; F. bilateral complete.

be bubbled or burped at frequent intervals, because air may be swallowed. If a cleft palate is present, the infant is unable to form a vacuum to maintain the suction necessary for feeding. The infant must be fed in an upright position, and the flow of milk should be directed to one side of the mouth to avoid choking. The degree of feeding difficulty depends on the size and type of defect; it is greatest in the child with a cleft palate. Newborns with less severe defects and intact lips can often successfully breastfeed because the breast may fill the cleft. Devices available for use with infants with cleft lip and palate include special nipples, compressible bottles, and syringe feeders.

Education, counseling, and emotional support for the parents is an important aspect of nursing care. This defect can be quite disfiguring. Parents need to be encouraged to ask questions and verbalize their anxieties and fears. Provide the parents with pamphlets that show photographs of infants both before and after surgical repairs. Parents must be taught to feed their infant in an upright position and to aim the nipple towards the intact part of the palate, while gently squeezing the bottle.

Surgical repair of the cleft lip is performed at approximately 3 months of age. Repair of the cleft palate is generally postponed until the infant is between 9 and 12 months of age. This delay allows time for the anatomic changes that normally occur in the palate contour (increase of the palate arch). Early surgery of a cleft palate seems to have a negative effect on facial growth, but the trend is toward closure during infancy because improved speech results. Preoperative teaching with parents should include information about the type of surgery being performed, postoperative care that the child will require, and how to use any appliances the infant needs. These children require multidisciplinary care through adolescence, including nursing care and specialist care, such as a pediatrician, audiologist, speech pathologist, otolaryngologist, plastic surgeon, orthodontist, and social worker (Guzzeta, Anderson, Eichelberger, Newman, Rouse, Schnitzer, Boyajian, & Tomaski, 1994).

Esophageal Atresia and Tracheoesophageal Atresia

Esophageal atresia (EA) and tracheoesophageal fistula (TEF) are uncommon anomalies in which the esophagus and trachea do not separate in a normal way. **Esophageal atresia** is a condition in which the esophagus ends in a blind pouch or narrows into a thin cord and is not connected to the stomach. During the 34th to 36th days of gestation, the trachea and esophagus ordinarily separate into two distinct tubes. Failure of this separation causes a **tracheoesophageal fistula** (TEF). TEF occurs in 1 in 4,500 births (Holland, Price, & Bensarb, 1998). The exact cause is unknown. These may be life-threatening anom-

alies of the esophagus and may occur together or singly. Figure 35-8 illustrates esophageal atresia.

Atresia is the congenital absence or closure of a normal body opening. EA can occur with or without a fistula (TEF) into the trachea. The most common esophageal atresia is a fistula between the distal esophagus and the trachea, which occurs in 86% of newborns born with *an esophageal defect*. Other types include esophageal atresia without a fistula (7.7%), H-type tracheoesophageal fistula without esophageal atresia (4.2%), esophageal atresia with a proximal fistula (0.8%), and atresia with proximal and distal fistulae (0.7%) (Holland, Price, & Bensard, 1998) (Figure 35-9). Infants born with this anomaly must be examined for other congenital anomalies, because 30% to 70% of affected infants have other malformations. CHD is the most common accompanying anomaly. Other potentially accompanying anomalies include vertebral malformations, atresias of the small intestine, imperforate anus, and genitourinary defects; the acronym for this syndrome is VATER, which stands for vertebral, anal, tracheoesophageal atresia or fistula, and renal anomalies. Some experts use the acronym VACTERL to delineate the same group of symptoms. The "C" stands for congenital heart defect and the "L" for limb deformities (Kenner, Lott, Flandermeyer, 1998).

Infants with EA and TEF may appear to be well immediately after birth. However, soon afterward, they present with copious oral secretions or are unable to swallow oral feedings. Signs and symptoms of esophageal atresia (with or without TEF) include drooling, choking, coughing, cyanosis, and regurgitation of food. Abdominal distention is a prominent feature in an infant with a distal fistula, because air is forced into the stomach.

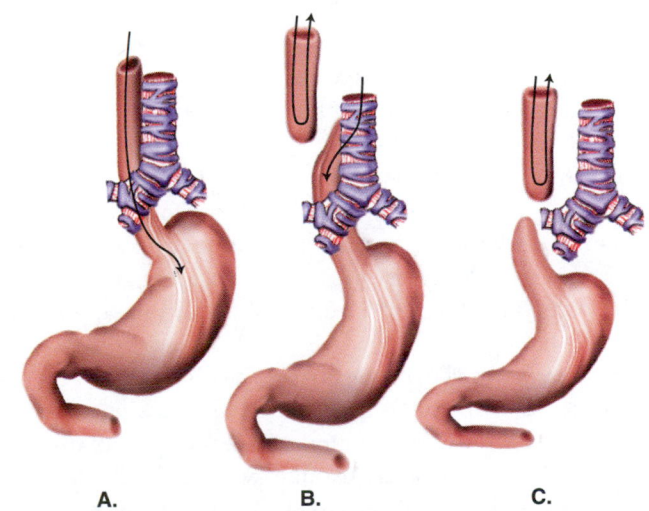

A.   B.   C.

Figure 35-8 A. Normal esophagus; B. tracheoesophageal fistula (esophagus ends in blind pouch, connects to trachea by fistula); C. congenital esophageal atresia (esophagus has two blind pouch ends with no communication to the trachea).

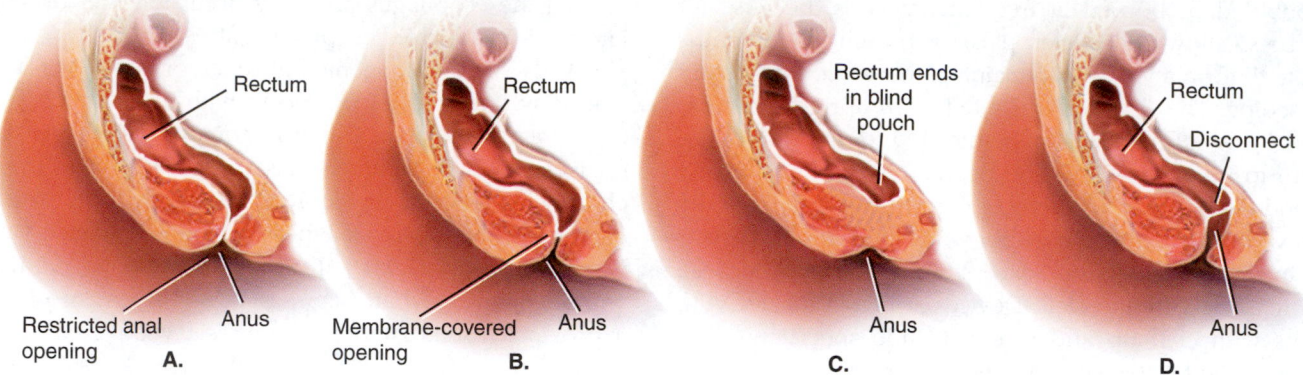

Figure 35-9 Imperforate anus. A. Anal opening is present but constricted; B. anus and rectum are normal but the anal opening is covered by a thin membrane; C. rectum ends in a blind pouch; D. rectum and anal canal are present but not connected.

Diagnosis of esophageal atresia is confirmed if a nasogastric catheter cannot be passed any further than 10 centimeters past the infant's nares, through the esophagus, and into the stomach. If a radiopaque catheter is used, an x-ray film reveals that the tube coils in the blind end (pouch) of the esophagus.

If the infant is stable, immediate primary surgical repair is done. If the infant is medically unstable, surgery is delayed until the infant's clinical status is stable and he or she can tolerate the surgical procedure.

After diagnosis is made and before surgery, nursing care of these infants includes positioning the infant in a 30-degree upright position to prevent gastroesophageal reflux; these infants should not be given anything orally. A catheter is placed in the upper esophageal pouch and connected to continuous low suction to remove secretions and prevent aspiration. The infant needs intravenous fluids to maintain fluid and electrolyte balance. Supplemental oxygen and intubation may be required if the infant experiences respiratory distress. Parents must be educated about the defect, the management plan, supported during this acute period, and kept informed about the care of the infant before and after surgery. Clarify and reinforce the physician's explanations about the malformation and the impending surgical repair. Encourage parents to ask questions and explain that the surgery is done in staged repairs. The first repair is provision of a gastrostomy and ligation of the fistula; the second is repair of the atresia, done several days later.

Surgery consists of closure of the fistula and anastomosis of the esophageal segments. Postoperative care involves the careful and continuous monitoring of the infant's cardiovascular and respiratory status and assessing for any potential complications. If the infant has a gastrostomy, feeding may be started in 48 hours. Oral feedings may be started in 5 to 10 days after the repair. The overall survival rate is 85% to 90%, with a good prognosis for a normal life.

Omphalocele and Gastroschisis

Omphalocele and gastroschisis are congenital defects in the abdominal wall. The incidence of omphalocele is 1 in 4,000 live births; gastroschisis occurs much less often than omphalocele, perhaps 1 in 10,000 births (Cunningham et al., 1997). The cause of these defects is unknown. An **omphalocele** is a defect covered by a peritoneal sac, located at the base of the umbilicus into which portions of the abdominal organs herniate. The peritoneal sac may contain both the small and large intestine, stomach, liver, spleen, and bladder. The peritoneal sac covering the defect may rupture during or after birth. Omphalocele develops during the 10th to 12th weeks of gestation and are often seen in conjunction with other cardiac, genitourinary, neurologic, or chromosomal anomalies.

This defect may be detected on an antenatal sonogram. If omphalocele is present, a vaginal delivery is still permitted, because the outcome is not any different than if the infant is delivered by cesarean section. If the diagnosis has not been made by sonogram, the defect is easily recognizable at the time of birth.

Gastroschisis is a condition in which the bowel herniates through an abdominal wall defect to the right of the umbilicus. In contrast to omphalocele, the contents are not contained in a sac, but instead the contents lie openly on the abdomen. Gastroschisis occurs in 1 in 4,000 to 10,000 live births (Quirk J. G. Jr, Fortney J, Collins H. B. 2nd, West J, Hassad S. J., Wagner C. 1996). This condition is often seen in small-for-gestational-age and preterm newborns and is rarely associated with other anomalies. Generally, there is a greater loss of fluid in the infant with gastroschisis than in the infant with omphalocele, unless the omphalocele is not covered by a layer of peritoneum. In utero, the intestine was allowed to float freely in amniotic fluid, so it may appear edematous and may be covered with black necrotic tissue.

Surgery is indicated for both ophalocele and gastroschisis. Preoperative care is similar for infants born with either defect. Immediate care is directed toward maintaining body heat and fluid and electrolyte balance and protecting the exposed abdominal organs. The exposed organs should be covered with a warm, sterile, saline-soaked gauze, which, in turn, should be covered with plastic wrap to contain body heat and prevent further trauma. The newborn should be positioned in the lateral position; the bowel should be supported to prevent injury. A nasogastric tube is inserted for gastric decompression. Intravenous fluids, volume expanders, and antibiotics should be ordered by the physician.

The surgical procedure to replace the organs in the abdominal cavity varies, depending on how large the defect is. If the defect is large, the surgery may need to be done in stages. A staged repair is done with a polymeric silicone (Silastic) pouch, which is used to suspend the viscera above the infant. Daily reduction maneuvers are done to return the suspended organs to the abdominal cavity. This staged reduction is generally done over 7 to 10 days. The infant then returns to surgery for closure of the abdominal wall (Kenner, Lott, Flandemeyer, 1998). If the defect is small, surgery to return the organs back into the abdominal cavity is performed as soon after birth as possible. With surgical treatment and nutritional support, the survival rate is more than 90% in affected infants (Rowe, 1995).

Parental support is extremely important. Parents need to be encouraged to hold their infant's hand and have as much physical contact as possible. The parents may experience a great deal of difficulty in accepting these disfiguring anomalies and in bonding with their newborn. The nurse must keep the parents informed about their newborn's condition, prognosis, physical appearance, and management plan. The nurse should assist and counsel parents who are trying to cope with this crisis.

Imperforate Anus

Imperforate anus refers to a group of congenital anomalies involving the rectum and anus. These anomalies result when the membrane separating the rectum from the anus fails to absorb during the seventh or eighth week of gestation. The condition occurs in 1 in 5,000 births and is 57% more common in males (Holland, Price, & Bensard, 1998). The anomalies are be classified by location, either high or low. In the low type, there may be stenosis of the anal opening or a thin transparent membrane may cover the normal anal opening. In the high type, the rectum ends in a blind pouch or there is no connection between the anus and the rectum (Figure 35-9). The necessary treatment and the prognosis are determined by the type of defect.

Approximately 20% to 75% of infants with an imperforate anus have accompanying anomalies. These anomalies are of the VATER or VACTERL variety (i.e., vertebral abnormalities, anal atresia, tracheoesophageal fistula with esophageal atresia, cardiac abnormalities and renal or radial limb abnormalities) (Kenner, Lott and Flandemeyer, 1998).

Visual inspection of the anal opening may lead the examiner to the diagnosis of imperforate anus. Additional clinical findings may include failure to pass a meconium stool and the inability of the rectum to allow insertion of a thermometer or a gloved small finger.

Surgery is done in stages if the anomaly is the high type. The infant requires a temporary colostomy in the interim. If the anomaly is of the low classification and a thin transparent membrane covers the anal opening, treatment consists of membrane excision, followed by daily dilation. Parents should be taught the dilation procedure.

Genitourinary System Anomalies

The urinary system begins to form during the fourth week of gestation, whereas first indications of the genitals appear during the fifth week. Defects in the genitourinary system are often not life-threatening but may be of great concern to the family, especially if the defect has involved formation of the genitalia. The anomalies can be surgically repaired with varying outcomes in regard to function and appearance. Some of the malformations may be a symptom of a much more complex disease.

Hypospadias

Hypospadias is a congenital anomaly in which the urethral meatus is located on the ventral surface of the glans penis instead of at the tip (Figure 35-10). This anomaly is

REFLECTIONS FROM A FATHER

"When my first son was born, I was absolutely on 'cloud nine'. The pregnancy, the birth, and our growth together as a couple had all been more than I could have ever hoped for. But when I looked at my son more closely, I noticed that his penis did not look right, because the opening was on the top rather than at the tip. I must admit that I was quite relieved to learn that this condition is easily repaired and will have no lasting negative effects on my son's growth and development."

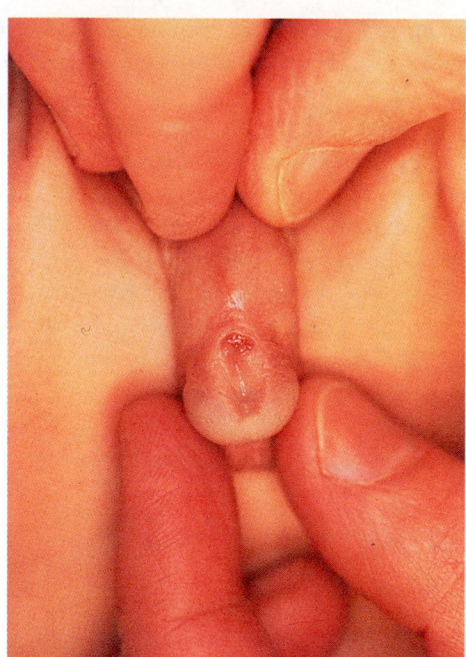

Figure 35-10 Hypospadias. (Courtesy of Dr. James Mandell, chief surgeon, Urology Department, Albany Medical College, Albany, NY.)

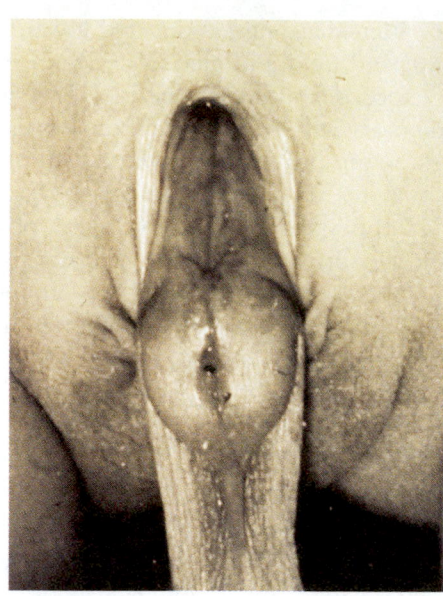

Figure 35-11 Epispadias. (Courtesy of Dr. James Mandell, chief surgeon, Urology Department, Albany Medical College, Albany, NY.)

fairly common, occurring in approximately 8 of 1000 male births (Angel, 1996). The exact cause is unknown, but it may be that hypospadias is inherited as a multifactorial problem. The sibling of an affected infant has an increased risk (14%) of also having this anomaly (Kaplan, 1994). Surgical repair is generally completed during the first year of life. The infant should not be circumcised before surgical repair because the foreskin is used, if necessary, for plastic surgery.

Epispadias

In **epispadias,** the urethral meatus is located on the dorsal surface of the penis (Figure 35-11). This is a rare anomaly, which occurs in only 1 of 100,000 live births (Kaplan, 1994). This condition often occurs with exstrophy of the bladder. Surgical repair is necessary and, as in infants with hypospadias, circumcision should not be done before the repair.

Exstrophy of the Bladder

Exstrophy of the bladder is an anomaly in which the anterior wall of the bladder and the lower portion of the abdominal wall are absent, causing the bladder to lie open and exposed on the lower abdomen. This defect is rare and occurs in only 1 of 25,000 live births (Kaplan, 1994). At birth, the bladder is visible in the suprapubic area and is red. Urine enters the bladder and can be seen draining onto the infant's skin. The exposed bladder should be kept

moist until surgical closure is completed. However, there is a difference of opinion on whether to cover the bladder or not; some physicians prefer to keep the bladder exposed, although others prefer to use a moist, sterile covering. Nursing care during this period before closure is aimed at preventing infection. Meticulous skin care around the bladder is required to prevent excoriation from the constant dripping of urine onto the infant's skin.

Surgical reconstruction is often done in two stages. The first stage is done within the first few hours after birth. The bladder and abdominal wall are surgically closed. The second surgical procedure involves creating a urethra, which is performed before the child goes to school, if possible.

Parents need support and education. They need understanding and guidance on how to accept their infant with such an obvious anomaly. They must be taught how to care for their infant at home until the final stage of the surgery is completed.

Ambiguous Genitalia

Even though parents may know the probable gender of their fetus from an ultrasonographic examination, gender is not certain until birth occurs. In rare cases, the gender of the newborn remains unclear at the time of birth. In these situations, it is imperative for the staff and physicians to be extremely cautious but to reassure the parents that the gender of their infant will be determined as soon as possible. Evaluation of the newborn with ambiguous genitalia must be treated as a medical emergency for many reasons. First, the ambiguous genitalia may be the result of several types of congenital adrenal hyperplasia that are life-threatening. Second, if the uncertainty of gender assignment is handled poorly, it can provoke long-term consequences for both the parents and the child (Moshang & Thornton, 1994).

Gender assignment should be achieved as soon as possible, preferably no later than age 2. However, gender determination within 3 to 6 months after birth is helpful in cases in which reconstructive surgery is necessary (Kenner, Lott, & Flandermeyer, 1998). Gender determination should only be done after careful review and consideration. The process of review should be initiated with a thorough maternal and family history, physical examination of the infant, and laboratory and radiographic studies. The mother should be asked about drugs that she took during the pregnancy, family history of a previous sibling who died during the first 10 days of life, or siblings who experienced precocious puberty. Positive responses from these questions might indicate congenital adrenal hyperplasia (Moshong & Thornton, 1994). The laboratory and radiographic evaluation consists of measurement of circulating hormones, analysis of the chromosomes (results are usually available in 2 to 3 days), and visualization of the internal organs (Kenner, Lott, & Flandermeyer, 1998).

Parental involvement is a critical consideration that the nurse must include in her plan of care. Parents require a great deal of support as they learn to deal with this situation. The nurse is responsible for coordination of care to ensure that the parents understand all the information they are given by various members of the health care team. Knowledge and understanding of basic neonatal embryology and sexual ambiguity can be beneficial to the nurse in identifying newborns with this disorder (Kenner, Lott, & Flandermeyer, 1998).

Musculoskeletal System Anomalies

Similar to many of the other systems, formation of the musculoskeletal system begins in the fourth week of gestation. This system includes development of the joints, muscles, and skeleton. Malformations are often relatively minor and, with proper recognition and treatment, the outcome is usually favorable.

Developmental Dysplasia of the Hip

Developmental dysplasia of the hip (DDH) was previously termed "congenital hip dislocation." DDH includes malformations of the hip involving varying degrees of deformity that may be present at birth, ranging from subluxation to complete dislocation. There are two basic types of DDH: developmental dislocation and teratogenesis. The more common of the two is the developmental dislocation, which is embryologically normal but is the result of mechanical forces in utero and the influence of maternal hormones, mainly estrogen, which relaxes tissues in preparation for birth. The infant's hip is generally dislocated in the perinatal period. The less common type of DDH, in which the hip is dislocated in the embryologic period of gestation has a teratogenic cause, seen in conjunction with malformation of the pelvis and hip (Griffin, 1994). Some affected infants show normal hip movement at birth, so the initial examination may be normal, but they later demonstrate abnormal hip development. Therefore, dysplastic hip screenings should be done at 2 weeks and 2, 4, 6, 9, and 12 months of age (Kenner, Lott, & Flandermeyer, 1998).

DDH occurs in 10 of 1,000 live births (Bennett, 1998). The cause is considered to be multifactorial, with genetic, hormonal, and environmental influences that predispose the hip joint to dislocation. The condition is approximately six times more common in girls than in boys. It is usually, but not always, unilateral, with the left hip being more commonly involved.

DDH must be detected in the neonatal period to enable early treatment and prevent complications. Ortolani's maneuver and Barlow's test are useful in making the diagnosis of DDH. These tests should be completed only by an experienced practitioner. Ortolani's maneuver determines whether one or both hips are dislocated (Figure 35-12). A positive result on Ortolani's maneuver is elicited when the hip is flexed at a 90-degree angle the leg is gently abducted, and an audible clunk is heard. In infants with DDH, Ortolani's maneuver elicits positive results until 8 weeks of age or longer (Griffin, 1994). Barlow's test determines whether the hip can be dislocated on manipulation. Positive results on Barlow's test occurs when the examiner flexes both hips and knees and slightly adducts the hips; a posterior-directed force on the knees causes the hip to dislocate (Bennett, 1998).

Secondary signs of DDH develop after 6 weeks of life, when the hip migrates laterally and superiorly (Figure 35-13). These signs are asymmetrical gluteal folds (higher on the affected side); limited abduction of the affected hip; and a femur that appears to be shorter on the affected side (Galeazzi's sign) (Griffin, 1994).

Treatment should be started as soon as possible after diagnosis to prevent any further deformity. Regardless of the type of hip dysplasia, the hips must be maintained in a flexed and abducted position. Methods used to maintain this position include triple diapering and an orthopedic splint, such as the Pavlik harness (Figure 35-14). The harness may be worn for the first 1–2 months of life. Frequently, a spontaneous relocation of the hip will occur in 3 to 4 weeks as a result of wearing the Pavlik harness (Cooperman & Thompson, 1997). The harness is effective

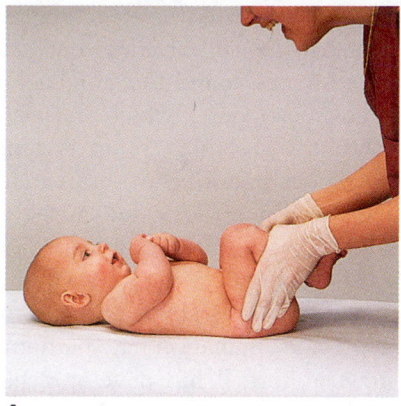

A.

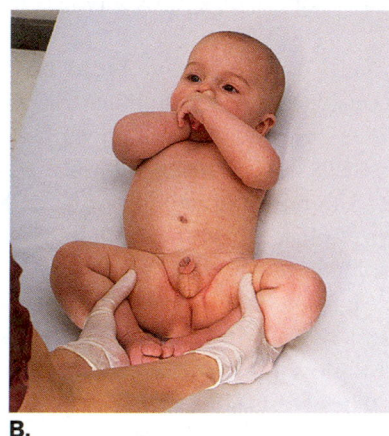

B.

Figure 35-12 Ortolani's maneuver. A. Hand placement; B. hip abduction.

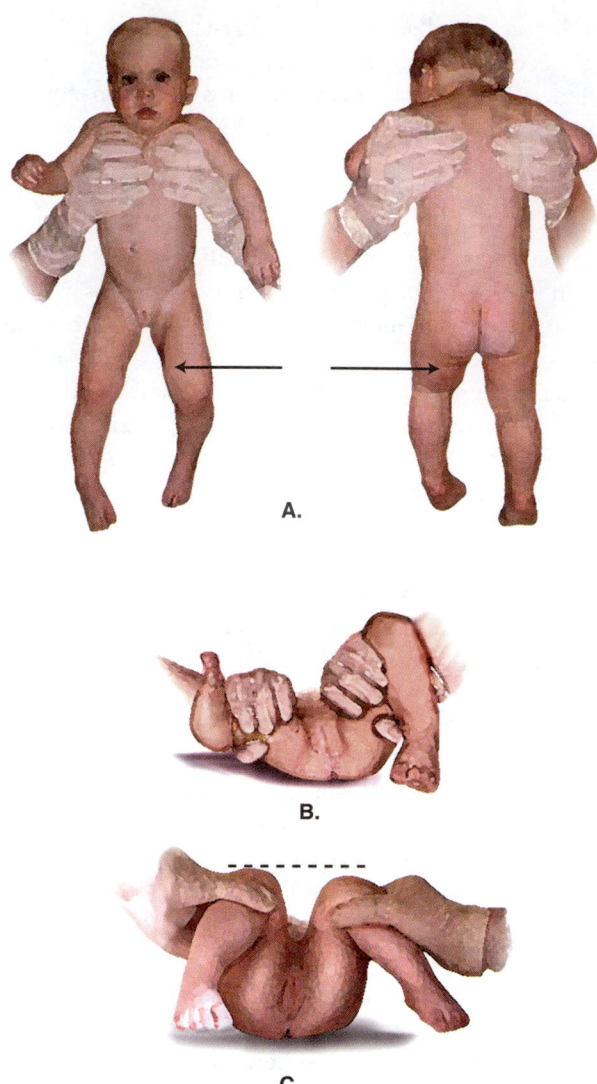

A.

B.

C.

Figure 35-13 Assessing for DDH. A. Thighs and gluteal folds show asymmetry; B. flexion shows limited hip abduction; C. knee height shows uneven level caused by shortened femur.

in 90% of cases. However, if the harness is ineffective in attempting to stabilize the hip, a spica cast may be applied to the hip or surgery may be necessary.

Parental support and teaching is an important part of the treatment plan. Parents must be educated about the

REFLECTIONS FROM FAMILIES

"Having our daughter in a Pavlik harness was a real challenge at first—especially the positioning, the diaper and clothing changes, and handling questions from curious observers. But then our 7-year-old son said, 'Hey, it looks like a slingshot to me,' and since then, we've had a more light-hearted view of the treatment and a more positive outlook about our daughter's future."

disorder, treatment management, and care of the infant in a harness or cast. Care should be directed toward preparing the parents for home care and assisting them in feeling comfortable holding and caring for their infant in an orthopedic device. The infant requires extensive follow-up with the orthopedist, and the nurse should stress keeping these follow-up visits.

Clubfoot

Clubfoot (talipes equinovarus) is the most common congenital deformity of the foot, in which portions of the foot and ankle are twisted out of a normal position (Figure 35-15). The foot is fixed in plantar flexion (downward) and is deviated medially (inward). Clubfoot is a musculoskeletal disorder that occurs twice as often in boys as in girls, with an overall incidence of 1 in 1,000 births (Coop-

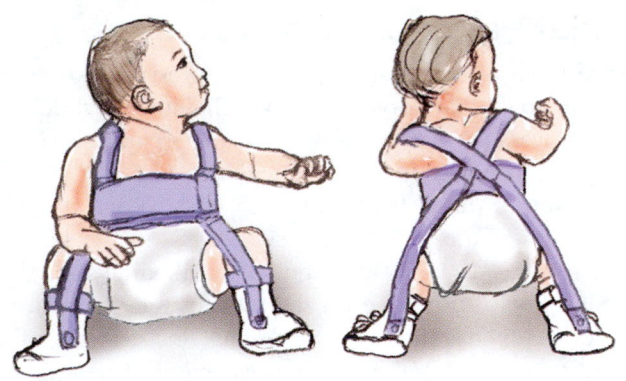

Figure 35-14 Infant in a Pavlik harness, used to treat developmental dysplasia of the hip.

erman & Thompson, 1997). The exact cause is unknown. This is a structural deformity that is easily recognized by its resistance to manual correction (Griffin, 1994).

Treatment is most successful when begun soon after birth, before the muscles and bones of the leg develop abnormally, causing shortening of the tendons. Nonsurgical treatment consists of gentle repeated manipulations of the foot, with serial castings done every few days for the first 1 to 2 weeks, then every week or two until correction of the foot is satisfactorily completed. Correction is usually completed in 6 to 8 weeks. To maintain the correction from serial castings, braces are usually worn for another 6 months, or longer. If conservative measures are unsuccessful in correcting the foot, surgical intervention is required during infancy.

Infants with this deformity are frequently placed in a cast while they are still in the newborn nursery. Nursing care is aimed toward supporting and educating the parents about this anomaly; nursing interventions include teaching the parents cast care, how to assess the toes to ensure adequate vascular circulation, how to handle the infant in a cast, and adhering to the follow-up treatment plan.

ACQUIRED DISORDERS

Conditions that result from environmental factors are referred to as acquired disorders. Although some disorders may be detected soon after birth, others may not become evident for several days. The longer an acquired disorder goes undetected and untreated, the greater the possibility of complications or long-term sequelae. Neonatal admission nurses must learn to carefully screen the maternal history for risk factors and must maintain up-to-date assessment skills. In addition, the nursing staff must remember to keep the parents of these neonates informed about the condition, treatment modalities, prognosis, and possible outcomes for infants with the disorder.

Trauma and Birth Injuries

In a difficult or traumatic delivery, certain birth injuries may occur. The injuries range from mild to life-threatening. A complete and thorough assessment of the neonate soon after birth allows the nurse to identify injuries sustained and develop an appropriate plan of care. In addition to meeting the specific needs of the neonate with a birth injury, nurses must also see to parental needs. The parents should be informed of their infant's condition, his or her special needs during the hospital stay and after discharge, and the possible outcomes.

A review of mortality rates indicates a steady decline in fetal deaths caused by birth injuries. Between 1981 and 1993, injury-related deaths decreased from 23.8 to 3.7 per 100,000 live births. Despite the significant decrease in mortality rates, birth injuries still rank as an important risk factor for neonatal morbidity (Fanaroff & Martin, 1997).

Fractures

Fractures often occur as the result of a difficult labor, breech deliveries, or large infants or when fetal distress is present and a rapid delivery is necessary. Common sites of fractures include the clavicle; long bones, such as the humerus and femur; and the skull. Fractures may not be detected immediately after birth because the infant may not display any signs of pain or the deformity may not be apparent. Definitive diagnoses for all fractures are determined by x-ray studies. During birth, the bone most often fractured is the clavicle. Fractured clavicles occur in at least 1.7% to 2.9% of term deliveries and more frequently on the right side (Fletcher, 1994). The break often occurs in the middle third of the bone; it is usually the result of dystocia in a vertex delivery. The newborn may be asymptomatic if the fracture is not displaced, and the fracture

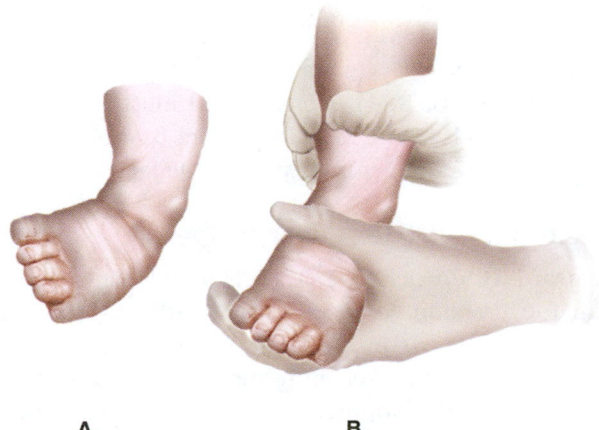

Figure 35-15 A. Talipes equinovarus (clubfoot); B. if the foot can be moved toward midline, the twisting is positional rather than congenital.

may not be detected until the infant is 2 to 3 weeks old. At that time, the infant develops a callus and mass over the fractured clavicle. Signs and symptoms of a fractured clavicle may include decreased mobility or immobility of the affected arm, crepitus along the involved clavicle, absence of the Moro reflex on the affected side, and crying by the infant when the arm is moved. Other than gentle handling to minimize pain, there is no medical or surgical treatment. The prognosis for complete recovery is good. Health care providers and the parents must be taught not to lift the infant up by the arms. If a fractured clavicle is suspected, the Scarf sign should not be assessed. Immobilization of the affected arm by immobilizing it close to the body (i.e., pinning sleeve to shirt or using a sling) may provide pain relief. The immobilization may be discontinued in 8 to 10 days when there is callus formation.

The second most often fractured bone is the humerus. These fractures result from a difficult delivery of the arms or shoulders during a vertex or breech delivery. The fracture is generally detected during delivery when the obstetrician hears and feels the humerus snap (Griffin, 1994). Signs and symptoms are the same as those of a fractured clavicle, with the exception that crepitus is not evident. The fractured arm should be immobilized in the adducted position with a splint or cast for 2 to 4 weeks, or until healing occurs.

Fractures of the femur also occur as the result of a difficult delivery. Deformity of the thigh, swelling, or immobility may be noted. Treatment involves traction, suspension, and casting for approximately 3 to 4 weeks (Mangurten, 1997).

The newborn's skull is extremely flexible and can withstand a great deal of molding; therefore, skull fractures are rare. The types of fractures that may occur are linear fractures and depressed fractures. Linear fractures, the most common, account for 70% of all skull fractures. This skull fracture generally has no signs or symptoms and does not require any special treatment, unless an intracranial hemorrhage has occurred. In depressed fractures, the skull becomes indented from the pressure exerted on the head by the pelvis or by forceps during delivery. Depressed fractures may require surgery if brain tissue is involved. Skull x-ray studies and CT scans are done to determine the site of fracture and to identify any potential complications.

The parents of newborns with fractures are often fearful of hurting their infant. To allay some of their fears, they should be taught how to handle and feed their infant and change diapers. Parents also should be taught the importance of follow-up care that includes additional x-rays films and CT scans, which may be necessary for several months after discharge to make sure that reunion of the bone occurs (Moe & Paige, 1998).

Facial Palsy or Paralysis

Facial palsy or paralysis results from pressure exerted on the seventh cranial nerve during a difficult vaginal delivery or from pressure of forceps, which causes paralysis on one side of the infant's face. The incidence of facial palsy in the newborn varies from 0.05% to 1.8% (Eng, 1994). In 75% of cases, the facial paralysis occurs on the left side (Moe & Paige, 1998). Usual signs of facial paralysis include inability to close the eye on the affected side, absence of wrinkles in the forehead during crying, and drawing of the mouth to one side when crying. No medical treatment is required, and the condition usually resolves within 3 weeks.

Brachial Paralysis or Palsy

Brachial palsy is a paralysis of the muscles involving the upper extremity that occurs as a result of injury to the brachial plexus during a prolonged and difficult labor, followed by a traumatic delivery. Brachial plexus injuries are estimated to occur at a rate of 0.5 to 1.9 per 1000 live births (Moe & Paige, 1998). The most common site of injury is at the fifth and sixth cranial nerve and is called Duchenne-Erb paralysis. This type of injury causes paralysis in the upper arm. Erb's paralysis usually results from the pulling or stretching of the shoulder away from the head during a difficult vertex or breech delivery. Clinical manifestations include a flaccid arm with the elbow extended and the hand internally rotated, an intact grasp reflex, absent or weak Moro reflex on the affected limb, and diminished or absent deep tendon reflexes on the affected arm.

Another type of injury that can occur from C8 to T1 is called Klumpke's palsy. This injury causes paralysis to the lower arm and hand. The incidence of Klumpke's paralysis is less than 2% of all cases. Treatment of brachial plexus injuries may include immobilization for 1 to 5 days, passive ROM exercises, and proper positioning of the affected arm and hand. In 88% to 92% of cases, full recovery is seen during the first year of life. Parents must be taught how to do passive ROM exercises and must be informed that these exercises are done to prevent further complications caused by contractures (Moe and Paige, 1998).

Intracranial Hemorrhage

Intracranial hemorrhage (ICH) is a collection of blood within the cranium. It results from birth trauma and is more likely to occur in the large, full-term newborn and spontaneously in the premature newborn, who is at highest risk for the development of ICH. There are different types of hemorrhage; the newborn can have one or more of these types. The most common types are subdural and subarachnoid hemorrhage.

Subdural hemorrhage (hematoma) is a collection of blood in the subdural space of the brain that results from lacerations of the large veins and sinuses that are frequently see in conjunction with a tear in the dura. Subdural hemorrhages occur less frequently now than in the past; they now account for less than 10% of all ICHs in the newborn because of improvements in obstetric monitoring and care. Subdural hemorrhages are a life-threatening condition because of their inaccessibility for aspiration by subdural tap (Fanaroff & Martin, 1997). Surgical evacuation of subdural clots may be necessary on an emergency basis.

Signs and symptoms include a decreased level of consciousness, seizures, and asymmetry of motor function. Diagnosis depends on results of a CT scan of the brain. If a subdural hemorrhage is confirmed, the prognosis is poor if the laceration is of the tentorium or falx; this diagnosis carries a mortality rate of 45%. The majority of infants with this type of laceration develop other complications, such as hydrocephalus. If the hemorrhage is of a lesser degree, 50% of the infants are neurologically normal at follow-up visits (Hill & Volpe, 1994).

Subarachnoid hemorrhage is the most common type of neonatal ICH. This type of hemorrhage in the full-term newborn is usually the result of trauma; in the premature infant, the hemorrhage results from hypoxia. Bleeding is of venous origin and is the result, more commonly, of smaller hemorrhages rather than massive ones. Diagnosis is confirmed by results of lumbar puncture and a CT scan of the brain. Signs of a subarachnoid hemorrhage include irritability, decreased level of consciousness, and seizures. Seizures are treated with anticonvulsant medications (Moe & Paige, 1998).

The nursing care of the newborn with ICH is generally supportive. Care includes monitoring of ventilatory and neurologic status; intravenous therapy to maintain fluid and electrolyte balance; observation and management of seizures; and prevention of increased ICP. The newborn should be handled minimally to promote rest and reduce stressors (Wong & Perry, 1998).

Because follow-up care varies, depending on the type and extent of hemorrhage, parent teaching must be individualized according to the prognosis for the infant's condition. Referral to local support groups may be beneficial.

Infants of Diabetic Mothers

Diabetes mellitus and gestational diabetes mellitus is increasing throughout the population. Gestational diabetes occurs in approximately 2% to 3% of pregnant women (Sills & Rapaport, 1994).

The **infant of a diabetic mother** (IDM) presents with a number of clinical problems. A better understanding of maternal and fetal metabolism, resulting in stricter meta-

bolic control, improved fetal surveillance, early delivery, and neonatal intensive care, has increased the survival rates for IDMs over the past few years (Kalhan & Saker, 1997). In recent years, perinatal mortality rates have decreased by 6% in IDMs, from more than 10% to less than 4% (Coustan, 1997).

The fetus is at risk for many problems when the mother has diabetes mellitus. Alteration in glucose metabolism affects the infant in utero and immediately after birth. One factor that determines how the fetus is affected is the severity and duration of the maternal diabetes. A positive outcome for the health of the fetus requires maintenance of normoglycemia in the pregnant woman with diabetes. Even with good control of the mother's glucose levels, problems can occur. Common problems observed in infants of diabetic mothers include macrosomia, respiratory distress syndrome, hypoglycemia, hypocalcemia, hypomagnesemia, hyperbilirubinemia, polycythemia, and congenital anomalies.

Macrosomatia

Macrosomatia is defined as a fetal weight above the 90th percentile for gestational age or a birth weight of more than 4,000 g (8 lb, 12.8 oz). Macrosomatia is a common characteristic of infants of diabetic mothers. The probability of insulin-dependent women giving birth to a macrosomatic infant is 20% to 30% (Ogata, 1994). Women with gestational diabetes have the same likelihood of bearing a macrosomatic infant as a woman with preexisting diabetes. The macrosomatic infant has a round chubby face, chubby body, and a plethoric appearance, which is related to polycythemia. The infant's internal organs (liver, spleen, and heart) are enlarged and amount of body fat is greater than normal. Much of this fat is deposited in the shoulders and intrascapular area. The IDM has normal brain growth, and the characteristic disproportion between head and shoulder size greatly contributes to dystocia and trauma during birth (Ogata, 1994).

Insulin is the hormone central to the development of macrosomatia. Late in pregnancy, when the mother's pancreas does not release enough insulin to meet the increasing needs, she becomes hyperglycemic. These high levels of maternal blood glucose cross through the placenta to the fetus, and the fetal pancreas responds by releasing large amounts of insulin. This increased production of insulin by the fetus stimulates the growth of insulin-sensitive tissues (i.e., adipose, muscle, and connective tissue), which causes macrosomatia (Fanaroff & Martin, 1997).

Respiratory Distress Syndrome

IDMs are at greater risk of developing respiratory distress syndrome (RDS) than normal full-term newborns. Fetal hyperinsulinemia adversely affects fetal lung maturation by inhibiting the development of enzymes necessary for the synthesis of the phospholipid components of surfactant. Fetal lung maturity in the normal full-term infant is evidenced by a lecithin-sphingomyelin (L/S) ratio of 2:1. But in the mother who has diabetes mellitus or gestational diabetes mellitus, it is recommended that the L/S ratio be 3:1 or more, or the amount of phosphatidyl glycerol in the amniotic fluid should be more than 3%, to confirm adequate lung maturity.

Hypoglycemia

The most common problem in an IDM at birth is **hypoglycemia** (i.e., blood glucose levels of less than 40 mg/dL). The infant's blood glucose level is high at the time of birth because of maternal hyperglycemia. Because of this elevated level of fetal blood glucose, the fetal pancreas responds by producing large quantities of insulin, causing a state of hyperinsulinemia. Even though there is a cessation of the maternal glucose supply when the cord is clamped, the infant is still in a hyperinsulinemic state. Hypoglycemia usually occurs during the first 3 hours after birth. The blood glucose level in the newborn is checked by heel stick after birth and again at frequent intervals, especially during the first 24 hours of life. Most IDMs are asymptomatic. Signs of hypoglycemia can include jitteriness and tremors, apnea, cyanosis, a high-pitched cry, lethargy, and tachypnea. Treatment includes providing early feedings (within 30 minutes after birth if bowel sounds are present) or the administration of intravenous glucose.

Hypocalcemia and Hypomagnesemia

Hypocalcemia and hypomagnesemia are metabolic problems seen in IDMs. **Hypocalcemia** is a blood calcium level of less than 7 mg/dL. It is one of the most common clinical problems that affect IDMs. Approximately 10% to 20% of IDMs experience hypocalcemia during the neonatal period. The cause is believed to be related to decreased concentrations of parathyroid hormone during the first four days of life (Ogata, 1994). Many infants with hypocalcemia are asymptomatic, but some may exhibit jitteriness, a high-pitched cry, irritability, seizures, and twitching. These symptoms may be indistinguishable from those of hypoglycemia, except that they generally occur between 24 and 36 hours after birth versus hypoglycemia, which occurs during the first 1 to 3 hours of life. To restore normal calcium levels, therapy is initiated by providing early feedings, intravenous calcium, or oral calcium supplements.

Reduced serum magnesium levels may occur in pregnant diabetic women and their infants. Hypomagnesemia in the newborn is believed to result from increased maternal losses of magnesium in the urine, which are charac-

teristic of diabetes. Magnesium deficiency may inhibit fetal parathyroid hormone secretion, which is associated with hypocalcemia (Barron, Lindheimer, & Davison, 2000).

Hyperbilirubinemia and Polycythemia

Hyperbilirubinemia, an elevated level of direct bilirubin in the blood, is a common finding that occurs in 20% to 25% of IDMs (Ogata, 1994). Many infants also have **polycythemia**, which results from an increased number of red blood cells, and plays a significant role in hyperbilirubinemia. An increased rate of erythrocyte breakdown results from changes in erythrocyte membrane composition, which, in turn, result from changes in maternal glucose availability (Ogata, 1994). This increased red blood cell breakdown, along with bruising suffered by the macrosomatic infant at birth, may contribute to high bilirubin levels.

Congenital Anomalies

The incidence of congenital malformations is two to four times higher in IDMs than in infants born to mothers who do not have diabetes (Ogata, 1994). The most common anomalies are cardiac and skeletal malformations and neural tube defects. In most anomalies related to diabetic pregnancies, the structural abnormalities have occurred before the eighth embryonic week. This reinforces the importance of women with diabetes monitoring their glucose levels before conception and delaying pregnancy until their glycosylated hemoglobin level is within the normal range (Coustan, 1997).

The incidence of congenital heart lesions in IDMs can be as much as five times that of infants of normoglycemic mothers. The most common lesions in the IDM are atrial or ventricular septal defects, transposition of the great vessels, and coarctation of the aorta (Fanaroff & Martin, 1997).

Skeletal malformations may include delayed ossification, osseous defects, caudal regression syndrome, and femur agenesis or hypoplasia. CNS anomalies include hydrocephalus, meningomyelocele, and anencephaly (Kenner, Amlung, Flandermayer, et al., 1998).

These infants may also present with abdominal distention, failure to pass meconium stool, and bile-stained vomitus, caused by a transient delay in the development of the left side of the colon. This condition is known as neonatal small left colon, or lazy colon syndrome. Normal bowel function develops in early infancy (Fanaroff & Martin, 1997).

Hyperbilirubinemia

Hyperbilirubinemia, or jaundice, is a common finding in all newborns. Hyperbilirubinemia is an excess of bilirubin in the blood, which causes jaundice. Bilirubin is formed from the breakdown of hemoglobin in the red blood cells. Jaundice results from deposits of the yellow pigment in bilirubin. Excess amounts of bilirubin are evidenced by a yellowish discoloration of the neonate's skin, mucous membranes, and sclera, termed **jaundice**. Jaundice proceeds in a cephalopedal progression, first appearing on the head and face and then progressing to the trunk and extremities. If jaundice is present, it may be observed by blanching the skin on the infant's forehead or over the bridge of the nose. If the skin blanches to a yellow hue, jaundice is present. In dark-skinned infants, the nurse may more easily detect jaundice by observing the color of the sclera and the buccal mucosa.

Hyperbilirubinemia may result from either physiologic or pathologic factors. Even though hyperbilirubinemia is a common clinical finding in the newborn, the normal physiologic jaundice process must be distinguished from the abnormal pathologic jaundice condition.

Physiologic Jaundice

Physiologic jaundice occurs in approximately 50% to 60% of full-term newborns and up to 80% of preterm newborns during the first week of life. It is a transient elevation of unconjugated bilirubin, which occurs after 24 hours of age, and is a normal physiologic process. The mean unconjugated bilirubin level in cord blood is 1.8 mg/dL. The full-term infant reaches peak bilirubin concentration levels of 6 to 7 mg/dL between 48 and 72 hours after birth. Increased bilirubin levels resolve without any intervention, declining to less than 2 mg/dL by 6 to 7 days after birth. Ethnic variability may also influence bilirubin levels during the first week of life. Asian and Native Americans have average peak serum bilirubin levels that are twice the level of other ethnic groups.

Pathologic Jaundice

Jaundice that is evident in the first 24 hours of life, a bilirubin level that rises more than 0.5 mg/dL per hour, or true hemolysis is considered **pathologic jaundice**. The most common cause of pathologic jaundice is blood group incompatibility, specifically ABO and Rh incompatibility. Other less common situations that may be seen in conjunction with pathologic jaundice in the newborn are maternal or fetal infections, swallowed maternal blood, maternal diabetes, fetal enzyme deficiencies, fetal enclosed hemorrhage (e.g., cephalhematoma or bruising), fetal polycythemia, fetal small-bowel obstruction, and fetal hypothyroidism.

Kernicterus

A possible complication of pathologic jaundice is kernicterus, also termed "bilirubin encephalopathy." **Kernicterus** is the excess accumulation of unbound, unconju-

gated bilirubin, which is deposited in brain tissues, particularly the basal ganglia. The excess bilirubin crosses the blood-brain barrier, causing yellow staining of the brain tissue, similar to its effect on the skin. Kernicterus causes varying degrees of neurologic damage. There is not a direct correlation between serum bilirubin levels and the severity of brain tissue damage. However, in the full-term healthy infant whose total serum bilirubin exceeds 25 mg/dL, the risk for kernicterus increases. Premature infants or infants with other medical complications are at risk for kernicterus at much lower serum bilirubin levels. Perinatal conditions can also influence the bilirubin-binding capacity of hemoglobin and increase the risk for kernicterus at lower serum bilirubin levels; these include hypoxia, acidosis, hypothermia, hypoglycemia, sepsis, and administration of certain medications (e.g., salicylates, sodium benzoate). Kernicterus usually becomes evident during the first 6 days of life. Early signs, which may be absent or present, include lethargy, poor feeding, temperature instability, hypotonia, and a high-pitched cry. Permanent neurologic sequelae in these children include ataxia, opisthotonos, deafness, seizures, and mental retardation (Blackburn, 1995).

ABO Incompatibility

ABO incompatibility occurs as a result of the mother and fetus having different blood groups. The mixing of maternal and fetal blood leads to hemolysis of fetal red blood cells. ABO incompatibility is the most common and mildest type of hemolytic disease; it rarely causes severe hemolytic problems, which would require an exchange transfusion. The incompatibility occurs when the fetal blood is type A, B, or AB and the mother is type O. The incompatibility arises because the mother does not have the fetal red blood cell antigen A or B and produces antibodies that cross the placenta to the fetus. This problem may occur in the first pregnancy, because mothers with type O blood already have naturally occurring anti-A and anti-B antibodies in their blood. There is no way of preventing ABO incompatibility.

Laboratory studies may be helpful in establishing a diagnosis of ABO incompatibility. Positive results on direct Coombs' test occurs in 3% of cases, but positive results in both direct and indirect Coombs' test occur in 80% of cases. The direct Coombs' test measures the presence of antibodies on the red blood cell surface, and the indirect test is a measurement of antibodies in the serum (Kenner, Amlung, & Flandermeyer, 1998).

Rh Incompatibility

Rh incompatibility is a hemolytic disease caused by the incompatibility of Rh factors in maternal and fetal blood. Rh incompatibility, or isoimmunization, occurs when the woman is Rh-negative and the fetus is Rh-positive. If both parents are Rh-negative, there is no hemolytic incompatibility with the infant and the infant is Rh-negative. Isoimmunization occurs when fetal blood cells escape and pass through the placenta into the maternal circulation. The fetal blood cells may pass into the maternal circulation as early as 8 weeks' gestation or during an abortion, amniocentesis, ectopic pregnancy, hydatidiform mole, abdominal trauma, or when the placenta separates during delivery. The woman may form protective antibodies against the fetal blood cells. The process by which the maternal immunologic system forms antibodies against fetal blood cells is termed "**maternal sensitization**." Usually, the woman becomes sensitized during the first pregnancy but does not form enough antibodies to adversely affect the infant. However, during subsequent pregnancies, antibodies form rapidly, resulting in lysis or destruction of fetal red blood cells.

Erythroblastosis fetalis is a condition in which there is vast destruction of fetal red blood cells by maternal antibodies, resulting in fetal anemia and hyperbilirubinemia. The severity of this condition depends on how well the infant can compensate for the destruction of red blood cells. However, the destruction of fetal red blood cells may be so severe that a marked hemolytic anemia develops and the blood does not have sufficient capacity to carry oxygen to the tissues. Fetal death or birth of an infant with hydrops fetalis may result from this condition (Ensher & Clark, 1994). **Hydrops fetalis** is the most severe form of fetal hemolytic disease: there is severe anemia resulting in hypoxia, cardiac decompensation, and hepatosplenomegaly.

The signs of Rh incompatibility in the newborn are jaundice, pallor, and enlargement of the liver and spleen. Jaundice becomes evident within the first 4 to 5 hours after birth and peaks when the infant is 3 or 4 days old (Blanchette, Doyle, Schmidt, & Zipursky, 1994).

Management of Rh incompatibilities focuses on prevention of the disease by administering Rh_o (D) immune globulin (RhoGAM) to the mother after delivery or abortion, if the infant was Rh-positive. This agent should be administered within 72 hours after delivery; this treatment should prevent the woman from producing antibodies to the fetal blood cells that entered her bloodstream during the delivery.

Management of Newborn Hyperbilirubinemia

The goal of managing the newborn with jaundice is to keep the serum bilirubin below neurotoxic levels. The most common treatment modalities are phototherapy and exchange transfusions.

Phototherapy is the use of ultraviolet light in the treatment of jaundice in the newborn (Figure 35-16).

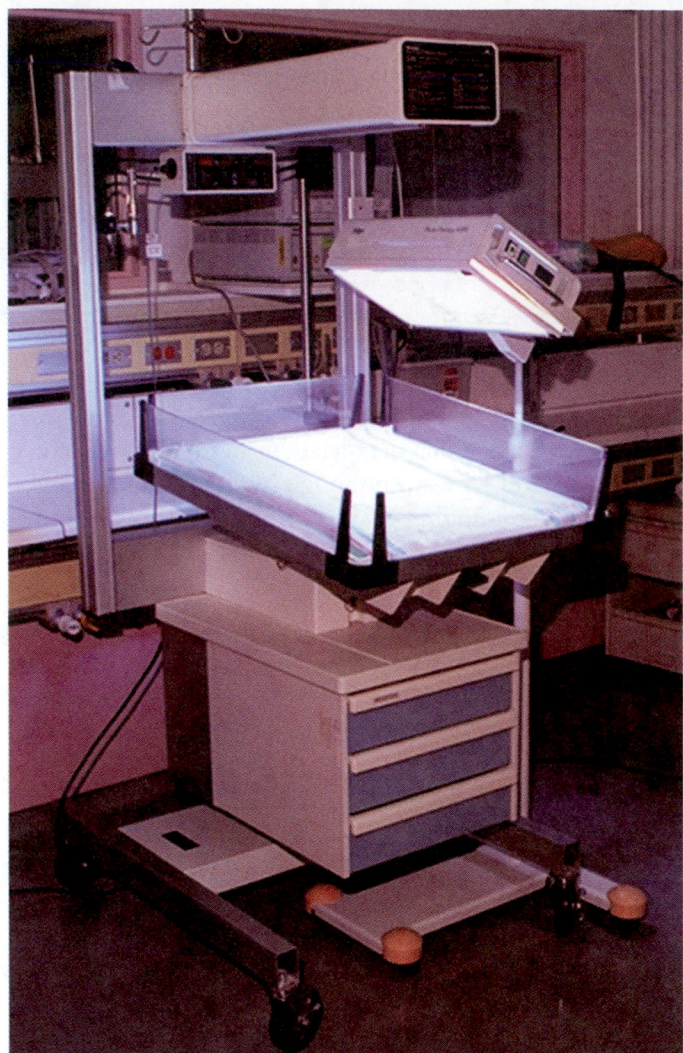

A.

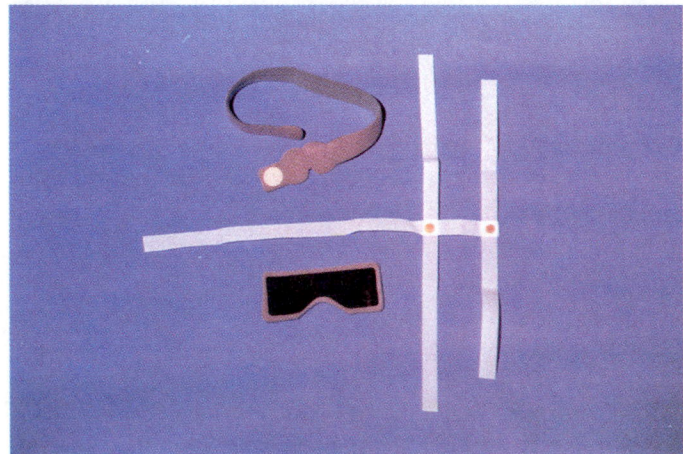

B.

Figure 35-16 A. Phototherapy, set-up for jaundiced newborn; B. phototherapy equipment including bilateral eye patches.

Phototherapy works by encouraging the liver to excrete bile in the form of unconjugated bilirubin. Blue or fluorescent bulbs are commonly used in phototherapy. The adverse effects of using phototherapy include dermal rash, lethargy, abdominal distention, possible eye damage, dehydration, thrombocytopenia, hypocalcemia, secretory diarrhea, and "bronze baby" syndrome (Kenner, Amlung, & Flandermeyer, 1998).

The prolonged exposure to ultraviolet light may cause retinal damage; therefore, it is extremely important to keep the infant's eyes shielded with eye patches when under the light. However, try to keep as much of the infant's skin exposed as possible. During oral feedings, the light and eye patches can be removed to provide sensory stimulation and interaction with the parents or care provider.

Infants undergoing phototherapy require close monitoring of their body temperature, fluid and electrolyte balance, and serum bilirubin concentration (lights should be turned off while drawing blood). The serum bilirubin levels must be checked frequently to ensure that phototherapy is effective.

If the infant is to receive phototherapy at home, the nurse is responsible for teaching the parents to record the infant's temperature, weight, and fluid intake; to weigh diapers; and to note the frequency of stools. Another method of phototherapy uses a fiberoptic blanket and is more convenient for home use.

If phototherapy is ineffective and the serum bilirubin level is rising to a level that may be neurotoxic, an exchange transfusion may be necessary. Exchange transfusions should lower the bilirubin level by 50% to 60%. During an exchange transfusion, the infant's antibody-coated red blood cells and excess bilirubin are removed and replaced by donor blood that contains noncoated red blood cells. Only small amounts of the infant's blood are removed and replaced at a time. The procedure is repeated until the infant's total blood volume has been diluted with the fresh blood. Exchange transfusions are considered safe, but complications may arise. The nurse must be alert for the following complications: bradycardia, arrhythmias, infection, thrombosis, hypocalcemia, and fluid overload.

NEONATAL INFECTIONS

Neonatal infections cause more than 30% of all neonatal deaths. Approximately 50% of neonatal mortalities that occur during the first 24 hours of life are attributed to infection (Kenner, Lott, Flandermeyer, 1998). Infection in the neonate can be caused by a variety of agents. Infection may be passed through the placenta to the baby during pregnancy or from exposure to organisms present in the vagina during birth or from the environment. Organisms that initially infect the mother and then are passed on

transplacentally to the fetus are referred to by the acronym TORCH (toxoplasmosis, other [gonorrhea, syphilis, varicella, parvovirus, HBV, and HIV], rubella, cytomegalovirus, and herpes simplex virus. (See STORCH, Chapter 21.) Major complications from infections include respiratory distress, shock, acidosis, disseminated intravascular coagulation (DIC), and meningitis (Kenner, Lott, & Flandermeyer, 1998).

Sepsis

Sepsis is a systemic bacterial, viral, or parasitic infection that invades the bloodstream of the newborn. It occurs either during or after birth in approximately 1 of 1000 full-term births (Ensher & Clark, 1994). Bacterial sepsis in the newborn is divided into two categories: early onset or late onset. Early onset sepsis occurs during the first few days of life and is generally caused by obstetric complications, such as prolonged or premature rupture of membranes, chorioamnionitis, peripartum maternal fever, fetal distress, or aspiration by the newborn. The microorganisms that usually cause the early-onset infection are from the maternal vaginal tract and include group B *Streptococcus species, Haemophilus influenza, Listeria monocytogenes, Escherichia coli,* and *S. pneumoniae.* Infants with early-onset sepsis have a high mortality rate.

Late-onset sepsis generally occurs after the first week of life. Bacteria that causes the late-onset sepsis include organisms acquired either from the mother's genital tract or by contact from humans and equipment (Merenstein, Adams, & Weisman, 1998). The bacteria that commonly cause late-onset sepsis include *Staphylococcus aureus, S. epidermidis, Pseudomonas* organisms, and group B beta-hemolytic Streptococci. The most common organisms for causing sepsis in the newborn is the group B *Streptococcus* species, which are acquired from the mother.

It is often difficult to distinguish sepsis in the neonate from other medical conditions because the symptoms of both early- and late-onset sepsis are vague and nonspecific. Because of the high mortality rate of sepsis, it is imperative for the nurse to observe and report to the physician any subtle changes that occur in the neonate's status.

The most accurate method of confirming bacterial sepsis is isolation of the bacteria from either the blood, CSF, or urine. Generally, the CSF is tested in the symptomatic newborn, because meningitis is a frequent cause of sepsis (Merenstein, Adams, & Weisman, 1998). Other tests include a complete blood cell (CBC) count with differential, C-reactive protein, erythrocyte sedimentation rate, total platelet count, and cultures (blood, urine, or CSF). A chest x-ray study detects pneumonia.

After obtaining the appropriate laboratory samples, antibiotic therapy is initiated. A broad-spectrum antibiotic, such as ampicillin in combination with an aminoglycoside, is commonly administered, pending culture and sensitivity results. Once the causative organism is determined and the antibiotic sensitivities are known, the least toxic antibiotic is administered for an appropriate period of time (Merenstein, Adams, & Weisman, 1998).

Before the advent of antibiotic therapy, the mortality rate from bacterial sepsis was 95% to 100%, but now, with antibiotics, the mortality rate has been reduced to less than 50%. The most common complications of bacterial sepsis are meningitis and septic shock. Bacterial meningitis affects 1 in 2,500 live births (Wong & Perry, 1998). The outcome of neonatal sepsis is influenced by early recognition, antibiotic therapy, and supportive care (Merenstein, Adams, & Weisman, 1998).

FAMILY EXPERIENCES

The nursing care of the family with a newborn who has a congenital disorder is extremely demanding and must involve a multidisciplinary team approach, including such specialists as nurse practitioners, surgeons, social workers, dieticians, physical therapists, and neurologists. The care must address the surgical and rehabilitative needs of the infants and the educational, psychosocial, and financial needs of the family.

In the early postpartum period, it is particularly challenging to work with the parents. At this time, parents are going through the shock and disappointment of having had a "less-than-perfect" child. They must first be given the time, opportunity, and support to go through the grief process. This process involves the parents experiencing shock, denial, anger, and depression before accepting the newborn and reorganizing the family. Nurses can best facilitate parental passage through the process by being accessible and keeping the lines of communication open between the parents and staff. Nurses should educate the family about the disorder and their infant's present and future health care needs. When they are ready, parents should be encouraged to touch and become involved in their infant's care.

NURSING PROCESS

Although not all congenital disorders can be predicted in the perinatal period, the nursing process provides a framework for nurses caring for families after the birth of an infant with an anomaly.

Assessment

Nursing assessment begins with a thorough review of the mother's history, including the family, past medical, psychosocial, previous obstetrical, and present prenatal history. Histories are reviewed to identify potential risk factors that alert the health care team to the possibility of a disorder in the fetus. As soon as the infant is delivered, the neonatal team must perform a physical assessment of the infant and its adaptation to extrauterine life. Initially, care is directed toward stabilization of the newborn and transport to the neonatal intensive care unit (NICU). Once the neonate with a disorder is stabilized in the NICU, attention is turned toward assessing the needs of the parents and family. Certain variables that may influence a family's ability to cope with the birth of a infant with a congenital or acquired disorder include age of the parents, culture, religion, and the support systems available to them. The nurse formulating the plan of care should assess the effect of these variables on the family and use that knowledge when providing information and communicating.

Nursing Diagnosis
Newborn

Care is individualized based on the disorder, the threat to survival, and family structure and coping abilities, but several general aspects of nursing care are common to most cases. Initially, nursing care is directed toward the stabilization and maintenance of life support. At this time, potential nursing diagnoses are:

Ineffective thermoregulation related to stress of condition and or birth defect

Ineffective breathing pattern related to oral pharyngeal secretions and/or structural anomalies

Decreased cardiac output related to decreased circulating oxygen secondary to a congenital cardiovascular defect

Should the infant survive the initial neonatal period, surgical correction of the birth defect is scheduled as soon as the infant's condition is stabilized. Postoperatively, potential nursing diagnoses are:

Risk for infection related to the immature immune system, lack of normal flora, environmental hazards, and open wounds

Impaired skin integrity related to structural anomalies and immobility

Imbalanced nutrition: less than body requirements, related to NPO status that is required by the structural anomaly

Pain related to procedures and treatments

Parents and Family

Grieving related to realization of present or future loss for family and or child and birth of a newborn with a defect

Ineffective coping (depression) related to perceived parental role failure and loss of a "perfect infant"

Deficient knowledge related to cause, management, and care of a newborn with a birth defect

Anxiety related to unpredictable outcomes or prognosis of impaired infant

Impaired parenting related to inadequate bonding, secondary to parent-child separation or failure to accept impaired child

Outcome Identification
Newborn

Sample targeted outcomes for the infant born with an anomaly might include:

Maintaining a core body temperature of 97.7°F to 99.5°F (36.5°C to 37.5°C)

Maintaining adequate gas exchange to support life

Demonstrating signs of adequate circulating oxygen

Exhibiting no signs of infection

Maintaining and/or demonstrating no further breakdown in skin integrity

Receiving adequate nutrients to support growth

Remaining free of, or displaying less frequent signs of, episodic pain.

Parents and Family

Anticipated outcomes of nursing care for the family might include that parents will:

Verbalize their feelings and concerns regarding their newborn's medical problems, prognosis, and outcome

Demonstrate an understanding of their infant's needs while participating in care

Show the beginnings of attachment and the development of a parent-infant bond

Planning
Newborn

After delivery, the infant born with a congenital or acquired anomaly is cared for in an NICU. There the infant is placed under a radiant heater, connected to a cardiac monitor, and oxygen is administered to maintain respiratory function. Care is directed towards stabilization and preparation for surgery if indicated.

Parents and Family

In addition to meeting the infant's needs, the nurse must also recognize and deal with the educational, emotional, and psychosocial needs of the parents and family. The nurse must function as educator, support person, and facilitator to the parents and family during all aspects of care for the infant born with a defect or disorder. The parents' feelings and reactions are carefully assessed, as is their ability to absorb and understand information regarding their infant's condition. Families need constant information, guidance, and support from the nursing staff to make decisions regarding the course of action to be taken.

Nursing Interventions

Preoperative interventions for the infant include temperature regulation, maintenance of respiratory and cardiovascular function, and management of fluid and electrolyte balance. Depending on the type of defect present, other potential nursing interventions may include the management of open lesions and gastric decompression with the insertion of an oral gastric tube.

Postoperatively, the infant returns to the NICU and must be continuously monitored and frequently assessed for changes in condition or the development of complications. Vital functions are maintained with oxygen or mechanical ventilation and monitored with a pulse oximeter and measurement of arterial blood gas levels. Other nursing interventions include maintaining a neutral thermal environment, administration of intravenous fluids and strict measurement of intake and output, daily weight, hourly vital signs, and blood glucose monitoring. The nurse also provides care of the surgical site, administers antibiotics, and provides pain relief for the promotion of comfort.

It is crucial that the nursing staff encourage and facilitate parent-infant bonding by encouraging parental involvement in the care of the infant. Touching, talking to, and holding the infant during visitation should be encouraged by the nurse.

Another important aspect of nursing care is the referral to appropriate community and national agencies for financial and psychological support. Nurses should familiarize themselves with available community services that provide support, assistance, and education to families with special needs or problems.

Evaluation
Newborn

The effectiveness of nursing interventions is determined by continuous assessment of the infant's condition and the evaluation of care. The following guidelines provide the basis by which to evaluate care and measure the degree of accomplishment of the expected outcomes.

Assess and monitor vital signs including body temperature hourly. Measure blood glucose levels at frequent intervals.

Case Study/Care Plan

INFANT OF A MOTHER WITH GESTATIONAL DIABETES

Rudy is a 4200 g (9 lb, 4 oz) male infant born via cesarean section at 38 weeks' gestation. His mother is a 27-year-old gravida 1, para 0, in whom gestational diabetes was detected at 28 weeks' gestation. His Apgar scores were: 7 at 1 minute (1 point off each for color, tone, and irritability); and 8 at 5 minutes (1 point off each for color and tone). Initial physical examination reveals the following: large for gestational age; blood glucose level, 38 mg/dL; heart rate, 156; respirations, 64/min with nasal flaring; gestational age, 37 weeks by Dubowitz scale; and apparent congenital anomalies or birth trauma, none.

Assessment

- 4200 g male
- IDM, LGA
- Apgar 7, 8
- HR 156, R 64

Nursing Diagnosis

Risk for injury related to hyperinsulinemia, secondary to gestational diabetes as evidenced by hypoglycemia.

Expected Outcome   Infant will maintain blood glucose levels that are within normal limits.

Planning   Discuss preferred feeding methods with parents.

Nursing Interventions	Rationales
1. Monitor glucose levels: at birth, on admission to the nursery, every 2 hours for the first 8 hours, and then every 4 hours for 24 hours. If glucose levels are abnormal, the testing should be repeated every 30 to 60 minutes until the infant has been stabilized	1. Hypoglycemia may be present without any observable signs.
2. Observe for signs of hypoglycemia (i.e., jitteriness and tremors, lethargy, apnea, cyanosis, tachypnea, and high-pitched cry).	2. These signs may indicate hypoglycemia, which generally develops 1 to 3 hours after birth.
3. Feed newborn early by providing glucose, breast milk, or formula.	3. Prevents or treats hypoglycemia that may develop 1 to 2 hours after birth.
4. Provide a neutral thermal environment.	4. Avoids cold stress, which increases metabolism, thereby causing rapid consumption of glucose.

Evaluation   Blood glucose levels are stabilized and remain above 40 mg/dL. No signs of hypoglycemia are evident. Axillary temperature remains between 97.6°F and 98°F (36.4°C and 36.7°C).

Nursing Diagnosis

Impaired gas exchange related to immature pulmonary system, secondary to maternal gestational diabetes.

Expected Outcome   Infant will demonstrate a normal respiratory status as evidenced by: a normal respiratory rate, rhythm, and depth; normal clear breath sounds; and arterial blood gas levels within the normal range.

Planning   Explain assessments and care to parents so that they will know what to expect.

(continued)

Nursing Interventions

1. Observe for signs of respiratory distress (i.e., nasal flaring, grunting, retractions, apnea, cyanosis).

2. Assess respiratory rate and effort and suction nasopharynx as needed.
3. Position infant on side with a rolled towel to the back.
4. Auscultate breath sounds every 3 to 4 hours as needed, assess infant for cyanosis, noting its relationship to activity.
5. Provide a neutral thermal environment.

Rationales

1. IDMs are at greater risk of developing respiratory distress because fetal hyperinsulinemia adversely affects fetal lung maturity.
2. Maintaining a clear airway will facilitate respiratory efforts.
3. Facilitates drainage of mucus.
4. Breath sounds and effectiveness of perfusion will indicate potential respiratory distress.

5. Prevents cold stress, which can increase the consumption of oxygen, leading to respiratory distress.

Evaluation   Respiratory rates are within normal limits (30 to 60 breaths per minute). No signs of respiratory distress are evident.

Nursing Diagnosis

Risk for injury related to hypocalcemia, secondary to maternal gestational diabetes.

Expected Outcome   Infant will maintain a calcium level between 7 mg/dL and 11 mg/dL.

Planning   Help parents understand the relationship between maternal gestational diabetes and the newborn's condition and required care.

Nursing Interventions

1. Monitor serum calcium levels.

2. Observe for signs of hypocalcemia (i.e., muscle twitching and jitteriness, irritability, seizures, and vomiting).
3. Administer calcium supplements as ordered by physician.

Rationales

1. Approximately 10% to 20% of IDMs experience hypocalcemia.
2. Hypocalcemia, generally occurs between 24 and 36 hours after birth.

3. Treats or prevents hypocalcemia.

Evaluation   No signs of hypocalcemia are evident and serum calcium levels remain above 7 mg/dL.

Assess respiratory function at frequent intervals: respiratory rate, breath sounds, skin color, and signs and symptoms of respiratory distress (nasal flaring, grunting, retractions).

Continuous pulse oximetry and frequent blood sampling for arterial blood gas (ABG) values provides valuable information about the oxygenation and ventilation status in the newborn.

Assess cardiovascular function and perfusion at frequent intervals: heart rate, blood pressure, rhythm, presence of murmur, capillary refill, skin color, and peripheral pulses.

Observe for signs and symptoms of infection.

Assess for signs of skin breakdown.

Strictly monitor infant's intake and output of fluids, maintain patency of infant's peripheral lines, and take body weight daily.

Observe infant's response to pain and pain relief interventions.

Parents and Family

Document all phone calls from parents and family received in the unit regarding infant's condition and progress.

Observe and document all visits from parents and family to the NICU.

Observe and document parent-infant interactions (i.e., talking to, holding, touching).

Document all parent teaching done (including CPR training).

Assess level of understanding of teaching done (i.e., return demonstration, question-and-answer).

Web Activities

- Search the Internet under some of the disorders discussed in this chapter, such as spina bifida. Are there support groups for families experiencing these conditions? What type of information is available? Do they also direct information to health care professionals?

- Search the Internet for government statistics on survival rates and quality-of-life issues for infants with the anomalies discussed in this chapter.

Key Concepts

- Genetic disorders are inherited defects passed down through generations; acquired disorders result from environmental factors.

- The most common anomalies affecting the CNS occur during the first 3 to 4 weeks' gestation, and many are detectable through prenatal diagnosis.

- Respiratory system anomalies are often life-threatening and require immediate intervention in the delivery room.

- There are more than 100 types of congenital heart defects, many with no known cause.

- Families need explicit instructions in feeding and caring for a newborn with a gastrointestinal anomaly, because special equipment, formulas, or techniques may be required.

- Many musculoskeletal anomalies, once detected, can be aggressively treated and have good prognoses.

- Birth injuries or trauma are often not evident at birth but are detected in the first few hours or days following delivery.

- Macrosomatia, or fetal weight above the 90th percentile, is a common characteristic of infants born to mothers with diabetes.

- Jaundice, or an elevated serum bilirubin level, occurs in more than half of all full-term newborns during the first week of life.

- Neonatal infections can have many causes and many characteristic complications, including respiratory distress, shock, acidosis, DIC, meningitis, and death.

Review Questions and Activities

Match the terms in Column I with a definition or statement from Column II.

Column I

_____ congenital disorder

_____ spina bifida

_____ meningocele

_____ myelomeningocele

_____ gastroschisis

_____ intracranial hemorrhage

_____ subdural hemorrhage

_____ phototherapy

Column II

a. Collection of blood within the cranium

b. Collection of blood in the subdural space of the brain

c. Results from genetic or prenatal environmental factors, or both

d. Contains meninges and CSF

e. Results from failure of the spinal cord to close

f. Exposure to an ultraviolet light

g. Abdominal wall defect to the right of the umbilicus, through which the abdominal organs herniate

h. Contains meninges, CSF, and neural tissue

Identify the following statements as true or false:

1. Hypocalcemia is defined as a calcium level of more than 7 mg/dL.
2. Hypoglycemia is defined as a blood glucose level of less than 60 mg/dL.
3. Physiologic jaundice generally occurs during the first 24 hours after birth.
4. Ortolani's maneuver and Barlow's test are useful in detecting clubfoot.
5. Hypospadias is a congenital anomaly in which the urethral meatus is located on the ventral surface of the glans penis.
6. Prenatal diagnosis of congenital diaphragmatic hernia can be made by antenatal ultrasound examination as early as 26 weeks' gestation.
7. Myelomeningocele is the most common form of spina bifida cystica.
8. Clinical manifestations of increased ICP include: widening sutures; bulging anterior fontanelle, high-pitched shrill cry, and the "setting sun" sign.

Study questions:

1. Differentiate physiologic from pathologic jaundice.
2. Provide four planning and implementation nursing actions for the infant at risk for injury related to hyperinsulinemia.
3. List five signs of respiratory distress in the newborn.
4. List seven signs of hypoglycemia in a newborn.
5. Describe the nursing care for an infant who is receiving phototherapy.

References

Angel, C. A. (1996). Urogenital abnormalities. *Rudolph's Pediatrics.* 20th ed. Stamford, CT: Appleton & Lange.

Barron, W. H., Linoheimer, M. D., & Davison, J. M. (2000). Medical disorders during pregnancy. 3rd ed. St. Louis: Mosby.

Bennett, J. T. (1998). Dysplasia of the hip. In Finberg, *Saunders' manual of pediatric practice.* Philadelphia: WB Saunders.

Blackburn, S. (1995). Hyperbilirubinemia and neonatal jaundice. *Neonatal Network,* 14: 7.

Blanchette, V., Doyle J., Schmidt, B., & Zipursky, A. (1994). Hematology. In Avery G, (Ed.). *Neonatology: Pathophysiology and management of the newborn.* Philadelphia: Lippincott.

Cooperman, D., & Thompson, G. H.. (1997). Neonatal orthopedics. In Fanaroff, A., & Martin, R. *Neonatal-perinatal medicine: Diseases of the fetus and newborn,* 6th ed. St Louis: Mosby.

Coniglio, J., Manzione, J., & Hengerer, A. (1988). Anatomic findings and management of choanal atresia and the CHARGE association. *Ann Oto Rhino Laryngol,* 97: 448.

Coustan, D. (1997). Diabetes in pregnancy. In Fanaroff A. & Martin R. *Neonatal-perinatal medicine: Diseases of the fetus and newborn.* 6th ed. St Louis: Mosby.

Eng, G. D. (1994). Neuromuscular Disease. In Avery G. (Ed.). *Neonatology: Pathophysiology and management of the newborn.* Philadelphia: Lippincott.

Ensher, G., & Clark, . (1994). *Newborns at risk: Medical care and psychoeducational intervention,* 2nd ed. Maryland: Aspen.

Fanaroff, A., & Martin, . (1997). Neonatal-perinatal medicine: Diseases of the fetus and newborn. 6th ed. St. Louis: Mosby.

Fletcher, M. (1994). Physical assessment and classification. In Avery G., (Eds.) *Neonatology: Pathophysiology and management of the newborn,* Philadelphia: Lippincott.

Golden, P. (1998). Symptoms of neurologic disorders. In Finberg, . *Saunders' manual of pediatric practice.* Philadelphia: WB Saunders.

Griffin, P. (1994). Orthopedics. In Avery, G., (Ed.) *Neonatology: Pathophysiology and management of the newborn.* Philadelphia: Lippincott.

Guzzetta, P., Anderson, K., Eichelberger, M., Newman, K., Rouse, T., Schnitzer, J., Boyajian, M., & Tomaski, S. (1994). General surgery. In Avery, G., (Ed.) *Neonatology: Pathophysiology and management of the newborn.* Philadelphia: Lippincott.

Hill, A., & Volpe, J. (1994). Neurologic disorders. In Avery, G., (Ed.) *Neonatology: Pathophysiology and management of the newborn.* Philadelphia: Lippincott.

Hoffman, J. (1995). Incidence of congenital heart disease: I. Postnatal incidence. *Pediatrics Cardiol* 6 (4): 103.

Holland, R., Price, F. N., & Bensaro, D. D. (1998). Neonatal surgery. In Merenstein, G., & Gardner, S. *Handbook of neonatal intensive care,* 4th ed. St. Louis: Mosby.

Kaplan, G. (1994). Structural abnormalities of the genitourinary system. In Avery, G., (Eds.) *Neonatology: Pathophysiology and management of the newborn.* Philadelphia: Lippincott.

Kalhan, ., & Saker, . (1997). Metabolic and endocrine disorders. In Fanaroff, A., & Martin, R. *Neonatal-perinatal medicine: Diseases of the fetus and newborn,* 6th ed. St. Louis: Mosby.

Kenner, C., Amlung, S., Flandermeyer, A. (1998). *Protocols in neonatal nursing,* Philadelphia: WB Saunders.

Kenner, C., Lott, J. W., Flandermeyer, A. A. (1998). *Comprehensive neonatal nursing: A physiologic perspective,* 2nd ed. Philadelphia: WB Saunders.

Mangurten, H. (1997). Birth injuries. In Fanaroff, A., & Martin, R. *Neonatal-perinatal medicine: Diseases of the fetus and newborn,* 6th ed. St Louis: Mosby.

Merenstein, G., Adams, K., & Weisman, L. (1998). Infection in the neonate. In Merenstein, G., & Gardner, S. *Handbook of neonatal intensive care.* St. Louis: Mosby.

Milhorat, T., & Miller, J. (1994). Neurosurgery. In Avery, G., (Ed.) *Neonatology: Pathophysiology and management of the newborn.* Philadelphia: Lippincott.

Miller, M. J., Fanaroff, A. A., & Martin, R. J. (1997). Respiratory disorders in preterm and term infants. In Fanaroff, A., & Martin R. *Neonatal-perinatal medicine: Diseases of the fetus and newborn.* 6th ed. St Louis: Mosby.

Moe, P., & Paige, P. (1998). Neurologic disorders. In Merenstein, G., & Gardner, S. *Handbook of neonatal intensive care.* St Louis: Mosby.

Moshang, T., & Thornton, P. (1994). Endocrine disorders. In Avery, G., (Eds.) *Neonatology: Pathophysiology and management of the newborn.* Philadelphia: Lippincott.

Ogata, E. (1994). Carbohydrate homeostasis. In Avery, G., (Ed.) *Neonatology: Pathophysiology and management of the newborn.* Philadelphia: Lippincott.

Paidas, M., & Cohen, A. (1994). Disorders of the central nervous system. *Seminars in Perinatology,* 18 (4), 226–282.

Quirk, J. G. Jr., Fortney, J., Collins, H. B. 2nd, West, J., Hassad, S. J., Wagner, C. (1996). Outcomes of newborn with gastroschisis: The effects of mode of delivery, site of delivery, and interval from birth to surgery. *American Journal of Obstetrics and Gynecology,* 174 (4), 1134–1140.

Rayburn, W. F., Stanley, J. R., Garrett, M. E. (1996). Periconceptual folate intake and neural tube defects. *J Am Coll Nutr,* 15 (2): 121.

Sills, I., & Rapaport, R. New-onset IDDM presenting with diabetic ketoacidosis in a pregnant adolescent. *Diabetes Care,* 17 (8), 904–905.

Shiminski-Maher, T., & Disabato, J. (1994). Current trends in the diagnosis and management of hydrocephalus in children. *J Pediat Nurse,* 9 (2): 74.

Wardinsky, T. (1994). Visual clues to diagnosis of birth defects and genetic disease. *Journal of Pediatric Health Care,* 8 (63).

Wong, D., & Perry, S. *Maternal child nursing care.* St Louis: Mosby.

Suggested Readings

American Academy of Pediatrics, American College of Obstetricians and Gynecologists. (1992). *Guidelines for perinatal care,* 3rd ed. Chicago: American Academy of Pediatrics.

Avery, G, (Ed.) (1994). *Neonatology: Pathophysiology and management of the newborn.* Philadelphia: Lippincott.

Beachy, P., & Deacon, J. (1992). *Core curriculum for neonatal intensive care nursing.* Philadelphia: WB Saunders.

Bekrman, R. E. (1992). *Nelson textbook of pediatrics,* 14th ed. Philadelphia: WB Saunders.

Gray, M. L. (1992). *Genitourinary disorders.* St Louis: Mosby.

Holmes, J. B. (1992). Prevention of neural tube defects. *Journal of Pediatrics,* 12 (6): 918–919.

Howell, K., & Kwon, I. (1998). Understanding gastroschisis: An abdominal wall defect. *Neonatal Network,* 17 (8).

Mattson, S., & Smith, J. (Ed.) (1992). *NAACOG core curriculum for maternal-newborn nursing.* Philadelphia: WB Saunders.

McClain, B., & Anand, K. (1996). Neonatal pain management. In Deshpande, J., & Tobias, J., (Eds.) *The pediatric pain handbook.* St Louis: Mosby.

Milas, M., Carlson, J., & Fink, S. (1996). Sources of support reported by mothers and fathers of infants hospitalized in an NICU. *Neonatal Network,* 15 (3): 45.

Richard M. (1991). Feeding the newborn with cleft lip and/or palate: The enlargement, stimulate, swallow, rest (ESSR) method. *Journal of Pediatric Nursing,* 6 (5): 317–321.

Shoppe, K. (1992). Developmental dysplasia of the hip, *Orthopedic Nursing,* 11 (5): 30–36.

Resources

Association of Women's Health, Obstetric, and Neonatal Nurses, www.awhonn.org

National Association of Neonatal Nurses, www.nann.org
Neonatal Network, www.neonatalnetwork.com

CHAPTER 36

Developmental Care of the Infant at Risk

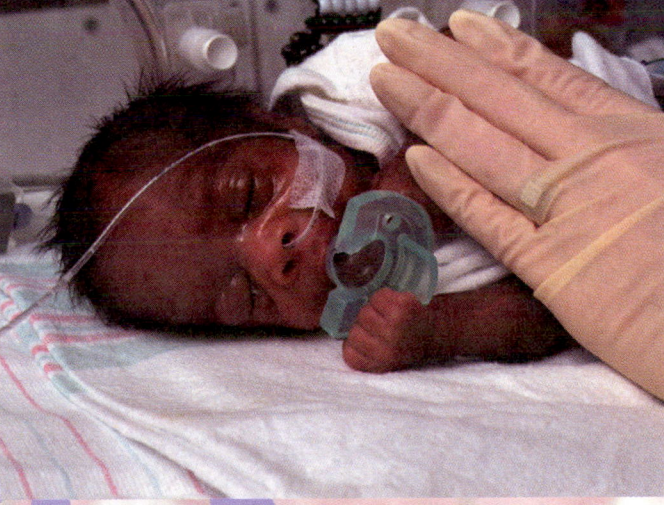

nderstanding the needs of high-risk neonates and their families is the first ingredient to providing effective and sensitive nursing care. Ask yourself the following:

- *How can I know if a baby is in distress if it cannot cry?*

- *Do I think all babies respond in the same ways, or are they as individual as are adults?*

- *Have I ever been in a neonatal intensive care unit (NICU)? How did it make me feel?*

- *How important do I think it is for parents to be fully involved in the care of their hospitalized infant?*

- *The NICU is a very high technology environment. How does that make me feel?*

- *Have I ever been in the presence of a critically ill infant? How did I feel?*

- *What do I know or believe about an infant's experience of suffering and pain?*

- *What are my ethical questions about aggressive technologic support of the critically ill infant?*

Key Terms

Developmental care   Macro-environment   Micro-environment   Standards of care
Facilitated tucking

Competencies

Upon completion of this chapter, the reader should be able to:

1. Discuss the history and philosophy of developmental care.
2. Explain the relationship of infant behaviors to the theories underlying developmental care.
3. Identify the elements of developmental care.
4. Apply the principles of developmental care to diverse clinical situations.
5. Use current standards of practice in the implementation of developmental care.
6. Discuss the research basis for developmental care.
7. Discuss the role of the family in the developmental care of the high-risk infant.

he premature birth of an infant continues to be a major challenge to the health care delivery system and families affected by this experience. The preterm birth rate in the United States increased in 1998 to 11.4% overall, with the rate for African Americans at 17.6% (Ventura et al., 2000). Despite major scientific breakthroughs in prenatal care and the technologically advanced care of the prematurely born infant, the U.S. infant mortality rates remain high compared with other developed countries (7.2 infant deaths per 1,000 births) and are disproportionately high for the African American population (14.3 infant deaths per 1,000 births) (Ventura et al., 2000). Prematurity or low birth weight is the second highest cause of infant mortality overall and the leading cause of infant death in the African American population (Ventura et al., 2000). In addition, as major advances in the medical care of these infants have resulted in the increasing survival of infants having very low and extremely low birth weights, the incidence of complications or morbidities secondary to premature birth has increased. Researchers and clinicians alike have focused attention on the environment of the intensive care nursery and caregiving practices surrounding the hospitalization period in an effort to provide optimal support for the healthy development of these infants. This focus has led to the development of new approaches to the care of the preterm infant aimed at improving developmental outcomes adapted to the individual infant, and emphasizing the inclusion of the family as a whole in their infant's care.

The term **developmental care** is used broadly to describe any infant care protocol designed to promote opti-

mal physical, cognitive, and emotional development in the first weeks or months of life. Whereas the protocols described as developmental care differ from one setting to another, they generally address issues of environmental light, sound, and temperature levels; infant position, containment, and handling strategies; nonnutritive sucking; feeding; and pain management. This chapter includes discussions of each of the individual developmental care strategies in common use, the effectiveness of a comprehensive developmental approach to infant care, and the role of families in the care of the infant at risk.

HISTORICAL DEVELOPMENT

Historically, the approach to the care of the infant at risk has evolved through three stages (Figure 36-1).

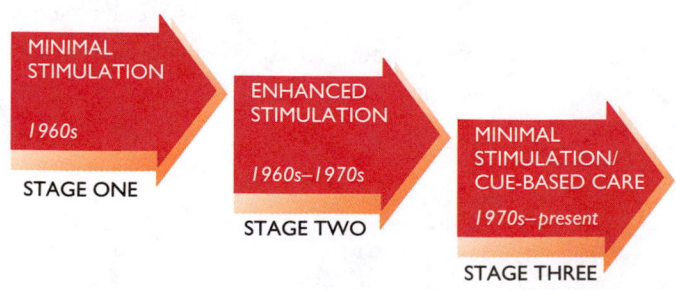

Figure 36-1 Historical overview of developmental care.

Stage 1

Before the early 1960s the standard of care for these infants was to maintain the infant in strict isolation, with minimal handling and little emphasis on the kind or amount of stimulation the infant received. The major concerns in infant care were protection of the infant, prevention of infection, and maintenance of a warm environment. Parents typically had little access to their infants for prolonged periods of time, and infants received little handling or interaction other than that necessary to provide care.

Stage 2

In the 1960s two concerns emerged related to the effects of these infant care practices. First, nurses and other caregivers began to be concerned about the effects of the long-term separation of the parent and infant on the baby's growth and development and on the development of the parent-infant relationship. Second, caregivers began to be concerned about the lack of sensory stimulation the hospital environment provided for the developing infant. This second concern was based on the observation that the sterile hospital environment did not provide the same richness of visual stimulation (pictures, toys, color), sound (music, mother's voice), touch (cuddling, caressing), or movement (rocking, walking with infant) that the home environment could offer. As a result, caregivers during this period began to focus on two things: increasing the involvement of parents by increasing visiting hours and encouraging them to participate in care, and enriching the infant's environment by placing pictures in the incubators, playing music for the baby, taping the parents' voices to play for the baby, and experimenting with the effects of touch through interventions such as infant massage. Research in this period emphasized issues of parent-infant attachment, the effects of early and prolonged separation on the development of the attachment relationship, and the effects of added stimulation on infant growth and development (Klaus & Kennell, 1982; Brazelton & Cramer, 1990).

Stage 3

The concept of the neonatal intensive care unit (NICU) began to evolve in the early 1970s, with the introduction of the continuous positive airway pressure (CPAP) technique (Gregory et al., 1971). The use of CPAP had the potential to dramatically increase the survival of the very premature infant but required specialized 24-hour care. This requirement provided the impetus for the development of the NICU. By the late 1970s, as CPAP and other life-saving technologies in hospital nurseries had begun to improve the survival rates of the very premature infant

(those weighing less than 1,500 g or born earlier than 32 weeks postconceptional age), the population of the intensive care nursery became increasingly younger and smaller. Caregivers of these vulnerable infants began to question how the intensive care environment affected the infants in their charge. They became aware that, rather than providing too little stimulation, the intensive care nursery was an environment of excessive and often inappropriate stimulation. For these babies, the high-technology intensive care nursery was characterized as an environment of continuous bright lights; loud, unexpected, and random sounds; and noxious, often painful, stimuli. The effort to provide developmentally appropriate care now focused on the need to protect the youngest and most vulnerable infants from excessive and often overwhelming environmental stimulation and to support their efforts to cope with those stimuli. The concept of individualized developmental care, as expressed in today's NICUs, has evolved from these concerns.

THEORETICAL FRAMEWORK FOR DEVELOPMENTAL CARE

One of the earliest proponents of modifying and individualizing the care of the premature infant to support optimal development was Heidelise Als. Als proposed a framework, or way of looking at infant development, which she identified as the synactive theory of neurobehavioral development (Als, 1986). This theory is based on four principles. First, infant development occurs in a way that is designed to best ensure the survival of the infant in the specific environment in which it exists. For example, healthy infants are born with a strong sucking reflex and need to suck, which supports their survival as a mechanism through which they are able to take in nutrition. Premature infants may not yet have developed a strong sucking reflex because the uterine environment in which they are developing does not require a sucking mechanism for the fetus to receive nutrients. In both cases the development of the fetus-infant is designed to support optimal functioning in the appropriate environment.

The second principle is that infants develop in continuous interaction with the environment around them. Before birth the fetus develops in interaction with the surrounding uterine environment. After birth, the infant continues to develop in interaction with the extrauterine environment. Therefore, prematurely born infants in hospital nurseries are developing in interaction with environments very different from the uterine environment in which they normally would be found.

The third developmental principle proposes that development occurs from global to discrete or from simple to complex. For example, as the infant's limbs develop, the arms develop as buds emerging from the body (global or simple development). As these arm buds grow they begin to differentiate into hands at the distal end, and finally, the fingers develop (discrete or complex development).

The fourth principle underlying Als' theory postulates that the developing organism (infant) seeks to maintain physiologic stability or balance in the presence of two powerful competing physiologic impulses, to explore or move out and to withdraw or avoid. Older infants exhibit these impulses, as they will eagerly explore their environment until a stranger comes too close, then will withdraw and move closer to their caregivers. Very immature prematurely born infants also actively respond to their external environment. Widening the eyes, raising the eyebrows, and softening the face are behaviors that may indicate interest and readiness to respond in the premature infant. If the stimuli become too powerful, the infant may withdraw by averting or closing the eyes or turning away from the stimuli. A prematurely born infant who is overwhelmed by environmental stimuli may show more extreme aversive reactions such as hiccoughing, spitting up, hyperextending the extremities, or demonstrating a brief period of apnea or bradycardia. Thus, Als postulates that infants develop in adaptation to their environment and in interaction with that environment. This development proceeds from global or undifferentiated states to discrete or differentiated states. As development occurs, the organism strives to maintain stability while both reaching out to explore and interact with the environment, and withdrawing or avoiding excessive stimuli.

INDIVIDUALIZED DEVELOPMENTAL CARE

Individualized Developmental Care refers to the modification of the nursery environment and caregiving practices to support the infant's optimal development. This approach to care includes the reduction of excessive environmental stimuli by lowering light and sound levels in the NICU; organizing caregiving activities to provide periods of rest and recovery for the infant; positioning the infant in a flexed, contained position; modifying caregiving practices based on an assessment of what the individual infant finds least distressing; and supporting the infant's efforts to provide self-comfort and maintain physiologic stability and organization.

In her theory, Als (1986) also proposes that infant neurobehavioral development occurs within five interrelated and interdependent subsystems and that through assessment of these subsystems the developmental status of the infant can be evaluated. These five subsystems are the autonomic, motor, state, attentional-interactive, and self-regulatory subsystems. The development of each of these subsystems includes infant behaviors that provide insight into the development of that subsystem. The first subsystem to develop is the autonomic subsystem. The stability and integration of the autonomic system can be assessed through respiratory patterns, heart rate responsiveness, skin color, and visceral responses (Als, 1986). The motor subsystem includes muscle tone, posture, and patterns of movement. The state subsystem refers to the infant's level of consciousness, ranging from deep sleep to awake and agitated. The attentional-interactive subsystem depends on the infant's ability to maintain a robust alert state and refers to the infant's readiness for social interaction. Finally, the self-regulatory subsystem refers to the infant's ability to maintain behavioral stability in the other subsystems or to initiate efforts to regain stability if it has been lost.

STANDARDS OF CARE

The term **standards of care** refers to formal guidelines for the care of clients developed by professional organizations. These guidelines describe or recommend the content, scope, and sequence of care activities that are considered appropriate, necessary, and sufficient for the care of a particular client population. Standards of care also may focus on a specific issue such as emergency transport of the high-risk infant. In general, formal standards of care should be viewed as a baseline or minimum criteria for directing care with the recognition that practice standards will change rapidly in some cases as new knowledge is generated. The American Nurses Association (ANA) has established general guidelines for clinical practice based on the nursing process (American Nurses Association, 1998). These guidelines direct practice in every area of nursing, focusing on the nursing process, nursing diagnosis, outcomes identification, nursing intervention, evaluation, and revision. In addition, in specialized areas of nursing practice, such as neonatal nursing, specialized professional groups may provide more specific practice guidelines.

In the 1990s, several professional groups began to focus on the need for formal guidelines to direct the implementation of developmental care. In 1999, the National Association of Neonatal Nurses (NANN) developed guidelines for the prevention, recognition, and management of neonatal pain. These guidelines reflected growing concern regarding the lack of appropriate pain management in the neonate, and represent an early and important step forward in changing practice in this area. In 2000, nursing care guidelines related to infant and family-centered developmental care also were developed by NANN. These guidelines include suggestions for interventions to facilitate the adaptation of the infant and family; modifications of the physical surroundings, including light and noise; and recommendations for handling the infant. In addition, the Physical and Developmental Environment of the High-Risk Infant Project (a national interdisciplinary project begun in 1993 and directed by Stanley Graven of the University of South Florida) began developing recommendations related to NICU light and sound levels and infant sleep, touch, and feeding practices for the very premature or high-risk infant. As these guidelines are developed, they are presented to major professional groups involved in the care of the high-risk infant for review and endorsement. When completed, these guidelines will represent the most definitive standards available for the developmental care of high-risk infants. In addition, Dr. Graven's group sponsors an annual conference for clinicians and researchers presenting the work of the study groups and related research.

In addition to guidelines specific to caregiving activities, professional organizations have developed standards of care for nursery design that have implications for developmental care activities. Guidelines related to the structural design of NICUs have been developed by the 4th Consensus Committee to Establish Recommended Standards for Newborn ICU Design (1999) developed under the auspices of the Physical and Developmental Environment of the High-Risk Infant Project, these guidelines have made recommendations specifically related to sound and light management in the NICU and have direct implications for the implementation of developmental care.

The specific recommendations from all of these guidelines are included in this chapter with the discussion of specific aspects of developmental care. It is important for the nurse beginning practice in the neonatal area to be aware of these guidelines and their contents and for all nurses in the neonatal area to ensure that their own practice is congruent with the best professional standard available.

ELEMENTS OF DEVELOPMENTAL CARE

The elements considered part of developmental care can and do vary somewhat among clinical sites. In general, however, these elements can be divided into those related to the total nursery environment, such as light and sound (macro-environment), and those related to the individual infant's environment or care experiences, such as positioning and handling (micro-environment). Each of the components discussed in this chapter has been studied individually and found to have important effects on infants.

In addition, the effectiveness of these components combined into comprehensive developmental care protocols will be discussed.

Macro-environment Components

The **macro-environment** of the high-risk infant is considered to be all of those elements that define the caregiving milieu, that is, the conditions that define the surrounding space in which caregiving occurs. This macro-environment has been found to have a major impact on the development of prematurely born and high-risk infants. The macro-environment is one aspect of the infant's neonatal experience in which nursing has a major responsibility. In this chapter the macro-environmental components to be discussed include the levels and patterns of NICU light and sound and temperature control.

Light

One element common to many developmental care protocols is the control of light levels in the infant's environment. Some protocols prescribe consistently dim lights throughout the 24-hour day, whereas others recommend regularly scheduled times when the lights are dimmed. The recommendation to dim environmental lighting in the NICU as part of a developmental care protocol is based on research related to the effects of light on the infant. NICU light levels and lighting patterns (i.e., same light level, random changes in light levels, and structured patterns of light-dark cycles over the 24 hour period) have been studied in terms of the effects of light levels on the incidence of retinopathy of prematurity (ROP); light patterns on the development of infant biologic rhythms; and on infant growth, behavior, and physiologic responses.

Nursery Light Levels and Patterns

Early articles related to light in the NICU focused on descriptions of the levels of lighting commonly found in these areas, sources of light, and patterns of lighting over time. The first studies describing lighting levels typically found in the NICU were published in the mid-1980s through 1990. Surveys of illumination levels in the NICUs of that time reported light levels of approximately 240 to 900 lux (approximately 24 to 90 ft-c) in the United Kingdom and illumination levels of 285 to 1485 lux (28 to 148 ft-c) in the United States (Robinson, Moseley, & Fielder, 1990; Landry, Scheidt, & Hammond, 1985; Glass et al., 1985). Peak light exposure for the infant was found to be associated with supplementary light sources such as phototherapy lamps (300 to 400 ft-c), treatment lamps (200 to 300 ft-c), and most dramatically, extensive direct window exposure supplementing artificial lighting (levels of up to

Critical Thinking

Light Patterns

The effects of light on human health have been the subject of much research. When you are thinking about the effects of lighting levels and patterns in the NICU, ask yourself how light affects you. Which kind of lighting is restful or quieting? When you are ill or tired, which kind of lighting do you prefer? What do you know about the effects of continuous lighting on adults? How do you think light levels affect sound levels?

1,024 ft-c have been reported) (Hamer, Dobson, & Mayer, 1984). Within hospitals, illumination levels were found to be highest in the areas of highest infant acuity and perhaps greatest infant vulnerability to negative effects of excessive illumination.

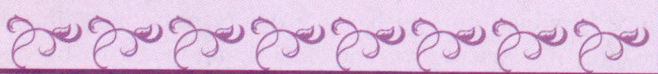

Nursing Alert

NICU DESIGN STANDARDS FOR LIGHT

Advocates for developmentally appropriate care for the hospitalized infant have long emphasized the importance of reduced light levels in the NICU; however, standard recommendations for NICU light levels have not been available. In 1999, the Consensus Committee to Establish Recommended Standards for Newborn ICU Design issued recommendations based on an analysis of existing research.

Recommendations for NICU lighting (Standards 14-16) include the following requirements: environmental light levels in the infant care areas should be adjustable from 1 to 60 footcandles; natural and artificial light sources should include a way they can be immediately darkened if necessary; artificial light sources should have visible spectrum distribution similar to daylight; and NICUs should be able to maintain environmental lighting in the 10 to 20 ft-c range, unless higher light levels are considered necessary for care delivery. (In 10 to 20 ft-c of light, the room would appear dim, all of the contents of the room would be clearly visible, and reading would be uncomfortable.)

---

*footcandle is a unit of illumination equal to 1 lumen per square foot.

In addition to documenting high levels of illumination, all of these studies indicated that the lighting levels within units tended to be consistent over time, demonstrating little structured diurnal variation (Robinson, Moseley, & Fielder, 1990; Landry, Scheidt, & Hammond, 1985). Documented temporal variability in illumination levels within units appeared to occur in a random pattern, with little or no predictability or temporal pattern. Some seasonal variability in illumination levels was noted as a function of direct window exposure (Landry, Scheidt, & Hammond, 1985).

A recent study by Lotas et al. (2001), surveyed 69 NICUs in the Southeastern United States to describe current lighting practices and assess changes in practice since the original research appeared. Nurse managers of the units were asked to describe their unit light levels as dim, moderate, or bright. A subset of NICUs in 18 surveyed hospital was then selected to be site visited for direct measurement of NICU lighting levels. For this subset, hospitals were grouped by their self-reported lighting group: low, moderate, and high lighting levels. Lighting levels obtained by direct measurement were then combined to provide a profile of lighting patterns within each of these groups. Light levels varied widely within each group, with little relationship between reported levels and measured levels. In fact, the lowest average daytime light levels were recorded in the group of hospitals self-identified as having high light levels. Overall, light levels ranged in all visited units from 25 to 68.05 ft-c throughout the 24-hour period of direct measurements. This represents a reduction in average light levels from those reported in earlier studies but demonstrates that many units still have lighting in excess of recommended levels.

Two limitations in all of these studies should be noted. The data are limited by variation in the instrumentation used in their collection and the calibration of those instruments. Many or most available light meters demonstrate a ±5% random error factor, and calibration processes usually include a ±10% random error factor. The potential cumulative error therefore is fairly high. The level of illumination for any particular infant in a nursery also may vary accord-

LUX

Lux is a metric unit of illumination equal to 1 lumen per square meter. Lumen refers to the unit of light flux emitted by a uniform source of one candela. Lux values can be converted to approximate footcandles by dividing by 10.

ing to placement of the incubator in relation to windows, overhead lighting, and other nursery equipment. The total light exposure of an infant also depends on factors such as the use of eye shields, frequency with which the fluorescent tubes are changed in both the phototherapy unit and rooms of the unit, and use of additional lighting for instrumentation and other procedures. The position of the infant's head also can influence light exposure. When the infant is in a side-lying position, the lower eye receives less light exposure than does the upper eye. The potential exists for infants lying in a supine position to be staring directly into the overhead lights. Therefore, illumination levels described for a NICU may or may not be representative of the conditions experienced by an individual infant, and comparisons between nurseries are difficult to make.

Effects of Nursery Light on the Visual System

Much of the concern about excessive light levels in the NICU environment has focused on the potential for damage to the developing visual system, most specifically regarding the incidence of ROP. ROP is a retinal neovascular disorder found commonly in prematurely born infants (Palmer et al., 1991). ROP varies in severity inversely with the gestational age of the infant, with infants over 31 weeks' gestation rarely developing the disease except in its mildest form. The condition usually heals with few or no sequelae; however, its most severe forms can lead to serious vision loss or, most extremely, complete blindness secondary to retinal detachment or severe retinal scarring. The primary factors associated with the development of ROP have been widely accepted to be the combination of retinal immaturity in the preterm infant and the high oxygen levels that may be part of the infant's treatment through the increase in oxygen free radicals in the retina (Hepner, Krause & Davis, 1949; Riley & Slater, 1969; Glass et al., 1985). However, excessive and precocious exposure of the immature retina to intense and continuous light in the NICU has been proposed as an important contributing factor. It has been hypothesized that energy from light striking the immature retina may cause a further increase in oxygen free radicals and, subsequently, an increase in retinal injury (Glass, 1988; Phelps & Watts, 1997). Some early clinical studies supported this hypothesis, reporting a significantly decreased incidence of ROP in infants who had been shielded from environmental light by dimming the room lights or shielding the incubators with thick covers (Glass et al., 1985; Ackerman, Sherwonit, & Williams, 1989). However, a meta-analysis completed in 1997 (Phelps & Watts, 1997). reviewed all randomized or quasi-randomized controlled trials that examined the effects of reduced light exposure to prematurely born infants on the incidence or severity of ROP. Only three studies qualified for this analysis (Locke & Reese, 1952; Lopes et al., 1997; Seiberth et al., 1994). The results of these three studies did not support

the hypothesis that reducing the preterm infant's exposure to environmental light would reduce the incidence of ROP. An additional six studies were reviewed that did not meet the inclusion criteria for the meta-analysis (Ackerman, Sherwonit, & Williams, 1989; Glass et al., 1985; Hepner, Krause, & Davis, 1949; Hommura et al., 1988; Locke & Reese, 1952; Repka et al., 1995). Even with the addition of these studies, no significant reduction in the incidence of ROP secondary to shielding the infant from environmental light could be documented.

Although current research does not document a relationship between nursery light levels and ROP incidence or severity, the samples in the existing studies are small and the data cannot be considered conclusive. Large controlled clinical trials are needed to definitively demonstrate the relationship of light exposure in the preterm infant and the development and severity of ROP. Other issues not well explored in the current research literature include the effects of excessive light levels or eye shielding on the subsequent development of visual processing and the relationship between gestational age and light levels optimal for infant visual development.

Nonvisual Effects of Nursery Light

In addition to concerns about the effects of excessive and precocious exposure to light on the developing visual system, caregivers also have explored the effects of light levels and patterns on other aspects of the functioning of the preterm infants. One major concern focuses on the effects of continuous lighting or random variation of lighting levels (both common NICU patterns) on the development of biologic rhythms (circadian or ultradian) in the infant. Biologic rhythms are controlled by the suprachiasmatic nucleus in the anterior hypothalamus, are thought to exist in all living beings, and serve the purpose of synchronizing and coordinating compatible physiologic functions and separating incompatible ones (Reppert, 1992; Moore-Ede, Sulzman, & Fuller, 1982). The dominant organizer of biologic rhythms in humans is the day-night cycle, with feeding patterns as additional organizers in the infant (Arendt, Minors, & Waterhouse, 1989). Physiologic functions considered to have a circadian pattern include heart and respiratory rates; temperature; sleep-wake cycles; and secretion of several hormones, including cortisol, adrenocorticotropic hormone (ACTH), and endorphins (Arendt, Minors, & Waterhouse, 1989; Moore-Ede, Sulzman, & Fuller, 1982). In addition, growth hormone, which does not exhibit a true circadian cycle, is strongly influenced by sleep-wake cycles, which are thought to have a circadian function.

In the human infant, early development of biologic rhythms occurs in the fetus and is thought to be determined predominantly by maternal biologic rhythms (Reppert, 1992). After birth, the development of circadian functions continues under the influence of the infant's environmental cues with light-dark cycles and feeding cycles. Circadian patterns in heart rate, body temperature, and sleep begin to emerge after the 3rd week of life (Hellbrugge, 1974; Tenreiro et al., 1991; Glotzbach, Edgar, & Ariagno, 1995). It is this development that may be disrupted if the preterm infant in the NICU environment receives inadequate or inappropriate environmental cues to develop normal circadian function.

A small number of studies have compared the effects of light-dark–cycled light with the effects of continuous bright lighting on the physiologic functioning of infants in the NICU (Mann et al., 1986; Blackburn & Patterson, 1991; Lotas & Medoff-Cooper, 2001). Six studies have compared infants maintained in a light-dark–cycled environment with infants maintained in continuous lighting (Mann et al., 1986; Blackburn & Patterson, 1991; Lotas & Medoff-Cooper, 2001; Miller et al., 1995; Shiroiwa, Kamiya, & Uchibori, 1986; Tenreiro et al., 1991). In four studies, the outcome variables included activity, heart rate, and respiratory rate (Blackburn & Patterson, 1991; Lotas & Medoff-Cooper, 2001; Shiroiwa, Kamiya, & Uchibori, 1986; Tenreiro et al., 1991). Blackburn and Patterson (1991) studied 18 infants cared for in continuous light compared with a light-dark environment and reported a significant reduction in heart rate and activity level, with longer periods of quiescence, although no differences in respiratory rate were noted. Lotas and Medoff-Cooper (2001) compared 18 infants assigned to either a nursery maintaining routine lighting or one maintaining light-dark cycles. These authors found a consistent decrease in heart and respiratory rates during the dark cycle in infants maintained in a light-cycled nursery; however, these findings were apparent only after infants had been in the light-cycled nursery for 3 weeks. The third study of 10 preterm infants achieved a decrease in illumination to the retina by blindfolding each infant for 10 hours in a 24-hour period. A reduction in infant movement and lower heart and respiratory rates were seen while the infants were blindfolded (Shiroiwa, Kamiya, & Uchibori, 1986). Although these findings should not be interpreted as support for the practice of routinely blindfolding infants, they do provide support for the premise that the intensity of nursery lighting may be an added stressor for infants and that reducing this stressor may contribute to increased physiologic stability.

Teneiro et al. (1991) examined the effects of continuous light initially, when infants were in the intensive care setting, followed by light-dark cycling, when infants were transferred to intermediate care areas. These authors reported increasing circadian rhythm development in temperature and heart rate once infants were placed in the light-cycled environment. It was noted, however, that all emerging biorhythms were unreliable. In addition, the timing of the light-cycled treatment coincided with concep-

tional ages when such rhythms might be expected to emerge.

Other studies focused on the effects of environmental light patterns on the development of infant sleep and activity patterns and on weight gain (Mann et al., 1986; Miller et al., 1995). Mann et al. (1986) studied the effects of light-dark cycles in the NICU on 41 healthy preterm infants. The 20 infants assigned to the light-cycled nursery were exposed to 12 hours of bright lighting and 12 hours of dim lighting. Infants in the control group were exposed to continuous bright lighting, which was the nursery routine. In the postdischarge follow-up, infants from the light-dark–cycled nursery were found to spend significantly more time sleeping (mean difference of 2 hours per day) and less time feeding (mean difference of 1 hour per day) and gained more weight (mean difference 0.5 kg) than did infants in the nursery with continuous light. Significant differences between the groups continued through the first year of life.

A recent study by Miller et al. (1995) examined 41 infants assigned to one of two intensive care rooms with either a continuous or day-night–cycled lighting pattern. Infants in the light-cycled group had greater weight gain, spent less time on assisted ventilation and under phototherapy, began oral feeding sooner, and had enhanced motor coordination as measured by the Brazelton Neonatal Behavioral Assessment Scale completed at discharge by an evaluator blind to the infant's lighting treatment. Whereas these studies use different methods, somewhat different lighting treatments, different populations of infants, and somewhat different outcomes and times for evaluation, they demonstrated similar findings in relation to significantly increased infant weight gain in the light-dark–cycled group.

These studies provide findings that are suggestive but not conclusive of the benefits of a light-cycled environment, at least for infants of 29 weeks' gestation or greater. Although these studies provide some contrast in findings, these differences are not necessarily contradictory. All report behaviors (i.e., increased alertness, sleep-wake organization, and improved physiologic stability) that may indicate an increase in infant neurobehavioral organization with reduced lighting. Some of the apparent contradictions in the findings of these studies may be related to the differences in lighting conditions used and in the timing and pattern of data collection; however, the extremely small sample size in each study makes data interpretation difficult. Changes in lighting levels also may have influenced other aspects of the environment, such as noise levels and staff activity, which were not documented. Furthermore, it should be emphasized that no studies have compared a light-dark–cycled nursery environment with a nursery environment with continuously dim lighting. These studies are further limited by lack of randomization in some and variations in light levels. Additionally, few data are available for extremely low birth weight infants.

Much research remains to be done to understand the effects of environmental light on the developing preterm infant. Although studies have shown that infant outcomes improve when light levels are reduced, at this time researchers have not documented the level of light that is most appropriate for the preterm infant, or whether the optimal light level varies for infants of different gestational ages. Definitive work on the effects of light-dark cycles compared with continuous light levels also remains to be done.

Recommendations for Practice

In the past, continuous lighting levels of 60 to 100 ft-c (approximately the light level in an office or classroom) were thought to be necessary to allow adequate evaluation of the infant's skin color and perfusion from any area of the NICU. Although, at this time there is no established standard for light levels in the NICU, within the concept of developmental care lower light levels (± 20 ft-c) are recommended. Current standards for NICU lighting recommend that light levels be adjustable over a range of 1 to 60 ft-c (Consensus Committee to Establish Recommended Standards for Nursery ICU Design, 1999). At this time no recommendation can be made for the implementation of light-dark cycles in the nursery. Specific strategies for reducing the effects of lighting on the infant in the NICU include the following:

- Avoid the use of overhead lights unless necessary. Use individual lighting at the infant's bedside for caregiving.

- Incubator covers can be used during times when the infant is at rest. Small, thin receiving-type blankets may not provide optimal light shielding for the infant. Opaque covers that cover the top and the sides of the incubator are preferable.

- Outside windows often are the source of the highest light levels in the NICU. When outside windows are present, opaque shades of some type should be available to allow modifications of light levels, and incubators should be placed away from direct sunlight.

- When overhead phototherapy lights are used, ensure that the infants in adjacent incubators are screened from any increase in light levels.

- Shield the infant's eyes when using treatment lights for procedures or caregiving. Place a screen between the treatment light and adjacent incubators to protect those infants from random light exposure.

- When the infant is placed in a supine or side-lying position with the face upward, ensure that the infant is not directly under an overhead light. Preterm infants may not have the ability to turn their heads away from the light or to adequately shield their eyes by closing them.

- Education of the family about the infant's development and caregiving needs should include explanations of the concerns about light levels and the precautions taken to protect the baby from excessive light. The nurse may help the family reflect on their own practices in relation to light levels in an infant's environment. Do they darken the room in which an infant is sleeping? Do they protect a baby's eyes from bright sunlight?

Sound

Over the past 3 decades researchers have repeatedly documented consistent sound levels of 50 to 90 dB in the NICU, with excursions to as high as 120 dB (Anagnostakis, Petmezakis, & Matsaniotis, 1980; Robertson & Philbin, 1996; Long, Lucey, & Philip, 1980; Thomas, 1989). For the purpose of comparison, 50 dB is about the sound level of light traffic and 90 dB is about that generated by light machinery (Figure 36-2). According to the Occupational Safety and Health Administration standards, 80 dB is the highest sound level that does not produce measurable damage, regardless of the duration of the sound, and 90 dB is the limit imposed in industrial standards as the highest safe level for an 8-hour period for adults. The NICU noise level also has been found to demonstrate little diurnal variation and fluctuations in sound; when fluctuations do occur, they are unpredictable (Thomas, 1989).

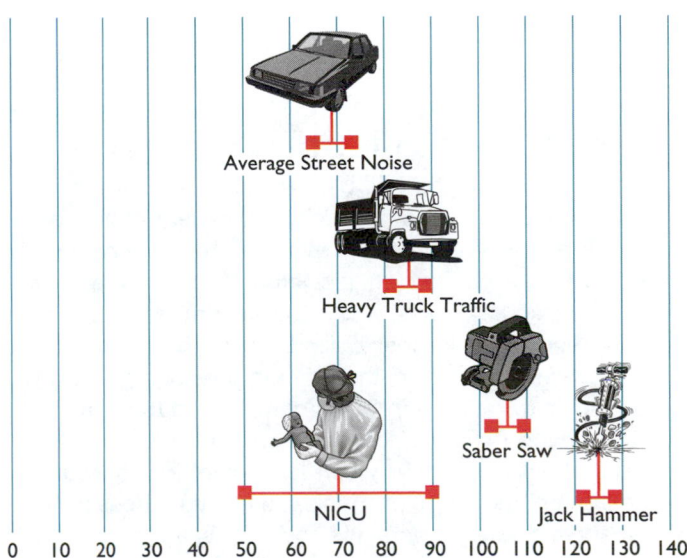

Figure 36-2 NICU sound levels (in dB) relative to other common environments.

Critical Thinking

Effects of Sound

Sound levels or sharp unexpected noises can negatively affect the sick or immature infant.

- How do you respond when you hear an unexpected sharp noise such as a car backfiring nearby or a door slamming? Do you startle?
- What happens to your heart rate and breathing?
- How do you feel when you have been in a very noisy environment for several hours?
- Do you think a premature or sick baby will respond differently or in the same way as you do?

Nursery Sound Levels and Patterns

In studies exploring the sources of sound in the NICU environment, researchers have identified both anticipated and unanticipated components of nursery sound. As expected, much of the sound present in the NICU is generated by the equipment used in the care of the infants, including incubators, oxygen monitoring devices, ventilators, and infusion pumps (Thomas, 1989). Furthermore, monitor alarms and telephones, as expected, contributed significantly to the high-amplitude sound excursions. Less expected, however, were findings demonstrating that most of the high-amplitude sound excursions, 70 dB or higher, were related to staff activities, including closing doors,

Nursing Alert

OTOTOXIC DRUGS IN THE NICU

Sound levels in the NICU have not been proved to have a negative effect on the development of hearing in the hospitalized preterm infant. Particular concern, however, is focused on the interaction of excessive ambient sound levels with ototoxic drugs the infant may receive while hospitalized. These drugs include but are not limited to the aminoglycosides, such as gentamicin, kanamycin, streptomycin, and tobramycin, when used for more than 5 days. An additional ototoxic effect may occur when loop diuretics (diuretics acting on the loop of Henle), such as furosemide, ethacrynic acid, bumetanide and others, are given with aminoglycosides. Nurses should be alert to the possible risks posed to infants by these drugs alone or in interaction with the NICU environment.

trash can lids, incubator ports or drawers; laughter; and conversation (Long, Lucey, & Philip, 1980).

Effects of Nursery Sound on Hearing

At this time no studies exist which definitively demonstrate that sensorineural hearing loss is associated with nursery noise levels. Approximately 8% to 9% of low birth weight infants develop clinically significant hearing loss (Pettigrew et al., 1988). This incidence has been attributed to multiple risk factors, including significant intraventricular hemorrhage, prolonged oxygen therapy, hyponatremia, the use of aminoglycoside antibiotics, incidence of asphyxia, and elevated serum bilirubin levels (Taeusch & Ballard, 1998). The toxic effect of excessive nursery noise levels has been proposed as another risk factor but has not been studied systematically in human infants. It should be noted, however, that the hearing loss found in these infants has been described as usually most marked in the high-frequency range (Pettigrew et al., 1988) and that much of the equipment-related sound in the infants environment, such as that from ventilators, incubators, and alarms, often is also in the high-frequency range (Thomas, 1989). It also is worth noting that infants with the greatest number of risk factors associated with sensorineural hearing loss are also likely to have the longest exposure to the ambient noise of the NICU.

A second area of concern related to the long-term effects of NICU noise on the low birth weight infant is whether, even in the absence of impairment of functional hearing, there may be some alteration in the infant's processing of auditory stimuli. The following may permanently influence the way in which auditory stimuli are processed and understood by the infant: the high level of continuous sound, or white noise, experienced by the infant in the incubator; lack of predictability or rhythmicity of NICU sound; and limited ability of the infant to associate a source, face, or event with the sounds heard. Certainly, the animal data describing developmental changes in the sensory and motor cortex secondary to altered sensory input support such a speculation, although the relationship has not been examined in human infants (Spinelli, 1990).

Effects of Nursery Sound on Infant Responses

The final group of studies examining the issue of sound in the NICU has focused on what the long-term and short-term outcomes of such sound may be for the infant in that environment. Researchers have examined the immediate responses of infants to noise in the nursery. Long et al. (1980) documented a repeated pattern of decreased transcutaneous oxygen tension, increased intracranial pressure, and increased heart and respiratory rates in two infants in response to sudden loud noise in the nursery. Gorski et al. (1983) described mottling, apnea, and bradycardia in preterm infants exposed to sharp excursions in sound such as telephones, monitor alarms, and conversation during medical rounds. Both studies provide support for the notion that nursery noise levels are a disorganizing influence on the neurologically immature low birth weight infant and raise speculation regarding the energy cost to the infant that these episodes represent.

Gaedki et al. (1969), in a related study of the effects of noise on the sleep patterns of term infants, reported that sound levels of greater than 70 dB were incompatible with infant sleep and sound levels of 55 dB aroused an infant from light sleep. Although this study has not been replicated with low birth weight infants, the reported sound levels are similar to those present in the NICU, suggesting that NICU noise may, in fact, interfere with the development of sleep and rest patterns in these infants. Alternatively, low birth weight infants in the NICU may be able to adapt to some degree to the continuous noise levels of their environment and therefore develop and maintain a pattern of sleep and rest.

Finally, a limited amount of research exists that suggests a relationship among ambient noise levels, infant stress, and endocrine responses. Early research using a rat model demonstrated measurable increases in ACTH secretion with increased stress, including sound levels as low as 68 dB (American Academy of Pediatrics Committee on Environmental Hazards, 1974). More recent research by Schanbert and Field (1987), using growth hormone secretion as a physiologic index of stress, reported that low birth weight infants stressed by handling manifested decreased growth hormone levels. Taken together these studies suggest that excessive noise levels may produce a stress response in infants, including alterations in endocrine function, and that one stress-related endocrine change in infants is a likely decrease in serum growth hormone levels. Certainly, each of these relationships is complex, measurement in human infants is difficult, and great caution must be used in extrapolating findings from animal studies to human infants. The premise that excessive noise in the NICU may contribute to poorer growth outcomes in infants, however, is worthy of further exploration.

Recommendations for Practice

A review of the research related to the effect of nursery sound on the developing low birth weight infant does provide support for realistic concern and justification for the modification of sound levels where possible, although it does not provide definitive evidence of any long-term effects of excessive sound. Several suggestions for sound reduction can be made:

- Some, though certainly not all, of the noxious noise is generated by staff activities that can be modified. NICU staff can begin to monitor activities, such as carrying on conversations with people across the room and loud laughing, to keep the associated noise levels to a minimum.

- Caregivers and families alike could be encouraged, when possible, to conduct conversations with one another away from the incubator or out of the caregiving area completely (Figure 36-3).

- Opening and closing doors and drawers and manipulating equipment can be done in ways that keep noise to a minimum. One source of noise could be minimized simply by depressing the latch on the incubator ports before closing them or applying some felt stripping around the incubator doors.

- Where possible, metal equipment such as wastebaskets could be replaced with plastic to reduce the associated noise level.

- Radios, intercoms, and other extraneous sound could be eliminated from the NICU.

- Equipment used in the nursery could be modified where possible to reduce the sound reaching the baby. Computer printers could be equiped with soundproofed covers. Telephones could be placed away from the caregiving area or equiped with flashers rather than ringers. Monitor alarms could be replaced with quieter audible alarms or flashing alarms.

- The use of carpeting and acoustical ceilings where possible can significantly reduce noise levels.

- When considering new or replacement equipment or other items for the nursery, the noise level generated by those items or equipment should be a primary consideration. Sound levels inside the incubator certainly are determined in large part by the noise of the machinery itself, and such noise levels should become part of the selection criteria.

- Specific guidelines for acceptable noise levels should be established for the NICU. These could be used as a standard when selecting nursery equipment and would serve to encourage manufacturers to design

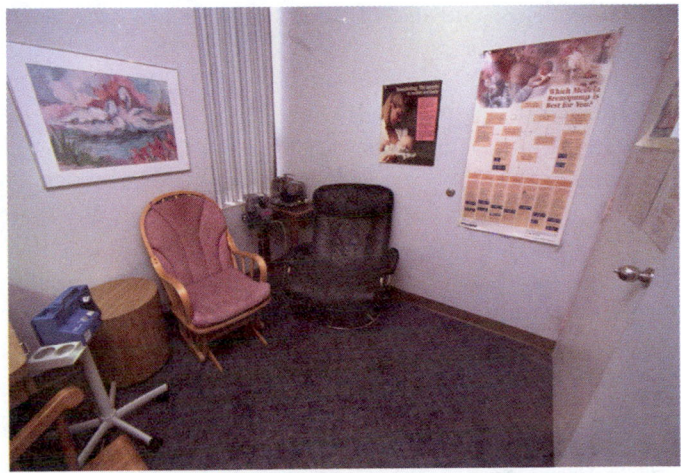

Figure 36-3 Many NICUs have a separate room in which families can spend quiet time with their newborn.

and develop quieter equipment for use in the NICU. Such guidelines also could be used to evaluate caregiving procedures.

Temperature

One of the earliest interventions known to improve survival in premature infants was maintaining them in a warm environment (Silverman, Sinclair, & Agate, 1966). Early strategies for keeping the infant warm included keeping the baby physically close to the parent and keeping the infant close to a heat source such as an oven, stove, or hot water bottle. Today, premature infants are maintained in incubators or on radiant warmers to support stabilization of body temperature until their own temperature-regulating mechanisms are adequate. These devices are designed to maintain infants in a *thermo-neutral environment,* that is, in an ideal environmental temperature in which infants, when quiet or asleep, can maintain their body temperature without increasing the metabolic rate above resting levels (Taeusch & Ballard, 1998). For premature infants, the range of environmental temperature fluctuation tolerated may be as little as 3.0°. Several factors make premature infants especially vulnerable to the effects of environmental temperatures. These infants have very little fat tissue, particularly brown adipose tissue, which plays a major role in heat production. Their larger body surface area to body mass ratio causes them to lose heat more rapidly than do full-term infants, older children, and adults. The increased permeability of their skin causes them to lose body water and heat more quickly than do older children and adults (Taeusch & Ballard, 1998).

In addition to the particular vulnerability of premature infants to heat loss, several external mechanisms interact to modify their thermal environment. These include the heat loss mechanisms of radiation, conduction, convection, and evaporation; heat maintenance strategies such as swaddling, wrapping, or otherwise covering the baby to avoid heat loss; and use of an external heat source, such as an incubator or radiant warmer, to provide heat to the infant.

Heat loss in the high-risk infant occurs primarily through the mechanisms of radiation, conduction, convection, and evaporation. Radiation is the major form of heat loss for infants in incubators. Heat loss through radiation refers to the transfer of body heat to cooler surfaces that surround infants but do not touch them, such as incubator walls, unit walls, and windows. The infant can become cold stressed through the loss of heat to cold walls and windows even when the incubator air is warm, or conversely, can become overheated in a cool incubator when the windows or room walls are too hot. Heat loss through conduction refers to the transfer of heat from the body core of the infant to the body surface and then to objects in direct contact with the infant such as mattresses, blankets, and scales. The colder the surface of the object is in relation to the baby, the greater the resulting heat loss. The process of convection refers to heat loss that occurs when heat generated in the body core is brought to the body surface, lost to the surrounding air by conduction, and finally, diffused away from the infant by moving air particles. The primary sources of heat loss by convection are drafts that touch the infant's skin or incubator walls. Evaporative heat loss increases as the humidity level of the air decreases. Evaporative heat loss also increases as the gestational age of the infant decreases owing to the extremely porous skin of the very immature infant. In these infants, evaporative heat loss may represent the greatest heat loss of any mechanism and presents a very real threat to the infant.

Recommendations for Practice

Understanding the sources of heat loss has enabled nurses to modify the infant's environment to minimize such losses. Some suggested interventions follow:

- Place incubators or radiant warmers away from external wall and windows and away from drafts.
- Use thermal shades on windows.
- Prewarm incubators and radiant warmers before placing the infant in them.
- Ensure use of double-walled incubators.
- Place warmed blankets on surfaces, such as scales, that will be in contact with the infant.
- Warm blankets before wrapping the infant.
- Avoid opening the incubator unnecessarily.
- Use the plastic sleeves on the portholes when caring for the baby. It also is important to teach families to use the sleeves on the portholes.
- Use side guards to protect the baby from air currents when using a radiant warmer.
- Keep infants in incubators swaddled (Figure 36-4).
- Keep the baby's head covered. Many nurseries use soft knit hats for this purpose.
- Replace wet blankets immediately with dry, warmed ones.
- Warm and humidify oxygen before administration.
- Prewarm solutions for the infant that are either applied externally or used internally such as intravenous medications.

Micro-environment Components

The second set of elements included in developmental care protocols are those specifically related to the environ-

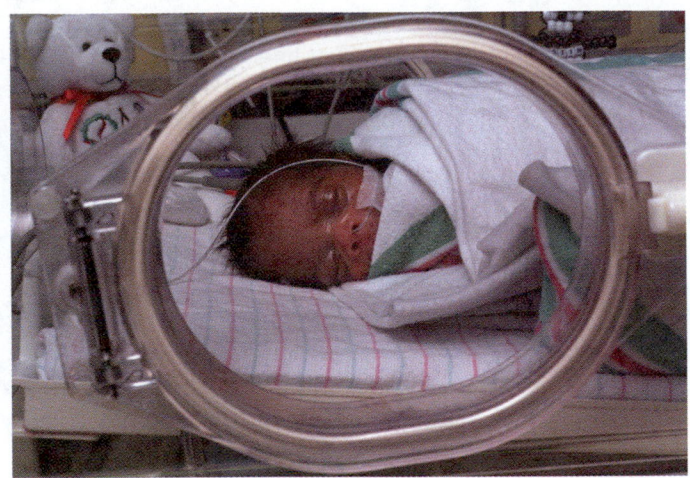

Figure 36-4 Infants in incubators should be swaddled comfortably to prevent heat loss.

ment or care experiences of the individual infant. As a group these components can be considered the **micro-environment** or individual sensory environment of the infant. The components of the micro-environment discussed in this chapter include positioning and containment strategies, handling and touching, nonnutritive sucking, and pain assessment and management.

Positioning and Containment Strategies

Current thought related to neonatal positioning in the NICU has evolved primarily from the study of the intrauterine posture of the fetus. The intrauterine environment is such that the fetus is aided in maintaining a position of flexion as well as midline posture. This flexed, midline position is important for normal motor development but also serves to facilitate hand-to-face and mouth behaviors, which provide opportunities for sucking and

---

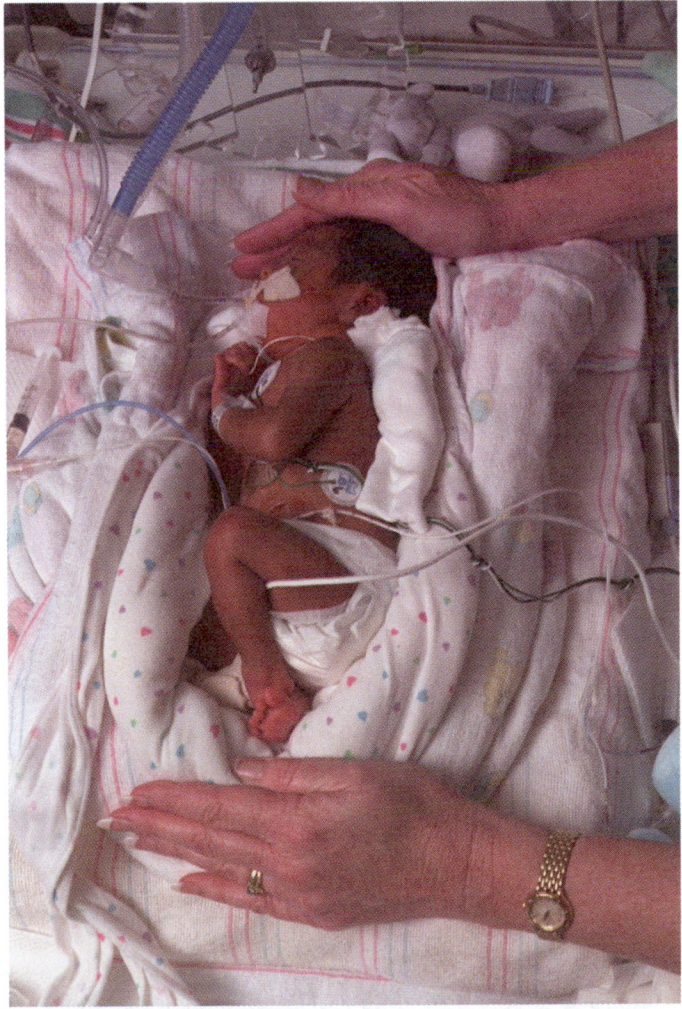

Figure 36-5 This premature infant is sleeping in the side-lying position; the nurse is containing the infant with her hands to offer a sense of warmth and security.

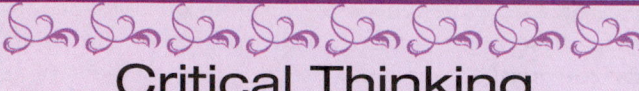

Critical Thinking

Positioning and Containment

Preterm infants are growing and developing in the hospital nursery environment during a period of time when they normally still would be growing and developing in their mother's uterus. It is this uterine environment that is most appropriate for the fetus and in which the fetus will grow and develop optimally. Think about how different the NICU environment is from the uterine environment. In the third trimester, the developing fetus would maintain a curled up flexed position, held there by the uterine walls. In contrast, in the NICU infants often are put in a supine, open position, which has been thought to make caregiving easier.

In the third trimester, the developing fetus also would feel the surrounding uterine walls as barriers or boundaries. As the fetus moves or kicks, the fetus impacts the uterine wall and feels the resistance and containment of that barrier. In contrast, in the NICU infants often are positioned in the center of the incubator or warmer bed, away from any barrier that could provide a sense of containment comparable with the uterine environment.

- How can the developmental care strategies for positioning and containment provide sensory input similar to that which infants would have received if they had remained in the uterus until gestational term?
- Which behavioral changes would you expect to see in preterm infants as you implement the positioning and containment strategies that are part of developmental care?

Nursing Tip

PRONE POSITION

Although the prone position often is preferred to enhance physiologic stability in preterm infants, you need to accustom infants to side- or supine-lying positions before discharge because these positions will be recommended to parents to reduce the risk for SIDS.

self-calming behaviors. Increasing evidence suggests that supportive positioning and handling of preterm neonates in the NICU may promote more normal motor development and minimize the chances of developing abnormal movement patterns (Fay, 1988; Jorgensen, 1993; Perez-Woods, Malloy, & Tse, 1992).

Historically, sick neonates have been cared for in the supine position to facilitate ease of physical assessments and accommodate medical interventions such as umbilical artery catheters and respiratory support devices. However, current research suggests that prone positioning may offer advantages over supine positioning for the sick neonate in terms of oxygenation, energy expenditure, and behavioral organization. Infants cared for in the prone position compared with those cared for in the supine position demonstrate increased oxygenation, tidal volume, and lung compliance; reduced energy expenditure; increased sleep time; and decreased behavioral disorganization (Fox, & Molesky, 1990; Lioy, & Maginello, 1988; Masterson, Zucker, & Schulze, 1987).

Developmentally supportive positioning also should prevent postural disorders common to chronically ill preterm neonates. One adverse effect of improper positioning is scapular retraction. In the NICU, scapular retraction may have an immediate impact on respiration and result in decreased hand-to-face or hand-to-mouth behaviors, leading to stress and avoidance behaviors in the

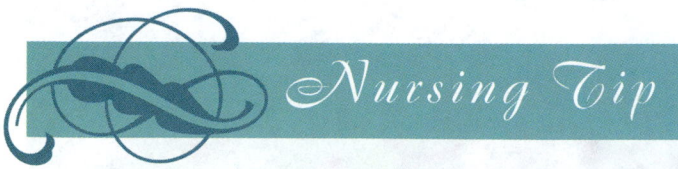

Client Education

Infant Positioning

When parents are present, talk with them as you position the baby. This is an opportunity to teach them how to position their infant and to practice positioning the baby with you there to support them. Talk with them about where the baby will sleep at home and how they will be able to position the baby with the supplies available to them in the home environment. A variety of positioning aids have become available on the commercial market to assist in developmentally supportive positioning, although many of these represent a significant expense. Point out to parents that although you may use some specialized equipment in the hospital, they will be able to position their baby appropriately using blanket rolls or small receiving blankets. Also discuss some of the concerns about using pillows and loose blankets in the crib with the infant (AAP, 2000).

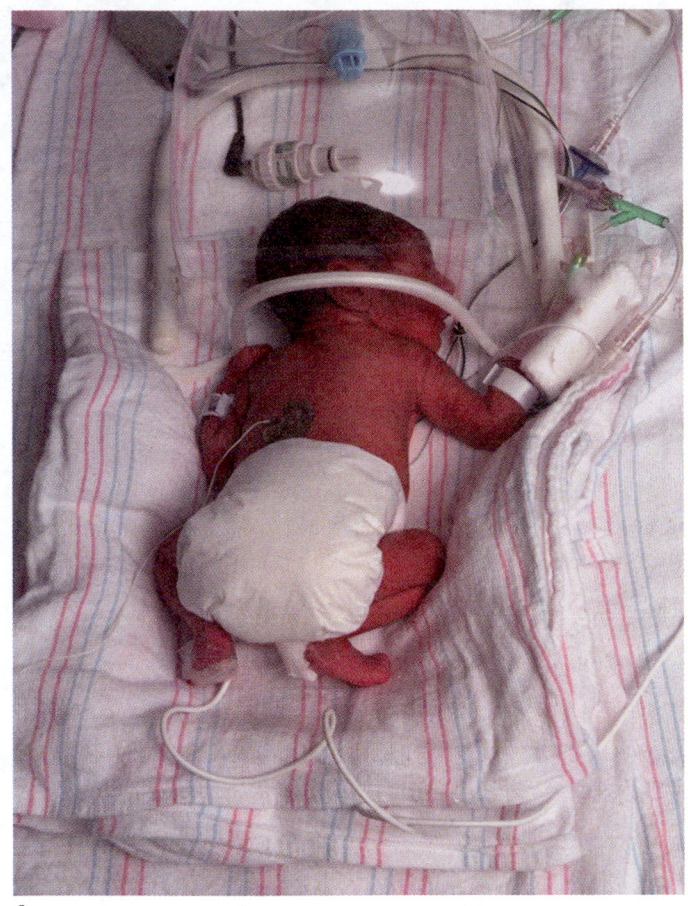

A.

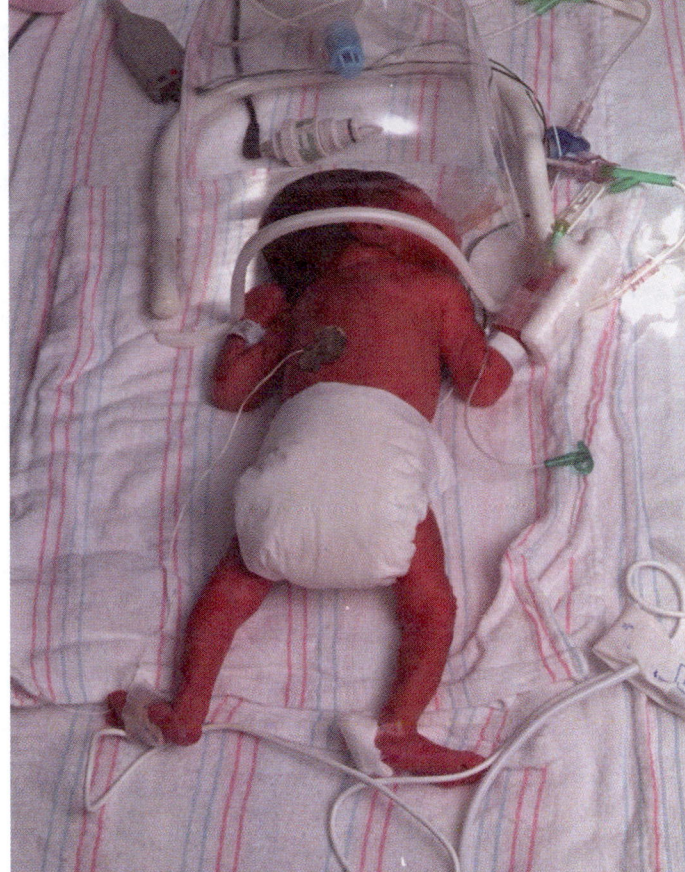

B.

NICU. Failure to promote shoulder rounding in preterm infants also may result in abnormal scapular retraction that may persist into early childhood, leading to delays in the achievement of normal developmental tasks (Georgieff & Bernbaum, 1986). Possible long-term effects of scapular abduction and retraction include difficulties in sitting without support, crawling, reaching for objects, and manipulating or transferring objects between hands.

External rotation and abduction of the hips is another postural disorder with potential adverse effects on long-term development. Prolonged supine or prone positioning of preterm neonates may result in excessive hip flexion and flattened frog-legged postures, which may ultimately interfere with normal movement patterns for gait and crawling (Downs et al., 1991).

Recommendations for Practice

The primary goal of supportive positioning for the preterm infant is to encourage a balance between flexion and extension (Figure 36-6). Careful attention also should be paid to maintaining body symmetry while enhancing midline

Figure 36-6 Developmental positioning of the preterm infant A. Prone, flexed (frog-legged position) B. Prone, extended position C. Supine position.

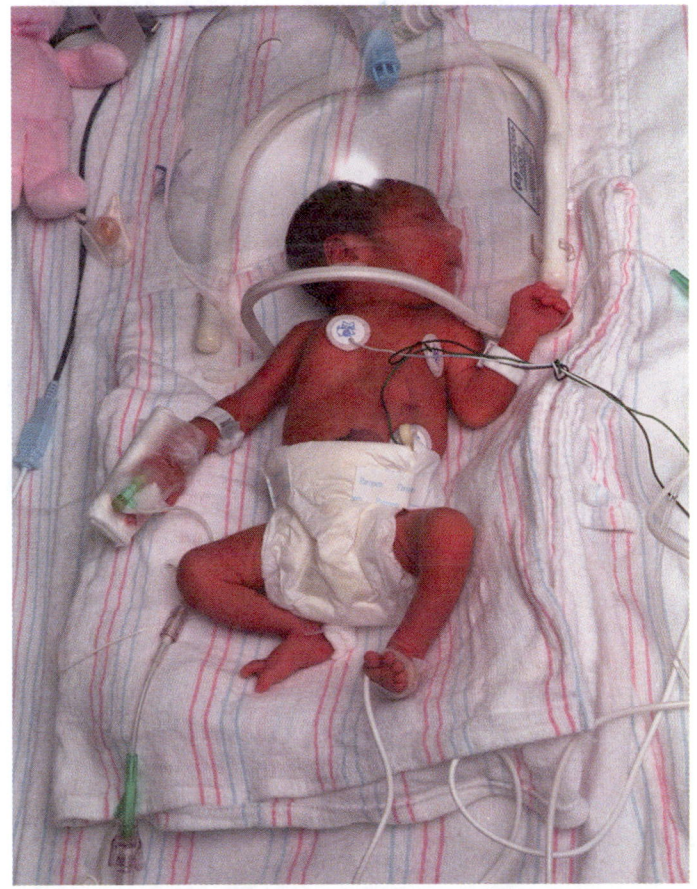

C.

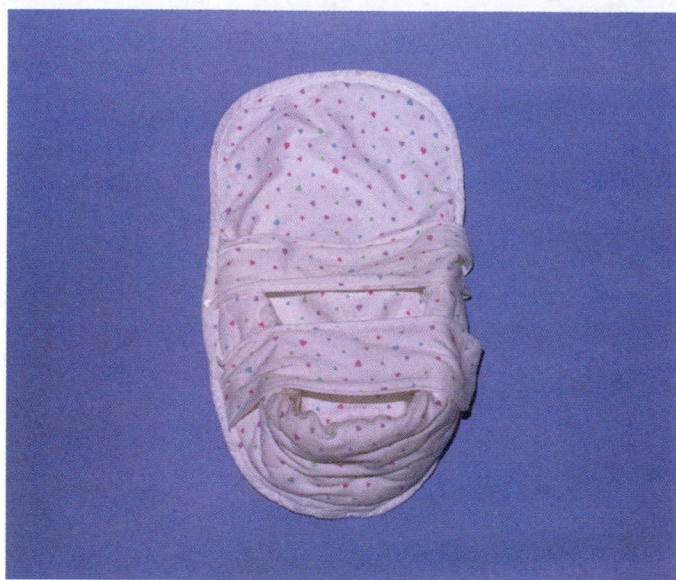

Figure 36-7 Swaddling-type bedding provides soft boundaries for the newborn.

orientation of extremities. Although sufficient research exists to promote prone positioning whenever possible in acute and chronically ill preterm neonates, the goals of developmentally supportive positioning can be accomplished in a variety of prone, lateral, and supine positions. Some developmentally supportive positioning interventions include the following:

- Provide boundaries that maintain the infant's position in flexion while allowing the infant adequate room for extension (Figure 36-7).
- Whenever possible, encourage side-lying positions for the acutely ill or recovering preterm infant.
- Provide midline orientation to facilitate hand-to-mouth activities and prevent shoulder retraction.
- To avoid head molding, use gel products or water pillows and reposition frequently.
- Use the smallest diaper available to prevent hip abduction.
- When positioning the infant in the prone position, prevent external hip rotation by placing a roll under the hips, thus supporting the pelvis and allowing the knees to be flexed and tucked in. An additional blanket roll that encircles the lower extremities and extends up to the upper thorax will provide opportunities for the infant to brace against as well as facilitate hand-to-mouth behaviors. To avoid hyperextension of the neck, the head should be kept in a neutral position or with the chin tucked slightly toward the chest.
- The side-lying position may be used to facilitate midline orientation and allow opportunities for the infant

to engage in sucking and self-calming behaviors. The infant can be properly positioned in the lateral position by placing a wedge or blanket roll behind the infant's back, with a folded sheet placed across the pelvis and tucked into the bedding. Doing so will facilitate flexion of extremities and maintain the trunk perpendicular to the bed surface. Neutral lower extremity positioning also may be facilitated by placing a soft roll between the infant's legs. Furthermore, a soft, thin blanket roll or small stuffed toy can be positioned at the anterior midline to encourage slight forward rounding of the spine and prevent of trunk arching. Finally, the head should be kept in midline or with the chin tucked slightly toward the chest.

- Supine positioning may be required for the provision of necessary medical care in the acutely ill preterm infant. In the supine position, the head, body, and feet can be supported midline, using soft blanket rolls positioned close to the infant. Lateral rolls should facilitate rounding of the shoulders by gently lifting and supporting the arms off the bed. A small roll under the knees will facilitate hip and knee flexion, thereby preventing hip abduction. Finally, a

Critical Thinking

Patterns of Caregiving

To provide optimal developmental support, any approach to caregiving must be embraced by all caregivers who come into contact with the infant. The care of the high-risk neonate involves the coordinated efforts of a full multidisciplinary team, including nurses, pharmacists, physicians, medicine, respiratory therapists, and X-ray technicians. Each member of the team has an important role in the care of the infant; however, all members may not be aware of the total demands on the infant's limited energy reserves. Neonatal nurses are in a key position to act as advocates for high-risk neonates to protect them from unnecessary handling or to structure the necessary care to provide for optimal rest and recovery.

- If you felt that the caregiving activities for an infant in your care were not allowing the infant to have periods of rest and recovery, how would you begin to modify those patterns?
- How would you work with caregivers from other disciplines in organizing the care activities of an infant?

blanket roll placed at the bottom of the feet will provide containment and improve muscle tone by providing a surface against which to flex.

Handling and Touching

Adequate rest is a primary prerequisite for optimal recovery of human beings experiencing acute and chronic con-

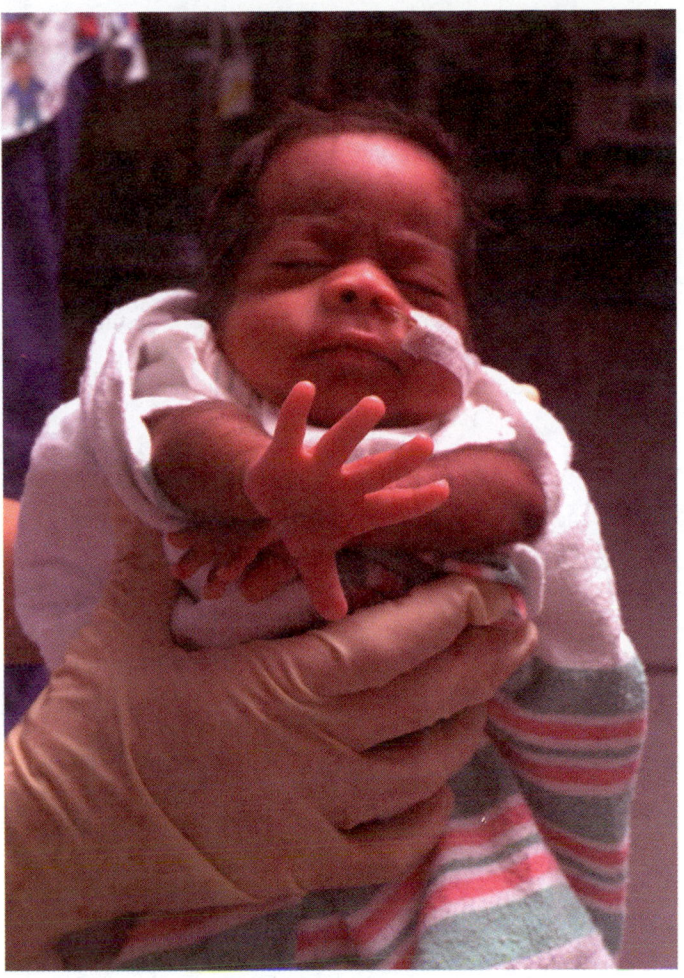

Figure 36-8 Finger splaying is a sign of distress.

ditions. Preterm infants in the NICU, however, often are subjected to frequent caregiving episodes. Indeed, the NICU is an environment in which the caregiving episodes are not only frequent but also intense, often painful or stressful, and involve multiple caregivers. Consistent with earlier reports, a recent study suggests that preterm infants are handled a mean of 113 times per 24 hours, with undisturbed rest periods ranging between 2 and 59 minutes (Appleton, 1997). In addition, the activity surrounding the infant may continue through the 24-hour period, with little variation in intensity.

Although most of the caregiving activities are a necessary part of medical care, some disruptions of the infant that occur daily in the NICU could be deemed unnecessary and poorly timed. For example, Appleton (1997) reported that increased infant disruptions occur surrounding the changing of nursing shifts in an attempt to "tidy" the infant's environment and make it aesthetically pleasing for other staff and parents. Although they seem routine to caregivers, such activities can be associated with deleterious effects on critically ill neonates. Adverse physiologic changes noted with handling include hypoxemia, tachycardia,

Client Education

Interpreting the Infant's Cues

One of the challenges for parents in caring for their preterm infant is to begin to understand the behavioral cues the baby provides. Infants born at full term provide many signals to adults around them that communicate when they are hungry, tired, or ready to interact. These babies cry robustly when hungry or uncomfortable and sleep quietly once they fall asleep. They make eye contact and maintain it, which parents may interpret variously as interest or liking. Parents often respond to such eye contact with deep wonderment and pleasure. In contrast, the preterm infant may produce behavioral cues that are much more ambiguous and difficult for parents to interpret. In the initial period, preterm infants may not be able to be either alertly awake or soundly asleep. Preterm infants often cannot produce the robust cry of the full-term infant to communicate distress. The effort to maintain eye contact with another person also may be overwhelmingly stressful to infants, causing them to avert their eyes (Figure 36-8). At times, parents may interpret this action as rejection or a lack of interest in them (the parents). They may feel that their presence is unimportant to the baby. From the parents' earliest visits to the baby, the nurse should use the opportunity to teach them about the baby's responses. Teach them the signs of stress in their baby and the ways the baby shows comfort and relaxation. For example, show them how the baby's vital signs become more stable, the extremities relax, and movements are smoother. Show them how to change their approach when the baby shows signs of stress, that is, parents' lowering their voices, touching the baby, or talking to the baby (but not doing both at the same time). By using opportunities to help parents get to know their infants throughout the hospitalization, an important part of the discharge planning process will be underway.

bradycardia, tachypnea, apnea, and increased intracranial pressures (Cooper Evans, 1991; Gorski, Hale, & Leonard, 1983; Long, Lucy, & Philip, 1980; Murdoch, & Darlow, 1984; Norris, Campbell, & Brenkert, 1982; Peters, 1992; Speidel, 1978). Frequent caregiver handling also has been associated with behavioral distress and may interfere with normal sleep patterns that are important for neurologic organization and growth (Appleton, 1997; Jorgensen, 1993; Wolke, 1987). Conversely, developmentally supportive handling allows for longer periods of sleep; results in earlier transition to oral feedings; and reduces hospital stays, with improved long-term outcomes (Lotas & Walden, 1996; Mann et al., 1986).

Organization of Care

Two strategies are necessary in reducing the infant's stress with handling during caregiving. First, all routine caregiving actions should be evaluated and unnecessary ones eliminated. Another strategy used by nurses to modify this continuous activity level is to cluster or group the infant's care in a way that protects some blocks of time for the baby to rest. This effort is based on two critical components: timing of caregiving and individualization of caregiving approaches to provide optimal rest and recovery for the infant. Neonatal nurses must coordinate the infant's care to decrease the frequency of disruptive contacts while providing periods of uninterrupted rest. To accomplish this, many NICUs have implemented hands-off times during which all nonemergency procedures are postponed to ensure infants an opportunity for undisturbed sleep. Caregiving activities are grouped together and typically timed to coincide with scheduled events such as feedings (Figure 36-9). Optimally, caregiving would also coincide with the infant's awake or more alert periods. Such clustering of care activities, although providing the infant with increased opportunities for undisturbed sleep, may not be tolerated by the acutely ill neonate. Since physiologically unstable infants may become easily stressed with handling, infant cues such as grimacing, changes in muscle tone, heart rate, respiratory rate, and color, should be used to evaluate the individual infant's tolerance for caregiving activities at a particular time. An infant's tolerance to handling may be observed through behavioral cues suggesting stress and disorganization (Table 36-1). Developmentally supportive caregiving individualizes care so that infant stress behaviors are minimized and self-regulatory behaviors facilitated.

Therapeutic Touch

Although the negative effects of excessive handling on preterm infants are well documented, several researchers have argued that certain kinds of supplemental touch therapies may be beneficial to preterm neonates. Some researchers have reported that supplemental tactile stimulation, such as infant massage, results in improved performance on developmental tests, increased growth and weight gain, early discharge, reduced behavioral distress, and improved parental bonding and attachment (Field et al., 1986; Field, Scafid, & Schanberg, 1987; Whitley, & Cowan, 1991; Nelson, Heitman, & Jennings, 1986; Booth, Johnson-Crowley, Barnard, 1985; Harrison and Woods, 1991; Paterson, 1990; Russell, 1993; White-Traut, & Hutchens Pate, 1987). These studies were performed with medically stable preterm infants, however, and the results should be extrapolated with caution to younger, sicker preterm neonates. Research in this area continues and should be evaluated carefully for inclusion in care protocols.

Other forms of touch have been found to be therapeutic in supporting or facilitating the infant in maintaining or regaining physiologic organization or stability when stressed, for example, the use of touching to provide gentle containment of the infant's extremities during a stressful procedure and allowing the infant to hold the caregiver's finger (Als, 1986). It is important to recognize that touching is a powerful stimulus that can be both stressful and

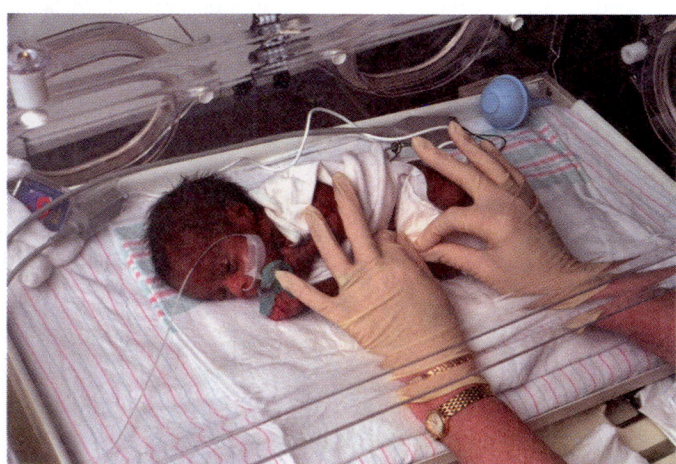

Figure 36-9 While this infant is awake, the nurse offers him a pacifier and schedules routine activities such as diaper changes.

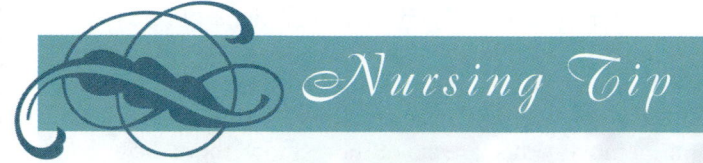

Nursing Tip

TOUCH THERAPIES

Therapeutic touch and healing touch are very different from infant massage because they may use very gentle tactile stimulation or even may provide no physical contact. These touch therapies may be useful in the high-risk neonate because they are less likely to cause overstimulation.

Table 36-1 Stress Signals and Self-Regulatory Behaviors for Autonomic, Motor, and State Subsystems of Functions

Subsystem	Behavior	Stress	Self-Regulatory
Autonomic	Respiratory	Irregular, slow, fast, pauses	Regular
	Color	Pale (gray), webbed, red, dusky, blue	Pink
	Instability-related patterns	Tremors, startles, twitches, yawning, sneezing	Absence of tremors, startles, twitches, yawning, sneezing
	Visceral and respiratory	Spitting up, gagging, hiccoughing, bowel movement grunting, sounds, sighing, gasping	Stable viscera as evidenced by absence of visceral and respiratory stress behaviors
Motor	General extremity and trunk	Flaccidity: arms, legs, postural hyperextension, arching, stretch-drown, diffuse squirming	Flexed, tucked arms and legs; well-regulated tone; trunk tucking; leg and foot bracing
	Face	Gape face, tongue extensions, grimacing; mouthing; frowning	Hand on face, suck searching, sucking
	Specific extremity movement	Finger splaying, airplaning, saluting, sitting on air, fisting	Hand clasping, foot clasping, hand-to-mouth, grasping, holding on
State	Sleep-Awake states	Diffuse sleep-awake states, eye floating, fussing; discharge; smiling	Clear, robust sleep states

Adapted from H. Als. (1982). Toward a synactive theory of development: Promise for the assessment and support of infant individuality, *Infant Mental Health Journal, 3*, (4), 237–238. Copyright 1982 Michigan Association for Infant Mental Health.

disorganizing, or soothing and organizing. Sensitive evaluation of the infant's individual response to a specific stimulus at a particular time is the most important skill for the nurse to develop in approaching the care of the preterm infant.

Kangaroo Care

In the early 1980s a concept of early mother-infant skin-to-skin touching referred to as kangaroo care began to be described in the literature. This practice was first reported from Bogota, Columbia, where clinicians described a decrease in infant mortality, morbidity, and infant abandonment when mothers were brought into the NICU and allowed to hold their diapered infants beneath their clothing, upright, between their breasts, with direct skin-to-skin contact (Rey and Martinez, 1983). Because of the resemblance of this practice to the way in which marsupial mothers hold and nurture their young, it became known as kangaroo care. The complete practice of kangaroo care includes both skin-to-skin contact with the infant placed vertically between the mother's breasts and self-regulatory breast-feeding (infant feeding as desired). One episode of kangaroo care may last a few minutes or 1 to 2 hours. Five categories of kangaroo care have been identified based on how long after the infant's birth the intervention is begun. Late kangaroo care usually is begun several days or weeks after birth when the infant has become physiologically stable. Intermediate kangaroo care begins within the first week of life while the infant is still unstable or may still be on a ventilator. Early kangaroo care is initiated in the first

day or hours of life in the infant who can be stabilized in a warmed incubator, with intravenous fluids and oxygen if necessary. Very early kangaroo care is initiated in the first hour of life in the delivery or recovery room. Finally, birth kangaroo care refers to placing the infant skin to skin on the mother's abdomen in the first minute after delivery (Anderson, 1999).

After the initial reports of kangaroo care appeared in the literature, researchers worldwide began to study this practice and evaluate its effects in rigorously controlled studies (Anderson, 1999). In these studies, positive effects on infants and on mother's and father's satisfaction were found. Infants receiving kangaroo care had longer and deeper sleep times compared with times when they were not receiving kangaroo care (Messmer et al., 1997). A study of 33 infants found that infants receiving early and intermediate kangaroo care had greater weight gain per week, fewer days of incubator care, shorter hospital stays, and were more frequently breast-fed on discharge than infants who were similar and had not received kangaroo care (Whalberg, 1991; Wahlberg, Afffonso, & Persson, 1992). In a recent study of 30 infants, researchers reported that infants receiving kangaroo care while undergoing a heel stick showed markedly reduced crying and grimacing compared with infants in the control group who experienced a heel stick without kangaroo care (Gray, Watt, & Blass, 2000). Infants in kangaroo care also did not show the dramatic increase in heart rate at the time of the heel stick that other infants commonly show. Other studies, while not documenting positive infant outcomes, have

REFLECTIONS FROM A MOTHER

"I couldn't think the first time they took me into the NICU to see my son. There were so many machines, so many people, so many other babies. All the babies were very quiet and still. When I saw my son I was terrified. He didn't look like I thought he would, like any other baby I had ever seen, or like me or like my husband. I didn't see how he could ever live or be normal. He was so small. I just felt helpless and wanted to cry. The nurses said the next time I came in I could hold him, but I didn't know if I wanted to. I knew I should feel something different—like other mothers do. I should be overwhelmed with love for him, but he didn't seem to be a part of me. I wanted to feel like a mother, but I couldn't. All I could do was cry. The nurses said that when I came back the second time I could do "kangaroo care" with him. They explained what I needed to do and said that I would hold my baby on my chest between my breasts. When I came back, the nurses had me stand by my baby's incubator while they picked him up, nestled him into my chest, and helped me sit down in a large comfortable chair. As he nestled in, they covered both of us with a soft warm blanket. He squirmed a little. I could feel him move against me—almost like when he was in the womb. Then he fell asleep. He looked very comfortable, and I wasn't afraid anymore. The nurse showed me how his heart rate, temperature, and everything else was stable—just like it should be. I just kept looking and looking at him. It was like I couldn't get enough of him. I think he has my husband's chin and my long fingers."

supported the safety of kangaroo care for the very premature infant (Bosque et al., 1995; de Leeuw et al., 1991; Ludington-Hoe et al., 1999; Moran et al., 1999). Kangaroo care has been implemented in nurseries throughout Europe, South America, and the United States.

Recommendations for Practice

Guidelines for appropriate handling of preterm infants are based on the characteristics of handling, the timing of caregiving activities, and individualizing care based on the infant's physiologic and behavioral responses to caregiving. Recommendations for handling of preterm neonates during caregiving are provided below:

Characteristics of Handling

- Use slow, gentle movements when handling the preterm infant.
- Use alerting techniques, that is, speaking softly to the infant or gently placing your hand on the infant, to prevent startling and signal the start of caregiving (Figure 36-10).
- Perform caregiving activities in an unhurried manner and allow time outs when the infant shows marked signs of stress.
- Provide extra caregiving hands or boundary support during difficult and uncomfortable procedures.
- Provide **facilitated tucking** with caregiving hands or boundary support until the infant settles after care, remaining at the bedside for at least 2 to 5 minutes after completion of any procedure.
- Bathe the infant while providing support with swaddling.

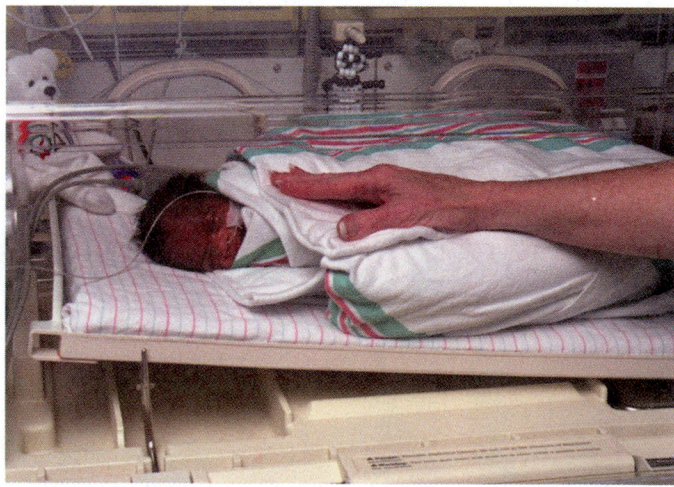

Figure 36-10 The nurse gently places a hand on the infant to signal the start of caregiving.

Research Highlight

Skin-to-Skin Contact is Analgesic in Healthy Newborns

Purpose

To determine whether skin-to-skin contact (kangaroo care) between mothers and their healthy full-term newborns reduced the pain experienced by infants during a heel stick.

Method

A sample of 30 healthy full-term newborns was randomly assigned to one of two groups. Infants in group one (experimental group) were held by their mothers in a kangaroo care protocol during a heel stick procedure. Infants in group two (control group) were swaddled in a crib during a heel stick procedure (standard protocol for the nursery). In both groups, the infants were positioned comfortably and left for 15 minutes to quiet. After 15 minutes, data collection began. The infants' faces were videotaped and heart rates monitored every 10 seconds for 2 minutes before the heel stick, during the heel stick procedure, and for a 3-minute recovery period after the procedure. Measures of pain response in the infants included heart rate changes, crying, and facial grimace.

Findings

Infants receiving kangaroo care demonstrated 82% less crying and 65% less grimacing than did infants maintained swaddled in their cribs. Infants receiving kangaroo care did not demonstrate a dramatic increase in heart rate at the time the heel was lanced as did the infants in the control group.

Nursing Implications

Kangaroo care appeared to provide a powerful analgesic effect for the infants in this study. When infants in the NICU need to have a painful procedure done, for example, an intravenous line insertion or a heel stick, arranging for the infant to be maintained in skin-to-skin contact can provide a nonpharmacologic approach to pain relief.

Gray, L., Watt, L., & Blass, E. (2000). Skin to skin contact is analgesic in healthy newborns. *Pediatrics, 105,* 1, 1–6.

- Perform caregiving with the infant in a prone or side-lying position to minimizing the need for repositioning, thereby reducing handling and stress.

- Weigh the infant while swaddled or in a containment device to maintain the infant's level of physiologic organization. The blanket or other containment device can be weighed separately so that its weight can be deducted from the infant's weight.

Timing of Care

- Time caregiving activities around the sleep-wake cycles of the infant.

- Protect periods of sleep, providing 2 to 3 hours of uninterrupted sleep.

- Use electronic monitoring devices for continuous display and routine assessment of physiologic parameters. Perform hands-on assessment of vital signs once per shift to correlate monitor readings, thereby minimizing infant handling.

- Cluster caregiving activities as much as possible without evoking a stress response in the infant.

- Gather all necessary supplies before disturbing the infant.

- Use signs at the bedside to remind all caregivers of scheduled touch times, thereby promoting periods of undisturbed sleep.

Evaluate Infant Responses

- Assess all caregiving activities for necessity, and avoid the use of routine procedures.

- Recognize stress behaviors, and use these in organizing the infant's care according to individual tolerance levels.

- Document and communicate an individualized plan of care based on infant behavioral cues of stress and self-regulation.

Recommendations for Kangaroo Care

- Kangaroo care is an important intervention for preterm and high-risk infants (Figure 36-11). Before initiating kangaroo care with a mother and infant, it is important that the nurse be thoroughly knowledgeable about the process and that the process be explained fully to the parent.

- In nurseries in which kangaroo care has not been initiated previously, an in-depth review of the literature, which is shared by the entire multidisciplinary team, would be an important first step.

- An in-service program by a clinician experienced in the use of kangaroo care would be an important step in preparing to implement this procedure in a nursery.

- Before implementing kangaroo care, ensure that you have a comfortable chair and, if possible, arrange for some privacy for the parent. A screen around the isolette can be used to provide some sense of private space.

- Arrange the timing of the kangaroo care in relation to other caregiving activities so that it is not necessary for anyone to interrupt the mother while she holds her baby.

- If the mother is planning to breast-feed, the period of kangaroo care can be an opportunity to initiate feeding. Evaluate for this before the beginning of kangaroo care.

- Kangaroo care also has been found to be beneficial for fathers in terms of facilitating their developing relationship with the baby. Offer the opportunity for kangaroo care to fathers when possible.

Nonnutritive Sucking

Nonnutritive sucking has been associated with numerous positive outcomes for preterm neonates (Figure 36-12). Positive benefits documented from nonnutritive sucking include improved oxygenation levels during gavage feedings and at rest, enhanced weight gain, earlier transition from gavage to oral feedings, increased levels of alertness before feedings, and shorter hospital stays (Bernbaum et al., 1983; McCain, 1992; Woodson, Drinkwin, & Hamilton, 1985). The benefits of nonnutritive sucking have been well documented; however, caregivers have noted that the smallest infants in the nursery who could benefit from nonnutritive sucking have difficulty owing to the size of most available pacifiers. Pacifiers designed for the term infant, and even those appropriately sized for the older premature infant (those born at 30 weeks' gestational age or older), may be too large for the younger preterm infant. Pacifiers, such as the Wee Thumbie, designed for very small preterm infants allow the nurse to provide important sucking opportunities for these babies. This pacifier was designed from developmental theories to simulate thumb sucking in utero. It has been tested on low-birth-weight infants (Engebretson & Wardell, 1997).

Recommendations for Practice

- Experiment with the available pacifiers to find the one best suited for an individual baby. Infants may demonstrate more effective sucking behavior with a particular size and style of pacifier.

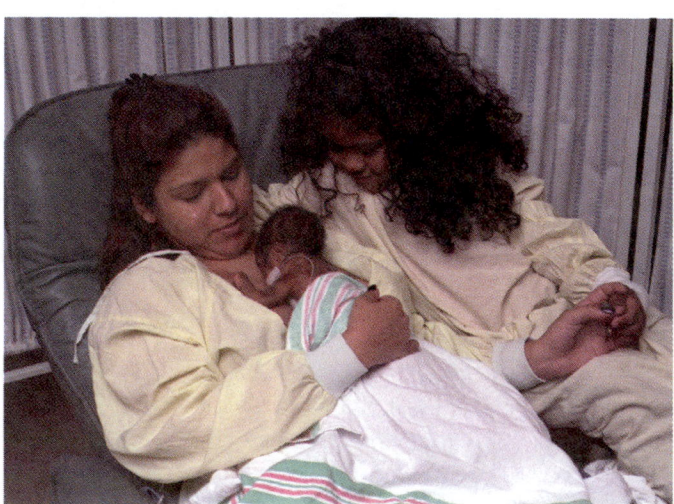

Figure 36-11 Preterm infants and their families benefit from kangaroo care.

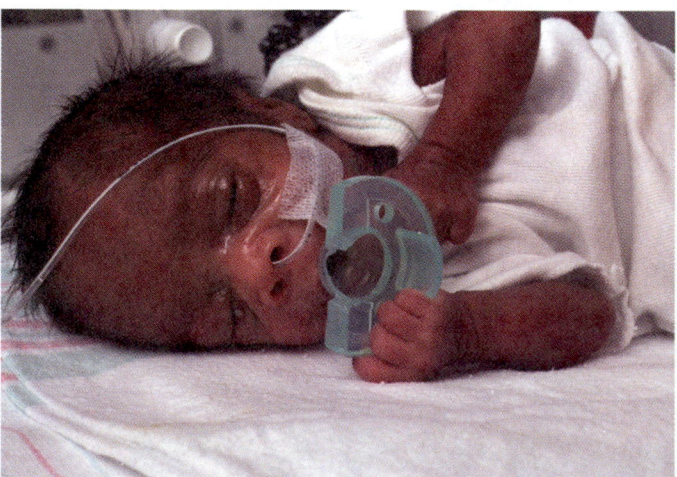

Figure 36-12 High-risk neonates can benefit from and find comfort in nonnutritive sucking.

Pain Assessment and Management

Preterm infants who require specialized neonatal care often are subjected to painful diagnostic and therapeutic procedures. Whereas pain may contribute to immediate physiologic instability and behavioral state changes, chronic, repeated pain experiences in the NICU also may result in adverse long-term developmental outcomes such as alterations in perceptions of pain in later childhood (Blackburn & Loper, 1992; Franck & Gregory, 1993; Porter, 1993; Corff et al., 1995; Grunau, Whitfield, & Petrie, 1994).

Accurate pain assessment is the first step to optimal pain management. Because pain is a multidimensional phenomenon, pain assessment should incorporate physiologic and behavioral measures. Many physiologic measures of pain have been studied in preterm neonates. The most evidence-based measures include increased heart rate and decreased oxygen saturation (Bozzette, 1993; Craig et al., 1993; McIntosh, van Veen, & Brameyer, 1994; Stevens, & Johnston, 1994; Stevens, Johnston, & Horton, 1993). Whereas physiologic measures provide greater objectivity in the assessment of pain responses, behavioral measures have been demonstrated to offer more specificity in terms of the pain experience, particularly facial actions. Brow bulge, eye squeeze, nasolabial furrow, and open mouth are the four most common facial patterns demonstrated by both preterm and full-term neonates (Bozzette, 1993; Grunau, Johnson, & Craig, 1990; Grunau, & Craig, 1987; Stevens, Johnston, & Horton, 1993; 1994).

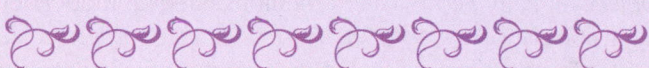

Critical Thinking

Nonnutritive Sucking

Infants in utero are able to bring their hands to their mouths by the middle of the second trimester. Often, sonograms taken during the second trimester show the fetus apparently sucking its thumb. Preterm infants, however, rarely show any spontaneous thumb sucking. Unlike in the watery uterine environment in which they can move freely and their flexed position helps bring their hands to their mouths, preterm infants in the NICU rarely are able to get their hands to their mouths. Think about it. If sucking often is seen on sonography in the second trimester, it must be a common behavior. If sucking is a common behavior in the developing fetus, is it just a chance occurrence or is it, in some way, important to fetal development? If it is important to fetal development, then is it important for the development of the preterm infant in the NICU? In studying this question, researchers have found that when preterm infants were given regular opportunities for nonnutritive sucking, they demonstrated more rapid weight gain and shorter hospital stays as well as changes in infant behavioral state and activity (Bernbaum et al., 1983; Field et al., 1982; Porter, & Anderson, 1979; McCain, 1992; Gill et al., 1988; Woodson, Drinkwin, & Hamilton, 1985).

* When infants are given bolus gavage feeding, nonnutritive sucking opportunities should be provided before initiation of the feeding and continued for a few minutes after the feeding is completed.
* When infants are continuously fed, nonnutritive sucking opportunities should be offered on a regular schedule such as 20 minutes every 3 to 4 hours.
* Nonnutritive sucking opportunities should be offered to even very immature infants who are not able to demonstrate a sustained organized suck. These early sucking behaviors may be important in stimulating the neurobehavioral development of the infant.
* Offer a pacifier to the infant who is fussy, restless, or irritable. Nonnutritive sucking is one of the mechanism infants use to calm and comfort themselves.
* Do not provide an empty nipple or one stuffed with cotton to the infant. Use only an approved pacifier that meets federal safety standards.

Critical Thinking

Pain in Neonates

In the past, it was thought that newborns were unable to experience pain sensations in the same way as do older children and adults.

* Have you ever watched a newborn when blood was being drawn through a heel stick? How did the baby respond?
* Have you ever had blood drawn or an injection? How did you respond?
* How was your response like or different from the response of the newborn infant?
* Ask yourself what you think is true about a newborn's response to pain.

Critical Thinking

Pain Management

Until just over a decade ago, myths regarding pain in neonates were pervasive in the NICU. Among the two most common myths were that the central nervous system of the preterm neonate was too immature to perceive pain that resulted from common neonatal therapies coupled with the myth that expounded the dangers of administering narcotics to neonates. Despite current evidence that neonates have the anatomic and functional capacity to perceive and respond to noxious stimuli, inadequate pain management practices continue to persist within the NICU. Think about it. Would you want to have a chest tube inserted without local and systemic analgesic? Does it make sense when medical care providers say they do not use local anesthesia to perform circumcisions on male infants because the infant cries more when immobilized on the circumcision board than when the prepuce is cut away from the glans penis?

The golden rule of pain management states that what is considered painful for older children and adults must be considered painful in neonates. Think about procedures that are commonly performed in neonates. Which strategies can you use to more effectively advocate for optimal pain management practices within the NICU?

Studies of full-term and preterm infants provide evidence that pain responses vary within the context in which pain is experienced. Therefore, the nurse also must consider contextual factors when assessing for pain in the neonate. Gestational age and behavioral state are the two most powerful contextual modifiers of the pain response in neonates (Craig et al., 1993; Grunau, & Craig, 1987; Johnston et al., 1993; Stevens, & Johnston, 1994; Stevens, Johnston, & Horton, 1993; 1994). For example, whereas term infants may respond to painful stimuli with crying and localized deliberate withdrawal responses, 26% to 90% of preterm neonates between 26 and 36 weeks postconceptional age will not cry in response to noxious stimuli (Johnston et al., 1995; Rushforth, & Levene, 1994; Stevens, Johnston, & Horton, 1994). Infants in awake or alert states also demonstrate a more robust reaction to painful stimuli than do infants in sleep states. Therefore, gestational age and behavioral state may contribute to a less vigorous response pattern, requiring the caregiver to be an astute observer. In order to provide optimal pain management

within the NICU, it must be assumed that what is painful to older children and adults is similarly painful to the preterm neonate who has limited behavioral capabilities to respond because of immaturity. It is particularly important to teach parents of hospitalized infants how to assess the pain cues of their child. Parents who are accustomed to seeing pain responses of full-term infants and older children may well not recognize the pain responses of a premature or sick baby.

Instruments for Pain Assessment in Infants

Several multidimensional instruments to assess pain in neonates have been published. The Pain Assessment Tool (PAT) is a multidimensional instrument designed for assessing postoperative pain in preterm and full-term neonates (Hodgkinson et al., 1994). The PAT includes four behavioral indicators of pain (posture and tone, sleep pattern, facial expression, and cry); four physiologic measures (respiration, heart rate, oxygen saturation, and blood pressure); color; and the nurses' perception of the neonate's pain. No psychometric properties of the instrument were reported. Bildner and Krechel (1996) developed the CRIES scale for assessing postoperative pain in preterm and full-term neonates. The acronym CRIES indicates five categories that are scored on a three-point scale (0, 1, 2) and includes *c*rying, *r*equires oxygen to maintain saturation greater than 95%, *i*ncreased vital signs, *e*xpression, and *s*leepless. The tool has moderately high interrater reliability ($r = 0.72$). Scores comparing the CRIES scale with the Objective Pain Score (OPS) demonstrated a moderately high correlation ($r = 0.73$; $P < 0.0001$) (Norden et al., 1991). Furthermore, scores were significantly lower after analgesic administration ($P < 0.0001$), suggesting that the measure has some beginning construct validity. The third instrument, the Premature Infant Pain Profile (PIPP), developed by Stevens et al. (1996), includes two physiologic indicators of pain (heart rate and oxygen saturation), three behavioral variables (brow bulge, eye squeeze, and nasolabial furrow), and two contextual factors (gestational age and behavioral state). The PIPP is scored on a point scale from zero to three. Content validity was established by careful review of the literature and by a panel of experts. Because the PIPP currently is the only multidimensional instrument that incorporates contextual factors that modify the pain response, it may serve to be a very useful instrument in assessing pain in preterm neonates in the NICU (Table 36-2).

Management Strategies

In the NICU, critically ill neonates are subjected to frequent painful procedures required for clinical monitoring and intervention. A study conducted by Barker and Rutter (1995) documented the alarming frequency in which painful invasive procedures were performed on infants from admission

Table 36-2 Premature Infant Pain Profile

Process	Indicator	0	1	2
Chart	Gestational age	36 weeks and more	32–35 weeks 6 days	28–31 weeks 6 days
Score 15 seconds immediately before event	Behavioral state	Active and awake Eyes open Facial movements	Quiet and awake Eyes open No facial movements	Quiet/sleep Eyes closed No facial movements
Record baseline heart rate Observe infant 30 seconds immediately after event	Maximum heart rate	0–4 bpm	5–14 bpm	15–24 bpm
Record baseline oxygen saturation Observe infant 30 seconds immediately after event	Minimum oxygen saturation	0–2.4% decrease	2.5%–4.9% decrease	5.0%–7.4% decrease
Observe infant 30 seconds immediately after event	Brow bulge	None 0%–9% of the time	Minimum 10%–39% of the time	Moderate 40%–69% of the time
Observe infant 30 seconds immediately after event	Eye squeeze	None 0%–9% of the time	Minimum 10%–39% of the time	Moderate 40%–69% of the time
Observe infant 30 seconds immediately event	Nasolabial furrow	None 0%–9% of the time	Minimum 10%–39% of the time	Moderate 40%–69% of the time

From B. Stevens, C. Johnston, P. Petryshen, & A. Taddio. (1996). "The premature infant pain profile: Development and validation" *The Clinical Journal of Pain, 12*, (1), 13–22. Copyright 1996, *The Clinical Journal of Pain.*

to discharge in one NICU setting. The study sample included 54 infants whose gestational ages ranged from 23 to 41 weeks, with a mean age of 33 weeks. The investigators reported 3,283 invasive procedures being performed, with increased frequency of procedures inversely related to gestational age and acuity of medical illness. One infant at 23 weeks' gestation and 560 g had 488 procedures performed during her hospital stay. Considering the long-term negative impact of frequent and prolonged pain in preterm infants, strategies to prevent pain in the NICU must be of paramount concern to health care providers in the NICU. The primary strategy to prevent pain in the high-risk neonate involves the change from protocol-based care to individualized strategic planning, which first evaluates the medical necessity of invasive procedures. This approach would promote caregiving techniques such as the minimal use of tape, use of noninvasive monitoring devices when possible, and tracheal suctioning on an as-needed basis only instead of as a routine procedure. Furthermore, for those procedures deemed medically necessary, careful coordination of painful procedures, such as grouping blood drawings, should be performed to minimize the number of heel sticks and venipunctures per day (Figure 36-13).

Another goal of pain management in infants is to minimize the intensity, duration, and physiologic cost of painful experiences. The intensity and duration of pain often can be minimized through the use of quick, efficient,

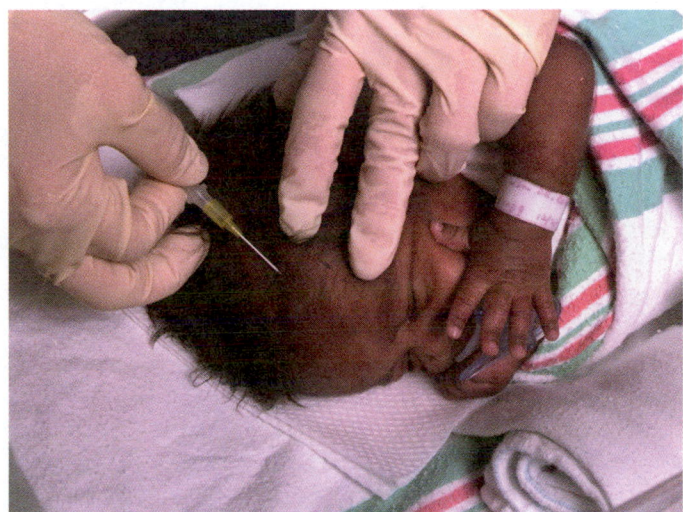

Figure 36-13 Offering a pacifier during a painful procedure, such as venipuncture, can help calm and reassure the infant.

and skilled execution of invasive procedures. This goal can be facilitated in units that routinely monitor the competence of their laboratory and nursing staff personnel or units that use only expert staff to attempt invasive procedures, such as intravenous placement, on the most unstable infants or those with a history of difficult intravenous access. Developmental care techniques discussed in this chapter may improve the infant's ability to cope with and recover from painful procedures. These techniques would include the strategies discussed to protect the infant from unacceptably high levels of noise, constant bright lights, and overstimulation and also would include clustering of care to allow the infant to rest sufficiently between procedures. For example, the physiologic cost of pain can be minimized by providing proper support to the neonate during a painful procedure. A study by Corff et al. (1995) reported that a technique known as *facilitated tucking,* which consists of generalized motoric containment of the arms and legs close to the infant's body while in a side-lying or supine position, resulted in significantly lower mean heart rates, shorter mean crying, shorter sleep disruption times, and fewer sleep-state changes after a painful heel stick procedure in infants than did motoric containment. Other interventions, such as swaddling, facilitating hand-to-mouth contact, nonnutritive sucking, and touch therapies, also may assist the infant in coping with noxious stimuli. Parents also can play an active role in relieving the stress of their infants in the NICU and should be encouraged to participate in the provision of nonpharmacologic comfort measures whenever possible.

Although the mechanism is unclear, preliminary studies suggest that sucrose may be effective in alleviating pain in certain situations. Blass and Hoffmeyer (1991) found that infants who were provided with a sucrose-flavored pacifier during heel lance and circumcision cried significantly less than did infants who did not have a pacifier or those who had a water-moistened pacifier.

Although nonpharmacologic measures may be used appropriately to manage pain in many circumstances in the NICU, pharmacologic agents should be used when severe or prolonged pain is assessed or anticipated (Agency for Health Care Policy and Research, 1993). Optimal treatment of pain in infants in the NICU often has been hindered by persistent fears of health care providers regarding safety, addiction, and respiratory depression associated with the administration of opioids. Although infants younger than 1 month of age and preterm infants generally metabolize pharmacologic agents more slowly and have prolonged elimination times of the drug from their systems, it is believed that analgesic and anesthetic agents can be administered with relative safety in the NICU. This is especially true given that equipment is present to monitor the physiologic status of the infant and equipment and personnel are immediately available for treatment with

naloxone and emergency airway management if the need arises (Agency for Health Care Policy and Research, 1993).

Opioid analgesics are considered the most effective agents to treat moderate to severe pain in neonates. A variety of analgesics is available. The most commonly used analgesics for neonates include morphine and fentanyl. Although the use of acetaminophen in neonates is limited by the constraints of the route of administration, acetaminophen may remain an option for treating mild pain in some infants. A summary of the routes of administration, recommended dosages for neonates, and side effects is provided in Table 36-3.

Although sedative and other adjuvant drugs often are used in combination with analgesics, no research is available regarding the efficacy or safety of combining these drugs in the neonatal population. It also must be remembered that sedatives have no analgesic effect and may depress the behavioral expression of pain. Therefore sedation should be used only if sedation—not pain relief—is required.

Although a few studies have reported on the efficacy of local anesthesia for invasive procedures in neonates, minimal research on the safety and efficacy of this pain management strategy is available to recommend its widespread use in the NICU. Some studies have investigated the use of a topical eutectic mixture of local anesthetics (lidocaine plus prilocaine [EMLA]) for painful diagnostic and

OPIOID USE IN INFANTS

Opioids remain the cornerstone of pharmacologic management of moderate to severe pain in neonates. Heath care professionals must examine their own personal beliefs about pain management in neonates and acknowledge the prevailing myths that may persist within the NICU in which they practice. Multidisciplinary focus groups may serve as a vehicle to open dialogue and discussions about current practices and to formulate strategies to improve pain management practices within the NICU. Nurses also must continue to systematically study the effectiveness of frequently used nonpharmacologic measures (cuddling, swaddling, touch, hands off periods, and nonnutritive sucking) to comfort infants undergoing minor painful procedures. As advocates for their small, preverbal clients, nurses must continue to play a major role in conducting research in the area of pain management for preterm infants.

Table 36-3 Drugs, Routes, Recommended Dosages, and Side Effects of Pharmacologic Pain Agents in Neonates

Drug	Routes*	Dosage	Frequency	Side Effects
Morphine	Intermittent IV	0.05–0.2 mg/kg over at least 5 min	As required (usually every 4 h)	• Respiratory depression • Hypotension • Ileus and delayed gastric emptying • Urine retention
	Continuous IV infusion	Loading dose 100 µg/kg over 1 h; then 0.01–0.03 mg/kg/h	Continuous	• Tolerance with prolonged use • Seizures
	IM, SQ	0.05–0.2 mg/kg		
Fentanyl	Intermittent IV	1–4 µg/kg slow IV push	As required (usually every 4 h)	• Respirator depression • Muscle rigidity • Seizures • Hypotension • Bradycardia
	Continuous IV infusion	1–5.0 µg/kg/h	Continuous IV	• Tolerance with prolonged use • Withdrawal symptoms after 5 days of continuous infusion
Acetaminophen	PO	10–15 mg/kg	Every 6–8 h	• Limited data in neonates • Liver toxicity • Rash
	PR	20–25 mg/kg	Every 6–8 h	• Fever • Thrombocytopenia • Leukopenia • Neutropenia

*IV–intravenous; IM–intramuscular; SQ–subcutaneous; PO–by mouth; PR–per rectum
From T. Young & O. Mangum. (1997). *NeoFax: A manual of drugs used in neonatal care.* Raleigh, NC: AcomPub (10th ed.). Copyright 1997 Thomas E. Young and O. Barry Mangum.

therapeutic superficial skin procedures, such as heel sticks in preterm infants and circumcisions in term infants (Fitzgerald, Millard, & McIntosh, 1989; Benini et al., 1993). The main potential problem with the use of EMLA in newborns younger than 3 months of age is the risk of methemoglobinemia because of the immaturity of the methemoglobin reductase enzyme in this age group (Taddio et al., 1995). Thus, until further research is performed to document the safety of using local anesthetics in high-risk neonates, systemic analgesics will remain the mainstay of therapy for pain management in the NICU.

Recommendations for Practice

The difficulty with pain measurement in preterm infants arises not from lack of empirical and clinical evidence to support that preterm infants do experience pain, but in the bedside practitioner's ability to accurately assess pain and to determine the potential impact of the experience on any given individual infant. Assessment of pain in the preverbal infant is entirely dependent on the caregiver's ability to properly evaluate pain and is a prerequisite for providing optimal pain management. Unfortunately, because of im-

maturity, clinical conditions or therapeutic programs, not all infants respond to pain with clear, robust behaviors. Thus, no single physiologic or behavioral measure should be used in isolation as an exclusive criterion to assess the presence and impact of pain in preterm infants. By combining physiologic and behavioral measures while considering contextual factors, health care providers can better assess pain in preterm infants. Better assessment can best be achieved through the use of a valid and reliable multidimensional pain instrument.

ASSESSMENT STRATEGIES IN DEVELOPMENTAL CARE

Developmental care focuses on individualizing care of high-risk neonates based on infant responses to caregiving and the environment. Healthy term infants have little difficulty in adapting to the extrauterine environment; however, high-risk neonates have a lower threshold for sensory input and often demonstrate difficulty in tolerating handling and interaction. Developmentally supportive care of the high-risk neonate involves modifying caregiving and structuring the infant's environment to support the infant's development and improve neurobehavioral organization. Since the late 1980s, several studies have demonstrated that modifying the care of preterm infants according to behavioral cues may achieve clinical outcomes such as reduced time on ventilation, earlier transition to nipple feeding, and shorter hospital stays (Lotas & Walden, 1996).

Critical to achieving these outcomes were periodic systematic assessments throughout the preterm infant's hospitalization that were used to tailor caregiving to the infant. While giving caregivers information about the infant's neurobehavioral organization, the periodic reassessments provided caregivers with opportunities for early intervention through developmentally based care plans.

One early developmental assessment tool was the Neonatal Behavioral Assessment Scale (NBAS). The NBAS is a comprehensive protocol designed to assess behavioral capabilities of healthy newborns from 36 to 44 weeks' postconceptional age (Brazelton, 1984). Infant behaviors are viewed within the context of a dynamic relationship with the evaluator and assess the infant through the continuum of sleep, arousal, and wakefulness. In this assessment, the evaluator provides a set of prescribed stimulation, activities, or tasks for the infant and assesses the infant's ability to perform and the amount of help or facilitation the infant needs to be successful. The type and amount of facilitation needed to elicit the infant's best performance is a reflection of the infant's organizational capabilities. To obtain a clinical description of infant behavior the NBAS uses clusters of behaviors, including habituation, orientation, motor performance, range of state, regulation of state, autonomic regulation, and reflexes.

After the development of the NBAS, the need for an assessment protocol designed for use with the preterm infant was identified. In response to this need, Als adapted the NBAS for the premature infant to develop the Assessment of Preterm Infant Behavior (APIB) (Als et al., 1982). The APIB consists of six sets of tasks or maneuvers that the evaluator presents to the infant. Each set of maneuvers moves from low-intensity stimulation to high-intensity stimulation. The evaluator observes the infant for behavioral signs of stress, the ability to maintain or regain stability in the face of stimulation, and the infant's need for and ability to use support or facilitation from the evaluator to maintain or regain stability throughout the assessment process. The APIB has been used clinically and in research to provide insight into the preterm infant's response to the NICU environment and caregiving activities.

A third developmental assessment tool, designed specifically for use in the NICU, is the Newborn Individualized Developmental Care Assessment Program (NIDCAP). The NIDCAP, developed by Als (1984), is designed to assess neurobehavioral organization by using systematic, naturalistic observations, that is, observations during rou-

tine caregiving. The assessment is designed for use with high-risk neonates who cannot tolerate the systematic handling and manipulation involved with other developmental assessment instruments such as the NBAS or APIB (Als, 1982). The infant is observed before, during, and after caregiving. Infant behaviors and measures of physiologic function are recorded systematically in 2-minute increments and provide the basis for specific recommendations of modifications to the infant's physical environment and direct caregiving. The NIDCAP encourages parental involvement and assists parents to recognize their infant's behavioral cues that indicate the need for time out as well as readiness for interaction.

RESEARCH SUPPORT FOR COMPREHENSIVE DEVELOPMENTAL CARE PROTOCOLS

Each of the care strategies discussed in this chapter has been shown to have value as an individual intervention for low birth weight infants. Substantial bodies of research exist supporting each of them. Both researchers and clinicians, however, have been interested in the effects of these interventions when combined in a comprehensive approach to developmental care. Comprehensive developmental care protocols are prescribed approaches to infant care that include all or most of the individual strategies described: low light and sound levels, careful maintenance of ambient temperatures, developmentally appropriate positioning and handling, protected periods for rest and sleep, pain relief, and nonnutritive sucking. However, only a few studies have tested this comprehensive approach (Table 36-4). All of these studies compared infants cared for using comprehensive developmental care protocols (the experimental group) with infants in routine nursery care (the control group). Each study evaluated the effect of a comprehensive developmental care protocol on the overall length of the infant's stay, length of time on oxygen therapy, age at which the infant was fed completely by bottle or breast, and developmental outcomes.

In evaluating the implications of these studies for clinical practice, it is important to assess the strengths and weaknesses of the methods used for each study, similarities and differences among the studies in both the methods used and findings, comparative risks and benefits to the infant in implementing the findings, and cost to the institution or third-party payer. All these studies are limited by their very small sample sizes. Two of the studies used randomized samples and quasi-experimental designs, which is a strength (Als et al., 1994; Fleisher et al., 1995). These studies differ from one another somewhat in the way they defined and implemented their developmental

Table 36-4 Summary of Developmental Studies

Study	Sample Size	N	Gestational Age	n	Birth Weight		Outcomes Reaching Significance at $P \leq 0.05$
Als, 1986	Experimental Control	8 8	Experimental Control	26.6 weeks 26.3 weeks	Experimental Control	879 g 831 g	• Fewer days on respirator • Fewer days on oxygen • Fewer days to complete bottle- or breast-feeding • Improved neurobehavioral organization at 1 mo post-EDC (APIB) • Improved performance on Bayley Scales at 3, 6, 9 mo post-EDC
Becker et al., 1991	Experimental Control	24 21	Experimental Control	29.0 weeks 28.3 weeks	Experimental Control	1,208 g 1,199 g	• Fewer days to first oral feedings • Fewer days to complete oral feedings • Reduced hospital days • Improved outcomes on BNAS at discharge • Decreased morbidity as measured by Minde's Neonatal Morbidity Scale
Becker at al., 1993							• Improved oxygen saturation levels at 30, 34 weeks' gestational age • Improved motor organization at 30, 32, 34 weeks' gestational age • Increased diffuse alert states at 34 weeks' gestational age
Als, 1994	Experimental Control	20 18	Experimental Control	27.1 weeks 26.5 weeks	Experimental Control	872 g 862 g	• Fewer days on oxygen • Fewer days to first bottle-feedings • Reduced incidence of IVH • Reduced incidence of severe BPI • Reduced hospital days • Younger age at hospital discharge • Reduced costs • Improved autonomic regulation, motor system functioning, self-regulatory abilities and visually evoked potential measures at 2 weeks' post-EDC • Improved Bayley mental and psychomotor development index scores and Kangaroo Paradigm Box scores at 9 mo post-EDC
Fleisher et al., 1995	Experimental Control	17 18	Experimental Control	26.5 weeks 26.1 weeks	Experimental Control	893 g 815 g	• Fewer days on positive pressure respiratory support • Improved neurodevelopmental outcome at 42 weeks' post-conceptual age
Subject numbers:	Experimental Control Total	69 65 134					

APIB–Assessment of Preterm Infant Behavior; BNBAS–Brazelton Neonatal Behavioral Assessment Scale; BPD–bronchopulmonary dysplasia; EDC–estimated date of confinement; IVH–intraventricular hemorrhage.

From M. J. Lotas & M. Walden. (1996). Individualized developmental care for very low birth weight infants: A critical review. *Journal of Obstetrics, Gynecologic, and Neonatal Nursing,* 684.

care protocols. They used different instruments to measure their variables. The nurses who cared for the babies in the studies differed in the kind or amount of training or preparation they had in the use of individualized developmental care approaches. Despite these differences, however, all studies reported similar findings. All studies reported significantly shorter hospital stays, a significantly reduced need for oxygen support, earlier progression to full bottle- or breast-feeding, and improved infant behavioral regulation for infants cared for using a comprehensive developmental care protocol. Thus, these infants received important benefits when compared with infants who received routine nursery care. No detrimental effects of developmental care on the babies were noted; therefore, no apparent risks to the baby can be identified in implementing comprehensive developmental care. The cost of training personnel to use the developmental care approach can be a major institutional expense; however, two studies documented that the savings in health care dollars from the reduced hospital stays more than offsets the cost of implementing the program, including personnel training Als et al. (1994) and Fleisher et al. (1995).

In summary, an analysis of the benefits, risks, and costs of implementing a comprehensive, individualized, developmental care protocol supports the recommendation that this approach to caregiving should be incorporated into standard practice in neonatal intensive care (Lotas & Walden, 1996). At the same time, however, it is critical that researchers continue to evaluate the effects of these interventions on long- and short-term health care outcomes of the premature infant.

FAMILIES AND THE HIGH-RISK INFANT

Parents play a vital role in shaping the future outcomes of their infants. When an infant is born prematurely and requires intensive care, parents often are not encouraged and facilitated to become active partners in the care of their infant. Parents often experience grief over the loss of a full-term healthy newborn and are frequently ambivalent about establishing an attachment to the preterm infant because they fear the infant will not survive or they fear the long-term prognosis. Parents with infants in the NICU often need the assistance of the health care team to participate more actively in decisions and in assuming care of their infant. Health care providers must provide opportunities for parents to interact with and care for their infant in developmentally supportive ways. Parental aspects of caregiving for the prematurely born infant can include temperature taking, oral care, diaper changes, and hand swaddling during periods of environmental or procedural stress (Figure 36-14). As the parents gain confidence in

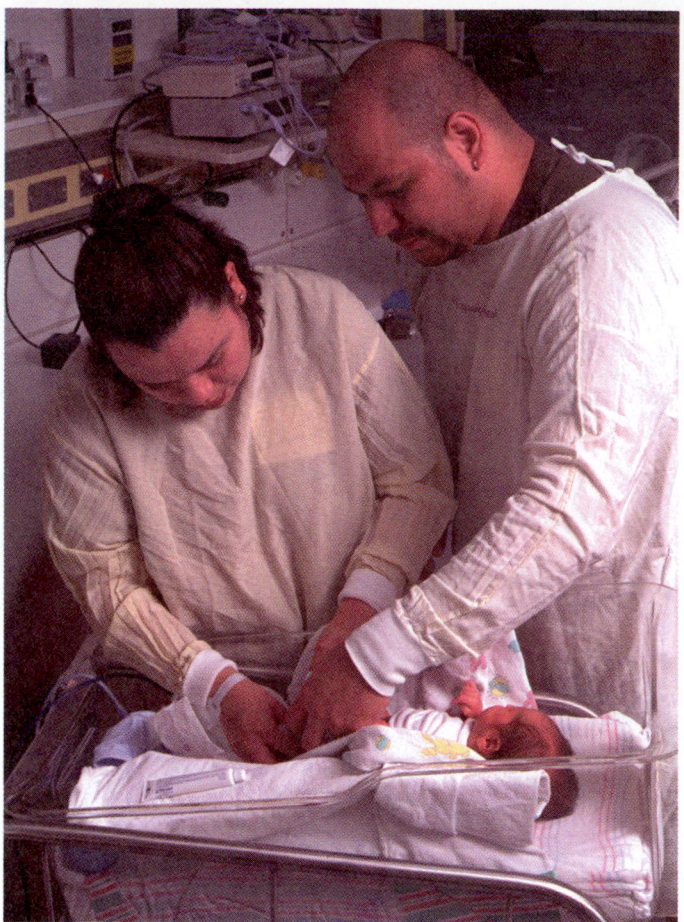

Figure 36-14 Parents of all newborns, especially premature or high-risk newborns, should be encouraged to bond with and care for their new baby.

caring for their infant and the infant's behavior reflects stability, parental caregiving can evolve to include more complicated tasks, as their infant's care requires.

A key component to parental caregiving in the NICU is helping parents to understand the behavior patterns of premature infants. Parents usually need assistance in interpreting their premature infant's behavior and becoming sensitive and responsive to subtle behavioral and physiologic cues. Parents should be educated to assess their infant for both time out behaviors and behaviors that support readiness for interaction. Parental education also should include developmentally supportive techniques such as clustering of care, strategies for gentle arousal of the infant for caregiving, and hand swaddling during procedures and periods of environmental stress. Assisting parents to learn appropriate interaction techniques with their preterm infant facilitates ongoing positive social interaction with their infant, allows the parents to contribute to their infant's recovery in a meaningful way, and may set the stage for parental confidence and competence in meeting

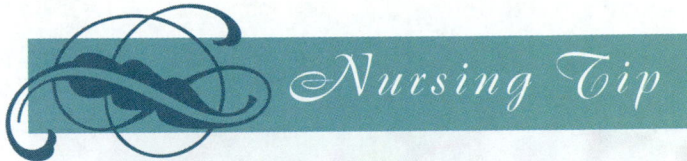

Critical Thinking

Role of Families

When preterm, small, or sick infants are admitted to the NICU, their survival depends on a combination of complex technology and highly skilled caregivers.

- How do you think parents feel when they come into this environment?
- Do you remember the first time you walked into any intensive care unit—adult, pediatric or neonatal?
- Did you understand what all of the equipment surrounding the patient was doing?
- Did you feel comfortable approaching the patient the first time?
- How important do you think it is that parents are able to be with their hospitalized newborn?
- Does it matter to the baby?
- Does it matter to the parents?
- Has one of your family members ever been critically ill and hospitalized?
- Was it important to you to be with your family member?
- Was it important for your family member to know you were there?
- What can we do as nurses to make parents feel more welcome in the NICU?

Nursing Tip

CHANGING ROLE OF THE NICU NURSE

One of the gaps in the care of the preterm or high-risk infant has been in the lack of support to families in making the transition from the hospital to the home with their infants. As infants have been discharged from NICUs younger, smaller, and with more complex care needs, the challenge to families has increased. NICUs are beginning to explore the efficacy and efficiency of having nurses from the intensive care environment work with the parents in preparation for discharge and then make home visits after the infant's discharge. The nurse, who is already familiar with the infant and the infant's care needs and with the parents (and they with the nurse), can provide support, consultation, and teaching to facilitate the family's adjustment to their new circumstances.

their infant's needs on discharge to home. As parents become increasingly involved in their infant's care, they can more actively participate in devising their infant's daily plan of care.

As the infant approaches being discharged, parents should be encouraged to assume more responsibility for the infant's care. In many units a special area is set aside for families to stay at the hospital for 24 to 48 hours before discharge and care for their babies with the support of the nursing staff. This opportunity allows the family to become comfortable with caring for the infant, when they have someone readily available to answer questions, and for the nurse to identify and address possible areas of concern before the infant's discharge. A particular focus at this time should be for the nurse and parents to discuss how each aspect of caregiving will be managed in the home environment. It is important to remember that parents may need some help in adapting the caregiving procedures

they see in the nursery to the situation they will face at home. When possible, a home visit before the infant's discharge will be invaluable in assisting parents to make this transition.

In addition to the routine care of the infant, discharge teaching should include discussions on how to evaluate the infant's signs and symptoms of illness. The nurse may need to teach the parents how to take a temperature and ensure that the parents have a thermometer in the home. Guidelines on when to call the clinic or pediatrician and when to go to the emergency room also are helpful. It is helpful to speak with parents about who they have available as a personal support system. Are extended family members, friends, or members of a church or other religious community available? If so it may be appropriate to involve that person in the teaching process in the hospital.

Finally, as the family leaves the hospital setting with their infant, it is important that they have been referred to all appropriate community resources. Referral should include information on a NICU follow-up clinic, a well baby clinic, or a private pediatrician; Special Supplemental Nutrition Program for Women, Infants, and Children (WIC) when appropriate; and parent support groups where available. Ideally, parents also should have access to professional advice by telephone. Many nurseries also provide routine telephone follow-up by nurses during the first few weeks after discharge.

Case Study/Care Plan

INFANT BORN AT 28 WEEKS' GESTATION

Nurses caring for preterm neonates can modify their care to facilitate the infant's growth and development by modifying the environment and initiating interventions that facilitate the infant's self regulatory action or have a calming effect on the infant. This requires careful monitoring of both the infant and the environment and continual adaptation of care. The following case study illustrates not only the nursing process, but within each diagnosis a specific illustration of the dynamic adaptation of the nursing interventions to the changes in the neonate and the environment.

At 2:08 a.m.: Kevin was born at 28 weeks' gestational age. His birth weight was 987 g and his Apgar scores were 5 (minus 1 for heart rate, 2 for color, 1 for respirations, 1 for muscle tone) at 1 minute; 8 (minus 1 for color, 1 for respirations) at 5 minutes. After being stabilized in the delivery room, Kevin was transported to the NICU in an incubator with free flow oxygen. On admission to the NICU, he was placed on a warmer bed, and oxygen therapy with nasal continuous positive airway pressure (NCPAP) was initiated. Routine cardiopulmonary monitoring and continuous pulse oximetry was begun. An umbilical venous catheter was placed to allow for the delivery of nutrients. Kevin's mother (Mrs. Jones) is a 29-year-old who had experienced two spontaneous abortions before the pregnancy with Kevin. Kevin's father, (Mr. Jones) a 32-year-old engineer was in the delivery room with his wife. Both parents deeply wanted a child and were highly anxious about Kevin's condition and prognosis.

10:00 a.m.: Kevin was lying in a supine position, wearing only a diaper. His heart rate and respiratory rate were labile, (HR 148-176 with excursions to 190+; RR 32-54 with excursions 72), with excursions in response to any loud, sharp, or unexpected noise in the environment. He also demonstrated repeated apneic periods of 15 to 20 seconds. He demonstrated frequent periodic twitching and tremors in both lower extremities. His brow was furrowed in a "frown" expression, and his color darkened and paled in response to activity around him. Kevin's parents came into the NICU. It was Kevin's mother's first time to see him, although the father was in the during the night.

Assessment

This preterm neonate is developmentally immature and unable to regulate and stabilize autonomic, motor, and sensory activity. He has exhibited signs of distress in response to environmental stimuli. Developmentally, it is crucial for him to conserve energy to maintain vital function and to grow.

Nursing Diagnosis

Inability to maintain neurobehavioral stability related to excessive environmental stimuli on the macro-environmental level.

Expected Outcomes The infant will exhibit physiologic stability as evidenced by the autonomic responses of heart rate, respirations, skin color, and a decrease in the motor signs of distress.

Planning Developmental care will be instituted. This entails careful monitoring and response to infant behavior and environmental events.

Nursing Interventions	Rationales
1. The nurse will modify the environment by moving the infant to an isolette with a cover and moving the isolette to a quiet area of the nursery.	1. This helps to isolate the neonate from some of the noise and light in the environment.

(continued)

2. The nurse will swaddle and position the infant in a flexed position if the infant shows signs of distress.

2. These positions and swaddling help the infant to self regulate and minimize the startle response that is very energy taxing.

Evaluation   Vital signs will be monitored and the infant will be carefully observed for signs of distress. (The following shows the dynamic monitoring and adaptation of the nursing process related to this diagnosis).

Nursing Diagnosis

Inability to maintain neurobehavioral stability in the face of excessive environmental stimuli secondary to gestational immaturity.

Expected Outcomes   The baby will increase physiologic stability as measured by: no HR excursions over 170 and no RR excursions over 60. Periodic breathing expected. No apneic pauses. No mottling is present. Skin remains pink. Reduced tremors of lower extremities. Hands remain in a relaxed posture. Face is relaxed.

Planning   Environment and caregiving activities will be evaluated for stimulating effect and timing.

Nursing Interventions	Rationales
1. Advocate for moving the infant to an isolette.	1. To reduce environmental stimuli to the baby.
2. Provide isolette cover to reduce light levels impacting the baby.	2. To reduce bright lights.
3. Create a quiet zone around the baby. Place signs around the isolette. Remind staff and visitors to lower their voices and minimize noise levels around the baby.	3. To reduce noise levels reduces stimuli.
4. Swaddle the infant to provide containment and flexion for extremities. Position the baby in a side-lying position, with limbs flexed. Provide support with blanket rolls.	4. This is a soothing position and makes the infant feel more secure, simulating the containment of the uterine environment.

Evaluation   Infant maintained HR between 154 and 162, with no excursions above 172; RR between 36 and 48, with no excursions above 54. Oxygen saturation stable between 97% and 99%. Apneic periods decreased; no tremors of lower extremities noted. Color, pink.

Assessment

In a period of 15 hours (6:45 a.m.–9:15 p.m., Kevin was approached for multiple caregiving activities. These included an examination by the resident, morning assessments by the primary care nurse, feeding by gavage, medical rounds, and a blood draw. Kevin was being handled or receiving some care for 45 minutes of each hour of the 15 hours, with no more than 15 minutes between any two activities to allow for recovery.

Nursing Diagnosis

Inability to maintain physiological stability in response to caregiving activities secondary to fatigue.

Expected Outcomes   Following caregiving events the infant will demonstrate:

- A rapid return to stable baseline HR, RR, and oxygen saturation.
- Decrease in apneic episodes.
- Continued baseline tone in the extremities and face.

(continued)

Planning The caregiving activities will be planned and grouped to avoid non-essential stimulation and allow the infant rest periods to destabilize. Reduce unnecessary noise or activity near the infant.

Nursing Interventions	Rationales
1. The nurse will group essential caregiving activities to allow for rest and recuperative periods. This also involves negotiating with other providers who care for the infant. The nurse will modify the environment to reduce noise and activity and allow rest time after feeding.	1. The excessive stimulation has created distress for this infant that is energy taxing and has disrupted autonomic function. The reduction of stimuli will allow the infant to restabilize vital functions.
2. Assess need and timing for each caregiving event.	2. Avoids unnecessary stimulation for handling.
3. Collaborate with the resident so that only one physical examination is performed in the early morning.	3. Minimize unnecessary simulation.
4. If infant tolerance allows based on cues exhibited, schedule feeding around the physical examination so that there is at least 1 hour of rest for the infant before medical rounds.	4. Allows for rest and energy exposure.
5. Negotiate with house staff to limit discussion at the bedside, stand away from the incubator when possible, and keep the handling of the baby to only the essentials.	5. Discuss unnecessary stimuli.

Evaluation The nurse continually monitors the infant for signs of stress and autonomic functioning. The process of limiting caregiving episodes and providing rest periods between caregiving or other interventions was effective in reducing the signs of stress in the infant. Following medical rounds, Kevin's HR was 156 bpm; RR, 42 rpm; color, normal; tone, normal. No apneic episodes were noted.

Kevin's parents are obviously distressed and fearful. On further discussion, neither parent has cared for babies and had no information about understanding the developmental issues with a preterm infant.

Assessment

The infant born at 28 weeks' conceptional age differs in important ways from the full-term infant the parents may have experienced in the past and whom they were preparing to parent. The preterm infant lacks the ability to express pleasure, distress, interest, and comfort with the same robust behaviors that are available to the full-term infant. The behaviors of the preterm infant that do communicate the infant's comfort, tolerance, and distress may not be recognized by parents. From the parents' first visits to the nursery the nurse can begin to teach them to recognize their baby's individual strengths, vulnerabilities, and ways of responding.

Nursing Diagnosis

Fear (parents) related to as evidenced by uncertainty about their baby in part secondary to a knowledge deficit regarding strengths and vulnerabilities of their infant and associated inability to understand infant behaviors and cues.

Expected Outcomes
- Parents will recognize positive signs in Kevin's condition.
- Parents will identify behaviors that indicate stress or comfort and stability in Kevin.
- Parents will identify Kevin's responses to environmental stimuli.

(continued)

- Parent's will identify the importance of their role in Kevin's recovery and development.

Planning   Nurses will use the time that the parents come to see Kevin to teach them about his development, the reason for medical and nursing interventions and encourage them to begin to care for Kevin in a manner that does not overstimulate him.

Nursing Interventions	Rationales
1. Stand quietly with with the parents and talk about what they are seeing. Explain some of the equipment and how you will be caring for Kevin. Talk about the purpose of swaddling, and how correct positioning can help aid breathing and improve motor stability.	1. Teaching the parents as care is given to Kevin allows spontaneous interaction, and the parents can ask questions.
2. When speaking with the parents, emphasize their importance to their baby—how much Kevin needs them.	2. Parents often feel displaced by the more knowledgeable health care professionals.
3. Support the parents in touching the baby's hand or face gently. Talk about some of the baby's individual characteristics, emphasizing strengths and qualities the parents would identify as normal.	3. These activities facilitate parent-infant attachment.
4. When the parents seem ready, introduce the idea of kangaroo care, emphasizing the importance of their closeness and touch for the baby.	4. This facilitates attachment.
5. When the parents are present during caregiving activities, use the opportunity to point out some of the baby's responses that indicate comfort, stress, or self-comforting behaviors used by the baby.	5. This facilitates the parents' understanding of infant behavior.

Evaluation   The parents continue to express concern about Kevin's progress but also are able to identify and take pleasure in indicators that show that he is progressing, that is, weight gain, more stable vital signs, better color, more self-comforting behaviors. Parents initiate opportunities to touch or hold Kevin and begin to ask about caregiving activities. Parents begin to express preferences about how things are done for their baby.

Web Activities

- Identify and evaluate five educational and support group resources for parents of premature infants.

- Explore the website of your state department of health for statistics on premature birth, infant mortality, and infant morbidity in your area. Which factors are associated with premature birth in your state? Explore health department data related to premature birth and maternal smoking, alcohol or drug use, maternal age, geographic location (rural versus urban counties), or ethnicity.

- Compare the statistics of your state on low-birth-weight incidence, teenage pregnancy, and infant mortality and morbidity rates with the goals outlined in "Healthy People 2010."

Key Concepts

🌸 Premature infants have special needs for care to assist with normal development.

🌸 The environment of the NICU is a factor that can enhance or detract from development of the high-risk neonate.

🌸 Even high-risk and preterm infants provide cues for caregivers when these infants experience stress.

🌸 The purpose of developmental care is to support the infant's neurobehavioral development and subsystems.

🌸 Developmental care is based on a thorough assessment of the neonate.

Review Questions and Activities

1. What are the common components of a comprehensive developmental care protocol?

2. What has research shown about the light levels in many NICUs?

3. What are the components of sound or noise in the NICU?

4. Identify three strategies for protecting infants from excessive light in the NICU.

5. Identify three strategies for reducing sound levels in the NICU.

6. Define the term *thermoneutral environment*.

7. Identify three strategies for maintaining body temperature in preterm infants.

8. Which characteristics of preterm infants make them particularly vulnerable to heat loss?

9. Define each of the four mechanisms of heat loss in the preterm infant, and identify one strategy for reducing heat loss through each mechanism.

10. What are the risks and benefits of care clustering to preterm infants?

11. What are the components of complete kangaroo care?

12. What are three benefits of kangaroo care as shown by research?

13. Identify three nonpharmacologic measures for providing pain management to preterm infants.

14. Identify three behaviors in preterm infants that may indicate pain or stress.

15. The Brazelton and the NIDCAP are two infant assessment strategies in common use. In which ways are they alike and in which ways do they differ?

References

Ackerman, B., Sherwonit, E., & Williams, J. (1989). Reduced incidental light exposure; Effect on the development of retinopathy of prematurity in low birth weight infants. *Pediatrics, 83,* 958–962.

Agency for Health Care Policy and Research (AHCPR). (1993). *Acute pain management in infants, children, and adolescents: Operative procedures.* (Publication No. 92-0020). Rockville, MD: Agency for Health Care Policy and Research.

Anagnostakis, D., Petmezakis, J., & Matsaniotis, N. (1980). Noise pollution in neonatal units: A potential health hazard. *Acta Paediatrica Scandanavia, 69,* 771–773.

Als, H. (1982). Toward a synactive theory of development: Promise for the assessment and support of infant individuality. *Infant Mental Health Journal, 3,* (4), 237–238.

Als, H. (1984). Newborn behavioral assessment. In W. J. Burns & J. V. Lavigne (Eds.). Progress in pediatric psychology. New York: Grune & Stratton.

Als, H. (1986). A synactive model of neonatal behavioral organization: Framework for the assessment of neurobehavioral development in the premature infant and for the support of infants and parents in the neonatal intensive care environment. *Physical and Occupational Therapy in Pediatrics, 6,* (3–4), 3–53.

Als, H., Lawhon, G., Duffy, F., McAnulty, G., Gibes-Grossman, R., & Blickman, J. (1994). Individualized developmental care for the very low birth weight preterm infant. *JAMA, 272,* 853–858.

Als, H., Lester, B. M., Tronick, E. Z., Brazelton, T. B. (1982). Assessment of preterm infant behavior (APIB). In H. E. Fitzgerald & M. Yogman (Eds.). Theory and research in behavioral pediatrics (Vol. 1, pp. 64–133). New York: Plenum Press.

American Academy of Pediatrics (AAP). (2000). *Changing concepts of sudden infant death syndrome: Implications for infant sleeping environment and sleep position* (RE9946.) American Academy of Pediatrics. Policy Statement *Pediatrics, 105,* (3), 650–656.

American Academy of Pediatrics Committee on Environmental Hazards. (1974). Noise Pollution: Neonatal Aspects. *Pediatrics, 54,* 476–479.

American Nurses Association (ANA). (1998). *Standards of clinical nursing practice* (2nd ed.). American Nurses Association.

Anderson, G. C. (1999). Kangaroo care of the premature infant. In E. Goldson (Ed.) *Nurturing the premature infant: Developmental interventions in the neonatal intensive care nursery.* New York: Oxford University Press.

Appleton, S. (1997). Touch or handling. *Midwives, 110,* (1317), 246.

Arendt, F., Minors, D., & Waterhouse, J. (Eds.), (1989). Basic concepts and implications. *Biological rhythms in clinical practice* (pp. 3–7). Boston, MA: Wright.

Barker, D., & Rutter Y. (1995). Analgesic effect of sucrose. Heel pricks were unnecessarily painful. *BMJ,* 16; 311, (7007), 1–747.

Becker, P., Grunwald, P., Moorman, J., Stuhr, S. (1991). Outcomes of developmentally supportive nursing care for very low birth weight infants. *Nursing Research, 40,* 224–229.

Becker, P., Grunwald, P., Moorman, J., Stuhr, S. (1993). Effects of developmental care on behavioral organization in very low birth weight infants. *Nursing Research, 42,* 214–220.

Bernbaum, J., Pereira, G., Watson, J., & Peckham, G. (1983). Non-nutritive sucking during gavage feeding enhances growth and maturation in preterm infants. *Pediatrics, 71,* (1), 41–45.

Benini, F., Johnston, C., Faucher, D., & Aranda, J. (1993). Topical anesthesia during circumcision in newborn infants. *JAMA, 270,* (7), 850–853.

Bildner, J., & Krechel, S. (1996). Increasing staff awareness of postoperative pain management in the NICU. *Neonatal Network, 15,* (1), 11–16.

Blackburn, S., & Loper, D. (1992). *Maternal, fetal, and neonatal physiology: A clinical perspective.* Philadelphia, PA: W. B. Saunders.

Blackburn, S., & Patterson, D. (1991). Effects of cycled light on activity state and cardiorespiratory function in preterm infants. *Journal of Perinatal-Neonatal Nursing, 4,* (4), 47–54.

Blass, E., & Hofmeyer, L. (1991). Sucrose as an analgesic for newborn infants. *Pediatrics, 87,* (2), 215–218.

Booth, C., Johnson-Crowley, N., & Barnard, K. (1985). Infant massage and exercise: Worth the effort? *MCN: American Journal of Maternal Child Nursing, 10,* 184–189.

Bosque, E., Brady, J., Affonso, D., & Wahlberg, V. (1995). Physiological measures of kangaroo versus incubator care in a tertiary-level nursery. *Journal of Obstetric, Gynecologic, and Neonatal Nursing, 24,* (3), 219–226.

Bozzette, M. (1993). Observation of pain behavior in the NICU: An exploratory study. *Journal of Perinatal and Neonatal Nursing, 7,* (1), 76–87.

Brazelton, T. B. (1984). *Neonatal behavioral assessment scale* (2nd ed.). Philadelphia, PA: J. B. Lippincott.

Brazelton, T. B., & Cramer, B. (1990). *The earliest relationship.* Reading, MA: Addison-Wesley.

Consensus Committee to Establish Recommended Standards for Newborn ICU Design. (1999). Recommended Standards for Newborn ICU Design. Physical and Developmental Environment of the High-Risk Infant Project.

Cooper Evans, J. (1991). Incidence of hypoxaemia associated with caregiving in premature infants. *Neonatal Network, 10,* (2), 17–24.

Corff, K., Seideman, R., Venkataraman, P., Lutes, L., & Yates, B. (1995). Facilitated tucking: A nonpharmacologic comfort measure for pain in preterm neonates. *Journal of Obstetric, Gynecologic, and Neonatal Nursing, 24,* (2), 143–147.

Craig, K., Whitfield, M., Grunau, R., Linton, J., & Hadjistavropoulos, H. (1993). Pain in the preterm neonate: Behavioural and physiological indices. *Pain, 52,* 287–299.

de Leeuw, R., Colin, E., Dunnebier, E., & Mirmiran, M. (1991). Physiological effects of kangaroo care in very small preterm infants. *Biology of the Neonate, 59,* 149–155.

Downs, J., Edwards, A., McCormick, D., & Stewart, A. (1991). Effect of intervention on development of hip posture in very preterm babies. *Archives of Disease in Childhood, 66,* 797–801.

Engebretson, J., & Wardell, D. (1997). Development of a pacifier for low-birth weight infants on nutritive sucking. *Journal of Obstetric, Gynecologic, and Neonatal Nursing, 6,* (6), 660–664.

Fay, M. (1988). The positive effects of positioning. *Neonatal Network, 6,* (5), 23–28.

Field, T., Ignatoff, M., Stringer, S., Brennan, J., Greenberg, R., Widmayer, S., & Anderson, G. (1982). Nonnutritive sucking during tube feeding: Effects on preterm neonates in an intensive care unit. *Pediatrics, 70,* 381–384.

Field, T., Schanberg, S., Scafidi, F., & Bauer, C. R., Vegan-Lahr, N., Garcia, R., Nystrom, J., Kuhn, C. M. (1986). Tactile/kinesthetic stimulation effects on preterm neonates. *Pediatrics, 77,* (5), 654–658.

Field, T., Scafidi, F., & Schanberg, S. (1987). Massage of preterm newborns to improve growth and development. *Pediatric Nursing, 13,* (6), 385–387.

Fielder, A., & Levere, M. (1992). Screening for retinopathy of prematurity. *Archives of Diseases in Childhood, 67,* (7), 860–867.

Fitzgerald, M., Millard, C., & McIntosh, N. (1989). Cutaneous hypersensitivity following peripheral tissue damage in newborn infants and it reversal with topical anesthesia. *Pain, 39,* 31–36.

Fleisher, B., Vandenberg, K., Constantinou, J., Heller, C., Benitz, W., Johnson, A., Rosenthal, A., & Stevenson, D. (1995). Individualized developmental care for very low birth weight premature infants. *Clinical Pediatrics, 34,* 523–529.

Fox, M., & Molesky, M. (1990). The effects of prone and supine positioning on arterial oxygen pressure. *Neonatal Network, 8,* (4), 25–29.

Franck, L., & Gregory, G. (1993). Clinical evaluation and treatment of infant pain in the neonatal intensive care unit. In N. Schechter, C. Berde, & M. Yaster (Eds.), *Pain in infants, children, and adolescents* (pp. 519–535). Baltimore, MD: Williams & Wilking.

Gaedki, R., Doiing, B., Keller, F., & Vogel, A. (1969). The noise level in a children's hospital and the wake-up threshold in infants. *Acta Pediatrica Scand, 58,* 164–170.

Georgieff, M., & Bernbaum, J. (1986). Abnormal shoulder girdle muscle tone in premature infants during their first 18 months of life. *Pediatrics, 77,* (5), 664–669.

Gill, N., Behnke, M., Conlon, M., McNeeley, J., & Anderson, G. (1988). Effect of nonnutritive sucking on behavioral state in preterm infants before feeding. *Nursing Research, 37,* 347–350.

Glass, P. (1988). Role of light toxicity in the developing retinal vasculature. [Review]. *Birth defects: Original Article Series, 24,* 103–117.

Glass, P., Avery, G., Subramanian, K., Keyes, M. P., Sostek, A. M. Friendly, D. S. (1985). Effect of bright light in the hospital environment on the incidence of retinopathy of prematurity. *New England Journal of Medicine, 313,* (7), 401–404.

Glotzbach, S. F., Edgar, D. M., & Ariagno, R. L. (1995). Biological rhythmicity in preterm infants prior to discharge from neonatal intensive care. *Pediatrics, 95,* (2), 231–237.

Gorski, P., Hale, W., & Leonard, C. (1983). Direct computer recording of premature infants and nursing care: Distress following two interventions. *Pediatrics, 72,* 198.

Gray, L., Watt, L., & Blass, E. (2000). Skin to skin contact is analgesic in healthy newborns. *Pediatrics, 105,* 1, 1–6.

Gregory, G., Kitterman, J., Phibbs, R., Tooley, W. H., & Hamilton, W. K. (1971). Treatment of the idiopathic respiratory distress syndrome with continuous, positive airway pressure. *New England Journal of Medicine, 284,* 1333.

Grunau, R., & Craig, K. (1987). Pain expression in neonates: Facial action and cry. *Pain, 28,* 395–410.

Grunau, R., Johnston, C., & Craig, K. (1990). Neonatal facial and cry responses to invasive and non-invasive procedures. *Pain, 42,* 295–305.

Grunau, R., Whitfield, M., & Petrie, J. (1994). Pain sensitivity and temperament in extremely low birth weight premature toddlers and preterm and full-term controls. *Pain, 58,* 341–346.

Hamer, R., Dobson, V., & Mayer, M. (1984). Absolute thresholds in human infants exposed to continuous illumination. *Investigative Ophthalmology and Visual Science, 25,* (4), 381–388.

Harrison, L., & Woods, S. (1991). Early parental touch and premature infants. *Journal of Obstetric, Gynecologic, and Neonatal Nursing, 20,* (4), 299–306.

Hellbrugge, T. (1974). The development of circadian and ultradian rhythms of premature and full-term infants. In L. Schevinng, F. Halberg, J. Pauly (Eds.). *Chronobiology* (pp. 339–341). Stuttgart: Georg Thieme.

Hepner, W., Krause, A., & Davis, M. (1949). Retrolental fibroplasias and light. *Pediatrics, 3,* 824–828.

Hodgkinson, K., Bear, M., Thorn, J., & Van Blaricum, S. (1994). Measuring pain in neonates: Evaluating an instrument and developing a common language. *The Australian Journal of Advanced Nursing, 12,* (1), 17–22.

Hommura, S., Usuki, Y., Takei, K., & Tsuboi, K., Sekine, Y., Fukuda, Y., Terauchi, M. (1988). Ophthalmic care of very low birth weight infants. Report 4. Clinical Studies on the influence of light on the incidence of retinopathy of prematurity. In D. Phelps & Watts, J. (1997). The Cochrane Library. Nippon Gauka Gakkai, 92, (3), 456–461 in Japanese.

Johnston, C., Steven, B., Craig, K., & Grunau, R. (1993). Developmental changes in pain expression in premature, full-term, two- and four-month-old infants. *Pain, 52,* 201–208.

Johnston, C., Stevens, B., Yang, F., & Horton, L. (1995). Differential response to pain by very premature neonates. *Pain, 61,* 471–479.

Jorgensen, K. (1993). *Developmental care of the premature infant: A concise overview.* S. Weymouth, USA: Developmental Care Division of Children's Medical Ventures.

Klaus, M., & Kennell, J. (1982). *Parent-infant bonding.* St. Louis, MO: Mosby.

Landry, R., Scheidt, P., & Hammond, R. (1985). Ambient light and phototherapy conditions of eight neonatal care units. *Pediatrics, 75,* (2 Pt. 2), 434–436.

Lioy, J., & Maginello, P. (1988). A comparison of prone and supine positioning in the immediate post extubation period of neonates. *Journal of Pediatrics, 112,* 982–984.

Locke, J., & Reese, A. (1952). Retrolental fibroplasia. The negative role of light, mydriatics and the opthalmoscopic examination in its etiology. *Archives of Ophthalmology, 48,* 44–47.

Long, J., Lucey, J., & Philip, A. (1980). Noise and hypoxemia in the intensive care nursery. *Pediatrics, 65,* 143–145.

Lotas, M., Seal, E., & Ambrose, B. (2001). NICU lighting levels and patterns revisited: A study in research utilization. Under Review.

Lotas, M., & Medoff-Cooper, B. (2001). Effects of light-dark cycles in the NICU environment on heart rate in the preterm infant. Under Review.

Lotas, M., & Walden, M. (1996). Individualized developmental care for very low birth weight infants: A critical review. *Journal of Obstetric, Gynecologic, and Neonatal Nursing, 25,* (8), 681–687.

Ludington-Hoe, S., Anderson, G., Simpson, S., Hollingsead, A., Argote, L., & Rey, H. (1999). Birth-related fatigue in 34–36 week preterm neonates: Rapid recovery with very early kangaroo (skin-to-skin) care. *Journal of Obstetric, & Gynecologic, and Neonatal Nursing, 28,* (1), 94–103.

Mann, N., Haddow, R., Stokes, L., Goodley, S., & Rutter, N. (1986). Effect of night and day on preterm infants in a newborn nursery: Randomised trial. *British Medical Journal, 293,* (15), 1265–1267.

Masterson, J., Zucker, C., & Schulze, K. (1987). Prone and supine positioning effects on energy expenditure and behaviour of low birth weight neonates. *Pediatrics, 80,* (5), 689–692.

McCain, G. (1992). Facilitating inactive awake states in preterm infants: A study of three interventions. *Nursing Research, 41,* (3), 157–160.

McIntosh, N., van Veen, I., & Brameyer, H. (1994). Alleviation of the pain of heel prick in preterm infants. *Archives of Disease in Childhood, 70,* F177–F181.

Messmer, P. R., Rodriguez, S., Adams, J., Wells-Gentry, J., Washburn, K., Zabaleta, L., & Abren, S. (1997). Effect of kangaroo care on sleep time for neonates. *Pediatric Nursing, 23,* (4), 408–414.

Miller, C., White, R., Whitman, T., O'Callaghan, M., & Maxwell, S. (1995). The effects of cycled versus noncycled lighting on growth and development in preterm infants. *Infant Behavior and Development, 18,* 87–95.

Moore-Ede, M., Sulzman, F., & Fuller, C. (1982). *The clocks that time us: Physiology of the circadian timing system.* Cambridge, MA: Harvard University Press.

Moran, M., Radzyminski, S., Higgins, K., Dowling, D., Miller, M., & Anderson, C. G. (1999). Maternal kangaroo (skin-to-skin) care in the NICU beginning 4 hours postbirth. *MCN; American Journal of Maternal Child Nursing, 24,* (2), 74–79.

Murdoch, D., & Darlow, B. (1984). Handling during neonatal intensive care. *Archives of Disease in Childhood, 59,* 957–961.

National Association of Neonatal Nurses (NANN). (1999). Position paper on pain management in infants (3019). NANN, Glenview, IL: www.nann.org.

National Association of Neonatal Nurses (NANN). (2000). Infant and family centered developmental care guidelines (2101). NANN, Glenview, IL:.

Nelson, D., Heitman, R., & Jennings, C. (1986). Effects of tactile stimulation on premature infant weight gain. *Journal of Obstetric, Gynecologic, and Neonatal Nursing, 15,* (3), 262–267.

Norden, J., Hannallah, R., Getson, P., O'Donnell, R., Kelliher, G., & Walker, N. (1991). Reliability of an objective pain scale in children. *Anesthesia and Analgesia, 72,* (4–6), S199.

Norris, S., Campbell, L., & Brenkert, S. (1982). Nursing procedures and alterations in transcutaneous oxygen tension in premature infants. *Nursing Research, 31,* (6), 330–336.

Palmer, E., Flynn, J., Hardy, R. J., & Phelps, D. L., & Phillips, C. I., Schaffer, D. B., Tung, B. (1991). Incidence and early course of retinopathy of prematurity. *Ophthalmology, 98,* (11) 1628–1640.

Paterson, L. (1990). Baby massage in the neonatal unit. *Nursing, 4,* (23), 19–21.

Perez-Woods, R., Malloy, M., & Tse, A. (1992). Positioning and skin care of the low birth weight neonate. *NAACOG's Clinical Issues in Perinatal and Women's Health, 3,* (1), 97–113.

Peters, K. (1992). Does routine nursing care complicate the physiologic status of the premature neonate with respiratory distress syndrome? *Journal of Perinatal-Neonatal Nursing, 6,* (2), 67–84.

Pettigrew, A., Edwards, D., & Henderson-Smart, D. (1988). Perinatal risk factors in preterm infants. *Medical Journal of Australia, 148,* (4), 174–177.

Phelps, D., & Watts, J. (1997). Early light reduction to prevent retinopathy of prematurity in very low birth weight infants. *The Cochrane Library, 3,* 1–11.

Porter, F. (1993). Pain assessment in children: Infants. In N. Schechter, C. Berde, & M. Yaster (Eds.). *Pain in infants, children, and adolescents* (pp. 87–96). Baltimore, MD: Williams, & Wilkins.

Porter, E., & Anderson, G. (1979). Non-nutritive sucking during tube feedings: Effect on clinical course in premature infants. *Journal of Obstetric, Gynecologic, and Neonatal Nursing, 8,* 265–272.

Repka, M., Fulton, A., Petersen, R., Robinson, J., & Simons, M. (1995). Retinopathy and light. Unpublished data.

Reppert, S. (1992). Pre-natal development of a hypothalamic biological clock. In Swaab, M., Hofman, M., Mirmiran, R., & van Leeuwen, F. (Eds.). *Progress in brain research,* (Vol. 93). New York: Elsevier Science Publishers.

Rey, E., & Martinez, H. (1983). Manejo Racional del Nino Prematuro. *Proceedings of the Conference I Curso de Medicina Fetal y Neonatal, Bogata, 1981.* Bogata, Columbia: Fundacion Vivar (Spanish). (Manuscript available in English from UNICEF, 3 UN Plaza, New York, NY, 10017.)

Riley, P., & Slater, T. (1969). Pathogenesis of retrolental fibroplasias. *Lancet, 2,* (614), 265.

Robertson, A., & Philbin, M. (1996). Studies of sound and auditory development. Paper presented at the Physical and Developmental Environment of the High Risk Neonate, January 31, 1996. Clearwater Beach, FL: University of South Florida College of Medicine.

Robinson, J., Moseley, M., & Fielder, A. (1990). Illuminance of neonatal units. *Archives of Diseases in Childhood, 65,* (7, Spec. No.), 679–682.

Russell, J. (1993). Touch and infant massage. *Paediatric Nursing, 5,* (3), 8, 10–11.

Schanbert, S., & Field, T. (1987). Sensory deprivation, stress and supplemental stimulation in the rat pup and the preterm neonate. *Child Development, 58,* 1431–1447.

Seiberth, V., Linderkamp, O., Knorz, M., & Liesenhoff, H. (1994). A controlled clinical trial of light and retinopathy of prematurity. *American Journal of Ophthalmology, 118,* 492–495.

Shiroiwa, Y., Kamiya, Y., & Uchiboi, S. (1986). Activity, cardiac and respiratory responses of blindfold preterm infants in a neonatal intensive care unit. *Early Human Development, 14,* 259–265.

Silverman, W., Sinclair, J., & Agate, F. (1966). The oxygen cost of minor changes in heat balance of small newborn infants. *Acta Paediatrica Scandinavia, 55,* 294.

Speidel, B. (1978). Adverse effects of routine procedures on preterm infants. *Lancet, 1,* 864–866.

Spinelli, D. (1990). Plasticity triggering experiences, nature and the dual genesis of brain structure and function. *Clinical Perinatology, 17,* 77–82.

Stevens, B., & Johnston, C. (1994). Physiological responses of premature infants to a painful stimulus. *Nursing Research, 43,* (4), 226–231.

Stevens, B., Johnston, C., & Horton, L. (1994). Factors that influence the behavioral pain responses of premature infants. *Pain, 59,* 101–109.

Stevens, B., Johnston, C., & Horton, L. (1993). Multidimensional pain assessment in premature neonates: A pilot study. *Journal of Obstetric, Gynecologic, and Neonatal Nursing, 22,* (6), 531–541.

Stevens, B., Johnston, C., Petryshen, P., & Taddio, A. (1996). The premature infant pain profile: Development and validation. *The Clinical Journal of Pain, 12,* (1), 13–22.

Taddio, A., Goldbach, M., Ipp, M., Stevens, B., & Koren, G. (1995). Effect of circumcision on pain responses during vaccination in male infants. *Lancet, 345,* 291–292.

Taeusch, W., & Ballard, R. (1998). *Avery's diseases of the newborn.* Philadelphia, PA: W. B. Saunders.

Tenreiro, S., Dowse, H., D'Souza, S., & Minors, D., Chiswick, M., Simms, D., & Waterhouse, J. (1991). The development of ultradian and circadian rhythms in premature babies maintained in constant conditions. *Early Human Development, 27,* 33–52.

Thomas, K. (1989). How the NICU environment sounds to a preterm infant. *MCN American of Maternal-Child Nursing, 14,* (4), 249–251.

Ventura, S. J., Martin, J. A., Curtin, S. C., Mathews, T., & Park, M. (2000). *Births: Final data for 1998.* U.S. Department of Health and Human Services, National Center for Health Statistics, Washington, DC: U.S. Government Printing Office.

Whalberg, V. (1991). The "Kangaroo method" and breastfeeding in low birth weight babies. *NU Nytt om U-landshalsovvard, 5,* 23–27.

Whalberg, V., Affonso, D., & Persson, B. (1992). A retrospective comparative study using the kangaroo method as a complement to standard incubator care. *European Journal of Public Health, 2,* (1), 34–37.

White-Traut, R., & Hutchens Pate, C. (1987). Modulating infant state in premature infants. *Journal of Pediatric Nursing, 2,* (2), 96–101.

Whitley, S., & Cowan, M. (1991). Developmental intervention in the newborn intensive care unit. *NAACOG's Clinical Issues in Perinatal and Women's Health Nursing, 2,* (1), 84–110.

Wolke, D. (1987). Environmental neonatology. *Archives of Disease in Childhood, 62,* 987–988.

Woodson, R., Drinkwin, J., & Hamilton, C. (1985). Effects of non-nutritive sucking on state and activity: Term-preterm comparisons. *Infant Behaviour and Development, 8,* (4), 435–441.

Young, T., & Mangum, O. (1997). NeoFax: A manual of drugs used in neonatal care (10th ed.). Raleigh, NC: Acorn Publishing.

Suggested Readings

American Academy of Pediatrics (AAP). (1992). *Guidelines for Perinatal Care,* (3rd ed.). Elk Grove Village, IL: American Academy of Pediatrics.

American Academy of Pediatrics (AAP). (1997). Noise: a hazard for the fetus and newborn (RE9728). American Academy of Pediatrics. Policy Statement *Pediatrics,* 100, (4).

Attia, J., Amiel-Tison, C., Mayer, M., Shnider, S., & Barrier, G. (1987). Measurement of postoperative pain and narcotic administration in infants using a new clinical scoring system. *Anesthesiology, 67,* (3A), A532.

Barr, R. (1992). Is this infant in pain? Caveats from the clinical setting. *American Pain Society Journal, 1,* (3), 187–190.

Elmore, S., Betrus, P., & Burr, R. (1994). Light, social zeitgebers, and the sleep-wake cycle in the entrainment of human circadian rhythms. *Research in Nursing and Health, 17,* 471–478.

Graven, S., Bowen, F., Brooten, D., Eaton, A., Graven, M., Hack, M., Hall, L., Hansen, N., Morrow, G., Oehler, J., Poland, R., Ram, B., Sauve, R., Taylor, P., Ward, S., & Sommers, J. (1992). The high risk infant environment: Part I. The role of the neonatal intensive care unit in the outcome of high-risk infants. *Journal of Perinatology, 12,* (2), 164–172.

Gunnar, M., Connors, J., Isenssee, J., & Wall, L. (1988). Adrenocortical activity and behavioral distress in human newborns. *Developmental Psychobiology, 21,* (4), 297–310.

Lawrence, J., Alcock, D., McGrath, P., Kay, J., MacMurray, S., & Dulberg, C. (1993). The development of a tool to assess neonatal pain. *Neonatal Network, 12,* (6), 59–66.

Lopes, J., Braz, R., Moreira, M., Motta, M., & (1997). A randomized trial of the effects of ambient light on the incidence of retinopathy of prematurity. *Pediatric Research, 41,* 954A.

Nading, J., & Landes, R. (1984). Oxygen tension changes due to non-nutritive sucking (NNS) during orogastric tube feeding. *Pediatric Research, 18,* (4), 206.

Rushforth, J., & Levene, M. (1994). Behavioral response to pain in healthy neonates. *Archives of Disease in Childhood, 70,* F174–F176.

Spears, H. (1986). *Drawing from the Newborn: Poems and drawings of infants in crisis.* Port Angeles, WA: Ben-Simon Publications.

Stevens, B., Johnston, C., & Grunau, R. (1995). Issues of assessment of pain and discomfort in neonates. *Journal of Obstetrics, Gynecologic, and Neonatal Nursing, 24,* (9), 849–855.

Resources

Information regarding kangaroo care can be obtained from Gene Cranston Anderson, PhD, RN, FAAN, Mellen Professor of Nursing, Frances Payne Bolton School of Nursing, Case Western Reserve University, 10900 Euclid Avenue, Cleveland, OH 44106-4904.

Information on prevention of SIDS and resources for parents can be obtained from www.aap.or/new/sids/reduceth.htm.

UNIT IX

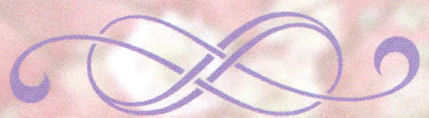

Special Considerations

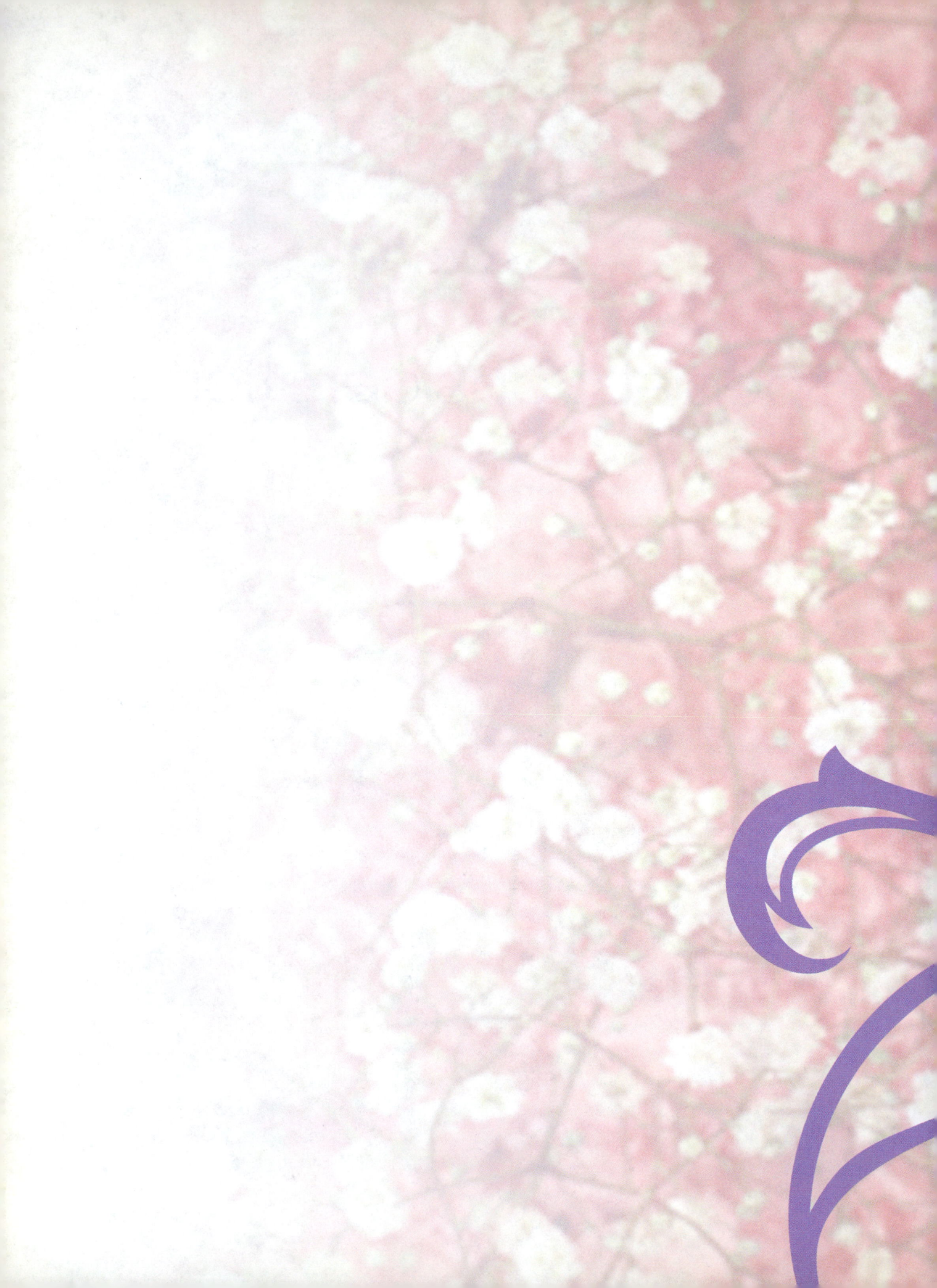

CHAPTER 37

Grief and the Family in the Perinatal Experience

The client sits alone in a darkened room. She has just been told that her baby has died in utero. As you enter, she says that she cannot believe this is happening. "This is my Christmas baby. They must be wrong. What will I do?"

As her nurse you will need to have an understanding of perinatal grief, a recognition of your own responses to death, and a knowledge of ways to best support a grieving parent.

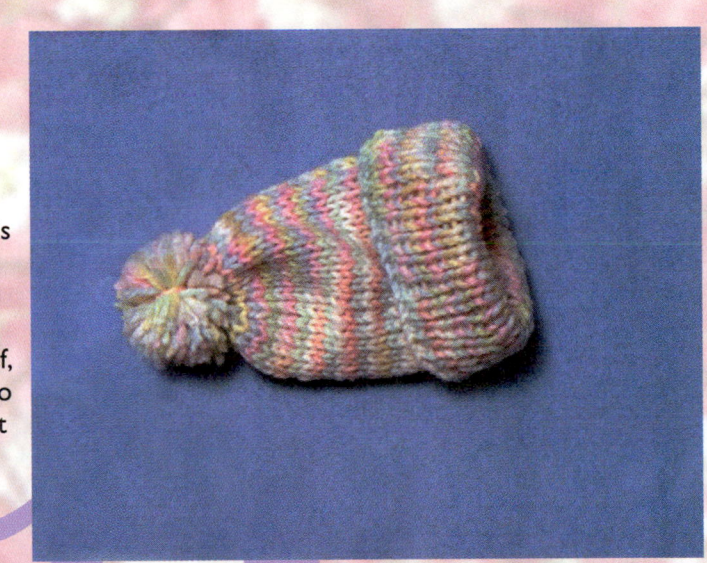

Key Terms

Anticipatory grieving	Dysfunctional grieving	Neonatal death	Reproductive loss
Attachment	Grief	Pathological grief	Sudden infant death
Chronic grief	Grief work	Relinquishment	syndrome (SIDS)

Competencies

Upon completion of this chapter, the reader should be able to:

1. Describe the phases of the perinatal bereavement process.
2. Analyze the behaviors that would be demonstrated by the bereaved mother and father.
3. Analyze assessment techniques for bereavement.
4. Describe five ways caregivers can support the emotional states of clients.
5. Compare unique aspects of gender grief, including the differences of inward and outward grief.
6. Demonstrate compassionate ways of presenting information and options to the person in crisis.

Perinatal nursing is an exciting and busy specialty that encompasses the best in working with clients as they begin their families. By definition, perinatal is the interval from about 28 weeks' gestation to about 28 days after birth (Anderson, 1998). Perinatal nurses work with clients in low- and high-risk obstetrics, at infertility clinics, and in the high-tech world of neonatal intensive care. Perinatal nurses work with clients during the physical and emotional adjustments of postpartum life.

An early miscarriage or the shattering experience of a death during the perinatal period also is part of perinatal nursing. The way in which caregivers support the client and family can make a profound difference in their grief work and their future health. The grieving parents are experiencing the death of their infant along with the end of all their hopes and dreams for that infant.

In the early 1900s, stillbirth, pregnancy loss, neonatal loss, and childhood death were commonplace. It was not unusual for a woman to lose half of her pregnancies and children. At that time, sterile technique was relatively new, and diseases and disorders that are easily controlled today by antibiotics, vaccines, and blood transfusions many times resulted in death. Family members grieving for an infant were supported by the community, and grieving mothers were supported by other women. The grieving process had a structure, for example, a particular color of clothing was to be worn and for a prescribed period. Members of the social structure knew their roles in bereavement. As science

and medicine advanced, labor and delivery moved into the hospital to be handled scientifically and the rate of perinatal death decreased dramatically. Today, it is unusual for problems to occur in pregnancy that result in the death of the infant (less than 1%). The reduced incidence of perinatal loss has, in turn, decreased the ability of clients and families to cope with this tragic event because they may never have experienced the death of a close family member.

When an unexpected death occurs, there is disappointment and loss of what could have been. A person's response to the loss results from a combination of factors: life experience, education, culture, traditions, and beliefs. The feeling of being in crisis and the need for support can depend on the type of loss being experienced and on the background and beliefs of the person.

PSYCHOLOGY OF LOSS

From the time of Freud, loss and bereavement were seen as a pathological experience. It was not until the work of David Peretz in the early 1970s that it became understood that there are different types of losses, all of which impact our lives. Losses take different forms; they may be sudden, gradual, traumatic, or not traumatic. Peretz (1970) has grouped losses into four categories:

1. The first and most obvious loss occurs through the death of a significant loved one or valued person or through separation, such as in divorce.

2. The second category is loss of some aspect of the "self"; that is, the overall mental representation or image a person has of the self is significantly altered. This type of loss includes ideas and feelings about worthiness, attractiveness, lovability, self-esteem, and status. It also includes physical aspects of the self. For example, part of the physical self can be lost by surgery, such as a hysterectomy, or in an accident, such as limb amputation. This type of loss also can be related to fantasies or expectations about a desired career or a pregnancy that failed to produce a healthy infant.

3. The third category is loss of external objects. External objects are personal possessions, such as money, property, and keepsakes. These losses can occur from, for example, difficult economic times, natural disasters, or robbery. During a pregnancy, the objects would include infant toys and clothing bought in preparation for the birth.

4. The last category of loss is loss that occurs during development. These losses are normal and occur naturally in the process of living. There is no real growth or change without loss (Simos, 1979). For example, a child loses the status of being the only child when a sibling arrives, young adults lose the close relationship with their parents when they move away from home and begin living independently, and women lose the physical ability to procreate at menopause.

The reaction to any loss is an individual one based on previous experience and shaped by traditions, culture, and spiritual beliefs. A client's perception of loss translates into grief. Because grief is an emotional rather than an intellectual or rational response the feelings often seem crazy, out of control, overwhelming, and all-consuming to the individual (Ewton, 1993). A supportive environment and an openness to discussion, about the meaning of the loss are most beneficial to parents when a perinatal death occurs.

Attachment

To understand loss, one must first understand **attachment**. British psychiatrist John Bowlby established the early work on attachment. His theory (1969) looks at how human beings create strong affectionate bonds with others and the strong emotional reaction that occurs when those bonds are threatened or broken. Bowlby believed that attachment behavior is distinct from feeding and sexual behavior; attachment behavior is seen in almost all species of mammals and has a role in survival.

Pregnancy is a maturational crisis; it is a time of loss of previous roles and a transition into new roles. Pregnancy is a time of planning for the future. Dreams, which may have had their basis in childhood, are about to be realized.

The loss of roles becomes overshadowed by the hopes for this new life and new family dynamic. At any point when the experience does not meet the expectations, there is a sense of loss, change, and transition.

Consider the four developmental tasks of pregnancy (Rubin, 1967) experienced by the mother and the emotions involved when a loss occurs at any of these stages. During the first 3 months thoughts turn inward as the pregnancy is validated. A woman's focus is on her changing body. A loss at this point can be seen as something wrong with her body, which was unable to support the pregnancy. From 4 to 6 months, a stage of fetal embodiment (a sense someone is really in there) occurs. The pregnant woman relies on her mate and reviews conflicts with her own mother. A pregnancy loss at this point may lead the woman to question her ability as a mother. Fetal distinction begins at 6 months when the mother views the baby as an individual distinct from herself. Because of this increasing sense of responsibility there is a keen interest in gathering information related to a healthy infant. When the infant dies at this point the pain of severed emotional ties is observed because, in most cases, the developed fetus is seen as a person.

Attachment begins in utero and is the basis for the emotional pain experienced by the mother regardless of whether she sees or holds her infant after the delivery. The fourth task, binding-in, occurs when she prepares to give up the baby to the birth process and usually begins at 8 to 9 months. Mothers report an empty feeling, anticipating a physical emptiness and a new set of responsibilities. When a death occurs at this stage the emptiness and pain of literally losing the baby can be devastating.

Technology has enabled parents to see the fetus at earlier stages (on ultrasonography). By talking about the meaning of the pregnancy and their hopes and plans for the child, parents exhibit signs of attachment. To experience attachment is to be vulnerable to grief. Once the delivery or procedure diagnosing the end of the pregnancy has occurred and the realization of the ending of these hopes and dreams begins, feelings of overwhelming sadness and emptiness occur.

REFLECTIONS FROM A CLIENT

"I can't believe this is true, that we've lost our baby. I want to go to sleep so that I can wake up and it will be ok. Half of my brain is screaming 'No!' while the other half is trying to list all the people to call and the things we need to do."

Grief

Grief is an intense and personal experience in response to a loss. Grief, as a response of sadness to a death, can have common characteristics, although the process is very individual. A person's response to a death or loss depends on culture, traditions, reaction to past losses, circumstances surrounding the death, and the perceived available support networks. Bowlby (1969, 1980) states that infants as young as 6 months can experience a grief reaction.

Freud's (1917) classic work was the first to connect mourning and depression. In "Mourning and melancholia," Freud separated patterns of mourning from the malignant features of melancholia, which differs from grief in that it brings with it a profound lowering of self-esteem not seen in mourning. Lindemann (1944), known best for his work with survivors of the Coconut Grove night club fire, followed the 32 survivors and the relatives of the 491 people who died in the fire. Lindemann was convinced that **pathologic grief** was a distortion of the normal bereavement process and was the first to suggest that a stoic response to death was abnormal behavior. He believed **grief work** must have three components: accepting the painful emotions involved, actively reviewing the experiences and events, and testing new patterns of interaction and role relationships. The behaviors found in normal grief work are listed in Box 37-1. Lindemann (1944) stated, "The duration of a grief reaction

REFLECTIONS FROM A CLIENT

"Seeing pregnant women or a newborn really tears me up. It should be me! Not that I wish anything bad for them, but why couldn't I be with my baby, too? I even find myself looking for babies that would be about the age of my baby having the same features, just so I could 'see' her again."

seems to depend on the success with which a person does the grief work." Lindemann's work was translated by Davidson (1979) to describe the response of the survivors-parents experiencing a perinatal death (Table 37-1).

The four stages identified by Davidson are shock and numbness, searching and yearning, disorientation, and reorganization. Shock and numbness also can occur when a prenatal diagnosis of a fatal disease or anomaly is made. Grieving parents report walking around "as if in a daze." After a birth and subsequent death, many times the mother may seem to be doing well at the wake; in reality, however, she is numb and is only responding to basic needs. According to Davidson, it is later, usually 3 weeks to 3 months, when she feels the full impact of the death and begins to realize what has occurred. By this time, the numbness has subsided and she is without the support of most family and friends.

As the shock and numbness stage comes to an end, searching and yearning begin. Davidson describes the searching and yearning phase as being characterized by restlessness, anger, guilt, and ambiguity. Searching is the need to identify what has happened and who and what was lost. There is yearning for what could have been. Every pregnant woman or infant the grieving mother sees is a reminder of what could have been. This also is a time for searching for details about the birth, diagnosis, and reasons for the death. Mothers report a physical ache in their arms from wanting to hold their infant, dreaming, and being preoccupied by "What if." The mother may be very sensitive to stimuli, restless, and impatient. Anger also is seen at this time. Anger is helpful because it is a real feeling and is a change from the numbness that was felt previously. The characteristics of searching and yearning peak around the time numbness has worn off and reappear with intensity at the anniversary of the death. The need to have questions answered and to gather mementos takes on renewed energy. It is an ideal time for parents to consider joining a group for support, to hear about the experiences of others, and to see how other parents are coping.

Box 37-1 Symptomatology of Normal Grief

- Acute grief: sensations of somatic distress occurring in waves and lasting 20 to 60 minutes
- Feeling of tightness in the throat
- Choking, with shortness of breath
- Need for sighing (recovering the oxygen level in the body)
- Empty feeling in the abdomen
- Lack of muscular power
- Intense subjective distress described as tension
- Frequent crying
- Slight sense of unreality
- Preoccupation with the image of the deceased
- Preoccupation with guilt ("If only . . .")
- Irritability and anger
- Restlessness
- Lack of energy

Lindemann, E. (1944). Symptomatology and management of acute grief. *American Journal of Psychiatry, 101,* 141–148.

Table 37-1 Normal Characteristics of Stages of Grief

Stage of Grief	Characteristics
Shock and numbness (24 h–3 wk)	• Resistance to stimuli and denial • Difficulty in making judgments • Impeded functioning • Emotional outbursts • Stunned feelings
Searching and yearning (3 wk–4 mo, with occasional recurrences)	• Extreme sensitivity to stimuli • Anger and guilt • Restlessness and impatience • Ambiguity • Testing of reality
Disorientation (intensity lifts by 7 mo)	• Disorganization • Depression and lowered self-esteem • Guilt • Anorexia • Awareness of reality and increasing acceptance of death
Reorganization (18–24 mo)	• Sense of release • Renewed energy and the ability to plan for the future • Better judgment • Stable eating and sleeping patterns • Stabilization of old relationships and formation of new ones

Davidson, G. W. (1979). *Understanding mourning*. Minneapolis, MN: Augsburg Publishing.

According to Davidson, just as the searching comes to an end, a sense of disorientation is felt. Disorientation usually occurs 5 to 6 months after the death and peaks just before the first anniversary. Clients may feel disorganized and depressed and may speak of feelings of guilt. This reaction is common; it is now that they are aware of the reality of the death and emptiness this loss has brought and no longer are testing what is true. This may be a time of weight loss or gain, difficulty with sleep patterns, and physical illness. Disorientation often diminishes after the grieving person has completed a cycle of "firsts" without the child they had expected; that is, they have experienced the first Mother's Day or Father's Day, Thanksgiving, birth and death anniversaries, and other significant dates. Experiencing these events is crucial to grief work and constitutes some of the most difficult moments in the grief work. If clients are in a support system at this point, the resources to help them through each of these significant dates are invaluable. During this time of disorientation, there has been a low-level sense of reorganization. The client may report a brief period of renewed energy, a "new normal." As the first 18 months pass, there is a sense of release and a pattern of stable eating and sleeping habits. This begins to occur because clients have survived the cycle of firsts and now have life experience without their "wished for" child. At the end of the second year, the client and family begin to understand what has happened and reconcile this into their lives. By no means are they over the death. They have only just begun to understand the impact of and will forever be changed by these events. They continually will strive to "keep it together" and at the same time understand there is something—someone—missing.

REFLECTIONS FROM A CLIENT

"When this first happened, I could not even catch my breath. I felt like I was drowning. Now I look back, and I can't imagine how I survived. I believe I am stronger for having had her. Her life does have meaning, and it will affect the rest of my life. I will never forget her. I am a different person now, with different expectations, especially about childbearing. I no longer believe that you get pregnant and then you have a healthy baby. I know there is so much more that happens—that can happen—and that it's a miracle to have a healthy baby!"

REFLECTIONS FROM A CLIENT

"I felt as if a weight had been lifted. I didn't miss her any less, it just was different. I didn't think of her with sadness every moment of the day. Now when I think of her, it may be about what we might have been doing if she were here. She's always in my heart. I'll always carry her with me."

Even though Davidson's research identified trends, it is important to remember that there can be wide variations between persons. Some parents report that the numbness is gone after the first 24 hours; others say it takes a few weeks. Most parents report a feeling of reorganization after all the first anniversaries have passed (around 18 to 24 months). Most parents find relief in understanding the complexity of grief and its variable reactions as well as the emotional and physical exhaustion that often accompanies grief. Consequently, it is important to assess individual personal responses to grief and to plan nursing interventions accordingly. Davidson used his findings in combination with the vision of Sr. Jane Marie Lamb to create the basis for the first international perinatal grief support program called SHARE Pregnancy and Infant Loss Support, Inc. This program has been a model for professionals and a critical link for families since the late 1970s.

Loss of a Dream

According to Peretz (1970), loss is simultaneously a real event and a perceptual or symbolic event. Perception clearly can create intense reactions. Some women who are committed to a vaginal birth but then must deliver by cesarean section react to this birth process as a loss. The woman perceives she has lost the experience of a normal vaginal birth. Parents often develop expectations or dreams about the pregnancy and infant. Even though the parents are unclear about the appearance of the child, they have aspirations and hopes attached to the child's future. When the pregnancy is terminated or when the infant dies, all of these hopes and dreams are crushed. They never will be fulfilled, and the parents experience great sadness around what might have been. This same sadness and emptiness can occur with each milestone that would have occurred if the child had lived. For example, first steps, the first day of kindergarten, graduations, and weddings remind parents of what could have been, and they revisit the loss at these times. It is helpful to talk about these dreams.

REPRODUCTIVE LOSS

Reproductive loss can include monthly menstruation for the infertile couple, miscarriage, preterm birth, birth of a child with an anomaly, death of one or more of a multiple gestation, intrauterine fetal death, neonatal death, relinquishment, and sudden infant death syndrome (SIDS). All of these losses result in the process of grief, which varies in length and intensity. Grief can cause physical and emotional distress and is a process of remembering. The nurse's role is to create a safe environment and provide support so the client or couple can recognize how this crisis will affect their lives and thus begin the work of grieving. The term *grief resolution* is a misnomer. It is inaccurate and leads to the false assumption that parents get over the loss of an infant. They will never get over the death of their dreams for the child. Parents will talk about an infant 10, 20, and even 40 years after the death as though the event happened yesterday. The nurse in different settings, over time, can help the survivors as they work through the grief and incorporate the meaning of this loss into their lives.

Nurses working with a family in crisis must be consistent, especially in the use of concepts and terminology. The ability to have common nomenclature and definitions is critical to education, discussion of issues, and understanding concerns related to perinatal loss and bereavement. Refer to the Key Terms section for common nomenclature.

Fetal Death

Even though fetal death through spontaneous abortion Carson (2000) is the most common reproductive loss (occurring in 2 out of every 15 pregnancies), historically our society has not recognized this event as being significant. Over the past 15 years, however, religious leaders and funeral directors have noted the move toward families wanting services and burial or cremation for their losses that have occurred before 20 weeks' gestation, whether or not there is an identifiable fetus. The client may not recognize the depth of the impact of this pregnancy loss because her support system has no outward expression of sympathy. Fetal loss that occurs in the first trimester also may symbolizes a loss of self because at this point in the pregnancy the fetus is not yet perceived as a separate person. Reconciliation of this loss occurs when the client or couple acknowledges that the outcome was not within their control.

Postmiscarriage distress is identified by perceived physical and emotional trauma at delivery and emotional distress related to poor follow-up (Lee & Slade, 1996). Because of the possibility that a follow-up program or support group would lessen the emotional distress, written resources and a telephone number to use when needed should be part of the discharge information.

Therapeutic abortion is the termination of a pregnancy by medical intervention owing to a fatal anomaly or risk to the mother's life. Two procedures are used. Dilatation and curettage (D&C), which is opening of the cervix and scraping of the uterine lining to empty the contents, can be done in the surgical suite of a labor and delivery unit. Dilatation and evacuation (D&E), in which suction is used to remove the products of conception, also is a surgical procedure. Regardless of the circumstance, a feeling of sadness and regret may be experienced. When an abnormality in the fetus is diagnosed, the client or couple are given a choice. If the mother's life is not in jeopardy, the choice is to end the pregnancy now or let nature take its course. The decision must be made quickly in most cases because test results usually are not available until around the time of fetal viability. Once beyond that point, most hospitals in most states will not permit a therapeutic abortion to be performed. Families who undergo elective abortion, for whatever reason, experience loss.

In addition to the termination of a pregnancy owing to a fatal diagnosis, some families who are grappling with the excitement and fears of a multiple pregnancy are faced with the decision of selective reduction to save the remaining fetuses. Whether multiple gestation is due to fertility drugs or naturally occurring, the human body is not structured to maintain multiple gestations. In many cases, the client will have complications, with preterm labor being the most common. In order to do the greatest good, a recommendation may be made to decrease the number of developing fetuses, to give the remaining babies the nutrition, circulation, and room they need to have better outcomes. When a decision of this magnitude must be made, it is critical to recognize there will be unanswered questions and the need for information. Written materials for the client to take home are beneficial because she may be unable to absorb and retain new information easily.

When a multiple pregnancy is progressing well and one (or more) fetus dies, either before or after birth, the grief response becomes more complex. The parents are attempting to attach to the surviving infants while grieving the loss of the one who has died. Bowlby (1980), who identified the tasks in attachment, said it is humanly impossible to attach to more than one human being at a time. When parents are attempting to attach to several infants and to grieve for the one who has died, their emotions are confusing. As they plan for the burial of the one who has died, the parents will have to work to get to know the surviving infants. The attachment process may be interrupted as the parents grieve. They may rationalize that the sibling died so that the others could live. Because this situation is unique, it calls for a specialized type of grief work. Support programs exist for families who experience a multiple gestation pregnancy in which not all infants survive.

Once fetal movement is felt, parents are filled with hope and expectation. They feel a level of comfort knowing there really is a separate living person in the mother's womb. Antepartum death at this point usually occurs suddenly and without warning. Spontaneous labor usually begins within 2 weeks of the death. When the death is diagnosed before delivery the knowledge that the fetus is dead will result in great emotional difficulty for the mother. She may be given the option of having labor induced. Because she has a sense of helplessness and disbelief, however, the mother may choose to wait until labor begins spontaneously. During labor, she has hope that everyone is wrong, resulting in the conflicting emotions of hope and dread. Her pain is heightened, and the need for pain management is critical. The mother staying alert during the delivery and being able to see her infant allows her to confirm what the infant looks like and to connect the infant with her family. Being able to see and touch the infant facilitates the grief work. Mementos of the infant's life inside the womb become precious. Ultrasonographic pictures may be the only tangible evidence of the infant's existence.

REFLECTIONS FROM A CLIENT

"They told us we had a choice! Therapeutic abortion or delivery of a dead fetus? What kind of a choice is that? We want our baby. At first we were in shock, but when they said we only had 3 days to decide, we had to pull ourselves together and ask some questions. Our questions were mainly about how sure they were and if there was anything that could be done to save our child. We never even asked about the procedure or thought about how we would feel after the procedure. What a terrible position to be in, to have to make this decision. No one else could truly understand the chaos churning inside us."

Loss of the Perfect Baby

Once the pregnancy test result is positive, a woman begins to plan. She knows the possible due date and begins to fantasize about her child's future. This trajectory of hopes and dreams that may extend into the child's adult years can be halted abruptly by the birth of an infant who does not meet parents' expectations or by the death of the

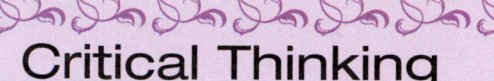

Critical Thinking

Fetal Demise

How do you feel about entering the room of a client whose infant is dying? Will your need to "make it better" cause you to use clichés or try to find a reason for parents? Will you choose to limit your contact with the client because of your discomfort? Or, can you sit down and listen to the family's story?

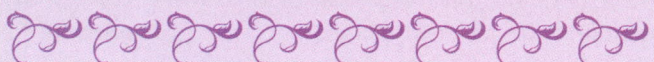

infant. Parents will grieve the loss of their expectations: a full-term healthy boy or girl with certain features. They also must grieve the loss of the idealized infant before they will be able to adapt and attach to the real child. Parents of premature infants and infants who have anomalies or deformities will ask themselves how a thing such as this could have happened. As the parents attempt to attach, they also have concerns that the child may not survive. The roller coaster of emotions may be overwhelming. Nurses can be most helpful by listening to parents without making judgments. The degree of their grief reaction may not be equal to the level of severity or critical state of the child. It is the personal meaning of the anomaly or the reaction to the shock of not having the child they imagined that will give form to the grief.

Once a child is born, parents are relieved. Even when the infant is born prematurely, parents believe something can be done to help their infant survive, especially since technology has improved so much in recent years. In many cases, something can be done. It must be remembered, however, that these parents have been thrown into the role of preterm parents without warning. It is frightening to see one's infant for the first time attached to equipment and wires. Most staff of neonatal intensive care units (NICUs) have a good working knowledge of what it takes to orient parents to the unit and the importance of getting them involved as early as possible as parents. Supporting the new mother to provide breast milk for her infant from the beginning—even thought it may be weeks before it can be used—helps foster the parental role. Care of the infant by parents continues to show results in the infant through improved weight gain and response to therapy. If the infant were to die in the NICU, the interdisciplinary care team would continue to work the with parents to assist them in making the transition from having the hope of taking their infant home to having the needs involved in the death of a child. The death of an infant will have a lifelong effect on the family. The care provided to them in the

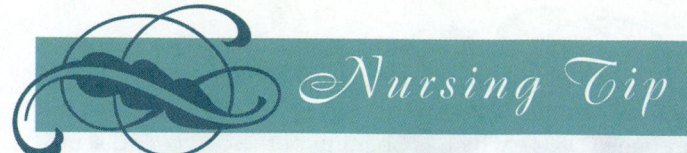

** Nursing Tip **

SPIRITUAL ASSESSMENT

Routinely include the chaplain in the admission process so that a spiritual assessment can be done. Valuable information gained related to the religious and cultural beliefs that surround birth and death will assist the nurse in planning care for families of infants in crisis.

hospital and the follow-up care during the first 18 months after the death will shape their future.

Sudden Infant Death

If the child is healthy at birth or is premature and survives the neonatal period, graduating from the NICU, the family will be given instructions on what to do to decrease the risk of SIDS. **Sudden infant death syndrome,** or **SIDS,** refers to any death of an infant that is unexpected and in which a thorough postmortem examination, medical history, and case study demonstrate adequate care before death (www:sidsalliance.org). Infants are most at risk for SIDS during the first 6 months of life. SIDS usually occurs during sleep, with no evidence of disease.

Relinquishment

Relinquishment refers to a mother's decision to give up her right to parent her child. Doing so may cause silent grieving that needs recognition. By carrying an infant to term, the feelings of attachment and detachment are simultaneous. A woman who goes through the birth process and then relinquishes her infant will experience a grief process that is prolonged and that may intensify over time

REFLECTIONS FROM A CLIENT

"Why me? All my friends are sexually active. Why was I the one to get pregnant? It's so unfair to me and my baby. I couldn't even look at a couple with a new baby without getting angry. I knew adoption was the right thing to do for my baby, but deep down I still did not want to give him up."

KEY ACTIONS FOR WORKING WITH MOTHERS WHO ARE RELINQUISHING

1. Prepare the birth parents for hospitalization and delivery. Explain their rights, discuss their options for contact with the child, and ensure that decisions and information are provided in written form. Include information on the grief process early in all discussions.

2. Validate the importance of the birth parents' roles. Recognize the birth mother's contribution to the child's life through caring for herself during the pregnancy and the work of delivery. Naming the infant is another way to validate the experience and give the birth parents someone for whom to grieve.

3. Encourage the birth parents to see, hold, and spend time in private with the baby. According to Roles (1997), one of the main regrets of parents who give up the right to parent their child is the decision not to see the infant.

4. Reconfirm the commitment to the adoption decision. Doubts that arise must be discussed immediately with the social worker or counselor before consent forms are signed. Parents need to understand the adoption law that rules the waiting period, that they have the opportunity to change their minds, and the irrevocability of the consent once the form is signed.

5. Assist the birth parents in creating memories. Just as it is recommended that mementos be created for parents grieving the death of an infant, the same rationale applies here.

6. Acknowledge the birth mother's role. Give ample opportunity during the postpartum period for the birth mother to discuss the pregnancy, labor, and birth, especially because the opportunity may be limited once she returns home.

7. Treat birth mothers with respect. When mothers are able to care for their infants for a short time after the birth, they may have less guilt in the future. When they choose this option, birth mothers will need the support, reassurance, and teaching provided to all new mothers.

8. Validate the significance of the loss. Be aware of the normal grief response and provide education about it to birth mothers. Offer resources that can be used immediately after discharge.

9. Be creative in ways the birth parents might say good-bye. There are booklets, such as a "Service in Giving a Child in Love," and "Given in Love," by Maureen Connelly from the Centering Corporation, that offer suggestions. Beginning to write in a journal or writing a letter to the adoptive parents and one to the child explaining why this choice was made and including the birth parents' medical histories can be helpful for all involved.

10. Encourage open dialogue and support. Refer the parents for family counseling.

11. Act as a neutral advocate. Facilitate information about issues, such as legal rights and rights to information, while birth mothers are in the hospital.

Adapted from Roles, P. (1997). Birth parents' grief: Relinquishing a baby for adoption. In J. R. Wood & J. L. Esposito (Eds.). *Loss during pregnancy or in the newborn period: Principles of care with clinical cases and analysis.* Pitman, NJ: Jannetti Publications.

(Davis, 1994; Askren & Bloom, 1999). This incomplete loss may contribute to the chronic aspect of the grief. The reasons for the relinquishment and the decision to have an open or closed adoption will be factors in the experience. The nurse caring for the woman at the time of relinquishment can be supportive by acknowledging the loss and the significance of the child to the birth mother. As the client goes through the labor and delivery process, the nurse should give her the opportunity to describe her decision to place the child for adoption. The nurse should work with the client to create mementos that have meaning for the birth mother. The nurse must recognize that the mother will experience shock as she goes through the confusing feelings of pride and joy when she give birth and the feelings of pain and sadness in the process of letting go.

The client may describe feelings of depression as the shock of relinquishing her infant diminishes. Everything will remind her of the infant that is no longer with her. Fatigue, sleep disturbances, and changes in eating habits are part of the grieving process. As described previously, anger and guilt occur during the searching and yearning stage. When a woman experiences anger while in the hospital, it may indicate a perceived lack of free choice, being overwhelmed by the legal issues, or the feeling of being rushed. When anger is noted, the social worker or chaplain can be an excellent source of support during this critical time.

Feelings of guilt are manifested by "If only." The mother may make statements such as, "If only I had made different decisions. . .," or, "If only I had listened, I would not be in this situation."

The birth mother recognizes that her choices are limited. She chooses to give her child the best chance possible and wants to be an advocate in the adoption process. Many choices follow the initial decision, including whether to see and hold the infant and receive mementos of the birth. The client needs to let go of the parental role and define what it means to be a birth parent. Despite the pain, she may feel a sense of release when the responsibilities of parenting are transferred to the adoptive parents, especially if she believes they are trustworthy and prepared. Because the grief process often is a lifelong experience, clients' reactions to relinquishment can differ greatly. In an open adoption, the birth mother is able to spend time with her child subsequent to the adoption and continue to know the decision she made was the best at the time. Thus, the birth mother continues her work to accept and reconcile her loss and incorporate its meaning into her life.

Because many birth mothers do not realize they will experience a normal grief reaction, an opportunity exists for education and preparation. Clients may have been told before delivery about grieving; however, a sense of denial exists that may hinder learning. Clients may experience **anticipatory grieving**, which is an emotional response based on the perception of a potential or expected loss. When clients are hospitalized and faced with the reality of the decision, it is important to have someone there to listen to them and to provide resources so that follow-up and support are available after discharge.

GRIEF RESPONSE

Supporting clients during the grieving process in the hospital is critical because it is a window of opportunity to assist the parents to begin a healthy grief process. The parents will be faced with learning a new role and decision-making at a time when they are in shock and least capable of making informed decisions. Flashbacks to painful moments when the problem was first diagnosed and the events surrounding the birth and death of the infant are very common. Flashbacks are an attempt by the grieving parent to put together more of the puzzle of what happened during the crisis. When assessing a grieving client, understand these are normal reactions. In addition, be aware of the signs and history that would put this client at risk. It is the responsibility of each caregiver throughout

the client's experience to make observations, document concerns, and access resources. Whether assessing a client in the doctor's office, the hospital, or as part of a community health visit, it is essential to include an assessment of the grief response. The nurse needs to understand that clients will not do their grief work sequentially but will move through the process, touching on each stage as needed. In the assessment, a discussion of the personal meaning of this pregnancy and the meaning of the loss for the client will help the nurse identify the client's progress in terms of the grieving process. With 20% of confirmed pregnancies ending in miscarriage and women stating that miscarriage is not perceived by medical staff as important or an emergency (Lee & Slade, 1996), it is little wonder that a woman would question herself. Self-esteem is diminished when no one confirms her reaction as being normal and a part of the grieving process.

DEPRESSION AND GRIEF WORK

The early assessment of women at risk for depression (Janssen, 1997) can be done during hospital admission. Symptoms of depression can be identified and incorporated into the plan of care (Table 37-2). Continued assessment of the risk for depression should be done as measured by the Munich Grief Scale, which assesses anxiety and depression from the time of the initial loss to 3 months after the loss. A post loss assessment also should be considered between 3 and 18 months to identify the progress of the grief work and the reorganization phase. This is the time when grieving parents can sense a level of release and have identified how the child's life and death can be incorporated into their lives.

Nursing Alert

POSTPARTUM RISK

Follow-up calls need documentation. When you hear something that sounds like a flat affect or hopelessness during a follow-up phone call following a perinatal loss, you need to document and act on the observation. "You mentioned, I am concerned, and I would like you to talk with someone. Are you willing?" If the concern is severe, do not hang up. Instead, ask to speak with a family member and suggest bringing the client to the emergency room. Contact social services or a nursing psychiatric liaison to support your efforts.

Table 37-2 Normal Grief and Depression Assessment

Normal Grief (Beutel)	Early Assessment of Women at Risk for Depression (Janssen)	Continued Assessment of Depression Risk (loss to 3 mo)	Postloss Assessment of Depression (3–18 mo)
• A state that changes with time • Note a process of confronting the loss • Gradual detachment from the person who died • Shock, preoccupation, resolution • Feelings of sadness • Feelings of loneliness • Feeling the world is empty • Positive social support	• Previous prenatal loss • No living children • Previous psychiatric problems • Longer length of gestation before loss • Older maternal age	• Verbalizing feelings of dejection • Irritation • Guilt • Alienation from others • Feelings of emptiness • Gloominess and despair • Sleep disturbances • Altered food intake • Loss and pain that may not be direct focus of attention	• No change in state • Dwelling on loss • Continued feelings of dejection, irritation, and guilt

Based on Beutel, M. Deckardt, R., Von Rad, M., & Weiner, H. (1995). Grief and depression after miscarriage: Their separation, antecedents, and course. *Psychosomatic Medicine, 57,* 517–526; and Janssen, H., Culsinier, C. J., Kees, P. (1997). A prospective study of risk factors predicting grief intensity following pregnancy loss. *Archives of General Psychiatry, 54,* 56–61.

DYSFUNCTIONAL GRIEVING

Dysfunctional grieving can be described as extended, unsuccessful emotional response to a perceived loss. Dysfunctional grieving is difficult to assess early in the grief process owing to the emotional and physical aspects of the normal process of grief. However, follow-up telephone calls, physician's office visits, and support group participation provide opportunities to assess the client for dysfunctional grieving.

Avoidance

Families and professionals alike can be well-meaning in their attempts to lessen the emotional pain of loss and death. The use of clichés in the hope of helping the bereaved feel better actually can cause more pain, upset, and anger. Trying to move the client past the pain by talking about the future and not talking about the experience is a disservice. Doing so gives the message that grief can be bypassed and life can continue as before, or that it is not appropriate to discuss what has happened and the associated feelings. The only way to get beyond grief is to experience it. If attempts are made to suppress the extreme emotional upset caused by the loss, the results can lead to pathological grief (Box 37-2). Nursing interventions should be supportive. The supportive intervention should be open to discussion, questions, and clarification of factual information. It also will help to focus on the individual client's emotional state. Teaching parents about grief work and what others have found to be helpful can open their eyes to what is ahead and allow for a good foundation from which they can progress.

Prolonged and Exaggerated Grief

Because there is no hard and fast rule for the length of time one should grieve, prolonged grief is difficult to recognize. As stated earlier, it takes at least 18 to 24 months before many clients feel a sense of reorganization. This

Box 37-2 Behaviors in Pathological Grief

- Overactivity without a sense of loss, or activities that bear a resemblance to those of the deceased.
- Symptoms belonging to those of the deceased.
- Initial episodes or exacerbations of diseases known to be associated with stress or psychosomatic conditions, such as ulcerative colitis, rheumatoid arthritis, and asthma.
- Alterations in relationships with friends and relatives owing to feelings of irritability and a marked desire to be left alone, which leads to progressive social isolation.
- Furious hostility against a specific person, particularly professionals, such as physicians and nurses.
- Affectivity and conduct resembling schizophrenic behavior often as a result of attempting to hide hostility.
- Lasting loss of social interaction patterns that also can include lack of decision-making and lack of initiative to participate in social activities without the intervention of a friend.
- Activities detrimental to personal economic and social existence, including spending large sums of money or engaging in activities, such as excessive drinking, leading to job loss.
- Agitated depression, including tension, agitation, insomnia, feelings of worthlessness, bitter self-accusation, and suicidal tendencies.

does not mean they have finished grieving. In fact, they are now able to recognize exaggerated grief, and they have some experience of what they need to do when they feel overwhelmed by the memory of their pregnancy loss or infant death. According to Janssen et al. (1997), the definition of complicated or pathological grief has not been universally established. Only 10% to 15% of mothers have an extreme response and meet the criteria for a psychiatric mood disorder. Within this group, a history of mental health problems was identified. The risk exists for an episode of major depressive disorder within 6 months after a miscarriage or infant death in women who were childless and those with a history of major depressive disorder (Carrera, Diez-Domingo, Montanana, Minguez, and Monleon, 1998). Clients may have an exaggerated response to a loss that is dependent on the definition of a so-called normal response. Keep in mind that culture and tradition play a role in a person's response to a crisis. The assessment for this situation is to recognize previous losses or

depressive reactions in an admission history, be available to listen, and create a plan to involve professionals able to respond to symptoms of depression that go beyond normal perinatal bereavement.

Multiple Losses

A situation that can exacerbate depression and serves as a red flag for the nurse is a history of multiple losses within a given time frame, usually a 12-month period. When thinking back to types of losses as discussed by Peretz, multiple losses can include the loss of other pregnancies or loss from a multiple gestation, or more commonly, the death of another family member or close friend. Multiple losses also can include other types of losses, such as job loss (for either the mother or father) or being involved in a natural disaster, burglary, or assault. When losses multiply or are "stacked" one on another, there is inadequate time and energy to appropriately grieve and work through each event before the next event occurs (Kowalski, 1996). Consequently, the coping mechanisms for subsequent losses are lacking and behaviors can become abnormal or pathological, with depression being a common occurrence. The intense feelings, search for understanding, and search for an answer to the question, "Why me?," complicate and confuse the perinatal loss situation, thus making the grief work much more difficult. Therefore, it is imperative that the nurse discover multiple losses in the admission assessment database. With this information, appropriate interventions can be developed.

Chronic Grief

The term **chronic grief** has been used to describe the prolonged and recurrent sorrow felt by parents whose child has a serious physical anomaly or mental disability but does not die at birth (Kowalski, 1987). Chronic grief also can occur after an infant's death and is predicted mainly by a lack of social support. According to Kay, Roman, & Schulte (1997), factors associated with the intensity of grief include previous poor adjustment to a death, loss of a planned pregnancy, not seeing the baby, marital problems, presence of a surviving twin, subsequent pregnancy within 5 months of the loss, and multiple losses within a short time.

Isolation

Because the death of a child and the associated hopes and dreams are very deep and personal experiences, it is not unusual for a woman to draw into herself, becoming physically and socially isolated. This isolation usually lasts for a brief period during which the client takes time for herself to try to understand what has happened. When a client continues to seek isolation and is preoccupied with the memory of the child who has died, there is need for intervention. Unless a caring family member brings the situation to the attention of a trained professional, the person may continue to move further away from contact with others.

SOCIOCULTURAL ISSUES

As parents and families respond to difficult and tragic events, the nurse observes the social network surrounding them that influences the experience. The funeral, a memorial, and prayer services are the sociocultural rites of passages associated with death. These transition rites benefit parents and their relationship to the social group rather than the infant. These rites are personal in their focus but societal in their consequences, and they are influenced by the cultural beliefs of each ethnic group. Through these rites of passage, the body is prepared for disposition and the bereaved are assisted through their process of shock and social reorientation. Such rites of passage make it possible for the entire social network to adjust to the loss of a human being. Through the shared experience, many times bonds are enhanced among members of the social network or family. Bereaved parents are in need of support from members of their social network. They need assurance that their feelings are understood and normal. Congruency in the perception of the loss between the parents and the social network facilitates the bereavement process (Kowalski, 1996). When there is incongruence or lack of common experience or beliefs, the network may be unable to provide support. In perinatal loss, members of the social group sometimes do not recognize the importance of the infant because they did not know the infant. A critical dividing point can arise when the bereaved parents are unable to share the experience with family or close friends. Some religions do not have a standard for recognizing the death of an unborn infant or one who dies before the first birthday, which may cause the parents to feel that their faith is not supporting their needs. Parents can seek a shared perspective of the death in other ways, including participation in bereavement support groups and attending an annual memorial service at which their child's life is recognized. Through a shared experience and common perspective, the healing process can begin. Failure to receive appropriate support may result in pathological avoidance of the intense emotions of acute grief.

Religious Practices and Spirituality

Spirituality is broader than religion. It is an important aspect of wellness and is indispensable in nursing care (Wright, 1998). *Spirituality* can be defined as the ability of the human person to decide how much he or she will adopt of the various physical, intellectual, social, political, and religious stimuli by which we are influenced, and thereby engage in a continual process of defining meaning. When spirituality is considered along with physical and psychological care, a more stable approach to grief support can be provided.

This perspective of loss and bereavement focuses on shared beliefs or, perhaps, a whole attitude or approach to one's very existence. Spirituality refers to the personal search for meaning and purpose in life, whereas religion refers to beliefs and practices associated with organized groups such as churches or synagogues (Fitchett & Handzo, 1998). Kowalski (1984) found that parents who were in a closely-knit religious congregation perceived the death of an infant in a similar way: "We may not understand why this tragedy occurred. However, God, who is all-knowing, understands. God loves us and will help and support us through this very difficult time; the parents and the baby will be reunited together in the afterlife."

Some Native American beliefs (Warrick, 1993) provide techniques for expressing fear and loss. In one Native American spiritual context, it is believed that everyone has *medicine,* that is, a healing energy that is always available and accessible. Within this spiritual context, a bereavement counselor is viewed as a friend whose function is to remind us that there is goodness in our hearts and the task is to bring forward that goodness.

It is important to include a spiritual assessment in the admission process, especially if a crisis has been identified. The spiritual assessment provides guidance as to the type of spiritual care needed and the ability to work from a recognized framework. Using the client's religious leader or the chaplain of the hospital, an assessment can help guide supportive action, such as relying on prayer for comfort or relaxation. Here are some examples. Muslims may request that the patient's bed face the Holy City of Mecca and that after death the body to be washed three times by a Muslim of the same sex as the one who has died. An Orthodox Jewish family may request the patient's bed sheets be buried with the body if they contain bodily fluids (Paulanka & Purnell, 1998). Again, some faiths do not have a prescribed way of dealing with the infant death.

Creating Memories and Finding Meaning

In perinatal loss, couples need ways to create memories. In harmony with their beliefs, a blessing, baptism, or naming ceremony can be created to recognize the infant-individual for whom they are grieving. If the ceremony is to be performed before the baby is born (or surgical procedure is begun), it can be done on the mother's abdomen. Prayers,

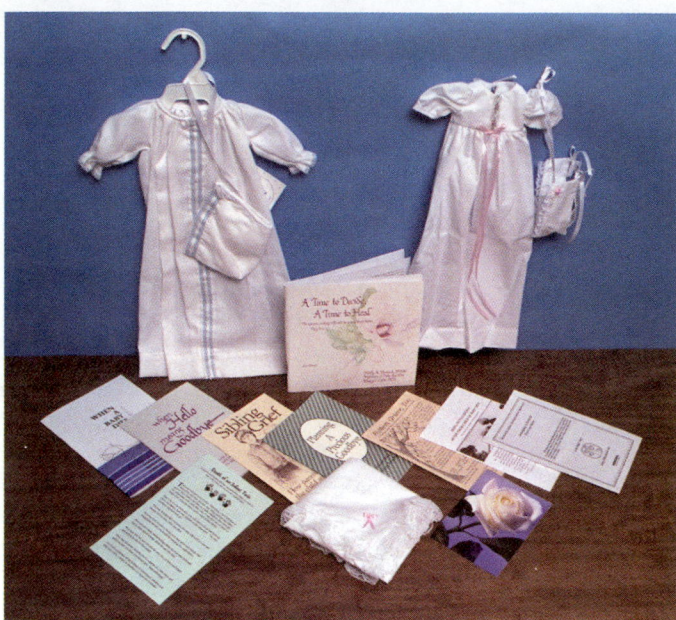

Figure 37-1 A memory kit may help grieving families preserve precious momentos of their baby.

chants, and readings can be done by the family in the informal setting of the client's room, chapel, or later in their place of worship. Resources to assist in planning a farewell service are available, such as *Bittersweet, Hello . . . Goodbye,* edited by Sr. Jane Marie Lamb (1988). These types of rituals are important to families who want to celebrate a life and keep the memory of these moments in their hearts forever (Figure 37-1).

EFFECTS OF LOSS ON THE FAMILY

Pregnancy loss is experienced by the woman as a loss of part of her being. In most cases, the father's grief is not the same as that of the mother. Immediately after pregnancy loss or infant death, a couple may feel a closeness created by the crisis. This is a survival mode that begins to fall apart as the differences in expectations surface. A father often will take on the active protector-provider role of planning the funeral, managing the household and returning to work. Being around people while performing all these functions allows him repeated opportunities to talk through the experience. Fathers receive reinforcement for this role of "doing" and for behaving with stoic strength. Yet, fathers often verbalize feelings of being left out when asked by co-workers how the woman is doing. They may feel that no one is asking about their feelings.

A woman experiencing a pregnancy loss feels an emptiness she cannot describe; her arms ache, and tears come easily. She may exhibit outward signs of grief, which

---

Client Education
Neonatal Loss

Because many couples separate or divorce after a perinatal loss, nurses can be instrumental in facilitating coping. It is often helpful to inform families of the following:

- That there are patterns of grieving, such as those described by Davidson.

- That individuals grieve according their own timetable.

- That the grieving process is not linear and many times a person may have conflicting feelings.

- That the mother and father may be experiencing different feelings at a given time and this sometimes leads to conflict. For example, one person is experiencing anger whereas the other is experiencing guilt.

- That men and women express their grief and feelings in gender-scripted ways. For example, women may be more comfortable expressing sadness and crying than men; conversely, men may be more comfortable expressing anger than women.

- That an understanding of these aspects of the grief process is the basis for the couple to communicate and support each other through the grieving process.

- That if there are other children in the family, their understanding and expression of grief and loss varies with their age.

- That resources are available to help the couple with grief and to help them work with their children.

can be very healthy because they are a safety valve for stress. When the mother is tearful, the father may try to maintain control. The differences are significant, and each wonders if the other will ever understand. They ask themselves questions, such as "Will she ever stop crying," and "Did he love or want this baby as much as I did, since he doesn't show his feelings?" Unless the couple is able to talk about and respect each other's differences, this conflict can escalate into a serious relationship problem.

To avoid this additional stress, the support team at the hospital can prepare the couple by identifying tasks that create a strong bond for their relationship. Reading materials that explain normal grief are helpful to guide expectations. Supporting the parents as they talk about the experience (each from their own perspective, without making the other person's viewpoint seem wrong), is a positive learning experience. It is very helpful to provide a list of resources parents can contact as needed that includes the support contact person at the hospital (nurse, chaplain, social worker, or physician), support group meetings in their area, and the names of professional counselors or therapists. Ideally, support will come from several sources: one's self, one's partner, and the community. Community includes people, activities, meditation, faith, self-help groups, education, and counseling (Simonton & Mathews-Simonton, 1978).

Issues of Intimacy and Communication

Owing to physical and emotional issues, intimacy can be difficult to re-establish after the ending of a pregnancy or death of a child. The woman is recovering from a vaginal delivery or surgical procedure. Many things can inhibit the desire for closeness: feeling tired; experiencing pain, cramping, or mood swings; and having breast tenderness. In some situations, sexual intercourse reminds the client of her infant and of how all this pain began, and deep sadness occurs. There can be a need for intense physical contact to escape the emotional pain temporarily. Because of the wide variations in needs, the focus must be on communicating the desire for intimacy because the partner may not be able to determine what would be fulfilling. In most cases, couples re-establish intimacy by holding each other and talking, actually scheduling quiet time together. Taking 5 minutes, five time a day to hold each other can go a long way toward renewing feelings of security at a time when the pervasive feeling is that of being out of control.

Gender Issues Related to the Grief Response

Although gender differences are not clear-cut, the responses of the man and woman can be influenced by tradition and cultural gender roles. As parents move beyond the initial period of shock and numbness, two types of physical reactions occur. The grieving person can be inwardly or outwardly bereaved. Persons who are *inwardly bereaved* do not find comfort in talking or crying with others. More effort is put into work, sports, and physical labor than ever before. They attempt to stay in control by staying busy and not thinking about the emptiness created by the loss. Clients who are *outwardly bereaved* appreciate speaking about what has happened and why, processing the information out loud. Tears, anger, signs of frustration,

and confusion are common. The outwardly bereaved show emotions and receive support when someone listens, especially if it is another grieving parent. The task at this point is education. Parents will need to identify which type of bereavement style each person exhibits and provide the appropriate support. Nurses also can help the parents understand the difference in grief copying styles and timetables, which will help parents support each other at a time when relationships can be strained.

Communication

When attempting to teach or communicate with grieving parents, nurse assessment of their roles within the family is a key caregiving point. When speaking with the woman as the client, keep in mind that if she is hesitant to share information or make decisions, it is not necessarily because she does not understand or cannot decide. It may be that in her culture, the male head of the family makes all decisions regarding the family, even if the woman does not agree. When speaking with a man, keep in mind that many men find it more comfortable to speak about emotional topics when they are occupied with something else. Talking may come much easier if, for example, the nurse walks with the man to get something to drink rather than sitting face to face and talking. To some men, especially when under stress, eye-to-eye contact is confrontational. In contrast, women generally want to look into your eyes and see the truth and when trying to comprehend the depth of what you are saying. Therefore, the method of delivery may be more important than the message itself. The grieving parents need to be made aware of the different communication styles. They also need to know that they cannot be everything to each other, especially during a crisis. They need to talk things out between themselves; however, they also need to discuss the issues on a different level, or with a different focus, with their friends. Communication problems sometime arise from persons being unaware of their true feelings. Only through talking in different social circles will meaning and understanding begin to surface.

Traditional support groups may not be helpful for the bereaved male. Chethik (2000) recognizes four categories of male bereavement. Doers are the most common who cope by walking, running, and building. Doing things allows for processing and a gradual release of energy. It would be difficult for these men to sit in a circle during a parent meeting and discuss how they feel. It is by doing that they begin to understand their feelings. For many men, self-esteem is reinforced with accomplishment. A father may see the death of his child as his failure. Unable to protect his family and unable to fix things, he may feel a loss of control. The woman may want him to fix things, to make things right. The result is anger. He is angry about the loss. He believes he is responsible for a solution and blames himself for causing the pain, or he feels guilty because her body must do all the work of the pregnancy and things are not going well. The failure may be in the form of genetic defects, inability to save the infant, inability to stop the birth process, or even inability to move God to work a miracle. He has a need to feel useful. To do so he searches for a solution, which may take the form of questioning. Given this information, the nurse can begin to help the couple understand there are differences and different needs during this crisis. In this way, the parents are educated to avoid the pitfalls of having expectations that cannot be fulfilled by the other.

Grandparents

Many couples express frustration when they speak of the response of their own parents to their loss. Yet, these are the persons from whom the grieving couple most expects to receive support and understanding. This may be problematic, however, because close family members also are grieving. A grandparent is experiencing the death of a grandchild and the pain of not being able to make things better for his or her own adult child. Grandparents are at a loss as they search for the right thing to say or do, and can be perceived as not caring when they do not talk about feelings or bring up the topic of this baby's death or pregnancy loss. Grandparents, other family members, and friends may try to minimize the pain by using clichés such as "You're young; you can have another baby" or "There probably was something wrong with the baby." These statements can cause confusion and anger because they send the message that *this* child is not important. The feelings of the parents may be hurt because they are attempting to make sense out of what has happened.

GRIEF PROCESS

Well-meaning family members can be guided to assist by recognizing the parents' need to experience the pain and tears to begin healthy grief. Part of the grief process includes telling the story of their pregnancy and infant's birth and subsequent death along with the tears. Grieving also includes the process of creating mementos and putting away baby items when the parents are ready, not when everyone else thinks they should be ready.

Parents will be able to receive the type of support from their family that will help them through the grief process if the staff educates the family on the importance of listening, limits of the parents ability to cope during the shock phase, individual nature of grief, and possible intensity of grief over the ensuing 18 to 24 months.

Siblings

Johnson (1989) states, "We fail to recognize that by teaching our children about death, we also teach them about life and joy." Death is part of life. Incorporating the teaching about death into everyday life best prepares children for when it happens to someone who is close to them. When children have the ability to name their emotions, feel included in the event, and feel they have family to talk with and feel secure with, then children will be able to move through the grief process (Table 37-3). When someone is very sick a child's first fear is of abandonment, especially when the focus is on the mother and the unborn baby. It is best to use words that are truthful, basic, and consistent. It is important to use the words *dead* and *died*. When parents try to make things better by saying, "God took our baby" or "The baby is sleeping," fear is instilled in children that they might also be taken. Information must be consistent and questions encouraged. When parents cry, it is important they share their feelings with their children. It can be a frightening feeling for a child to see their parents upset, and sharing the feelings can bring a sense of security to the situation. When parents are emotionally unable to support their surviving children, a plan needs to be made for a trusted relative or family friend to stay with the children during the critical moments at the hospital or, in the case of the infant's death, accompany the children to services acknowledging the death.

A child of any age can be part of saying goodbye. Vining (1982) said it simply in the booklet "Grief": "the visitation is a social release of the body; the funeral is the spiritual release; and the burial is the physical release." With this in mind, staff can support parents in their decision to allow the surviving children to stay with the family during any ceremony. Children can also confirm the tangible part of death at the funeral. If it is an open-casket service, they can see that the body is not working. They can draw a picture, write a letter, or bring a flower to be put in the casket with the baby.

Many families look for ways other than a private burial to celebrate their infant's existence. Suggestions range from attending an annual memorial service to donating a tree in their child's name or naming a star. The celebration can be as creative and personal as parents like, and this is a project with which children can help. According to Bluebond-Langer (1978), adequate information and support allows for integration and synthesis of information,

Table 37-3 Stages of Infant and Child Development Related to Death

Age	Concept of Death	Developmental Factors
Infant (birth to 2 years)	No concept of death.	Birth–6 mo: separation anxiety is not operative. 6 mo–2 ys: strong ties between infant and mother; not okay with substitute. Death is seen as separation. Can sense sorrow and pain in others; will respond with distress.
Toddler	Death is seen as separation. No concept of permanence.	2–3-year-old: not upset with sight of a dead animal. Objects that disappear are not considered gone.
Preschool age	Distressed at separation not death.	May respond with anger. Awareness that death occurs, especially from television. Play includes car crashes and gun play. Believes thoughts can make someone die. Magical thinking–operational stage. 5–6-year-old: can talk about death but not permanence. Believe death is temporary and reversible. Can be frightened when anesthesia is referred to as being "put to sleep."
School age (5 to 9 years old)	Sees death as permanent but not inevitable and not related to themselves.	5–7-year-old: needs to have repeated opportunities to talk. Will understand more information with each interaction. 7–9-year-old: may be curious about death. 7–11-year-old: identifies concrete causes for death (guns, poison, cancer) but is unable to incorporate into own experience.
9 to 10 years old	Believes it could happen to anyone.	Incorporates the experiences of others.
11 to 15 years old	Adultlike understanding but also into risk-taking.	Can verbalize consequences associated with high-risk activity. Belief in invincibility and that death happens to others.
Adolescent	Recognizes death as a fact of life. Meaning of life and death will vary with the individual.	Intellectual understanding does not mean emotional understanding. Intense concern with body image. Any threat to existence is a threat to identity. Can romanticize the death experience or see it as an escape.

which is the key to understanding. Understanding is not a function of age or intellectual ability.

Asking questions is how children learn, and thus they will ask many questions when a family has an infant who has died. Basic and consistent answers will best serve their long-term needs. When a parent looks to the nurse for suggestions, the nurse should respond that the goal is to stress that the child did not do or think anything that caused the infant's death. The reaction to the death will depend on the child's developmental stage. Preschoolers may believe that a wish made this happen. Allowing them to play is the best way for children to work out some of their feelings. As they play, they will come back to their parents with questions. When the questions are answered the same way each time, the young child will begin to comprehend the information over time and will feel a sense of security. It is comforting for a child to hear that it is uncommon for a baby to die and that death usually comes to those who are

very old and have lived a long life. Children also need reassurance that their parents are healthy. It also is important to explain that the baby died because his or her body was too little or too sick to survive.

School-aged children need to be an integral part of what is happening with the baby to decrease their feelings of abandonment. They are developing a sense of permanence, and they can be angry because of the unfairness of it all. They can display anger toward the baby for being sick and taking so much of their parents' time and energy, or anger toward the parents for not spending time together. When children are involved and supported in the knowledge that their feelings are normal, they will be a great source of comfort to their parents. The school-aged child may benefit from learning how to use a journal or art to express their feelings. Some children are able to write a letter to the baby and in that way release some of their emotions.

The teenaged and adolescent years are full of turmoil. When a crisis occurs during this time of major change, the focus is on finding a safe place where teenagers can work out their feelings and the meaning of what is going on with their family. Their feelings are deep and often confusing. A special time set aside to do something with their parents and a time for them to be with the dying baby or involved in the planning of the ceremony can be helpful. Whether tears, resentment, anger, or silence is exhibited during this time, adolescents need reassurance and comfort.

CARE FOR THE GRIEVING FAMILY

Over the past 25 years both research and anecdotal stories of bereaved families have appeared in the literature. In Kavanaugh's (1997) research, behaviors that are perceived by the parents as supportive include accepting parents' feelings and behaviors, being there, and sharing the experience. Families expect they will receive competent care, accurate information, and special attention (Figure 37-2). The continuum of care in supporting a grieving family begins wherever the crisis is first identified and follows the client through the experience. Having some type of structure available during a time of feeling out of control, can be reassuring for all parties involved. This holds true for families receiving a fatal prenatal diagnosis and those ex-

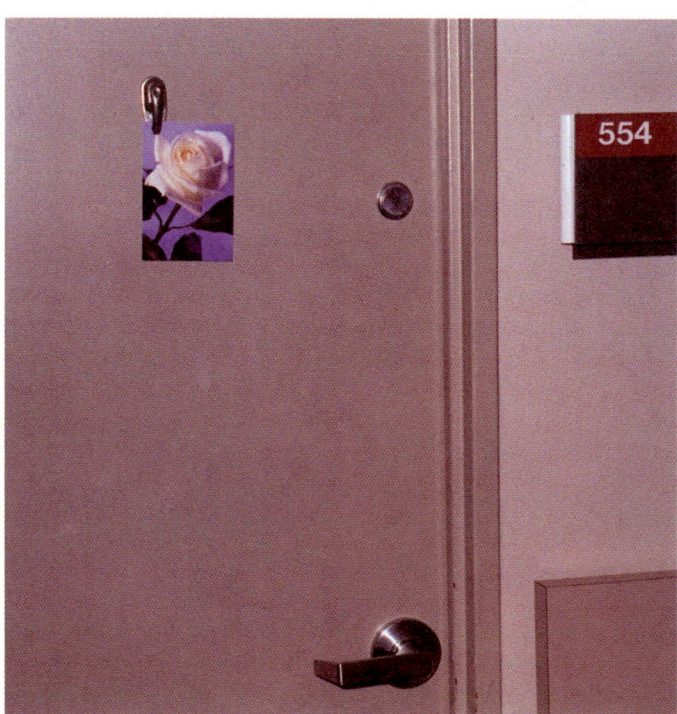

Figure 37-2 Placing a rose or card on the door of a client who has suffered a neonatal loss is a gentle reminder to staff of the need for sensitive care.

Nursing Tip

CARING FOR A BEREAVED FAMILY

Many of the behaviors that began in the initial crisis period must continue through the continuum of care. The following are tips for nursing care of a bereaved family:

● Recognize the initial confusion and shock.

● Provide ample time for taking-in the information.

● Repeat information as needed. Encourage parents to repeat or summarize what they have heard. Prepare written information.

● Prepare other health care workers and support their work with parents in a caring way whenever they need care in an area of the facility other than the obstetrics.

● Help parents with the logistics of admission to the facility.

● Acknowledge the difficulty in concentrating and understanding.

● Encourage the presence of a support person.

● Identify important cultural and spiritual practices.

● Provide opportunities for the client to tell her story.

● Recognize the unique aspects of the infant that binds the infant to the family, and treat the infant with respect.

● Identify and address fears as defined by the client.

● Be attentive during labor even though the baby cannot be saved.

● Provide comfort measures, such as music, massage, whirlpool baths, and family support.

● Support the client to experience the many emotions that may arise during labor.

● Refrain from comments that attempt to fix or minimize the parents' experience.

● Facilitate holding the baby as the parents desire.

● Create mementos consistent with hospital practices.

● Support sharing the experience with other family members.

● Discuss options regarding funeral or memorial services.

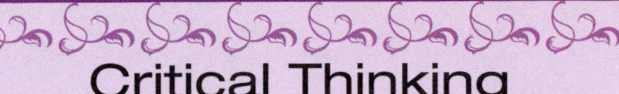

Critical Thinking

Grief Process

Many parents experiencing the death of an infant are in shock emotionally. They initially think it would be easier not to see and hold their baby, have a photograph, name their baby, or have a private burial.

- Do you think these activities can assist the parents in their grief process by identifying the infant?
- How would you assist them to recognize the importance of mementos and rituals in their grief process and still support their needs?

periencing a stillbirth or neonatal death. Woods (1997) states: "Patients have expectations that their physician will supply answers to the following questions: What does this horrific information you have provided mean; how did you arrive at this terrible conclusion; is my own health at risk/(spouse) is my wife at risk; do we know everything we need to know; what are my options; how quickly do I need to make decisions; in what order must these decisions be made; how will I respond to questions from my family; how will I tell my children?" Another question might be "what if you are wrong?"

Bereavement Program

It is important to come together as a community to recognize the children who have died and the hopes and dreams carried by their parents. An annual memorial service or walk to remember that is sponsored by the hospital is an excellent way for families and staff to come together to recognize the life and death that occurred at the hospital. It also allows staff to reconnect with families and see how they are progressing with their grief work after the hospital experience.

The knowledge gained from families' input is invaluable to learning. The follow-up mechanism of a bereavement program, such as support groups where staff are invited to attend, follow-up phone calls, feedback from doctor's offices, and letters from families that are shared routinely with staff, becomes an important learning tool. This feedback can be both oral and written and can be used as the starting point for quality improvement projects. Knowing the parents' pain did not end when they left the hospital and hearing what parents have done to reconcile this death into their lives gives the staff the opportunity to

REFLECTIONS FROM FAMILIES

"I will never forget the nurse who came in and spent time with us. I know she had other patients and it probably would have been easy to say she was busy. I feel she spent quality time with us by listening to us, allowing us to piece together what happened, and even crying with us. She validated that what happened was very significant and that our baby was very precious. No matter what the gestation or diagnosis, he still was our baby."

improve actions taken in the hospital during the crisis. Families do not easily forget the face or name of the nurse who helped them through the beginning of their nightmare, nor do they forget what was helpful and not helpful during that time. Take every chance to learn the client's perception of the experience because it can be very different from how you perceived the hospital stay. Box 37-3 lists the rights of parents, siblings, and the baby when an infant dies. The rights were developed by the Perinatal Bereavement Team at Women's College, Toronto, Canada, and adapted by the SHARE Pregnancy and Infant Loss Support, Inc. They are used worldwide to guide care and set standards (Levine, 1998).

Care for the Caregivers

One of the most difficult things nurses are required to do is to stay focused in the moment with someone who is experiencing intense psychological pain. Seldom is this pain more intense than at the death of a loved one, particularly a child. There is grieving for the loss of a significant human being, the newborn baby. There also is loss of all

REFLECTIONS FROM A NURSE

"The death of a child is a fire in the mind—a fire that burns a long time, for no other loss is so difficult to accept; no other loss feels so utterly un-natural. It is a loss beyond comprehension."

Box 37-3 The Rights of Parents and Baby when an Infant Dies

Rights of Parents when a Baby Dies

- To be given the opportunity to see, hold, and touch their baby at any time before or after death within reason.
- To have photographs taken of their baby and made available or held in security until the parents wish to see them.
- To be given as many mementos as possible, that is, the crib card, baby beads, ultrasound pictures and photographs, a lock of hair, feet prints and handprints, and a record of the baby's weight and length.
- To name their child and bond with their child.
- To observe cultural and religious practices.
- To be cared for by an empathetic staff who respects their feelings, thoughts, beliefs, and individual requests.
- To be with each other as much as possible throughout the hospitalization.
- To be informed of the grieving process.
- To be given time alone with their baby, allowing for individual needs.
- To request an autopsy. In case of miscarriage, to request to have or not have an autopsy or pathology examination performed as determined by applicable law.
- To have information presented in terminology understandable to the parents regarding their baby's status and cause of death, including autopsy and pathology reports and medical records.

- To plan a farewell ritual, burial, or cremation in compliance with local and state regulations and according to their personal beliefs, religious beliefs, or cultural traditions.
- To be provided with information about support resources that assist in the healing process, that is, support groups, counseling, reading materials, and perinatal loss newsletters.

Rights of the Baby

- To be recognized as a person who was born and died.
- To be named.
- To be seen, touched, and held by the family.
- To have the ending of life acknowledged.
- To be put to rest with dignity.

Rights of Children when a Sibling Dies

- To be acknowledged as persons who have feelings that need to be expressed.
- To be given the choice to see and hold the baby before and after the death within reason.
- To have the option of being considered in the choices parents make.
- To be informed about the feelings of grief in our terms, giving us the choice of a support group or counselor.
- To be recognized by our society that we will always love and miss our sibling.

Lammert, C. (1991). Rights of children when a sibling dies. *SHARE Pregnancy and Infant Loss Support, Inc., 1,* (3).

---

the hopes and dreams that surrounded the child. There is grieving for the loss of the future because children, in many respects, are our future and our link to immortality.

Nursing Responses

Working with families suffering the intense pain of a death can stimulate memories of nurses' own losses. When the loved one is a newborn infant or a wanted pregnancy, multiple aspects of bereavement occur simultaneously. There are several perspectives from which death and grief in pregnancy reproduction can be considered. Ontology is the science of "being," focusing on "what is," concentrat-

ing on the present moment rather than the past or the future. From an ontological perspective, focusing on the present is time spent without judgment but focused on possibilities. From this point of view, persons always have choice. We choose our responses to any given situation, including the death of a newborn. During a career, a nurse can observe families and persons who spiral into depression partly because of their feelings of helplessness as they attempt to cope with a loss. The professional nurse can educate clients about choices, reality, acceptance, pain and suffering, and forgiveness of self and others in association with the loss of a much desired pregnancy (Kowalski, 1996).

Supporting the Caregivers

Because the nursing staff often internalizes losses suffered by clients and these events bring up past experiences, a feeling of being out of control and unable to help can result. Putting the client in a room at the end of the hall and closing the door to give her privacy is one way the nursing staff attempts to avoid an uncomfortable interaction with a grieving client. In contrast, a nurse may be unable to accept death and thus attempt to prolong life by encouraging heroic interventions. These actions usually only serve to prolong death. According to Karen Soto, "There is an arrogance in Western Medicine that we can cure everything, that we have the cure-all and the quick fix for every illness. But we don't. Death is a welcome rest and source of comfort for some and we need to be gracious about that invaluable experience we will all have one day" (Soto, 1996).

Companioning as a Support Technique

Traditional bereavement care is based on the medical model in which grief is seen as an illness that demands a cure. In this model, we get a sense nurses are the experts and must fix what is wrong. This type of thinking sets up expectations that clients will recover from grief, let go, and return to normal. The more a nurse experiences death and grief with families, the clearer it becomes that this is not what happens. As educators, nurses are not experts in this family's grief experience. When it comes to death, nurses cannot direct or guide but can bring knowledge and experience. They can support parents to begin their journey through grief instead of trying to script parents' experiences. It is a very individual and lonely journey.

Alan Wolfelt (1998) speaks of a growth-oriented model that focuses on "companioning." As companions, nurses can learn to be present with a person's pain, respect disorder, listen to their heart, be still, and walk alongside the grieving person. In Wolfelt's model, growth means change, never returning to the old self. It means encountering pain and experiencing it in doses, yet having a safe place to retreat and acknowledge the pain and growth. A new inner balance is sought that has no end point. It allows us to explore and challenge our assumptions about life while actualizing the loss and fueling the potential within.

This broad approach to grief support allows the nurse the freedom not to have all the answers. As a member of a team, which includes the family, nurses can provide resources; however, but most importantly, they must let go of the dependency of "doing" (the focus of high-tech) and look to the idea of companioning of "being" (high-touch) with families. The opportunity to listen with the heart, one example of being, is almost a lost art as we depend more and more on machines to tell us what is happening with clients. By listening and empathizing with the crisis that is occurring inside these grieving parents, the nurse has the responsibility to create a safe place where they can touch the pain and not feel as though the nurse needs to eliminate the pain—to fix it. The sense of loss of control, disorder, and confusion in grief work, needs to be acknowledged. From these depths will come a higher functioning person, one that can experience healing. The nurse can use compassionate caring to discover the gift of silence, recognizing there is so much going on within the newly bereaved that often they have no ability or energy to speak. There is no expectation for the nurse to fill the silence. Just being still and paying attention can support parents who may fear being alone during this tragedy and give them the space to express their feelings and their experience without interruption.

Staff Education and Support

Few nursing care situations produce more anxiety than being left alone with a grieving patient or family. The first few times a nurse cares for such a client, an experienced nurse or the bereavement resource person should be present. The nurse needs to feel supported to sort through the feelings and responses stimulated by working with parents in intense psychological pain who are in shock and denial. An overview of the bereavement program also should be included in new staff orientation for nurses and physicians. This overview could include the philosophy and goals of the program; the process used to support families (such as checklists, books, consultants, and mementos); and most importantly, an organized opportunity to discuss concerns and past experiences.

Ongoing education and support for staff, even in tertiary care centers in which death may occur more frequently, is pivotal to the well-being of the staff. An example of supportive education is a discussion that focuses on case studies and ethical issues emphasizing difficult situations. Key points in these discussions might include those found in Box 37-4.

Care Team

Identify key unit and hospital support team members. The ideal goal is to minimize the number of staff who interact with the family. A bereavement resource person can work through the main team members by coaching them or joining them when time does not allow for coaching. Team members can include the bedside nurse and physician, the chaplain or family's religious representative, the social worker or counterpart, a close friend or family member, the parents, and the dying child or baby. Each member of the team can assist the family at different times with

Box 37-4 Key Discussion Points in an Educational Session after a Stillborn or Newborn Loss

- Never underestimate the supportive power of your peers.
- Offer opportunities to express emotions and gain an understanding of the management of the case.
- Schedule debriefing sessions as close as possible to a major incident.
- Encourage staff to hear all sides of the situation without judgment.
- Work to establish feelings of trust and support.
- Recognize your own response regarding how you can learn and grow from the experience.
- Work to build confidence in the staff in supporting grieving parents.
- Perform an annual review of the program, philosophy, and goals, with input from staff.
- Create a clinical competency that ensures all staff, including the nurse, doctor, social workers and chaplains, have a basic understanding of perinatal grief.

different information. One of the nurse's most important roles is to slow the pace of the events (such as decisions, information, and phone calls) and involve the family to ensure understanding of each aspect of the process they are experiencing. Recognize that what professionals see during the hospital stay is only a glimpse of what has occurred and how families are responding. For the care team to be able to acknowledge the intensity of the crisis, ongoing education of staff and the use of resources are necessary.

Ideally, the members of the team should meet the client before she is in advanced labor or before the surgical procedure occurs. Thus, the work to be done after the delivery or death of the baby will not be complicated by introducing new personnel. In the delivery room, recognize the unique aspect of the birth when a child has died or when lethal anomalies have been discovered. Heavy sedation will compound the psychological needs of the grieving parent and delay the reality. In turn, the grief response will be delayed. Remember that the mother needs to say hello and goodbye at the same time. No limit should be placed on the time the mother spends with her infant. She needs to be included in bathing and dressing the infant. Depending on the mother's customs and beliefs, there may be very specific procedures for this part of the care of the body. Remember that the mother will never

NON–ENGLISH-SPEAKING CLIENTS

A one-page information sheet in bulleted format that highlights the most important issues a parent might face must be available for your non–English-speaking clients. Examples of content follow: a policy on finding an interpreter; types of questions they can expect to be asked; burial options; policy on photographs; religious and spiritual resources. This document needs to be translated by a certified individual or company (or preprinted booklets can be used). When you use a member of the client's family or staff as the interpreter, always document the person's name and relationship to the client in your notes. Include the chaplain, social worker, and grief support person in the plan of care.

have another opportunity to do these things for her infant. Include a private place where family can join her to help share her grief. Having family members present also will make the transition to home easier because she will know that others saw her baby.

Allowing the mother to go home soon after a D&E or D&C does not provide the best support to the family. They have little to no time to process what has happened, ask questions, and learn about the grief process. At the very least, each family needs to leave the hospital with a phone number for a support program, an appointment for medical follow-up, and instructions written in understandable language. To be consistent, many hospitals have gone to a task checklist or a set of guidelines. For examples of these lists see the following references: Brost & Kenny, 1992; Calhoun, 1994; Hutti, 1988; Lawson, 1990; 1988; Mueller, 1991; Null, 1989; Rosas & Rosas, 1987; Ryan, Corte-Arsenault, & Sugarman, 1991; Weinfield, 1990; Welch, 1991; Wheeler & Limbo, 1990; Woods & Esposito, 1987.

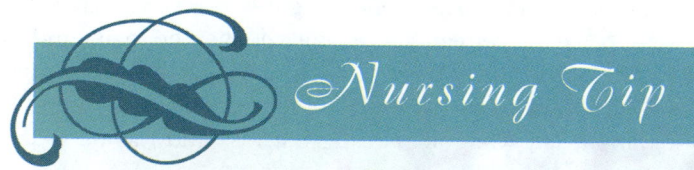

PRENATAL DEATH

If the pregnancy ended at 10 to 16 weeks' gestation or the infant was stillborn, the infant can be viewed. Care must be taken owing to the delicate nature of the fetal tissue. Many hospital programs have a special cradle or basket to bring the infant to the parents for viewing.

NURSING PROCESS

Implementation of the nursing process is very useful in working with bereaved parents and their family and friends. The nursing process provides a structure to make certain that all steps in caring for a family experiencing loss are addressed. The following is an example of the process to help nurses begin thinking in this way about perinatal loss.

Assessment

When making an assessment, the nursing history is the first step. The areas that are important can be discovered by asking the following:

- Did the parents have days or even hours of advanced warning that the baby was dead or very ill? Are there medical complications for the mother?

- Was the pregnancy wanted or unwanted? When a pregnancy is unwanted, one or both parents can exhibit a combination of guilt and relief that appears different from the feelings exhibited in a planned pregnancy.

- Were there multiple losses? Parents who have had other pregnancy losses or other significant losses often feel overwhelmed and lack fundamental coping mechanisms.

- How do their religious beliefs or culture support them? Parents who have very strong religious or cultural beliefs often have a structure of support that can be very helpful.

- Are there close friends or family who share the same culture or beliefs, and are they able to help? Seek information from family and friends regarding beliefs and customs.

- What are the size and type of social connections within the network of friends and family that surround the parents? What is the relationship between the infant's mother and father? These relationships can make a huge difference in how parents handle the loss and progress through the bereavement process.

- Do the parents, family, and friends express their feelings regarding the loss? Does evidence exist of anger, tears, guilt, sadness, shock, and numbness?

Nursing Diagnosis

Problems need to be identified on an individual basis because each family unit will cope with loss differently. Examples of some general nursing diagnosis include the following:

- Fear related to the initial diagnosis of infant death as evidenced by increased tension and expression of horror or dread.

- Ineffective coping related to gender differences in coping strategies, uncertainty, inadequate social support, a high degree of threat, or disturbance in the pattern of tension release as evidenced by a lack of goal-directed behavior, poor concentration, destructive behavior toward self or others, or fatigue.

- Spiritual distress related to perinatal loss as evidenced by energy-consuming anxiety, physical or psychological stress, loss of a loved one, or poor relationships.

- Health-seeking behaviors related to effective managing of adaptive tasks by the family as evidenced by the family moving in the direction of a health-promoting and enriching lifestyle that supports maturational processes.

Outcome Identification/Planning

Planning for desired outcomes must be constructed with the participation of the mother and her partner. Planning also could involve friends and family:

- Mother and father will be able to work through the bereavement process, each at their own pace, with understanding and support for one another.

- At 1 or 2 years after the loss, the parents will be able to identify positive growth for themselves from the experience.

Nursing Intervention

The nurse needs to take the following actions with the client and her partner:

- Physical care. After delivery, the mother has the same needs as does a mother whose baby was born alive. Do not forget breast engorgement because there is not an infant to empty the breasts. Sleeping medication is

Web Activities

- Develop a plan of care for a family with a single parent, siblings, and grandparents who are coping with a perinatal loss.
- Visit three of the grief websites listed in this chapter. Compare the information they offer for families and health care provided.

Case Study/Care Plan

CLIENT EXPERIENCING INTRAUTERINE FETAL DEMISE

Bonnie is registered nurse in a labor and delivery ward of a busy county hospital. She has her bachelor's degree and has been working on this particular ward for 2 years. Her morning assignment includes care of a laboring patient, Mrs. Kay, a 29-year-old Caucasian American, gravida 1, para 0, with an intrauterine fetal demise (IUFD) at 36 weeks' gestation. Mrs. Kay entered the hospital last night at 3 a.m. with complaints of contractions. She and her husband were not aware there was a problem with the baby because her pregnancy had been without complications. Mrs. Kay was diagnosed with a term IUFD shortly after admission. Owing to the rapid progression of her labor, Mrs. Kay has not had much time to grieve. She currently dilated at 6 cm. The report from the night shift reveals that Mrs. Kay received intravenous Demerol, which had been controlling her pain until the last 30 minutes or so when she started becoming restless. No support services were activated because the admission had been in the middle of the night. Mr. and Mrs. Kay are new to the area; all their family and friends live 500 miles away. Although their immediate families have been notified, there are no plans for them to come at this time.

Assessment

Mrs. Kay lay in the labor bed staring out of the window. Her face is stained with tears. Her husband is sitting quietly with his hand on hers, and there is no verbal communication between the two. Her contractions are coming every 3 minutes, and she breathes hard and cries out with each contraction. Between contractions, Mrs. Kay tells Bonnie that she is in terrible pain and that she is frightened about delivering the baby. Mrs. Kay also states that she and her husband would like to see a member of the clergy.

Nursing Diagnosis

Pain as related to contractions associated with active labor as evidenced by crying out and an accelerated respiratory rate.

Expected Outcomes The client-family will be able to manage the pain experience through partner support, breathing techniques, and medications.

Planning Pain management and support are interventions aimed at assisting the client now.

Nursing Interventions	Rationales
1. Use pain medications that do not alter alertness.	1. Although the client may feel distressed at this particular time, mind altering medications will only prolong the grieving process. The woman also may grieve the inability to remember her baby.

Evaluation As is the healing process, evaluation is ongoing. Management of pain in the intrapartum period while soothing fears and anxiety may be monitored by the labor nurse. Effective management of the client may be evidenced by the client stating she has little pain or is pain-free while also monitoring mental alertness.

(continued)

not usually helpful because it dulls the feelings and delays coping until after the client has left the hospital, when she cannot receive help as easily.

❧ Psychological and emotional care. Keep parents and families informed and together. Support seeing and holding the infant and create memories, including photographs and mementos. Support decision-making regarding paperwork and disposition of the infant's body. Encourage choices and an increased sense of control. Listen.

❧ Educational care. Provide educational pamphlets and booklists. Discuss the bereavement process.

Nursing Diagnosis

Fear related to delivering a dead infant, as evidenced by the client's apprehension and increased tension.

Expected Outcomes The couple supports each other through the labor process, with help of the nurse, clergy, physician, and other support members.

Planning The nurse must plan interventions aimed at assisting the client and family with immediate and future needs.

Nursing Interventions	Rationales
1. Use coaching techniques for labor and encourage use. Speak softly and respectfully.	1. The client's response during labor usually is focused on what is happening from moment to moment. By providing support, encouragement, and direction, the nurse may help ease the client's anxiety and fear.

Evaluation Levels of anxiety and fear may be monitored by verbal and nonverbal cues from the client and family.

Nursing Diagnosis

Spiritual distress related to perinatal loss as evidenced by energy-consuming anxiety, psychological stress, and loss of a loved one.

Expected Outcomes Work through the grieving process at their own pace with understanding and support for each other.
Identify positive growth for themselves from the experience.

Planning Consultations with the clergy and grief counselor may assist the client and family in the near future.

Nursing Interventions	Rationales
1. Follow institution guidelines to create momentos: footprints, photographs, and certificates.	1. Momentos are helpful in assisting the family move through the grieving process. Parents may desire to look at these reminders of their baby for years to come.

Evaluation The family is meeting with a grief counselor and or clergy; this is just the first step in a long journey.

Encourage questions. Address issues, such as burial arrangements, funeral, or memorial service; and telling the other children, family, friends and strangers who know the mother was pregnant. Identify the available resources, such as support groups, reading materials, and websites.

- Follow-up. With much briefer hospital stays today than in the past, follow-up is even more important. It is critical to have a physician follow-up visit scheduled.

There may be community follow-up available with a public health nurse. Some facilities have a perinatal loss clinic in which clients receive special attention.

Evaluation

Ongoing evaluation of the bereavement process is important. Encourage couples to seek help and support. Facilities that have a significant volume of deliveries need a nurse or social worker who is responsible for follow-up phone calls to see how the couple is managing. Issues, such as subsequent pregnancy, need extensive discussion as to when, where, and how it fits into the bereavement process. It is evident from the previous example that working with families experiencing loss is not easy. Doing so requires thoughtfulness and strong communication and listening skills.

Key Concepts

- Nursing care and support for parents and families when a pregnancy ends or a baby dies, constitutes a difficult nursing intervention in an environment that is supposed to be happy, exciting, and focused on new life.

- Understanding the theories of loss and attachment and how they relate to reproductive loss can assist the nurse in planning care for the grieving family.

- The concepts of gender differences and cultural variations have major impacts on reaction to the loss.

- When caring for clients at any point during a reproductive loss, it is the individualization of the plan that will give the family the best opportunity to successfully grieve the loss.

- Using resources that include hospital policies and staff, support programs, written materials, and websites will best prepare the caregiver when the opportunity arises to care for a grieving client.

- Reproductive loss can be meaningful, growth-producing and may have positive aspects when the nursing staff can look at this death and loss and create the best possible experience for this family, given the intensely painful situation.

Review Questions and Activities

1. There are some identifiable phases in the bereavement process that always occur in the same order, one step at a time. True or False?

   The correct response is false.

2. Saying. "I know how you feel," will help the family to know that you care and will ease the expression of their grief. True or False?

   The correct response is false.

3. Mementos and pictures are important for grieving parents. True or False?

   The correct response is true.

4. Parents should be encouraged to join an infant loss support group. True or False?

   The correct response is true.

5. List three feelings that parents may display in response to their loss.

6. List five ways that caregivers can be sensitive to the emotions and needs of parents.

7. List the four phases of the grief process as described in this chapter.

8. Which of the following would not express a feeling parents may have regarding their loss?
   a. Anger
   b. Guilt
   c. Easy decision making
   d. Loss of control

   The correct response is c.

9. Construct an active listening exercise to stress the importance of listening to rather than talking with bereaved parents. For example, practice in dyads what it feels like to dominate the conversation, not listen to the other person, and interrupt. Then practice empathetic listening.

10. Build a case example (preferably one that has happened to the instructor or someone in the class) and then conduct a debriefing, educational meeting, or discussion of staff response to the example using the guidelines in Box 37-4.

References

Askren, H. A., & Bloom, K. C. (1999). Postadaptive reactions of the relinquishing mother: A review. *Journal of Obstetric, Gynecologic, and Neonatal Nursing, 28,* (4), 395–400.

Bowlby, J. (1969). *Attachment and loss: Vol. I.* New York: Basic Books.

Bowlby, J. (1980). *Attachment and loss: Vol. II*. New York: Basic Books.

Beutel, M., Deckardt, R., Von Rad, M., & Weiner, H. (1995). Grief and depression after miscarriage: Their separation, antecedents, and course. *Psychosomatic Medicine, 57,* 517–526.

Bluebond-Langer, M. (1978). *The private worlds of dying children* (p. 54). Princeton, NJ: Princeton University Press.

Carerra, L., Diez-Domingo, J., Montanana, V. Monleon, S. J., & Minguez, J. (1998). Depression in women suffering from perinatal loss. *International Journal of Obstetrics and Gynecology, 62,* (2), 149–153.

Carson, S. A. (2000). Spontaneous Abortion in S. Ransom Ed. Practical Strategies in Obstetrics & Gynecology.

Chethik, N. (2000). Reaching bereaved men requires innovation. *The Forum, 26,* (5), 4–5.

Connelly, M. (1990). *Given in love-for mothers who are choosing an adoption plan*. Omaha, NE: Centering Corp.

Davidson, G. W. (1979). *Understanding death of the wished-for child*. Springfield, IL: OGR Service Corp.

Davidson, G. W. (1984). *Understanding mourning*. Minneapolis, MN: Augsburg Publishing.

Davis, C. E. (1994). Separation loss in relinquishing birth mothers. *The International Journal of Psychiatric Nursing Research, 1,* (2), 63–70.

Fitchett, G., & Handzo, J. (1998). Spiritual assessment, screening and intervention In J. Holland (Ed.). *Psycho-oncology* (pp. 790–808). New York: Oxford University Press.

Freud, S. (1917). Mourning and melancholia. In *The standard edition of the complete psychological works of Sigmund Freud* (Vol. XIV). London: Hogarth Press.

Janssen, H., Culsinier, C. J., Kees, P. (1997). A prospective study of risk factors predicting grief intensity following pregnancy loss. *Archives of General Psychiatry, 54,* 56–61.

Johnson, J. (1989). Guiding children through grief. *Mothering,* Spring 89, 29.

Kavanaugh, K. (1997). Parents experiences surrounding the death of a newborn whose birth is at the margin of viability. *Journal of Obstetric, Gynecologic, and Neonatal Nursing, 26,* 43–51.

Kay, J., Roman, B., & Schulte, H. (1997). Pregnancy loss and the grief process. In: J. R. Woods, Jr., & J. L. E. Woods (Eds.). *Loss during pregnancy or in the newborn period*. Pitman, NJ: Jannetti Publications.

Kowalski, K. (1984). Perinatal loss and bereavement. In L. Sonstegard, K. Kowalski, & B. Jennings (Eds.). *Women's health: Crisis and illness in childbearing*. Orlando, FL: Grune & Stratton.

Kowalski, K. (1987). Perinatal Loss and Bereavement. In: L. J. Sonstegard, K. Kowalski, & B. Jennings (Eds.). *Women's health: Crisis and illness in childbearing,* Vol. 3. New York: Grune & Stratton.

Kowalski, K. (1996). Loss and Bereavement: Psychological, Sociological, Spiritual and Ontological Perspectives. In K. R. Simpson & P. A. Creehan (Eds.). *AWHONN's perinatal nursing*. Washington, DC: Association of Women's Health, Obstetric, and Neonatal Nurses.

Lamb, J. M. Ed. (1988). *Bittersweet; Hello . . . goodbye: A resource in planning farewell rituals when a baby dies*. Belleville, IL: National Share Office.

Lammert, C. (1991). Rights of children when a sibling dies. *SHARE Pregnancy and Infant Loss Support, Inc., 1,* (2).

Lee, C., & Slade, P. (1996). Miscarriage as a traumatic event: A review of the literature and new implications for intervention. *Journal of Psychosomatic Research, 40,* (3), 235–244.

Levine, S. 1998. Who dies? An investigation of conscious living and conscious dying. In C. Farella (Ed.). "The Many Faces of Grief", *Nursing Spectrum*.

Lindemann, E. (1944). Symptomatology and management of acute grief. *American Journal of Psychiatry, 101,* 141–148.

Peretz, D. (1970). Development, object relationships and loss. In B. Schoenberg, A. C. Karr, D. Peretz, & A. H. Kutschner (Eds.). *Loss and grief: Psychological management in medical practice*. New York: Columbia University.

Paulanka, B., & Purnell, L. (1998). Transcultural healthcare: A culturally competent approach. Philadelphia, PA: F. A. Davis.

Roles, P. (1997). Birth parents' grief: Relinquishing a baby for adoption. In J. R. Wood & J. L. Esposito (Eds.). *Loss during pregnancy or in the newborn period: Principles of care with clinical cases and analysis*. Pitman, NJ: Jannetti Publications.

Rubin, R. (1967). Attainment of the maternal role, Part 1. *Processes, Nursing Research, 16,* (3), 237–245.

Simonton, O. C., & Mathews-Simonton, S. M. (1978). *Getting well again*.

Simos, B. G. (1979). *A time to grieve*: Loss as a universal human experience. New York: Family Service Association of America.

Vining, E. (1982). *Saying goodbye* (p. 10). Omaha, NE: Centering Corp.

Warrick, C. (1993). Healing Native American spirituality helps kids deal with grief: Interview with Steve Sunderland. *Cincinnati Post,* p. 1b.

Wolfelt, A. (1998). Keynote Address. 20th Annual Conference-Association for Death Education and Counseling. 3/19-22/98. Chicago, IL.

Woods, Jr., J. J. (1997). Pregnancy loss counseling: The challenge to the obstetrician. In J. R. Woods, Jr., & J. L. Woods (Eds.). *Loss during pregnancy or in the newborn period* (p. 84). Pitman, NJ: Jannetti Publications.

Wright, K. B. (1998). Professional, ethical and legal implications for spiritual care. *Nursing Image, 30,* (1), 81.

Suggested Readings

American Academy of Pediatrics & American College of Gynecologists. (1997). *Guidelines for perinatal care* (4th ed.). Elk Grove, IL: American Academy of Pediatrics and American College of Gynecologists.

Anderson, K. (Ed.). (1998). *Mosby's medical, nursing and allied health dicitionery,* (5th ed.). Chicago, IL: Mosby.

Association of Women's Health, Obstetric, and Neonatal Nurses (AWHONN) Committee on Practice. (1997). *Guidelines for providing care to the family experiencing perinatal loss and fetal death*. Washington, DC: Association of Women's Health, Obstetric, and Neonatal Nurses.

Attig, T. (1996). *How we grieve. Relearning the world.* New York: Oxford University Press.

Barnum, B. (1996). The challenge of providing nursing care for the dying: An interview with K. Soto, R. Whyte. *Nursing Leadership Forum, 2,* (1), 35.

Borg, S., & Lasker, J. (1981). *When pregnancy fails: Families coping with miscarriage, stillbirth and infant death.* Boston, MA: Beacon Press.

Bowlby, J., & Parkes, C. M. (1970). Separation and loss within the family. In E. J. Anthony & C. Koupernik (Eds.). *The child in his family.* New York: John Wiley.

Bryan, E. M. (1991). Perinatal bereavement after the loss of one twin. *Journal of Perinatal Medicine, 19,* (suppl) 241–245.

Calhoun, L. K. (1994). Parents' perceptions of nursing support following neonatal loss. *Journal of Perinatal and Neonatal Nursing, 8,* (2), 57–66.

Callahan, D. (1995). Frustrated mastery: The cultural context of death in America. *Western Journal of Medicine, 163,* (3), 226–230.

Chez, R. (1995). Acute grief and mourning: One obstetricians experience. *Obstetrics and Gynecology, 85,* (6), 1059–1061.

Conley, B. H. (1986). *Handling the holidays.* Elburn, IL: Thumb Printing.

Davis, D. L. (1996). *Empty cradle, broken heart: Surviving the death of your baby* (rev. ed.). Golden, CO: Fulcrum Publications.

DeFrain, J., Taylor, J., & Ernst, L. (1982). *Coping with sudden infant death.* Lexington, MA: Lexington Books.

Ewton, D. S. (1993). A Perinatal Loss Follow-up Guide for Primary Care. *Nurse Practitioner, 18,* (12), 30–36.

Fertel, P., Holowinsky, S., Lams, P., Winterstein, M. (1988). *Difficult decisions for families who unborn baby has a serious problem.* Omaha, NE: Centering Corp.

Gatlin, S. (1987). Some psychosocial ramifications of abortions for genetic reasons. *Journal of Perinatology, 5,* (4).

Grollman, E. (1967). *Explaining death to children* (p. 102). Boston, MA: Beacon Press.

Gunderson, J. M., & Harris, D. E. (Eds.). (1990). *Quietus: a story of stillbirth.* Omaha, NE: Centering Corp.

Harrigan, R., Naber, M. M., Jensen, K. A. (1993). Perinatal grief: Response to the loss of an infant. *Neonatal Network, 12,* (5), 25–31.

Hendel, J. (1989). The death of a twin. *Bereavement Magazine,* July/August 34–35.

Hinnells, J. R.(Ed.). (1984). *The facts on file dictionary of religions.* New York: Facts on File Inc.

Hutti, M. H. (1998). A quick reference table of interventions to assist families to cope with pregnancy loss or perinatal death. *Birth: Issues in Perinatal Care and Education, 15,* 33–35.

Ilse, S., & Furrh, C. B. (1988). Development of a comprehensive follow-up care plan after perinatal and neonatal loss. *Journal of Perinatal and Neonatal Nursing, 2,* (2), 23–33.

Kennel, J. H., Slyter, S. H., & Klaus, M. H. (1970). The mourning response of parents to the death of a newborn infant. *New England Journal of Medicine, 283,* 334.

Kimble, D. L. (1991). Neonatal death: A descriptive study of father's expectations. *Neonatal Network, 9,* (8), 45–49.

Klass, D., Silverman, P. R., & Nickman, S. L. (Eds.). (1996). *County bonds: new understanding of grief.* Washington, DC: Taylor and Francis.

Klaus, M. H., & Kennel, J. H. (1976). *Maternal infant bonding.* St. Louis, MO: Mosby.

Knapp, R. J., & Peppers, L. (1980). *Motherhood and mourning: Perinatal death* (pp. 74–79). New York: Praeff.

Kowalski, K. (1983). *A bereaved parents group: An ethnographic study.* Unpublished comprehensive examination paper, Boulder, CO: University of Colorado.

Kushner, H. S. (1981). *When bad things happen to good people.* New York: Collier Books.

Lake, M. F., Knuppel, R. A., & Angel, J. L. (1987). The rationale for supportive care after perinatal death. *Journal of Perinatology, 7,* (2), 85–89.

Labun, E. (1988). Spiritual care: An element in nursing care planning. *Journal of Advanced Nursing, 13,* 314–320.

Larson, D. G. (1993). *The helper's journey: Working with people facing grief, loss and life threatening illness.* IL: Research Press.

Lasker, J. N., & Toedter, L. J. (1994). Satisfaction with hospital care and interventions after pregnancy loss. *Death Studies, 18,* 41–64.

Lawson, L. V. (1990). Culturally sensitive support for grieving parents. *Maternal-Child Nursing, 15,* 76–79.

Leon, I. G. (1992). Perinatal loss: A critque of current hospital practices. *Clinical Pediatrics, 31,* (6), 366–374.

Leoni, L. C. (1997). The nurse's role: Care of patients after pregnancy loss. In J. R. Woods Jr., & J. L. E. Woods (Eds.). *Loss during pregnancy or in the newborn period* (pp. 361–386). Pitman, NJ: Jannetti Publications.

Lindemann, E. (1979). Beyond grief: Studies in crisis intervention. New York: Jason Aronson.

Linn, E. (1986). *I Know Just How you Feel. . . . Avoiding the cliches of grief.* Incline Village, NV: Publisher's Mark.

Minnick, M. A., Delp, K. J., & Ciotti, M. C. (1994). *A time to decide, a time to heal: For parents making difficult decisions about babies they love* (4th ed.). St. John, MI: Pineapple Press.

Outerbridge, E. (1983). Support for parents experiencing parinatal loss. *Canadian Medical Association, 129,* 335.

Parkes, C. M. (1979). *Bereavement: Studies of grief in adult life.* New York: International University Press.

Pettigrew, J. (1990). Intensive care nursing: The ministry of presence. *Critical Care Clinics of North America, 2,* (3), 502–508.

Pine, V. (1986). In T. Rando (Ed.). *Loss and anticipatory grief.* Lexington, MA: Lexington Books.

Primeau, M. R., & Lamb, J. M. (1995). When A Baby Dies. *Journal of Obstetrics, Gynecology, and Neonatal Nursing, 24,* 206–208.

Rando, T. (1984). *Grief, dying and death: Clinical interventions for caregivers* (p. 443). Champaign, IL: Research Press.

Rando, T. A. (1986). *Loss and anticipatory grief.* Lexington, MA: Lexington Books.

Rando, T. A. (1986). *Parental loss of a child.* Champaign, IL: Research Press.

Schaeffer, D., & Lyons, C. (1986). *How do we tell the children?* New York: Newmarket Press.

Schiff, H. S. (1977). *The bereaved parent.* New York: Penguin Books.

Speck, W. T., & Kennell, J. H. (1980). Management of perinatal death. *Pediatrics in Review, 2,* (2), 59–62.

Stevenson, R., & Stevenson, E. P. (1996). Teaching students about death: A comprehensive resource for educators and parents (p. 2). Philadelphia, PA: The Charles Press.

Toedter, L. J., Lasker, J. N., & Alhadeff, J. M. (1988). The perinatal grief scale: Development of initial validation. *American Journal of Orthopsychiatry, 58,* 435–449.

Tizard, J. P. M. (1976). Mourning made easier if parents can view body of neonate. *Obstetrics and Gynecology News, 11,* (21), 35.

Williamson, W. B. (1992). An encyclopedia of religions in the U.S.: One hundred religious groups speak for themselves. (Ed.). New York: Crossroads.

Wilson, A. L., Soule, D. J., & Fenton, L. J. (19xx). The next baby: Parents' response to perinatal experiences subsequent to a stillborn. *Journal of Perinatology, 8.*

Wheeler, S. R., & Pike, M. M. (1992). *Goodbye my child: A gentle guide for parents whose child has died.* Omaha, NE: Centering Corp.

Wolfelt, A. (1997). *The journey through grief: Reflections on healing.* Fort Collins, CO: The Center for Loss and Life Transition.

Worden, W. (1991). *Grief counseling and grief therapy: A handbook for the mental health practitioner.* New York: Springer Press.

Zeanan, C., Darley, J. V., Rosenblatt, M. J., & Saller, D. N. (1993). Do women grieve after terminating pregnancies because of fetal anomalies? A controlled investigation. *Obstetrics and Gynecology, 82,* 270–275.

Resources

National Organizations: Parents experiencing perinatal death

Association of Death Educators and Counselors (ADEC), Professional organization and certification, 683 Prospect Ave, Hartford, CT 06105-4298

Bereaved Parents of the USA, National Headquarters, PO Box 95, Park Forest, IL 60466

Bereavement Services—RTS, Gundersen Lutheran Medical Center, 1910 South Ave., LaCross, WI 54601, 800-362-9567, x4767

Center for Loss in Multiple Births (CLIMB), P.O. Box 1064, Palmer, AK 99645, 907-746-6123

The Centering Corporation (books and videos), 1531 N. Saddle Creek Rd., Omaha, NE 68104, 402-553-1200

National Funeral Directors Association (NFDA), Marketplace (books and videos), 11121 W. Oklahoma Ave., Milwaukee, WI 53227-0496, 800-228-6332

National Organization for Rare Disorders (NORD), 800-999-6673

Paraclete Press & Paraclete Video Productions (book and videos), PO Box 1568, Orleans, MA 02653, 800-451-5006

Pregnancy and Infant Loss Center of Minnesota (PILC), 1421 E. Wayzata Blvd., Suite 70, Wayzata, MN 55391, 952-473-9372

Resolve, Inc. Infertility, 1310 Broadway, Somerville, MA 02144-1731

SHARE, Pregnancy & Infant Loss Support, Inc., St. Joseph Health Center, 300 First Capital Drive, St. Charles, MO 63301-2893, 800-821-6819, www.NationalSHAREoffice.com

Sidelines National Support Network, PO Box 1808, Laguna Beach, CA 92652, 714-497-2265

SIDS Alliance, 1314 Bedord Ave., Suite 210, Baltimore, MD 21208, 800-221-SIDS

The Compassionate Friends (TCF) National Office, PO Box 3696, Oak Brook, IL 60522-3696, 630-990-0010, www.Compassionatefriends.org, e-mail: TCF National@prodigy.com

The Self-Help Center, A Division of the Mental Health Association of Illinois, 312-368-9070

Wisconsin Stillbirth Service Program: Life and Death before Birth
For professional use
#1: Stillbirth, 23 minutes
#2: Justification for stillbirth assessment and evaluation, 21 minutes
#3: Practical guide to stillbirth evaluation, 21 minutes
#4: Summarization data of the 10-year study, 17 minutes
#5: Case studies of evaluations

Pediatrics Bereavement Support Groups

Centers and Publications

The Bobbi Burrow: A Center for Grieving Children of all Ages, 403 Walnut Street, St. Charles, IL 60174, 603-513-8327

The Compassionate Friends, Inc., P.O. Box 3696, Oak Brook, IL 60522-3696, 630-990-0010, Theresa Goodrich

The Dougy Center: The National Center for Grieving Children and Families, 3909 S.E. 52nd Ave., P.O. Box 86852, Portland, OR 97286, Phone: 503-775-5683, Fax: 503-777-3097, www.dougy.org

Just for Us: A Bereavement Newsletter for Children and Teens, St. Mary's Hospital for Children, 29-01 216th St., Bayside, New York, 11360, 212-281-8810

Marcie's Place: A Camp for Grieving Children, P.O. Box 1855, Evanston, IL 60204-1855, 773-509-0983

Suggested Readings for Children

Brown, L. K., & Brown, M. (1996). *When dinosuars die: A guide to understanding death.* Boston, MA: Little, Brown.

Buscalia, L. (1983). *The fall of Freddy the leaf.*

Coh, J. (1987). *I had a friend named Peter: Talking to children about the death of a friend.* New York: Morrow Junior Books.

Cohn, J. (1994). *Molly's rosebush.* Morton Grove, IL: Whitman & Co. ISBN #08075-5213-5

Collins, P. L. (1990). *Waiting for baby Joe.* ICEA Publication #FC9201.

Dodge, N. C. (1984). *Thump's story: A story of love and grief shared by Thumpy, the Bunny.* Springfield, IL: Prairie Lark Press.

Grollman, E. A. (1970). *Talking about death: A dialogue between parent and child.* Boston, MA: Beacon Press.

Gryte, M. (1988). *No new baby.* ICEA Publication FC#8811.

Johnson, J., & Johnson, M. (1982). *Where's Jess.*

O'Connor, J. (1997). *Heaven's not a crying place: Teaching your child about funerals, death and the life beyond.* Grand Rapids, MI: Baker Book House.

O'Toole, D. (1988). *Aarvy Aardvark finds hope.* Burnsville, NC: Celo Press.

Palmer, P. (1994). *I wish I could hold your hand: A child's guide to grief and loss.* San Luis, CA: Impact Publishers.

Roberts, J., & Johnson, J. (1994). *Thank-you for coming to say goodbye.* Omaha, NE: Centering Corp.

Rofes, Eric (1985). *The kid's book about death and dying.* Boston, MA: Little, Brown.

Sanford, D. (1986). *It must hurt a lot: A child's book about death.* Multnomah Press.

Sims, A. (1986). *Am I still a big sister?* Big A & Company.

Skeie, E. (19xx). *Summerland: A story about death and hope.* Elgin, IL: Brethren Press.

Slater, R. C. (1978). *Tell me, papa.* Omaha, NE: Centering Corp.

Van-Si, L. and Powers, L. (1994). *Helping children heal from loss: A keepsake book of special memories.* Portland State University/Continuing Education Press.

Viorst, J. (1971). *The tenth good thing about Barney* New York: Atheneum Press.

White, E. B. (1952). *Charlotte's web.* New York: Harper.

Wolfelt, A. (1994). *Sarah's journey: One child's experience with the death of her father.* Center for Loss and Life Transition.

Grief Websites

Achoo: www.achoo.com

American Board of Pediatric Ethics: www.abd.org/bioethix.htm

American Medical Association: www.ama-assn.org

Association of Women's Health, Obstetric, and Neonatal Nurses (AWHONN): www.awhonn.org

Bereavement and hospice directory: www.ubalt.edu/www/bereavement

Care plans, library, forum, and tips on patient education: www.rncentral.com

Centers for Disease Control and Prevention: www.cdc.gov

The Changing Face of Women's Health: www.whealth.org/exhibit

Child Trends: www.childtrends.org

Citizens for Sensitive Care following the Loss of a Pregnancy: www.petitionpetition.com

Cremation Society: locations: www.cremation.org

DeathNET: choices in dying: www.rights.org/deathnet

Dos and don'ts of Grief Support: www.pw2.netcom.com/~jcaccia/dosdonts.html

The Dougy Center: The National Center for Grieving Children and Families: www.dougy.org

For Women: www.4women.gov

Grief net website linking to support groups: www.grotmet.org

GriefNet: http://rivendell.org/supportgroups.htm

Growth House: directory, end of life care: www.growthhouse.org

Health Finder: www.healthfinder.gov

Health Web: evaluated and annotated links to health-related resources: www.healthweb.org

Hospice Hands: global and multicultural: http://hospice-cares.com

Hospital Web: information on hospitals: http://neuro-www.mgh.harvard.edu/hospitalweb.shtm

Information for medical and caregiving professionals on how to assist grieving families: www.fortunecity.com/millenium/babar/log/propage/html

The Internet Cremation: www.cremation.org

Kids' Health: www.kidshealth.org

Library of Congress: access to catalogues and databases: http://lcweb.loc.gov

Mayo Health: www.mayohealth.org

MedNet Interactive: www.mednet-i.com

National Library of Medicine: www.nlm.nih.gov

National Public Radio: The End of Life—Exploring Death in America: www.npr.org/programs/death

The NLM PubMed Project: www.ncbi.nlm.nih.gov

OncoLink: University of Pennsylvania Cancer Center: www.oncolink.upenn.edu

Office of Minority Health Resource Center: www.omhrc.gov

Pregnancy and Infant Loss: www.pilc.org

Reincarnation International: www.dircon.co.uk/reincarn

The Robert Wood Johnson Foundation: Last Acts: www.lastacts.org

SA/VE: Suicide Awareness/Voices of Education: www.save.org

Soros Foundation: Project on Death in America: www.soros.org/death.htm

United Kingdom–based Child Bereavement Trust Center of Minnesota: www.childbereavement.org.uk

University of Toronto Joint Centre for Bioethics: www.utoronto.ca.jcb

Webster's Death, Dying and Grief Guide: www.katsden.com/death/index.htm

Wisconsin Stillbirth Service Program: www.wisc.edu/wissp

World Wide Nurse Network: www.wnurse.com

You are Not Alone website: general resources: www.teleama.com/~jaff7

CHAPTER 38

Community and Home Health Care Nursing for the High-Risk Infant

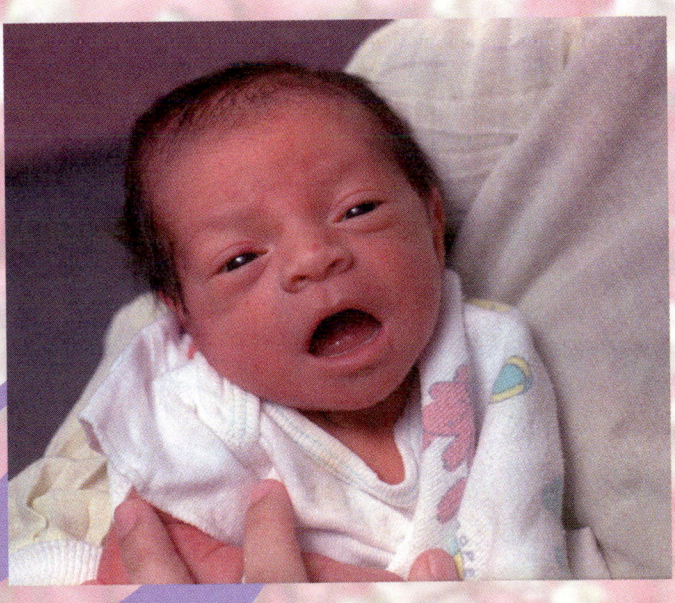

Current health care practices have forced nurses to focus on creating new ways to provide high-quality care while keeping down costs. Health care delivered during home visits can significantly benefit high-risk infants and their families. These benefits are evidenced by improvements in maternal health, mother-infant interaction, infant health and development, and overall family function. Home health care nurses need to take the lead in delivering health care in the home to promote continuity of care for high-risk infants. This type of intervention is important in the health care surveillance and maintenance of high-risk infants and their families.

Key Terms

Barrier to service
  utilization

Follow-up services

Home care

Home care nursing

Competencies

Upon completion of this chapter, the reader should be able to:

1. Discuss the significance of home care in the present health care delivery system.
2. Describe the nurse's role in home care to promote and maintain the health of infants and families.
3. Discuss a nursing model with application to the home care of infants and their caregivers.
4. Explore significant factors in the environment that influence the health of infants.
5. Apply the nursing process to home care.
6. Discuss the standards of care for home visiting of high-risk infants.

One of the most heartening indicators of the improvement in health in the United States during the 20th century has been the steady decrease in the infant mortality rate. Between 1950 and 1987, the U.S. infant mortality rate decreased from 29.2 per 1,000 live births to 10.1; the rate in 1998 was 7.2. The U.S. international ranking is 26, which indicates that the infant mortality rate is higher in the United States than in many other countries worldwide. The continuing disparities between minority and majority populations represent a major health challenge. In 1987, the mortality rate for African American infants was still more than twice that of Caucasian infants. The infant mortality rate in 1998 was 6 for Caucasians and 14.3 for African Americans. Neonatal deaths were 4.8 overall, 4.0 for Caucasians and 9.5 for African Americans based on a denominator of 1,000 live births.

Infant mortality rates provide a summary measure of the effect of major health threats to the developing fetus and newborn baby. For every 10 babies who die, however, 990 live. Some of those who live have been harmed, often permanently, by unhealthy beginnings. In the United States, complications of prematurity account for more than 70% of fetal & neonatal deaths annually in infants without anomalies (Colombo & Ians, 2000). The quality, not just the quantity, of their lives is a function of health during the prenatal and infant periods. Although overall infant mortality rates have declined, there has been no improvement in preterm birth rates (American College of Obstetricous and Gynecologists [ACOG] 1995). The incidence of preterm births also has increased from 9.4% in 1981 to 11.9% in 1997 (a 20% increase) (Ventura, Martin, Curtin, Mathews, & Park 1998).

Technology has contributed significantly to the improved prospects for infant survival over the past several decades. Neonatal intensive care, new surgical techniques, and other medical interventions save lives and overcome conditions that formerly guaranteed lifelong disability. Opportunities for primary prevention offer new frontiers for improving infant health in the coming years. Some opportunities will result from breakthroughs in understanding the genetic origins of human diseases; most will be in areas of personal lifestyle and use of existing health interventions.

ECONOMICS AND HOME HEALTH CARE

The 1990s marked the transition from hospital-based care to home care for chronic conditions (Stutts, 1994). In neonatal medicine, this move to home care was directed by motivation for health. The goals of health care providers are to assist families in identifying health needs and in developing problem-skills using the family's own resources. To meet these goals the nurse needs to identify the family's perception of healthy or unhealthy practices, which greatly influences participation in health-promoting activities. Age, gender, educational level, cultural orientation, financial status, and occupation influence health perception. If parents believe the infant is more susceptible to a health problem they will become more motivated to adopt the behavior (Pennacchia, 1994).

The family as the unit of care has long been the focus of home care nurses. In **home care nursing**, nurses deliver care in the home environment. Many clients who receive home health care would not be able to remain in their homes if it were not for family members who devote themselves to their care (Bradley & Alpers, 1996). Therefore, the basic and most important approach when addressing health promotion and disease prevention issues with a client is through their family. According to McCarthy (1994) it is in families that children and adults are nurtured, provided for, and taught about health values by word and example. It is in families that an individual is socialized and first learns to make choices that promote personal physical and emotional health.

The nurse's role is to help the parents recognize the infant's susceptibility and the potential consequences when good-quality health practices are not used. The nurse must work within the family's health perception framework to become acquainted with the characteristics that strongly influence the infant's health. Unless caregivers meet their own needs, they will be less able to meet their infant's physical and mental needs (Janosik & Green, 1992). The nurse supports the parents, building up their parental confidence and self-esteem, providing information in meeting the infant's needs, and reinforcing their health perception and management patterns (Pennacchia, 1994).

The nursing process guides and supports the family and nurse during the development of a plan that will enhance wellness or solve problems or potential problems. This process and encounter can occur in multiple settings. Home care services have become a rapidly expanding and popular area of health care in the past 5 years. The home is a natural environment for all families. Members of different age groups—infants, children, and older persons—are apt to be more readily available in the home. The home health care nurse also can observe firsthand the physical environment during the home visit. The nurse can see the whole family as a unit, observing mealtime rituals, roles of family members, and interpersonal interactions. Including each member of the family in the visit will provide the nurse with a broader perspective than will observing and interviewing an isolated member. During the home visit the nursing process is carried out *with* the family and not *for* the family; the family becomes a partner with the nurse in all phases of the process (McCarthy, 1994).

Using a systems perspective when working with a family to enhance health promotion and disease prevention, the nurse's role includes the following tasks (McCarthy, 1994):

- To become aware of family attitudes and behaviors toward health promotion and disease prevention
- To serve as a role model for the family
- To collaborate with family members in assessing, improving, enhancing, and evaluating their current health practices

- To assist the family in growth and development behaviors
- To assist the family in identifying risk-taking behaviors
- To assist the family in decision-making regarding lifestyle choices
- To provide reinforcement for positive health behaviors
- To assist the family in learning behaviors that promote health and prevent disease
- To serve as a liaison for referral or collaboration between community resources and the family

The home care nurse should enter the relationship with an open approach to assess the norms and expectations of family members, communication patterns, decision-making patterns (collectively or individually), and how family members address each other's needs. Employing the nursing process and a systems perspective when working with families during home care helps the nurse and family strive for optimal levels of health promotion and disease prevention (McCarthy, 1994).

MULTICULTURAL DIVERSITY IN HOME HEALTH CARE

The issue of cultural influence is relevant when working with clients and families, even with families of the same cultural background as the home nurse. Persons in a nurse-client relationship should respect each other and appreciate each other's diversity. Cultural influences can directly affect the health care practices clients turn to for healing. For example, a person may turn to an alternative health care practitioner because of a language barrier, lack of trust, and lack of satisfaction with the treatment plan provided by the Western medical or nurse practitioner. Therefore, culturally competent nursing care promotes the well-being of the infant and family and should be a major component of providing family-centered home care services (Ahmann, 1996). Cultural traditions provide a sense of security that families refer to for guidance, comfort, and dealing with stressful situations, that is, the health-illness of their infant.

A **barrier to service utilization** is any real or perceived deterrent that prevents or delays use of available health care. These barriers may have underpinnings of social or cultural influences. According to Spector (1994) innumerable barriers of a social nature, including poverty, language, and transportation, restrict infants and their families from using health care services in ordinary and expected ways. The major factor is poverty because it restricts a person's access to these services. Other barriers

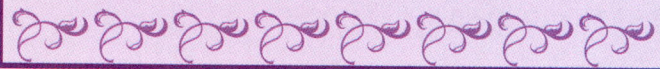

Critical Thinking

Foster Care Practices

EM is a Caucasian male born at 26 weeks' gestational age to a mother who uses cocaine. His urine drug screening test was positive for cocaine. Child protective services placed EM in foster care after hospital discharge. EM was released to an African American foster mother at 7 months of age. The foster mother could not participate in his care during the hospital stay. EM's medical history includes having a gastric tube in place for feeding and apnea of prematurity for which he remains on an apnea monitor and medication.

- What are some of the cultural issues related to an African American foster parent raising a Caucasian infant or vice versa?
- What are some American cultural values reflected in the process of placing this infant in a foster home?

may include lack of childcare, inconvenience, provider characteristics, immigration status, and failure to work within a person's belief system.

Nurses must be aware of and sensitive to cultural factors that influence the client and family in seeking health care services. Moreover, the nurse should be aware of these influences when assessing a community, family, and client. A cultural assessment provides a database from which the home care nurse can obtain an idea of the client's attitudes, values, and beliefs about the world. If culture provides standards for behavior, then home health nurses should assess their own culture of health care both from the viewpoint of the culture of origin (what they were taught to believe when growing up) and from that of the system into which they have been socialized. Home health care nurses need to explore values because they form the basis for behavior (Ahmann, 1996).

HISTORY OF HOME CARE

During the early 1900s demographic changes in the United States influenced the development of the visiting nurse. Many new child and family services were developed and implemented to address the issues associated with urbanization, immigration, poverty, contagious diseases, unhealthy living conditions, and high infant mortality rates. During this time period, it was felt that environmental conditions were major contributors to personal problems and

illness. Consequently, strong efforts were directed at changing poor social conditions, particularly those contributing to illness, accidents, and infant mortality. The role of the visiting nurse continued to develop and expand, and two additional roles for service were developed: visiting teachers and social workers (Wasik, Bryant, & Lyons, 1990).

Visiting nurses also addressed preventive care in their efforts to provide home health care. By 1910, most large urban visiting nurse associations had developed and implemented preventive programs for infants, children, mothers, and patients with tuberculosis (Buhler-Wilkerson, 1985). Voluntary and publicly funded institutions, however, dominated public health and prevention efforts and voiced that these issues were in their domain. Moreover, these institutions objected to visiting nurses' involvement in prevention. Buhler-Wilkerson (1985) reported that this assertion and possession of health care preventive efforts outraged nursing leaders. Visiting nurses, they insisted, had taken the lead to teach prevention and hygiene and had, in fact, "blazed the trail" for all health department preventive program. Although debate over the roles of visiting and public health nurses in the community continued to evolve, in practice, both groups of nurses were actively involved in home care throughout the 20th century. Today, home visiting and public health nurses continue to have a strong presence in the community health arena.

The Family Preservation and Support Act of 1993 was the first major change in Title IV-B of the Social Security Act since the enactment of the Adoption Assistance and Child Welfare Act of 1980. The Family Preservation and Support Act of 1993 provides federal funding through the states for services to strengthen and support families to enable them to provide a safe and nurturing environment for their children. Services are aimed at prevention to reduce the risks of out-of-home placement and family disintegration. Through the Home Visiting for At-Risk Families (HVAF) state health planning initiative, the Maternal and Child Health Bureau (on behalf of the Health Resources and Services Administration) and the Children's Bureau (on behalf of the Administration for Children and Families) have come together to stimulate and support coordinated planning for family preservation and to support the development of systems of care that will focus on prevention and address the range of health, social, and related concerns facing families (National Center for Education in Maternal and Child Health, 1995).

RESEARCH ON HOME VISITING PROGRAMS

Olds and Kitzman (1990; 1993) provided a comprehensive review of home visitation programs. In 1993, the *Future of Children: Home Visiting* analyzed 31 randomized trials of

Research Highlight

Home Visitation and Parenting Skills

Purpose

To examine the outcomes of home visits by nurses to teach parenting skills.

Methods

Sixty-one low income, first-time adolescent and nonadolescent mothers were enrolled. Mothers were single, with a mean age of 18.5 years, predominantly Caucasian, having a low educational level, unemployed, and were living with at least one parent or sibling or with their husband. Each participant was enrolled in the Parent Education/Home Visitation Program that consisted of weekly in-home education sessions over a 6-month period. A trained female "parent educator" conducted the sessions targeted at enhancing the development of the parent and child and fostering the parent-child relationship. Outcomes were based on six variables, that is, parenting developmental expectations, parenting skill knowledge of empathy, role reversal, corporal punishment, safety of the home, and community agency involvement, in four areas:

1. Parent's knowledge level of appropriate developmental expectations.
2. Parent's knowledge of appropriate parenting skills.
3. Safety of the home.
4. Use of community resources.

Findings

The results indicated that the mothers had significant improvement in five of the six outcomes (all but corporal punishment). After 6 months it also was noted that adolescent mothers, compared with nonadolescent mothers, improved their scores (adolescents had lower scores than did nonadolescents at the beginning of the study) for empathy and child-parent roles.

Nursing Implications

Nursing research has shown that home health care visits to mother-infant dyads are effective in promoting support for the physiologic, behavioral-psychosocial, and family aspects of parenting. The most successful of these programs include use of nurses, structured teaching of maternal skills for infant care, long-term follow-up, additional comprehensive services and resources, flexibility and variety in outreach methods, and maternal focused support and recognition. Although not consistently supported in research, infant outcomes have purported to promote development and intelligence; improve responsiveness and interaction with mothers; yield fewer emergency room visits and fewer days of hospitalization; and result in fewer problems with temperament and behavior. Clients were also more likely to have safer homes and increased child use of health care. Research and clinical experience uphold the belief that women, and their children, at highest risk (those of low income with poor self-esteem who are young, unmarried, poorly educated, unemployed, and involved in domestic violence or abuse) show the greatest need and have the best outcomes.

Culp, A. M., Culp, R. E., Blankemeyer, M., Passmark, L. (1998). Parent Education/Home Visitation Program: Adolescent and non-adolescent mother comparison after six months of intervention. *Infant Mental Health Journal, 19,* (2), 111–123.

home visiting programs. The review was divided into five major sections: prenatal programs, programs to improve the health and development of low-birth-weight or preterm infants and their parents, programs for children from families at social or economic risk, programs designed for children with developmental disabilities or chronic illnesses, and programs that evaluated program costs and savings. Some of the noteworthy conclusions follow:

- Home visiting can promote the development of preterm and low-birth-weight infants for those families who remain enrolled in these programs.

- Teenagers who are members of families with low income and unmarried teenagers are responsive to home visiting programs.

- Programs that had professionals (nurses) or highly trained staff should positive effects on children's intellectual functioning.

- Professionals (nurses) and comprehensive service models produced a greater chance of influencing the quality of parental caregiving.

- The positive effects of home visiting were greatest for those at highest psychosocial risk.

- Mothers valued the nurses as home visitors because nurses addressed concerns mothers' about child health.

- Flexible programs (that allowed the frequency of contact to be adjusted to the family's specific needs) proved more successful than did programs that were inflexible.

The implications of this review by Olds and Kitzman are that not only is further research necessary but, with the increase in vulnerable families, systematic understanding of which preventative strategies are most effective is more important to uncover.

BARNARD'S NURSING MODEL

The Barnard Parent-Child Interaction Theory can be used as a foundation when working with high-risk infants and their mothers. The theory was developed from earlier work by Barnard on the Nursing Child Assessment Project, a longitudinal study that examined the developmental outcomes of children prenatally and postnatally at 1 month, 8 months, 1 year, 2 years, and 7 years (Barnard and Kelly, 1990). The three concepts of Barnard's theory are the mother, child, and environment. The mother is required to adapt to the infant's needs and demands and to use positive and negative feedback with her verbal and nonverbal cues. The infant, in turn, is required to respond to the mother through changing its behavior. The environment includes animate (other peo-

ple and animals), inanimate (toys, sounds, and objects), and the surrounding milieu. This important interaction between the three components assert a major influence on the infant (Barnard & Eyres, 1979).

Barnard describes this mother-infant interaction as a dialogue or a mutually adaptive "waltz" between partners (Barnard, 1976). If the cues (verbal and nonverbal behavior) given by the infant are not clear or the mother is unable to recognize the cues, the health of the infant is affected, resulting in poor development and developmental delays. For example, research that investigates parent interaction links synchronous mother-infant interaction with positive developmental outcomes (Barnard, 1997).

This middle range theory deals with the mother-infant-environment relationship and suggests that the relationship between the mother and the infant will directly affect the health of the infant. The Barnard model is based on various disciplines, including medicine, child development, psychology, and sociology. The theory is testable, and several tools have been derived from the model, for example, the Nursing Child Assessment Feeding Scale and Nursing Child Assessment Teaching Scale.

Barnard also developed a program called Keys to Caregiving to present up-to-date information about infant behavior, describe the impact of caregiving, and aid nurses in translating this information to parents. For example, one of the earliest forms of infant communication occurs during feeding. It is during this interaction that Barnard focuses her attention on promoting positive caregiving behaviors. Her research has demonstrated that the absence of these skills by either partner (mother or infant) has a major impact on the nature of the caregiver-infant interaction pattern and later development (Barnard, 1980). This example illustrates how theory and research provide the foundation for nursing practice.

MULTIDISCIPLINARY TEAM APPROACH TO HOME HEALTH CARE

Collaboration in the assessment process, as an in-service provision, has two areas: collaboration between the family and the nurse or other professionals (parent-professional collaboration) and collaboration between the many disciplines that may be involved in the care of the infant and family (multidisciplinary collaboration).

To best meet the needs of the infant-child and family, care must be planned that reflects the family's values, goals, and priorities. To accomplish this plan of care, a central aspect of the assessment process is for family members to identify their needs or problems and strengths or resources. Involving families in the assessment process may be new to many nurses; however, active participation of the family members in developing the plan of care ensures a plan that meets their needs (Ahmann & Floyd, 1996).

The nurse brings special experience and expertise to the collaborative effort. This expertise can be shared with the family in a way that can foster collaboration. The nurse can share observations, comments, and knowledge with the family in a neutral manner, that is, without value judgment and without subverting the family's central decision-making role (Bond, Phillips, & Rollins, 1994). An essential part of the assessment process is assisting the family in determining whether the infant-child or family may need additional services and disciplines not originally prescribed as part of the plan of care. Such services might include those of a social worker; a physical, occupational, or speech therapist; or a registered dietitian. Each home care agency should have preestablished criteria that can guide the nurse in deciding when such referrals are appropriate for more in-depth assessment or intervention.

As the team extends beyond the nurse and family, multidisciplinary collaboration becomes crucial. Jointly defining initial goals for the client followed by providing consistent communication among disciplines will benefit the family and staff in many ways. Close collaboration will result in more rapid attainment of goals and a higher level of desired client outcomes. Joint visits and team conferencing are two ways multidisciplinary collaboration can be facilitated (Ahmann & Floyd, 1996). Home visits by multidisciplinary teams significantly benefit the infant and family by providing education, emotional support, preventive care, and information on community resources.

Home visits for infants and families that are in high-risk environments provide not only continuity of care after hospital discharge but also play a major role in the successful development of these infants and families (Kang et al., 1995; Olds et al., 1995; Starn, 1992).

Nursing Guidelines and Recommendations for Home Health Care

The Association of Women's Health, Obstetric, and Neonatal Nurses (AWHONN) has set forth standards and guidelines for the home care of women and newborns. These guidelines state that care in the home provides an opportunity for clients to receive technical and psychological support for their particular need or problem in a familiar, noninstitutional setting. Care in the home is designed to help the client achieve an optimal level of health. The importance of considering the mother or newborn as a whole person is underscored in the home care environment. Care often is provided by a multidisciplinary team, with the nurse coordinating the components (AWHONN, 1998). This association defines **home care** as the provi-

sion of technical, psychological, and other therapeutic support in the client's home environment rather than in an institution. The scope of nursing care delivered within the home setting is necessarily limited to practices deemed safe and appropriate to be carried out in an environment that is physically separated from a health care institution and its resources.

The guidelines for providing home care to mothers and their newborns include the following:

- Women and newborns are given the same level of nursing care and expertise in the home as would be expected in an inpatient setting.

- The plan of care for the client is developed collaboratively with the nurse, health care provider, and family members, taking into consideration the various aspects of the home life.

- Nursing practice in a home care setting is consistent with federal and state regulations or Canadian provincial regulations that direct home care practice. The nurse demonstrates practice competence through formalized orientation and ongoing clinical education and performance evaluation in the respective home care agency. Standards for practice from key specialty organizations (such as AWHONN, the American College of Obstetricians and Gynecologists [ACOG], American Academy of Pediatrics [AAP], and Intravenous Nurse Society [INS]) provide the basis for clinical protocols and pathways and organizational programs in home care practice. The joint Commission on Accreditation of Healthcare Organizations (JCAHO) provides criteria for home care operations.

- The client's physiologic needs are the focus for planning. In addition, the client's social, spiritual, and psychological needs and the needs of the family are assessed and included in the plan of care. Many factors beyond those of hospital care are considered. The nurse's responsibilities may include the following:

  —Planning for comprehensive home health services, 24 hours a day, 7 days a week, with clients and families.

  —Supervising rehabilitation specialists who provide client services.

  —Acting as a coordinator in communicating a plan of care between clients and primary care providers.

  —Recording and communicating clients' responses to the plan of care and family support of the care.

  —Acting as a liaison with ancillary health care providers.

  —Developing and supervising a written plan of care for the homemaker or home health aide.

—Acting as an advocate for clients by promoting informed decision-making regarding care and orienting, supervising, and evaluating persons on the home health team as appropriate.

Home health care for mothers, infants, and families may require creative use of resources and adaptation of the more traditional methods of teaching and learning, especially in light of the limited technologic resources in the home (AWHONN, 1998).

The Council on Child and Adolescent Health, representing the AAP, published a policy statement in 1998 on *The Role of Home Visitation Programs in Improving Health Outcomes for Children and Families* (AAP, 1998). In this publication, cited and endorsed were a clear recognition of the postnatal effects of home visiting (improved maternal-child interaction, maternal satisfaction, and higher developmental quotients in infants visited), the long-term benefits (fewer maternal behavioral impairments attributable to alcohol and drug abuse), and elements of what constitutes a successful home visiting program. The recommendations of the Council included full support of home visiting programs, support for the use of home visitors as integral and active members of the health care team, and encouragement of early referral of known high-risk parents.

NURSING ROLE IN THE HOME HEALTH CARE OF THE HIGH-RISK INFANT

Home health visits are made by nurses from different disciplines. The purpose of home visits is to provide nursing care to clients and families in the home. The specific objectives and services provided by nurses vary depending on the type of agency providing services and the population served (Lyon, Bolla, & Nies, 1997). Historically, home visits were provided by community health nurses who were employed by public health departments, visiting nurse associations, and home health care agencies. These home visits focused on the investigation of chronic and communicable diseases. More recently, home visiting programs have expanded so that the major focus is on the health outcomes of the mother, infant, and family.

Home care nursing is in its early developmental stage and is getting stronger. Home care nurses practice under the direction of standards set by the American Nurses Association (ANA). Home health care nurses also can become certified in home care as nursing generalists. Many nurses are joining the home health care arena, and more research is being conducted to guide their practice (Humphrey, 1996).

The number of home health care agencies certified by Medicare increases annually. Downsizing continues in many hospitals. Nurses leave acute care settings seeking employment in home health care. Nurses are attracted to home care by flexible schedules and competitive salaries. The challenge to the home health care management staff is to recruit and orient nurses with varied levels of educational preparation to assume the responsibilities as home health care nurses in today's environment of rapid change (Ark & Nies, 1996). Home health care nurses need to be more knowledgeable and experienced in dealing with various factors specific to home health care, for example, family structure, folk medicine, and cultural differences. Moreover, home health care nurses develop their interventions based on the community resources available.

The focus of all home visits is on the infant for whom the referral is received. The home health care nurse makes an assessment of the interaction between the infant and family then provides education and intervention. The nurse then evaluates how the infant and family interact as part of an aggregate group in the community. The need for referrals for community services is identified by the home health care nurse and made as necessary (Lyon, Bolla, & Nies, 1997).

HOME VISIT PREPARATION

Once the high-risk infant is discharged from the hospital, special care needs do not stop. Many of these infants have needs that exceed routine well-child care. Special attention must be given to their growth and nutrition, immunizations, vision and hearing, and sequelae of illnesses experienced during the neonatal period. Premature infants have an increased likelihood of long-term sequelae and continuing medical problems compared with term infants; however, many of the issues discussed specifically about prematurity also apply to term infants (Bernbaum, 1994).

Critical Thinking

Organizing Home Health Care for the Infant

When you begin home visits to a family, the following questions should be addressed:

- What is the extent of the medical and nursing care needed?
- In what time frame is the care needed (e.g., the entire day or night, or only during the waking hours)?
- What are the physical, social, and emotional needs of the parents and family?
- What are the teaching needs of the family?

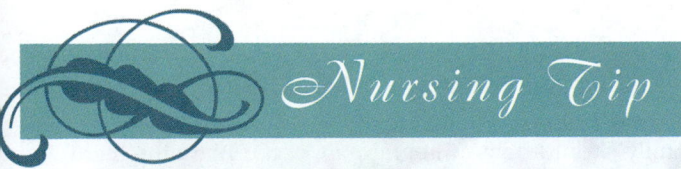

SAFETY FOR HOME HEALTH CARE VISITS

Here are some safety tips for the home health care nurse (Humphrey and Milone-Nuzzo, 1996):

- Know where you are going and how to get there.
- Avoid walking down alleys or on private property to and from a client's residence.
- Avoid carrying a purse or pocketbook.
- Park as close as possible to the client's home.
- Dress appropriately.
- If you have fears about your safety while in the home (e.g., if you feel threatened by someone who is intoxicated or if weapons are evident) leave the home.
- If pets are bothersome during the home visit, insist that they be put in another room.
- Know the telephone numbers of your agency, the local police, and the fire department.
- Keep your nursing bag within your sight.
- Do not attempt to break up a domestic argument.
- Never walk into a home uninvited.

The first home visit is important for several reasons. First, it is the beginning of the relationship between the home health care nurse and the family. In all likelihood, the first visit will set the tone of the relationship and thus influence subsequent visits. Second, in most agencies, the first home visit requires the most documentation (e.g., permission forms, insurance information, and medical history). Third, the first home visit must include an immediate assessment of the infant's status and safety at home. Fourth, nursing interventions, including teaching and direct care, may be required on the first home visit (Ahmman & Floyd, 1996).

TRANSITION FROM HOSPITAL TO HOME HEALTH CARE

The transition of care from the hospital to home for high-risk infants has been advanced by the increased availability of new technologies for use in the home (such as ventilators, infusion pumps, and apnea monitors) and supported by the need for health care cost containment and an increase in patient knowledge and participation in

self-care. Home care of the high-risk infant has many advantages compared with hospitalization. Such as paranatal education, social support, and linkage with community services. Home care allows for a normal environment-patient interaction and minimizes family disruption (Kenner & Bagwell, 1998).

High-risk infants have many conditions with the potential for long-term sequelae, accounting for the morbidity in this population. Having an infant who might remain dependent on technology for survival impacts the entire family unit. The normal progression and emotional preparation for parenting has been interrupted by the infant's illness. Moreover, the family also has the fears that accompany having a family member who is seriously ill or at high risk for future illnesses. Parents may exhibit feelings of helplessness, anger, grief, and depression. These feelings along with the financial burden of care may exhaust the family's financial, emotional, and physical resources. Consequently, the parent-infant interaction may be altered. Home health care helps identify issues surrounding the parent-infant relationship, helps parents deal with the illness, and supports parents caring for high-risk infants (Fleming et al., 1994).

Discharge and Home Health Care Planning

Admission of an infant to the neonatal intensive care unit (NICU) places the infant and family at risk. Because this high-risk situation will trigger others, careful discharge planning is important. Continuity of care that is directed by discharge planning can minimize fragmentation, help avoid repetition and delay, and ensure information about essential community resources is provided. By using a comprehensive discharge plan the nurse will help ensure that the family is adequately prepared to care for the infant at home. This plan should include organized **follow-up services** (health care services provided after discharge from the hospital) for the infant and family. Many high-risk infants have needs that are far from routine, in addition to requiring well-care. Attention should be given to the infant's growth and nutrition, immunizations, vision and hearing, and illnesses that may occur during the neonatal period (Bernbaum, 1994).

An accurate and detailed assessment is the basis for optimal care. The consistency of care from hospital to home provided by a primary care team enables these assessments to be comprehensive and highly individualized. Beginning with admission, the team identifies problems or needs that require special planning, intervention, teaching, or follow-up. Before hospital discharge, the needs of the infant, family, and environment once again are assessed (Cox, 1996). The results of the assessment should be clearly communicated to the nurse who will provide the home

Client Education

Information to Help Parents Understand their Infant's Behaviors

- Infant temperament: Infants have different temperaments that are expressed immediately after birth. These are stable characteristics and are a part of the infant's personality. Parents can benefit from a discussion regarding temperament.

- Crying: Infants express their needs and emotions through crying. Infants expend large amounts of energy while crying. Parents can benefit from learning to distinguish different cries and methods of calming the infant.

- Poor feeding habits: High-risk infants may have difficulty feeding after they go home. Nurses may need to help the family employ special feeding techniques.

health care. Ideally, the home visit should be part of a team effort. The following is a discharge planning checklist:

- The infant's medical issues are well defined.
- Medications are labeled clearly and verified before being sent home with the family.
- The home visiting nurse and family members have been given clear instructions on the use of required monitoring devices.
- Special formulas and diet have been explained to the nurse and family members.
- Instructions and demonstrations on specialized needs (e.g., shunts, gastrostomy, and home oxygen) have been given to the nurse and family.

The following should be performed before the infant is discharged:

- Metabolic screening
- Hearing evaluation
- Ophthalmologic examination
- Developmental assessment
- Blood tests for hematocrit level, reticulocyte count, and levels of theophylline and anticonvulsants
- Continuing evaluation of or serial physical examinations for medical conditions such as chronic lung disease and birth asphyxia

Every family has the right to discharge planning. Some infants will require relatively simple preparation for dis-

charge, with a focus on well-infant care and routine medical follow-up. A more complex level of planning, however, may be required for infants who have special needs. The family should be an integral part of the planning team. Including the family will improve the appropriateness of the assessment and the likelihood that the plan is realistic and can be implemented effectively (Cox & Ahmann, 1996).

Follow-up Care for the High-Risk Infant

Follow-up programs should be an integral extension of every NICU. Specialized care must be available for problems of growth, development, and chronic disease and is best provided within the setting of a neonatal follow-up program. The follow-up care initially should be provided by the neonatologist, pediatrician, nurse practitioner, developmental specialist, and community health nurse. This initial continuity of care is important to reassure the family that the same persons responsible for the life-saving decisions are continuing to assume responsibility during the child's adaptation to home life. Furthermore, even if the neonatal staff members do not continue the follow-up for a long period, they will benefit greatly by maintaining contact with the infants leaving the nursery and recognizing the sequelae of early neonatal interventions. Growth (height, weight, and head circumference), neurologic development, psychomotor development, vision, and hearing should be sequentially assessed (Hack et al., 1994).

Follow-up care after hospital discharge provides the opportunity for assessment of the infant and identification of actual or potential problems (Box 38-1). Follow-up care allows the experienced neonatal registered nurse to teach,

Box 38-1 Successful Follow-up Outcomes

- Decrease in the number of rehospitalizations during the first year of life.
- Decrease in the number of emergency room visits during the first year of life.
- Decrease in the number of acute care visits and calls to the primary care provider.
- Positive growth patterns.
- Positive integration of the neonate into the family unit.
- Client and caregiver satisfaction.
- Client and caregiver competence and confidence.
- Absence of child abuse and neglect.
- Neurobehavioral and motor stability, with positive progress toward developmental milestones.

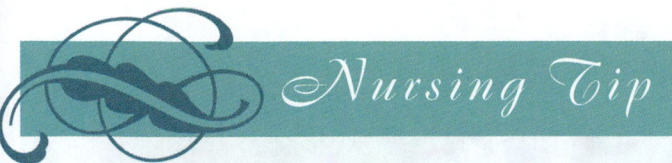

Nursing Tip

INTERVENTIONS TO ENHANCE PARENT-INFANT INTERACTION DURING HOME HEALTH CARE VISIT

You should do the following:

- Encourage eye-to eye contact during feeding and playing with the infant.
- Discuss the importance of stimulation during "social time."
- Identify the infant's attributes and unique qualities.
- Demonstrate appropriate feeding positions.

provide a role model, and assess parent-infant interactions. Follow-up care promotes the transition from hospital to home. Parent satisfaction with health care is increased when individualized follow-up care is planned and coordinated before discharge. Since 1986, Brooten's team of researchers has advocated long-term follow-up for these neonates and families (extending up to 18 months after discharge) by registered nurses with a master's degree. In today's health care structure of health maintenance organization and health alliances, such long-term visitation may not be feasible or necessary (Brooten et al., 1996). However, an experienced neonatal home care nurse should perform home visits. Ideally, a home visit should be made before the neonate is discharged from the hospital.

Infants at the highest risk for later neurodevelopmental problems include those who have had severe asphyxia, severe intraventricular or other intracranial hemorrhage, menigitis, seizures, respiratory failure resulting from pneumonia, persistent fetal circulation, severe respiratory distress syndrome, multisystem congenital malformations, and those born with very low birth weight (less than 1500 g) (Hack, Klein, & Taylor, 1995).

THE HOME HEALTH CARE VISIT

The first home health care visit in the postdischarge period should occur within 24 to 48 hours. This visit should include physical, developmental, nutritional, and social-environmental assessments; obtaining blood for laboratory tests; specific teaching; and referrals.

Physical Assessment

Assessment by systems should follow this sequence (Humphrey & Milone-Nuzzo, 1996):

Nursing Alert

RED FLAGS DURING HOME HEALTH CARE VISITS

During the home visit you should be alert for any red flags specific to the overall health of the infant. *Red flags* refer to the physical, emotional, or social aspect of infant behavior or appearance that requires attention or further investigation. Red flags provide clues to possible problems: social, emotional, growth and development problems; inadequate nutrition; parenting difficulties; environmental (safety) concerns; illness; and abuse and neglect. Some general red flags regarding health might include the following:

- Vomiting
- Diarrhea
- Slow development
- Noted change in any behavior (e.g., sleep and appetite)
- Constant crying
- Weight change
- Feeding difficulties
- Color changes
- Less responsiveness
- Stiff or limp (muscle tone)

1. Weight
2. Length
3. Head circumference
4. Thermal stability
5. Fontanel: size and shape
6. Vital signs, peripheral pulses, and ausculation of heart and lung sounds
7. Color: dusky, pale, cyanotic, or jaundiced (validated with pulse oximetry when indicated)
8. Sleep-wake cycles

Developmental Assessment

A development assessment or screening should always be included in follow-up care of the infant. We recommend the use of the Bayley Infant Neurodevelopmental Screen (BINS) initiated at 3 to 4 months corrected age. The Bayley Screen needs to be administered and interpreted by trained personnel. In order to evaluate the development of parent-child interaction as it unfolds, Barnard suggests the use of Nursing Child Assessment Satellite Training (NCAST

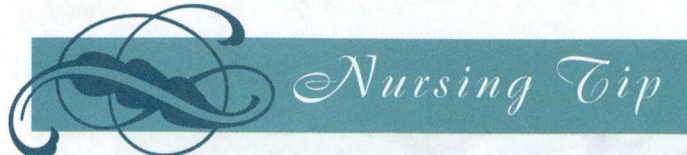
NURSING ASSESSMENT

The following questions are helpful in conducting a nutritional assessment:

- Is thrush present?
- Does the caregiver prop a bottle in the crib?
- How are utensils, bottles, and equipment sterilized or cleaned?
- Is a pacifier used? If so, how is it cleaned?

scales), particularly feeding and teaching, to support parent-child interaction. Both the BINS and NCAST scales are reliable and valid measures for positive infant growth and development and positive parenting. These scales provide outcomes data for the problems and development of interventions, and a method for outcomes to be evaluated.

Nutritional Assessment

A nutritional assessment will include the following:

- Assessment of breast-feeding, bottle-feeding, or alternative method of feeding
- Assessment of formula preparation
- Assessment of breast-feeding technique, breast care, pumping, and storage of breast milk
- With any feeding method (enteral, parenteral, or both), the following must be assessed: the volume being delivered; success of the feeding; frequency of feedings; urinary and stooling patterns; indications of intolerance; and most importantly, weight gain.

Social and Environmental Assessment

Social and environmental assessment helps identify potential health risks and barriers that may pose problems for the infant or family. Areas to assess include the following:

- Parent or caregiver interaction with the infant, ideally through the use of the NCAST scale, otherwise by observing the caregiver's handling of the neonate and sensitivity to stability and stress cues
- Parent or caregiver coping skills
- Availability of support such as community, financial, extended family, home care professionals, equipment companies, and employers

Client Teaching
The High-Risk Infant

Parents of high-risk infants often have the need to learn about parenting and general infant care as well as infant medical needs and procedures. The following are some teaching ideas for families of high-risk infants:

- General infant care: bathing; cord care; circumcision care; feeding techniques; nutritional needs; how to dress the infant for weather changes; sleep-wake patterns; a supportive environment; infant stability and stress cues; growth spurts, that is, what to do and when to expect them
- General safety issues, including crib safety
- Recommended sleeping positions and association with the prevention of sudden infant death syndrome (SIDS)
- Signs and symptoms of dehydration, fever, hypothermia, infection, or other illnesses
- Urination and stooling patterns, including the differences between bottle-fed and breast-fed infants
- When and whom to call for health care needs
- Care procedures needed for the neonate, for example, medication or special feeding administration
- Use and troubleshooting of home durable medical equipment and supplies
- Available community resources
- Possible sources for referrals
- Need for primary care follow-up, which includes routine physical examinations, immunization schedules, eye and hearing examinations, and appropriate speciality care
- Information about help available on a 24-hour basis
- Use of a car seat and current recommendations
- Sibling issues

- Home safety, including the availability of utility priorities: electricity, running water, sanitation, heat, and telephone services
- Parent or caregiver knowledge of infant care, safety, and specialized needs

* Parents' or caregivers' plans for infant care in their absence

Laboratory Tests

Laboratory tests will include tests as ordered by the primary care provider (the neonatologist, pediatrician, or nurse practitioner). These tests may include blood samples for serum bilirubin levels, serum levels to monitor drug therapy, neonatal screening tests, and others as indicated.

Referrals

The home health care visit often highlights the family's need for referrals to and information about resources and other agencies. Some of these referrals might include the following for infants with special needs:

* Social service agencies can help with financial or psychological adaptation.
* Occupational therapists and nutritionists provide support for infants with feeding problems.
* Nurses or occupational therapists with special education can help with the infant's developmental care.
* Lactation consultants can work with mothers of preterm and high-risk infants regarding breast-feeding.
* Breast-feeding support groups, such as La Leche League, can help parents.
* Support groups, such as the March of Dimes, can provide a listing of support groups for parents.

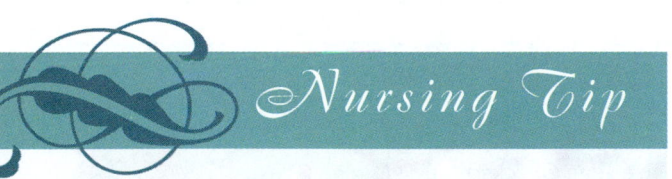

DEVELOPING A TEACHING PLAN

Before the home health care nurse can develop a teaching plan, the following assessments should be made:

* Level of knowledge of material to be taught
* Ability to address the cultural, social, and religious factors regarding the client
* Knowledge of the socioeconomic status of the client
* Awareness that the learning needs of the client are important
* Ability or level of the home nurse's skill in teaching
* Importance of evaluating client understanding before completing teaching tasks

* Paraprofessional help, such as homemakers and providers of respite care, can be contacted through social service agencies.
* Equipment companies for technical support can be accessed through the hospital or nurse home visiting agency.
* Early intervention programs may be helpful for long-term education of the child.
* Professional therapists, such as occupational, physical, and speech therapists, often are a part of interdisciplinary teams working with high-risk infants.
* Family and grief counselors may be found through social service agencies.

Recording the Visit

The home visit record documents the maternal medical history, the physical and developmental assessments, client needs, services provided, and follow-up recommendations and appointments. Home care records often are forms in triplicate, with one copy going to the client, one kept on file at the home health care agency, and one for the nurse's records. Complete and accurate documentation is necessary because these records are a part of the client's permanent medical record. Figure 38-1 shows an example of a home visit record.

PROGRAMS FOR THE INFANT AND FAMILY WITH SPECIAL NEEDS

Selected special needs situations and potential programs are discussed.

Home Health Care for the Infant Exposed to Drugs

It is difficult to determine the actual number of women who use alcohol or drugs before and during pregnancy and, thus, the number of infants exposed to alcohol or drugs in utero. Currently, identification of alcohol and drug use by pregnant women is primarily based self-reporting and sporadic testing at the time of delivery. Self-reporting is an unreliable method, and drug screening of pregnant women is not done routinely (Sackoff et al., 1992; Donaldson & Ahmann, 1996). According to Dungy-Poythress (1995), toxicology testing for most drugs can detect substances only for a short time after use. Thus, frequency, dosage, and gestational timing of drug use often are not addressed reliably. Confounding variables also often exist and include polysubstance abuse, absence of or poor prenatal care, poor general health, and nutritional

Date _____

Case Manager _____

RN _____

Name _____ Sex _____ Date of Birth _____

History:

    Type of Delivery _____ Complications _____

    Neonatal Complications _____

    Apgar Score _____ Gestational Age _____

    Birth Weight _____ Head Circumference _____ Length _____

Present:

    Age _____ Weight _____ FOC _____ Length _____

    Temperature _____ Heart Rate _____ Respiratory Rate _____

    Medications _____ Allergies _____

    Recent Illnesses/Hospitalizations _____

    Immunizations Needed _____

    Oxygen: Y   N   Apnea Monitor: Y   N

    Feedings _____

Physical Examination:

    General _____

    Head, Ears, Eyes, Nose, Throat _____

    Cardiovascular _____

    Respiratory _____

    GI/GU _____

    Extremities _____

    Neuro/Reflexes _____

Developmental Screening:

    Holds Head Erect: Y   N   Passive Muscle Tone Checked: Y   N

    Rolls from Prone: Y   N   Rolls from Supine: Y   N

    Sits with Assistance: Y   N   Sits Alone: Y   N

    Walks with Assistance: Y   N   Walks Alone: Y   N

    Communication: Smiles: Y   N   Coos: Y   N

    Words _____

Dates:

    Next Clinic Visit _____ Next Developmental Clinic Visit _____

    Next Home Visit _____

    Impression/Plans _____

    _____

    _____

Figure 38-1 Home visit record

deficiencies. All these factors contribute to the difficulty of studying the effects on infants of alcohol and drug use during pregnancy; however, national and regional studies conducted over the past few years continue to document an increasing number of women of childbearing age who regularly use substances, such as cocaine, alcohol, and marijuana, and continue to do so during pregnancy (Chasnoff, Landress, & Barrett, 1990; Mathias, 1995).

The health care problems associated with alcohol or drug abuse during pregnancy include spontaneous abortion, low birth weight, premature birth, small for gestational age growth parameters, central nervous system damage, teratogenic effects, withdrawal effects, and an increased incidence of SIDS (Davis, 1993; Kelley, 1992; Famularo, Kinscherff, & Fenton, 1992).

Ideally, the process of identification, intervention, referral, and treatment of a mother's substance abuse problem begins prenatally, with a focus on the current pregnancy. Unfortunately, substance abuse usually is identified after delivery of the infant by a positive result on urine drug screening or by maternal self-reporting. At this point, child protective services usually are called and several options are evaluated and discussed. The infant can be discharged in the care of the parents or a close relative, or can be placed in a foster home. The history and type of drug use, family support, and the mother's willingness to seek drug treatment generally are the determining factors in placement of the infant (Donaldson & Ahmann, 1996).

The infant may be discharged to a relative, frequently the maternal grandmother, which may create a problem if the mother lives in the same household. An unhealthy environment for the infant and mother may continue. According to Donaldson & Ahmann (1996), recognizing unsafe and undesirable living conditions owing to a current alcohol or drug problem in the home is an important nursing intervention. Signs causing concern may include the following:

- An unkempt house
- Little or no food in the refrigerator
- Signs of illicit drug paraphernalia, alcohol use, and tobacco use
- Signs of personal hygiene neglect
- Signs of maternal depression such as a flat affect, excessive sleeping, and crying
- Mother's harsh or derogatory language when talking to or about the infant
- Lack of attention to the infant's needs
- Poor maternal-infant interaction

Donaldson & Ahmann (1996) suggest that the approach to working with mothers who abuse substances should be a three-pronged one:

1. Support the mother and assist in referring her for treatment.
2. Identify the special needs of the infant.
3. Provide special training and support to caregivers as needed.

Programs that provide a comprehensive approach to families of infants and young children of mothers who abuse substances are described next.

CRADLES Integrated Children's Project

Infants exposed to drugs in utero are the primary beneficiaries of an innovative project by the Houston Council on Alcoholism and Drug Abuse (HCADA) called CRADLES. CRADLES works in a collaborative effort with the Harris County Hospital District and its own coalition comprised of other community institutions and agencies in Harris County dedicated to the well-being of children. CRADLES is a four-pronged project that provides intensive case management through regular in-home visits to assist specific clients, that is, infants exposed to substances, and their caregivers and families. Clients are assigned from the Harris County Hospital District (Ben Taub General Hospital and Lyndon B. Johnson General Hospital) after an assessment by an alcohol and drug abuse counselor from HCADA who is licensed by the state.

The mission of CRADLES is to enhance the overall development of infants through strengthening the family unity with the intent to impact the transgenerational nature of drug abuse (Box 38-2). The foundation of the project is the regular in-home visits with the family using an intensive case management model designed to provide information about access to needed resources. These resources include access to medical, psychiatric, and emotional care; treatment for substance abuse and dependence; relapse prevention; education; various types of therapy; and job training. Also included are the necessities of daily living such as housing, food, and transportation. To ensure that the needs of the clients are met, case managers and parents-caregivers work together to create and maintain a plan of action known as the Individual Family Service Plan (IFSP). The plan, a viable working document, is revised over time as goals are met and as needs change. Clients who, for a variety of reasons, do not meet the criteria for inclusion in the intensive regular home visit but whose mothers are using or abusing substances are followed by the hospital counselor on a supportive basis.

During the home visit the nurse should gather information to develop a plan for the mother-infant dyad by asking the mother questions and by observation. The role of the nurse working in collaboration with CRADLES case managers is to:

- Monitor and advise on the overall health status of the infant.
- Assess, record, and monitor growth and development.
- Offer anticipatory guidance on all aspects of the infant's health.
- Evaluate and recommend basic infant nutritional needs.
- Document health interventions and their outcomes.
- Advise parents-caregivers on issues relevant to optimal infant care practices and provide opportunities for parents to raise issues pertaining to health issues.
- Offer a written evaluation and suggestions to case managers for each home visit.
- Act as a liaison between health care professionals and case managers.
- Provide a means of continuity of health care.

A second important part of the project is the weekly curriculum-based parenting classes conducted simultaneously with play therapy and childcare. Two parenting groups are offered simultaneously with a social hour to encourage interaction with parents-caregivers who also are caring for infants exposed to drugs in utero while maintaining their own sobriety. Childcare is offered during the parenting classes with the purpose of enhancing age-appropriate social development and behavior. Art-play therapy is organized and implemented aimed at helping younger siblings (who also may have been exposed to substances in utero) attain and maintain age-appropriate social development and behavior.

Curriculum-based parenting classes include the following:

- One weekly closed parenting class in English during the day
- One weekly parenting class in Spanish during the day that is open to the community
- One weekly parenting class in English in the evening that is open to the community

During the parenting classes and while older siblings are in play therapy, another important aspect of the overall project takes place with the infant's younger siblings, that is, purposeful childcare. Purposeful childcare is planned to aid social development for toddlers (aged 1 to 3 years) and infants (from birth to 1 year of age). Moreover, a part of this purposeful childcare includes a counselor in training and invited retirees from various churches and organizations who serve as grandparents and role models.

Massage is demonstrated and taught to parents-caregivers as a method to enhance interaction between parents-caregivers and infants. Massage also serves as a way to calm the baby and, incidentally and simultaneously, the parent-caregiver. Three consultants also are involved with the project: a licensed massage therapist who works with these infants and families, an art-play therapist in charge of the art-play therapy aspect of the project, and a clinical developmental specialist with experience in the area of program development and evaluation who is responsible for the quality control of outcomes measured data.

Healthy Families Alexandria

Healthy Families Alexandria (HFA) adapted the Hawaii Healthy Start model, which also served as the primary model for the Healthy Families America approach to comprehensive and intensive home visit services. The National Committee to Prevent Child Abuse (NCPCA) actively promotes the Healthy Families America approach.

The Alexandria program provides outreach and supportive services to prenatal women and serves a significant number of teenage mothers as well as a highly diverse, multicultural population. Prenatal women and first-time mothers with infants no older than 2 months of age are referred and screened for voluntary enrollment until the child is 3 years old. The HFA model provides systematic and proactive early identification of at-risk families and home-based visiting and case management services delivered by trained, largely paraprofessional, family support workers.

Building on its successful adaptation of Hawaii's model in adjacent Fairfax County, Northern Virginia Family

Service designed HFA to address the needs of some of Alexandria's at-risk population. The HFA model incorporates 12 critical elements that reflect over 20 years of research on the structure, organization, staff, and activities of effective home visit programs (as summarized by NCPCA):

1. Initiate services prenatally or at birth.

2. Use a standardized assessment process and tool to identify families in need of services.

3. Offer services voluntarily and in a positive manner to build family trust.

4. Offer services intensely (at least once a week) with well-defined criteria for changing intensity of services and over the long term (3 to 5 years).

5. Offer culturally competent services with staff and materials that reflect the cultural, linguistic, geographic, racial, and ethnic diversity of the population served.

6. Focus on supporting the parent as well as parent-child interaction and child development.

7. Link all families with a medical provider to ensure optimal health and development and to other services, depending on family needs.

8. Limit staff case loads so that home visitors have adequate time with each family.

9. Select staff who have the appropriate personal characteristics (who are nonjudgmental, compassionate, and have the ability to establish a trusting relationship), willingness to work with culturally diverse communities, and the skills to do the job.

10. Select staff whose education or experience enables them to handle the experiences they will encounter in working with at-risk families and have them receive basic training.

11. Have staff receive intensive training specific to their role to understand the essential components of family assessment and home visitation.

12. Ensure that staff receive ongoing and effective supervision so they can develop realistic and effective plans to empower families to meet their objectives, work effectively with families who may not be making progress, and discuss their concerns to solve problems and avoid stress-related burnout.

Healthy Families Alexandria has four primary goals:

1. Ensure adequate prenatal care as prescribed by the mother's medical provider or the ACOG.

2. Ensure preventive well-care as prescribed by the child's medical provider or the AAP and advanced optimal child development (e.g., well-care visits, immunizations, and developmental assessments).

3. Improve new mothers' knowledge of their child's needs and behaviors and enhance parent-child interaction, bonding, and parenting skills.

4. Prevent child abuse and neglect among enrollees.

PUBLIC HEALTH PROGRAMS FOR INFANTS AND CHILDREN

Programs focused on young children and women with children are covered.

Early Childhood Intervention (Birth to 3 Years)

Parents want their children to grow, learn, and reach their potential. Some children with disabilities or developmental delays face unique challenges and need extra help. This extra help is called early childhood intervention. Early childhood intervention (ECI) programs work with more than 20,000 families a year whose children need help growing and learning. ECI staff and families become partners during these important first 3 years of the child's life (Early Childhood Intervention, 1997).

Early Childhood Intervention, which will celebrate 20 years of service in 2002, teaches families how to help their children reach their potential through education and therapy services. There are 71 local ECI programs that serve more than 23,000 children a year. In fiscal year 1997, ECI received $42 million in state and federal funds. Anyone can refer a family with a child under the age of 3 years who has a disability or suspected developmental delays. The child should be referred as soon as you or the family has a concern about the child's development. A diagnosis is not needed for referral. Federal law requires that professionals refer children for services within 2 working days. ECI provides needed support to families who are beginning to learn about their child's disability or delays. Early identification of children with problems helps minimize and prevent future problems. Local programs conduct free developmental screenings, assess children for developmental delays, and determine eligibility. Once a child is enrolled, a family plan will begin. If the child is not eligible for ECI, staff will refer the family to other resources.

The services of ECI may include the following:

- Assisstive technology
- Occupational therapy
- Physical therapy
- Psychological therapy
- Service coordination

- Social work
- Special instruction
- Speech and language therapy
- Transportation
- Vision
- Nursing
- Nutrition
- Audiology
- Early identification, screening and assessment
- Family counseling
- Family education
- Home visits
- Medical (only diagnostic or evaluation services)

Services are provided individually or with other children, depending on how the child would benefit most. Services are delivered in the home; in community-based areas; and in settings with children who do not have delays in their development, such as the child's day-care program. All services are free. To allow more children to be served, ECI will bill Medicaid or ask for permission to bill the health care insurance provider for covered services.

Women, Infants, and Children (WIC) Nutritional Program

The Special Supplemental Nutrition Program for Women, Infants, and Children (WIC) receives funding from the federal Maternal Child Health Block Grant, which is administered by the Public Health Department. The WIC program is a prevention-orientation program that provides nutritional assessment, counseling, and supplemental food to clients in the following categories: pregnant women, non–breast-feeding women, breast-feeding women, infants, and children up to 5 years of age. For families to be eligible for WIC they must meet income guidelines, be considered a nutritional risk (e.g., iron deficiency, low birth weight, and inadequate weight gain), have a medical referral form completed by a health care provider outlining the infant's medical history, and participate in reevaluation and recertification in the program every 6 months. The WIC program has higher income guidelines than does any other federal program, and families should be encouraged to apply.

Zahr and Montijo (1993) evaluated the effectiveness of home visiting in a total of 40 very low-birth-weight infants. All infants in this study required further nursing care after being discharged from NICU. Nursing care was provided for 8 to 24 hours daily initially and was reduced as the infant became more stable or the parents become more competent to provide care. Most of the infants were dis-

charged from the NICU on apnea monitors; pulse oximeters; oxygen therapy; total parenteral nutrition; and a variety of medications such as antibiotics, cardiac drugs, and theophylline. The findings of this study suggest that home care of sick, premature infants by trained nursing personnel can reduce the frequency of medical resource use. The mean number of emergency room visits for this sample of very low-birth-weight infants was lower than the average of emergency room visits reported for infants in earlier studies. All minor illnesses were taken care of by the nurses who provided home care, and there were no reported visits to physicians' offices for such illnesses.

NURSING IMPLICATIONS

While an assessment is essential at the onset of providing home care services, in reality, assessment is an ongoing process, extending over the entire period of working with a family (Ahmann, 1996). Care must be flexible enough to respond to the infant's or child's changing health and developmental needs, multidisciplinary input, and the family's changing priorities (Ahmann & Floyd, 1996).

In some cases, nurses may not be the exclusive providers of care during a home visit program. The plan of care is used as a guide to the provider of care, whether the provider is the nurse, client, or family members. The implementation phase also includes recording the client care on the appropriate documents (Humphrey & Milone-Nuzzo, 1996). The nurse should have a plan for each home visit that addresses one or more aspects of the overall plan of care. Throughout each home visit, the information elicited from parents and other caregivers, with the nurse's skilled observations and assessments, will provide the basis on which the nurse, other disciplines, and family update the plan of care (Ahmann & Floyd, 1996).

Regular evaluation and refinement of the care plan are essential from one visit to the next. Periodically, a more

Web Activities

- The continuum Pediatric Homecare Team is a resource center for home care nurses. Visit the website at www.continuum-nursing.com to determine which resources are offered regarding developing a home visit program.
- Visit Building Blocks Pediatric Home Health Services at www.care4kids.com for useful information and links for nurses and families.

formal review of the entire plan of care, including re-assessment of the goals, is advised. This process should include the nurse, family, and other key providers (Ahmann & Floyd, 1996).

The nurse can encourage the client and family to actively participate in all phases of care. Continuity of care is ensured through a systematic process of delivering care to clients and an organized and complete home visit record. Accurate communication justifies coverage to third-party payers and also allows the nurse and agency to document care that stands up legally and against standards and regulations.

Key Concepts

- Health promotion is one of the key components of home care.

- Home care is a cost-effective method of meeting health care needs.

- The nurse brings unique skills to the provision of home care.

- Client care is so complex that even home care requires a multidisciplinary team of providers.

- The Barnard nursing model of infant care is applicable to home care.

- Preparing for the home visit and following the steps of the nursing process are appropriate for home care.

- Nurses should be familiar with professional standards for home care.

Review Questions and Activities

1. The health care system is changing, and nurses must take the lead to adapt their health care delivery in the following way:
   a. Provide high-cost health care
   b. Provide health care directly to the community
   c. Provide generic health care to all clients
   d. Provide high-technology health care to high-risk infants

   The correct answer is b.

2. Health care promotion strategies for the high-risk infant in the community include the following except:
   a. Growth and development
   b. Sleep-wake patterns
   c. Religious preference
   d. Safety and nutrition

   The correct answer is c.

3. Barriers to health care use when working with a family from the same cultural background as the home visiting nurse might include the following:
   a. Poverty, social nature, values, and belief systems
   b. Family structure, high school attended, and number of children in the family
   c. Age, food preference, and nutritional status
   d. Coping skills, music preference, and a history of mental health illness

   The correct answer is a.

4. A nursing model for working with high-risk infants and their mothers helps the home visiting nurse to:

   a. Better organize time during the home visit
   b. Provide a foundation for the home visit
   c. Enhance the multipurpose approach
   d. Support safety during the home visit

   The correct answer is b.

5. Follow-up care of the high-risk infant in the community helps the home visiting nurse:
   a. Decrease long-term sequelae owing to medical conditions
   b. Increase job opportunities for home visiting nurses
   c. Promote medical consequences in the high-risk infant
   d. Help doctors in the delivery of health care

   The correct answer is a.

6. Priority assessment and screening should always be included in a home visit because they evaluate the following except:
   a. Feeding practices and techniques
   b. Parent-infant interactions
   c. Financial status
   d. General infant care practices

   The correct answer is c.

7. An important issue the nurse must address during a home visit is to:
   a. Ensure the family has gas money
   b. Provide a ride for the mother and infant to the clinic

c. Promote extended family interaction

d. Recommend referrals to community resources

The correct answer is d.

8. A successful home visiting program for the high-risk infant results in the following outcomes except:

a. Positive growth patterns

b. Decrease in the number of emergency room visits during the first year of life

c. Parent-caregiver satisfaction

d. Increase reporting to child protective services

The correct answer is d.

References

American Academy of Pediatrics. (1998). Policy Statement: The Role of Home Visitation Programs in Improving Health Outcomes for Children and Families (RE97-34) *Pediatrics, 101,* (3), 486–489.

American College of Obstetricians & Gynecologist. (1995). Preterm labor. *ACOG Technical Bulletin #206.* Washington, D.C.: ACOG.

Ahmann, E. (1996). Family-centered home care. In Ahmann E. (Ed.). *Home care for the high-risk infant* (2nd ed.). Gaithersburg, MD: Aspen.

Ahmann, E., & Floyd, C. (1996). The nursing intake process and the plan of care. In Ahmann E. (Ed.). *Home care for the high-risk infant* (2nd ed.). Gaithersburg, MD: Aspen.

Ark, P. D., & Nies M. (1996). Knowledge and skills of the home healthcare nurse. *Home Healthcare Nurse, 14,* (4), 292–297.

Association of Women's Health, Obstetric and Neonatal Nurses (AWHONN). (1998). *Guidelines for home care of women and newborns. Standards and guidelines* (5th ed.). Chicago, IL: Association of Women's Health, Obstetric, and Neonatal Nurses.

Barnard, K. E. (1976). *NCAST II learners resource manual.* Seattle, WA: NCAST Publications.

Barnard, K. E. (1980). Sleep behavior of infants-is-it-important? In K. E. Barnard (Ed.). *Nursing child assessment sleep/activity manual.* Seattle, WA: NCAST Publications.

Barnard, K. E. (1997). *Influencing parent-child assessment satellite training: Learning resource manual.* Seattle, WA: NCAST Publications.

Barnard, K. E., & Eyres, S. J. (1979). *Child health assessment part 2: The first year of life.* Hyattville, MD: U.S. Department of Health, Education and Welfare.

Barnard, K. E., & Kelly, J. F. (1990). Assessment of parent-child interaction. In S. J. Meisels & J. Shonkoff (Eds.). *Handbook of early childhood intervention.* Cambridge, MA: Cambridge University Press.

Bernbaum, J. C. (1994). Medical care after discharge. In G. B. Avery, M. A. Fletcher, & M. G. MacDonald (Eds.). *Neonatology: Pathophysiology and management of the newborn* (4th ed.). Philadelphia, PA: J. B. Lippincott.

Colombo, D. F., & Ians, J. D. (2000). Preterm birth. In *Practical Strategies in Obstetrics and Gynecology* Scott B. Rausen (Ed.). Philadelphia: W. B. Saunders.

Bond, N., Phillips, P., & Rollins, J. A. (1994). Family-centered care at home for families with children who are technology-dependent. *Pediatric Nursing, 20,* (2), 123–130.

Bradley, P. J., Alpers, R. (1996). Home healthcare nurses should regain their family focus. *Home Healthcare Nurse, 14,* (4), 281–288.

Brooten, D., Naylor, M., Brown, L., York, R., Hollingsworth, A., Cohens, S., Ronloli, & M., Jacobsen, B. (1996). Profile of post-discharge rehospitalization and acute care visits for seven patient groups. *Public Health Nursing, 13,* (2), 129–134.

Buhler-Wilkerson, K. (1985). Public health nursing: In sickness or in health. *American Journal of Public Health, 75,* (10), 1155–1167.

Center for Disease Control/National Center for Health Statistics. (2000). Infant Mortality http://www.cdc.gov/nchs/fastats/informt.htm accessed 3/01).

Chasnoff, I. J., Landress, H. J., & Barrett, M. E. (1990). The prevalence of illicit drug or alcohol use during pregnancy and discrepancies in mandatory reporting in Pinellas county, Florida. *New England Journal of Medicine, 322,* 1202–1206.

Cox, M., & Ahmann, E. (Eds.). (1996). Discharge planning for the high risk infant. In *Home Care for the High-Risk Infant* (2nd ed.). Gaithersburg, MD: Aspen.

Culp, A. M., Culp, R. E., Blankemeyer, M., & Passmark, L. (1998). Parent Education/Home Visitation Program: Adolescent and non-adolescent mother comparison after six months of intervention. *Infant Mental Health Journal, 19,* (2), 111–123.

Donaldson, P. A., & Ahmann, E. (Eds.). (1996). Caring for substance-abusing mothers and their infants. *In home care for the high-risk infant* (2nd ed.). Gaithersburg, MD: Aspen.

Davis, J. H. (1993). Evaluation of novice home visitor preparation strategies. *Journal of Community Health Nursing, 10,* (4), 249–258.

Dungy-Poythress, L. J. (1995). Cocaine effects on pregnancy and infant outcome: Do we really know how bad it is? *Journal of the Association for Academic Minority Physicians, 6,* (1), 46–50.

Early Childhood. Greater Gulf Coast Interagency Infant Task Force, (1997).

Education of the Handicapped Act Amendments of 1986, PL 99-457, 20 U.S.C. 1400 et seq. March of Dimes, Houston, TX: Chapter.

Fleming, J., Challela, M., Eland, J., Hornick, R., Martinson, I., Nativio, D., Nokes, K., Riddle, I., & Steele, N. (1994). Impact on the family of children who are technology dependent and care for in the home. *Pediatric Nursing, 20,* (4), 379–387.

Hack, M., Klein, N., & Taylor, G. (1995). Long-term developmental outcomes of low birth weight infants. *The Future of Children, 5,* 176–196.

Hack, M., Taylor, G., Klein, N., Eiben, R., Schatschneider, C., & Mercuri-Minicti, N. (1994). School-age outcomes in children with birth weights under 750 g. *New England Journal of Medicine, 331,* (12), 753–759.

Humphrey, C. J. (1996). Editorial: We've all got to stick together! *Home Healthcare Nurse, 14,* (4), 236.

Humphrey, C. J., & Milone-Nuzzo, P. (1996). The specialty of home care nursing. In *Orientation to Home Care Nursing* (pp. 21–169). Gaithersburg, MD: Aspen.

Janosik, E., & Green, E. (1992). Family life: Process and practice. Boston, MA: Jones & Barlett.

Kang, R., Barnard, K., Hammond, M., Oshio, S., Spencer, C., Thibodeaux, B., & Williams, J. (1995). Preterm infant follow-up project: A multi-site field experiment of hospitals and home intervention programs for mothers and preterm infants. *Public Health Nursing, 12,* (3), 171–200.

Kelley, S. J. (1992). Parenting stress and child maltreatment in drug-exposed children. *Child Abuse and Neglect, 16,* 317–328.

Kenner, C., & Bagwell, G. A. (1998). Assessment and management of the transition to home. In C. Kenner, J. W. Lott, & A. A. Flandermeyer (Eds.). *Comprehensive neonatal nursing: A physiologic perspective* (2nd ed.). Philadelphia, PA: W. B. Saunders.

Lyon, J. C., Bolla, C. D., & Nies, M. A. (1997). The home visit and home health care. In J. M. Swanson & M. A. Nies (Eds.). *Community health nursing: Promoting the health of aggregates.* Philadelphia, PA: W. B. Saunders.

Mathias, R. (1995). NIDA survey provides first national data on drug use during pregnancy. *Women & Drug Abuse,* 6–7.

McCarthy, N. C. (1994). Health promotion and the family. In C. K. Edelman, & C. L. Mandle (Eds.). *Health promotion throughout the lifespan.* St. Louis, MO: Mosby.

National Center for Education in Maternal and Child Health (NCEMCH). (1995). *Home visiting for at-risk families: Abstracts of active projects FY 1995.* Arlington, VA: National Center for Education in Maternal and Child Health.

Olds, D. L., Henderson, C. R., Kitzman, H., & Cole, R. (1995). Effects of prenatal and infancy nurse home visitation on surveillance of child maltreatment. *Pediatrics, 95,* (3), 365–372.

Olds, D. L., & Kitzman, H. (1990). Can home visitation improve the health of women and children at environmental risk? *Pediatrics, 86,* (1), 108–166.

Olds, D. L., & Kitzman, H. (1993). Review of research on home visiting for pregnant women and parents of young children. *The Future of Children: Home Visiting, 3,* (3), 53–92.

Pennacchia, S. (1994). Infancy. In C. L. Edelman & C. L. Mandle (Eds.). *Health promotion Throughout the Lifespan.* St. Louis, MA: Mosby.

Sackoff, J., Kline, J., Kinney, A., & Grunebaum, A. (1992). Cocaine use in obstetric patients unreported. *American Journal of Public Health, 82,* 1043–1045.

Spector, R. E. (1994). Sociocultural issues related to child health care. In S. J. Kelley (Eds.). *Pediatric Emergency Nursing,* 53–65. Norwalk, Conn: Appleton Lange.

Starn, J. R. (1992). Community health nursing visits for at-risk women and infants. *Journal of Community Health Nursing, 9,* (2), 103–110.

Stutts, A. L. (1994). Selected outcomes of technology dependent children receiving home care and prescribed child care services. *Pediatric Nursing, 20,* (5), 501–507.

Wasik, B. H., Bryant, D. M., & Lyons, C. M. (1990). *Home visiting: Procedures for helping families.* Newbury Park, CA: Sage Publications.

Zahr, L. K., & Montijo, J. (1993). The benefits of home care for sick premature infants. *Neonatal Network, 12,* (1), 33–37.

Suggested Readings

Ahmann, E. (1994). "Chunky stew": Appreciating cultural diversity while providing health care for children. *Pediatric Nursing, 20,* (3), 320–324.

Ahmann, E. (1994). Thinking critically about family-centered home care nursing. *Pediatric Nursing, 20,* (6), 588–590.

Allen, M. C. (1998). Outcome and follow-up of high-risk infants. In H. W. Taeusch & R. A. Ballard (Eds.). *Avery's diseases of the newborn* (7th ed.). Philadelphia, PA: J. B. Lippincott.

American Academy of Pediatrics (AAP). (1998). Hospital discharge of the high-risk neonate-proposed guidelines. Committee on Fetus and Newborn. *Pediatrics, 102,* (2).

American Nurses Association (ANA). (1980). *A conceptual model of community health nursing practice.* Kansas City, MO: American Nurses Association.

American Nurses Association (ANA). (1986). *Standards of home health nursing practice.* Washington, DC: American Nurses Association.

Baginski, Y. (1994). Roadblocks to home care. *Continuing Care Magazine, 12,* (4), 16–29.

Bennett, F. C. (1994). Developmental outcome. In G. B. Avery, M. A. Fletcher, & M. G. MacDonald (Eds.). *Neonatology: Pathophysiology and management of the newborn* (4th ed.). Philadelphia, PA: J. B. Lippincott.

Bernbaum, J. C., Gerdes, M., & Spitzer, A. R. (1996). Follow-up of the high-risk infant. In A. R. Spitzer (Ed.). *Intensive care of the fetus and neonate.* St. Louis: Mosby.

Black, M. M., & Teti, L. O. (1997). Promoting mealtime communication between adolescent mothers and their infants through videotape. *Pediatrics, 99,* (3), 432–435.

Braveman, P., Miller, C., Egerter, S., Bennett, T., English, P., Katz, P., & Showstack, J. (1996). Health service use among low-risk newborns after early discharge with and without home visiting. *Journal of the American Board of Family Practice, 9,* (4), 298–300.

Brown, K. A., & Sauve, R. S. (1994). Evaluation of a caregiver education program: Home oxygen therapy for infants. *Journal of Obstetric, Gynecologic, and Neonatal Nursing, 23,* (5), 429–435.

Chestnut, M. A. (1998). *High-risk newborn home care manual.* Philadelphia, PA: J. B. Lippincott.

Famularo, R., Kinscherff, R., & Fenton, T. (1992). Parental substance abuse and the nature of child maltreatment. *Child Abuse and Neglect, 16,* 475–483.

Fobes, D. A. (1996). Clarification of the constructs of satisfaction and dissatisfaction with home care. *Public Health Nursing, 13,* (6), 337–385.

Gibson, C. H. (1995). The process of empowerment in mothers of chronically ill children. *Journal of Advanced Nursing, 21,* (6), 1201–1210.

Hack, M. (1997). Follow-up for high risk neonates. In A. A. Fanaroff, & R. J. Martin (Eds.). *Neonatal-perinatal medicine: Diseases of the fetus and infant* (6th ed.). St. Louis, MO: Mosby.

Humphrey, C. (1994). *Home care nursing handbook*. Gaithersburg, MD: Aspen.

Jenkins, R. (1996). Grieving the loss of the fantasy child. *Home Healthcare Nurse, 14,* (9), 691–695.

Kamerman, S. B., & Kahn, A. J. (1993). Home health visiting in Europe. *The Future of Children, 3,* 39–52.

Murphy, K. E. (1997). Parenting a technology assisted infant: Coping with occupational stress. *Social Work in Health Care, 24,* (3–4), 113–126.

National Association of Neonatal Nurses (NANN). (1997). Position statement on neonatal follow-up. care of the high risk neonate. *Neonatal Network: The Journal for Neonatal Nursing, 16,* (6), 68–70.

da, S. D., & O'Grady, R. (1994). Public health nursing services for drug-exposed infant and mother: A pilot study. *Journal of Community Health Nursing, 11,* (3), 165–175.

Patterson, J. M., Leonard, B. J., & Titus, J. C. (1994). Caring for medically fragile children at home: The parent-professional relationship. *Journal of Pediatric Nursing, 9,* (2), 98–106.

Peter, C. G., Murdock, B., & Chapin, R. (1995). Home care for children dependent on medical technology: The family perspective. *Social Work in Health Care, 21,* (1), 5–22.

Schieber, G. J., Poullier, J. P., & Greenwald, L. M. (1991). Health care systems in twenty-four countries. *Health Affairs (Millwood), 10,* 22–38.

Stanhope, M., & Lancaster, J. (1996). *Community health nursing: Process and practice for promoting health*. Boston, MA: Mosby.

U.S. Department of Commerce/International Trade Administration. (1990). U.S. Industrial Outlook. Washington, DC, U.S. Government Printing Office.

U.S. Department of Health and Human Services (DHHS). (1990). *Healthy people 2000*. Washington, DC: U.S. Government Printing Office.

U.S. Department of Health and Human Services (DHHS). (2000). *Healthy people 2010*. Washington, DC: U.S. Government Printing Office.

Ventima S. J., Martin, J. A. Curtin S. C., Matthews, T. J. & Park (2000). National Vital Statistic Reporting Vol 38 J. www.edc.gov.nvsr Accessed 3-22-01.

Warhola, C. F. (1980). *Planning for home health services: A resource handbook*. U.S. Department of Health and Human Services. Washington, DC: U.S. Government Printing Office.

Youngbult, J. M., Brennan, P. F., & Swegart, L. A. (1994). Families with medically fragile children: An exploratory study. *Pediatric Nursing, 20,* (5), 463–468.

Zelle, R. S. (1995). Follow-up of at risk infants in the home setting: Consultation model. *Journal of Obstetric, Gynecologic, and Neonatal Nursing, 24,* (1), 51–55.

Resources

Association for the Care of Children's Health, 7910 Woodmont Avenue, Suite 300, Bethesda, MD 20814, 301-654-6549

Child Welfare League of America, 440 First Street, NW, Third Floor, Washington, DC 20001, 202-638-2953, cwla.org

National Association of Pediatric Home and Community Care, 21 North Quinsigamond Avenue, Shrewsbury, MA 01545, 508-856-1908, dorothy.page@banyan.unmed.edu

National Association of Pediatric Nurses Associates and Practitioners, 1101 Kings Highway N., Suite 206, Cherry Hill, NJ 08034, 856-667-1773, napnap.orgNational Easter Seal Society, 230 West Monroe Street, Suite 1800, Chicago, IL 60606, 312-726-6200 or 800-2221-6827

National Information Center for Children and Youth with Disabilities, P.O. Box 1492, Washington, DC 20013, 202-844-8200 or 800-695-0285

Parents Helping Parents, Inc., 3041 Olcott Street, Santa Clara, CA 95054, 480-727-5775

APPENDIX A
STANDARDS OF HOLISTIC NURSING PRACTICE

The American Holistic Nurses Association (AHNA) Standards of Holistic Nursing Practice:

- are used in conjunction with the American Nurses Association Standards of Practice and the specific specialty standards where holistic nurses practice.
- contain five core values that are followed by a description and standards of practice action statements. Depending on the setting or area of practice, holistic nurses may or may not use all of these action statements.
- draw on modalities derived from a number of explanatory models, of which biomedicine is only one model.
- reflect the diverse nursing activities in which holistic nurses are engaged.
- serve holistic nurses in personal life, clinical and private practice, education, research, and community service.

CORE VALUE 1: HOLISTIC PHILOSOPHY AND EDUCATION

Holistic Philosophy

Holistic nurses develop and expand their conceptual framework and overall philosophy in the art and science of holistic nursing to model, practice, teach, and conduct research in the most effective manner possible.

Standards of Practice

Holistic nurses:

- recognize the person's capacity for self-healing and the importance of supporting the natural development and unfolding of that capacity.
- support, share, and recognize expertise and competency in holistic nursing practice that is used in many diverse clinical and community settings.
- participate in person-centered care by being a partner, coach, and mentor who actively listens and supports others in reaching personal goals.
- focus on strategies to bring harmony, unity, and healing to the nursing profession.
- communicate with traditional health care practitioners about appropriate referrals to other holistic practitioners when needed.
- interact with professional organizations in a leadership or membership capacity at local, state, national, and international levels to further expand the knowledge and practice of holistic nursing and awareness of holistic health issues.

Holistic Education

Holistic nurses acquire and maintain current knowledge and competency in holistic nursing practice.

Standards of Practice

Holistic nurses:

- participate in activities of continuing education and related fields that have relevance to holistic nursing practice.
- identify areas of knowledge from nursing and various fields such as biomedical, epidemiology, behavioral medicine, cultural and social theories.
- continually develop and standardize holistic nursing guidelines, protocols, and practice to promote

competency in holistic nursing practice and assure quality of care to individuals.

- use the results of quality care activities to initiate change in holistic nursing practice.
- may seek certification in holistic nursing as one means of advancing the philosophy and practice of holistic nursing.

CORE VALUE 2: HOLISTIC ETHICS, THEORIES, AND RESEARCH

Holistic Ethics

Holistic nurses hold to a professional ethic of caring and healing that seeks to preserve wholeness and dignity of self, students, colleagues, and the person who is receiving care in all practice settings, be it in health promotion, birthing centers, acute or chronic care facilities, end-of-life care centers, and in homes.

Standards of Practice

Holistic nurses:

- identify the ethics of caring and its contribution to unity of self, others, nature, and God/Life Force/Absolute/Transcendent as central to holistic nursing practice.
- integrate the standards of holistic nursing practice with applicable state laws and regulations governing nursing practice.
- engage in activities that respect, nurture, and enhance the integral relationship with the earth, and advocate for the well-being of the global community's economy, education, and social justice.
- advocate for the rights of patients to have educated choices regarding their plan of care.
- participate in peer evaluation to ensure knowledge and competency in holistic nursing practice.
- protect the personal privacy and confidentiality of individuals, especially with health care agencies and managed care organizations.

Holistic Theories

Holistic nurses recognize that holistic nursing theories provide the framework for all aspects of holistic nursing practice and transformational leadership.

Standards of Practice

Holistic nurses:

- strive to use nursing theories to develop holistic nursing practice and transformational leadership.
- interpret, use, and document information relevant to a person's care according to a theoretical framework.

Holistic Research

Holistic nurses provide care and guidance to persons through nursing interventions and holistic therapies consistent with research findings and other sound evidence.

Standards of Practice

Holistic nurses:

- use available research and evidence from different explanatory models to mutually create a plan of care with a person.
- use expert clinical judgment to select appropriate interventions.
- discuss holistic application to clinical situations where rigorous research has not been done.
- create an environment conducive to systematic inquiry into healing and health issues by engaging in research or supporting and utilizing the research of others.
- disseminate research findings at meetings and through publications to further develop the foundation and practice of holistic nursing.
- provide consultation services on holistic nursing interventions to persons and communities based on research.

CORE VALUE 3: HOLISTIC NURSE SELF-CARE

Holistic Nurse Self-Care

Holistic nurses engage in self-care and further develop their own personal awareness as being an instrument of healing to better serve self and others.

Standards of Practice

Holistic nurses:

- recognize that a person's body-mind-spirit has healing capacities that can be enhanced and supported through self-care practices.

- identify and integrate self-care strategies to enhance their physical, psychological, sociological, and spiritual well-being.
- recognize and address at-risk health patterns and begin the process of change.
- consciously cultivate awareness and understanding about the deeper meaning, purpose, inner strengths, and connections with self, others, nature, and God/Life Force/Absolute/Transcendent.
- use clear intention to care for self and to seek a sense of balance, harmony, and joy in daily life.
- participate in the evolutionary holistic process with the understanding that crisis creates opportunity in any setting.

CORE VALUE 4: HOLISTIC COMMUNICATION, THERAPEUTIC ENVIRONMENT, AND CULTURAL DIVERSITY

Holistic Communication

Holistic nurses engage in holistic communication to ensure that each person experiences the presence of the nurse as authentic and sincere; there is an atmosphere of shared humanness that includes a sense of connectedness and attention reflecting the individual's uniqueness.

Standards of Practice

Holistic nurses:

- develop an awareness of the most frequently encountered challenges to holistic communication.
- increase therapeutic and cultural competence skills to enhance their effectiveness through listening to themselves and others.
- explore with each person those strategies that can assist her/him, as desired, to understand the deeper meaning, purpose, inner strengths, and connections with self, others, nature, and God/Life Force/Absolute/Transcendent.
- recognize that holistic communication and awareness of individuals is a continuously evolving multilevel exchange that offers itself through dreams, images, symbols, sensations, meditations, and prayers.
- respect the person's health trajectory which may be incongruent with conventional wisdom.

Therapeutic Environment

Holistic nurses recognize that each person's environment includes everything that surrounds the individual, both the external and the internal (physical, mental, emotional, and spiritual) as well as patterns not yet understood.

Standards of Practice

Holistic nurses:

- promote environments conducive to experiencing healing, wholeness, and harmony, and care for the person in as healthy an environment as possible.
- work toward creating organizations that value sacred space and environments that enhance healing.
- integrate holistic principles, standards, policies, and procedures in relation to environmental safety and emergency preparedness.
- recognize that the well-being of the ecosystem of the planet is a prior determining condition for the well-being of the human.
- promote social networks and social environments where healing can take place.

Cultural Diversity

Holistic nurses recognize each person as whole, being of body-mind-spirit, and mutually create a plan of care consistent with cultural backgrounds, health beliefs, sexual orientation, values, and preferences.

Standards of Practice

Holistic nurses:

- assess and incorporate the person's cultural practices, values, beliefs, meanings of health, illness, and risk behaviors in care and health education.
- use appropriate community resources and experts to extend their understanding of different cultures.
- assess for discriminatory practices and change as necessary.
- identify discriminatory health care practices as they impact the person and engage in effective nondiscriminatory practices.

CORE VALUE 5: HOLISTIC CARING PROCESS

Assessment

Each person is assessed holistically, using appropriate traditional and holistic methods while the uniqueness of the person is honored.

Standards of Practice

Holistic nurses:

- use an assessment process, including appropriate traditional and holistic methods, to systematically gather information.
- value all types of knowing, including intuition, when gathering data from a person and validate this intuitive knowledge with the person when appropriate.

Patterns/Problems/Needs

Each person's actual and potential patterns/problems/needs/life processes related to health, wellness, disease, or illness, which may or may not facilitate well-being, are identified and prioritized.

Standards of Practice

Holistic nurses:

- assist the person to access inner wisdom that can provide opportunities to enhance and support growth, development, and movement towards health and well-being.
- collect data and collaborate with the person and health care team members as appropriate to identify and record a list of actual and potential patterns/problems/needs.
- use collected data to formulate an etiology of the person's identified actual or potential patterns/problems/needs.
- make referrals to other holistic practitioners or traditional therapists when appropriate.

Outcomes

Each person's actual or potential patterns/problems/needs have appropriate outcomes specified.

Standards of Practice

Holistic nurses:

- honor the person in all phases of her/his healing process regardless of expectations or outcomes.
- identify and partner with the person to specify measurable outcomes and realistic goals.

Therapeutic Care Plan

Each person engages with the holistic nurse to mutually create an appropriate plan of care that focuses on health promotion, recovery, restoration, or peaceful dying so that the person is as independent as possible.

Standards of Practice

Holistic nurses:

- partner with the person in a mutual decision process to create a health care plan for each pattern/problem/need/opportunity to enhance health and well-being.
- help a person identify areas for education to make decisions about life choices in a conscious, informed manner that empowers the person to maintain her/his uniqueness and independence.
- offer self-assessment tools, word associations, storytelling, dreams, and journals as appropriate.
- use skills of cultural competence and communicate acceptance of the person's values, beliefs, culture, religion, and socioeconomic background.
- assist the person in recognizing at-risk patterns/problems/needs for potential or existing health situations (e.g., personal habits, personal and family health history, age-related risk factors), and also assist in recognizing opportunities to enhance well-being.
- engage the person in problem-solving dialogue in relation to living with changes secondary to illness and treatment.

Implementation

Each person's plan of holistic care is prioritized and holistic nursing interventions are implemented accordingly.

Standards of Practice

Holistic nurses:

- implement the mutually created plan of care within the context of assisting the person towards the higher potential of health and well-being.

- support and promote the person's capacity for the highest level of participation and problem-solving in the plan of care and collaborate with other health team members when appropriate.
- use holistic nursing skills in implementing care, including cultural competency and all ways of knowing.
- advocate that the person's plan, choices, and unique healing journey be honored.
- provide care that is clear about and respectful of the economic parameters of practice, balancing justice with compassion.

Evaluation

Each person's responses to holistic care are regularly and systematically evaluated and the continuing holistic nature of the healing process is recognized and honored.

Standards of Practice

Holistic nurses:

- collaborate with the person and with other health care team members when appropriate in evaluating holistic outcomes.
- explore with the person her/his understanding of the cause of any significant deviation between the responses and the expected outcomes.
- mutually create with the person and other team members a revised plan, if needed.

APPENDIX B
ABBREVIATIONS, ACRONYMS, AND SYMBOLS

AA	Alcoholics Anonymous		ARBD	Alcohol Related Birth Defects
AA	arachidonic acid		AROM	artificial rupture of membranes
AANA	American Association of Nurse Anesthetists		ART	assistive reproduction technology
AAP	American Academy of Pediatrics		AUB	abnormal uterine bleeding
ABC	airway breathing circulation		AWHONN	Association of Women's Health, Obstetric, and Neonatal Nurses
ABG	arterial blood gas		AZT	zidovudine
ACE	angiotensin-converting enzyme		β-hCG	β-human chorionic gonadotropin
ACOG	American College of Obstetricians and Gynecologists		BBT	basal body temperature
ACS	American Cancer Society		BINS	Bayley Infant Neurodevelopmental Screen
ACTG	AIDS Clinical Trial Group		BMC	bone mineral content
ADH	antidiuretic hormone		BMD	bone mineral density
ADOPE	age, diabetes, obesity, postterm, excessive		BMR	basal metabolic rate
AFDC	Aid to Families with Dependent Children		BNE	Board of Nursing Examiners
AFP	alpha-fetoprotein		BP	blood pressure
AFV	amniotic fluid volume		bpm	beats per minute
AGA	appropriate for gestational age		BPP	biophysical profile
AHCPR	Agency for Health Care Policy and Research		BRP	bed rest bathroom privileges
AHNA	American Holistic Nurses Association		BSE	breast self-examination
AHPA	American Herbal Products Association		BUBBLE-HE	breasts, uterus, bladder, bowel, lochia, episiotomy, Homan's Sign, emotional status
AHRQ	Agency for Healthcare Research and Quality		BUN	blood urea nitrogen
AI	adequate intake		Ca	calcium
AICR	American Institute for Cancer Research		CAM	complementary and alternative medicine
AIDS	acquired immunodeficiency syndrome		CBC	complete blood count
AMA	American Medical Association		CCES	Council of Childbirth Education Specialists
ANA	American Nurses Association		CDC	Centers for Disease Control and Prevention
ANAD	Anorexia Nervosa and Associated Disorders		CDH	congenital diaphragmatic hernia
ANDMCN	American Nursing Division of Maternal Child Nursing		CF	cystic fibrosis
			C-H	crown-heel
ANRED	Anorexia Nervosa and Related Eating Disorders		CHARGE	coloboma, heart disease, choanal atresia, retardation (physical and mental), genital hypoplasia, ear anomalies
ANS	autonomic nervous system			
AOA	Administration on Aging		CHD	congenital heart defect
APIB	Assessment of Premature Infant Behavior		CHD	coronary heart disease
APN	advanced practice nurse		CHF	congestive heart failure
APS	Adult Protective Services		CHO	carbohydrate

CIMS	Coalition for Improved Maternity Services		EDD	expected date of delivery
CIS	Communities in Schools		EDNP	energy-dense, nutrient-poor
cm	centimeter		EEG	electroencephalogram
CMV	cytomegalovirus		EFM	electronic fetal monitoring
CNM	Certified Nurse Midwife		EFNEP	Expanded Food and Nutrition Education Program
CNS	central nervous system		EIP	early intervention program
CO_2	carbon dioxide		ELISA	enzyme-linked immunosorbent assay
COC	combined oral contraceptive		EMLA	eutectic mixture of local anesthetics
COPD	chronic obstructive pulmonary disease		ER	estrogen receptors
CPAP	continuous positive airway pressure		ERT	estrogen replacement therapy
CPD	cephalopelvic disproportion		ESPGN	European Society of Pediatric Gastroenterology and Nutrition
CPR	cardiopulmonary resuscitation		ET	embryo transfer
CPS	Canadian Paediatric Society		FAE	fetal alcohol effects
C-R	crown-rump		FAS	fetal acoustic stimulation
CRNA	Certified Registered Nurse Anesthetist		FAS	Fetal Alcohol Syndrome
CRS	congenital rubella syndrome		FCMC	family-centered maternity care
CSF	cerebrospinal fluid		FDA	Food and Drug Administration
CST	contraction stress test		FFN	fetal fibronectin
CT	complementary therapy		FH	familial hypercholesterolemia
CT	computerized tomography		FHR	fetal heart rate
CVD	cardiovascular disease		FHT	fetal heart tone
CVS	chorionic villus sampling		FMC	fetal movement counting
D & C	dilation and curettage		FOBT	fecal occult blood test
D & E	dilation and evacuation		FOC	frontal-occipital-circumference
DDH	developmental dysplasia of the hip		FPAL	full-term deliveries/preterm deliveries/abortions/living children
DDT	dichlorodiphenyltrichloroethane		FSE	fetal scalp electrode
DES	diethylstilbestrol		FSH	follicle-stimulating hormone
DFE	dietary folate equivalent		ftc	footcandle
DHA	docosahexaenoic acid		g	gram
DHHS	Department of Health and Human Services		G6PD	glucose-6-phosphate dehydrogenase
DIC	disseminated intravascular coagulation		GAO	General Accounting Office
dL	deciliter		GBS	group B *Streptococcus*
DMD	Duchenne muscular dystrophy		GCT	genetic counseling team
DMPA	depot medroxyprogesterone acetate		GFR	glomerular filtration rate
DMPA	Depo-Provera		GI	gastrointestinal
DNA	deoxyribonucleic acid		GIFT	gamete intra-fallopian transfer
DO	Doctor of Osteopathy		gm	gram
DRI	Dietary Reference Intake		GNP	gross national product
DRV	daily reference value		GnRH	gonadotropin releasing hormone
DSHEA	Dietary Supplement Health and Education Act		H & H	hematocrit and hemoglobin
DTR	deep tendon reflex		HbeAg	hepatitis B e antigen
DUB	dysfunctional uterine bleeding		HBIG	hepatitis B immune globulin
DV	daily value		HBsAg	hepatitis B surface antigen
EA	esophageal atresia		HC/AC	head-abdomen circumference
ECG	electrocardiogram		HCADA	Houston Council on Alcoholism and Drug Abuse
ECI	Early Childhood Intervention		hCG	human chorionic gonadotropin
ECMO	extracorporeal membrane oxygenation		Hct	hematocrit
EDB	expected date of birth			
EDC	expected date of confinement			

HDL	high-density lipoprotein	IUD	intrauterine device
HDN	hemolytic disease of the newborn	IUFD	intrauterine fetal demise
HEENT	head, ears, eyes, nose, and throat	IUGR	intrauterine growth restriction
HELLP	hemolysis, elevated liver enzymes, low platelets	IUPC	intrauterine pressure catheter
HexA	hexosaminidase	IV	intravenous
HFA	Healthy Families Alexandria	IVF	in vitro fertilization
Hgb	hemoglobin	IVH	intraventricular hemorrhage
HGH	Human Growth Hormone	IWL	insensible water loss
HGP	Human Genome Project	JCAHO	Joint Commission on Accreditation of Healthcare Organizations
HGPRT	hypoxanthine-guanine phosphoribosyl-transferase	JOGNN	Journal of Obstetric, Gynecologic, and Neonatal Nursing
HHCC	Home Health Care Classification	KC	kangaroo care
HIV	human immunodeficiency virus	kg	kilogram
HMG	hydroxymethylglutaryl	LAM	lactational amenorrhea method
HMO	health maintenance organization	lb	pound
HNC	holistic nurse certification	LBW	low birth weight
HNC	Holistic Nurse Certified	LDL	low-density lipoprotein
hPL	human placental lactogen	LDR	labor, delivery, recovery
HPV	human papillomavirus	LDRP	labor, delivery, recovery, postpartum
HRT	hormone replacement therapy	LEEP	Loop Electrosurgical Excision Procedure
HSV	herpes simplex virus		
HT	Healing Touch	LGA	large for gestational age
HTI	Healing Touch International	LH	luteinizing hormone
HTLV-1	human T-cell leukemia virus type 1	LLI	LaLeche League International
HVAF	Home Visiting for At-Risk Families	LMA	left-mentum-anterior
IBFAN	International Breastfeeding Association	LMP	last menstrual period
ICEA	International Childbirth Education Association	LMP	left-mentum-posterior
		LMT	left-mentum-transverse
ICH	intracranial hemorrhage	LOA	left-occiput-anterior
ICSI	intracytoplasmic sperm injection	LOP	left-occiput-posterior
ICU	intensive care unit	LOT	left-occiput-transverse
IDDM	insulin-dependent diabetes mellitus	LSA	left-sacrum-anterior
IDM	infant of a diabetic mother	LSP	left-sacrum-posterior
IF	intrinsic factor	LST	left-sacrum-transverse
IFSP	Individual Family Service Plan	LTV	long-term variability
IgA	immunoglobulin A	μg	microgram
IgE	immunoglobulin E	m	meter
IgG	Immunoglobulin G	MAI	Maternal Attachment Inventory
IICP	increased intracranial pressure	MCV	mean corpuscular volume
ILCA	International Lactation Consultants Association	Mg	magnesium
		mg	milligram
ILP	interstitial lymphocytic pneumonia	MI	myocardial infarction
IM	intramuscular	mL	milliliter
IMR	infant mortality rate	mmHg	millimeters of mercury
in	inch	MNF	multiple neurofibromatosis
IOM	Institute of Medicine	MPA/E2C	medroxy progesterone and estradiol cypionate
IQ	intelligence quotient		
ISONG	International Society of Nurses in Genetics	MPS	mucopolysaccharide accumulation
		MRFIT	Multiple Risk Factor Intervention Trial
ITP	idiopathic thrombocytopenic purpura	MRI	magnetic resonance imaging

MSAFP	maternal serum alpha-fetoprotein
MSDS	Material Safety Data Sheet
MVU	Montivideo Unit
NAACOG	Nurses Association of the American College of Obstetricians and Gynecologists
NANBH	non-A, non-B hepatitis
NANDA	North American Nursing Diagnosis Association
NANN	National Association of Neonatal Nurses
NAS	National Academies of Science
NBAS	Neonatal Behavioral Assessment Scale
NCAST	Nursing Child Assessment Satellite Training
NCCAM	National Center for Complementary and Alternative Medicine
NCEA	National Center for Elder Abuse
NCHPEG	National Coalition for Health Professional Education in Genetics
NCHS	National Center for Health Statistics
NCPAP	nasal continuous positive airway pressure
NCPCA	National Committee to Prevent Child Abuse
NE	niacin equivalent
NEC	necrotizing enterocolitis
NHANES	National Health and Nutrition Examination Society
NIC	Nursing Intervention Classification
NICU	neonatal intensive care unit
NIDCAP	Newborn Individualized Developmental Care Assessment Program
NIH	National Institutes of Health
NIHF	nonimmune hydrops fetalis
NIPS	Neonatal Infant Pain Scale
NLN	National League for Nursing
NMDS	nursing minimum data set
NRC	National Research Council
NSAID	nonsteroidal anti-inflammatory drug
NST	nonstress test
NTD	neural tube defect
NVP	nausea and vomiting of pregnancy
O_2	oxygen
OAM	Office of Alternative Medicine
OCA	oral contraceptive agents
OCP	oral contraceptive pill
OI	osteogenesis imperfecta
OMAR	Office of Medical Applications and Research
OMH	Office of Minority Health
ORWH	Office of Research on Women's Health
OSHA	Occupational Safety and Health Administration
OTC	over-the-counter
oz	ounce
P	phosphorus
PAI	Prenatal Attachment Inventory
PaO_2	partial pressure of oxygen
PAT	Pain Assessment Tool
PBB	polybromated biphenyl
PCA	patient-controlled analgesia
PCB	polychlorinated biphenyl
PCO_2	partial pressure of carbon dioxide
PCOS	polycystic ovary syndrome
PCP	*Pneumocystis carinii* pneumonia
PCR	polymerase chain reaction
PDA	patent ductus arteriosis
PDR	Physicians' Desk Reference
PEEP	positive end expiratory pressure
PEPI	postmenopausal estrogen/progestin interventions
PG	phosphatidylglycerol
PGE_2	prostaglandin E_2
PGIS	Perinatal Grief Intensity Scale
PHS	Public Health Service
PID	pelvic inflammatory disease
PIH	pregnancy-induced hypertension
PIPP	Premature Infant Pain Profile
PKU	phenylketonuria
PLISSIT	permission, limited information, specific suggestions, intensive therapy
PMI	point of maximum impulse
PMS	premenstrual syndrome
PNI	psychoneuroimmunology
PO_2	partial pressure of oxygen
POS	point of service
PPHN	persistent pulmonary hypertension of the newborn
PPO	preferred provider organization
PPROM	preterm premature rupture of membranes
PPT	partial prothrombin time
PROM	premature rupture of membranes
PT	prothrombin time
PTL	preterm labor
PTSD	Post-Traumatic Stress Disorder
PTT	partial thromboplastin time
PTU	propylthiouracil
PUBS	percutaneous umbilical blood sampling
PUPPP	pruritic urticarial papules and plaques of pregnancy
PVR	pulmonary vascular resistance

RBC	red blood cell
RD	registered dietitian
RDA	recommended daily allowance
RDI	Reference Daily Intake
RDS	respiratory distress syndrome
REEDA	redness, edema, ecchymosis, discharge, approximation
Rh	rhesus factor
RH_0GAM	Rh_O (D) immune globulin
RMA	right-mentum-anterior
RMP	right-mentum-posterior
RMT	right-mentum-transverse
RNA	ribonucleic acid
ROA	right-occiput-anterior
ROM	range of motion
ROM	rupture of membranes
ROP	retinopathy of prematurity
ROP	right-occiput-posterior
ROT	right-occiput-transverse
RSA	right-sacrum-anterior
RSP	right-sacrum-posterior
RST	right-sacrum-transverse
RUQ	right upper quadrant
SC disease	sickle cell-hemoglobin C disease
SCD	sickle-cell disease
SDA	specific dynamic action
SGA	small for gestational age
SIDS	sudden infant death syndrome
sIgA	secretory immunoglobulin A
SLE	systemic lupus erythematosus
SOAP	subjective, objective, assessment, plan
SQ	subcutaneous
SS disease	sickle cell disease
STD	sexually transmitted disease
STORCH	syphilis, toxoplasmosis, other infections, rubella, cytomegalovirus, herpes
STV	short term variability
SVE	sterile vaginal examination
TB	tuberculosis
TC	total cholesterol
TCM	traditional Chinese medicine
TEF	tracheoesophageal fistula
TENS	transcutaneous electrical nerve stimulation
THF	tetrahydrofolate
TNM	tumor, nodal involvement, and metastasis
TOLAC	trial of labor after cesarean
TORCH	toxoplasmosis, other (gonorrhea, syphilis, varicella, Parvovirus, HBV, and HIV), rubella, Cytomegalovirus, and herpes simplex virus
TPR	temperature, pulse, respirations
TRH	thyrotropin-releasing hormome
TSD	Tay-Sachs disease
TSH	thyroid-stimulating hormone
TT	Therapeutic Touch
TTN	transient tachypnea of the newborn
UAP	unlicensed assistive personnel
UC	uterine contraction
uE_3	unconjugated estrogen
UIL	upper intake level
UNAIDS	Joint United Nations Programme on HIV/AIDS
UNICEF	United Nation's Children's Fund
US	ultrasonography
USDA	United States Department of Agriculture
USDA/FCS	United States Department of Agriculture, Food, and Consumer Service
USDHHS	United States Department of Health and Human Services
USFDA	United States Food and Drug Administration
USP	United States Pharmacopoeia
USPSTF	United States Preventive Services Task Force
UTI	urinary tract infection
VACTERL	vertebral, anal, congenital heart defect, tracheoesophageal atresia or fistula, renal anomalies, and limb deformities
VATER	vertebral, anal, tracheoesophageal atresia or fistula, and renal anomalies
VBAC	vaginal birth after cesarean
VDRL	Venereal Disease Research Laboratory
VLBW	very low birth weight
VNA	Visiting Nurse Association
VNS	Visiting Nurse Service
VPS	ventricular peritoneal shunt
VSD	ventricular septal defect
VZIG	varicella-zoster immune globulin
WABA	World Alliance for Breastfeeding Action
WBC	white blood cell
WHO	World Health Organization
WIC	Women, Infants, and Children
YRBSS	Youth Risk Behavior Surveillance System
ZDV	zidovudine

GLOSSARY

A

ABO incompatibility   Condition that occurs when the blood types of the mother and fetus do not match.

Accretion   Growth in size, especially by addition or accumulation.

Acquaintance rape   Sexual assault that occurs when a perpetrator with whom the victim has had a previous nonviolent relationship uses deceit and coercion to obtain sex.

Acquired disorder   Condition resulting from environmental factors, rather than genetic circumstances.

Acupressure   Application of pressure along certain meridians of the skin.

Acupuncture   Insertion of needles into the skin along certain meridians.

Adolescence   Period of life beginning with the appearance of secondary sex characteristics and ending with the cessation of growth, approximately 11 to 18 years of age; passage from childhood to maturity.

Adolescent pregnancy   Pregnancy in girls, ages 11 to 19.

Adult maltreatment syndrome   ICD-9 diagnostic code category for the adult who is abused.

Advanced reproductive age   Women between ages 45 and 50 who are perimenopausal or postmenopausal.

Allantois   Small diverticulum of the yolk sac.

Allele   Alternative expressions of a gene at a given locus.

Allopathy   Traditional or established medical or surgical procedures, both invasive and noninvasive, used in the diagnosis and treatment of mental or physical illnesses.

Alpha-fetoprotein (AFP)   Protein produced by the developing fetus that can be used as a marker for neural-tube defects (increased AFP) and Down syndrome (decreased AFP).

Alternative therapies   Therapies used instead of conventional biomedicine.

Alveoli   Secretory units of the mammary gland in which milk production takes place.

Amenorrhea   The absence of menstruation for 3 or more months in women who have established menstrual cycles.

Amniocentesis   Prenatal diagnostic procedure that consists of withdrawal of a small sample of amniotic fluid for genetic analysis of embryonic cells.

Amnion   Inner membrane of the two fetal membranes; it forms the sac in which the fetus and the amniotic fluid are contained.

Amniotic fluid   Fluid surrounding the developing fetus during pregnancy; formed from maternal serum and fetal urine.

Amylophagia   Ingestion of nonfood substances, such as laundry starch or cornstarch.

Analgesia   Relief of pain.

Anencephalus   Complete or partial absence of the cerebral hemispheres and the skull overlying the brain.

Anencephaly   Fatal condition in which a baby is born with a severely underdeveloped brain and skull and dies shortly after birth.

Anesthesia   Absence of sensation.

Anesthesiologist   Physician who has completed a post-graduate residency in anesthesia.

Aneuploidy   Abnormal chromosome pattern, in which the total number of chromosomes is not a multiple of the haploid number (n=23).

Anorexia nervosa   Condition of self-starvation motivated by excessive concern with weight and an irrational fear of becoming fat.

Anovulatory   Lack of ovulation.

Anovulatory cycle   Menstrual cycle in which no ovum is discharged.

Antioxidant   A substance that slows down the oxidation of hydrocarbons, oils, fats, etc. and thus helps to check deterioration.

Antiretroviral therapy   Course of medications used to suppress HIV replication and viral load.

Areola   Pigmented ring of tissue surrounding the nipple.

Asphyxia   Interference with gas exchange, resulting in decreased oxygen delivery (hypoxemia), accumulation of carbon dioxide (hypercapnia), development of respiratory and metabolic acidosis, and inadequate perfusion of the tissues and major organs (ischemia).

Assault   The intentional act of inflicting physical injury on another person.

Attachment   Process of connecting with another human being over time.

Autonomy   An individual's ability to hold a particular view, make choices, and undertake actions based on values and beliefs.

Autosome   The 22 pairs of chromosomes that do not greatly influence sex determination at conception; excludes the sex chromosomes, X and Y.

Ayurvedic medicine   Traditional medicine of India, meaning knowledge of life or science of longevity.

B

Ballottement   Rebounding of the floating fetus against the examiner's fingers.

Barrier to service utilization   Any deterrent either real or perceived, that presents or delays use of available health care.

Basal metabolism Energy used to support body functions while the body is at rest.

Behavioral medicine Branch of medicine that focuses on behavior, and the cognition, emotion, motivation and biobehavioral interactions.

Behavioral state Continuum of levels of consciousness, encompassing quiet sleep, drowsiness, wakeful attentiveness, and hyperalert, agitated, or crying states.

Beneficence The practice of doing good, which may include prevention of harm, removal of evil, or promotion of good.

Binge eating An eating disorder of periodic binge eating (several thousand calories) not normally followed by vomiting, the use of laxatives, or excessive exercise.

Bioavailability Rate at which a nutrient enters the bloodstream and is circulated to specific organs or tissues.

Biomedicine The scientific-based professional medicine that is taught in medical schools and is generally practiced in the United States and Canada.

Biophysical profile (BPP) Noninvasive, dynamic assessment of the fetus and the fetal environment.

Birth rate Number of births per 1,000 population.

Blastocyst Mammalian conceptus in the post-morula stage; consists of the trophoblast and an inner cell mass; develops into the embryo.

Blended family Family formed through remarriage.

Body mass index (BMI) Ratio that defines the relationship between height and weight. BMI is calculated by the formula: $BMI = weight (kg)/height (m^2) \times 100$, or $weight (lb) \times 700/height (in^2)$.

Botanicals All parts of plants that have medicinal value: roots, rhizomes, leaves, stems, and flowers.

Brachial palsy Paralysis of the muscles involving the upper extremity; occurs as a result of a prolonged and difficult labor followed by a traumatic delivery.

Braxton-Hicks contractions Intermittent painless contractions of the uterus, observed throughout pregnancy; also known as false labor.

Bulimia nervosa Condition characterized by bingeing, or excessive consumption of calories over a short period of time, and purging by self-induced vomiting, use of laxatives or diuretics or both, excessive exercise or periods of severe caloric restriction.

C

Calorie Amount of energy needed to raise the temperature of 1/kg of water (about 4 cups) 1°C.

Calorimetry Measurement of the quantity of heat; used for measuring the energy produced by food when oxidized in the body.

Capacitation Process by which the spermatozoon (sperm) is capable of penetrating the ovum.

Carcinoma in situ Cancer that involves only the cells of the organ in which it began and has not spread to any other tissue.

Carotenoids Pigments in fruits and vegetables, which include alphacarotene, beta-carotene, lycopene, lutein, and many other compounds.

Case management, care coordination Process of coordinating care and services to assure that clients receive appropriate care and services in a timely manner.

Categorical imperative Supreme rule that governs actions.

Certified Registered Nurse Anesthetist (CRNA) Advanced practice nurse, graduated from an accredited program of nurse anesthesia education who has passed the National Certification Examination.

Cervical cancer Neoplasm of the uterine cervix.

Cervical infection Inflammation of the cervix caused by a microorganism or foreign body.

Chadwick's sign Dark blue or purple coloration of vaginal mucous membranes during pregnancy.

Chi A concept in Oriental medicine that refers to the subtle material or energy that influences physiologic function and maintains the health and vitality of the individual.

Chi gong The oriental practice of "working the chi", or exercises to maintain health and vitality.

Child abuse Physical or mental injury, sexual abuse, exploitation, negligent treatment, or maltreatment of a child.

Chloasma Brownish pigmentation of the face, commonly called "mask of pregnancy."

Choanal atresia A bony or membranous separation between the nose and the pharynx.

Chorion Outermost portion of the fetal membrane; composed of trophoblast and mesoderm lining; develops villi and becomes vascularized; forms the fetal portion of the placenta.

Chorionic villi Vascular protrusions along the chorion.

Chorionic villus sampling (CVS) Procedure to obtain fetal cells in the first trimester of the developing pregnancy.

Chromosome Filament-like nuclear structure, consisting of chomatin, which stores genetic information as base sequences in DNA and whose number is constant in each species.

Civil law Rule protecting individuals, which punishes wrongs against the individual.

Clastogen Agent capable of producing chromosome breakage.

Cleft lip Congenital fissure or elongated opening of the lip.

Cleft palate Congenital fissure in the palate.

Clubfoot (talipes eqinovarus) Congenital deformity in which portions of the foot and ankle are twisted out of normal position.

Code Definition of professional obligations and responsibilities, expected of practitioners by society.

Cognitive development Age-related development of intellectual reasoning and perception.

Cohabitation Couple living together without entering into marriage.

Colostrum A yellowish, protein-rich fluid, secreted from the breast during pregnancy and for 3 to 4 days following delivery.

Communal family Group of individuals, couples, or families living together and jointly carrying out family functions.

Complementary therapies Therapies used in addition *to* or as an *adjunct* to biomedicine for the promotion of health and well being.

Congenital disorder Anomaly present at birth; results from genetic or prenatal environmental factors, or both.

Congenital heart defect A structural abnormality or defect of the heart that is present at birth.

Contraction stress test (CST) Evaluation of uterine contractions for the purpose of assessing fetal response.

Corona radiata   Layer of cells surrounding the zona pellucida of the ovum.

Corpus luteum   Yellow glandular mass in the ovary formed by an ovarian follicle that has matured and discharged its ovum.

Cost-benefit analysis   Process of measuring the cost of doing something against the outcome in monetary terms.

Cost-effectiveness analysis   Process of comparing the cost of doing something and measuring the outcomes in non-monetary terms.

Cotyledons   Subdivisions along the uterine surface of the placenta.

Couvade   Physical symptoms experienced by an expectant father during pregnancy; also the ritualistic behaviors he performs during labor and birth.

Criminal law   Rule that addresses public concerns and punishes the wrongs that threaten a group or society.

Crisis   Situation in which the balance in individual or family life is disrupted and new coping strategies must be developed.

Critical thinking   Formal and structured type of reasoning that is used in nursing as the foundation for sound clinical judgement.

Cultural competence   Process of integrating cultural awareness in the delivery of culturally appropriate clinical care.

Cultural competence continuum   Progressive description of the ability of an individual or institution to respond to the individual, culturally specific needs of people.

Culture   An individual's way of looking at life, encompassing the person's feelings, beliefs, attitudes, and practices in dealing with family, community, and society.

Cytogenetics   The study of chromosomes, with special focus on chromosome abnormalities.

Cytotrophoblast   Inner layer of the trophoblast; also referred to as Langhan's layer.

D

Daily Reference Values (DRVs)   Standards for daily intake of total fat, saturated fat, cholesterol, total carbohydrate, dietary fiber, and protein.

Date rape   Assault between a dating couple without consent of one of the participants.

Decidua   Term applied to the endometrium during pregnancy.

Decidua basalis   Portion on which the implanted ovum rests.

Decidua capsularis   Portion directly overlaying the implanted ovum.

Decidua vera   Decidua exclusive of the area occupied by the implanted ovum.

Deletion   Loss of chromosomal material.

Deontology   Form of ethical reasoning that focuses on duty; right actions are those that fulfill duty.

Dermatome   The area of the body innervated through a specific spinal nerve.

Desire phase   First phase of human sexual response in which a person develops a motivation or intention to be sexual.

Developmental care   Infant care protocol designed to promote optimal physical, cognitive, and emotional development in the first weeks or months of life.

Developmental crisis   Adjustment of an individual to new stages of development.

Developmental dysplasia of the hip (DDH)   Malformation of the hip involving varying degrees of deformity, ranging from subluxation to complete dislocation, that may be present at birth.

Developmental tasks   Competencies in psychosocial development related to identity formation, sexual identity, vocational identity, and autonomy and independence.

Diaphragmatic hernia   Condition in which the diaphragm fails to close during the seventh or eighth week, allowing the abdominal organs to be displaced into the left chest.

Dietary Guidelines for Americans   Guidance on diet and health for the general population with practical recommendations that meet nutritional requirements, promote health, support an active lifestyle, and reduce the risk of chronic disease.

Dilemma   Choice between two equally unsatisfactory alternatives.

Diploid   Cell that contains two copies of each chromosome; the diploid number (2n) in humans is 46.

Disease prevention   Activities taken to prevent the onset of a disease or disorder.

Doctrine of the golden mean   Virtues at the midpoint between extremes of less desirable characteristics.

Dominant   Allele that is phenotypically expressed in single copy (heterozygote), as well as in double copy (homozygote).

Doppler blood studies   Measurement of blood flow velocity and direction in major fetal and uterine structures; also known as umbilical vessel velocimetry.

Dosha   A term used in Ayurvedic medicine referring to metabolic types of people.

Ductus arteriosus   Fetal shunt that connects the pulmonary artery to the descending aorta.

Ductus venosus   Fetal shunt passing through the liver that connects the umbilical vein to the inferior vena cava.

Due care   Legal and ethical standards of performance by which nursing professionals are expected to abide.

Dyads   Group of two people.

Dysfunctional uterine bleeding (DUB)   Any significant deviation from the usual menstrual pattern; also known as abnormal uterine bleeding (AUB).

Dysmenorrhea   Painful menses or cramping with menstruation.

Dyspareunia   Painful sexual intercourse.

E

ECMO   Extracorporeal membrane oxygenation, a method of cardiopulmonary bypass therapy.

Ecologic environment   Combined social context in which a family resides.

Elderly primigravida   Woman over age 35 who is pregnant for the first time.

Embryo   Period of human development from the second week until the eighth week after fertilization; period characterized by cell differentiation and hyperplasic growth.

Embryo transfer (ET)   Transfer of an externally fertilized egg in embryonic stage by transcervical or other methods.

Empowering   A therapeutic approach that encourages the family to actively participate in the solution to their problems, and acknowledge that capacity.

Empowerment   Process of assisting clients to care for themselves.

Enablement   Process of assisting clients in locating needed services and resources.

Enabling   The approach to interventions that allow competencies to develop in the client.

Encephalocele   Herniation of the brain and meninges through a skull defect.

Endometrial cancer   Malignant neoplasm of the uterine lining.

Endometriosis   Chronic disorder caused by implantation of endometrial tissue outside the uterus.

Endometrium   Cellular lining of the uterus that is shed monthly at the time of menses.

***En-face* positioning**   Face-to-face positioning between parent and newborn.

Engorgement   The process of swelling of the breast tissue due to vascular congestion following delivery and preceding lactation.

Engrossment   Process characterized by intense parental interest in the newborn.

Enhancement   Process of building on a client's existing strengths in order to increase capacity for problem solving and self-care.

Epidural   A technique used to produce analgesia or anesthesia of the lower body by placing opioid and/or local anesthetic within the epidural space, which then diffuses into the nerve roots as they exit the dura.

Epispadias   Condition in which the urethral meatus is located on the dorsal surface of the penis.

Erythroblastosis fetalis   Vast destruction of fetal red blood cells by maternal antibodies, resulting in fetal anemia.

Esophageal atresia   Condition in which the esophagus ends in a blind pouch or narrows into a thin cord and is not connected to the stomach.

Estrogen   Female sex hormone produced primarily by the ovary and stored in fat cells.

Estrogen deficiency vulvovaginitis   Vulvo vaginal burning related to estrogen decline.

Ethic of care   Perspective that recognizes the personal concerns and vulnerabilities of clients in health and illness.

Ethics   Rules and principles that can be used for resolving ethical dilemmas.

Ethnic group   Community of people who share the same cultural and social beliefs, which have been passed from one generation to another.

Euploid   Cell (and, by extension, an individual) whose chromosome number is a multiple of 23.

Evidence-based practice   Systematic approach to finding, appraising and judiciously using research results as a basis for clinical decisions.

Excitement phase   Phase of the human sexual response in which physical and emotional changes take place in the person to increase interest in intercourse.

Exstrophy of the bladder   Anomaly in which the anterior wall of the bladder and lower portion of the abdominal wall are absent, causing the bladder to lie open and exposed on the lower abdomen.

Extended family   Family which includes generations beyond the parents and their children, such as grandparents or aunts and uncles; or two or more nuclear families together.

Extrauterine life   Life outside of the uterus following birth.

F

Facial palsy   Paralysis of one side of the face.

False discharge   Fluid appearing on the nipple or areolar surface that is not secreted by breast tissue.

Family   Group of adults and children linked by biological, kinship, or social bonds.

Family boundaries   The demarcations between individuals within a family and between the family and the rest of society.

Family dynamics   Concept from psychology that refers to the patterns in the interrelationships within the family.

Family structure   Configuration of the family unit, including who is in the family and their relationship to each other.

Femicide   Homicide of women.

Fertility rate   Number of births per 1,000 women of ages 15 to 44.

Fertilization   Process by which the male's sperm unites with the female's ovum.

Fetal circulation   The pathway of blood circulation in the fetus.

Fetal fibronectin (fFN) testing   Screening procedure for the prediction of preterm labor.

Fetal movement counting (FMC)   Daily maternal assessment of fetal activity by counting the number of fetal movements within a specified time period.

Fetal tissue sampling   Direct biopsy of fetal tissue.

Fibroadenoma   Painless solid breast mass or tumor.

Fibrocystic changes   Hormonal age-related changes, most commonly involving cyst formation and thickening of breast tissue.

Fibroid tumor   Benign tumor arising in the myometrium, which can protrude into the uterine cavity, bulge through the outer uterine layer, or grow within the myometrium.

Fidelity   Quality of being faithful.

Fimbriae   Fine hair-like structures.

Follicle stimulating hormone (FSH)   Hormone produced by the anterior pituitary whose function is to stimulate the ovary to prepare a mature ovum for release.

Follicular phase   Phase of the ovarian cycle in which a follicle becomes mature and prepared for ovulation.

Follow-up services   Health care services provided following hospital discharge.

Food Guide Pyramid   Translation of the Dietary Guidelines for Americans into practical eating portions and, if foods are chosen carefully, they also meet the Recommended Daily Allowances (RDA) and Dietary Reference Intakes (DRI).

Foramen ovale   An opening in the septum between the right and the left atria of the fetal heart.

Foremilk   Thin watery breastmilk secreted at the beginning of a feeding.

G

Galactopoiesis   The maintenance of established lactation.

Galactorrhea   White discharge from the nipples.

Gamete   Mature reproductive cell; spermatozoon or ovum.

Gametogenesis   Series of mitotic and meiotic divisions that occurs in the gonads and leads to the production of gametes; in males, spermatogenesis, and in females, oogenesis.

Gastroschisis   Abdominal wall defect to the right of the umbilicus through which the abdominal organs herniate.

Gene   Segment of nucleic acid that contains genetic information necessary to control a certain function, such as the synthesis of a polypeptide (structural gene); also referred to as a site, or locus, on a chromosome.

General anesthesia   Loss of sensation from the entire body secondary to loss of consciousness produced by intravenous and/or inhalation anesthetic agents.

Genetic counseling   Process by which genetic information is given to clients and their families.

Genetic disorder   Inherited defect that is transmitted from generation to generation.

Genotype   Genetic constitution of an individual at any given locus.

Geophagia   Ingestion of nonfood substances, such as dirt or clay.

Germ cells   Precursors of the ova.

Goals   Broad statements of a desired outcome.

Gonadal   Pertaining to the ovaries in the female and the testes in the male.

Gonadotropin-releasing hormone (Gm-RH)   Neurohormone released by the hypothalamus that acts on the pituitary to stimulate the release of follicle-stimulating hormone, luteinizing hormone, thyroid stimulating hormone, and prolactin.

Goodell's sign   Marked softening of the cervix in early pregnancy.

Graafian follicle   Fully mature ovum and surrounding elements just before ovulation.

H

Habituation   A newborn's ability to alter response to a repeated stimulus by decreasing and finally eliminating the response after repetitions of the stimulus.

Haploid   Cell that contains one copy of each chromosome; the haploid number (n) in humans is 23.

Harm   Interference with the mental or physical well-being of others.

Healing   To make whole and incorporates physical, psychological, social, spiritual and environmental health and may or may not include cure.

Health care informatics   Integration of computer science, information science and various health care professionals involved in collecting, processing and managing data.

Health promotion   Process, action, program, or endeavor to obtain the goal of complete physical, mental, and social well-being.

Hegar's sign   Softening of the isthmus of the uterus in pregnancy.

Heme iron   A type of iron from animal sources, which constitutes about half of the iron available from animal sources.

Hemizygous   Condition in which an allele is present in a single copy.

Hemochromatosis   Rare genetic defect in iron metabolism, in which excess iron is deposited in the tissues, causing abnormal skin pigmentation, hepatic cirrhosis and decreased carbohydrate tolerance, which eventually ends in multiple-organ failure.

Hemosiderosis   Iron storage disorder that results in iron toxicity.

Herbs   Leafy plants that do not have woody stems.

Heterozygote   Individual who has two different alleles at a given locus on a pair of homologous chromosomes.

Hindmilk   Thicker, high-fat breastmilk, secreted at the end of a feeding.

Holism   Philosophy of integration of body, mind and spirit within a dynamic environment.

Home care   Provision of technical, psychological, and other therapeutic support in the client's home environment rather than in an institution.

Home care nursing   Delivery of nursing care in the home environment.

Home visit   Visit occurring in the family's place of residence or in any such facility where a family may be housed, such as a homeless shelter, group home, church or halfway house.

Homologous   Refers to chromosomes with matching genes, or to those genes individually.

Homozygote   Individual who has a pair of identical alleles at a given locus.

Human chorionic gonadotropin (hCG)   Hormone secreted by the corpus luteum of the ovary after conception.

Human immunodeficiency virus (HIV) and acquired immunodeficiency syndrome (AIDS)   Retrovirus that causes progressive and severe impairment of the body's natural immunologic function, resulting in serious opportunistic infections, various cancers, and eventual death (AIDS).

Human placental lactogen (hPL)   Produced by the syncytiotrophoblast cell as early as 3 weeks after ovulation and is detectable in the maternal serum at 4 weeks after fertilization.

Hydrocele   Collection of serous fluid in the scrotum.

Hydrocephaly   Condition that results from an excess accumulation of cerebrospinal fluid (CSF) in the ventricles of the brain, caused by an imbalance between CSF production and absorption.

Hydrops fetalis   Severe form of fetal hemolytic disease; severe anemia results in hypoxia, cardiac decompensation, and hepatosplenomegaly.

Hyperbilirubinemia   Elevated level of bilirubin in the blood.

Hyperemesis gravidarum   Severe vomiting during pregnancy.

Hypocalcemia   A low level of calcium in the blood; (less than 7 mg/dL).

Hypochromic anemia   Anemia characterized by red blood cells lacking in color.

Hypoglycemia   A less than normal amount of glucose in the blood; in the newborn, a plasma glucose level of less than 40 mg/dL.

Hypophyseal-pituitary-ovarian axis   Transport mechanism of gonadotropin-releasing hormone from the hypothalamus that stimulates the release of gonadotropins from the anterior pituitary that, in turn, causes stimulation of the ovaries to release estrogen and progesterone.

Hypospadias Congenital anomaly in which the urethral meatus is located on the ventral surface of the glans penis instead of at the end.

Hypothalamic-pituitary-gonadal axis Triad of the hypothalamus, pituitary, and ovaries that must function in synchrony for conception to occur.

Hypothermia Rectal or axillary temperature below 97.0°F.

Hypovolemia Decreased circulating blood volume.

I

Imperforate anus A group of anatomic anomalies of the rectum and anus.

Implantation Embedding of the fertilized ovum into the endometrium.

Impotence Inability of the male to achieve or maintain an erection.

Incest Sexual relations between blood relatives or surrogate family members.

Infant of a diabetic mother (IDM) Infant born to a mother who has diabetes mellitus.

Infertility Diminished or absent ability to produce an offspring despite regular unprotected intercourse for 1 year.

Informed consent Information regarding treatment procedures are given to clients, and their consent is secured.

Insoluble fiber Fiber that resists absorption into the body.

Integrated medicine Provision of health care services combining both biomedical and complementary medicine.

Interdisciplinary teams Health care that is delivered by individuals from various disciplines that share responsibility, authority and decision making.

Intracranial hemorrhage Collection of blood within the cranium.

Intrathecal A technique used to produce analgesia of the lower body by placing a small amount of opioid drug into the cerebral spinal fluid.

Invasive breast cancer Cancer that has extended beyond the local epithelium and has the potential to spread from the breast to other parts of the body.

Invasive cancer Cancer that has spread or infiltrated beyond the original site or organ.

J

Jaundice Accumulation of bilirubin; produces a yellow discoloration of the newborn's skin, mucous membranes, and sclera.

Justice Division of benefits and burdens in society.

K

Kangaroo care Skin to skin contact between mother and infant.

Karyotype Chromosome constitution of an individual, represented by a laboratory-made display in which chromosomes are arranged by size and centromere position.

Kernicterus Excess accumulation of unbound, unconjugated bilirubin, deposited in brain tissues, especially the basal ganglia.

L

La Leche League International organization that promotes breastfeeding.

Lactation consultant Specially trained health care provider whose primary focus is providing breastfeeding assistance to help new mothers in establishing breastfeeding.

Lactational discharge Any secretory discharge occurring as a physiologic response to the normal hormonal stimulation of pregnancy, postpartum, or after weaning.

Lactogenesis The process of milk production 2-5 days postpartum.

Langhan's layer Inner layer of the trophoblast; also referred to as the cytotrophoblast.

Lanugo Downy hair that is present on the fetus between the 20th week and birth.

Latching-on Proper attachment of the infant to the breast for feeding.

Law Rules governing human behavior that represent the minimum standard of morality.

Let-down reflex Milk ejection from the breast triggered by nipple stimulation or emotional response to the infant.

Letting-go phase Final phase of maternal adjustment characterized by role attainment and relationship adjustment.

Leydig cells Interstitial tissue cells of the testes that produce testosterone.

Liability Accountability for professional conduct according to standards that have been set.

Libido Conscious or unconscious sexual desire.

Life expectancy Average number of years for which a group of individuals of the same age are expected to live.

Linea nigra Dark line of pigmentation that extends from the symphysis pubis to the umbilicus, at midline on the abdomen during pregnancy.

Local anesthetic Class of drugs that produce reversible blockade of electrical impulses along nerve fiber.

Local infiltration anesthesia Loss of sensation in a small area due to blockade of neural impulses as a result of infiltration of tissue with an anesthetic drug such as lidocaine.

Localized breast cancer Cancer that has not metastasized, is usually less than 2 cm in size, is considered noninvasive beyond the breast, and has the best outcome.

Luteal phase Phase of the ovarian cycle after ovulation when the corpus luteum secretes hormones to prepare the uterine endometrium for implantation until the placenta matures and assumes the function of providing nutrients for the embryo.

Luteinizing hormone (LH) Anterior pituitary hormone whose surge occurs immediately before ovulation and is responsible for release of the ovum.

M

Macro-environment Elements that define the caregiving milieu, that is, conditions that define the surrounding space in which caregiving occurs.

Macronutrients Any of the chemical elements, such as carbon, required in relatively large quantities for growth.

Macrosomatia Birth weight above the 90th percentile for gestational age, or a birth weight of more than 4 kg (8 lb, 12.8 oz).

Magnetic resonance imaging (MRI)   Noninvasive diagnostic tool that provides high-resolution cross-sectional images of fluid-filled soft tissues.

Malpractice   Negligence involving the actions of professionals.

Managed care   Health care plans with a selected list of providers and institutions from which the recipient is entitled to receive health care that is reimbursed by the insurer.

Mastectomy   Excision (removal) of the breast.

Mastitis   Infection in the breast, usually confined to a milk duct, characterized by influenza-like symptoms and redness and tenderness in the infected breast.

Material principles of justice   Guidelines that can be used to justify the distribution of benefits.

Maternal sensitization   Process by which the maternal immunologic system forms antibodies against fetal blood cells.

Maternal serum–α-fetoprotein (MS-AFP) testing   Screen of maternal blood for the presence and volume of alpha-feto protein (AFP).

Maternal-infant bonding   The forming of an emotional attachment between mother and newborn.

Mature milk   Breast milk that contains 10% solids for energy and growth.

Meconium   Initial stool developed in the fetus; it is viscid, sticky, dark in color, sterile, and odorless.

Meconium staining   Staining of the newborn's skin and nails; results from fetal passage of stool in utero.

Medical model   Biomedical approach to health care that is oriented to treating specific diagnosis and focused on physical problems.

Meiosis   Process by which germ cells divide and decrease their chromosomal number by half.

Menarch   Establishment or beginning of the menstrual function.

Menarche   Initiation of the first menses.

Meningocele   Spinal cord defect in which an external sac that protrudes through the defect and contains meninges and cerebrospinal fluid.

Menopause   Natural or surgically imposed cessation of menses.

Menses   Monthly bleeding from the lining of the uterus.

Menstrual phase   Phase of the menstrual cycle when a woman experiences vaginal bleeding.

Meridian   In Oriental medicine, the channels or pathways in the body through which Chi travels.

Mesenchyme   Meshwork of embryonic connective tissue that forms the connective tissue of the body, blood vessels, and lymph vessels.

Metastatic breast cancer   Breast cancer that is found in parts of the body in addition to the breasts.

Microcephaly   A small brain in a normally well-formed head.

Microcytic anemia   Anemia characterized by red blood cells of small size.

Micro-environment   Elements that are specifically related to the individual infant's environment or care experiences.

Micronutrients   Any of the chemical elements, such as iron, required in minute quantities for growth.

Mitosis   Process in which body cells duplicate themselves and then separate into two new daughter cells.

Mittelschmerz   Abdominal pain occurring at the time of ovulation.

Monosomy   Aneuploid condition of having a chromosome represented by a single copy in a somatic cell, i.e., the absence of a chromosome from a given pair.

Morbidity rate   Ratio of the number of cases of a disease or a condition to a given population.

Mortality rate   Ratio of the number of deaths in various categories to a given population.

Morula   Solid mass of cells formed by cleavage of a fertilized ovum.

Mosaicism   Condition that results in an individual (mosaic) with two or more genetically different cell populations.

Moxibustion   In Oriental medicine, the burning of herbs near the skin in order to affect movement of Chi.

Multifactorial   Resulting from interactions between genetic and environmental factors.

Mutation   Abrupt genetic alteration in an individual, which is transmitted to the offspring.

Myelomeningocele   Spinal cord defect in which part of the spinal cord is herniated into the external sac, which contains meninges, cerebrospinal fluid, and neural tissue.

N

Neglect   Withholding of essential components of daily living, such as food, clothing, medications, and shelter.

Negligence   Unintentional wrong caused by failure to act as a reasonable person would under similar circumstances.

Neurohormonal   Pertaining to hormones formed by neurosecretory cells and liberated by nerve impulses.

Neutral thermal environment   A set of environmental conditions created to maintain the normal body temperature; minimizes oxygen consumption and caloric expenditure.

Nipple discharge   Fluid produced by and accumulating within a secretory unit of the breast, exiting through the nipple.

Nondisjunction   Failure of homologous chromosomes, or chromatids, to separate properly during anaphase meiosis I and II, or mitosis, resulting in daughter cells with unequal chromosome numbers; meiotic nondisjunction may result in gametes with abnormal chromosome number, which upon fertilization may produce aneuploidy; mitotic nondisjunction that occurs in a developing embryo may result in mosaicism.

Nonheme iron   Dietary iron from foods other than meats, in which the iron is not bound in the hemoglobin molecule; comprises half of the iron found in animal sources and all of the iron found in plant sources, including grains and cereals.

Nonmaleficence   Acting to prevent harm to others.

Nonstress test (NST)   Evaluation of fetal heart rate in response to an increase in either spontaneous or stimulated fetal activity.

Nuchal cord   Umbilical cord encircling the fetal neck.

Nuclear family   Family composed of two generations, parents and their children.

Nutrition Facts Food Label   Labeling on processed packaged foods that lists credible health and nutrient content claims, standardized serving sizes, and the Percent Daily Values (DV), based on a 2000-calorie diet.

O

Obesity   Body weight of 20% or more over ideal body weight.

Objectives   Specific short-term achievements expected to result in the accomplishment of the goal. These are generally written in specific measurable outcomes.

Omphalocele   Defect covered by a peritoneal sac at the base of the umbilicus, into which portions of the abdominal organs herniate.

Opioid   A type of drug which binds to opioid receptors and produces a degree of analgesia. Morphine and Demerol are two drugs of this type.

Organogenesis   Development of organs.

Orgasmic phase   Phase of the human sexual response after the plateau phase in which immense sexual tension is released.

Osteoporosis   Progressive bone loss, increased bone fragility, and increased risk for bone fractures, which occurs in post-menopausal women.

Ovarian cancer   Malignant neoplasm of the ovary.

Ovulation   Release of a mature ovum in preparation for conception.

Oxytocin   Hormone produced by the posterior pituitary that stimulates uterine contractions and the release of milk from the mammary glands.

P

Pagophagia   Ingestion of nonfood substances, such as ice and ice frost.

Parenteral   Administration of drug via intramuscular or intravenous routes.

Paternalism   Interference in the liberty of a person, in which the interference is justified by promoting the well-being of that individual.

Pathologic discharge   Results from pathologic conditions affecting the hypothalamic-pituitary axis, prolactin levels, or breast diseases that affect both breasts.

Pathologic jaundice   Jaundice of the newborn caused by the excessive breakdown of red blood cells as a result of hematologic incompatibility.

Pedigree (genogram)   Diagram that describes family relationships and gender, disease status, and other relevant information about a family.

Pelvic inflammatory disease (PID)   Inflammation of the uterus, fallopian tubes, or ovaries caused by ascent of vaginal flora or bacteria.

Pelvic relaxation   The loss of muscle support of the pelvic organs.

Percutaneous umbilical blood sampling (PUBS)   Evaluation technique that provides direct access to the fetal circulation and involves direct aspiration of fetal blood.

Perimenopause   Time period before the cessation of menses.

Perpetrator   Person accused of a criminal offense.

Persistent pulmonary hypertension   A condition caused by a sustained elevation in pulmonary vascular resistance after birth, preventing the transition to the normal extrauterine circulatory pattern.

Phenotype   Any observable or measurable expression of gene function.

Phototherapy   Ultraviolet light used for treatment of jaundice in the newborn.

Physiologic anemia of pregnancy   Disproportionate increase of the plasma volume compared with the red blood cell volume, resulting in a lower-than-normal hemoglobin level and hematocrit during pregnancy.

Physiologic discharge   Result of physiologic conditions affecting all breast tissue equally, involving secretory tissue in each breast and resulting in milky white or multicolored fluid.

Physiologic jaundice   Benign form of jaundice that usually occurs after the third day of life and is caused by the normal breakdown of superfluous red blood cells.

Phytochemicals   Plant-based chemicals.

Phytotherapy   The therapeutic use of plants, often referring to herbal remedies.

Pica   Psychobehavioral disorder that manifests as persistent ingestion of substances having little or no nutritional value or craving of unnatural articles as food during pregnancy.

Plateau phase   Phase of human sexual response occurring just before orgasm.

Plumbism   Ingestion of nonfood substances, such as lead paint flakes.

Polycystic ovary syndrome   Endocrine disorder characterized by long-term anovulation and an excess of androgens circulating in the blood; characterized by formation of cysts in the ovaries, a process related to the failure of the ovary to release an ovum.

Polycythemia   Increased number of red blood cells.

Polygenic   Referring to a trait whose phenotypic expression results from the cooperation of various genes.

Postnatal circulation   The normal extrauterine circulatory pattern of blood flow through the heart, lungs, and body.

Prana   A term used in Ayurvedic medicine referring to vital energy.

Precocious   Developing maturity very early or rapidly.

Premature ovarian failure   Failure of ovarian estrogen production and ovulation after menarche and before age 40, in which the woman experiences the symptoms of menapause.

Premenstrual syndrome   Cyclic cluster of behavioral, emotional, and physical symptoms, which occur during the luteal phase of the menstrual cycle and are of sufficient severity to interrupt normal activity.

Preterm   An infant born at less than 38 weeks' gestation.

Prima facie   A conditional duty that can be overridden by a more stringent duty.

Primary amenorrhea   Absence of menarche until age 16 or absence of the development of secondary sex characteristics and menarche until age 14.

Primary apnea   A self-limited condition characterized by absence of respiration; occurs in the early stage of asphyxia.

Primary dysmenorrhea   Painful menses from uterine causes but without pelvic pathology; usually occurs within 3 years of onset of menstrual cycling.

Proactive   Development of capacity to deal with stressors prior to a crises.

Proband   Clinically identified person who displays the characteristics or features of a disease; also referred to as index case, or propositus (fem, proposita).

Progesterone Antiestrogenic hormone produced by the corpus luteum of the ovary that assists in maintenance of pregnancy through implantation.

Prolactin Hormone from the pituitary gland that triggers milk production in response to tactile stimulation of the breast.

Proliferative phase Phase of the menstrual cycle in which the endometrium becomes prepared for implantation.

Prostaglandins Class of hormones found in many tissues that affects vasodilation, constriction, and uterine smooth muscle.

Pseudomenstruation Pinkish-white mucoid vaginal discharge noted shortly after birth owing to maternal transfer of estrogen.

Puberty Period in which the secondary sex characteristics begin to develop and the capability of sexual reproduction is attained; onset of the process of physical maturity.

Pudendal block A technique using local anesthesia to block transmission through the pudendal nerves.

Pulmonary vascular resistance Resistance in the pulmonary vascular bed against which the right ventricle must eject blood.

Q

Quickening First fetal movement, felt by the mother; usually noticed at about 18 to 20 weeks' gestation.

R

Race A group of people defined by similar physical features, such as skin color, facial features, and texture of body hair.

Rape Nonconsensual sexual penetration of another by force or threat of force.

Recessive Allele whose phenotypic expression occurs in homozygous or hemizygous conditions.

Recommended Dietary Allowances (RDA) Average daily nutrient intake levels recommended for healthy Americans.

Reconstituted family Family formed through remarriage.

Reducing agent Any substance that reduces another substance, or brings about reduction, and is itself oxidized in the process.

Reference Daily Intakes (RDIs) Standard that addresses the vitamin and mineral content of foods.

Refractory period Period of time after orgasm when the human is incapable of further sexual activity.

Regional anesthesia Loss of sensation from a large area of the body due to blockade of neural impulses.

Relactation Reinstitution of lactation after it has been discontinued.

Renal solute load The sum of solutes that must be excreted by the kidneys.

Resolution phase Phase of human sexual response when the physiologic changes in the body that occur as a result of sexual activity return to normal.

Resuscitation Basic emergency procedure used for life support, consisting of airway management, positive pressure ventilation, chest compressions, medication, and thermal support.

Rh incompatibility (isoimmunization) Hemolytic disease caused by the incompatibility of Rh factors in maternal and fetal blood.

Risk assessment Process of examining the risk factors that may place an individual at risk for disease.

Role attainment Completing the developmental tasks of a new social role.

Role mastery Successful attainment of developmental tasks.

Role transition Process of adopting new behaviors to accomplish change and developmental tasks.

Rooting reflex Normal response of the newborn to move toward whatever touches the area around the mouth.

S

Screening A test or examination to detect the most characteristic sign or signs of a disorder or disease that may require further investigation.

Secondary amenorrhea Absence of menses for at least 6 months or for three cycles, after previously experiencing menstrual cycles.

Secondary apnea An abnormal condition that occurs in the late stages of asphyxia in which respiration is absent and does not resume spontaneously without resuscitation.

Secondary dysmenorrhea Painful menses accompanied by a pathologic process.

Secretory phase Phase of the menstrual cycle that occurs after ovulation and before menstruation.

Seminiferous tubules Tubules that carry semen from the testes.

Sepsis Systemic bacterial, viral, or parasitic infection that invades the bloodstream.

Serial monogamy Practice of having one sexual partner at a time but several partners during a lifetime.

Seroconversion Conversion of the blood serum from negative to positive for any infecting agent.

Sexual dysfunction Related to a disorder of one of the phases of human sexual response.

Sexual maturation Establishment of menstruation and ovulation in females and the development of spermatogenesis in males.

Situational crisis Event or situation that occurs in a personal or a family life, which requires the adaptation or acquisition of new coping mechanisms.

Sleep-wake cycle Stages of newborn sleep pattern.

Social assets Assets or benefits to ones health that are related to one's social position and socioeconomic status.

Soluble fiber Fiber that binds bile acids and coats the intestines, thus inhibiting absorption.

Somite One of the paired segments along the neural tube of the embryo.

Spermatogenesis Entire process of development and maturation of sperm cells.

Spermatozoa Male gamete or sex cell.

Spermatozoon Mature male germ cell (sperm); spermatozoa (plural).

Spina bifida Congenital defect in which the spinal canal does not close and protrudes from the back.

Spinnbarkeit Stringy elastic character of cervical mucus at time of ovulation.

Stalking "A course of conduct directed at a specific person that involves repeated visual or physical proximity, nonconsensual communication, violence toward property, verbal, written or implied threats, or a combination thereof" (Tjaden & Thoennes, 1998, p. 2).

Standards of care Documents developed by members of a profession to establish a mutually adopted level of practice.

STORCH An acronym used to describe a titer for syphilis, toxoplasmosis, other, rubella, cytomegalovirus, and herpes.

Stranger rape Nonconsensual sexual experience between a victim and assailant who are strangers.

Stress incontinence Involuntary discharge of urine with a cough, sneeze, or laughter owing to the loss of muscular support at the neck of the urethra.

Stressor Illness, that may result in change.

Striae gravidarum Pinkish or darkened streaks, resulting from stretching of the skin during pregnancy that occurs predominantly on the breasts and abdomen.

Subarachnoid hemorrhage Collection of blood in the subarachnoid space of the brain.

Subdural hemorrhage Collection of blood in the subdural space of the brain.

Supine hypotension Condition of reduced blood flow to the right atrium when the pregnant woman lies in a supine position.

Surfactant Complete lipoprotein that reduces the surface tension of pulmonary fluids, allowing the exchange of gases in the alveoli of the lungs.

Syncytiotrophoblast Outer layer of the trophoblast.

Systemic vascular resistance Resistance against which the left ventricle must eject its stroke volume with each heart beat.

T

Taking-hold phase Second phase of maternal adjustment, characterized by an increased readiness to be involved with the newborn.

Taking-in phase Initial, early period of maternal adjustment, characterized by basic maternal needs for food, care, and comfort.

Tanner Stages Five stages of female and male physiologic development.

Teratogen Environmental substance that can cause physical defects in the developing embryo and fetus.

Testosterone Most potent naturally occurring androgen (male) hormone that is made in the testes, ovary, and adrenal cortex.

Thelarche Beginning of the development of the breasts at puberty, with prominence of glandular tissue behind the nipples. The first sign of puberty.

Thermoregulation The control of heat production and heat loss, specifically the maintenance of body temperature through physiologic mechanisms activated by the hypothalamus.

Tort Civil wrong that may be caused either intentionally or unintentionally.

Tracheoesophageal fistula Condition in which the trachea and esophagus are abnormally connected.

Transient tachypnea of the newborn Mild, self-limited respiratory disorder, characterized by an increased respiratory rate and mild cyanosis and thought to be related to delayed resorption of fetal lung fluid.

Transitional milk Milk produced at the end of colostrum production and immediately before mature milk comes in the breast.

Translocation Misplacement of genetic material from one chromosome to another.

Trisomy Aneuploid condition caused by the presence of an extra chromosome, which is added to a given chromosome pair and results in a total number of 47 chromosomes per cell; Down syndrome is the most common human autosomal trisomy.

Trophoblast cells Peripheral cells of the blastocyst that attach the fertilized ovum to the uterine wall and develop into the placenta and membranes.

U

Ultrasonography Use of high-frequency (>20,000 Hz) sound waves to detect differences in tissue density and to visualize outlines of structures within the body.

Universalizability Rule used to guide actions that could be followed in all other similar situations.

Upper intake level (UL) Maximum level of daily nutrient intake.

Urge incontinence Inability to postpone urination for more than a few minutes once the need to urinate is sensed. The bladder is unable to empty normally and becomes distended, which results in an uncontrolled loss of urine.

Utilitarianism Type of ethical thinking focusing on the consequences of actions; actions are right if they bring about the best possible outcomes and the least bad effects for the greatest number of persons.

V

Vaginal infection Inflammation of the vagina caused by a microorganism or foreign body.

Vaginismus Painful spasms of the muscles of the introitus that prevent penetration.

Varicocele Abnormal blood vessel in the scrotum.

Vegan Vegetarian who consumes no animal products.

Veracity Truthfulness.

Vertical transmission Transmission of HIV by the mother to the fetus or neonate during pregnancy, delivery, and postnatally, during breastfeeding.

Virtue Character trait that is valued.

Virtue ethics The way in which personal characteristics of the moral agent or person guide moral action.

Vitalism A term used in 19th Century Europe and America referring to a type of vital energy or life force.

W

Weaning Process of discontinuing breastfeeding and accustoming an infant to another feeding method.

Wet nurse   Woman who breastfeeds for pay infants who are not her own.

Wharton's jelly   Soft, jelly-like substance of the umbilical cord.

Wife rape   Forced sexual experience with a common-law or legally married spouse.

Z

Zona pellucida   Transparent, noncellular layer surrounding the ovum.

Zygote   Cell resulting from the union of the ovum and spermatozoon.

INDEX